DORLAND'S MEDICAL DICTIONARY

Shorter Edition

DORLAND'S MEDICAL DICTIONARY

Shorter Edition

INTRODUCTION BY
Franz J. Ingelfinger
Editor Emeritus, *New England Journal of Medicine*

With 16 pages of color illustrations on
Highlights of Structures and Function in the Human Body

Abridged from the 25th Edition of
Dorland's Illustrated Medical Dictionary

The Saunders Press

W. B. SAUNDERS COMPANY
PHILADELPHIA • LONDON • TORONTO

THE SAUNDERS PRESS
W. B. Saunders Company
West Washington Square
Philadelphia, Pa. 19105

Distributed by: Holt, Rinehart & Winston
Trade Sales Department
383 Madison Avenue
New York, N.Y. 10017

MADE IN THE UNITED STATES OF AMERICA
AT THE PRESS OF W. B. SAUNDERS COMPANY
WBS—ISBN 0-7216-3142-8
HRW—ISBN 0-03-056744-0

LIBRARY OF CONGRESS CATALOG CARD NUMBER: 79-67113

Print No.:   9   8   7   6   5   4   3   2   1

INTRODUCTION

by

Franz J. Ingelfinger, M.D.

Distinguished Physician, Veterans Administration
Bedford, Massachusetts
and
Editor Emeritus,
New England Journal of Medicine

Americans have become deeply — some would say obsessively — concerned with health. Moreover, not only doctors, nurses, and other health-care personnel, but also clergymen, lawyers, politicians, philosophers, teachers, physicists, and chemists are held responsible for the maintenance and preservation of health. Indeed, in view of the recent emphasis on self-care and improved lifestyles, one may argue that the entire population between early adolescence and late senility is expected to attend to its own well-being. That the health care system is being concocted by such a jumble of cooks is worrisome and, unless there is some common means of communication, conditions may become more chaotic than they already are.

The basic means of communication is language, and in discussions dealing with health and health care the language of the physician unfortunately must be the common linguistic bond — "unfortunately," because so many medical terms are difficult and not part of our everyday language. If a new disease, *physiologic* mechanism, or mechanical device is discovered in the field of medicine, the chances are that it will be given a ponderous name, and the name selected is usually derived from Greek or Latin rather than Anglo-Saxon roots. *Acrohypothermy,* for example, merely means cold hands and feet. Why do we not express *ultrasonography (echography),* a diagnostic device using the principles of radar, for example, in words that are probably Anglo-Saxon in derivation, such as "sound-rebound?" The answer is simply that scientific processes are traditionally expressed by words etymologically related to Greek and Latin. In fact, Professor Sir George Pickering, a famous elderly English physician, has deplored the disappearance of Latin from the education of doctors, since he maintains that knowledge of Latin is the feature "which distinguished the learned professions from other vocations." So, if a new recording device is developed, it is almost automatic that its name will end with the syllables "-graphy."

Whatever the reasons, whether etymological tradition or artificial elitism, medicine has employed and developed an ultra-jargon that is far more difficult to understand, far more elaborate, and far more difficult to spell correctly than the jargon of most other professions or trades.

A language of such size and complexity as medicine's obviously requires a standard reference, a dictionary. The first technical dictionary devoted to medicine and written in English was published in England under the name *Physical Dictionary* in 1684. In fact, however, it was a translation from a dictionary written in Latin and compiled by Stephen Blankaart, a Dutchman. The first bona fide English *Medical Dictionary* was the work of Robert James (1743). Nearly a century later the American physician Robley Dunglison put out in 1833 his *New Dictionary of Medical Sciences and Literature*. In 1898, the W. B. Saunders Company began to publish *Dorland's Illustrated Medical Dictionary,** which has become probably the most widely used of the several American medical dictionaries now on the market.

Some comprehensive medical dictionary, such as *Dorland's,* is essential to provide doctors, dentists, nurses, hospital administrators, and lawyers dealing in medical matters with definitions, correct spellings, and pronunciations. The same book should be available to medical secretaries to help them with the spelling of these technical terms, and also to radio or TV announcers, whose pronunciation of medical terms sometimes verges on the ludicrous. But the regular *Dorland's* is a bulky volume listing about 100,000 items; it is far too comprehensive to be useful to the literate laity who have become interested — and intensely so — in medicine. For this vast population the W. B. Saunders Company has now prepared a "*Shorter Edition*," an abridged version of the regular *Dorland's*. In this Introduction I have italicized some of the medical terms commonly used in the media but also defined in this shorter *Dorland's*.

The reasons for the general explosion of interest in medicine and related matters are many. Medicine, in all its ramifications, has become Big News. Hardly a day passes without some medical event being reported in the daily press or in the many TV or radio news broadcasts. Sometimes the event is to the credit of medicine, more often to medicine's discredit, but usually it is cast in the most sensational terms possible.

Technologic Advances

Technology is said to be at the base of much of the trouble that society is having with medicine, and vice versa. Many feel that technology has gone too far. "No More Nukes," chant those who protest nuclear power. Several years ago a group of scientists questioned the advances of medical power and especially the technique of *gene* splitting and then recombining the split chains of *deoxyribonu-*

---

*When the book by W. A. Newman Dorland, M.D., was first published by Saunders it was entitled *The American Illustrated Medical Dictionary* and continued under that title until 1957, when, for the 23rd edition, the title was changed to the present one.

cleic acid into new genetic material, possibly producing new and uncontrollable viruses. Some people even feared that the gene-splitters and recombiners were Frankensteins, about to produce horrendous monsters. The dangers seem less now, but genetic manipulations have occasioned much debate, not only among scientists but also among concerned laity. Indeed, controls of research on recombinant DNA have been imposed by both federal and state governments, and regulations have been formulated by committees of laymen as well as by scientists. The potential dangers of recombinant DNA of course made the headlines and are still making them from time to time. A convenient technical dictionary is almost essential for any nonbiologist who wants to understand the pertinent news stories.

A less sensational but nevertheless crucial question is whether the government should underwrite a program for designing an artificial heart, and private entrepreneurs are still making efforts along this line. Without some guide describing the rather complex arrangement of the heart's chambers (*atria* and *ventricles*), the average citizen will have a hard time understanding the pros and cons of searching for a workable artificial heart.

Making a successful artificial heart requires considerable basic research, but clinical research as applied to the heart is also very much in the news. *Angina pectoris* is one of the most common complaints of cardiac patients, but surgeons appear to have found a way of ameliorating this condition. They certainly can relieve the pain of most angina patients (except those with *Prinzmetal's angina*) by *coronary artery* bypass procedures, in which a segment or segments of the patient's *veins* are used to fashion a channel bypassing the *stenotic* or *occluded* coronary artery (or arteries). Whether these bypass operations prolong life is still a controversial issue, even though some 500,000 bypasses already have been performed in the United States. Surely, if the procedure remains as popular as it now is, a diagram of the coronary circulation in the next edition of this shorter *Dorland's* is warranted.

Surgical skills are also blossoming in other directions. By means of *microsurgery*, anastomoses can be performed between tiny vessels, and nerves can be reconnected so that the implantation of severed limbs or digits is now possible. Unimaginably delicate operations on the eye have also become feasible by microsurgical methods.

Another biomedical advance that is burgeoning is that of *transplantation*. Transplantation requires fine surgical skills, but these usually can be developed. The more serious problem is *rejection* of the transplanted organ because of the lack of *histocompatibility*. Thus, the basic discipline of *immunology* must be studied to enhance, when desired, *immunosuppression*. Transplantation of living organs also raises ethical issues, which are discussed later in this Introduction.

Immunologic principles were also used to devise the *radioimmunoassay*, a Nobel Prize–winning achievement. If, for example, the concentration of *insulin* in plasma is to be measured, an *antibody* to insulin is prepared and allowed to react with radioactively labeled insulin. The *antigen-antibody* complex is then exposed to the biological sample to be tested. The labeled insulin is displaced from the complex in proportion to the amount of unlabeled insulin in the sample being assayed. The amount of *radioactivity* freed thus provides indirect quantification of the insulin present in the unknown. By this method, tiny concentrations — *nanograms, picograms,* and *femtograms* — of a given substance can be determined in the blood or other body fluids. Measurement of the concentrations of such substances in the blood, urine, or *cerebrospinal fluid* is revealing that some of them exert unexpected *hormonal* functions.

Other tests that have been developed and get into the news utilize *light* or *electron microscopes,* or a variety of other modifications of the microscope, to examine tissues for early signs of neoplastic changes. The best known and most discussed of such tests is the *Papanicolaou (Pap)* test to search for *malignant* or *premalignant* changes in the *cervix,* the exit passage of the *uterus.* How often should a woman have a Pap test? How reliable are they? At what ages should women have Pap tests? Questions of this type are constantly debated not only in medical but also in lay publications. Indeed, questions of this type are also frequently argued on TV. Equally controversial and equally publicized is the use of *mammography* to search for signs of *neoplasm* in the female breast.

In most "developed" countries, *vaccination* has come to be accepted as an effective means of preventing diseases such as *pertussis, rubeola,* and *rubella.* Although there always have been opponents of inoculation of attenuated or killed infective agents into human beings to induce specific immunities (see, for example, Bernard Shaw's preface to "The Doctor's Dilemma"), the fantastic success of the *Salk* and *Sabin vaccines* for *poliomyelitis* gave the practice of vaccination a tremendous boost. On the other hand, the ill-advised attempt in 1977 to vaccinate most of the United States population against swine *flu,* an attempt possibly responsible for some cases of *Guillain-Barré syndrome,* heightened the public's distrust of immunologic means of preventing disease. Thus, vaccination has been and will continue to be an issue of public interest for reasons of safety, effectiveness, religion, and moral convictions.

Technology has also made available to doctors an entirely new arsenal of mechanical diagnostic equipment. *Ultrasonography* is being widely used to delineate internal structures and their abnormalities, and a new radiologic technique, computerized tomography (CAT scanner), produces a cross-sectional shadow picture of the part of the body under examination. By means of *angiography* the details of the vascular supply of organs can be revealed. *Radionuclides* of various types have been devised for diagnostic purposes. After intravascular injection, these substances accumulate in specific organs and produce, by their radioactive properties, *scintiscans* (or simply "scans"), which reveal space-occupying lesions or other abnormalities. Finally, developments in *fiberoptics* have made possible transmission of images through bundles of flexible tubing. As a result, the interior of nearly all hollow organs of the body can now be viewed directly by a variety of specially designed instruments, such as the *gastroscope* and the *bronchoscope.*

Technological innovations such as these often make headlines because of the medical advances the new technology makes possible. But of similar if not greater news appeal are the disadvantages the new technology brings with it.

The Dangers of Technology

One major concern is that many of the new procedures are not entirely safe. Blood tests are, of course, not very harmful (except that the quantity of tests and their frequent repetition may literally drain off much of the patient's blood), and ultrasonography has so far proved so safe that it is one of the few procedures to which a fetus can be exposed. Most of the other technologic innovations in medicine, however, are invasive in that needles or *catheters* are inserted into the body, thus introducing the dangers of bleeding, infection, or accidental penetration of the walls of an organ. Other new diagnostic means require additional exposure to *radiation* or the injection of substances to which the patient may have a serious and sometimes lethal reaction. Nor is any test invariably reliable. Indeed, the dependability of various scanning procedures, of ultrasonography, and of various radiologic refinements is still being evaluated.

Another problem with the elaborate testing procedures fashioned by technologic ingenuity is their expense. Medical costs, along with the general trend, continue to soar upwards, and the introduction of new tests costing up to $1,000 each does not help matters. Because of their cost, both in dollars and patient safety, a major attempt is being made to control the number of new instruments that can be installed and to reduce the number of tests — often repeated — that doctors may request. Many of these attempts are being made by consumer groups, others by legislators, and still others by "certificate of need" committees. These committees, which have many lay members, are supposed to prohibit the purchase and installation of expensive laboratory equipment if, in the committees' opinion, a given region already has its quota of necessary instruments. Actually, legislation and regulations of this type evoke bitter arguments about "interference with medical practice" and hence are a constant source of angry statements, editorials, and magazine articles directed at the public.

After all, American medical expenses, amounting currently to $200 billion per year, are second only to the dollars spent for military defense, and it is thus unavoidable that medicine and its many ancillary activities are very much in the public eye. Anyone who would vote intelligently on the needs of hospitals, medical schools, or clinics must to some degree understand medical terms.

Elsewhere I have argued that technology is being misused if the doctor and the public seek 100 percent accuracy in their diagnostic efforts: "Let us assume that, for a particular patient, a doctor who uses conventional methods of diagnosis and supplements them with one modern technique can establish a diagnosis that has a 95 percent chance of being correct. Adding a second modern procedure may raise this level of confidence to 97 percent, a third to 98 percent, a fourth to 98.6 percent, and a fifth to 99.2 percent.

"As more and more modern tests are used, the likelihood of a correct diagnosis gradually approaches 100 percent, but the increments between each new level of confidence diminish rapidly, whereas the costs increase linearly. Each small gain in accuracy costs money and time, ties up scarce resources, and, most important, impairs the patient's health and comfort disproportionately.

"From a long-term viewpoint, the millions of dollars spent on the battery of modern tests aimed at the will-o'-the-wisp of 100 percent diagnostic accuracy make a major contribution to the inflationary prices of health care. After 95 percent diagnostic confidence is achieved, the ratio of the benefits of a diagnostic procedure to its cost decreases rapidly, and I therefore propose that, on the average, the individual is better served if the goal is pegged at 95 percent diagnostic accuracy rather than at 100 percent."

The Influence of Technology

Up to this point, I have mentioned some of the pros and cons of specific advances of medical diagnosis, *therapeutics,* and instrumentation. Technology, however, has also influenced the general character of medical practice, and many find this influence deplorable. In the late sixties and early seventies, medical planners and pedagogues feared a shortage of physicians which, in turn, would add to the high cost of medical care and would accentuate the lack of access to such care by the impoverished population in inner cities and rural areas. Annual graduates of American medical schools numbered about 8,000 at that time. Now, in response to public pressures and carrot-and-stick tactics by the government, about 14,000 students receive their M.D. degrees annually in the United States — almost too many, some federal officials now maintain. Yet the poor still lack the care that the wealthy receive.

One of the many reasons for the continuing problem of health care is the influence of technologic developments. As new diagnostic and therapeutic devices become available, physicians with special skills to apply these new devices and to interpret their results must be trained. In other words, technology spawns specialization, and the devotees of specialization congregate in medical centers or settle in affluent suburbs and do not treat the population at large.

Furthermore, technology enhances the lures of specialization — higher incomes, less work, and greater intellectual stimulation — and thus counters the strong efforts being made by government, foundations, and educators to interest a greater proportion of medical graduates in general practice. Technologic advances unfortunately are partly responsible for the difficulties encountered in the attempt to obtain a better distribution of doctors with respect to what and where they practice.

But the most serious charge to which technology is subject is the change it has brought about in doctor-patient relations. The "good old doc" of a century ago might have done much harm in his ignorance (perhaps no more so than his late twentieth century coldly scientific counterpart), but at least the old version and his patients must have known each other better. The old model went to patients' homes and became acquainted with them and their families. He must have talked to his patients a good deal and relaxed their fears and stresses without encumbering himself with the label "psychiatrist." Today's physician can't make house calls, even if he wants to. The elaborate facilities he needs (and must use if he is to avoid the malpractice litigation) and the laboratory aids that are the cornerstones of his diagnostic approach may be available only in or near his office or in a hospital emergency room. Once he and the patient meet, the time required for tests diminishes the time left for talking and getting acquainted. Many a modern doctor's practice is molded to satisfy technologic demands.

Above all, the doctor has lost the precious opportunity to detail to the patient the reasons for the actions of nameless and sometimes faceless personnel, the reasons for the seemingly endless *venipunctures,* and the reasons for the many exhausting trips to various technical laboratories for special examinations. The same technical obstacles to adequate physician-patient relations may explain why many patients go home without really understanding how the doctor interpreted their symptoms, the nature of the diagnosis, and the need for taking certain medicines. Doctors, in turn, assert that the patient who does not follow instructions is noncompliant.

Under the pressures of the "technologic imperative," intimacy between doctor and patient is thwarted, and distrust may displace confidence. Unavoidably, technology has made medical practice more accurate but less humanistic. If patients had the opportunity of becoming better acquainted with medical "lingo," the decline in good doctor-patient relations might be mitigated.

Another adverse effect of technologic sophistication is that the promises of new diagnostic apparatus, of new drugs, and of new surgical interventions are oversold to the public, usually by the news media, occasionally by physicians, but particularly by organizations and institutions whose business it is to solicit contributions to fight and "conquer" certain diseases. If only enough money were at hand, the solicitors imply, this or that disease could be eradicated. But the fantastic accomplishments do not materialize, and the public, and especially those with diseases on behalf of which special support is sought, become disillusioned and sometimes bitter. As a reaction against what they perceive as failures of medicine, many people turn to "wonder drugs" such as Laetrile or join quasi-evangelical movements in the hope of obtaining the relief that standard modern medicine apparently cannot provide. The active involvement of the public at large in such activities obviously leads to exposure to a wide variety of medical terms.

Drugs

Oliver Wendell Holmes' indictment of *polypharmacy* was well taken about 120 years ago: "I firmly believe that if the whole *materia medica,* as now used, could be sunk to the bottom of the sea, it would be all the better for mankind — and all the worse for the fishes." However, the doctors' dependence on drugs and the public's desire for them continue unabated. Many hospitalized patients receive between 10 and 15 different medications daily. New drugs are being developed constantly: new *antibiotics* to replace those to which microorganisms have become resistant, new antiviral agents, new *immunosuppressive* substances to protect transplanted organs, potent drugs to be used in the *chemotherapy* of neoplastic diseases, and innumerable additional *tranquilizers* or *stimulants.* New and potent drugs, however, bring with them new and serious adverse effects. A constant dispute is thus promoted between those who advocate more and those who argue for less drug use. On one side are the consumer groups, who insist that ours is an overmedicated society; on the other are pharmaceutical companies, many physicians, and some economists who believe that drug use in this country is too restricted. As an often criticized mediator in this dispute, the Federal Drug Administration establishes regulations, many of which are deeply resented, concerning the allowable use of prescription drugs. Obviously the public is interested in the decisions of the FDA and their consequences.

Prescription drugs usually have three names. One indicates the chemical composition of the drug, the second is the *generic* name, and the third may be a brand name selected by a pharmaceutical company to sell a drug that it manufactures or distributes. Brand names usually are pronounceable and easily remembered; generic names tend to be more difficult. The generic name for the tranquilizer *Librium,* for example, is *chlordiazepoxide.* A drug sold under a brand name is, as a rule, more expensive than the same drug sold under its generic name. The big pharmaceutical companies insist that their products with brand names tend to be more standardized and dependable than generically named products. Whether or not this claim is true is another subject of continuing controversy, but more and more states now have laws that require doctors or pharmacists or both to acquaint patients with the availability of generic products that usually are far cheaper than the brand name product the doctor tends to prescribe.

Acronyms and Other Initials

Another obstacle to public understanding of medical language is medicine's propensity to use initials; only government appears able to outdo medicine in this practice. Sometimes both government and medicine make use of the same initials: *NHI* and *NIH,* for example, which are confusingly similar but represent important entities that are entirely different, namely, *N*ational *H*ealth *I*nsurance and *N*ational *I*nstitutes of *H*ealth. This dictionary will help to allay the confusion.

Medical Ethics

Medical ethics used to deal with the behavior of doctors: the practice of fee-splitting, criticism of other doctors, and violating patient confidentiality. In retrospect, these topics might be called medical etiquette rather than ethics, especially when compared with the life-and-death issues that constitute today's medical ethics.

One of the major tasks of today's medical ethics is to weigh duration versus quality of life. Because of technical skills and equipment, doctors can keep patients "alive" (with circulating blood and *pulmonary* gas exchange) for long periods. But is it worthwhile — especially if the patient is permanently *comatose,* afflicted with brain death, or suffering unremitting and progressive agonies? Should a fetus be kept alive by heroic means if he or she is destined to become and stay a hopeless imbecile? When is it allowable to take an organ for transplantation from a patient considered to have brain death? Is "brain death" a viable concept anyhow? Innumerable questions of this type, involving the profoundest philosophic concepts, are increasingly harrassing doctors, families, and ethicists.

Another ethical problem is generated by research. In a way, scientific progress in medicine (if we want any more progress) eventually depends on doing research in humans, but what kind of research is allowable on what kind of patient, i.e., on prisoners, minors, or mental incompetents? And confidentiality has become a much more serious issue in view of all the information now demanded by government and commerce.

In trying to settle such issues, many nonmedical professionals have become involved: philosophers, clergymen, ordinary citizens, and, above all, lawyers and the courts. To them some source of medical definitions is essential.

Self-Care

It is voguish today to insist that the layman know more about his body and his health, that he should question doctors rather than accept their authoritarian pronouncements, that he should observe proper dietary habits, and that he should adopt a beneficial lifestyle to protect his own health. Thus words such as *carbohydrate, cholesterol,* and *fatty acids* are constantly mentioned in TV or newspaper advertising that promotes certain food products. At the same time, some food additives, such as flavors, preservatives, and color, are attacked as *carcinogenic.* Since evidence of their carcinogenicity is often indirect or based on the effect of massive doses given to small laboratory animals over long periods of time, the decision that a certain food additive may be harmful may induce violent public debate.

The philosophy underlying our health care is also criticized. It is said to be "crisis-oriented" in the sense that the patient seeks and obtains care after he has begun to feel ill. Medicine, say these critics, should be prevention-oriented. In this context, education of the public in medical matters and maintenance of beneficial lifestyles are important. So is reduction of public exposure to health hazards. In the pursuit of this goal, it is ironic that millions of hours and dollars are spent trying to prove or disprove that a certain substance under rare conditions might be carcinogenic, but little is done to decrease the greatest man-made health hazard, namely, automobile accidents.

As part of the campaign to prevent disease rather than to treat it, certain measures cause little disagreement: adequate nutrition, sanitary living conditions, and vaccinations known to be effective are endorsed by most professionals and nonprofessionals. Less agreement exists with respect to so-called periodic checkups. Yet it may prove beneficial to the public and cost-effective in an overall way to carry out *urinalyses, hematologic* studies, tests for fresh and occult blood in the *feces,* and blood pressure measurements on a regular basis. These tests are neither dangerous nor expensive. Whether more elaborate tests, such as *electrocardiograms, barium* or *contrast enemas, proctosigmoidoscopies,* or chest x-rays should be performed on a routine basis is much more questionable. All too often a test carried out as part of a checkup program misses the early manifestations of a disease and thus actually encourages a false sense of security. At the other end of the scale, nearly everyone agrees that dangerous and invasive tests are only indicated when a patient has a given set of *symptoms* or findings. Whether routine survey tests will save money in the long run is also a hotly disputed matter.

Environmental Pollution

Similarly newsworthy are charges of pollution by the discharge of poisonous, radioactive, or other carcinogenic wastes into the air or into bodies of water. Dumping of noxious substances is said to be widely practiced and leads to public accusations and denials concerning the health hazards involved.

Conclusion

In this Introduction I have tried to show how the public is getting increasingly involved in health care — sometimes for the sake of the individual and sometimes to establish public policy. "Establishing public policy" means politics, and in a sense almost every aspect of American medicine has become politicized. Each of the topics mentioned in this essay was formerly handled by an authoritarian medical profession. Now the laity has introduced itself into the decision-making process, and when decisions are made by the public at large, the process becomes increasingly political.

Many of our citizens stay out of politics, but a passive attitude in medical matters is deplorable. If a citizen wants to play a role in the broad affairs of medicine, he must perforce become acquainted with the language of medicine — with many of the words, in brief, that he will find in this *Dorland's Shorter Edition*.

The reader can also have some fun picking up some words from this handy technical dictionary. If his or her spouse grinds his or her teeth at night, the spouse can justifiably request, "Darling, I wish you would get over that *bruxism*."

CONTENTS

NOTES ON THE USE
OF THIS BOOK

ARRANGEMENT OF ENTRIES

All terms in this Dictionary are listed in one alphabetical sequence except the open compound terms, which are listed as subentries under the principal word (the *noun*). Thus, for example, acetic acid, amino acid, ribonucleic acid, and other acids will be found as subentries under the main entry *acid*. Addison's disease, collagen disease, Raynaud's disease, etc., are subentries under *disease*. Interstitial pneumonia, primary atypical pneumonia, lobar pneumonia, etc., are subentries under *pneumonia*, and so on.

In all subentries, the noun (main entry) is repeated in abbreviated form (e.g., *a.* for acid, *d.* for disease). Subentries that are plural in form are indicated by adding an apostrophe and *s* to the abbreviation of the noun. Thus, under *body*, the subentry *Aschoff's b's* is read Aschoff's bodies, *ketone b's* is read ketone bodies, etc.

PRONUNCIATION

The pronunciation of words is indicated by a phonetic respelling which appears in parentheses immediately following each main entry. These phonetic respellings, devised for ease of interpretation, are presented with a minimum of diacritical markings. The basic rule is this: An unmarked vowel ending a syllable is long; an unmarked vowel in a syllable ending with a consonant is short. By the same token, a long vowel in a syllable ending with a consonant is indicated by a macron (ā, ē, ī, ō, and ū): for example, ah-bāt′ (abate), lēd (lead), bīl (bile), hor′mōn (hormone), and am′pūl (ampule). A short vowel that constitutes or ends a syllable is indicated by a breve (ĕ, ĭ, ŏ, or ŭ): for example, ĕ-fu′zhun (effusion), ĭ-mu′nĭ-te (immunity), and ŏ-fish′al (official).

The syllable *ah* is used to represent the sound of *a* in open unaccented syllables (ah-pof′ĭ-sis, ah-tak′se-ah) and to indicate a broader *a* sound in syllables ending with a consonant, as in fahr′mah-se (pharmacy).

The primary accent in a word is indicated by a boldface, single accent, the secondary accent by a light face, double accent.

When, on successive words, the first syllables are pronounced in the same way, these syllables are given in the phonetic respelling of only the first of the sequence of terms. If the accent varies or other change occurs in the pronunciation of these syllables, even when they involve the same letters, the entire pronunciation is indicated in the phonetic respelling. For example:

> **ichthyophagous** (ik″the-of′ah-gus)
> **ichthyosarcotoxin** (ik″the-o-sar″ko-tok′sin)
> **ichthyosarcotoxism** (-sar″ko-tok′sizm)
> **ichthyosis** (ik″the-o′sis)
> **ichthyotoxin** (ik″the-o-tok′sin)

The qualities of compactness and convenience have been achieved by careful selection of terms and by concision of definitions insofar as brevity permits accuracy, clearness, and understanding. To further conserve space and, at the same time, to enhance the usefulness of this book, adjectival forms of many words are given on the noun entries (e.g., **allele** . . . **allelic,** adj.; **allergen** . . . **allergenic,** adj.). In similar fashion, irregular plural forms are given on the singular forms (e.g., **epiphysis** . . . pl. *epiphyses*). When, however, such forms may not be readily recognizable they are also given as separate entries (e.g., **viscera** . . . plural of *viscus*).

COMBINING FORMS IN MEDICAL TERMINOLOGY*

The following is a list of combining forms encountered frequently in the vocabulary of medicine. A dash or dashes are appended to indicate whether the form usually precedes (as *ante-*) or follows (as *-agra*) the other elements of the compound or usually appears between the other elements (as *-em-*). Following each combining form, the first item of information is the Greek or Latin word, or both a Greek and a Latin word, from which it is derived. Those words that are not printed in Greek characters are Latin. Information necessary to an understanding of the form appears next in parentheses. Then the meaning or meanings of the word are given, followed where appropriate by reference to a synonymous combining form. Finally, an example is given to illustrate the use of the combining form in a compound English derivative.

a-   *a-* (*n* is added before words beginning with a vowel) negative prefix. Cf. in-³. *ametria*

ab-   *ab* away from. Cf. apo-. *abducent*

abdomin-   *abdomen, abdominis. abdominoscopy*

ac-   See ad-. *accretion*

acet-   *acetum* vinegar. *acetometer*

acid-   *acidus* sour. *aciduric*

acou-   ἀκούω hear. *acouesthesia*. (Also spelled acu-)

acr-   ἄκρον extremity, peak. *acromegaly*

act-   *ago, actus* do, drive, act. *reaction*

actin-   ἀκτίς, ἀκτῖνος ray, radius. Cf. radi-. *actinogenesis*

acu-   See acou-. *osteoacusis*

ad-   *ad* (*d* changes to *c, f, g, p, s,* or *t* before words beginning with those consonants) to. *adrenal*

aden-   ἀδήν gland. Cf. gland-. *adenoma*

adip-   *adeps, adipis* fat. Cf. lip- and stear-. *adipocellular*

aer-   ἀήρ air. *anaerobiosis*

aesthe-   See esthe-. *aesthesioneurosis*

af-   See ad-. *afferent*

ag-   See ad-. *agglutinant*

-agogue   ἀγωγός leading, inducing. *galactagogue*

-agra   ἄγρα catching, seizure. *podagra*

alb-   *albus* white. Cf. leuk-. *albocinereous*

alg-   ἄλγος pain. *neuralgia*

all-   ἄλλος other, different. *allergy*

alve-   *alveus* trough, channel, cavity. *alveolar*

amph-   See amphi-. *ampheclexis*

amphi-   ἀμφί (*i* is dropped before words beginning with a vowel) both, doubly. *amphicelous*

amyl-   ἄμυλον starch. *amylosynthesis*

an-¹   See ana-. *anagogic*

an-²   See a-. *anomalous*

ana-   ἀνά (final *a* is dropped before words beginning with a vowel) up, positive. *anaphoresis*

ancyl-   See ankyl-. *ancylostomiasis*

andr-   ἀνήρ, ἀνδρός man. *gynandroid*

angi-   ἀγγεῖον vessel. Cf. vas-. *angiemphraxis*

ankyl-   ἀγκύλος crooked, looped. *ankylodactylia*. (Also spelled ancyl-)

*Compiled by Lloyd W. Daly, A. M., Ph.D., Litt. D., Allen Memorial Professor of Greek, University of Pennsylvania.

ant-   See anti-. *ant*ophthalmic

ante-   *ante* before. *ante*flexion

anti-   ἀντί (*i* is dropped before words beginning with a vowel) against, counter. Cf. contra-. *anti*pyogenic

antr-   ἄντρον cavern. *antr*odynia

ap-¹   See apo-. *ap*heter

ap-²   See ad-. *ap*pend

-aph-   ἅπτω, ἀφ- touch. dys*aph*ia. (See also hapt-)

apo-   ἀπό (*o* is dropped before words beginning with a vowel) away from, detached. Cf. ab-. *apo*physis

arachn-   ἀράχνη spider. *arachn*odactyly

arch-   ἀρχή beginning, origin. *arch*enteron

arter(i)-   ἀρτηρία elevator (?), artery. *arteri*osclerosis, peri*arter*itis

arthr-   ἄρθρον joint. Cf. articul-. syn*arthr*osis

articul-   *articulus* joint. Cf. arthr-. dis*articul*ation

as-   See ad-. *as*similation

at-   See ad-. *at*trition

aur-   *auris* ear. Cf. ot-. *aur*inasal

aux-   αὔξω increase. enter*aux*e

ax-   ἄξων or *axis* axis. *ax*ofugal

axon-   ἄξων axis. *axon*ometer

ba-   βαίνω, βα- go, walk, stand. hypno*ba*tia

bacill-   *bacillus* small staff, rod. Cf. bacter-. actino*bacill*osis

bacter-   βακτήριον small staff, rod. Cf. bacill-. *bacter*iophage

ball-   βάλλω, βολ- throw. *ball*istics. (See also bol-)

bar-   βάρος weight. pedo*bar*ometer

bi-¹   βίος life. Cf. vit-. aero*bi*c

bi-²   *bi*- two (see also di-¹). *bi*lobate

bil-   *bilis* bile. Cf. chol-. *bil*iary

blast-   βλαστός bud, child, a growing thing in its early stages. Cf. germ-. *blast*oma, zygoto*blast*.

blep-   βλέπω look, see. hemia*blep*sia

blephar-   βλέφαρον (from βλέπω; see blep-) eyelid. Cf. cili-. *blephar*oncus

bol-   See ball-. em*bol*ism

brachi-   βραχίων arm. *brachi*ocephalic

brachy-   βραχύς short. *brachy*cephalic

brady-   βραδύς slow. *brady*cardia

brom-   βρῶμος stench. podo*brom*idrosis

bronch-   βρόγχος windpipe. *bronch*oscopy

bry-   βρύω be full of life. em*bry*onic

bucc-   *bucca* cheek. disto*bucc*al

cac-   κακός bad, abnormal. Cf. mal-. *cac*odontia, arthro*cac*e. (See also dys-)

calc-¹   *calx, calcis* stone (cf. lith-), limestone, lime. *calc*ipexy

calc-²   *calx, calcis* heel. *calc*aneotibial

calor-   *calor* heat. Cf. therm-. *calor*imeter

cancr-   *cancer, cancri* crab, cancer. Cf. carcin-. *cancr*ology. (Also spelled chancr-)

capit-   *caput, capitis* head. Cf. cephal-. de*capit*ator

caps-   *capsa* (from *capio;* see cept-) container. en*caps*ulation

carbo(n)-   *carbo, carbonis* coal, charcoal. *carbo*hydrate, *carbon*uria

carcin-   καρκίνος crab, cancer. Cf. cancr-. *carcin*oma

cardi-   καρδία heart. lipo*cardi*ac

cary-   See kary-. *cary*okinesis

cat-   See cata-. *cat*hode

cata-   κατά (final *a* is dropped before words beginning with a vowel) down, negative. *cata*batic

caud-   *cauda* tail. *caud*ad

cav-   *cavus* hollow. Cf. coel-. con*cav*e

cec-   *caecus* blind. Cf. typhl-. *cec*opexy

cel-¹   See coel-. amphi*cel*ous

cel-²   See -cele. *cel*ectome

-cele   κήλη tumor, hernia. gastro*cele*

cell-   *cella* room, cell. Cf. cyt-. *cell*iferous

cen-   κοινός common. *cen*esthesia

cent-   *centum* hundred. Cf. hect-. Indicates fraction in metric system. [This exemplifies the custom in the metric system of identifying fractions of units by stems from the Latin, as centimeter, decimeter, millimeter, and multiples of units by the similar stems from the Greek, as hectometer, decameter, and kilometer.] *cent*imeter, *cent*ipede

cente-   κεντέω puncture. Cf. punct-. entero*cente*sis

centr-   κέντρον or *cenrum* point, center. neuro*centr*al

cephal-   κεφαλή head. Cf. capit-. en*cephal*itis

cept-   *capio, -cipientis, -ceptus* take, receive. re*cept*or

cer-   κηρός or *cera* wax. *cer*oplasty, *cer*omel

cerat-   See kerat-. a*cerat*osis

cerebr-   *cerebrum.* *cerebr*ospinal

cervic-   *cervix, cervicis* neck. Cf. trachel-. *cervic*itis

chancr-   See cancr-. *chancr*iform

cheil-   χεῖλος lip. Cf. labi-. *cheil*oschisis

cheir-   χείρ hand. Cf. man-. macro*cheir*ia. (Also spelled chir-)

chir-   See cheir-. *chir*omegaly

chlor-   χλωρός green. a*chlor*opsia

chol-   χολή bile. Cf. bil-. hepato*chol*angeitis

chondr-   χόνδρος cartilage. *chondr*omalacia

chord-   χορδή string, cord. peri*chord*al

chori-   χόριον protective fetal membrane. endo*chori*on

chro-	χρώς color. poly*chro*matic	cyst-	κύστις bladder. Cf. vesic-. nephrocystitis
chron-	χρόνος time. syn*chron*ous		
chy-	χέω, χυ- pour. ec*chy*mosis	cyt-	κύτος cell. Cf. cell-. plasmo*cyt*oma
-cid(e)	caedo, -cisus cut, kill. infanti*cide*, germi*cid*al	dacry-	δάκρυ tear. *dacry*ocyst
cili-	cilium eyelid. Cf. blephar-. super*cili*ary	dactyl-	δάκτυλος finger, toe. Cf. digit-. hexa*dactyl*ism
cine-	See kine-. auto*cine*sis	de-	de down from. *de*composition
-cipient	See cept-. in*cipient*	dec-¹	δέκα ten. Indicates multiple in metric system. Cf. dec-². *deca*gram
circum-	circum around. Cf. peri-. *circum*ferential		
-cis-	caedo, -cisus cut, kill. ex*cis*ion	dec-²	decem ten. Indicates fraction in metric system. Cf. dec-¹. *deci*para, *deci*meter
clas-	κλάω, κλασ- break. cranio*clas*t		
clin-	κλίνω bend, incline, make lie down. *clin*ometer	dendr-	δένδρον tree. neuro*dendr*ite
clus-	claudo, -clusus shut. Maloc*clus*ion	dent-	dens, dentis tooth. Cf. odont-. inter*dent*al
co-	See con-. *co*hesion	derm(at)-	δέρμα, δέρματος skin. Cf. cut-. endo*derm*, *derm*atitis
cocc-	κόκκος seed, pill. gono*cocc*us		
coel-	κοῖλος hollow. Cf. cav-. *coel*enteron. (Also spelled cel-)	desm-	δεσμός band, ligament. syn*desm*opexy
col-¹	See colon-. *col*ic	dextr-	dexter, dextr- right-hand. ambi*dextr*ous
col-²	See con-. *col*lapse		
colon-	κόλον lower intestine. *colon*ic	di-¹	di- two. *di*morphic. (See also bi-²)
colp-	κόλπος hollow, vagina. Cf. sin-. endo*colp*itis	di-²	See dia-. *di*uresis.
com-	See con-. *com*masculation	di-³	See dis-. *di*vergent.
con-	con- (becomes co- before vowels or h; col- before l; com- before b, m, or p; cor- before r) with, together. Cf. syn-. *con*traction	dia-	διά (a is dropped before words beginning with a vowel) through, apart. Cf. per-. *dia*gnosis
		didym-	δίδυμος twin. Cf. gemin-. epi*didym*al
contra-	contra against, counter. Cf. anti-. *contra*indication	digit-	digitus finger, toe. Cf. dactyl-. *digit*igrade
copr-	κόπρος dung. Cf. sterco-. *copr*oma	diplo-	διπλόος double. *diplo*myelia
cor-¹	κόρη doll, little image, pupil. iso*cor*ia	dis-	dis- (s may be dropped before a word beginning with a consonant) apart, away from. *dis*location
cor-²	See con-. *cor*rugator		
corpor-	corpus, corporis body. Cf. somat-. intra*corpor*al	disc-	δίσκος or discus disk. *disc*oplacenta
cortic-	cortex, corticis bark, rind. *cortic*osterone	dors-	dorsum back. ventro*dors*al
cost-	costa rib. Cf. pleur-. inter*cost*al	drom-	δρόμος course. hemo*drom*ometer
crani-	κρανίον or cranium skull. peri*crani*um	-ducent	See duct-. ad*ducent*
creat-	κρέας, κρεατ- meat, flesh. *creat*orrhea	duct-	duco, ducentis, ductus lead, conduct. ovi*duct*
-crescent	cresco, crescentis, cretus grow. ex*crescent*	dur-	durus hard. Cf. scler-. in*dur*ation
cret-¹	cerno, cretus distinguish, separate off. Cf. crin-. dis*cret*e	dynam(i)-	δύναμις power. *dynam*oneure, neuro*dynam*ic
cret-²	See -crescent. ac*cret*ion	dys-	δυσ- bad, improper. Cf. mal-. *dys*trophic. (See also cac-)
crin-	κρίνω distinguish, separate off. Cf. cret-¹. endo*crin*ology	e-	e out from. Cf. ec- and ex-. *e*mission
crur-	crus, cruris shin, leg. brachio*crur*al	ec-	ἐκ out of. Cf. e-. *ec*centric
cry-	κρύος cold. *cry*esthesia	-ech-	ἔχω have, hold, be. syn*ech*otomy
crypt-	κρύπτω hide, conceal. *crypt*orchism	ect-	ἐκτός outside. Cf. extra-. *ect*oplasm
cult-	colo, cultus tend, cultivate. *cult*ure	ede-	οἰδέω swell. *ede*matous
cune-	cuneus wedge. Cf. sphen-. *cune*iform	ef-	See ex-. *ef*florescent
		-elc-	ἕλκος sore, ulcer. enter*elc*osis. (See also helc-)
cut-	cutis skin. Cf. derm(at)-. sub*cut*aneous	electr-	ἤλεκτρον amber. *electr*otherapy
cyan-	κύανος blue. antho*cyan*in	em-	See en-. *em*bolism, *em*pathy, *em*phlysis
cycl-	κύκλος circle, cycle. *cycl*ophoria		

-em-   αἷμα blood. anemia. (See also hem(at)-)

en-   ἐν (n changes to m before b, p, or ph) in, on. Cf. in-². encelitis

end-   ἔνδον inside. Cf. intra-. endangium.

enter-   ἔντερον intestine. dysentery

ep-   See epi-. epaxial

epi-   ἐπί (i is dropped before words beginning with a vowel) upon, after, in addition. epiglottis

erg-   ἔργον work, deed. energy

erythr-   ἐρυθρός red. Cf. rub(r)-. erythrochromia

eso-   ἔσω inside. Cf. intra-. esophylactic

esthe-   αἰσθάνομαι, αἰσθη- perceive, feel. Cf. sens-. anesthesia

eu-   εὖ good, normal. eupepsia

ex-   ἐξ or ex out of. Cf: e-. excretion

exo-   ἔξω outside. Cf. extra-. exopathic

extra-   extra outside of, beyond. Cf. ect- and exo-. extracellular

faci-   facies face. Cf. prosop-. brachiofaciolingual

-facient   facio, facientis, factus, -fectus make. Cf. poie-. calefacient

-fact-   See facient-. artefact

fasci-   fascia band. fasciorrhaphy

febr-   febris fever. Cf. pyr-. febricide

-fect-   See -facient. defective

-ferent   fero, ferentis, latus bear, carry. Cf. phor-. efferent

ferr-   ferrum iron. ferroprotein

fibr-   fibra fibre. Cf. in-¹. chondrofibroma

fil-   filum thread. filiform

fiss-   findo, fissus split. Cf. schis-. fission

flagell-   flagellum whip. flagellation

flav-   flavus yellow. Cf. xanth-. riboflavin

-flect-   flecto, flexus bend, divert. deflection

-flex-   See -flect-. reflexometer

flu-   fluo, fluxus flow. Cf. rhe-. fluid

flux-   See flu-. affluxion

for-   foris door, opening. perforated

-form   forma shape. Cf. -oid. ossiform

fract-   frango, fractus break. refractive

front-   frons, frontis forehead, front. nasofrontal

-fug(e)   fugio flee, avoid. vermifuge, centrifugal

funct-   fungor, functus perform, serve, function. malfunction

fund-   fundo, fusus pour. infundibulum

fus-   See fund-. diffusible

galact-   γάλα, γάλακτος milk. Cf. lact-. dysgalactia

gam-   γάμος marriage, reproductive union. agamont

gangli-   γάγγλιον swelling, plexus. neurogangliitis

gastr-   γαστήρ, γαστρός stomach. cholangiogastrostomy

gelat-   gelo, gelatus freeze, congeal. gelatin

gemin-   geminus twin, double. Cf. didym-. quadrigeminal

gen-   γίγνομαι, γεν-, γον- become, be produced, originate, or γεννάω produce, originate. cytogenic

germ-   germen, germinis bud, a growing thing in its early stages. Cf. blast-. germinal, ovigerm

gest-   gero, gerentis, gestus bear, carry. congestion

gland-   glans, glandis acorn. Cf. aden-. intraglandular

-glia   γλία glue. neuroglia

gloss-   γλῶσσα tongue. Cf. lingu-. trichoglossia

glott-   γλῶττα tongue, language. glottic

gluc-   See glyc(y)-. glucophenetidin

glutin-   gluten, glutinis glue. agglutination

glyc(y)-   γλυκύς sweet. glycemia, glycyrrhizin. (Also spelled gluc-)

gnath-   γνάθος jaw. orthognathous

gno-   γιγνώσκω, γνω- know, discern. diagnosis

gon-   See gen-. amphigony

grad-   gradior walk, take steps. retrograde

-gram   γράφω, γραφ- + -μα scratch, write, record. cardiogram

gran-   granum grain, particle. lipogranuloma

graph-   γράφω scratch, write, record. histography

grav-   gravis heavy. multigravida

gyn(ec)-   γυνή, γυναικός woman, wife. androgyny, gynecologic

gyr-   γῦρος ring, circle. gyrospasm

haem(at)-   See hem(at)-. haemorrhagia, haematoxylon

hapt-   ἅπτω touch. haptometer

hect-   ἑκτ- hundred. Cf. cent-. Indicates multiple in metric system. hectometer

helc-   ἕλκος sore, ulcer. helcosis

hem(at)-   αἷμα, αἵματος blood. Cf. sanguin-. hemangioma, hematocyturia. (See also -em-)

hemi-   ἡμι- half. Cf. semi-. hemiageusia

hen-   εἷς, ἑνός one. Cf. un-. henogenesis

hepat-   ἧπαρ, ἥπατος liver. gastrohepatic

hept(a)-   ἑπτά seven. Cf. sept-². heptatomic, heptavalent

hered-   heres, heredis heir. heredoimmunity

hex-¹   ἕξ six. Cf. sex-. hexyl-. An a is added in some combinations.

hex-²   ἔχω, ἑχ- (added to σ becomes ἑξ-) have, hold, be. cachexy

hexa-   See hex-¹. hexachromic

hidr- ἱδρώς sweat. hyperhidrosis

hist- ἱστός web, tissue. histodialysis

hod- ὁδός road, path. hodoneuromere. (See also od- and -ode[1])

hom- •ὁμός common, same. homomorphic

horm- ὁρμή impetus, impulse. hormone

hydat- ὕδωρ, ὕδατος water. hydatism

hydr- ὕδωρ, ὑδρ- water. Cf. lymph-. achlorhydria

hyp- See hypo-. hypaxial

hyper- ὑπέρ above, beyond, extreme. Cf. super-. hypertrophy

hypn- ὕπνος sleep. hypnotic

hypo- ὑπό (o is dropped before words beginning with a vowel) under, below. Cf. sub-. hypometabolism

hyster- ὑστέρα womb. colpohysteropexy

iatr- ἰατρός physician. pediatrics

idi- ἴδιος peculiar, separate, distinct. idiosyncrasy

il- See in-[2], [3]. illinition (in, on), illegible (negative prefix)

ile- See ili- [ile- is commonly used to refer to the portion of the intestines known as the ileum]. ileostomy

ili- ilium (ileum) lower abdomen, intestines [ili- is commonly used to refer to the flaring part of the hip bone known as the ilium]. iliosacral

im- See in-[2], [3]. immersion (in, on), imperforation (negative prefix)

in-[1] ἴς, ἰνός fiber. Cf. fibr-. inosteatoma

in-[2] in (n changes to l, m, or r before words beginning with those consonants) in, on. Cf. en-. insertion

in-[3] in- (n changes to l, m, or r before words beginning with those consonants) negative prefix. Cf. a-. invalid

infra- infra beneath. infraorbital

insul- insula island. insulin

inter- inter among, between. intercarpal

intra- intra inside. Cf. end- and eso-. intravenous

ir- See in-[2], [3]. irradiation (in, on), irreducible (negative prefix)

irid- ἴρις, ἴριδος rainbow, colored circle. keratoiridocyclitis

is- ἴσος equal. isotope

ischi- ἰσχίον hip, haunch. ischiopubic

jact- iacio, iactus throw. jactitation

ject- iacio, -iectus throw. injection

jejun- ieiunus hungry, not partaking of food. gastrojejunostomy

jug- iugum yoke. conjugation

junct- iungo, iunctus yoke, join. conjunctiva

kary- κάρυον nut, kernel, nucleus. Cf. nucle-. megakaryocyte. (Also spelled cary-)

kerat- κέρας, κέρατος horn. keratolysis. (Also spelled cerat-)

kil- χίλιοι one thousand. Cf. mill-. Indicates multiple in metric system. kilogram

kine- κινέω move. kinematograph. (Also spelled cine-)

labi- labium lip. Cf. cheil-. gingivolabial

lact- lac, lactis milk. Cf. galact-. glucolactone

lal- λαλέω talk, babble. glossolalia

lapar- λαπάρα flank. laparotomy

laryng- λάρυγξ, λάρυγγος windpipe. laryngendoscope

lat- fero, latus bear, carry. See -ferent. translation

later- latus, lateris side. ventrolateral

lent- lens, lentis lentil. Cf. phac-. lenticonus

lep- λαμβάνω, ληπ- take, seize. cataleptic

leuc- See leuk-. leucinuria

leuk- λευκός white. Cf. alb-. leukorrhea. (Also spelled leuc-)

lien- lien spleen. Cf. splen-. lienocele

lig- ligo tie, bind. ligate

lingu- lingua tongue. Cf. gloss-. sublingual

lip- λίπος fat. Cf. adip-. glycolipin

lith- λίθος stone. Cf. calc-[1]. nephrolithotomy

loc- locus place. Cf. top-. locomotion

log- λέγω, λογ- speak, give an account. logorrhea, embryology

lumb- lumbus loin. dorsolumbar

lute- luteus yellow. Cf. xanth-. luteoma

ly- λύω loose, dissolve. Cf. solut-. keratolysis

lymph- lympha water. Cf. hydr-. lymphadenosis

macr- μακρός long, large. macromyeloblast

mal- malus bad, abnormal. Cf. cac- and dys-. malfunction

malac- μαλακός soft. osteomalacia

mamm- mamma breast. Cf. mast-. submammary

man- manus hand. Cf. cheir-. maniphalanx

mani- μανία mental aberration. manigraphy, kleptomania

mast- μαστός breast. Cf. mamm-. hypermastia

medi- medius middle. Cf. mes-. medifrontal

mega- μέγας great, large. Also indicates multiple (1,000,000) in metric system. megacolon, megadyne. (See also megal-)

megal- μέγας, μεγάλου great, large. acromegaly

mel- μέλος limb, member. symmelia

melan- μέλας, μέλανος black. hippo-melanin

men- μήν month. dysmenorrhea

mening- μῆνιγξ, μήνιγγος membrane. encephalomeningitis

ment- mens, mentis mind. Cf. phren-, psych- and thym-. dementia

mer- μέρος part. polymeric

mes- μέσος middle. Cf. medi-. mesoderm

met- See meta-. metallergy

meta- μετά (a is dropped before words beginning with a vowel) after, beyond, accompanying. metacarpal

metr-¹ μέτρον measure. stereometry

metr-² μήτρα womb. endometritis

micr- μικρός small. photomicrograph

mill- mille one thousand. Cf. kil-. Indicates fraction in metric system. milligram, millipede

miss- See -mittent. intromission

-mittent mitto, mittentis, missus send. intermittent

mne- μιμνήσκω, μνη- remember. pseudomnesia

mon- μόνος only, sole. monoplegia

morph- μορφή form, shape. polymorphonuclear

mot- moveo, motus move. vasomotor

my- μῦς, μυός muscle. inoleiomyoma

-myces μύκης, μύκητος fungus. myelomyces

myc(et)- See -myces. ascomycetes, streptomycin

myel- μυελός marrow. poliomyelitis

myx- μύξα mucus. myxedema

narc- νάρκη numbness. toponarcosis

nas- nasus nose. Cf. rhin-. palatonasal

ne- νέος new, young. neocyte

necr- νεκρός corpse. necrocytosis

nephr- νεφρός kidney. Cf. ren-. paranephric

neur- νεῦρον nerve. esthesioneure

nod- nodus knot. nodosity

nom- νόμος (from νέμω deal out, distribute) law, custom. taxonomy

non- nona nine. nonacosane

nos- νόσος disease. nosology

nucle- nucleus (from nux, nucis nut) kernel. Cf. kary-. nucleide

nutri- nutrio nourish. malnutrition

ob- ob (b changes to c before words beginning with that consonant) against, toward, etc. obtuse

oc- See ob-. occlude.

ocul- oculus eye. Cf. ophthalm-. oculomotor

-od- See -ode¹. periodic

-ode¹ ὁδός road, path. cathode. (See also hod-)

-ode² See -oid. nematode

odont- ὁδούς, ὁδόντος tooth. Cf. dent-. orthodontia

-odyn- ὀδύνη pain, distress. gastrodynia

-oid εἶδος form. Cf. -form. hyoid

-ol See ole-. cholesterol

ole- oleum oil. oleoresin

olig- ὀλίγος few, small. oligospermia

omphal- ὀμφαλός navel. periomphalic

onc- ὄγκος bulk, mass. hematoncometry

onych- ὄνυξ, ὄνυχος claw, nail. anonychia

oo- ᾠόν egg. Cf. ov-. perioothecitis

op- ὁράω, ὀπ- see. erythropsia

ophthalm- ὀφθαλμός eye. Cf. ocul-. exophthalmic

or- os, oris mouth. Cf. stom(at)-. intraoral

orb- orbis circle. suborbital

orchi- ὄρχις testicle. Cf. test-. orchiopathy

organ- ὄργανον implement, instrument. organoleptic

orth- ὀρθός straight, right, normal. orthopedics

oss- os, ossis bone. Cf. ost(e)-. ossiphone

ost(e)- ὀστέον bone. Cf. oss-. enostosis, osteanaphysis

ot- οὖς, ὠτός ear. Cf. aur-. parotid

ov- ovum egg. Cf. oo-. synovia

oxy- ὀξύς sharp. oxycephalic

pachy(n)- παχύνω thicken. pachyderma, myopachynsis

pag- πήγνυμι, παγ- fix, make fast. thoracopagus

par-¹ pario bear, give birth to. primiparous

par-² See para-. parepigastric

para- παρά (final a is dropped before words beginning with a vowel) beside, beyond. paramastoid

part- pario, partus bear, give birth to. parturition

path- πάθος that which one undergoes, sickness. psychopathic

pec- πήγνυμι, πηγ- (πηκ- before τ) fix, make fast. sympectothiene. (See also pex-)

ped- παῖς, παιδός child. orthopedic

pell- pellis skin, hide. pellagra

-pellent pello, pellentis, pulsus drive. repellent

pen- πένομαι need, lack. erythrocytopenia

pend- pendeo hang down. appendix

pent(a)- πέντε five. Cf. quinque-. pentose, pentaploid

peps- πέπτω, πεψ- (before σ) digest bradypepsia

pept- πέπτω digest. dyspeptic

per- per through. Cf. dia-. pernasal

peri- περί around. Cf. circum-. periphery

pet- peto seek, tend toward. centripetal

pex- πήγνυμι, πηγ- (added to σ becomes πηξ-) fix, make fast. hepatopexy

pha-   φημί, φα- say, speak. dysphasia
phac-   φακός lentil, lens. Cf. lent-. phacosclerosis. (Also spelled phak-)
phag-   φαγεῖν eat. lipophagic
phak-   See phac-. phakitis
phan-   See phen-. diaphanoscopy
pharmac- φάρμακον drug. pharmacognosy
pharyng- φάρυγξ, φαρυγγ- throat. glossopharyngeal
phen-   φαίνω, φαν- show, be seen. phosphene
pher-   φέρω, φορ- bear, support. periphery
phil-   φιλέω like, have affinity for. eosinophilia
phleb-   φλέψ, φλεβός vein. periphlebitis
phleg-   φλέγω, φλογ- burn, inflame. adenophlegmon
phlog-   See phleg-. antiphlogistic
phob-   φόβος fear, dread. claustrophobia
phon-   φωνή sound. echophony
phor-   See pher-. Cf. -ferent. exophoria
phos-   See phot-. phosphorus
phot-   φῶς, φωτός light. photerythrous
phrag-   φράσσω, φραγ- fence, wall off, stop up. Cf. sept-¹. diaphragm
phrax-   φράσσω, φραγ- (added to σ becomes φραξ-) fence, wall off, stop up. emphraxis
phren-   φρήν mind, midriff. Cf. ment-. metaphrenia, metaphrenon
phthi-   φθίνω decay, waste away. ophthalmophthisis
phy-   φύω beget, bring forth, produce, be by nature. nosophyte
phyl-   φῦλον tribe, kind. phylogeny
-phyll   φύλλον leaf. xanthophyll
phylac-   φύλαξ guard. prophylactic
phys(a)- φυσάω blow, inflate. physocele, physalis
physe-   φυσάω, φυση- blow, inflate. emphysema
pil-   pilus hair. epilation
pituit-   pituita phlegm, rheum. pituitous
placent- placenta (from πλακοῦς) cake. extraplacental
plas-   πλάσσω mold, shape. cineplasty
platy-   πλατύς broad, flat. platyrrhine
pleg-   πλήσσω, πληγ- strike. diplegia
plet-   pleo, -pletus fill. depletion
pleur-   πλευρά rib, side. Cf. cost-. peripleural
plex-   πλήσσω, πληγ- (added to σ becomes πληξ-) strike. apoplexy
plic-   plico fold. complication
pne-   πνοιά breathing. traumatopnea
pneum(at)- πνεῦμα, πνεύματος breath, air. pneumodynamics, pneumatothorax
pneumo(n)- πνεύμων lung. Cf. pulmo(n)-. pneumocentesis, pneumonotomy

pod-   πούς, ποδός foot. podiatry
poie-   ποιέω make, produce. Cf. -facient. sarcopoietic
pol-   πόλος axis of a sphere. peripolar
poly-   πολύς much, many. polyspermia
pont-   pons, pontis bridge. pontocerebellar
por-¹   πόρος passage. myelopore
por-²   πῶρος callus. porocele
posit-   pono, positus put, place. repositor
post-   post after, behind in time or place. postnatal, postoral
pre-   prae before in time or place. prenatal, prevesical
press-   premo, pressus press. pressoreceptive
pro-   πρό or pro before in time or place. progamous, procheilon, prolapse
proct-   πρωκτός anus. enteroproctia
prosop-   πρόσωπον face. Cf. faci-. diprosopus
pseud-   ψευδής false. pseudoparaplegia
psych-   ψυχή soul, mind. Cf. ment-. psychosomatic
pto-   πίπτω, πτω- fall. nephroptosis
pub-   pubes & puber, puberis adult. ischiopubic. (See also puber-)
puber-   puber adult. puberty
pulmo(n)- pulmo, pulmonis lung. Cf. pneumo(n)-. pulmolith, cardiopulmonary
puls-   pello, pellentis, pulsus drive. propulsion
punct-   pungo, punctus prick, pierce. Cf. cente-. punctiform
pur-   pus, puris pus. Cf. py-. suppuration
py-   πύον pus. Cf. pur-. nephropyosis
pyel-   πύελος trough, basin, pelvis. nephropyelitis
pyl-   πύλη door, orifice. pylephlebitis
pyr-   πῦρ fire. Cf. febr-. galactopyra
quadr-   quadr- four. Cf. tetra-. quadrigeminal
quinque- quinque five. Cf. pent(a)-. quinquecuspid
rachi-   ῥαχίς spine. Cf. spin-. encephalorachidian
radi-   radius ray. Cf. actin-. irradiation
re-   re- back, again. retraction
ren-   renes kidneys. Cf. nephr-. adrenal
ret-   rete net. retothelium
retro-   retro backwards. retrodeviation
rhag-   ῥήγνυμι, ῥαγ- break, burst. hemorrhagic
rhaph-   ῥαφή suture. gastrorrhaphy
rhe-   ῥέω flow. Cf. flu-. diarrheal
rhex-   ῥήγνυμι, ῥηγ- (added to σ becomes ῥηξ-) break, burst. metrorrhexis

rhin-   ῥίς, ῥινός nose. Cf. nas-. basi-
         rhinal

rot-   rota wheel. rotator

rub(r)- ruber, rubri red. Cf. erythr-.
         bilirubin, rubrospinal

salping- σάλπιγξ, σάλπιγγος tube,
         trumpet. salpingitis

sanguin- sanguis, sanguinis blood. Cf.
         hem(at)-. sanguineous

sarc-   σάρξ, σαρκός flesh. sarcoma

schis-   σχίζω, σχιδ- (before τ or added
         to σ becomes σχισ-) split.
         Cf. fiss-. schistorachis,
         rachischisis

scler-   σκληρός hard. Cf. dur-. sclero-
         sis

scop-   σκοπέω look at, observe. endo-
         scope

sect-   seco, sectus cut. Cf. tom-.
         sectile

semi-   semi- half. Cf. hemi-. semi-
         flexion

sens-   sentio, sensus perceive, feel.
         Cf. esthe-. sensory

sep-   σήπω rot, decay. sepsis

sept-¹   saepio, saeptus fence, wall off,
         stop up. Cf. phrag-. naso-
         septal

sept-²   septem seven. Cf. hept(a)-.
         septan

ser-   serum whey, watery substance.
         serosynovitis

sex-   sex six. Cf. hex-¹. sexdigitate

sial-   σίαλον saliva. polysialia

sin-   sinus hollow, fold. Cf. colp-.
         sinobronchitis

sit-   σῖτος food. parasitic

solut-   solvo, solventis, solutus loose,
         dissolve, set free. Cf. ly-.
         dissolution

-solvent See solut-. dissolvent

somat-   σῶμα, σώματος body. Cf. corpor-.
         psychosomatic

-some   See somat-. dictyosome

spas-   σπάω, σπασ- draw, pull. spasm,
         spastic

spectr- spectrum appearance, what is
         seen. microspectroscope

sperm(at)- σπέρμα, σπέρματος seed. sper-
         macrasia, spermatozoon

spers-   spargo, -spersus scatter. dis-
         persion

sphen-   σφήν wedge. Cf. cune-. sphenoid

spher-   σφαῖρα ball. hemisphere

sphygm- σφυγμός pulsation. sphygmo-
         manometer

spin-   spina spine. Cf. rachi-. cere-
         brospinal

spirat- spiro, spiratus breathe. in-
         spiratory

splanchn- σπλάγχνα entrails, viscera.
         neurosplanchnic

splen-   σπλήν spleen. Cf. lien-. splen-
         omegaly

spor-   σπόρος seed. sporophyte, zygo-
         spore

squam-   squama scale. desquamation

sta-   ἵστημι, στα- make stand, stop.
         genesistasis

stal-   στέλλω, σταλ- send. peristalsis.
         (See also stol-)

staphyl- σταφυλή bunch of grapes, uvula.
         staphylococcus, staphylec-
         tomy

stear-   στέαρ, στέατος fat. Cf. adip-.
         stearodermia

steat-   See stear-. steatopygous

sten-   στενός narrow, compressed.
         stenocardia

ster-   στερεός solid. cholesterol

sterc-   stercus dung. Cf. copr-. sterco-
         porphyrin

sthen-   σθένος strength. asthenia

stol-   στέλλω, στολ- send. diastole

stom(at)- στόμα, στόματος mouth, orifice.
         Cf. or-. anastomosis, stomato-
         gastric

strep(h)- στρέφω, στρεπ- (before τ) twist.
         Cf. tors-. strephosymbolia,
         streptomycin. (See also
         stroph-)

strict- stringo, stringentis, strictus
         draw tight, compress, cause
         pain. constriction

-stringent See strict-. astringent

stroph- στρέφω, στροφ- twist. an-
         astrophic. (See also
         strep(h)-)

struct- struo, structus pile up (against).
         obstruction

sub-   sub (b changes to f or p before
         words beginning with those
         consonants) under, below.
         Cf. hypo-. sublumbar

suf-   See sub-. suffusion

sup-   See sub-. suppository

super-   super above, beyond, extreme.
         Cf. hyper-. supermotility

sy-   See syn-. systole

syl-   See syn-. syllepsiology

sym-   See syn-. symbiosis, symmetry,
         sympathetic, symphysis

syn-   σύν (n disappears before s,
         changes to l before l, and
         changes to m before b, m, p,
         and ph) with, together. Cf.
         con-. myosynizesis

ta-   See ton-. ectasis

tac-   τάσσω, ταγ- (τακ- before τ)
         order, arrange. atactic

tact-   tango, tactus touch. contact

tax-   τάσσω, ταγ- (added to σ be-
         comes ταξ-) order, arrange.
         ataxia

tect-   See teg-. protective

teg-   tego, tectus cover. integument

tel-   τέλος end. telosynapsis

tele-   τῆλε at a distance. teleceptor

tempor- tempus, temporis time, timely
         or fatal spot, temple. tempo-
         romalar

ten(ont)- τένων, τένοντος (from τείνω
         stretch) tight stretched band.
         tenodynia, tenonitis, tenon-
         tagra

tens-   *tendo, tensus* stretch. Cf. ton-. ex*tens*or

test-   *testis* testicle. Cf. orchi-. *test*itis

tetra-   τετρα- four. Cf. quadr-. *tetrag*enous

the-   τίθημι, θη- put, place. syn*the*sis

thec-   θήκη repository, case. *thec*ostegnosis

thel-   θηλή teat, nipple. *thel*erethism

therap-   θεραπεία treatment. hydro*therap*y

therm-   θέρμη heat. Cf. calor-. dia*therm*y

thi-   θεῖον sulfur. *thi*ogenic

thorac-   θώραξ, θώρακος chest. *thorac*oplasty

thromb-   θρόμβος lump, clot. *thromb*openia

thym-   θυμός spirit. Cf. ment-. dys*thym*ia

thyr-   θυρεός shield (shaped like a door θύρα). *thyr*oid

tme-   τέμνω, τμη- cut. axono*tme*sis

toc-   τόκος childbirth. dys*toc*ia

tom-   τέμνω, τομ- cut. Cf. sect-. ap pendec*tom*y

ton-   τείνω, τον- stretch, put under tension. Cf. tens-. peri*ton*eum

top-   τόπος place. Cf. loc-. *top*esthesia

tors-   *torqueo, torsus* twist. Cf. strep-. ex*tors*ion

tox-   τοξικόν (from τόξον bow) arrow poison, poison. *tox*emia

trache-   τραχεῖα windpipe. *trache*otomy

trachel-   τράχηλος neck. Cf. cervic-. *trachel*opexy

tract-   *traho, tractus* draw, drag. pro*tract*ion

traumat-   τραῦμα, τραύματος wound. *traumat*ic

tri-   τρεῖς, τρία or *tri-* three. *tri*gonid

trich-   θρίξ, τριχός hair. *trich*oid

trip-   τρίβω rub. en*trip*sis

trop-   τρέπω, τροπ- turn, react. sito*trop*ism

troph-   τρέφω, τροφ- nurture. a*troph*y

tuber-   *tuber* swelling, node. *tuber*cle

typ-   τύπος (from τύπτω strike) type. a*typ*ical

typh-   τῦφος fog, stupor. adeno*typh*us

typhl-   τυφλός blind. Cf. cec-. *typhl*ectasis

un-   *unus* one. Cf. hen-. *un*ioval

ur-   οὖρον urine. poly*ur*ia

vacc-   *vacca* cow. *vacc*ine

vagin-   *vagina* sheath. in*vagin*ated

vas-   *vas* vessel. Cf. angi-. *vas*cular

vers-   See vert-. in*vers*ion

vert-   *verto, versus* turn. di*vert*iculum

vesic-   *vesica* bladder. Cf. cyst-. *vesic*ovaginal

vit-   *vita* life. Cf. bi-¹. de*vit*alize

vuls-   *vello, vulsus* pull, twitch. con*vuls*ion

xanth-   ξανθός yellow, blond. Cf. flav- and lute-. *xanth*ophyll

-yl-   ὕλη substance. cacod*yl*

zo-   ζωή life, ζῷον animal. micro*zo*aria

zyg-   ζυγόν yoke, union. *zyg*odactyly

zym-   ζύμη ferment. en*zym*e

DORLAND'S MEDICAL DICTIONARY

Shorter Edition

THE HUMAN BODY
HIGHLIGHTS of STRUCTURE and FUNCTION

SKELETAL SYSTEM

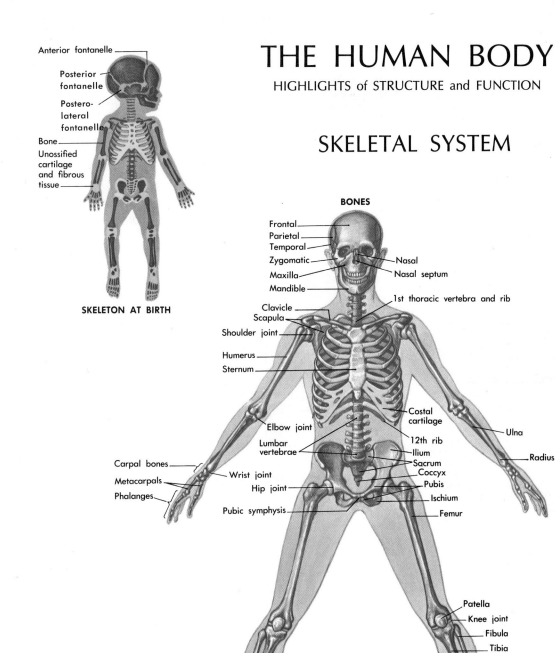

Anterior fontanelle

Posterior fontanelle

Postero-lateral fontanelle

Bone

Unossified cartilage and fibrous tissue

SKELETON AT BIRTH

BONES

Frontal
Parietal
Temporal
Zygomatic
Maxilla
Mandible

Nasal
Nasal septum

1st thoracic vertebra and rib

Clavicle
Scapula
Shoulder joint

Humerus
Sternum

Costal cartilage

12th rib
Ilium
Sacrum
Coccyx

Elbow joint

Lumbar vertebrae

Carpal bones
Metacarpals
Phalanges

Wrist joint

Hip joint

Pubic symphysis

Ulna

Radius

Pubis
Ischium
Femur

Patella
Knee joint
Fibula
Tibia

Tarsal bones
Metatarsals
Phalanges

Ankle joint

Designed by
WILLIAM A. OSBURN, M.M.A.
Artwork by
ELLEN COLE
ROBERT DEMAREST
GRANT LASHBROOK
WILLIAM OSBURN

W. B. SAUNDERS COMPANY
Philadelphia — London — Toronto

Plate 1

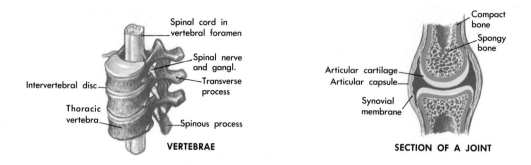

Spinal cord in vertebral foramen

Spinal nerve and gangl.

Transverse process

Intervertebral disc

Thoracic vertebra

Spinous process

VERTEBRAE

Compact bone

Spongy bone

Articular cartilage

Articular capsule

Synovial membrane

SECTION OF A JOINT

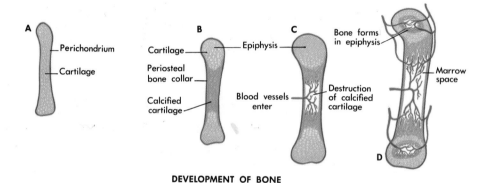

A

Perichondrium

Cartilage

B

Cartilage

Periosteal bone collar

Calcified cartilage

Epiphysis

C

Blood vessels enter

Destruction of calcified cartilage

Bone forms in epiphysis

Marrow space

D

DEVELOPMENT OF BONE

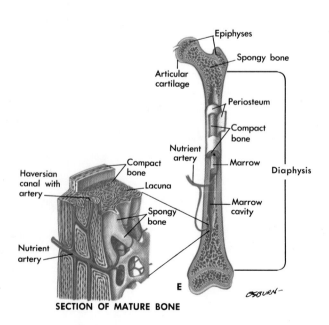

Epiphyses

Spongy bone

Articular cartilage

Periosteum

Compact bone

Nutrient artery

Marrow

Diaphysis

Compact bone

Haversian canal with artery

Lacuna

Spongy bone

Marrow cavity

Nutrient artery

E

OSBURN

SECTION OF MATURE BONE

Plate 2

SKELETAL MUSCLES

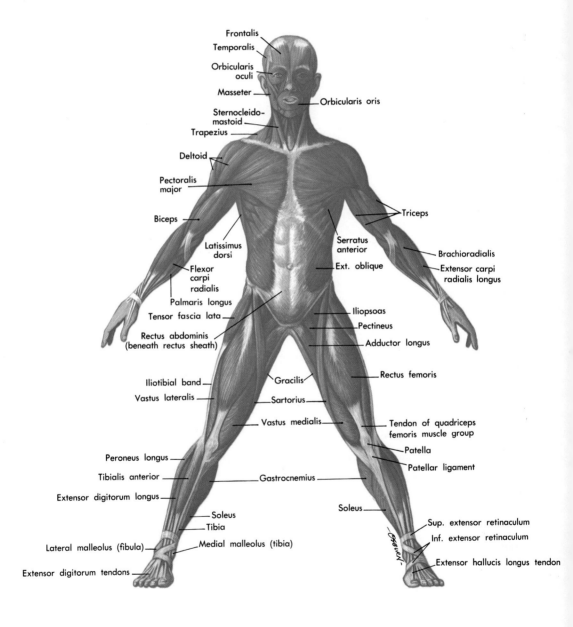

Frontalis
Temporalis
Orbicularis oculi
Masseter
Orbicularis oris
Sternocleido- mastoid
Trapezius
Deltoid
Pectoralis major
Triceps
Biceps
Serratus anterior
Latissimus dorsi
Brachioradialis
Ext. oblique
Flexor carpi radialis
Extensor carpi radialis longus
Palmaris longus
Tensor fascia lata
Iliopsoas
Pectineus
Rectus abdominis (beneath rectus sheath)
Adductor longus
Rectus femoris
Iliotibial band
Gracilis
Vastus lateralis
Sartorius
Vastus medialis
Tendon of quadriceps femoris muscle group
Patella
Peroneus longus
Patellar ligament
Tibialis anterior
Gastrocnemius
Extensor digitorum longus
Soleus
Soleus
Tibia
Sup. extensor retinaculum
Lateral malleolus (fibula)
Medial malleolus (tibia)
Inf. extensor retinaculum
Extensor hallucis longus tendon
Extensor digitorum tendons

Plate 3

HOW A MUSCLE PRODUCES MOVEMENT

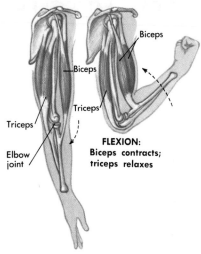

Biceps

Biceps

Triceps

Triceps

Triceps

Elbow
joint

Elbow joint

FLEXION:
Biceps contracts;
triceps relaxes

EXTENSION:
Triceps contracts;
biceps relaxes

HOW A MUSCLE ATTACHES TO BONE

Penetrating fibers — Periosteum

Muscle fiber
Int. perimysium
Ext. perimysium
Muscle fasciculus

Tendon

The connective tissue which surrounds
the muscle fibers and bundles may (1)
form a tendon which fuses with the
periosteum, or (2) may fuse directly
with the periosteum without forming
a tendon.

HOW A MUSCLE CONTRACTS

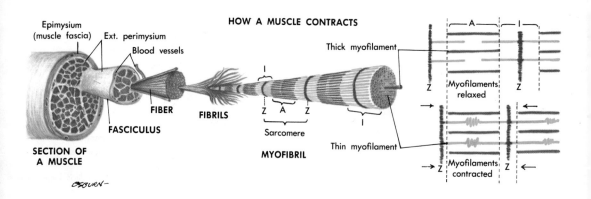

Epimysium
(muscle fascia)   Ext. perimysium

Blood vessels

Thick myofilament

FIBER

FIBRILS

FASCICULUS

Z A Z

Sarcomere

MYOFIBRIL

SECTION OF
A MUSCLE

Thin myofilament

A — I

Z

Myofilaments
relaxed

Z

Myofilaments
contracted

Z

Z

OSBURN—

Plate 4

RESPIRATION AND THE HEART

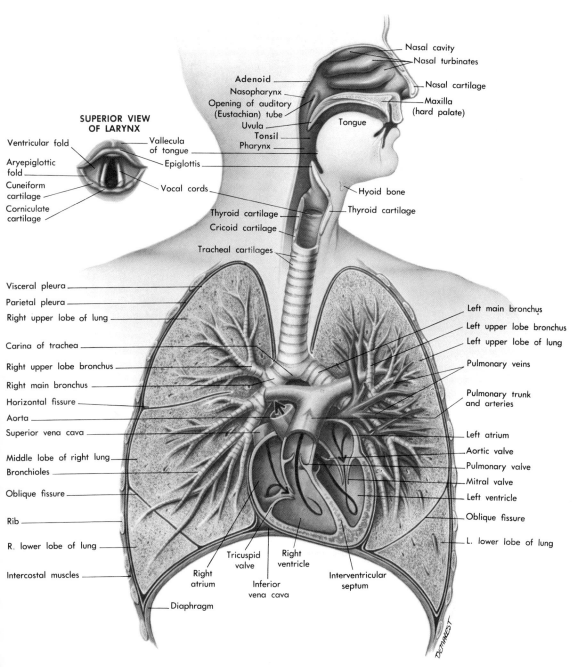

SUPERIOR VIEW OF LARYNX

Ventricular fold
Aryepiglottic fold
Cuneiform cartilage
Corniculate cartilage
Vallecula of tongue
Epiglottis
Vocal cords

Nasal cavity
Nasal turbinates
Nasal cartilage
Maxilla (hard palate)
Adenoid
Nasopharynx
Opening of auditory (Eustachian) tube
Uvula
Tonsil
Pharynx
Tongue

Thyroid cartilage
Cricoid cartilage
Tracheal cartilages

Hyoid bone
Thyroid cartilage

Visceral pleura
Parietal pleura
Right upper lobe of lung

Carina of trachea

Right upper lobe bronchus
Right main bronchus
Horizontal fissure
Aorta
Superior vena cava

Middle lobe of right lung
Bronchioles

Oblique fissure

Rib

R. lower lobe of lung

Intercostal muscles

Left main bronchus
Left upper lobe bronchus
Left upper lobe of lung
Pulmonary veins
Pulmonary trunk and arteries
Left atrium
Aortic valve
Pulmonary valve
Mitral valve
Left ventricle
Oblique fissure
L. lower lobe of lung

Right atrium
Tricuspid valve
Right ventricle
Inferior vena cava
Interventricular septum
Diaphragm

Plate 5

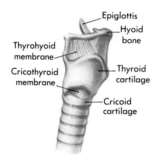

Epiglottis

Hyoid bone

Thyrohyoid membrane

Cricothyroid membrane

Thyroid cartilage

Cricoid cartilage

LATERAL VIEW OF THE LARYNX

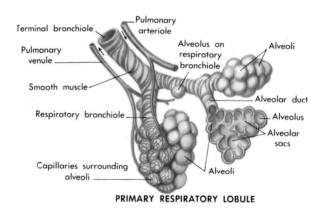

Terminal bronchiole

Pulmonary arteriole

Pulmonary venule

Alveolus on respiratory bronchiole

Alveoli

Smooth muscle

Alveolar duct

Respiratory bronchiole

Alveolus

Alveolar sacs

Capillaries surrounding alveoli

Alveoli

PRIMARY RESPIRATORY LOBULE

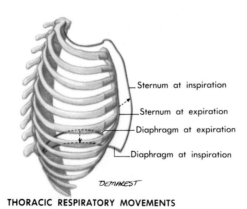

Sternum at inspiration

Sternum at expiration

Diaphragm at expiration

Diaphragm at inspiration

DEMAREST

THORACIC RESPIRATORY MOVEMENTS

Plate 6

BLOOD VASCULAR SYSTEM

VEINS

STRUCTURE

Tunica intima:
Endothelium

Tunica media:
Circular smooth
muscle and
elastic tissue

Tunica
adventitia:

White
fibrous
connective
tissue

VEINS

Int. jugular

Sup. vena cava
Subclavian
Intercostal

Hepatic
Median
cubital
Portal
Renal
Sup. mesen.
Inf. mes.

Inf.
vena
cava

Valve open

Muscle
contracted

Valve closed

Muscle
relaxed

Ext. iliac
Femoral

Greater
saphenous

Popliteal

Peroneal

Valve
open

Dorsal venous
arch of foot

from venule

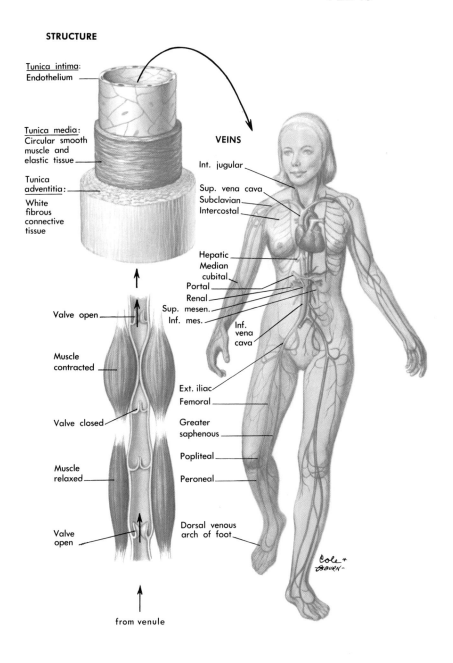

Cole +
OSBURN

Plate 7

STRUCTURE

ARTERIES

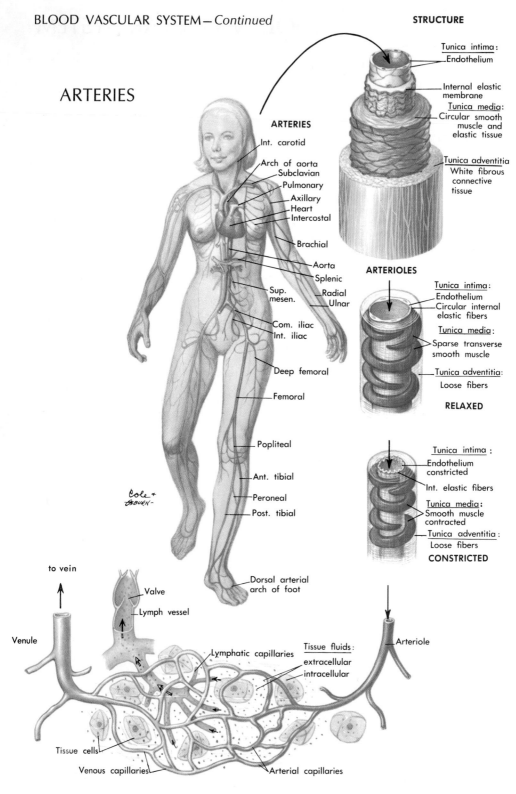

ARTERIES

Int. carotid
Arch of aorta
Subclavian
Pulmonary
Axillary
Heart
Intercostal
Brachial
Aorta
Splenic
Sup. mesen.
Radial
Ulnar
Com. iliac
Int. iliac
Deep femoral
Femoral
Popliteal
Ant. tibial
Peroneal
Post. tibial
Dorsal arterial arch of foot

Tunica intima:
Endothelium
Internal elastic membrane
Tunica media:
Circular smooth muscle and elastic tissue
Tunica adventitia
White fibrous connective tissue

ARTERIOLES

Tunica intima:
Endothelium
Circular internal elastic fibers
Tunica media:
Sparse transverse smooth muscle
Tunica adventitia:
Loose fibers

RELAXED

Tunica intima :
Endothelium constricted
Int. elastic fibers
Tunica media:
Smooth muscle contracted
Tunica adventitia :
Loose fibers

CONSTRICTED

to vein
Valve
Lymph vessel
Venule
Lymphatic capillaries
Tissue fluids:
extracellular
intracellular
Arteriole
Tissue cells
Venous capillaries
Arterial capillaries

A CAPILLARY BED

Cole + OSBURN-

Plate 8

DIGESTIVE SYSTEM

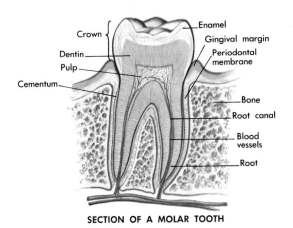

Crown {
Enamel
Gingival margin
Dentin
Periodontal membrane
Pulp
Cementum
Bone
Root canal
Blood vessels
Root

SECTION OF A MOLAR TOOTH

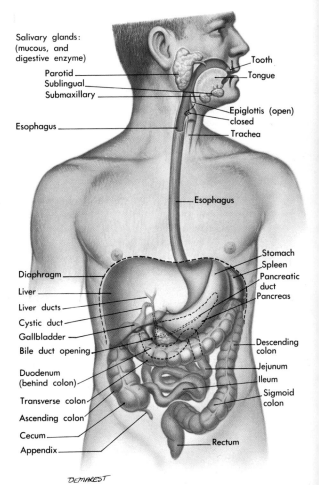

Salivary glands: (mucous, and digestive enzyme)
Parotid
Sublingual
Submaxillary
Esophagus
Tooth
Tongue
Epiglottis (open)
closed
Trachea
Esophagus
Diaphragm
Liver
Liver ducts
Cystic duct
Gallbladder
Bile duct opening
Duodenum (behind colon)
Transverse colon
Ascending colon
Cecum
Appendix
Stomach
Spleen
Pancreatic duct
Pancreas
Descending colon
Jejunum
Ileum
Sigmoid colon
Rectum

DEMAREST

Plate 9

DIGESTIVE SYSTEM — *Continued*

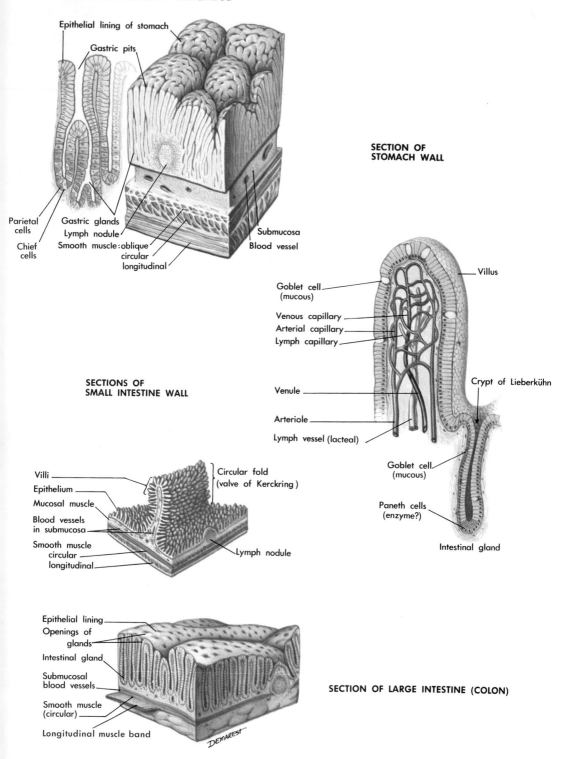

Epithelial lining of stomach

Gastric pits

SECTION OF STOMACH WALL

Parietal cells

Chief cells

Gastric glands

Lymph nodule

Smooth muscle: oblique
circular
longitudinal

Submucosa

Blood vessel

SECTIONS OF SMALL INTESTINE WALL

Villus

Goblet cell (mucous)

Venous capillary

Arterial capillary

Lymph capillary

Crypt of Lieberkühn

Venule

Arteriole

Lymph vessel (lacteal)

Goblet cell (mucous)

Villi

Epithelium

Mucosal muscle

Blood vessels in submucosa

Smooth muscle
circular
longitudinal

Circular fold (valve of Kerckring)

Lymph nodule

Paneth cells (enzyme?)

Intestinal gland

Epithelial lining

Openings of glands

Intestinal gland

Submucosal blood vessels

Smooth muscle (circular)

Longitudinal muscle band

SECTION OF LARGE INTESTINE (COLON)

DEMAREST

Plate 10

GENITOURINARY SYSTEM

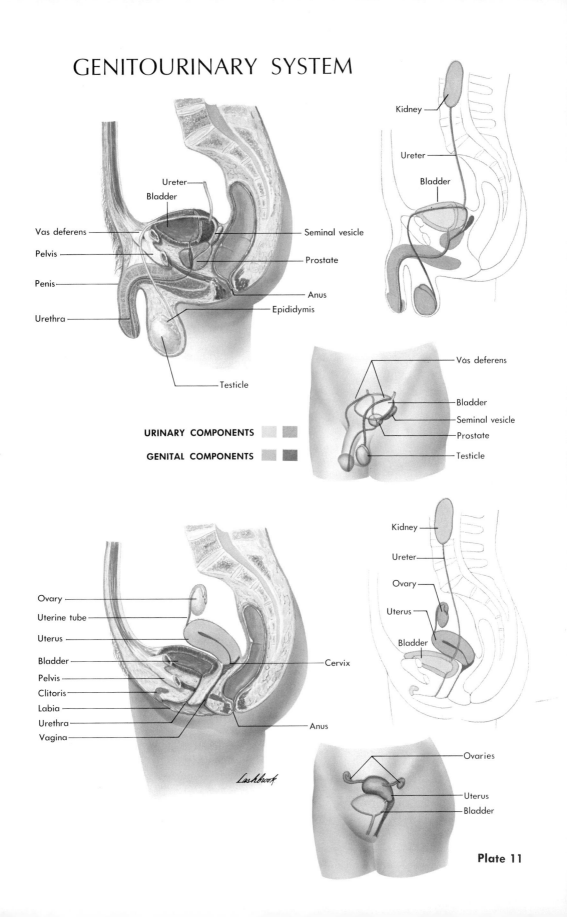

Kidney

Ureter

Bladder

Ureter
Bladder

Vas deferens
Pelvis
Penis
Urethra

Seminal vesicle
Prostate

Anus
Epididymis

Testicle

URINARY COMPONENTS

GENITAL COMPONENTS

Vas deferens

Bladder
Seminal vesicle
Prostate
Testicle

Kidney
Ureter
Ovary
Uterus
Bladder

Ovary
Uterine tube
Uterus
Bladder
Pelvis
Clitoris
Labia
Urethra
Vagina

Cervix

Anus

Lashbook

Ovaries

Uterus
Bladder

Plate 11

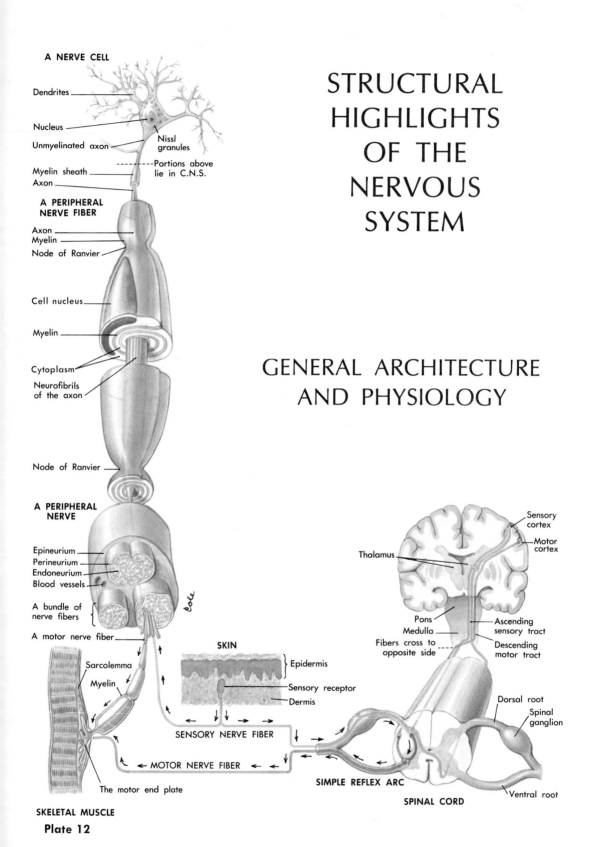

STRUCTURAL HIGHLIGHTS OF THE NERVOUS SYSTEM

GENERAL ARCHITECTURE AND PHYSIOLOGY

A NERVE CELL

Dendrites

Nucleus

Unmyelinated axon

Nissl granules

Portions above lie in C.N.S.

Myelin sheath

Axon

A PERIPHERAL NERVE FIBER

Axon

Myelin

Node of Ranvier

Cell nucleus

Myelin

Cytoplasm

Neurofibrils of the axon

Node of Ranvier

A PERIPHERAL NERVE

Epineurium

Perineurium

Endoneurium

Blood vessels

A bundle of nerve fibers

A motor nerve fiber

Sarcolemma

Myelin

SKIN

Epidermis

Sensory receptor

Dermis

SENSORY NERVE FIBER

← MOTOR NERVE FIBER ←

The motor end plate

SKELETAL MUSCLE

Plate 12

Sensory cortex

Motor cortex

Thalamus

Pons

Medulla

Fibers cross to opposite side

Ascending sensory tract

Descending motor tract

Dorsal root

Spinal ganglion

SIMPLE REFLEX ARC

Ventral root

SPINAL CORD

BRAIN AND SPINAL NERVES

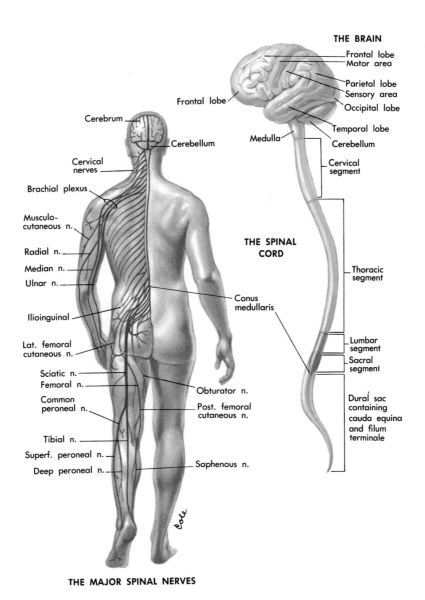

THE BRAIN

Frontal lobe
Motor area
Parietal lobe
Sensory area
Occipital lobe
Temporal lobe
Cerebellum

Frontal lobe

Medulla

Cervical
segment

Cerebrum

Cerebellum

Cervical
nerves

Brachial plexus

Musculo-
cutaneous n.

**THE SPINAL
CORD**

Radial n.

Median n.

Ulnar n.

Thoracic
segment

Ilioinguinal

Conus
medullaris

Lat. femoral
cutaneous n.

Lumbar
segment

Sciatic n.

Sacral
segment

Femoral n.

Common
peroneal n.

Obturator n.

Post. femoral
cutaneous n.

Dural sac
containing
cauda equina
and filum
terminale

Tibial n.

Superf. peroneal n.

Deep peroneal n.

Saphenous n.

THE MAJOR SPINAL NERVES

Plate 13

AUTONOMIC NERVES

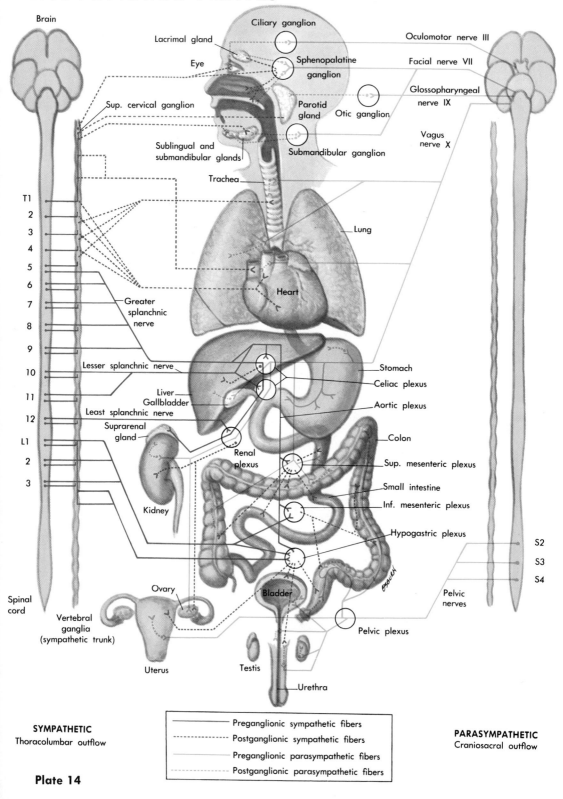

Brain

Ciliary ganglion

Lacrimal gland

Eye

Oculomotor nerve III

Sphenopalatine ganglion

Facial nerve VII

Glossopharyngeal nerve IX

Sup. cervical ganglion

Parotid gland

Otic ganglion

Vagus nerve X

Sublingual and submandibular glands

Submandibular ganglion

Trachea

T1
2
3
4

Lung

5
6
7

Heart

8
9

Greater splanchnic nerve

10
11
12

Lesser splanchnic nerve

Liver
Gallbladder

Stomach

Celiac plexus

Aortic plexus

Least splanchnic nerve

Suprarenal gland

L1
2
3

Renal plexus

Colon

Sup. mesenteric plexus

Small intestine

Inf. mesenteric plexus

Kidney

Hypogastric plexus

S2
S3
S4

Spinal cord

Ovary

Bladder

Pelvic nerves

Vertebral ganglia (sympathetic trunk)

Pelvic plexus

Uterus

Testis

Urethra

SYMPATHETIC
Thoracolumbar outflow

——————	Preganglionic sympathetic fibers
- - - - - -	Postganglionic sympathetic fibers
——————	Preganglionic parasympathetic fibers
- - - - - -	Postganglionic parasympathetic fibers

PARASYMPATHETIC
Craniosacral outflow

Plate 14

ORGANS OF SPECIAL SENSE

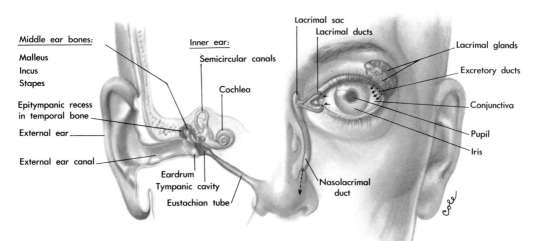

Middle ear bones:

Malleus
Incus
Stapes

Epitympanic recess
in temporal bone

External ear

External ear canal

Inner ear:

Semicircular canals

Cochlea

Eardrum
Tympanic cavity

Eustachian tube

THE ORGAN OF HEARING

Lacrimal sac
Lacrimal ducts

Lacrimal glands

Excretory ducts

Conjunctiva

Pupil

Iris

Nasolacrimal
duct

THE LACRIMAL APPARATUS AND THE EYE

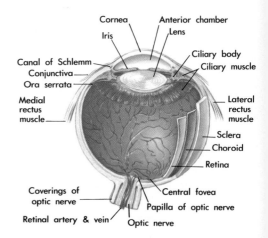

HORIZONTAL SECTION OF THE EYE

Cornea

Iris

Canal of Schlemm
Conjunctiva
Ora serrata
Medial
rectus
muscle

Anterior chamber
Lens

Ciliary body
Ciliary muscle

Lateral
rectus
muscle

Sclera
Choroid
Retina

Coverings of
optic nerve

Retinal artery & vein

Central fovea
Papilla of optic nerve
Optic nerve

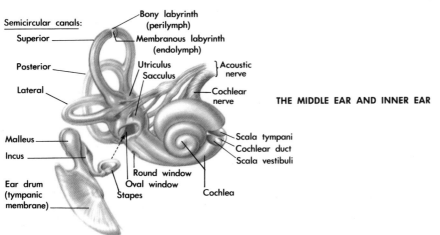

Semicircular canals:

Superior

Posterior

Lateral

Malleus

Incus

Ear drum
(tympanic
membrane)

Bony labyrinth
(perilymph)
Membranous labyrinth
(endolymph)

Utriculus
Sacculus

Round window
Oval window
Stapes

Acoustic
nerve

Cochlear
nerve

Scala tympani
Cochlear duct
Scala vestibuli

Cochlea

THE MIDDLE EAR AND INNER EAR

Plate 15

PARANASAL
SINUSES

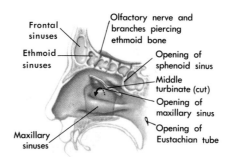

SAGITTAL SECTION OF THE NOSE

Frontal sinuses

Olfactory nerve and branches piercing ethmoid bone

Ethmoid sinuses

Opening of sphenoid sinus

Middle turbinate (cut)

Opening of maxillary sinus

Maxillary sinuses

Opening of Eustachian tube

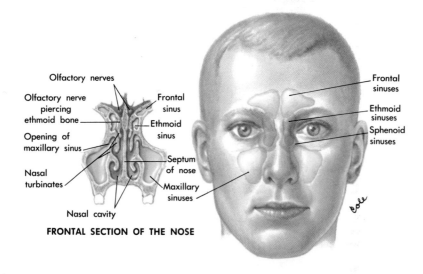

Olfactory nerves

Olfactory nerve piercing ethmoid bone

Opening of maxillary sinus

Nasal turbinates

Frontal sinus

Ethmoid sinus

Septum of nose

Maxillary sinuses

Nasal cavity

Frontal sinuses

Ethmoid sinuses

Sphenoid sinuses

FRONTAL SECTION OF THE NOSE

Plate 16

A

A symbol, *mass number.*

A or Å symbol, *angstrom* or *Angström unit.*

A. absorbance; accommodation; ampere; anode (anodal); anterior; axial; total acidity.

A₂ aortic second sound; both ears.

a [L.] *arteria* (artery); atto.

a- word element [L.], *without; not.*

A.A. achievement age; Alcoholics Anonymous.

a̅a̅ [L. pl.] *arteriae* (arteries).

aa ana (*of each*).

A.A.A. American Academy of Allergy; American Association of Anatomists.

A.A.A.S. American Association for the Advancement of Science.

A.A.B.B. American Association of Blood Banks.

A.A.C.P. American Academy for Cerebral Palsy.

A.A.D.P. American Academy of Denture Prosthetics.

A.A.D.R. American Academy of Dental Radiology.

A.A.D.S. American Academy of Dermatology and Syphilology; American Association of Dental Schools.

A.A.E. American Association of Endodontists.

A.A.F.P. American Academy of Family Physicians.

A.A.G.P. American Academy of General Practice.

A.A.I. American Association of Immunologists.

A.A.I.D. American Academy of Implant Dentures.

A.A.I.N. American Association of Industrial Nurses.

A.A.M.A. American Association of Medical Assistants.

A.A.M.R.L. American Association of Medical Record Librarians.

A.A.O. American Association of Orthodontists.

A.A.O.O. American Academy of Ophthalmology and Otolaryngology.

A.A.O.P. American Academy of Oral Pathology.

A.A.O.S. American Academy of Orthopedic Surgeons.

A.A.P. American Academy of Pediatrics; American Academy of Pedodontics; American Academy of Periodontology; Association for the Advancement of Psychotherapy; Association of American Physicians.

A.A.P.B. American Association of Pathologists and Bacteriologists.

A.A.P.M.R. American Academy of Physical Medicine and Rehabilitation.

A.A.P.S. American Association of Plastic Surgeons.

A.B. [L.] *Artium Baccalaureus* (Bachelor of Arts).

ab [L.] *from.*

ab- word element [L.], *from; off; away from.*

abacterial (a″bak-te′re-al) free from bacteria.

abarognosis (ah-bar″og-no′sis) loss of sense of weight.

abarthrosis (ab″ar-thro′sis) abarticulation.

abarticular (ab-ar-tik′u-ler) not affecting a joint; at a distance from a joint.

abarticulation (ab-ar-tik″u-la′shun) 1. synovial joint. 2. dislocation of a joint.

abasia (ah-ba′ze-ah) inability to walk. aba′sic, abat′ic, adj. a.-asta′sia, astasia-abasia. a. atac′tica, abasia with uncertain movements, due to a defect of coordination. choreic a., abasia due to chorea of the legs. paralytic a., abasia due to paralysis of leg muscles. paroxysmal trepidant a., abasia due to spastic stiffening of the legs on attempting to stand. spastic a., paroxysmal trepidant a. trembling a., a. trep′idans, abasia due to trembling of the legs.

abatement (ah-bāt′ment) decrease in severity of a pain or symptom.

abdomen (ab-do′men) that part of the body lying between the thorax and the pelvis, and containing the abdominal cavity and viscera. acute a., an acute intra-abdominal condition of abrupt onset, usually associated with pain due to inflammation, perforation, obstruction, infarction, or rupture of abdominal organs, and usually requiring emergency surgical intervention. carinate a., navicular a., scaphoid a. a. obsti′pum, congenital shortness of the rectus abdominis muscle. scaphoid a., one whose anterior wall is hollowed, occurring in children with cerebral disease. surgical a., acute a.

abdomin(o)- word element [L.], *abdomen.*

abdominal (ab-dom′ĭ-nal) pertaining to the abdomen.

abdominocentesis (ab-dom″ĭ-no-sen-te′sis) surgical puncture of the abdomen.

abdominocystic (-sis′tik) pertaining to the abdomen and gallbladder.

abdominohysterectomy (-his″ter-ek′to-me) hysterectomy through an abdominal incision.

abdominohysterotomy (-his″ter-ot′o-me) hysterotomy through an abdominal incision.

abdominoscopy (ab-dom″ĭ-nos′ko-pe) examination of the abdominal cavity.

abdominovaginal (ab-dom″ĭ-no-vaj′ĭ-nal) pertaining to the abdomen and vagina.

abducens (ab-du′senz) [L.] drawing away.

abducent (ab-du′sent) abducting.

abduct (ab-dukt′) to draw away from the median plane, or (the digits) from the axial line of a limb.

1

abduction (ab-duk'shun) the act of abducting; the state of being abducted.

abductor (ab-duk'tor) that which abducts.

aberratio (ab''er-a'she-o) [L.] aberration.

aberration (ab-er-a'shun) 1. deviation from the normal or usual. 2. unequal refraction or focalization of a lens. **chromatic a.,** unequal refraction of light rays of different wavelength, producing a blurred image with fringes of color. **chromosomal a.,** loss, gain, or exchange of genetic material in the chromosomes of a cell, resulting in a deletion, duplication, inversion, or translocation of genes. **dioptric a.,** spherical a. **distantial a.,** blurring of vision for distant objects. **mental a.,** unsoundness of mind of mild degree, not affecting intelligence. **spherical a.,** inherent inability of a spherical lens to bring all rays of light to a single focus.

abetalipoproteinemia (a-ba''tah-lip''o-pro''te-in-e'me-ah) a hereditary syndrome marked by a lack of β-lipoproteins in the blood and by acanthocytosis, hypocholesterolemia, progressive ataxic neuropathy, atypical retinitis pigmentosa involving the macula, and malabsorption.

abionergy (ab''e-on'er-je) abiotrophy.

abiosis (ab-e-o'sis) absence or deficiency of life. **abiot'ic,** adj.

abiotrophy (ab-e-ot'ro-fe) progressive loss of vitality of certain tissues or organs leading to disorders or loss of function; applied especially to degenerative hereditary diseases of late onset, e.g., Huntington's chorea.

abirritant (ab-ir'i-tant) 1. diminishing irritation; soothing. 2. an agent that relieves irritation.

abirritation (ab-ir''i-ta'shun) diminished irritability; atony.

ablactation (ab''lak-ta'shun) weaning or cessation of milk secretion.

ablate (ab-lāt') to remove, especially by cutting.

ablatio (ab-la'she-o) [L.] ablation.

ablation (ab-la'shun) 1. separation or detachment; extirpation; eradication. 2. removal, especially by cutting.

ablepharia (a''blef-a're-ah) congenital reduction or absence of the eyelids. **ableph'arous,** adj.

ablepharon (a-blef'ah-ron) ablepharia.

ablepsia (a-blep'se-ah) blindness.

abluent (ab'lu-ent) 1. detergent; cleansing. 2. a cleansing agent.

abmortal (ab-mor'tal) situated or directed away from a dead or injured part; applied especially to electric currents set up in injured tissue.

abnerval (ab-ner'val) passing from a nerve through a muscle; said of electric currents.

abnormality (ab''nor-mal'i-te) 1. the state of being abnormal. 2. a malformation.

abomasitis (ab''o-ma-si'tis) inflammation of the abomasum.

abomasum (ab''o-ma'sum) the fourth stomach of ruminants.

aborad (ab-o'rad) away from the mouth.

aboral (ab-o'ral) opposite to, or remote from, the mouth.

abort (ah-bort') to arrest prematurely a disease or developmental process; to expel the products of conception before the fetus is viable.

abortifacient (ah-bor''ti-fa'shent) 1. causing abortion. 2. an agent that induces abortion.

abortion (ah-bor'shun) 1. expulsion from the uterus of the products of conception before the fetus is viable. 2. premature arrest of a natural or morbid process. **artificial a.,** induced a. **contagious a.,** infectious a. **criminal a.,** induced abortion performed illegally. **enzootic a. of ewes,** abortion in ewes, usually late in the gestation period, caused by a strain of *Chlamydia.* **equine virus a.,** see under *rhinopneumonitis.* **habitual a.,** spontaneous abortion occurring in three or more successive pregnancies, at about the same level of development. **incomplete a.,** abortion with retention of parts of the products of conception. **induced a.,** abortion brought on intentionally by medication or instrumentation. **inevitable a.,** abortion which cannot be averted. **infectious a.,** 1. a disease of cattle due to *Brucella abortus,* causing premature loss of the developing calf. 2. an infectious disease of horses due to *Salmonella abortusequi* and of sheep due to *S. abortusovis.* **missed a.,** retention in the uterus of an abortus that has been dead for at least four weeks. **septic a.,** a serious infection of the uterus leading to generalized infection; it more commonly occurs after criminal abortion and often results in death of the mother. **spontaneous a.,** abortion occurring naturally. **therapeutic a.,** interruption of pregnancy by artificial means for medical considerations. **threatened a.,** signs of premature expulsion of the products of conception.

abortionist (ah-bor'shun-ist) one who makes a business of inducing criminal abortions.

abortive (ah-bor'tiv) 1. incompletely developed. 2. abortifacient.

abortus (ah-bor'tus) a dead or nonviable fetus (weighing less than 500 gm. at birth).

abrachia (ah-bra'ke-ah) congenital absence of the arms.

abrachiocephalia (ah-bra''ke-o-se-fa'le-ah) congenital absence of the head and arms.

abrachius (ah-bra'ke-us) a fetus without arms.

abrasio (ah-bra'se-o) [L.] abrasion. **a. cor'neae,** the scraping off of corneal excrescences. **a. den'tium,** wearing away of tooth substance.

abrasion (ah-bra'zhun) 1. a rubbing or scraping off; see also *planing.* 2. a rubbed or scraped area on skin or mucous membrane. **dental a.,** the wearing away of tooth structure due to mechanical action other than mastication.

abrasive (ah-bra'siv) 1. causing abrasion. 2. an agent that produces abrasion.

abreaction (ab''re-ak'shun) the process of releasing anxiety and tension by recalling to awareness and emotionally reliving the stressful situation which produces the symptoms and which has been forgotten (repressed) because it was consciously intolerable; *catharsis* is the method by which this is achieved.

abruptio (ah-brup'she-o) [L.] separation. **a.**

placen'tae, premature detachment of the placenta.

abscess (ab'ses) a localized collection of pus in a cavity formed by disintegration of tissues. **alveolar a.,** a localized suppurative inflammation of tissues about the apex of a tooth root. **amebic a.,** one caused by *Entamoeba histolytica,* usually hepatic. **anorectal a.,** one involving the anorectum. **appendiceal a., appendicular a.,** one resulting from perforation of an acutely inflamed appendix. **Bezold's a.,** subperiosteal abscess of the temporal bone. **Brodie's a.,** a roughly spherical region of bone destruction, filled with pus or connective tissue, usually in the metaphyseal region of long bones and caused by *Staphylococcus aureus* or *S. albus.* **cold a.,** one of slow development and with little inflammation, usually tuberculous. **diffuse a.,** a collection of pus not enclosed by a capsule. **miliary a.,** one of a set of small multiple abscesses. **milk a.,** abscess of the breast occurring during lactation. **Pautrier's a.,** focal collections of reticular cells in the epidermis. **perianal a.,** one adjacent to the anal canal. **peritonsillar a.,** an abscess in the connective tissue of the tonsil capsule, resulting from suppuration of the tonsil. **phlegmonous a.,** one associated with acute inflammation of the subcutaneous connective tissue. **primary a.,** one formed at the seat of the infection. **ring a.,** a ring-shaped purulent infiltration at the periphery of the cornea. **scrofulous a.,** tuberculous a. **shirt-stud a.,** one separated into two cavities connected by a narrow channel. **stitch a.,** one developed about a stitch or suture. **strumous a.,** tuberculous a. **thecal a.,** one arising in a sheath, as in a tendon sheath. **tuberculous a.,** one due to infection with tubercle bacilli. **vitreous a.,** an abscess of the vitreous humor of the eye due to infection, trauma, or foreign body. **wandering a.,** one that burrows into tissues and finally points at a distance from the site of origin. **web-space a.,** one in the loose connective tissue and fat at the base of the fingers.

abscissa (ab-sis'ah) the horizontal line in a graph along which are plotted the units of one of the factors considered in the study, as time in a time-temperature study.

abscission (ab-sish'un) removal by cutting.

abscopal (ab-sko'p'l) pertaining to the effect that irradiation of a tissue has on a nonirradiated tissue.

Absidia (ab-sid'ĭ-ah) a genus of fungi (order Mucorales), including *A. corymbif'era,* which may cause mycosis in man, and *A. ramo'sa,* which grows on bread and decaying vegetation and causes otomycosis and sometimes mucormycosis.

absinthe (ab'sinth) an extract of absinthium and other bitter herbs, containing 60% alcohol; prolonged ingestion causes nervousness, convulsions, trismus, amblyopia, optic neuritis, and mental deterioration.

absorbance (ab-sor'bans) in radiology, a measure of the ability of a medium to absorb radiation, expressed as the logarithm of the quotient of the intensity of the radiation entering the medium divided by that leaving it.

absorbefacient (ab-sor″bĕ-fa'shent) 1. causing absorption. 2. an agent that promotes absorption.

absorben (ab-sor'ben) an antigen used to adsorb homologous antibodies from antiserum.

absorbent (ab-sorb'ent) 1. able to take in, or suck up and incorporate. 2. a tissue structure involved in absorption. 3. a substance that absorbs or promotes absorption.

absorptiometer (ab-sorp″she-om'ĕ-ter) 1. an apparatus for determining the amount of gas absorbed by a fluid. 2. a device for measuring the layer of liquid absorbed between two glass plates; used as a hematoscope.

absorption (ab-sorp'shun) 1. the uptake of substances into or across tissues. 2. in psychology, devotion of thought to one object or activity only. 3. in radiology, uptake of energy by matter with which the radiation interacts. **intestinal a.,** the uptake from the intestinal lumen of fluids, solutes, proteins, fats, and other nutrients into the intestinal epithelial cells, blood, lymph, or interstitial fluids.

absorptive (-tiv) capable of absorbing; involving absorption.

abstergent (ab-ster'jent) 1. cleansing or detergent. 2. a cleansing agent.

abstinence (ab'stĭ-nens) a refraining from the use of or indulgence in food, stimulants, or sexual intercourse.

abstraction (ab-strak'shun) 1. the mental process of forming abstract ideas. 2. the withdrawal of any ingredient from a compound. 3. malocclusion in which the occlusal plane is further from the eye-ear plane, causing lengthening of the face; cf. *attraction* (2).

abtropfung (ahb-trop'foong) the proliferative transition of theques of nevus cells from the epidermis down into the dermis.

abulia (ah-bu'le-ah) loss or deficiency of will power, initiative, or drive. **abu'lic,** adj.

abulomania (ah-bu″lo-ma'ne-ah) mental disorder characterized by lack of will power and indecisiveness.

abutment (ah-but'ment) a supporting structure to sustain lateral or horizontal pressure, as the anchorage tooth for a fixed or removable partial denture.

A.C. air conduction; alternating current; anodal closure; axiocervical.

Ac chemical symbol, *actinium.*

a.c. [L.] *an'te ci'bum* (before meals).

A.C.A. American College of Angiology; American College of Apothecaries.

acacia (ah-ka'shah) the dried gummy exudate from stems and branches of species of *Acacia,* prepared as a mucilage or syrup, and used as a pharmaceutical aid.

acalcicosis (ah-kal″sĭ-ko'sis) a condition due to deficiency of calcium in the diet.

acalculia (a″kal-ku'le-ah) inability to do mathematical calculations.

acampsia (a-kamp'se-ah) rigidity of a part or limb.

acanth(o)- word element [Gr.], *sharp spine; thorn.*

acantha (ah-kan′tha) 1. the spine. 2. a spinous process of a vertebra.

acanthaceous (ak″an-tha′shus) bearing prickles.

acanthamebiasis (ah-kan″thah-me-bi′ah-sis) infection with *Acanthamoeba castellani.*

Acanthamoeba (-me′bah) a genus of amebas of the order Amoebida, including *A. castella′ni,* which ordinarily inhabits moist soil or water, but has been found as an opportunistic parasite of man, causing a fatal meningoencephalitis.

acanthesthesia (a-kan″thes-the′ze-ah) perverted sensation of a sharp point pricking the body.

acanthion (ah-kan′the-on) a point at the base of the anterior nasal spine.

Acanthocephala (ah-kan″tho-sef′ah-lah) a phylum of elongate, mostly cylindrical organisms (thorny-headed worms) parasitic in the intestines of all classes of vertebrates; in some classifications, considered to be a class of the phylum Nemathelminthes.

acanthocephaliasis (-sef″ah-li′ah-sis) infection with worms of the phylum Acanthocephala.

acanthocephalous (-sef′ah-lus) pertaining to or caused by worms of the phylum Acanthocephala.

Acanthocephalus (-sef′ah-lus) a genus of parasitic worms (phylum Acanthocephala).

Acanthocheilonema (-ki″lo-ne′mah) a genus of long, threadlike worms. **A. per′stans,** *Dipetalonema perstans.*

acanthocyte (ah-kan′tho-sīt) a distorted erythrocyte with protoplasmic projections giving it a "thorny" appearance; seen in abetalipoproteinemia.

acanthocytosis (ah-kan″tho-si-to′sis) the presence in the blood of acanthocytes, characteristically seen in abetalipoproteinemia.

acantholysis (ah″kan-thol′ĭ-sis) dissolution of the intercellular bridges of the prickle-cell layer of the epidermis. **acantholyt′ic,** adj.

acanthoma (ak″an-tho′mah) a tumor composed of epidermal or squamous cells.

acanthorrhexis (ah-kan″tho-rek′sis) rupture of the intercellular bridges of the prickle-cell layer of the epidermis, as in blisters caused by severe edema of the skin.

acanthosis (ak″an-tho′sis) diffuse hyperplasia and thickening of the prickle-cell layer of the epidermis. **acanthot′ic,** adj. **a. ni′gricans,** diffuse acanthosis with gray or black pigmentation, chiefly in body folds, occurring in an adult form (often associated with visceral carcinoma) and in a mild, juvenile nevoid form (related to obesity or endocrine disturbances).

acanthrocyte (ah-kan′thro-sīt) acanthocyte.

acanthrocytosis (ah-kan″thro-si-to′sis) acanthocytosis.

acapnia (ah-kap′ne-ah) decrease of carbon dioxide in the blood; hypocapnia. **acap′nic,** adj.

acarbia (ah-kar′be-ah) decrease of bicarbonate in the blood.

acardia (ah-kar′de-ah) congenital absence of the heart.

acardiacus (ah″kar-di′ah-kus) [L.] having no heart.

acardius (ah-kar′de-us) an imperfectly formed twin fetus without a heart and invariably lacking other body parts.

acariasis (ak″ah-ri′ah-sis) infestation with mites.

acaricide (ah-kar′ĭ-sīd) 1. destructive to mites. 2. an agent that destroys mites.

acarid (ak′ah-rid) a tick or mite of the order Acarina.

acaridiasis (ah-kar″ĭ-di′ah-sis) acariasis.

Acarina (ak″ah-ri′nah) an order of arthropods (class Arachnida), including mites and ticks.

acarinosis (ah-kar″i-no′sis) any disease caused by mites; acariasis.

acarodermatitis (ak″ah-ro-der″mah-ti′tis) any skin inflammation caused by mites (acarids). **a. urticarioi′des,** grain itch.

acarologist (ak″ah-rol′o-jist) a specialist in acarology.

acarology (ak″ah-rol′o-je) the scientific study of mites and ticks.

acarophobia (ak″ah-ro-fo′be-ah) morbid dread of mites or of small objects.

Acarus (ak′ah-rus) a genus of small mites. **A. folliculo′rum,** *Demodex folliculorum.* **A. scab′iei,** *Sarcoptes scabiei.* **A. si′ro,** a mite that causes vanillism in vanilla pod handlers.

acaryote (ah-kār′e-ōt) 1. non-nucleated. 2. a non-nucleated cell.

acatalasemia (a″kat-ah-la-se′me-ah) acatalasia.

acatalasia (-la′ze-ah) a rare hereditary disease seen mostly in the Japanese, marked by congenital absence of catalase; it may be associated with recurrent infections of oral structures.

acatamathesia (a-kat″ah-mah-the′ze-ah) 1. loss or impairment of the power to understand speech. 2. impairment of any one of the perceptive faculties, due to a central lesion.

acataphasia (-fa′ze-ah) speech disorder, with inability to express one's thoughts in a connected manner, due to a central lesion.

acathexia (ak″ah-thek′se-ah) inability to retain bodily secretions. **acathec′tic,** adj.

acathexis (-sis) a mental disturbance in which certain things, such as objects, ideas, and memories, that ordinarily have great significance to an individual arouse no emotional response.

acaudal (a-kaw′dal) acaudate.

acaudate (a-kaw′dāt) lacking a tail.

A.C.C. American College of Cardiology; anodal closure contraction.

accelerator (ak-sel″er-a′tor) [L.] 1. an agent or apparatus that increases the rate at which something occurs or progresses. 2. any nerve or muscle that hastens the performance of a function. **linear a.,** an apparatus for the acceleration of subatomic particles. **serum prothrombin conversion a.,** coagulation Factor VII. **serum thrombotic a.,** a factor in serum which has procoagulant properties and the ability to induce blood coagulation.

acceptor (ak-sep′tor) a substance which unites

with another substance; specifically, one that unites with hydrogen or oxygen in an oxidoreduction reaction and so enables the reaction to proceed.

accessory (ak-ses′o-re) supplementary; affording aid to another similar and generally more important thing.

accident prone (ak′sĭ-dent prōn) specially susceptible to accidents owing to psychological factors.

accipiter (ak-sip′ĭ-ter) a facial bandage with tails like the claws of a hawk.

acclimation (ak-lĭ-ma′shun) the process of becoming accustomed to a new environment.

acclimatization (ah-kli″mah-ti-za′shun) acclimation.

accommodation (ah-kom″o-da′shun) adjustment, especially of the eye for seeing objects at various distances. **absolute a.,** the accommodation of either eye separately. **histologic a.,** changes in morphology and function of cells following changed conditions. **negative a.,** adjustment of eye for long distances by relaxation of the ciliary muscles. **positive a.,** adjustment of eye for short distances by contraction of the ciliary muscles.

accommodometer (ah-kom″ŏ-dom′ĕ-ter) an instrument for measuring accommodative capacity of the eye.

accouchement (ah-kōōsh-maw′) [Fr.] delivery; labor. **a. forcé,** rapid forcible delivery by one of several methods; originally, rapid dilatation of the cervix with the hands, followed by version and extraction of the fetus.

accrementition (ak″re-men-tish′un) growth by addition of similar tissue.

accretion (ah-kre′shun) 1. growth by addition of material. 2. accumulation. 3. adherence of parts normally separated.

aceclidine (as-sek′lĭ-dēn) a cholinergic, C_9H_{15}-NO_2.

acedapsone (as″ĕ-dap′sŏn) a dapsone derivative, $C_{16}H_{16}N_2O_4S$, having antimalarial and leprostatic activities.

acellular (a-sel′u-lar) not cellular in structure.

acelomate (ah-se′lo-māt) having no coelom or body cavity.

acelous (a-se′lus) not concave on either surface; said of vertebrae of certain animals.

acenesthesia (ah-sen″es-the′ze-ah) loss of sense of well-being or physical existence.

acenocoumarol (ah-se″no-koo′mah-rol) an anticoagulant.

acentric (a-sen′trik) 1. not central; not located in the center. 2. lacking a centromere, so that the chromosome will not survive cell divisions.

acephalobrachia (ah-sef″ah-lo-bra′ke-ah) congenital absence of the head and arms.

acephalocardia (-kar′de-ah) congenital absence of the head and heart.

acephalocardius (-kar′de-us) a fetus without a head or heart.

acephalochiria (-ki′re-ah) congenital absence of the head and hands.

acephalocyst (ah-sef′ah-lo-sist″) a sterile echinococcus cyst.

acephalogaster (ah-sef″ah-lo-gas′ter) a fetus without a head or stomach.

acephalogastria (-gas′tre-ah) congenital absence of the head, chest, and upper part of the abdomen.

acephalopodia (-po′de-ah) congenital absence of the head and feet.

acephalopodius (-po′de-us) a fetus without a head or feet.

acephalorachia (-ra′ke-ah) congenital absence of the head and spinal column.

acephalostomia (-sto′me-ah) congenital absence of the head, with a mouth aperture on the upper aspect of the body.

acephalothoracia (-tho-ra′se-ah) congenital absence of the head and thorax.

acephalous (ah-sef′ah-lus) headless.

acephalus (ah-sef′ah-lus) a headless monster.

acerin (ah′ser-in) an extract from the dried fruit of the Norway maple, *Acer plantanoides,* effective against *Escherichia coli* and the vaccinia virus.

acerola (ah-sĕ-ro′lah) the West Indian cherry fruit, thought to be the richest natural source of vitamin C.

acervuline (ah-ser′vu-lĭn) aggregated; heaped up; said of certain glands.

acervulus (ah-ser′vu-lus), pl. *acer′vuli*[L.] gritty matter in or near the pineal body, the choroid plexus, and other parts of the brain. **a. cer′ebri,** acervulus.

acetabular (as″ĕ-tab′u-ler) pertaining to the acetabulum.

acetabulectomy (as″ĕ-tab″u-lek′to-me) excision of the acetabulum.

acetabuloplasty (as″ĕ-tab′u-lo-plas″te) plastic repair of the acetabulum.

acetabulum (as″ĕ-tab′u-lum) the cup-shaped cavity on the lateral surface of the hip bone, receiving the head of the femur. **sunken a.,** Otto pelvis.

acetal (as′ĕ-tal) an organic compound formed by a combination of an aldehyde with an alcohol.

acetaldehyde (as″et-al′de-hīd) a colorless, volatile, flammable liquid, CH_3CHO, used in the manufacture of acetic acid, perfumes, and flavors.

acetaminophen (as″et-am′ĭ-no-fen″) an analgesic, $C_8H_9NO_2$.

acetanilid (as″ĕ-tan′ĭ-lid) a colorless crystalline powder, C_8H_9NO; analgesic and antipyretic.

acetannin (as″ĕ-tan′in) acetyltannic acid.

acetarsol (as″et-ar′sol) acetarsone.

acetarsone (as″et-ar′sŏn) an arsenical, $C_8H_{10}As$-NO_3, used in amebic dysentery and trichomonas vaginitis.

acetate (as′ĕ-tāt) any salt of acetic acid.

acetazolamide (as″et-ah-zol′ah-mīd) a renal carbonic anhydrase inhibitor, $C_4H_6N_4O_3S_2$, used as a diuretic in the treatment of carbon dioxide retention in chronic lung disease and to reduce intraocular pressure in glaucoma. **sodium a.,** a form suitable for parenteral use.

Acetest (ah′sĕ-test) trademark for reagent tablets containing sodium nitroprusside, aminoacetic acid, disodium phosphate, and lactose. A drop of urine is placed on a tablet on a sheet of white paper; if significant quantities of acetone are present the tablet changes from a purple tint (1+), to lavender (2+), to moderate purple (3+), or to deep purple (4+).

acetic (ah-se'tik, ah-set'ik) pertaining to vinegar or its acid; sour.

acetimeter (as''ĕ-tim'ĕ-ter) an instrument for measuring the acetic acid in a fluid.

acetin (as'ĕ-tin) a glyceryl acetate, $C_3H_5(C_2H_3O_2)_3$.

Acetobacter (ah-se''to-bak'ter) a genus of schizomycetes (family Pseudomonadaceae) important in completion of the carbon cycle and in production of vinegar.

acetohexamide (as''ĕ-to-heks'ah-mīd) an oral hypoglycemic, $C_{15}H_{20}O_4S$.

acetoin (ah-set'o-in) a liquid ketone product of carbohydrate fermentation.

acetokinase (as''ĕ-to-ki'nās) acetate kinase.

acetometer (as''ĕ-tom'ĕ-ter) acetimeter.

acetone (as'ĕ-tōn) a compound, $CH_3 \cdot CO \cdot CH_3$, with solvent properties and characteristic odor, obtained by fermentation or produced synthetically; one of the ketone bodies produced in abnormal amounts in diabetes mellitus. It is used as a solvent for fats, resins, rubber, and plastic and to cleanse the skin before injections and vaccinations.

acetonemia (as''ĕ-to-ne'me-ah) ketonemia.

acetonitrile (-ni'trīl) methyl cyanide, CH_3CN, a poisonous colorless acid.

acetonuria (-nu're-ah) ketonuria.

aceto-orcein (-or'se-in) orcein dissolved in acetic acid, used in making squash preparations of polytene chromosomes.

acetophenazine (-fen'ah-zēn) a mildly sedative substance, $C_{23}H_{29}N_3O_2S \cdot 2C_4H_4O_4$, whose maleate salt is used as a tranquilizer.

acetophenetidin (-fĕ-net'ĭ-din) phenacetin.

acetous (as'ĕ-tus) pertaining to, producing, or resembling acetic acid.

acetphenarsine (as''et-fen-ar'sēn) acetarsone.

acetphenetidine (-fĕ-net'ĭ-din) phenacetin.

acetyl (as'ĕ-til) the monovalent radical, CH_3CO, a combining form of acetic acid. **a. peroxide,** a thick liquid, $(C_2H_3O)_2O_2$; a powerful oxidizing agent. **a. sulfisoxazole,** a sulfanilamide used as an antimicrobial.

acetylaminobenzine (as''ĕ-til-am''ĭ-no-ben'zēn) acetanilid.

acetylaniline (-an'ĭ-līn) acetanilid.

acetylation (ah-set''ĭ-la'shun) introduction of an acetyl radical into an organic molecule.

acetyl-beta-methylcholine (as''ĕ-til-ba''tah-meth''il-ko'lēn) methacholine.

acetylcarbromal (-kar-bro'mal) a sedative, $(C_2H_5)_2CBrCONHCONHCOCH_3$.

acetylcholine (-ko'lēn) an acetic acid ester of choline, $CH_3 \cdot CO \cdot O \cdot CH_2 \cdot N(CH_3)_3 \cdot OH$, normally present in many body tissues; used as a parasympathomimetic.

acetylcholinesterase (-ko''lin-es'ter-ās) an enzyme present in nervous tissue, muscle, and red cells that catalyzes the hydrolysis of acetylcholine to choline and acetic acid.

acetyl-CoA acetylcoenzyme A.

acetylcoenzyme A (-ko-en'zīm) an important intermediate in the citric acid (Krebs') cycle and the chief precursor of lipids; it is formed from glucose via pyruvate and by the degradation of fatty acids and of amino acids.

acetylcysteine (-sis'te-in) a compound, $C_5H_9NO_3S$, with mucolytic properties, used as an adjuvant in various bronchopulmonary disorders.

acetyldigitoxin (-dij''ĭ-tok'sin) a digitalis derivative, $C_{43}H_{66}O_{14}$, used as a cardiotonic.

acetylene (ah-set'ĭ-lēn) 1. a colorless, combustible gas, C_2H_2, with a garlic-like odor. 2. the type of a class of unsaturated (triple bonded) organic compounds.

acetylphenylhydrazine (as''ĕ-til-fen''il-hi'drah-zēn) an erythrocyte depressant, $C_8H_{10}N_2O$, which has been used in polycythemia vera.

acetylstrophanthidin (-stro-fan'thĭ-din) a synthetic fast-acting digitalis-like preparation.

acetyltransferase (-trans'fer-ās) any of a group of enzymes that catalyze the transfer of an acetyl group from one substance to another.

A.C.G. American College of Gastroenterology.

AcG accelerator globulin (coagulation Factor V).

ACh acetylcholine.

A.C.H.A. American College of Hospital Administrators.

achalasia (ak''ah-la'ze-ah) failure to relax of smooth muscle fibers at any junction of one part of the gastrointestinal tract with another, especially failure of the esophagogastric sphincter to relax with swallowing, due to degeneration of ganglion cells in the wall of the organ; the thoracic esophagus also loses its normal peristaltic activity and becomes dilated (megaesophagus).

Achatina (ak''ah-ti'nah) a genus of very large land snails, including *A. fuli'ca,* which serves as an intermediate host of *Angiostrongylus cantonensis.*

AChE acetylcholinesterase.

ache (āk) 1. to suffer a continuous pain. 2. a continuous, fixed pain, as distinguished from twinges.

acheilia (ah-ki'le-ah) congenital absence of one or both lips. **achei'lous,** adj.

acheiria (ah-ki're-ah) 1. congenital absence of one or both hands. 2. sense as of the loss of the hands, seen in hysteria.

acheiropodia (ah-ki''ro-po'de-ah) congenital absence of both hands and feet.

achillobursitis (ah-kil''o-ber-si'tis) inflammation of the bursae about the Achilles tendon.

achillodynia (-din'e-ah) pain in the Achilles tendon or its bursa.

achillorrhaphy (ak''il-lor'ah-fe) suturing of the Achilles tendon.

achillotenotomy (ah-kil''o-ten-ot'o-me) surgical division of the Achilles tendon.

achlorhydria (a''klōr-hi'dre-ah) absence of hydrochloric acid from gastric secretions. **achlorhy'dric,** adj.

achloropsia (ah''klo-rop'se-ah) inability to distinguish green colors.

acholia (a-ko′le-ah) lack or absence of bile secretion. **acho′lic**, adj.

acholuria (ah″ko-lu′re-ah) lack of bile pigments in the urine.

achondrogenesis (a-kon″dro-jen′ĕ-sis) a hereditary disorder characterized by hypoplasia of bone, resulting in markedly shortened limbs; the head and trunk are normal.

achondroplasia (-pla′ze-ah) a hereditary, congenital disorder of cartilage formation, leading to a type of dwarfism. **achondroplas′tic**, adj.

Achorion (ah-ko′re-on) *Trichophyton*.

achrestic (a-kres′tik) caused not by absence of a necessary substance, but by inability to utilize such a substance.

achromasia (ak″ro-ma′se-ah) 1. lack of normal skin pigmentation. 2. the inability of tissues or cells to be stained.

achromat (a′kro-mat) a person who is color blind.

achromate (ah-kro′māt) achromat.

Achromatiaceae (ah-kro″mah-ti-a′se-e) a family of schizomycetes (order Beggiatoales) whose cells lack photosynthetic pigments.

achromatic (ak″ro-mat′ik) 1. producing no discoloration. 2. staining with difficulty. 3. pertaining to achromatin. 4. refracting light without decomposing it into its component colors. 5. pertaining to or characterized by complete lack of color vision.

achromatin (ah-kro′mah-tin) the faintly staining groundwork of a cell nucleus.

achromatism (ah-kro′mah-tizm) 1. the quality or the condition of being achromatic. 2. achromatopia.

Achromatium (ah″kro-ma′te-um) a genus of schizomycetes (family Achromatiaceae).

achromatolysis (ak″ro-mah-tol′ĭ-sis) disorganization of cell achromatin.

achromatophil (ak″ro-mat′o-fil, a″kro-mat′o-fil) 1. not easily stainable. 2. an organism or tissue that does not stain easily.

achromatopia (ah″kro-mah-to′pe-ah) defective visual perception of colors. **achromatop′ic**, adj.

achromatopsia (ah-kro″mah-top′se-ah) achromatopia.

achromatosis (-to′sis) 1. deficiency of pigmentation in the tissues. 2. lack of staining power in a cell or tissue.

achromatous (a-kro′mah-tus) colorless.

achromaturia (a-kro″mah-tu′re-ah) colorless state of the urine.

achromia (a-kro′me-ah) absence of normal color; specifically, a condition of erythrocytes in which their centers are paler than normal (*central a.*). **achro′mic**, adj.

Achromobacter (a-kro″mo-bak′ter) a genus of schizomycetes (family Achromobacteraceae) found in soil or in fresh or salt water.

Achromobacteraceae (-bak″tĕ-ra′se-e) a family of schizomycetes (order Eubacteriales) generally found in soil or in fresh or salt water.

achromocyte (a-kro′mo-sīt) a red cell artifact in the shape of a quarter moon which stains more faintly than intact red cells.

achromophil (-fil) achromatophil.

Achromycin (ak″ro-mi′sin) trademark for preparations of tetracycline.

achroodextrin (a-kro″o-deks′trin) a kind of low-molecular-weight dextrin not colored by iodine.

achylia (ah-ki′le-ah) absence of hydrochloric acid and pepsinogens (pepsin) in the gastric juice (*gastric a.*).

achylous (ah-ki′lus) deficient in chyle.

achymia (ah-ki′me-ah) imperfect, insufficient, or absence of chyme formation.

acicular (ah-sik′u-lar) needle-shaped.

aciculum (ah-sik′u-lum) a bent, finger-like structure observed in certain flagellates.

acid (as′id) 1. sour. 2. a substance which forms hydrogen ions in solution and from which hydrogen may be displaced by a metal when a salt is formed. **abietic a.**, $C_{20}H_{30}O_2$, prepared by isomerization of rosin. **acetic a.**, a saturated fatty acid, CH_3COOH, the characteristic component of vinegar; used in solutions of various strengths, as *dilute acetic acid* (6%) and *glacial acetic acid* (99.4%). Its salts (*potassium* and *sodium acetate*) are used as urinary and systemic alkalizers. **acetoacetic a.**, $CH_3 \cdot CO \cdot CH_2 \cdot COOH$, one of the ketone bodies formed in the metabolism of certain substances and present in increased amounts in various pathologic states. **acetrizoic a.**, an acid, $C_9H_6I_3NO_3$; its sodium salt (*sodium acetrizoate*) is used as an x-ray contrast medium. **acetylsalicylic a.**, aspirin. **acetyltannic a.**, a yellowish or grayish white powder; astringent and antidiarrheal. **adenylic a.**, a component of nucleic acid, consisting of adenine, ribose, and phosphoric acid, found in muscle, yeast, and other material. **adipic a.**, a crystalline acid, $COOH(CH_2)_4 \cdot COOH$, obtained by oxidizing certain fats with nitric acid and made commercially by oxidation of cyclohexanol; used in manufacturing resins and nylon. **alginic a.**, a hydrophilic, colloidal carbohydrate acid from seaweeds; its sodium salt (*sodium alginate*) is used as a suspending agent and, for its emulsifying, stabilizing, thickening, and water-binding qualities, in foods, medicines, and cosmetics. **amino a.**, one of a class of organic compounds containing the amino (NH_2) and the carboxyl ($COOH$) group, occurring naturally in plant and animal tissues and forming the chief constituents of protein; many of them are necessary for human and animal growth and nutrition and hence are called essential amino acids. **amino a., essential**, one that is essential for optimal growth or nitrogen equilibrium. **aminoacetic a.**, a nonessential amino acid, H_2NCH_2COOH, derived from many proteins; used as an antacid and dietary supplement. **aminobenzoic a., p-aminobenzoic a.**, para-aminobenzoic a. **aminocaproic a.**, epsilon-aminocaproic acid; a nonessential amino acid that is an inhibitor of plasminogen and plasmin and indirectly of fibrinolysis; used as a hemostatic. **aminohippuric a.**, the *N*-acetic acid of para-aminobenzoic acid, $C_9H_{10}N_2O_3$, used as a pharmaceutic aid; its sodium salt (*sodium aminohippurate*) is used to measure the effective renal plasma flow and to determine the functional capacity of the tubular excretory mechanism. **aminosalicylic a.,** para-aminosalicylic acid (PAS); an acid, $NH_2 \cdot \cdot C_6H_3 \cdot OH \cdot COOH$, with antibacterial properties, whose salts (*calcium, potassium,* and *sodium aminosalicylate*) are used as tuberculostatics. **anthranilic a.,** a crystalline acid, $NH_2 \cdot C_6H_4COOH$, whose cadmium salt is used as an ascaricide in swine. **arachic a., arachidic a.,** a saturated fatty acid, $C_{19}H_{39}COOH$, occurring in peanut oil. **arachidonic a.,** a polyunsaturated essential fatty acid, $C_{19}H_{39}COOH$; a constituent of lecithin and a source of some prostaglandins. **argininosuccinic a.,** an amino acid normally formed in the ornithine cycle of urea formation in the liver, but not normally present in the urine. **arsenous a.,** arsenic trioxide. **ascorbic a.,** vitamin C, $C_6H_8O_6$, found in many vegetables and fruits, and an essential element in the diet of man and many other animals; deficiency produces scurvy. Its sodium salt (*sodium ascorbate*) is used in solution for parenteral administration. **aspartic a.,** a nonessential, natural dibasic amino acid, $COOH \cdot CH(NH_2) \cdot CH_2 \cdot \cdot COOH$, involved in transamination reactions, the ornithine cycle, and the formation of carnosine, anserine, purines, and pyrimidines. **barbituric a.,** $C_4H_4N_2O_3$, the parent substance of barbiturates. **benzoic a.,** a crystalline acid, C_6H_5COOH, from benzoin and other resins and from coal tar; used as an antifungal agent and as a germicide. Its sodium salt (*sodium benzoate*) is also used as an antifungal agent, and may be used as a test for liver function. **beta-hydroxybutyric a.,** beta-oxybutyric a. **beta-ketobutyric a.,** acetoacetic a. **beta-oxybutyric a.,** $CH_3CHOH \cdot CH_2COOH$, one of the ketone bodies, occurring in the urine in diabetic ketoacidosis and in starvation due to incomplete fatty acid oxidation. **bile a's,** steroid acids of the bile formed in the liver, usually occurring in conjugate form, e.g., glycocholic acid, and metabolically derived from cholesterol. **boric a.,** a crystalline powder, H_3BO_3, used as a buffer. Its sodium salt (*sodium borate,* or *borax*) is used as an alkalizing agent in pharmaceuticals. **butyric a.,** a saturated fatty acid, C_3H_7COOH, found in butter, sweat, feces, and urine, and in traces in the spleen and blood. **cacodylic a.,** a crystalline compound, $(CH_3)_2ASO \cdot OH$, used as a herbicide. **caffeic a.,** a crystalline acid, $C_9H_8O_4$, from coffee. **camphoric a.,** a crystalline acid, $C_{10}H_{16}O_4$, from camphor, which may stimulate the respiratory center. **camphoronic a.,** an antiseptic compound, $C_9H_{14}O_6$, obtained by oxidation of camphoric acid. **capric a.,** a rancid-smelling saturated fatty acid, $C_9H_{19}COOH$, in butter, coconut oil, etc. **caproic a.,** a saturated fatty acid, $C_5H_{11}COOH$, in milk fat and some plant oils, used in manufacture of artificial flavors. **caprylic a.,** a saturated fatty acid, C_7H_5COOH, found in goat- and cow-milk fat and in some seed oils; used in manufacture of perfumes. **carbamic a.,** NH_2COOH, the parent acid of urethan. **carbolic a.,** phenol. **carbonic a.,** an aqueous solution of carbon dioxide, H_2CO_3. **carminic a.,** the active principle of carmine and cochineal, $C_{22}H_{20}O_{13}$. **carnaubic a.,** a saturated fatty acid, $C_{23}H_{47}COOH$, found in carnauba wax and wool fat. **cerebronic a.,** the principal hydroxy acid from the brain, $C_{24}H_{48}O_3$, a constituent of sphingomyelin. **cerotic a.,** a saturated fatty acid, $C_{25}H_{51}COOH$, found in beeswax and other insect and plant waxes. **cevitamic a.,** ascorbic a. **chaulmoogric a.,** an unsaturated fatty acid, $C_{18}H_{32}O_2$, from chaulmoogra oil; see also *ethyl chaulmoograte.* **chenodeoxycholic a.,** the third most abundant acid of human bile, $C_{23}H_{37}(OH)_2COOH$; it has gallstone-dissolving properties. **chloroacetic a.,** an acid in which the three hydrogen atoms of acetic acid are wholly or partly replaced by chlorine. **cholic a.,** an acid, $C_{24}H_{40}O_5$, formed in the liver from cholesterol; it plays, with other bile acids, an important role in digestion. **chondroitic a., chondroitin sulfuric a.,** a compound of high molecular weight in skin and connective tissue and, combined with collagen, constituting 20–40 per cent of cartilage. **chromic a.,** a dibasic acid, H_2CrO_4. **chrysophanic a.,** a yellow crystalline acid, $C_{15}H_{10}O_4$, present in cascara sagrada, senna, rhubarb, and certain⋅ lichens, and in chrysarobin, whose therapeutic properties it shares. **cinnamic a.,** a crystalline acid, $C_6H_5(CH)_2COOH$, from cinnamon, storax, the balsams, and other aromatic resins. **citric a.,** a crystalline acid, $C_6H_8O_7$, from citrus fruits and other plant and animal sources or produced by fermentation of sugars; it is antiscorbutic, refrigerant, and diuretic. Used as a flavoring agent or vehicle. Its sodium salt (*sodium citrate*) is used chiefly as an anticoagulant for blood that is to be fractionated or stored; its potassium salt (*potassium citrate*) is used in potassium deficiencies and as a systemic alkalizer, sudorific, diuretic, and expectorant. **clofenamic a.,** an anti-inflammatory agent, $C_{13}H_9ClNO_2$. **clorazepic a.,** an acid, $C_{16}H_{13}ClN_2O$, the dipotassium salt of which is a minor tranquilizer. **cresylic a.,** cresol. **cromoglycic a.,** acid whose disodium salt (*sodium cromolyn*) is used as a bronchodilator. **cyanic a.,** a highly vesicant acid, $H \cdot CNO$. **cyclamic a.,** an acid, $C_6H_{17}NO_3S$; its salts (*calcium* and *sodium cyclamate*) were once widely used as synthetic sweetening agents; now available only by prescription in the U.S. **cysteic a.,** an intermediate product in the oxidation of cysteine to taurine. **cytidylic a.,** a pyrimidine nucleotide constituent of ribonucleic acid. **dehydrocholic a.,** an acid, $C_{24}H_{34}O_5$, formed by oxidation of cholic acid and derived from natural bile acids. **deoxyadenylic a.,** a purine nucleotide constituent of deoxyribonucleic acid. **deoxycholic a.,** one of the bile acids, capable of forming soluble, diffusible complexes with fatty acids. **deoxycytidylic a.,** a pyrimidine nucleotide constituent of deoxyribonucleic acid. **deoxyguanylic a.,** a purine nucleotide constituent of deoxyribonucleic acid. **deoxyribonucleic a. (DNA),** a nucleic acid that on hydrolysis yields adenine, guanine, cytosine, thymine, deoxyribose, and phosphoric acid; it is the carrier of genetic information for all organisms except RNA viruses. See *Watson-Crick helix.* **diacetic a.,** acetoacetic a. **diallylbarbituric a.,** allobarbital. **2,4-diaminobutyric a.,** a naturally occurring amino acid discovered in 1948. **2,6-diaminopimelic a.,** a naturally occurring amino acid discovered in 1950. **diatrizoic a.,** an acid, $C_{11}H_9I_3N_2O_4$, the meglumine and sodium salts of which are used as diagnostic radiopaque media. **edetic a.,** ethylenediaminetetraacetic acid (EDTA); an acid, $C_{10}H_{16}N_2O$, whose salts are strong chelating agents; see *edetate.* **ethacrynic a.,** a powerful diuretic, $C_{13}H_{12}Cl_2O_4$, administered orally or parenterally, effective in promoting sodium and chloride excretion. **ethylenediaminetetraacetic a. (EDTA),** a chelating agent; see *edetate.* **fatty a.,** any monobasic aliphatic acid containing only carbon, hydrogen, and oxygen, which combines with glycerin to form fat. **fatty a., essential,** an unsaturated fatty acid that cannot be formed in the body and therefore must be provided by the diet; the most important are linoleic acid, linolenic acid, and arachidonic acid. **filicic a.,** an acid, $(CH_3)_2C_6HO(OH)_2$, from male fern. **fluoroacetic a.,** a metabolic poison from *Chailletia cymosa,* a tree of South Africa, which blocks the tricarboxylic acid cycle, causing convulsions and ventricular fibrillation. **folic a.,** one of the vitamins of the B group, $C_{19}H_{19}N_7O_6$, found in green vegetables, liver, and yeast, and produced synthetically (pteroylglutamic acid); it is an essential growth factor for many organisms, and has hematopoietic influence in certain macrocytic anemias. **folinic a.,** a folic acid derivative, $C_{20}H_{23}N_7O_7$, necessary for the growth of *Leuconostoc citrovorum;* used in treating megaloblastic anemias not due to vitamin B_{12} deficiency and in folic acid deficiency, and as an antidote to toxic effects of folic acid antagonists. **formic a.,** colorless, pungent liquid with vesicant properties, HCOOH, from nettles and ants and other insects; derivable from oxalic acid and from glycerin and from the oxidation of formaldehyde. **formiminoglutamic a.,** a product in the metabolism of histidine which accumulates in the urine of humans and rats deficient in folic acid. **a. fuchsin,** see under *fuchsin.* **fumaric a.,** an unsaturated dibasic acid, $C_4H_4O_4$; it is the *trans*-isomer of maleic acid and an intermediate in the tricarboxylic acid cycle. **fusidic a.,** a fermentation product of *Fusidium coccineum,* $C_{31}H_{48}O_6$; used as an antibiotic. **gallic a.,** a crystalline acid, $C_7H_6O_5$, usually obtained from nutgalls and tannic acid. **gallotannic a.,** tannic a. **glucoascorbic a.,** an analogue of ascorbic acid, COOH, which competitively inhibits the latter. **gluconic a.,** $CH_2OH(CHOH)_4COOH$, an intermediate product formed in biosynthesis of pentoses. **glucuronic a.,** an acid, $C_6H_{10}O_7$, formed by oxidation of glucose in animal metabolism and found in urine combined with camphor, chloroform, chloral, and other aromatic bodies. **glutamic a.,** a crystalline dibasic nonessential amino acid, $C_5H_9NO_4$, widely distributed in proteins; its hydrochloride salt is used as a gastric acidifier. The monosodium salt of L-glutamic acid (*sodium glutamate*) is used in treating encephalopathies associated with hepatic disease, and to enhance the flavor of foods and tobacco. **glutaric a.,** $C_5H_8O_4$, occurring in various natural products. **glyceric a.,** CH_2-$OH \cdot CHOH \cdot COOH$, an intermediate product in the transformation in the body of carbohydrate

to lactic acid, formed by oxidation of glycerol. **glycocholic a.,** a conjugated form of one of the bile acids that yields glycine and cholic acid on hydrolysis. **glycolic a.,** $CH_2OH \cdot COOH$, formed by electrolytic reduction of oxalic acid or by the action of sodium hydroxide on monochloroacetic acid; used in pH control. Also produced in the body as an intermediate product in the conversion of serine to glycine. **glyoxylic a.,** $CHO \cdot COOH$, formed in the oxidative deamination of glycine. **guanidinoacetic a.,** an intermediate product in the synthesis of creatine. **guanidinosuccinic a.,** a metabolite first found in the urine of uremic patients, which at high levels inhibits platelet aggregation. **haloid a.,** one containing no oxygen, but composed of hydrogen and a halogen element. **helvolic a.,** an antibiotic, $C_{32}H_{42}O_8$, from *Aspergillus fumigatus* and *A. fumigatus* var. *helvola;* used as an antimicrobial. **hippuric a.,** $C_6H_5 \cdot CO \cdot NH \cdot$-$CH_2 \cdot COOH$, formed by conjugation of benzoic acid and glycine. **homogentisic a.,** an intermediate product of the metabolism of tyrosine and phenylalanine, which is ultimately metabolized to acetone; see also *alkapton bodies* and *alkaptonuria.* **homovanillic a.,** a major terminal urinary metabolite, converted from dopa, dopamine, and norepinephrine. **hyaluronic a.,** a sulfate-free mucopolysaccharide in the intercellular substance of various tissue, especially the skin; also isolated from the vitreous humor, synovial fluid, umbilical cord, etc. **hydnocarpic a.,** an unsaturated fatty acid, $C_{16}H_{28}O_2$, from chaulmoogra (hydnocarpus) oil; see also *ethyl chaulmoograte.* **hydriodic a.,** a gaseous haloid acid, HI; its aqueous solution and its syrup have been used as alteratives. **hydrobromic a.,** a gaseous haloid acid, HBr. **hydrochloric a.,** HCl, a normal constituent of gastric juice in man and other animals. **hydrocyanic a.,** hydrogen cyanide. **hydrofluoric a.,** a gaseous haloid acid, HF, extremely poisonous and corrosive. **hydrosulfuric a.,** hydrogen sulfide. **hydroxybutyric a.,** a poisonous acid, CH_3-$CHOHCH_2COOH$, found in the urine and the blood in diabetes. **5-hydroxyindoleacetic a.,** a product of serotonin metabolism present in cerebrospinal fluid and in increased amount in the urine in carcinoid. **hypochlorous a.,** an unstable compound, HClO, with disinfectant and bleaching action; its sodium salt (*sodium hypochlorite*) is used in solution as a disinfectant. **hypophosphoric a.,** H_2PO_3; its salts are hypophosphates. **hypophosphorous a.,** a toxic, monobasic acid with strong reducing properties, H_3PO_2, which forms hypophosphites; used in 30 to 32% and 50% solutions. **indigotindisulfonic a.,** $C_{16}H_8N_2O_2(SO_3H)_2$, from indigo blue; its disodium salt (*indigo carmine*) is used as a stain in histology and as a test for renal function. **inorganic a.,** any acid containing no carbon atoms. **inosinic a.,** a mononucleotide constituent of muscle, made up of hypoxanthine, ribose, and phosphoric acid. **iodic a.,** a monobasic acid, HIO_3, formed by oxidation of iodine with nitric acid or chlorates, which has strong acid and reducing properties. **iodoalphionic a.,** an iodine compound, $C_{15}H_{12}I_2O_3$; used as a radiopaque medium in cholecystography. **iodogorgoic a.,** 3,5-diiodotyrosine. **iopa-noic a.,** $C_{11}H_{12}I_3NO_3$; used as a radiopaque medium in cholecystography. **iophenoxic a.,** C_{11}-$H_{11}I_3O_3$; used as a radiopaque medium in cholecystography. **iothalamic a.,** $C_{11}H_9I_3N_2O_4$; its meglumine and sodium salts are used as diagnostic radiopaque media. **isolysergic a.,** C_{16}-$H_{16}N_2O_2$, one of the main cleavage products of hydrolysis of the alkaloids characteristic of ergot, and the parent compound of the ergotinine group of alkaloids. **keto a's,** compounds containing the groups CO and COOH. **kynurenic a.,** a crystalline acid, $C_9H_5N(OH)COOH$, metabolite of tryptophan found in microorganisms and in the urine of normal mammals. **lactic a.,** $CH_3CHOHCOOH$, a compound formed in the body in anaerobic metabolism of carbohydrate; also produced by bacterial action in milk. The sodium salt of racemic or inactive lactic acid (*sodium lactate*) is used as an electrolyte and fluid replenisher. **lauric a.,** $C_{12}H_{24}O_2$, found in many vegetable oils, especially laurel seed oil and coconut oil, and in milk fat. **levulinic a.,** $C_5H_8O_3$, formed by the action of heat and acid on carbohydrates. **lignoceric a.,** a saturated fatty acid, $C_{23}H_{47}COOH$, found in wood tar, various cerebrosides, and in small amounts in most natural fats. **linoleic a.,** a doubly unsaturated fatty acid, $C_{18}H_{32}O_2$, the most abundant such acid in various vegetable oils. **lipoic a.,** a bacterial growth factor present in the water-soluble fraction of liver and yeast, necessary for the oxidative decarboxylation of pyruvic acid by *Streptococcus fecalis* and for the growth of *Tetrahymena gelii*, and replacing acetate for the growth of *Lactobacillus casei*. **lithic a.,** uric a. **lysergic a.,** a constituent of ergot alkaloids, $C_{16}H_{16}N_2O_2$, obtained by hydrolysis; see *lysergide*. **lysergic a. diethylamide,** lysergide. **malic a.,** a crystalline acid, $C_4H_6O_5$, from juices of many fruits and plants, and an intermediary product of carbohydrate metabolism. **maleic a.,** an unsaturated dibasic acid, $C_4H_4O_4$; the *cis*-isomer of fumaric acid. **mandelic a.,** $C_8H_8O_3$, from amygdalin; used, usually as the ammonium, calcium, or sodium salt, as a urinary antiseptic. **meconic a.,** a crystalline compound, $C_7H_4O_7$, from opium. **metaphosphoric a.,** a glassy solid, HPO_3, used as a test for albumin in urine and as a reagent for chemical analysis. **mucic a.,** a tetrahydroxy dibasic acid, COOH-$(CHOH)_4COOH$, produced by oxidizing galactose or any carbohydrate containing galactose. **muriatic a.,** hydrochloric a. **myristic a.,** a saturated fatty acid, $C_{14}H_{28}O_2$, found in spermaceti, nutmeg butter, and other fats. **nalidixic a.,** a synthetic antibacterial agent, $C_{12}H_{12}N_2O_3$, used in the treatment of genitourinary infections caused by gram-negative organisms. **nervonic a.,** an unsaturated fatty acid, $C_{23}H_{45}$-COOH, from nervone. **neuraminic a.,** a 9-carbon aminosugar acid, one of the sialic acids. **nicotinic a.,** niacin. **nitric a.,** a colorless liquid, HNO_3, which fumes in moist air and has a characteristic choking odor; used as a cauterizing agent. Its potassium salt (*potassium nitrate*) is used in potassium deficiencies and as a diuretic; its sodium salt (*sodium nitrate*) as a reagent. **nitrohydrochloric a.,** a yellow, fuming mix-

ture of nitric and hydrochloric acids. **nitrous a.,** an unstable weak acid, HNO_2, with which free amino groups react to form hydroxyl groups and liberate gaseous nitrogen; used in the determination of urea, the N_2, being collected and measured. Its salts (*sodium nitrite* and sometimes *potassium nitrite*) are used for the relief of pain in certain conditions. **nucleic a's,** high-molecular-weight polymeric substances composed of nucleotides which constitute the acidic groups of the nucleoproteins and contain phosphoric acid, sugars, and purine and pyrimidine bases; see *deoxyribonucleic a.* and *ribonucleic a.* **oleic a.,** an unsaturated fatty acid, C_{17}-$H_{33}COOH$, found in animal and vegetable fats. **organic a.,** any acid containing the carboxyl group, COOH. **orthophosphoric a.,** phosphoric a. **osmic a.,** 1. a dibasic acid, H_2OsO_4, forming osmates. 2. osmium tetroxide. **oxalic a.,** a poisonous dibasic acid, $(COOH)_2 \cdot 2H_2O$, found in various fruits and vegetables, and formed in metabolism of ascorbic acid; used as a chemical reagent in pharmacy, industry, and the arts. **palmitic a.,** a saturated fatty acid, $C_{15}H_{31}$-COOH, from animal and vegetable fats; see also *stearic a.* **palmitoleic a.,** an unsaturated fatty acid, $C_{15}H_{29}COOH$, found in various oils. **pangamic a.,** an amino derivative of glucuronic acid, $C_{10}H_{19}O_8N$. **pantothenic a.,** a vitamin of the B complex, $C_9H_{17}O_5N_5$, widely distributed in foods and tissues, and essential for normal growth and development of rats and chicks; available as *calcium pantothenate*, the dextrorotatory salt, and as *racemic calcium pantothenate*, a mixture of dextrorotatory and levorotatory isomers. **para-aminobenzoic a.,** $NH_2 \cdot C_6H_4 \cdot COOH$, considered to be associated with or a member of the B group of vitamins; it is a growth factor for certain organisms. It is used as a sunscreen agent and in bacterial culture media. Abbreviated PABA. **pectic a.,** a polysaccharide, $C_{32}H_{48}O_{32}$, from pectin. **penicillic a.,** an antibiotic substance, $C_8H_{10}O_4$, isolated from cultures of various species of *Penicillium* and *Aspergillus*. **perchloric a.,** a colorless volatile liquid, $HClO_4$, which can cause powerful explosions in the presence of organic matter or anything reducible. **persulfuric a.,** an oxidized form of sulfuric acid. **phenic a.,** phenol. **phenyllactic a.,** an acid excreted in the urine in phenylketonuria. **phenylpyruvic a.,** C_6H_5-$CH_2COCOOH$, an intermediary product in the metabolism of phenylalanine. **phosphatidic a.,** any compound formed by esterification of three hydroxyl groups of glycerol with two fatty acid groups and one phosphoric acid group; found widely in animals and plants. **phosphoric a.,** a crystalline acid, H_3PO_4, formed by the oxidation of phosphorus; its salts are called phosphates. **phosphorous a.,** H_3PO_3; its salts are called phosphites. **phytic a.,** the hexaphosphoric acid ester of inositol, found in many plants and microorganisms and in animal tissues. **picric a.,** trinitrophenol. **pimelic a.,** $HOOC(CH_2)_5COOH$, formed in oxidation of unsaturated fats. **polyunsaturated fatty a's,** acids with abundant unsaturated bonds; in large amounts in diets, they tend to lower plasma cholesterol levels. **propionic a.,** CH_3-

$CH_2 \cdot COOH$, found in chyme and sweat, and one of the products of bacterial fermentation of wood pulp waste; its salts (*calcium* and *sodium propionate*) are used as local antifungals, and to inhibit mold growth in bakery and dairy products. **pteroylglutamic a.,** a form of folic acid. **pyrophosphoric a.,** a crystalline acid, $H_4P_2O_7$, one of the forms of phosphoric acid. **pyruvic a.,** $CH_3 \cdot CO \cdot COOH$, formed in the body in aerobic metabolism of carbohydrate; also formed by dry distillation of tartaric acid. **quinic a.,** a crystalline compound, $C_7H_{12}O_6$, from cinchona bark, coffee, cranberries, and many other plants; in man, largely transformed into benzoic acid and excreted as hippuric acid. **ribonucleic a. (RNA),** a nucleic acid found in all living cells, which on hydrolysis yields adenine, guanine, cytosine, uracil, ribose, and phosphoric acid; *messenger RNA* is an RNA fraction which transfers information from DNA to the protein-forming system of the cell; *ribosomal RNA* comprises about half the substance of ribosomes; *transfer RNA* (soluble RNA) is an RNA fraction which combines with one amino acid species, transferring it from activating enzyme to ribosome. **rosolic a.,** aurin. **saccharic a.,** a dibasic acid formed by the action of nitric acid on dextrose or on carbohydrates containing dextrose. **salicylic a.,** a crystalline acid, $C_7H_6O_3$, used as a topical keratolytic; its sodium salt is used as an analgesic and antipyretic. **salicyluric a.,** a compound of glycol and salicylic acid, found in urine after administration of salicylic acid. **sarcolactic a.,** a dextrorotatory form of lactic acid, found in muscle. **shikimic a.,** a compound originally isolated from Japanese anise; it is a precursor in the biosynthesis of several aromatic compounds, including phenylalanine and tyrosine. **sialic a's,** a group of acetylated derivatives of neuraminic acid which occur in a number of mucopolysaccharides and glycolipids. **stannic a.,** a vitreous acid of tin, H_2SnO_3, forming stannates. **stearic a.,** a saturated fatty acid, $C_{17}H_{35}COOH$, from animal and vegetable fats; a pharmaceutical preparation of solid acids from fats, consisting chiefly of stearic acid and palmitic acid, is used in glycerin suppositories. **succinic a.,** $COOH(CH_2)_2COOH$, from amber, lichens, fossils, and certain hydatid cysts; it is an intermediate in the tricarboxylic acid cycle. **sulfanilic a.,** a crystalline compound, $C_6H_7NSO_3 \cdot H_2O$, used as a reagent. **sulfuric a.,** an oily, highly caustic, poisonous acid, H_2SO_4, widely used in chemistry, industry, and the arts. **sulfurous a.,** 1. a solution of sulfur dioxide in water, H_2SO_3; used as a reagent. 2. sulfur dioxide. **tannic a.,** $C_{76}H_{52}O_{46}$, from the bark and fruit of many plants, usually obtained from nutgalls; used as an astringent. **tartaric a.,** $C_4H_6O_6$, from the lees of wine and from various plants, used in baking and tanning, and as a chemical reagent. **taurocholic a.,** a bile acid, $C_{26}H_{45}NSO_7$; when hydrolyzed, it splits into taurine and cholic acid. **ternary a.,** one containing three distinct radicals. **tetrahydrofolic a.,** the coenzyme of folic acid, being a reduced folic acid with four hydrogen atoms attached; in dissociated form, called *tetrahydrofolate*. **thiobarbituric a.,** a condensation of malonic acid and thiourea, $C_8H_4N_2O_2S$, differing from barbituric acid only by the presence of a sulfur atom instead of an oxygen atom at the number 2 carbon. It is the parent compound of a class of drugs, the thiobarbiturates, which are analogous in their effects to barbiturates. **thymic a.,** thymol. **thymonucleic a.,** deoxyribonucleic a. **trichloroacetic a.,** $C_2HCl_3O_2$, used as a caustic. **triiodoethionic a.,** iophenoxic a. **undecylenic a.,** an unsaturated fatty acid, $C_{11}H_{20}O_2$; antifungal agent. **uric a.,** a crystalline acid, $C_5H_4N_4O_3$, present in blood and urine, the chief end-product of nitrogen metabolism in man. **uridylic a.,** a pyrimidine nucleotide constituent of ribonucleic acid. **urocanic a.,** an intermediate metabolite of histamine, $C_6H_6N_2O_2$, convertible normally to glutamic acid. **ursolic a.,** ursone. **vanillylmandelic a.,** an excretory product of the catecholamines, used as a test for epinephrine metabolism. **xanthurenic a.,** $C_9H_5N(OH)_2COOH$, a metabolite of L-tryptophan, present in normal urine and in increased amounts in vitamin B_6 deficiency.

acidaminuria (as″id-am″ĭ-nu′re-ah) aminoaciduria.

acidemia (as″ĭ-de′me-ah) abnormal acidity of the blood. **argininosuccinic a.,** the presence in the blood of argininosuccinic acid. **isovaleric a.,** an inborn error of leucine metabolism characterized by high levels of isovaleric acid in the blood, periodic acidosis with coma, objectionable body odor, and psychomotor retardation. **propionic a.,** an excess of propionic acid in the blood, due to failure of activity of propionyl-CoA carboxylase and characterized by ketosis, acidosis, and hyperglycinemia and, in the absence of dietary controls, by developmental retardation, ECG abnormalities, and osteoporosis.

acid-fast (as′id-fast) not readily decolorized by acids after staining.

acidic (ah-sid′ik) of or pertaining to an acid; acid-forming.

acidifiable (ah-sid″ĭ-fi′ah-b'l) capable of being made acid.

acidifier (ah-sid′ĭ-fi″er) an agent that causes acidity; a substance used to increase gastric acidity.

acidify (-ĭ-fi) to make sour; to convert into an acid.

acidimeter (as″ĭ-dim′ĕ-ter) an instrument for performing acidimetry.

acidimetry (-ĕ-tre) determination of the amount of free acid in a liquid.

acidity (ah-sid′ĭ-te) the quality of being acid; the power to unite with positively charged ions or with basic substances.

Acidol (a′sĭ-dol) trademark for a preparation of betaine.

acidology (as″ĭ-dol′o-je) the science of surgical appliances.

acidophilic (as″ĭ-do-fil′ik) 1. easily stained with acid dyes. 2. growing best on acid media.

acidophilism (as″ĭ-dof′ĭ-lizm) the state produced by acidophilic adenoma of the hypophysis, resulting in acromegaly.

acidosis (as″ĭ-do′sis) a pathologic condition resulting from accumulation of acid in, or loss of base from, the body. **acidot′ic,** adj. **compensated a.,** a condition in which the compensatory mechanisms have returned the pH toward normal. **diabetic a.,** metabolic acidosis produced by accumulation of ketones in uncontrolled diabetes mellitus. **hypercapnic a.,** respiratory a. **hyperchloremic a.,** metabolic acidosis accompanied by elevated plasma chloride. **metabolic a.,** a disturbance in which the acid-base status shifts toward the acid because of loss of base or retention of noncarbonic, or fixed (nonvolatile), acids. **nonrespiratory a.,** metabolic a. **renal hyperchloremia a.,** renal tubular a. **renal tubular a.,** metabolic acidosis resulting from impairment of renal function. **respiratory a.,** a state due to excess retention of carbon dioxide in the body. **starvation a.,** metabolic acidosis due to accumulation of ketone bodies which may accompany a caloric deficit. **uremic a.,** the condition in chronic renal disease in which the ability to excrete acid is decreased, causing acidosis.

acidulated (ah-sid′u-lāt″ed) rendered acid in reaction.

acidulous (-u-lus) somewhat acid.

acidum (as′ĭ-dum) [L.] acid.

aciduria (as″ĭ-du′re-ah) the presence of acid in the urine. **beta-aminoisobutyric a.,** excessive excretion of β-aminoisobutyric acid in the urine; it occurs as a benign genetic metabolic variant and in certain illnesses. **orotic a.,** a hereditary disorder in which a defect in the metabolism of pyrimidines is associated with excessive excretion of orotic acid in the urine, with megaloblastic anemia, crystalluria, and frequently physical and mental retardation.

aciduric (as″ĭ-du′rik) capable of growing in extremely acid media; said of bacteria.

acinesia (as″ĭ-ne′ze-ah) akinesia.

acinetic (as″ĭ-net′ik) akinetic.

aciniform (ah-sin′ĭ-form) shaped like an acinus, or grape.

acinitis (as″ĭ-ni′tis) inflammation of the acini of a gland.

acinose (as′ĭ-nōs) made up of acini.

acinous (as′ĭ-nus) shaped like a grape.

acinus (as′ĭ-nus), pl. *ac′ini* [L.] a small saclike dilatation, particularly one found in various glands; see also *alveolus.*

acladiosis (ah-klad″e-o′sis) an ulcerative dermatomycosis caused by *Acladium castellani.*

Acladium (ah-kla′de-um) a genus of fungi sometimes infecting man.

aclasia (ah-kla′ze-ah) aclasis.

aclasis (ak′lah-sis) pathologic continuity of structure, as in enchondromatosis. **diaphyseal a.,** enchondromatosis.

aclastic (a-klas′tik) 1. pertaining to or characterized by aclasis. 2. not refracting.

acleistocardia (ah-klīs″to-kar′de-ah) an open state of the foramen ovale of the fetal heart.

acme (ak′me) the critical stage or crisis of a disease.

acne (ak′ne) an inflammatory disease of the skin with the formation of an eruption of papules or pustules; more particularly, acne vulgaris. **beatle a.,** seborrheic dermatitis. **bromide a.,** an acneiform eruption without comedones, one of the most constant symptoms of brominism. **a. congloba′ta, conglobate a.,** severe acne with many comedones, marked by suppuration, cysts, sinuses, and scarring. **a. indura′ta,** a progression of papular acne, with deep-seated and destructive lesions that may produce severe scarring. **keloid a.,** keloid folliculitis. **a. kerato′sa,** acne marked by horny conical plugs, typically at the angles of the mouth, which become inflamed. **a. necrot′ica milia′-ris,** a rare and chronic form of folliculitis of the scalp, occurring principally in adults, with formation of tiny superficial pustules which are destroyed by scratching; see also *a. variolifor-mis.* **a. papulo′sa,** acne vulgaris with the formation of papules. **premenstrual a.,** acne of a cyclic nature, appearing shortly before (rarely after) the onset of menses. **a. rosa′cea,** rosacea. **tropical a., a. tropica′lis,** a severe and extensive form of acne occurring in hot, humid climates, with nodular, cystic, and pustular lesions chiefly on the back, buttocks, and thighs; conglobate abscesses frequently form, especially on the back. **a. variolifor′mis,** a rare condition with reddish-brown, papulopustular umbilicated lesions, usually on the brow and scalp; probably a deep variant of acne necrotica miliaris. **a. vulga′ris,** chronic acne, usually occurring in adolescence, with comedones, papules, nodules, and pustules on the face, neck, and upper part of the trunk.

acnegenic (ak″nĕ-jen′ik) producing acne.

acneiform (ak-ne′ĭ-form) resembling acne.

acnitis (ak-ni′tis) papulonecrotic tuberculid.

acoelomate (a-se′lo-māt) without a coelom or body cavity; an animal lacking a body cavity.

A.C.O.G. American College of Obstetricians and Gynecologists.

aconite (ak′o-nīt) a poisonous drug from the dried tuberous root of *Aconitum napellus,* containing several closely related alkaloids, the principal one being aconitine.

aconitine (ah-kon′ĭ-tin) a poisonous alkaloid, $C_{34}H_{47}O_{11}N$, the active principle of aconite.

acorea (ah″ko-re′ah) absence of the pupil.

acoria (ah-ko′re-ah) excessive ingestion of food, not from hunger but due to loss of the sensation of satiety.

acortan (a-kor′tan) corticotropin.

acouesthesia (ah-koo″es-the′ze-ah) acoustic sensibility.

acoumeter (ah-koo′mĕ-ter) an instrument for measuring hearing power.

acousmatamnesia (ah-koos″mat-am-ne′ze-ah) failure of the memory to call up images of sounds.

acoustic (ah-koos′tik) relating to sound or hearing.

acoustics (-tiks) the science of sound or of hearing.

acoustogram (-to-gram) the graphic tracing of the curves of sounds produced by motion of a joint.

A.C.P. American College of Pathologists; American College of Physicians; Animal Care Panel, Inc.

acquired (ah-kwīrd′) incurred as a result of factors acting from or originating outside the organism; not inherited.

acquisition (ah″kwĭ-zĭ′shun) in psychology, the period in learning during which progressive increments in response strength can be measured. Also, the process involved in such learning.

A.C.R. American College of Radiology.

acragnosis (ak″rag-no′sis) acroagnosis.

acral (a′kral) pertaining to or affecting the extremities.

acrania (ah-kra′ne-ah) congenital absence of part or all of the cranium. **acra′nial,** adj.

acranius (a-kra′ne-us) a monster exhibiting acrania.

acridine (ak′rĭ-dēn) an alkaloid of anthracene, CH:(C₆H₄)₂:N, used in the synthesis of dyes and drugs.

acriflavine (ak″rĭ-fla′vin) a deep orange, granular powder, used as a topical and urinary antiseptic. **a. hydrochloride,** a brownish red crystalline acridine dye; used as an antiseptic and germicide.

acrisorcin (ak″rĭ-sor′sin) a topical antifungal agent, C₁₃H₁₀N₂·C₁₂H₁₈O₂, used in the treatment of tinea versicolor.

acritical (a-krit′ĭ-kal) having no crisis.

acro- word element [Gr.], *extreme; top; extremity.*

acroagnosis (ak″ro-ag-no′sis) lack of sensory recognition of a limb; lack of acrognosis.

acroanesthesia (-an″es-the′ze-ah) anesthesia of the extremities.

acroarthritis (-ar-thri′tis) arthritis of the extremities.

acroblast (ak′ro-blast) Golgi material in the spermatid from which the acrosome arises.

acrobrachycephaly (ak″ro-brak″e-sef′ah-le) abnormal height of the skull, with shortness of its anteroposterior dimension. **acrobrachycephal′ic,** adj.

acrocentric (-sen′trik) having the centromere toward one end of the replicating chromosome so that one arm is much longer than the other.

acrocephalia (-sĕ-fa′le-ah) oxycephaly.

acrocephalic (-sĕ-fal′ik) oxycephalic.

acrocephalopolysyndactyly (-sef″ah-lo-pol″e-sin-dak′tĭ-le) acrocephalosyndactyly with polydactyly as an additional feature.

acrocephalosyndactyly (-sin-dak′tĭ-le) oxycephaly associated with webbing of the fingers and toes (syndactyly).

acrocephaly (-sef′ah-le) oxycephaly.

acrochordon (-kor′don) a pedunculated skin tag, occurring principally on the neck, eyelids, upper chest, and axillae in women of middle age or older.

acrocinesis (-si-ne′sis) acrokinesia.

acrocontracture (-kon-trak′tūr) contracture of the muscles of the hand or foot.

acrocyanosis (-si″ah-no′sis) cyanosis of the extremities with mottled blue or red discoloration of the skin of the digits, wrists, and ankles, and

with profuse sweating and coldness of the digits.

acrodermatitis (-der″mah-ti′tis) inflammation of the skin of the hands or feet. **chronic atrophic a., a. chron′ica atroph′icans,** chronic, idiopathic inflammation of the skin, usually of the extremities, leading to atrophy of the skin. **a. contin′ua, continuous a.,** chronic inflammation of the extremities, in some cases becoming generalized. **enteropathic a., a. entero-path′ica,** a hereditary disorder of infancy, with a vesiculopustulous dermatitis preferentially located periorificially and on the head, elbows, knees, hands, and feet, associated with gastrointestinal disturbances, chiefly manifested by diarrhea, and total alopecia. **Hallopeau's a.,** a. continua. **infantile lichenoid a., infantile papular a., a. papulo′sa infan′tum,** Gianotti-Crosti syndrome. **a. per′stans,** a. continua.

acrodermatosis (-der″mah-to′sis) any disease of the skin of the hands and feet.

acrodolichomelia (-dol″ĭ-ko-me′le-ah) abnormal length of hands and feet.

acrodynia (-din′e-ah) a disease of infancy and early childhood marked by pain and swelling in, and pink coloration of, the fingers and toes and by listlessness, irritability, failure to thrive, profuse perspiration, and sometimes scarlet coloration of the cheeks and tip of the nose.

acrodysplasia (-dis-pla′se-ah) acrocephalosyndactyly.

acroesthesia (-es-the′ze-ah) 1. exaggerated sensitiveness. 2. pain in the extremities.

acrognosis (ak″rog-no′sis) sensory recognition of the limbs.

acrohypothermy (ak″ro-hi′po-ther″me) abnormal coldness of the hands and feet.

acrokeratosis (-ker″ah-to′sis) a condition involving the skin of the extremities, with the appearance of horny growths. **a. verrucifor′-mis,** a condition resembling epidermodysplasia verruciformis, but with the lesions appearing chiefly on the palms and soles, and not on the face.

acrokinesia (-ki-ne′se-ah) abnormal motility or movement of the extremities. **acrokinet′ic,** adj.

acrolein (ak-ro′le-in) a volatile liquid, C₃H₄O, from decomposition of glycerin.

acromacria (ak″ro-mak′re-ah) arachnodactyly.

acromania (-ma′ne-ah) mania characterized by great motor activity.

acromegaly (-meg′ah-le) abnormal enlargement of the extremities of the skeleton—nose, jaws, fingers, and toes—caused by hypersecretion of the pituitary growth hormone after maturity.

acromelalgia (-mel-al′je-ah) erythromelalgia.

acrometagenesis (-met″ah-jen′ĕ-sis) undue growth of the extremities.

acromicria (-mi′kre-ah) abnormal hypoplasia of the extremities of the skeleton—nose, jaws, fingers, and toes.

acromio- word element [Gr.], *acromion.*

acromioclavicular (ah-kro″me-o-klah-vik′u-lar) pertaining to the acromion and clavicle.

acromiohumeral (-hu′mer-al) pertaining to the acromion and humerus.

acromion (ah-kro′me-on) the lateral extension of the spine of the scapula, forming the highest point of the shoulder. **acro′mial,** adj.

acromionectomy (ah-kro″me-on-ek′to-me) resection of the acromion.

acromiothoracic (ah-kro″me-o-tho-ras′ik) pertaining to the acromion and thorax.

acromphalus (ah-krom′fah-lus) 1. bulging of the navel; sometimes a sign of umbilical hernia. 2. the center of the navel.

acromyotonia (ak″ro-mi″o-to′ne-ah) myotonia of the extremities.

acronarcotic (-nar-kot′ik) acrid and narcotic.

acroneurosis (-nu-ro′sis) any neuropathy of the extremities.

acronine (a′kro-nēn) an antineoplastic agent, $C_{20}H_{19}NO_3$.

acronym (ak′ro-nim) a word formed by the initial letters of the principal components of a compound term, as *rad* from *r*adiation *a*bsorbed *d*ose.

acro-osteolysis (ak″ro-os″te-ol′ĭ-sis) osteolysis involving the distal phalanges of the fingers and toes.

acropachy (ak′ro-pak″e) clubbing of the fingers and toes.

acropachyderma (ak″ro-pak″e-der′mah) thickening of the skin over the face, scalp, and extremities, clubbing of the extremities, and deformities of the long bones; usually associated with acromegaly.

acroparalysis (-pah-ral′ĭ-sis) paralysis of the extremities.

acroparesthesia (-par″es-the′ze-ah) 1. paresthesia of the digits. 2. a disease marked by attacks of tingling, numbness, and stiffness in the extremities, chiefly the fingers, hands, and forearms, sometimes with pain, skin pallor, or slight cyanosis.

acropathology (-pah-thol′o-je) pathology of diseases of the extremities.

acropathy (ak-rop′ah-the) any disease of the extremities.

acrophobia (ak″ro-fo′be-ah) morbid fear of heights.

acroposthitis (-pos-thi′tis) inflammation of the prepuce.

acropurpura (-pur′pu-rah) purpura affecting the extremities, especially the digits.

acroscleroderma (-skle″ro-der′mah) acrosclerosis.

acrosclerosis (-skle-ro′sis) a combination of Raynaud's disease and scleroderma of the distal parts of the extremities, especially of the digits, and of the neck and face, particularly the nose.

acrosome (ak′ro-sōm) the caplike investment of the anterior half of the head of a spermatozoon.

acrotism (ak′ro-tizm) absence or imperceptibility of the pulse. **acrot′ic,** adj.

acrotrophoneurosis (ak″ro-trof″o-nu-ro′sis) trophoneurotic disturbance of the extremities.

A.C.S. American Cancer Society; American Chemical Society; American College of Surgeons.

A.C.S.M. American College of Sports Medicine.

ACTH adrenocorticotropic hormone; see *corticotropin.*

Actidil (ak′tĭ-dil) trademark for preparations of triprolidine.

actin (ak′tin) a muscle protein localized in the I band of the myofibrils; acting along with myosin, it is responsible for contraction and relaxation of muscle.

acting out (ak′ting owt) the behavioral expression of hidden emotional conflicts, such as hostile feelings, in various kinds of neurotic behavior, as a defense pattern analogous to somatic conversion.

actinic (ak-tin′ik) producing chemical action; said of rays of light beyond the violet end of the spectrum.

actinism (ak′tĭ-nizm) the chemical property of light rays.

actinium (ak-tin′e-um) a chemical element (*see table*), at. no. 89, symbol Ac.

actino- word element [Gr.], *ray; radiation.*

actinobacillosis (ak″tĭ-no-bas″ĭ-lo′sis) an actinomycosis-like disease of domestic animals caused by *Actinobacillus ligniere′sii,* in which the bacilli form radiating structures in the tissues; sometimes seen in man.

Actinobacillus (-bah-sil′us) a genus of schizomycetes (family Brucellaceae) capable of infecting cattle, but rarely man. **A. mal′lei,** *Pseudomonas mallei.* **A. ligniere′sii,** the causative agent of actinobacillosis.

actinochemistry (-kem′is-tre) the chemistry of radiant energy.

actinocutitis (-ku-ti′tis) radiodermatitis.

actinodermatitis (-der″mah-ti′tis) radiodermatitis.

actinogen (ak-tin′o-jen) any radioactive substance.

actinogenesis (ak″tĭ-no-jen′ĕ-sis) the formation or production of actinic rays.

actinogenic (-jen′ik) producing rays, especially actinic rays.

actinology (ak″tĭ-nol′o-je) 1. the study of radiant energy. 2. the science of the chemical effects of light.

actinolyte (ak-tin′o-līt) an apparatus for concentrating the rays of electric light in phototherapy.

Actinomadura (ak″tĭ-no-mad′ŭ-rah) a genus of schizomycetes (family Actinomycetaceae), including *A. madu′rae,* the cause of maduromycosis in which the granules in the discharged pus are white, and *A. pelletier′ii,* the cause of maduromycosis in which the granules are red.

actinometer (ak″tĭ-nom′ĕ-ter) 1. an instrument for measuring the intensity of actinic effects. 2. an apparatus for measuring the penetrating power of actinic rays.

Actinomyces (ak″tĭ-no-mi′sēz) a genus of schizomycetes (family Actinomycetaceae). **A. baudet′ii,** an etiologic agent of actinomycosis in cats and dogs. **A. bo′vis,** a gram-positive microorganism causing actinomycosis in cattle. **A. israe′lii,** a species parasitic in the mouth, proliferating in necrotic tissue; it is the cause of some cases of human actinomycosis.

actinomyces (-mĭ′sēz) an organism of the genus *Actinomyces*. **actinomycet′ic,** adj.

Actinomycetaceae (-mi″sě-ta′se-e) a family of schizomycetes (order Actinomycetales).

Actinomycetales (-mi″sě-ta′lēz) an order of schizomycetes made up of elongated cells having a definite tendency to branch.

actinomycete (-mĭ′sēt) any member of the order Actinomycetales. **actinomycet′ic,** adj.

actinomycin (-mĭ′sin) a family of antibiotics from various species of *Streptomyces*, which are active against bacteria and fungi; it includes the antineoplastic agents cactinomycin (actinomycin C) and dactinomycin (actinomycin D).

actinomycoma (-mi-ko′mah) a tumor-like reactive lesion due to actinomycetes.

actinomycosis (-mi-ko′sis) an infectious disease caused by *Actinomyces*, marked by indolent inflammatory lesions of the lymph nodes draining the mouth, by intraperitoneal abscesses, or by lung abscesses due to aspiration. **actinomycot′ic,** adj.

actinon (ak′tĭ-non) a radioactive isotope of radon, symbol An.

actinoneuritis (ak″tĭ-no-nu-ri′tis) radioneuritis.

Actinoplanaceae (-plah-na′se-e) a family of schizomycetes (order Actinomycetales).

Actinoplanes (-pla′nēz) a genus of schizomycetes (family Actinoplanaceae).

actinotherapy (-ther′ah-pe) treatment of disease with ultraviolet or actinic rays.

actinotoxemia (-tok-se′me-ah) radiation sickness.

actinotoxin (-tok′sin) a crude poison derived from alcoholic extracts of the tentacles of sea anemones.

action (ak′shun) the accomplishment of an effect, whether mechanical or chemical, or the effect so produced. **ac′tive,** adj. **cumulative a.,** the sudden and markedly increased action of a drug after administration of several doses. **reflex a.,** involuntary response to a stimulus conveyed to the nervous system by passage of excitation potential from a receptor to a muscle or gland, over a system of neurons without the necessity of volition. **specific dynamic a.,** increased metabolic rate produced by the ingestion and assimilation of food.

activator (ak″tĭ-va′tor) a substance that makes another substance active or that renders an inactive enzyme capable of exerting its proper effect. **plasminogen a.,** a substance that activates plasminogen and converts it into plasmin. **tissue a.,** fibrinokinase.

activity (ak-tiv′ĭ-te) the quality or process of exerting energy or of accomplishing an effect. **displacement a.,** irrelevant activity produced by an excess of one of two conflicting drives in a person. **enzyme a.,** the catalytic effect exerted by an enzyme, expressed as units per milligram of enzyme (*specific a.*) or as molecules of substrate transformed per minute per molecule of enzyme (*molecular a.*). **optical a.,** the ability of a chemical compound to rotate the plane of polarization of plane-polarized light.

actometer (ak-tom′ě-ter) a device for measuring activity, as in hyperkinesis, as reflected in locomotion in the horizontal plane.

actomyosin (ak″to-mi′o-sin) the system of actin filaments and myosin particles constituting muscle fibers and responsible for the contraction and relaxation of muscle.

acufilopressure (ak″u-fi′lo-presh″er) a combination of acupressure and ligation.

acuity (ah-ku′ĭ-te) clarity or clearness, especially of vision.

acumeter (ah-koo′mě-ter) acoumeter.

acuminate (ah-ku′mĭ-nāt) sharp-pointed.

acupressure (ak″u-presh′er) compression of a bleeding vessel by inserting needles into adjacent tissue.

acupuncture (-pungk′chūr) the Chinese practice of piercing specific areas of the body along peripheral nerves with fine needles to relieve pain, to induce surgical anesthesia, and for therapeutic purposes.

acus (a′kus) a needle or needle-like process.

acute (ah-kūt′) 1. sharp. 2. having severe symptoms and a short course.

acutorsion (ak″u-tor′shun) twisting of a blood vessel with a needle to control bleeding.

acyanoblepsia (ah-si″ah-no-blep′se-ah) inability to distinguish blue tints.

acyanopsia (ah-si″ah-nop′se-ah) acyanoblepsia.

acyanotic (ah-si″ah-not′ik) characterized by absence of cyanosis.

acyesis (ah″si-e′sis) 1. sterility in woman. 2. absence of pregnancy.

Acylanid (as″il-an′id) trademark for a preparation of acetyldigitoxin.

acylase (as′ĭ-lās) any enzyme that catalyzes the hydrolysis of acylated amino acids.

acylmutase (as″il-mu′tās) an enzyme of the isomerase class that catalyzes the intermolecular transfer of acyl groups.

acylphosphatase (-fos′fah-tās) acylphosphate hydrolase: an enzyme occurring in muscle, liver, and kidney that catalyzes the hydrolysis of an acyl phosphate to an anion and an orthophosphate.

acyltransferase (-trans′fer-ās) any of a group of enzymes that catalyze the transfer of an acyl group from one substance to another.

acystia (a-sis′te-ah) congenital absence of the bladder.

acystinervia (ah-sis″tĭ-ner′ve-ah) .paralysis of the bladder.

A.D. [L.] *au′ris dex′tra* (right ear).

ad [L.] preposition, *to.*

ad. [L.] *adde* (add).

A.D.A. American Dental Association; American Diabetes Association; American Dietetic Association.

adactylia (a″dak-til′e-ah) adactyly.

adactyly (a″dak′tĭ-le) congenital absence of fingers or toes. **adac′tylous,** adj.

Adam's apple (ad′amz ap″′l) a subcutaneous prominence on the front of the neck produced by the thyroid cartilage of the larynx.

adamantine (ad″ah-man′tin) pertaining to the enamel of the teeth.

adamantinoma (ad″ah-man″tĭ-no′mah) ameloblastoma.

adamantoblast (ad″ah-man′to-blast) ameloblast.

adamantoblastoma (ad″ah-man″to-blas-to′-mah) ameloblastoma.

adamantoma (ad″ah-man-to′mah) ameloblastoma.

adaptation (ad″ap-ta′shun) 1. the adjustment of an organism to its environment, or the process by which it enhances such fitness. 2. immunization. 3. the normal ability of the eye to adjust itself to variations in the intensity of light; the adjustment to such variations. 4. the decline in the frequency of firing of a neuron, particularly of a receptor, under conditions of constant stimulation. 5. in dentistry, (*a*) the proper fitting of a denture, (*b*) the degree of proximity and interlocking of restorative material to a tooth preparation, (*c*) the exact adjustment of bands to teeth. 6. in microbiology, the adjustment of bacterial physiology to a new environment. **color a.,** 1. changes in visual perception of color with prolonged stimulation. 2. adjustment of vision to degree of brightness or color tone of illumination. **dark a.,** adaptation of the eye to vision in the dark or in reduced illumination. **enzymatic a.,** inducible enzyme synthesis. **genetic a.,** the natural selection of the progeny of a mutant better adapted to a new environment; especially seen in the development of microbes resistant to chemotherapeutic agents or to other inhibitors of growth (drug resistance). **light a.,** adaptation of the eye to vision in the sunlight or in bright illumination (photopia), with reduction in the concentration of the photosensitive pigments of the eye. **phenotypic a.,** a change in the properties of an organism, without any change in genotype, in response to a change in the environment. In microbiology, especially the formation of specific enzymes required for the utilization of new foodstuffs (induced enzyme formation), or a change in cell size and composition with variation in growth rate. **photopic a.,** light a. **retinal a.,** the adjustment of the photoreceptor cell of the eye to the surrounding illumination. **scotopic a.,** dark a.

adapter (ah-dap′ter) a device for connecting parts of an instrument or apparatus.

adaptometer (ad″ap-tom′ĕ-ter) an instrument for measuring the time required for retinal adaptation, i.e., for regeneration of the visual purple; used in detecting night blindness, vitamin A deficiency, and retinitis pigmentosa. **color a.,** an instrument to demonstrate adaptation of the eye to color or light.

adder (ad′er) 1. *Vipera berus.* 2. any of many venomous snakes of the family Viperidae, such as the puff adder and European viper.

addict (ad′dikt) a person exhibiting addiction.

addiction (ah-dik′shun) physiologic or psychologic dependence on some agent (e.g., alcohol, drug), with a tendency to increase its use.

addisonism (ad′ĭ-son-izm″) symptoms seen in pulmonary tuberculosis, consisting of debility and pigmentation, resembling Addison's disease.

additive (ad′ĭ-tiv) 1. characterized by addition; see also under *effect.* 2. a substance added to another substance to improve its appearance, increase its nutritional value, etc.

adduct (ad-dukt′) to draw toward the median plane or (in the digits) toward the axial line of a limb.

adduction (ad-duk′shun) the act of adducting; the state of being adducted.

adductor (ad-duk′tor) that which adducts.

adelomorphous (ah-del″o-mor′fus) of indefinite form.

adenalgia (ad″ĕ-nal′je-ah) pain in a gland.

adenase (ad′ĕ-nās) a deaminizing enzyme of the spleen, liver, and pancreas that converts adenine into hypoxanthine and ammonia.

adenasthenia (ad″en-as-the′ne-ah) deficient glandular activity.

adendric (ah-den′drik) adendritic.

adendritic (ah″den-drit′ik) lacking dendrites.

adenectomy (ad″ĕ-nek′to-me) excision· of a gland.

adenectopia (ad″ĕ-nek-to′pe-ah) malposition or displacement of a gland.

adenia (ah-de′ne-ah) chronic enlargement of the lymphatic glands; see also *lymphoma.*

adeniform (ah-den′ĭ-form) resembling a gland, especially in shape.

adenine (ad′ĕ-nēn) a white, cystalline base, $C_5H_5N_5$, found in plant and animal tissues as one of the purine base constituents of DNA and RNA; it is one of the decomposition products of nuclein. **a. arabinoside,** a purine analogue that inhibits viral replication, probably by its effect on DNA polymerase. **a. hypoxanthine,** a leukomaine, $C_5H_5N_5 + C_4H_4N_4O$, a compound of adenine and hypoxanthine.

adenitis (ad″ĕ-ni′tis) inflammation of a gland. **cervical a.,** a condition characterized by enlarged, inflamed, and tender lymph nodes of the neck; seen in certain infectious diseases of children, such as acute throat infections. **phlegmonous a.,** inflammation of a gland and the surrounding connective tissue.

adenization (ad″ĕ-ni-za′shun) assumption by other tissue of an abnormal glandlike appearance.

adeno- word element [Gr.], *gland.*

adenoacanthoma (ad″ĕ-no-ak″an-tho′mah) adenocarcinoma in which some of the cells exhibit squamous differentiation.

adenoameloblastoma (-ah-mel″o-blas-to′mah) an odontogenic tumor with formation of ductlike structures in place of or in addition to a typical ameloblastic pattern.

adenoblast (ad′ĕ-no-blast″) embryonic forerunner of gland tissue.

adenocarcinoma (ad″ĕ-no-kar″sĭ-no′mah) carcinoma derived from glandular tissue or in which the tumor cells form recognizable glandular structures. **alveolar c.,** adenocarcinoma composed of cells arranged in the form of alveoli. **mucinous a.,** see under *carcinoma.*

adenocele (ad′ĕ-no-sēl″) a cystic adenomatous tumor.

adenocellulitis (ad″ĕ-no-sel″u-li′tis) inflammation of a gland and the tissue around it.

adenochondroma (-kon-dro′mah) a tumor containing both glandular and cartilaginous elements.

adenocyst (ad′ĕ-no-sist″) adenocystoma.

adenocystoma (ad″ĕ-no-sis-to′mah) adenoma in which there is cyst formation. **papillary a. lymphomato′sum,** a cystic tumor containing epithelial and lymphoid tissue, found in the regions of the submaxillary and parotid glands.

adenocyte (ad′ĕ-no-sīt″) a mature secretory cell of a gland.

adenodynia (ad″ĕ-no-din′e-ah) pain in a gland.

adenoepithelioma (-ep″ĭ-the″le-o′mah) a tumor composed of glandular and epithelial elements.

adenofibroma (-fi-bro′mah) a tumor composed of glandular and fibrous structures.

adenogenous (ad″ĕ-noj′ĕ-nus) originating from glandular tissue.

adenography (ad″ĕ-nog′rah-fe) roentgenography of the glands.

adenohypophysectomy (ad″ĕ-no-hi-pof″ĭ-sek′-to-me) excision of the glandular portion (the adenohypophysis) of the pituitary gland.

adenohypophysis (-hi-pof′ĭ-sis) the anterior (or glandular) lobe of the pituitary gland. **adenohypophys′eal,** adj.

adenoid (ad′ĕ-noid) 1. resembling a gland. 2. (pl.) hypertrophy of the adenoid tissue (pharyngeal tonsil) that normally exists in the nasopharynx of children.

adenoidectomy (ad″ĕ-noid-ek′to-me) excision of adenoids.

adenoiditis (-i′tis) inflammation of the adenoids.

adenolipoma (ad″ĕ-no-lĭ-po′mah) a tumor composed of both glandular and fatty tissue elements.

adenolipomatosis (-lip″o-mah-to′sis) the formation of numerous adenolipomas in the neck, axilla, and groin.

adenolymphitis (-lim-fi′tis) lymphadenitis.

adenolymphocele (-lim′fo-sēl) lymphadenocele.

adenolymphoma (-lim-fo′mah) papillary adenocystoma lymphomatosum.

adenoma (ad″ĕ-no′mah) a benign epithelial tumor in which the cells form recognizable glandular structures or in which the cells are derived from glandular epithelium. **acidophilic a.,** a tumor, usually in the anterior lobe of the pituitary gland, whose cells stain with acid dyes. **basophilic a.,** a tumor of the anterior lobe of the pituitary gland whose cells stain with basic dyes. **bronchial a′s,** adenomas situated in the submucosal tissues of large bronchi; sometimes composed of well differentiated cells and usually circumscribed, these tumors have two histologic forms: carcinoid and cylindroma. Although termed "adenomas," these tumors are now recognized as being of low grade malignancy. **chromophobe a., chromophobic a.,** a tumor of the anterior lobe of the pituitary gland whose cells do not readily stain with either acid

or basic dyes. **eosinophil a.,** a tumor of the eosinophilic cells of the anterior lobe of the pituitary gland. **malignant a.,** adenocarcinoma. **sebaceous a.,** hypertrophy or benign hyperplasia of a sebaceous gland. **a. seba′ceum,** nevoid hyperplasia of sebaceous glands, forming multiple yellow papules or nodules on the face. **villous a.,** a large soft papillary polyp on the mucosa of the large intestine.

adenomalacia (ad″ĕ-no-mah-la′she-ah) undue softness of a gland.

adenomatoid (ad″ĕ-no′mah-toid) resembling adenoma.

adenomatosis (ad″ĕ-no″mah-to′sis) the development of numerous adenomatous growths. **polyendocrine a.,** a rare syndrome in which there are adenomas or hyperplasia of more than one endocrine tissue; common sites are the anterior pituitary gland, the islets of Langerhans, and the parathyroid. The Zollinger-Ellison syndrome may occur in affected families.

adenomatous (ad″ĕ-no′mah-tus) pertaining to adenoma or to nodular hyperplasia of a gland.

adenomere (ad′ĕ-no-mēr) the blind terminal portion of the glandular cavity of a developing gland, becoming the functional portion of the organ.

adenomyofibroma (ad″ĕ-no-mi″o-fi-bro′mah) a fibroma containing both glandular and muscular elements.

adenomyoma (-mi-o′mah) see *adenomyosis.*

adenomyomatosis (-mi″o-mah-to′sis) the formation of multiple adenomyomatous nodules in the tissues around or in the uterus.

adenomyomatous (-mi-o′mah-tus) pertaining to or resembling adenomyoma.

adenomyometritis (-mi″o-mĕ-tri′tis) adenomyosis.

adenomyosarcoma (-sar-ko′mah) a mixed mesodermal tumor containing striated muscle cells.

adenomyosis (-mi-o′sis) benign ingrowth of the endometrium into the uterine musculature, sometimes with overgrowth of the latter; if the lesion forms a circumscribed tumor-like nodule, it is called *adenomyoma.* **a. subbasa′lis,** a bandlike, usually diffuse and superficial invasion of the myometrium by epithelial elements, accompanied by small clusters of endometrial stromal cells.

adenoncus (ad″ĕ-nong′kus) enlargement of a gland.

adenopathy (ad″ĕ-nop′ah-the) enlargement of glands, especially of the lymph nodes.

adenopharyngitis (ad″ĕ-no-far″in-ji′tis) inflammation of the adenoids and pharynx, usually involving the tonsils.

adenophlegmon (-fleg′mon) phlegmonous adenitis.

adenosarcoma (-sar-ko′mah) a mixed tumor composed of both glandular and sarcomatous elements.

adenosclerosis (-skle-ro′sis) hardening of a gland.

adenosine (ah-den′o-sēn) a nucleoside consisting of adenine and the pentose sugar D-ribose.

a. 3′:5′-cyclic phosphate, cyclic AMP; a cyclic nucleotide participating in the activities of many hormones, including catecholamines, ACTH, vasopressin, etc.; because it is formed from ATP by the action of adenyl cyclase, which in turn is stimulated by the interaction of the aforementioned hormones with the plasma membrane of target cells, it has been called the "second messenger" in a mechanism of hormone action. **a. diphosphate (ADP),** a product containing two phosphoric acids, formed by hydrolysis of adenosine triphosphate, with release of one high-energy bond. **a. monophosphate (AMP),** adenosine containing only one phosphoric acid. **a. phosphate,** any of the three interconvertible compounds in which adenosine is attached through its ribose group to one (a. monophosphate), two (a. diphosphate), or three (a. triphosphate) phosphoric acid molecules. **a. 3′-phosphate,** see *adenylic acid.* **a. 5′-phosphate,** see *adenylic acid.* **a. triphosphate (ATP),** a compound containing three phosphoric acids, with one low- and two high-energy bonds; it occurs in all cells, where it represents energy storage.

adenosis (ad″ĕ-no′sis) 1. any disease of a gland. 2. the abnormal development of a gland.

adenotome (ad′ĕ-no-tōm″) an instrument for excision of adenoids.

adenotomy (ad″ĕ-not′o-me) 1. anatomy, incision, or dissection of glands. 2. incision of adenoids.

adenotonsillectomy (ad″ĕ-no-ton″sil-lek′to-me) removal of the tonsils and adenoids.

adenovirus (-vi′rus) any of a large group of viruses causing disease of the upper respiratory tract and conjunctiva, and also present in latent infections in normal persons; many induce malignancy in certain species.

adenylate (ah-den′ĭ-lāt) adenylic acid, or any salt of adenylic acid. **a. kinase,** ATP:AMP phosphotransferase; an enzyme occurring in muscle, heart, brain, and liver that converts AMP and ATP to two molecules of ADP.

adenylyl (ad′ĕ-nĭ-lil) the radical of adenylic acid with one H ion removed.

adequacy (ad′ĕ-kwah-se) the state of being sufficient for a specific purpose. **velopharyngeal a.,** sufficient functional closure of the velum against the postpharyngeal wall so that air and hence sound cannot enter the nasopharyngeal and nasal cavities.

adermia (ah-der′me-ah) congenital defect or absence of the skin.

adermogenesis (ah-der″mo-jen′ĕ-sis) imperfect development of skin.

ADH antidiuretic hormone.

adherence (ad-hēr′ens) the act or quality of sticking to something. **immune a.,** a complement-dependent phenomenon in which antigen-antibody complexes or particulate antigens coated with antibody (e.g., antibody-coated bacteria) adhere to red blood cells when complement component C3 is bound. It is a sensitive detector of complement-fixing antibody.

adhesion (ad-he′zhun) 1. the property of remaining in close proximity. 2. the stable joining of parts to one another, which may occur abnormally. 3. a fibrous band or structure by which parts abnormally adhere. **primary a.,** healing by first intention. **secondary a.,** healing by second intention.

adhesiotomy (ad-he″ze-ot′o-me) surgical division of adhesions.

adhesive (ad-he′siv) 1. sticky; tenacious. 2. a substance that causes close adherence of adjoining surfaces.

A.D.I. American Documentation Institute.

adiadochokinesia (ah-di″ah-do″ko-ki-ne′ze-ah) inability to perform fine, rapidly repeated, coordinated movements.

adiaphoria (-fo′re-ah) nonresponse to stimuli as a result of previous similar stimuli; see also *refractory period.*

adiathermancy (-ther′man-se) imperviousness to heat rays.

adiospiromycosis (ad″ĭ-o-spi″ro-mi-ko′sis) a pulmonary disease of many species of rodents throughout the world and rarely of man, due to inhalation of spores produced by the fungus *Emmonsia parva* or *E. crescens,* and marked by the presence of huge spherules (adiospores) without endospores in the lungs.

adiospore (ad′ĭ-o-spōr″) a spore produced by the soil fungi *Emmonsia parva* and *E. crescens;* see *adiospiromycosis.*

adipectomy (ad″ĭ-pek′to-me) excision of adipose tissue.

adiphenine (ad″ĭ-fen′ēn) an anticholinergic C_{20}-$H_{25}NO_2$; used as an antispasmodic in the form of the hydrochloride salt.

adipic (ah-dip′ik) pertaining to fat.

adip(o)- word element [L.], *fat.*

adipocele (ad′ĭ-po-sēl″) a hernia containing fat.

adipocellular (ad″ĭ-po-sel′u-ler) composed of fat and connective tissue.

adipocere (ad′ĭ-po-sēr″) a waxy substance formed during decomposition of dead animal bodies, consisting mainly of insoluble salts of fatty acids.

adipofibroma (ad″ĭ-po-fi-bro′mah) a lipoma with fibrous elements.

adipogenic (-jen′ik) producing fat or fatness.

adipogenous (ad″ĭ-poj′ĕ-nus) adipogenic.

adipokinesis (ad″ĭ-po-ki-ne′sis) the mobilization of fat in the body. **adipokinet′ic,** adj.

adipokinin (-ki′nin) a hormone from the anterior pituitary which accelerates mobilization of stored fat.

adipolysis (ad″ĭ-pol′ĭ-sis) the digestion of fats. **adipolyt′ic,** adj.

adiponecrosis (ad″ĭ-po-nĕ-kro′sis) necrosis of fatty tissue. **a. subcuta′nea neonato′rum,** subcutaneous fat necrosis of the newborn.

adipopexis (-pek′sis) the fixation or storing of fats. **adipopec′tic,** adj.

adipose (ad′ĭ-pōs) pertaining to fat; fatty; fat.

adiposis (ad″ĭ-po′sis) 1. obesity; excessive accumulation of fat. 2. fatty change in an organ or tissue. **a. cerebra′lis,** cerebral adiposity. **a. doloro′sa,** a disease, usually of women, marked by painful localized fatty swellings and by various nerve lesions; death may result from pulmonary complications. **a. hepat'ica,** fatty change in the liver. **a. tubero'sa sim'plex,** a disorder resembling adiposis dolorosa, marked by fatty masses, which may be painful to pressure, in the subcutaneous tissue.

adipositis (ad"ĭ-po-si'tis) panniculitis.

adiposity (ad"ĭ-pos'ĭ-te) the state of being fat; obesity. **cerebral a.,** fatness due to cerebral disease, especially of the hypothalamus. **pituitary a.,** obesity due to pituitary insufficiency.

adiposuria (ad"ĭ-po-su're-ah) the occurrence of fat in the urine.

adipsia (a-dip'se-ah) absence of thirst, or abnormal avoidance of drinking.

aditus (ad'ĭ-tus), pl. *ad'itus* [L.] in anatomic nomenclature, an approach or entrance to an organ or part.

adjuvant (ad'joo-vant) 1. assisting or aiding. 2. a substance which, administered with a drug or antigen, enhances its pharmacologic effect or its antigenicity. **Freund's a.,** a water-in-oil emulsion incorporating antigen, in the aqueous phase, into light-weight paraffin oil with the aid of an emulsifying agent. On injection, this mixture (*Freund's incomplete a.*) induces strong persistent antibody formation. The addition of killed, dried mycobacteria, e.g., *Mycobacterium butyricum,* to the oil phase (*Freund's complete a.*) elicits cell-mediated immunity (delayed hypersensitivity), as well as humoral antibody formation.

adjuvanticity (ad"ju-van-tĭ'sĭ-te) the ability to modify the immune response.

adnerval (ad-ner'val) 1. situated near a nerve. 2. toward a nerve, said of electric current that passes through muscle toward the entrance point of a nerve.

adneural (ad-nu'ral) adnerval.

adnexa (ad-nek'sah) [L., pl.] appendages or accessory structures of an organ, as the appendages of the eye (*a. oc'uli*), including the eyelids and lacrimal apparatus, or of the uterus (*a. u'teri*), including the uterine tubes and ligaments and ovaries. **adnex'al,** adj.

adnexogenesis (ad-nek"so-jen'ĕ-sis) the embryonic development of the adnexa.

adolescence (ad"o-les'ens) the period between puberty and the completion of physical growth, roughly from 11 to 19 years of age. **adoles'cent,** adj.

adoral (ad-o'ral) toward or near the mouth.

ADP adenosine diphosphate.

adren(o)- word element [L.], *adrenal gland.*

adrenal (ah-dre'nal) 1. near the kidney. 2. an adrenal gland.

adrenalectomy (ah-dre"nah-lek'to-me) excision of one or both adrenal glands.

Adrenalin (ah-dren'ah-lin) trademark for epinephrine.

adrenaline (-ah-lēn) official British Pharmacopoeia name for epinephrine.

adrenalinemia (ah-dren"ah-lin-e'me-ah) the presence of epinephrine in the blood.

adrenalinuria (-u're-ah) the presence of epinephrine in the urine.

adrenalism (ah-dren'ah-lizm) ill health due to adrenal dysfunction.

adrenalitis (ah-dre"nal-i'tis) inflammation of the adrenal glands.

adrenalopathy (-op'ah-the) any disease of the adrenal glands.

adrenergic (ad"ren-er'jik) sympathomimetic: activated or transmitted by epinephrine; said of those nerve fibers that liberate epinephrine (sympathin) at a synapse when a nerve impulse passes, i.e., the sympathetic fibers. Also, any agent that produces such an effect.

adrenic (ah-dren'ik) pertaining to the adrenal glands.

adrenoceptor (ah-dre"no-sep'tor) adrenergic receptor.

adrenocortical (-kor'tĭ-kal) pertaining to or arising from the cortex of the adrenal gland.

adrenocorticohyperplasia (-kor"tĭ-ko-hi"per-pla'ze-ah) adrenal cortical hyperplasia.

adrenocorticomimetic (-mi-met'ik) having effects similar to those of hormones of the adrenal cortex.

adrenocorticotrophic (-trof'ik) corticotropic.

adrenocorticotrophin (-trof'in) corticotropin.

adrenocorticotropic (-trōp'ik) corticotropic.

adrenocorticotropin (-trōp'in) corticotropin.

adrenoglomerulotropin (-glo-mer"u-lo-tro'-pin) a hormone alleged to stimulate production of aldosterone by the adrenal cortex.

adrenolytic (-lit'ik) inhibiting the action of the adrenergic nerves or the response to epinephrine.

adrenomegaly (-meg'ah-le) enlargement of one or both of the adrenal glands.

adrenopathy (ad"ren-op'ah-the) adrenalopathy.

adrenoreceptor (ah-dre"no-re-sep'tor) adrenergic receptor.

adrenotoxin (-tok'sin) any substance that is toxic to the adrenal glands.

adriamycin (a"dre-ah-mi'sin) an antibiotic used in conjunction with dimethyl triazeno imidiazole carboxamide (DIC) as an antineoplastic.

Adroyd (ad'roid) trademark for a preparation of oxymetholone.

adsorb (ad-sorb') to attract and retain other material on the surface.

adsorbent (-ent) 1. pertaining to or characterized by adsorption. 2. a substance that attracts other materials or particles to its surface. **gastrointestinal a.,** a substance, usually a powder, taken to adsorb gases, toxins, and bacteria in the stomach and intestines.

adsorption (ad-sorp'shun) the action of a substance in attracting and holding other materials or particles on its surface.

adtorsion (ad-tor'shun) conclination.

adult (ah-dult') having attained full growth or maturity, or an organism that has done so.

adulterant (ah-dul'ter-ant") a substance used as an addition to another for sophistication or adulteration.

adulteration (ah-dul"ter-a'shun) addition of an impure, cheap, or unnecessary ingredient to cheat, cheapen, or falsify a preparation; in legal terminology, incorrect labeling, including dosage not in accordance with the label.

adumbration (ah″dum-bra′shun) a geometric lack of sharpness; an inherent property of the focal spot which causes the production of double images. In radiology, the giving forth of a shadow.

advancement (ad-vans′ment) surgical detachment, as of a muscle or tendon, followed by reattachment at an advanced point; chiefly done with an eye muscle for correction of strabismus. **capsular a.**, attachment of the capsule of Tenon in front of its normal position.

adventitia (ad″ven-tish′e-ah) the outer coat of an organ or structure, especially the outer coat of an artery.

adventitious (ad″ven-tish′us) 1. accidental or acquired; not natural or hereditary. 2. found out of the normal or usual place.

adynamia (ad″ĭ-na′me-ah) lack or loss of normal or vital powers; asthenia. **adynam′ic**, adj.

Aedes (a-e′dēz) a genus of mosquitoes, including approximately 600 species; some are vectors of disease, others are pests. It includes A. aegyp′ti, a vector of yellow fever and dengue.

A.E.E.G.S. American Electroencephalographic Society.

aeg- for words beginning thus, see those beginning eg-.

A.E.L. American Electronics Laboratories.

aer(o)- word element [Gr.], air; gas.

aeration (a″er-a′shun) 1. the exchange of carbon dioxide for oxygen by the blood in the lungs. 2. the charging of a liquid with air or gas.

aeriform (ār′ĭ-form, a-er′ĭ-form) resembling air; gaseous.

Aerobacter (a″er-o-bak′ter) a genus of schizomycetes (order Eubacteriales, tribe Escherichieae), which ferment glucose and lactose to produce acid and gas; it includes two species, A. aero′genes and A. cloa′cae.

aerobe (a′er-ōb) a microorganism that lives and grows in the presence of free oxygen. **aero′bic**, adj. **facultative a.**, one that can live in the presence of oxygen, but does not require it. **obligate a.**, one that cannot live without oxygen.

aerobiology (a″er-o-bi-ol′o-je) the study of the distribution of living organisms (microorganisms) by the air.

aerobiosis (-bi-o′sis) life requiring free oxygen.

aerocele (a′er-o-sēl″) a tumor formed by air filling an adventitious pouch. **epidural a.**, a collection of air between the dura mater and the wall of the spinal column.

aerocolpos (a″er-o-kol′pos) distention of the vagina with gas.

aerodermectasia (-der″mek-ta′ze-ah) subcutaneous emphysema, which may be spontaneous, traumatic, or surgical in origin.

aerodontalgia (-don-tal′je-ah) pain in the teeth due to lowered atmospheric pressure at high altitudes.

aerodontics (-don′tiks) the branch of dentistry concerned with effects on the teeth of high-altitude flying.

aerodynamics (-di-nam′iks) the science of air and gases in motion.

aeroembolism (-em′bo-lizm) obstruction of a blood vessel by air or gas.

aeroemphysema (-em″fĭ-ze′mah) pulmonary emphysema and edema with collection of nitrogen bubbles in the lung tissues; due to excessively rapid atmospheric decompression.

aerogen (a′er-o-jen″) a gas-producing bacterium.

aerogenesis (a″er-o-jen′ĕ-sis) formation or production of gas. **aerogen′ic**, adj.

aerogram (a′er-o-gram″) roentgenogram of an organ after injection with air or gas.

aerometer (a″er-om′ĕ-ter) an instrument for estimating gaseous density.

Aeromonas (a″er-o-mo′nas) a genus of schizomycetes (family Pseudomonadaceae), usually found in water, some being pathogenic for fish and amphibians.

aeroneurosis (-nu-ro′sis) a functional nervous disorder occurring in pilots.

aero-otitis (-o-ti′tis) barotitis.

aeropathy (a″er-op′ah-the) any disease due to change in atmospheric pressure, e.g., decompression sickness.

aeroperitonia (a″er-o-per″ĭ-to-ne′ah) pneumoperitoneum.

aerophagia (-fa′je-ah) habitual swallowing of air.

aerophilic (-fil′ik) requiring air for proper growth.

aerophilous (a″er-of′ĭ-lus) aerophilic.

aerophobia (a″er-o-fo′be-ah) 1. morbid dread of drafts of air. 2. morbid dread of being up in the air.

aerophyte (a′er-o-fīt″) any plant organism that lives upon air.

aeropiesotherapy (a″er-o-pi-e″so-ther′ah-pe) treatment by compressed or rarefied air.

Aeroplast (a′er-o-plast″) trademark for vibesate.

aeroplethysmograph (a″er-o-plĕ-thiz′mo-graf) an apparatus for measuring respiratory volumes by recording changes in body volume.

aerosinusitis (-si″nus-i′tis) barosinusitis.

aerosol (a′er-o-sol″) a colloid system in which solid or liquid particles are suspended in a gas, especially a suspension of a drug or other substance to be dispensed in a fine spray or mist.

Aerosporin (a″er-o-spōr′in) trademark for a preparation of polymyxin B sulfate.

aerostatics (-stat′iks) the science of air or gases in equilibrium.

aerotaxis (-tak′sis) movement of an organism in response to the presence of molecular oxygen.

aerotitis (-ti′tis) barotitis. **a. me′dia**, barotitis media.

aerotonometer (-to-nom′ĕ-ter) a device used in measuring the tension of blood gases.

A.E.S. American Encephalographic Society; American Epidemiological Society.

aes-, aet- for words beginning thus, see also those beginning es-, et-.

Æsculapius (es″cu-la′pe-us) the god of healing

in Roman mythology; see also *caduceus*, and under *staff*.

afebrile (a-feb′rĭl) without fever.

affect (af′ekt) a freudian term for the feeling of pleasantness or unpleasantness evoked by a stimulus; also the emotional complex associated with a mental state; the feeling experienced in connection with an emotion.

affection (ah-fek′shun) 1. a state of emotion or feeling. 2. a morbid condition or diseased state.

affective (ah-fek′tiv) pertaining to or resulting from emotions or feelings.

afferent (af′er-ent) conducting toward a center or specific site of reference.

affinin (af′ĭ-nin) a lipid amide obtained from the plant *Heliopsis longipes*, having insecticidal and local anesthetic properties; the plant is used in Mexico as a dental analgesic.

affinity (ah-fin′ĭ-te) attraction; a tendency to seek out or unite with another object or substance. **chemical a.**, 1. the force that unites atoms into molecules. 2. the tendency of substances to react with one another. **elective a.**, the force that causes union of a substance with one substance rather than another.

afibrinogenemia (a-fi″brin-o-jĕ-ne′me-ah) deficiency or absence of fibrinogen in the blood. **congenital a.**, an uncommon hemorrhagic coagulation disorder, probably transmitted by an autosomal recessive gene, and characterized by complete incoagulability of the blood.

aflatoxicosis (af″lah-tok″sĭ-ko-sis) poisoning by aflatoxin.

aflatoxin (-tok′sin) a toxin, $C_{17}H_{12}O_6$, produced by *Aspergillus flavus* and *A. parasiticus*, molds which contaminate ground nut seedlings; it produces aflatoxicosis (x disease), with high mortality rates, in fowl and other farm animals fed with infected ground nut meal.

afterbirth (af′ter-berth″) the placenta and membranes delivered from the uterus after childbirth.

afterbrain (-brān″) metencephalon.

afterhearing (af″ter-hēr′ing) perception of aftersounds.

afterimage (-im′ij) a retinal impression remaining after cessation of the stimulus causing it.

afterpains (af′ter-pānz″) cramplike pains that follow expulsion of the placenta, due to uterine contractions.

afterperception (af″ter-per-sep′shun) perception of aftersensations.

aftersensation (-sen-sa′shun) sensation persisting after cessation of the stimulus which caused it.

aftersound (af′ter-sownd″) sensation of a sound after cessation of the stimulus causing it.

aftertaste (-tāst″) a taste continuing after the substance producing it has been removed.

Ag chemical symbol, *silver* [L. *argentum*]; antigen.

A.G.A. American Geriatrics Association.

agalactia (ag″ah-lak′she-ah) absence or failure of secretion of milk.

agametic (a″gah-met′ik) devoid of germ cells; not possessing gametes.

agammaglobulinemia (a″gam-mah-glob″u-lin-e′me-ah) an immunological deficiency state in which there is an extremely low level of generally all classes of gamma globulins in the blood, resulting in heightened susceptibility to infectious diseases. **Swiss type a.**, a lethal form with associated alymphocytosis and aplasia of the thymus, first recognized in Switzerland.

agamogenesis (ag″ah-mo-jen′ĕ-sis) schizogony.

aganglionic (a-gang″gle-on′ik) lacking ganglion cells.

aganglionosis (a-gang″gle-on-o′sis) congenital absence of parasympathetic ganglion cells.

agar (ag′ar) a dried hydrophilic, colloidal substance extracted from various species of red algae; used in solid culture media for bacteria and other microorganisms, as a bulk laxative, in making emulsions, and as a supporting medium for immunodiffusion and immunoelectrophoresis.

Agarbacterium (ag″ar-bak-te′re-um) a genus of schizomycetes (family Achromobacteraceae) which digest agar; primarily found on decomposing seaweed and in sea water.

agaric (ah-gar′ik) 1. any mushroom, more especially any species of *Agaricus*. 2. the tinder or punk prepared from dried mushrooms.

agastric (ah-gas′trik) having no alimentary canal.

age (āj) 1. the duration, or the measure of time of the existence of a person or object. 2. to undergo change as a result of passage of time. **achievement a.**, the age of a person expressed as the chronologic age of a normal person showing the same proficiency in study. **chronologic a.**, the actual measure of time elapsed since a person's birth. **mental a.**, the age level of mental ability of a person as gauged by standard intelligence tests.

agenesia (ah″jĕ-ne′ze-ah) 1. imperfect development. 2. sterility or impotence.

agenesis (a-jen′ĕ-sis) absence of an organ due to nonappearance of its primordium in the embryo; imperfect development of a part. **gonadal a.**, complete failure of gonadal development; see *Turner's syndrome*. **nuclear a.**, Möbius' syndrome. **ovarian a.**, failure of development of the ovaries; see *Turner's syndrome*.

agenitalism (a-jen′ĭ-tal-izm″) a condition due to lack of secretion of the testes or ovaries.

agenosomia (ah-jen″o-so′me-ah) congenital absence or imperfect development of the genitals and eventration of the lower part of the abdomen.

agent (a′jĕnt) something capable of producing an effect. **adrenergic blocking a.**, one that inhibits response to sympathetic impulses by blocking the alpha or beta receptor sites of effector organs. **alkylating a.**, any hydrocarbon derivative whose functional group may be replaced in a chemical reaction in which the hydrocarbon fragment is attached to another organic molecule. **blocking a.**, an agent that inhibits the response of effector organs to neural impulses of the autonomic nervous system; it may be an adrenergic or anticholinergic blocking agent. **chelating a.**, a compound which combines with metals to form weakly dissociated complexes in which the metal is part of a ring; used to extract certain elements from a system. **chimpanzee coryza a.,** respiratory syncytial virus. **Eaton a.,** *Mycoplasma pneumoniae.* **fixing a's,** agents, such as formalin, alcohol, acids, salts of heavy metals, or mixtures of these, which precipitate the proteins of cells or tissues and render them insoluble. **levigating a.,** material used for moistening a solid before reducing it to a powder. **mammary tumor a., mouse mammary tumor a.,** one of the factors, the virus factor, involved in mammary tumor production in mice; transmitted to offspring through the mother's milk. **progestational a's,** a group of hormones secreted by the corpus luteum and placenta and, in small amounts, by the adrenal cortex, including progesterone, Δ^4-3-ketopregnene-20(α)-ol, and Δ^4-3-ketopregnene-20(β)-ol; agents having progestational activity are also produced synthetically. **reducing a.,** an agent that causes chemical reduction. **surface-active a.,** a substance that exerts a change on the surface properties of a liquid, especially one, such as a detergent, that reduces its surface tension; see also *surfactant.*

ageusia (ah-gu'ze-ah) lack or impairment of the sense of taste. **ageu'sic,** adj.

agger (aj'er), pl. *ag'geres* [L.] an eminence or elevation. **a. na'si,** an elevation between the anterior margin of the middle concha and the inner surface of the dorsum of the nose.

agglutinable (ah-gloo'tĭ-nah-b'l) capable of agglutination.

agglutinant (ah-gloo'tĭ-nant) 1. promoting union by adhesion. 2. a tenacious or gluey substance that holds parts together during the healing process.

agglutination (ah-gloo''tĭ-na'shun) 1. aggregation of suspended cells into clumps or masses, especially the clumping together of bacteria exposed to specific immune serum. 2. the process of union in wound healing. **agglutina'tive,** adj. **group a.,** agglutination of members of a group of biologically related organisms or corpuscles by an agglutinin specific for that group. **intravascular a.,** clumping of particulate elements within the blood vessels; used conventionally to denote red blood cell aggregation.

agglutinator (ah-gloo'tĭ-na''tor) an agglutinin.

agglutinin (ah-gloo'tĭ-nin) an antibody in serum which, when combined with its homologous antigen, causes the antigen elements to adhere to one another in clumps. **anti-Rh a.,** an agglutinin not normally present in human plasma, which may be produced in Rh-negative mothers carrying an Rh-positive fetus, or after transfusion of Rh-positive blood into an Rh-negative patient. **chief a.,** the specific immune agglutinin in the blood of an animal immunized against an infectious disease agent. **cold a.,** one that acts only at relatively low temperatures (0°–20° C.). **group a.,** one which has a specific action on certain organisms, but will agglutinate other species as well. **H a.,** one that is specific for flagellar antigens of the motile strain of a microorganism. **immune a.,** a specific agglutinin found in the blood after recovery from the disease or injection with the microorganism causing the disease. **incomplete a.,** one that at appropriate concentrations fails to agglutinate the homologous antigen. **leukocyte a.,** one that is directed against neutrophilic and other leukocytes. **major a.,** chief a. **minor a.,** partial a. **normal a.,** a specific agglutinin found in the blood of an animal or of man that has neither had associated disease nor been injected with the causative associated organism. **O a.,** one that is specific for somatic antigens of a microorganism. **partial a.,** one present in agglutinative serum which acts on organisms closely related to the specific antigen, but in a lower dilution. **platelet a.,** one that is directed against platelets. **warm a.,** an antibody that reacts best at 37° C., usually without producing agglutination.

agglutinogen (ag''loo-tin'o-gen) any substance that stimulates the production of agglutinin.

agglutinogenic (ah-gloo''tĭ-no-jen'ik) pertaining to the production of agglutinin; producing agglutinin.

agglutinophilic (ah-gloo''tĭ-no-fil'ik) agglutinating easily.

aggregation (ag-re-ga'shun) 1. massing or clumping of materials together. 2. a clumped mass of material. **familial a.,** the occurrence of more cases of a given disorder in close relatives of a person with the disorder than in control families. **platelet a.,** a clumping together of platelets induced by various agents (e.g., thrombin) as part of the mechanism leading to thrombus formation.

aggregen (ag'rĕ-jen) an organized mass of mammalian cells growing in agitated culture, resembling an aggregate in having a continuous layer of peripheral cells forming a smooth surface, but having the capacity to fragment to form daughter aggregens.

aggression (ah-gresh'un) behavior leading to self-assertion, which may arise from innate drives and/or a response to frustration, and may be manifested by destructive and attacking behavior, by covert attitudes of hostility and obstructionism, or by self-expressive drive to mastery.

aging (āj'ing) the gradual structural changes that occur with the passage of time, that are not due to disease or accident, and that eventually lead to increased probability of death as the organism grows older.

agitated (aj'ĕ-tāt''ed) marked by restlessness and increased activity intermingled with anxiety, fear, and tension.

aglaucopsia (ah''glaw-kop'se-ah) inability to distinguish green tints.

aglossia (ah-glos'e-ah) congenital absence of the tongue.

aglossostomia (ah''glos-o-sto'me-ah) congenital absence of the tongue and mouth opening.

aglucone (a-gloo'kōn) aglycone.

aglutition (ag''loo-tish'un) inability to swallow.

aglycemia (a''gli-se'me-ah) absence of sugar from the blood.

aglycone (a-gli'kōn) the noncarbohydrate portion of a glycoside molecule.

aglycosuric (ah-gli″ko-su′rik) free from glycosuria.

agnathia (ag-na′the-ah) congenital absence, total or virtual, of the lower jaw.

agnathus (ag′nah-thus) a fetus exhibiting agnathia.

agnogenic (ag″no-jen′ik) of unknown origin.

agnosia (ag″no′ze-ah) inability to recognize the import of sensory impressions; the varieties correspond with several senses and are distinguished as *auditory (acoustic), gustatory, olfactory, tactile,* and *visual.* **finger a.,** loss of ability to indicate one's own or another's fingers. **time a.,** loss of comprehension of the succession and duration of events.

-agogue word element [Gr.], *something which leads or induces.*

agomphiasis (ah″gom-fi′ah-sis) absence of the teeth.

agonad (ah-go′nad) an individual having no sex glands.

agonadal (ah-gon′ah-dal) having no sex glands; due to absence of sex glands.

agonadism (ah-go′nah-dizm) the condition of being without sex glands.

agonal (ag′ŏ-nal) 1. pertaining to the death agony; occurring at the moment of or just before death. 2. pertaining to terminal infection.

agonist (ag′o-nist) a muscle which in contracting to move a part is opposed by another muscle (the antagonist).

agony (ag′o-ne) 1. death struggle. 2. extreme suffering.

agoraphobia (ag″o-rah-fo′be-ah) morbid dread of open spaces.

-agra word element [Gr.], *attack; seizure.*

agrammatism (a-gram′ah-tizm) inability to speak grammatically due to a disorder of the language center of the brain.

agranulocytosis (a-gran″u-lo-si-to′sis) a symptom complex characterized by a marked decrease in the number of granulocytes and by lesions of the throat and other mucous membranes, of the gastrointestinal tract, and of the skin.

agranuloplastic (-plas′tik) forming nongranular cells only; not forming granular cells.

agranulosis (a-gran″u-lo′sis) agranulocytosis.

agraphia (a-graf′e-ah) inability to express thoughts in writing, due to a lesion of the cerebral cortex. **agraph′ic,** adj.

agria (ag′re-ah) an obstinate pustular eruption.

Agrobacterium (ag″ro-bak-te′re-um) a genus of schizomycetes found in soil or in the roots or stems of plants.

A.G.S. American Geriatrics Society.

ague (a′gu) 1. malarial fever, or any other severe recurrent symptom of malarial origin. 2. a chill.

agyria (ah-ji′re-ah) a malformation in which the gyri of the cerebral cortex are not normally developed and the brain is usually small.

A.H.A. American Heart Association; American Hospital Association.

AHF antihemophilic factor (coagulation Factor VIII; see under *factor*).

AHG antihemophilic globulin (coagulation Factor VIII; see under *factor*).

ahistidasia (ah-his″tĭ-da′ze-ah) absence of histidase activity; see *histidinemia.*

A.H.P. Assistant House Physician.

A.H.S. Assistant House Surgeon.

A.I. artificial insemination.

A.I.C. Association des Infirmières Canadiennes.

aichmophobia (āk″mo-fo′be-ah) morbid dread of pointed instruments.

A.I.D. artificial insemination (donor semen).

aid (ād) help or assistance; by extension, applied to any device by which a function can be improved or augmented, as a hearing aid. **first a.,** emergency assistance and treatment of an injured or ill person before regular surgical or medical therapy can be obtained. **pharmaceutic a., pharmaceutical a.,** see under *necessity.*

A.I.H. American Institute of Homeopathy; artificial insemination (husband's semen).

A.I.H.A. American Industrial Hygiene Association.

ailment (āl′ment) any disease or affection of the body, especially a slight or minor disorder.

ailurophobia (i-lu″ro-fo′be-ah) morbid fear of cats.

A.I.N. American Institute of Nutrition.

ainhum (ān′hum, i′num) a condition of unknown origin, occurring chiefly in dark-skinned races in the tropics, in which linear constriction of a toe, especially the fifth one, leads to gradual spontaneous amputation.

air (ār) the gaseous mixture which makes up the atmosphere. **alveolar a.,** air in the lungs, varying in volume (during normal respiration) from the functional residual capacity at the end of expiration to the functional residual capacity plus tidal volume at the end of inspiration. **factitious a.,** nitrous oxide. **reserve a.,** see *expiratory* and *inspiratory reserve volume.* **residual a.,** see under *volume.* **tidal a.,** see under *volume.*

airway (ār′wa) 1. the passage by which air enters and leaves the lungs. 2. a tube for securing unobstructed respiration.

akaryocyte (ah-kar′e-o-sīt″) a non-nucleated cell, e.g., an erythrocyte.

akaryote (ah-kar′e-ōt) 1. non-nucleated. 2. a non-nucleated cell.

akatamathesia (ah-kat″ah-mah-the′ze-ah) inability to understand.

akathisia (ak″ah-the′ze-ah) a condition marked by motor restlessness, ranging from anxiety to inability to lie or sit quietly or to sleep, as seen in toxic reactions to phenothiazines.

akinesia (a″ki-ne′ze-ah) absence or poverty of movements. **akinet′ic,** adj. **a. al′gera,** Möbius' syndrome.

akinesthesia (ah-kin″es-the′ze-ah) absence of movement sense.

Akineton (a″ki-ne′ton) trademark for preparations of biperiden.

Al chemical symbol, *aluminum.*

A.L.A. American Laryngological Association.

Ala alanine.

ala (a′lah), pl. *a′lae* [L.] a winglike process. **a′late**, adj. **a. mag′na, a. ma′jor**, the great wing of the sphenoid bone. **a. mi′nor**, the lesser wing of the sphenoid bone. **a. na′si**, the cartilaginous flap on the outer side of either nostril. **a. par′va**, a. minor.

alactasia (ah-lak-ta′se-ah) a genetically determined condition marked by malabsorption of lactose due to deficiency of lactase; it is very rare in infants of any race, but is common in nonwhite adults.

alalia (ah-la′le-ah) impairment of the ability to speak.

alanine (al′ah-nēn, al′ah-nin) a natural amino acid occurring in two forms: alpha-alanine, $CH_3CH(NH_2)\cdot COOH$, and beta-alanine, $CH_2NH_2\cdot CH_2COOH$.

alar (a′lar) pertaining to an ala, or wing.

alastrim (ah-las′trim) variola minor.

alba (al′bah) [L.] white.

Albamycin (al′bah-mi″sin) trademark for preparations of novobiocin.

albedo (al-be′do) [L.] whiteness. **a. ret′inae**, paleness of the retina due to edema caused by transudation of fluid from the retinal capillaries.

albicans (al′bĭ-kans) [L.] white.

albiduria (al″bĭ-du′re-ah) the discharge of white or pale urine.

albinism (al′bĭ-nizm) congenital absence, either total or partial, of normal pigmentation in the body (hair, skin, eyes) due to a defect in melanin precursors.

albino (al-bi′no) a person affected with albinism.

albinoidism (al-bĭ-noid′izm) deficiency of pigment in the hair, skin, and eyes, but not to the degree seen in albinism.

albinuria (al″bĭ-nu′re-ah) albiduria.

albuginea (al″bu-jin′e-ah) 1. a tough, whitish layer of fibrous tissue investing a part or organ. 2. the tunica albuginea. **a. oc′uli**, sclera. **a. ova′rii**, the outer layer of the ovarian stroma. **a. pe′nis**, the outer envelope of the corpora cavernosa.

albumen (al-bu′men) albumin.

albumin (al-bu′min) a protein found in nearly all animal and many vegetable tissues, characterized by being soluble in water and coagulable by heat. **acid a.**, albumin altered by action of acid. **alkali a.**, albumin which has been treated with alkali. **circulating a.**, that found in the body fluids. **derived a.**, albumin denatured by chemical action. **egg a.**, albumin of egg whites. **iodinated** [131]**I serum a.**, normal human serum albumin treated with iodine-131, used for measuring blood volume and cardiac output. **native a.**, any albumin normally present in the body. **normal human serum a.**, a sterile preparation of serum albumin obtained by fractionating blood from healthy human donors; used in the prevention and treatment of shock and in the treatment of hypoproteinemia. **radioiodinated serum a.**, iodinated ^{131}I serum a. **serum a.**, albumin of the blood. **a. tannate**, an astringent powder containing about 50% tannic acid combined with protein; used in diarrhea. **vegetable a.**, albumin of vegetable tissue.

albuminate (al-bu′mĭ-nāt) albumin denatured by a base or an acid.

albuminaturia (al-bu″mĭ-nah-tu′re-ah) proteinuria in which there is an excess of albuminates in the urine.

albuminimeter (-nim′ĕ-ter) an instrument for determining the proportion of albumin present, as in the urine.

albuminocholia (-no-ko′le-ah) presence of protein in the bile.

albuminoid (al-bu′mĭ-noid) 1. resembling albumin. 2. a scleroprotein.

albuminolysin (al-bu″mĭ-nol′ĭ-sin) 1. a lysin which splits up albumins. 2. anaphylactin.

albuminolysis (-nol′ĭ-sis) the splitting up of albumins.

albuminometer (-nom′ĕ-ter) albuminimeter.

albuminoptysis (-nop′tĭ-sis) albumin in the sputum.

albuminous (al-bu′mĭ-nus) charged with or resembling albumin.

albuminuretic (al-bu″min-u-ret′ik) pertaining to, characterized by, or promoting albuminuria; also, an agent that promotes albuminuria.

albuminuria (al-bu″mĭ-nu′re-ah) presence in the urine of serum albumin; see *proteinuria*. **albuminu′ric**, adj.

Albumisol (al-bu′mĭ-sol) trademark for a preparation of normal human serum albumin.

albumoscope (al-bu′mo-skōp) an instrument for determining the presence and amount of albumin in the urine.

Alcaligenes (al″kah-lij′ĕ-nēz) a genus of schizomycetes (family Achromobacteraceae) found in the intestinal tract of vertebrates or in dairy products.

alcapton (al-kap′ton) see *alkapton bodies*, under *body*.

alcaptonuria (al-kap″to-nu′re-ah) alkaptonuria.

alcohol (al′ko-hol) 1. ethanol or ethyl alcohol: a colorless, volatile liquid, C_2H_6O, obtained by fermentation of carbohydrates by yeast; it is used in beverages, and as a topical anti-infective and solvent. 2. any compound of a hydrocarbon with hydroxyl (OH). **absolute a.**, dehydrated a. **benzyl a.**, a colorless liquid, $C_6H_5\cdot CH_2\cdot OH$, used as a bacteriostatic in solutions for injection; also applied topically as a local anesthetic. **cetyl a.**, a solid alcohol, $C_{16}H_{34}O$, used as an emulsifying and stiffening agent. **dehydrated a.**, an extremely hygroscopic, transparent, colorless, volatile liquid, containing 99.5% by volume of C_2H_5OH. **denatured a.**, alcohol rendered unfit for human consumption. **ethyl a.**, ordinary alcohol ($CH_3\cdot CH_2OH$). **isopropyl a.**, transparent, colorless, volatile liquid, $CH_3CHOH\cdot CH_3$, used as a solvent. **isopropyl rubbing a.**, a preparation containing between 68% and 72% isopropyl alcohol in water, used as a rubefacient. **methyl a.**, methanol. **nicotinyl a.**, an alcohol, C_6H_7NO, used as a peripheral vasodilator in vasospastic conditions. **phenylethyl a.**, a colorless liquid, $C_8H_{10}O$, used as a bacteriostatic and preservative. **primary a.**, one containing the monovalent carbinol group, $—CH_2OH$. **propyl a.**, a colorless fluid of alcoholic taste and fruity odor; used as a solvent. **rubbing a.,** a preparation of acetone, methyl isobutyl ketone, and 68.5% to 71.5% ethyl alcohol; used as a rubefacient. **secondary a.,** one containing the divalent group, $=CHOH$. **stearyl a.,** a mixture of solid alcohols, consisting chiefly of $CH_3(CH_2)_{16}CH_2$-OH; used as an ingredient of various pharmaceutic or cosmetic preparations. **tertiary a.,** one containing the trivalent group, $\equiv COH$. **wood a.,** methanol.

alcoholic (al″ko-hol′ik) 1. containing or pertaining to alcohol. 2. a person suffering from alcoholism.

alcoholism (al′ko-hol″izm) a behavioral disorder manifested by excessive consumption of alcoholic beverages to an extent that interferes with the patient's health and economic functioning; some degree of habituation, dependence, or addiction is implied. **acute a.,** simple drunkenness, a transient condition due to excessive intake of ethyl alcohol, with depression of the centers of the nervous system. **chronic a.,** long-continued, excessive intake of ethyl alcohol, characterized by various conditions, including anorexia, diarrhea, weight loss, mental deterioration, personality changes, peripheral neuropathy, and fatty deterioration of the liver.

alcoholize (al′ko-hol-īz″) 1. to treat with alcohol. 2. to transform into alcohol.

alcoholometer (al″ko-hol-om′ĕ-ter) instrument for determining amount of alcohol present.

alcoholuria (-u′re-ah) the presence of alcohol in the urine.

alcoholysis (al″ko-hol′ĭ-sis) decomposition of a compound due to the incorporation and splitting of alcohol.

Aldactazide (al-dak′tah-zīd) trademark for a preparation of spironolactone with hydrochlorothiazide.

Aldactone (al-dak′tōn) trademark for a preparation of spironolactone.

aldehyde (al′dĕ-hīd) 1. a chemical compound derived from primary alcohols by oxidation and containing the monovalent —CHO. 2. acetaldehyde. **acetic a.,** acetaldehyde. **cinnamic a.,** a colorless aldehyde, $C_6H_5(CH)_2CHO$, from oil of cinnamon; used in flavors and perfumes.

aldehyde-lyase (-li′ās) a group of lyases that catalyze the removal of an aldehyde group.

aldolase (al′do-lās) an enzyme in muscle extract that acts as a catalyst in the production of dihydroxyacetone phosphate and glyceraldehyde phosphate from fructose 1,6-diphosphate.

aldopentose (al″do-pen′tōs) any of a class of sugars containing five carbon atoms and an aldehyde group (—CHO).

aldose (al′dōs) a sugar containing an aldehyde group (—CHO).

aldosterone (al-dos′ter-ōn) a mineralocorticoid, the principal electrolyte-regulating steroid hormone secreted by the adrenal cortex.

aldosteronism (-izm″) hyperaldosteronism.

aldrin (al′drin) a chlorinated naphthalene derivative used as an insecticide.

alecithal (ah-les′ĭ-thal) without yolk; applied to eggs with very little yolk; see under *ovum.*

aleukemia (ah″lu-ke′me-ah) 1. absence or deficiency of leukocytes in the blood. 2. aleukemic leukemia.

aleukemic (ah″lu-ke′mik) characterized by aleukemia.

aleukia (ah-lu′ke-ah) leukopenia; absence of leukocytes from the blood. **alimentary toxic a.,** a form of mycotoxicosis associated with the ingestion of grain that has overwintered in the field; abbreviated ATA. **a. hemorrha′gica,** an accessory or auxiliary term which actually refers to the condition of aplastic anemia.

aleukocytic (ah-lu″ko-sit′ik) showing no leukocytes.

aleukocytosis (-si-to′sis) deficiency in the proportion of white cells in the blood; leukopenia.

alexia (ah-lek′se-ah) inability to read; see *word blindness.* **cortical a.,** a form of sensory aphasia due to lesions of the left gyrus angularis. **motor a.,** alexia in which the patient understands what he sees written or printed, but cannot read it aloud. **musical a.,** loss of the ability to read music. **optical a.,** word blindness. **subcortical a.,** a form due to interruption of the connection between the optic center and the gyrus angularis.

alexic (ah-lek′sik) 1. pertaining to alexia. 2. having the properties of an alexin.

alexin (ah-lek′sin) a nonspecific thermolabile substance which in the presence of specific sensitizer exerts a lytic action on bacteria and other cells; see also *complement.*

aleydigism (ah-li′dig-izm) absence of secretion of the interstitial cells of Leydig.

Alflorone (al′flo-rōn) trademark for preparations of fludrocortisone.

ALG antilymphocyte globulin.

alga (al′gah), pl. *al′gae* [L.] an individual organism of the algae.

algae (al′je) a group of plants, including the seaweeds and many unicellular marine and fresh-water plants, most of which contain chlorophyll and account for about 90% of the earth's photosynthetic activity. **al′gal,** adj.

algefacient (al″jĕ-fa′shent) cooling or refrigerant.

algesia (al-je′ze-ah) sensitiveness to pain; hyperesthesia. **alge′sic, alget′ic,** adj.

algesimeter (al″jĕ-sim′ĕ-ter) an instrument used in measuring the sensitiveness to pain as produced by pricking with a sharp point.

algesimetry (-ĕ-tre) measurement of sensitivity to pain.

algesthesia (al″jes-the′ze-ah) pain sensibility; algesthesis.

algesthesis (-sis) the perception of pain; a painful sensation.

-algia word element [Gr.], *pain.*

algicide (al′jĭ-sīd) 1. destructive to algae. 2. an agent which destroys algae.

algid (al′jid) chilly; cold.

alginate (al′jĭ-nāt) a salt of alginic acid; certain alginates have been used as foam, clot, or gauze for absorbable surgical dressings, and others are useful as materials for dental impressions.

algo- word element [Gr.], *pain; cold.*

algogenic (al″go-jen′ik) 1. causing pain. 2. lowering the temperature.

algology (al-gol′o-je) phycology.

algometer (al-gom′ĕ-ter) a device used in testing the sensitiveness of a part to pain.

algometry (-ĕ-tre) measurement of the sensitivity to painful stimuli.

algophobia (al″go-fo′be-ah) morbid dread of pain.

algor (al′gor) chill or rigor; coldness. **a. mor′tis,** the gradual decrease of body temperature after death.

Alidase (al′ĭ-dās) trademark for a preparation of hyaluronidase for injection.

alienia (ah″li-e′ne-ah) absence of the spleen.

alienism (āl′yen-izm) 1. mental disorder. 2. the practice of forensic psychiatry.

alienist (-ist) 1. former term for a psychiatrist. 2. a forensic psychiatrist.

aliform (al′ĭ-form) shaped like a wing.

aliment (al′ĭ-ment) food; nutritive material.

alimentary (al″ĭ-men′tar-e) pertaining to food or nutritive material or to the organs of digestion.

alimentation (-men-ta′shun) giving or receiving of nourishment. **rectal a.,** feeding by injection of nutriment into the rectum.

alimentotherapy (-men″to-ther′ah-pe) treatment by systematic feeding.

alinasal (-na′zal) pertaining to either ala of the nose.

aliphatic (-fat′ik) pertaining to an oil; having an open-chain (carbohydrate) structure.

aliquot (al′ĭ-kwot) the part of a number which will divide it without a remainder; e.g., 2 is an aliquot of 6. By extension, any portion bearing a known quantitative relationship to a whole or to other portions of the same whole, as an aliquot portion of a solution; a sample of a whole taken to determine the quantitative composition of the whole.

alisphenoid (al-ĭ-sfe′noid) 1. pertaining to the great wing of the sphenoid. 2. a cartilage of the fetal chondrocranium on either side of the basisphenoid; later in development it forms the greater part of the great wing of the sphenoid.

alizarin (ah-liz′ah-rin) a red crystalline dye, C_{14}-H_8O_4, prepared synthetically or obtained from madder; its compounds are used as indicators.

alkalemia (al″kah-le′me-ah) increased pH (abnormal alkalinity) of the blood.

alkalescent (-les′ent) having a tendency to alkalinity.

alkali (al′kah-li) any one of a class of compounds which form salts with acids and soaps with fats. **caustic a.,** any solid hydroxide of a fixed alkali. **fixed a.,** any alkali except ammonium.

alkalimeter (al″kah-lim′ĕ-ter) an instrument for performing alkalimetry.

alkalimetry (-lim′ĕ-tre) measurement of the alkalis present in any substance.

alkaline (al′kah-līn) having the reactions of an alkali.

alkalinity (al″kah-lin′ĭ-te) the quality of being alkaline.

alkalinuria (-lin-u′re-ah) an alkaline condition of the urine.

alkalitherapy (-li-ther′ah-pe) treatment with alkalis.

alkalization (-za′shun) the act of making alkaline.

alkalizer (-līz′er) an agent that causes alkalization.

alkaloid (al′kah-loid) any of a group of organic basic substances found in plants, many of which are pharmacologically active, e.g., atropine, caffeine, morphine, nicotine, quinine, and strychnine. Also applied to synthetic substances, such as procaine, having structures similar to plant alkaloids.

alkalosis (al″kah-lo′sis) a pathologic condition due to accumulation of base in, or loss of acid from, the body. **alkalot′ic,** adj. **altitude a.,** increased alkalinity in blood and tissues due to exposure to high altitudes. **compensated a.,** a condition in which compensatory mechanisms have returned the pH toward normal. **hypokalemic a.,** metabolic alkalosis associated with a low serum potassium level. **metabolic a.,** a disturbance in which the acid-base status shifts toward the alkaline side because of retention of base or loss of noncarbonic, or fixed (nonvolatile), acids. **respiratory a.,** a state due to excess loss of carbon dioxide from the body.

alkanet (al′kah-net) the reddish dye-containing root of the herb *Alkanna tinctoria,* used as a coloring agent.

alkannin (al-kan′in) the red dye principle from alkanet.

alkapton (al-kap′tōn) see under *body.*

alkaptonuria (al-kap″to-nu′re-ah) excretion in the urine of alkapton bodies (most commonly homogentisic acid) as a result of a genetic disorder of phenylalanine-tyrosine metabolism, characterized by darkening of the urine when left standing, or on addition of alkali; it is the precursor of ochronosis. **alkap′tonuric,** adj.

alkavervir (al″kah-ver′vir) a yellow powdery mixture of alkaloids extracted from *Veratrum viride;* rarely used to lower blood pressure.

alkyl (al′kil) a monovalent radical of the general formula C_nH_{2n+1}, formed when an aliphatic hydrocarbon loses one hydrogen atom.

alkylate (al′kĭ-lāt) to treat with an alkylating agent.

alkylation (al″kĭ-la′shun) the substitution of an alkyl group for an active hydrogen atom in an organic compound.

all(o)- word element [Gr.], *other; deviating from normal.*

allachesthesia (al″ah-kes-the′ze-ah) allesthesia.

allantiasis (al″an-ti′ah-sis) sausage poisoning; botulism from improperly prepared sausages.

allantochorion (ah-lan″to-ko′re-on) the allantois and chorion as one structure.

allantoicase (al″an-to′ĭ-kās) an enzyme that converts the allantoic acid formed by allantoinase from allantoin, producing glyoxylic acid and urea.

allantoid (ah-lan′toid) 1. resembling the allantois. 2. sausage-shaped.

allantoin (ah-lan′to-in) a crystalline substance, $C_4H_6N_4O_3$, found in allantoic fluid, fetal urine, and many plants, and as a urinary excretion product of purine metabolism in most mammals but not in man or the higher apes; used topically to promote wound healing.

allantoinuria (ah-lan″to-ĭ-nu′re-ah) the presence of allantoin in the urine.

allantois (ah-lan′to-is) a ventral outgrowth of the embryos of reptiles, birds, and mammals. In man, it is vestigial except that its blood vessels give rise to those of the umbilical cord. **allanto′ic**, adj.

allele (ah-lēl′) one of two or more alternative forms of a gene at corresponding sites (loci) on homologous chromosomes, which determine alternative characters in inheritance. 2. one of two or more contrasting characters transmitted by alternative genes. **allel′ic**, adj. **multiple a′s**, alleles of which there are more than two alternative forms possible at any one locus. **silent a.**, one that produces no detectable effect.

allelochemics (al-le″lo-kem′iks) chemical interactions between species, involving release of active chemical substances, such as scents, pheromones, and toxins.

allelomorph (ah-le′lo-morf) allele. **allelomor′phic**, adj.

allelotaxis (ah-le″lo-tak′sĭs) development of an organ from several embryonic structures.

allergen (al′ler-jen) 1. a substance capable of inducing allergy or hypersensitivity. 2. the purified protein(s) of some food, bacterium, or pollen, used to test hypersensitivity to certain substances. **allergen′ic**, adj.

allergid (-jid) a papular or nodular allergic skin reaction.

allergist (-jist) a physician specializing in the diagnosis and treatment of allergies.

allergization (al″ler-ji-za′shun) active sensitization by introduction of allergens into the body.

allergize (-jīz) to subject to sensitization; to make allergic.

allergy (al′ler-je) a hypersensitive state acquired through exposure to a particular allergen, reexposure bringing to light an altered capacity to react. **aller′gic**, adj. **atopic a.**, atopy. **bacterial a.**, specific hypersensitiveness to a particular bacterial antigen. **bronchial a.**, see *asthma*. **cold a.**, a condition manifested by local and systemic reactions, mediated by histamine, which is released from mast cells and basophils as a result of exposure to cold. **contact a.**, hypersensitiveness marked by an eczematous reaction to contact between the epidermis and the allergen. **delayed a.**, an allergic response appearing hours or days after application or absorption of an allergen; it includes contact dermatitis and bacterial allergy. **drug a.**, an allergic reaction occurring as the result of unusual sensitivity to a drug. **endocrine a.**, allergy to an endogenous hormone. **food a.**, **gastrointestinal a.**, allergy, usually manifested by a skin reaction, in which the ingested antigens include food as well as drugs. **hereditary a.**, atopy.

immediate a., an allergic response appearing within a short time, i.e., from a few minutes up to an hour, after application or absorption of an allergen; it includes anaphylaxis and atopy. **induced a.**, that resulting from the injection of or contact with an antigen, or infection with a microorganism, as contrasted with hereditary allergy. **latent a.**, that not manifested by symptoms but which may be detected by tests. **nonatopic a.**, one of two general groups of clinical allergies, including contact dermatitis and some food and drug allergies; cf. *atopy*. **normal a.**, induced a. **pathologic a.**, hereditary a. **physical a.**, a condition in which the patient is sensitive to the effects of physical agents, such as heat, cold, light, etc. **physiologic a.**, induced a. **pollen a.**, hay fever. **polyvalent a.**, see *pathergy* (2). **spontaneous a.**, atopy.

allesthesia (al″es-the′ze-ah) sensation of touch experienced at a point remote from the point touched.

allethrin (al′ĕ-thrin) an insecticide, $C_{19}H_{26}O_3$.

alligator boy (al′ĭ-ga″tor boi) a child with severe ichthyosis.

alloantigen (al″o-an′tĭ-jen) isoantigen.

allobarbital (-bar′bĭ-tal) a hypnotic and sedative, $(C_3H_5)_2C(CO \cdot NH)_2CO$.

allocheiria (-ki′re-ah) allesthesia.

allochroism (-kro′izm) change or variation in color, as in certain minerals.

allochromasia (-kro-ma′ze-ah) change in color of hair or skin.

allocytophilic (-si″to-fil′ik) having an affinity for cells derived from the same species.

allodiploid (-dip′loid) 1. characterized by allodiploidy. 2. an individual or cell exhibiting allodiploidy.

allodiploidy (-dip′loi-de) the state of having two sets of chromosomes derived from different ancestral species.

alloeroticism (-ĕ-rot′ĭ-sizm) sexuality directed to another.

alloerotism (-er′o-tizm) alloeroticism.

allogeneic (-jĕ-ne′ik) 1. having cell types that are antigenically distinct. 2. in transplantation biology, denoting individuals (or tissues) that are of the same species but antigenically distinct. NOTE: In contrast, *syngeneic* (or *isogeneic*) refers to individuals having identical genotypes, and *xenogeneic* to individuals of different species, which by definition have different genotypes.

allogenic (-jen′ik) allogeneic.

allograft (al′o-graft) a graft between animals of the same species, but of different genotype.

alloimmune (al″o-im-mūn′) specifically immune to an allogeneic antigen.

allolalia (-la′le-ah) any defect of speech of central origin.

allomerism (ah-lom′er-izm) change in chemical constitution without change in crystalline form.

allomorphism (al″o-mor′fizm) change in crystalline form without change in chemical constitution.

allopathy (al-lop′ah-the) a system of therapeutics based on the production of a condition incompatible with or antagonistic to the condition being treated.

alloplasia (al″o-pla′ze-ah) heteroplasia.

alloplast (al′o-plast) an inert foreign body used for implantation into tissue.

alloplastic (-plas″tik) pertaining to or characterized by alloplasty; pertaining to an alloplast.

alloplasty (-plas″te) direction of the libido away from self to other people or objects.

alloploid (-ploid) 1. characterized by alloploidy. 2. an individual or cell characterized by alloploidy.

alloploidy (al″o-ploi′de) the state of having any number of chromosome sets derived from different ancestral species.

allopolyploid (-pol′e-ploid) 1. characterized by allopolyploidy. 2. an individual or cell characterized by allopolyploidy.

allopolyploidy (-pol′e-ploi″de) the state of having more than two sets of chromosomes derived from different ancestral species.

allopsychic (-si′kik) pertaining to the mind in its relation to the external world.

allopurinol (-pu′rin-ol) an isomer of hypoxanthine, capable of inhibiting xanthine oxidase and thus of reducing serum and urinary levels of uric acid; used in the treatment of gout.

allorhythmia (-rith′me-ah) irregularity of the heart beat or pulse that recurs regularly.

all-or-none the heart muscle, under whatever stimulation, will contract to the fullest extent or not at all; in other muscles and in nerves, stimulation of a fiber causes an action potential to travel over the entire fiber, or not to travel at all.

allosome (al′o-sōm) a foreign constituent of the cytoplasm which has entered from outside the cell.

allosteric (al″o-ster′ik) denoting a macromolecule (an enzyme) whose reactivity with another molecule is altered by combination with a third molecule; also, denoting the enzyme inhibition exercised by such alteration. See also under *site.*

allotherm (al′o-therm) 1. poikilotherm. 2. heterotherm.

allotope (-tōp) a site on the constant or nonvarying portion of an antibody molecule that can be recognized by a combining site of other antibodies.

allotriogeustia (ah-lot″re-o-jōōs′te-ah) perverted sense of taste.

allotropic (al″o-trop′ik) 1. exhibiting allotropism. 2. concerned with others; said of a type of personality that is more preoccupied with others than with oneself.

allotropism (ah-lot′ro-pizm) existence of an element in two or more distinct forms.

allotropy (-ro-pe) allotropism.

allotype (al′o-tīp) any of the alternative characters controlled by allelic genes. **allotyp′ic,** adj.

allotypy (al″o-ti′pe) the genetically controlled property, in proteins, of existing in antigenically distinguishable forms in different members of the same species.

alloxan (ah-lok′san) an oxidized product of uric acid, $C_4H_2N_2O_4$, which tends to destroy the islet cells of the pancreas, thus producing diabetes. It has been obtained from intestinal mucus in diarrhea and has been used in nutrition experiments and as an antineoplastic.

alloxantin (al″oks-an′tin) a derivative of alloxan and dialuric acid, obtained by reduction.

alloxazine (ah-lok′sah-zēn) an isomer of isoalloxazine, $C_{10}H_6N_4O_2$, which is allied to riboflavin.

alloxuremia (ah-lok″su-re′me-ah) the presence of purine bases in the blood.

alloxuria (al″oks-u′re-ah) presence of purine bases in the urine. **alloxu′ric,** adj.

alloy (al′oi) a solid mixture of two or more metals or metalloids that are mutually soluble in the molten condition.

all-*trans* retinal see *retinal* (2).

allyl (al′il) a univalent radical, $CH_2:CH\cdot CH_2$.

alochia (ah-lo′ke-ah) absence or supression of the lochia.

aloe (al′o) the dried juice of leaves of various species of *Aloe,* used in pharmaceutical preparations.

aloe-emodin (-em′o-din) a compound, $C_{15}H_{10}O_5$, occurring in the free state and as a glycoside in rhubarb, senna leaves, and in various species of *Aloe;* used as a laxative.

alogia (ah-lo′je-ah) inability to speak, due to a central lesion.

aloin (al′o-in) a mixture of active principles from aloe, having cathartic properties.

alopecia (al″o-pe′she-ah) baldness; absence of hair from skin areas where it is normally present. **a. area′ta,** hair loss, usually reversible, in sharply defined areas, usually involving the beard or scalp. **a. cap′itis tota′lis,** loss of all the hair from the scalp. **cicatricial a., a. cicatrisa′ta,** irreversible loss of hair associated with scarring, usually on the scalp. **congenital a., a. congenita′lis,** congenital absence of hair, usually from the scalp. **a. generalisa′ta,** 1. a. universalis. 2. a. totalis. **a. limina′ris,** hair loss at the hairline along the front and back margins of the scalp, due to trauma or pressure. **male pattern a.,** loss of scalp hair genetically determined and androgen-dependent, beginning with frontal recession and progressing symmetrically to leave ultimately only a sparse peripheral rim of hair. **a. medicamento′sa,** hair loss due to ingestion of a drug. **a. symptomat′ica,** loss of hair due to systemic or psychogenic causes, or to other stress. **a. tota′lis,** loss of hair from the entire scalp. **a. universa′lis,** loss of hair from the entire body.

aloxidone (ah-lok′sĭ-dōn) an anticonvulsant, $C_7H_9NO_3$.

alpha (al′fah) first letter of the Greek alphabet, α; used in names of chemical compounds to distinguish the first in a series of isomers, or to indicate position of substituting atoms or groups.

alphadione (al″fah-di′ōn) a steroid anesthetic, a combination of two steroids which are structurally similar to progesterone.

Alphadrol (al'fah-drol) trademark for a preparation of fluprednisolone.

alphalytic (al''fah-lit'ik) blocking the α-adrenergic receptors of the sympathetic nervous system; also, an agent that so acts.

alphamimetic (-mi-met'ik) stimulating or mimicking the stimulation of the α-adrenergic receptors of the sympathetic nervous system; also, an agent that so acts.

alphanaphthol (-naf'thol) a form of naphthol, $C_{10}H_7H$, used in microscopy.

alphaprodine (-pro'dēn) a narcotic analgesic, $C_{16}H_{23}NO_2$; used as the hydrochloride salt.

A.L.R.O.S. American Laryngological, Rhinological, and Otological Society.

ALS antilymphocyte serum.

alseroxylon (al''ser-ok'sĭ-lon) a purified extract of *Rauwolfia serpentina*, containing reserpine and other amorphous alkaloids; used as a tranquilizer and sedative.

alter (awl'ter) to castrate, as housepets or livestock.

alternans (awl-ter'nanz) [L.] alternating or alternation, as in pulsus alternans (alternating strength of the pulse). **electrical a.,** alternating variations in the amplitude of electrocardiographic waves. **a. of the heart,** alternating strength in the heart beat or pulse. **pul'sus a.,** the presence of alteration of intensity of heart sounds, indicating left ventricular failure.

alternation (awl''ter-na'shun) the regular succession of two opposing or different events in turn. **a. of generations,** alternate sexual and asexual reproduction, one generation reproducing sexually, the next asexually.

alum (al'um) a crystalline substance, ammonium alum, $AlNH_4(SO_4)_2 \cdot 12H_2O$, or potassium alum, $AlK(SO_4)_2 \cdot 12H_2O$; used topically as an astringent and styptic. **exsiccated a.,** alum dried by heat, a white odorless powder, $AlNH_4$-$(SO_4)_2$ or $AlK(SO_4)_2$.

alumina (ah-loo'mĭ-nah) aluminum oxide, Al_2-O_3.

aluminosis (ah-loo''mĭ-no'sis) pneumoconiosis due to the presence of aluminum-bearing dust in the lungs.

aluminum (ah-loo'mĭ-num) a chemical element (*see table*), at. no. 13, symbol Al. **a. chloride,** $AlCl_3 \cdot 6H_2O$, used topically as an astringent solution, and as an antiperspirant. **a. phosphate** $AlPO_4$, used with calcium sulfate and sodium silicate in dental cements, and in pharmacy as the gel. **a. subacetate,** a compound used as an astringent when diluted with water. **a. sulfate,** $Al_2(SO_4)_3 \cdot 18H_2O$, used as an astringent and antiperspirant.

Alurate (al'ūr-āt) trademark for a preparation of aprobarbital.

alveolectomy (al''ve-o-lek'to-me) surgical excision of part of the alveolar process.

alveolitis (-li'tis) inflammation of an alveolus.

alveoloclasia (-lo-kla'ze-ah) disintegration or resorption of the inner wall of a tooth alveolus.

alveolodental (-lo-den'tal) pertaining to a tooth and its alveolus.

alveoloplasty (al-ve'o-lo-plas''te) surgical alteration of the shape and condition of the alveolar process, in preparation for denture construction.

alveolotomy (al''ve-o-lot'o-me) incision of the alveolar process.

alveolus (al-ve'o-lus), pl. *alve'oli* [L.] a small saclike dilatation; see also *acinus.* **alve'olar,** adj. **dental alveoli,** the cavities or sockets of either jaw, in which the roots of the teeth are embedded. **pulmonary alveoli,** small outpocketings of the alveolar ducts and sacs and terminal bronchioles through whose walls the exchange of carbon dioxide and oxygen takes place between alveolar air and capillary blood; see Plate VII.

alverine (al've-rēn) an anticholinergic, C_{20}-$H_{27}N$; used as a smooth muscle relaxant and antispasmodic in the form of the citrate salt.

alveus (al've-us), pl. *al'vei* [L.] a canal or trough.

Alvodine (al'vo-dīn) trademark for a preparation of piminodine.

alymphia (ah-lim'fe-ah) absence or lack of lymph.

alymphocytosis (a-lim''fo-si-to'sis) deficiency or absence of lymphocytes from the blood; lymphopenia.

alymphoplasia (-pla'ze-ah) failure of development of lymphoid tissue. **thymic a.,** congenital agammaglobulinemia in which there is thymic hypoplasia, sparsity of lymphocytes in the thymus, spleen, lymph nodes, and intestines, absence of plasma cells, and absence of Hassall's corpuscles.

A.M. amperemeter; [L.] ante meridiem (*before noon*); meter angle.

Am chemical symbol, *americium.*

A.M.A. Aerospace Medical Association; American Medical Association; Australian Medical Association.

amacrine (am'ah-krīn) 1. without long processes. 2. any of a group of branched retinal structures regarded as modified nerve cells.

Amadil (am'ah-dil) trademark for a preparation of acetaminophen.

amalgam (ah-mal'gam) an alloy of two or more metals, one of which is mercury. **emotional a.,** an unconscious attempt to bind, neutralize, deny, or counteract anxiety.

Amanita (am''ah-ni'tah) a genus of mushrooms, some of which are poisonous and others edible; ingestion of *A. phalloi'des, A. musca'ria, A. pantheri'na, A. ver'na,* and others, is manifested by nausea, vomiting, abdominal pain, and diarrhea, followed by a period of improvement, and culminating in signs and symptoms of severe hepatic, renal, and central nervous system damage.

amaranth (am'ah-ranth) a dark red-brown coloring agent, $C_{20}H_{11}N_2Na_3O_{10}S_3$, used in food, cosmetics, and drugs.

amastia (ah-mas'te-ah) congenital absence of one or both mammary glands.

amastigote (ah-mas'tĭ-gōt) the nonflagellate, intracellular, morphologic stage in the development of certain hemoflagellates, resembling the typical adult form of *Leishmania.*

amaurosis (am″aw-ro′sis) blindness, especially that occurring without apparent lesion of the eye. **amaurot′ic,** adj. **a. congen′ita of Leber, Leber's congenital a.,** hereditary blindness, occurring at or shortly after birth, associated with an atypical form of diffuse pigmentation and commonly with optic atrophy and attenuation of the retinal vessels. **a. fu′gax,** transient monocular or partial blindness.

ambenonium (am″bĕ-no′ne-um) a cholinergic, $C_{28}H_{42}N_4O_2$; the chloride salt is used to treat symptoms of muscular weakness and fatigue in myasthenia gravis.

ambidextrous (am″bĭ-deks′trus) able to use either hand with equal dexterity.

ambilateral (-lat′er-al) pertaining to or affecting both sides.

ambilevous (-le′vus) unable to use both hands with equal dexterity.

ambiopia (am″be-o′pe-ah) diplopia.

ambisexual (am″bĭ-seks′u-al) denoting sexual characteristics common to both sexes, e.g., pubic hair.

ambivalence (am-biv′ah-lens) simultaneous existence of conflicting emotional attitudes toward a goal, object, or person. **ambiv′alent,** adj.

amblyacousia (am″ble-ah-ku′se-ah) dullness of hearing.

amblyaphia (-a′fe-ah) bluntness or dullness of the sense of touch.

amblygeustia (-go͞os′te-ah) dullness of the sense of taste.

Amblyomma (-om′mah) a genus of hard-bodied ticks of worldwide distribution. **A. america′num,** the Lone Star tick, found in southern and southwestern United States, Central America, and Brazil; a vector of Rocky Mountain spotted fever. **A. cajennen′se,** a common pest of domestic animals and man in the southern United States, Central and South America, and the West Indies; a vector of Rocky Mountain spotted fever. **A. macula′tum,** the Gulf Coast tick, infesting cattle in southwestern United States and Central and South America; its bite causes painful sores that serve as sites of screwworm infections and secondary bacterial and fungal infections.

amblyopia (-o′pe-ah) dimness of vision without detectable organic lesion of the eye. **amblyop′ic,** adj. **color a.,** dimness of color vision due to toxic or other influences. **a. ex anop′sia,** that resulting from long disuse.

amblyoscope (am′ble-o-skō″) an instrument for training an amblyopic eye to take part in vision and for measuring and increasing fusion of the eyes.

ambo (am′bo) ambon.

amboceptor (am′bo-sep″tor) hemolysin, particularly its double receptors, the one combining with the blood cell, the other with complement.

Ambodryl (am′bo-dril) trademark for preparations of bromodiphenhydramine.

ambon (am′bon) the fibrocartilaginous ring forming the edge of the socket in which the head of a long bone is lodged.

ambulant (am′bu-lant) ambulatory.

ambulatory (am′bu-lah-tor″e) walking or able to walk; not confined to bed.

ameba (ah-me′bah), pl. *ame′bae, ame′bas* [L.] a minute protozoon (class Rhizopoda, subphylum Sarcodina), occurring as a single-celled nucleated mass of protoplasm that changes shape by extending cytoplasmic processes (pseudopodia), by means of which it moves about and absorbs food; most amebae are free-living but some parasitize man. **ame′bic,** adj.

amebiasis (am″ĕ-bi′ah-sis) infection with amebas, especially with *Entamoeba histolytica,* the causative agent of amebic dysentery.

amebicide (ah-me′bĭ-sīd) an agent that is destructive to amebae.

amebiform (-form) ameboid.

amebocyte (ah-me′bo-sīt) any cell showing ameboid movement.

ameboid (ah-me′boid) resembling an ameba in form or movement.

ameboma (am″ĕ-bo′mah) a tumor-like mass caused by granulomatous reaction in the intestines in amebiasis.

amebula (ah-meb′u-lah) the motile ameboid stage of spores of certain sporozoa.

ameburia (am″ĕ-bu′re-ah) the presence of amebae in the urine.

amelia (ah-me′le-ah) congenital absence of a limb or limbs.

amelification (ah-mel′ĭ-fĭ-ka′shun) the development of enamel cells into enamel.

ameloblast (ah-mel′o-blast) a cell which takes part in forming dental enamel.

ameloblastoma (ah-mel″o-blas-to′mah) a true neoplasm of tissue of the type characteristic of the enamel organ, but which does not differentiate to the point of enamel formation. **melanotic a.,** melanotic neuroectodermal tumor. **pituitary a.,** craniopharyngioma.

** amelodentinal** (am″ĕ-lo-den′tĭ-nal) pertaining to dental enamel and dentin.

amelogenesis (ah-mel′o-jen′ĕ-sis) the formation of dental enamel. **a. imperfec′ta,** a hereditary condition resulting in defective development of dental enamel, marked by a brown color of the teeth; due to improper differentiation of the ameloblasts.

amelogenic (am″ĕ-lo-jen′ik) forming enamel.

amelus (am′ĕ-lus) an individual exhibiting amelia.

amenorrhea (a-men″o-re′ah) absence or abnormal stoppage of the menses. **amenorrhe′al,** adj. **primary a.,** failure of menstruation to occur at puberty. **secondary a.,** cessation of menstruation after it has once been established at puberty.

amensalism (a-men′sal-izm) symbiosis in which one population (or individual) is adversely affected and the other is unaffected.

amentia (a-men′she-ah) 1. congenital mental retardation of varying extent. 2. a mental disorder characterized by marked mental confusion. **nevoid a.,** Sturge-Weber syndrome.

americium (am″er-ish′e-um) chemical element (*see table*), at. no. 95, symbol Am.

amethocaine (ah-meth′o-kān) tetracaine.

ametria (ah-me′tre-ah) congenital absence of the uterus.

ametrometer (am″ĕ-trom′ĕ-ter) an instrument for measuring the degree of ametropia.

ametropia (am″ĕ-tro′pe-ah) a condition of the eye in which images fail to come to a proper focus on the retina, due to a discrepancy between the size and refractive powers of the eye. **ametrop′ic,** adj.

amicrobic (ah″mi-kro′bik) not produced by microbes.

amicron (ah-mi′kron) a colloid particle so small (10^{-7} cm. in diameter) that it is just visible with the ultramicroscope.

amidase (am′ĭ-dās) a deamidizing enzyme.

amide (am′īd) any compound derived from ammonia by substitution of an acid radical for hydrogen, or from an acid by replacing the —OH group by —NH$_2$.

amidine-lyase (am′ĭ-dēn-li′ās) an enzyme that catalyzes the removal of an amindino group, as from L-argininosuccinate to form fumarate and L-arginine.

amido (am′ĭ-do) the monovalent radical NH$_2$ united with an acid radical.

amido-ligase (-li′gās) any enzyme that catalyzes the coupling of two molecules, with glutamine acting as an ammonia donor.

amidopyrine (am″ĭ-do-pi′rēn) aminophenazone.

Amigen (am′ĭ-jen) trademark for protein hydrolysate preparation for intravenous injection.

amimia (a-mim′e-ah) loss of the power of expression by the use of signs or gestures.

aminacrine (am″in-ak′rin) an amino derivative of acridine, C$_{13}$H$_{10}$N$_2$, the hydrochloride salt, effective against many gram-negative and gram-positive bacteria, is used as a topical anti-infective.

amine (am′in, ah-mēn) an organic compound containing nitrogen; any of a group of compounds formed from ammonia by replacement of one or more hydrogen atoms by organic radicals. **catechol a.,** catecholamine.

amino (am′ĭ-no, ah-me′no) the monovalent radical NH$_2$, when not united with an acid radical.

aminoacidemia (am″ĭ-no-as″ĭ-de′me-ah) an excess of amino acids in the blood.

aminoacidopathy (-as″ĭ-dop′ah-the) any of a group of disorders due to a defect in an enzymatic step in the metabolic pathway of one or more amino acids or in a protein mediator necessary for transport of certain amino acids into or out of cells.

aminoaciduria (-as″ĭ-du′re-ah) an excess of amino acids in the urine.

aminoacylase (-as″ĭ-lās) an enzyme in the kidney that catalyzes the hydrolysis of hippuric acid to benzoic acid and glycine.

aminoglutethimide (-gloo-teth″ĭ-mīd) an anticonvulsant, C$_{13}$H$_{16}$N$_2$O$_2$, used in the treatment of epilepsy.

aminohippurate (-hip′u-rāt) any salt of aminohippuric acid.

aminolysis (am″ĭ-nol′ĭ-sis) reaction with an amine, resulting in the addition of (or substitution by) an imino group —NH—.

aminometradine (am″ĭ-no-met′rah-dēn) a diuretic, C$_{19}$H$_{13}$N$_3$O$_2$.

aminometramide (-met′rah-mīd) aminometradine.

aminopentamide (-pen′tah-mīd) an anticholinergic, C$_{19}$H$_{24}$N$_2$O.

aminophenazone (-fen′ah-zōn) an antipyretic and analgesic, C$_{13}$H$_{17}$N$_3$O.

aminopherase (am″ĭ-nof′er-ās) transaminase.

aminophylline (am″ĭ-no-fil′in) a bronchial smooth muscle relaxant, respiratory stimulant, and diuretic, C$_{16}$H$_{25}$N$_{10}$O$_4$.

aminopolypeptidase (-pol″e-pep′tĭ-dās) an enzyme which splits off free amino groups from a polypeptide.

aminopterin (am″in-op′ter-in) a folic acid antagonist, C$_{19}$H$_{20}$N$_8$O$_5$, used in the treatment of leukemia, and as a rodenticide.

aminopyrine (am″ĭ-no-pi′rēn) aminophenazone.

aminosalicylate (-sal″ĭ-sil′āt) any salt of aminosalicylic acid.

Aminosol (ah-me′no-sol) trademark for an amino acid preparation for intravenous injection.

aminotrate (am′ĭ-no-trāt″) any of a group of compounds composed of proteins and vitamins, used as a food supplement.

aminuria (am″ĭ-nu′re-ah) an excess of amines in the urine.

amiphenazole (ah-mĭ-fen′ah-zol) a respiratory stimulant, C$_9$H$_9$N$_3$S, used as the hydrochloride salt.

amisometradine (am-i″so-met′rah-dēn) a diuretic, C$_9$H$_{13}$N$_3$O$_2$.

amithiozone (am″ĭ-thi″ŏ-zōn) thiacetazone.

amitosis (am″ĭ-to′sis) direct cell division, i.e., the cell divides by simple cleavage of the nucleus without formation of spireme spindle figures or chromosomes. **amitot′ic,** adj.

amitriptyline (am″ĭ-trip′tĭ-lēn) an antidepressant, C$_{20}$H$_{23}$N, used as the hydrochloride salt.

ammeter (am′me-ter) an instrument for measuring in amperes or subdivisions of amperes the strength of a current flowing in a circuit.

ammoaciduria (am″o-as″ĭ-du′re-ah) an excess of ammonia and amino acids in the urine.

ammonemia (ah″mo-ne′me-ah) an abnormal condition marked by the presence of ammonia or its compounds in the blood.

ammonia (ah-mo′ne-ah) a colorless alkaline gas with a pungent odor and acrid taste, NH$_3$.

ammonia-lyase (-li′ās) any of a group of lyases that catalyze the removal of ammonia by cleaving a C—N bond.

ammoniated (ah-mo′ne-āt″ed) treated or combined with ammonia.

ammoniemia (ah-mo″ne-e′me-ah) ammonemia.

ammonium (ah-mo′ne-um) the hypothetical radical, NH$_4$, forming salts analogous to those of the alkaline metals. **a. carbonate,** a mixture of NH$_4$HCO$_3$ (ammonium bicarbonate) and NH$_4$COONH$_4$ (ammonium carbamate), used as a stimulant, as in smelling salts, and as an expectorant. **a. chloride,** crystalline compound, NH_4Cl, used as a systemic acidifier.

ammoniuria (ah-mo″ne-u′re-ah) excess of ammonia in the urine.

ammonolysis (am″o-nol′ĭ-sis) a process analogous to hydrolysis, but in which ammonia takes the place of water.

ammonotelic (ah-mo″no-tel′ik) having ammonia as the chief excretory product of nitrogen metabolism, as in fresh-water fishes.

amnalgesia (am″nal-je′ze-ah) abolition of pain and memory of a painful procedure by the use of drugs or hypnosis.

amnesia (am-ne′zhe-ah) pathologic impairment of memory. **amnes′tic,** adj. **anterograde a.,** amnesia for events occurring subsequent to the episode precipitating the disorder. **auditory a.,** auditory aphasia. **immunologic a.,** the failure of the anamnestic immunologic response to antigens. **retrograde a.,** amnesia for events occurring prior to the episode precipitating the disorder. **visual a.,** see under *aphasia.*

amniocele (am′ne-o-sēl″) omphalocele.

amniocentesis (am″ne-o-sen-te′sis) surgical transabdominal or transcervical penetration of the uterus for aspiration of amniotic fluid.

amniochorial (-ko′re-al) pertaining to the amnion and chorion.

amniogenesis (-jen′ĕ-sis) the development of the amnion.

amniography (am″ne-og′rah-fe) roentgenography of the gravid uterus.

amnion (am′ne-on) the extraembryonic membrane of birds, reptiles, and mammals, which lines the chorion and contains the fetus and the amniotic fluid. **amnion′ic, amniot′ic,** adj. **a. nodo′sum,** a nodular condition of the fetal surface of the amnion, observed in oligohydramnios associated with absence of the kidneys of the fetus.

amnionitis (am″ne-o-ni′tis) inflammation of the amnion.

amniorrhea (-re′ah) escape of the amniotic fluid.

amniorrhexis (-rek′sis) rupture of the amnion.

amnioscope (am′ne-o-skōp″) an endoscope that, by passage through the maternal abdominal wall into the amniotic cavity, permits direct visualization of the fetus and amniotic fluid.

amnioscopy (am″ne-os′ko-pe) observation of the fetus by means of the amnioscope.

amniote (am′ne-ōt) any animal that develops an amnion.

amniotome (am′ne-o-tōm″) an instrument for cutting the fetal membranes.

amniotomy (am″ne-ot′o-me) surgical rupture of the fetal membranes to induce labor.

amobarbital (am″o-bar′bĭ-tal) a hypnotic and sedative, $C_{11}H_{18}N_2O_3$, having a short to intermediate action; also used as the sodium salt.

amodiaquine (-di′ah-kwin) a drug, $C_{20}H_{22}Cl-N_3O$, used as the hydrochloride salt in treatment of malaria, especially falciparum malaria, and of amebic abscess.

Amoeba (ah-me′ba) a genus of amebae.

amoeba (ah-me′bah) ameba.

amolanone (ah-mo′lah-nōn) a drug, $C_{20}H_{23}NO_2$, having anticholinergic and anesthetic properties.

amorph (a′morf) an inactive mutant gene.

amorphia (ah-mor′fe-ah) the fact or quality of being amorphous.

amorphic (ah-mor′fik) amorphous; in genetics, almost completely inactive.

amorphism (ah-mor′fizm) amorphia.

amorphous (ah-mor′fus) having no definite form; shapeless; having no specific orientation of atoms; in pharmacy, not crystallized.

amotio (ah-mo′she-o) [L.] a removing. **a. ret′inae,** detachment of the retina.

AMP adenosine monophosphate. **cyclic AMP,** adenosine 3′:5′-cyclic phosphate.

amp. ampere, ampule.

ampere (am′pēr) unit of electric current strength, the current yielded by one volt of electromotive force against one ohm of resistance.

amperemeter (-me″ter) an instrument for measuring amperage.

Amphedroxyn (am″fe-drok′sin) trademark for a preparation of methamphetamine.

amphetamine (am-fet′ah-mēn) a synthetic, powerful central nervous system stimulant, $C_6H_5CH_2CHNH_2CH_3$, most commonly used as the sulfate salt. Abuse may lead to dependence.

amphi- word element [Gr.], *both; on both sides.*

amphiarkyochrome (am″fi-ar′ke-o-krōm″) a nerve cell with peculiar staining qualities.

amphiarthrosis (-ar-thro′sis) a joint permitting little motion, the opposed surfaces being connected by fibrocartilage, as between vertebrae.

amphiaster (am′fi-as″ter) the double star figure formed by achromatin fibers in karyokinesis.

Amphibia (am-fib′e-ah) a class of vertebrates, including frogs, toads, newts, and salamanders, capable of living both on land and in water.

amphiblastula (am″fi-blas′tu-lah) a blastula with unequal blastomeres.

amphibolic (-bol′ik) 1. uncertain. 2. having both an anabolic and a catabolic function.

amphicelous (-se′lus) concave at both ends.

amphicentric (-sen′trik) beginning and ending in the same vessel.

amphichroic (-kro′ik) exhibiting two colors; affecting both red and blue litmus.

amphichromatic (-kro-mat′ik) amphichroic.

amphicytula (-sit′u-lah) a fertilized telolecithal ovum.

amphidiarthrosis (-di″ar-thro′sis) a joint having the nature of both ginglymus and arthrodia, as that of the lower jaw.

amphigastrula (-gas′troo-lah) the gastrula resulting from unequal segmentation, the cells of the two hemispheres being of unequal size.

amphigonadism (-gon′ah-dizm) possession of both ovarian and testicular tissue.

amphimorula (-mor′u-lah) the morula resulting from unequal segmentation, the cells of the two hemispheres being of unequal size.

amphistome (am-fis′tōm) a fluke having the ventral sucker near the posterior end, usually found in the rumen or intestine of herbivorous mammals.

amphitrichous (am-fit′rĭ-kus) having flagella at each end.

amphocyte (am′fo-sīt) a cell staining with either acid or basic dyes.

ampholyte (-līt) an organic or inorganic substance capable of acting as either an acid or a base.

amphomycin (am″fo-mi′sin) an antibiotic substance produced by *Streptomyces canus.*

amphophil (am′fo-fil) an amphophilic cell or element.

amphophilic (am″fo-fil′ik) staining with either acid or basic dyes.

amphoric (am-for′ik) pertaining to a bottle; resembling the sound made by blowing across the neck of a bottle.

amphoteric (am″fo-ter′ik) having opposite characters; capable of acting as both an acid and a base; capable of neutralizing either bases or acids.

amphotericin B (-ter′ĭ-sin) an antibiotic derived from strains of *Streptomyces nodosus;* used in cryptococcal meningitis and systemic fungal infections.

amphotericity (-ter-is′ĭ-te) the quality of being amphoteric.

amphoterism (am-fo′ter-izm) the possession of both acid and basic properties.

amphotony (am-fot′o-ne) tonicity of the sympathetic and parasympathetic nervous systems.

ampicillin (amp″ĭ-sil′in) a semisynthetic, acid-resistant penicillin, $C_{16}H_{19}N_3O_4S$, used as an antibacterial against gram-negative bacteria and nonpenicillinase-producing strains of *Escherichia coli.*

amplification (am″plĭ-fĭ-ka′shun) the process of making larger, as the increase of an auditory stimulus, as a means of improving its perception.

amplitude (am′plĭ-tūd) largeness, fullness; wideness in range or extent. **a. of accommodation,** amount of accommodative power of the eye.

amprotropine (am″pro-tro′pēn) an anticholinergic, $C_{18}H_{29}NO_3$; the phosphate salt is used as an antispasmodic.

ampule (am′pūl) a small, hermetically sealed glass flask, e.g., one containing medication for parenteral administration.

ampulla (am-pul′ah), pl. *ampul′lae* [L.] a flask-like dilatation of a tubular structure, especially of the expanded ends of the semicircular canals of the ear. **ampul′lar,** adj. **a. chy′li,** cisterna chyli. **a. duc′tus deferen′tis,** the enlarged and tortuous distal end of the ductus deferens. **Henle's a.,** a. ductus deferentis. **hepatopancreatic a., a. hepatopancreat′ica,** the dilatation formed by junction of the common bile duct and the pancreatic duct proximal to their opening into the lumen of the duodenum. **ampul′lae lactif′erae,** lactiferous sinuses. **Lieberkühn's a.,** the blind termination of lacteals in the villi of the intestines. **ampul′lae membrana′ceae,** the dilatations at one end of each of the three semicircular ducts.

ampul′lae os′seae, the dilatations at one of the ends of the semicircular canals. **phrenic a.,** the dilatation at the lower end of the esophagus. **rectal a., a. rec′ti,** the dilated portion of the rectum just proximal to the anal canal. **a. of Thoma,** one of the small terminal expansions of an interlobar artery in the pulp of the spleen. **a. of uterine tube,** the thin-walled, almost muscle-free, midregion of the uterine tube; its mucosa is greatly plicated. **a. of vas deferens,** a. ductus deferentis. **a. of Vater,** hepatopancreatic a.

amputation (am″pu-ta′shun) removal of a limb or other appendage of the body. **Chopart's a.,** amputation of the foot by a midtarsal disarticulation. **closed a.,** one in which flaps are made from the skin and subcutaneous tissue and sutured over the end of the bone. **congenital a.,** absence of a limb at birth, attributed to constriction of the part by an encircling band during intrauterine development. **consecutive a.,** an amputation during or after the period of suppuration. **a. in contiguity,** amputation at a joint. **a. in continuity,** amputation of a limb elsewhere than at a joint. **diaclastic a.,** amputation in which the bone is broken by an osteoclast and the soft tissues divided by an écraseur. **double-flap a.,** one in which two flaps are formed. **Dupuytren's a.,** amputation of the arm at the shoulder joint. **elliptical a.,** one in which the cut has an elliptical outline. **flap a.,** closed a. **flapless a.,** guillotine a. **Gritti-Stokes a.,** amputation of the leg through the knee, using an oval anterior flap. **guillotine a.,** one performed rapidly by a circular sweep of the knife and a cut of the saw, the entire cross-section being left open for dressing. **Hey's a.,** amputation of the foot between the tarsus and metatarsus. **interpleviabdominal a.,** amputation of the thigh with excision of the lateral portion of the pelvic girdle. **interscapulothoracic a.,** amputation of the arm with excision of the lateral portion of the shoulder girdle. **intrauterine a.,** congenital a. **Larrey's a.,** amputation at the shoulder joint. **Lisfranc's a.,** 1. Dupuytren's a. 2. amputation of the foot between the metatarsus and tarsus. **oblique a.,** oval a. **open a.,** guillotine a. **oval a.,** one in which the incision consists of two reversed spirals. **Pirigoff's a.,** amputation of the foot at the ankle, through the malleoli of the tibia and fibula. **pulp a.,** pulpotomy. **racket a.,** one in which there is a single longitudinal incision continuous below with a spiral incision on either side of the limb. **root a.,** removal of one or more roots from a multirooted tooth, leaving at least one root to support the crown; when only the apex of a root is involved, it is called *apicoectomy.* **spontaneous a.,** loss of a part without surgical intervention, as in leprosy, etc. **Stokes' a.,** Gritti-Stokes a. **subperiosteal a.,** one in which the cut end of the bone is covered by periosteal flaps. **Syme's a.,** disarticulation of the foot with removal of both malleoli. **Teale's a.,** amputation with short and long rectangular flaps. **traumatic a.,** amputation of a part by accidental injury. **Tripier's a.,** amputation of the foot through the calcaneus.

A.M.R.L. Aerospace Medical Research Laboratories.

A.M.S. American Meteorological Society.

Amsustain (am′sus-tān) trademark for a preparation of dextroamphetamine.

amu atomic mass unit.

amusia (a-mu′ze-ah) loss of ability to produce (*motor a.*) or to recognize (*sensory a.*) musical sounds.

A.M.W.A. American Medical Women's Association; American Medical Writers' Association.

amyelia (a″mi-e′le-ah) congenital absence of the spinal cord.

amyelinic (ah-mi″ĕ-lin′ik) without myelin.

amyelonic (-lon′ik) 1. having no spinal cord. 2. having no marrow.

amyelotrophy (-lot′ro-fe) atrophy of spinal cord.

amyelus (ah-mi′ĕ-lus) a fetus with no spinal cord.

amygdala (ah-mig′dah-lah) an almond-shaped structure, as the amygdala of the brain.

amaygdalin (-lin) a glycoside, $C_{20}H_{27}NO_{11}$, found in almonds and other members of the same family.

amygdaline (-līn) 1. like an almond. 2. pertaining to a tonsil; tonsillar.

amygdalolith (-lo-lith″) calculus in a tonsil.

amyl (am′il) the radical C_5H_{11}. **a. nitrite**, an inflammable liquid, $C_5H_{11}NO_2$, inhaled as a vapor during pain of heart disease; used also to relieve pain of angina, and in cyanide poisoning.

amyl(o)- word element [Gr.], *starch.*

amylaceous (am″ĭ-la′shus) composed of or resembling starch.

amylase (am′ĭ-lās) an enzyme that catalyzes the hydrolysis of starch into simpler compounds. The *α-amylases* occur in animals and include pancreatic and salivary amylase; the *β-amylases* occur in higher plants.

amylene (am′ĭ-lēn) a flammable liquid hydrocarbon, C_5H_{10}, having anesthetic properties, but too dangerous for use. **a. hydrate**, a liquid, $C_5H_{12}O$, used as a solvent, as a vehicle in pharmacy, and as a hypnotic.

amylobarbitone (am″ĭ-lo-bar′bĭ-tōn) amobarbital.

amylodextrin (-deks′trin) a compound formed during the change of starch into sugar.

amylogenesis (-jen′ĕ-sis) the formation of starch. **amylogen′ic**, adj.

amyloid (am′ĭ-loid) 1. starchlike; amylaceous. 2. an optically homogeneous, waxy, translucent material, probably a glycoprotein, bearing a superficial resemblance to starch and deposited intercellularly in a variety of pathologic conditions; see *amyloidosis.*

amyloidosis (am″ĭ-loi-do′sis) extracellular deposition of amyloid in tissues; when sufficiently advanced, the accumulations obliterate the parenchyma of affected organs. The disease may be primary (of unknown cause), secondary to chronic diseases (e.g., tuberculosis and rheumatoid arthritis), or hereditary, as in familial Mediterranean fever. It may affect the abdominal viscera, the heart, the nervous system, the skin (see *lichen amyloidosus*), etc.

amylolysis (am″ĭ-lol′ĭ-sis) digestive change of starch into sugar.

amylolytic (am″ĭ-lo-lit′ik) pertaining to, marked by, or promoting amylolysis.

amylopectin (-pek′tin) the insoluble constituent of starch; the soluble constituent is amylose.

amylopectinosis (-pek′tĭ-no″sis) glycogenosis (type IV) in which deficiency of the brancher enzyme amylo-1:4,1:6-transglucosidase results in cirrhosis of the liver, hepatosplenomegaly, and progressive hepatic failure and death.

amylopsin (am″ĭ-lop′sin) α-amylase occurring in the pancreas.

amylorrhea (am″ĭ-lo-re′ah) presence of excessive starch in the stools.

amylorrhexis (-reks′is) the enzymatic splitting of starch.

amylose (am′ĭ-lōs) 1. any carbohydrate other than a glucose or saccharose. 2. the soluble constituent of starch, as opposed to amylopectin.

amylosuria (am″ĭ-lo-su′re-ah) the presence of amylose in the urine.

amyluria (am″ĭ-lu′re-ah) an excess of starch in the urine.

amyoplasia (ah-mi″o-pla′ze-ah) lack of muscle formation or development. **a. congen′ita**, generalized lack in the newborn of muscular development and growth, with contracture and deformity at most joints.

amyostasia (-sta′ze-ah) a tremor of the muscles.

amyosthenia (ah-mi″os-the′ne-ah) deficient muscular strength.

amyosthenic (-then′ik) 1. characterized by amyosthenia. 2. an agent that diminishes muscular power.

amyotaxy (ah-mi′o-tak″se) ataxia.

amyotonia (a-mi″o-to′ne-ah) atonic condition of the muscles. **a. congen′ita**, any of several rare congenital diseases marked by general hypotonia of the muscles.

amyotrophia (ah-mi″o-tro′fe-ah) amyotrophy.

amyotrophy (ah″mi-ot′ro-fe) muscular atrophy. **amyotroph′ic**, adj. **diabetic a.**, a painful condition, rarely associated with diabetes, with progressive wasting and weakening of muscles, usually limited to the muscles of the pelvic girdle and thigh. **neuralgic a.**, atrophy and paralysis of the muscles of the shoulder girdle, with pain across the shoulder and upper arm.

Amytal (am′ĭ-tal) trademark for preparations of amobarbital.

amyxia (ah-mik′se-ah) absence of mucus.

amyxorrhea (a-mik″sŏ-re′ah) absence of mucous secretion.

An chemical symbol, *actinon.*

An. anisometropia; anode.

A.N.A. American Neurological Association; American Nurses' Association.

ana (an′ah) [Gr.] of each.

ana- word element [Gr.], *upward; again; backward; excessively.*

anabasis (ah-nab′ah-sis) the stage of increase in a disease. **anabat′ic**, adj.

anabiosis (an″ah-bi-o′sis) restoration of the vital processes after their apparent cessation; bringing back to consciousness. **anabiot′ic,** adj.

anabolergy (an″ah-bol′er-je) energy expended in anabolism.

anabolin (an-nab′o-lin) anbolite.

anabolism (-lizm) the constructive process by which living cells convert simple substances into more complex compounds, especially into living matter. **anabol′ic,** adj.

anabolite (-līt″) any product of anabolism.

anachoresis (an″ah-ko-re′sis) preferential collection or deposit of particles at a site, as of bacteria or metals that have localized out of the blood stream in areas of inflammation. **anachoret′ic,** adj.

anacidity (-sid′ĭ-te) lack of normal acidity. **gastric a.,** achlorhydria.

anaclisis (-kli′sis) the state of leaning against or depending on something; in psychoanalysis, the development of the infant's love for his mother from his original dependence on her care. **anaclit′ic,** adj.

anacousia (-koo′ze-ah) anakusis.

anacrotism (ah-nak′rŏ-tizm) a pulse anomaly evidenced by the presence of a prominent notch on the ascending limb of the pulse tracing. **anacrot′ic,** adj.

anadipsia (an″ah-dip′se-ah) intense thirst.

anadrenalism (-dre′nal-izm) absence or failure of adrenal function.

Anadrol (an′ah-drol) trademark for a preparation of oxymetholone.

anaerobe (an-a′er-ōb) an organism that lives and grows in the absence of molecular oxygen. **anaero′bic,** adj. **facultative a.,** a microorganism that can live and grow with or without molecular oxygen. **obligate a.,** a microorganism that can grow only in the complete absence of molecular oxygen; some are killed by oxygen.

anaerobiosis (an-a″er-o-bi-o′sis) life only in the absence of molecular oxygen. **anaerobiot′ic,** adj.

anaerogenic (-jen′ik) 1. producing little or no gas. 2. suppressing the formation of gas by gas-producing bacteria.

anaerosis (an″a-er-o′sis) interruption of respiratory function.

anagen (an′ah-jen) the first phase of the hair cycle, during which synthesis of hair takes place.

anakatadidymus (an″ah-kat″ah-did′ĭ-mus) a twin monster separate above and below, but united in the middle.

anakusis (-ku′sis) total deafness.

anal (a′nal) relating to the anus.

analbuminemia (an″al-bu″mĭ-ne′me-ah) absence or deficiency of serum albumins.

analeptic (an″ah-lep′tik) a drug that acts as a restorative, such as caffeine, etc.

Analexin (an″ah-lek′sin) trademark for preparations of phenyramidol.

analgesia (an″al-je′ze-ah) absence of sensibility to pain, particularly the relief of pain without loss of consciousness. **a. al′gera,** spontaneous pain in a denervated part. **audio a.,** audioanalgesia. **continuous caudal a.,** continuous injection of an anesthetic solution into the sacral and lumbar plexuses within the epidural space to relieve the pain of childbirth; also used in general surgery to block the pain pathways below the navel. **a. doloro′sa,** a. algera. **infiltration a.,** paralysis of the nerve endings at the site of operation by subcutaneous injection of an anesthetic. **paretic a.,** loss of the sense of pain accompanied by partial paralysis. **relative a.,** in dental anesthesia, a maintained level of conscious-sedaton, short of general anesthesia, in which the pain threshold is elevated; usually induced by inhalation of nitrous oxide and oxygen. **surface a.,** local analgesia produced by an anesthetic applied to the surface of such mucous membranes as those of the eye, nose, urethra, etc.

analgesic (-je′sik) 1. relieving pain. 2. pertaining to analgesia. 3. an agent that relieves pain without causing loss of consciousness.

Analgesine (-je′sin) trademark for a preparation of antipyrine.

analgetic (-jet′ik) analgesic.

analgia (an-al′je-ah) painlessness. **anal′gic,** adj.

anallergic (an″ah-ler′jik) not allergic; not causing anaphylaxis or hypersensitivity.

analogous (ah-nal′o-gus) resembling or similar in some respects, as in function or appearance, but not in origin or development.

analogue (an′ah-log) 1. a part or organ having the same function, but of different evolutionary origin. 2. a chemical compound having a structure similar to that of another but differing from it in respect to a certain component; it may have similar or opposite action metabolically.

analogy (ah-nal′o-je) the quality of being analogous; resemblance or similarity in function or appearance, but not in origin or development.

analysand (ah-nal′ĭ-sand) a person undergoing psychoanalysis.

analysis (ah-nal′ĭ-sis) 1. separation into component parts; the act of determining the component parts of a substance. 2. psychoanalysis. **analyt′ic,** adj. **bite a.,** occlusal a. **gasometric a.,** analysis by measurement of the gas evolved. **gravimetric a.,** quantitative a. **occlusal a.,** study of the relations of the occlusal surfaces of opposing teeth. **organic a.,** analysis of animal and vegetable tissues. **proximate a.,** determination of the simpler constituents of a substance. **qualitative a.,** determination of the nature of the constituents of a compound. **quantitative a.,** determination of the proportionate quantities of the constituents of a compound. **ultimate a.,** resolution of a substance into its component elements. **vector a.,** analysis of a moving force to determine both its magnitude and its direction, e.g., analysis of the scalar electrocardiogram to determine the magnitude and direction of the electromotive force for one complete cycle of the heart. **volumetric a.,** quantitative analysis by measuring volumes of liquids.

analyzer (an″ah-līz′er) 1. a Nicol prism attached to a polarizing apparatus which extinguishes the ray of light polarized by the polarizer. 2.

Pavlov's name for a specialized part of the nervous system which controls the reactions of the organism to changing external conditions. 3. a nervous receptor together with its central connections, by means of which sensitivity to stimulations is differentiated.

anamnesis (an″am-ne′sis) 1. the faculty of memory. 2. the past history of a patient and his family.

anamnestic (-nes′tik) 1. pertaining to anamnesis. 2. aiding the memory. 3. see under *response*.

anamniote (an-am′ne-ōt″) any animal that develops no amnion, including fishes and amphibians.

anamniotic (an″am-ne-ot′ik) having no amnion.

ananabolic (an″an-ah-bol′ik) characterized by absence of anabolism.

ananaphylaxis (an-an″ah-fĭ-lak′sis) antianaphylaxis.

anaphase (an′ah-fāz) the third stage of division of the nucleus in either meiosis or mitosis.

anaphia (an-a′fe-ah) lack or loss of the sense of touch.

anaphoria (an″ah-fo′re-ah) the tendency to tilt the head downward, with the visual axes deviating upward, on looking straight ahead.

anaphrodisia (an″af-ro-diz′e-ah) absence or loss of sexual desire.

anaphrodisiac (-diz′e-ak) 1. repressing sexual desire. 2. a drug that represses sexual desire.

anaphylactin (an″ah-fĭ-lak′tin) the antibody in anaphylaxis; it is formed after the first injection of the foreign protein (antigen) and interacts with it on the second injection.

anaphylactogen (-fĭ-lak′to-jen) any substance that produces anaphylaxis.

anaphylactogenesis (-fĭ-lak″to-jen′ĕ-sis) the production of anaphylaxis. **anaphylactogen′ic**, adj.

anaphylatoxin (-fil″ah-tok′sin) a substance produced in blood serum during complement fixation which serves as a mediator of inflammation by inducing mast cell degranulation and histamine release; on injection into animals, it causes anaphylactic shock.

anaphylaxin (-fĭ-lak′sin) anaphylactin.

anaphylaxis (-fĭ-lak′sis) 1. exaggerated reaction of an organism to a foreign protein or other sustance to which it has previously become sensitized. 2. anaphylactic shock. **anaphylac′tic**, adj. **acquired a.,** that in which sensitization is known to have been produced by administration of a foreign protein. **active a.,** that produced by injection of a foreign protein. **antiserum a.,** passive a. **cutaneous a., active,** localized anaphylaxis in the form of the wheal and flare reaction on injection of antigen into the skin of a sensitized subject; used as a test for allergy to pollen. **cutaneous a., passive (PCA),** localized anaphylaxis passively transferred by intradermal injection of an antibody and, after a latent period (about 24 to 72 hours), intravenous injection of the homologous antigen and Evans blue dye; blueing of the skin at the site of the intradermal injection is evidence of the permeability reaction. Used in studies of antibodies causing immediate hypersensitivity re-

actions. **cytotoxic a.,** that following the injection of antibodies specific for natural antigenic constituents of the body cell surfaces. **cytotropic a.,** that mediated by antibodies which have become attached to cell receptors following a latent period. **heterologous a.,** passive anaphylaxis induced by transfer of serum to one animal from an animal of a different species. **homologous a.,** passive anaphylaxis induced by transfer of serum to one animal from an animal of the same species. **indirect a.,** that induced by an animal's own antigen modified in some way. **local a.,** that confined to a limited area, e.g., cutaneous anaphylaxis. **passive a.,** that resulting in a normal person from injection of serum of a sensitized person. **reverse a.,** that following injection of antigen, succeeded by injection of antiserum.

anaplasia (an″ah-pla′ze-ah) loss of differentiation of cells (dedifferentiation) and of their orientation to one another and to their axial framework and blood vessels, a characteristic of tumor tissue.

Anaplasma (-plaz′mah) a genus of microorganisms (family Anaplasmataceae), including *A. margina′le*, the etiologic agent of gallsickness.

Anaplasmataceae (-plaz″mah-ta′se-e) a family of microorganisms (order Rickettsiales).

anaplasmosis (-plaz-mo′sis) infection with *Anaplasma*, as in gallsickness.

anaplastic (-plas′tik) 1. restoring a lost or absent part. 2. characterized by anaplasia.

anapophysis (-pof′ĭ-sis) an accessory vertebral process.

anaptic (an-ap′tik) marked by anaphia.

anarithmia (an″ah-rith′me-ah) inability to count, due to a central lesion.

anarthria (an-ar′thre-ah) severe dysarthria resulting in speechlessness. **a. litera′lis,** stuttering.

anasarca (an″ah-sar′kah) generalized massive edema.

anastalsis (-stal′sis) reversed peristalsis.

anastaltic (-stal′tik) styptic; astringent.

anastole (ah-nas′to-le) retraction, as of the edges of a wound.

anastomosis (ah-nas″to-mo′sis) 1. communication between vessels by collateral channels. 2. surgical, traumatic, or pathological formation of an opening between two normally distinct spaces or organs. **anastomot′ic,** adj. **arteriovenous a.,** one between an artery and a vein. **crucial a.,** an arterial anastomosis in the upper part of the thigh. **heterocladic a.,** one between branches of different arteries. **intestinal a.,** establishment of a communication between two formerly distant portions of the intestine. **a. of Riolan,** anastomosis of the superior and inferior mesenteric arteries. **Roux-en-Y a.,** any Y-shaped anastomosis in which the small intestine is included.

anastral (an-as′tral) lacking, or pertaining to the lack of, an aster.

anat. anatomy.

anatomic (an″ah-tom′ik) anatomical.

anatomical (-tom′ĕ-kal) pertaining to anatomy, or to the structure of the body.

anatomist (ah-nat′o-mist) one skilled in anatomy.

anatomy (-o-me) the science of the structure of living organisms. **applied a.,** anatomy as applied to diagnosis and treatment. **comparative a.,** comparison of the structure of different animals and plants, one with another. **developmental a.,** structural embryology. **gross a.,** that dealing with structures visible with the unaided eye. **macroscopic a.,** gross a. **microscopic a.,** histology. **morbid a., pathologic a.,** that of diseased tissues. **radiological a.,** the study of the anatomy of tissues based on their visualization on x-ray films. **special a.,** the study of particular organs or parts. **topographic a.,** the study of parts in their relation to surrounding parts. **veterinary a.,** the anatomy of domestic animals. **x-ray a.,** radiologic a.

anatriptic (an″ah-trip′tik) a medicine applied by rubbing.

anatrophic (-trof′ik) correcting or preventing atrophy; also, an agent that so acts.

anatropia (-tro′pe-ah) upward deviation of the visual axis of one eye when the other eye is fixing. **anatrop′ic,** adj.

anchorage (ang′kŏ-rij) fixation, e.g., surgical fixation of a displaced viscus or, in operative dentistry, fixation of fillings or of artificial crowns or bridges. In orthodontics, the support used for a regulating apparatus.

anchylo- for words beginning thus, see those beginning *ankylo-*.

ancipital (an-sip′ĭ-tal) two-edged or two-headed.

anconad (ang′ko-nad) toward the elbow or olecranon.

anconagra (ang″ko-nag′rah) gout of the elbow.

anconal (ang′ko-nal) anconeal.

anconeal (ang-ko′ne-al) pertaining to the elbow.

anconitis (an″ko-ni′tis) inflammation of the elbow joint.

ancylo- for words beginning thus, see also those beginning *ankylo-*.

Ancylostoma (an″sĭ-los′to-mah, an″kĭ-) a genus of hookworms (family Ancylostomidae). **A. america′num,** *Necator americanus.* **A. brazilien′se,** a species parasitizing dogs and cats in tropical areas; its larvae may cause creeping eruption in man. **A. cani′num,** the common hookworm of dogs and cats; its larvae may cause creeping eruption in man. **A. ceylon′icum,** A. *brazilien′se.* **A. duodena′le,** the common European or Old World hookworm, parasitic in the small intestine, producing the condition known as *hookworm disease.*

ancylostomiasis (an″sĭ-los″to-mi′ah-sis, an″ki-) infection with hookworms; see *hookworm disease.* **a. brazilien′sis,** larva migrans.

Ancylostomidae (an″sĭ-lo-sto′mĭ-de, an″kĭ-lo-) a family of nematode parasites having two ventrolateral cutting plates at the entrance to a large buccal capsule, and small teeth at its base; the hookworms.

ancyroid (an′sĭ-roid) anchor-shaped.

andr(o)- word element [Gr.], *male; masculine.*

androblastoma (an″dro-blas-to′mah) 1. a rare benign tumor of the testis histologically resembling the fetal testis; there are three varieties: diffuse stromal, mixed (stromal and epithelial), and tubular (epithelial). The epithelial elements contain Sertoli cells, which may produce estrogen and thus cause feminization. 2. arrhenoblastoma.

androgen (an′dro-jen) any substance, e.g., androsterone and testosterone, that stimulates male characteristics. **androgen′ic,** adj.

androgenicity (an″dro-jĕ-nis′ĭ-te) the quality of exerting a masculinizing effect.

android (an′droid) resembling a man.

andromerogon (an″dro-mer′o-gon) an organism produced by andromerogony and containing only the paternal set of chromosomes.

andromerogony (-mer-og′o-ne) development of a portion of a fertilized ovum containing the male pronucleus only.

androphilic (-fil′ik) anthropophilic.

androphobia (-fo′be-ah) morbid dread of the male sex.

androstane (an′dro-stān) the hydrocarbon nucleus, $C_{19}H_{32}$, from which androgens are derived.

androstanediol (an″dro-stān′de-ol) an androgen, $C_{19}H_{32}O_2$.

androstanedione (-stān′de-ōn) an androgen, $C_{19}H_{28}O_2$, formed in the testes.

androstene (an′dro-stēn) cyclic hydrocarbon, $C_{19}H_{30}$, forming the nucleus of testosterone and certain other androgens.

androstenediol (an″dro-stēn′de-ol) a crystalline androgenic steroid, $C_{19}H_{30}O_2$.

androsterone (an-dros′ter-ōn) an androgenic hormone, $C_{19}H_{30}O_2$, occurring in urine or prepared synthetically.

-ane word termination denoting (1) a saturated open-chain hydrocarbon (C_nH_{2n+2}); (2) an organic compound in which hydrogen has replaced the hydroxyl group.

anechoic (an-ĕ-ko′ik) without echoes; said of a chamber for measuring the effects of sound.

anectasis (an-ek′tah-sis) congenital atelectasis due to developmental immaturity.

Anectine (an-ek′tin) trademark for preparations of succinylcholine.

anelectrotonus (an″e-lek-trot′ŏ-nus) lessened irritability of a nerve at the anode during passage of electric current.

anemia (ah-ne′me-ah) reduction below normal of the number of erythrocytes, quantity of hemoglobin, or the volume of packed red cells in the blood; a symptom of various diseases and disorders. **achrestic a.,** megaloblastic anemia morphologically resembling pernicious anemia, but with multiple other causes. **aplastic a.,** that resistant to therapy and characterized by absence of regeneration of red blood cells. **Cooley's a.,** see *β-thalassemia,* under *thalassemia.* **drepanocytic a., Dresbach's a.,** sickle cell a. **equine infectious a.,** a viral disease of equines, with recurring malaise and abrupt temperature rises, weight loss, edema, and anemia; transmission to man has been suggested, in whom it causes anemia, neutropenia, and relative lymphocytosis. **hemolytic a.,** that due to shortened survival of mature erythrocytes and inability of the bone marrow to compensate for their decreased life span; it may be hereditary or acquired, as that resulting from infection or chemotherapy or occurring as part of an autoimmune process. **hypochromic a.,** that in which the decrease in hemoglobin is proportionately much greater than the decrease in number of red blood cells. **hypoplastic a.,** that due to varying degrees of erythrocytic hypoplasia without leukopenia or thrombocytopenia. **hypoplastic a., congenital, 1.** idiopathic progressive anemia occurring in the first year of life, without leukopenia and thrombocytopenia; it is unresponsive to hematinics and requires multiple blood transfusions to sustain life. **2.** Fanconi's syndrome (1). **iron deficiency a.,** a form characterized by low or absent iron stores, low serum iron concentration, low transferrin saturation, elevated transferrin, low hemoglobin concentration or hematocrit, and hypochromic, microcytic red blood cells. **Lederer's a.,** an acute hemolytic anemia of short duration and unknown etiology, possibly autoimmune. **macrocytic a.,** a group of anemias, of varying etiologies, marked by larger than normal red cells, absence of the customary central area of pallor, and an increased mean corpuscular volume and mean corpuscular hemoglobin. **Mediterranean a.,** see *β-thalassemia,* under *thalassemia.* **megaloblastic a.,** that marked by the presence of megaloblasts in the bone marrow. **microcytic a.,** that marked by decrease in size of the red cells. **miner's a.,** hookworm disease. **myelopathic a., myelophthisic a.,** leukoerythroblastosis. **normochromic a.,** that in which the hemoglobin content of the red cells as measured by the MCHC is in the normal range. **normocytic a.,** that marked by a proportionate decrease in the hemoglobin content, the packed red cell volume, and the number of erythrocytes per cubic millimeter of blood. **pernicious a.,** megaloblastic anemia, most commonly affecting adults, due to failure of the gastric mucosa to secrete adequate and potent intrinsic factor, resulting in malabsorption of vitamin B_{12}. **a. pseudoleuke′mica infan′tum,** a syndrome caused by many factors, e.g., malnutrition, chronic infection, malabsorption, etc., with anisocytosis, poikilocytosis, peripheral red cell immaturity, leukocytosis, lymphadenopathy, and hepatosplenomegaly; once considered to be a specific entity in children under age 3. **refractory a.,** aplastic a. **scorbutic a.,** anemia due to deficiency of ascorbic acid. **sickle cell a.,** a genetically determined defect of hemoglobin synthesis, occurring almost exclusively in Negroes, characterized by the presence of sickle-shaped erythrocytes in the blood, arthralgia, acute adominal pain, ulcerations of the legs, and homozygosity for S hemoglobin. **sideremic a.,** a heterogeneous group of anemias with multiple etiologies, marked by normal or increased levels of iron in the plasma and tissues, but in which the iron is not utilized. **sideroblastic a.,** a heterogeneous group of anemias with diverse clinical manifestations and with multiple causes each involving a derangement in the final pathway of heme synthesis, in which iron

stores of the reticuloendothelial tissues are almost always increased and bone marrow normoblasts contain iron (sideroblasts). **siderochrestic a.,** sideroblastic a. **sideropenic a.,** a group of anemias marked by low levels of iron in the plasma; it includes iron deficiency anemia and the anemia of chronic disorders. **spherocytic a.,** hereditary spherocytosis. **splenic a., a. splen′ica,** congestive splenomegaly.

anemic (ah-ne′mik) pertaining to anemia.

anemophilous (an″em-of′ĭ-lus) fertilized by wind-borne pollen; said of certan flowers.

anemophobia (an″ĕ-mo-fo′be-ah) morbid fear of wind or draughts.

anencephaly (an″en-sef′ah-le) congenital absence of the cranial vault, with the cerebral hemispheres completely missing or reduced to small masses. **anancephal′ic,** adj.

anenzymia (an″en-zi′me-ah) a morbid condition due to absence of an enzyme normally present in the body. **a. catala′sea,** acatalasia.

anergasia (an″er-ga′ze-ah) lack of functional activity; a psychosis associated with a structural lesion of the central nervous system. **anerga′sic,** adj.

anergy diminished reactivity to specific antigen(s). **aner′gic,** adj.

anerythroplasia (an″ĕ-rith″ro-pla′ze-ah) absence of erythrocyte formation. **anerythroplas′tic,** adj.

anerythropoiesis (-poi-e′sis) deficient production of erythrocytes.

anerythropsia (an″er-ĭ-throp′se-ah) inability to distinguish red colors.

anesthecinesia (an-es″the-sĭ-ne′ze-ah) combined sensory and motor paralysis.

anesthesia (an″es-the′ze-ah) loss of feeling or sensation, especially the loss of pain sensation induced to permit the performance of surgery or other painful procedures. **basal a.,** narcosis produced by preliminary medication so that the inhalation of anesthetic necessary to produce surgical anesthesia is greatly reduced. **block a.,** see *regional a.,* and see *block.* **bulbar a.,** that due to a lesion of the pons. **caudal a.,** anesthesia produced by injection of a local anesthetic into the caudal or sacral canal. **central a.,** that due to disease of the nerve centers. **cerebral a.,** that due to a cerebral lesion. **closed a.,** that produced by continuous rebreathing of a small amount of anesthetic gas in a closed system with an apparatus for removing carbon dioxide. **conduction a.,** regional a. **crossed a.,** see under *hemianesthesia.* **dissociated a., dissociation a.,** loss of perception of certain stimuli while that of others remains intact. **doll's head a.,** anesthesia of the head, neck, and upper part of the chest. **a. doloro′sa,** analgesia algera. **electric a.,** that induced by passage of an electric current. **endotracheal a.,** that produced by introduction of a gaseous mixture through a tube inserted into the trachea. **epidural a.,** that produced by injection of the anesthetic between the vertebral spines and beneath the ligamentum flavum into the extradural space. **frost a.,** abolition of feeling or sensation as a result of topical refrigeration produced by a jet of a highly volatile liquid. **gauntlet a.,** that from the wrist to fingertips. **general a.,** a state of unconsciousness and insusceptibility to pain, produced by administration of anesthetic agents by inhalation, intravenously, intramuscularly, rectally, or via the gastrointestinal tract. **girdle a.,** that in a zone encircling the hips. **gustatory a.,** ageusia. **infiltration a.,** local anesthesia produced by injection of the anesthetic solution in the area of terminal nerve endings. **inhalation a.,** that produced by the inhalation of vapors of a volatile liquid or gaseous anesthetic agent. **insufflation a.,** that produced by blowing a mixture of gases or vapors into the respiratory tract through a tube. **intraoral a.,** that within the oral cavity produced by injection, spray, pressure, etc. **local a.,** that confined to a limited area. **lumbar epidural a.,** that produced by injection of the anesthetic into the epidural space at the second or third lumbar interspace. **mental a.,** inability to recognize and identify sensory stimuli. **mixed a.,** that produced by use of more than one anesthetic agent. **muscular a.,** loss of the muscular sense. **olfactory a.,** anosmia. **open a.,** general inhalation anesthesia utilizing a cone; there is no significant rebreathing of expired gases. **partial a.,** that with retention of some degree of sensibility. **peripheral a.,** that due to changes in the peripheral nerves. **rectal a.,** that induced by introduction of the anesthetic agent into the rectum. **refrigeration a.,** local anesthesia produced by applying a tourniquet and chilling the part to near freezing temperature. **regional a.,** insensibility of a part induced by interrupting the sensory nerve conductivity of that region of the body; it may be produced by (1) *field block,* encircling the operative field by means of injections of a local anesthetic; or (2) *nerve block,* making injections in close proximity to the nerves supplying the area. **saddle-block a.,** that produced in a region corresponding roughly with the areas of the buttocks, perineum, and inner aspects of the thighs which impinge on the saddle in riding, by introducing the anesthetic low in the dural sac. **segmental a.,** loss of sensation caused by lesions of nerve roots. **spinal a.,** 1. that produced by injection of a local anesthetic into the subarachnoid space around the spinal cord. 2. loss of sensation due to a spinal lesion. **splanchnic a.,** regional anesthesia for visceral operation by injection of anesthetic agent into the region of the semilunar ganglia. **surgical a.,** that degree of anesthesia at which operation may safely be performed. **tactile a.,** loss or impairment of the sense of touch. **thermal a., thermic a.,** loss of the temperature sense. **topical a.,** that produced by application of a local anesthetic directly to the area involved, as to the oral mucosa or the cornea. **transsacral a.,** spinal anesthesia produced by injection of the anesthetic into the sacral canal and about the sacral nerves through each of the posterior sacral foramina. **twilight a.,** twilight sleep. **unilateral a.,** hemianesthesia. **visceral a.,** loss of visceral sensations.

anesthesimeter (an″es-thĕ-sim′ĕ-ter) 1. an instrument for testing degree of anesthesia. 2. a device for regulating the amount of anesthetic given.

Anesthesin (ah-nes′thĕ-sin) trademark for a preparation of benzocaine.

anesthesiologist (an″es-the″ze-ol′o-jist) a physician who specializes in anesthesiology.

anesthesiology (-ol′o-je) that branch of medicine which studies anesthesia and anesthetics.

anesthetic (an″es-thet′ik) 1. pertaining to, characterized by, or producing anesthesia. 2. an agent that produces anesthesia.

anesthetist (ah-nes′thĕ-tist) a person trained in administering anesthetics.

anesthetization (-ti-za′shun) production of anesthesia.

anethole (an′ĕ-thōl) a flavoring agent for drugs, $C_{10}H_{12}O$, from anise and fennel oils and other sources, or prepared synthetically.

anetoderma (ah-ne″to-der′mah) looseness and atrophy of the skin.

aneuploid (an′u-ploid) 1. characterized by aneuploidy. 2. an individual or cell characterized by aneuploidy.

aneuploidy (an″u-ploi′de) any deviation from an exact multiple of the haploid number of chromosomes, whether fewer or more.

aneurin (ah-nu′rin) thiamine hydrochloride.

aneurysm (an′u-rizm) a sac formed by localized dilatation of an artery or vein. **aneurys′mal,** adj. **aortic a.,** aneurysm of the aorta. **arteriovenous a.,** abnormal communication between an artery and a vein in which the blood flows directly into a neighboring vein or is carried into the vein by a connecting sac. **atherosclerotic a.,** one arising as a result of weakening of the tunica media in severe atherosclerosis. **berry a.,** a small saccular aneurysm of a cerebral artery, usually at the junction of vessels in the circle of Willis, having a narrow opening into the artery. **cirsoid a.,** racemose a. **compound a.,** one in which some of the layers of the wall of the vessel are ruptured and some merely dilated. **dissecting a.,** one in which rupture of the inner coat has permitted blood to escape between layers of the vessel wall. **false a.,** one in which the entire wall is injured and the blood is retained in the surrounding tissues; a sac communicating with the artery (or heart) is eventually formed. **fusiform a.,** a spindle-shaped arterial aneurysm in which the distention affects the entire circumference of the artery. **mixed a.,** compound a. **racemose a.,** dilatation and tortuous lengthening of the blood vessels. **saccular a., sacculated a.,** a distended sac affecting only part of the arterial circumference. **spurious a.,** false a. **syphilitic a.,** aortic aneurysm occurring in cardiovascular syphilis. **varicose a.,** one in which an intervening sac connects the artery with contiguous veins.

aneurysmectomy (an″u-riz-mek′to-me) excision of an aneurysm.

aneurysmoplasty (an″u-riz′mo-plas″te) plastic repair of the affected artery in the treatment of aneurysm.

aneurysmorrhaphy (an″u-riz-mor′ah-fe) suture of an aneurysm.

aneurysmotomy (-mot′o-me) incision of an aneurysm.

anfractuous (an-frak′tu-us) convoluted, sinuous, or tortuous.

angi(o)- word element [Gr.], *vessel (channel)*.

angiasthenia (an″je-as-the′ne-ah) loss of tone in the vascular system.

angiectasis (-ek′tah-sis) gross dilatation and, often, lengthening of a blood vessel. **angiectat′ic,** adj.

angiectomy (-ek′to-me) excision or resection of a vessel.

angiectopia (-ek-to′pe-ah) abnormal position or course of a vessel.

angiitis (-i′tis) inflammation of the coats of a vessel, chiefly blood or lymph vessels; vasculitis.

angina (an-ji′nah, an′jĭ-nah) spasmodic, choking, or suffocating pain; used almost exclusively to denote angina pectoris. **an′ginal,** adj. **agranulocytic a.,** agranulocytosis. **a. cru′ris,** intermittent claudication. **intestinal a.,** generalized cramping abdominal pain occurring shortly after a meal and persisting for one to three hours, due to ischemia of the smooth muscle of the bowel. **a. inver′sa,** a variant form of angina pectoris in which there is elevation, rather than depression, of the RS-T interval of the electrocardiogram. **a. laryn′gea,** laryngitis. **a. ludovi′ci, a. ludwig′ii, Ludwig's a.,** diffuse purulent inflammation of the floor of the mouth, usually due to streptococcal infection. **a. parotid′ea,** mumps. **a. pec′toris,** paroxysmal pain in the chest, usually due to interference with the supply of oxygen to the heart muscle, and precipitated by excitement or effort. **Plaut's a.,** necrotizing ulcerative gingivostomatitis. **Prinzmetal's a.,** a variant of angina pectoris in which the attacks occur during rest, exercise capacity is well preserved, and attacks are associated electrocardiographically with elevation of the ST-segment. **streptococcus a.,** that due to streptococci. **a. tonsilla′ris,** peritonsillar abscess. **a. trachea′lis,** croup. **variant a. pectoris,** Prinzmetal's a.

anginoid (an′jĭ-noid) resembling angina.

anginophobia (an″jĭ-no-fo′be-ah) morbid dread of angina pectoris.

anginose (an′jĭ-nōs) characterized by angina.

angioblast (an′je-o-blast″) 1. the earliest formative tissue from which blood cells and blood vessels arise. 2. an individual vessel-forming cell. **angioblast′ic,** adj.

angioblastoma (an″je-o-blas-to′mah) a term applied to certain blood-vessel tumors of the brain: those arising in the cerebellum (*cerebellar a.*) may be cystic and associated with von Hippel-Lindau disease; also, a blood-vessel tumor arising from the meninges of the brain or spinal cord (angioblastic meningioma).

angiocardiogram (-kar′de-o-gram) the film produced by angiocardiography.

angiocardiography (-kar″de-og′rah-fe) radiography of the heart and great vessels after introduction of an opaque contrast medium into a blood vessel or a cardiac chamber.

angiocardiokinetic (-kar″de-o-ki-net′ik) affecting the movements of the heart and blood vessels; also, an agent that affects such movements.

angiocardiopathy (-kar″de-op′ah-the) disease of the heart and blood vessels.

angiocarditis (-kar-di′tis) inflammation of the heart and blood vessels.

angiochondroma (-kon-dro′mah) chondroma with excessive development of blood vessels.

angioedema (-ĕ-de′mah) angioneurotic edema.

angioendothelioma (-en″do-the″le-o′mah) hemangioendothelioma.

angiofibroma (-fi-bro′mah) an angioma containing fibrous tissue. **nasopharyngeal a.,** a relatively benign tumor of the nasopharynx composed of fibrous connective tissue with abundant endothelium-lined vascular spaces, usually occurring during puberty, most commonly in boys. It is marked by nasal obstruction which may become total, adenoid speech, discomfort in swallowing, and auditory tube obstruction.

angiogenesis (-jen′ĕ-sis) development of blood vessels in the embryo.

angiogenic (-jen′ik) 1. pertaining to angiogenesis. 2. of vascular origin.

angioglioma (-gli-o′mah) a very vascular form of glioma.

angiogram (an′je-o-gram) a roentgenogram of a blood vessel filled with contrast medium.

angiography (an″je-og′rah-fe) roentgenography of the blood vessels after introduction of a contrast medium.

angiohemophilia (an″je-o-he″mo-fil′e-ah) a congenital hemorrhagic diathesis with bleeding from the skin and mucosal surfaces, due to abnormal blood vessels with or without platelet defects or deficiencies of blood coagulation Factor VIII or IX.

angiohyalinosis (-hi″ah-lĭ-no′sis) hyaline degeneration of the walls of blood vessels.

angioid (an′je-oid) resembling blood vessels.

angiokeratoma (an″je-o-ker″ah-to′mah) a skin disease in which telangiectasis or warty growths occur in groups, together with epidermal thickening. **a. circumscrip′tum,** a rare form with discrete papules and nodules usually localized to a small area on the leg or trunk. **a. cor′poris diffu′sum,** a hereditary disorder of phospholipid metabolism affecting many of the body systems, chiefly the blood vessels, marked by purpuric cutaneous lesions, associated with cardiovascular disease, renal abnormalities, and hypertension.

angiokinetic (-ki-net′ik) vasomotor.

angiolipoleiomyoma (-lip″o-li″o-mi-o′mah) see *angiomyolipoma.*

angiolipoma (-lĭp-o′mah) a tumor composed of adipose tissue and blood vessels.

angiolith (an′je-o-lith″) a calcareous deposit in the wall of a blood vessel. **angiolith′ic,** adj.

angiology (an″je-ol′o-je) the scientific study of the vessels of the body; also, the sum of knowledge relating to the blood and lymph vessels.

angiolupoid (an″je-o-lu′poid) a granuloma occurring chiefly on the side of the nose, consisting of small, oval red plaques with telangiectases over the surface.

angiolysis (an″je-ol′ĭ-sis) retrogression or obliteration of blood vessels, as in embryologic development.

angioma (an″je-o′mah) a tumor whose cells tend to form blood vessels (hemangioma) or lymph vessels (lymphangioma); a tumor made up of blood vessels or lymph vessels. **angiom′atous,** adj. **a. caverno′sum, cavernous a.,** see under *hemangioma.* **cherry a's,** bright red, circumscribed, round or oval angiomas, 2 to 6 mm. in diameter, containing many vascular loops, due to a telangiectatic vascular disturbance, usually seen on the trunk but may appear on other areas of the body, as in angioma serpiginosum, and occurring in most of the middle-aged and elderly. **hereditary hemorrhagic a.,** see under *telangiectasia.* **senile a's,** cherry a's. **a. serpigino′sum,** a skin disease marked by minute vascular points arranged in rings on the skin. **telangiectatic a.,** one made up of dilated blood vessels.

angiomatosis (an″je-o-mah-to′sis) a diseased state of the vessels with formation of multiple angiomas. **cerebroretinal a.,** von Hippel-Lindau disease. **encephalofacial a., encephalotrigeminal a.,** Sturge-Weber syndrome. **hemorrhagic familial a.,** hereditary hemorrhagic telangiectasia. **a. of retina,** von Hippel's disease. **retinocerebral a.,** von Hippel-Lindau disease.

angiomegaly (-meg′ah-le) enlargement of blood vessels, especially a condition of the eyelid marked by great increase in its volume.

angiomyolipoma (-mi″o-lĭ-po′mah) a benign tumor containing vascular, adipose, and muscle elements, occurring most often in the kidney with smooth muscle elements (angiolipoleiomyoma) in association with tuberous sclerosis, and considered to be a hamartoma.

angiomyoma (-mi-o′mah) a hamartoma composed of blood vessels and smooth muscle.

angiomyoneuroma (-mi″o-nu-ro′mah) glomangioma.

angiomyosarcoma (-mi″o-sar-ko′mah) a tumor composed of elements of angioma, myoma, and sarcoma.

angioneurectomy (-nu-rek′to-me) excision of vessels and nerves.

angioneuroma (-nu-ro′mah) glomangioma.

angioneuromyoma (-nu″ro-mi-o′mah) glomangioma.

angioneuropathy (-nu-rop′ah-the) any neuropathy primarily affecting the blood vessels; a disorder of the vasomotor system, as angiospasm or vasomotor paralysis. **angioneuropath′ic,** adj.

angionoma (-no′mah) ulceration of blood vessels.

angioparalysis (-pah-ral′ĭ-sis) vasomotor paralysis.

angioparesis (-pah-re′-sis) vasomotor paralysis.

angiopathy (an″je-op′ah-the) any disease of the vessels.

angioplasty (an′je-o-plas″te) surgery of blood vessels.

angiopoiesis (an″je-o-poi-e′sis) the formation of blood vessels. **angiopoiet′ic,** adj.

angiopressure (-presh′ūr) the application of pressure to a blood vessel to control hemorrhage.

angiorhigosis (-ri-go′sis) rigidity of blood vessels.

angiorrhaphy (an″je-or′ah-fe) suture of a vessel or vessels.

angiosarcoma (an″je-o-sar-ko′mah) hemangiosarcoma.

angiosclerosis (-skle-ro′sis) hardening of the walls of blood vessels.

angioscope (an′je-o-skōp″) a microscope for observing the capillaries.

angioscotoma (an″je-o-sko-to′mah) a scotoma, or defect in the usual field, caused by shadows of the retinal blood vessels.

angioscotometry (-sko-tom′ĕ-tre) the plotting or mapping of an angioscotoma; done particularly in diagnosing glaucoma.

angiospasm (an′je-o-spazm″) spasmodic contraction of the walls of a blood vessel. **angiospas′tic,** adj.

angiostaxis (an″je-o-stak′sis) hemorrhagic diathesis.

angiostenosis (-ste-no′sis) narrowing of the caliber of a vessel.

angiosteosis (an″je-os″te-o′sis) ossification or calcification of a vessel.

angiostrongyliasis (an″je-o-stron″jĭ-li′ah-sis) infection with *Angiostrongylus cantonensis.*

Angiostrongylus (-stron′jĭ-lus) a genus of nematode parasites. **A. cantonen′sis,** the rat lungworm of Australia and many Pacific islands, including Hawaii; human infection—thought to be due to ingestion of larvae in intermediate hosts, e.g., freshwater crabs—results in migration of the larval worms to the central nervous system, where they provoke eosinophilic meningoencephalitis. **A. vaso′rum,** a species parasitic in the pulmonary arteries of dogs.

angiostrophe, angiostrophy (an″je-os′tro-fe) twisting of a vessel to arrest hemorrhage.

angiotelectasis (an″je-o-tel-ek′tah-sis) dilatation of the minute arteries and veins.

angiotensin (-ten′sin) a polypeptide formed by action of renin and angiotensinogen in blood plasma. The inactive form, angiotensin I, is in turn acted upon by a peptidase to form angiotensin II, a vasopressor and stimulator of aldosterone secretion by the adrenal cortex. **a. amide,** $C_{49}H_{70}N_{14}O_{11}$, used as a vasopressor.

angiotensinase (-ten′sĭ-nās) any of a group of peptidases in plasma and tissues that inactivate angiotensin.

angiotensinogen (-ten′sin-o-jen) a serum α_2-globulin secreted in the liver which, on hydrolysis by renin, gives rise to angiotensin.

angiotitis (-ti′tis) inflammation of the vessels of the ear.

angiotome (an′je-o-tōm″) one of the segments of the vascular system of the embryo.

angiotomy (an″je-ot′o-me) incision or severing of a blood or lymph vessel.

angiotonase (an″je-o-to′nās) an enzyme formed by the kidneys that inactivates angiotensin.

angiotonic (-ton′ik) increasing vascular tension.

angiotonin (-to′nin) angiotensin.

angiotribe (an′je-o-trīb″) a strong forceps in which pressure is applied by means of a screw; used to crush tissue containing an artery in order to check hemorrhage from the vessel.

angiotripsy (-trip″se) hemostasis by means of an angiotribe.

angiotrophic (an″je-o-trof′ik) pertaining to nutrition of vessels.

angle (ang′g′l) 1. the space or figure formed by two diverging lines, measured as the number of degrees one would have to be moved to coincide with the other. 2. the point at which two intersecting borders or surfaces converge. **acromial a.,** the subcutaneous bony point at which the lateral border becomes continuous with the spine of the scapula. **alpha a.,** that formed by intersection of the visual axis with the optic axis. **axial a.,** any line angle parallel with the long axis of a tooth. **cardiodiaphragmatic a.,** that formed by the junction of the shadows of the heart and diaphragm in posteroanterior roentgenograms of the chest. **cavity a's,** those formed by the junction of two or more walls of a tooth cavity. **costovertebral a.,** that formed on either side of the vertebral column between the last rib and the lumbar vertebrae. **filtration a.,** a narrow recess between the sclerocorneal junction and the attached margin of the iris, at the periphery of the anterior chamber of the eye; it is the principal exit site for the aqueous fluid. **iridocorneal a., a. of iris,** filtration a. **a. of jaw,** the junction of the lower edge of the lower jaw with the posterior edge of its ramus. **kappa a.,** that between the pupillary axes. **line a.,** an angle formed by the junction of two planes; in dentistry, the junction of two surfaces of a tooth or of two walls of a tooth cavity. **Louis' a., Ludwig's a.,** that between manubrium and gladiolus. **meter a.,** a unit of convergence of the eye: that amount of convergence required for binocular fixation of an object at 1 meter, using 1 diopter of accommodation. **optic a.,** visual a. **point a.,** one formed by the junction of three planes; in dentistry, the junction of three surfaces of a tooth, or of three walls of a tooth cavity. **a. of pubis,** that formed by the conjoined rami of the ischial and pubic bones. **sternoclavicular a.,** that between the sternum and the clavicle. **subpubic a.,** a. of pubis. **tooth a's,** those formed by two or more tooth surfaces. **visual a.,** that between two lines passing from the extremities of an object seen, through the nodal point of the eye, to the corresponding extremities of the image of the object seen. **Y a.,** that between the radius fixus and the line joining the lambda and inion.

angstrom (ang′strom) a unit of linear measurement, equivalent to 0.1 millimicron (10^{-7} mm.); abbreviated A or Å.

angulation (ang″gu-la′shun) 1. formation of a sharp obstructive bend, as in the intestine, ureter, or similar tubes. 2. deviation from a straight line, as in a badly set bone.

angulus (ang′gu-lus) [L.] angle; used in names of anatomic structures or landmarks. **a. infectio′sus,** perlèche. **a. i′ridis,** filtration angle. **a. Ludovi′ci,** Louis' angle. **a. mandib′ulae,** angle of jaw. **a. oc′uli,** the canthus of the eye. **a. o′ris,** the angle at either side of the mouth formed by the juncture of the upper and lower lip. **a. pu′bis,** angle of pubis. **a. ster′ni,** Louis' angle. **a. veno′sus,** the angle at the junction of the internal jugular vein and the subclavian vein.

anhedonia (an″he-do′ne-ah) inability to experience pleasure in normally pleasurable acts.

anhidrosis (an″hĭ-dro′sis) abnormal deficiency of sweat.

anhidrotic (an″hĭ-drot′ik) 1. checking the flow of sweat. 2. an agent which suppresses perspiration.

anhydrase (an-hi′drās) an enzyme that catalyzes the removal of water from a compound. **carbonic a.,** an enzyme that catalyzes the decomposition of carbonic acid into carbon dioxide and water, facilitating the transfer of carbon dioxide from tissues to blood and from blood to alveolar air.

anhydration (an″hi-dra′shun) dehydration.

anhydremia (an″hi-dre′me-ah) deficiency of water in the blood.

anhydride (an-hi′drĭd) any compound derived from a substance, especially an acid, by abstraction of a molecule of water. **chromic a.,** chromic acid (2).

anhydrous (an-hi′drus) containing no water.

anianthinopsy (an″e-an″thĭ-nop′se) inability to distinguish violet tints.

anideus (ah-nid′e-us) holoacardius amorphus.

anidrosis (an″ĭ-dro′sis) anhidrosis.

anileridine (an″ĭ-ler′ĭ-dēn) a narcotic analgesic, $C_{22}H_{28}N_2O_2$.

anilide (an′ĭ-līd) any compound formed from aniline by substituting a radical for the hydrogen of NH_2.

aniline (an′ĭ-lēn) an oily liquid, $C_6H_5NH_2$, from coal tar and indigo or prepared by reducing nitrobenzene; the parent substance of colors or dyes derived from coal tar. It is an important cause of serious industrial poisoning associated with bone marrow depression as well as methemoglobinemia.

anilinism, anilism (an′ĭ-lin-izm; an′ĭ-lizm) poisoning by exposure to aniline.

anility (ah-nil′ĭ-te) 1. the state of being like an old woman. 2. imbecility.

anima (an′i-mah) 1. the soul. 2. Jung's term for the unconscious, or inner being, of the individual, as opposed to the personality he presents to the world (persona). In psychoanalysis, the more feminine soul or inner being of a man; cf. *animus.*

animal (an′ĭ-mal) 1. a living organism having sensation and the power of voluntary movement and requiring for its existence oxygen and organic food. 2. of or pertaining to such an organism. **control a.,** an untreated animal otherwise identical in all respects to one that is used for purposes of experimentation, used for checking results of treatment. **Houssay a.,** an experimental animal deprived of both hypophysis (pituitary gland) and pancreas. **hyperphagic a.,** an experimental animal in which the cells of the ventromedial nucleus of the hypothalamus have been destroyed, abolishing its awareness of the point at which it should stop eating; excessive eating and savageness characterize such an animal. **Long-Lukens a.,** an experimental animal deprived of the pancreas and adrenal glands. **spinal a.,** one whose spinal cord has been severed, cutting off communication with the brain.

animalcule (an″ĭ-mal′kūl) a minute animal organism.

animation (an″ĭ-ma′shun) the quality of being full of life. **suspended a.,** temporary suspension or cessation of the vital functions.

animus (an′ĭ-mus) in psychoanalysis, the more male soul or inner being of a woman; cf. *anima.*

anion (an′i-on) an ion carrying a negative charge; the element which in electrolysis passes to the positive pole.

aniridia (an″ĭ-rid′e-ah) congenital absence of the iris.

aniseikonia (an″ĭ-si-ko′ne-ah) inequality of the retinal images of the two eyes.

anisindione (an″is-in-dĭ′ōn) an anticoagulant, $C_{16}H_{12}O_3$.

aniso- word element [Gr.], *unequal.*

anisochromatic (an-i″so-kro-mat′ik) not of the same color throughout.

anisocoria (-ko′re-ah) inequality in size of the pupils of the eyes.

anisocytosis (-si-to′sis) presence in the blood of erythrocytes showing excessive variations in size.

anisodactyly (-dak′tĭ-le) a condition in which the corresponding digits are of unequal length. **anisodac′tylous,** adj.

anisogamete (-gam′ēt) a gamete differing in size and structure from the one with which it unites. **anisogamet′ic,** adj.

anisogamy (an″i-sog′ah-me) conjugation of gametes differing in size and structure.

anisognathous (-nah-thus) having jaws (maxilla and mandible) of unequal width.

anisokaryosis (an-i″so-kar″e-o′sis) inequality in the size of the nuclei of cells.

anisomastia (-mas′te-ah) inequality in size of the breasts.

anisomelia (-me′le-ah) inequality between paired limbs.

anisometropia (-mě-tro′pe-ah) inequality in refractive power of the two eyes. **anisometrop′ic,** adj.

anisopiesis (-pi-e′sis) variation or inequality in the blood pressure as registered in different parts of the body.

anisopoikilocytosis (-poi″kĭ-lo-si-to′sis) the presence in the blood of erythrocytes of varying sizes and abnormal shapes.

anisospore (an-i′so-spōr) 1. an anisogamete of organisms reproducing by spores. 2. an asexual spore produced by heterosporous organisms.

anisosthenic (an-i″sos-then′ik) not having equal power; said of muscles.

anisotonic (an-i″so-ton′ik) 1. varying in tonicity or tension. 2. having different osmotic pressure; not isotonic.

anisotropic (-trop′ik) 1. having unlike properties in different directions. 2. doubly refracting, or having a double polarizing power.

anistotropy (an″i-sot′ro-pe) the quality of being anisotropic.

anisuria (an″i-su′re-ah) alternating oliguria and polyuria.

ankle (ang′k'l) the region of the joint between leg and foot; the tarsus. Also, the ankle joint.

ankylo- word element [Gr.], *bent; crooked; in the form of a loop; adhesion.*

ankyloblepharon (ang″kĭ-lo-blef′ah-ron) adhesion of the ciliary edges of the eyelids to each other.

ankylocheilia (-ki′le-ah) adhesion of the lips to each other.

ankyloglossia (-glos′e-ah) tongue-tie. **a. superior,** extensive adhesion of the tongue to the palate, associated with deformities of hands and feet.

ankylopoietic (-poi-et′ik) producing ankylosis.

ankylosed (ang′kĭ-lōsd) fused or obliterated, as an ankylosed joint.

ankylosis (ang″kĭ-lo′sis) immobility and consolidation of a joint due to disease, injury, or surgical procedure. **ankylot′ic,** adj. **artificial a.,** arthrodesis. **bony a.,** union of the bones of a joint by proliferation of bone cells, resulting in complete immobility; true a. **extracapsular a.,** that due to rigidity of structures outside the joint capsule. **false a.,** fibrous a. **fibrous a.,** reduced joint mobility due to proliferation of fibrous tissue. **intracapsular a.,** that due to disease, injury, or surgery within the joint capsule. **spurious a.,** fibrous a. **true a.,** bony a.

ankylotia (-lo′she-ah) closure of external meatus of ear.

ankyroid (ang′kĭ-roid) hook-shaped.

anlage (ahn′lah-geh), pl. *anla′gen* [Ger.] primordium.

anneal (an-nēl′) to soften a material, as a metal, by controlled heating and cooling, to make its manipulation easier.

annectent (an-nek′tent) connecting; joining together.

annelid (ah′nel-id) any member of Annelida.

Annelida (ah-nel′ĭ-dah) a phylum of metazoan invertebrates, the segmented worms, including leeches.

annular (an′u-lar) ring-shaped.

annulorrhaphy (an″u-lor′ah-fe) closure of a hernial ring or defect by sutures.

annulus (an′u-lus), pl. *an′nuli* [L.] a small ring or encircling structure; spelled also *anulus* [NA].

anococcygeal (a″no-kok-sij′e-al) pertaining to the anus and coccyx.

anode (an′ōd) the positive electrode or pole to which negative ions are attracted. **ano′dal,** adj.

anodontia (an″o-don′she-aḷ) congenital absence of some or all of the teeth.

anodyne (an′o-dīn) 1. relieving pain. 2. a medicine that eases pain.

anodynia (an″o-din′e-ah) freedom from pain.

anoia (ah-noi′ah) idiocy.

anomalopia (ah-nom″ah-lo′pe-ah) a slight anomaly of visual perception. **color a.,** a minor deviation of color vision, without loss of ability to distinguish the four primary colors.

anomaloscope (ah-nom′ah-lo-skōp″) an apparatus used to detect anomalies of color vision.

anomaly (ah-nom′ah-le) marked deviation from normal, especially as a result of congenital or hereditary defects. **anom′alous,** adj. **Alder's a.,** a hereditary condition in which all leukocytes, but mainly those of the myelocytic series, contain coarse, azurophilic granules. **Axenfeld's a.,** see under *syndrome.* **Chédiak-Higashi a.,** see under *syndrome.* **developmental a.,** a defect resulting from imperfect embryonic development. **Ebstein's a.,** a malformation of the tricuspid valve, usually associated with an atrial septal defect. **Pelger's nuclear a., Pelger-Huët nuclear a.,** a hereditary or acquired defect in which the nuclei of neutrophils and eosinophils appear rodlike, spherical, or dumbbell-shaped; the nuclear structure is coarse and lumpy. **Poland's a.,** see under *syndrome.* **Rieger's a.,** see under *syndrome.*

anomia (ah-no′me-ah) loss of power of naming objects or of recognizing names.

anonychia (an″o-nik′e-ah) congenital absence of a nail or nails.

anoopsia (an″o-op′se-ah) hypertropia.

Anopheles (ah-nof′ĕ-lēz) a widely distributed genus of mosquitoes, comprising over 300 species, many of which are vectors of malaria; some are vectors of *Wuchereria bancrofti.*

anophthalmia (an″of-thal′me-ah) a developmental anomaly characterized by complete absence of the eyes (rare) or by the presence of vestigial eyes.

anophthalmos (an″of-thal′mos) anophthalmia.

anoplasty (a′no-plas″te) plastic or reparative surgery of the anus.

anopsia (an-op′se-ah) 1. nonuse or suppression of vision in one eye. 2. hypertropia.

anorchid (an-or′kid) a person with no testes or with undescended testes.

anorchism (an-or′kizm) congenital absence of one or both testes.

anorectic (an″o-rek′tik) 1. pertaining to anorexia. 2. an agent that diminshes the appetite.

anorectocolonic (a″no-rek″to-ko-lon′ik) pertaining to the anus, rectum, and colon.

anorectum (-rek′tum) the anus and rectum considered as a single unit. **anorec′tal,** adj.

anoretic (an″o-ret′ik) anorectic.

anorexia (-rek′se-ah) lack or loss of appetite for food. **a. nervo′sa,** loss of appetite due to emotional reasons, leading to emaciation.

anorexic (-rek′sik) anorectic.

anorexigenic (-rek″sĭ-jen′ik) 1. producing anorexia. 2. an agent that diminishes or controls the appetite.

anorthography (an″or-thog′rah-fe) loss of the ability to write.

anorthopia (-tho′pe-ah) asymmetrical or distorted vision.

anorthosis (-tho′sis) absence of penile erectility.

anoscope (a′no-skōp) a speculum for examining the anal canal and lower rectum.

anoscopy (a-nos′ko-pe) examination of the anal canal with an anoscope.

anosigmoidoscopy (a″no-sig″moi-dos′ko-pe) endoscopic examination of the anus, rectum, and sigmoid colon. **anosigmoidoscop′ic,** adj.

anosmia (an-oz′me-ah) absence of the sense of smell. **anos′mic, anosmat′ic,** adj.

anosognosia (an″o-sog-no′zhe-ah) loss of ability to recognize or to acknowledge bodily defect, usually associated with lesions of the nondominant hemisphere and resultant left hemiparesis. **anosogno′sic,** adj.

anospinal (a″no-spi′nal) pertaining to the anus and spinal cord.

anostosis (an″os-to′sis) defective formation of bone.

anotia (an-o′she-ah) congenital absence of the external ears.

anotus (an-o′tus) a fetus without ears.

anovaginal (a″no-vaj′ĭ-nal) pertaining to or communicating with the anus and vagina.

anovarism (an-o′var-izm) absence of the ovaries.

anovesical (a″no-ves′ĭ-kal) pertaining to the anus and bladder.

anovular (an-ov′u-lar) not associated with ovulation.

anovulatory (an-ov′u-lah-tor″e) anovular.

anoxemia (an″ok-se′me-ah) reduction in oxygen content of the blood below normal levels. **anoxe′mic,** adj.

anoxia (an-ok′se-ah) absence or deficiency of oxygen, as reduction of oxygen in body tissues below physiologic levels. **anox′ic,** adj. **altitude a.,** that due to reduced oxygen pressure at high altitudes. **anemic a.,** that due to decrease in amount of hemoglobin or number of erythrocytes in the blood. **anoxic a.,** that due to interference with the oxygen supply. **histotoxic a.,** that resulting from diminished ability of cells to utilize available oxygen. **stagnant a.,** that due to interference with the flow of blood and its transport of oxygen.

ansa (an′sah), pl. *an′sae*[L.] a looplike structure. **a. cervica′lis,** a nerve loop in the neck that supplies the infrahyoid muscles. **a. hypoglos′si,** a. cervicalis. **a. lenticula′ris,** a small nerve fiber tract arising in the globus pallidus and joining the anterior part of the ventral thalamic nucleus. **an′sae nervo′rum spina′lium,** loops of spinal nerves joining the ventral roots of the spinal nerves. **a. peduncula′ris,** a complex grouping of nerve fibers connecting the amygdaloid nucleus, piriform area, and anterior hypothalamus, and various thalamic nuclei. **a. subcla′via, a. of Vieussens,** nerve filaments passing around the subclavian artery to form a loop connecting the middle and inferior cervical ganglia. **a. vitelli′na,** an embryonic vein from the yolk sac to the umbilical vein.

Ansolysen (an″so-li′sen) trademark for preparations of pentolinium.

Antabuse (an'tah-būs) trademark for a preparation of disulfiram.

antacid (ant-as'id) counteracting acidity; an agent that so acts.

antagonism (an-tag'o-nizm'') opposition or contrariety between similar things, as between muscles, medicines, or organisms; cf. *antibiosis*.

antagonist (an-tag'o-nist) 1. a muscle that counteracts the action of another muscle, its agonist. 2. a substance that tends to nullify the action of another, as of an enzyme, hormone, or drug. 3. a tooth in one jaw that articulates with one in the other jaw.

antarthritic (ant''ar-thrit'ik) alleviating arthritis; an agent that so acts.

antazoline (ant-az'o-lēn) an antihistaminic, $C_{17}H_{19}N_3$, used as the hydrochloride and phospate salts.

ante (an'te) [L.] *before.*

ante- word element [L.], *before* (in time or space).

antebrachium (an''te-bra'ke-um) the forearm. **antebra'chial**, adj.

antecedent (-se'dent) a precursor. **plasma thromboplastin a. (PTA)**, coagulation Factor XI.

antecurvature (-ker'vah-tūr) a slight anteflexion.

antefebrile (-feb'rīl) preceding fever.

anteflexion (-flek'shun) 1. abnormal forward bending of an organ or part. 2. the normal forward curvature of the uterus.

ante mortem (an'te mor'tem) [L.] before death.

antemortem (an''te-mor'tem) performed or occurring before death.

antenna (an-ten'ah) either of the two lateral appendages on the anterior segment of the head of arthropods.

Antepar (an'tĕ-par) trademark for preparations of piperazine.

antepartal (an''te-par'tal) occurring before childbirth, with reference to the mother.

ante partum (an'te par'tum) [L.] before parturition.

antepartum (an''te-par'tum) antepartal.

antephase (an'te-fāz) the portion of interphase immediately preceding mitosis (or meiosis) when energy is being produced and stored for mitosis (or meiosis) and chromosome reproduction is taking place.

antepyretic (an''te-pi-ret'ik) occurring before the stage of fever.

anterior (an-te're-or) situated at or directed toward the front; opposite of posterior.

antero- word element [L.], *anterior; in front of.*

anteroclusion (an''ter-o-kloo'zhun) mesioclusion.

anterograde (an'ter-o-grād'') extending or moving forward.

anteroinferior (an''ter-o-in-fe're-or) situated in front and below.

anterolateral (-lat'er-al) situated in front and to one side.

anteromedian (-me'de-an) situated in front and toward the median plane.

anteroposterior (-pos-te're-or) directed from the front toward the back.

anterosuperior (-su-pe're-or) situated in front and above.

anteversion (an''te-ver'zhun) the tipping forward of an entire organ.

anthelix (ant'he-liks) the semicircular ridge on the flap of the ear, anteroinferior to the helix.

anthelmintic (ant''hel-min'tik) 1. destructive to worms. 2. an agent destructive to worms.

anthelone (ant-he'lōn) see *enterogastrone* (anthelone E) and *urogastrone* (anthelone U).

anthocyanin (an''tho-si'ah-nin) any of a class of glycoside pigments of blue, red, and violet flowers.

anthracene (an'thrah-sēn) 1. a crystalline hydrocarbon, $C_{14}H_{10}$, from coal tar. 2. a ptomaine from *Bacillus anthracis*.

anthracoid (an'thrah-koid) resembling anthrax or a carbuncle.

anthracometer (an''thrah-kom'ĕ-ter) an instrument for measuring carbon dioxide in the air.

anthraconecrosis (an''thrah-ko-nĕ-kro'sis) degeneration of tissue into a black mass.

anthracosilicosis (-sil''ĭ-ko'sis) a combination of anthracosis and silicosis.

anthracosis (an''thrah-ko'sis) pneumoconiosis, usually asymptomatic, due to deposition of coal dust in the lungs.

anthracotherapy (an''thrah-ko-ther'ah-pe) treatment with charcoal.

anthralin (an'thrah-lin) a compound, $C_{14}H_{10}O_3$, used topically in eczema and psoriasis.

anthramycin (an-thrah-mi'sin) an antineoplastic, $C_{16}H_{17}N_3O_4$, produced by *Streptomyces refuineus* var. *thermotolerans*.

anthraquinone (an''thrah-kwin'ōn) a yellow substance, $C_{14}H_8O_2$, from anthracene.

anthrax (an'thraks) an often fatal, infectious disease of ruminants due to ingestion of spores of *Bacillus anthracis* in soil; acquired by man through contact with contaminated wool or other animal products or by inhalation of airborne spores. **acute a.,** a usually rapidly fatal form with high fever, death occurring in a day or two. **apoplectic a.,** fulminant anthrax, so called because the symptoms resemble those of cerebral apoplexy **chronic a.,** a persistent form with local lesions confined to the tongue and throat. **cutaneous a.,** that due to inoculation of *Bacillus anthracis* into superficial wounds or abrasions of the skin, producing a black crusted pustule on a broad zone of edema. **industrial a.,** anthrax in man due to contact with wool, hair, hides, or other material from infected animals. **intestinal a.,** a severe form in which the intestine is affected. **localized a.,** cutaneous a. **pulmonary a.,** anthrax of the lungs due to inhalation of dust or animal hair containing anthrax spores; an occupational disease usually affecting those who handle and sort wools and fleeces. **symptomatic a.,** blackleg; a disease of sheep, cattle, and goats marked by emphysematous and subcutaneous swellings and nodules, due to *Clostridium chauvoei* and sometimes *C. septicum.*

anthropo- word element [Gr.], *man (human being)*.

anthropocentric (an″thro-po-sen′trik) with a human bias; considering man the center of the universe.

anthropoid (an′thro-poid) resembling man; the anthropoid apes are tailless apes, including the chimpanzee, gibbon, gorilla, and orang-utan.

Anthropoidea (an″thro-poi′de-ah) a suborder of Primates, including monkeys, apes, and man.

anthropokinetics (an″thro-po-ki-net′iks) study of the total human being in action, including biological and physical, psychologic and sociologic aspects.

anthropology (an″thro-pol′o-je) the science that treats of man, his origins, historical and cultural development, and races.

anthropometer (-pom′ĕ-ter) an instrument designed for measuring various body dimensions.

anthropometry (-pom′ĕ-tre) the science dealing with measurement of the size, weight, and proportions of the human body. **anthropomet′ric,** adj.

anthropomorphism (an″thro-po-mor′fizm) the attribution of human characteristics to nonhuman objects.

anthropophilic (-fil′ik) preferring man to animals; said of mosquitoes.

anthropozoonosis (-zo″o-no′sis) a disease of either animals or man that may be transmitted from one to the other.

anthysteric (ant″his-ter′ik) antihysteric.

anti- word element [Gr.], *counteracting; effective against.*

antiabortifacient (an″tĭ-ah-bor″tĭ-fa′shent) 1. preventing abortion or promoting gestation. 2. an antiabortifacient agent.

antiadrenergic (-ah-dren-er″jik) 1. sympatholytic: opposing the effects of impulses conveyed by adrenergic postganglionic fibers of the sympathetic nervous system. 2. an antiadrenergic agent.

antiagglutinin (-ah-gloo′tĭ-nin) a substance that opposes the action of an agglutinin.

antialbumin (-al-bu′min) a precipitin from albumin.

antialexin (-ah-lek′sin) a substance which opposes the action of alexin (complement).

antiamebic (-ah-me′bik) 1. destroying or suppressing the growth of amebas. 2. an agent having such properties.

antiamylase (-am′ĭ-lās) a substance counteracting the action of amylase.

antianaphylactin (-an″ah-fi-lak′tin) an antibody which counteracts anaphylactin.

antianaphylaxis (-an″ah-fi-lak′sis) a condition in which the anaphylaxis reaction does not occur because of free antigens in the blood; the state of desensitization to antigens.

antiandrogen (-an′dro-jen) any substance capable of inhibiting the biological effects of androgenic hormones.

antianemic (-ah-ne′mik) 1. counteracting anemia. 2. an agent that so acts.

antiantibody (-an′tĭ-bod″e) an immunoglobulin formed in the body after administration of anti-body acting as immunogen, and which interacts with the latter.

antiarrhythmic (-ah-rith′mik) 1. preventing or alleviating cardiac arrhythmias. 2. an agent that so acts.

antiarthritic (-ar-thrit′ik) antarthritic.

antibacterial (-bak-te′re-al) destroying or suppressing growth or reproduction of bacteria; also, an agent having such properties.

antibechic (-bek′ik) 1. relieving cough. 2. an agent that relieves cough.

antibiosis (-bi-o′sis) an antagonist association between organisms based on the production of an antibiotic.

antibiotic (-bi-ot′ik) a chemical substance produced by a microorganism, which has the capacity to inhibit the growth of or to kill other microorganisms; antibiotics sufficiently nontoxic to the host are used in the treatment of infectious diseases. **broad-spectrum a.,** one effective against a wide range of bacteria. **macrolide a.,** one characterized by a lactone ring, a ketone function, commonly an α-β unsaturated system, and a deoxyamino sugar containing a dimethylamino group. **polyene a.,** one having the general structure $(CH=CH)_n$, and containing large lactone rings; active againt a variety of fungi.

antibiotin (-bi′o-tin) avidin.

antiblennorrhagic (-blen″o-raj′ik) 1. preventing or relieving gonorrhea. 2. an agent that so acts.

antibody (an′tĭ-bod″e) an immunoglobulin molecule having a specific amino acid sequence by virtue of which it interacts only with the antigen that induced its synthesis in lymphoid tissue, or with antigen closely related to it; antibodies are classified according to their mode of action as agglutinins, bacteriolysins, hemolysins, opsonins, precipitins, etc. See *immunoglobulin.* **anaphylactic a.,** a substance formed as a result of the first injection of an anaphylactogen and responsible for the anaphylactic symptoms following the second injection of the same anaphylactogen. **blocking a.,** one which has the same specificity as one from another source and interferes with the reactivity of the other by combining available epitopes. **cytophilic a., cytotropic a.,** any of a class of antibodies that attach to tissue cells (such as mast cells and basophils) through their Fc segments to induce the release of histamine and other vasoconstrictive amines important in immediate hypersensitivity reactions. In man this antibody, also known as *reagin,* is of the immunoglobulin class IgE. Cytotropic antibodies derived from the same species are called *homocytotropins,* or *homocytotropic* or *allocytophilic a's;* those from different species, *heterocytotropins,* or *heterocytotropic* or *xenocytophilic a's.* **Forssman a.,** an antibody produced by injecting rabbits with sheep erythrocytes, saline solutions containing guinea pig kidney, or other tissues containing Forssman antigen. **inhibiting a.,** blocking a. **neutralizing a.,** one which, on mixture with the homologous infectious agent, reduces the infectious titer. **Prausnitz-Küstner a's,** homocytotropic antibodies of the immunoglobulin class IgE responsible for cutaneous anaphylaxis; abbreviated P-K a's. See *reagin*. **protective a.,** one responsible for immunity to an infectious agent observed in passive immunity. **reaginic a.,** reagin. **7S a's,** those with a sedimentation coefficient of 7S, inluding all those of immunoglobulin classes IgG and IgD and some of class IgA. **sensitizing a.,** anaphylactic a.

antibrachium (an″tĭ-bra′ke-um) antebrachium, or forearm.

anticalculous (-kal′ku-lus) suppressing the formation of calculi.

anticariogenic (-kār″e-o-jen′ik) effective in suppressing caries production.

anticarious (-ka′re-us) anticariogenic.

anticheirotonus (-ki-rot′o-nus) spasmodic flexion of the thumb.

anticholesteremic (-ko-les″ter-e′mik) promoting a reduction of cholesterol levels in the blood; also, any agent that so acts, e.g., the sitosterols and clofibrate.

anticholinergic (-ko″lin-er′jik) parasympatholytic: blocking the passage of impulses through the parasympathetic nerves; also, an agent that so acts.

anticholinesterase (-ko″lin-es′ter-ās) a substance that inhibits the action of cholinesterase.

anticlinal (-kli′nal) sloping or inclined in opposite directions.

anticoagulant (-ko-ag′u-lant) 1. acting to prevent clotting of blood. 2. any substance which suppresses, delays, or nullifies blood coagulation. **circulating a.,** a substance in the blood which inhibits normal blood clotting and may cause a hemorrhagic syndrome.

anticoagulin (-ko-ag′u-lin) a substance that suppresses, delays, or nullifies coagulation of the blood.

anticodon (-ko′don) a triplet of nucleotides in transfer RNA that is complementary to the codon in messenger RNA which specifies the amino acid.

anticomplement (-kom′plĕ-ment) a substance that counteracts a complement.

anticonvulsant, anticonvulsive (-kon-vul′-sant; -kon-vul′siv) 1. inhibiting convulsions. 2. an agent that suppresses convulsions.

anticus (an-ti′kus) [L.] anterior.

anticytolysin (an″tĭ-si-tol′ĭ-sin) a substance that counteracts cytolysin.

anticytotoxin (-si″to-tok′sin) a substance that counteracts cytotoxin.

antidepressant (-de-pres′sant) preventing or relieving depression; also, an agent that so acts.

antidiarrheal (-di″ah-re′al) counteracting diarrhea; also, an agent that so acts.

antidinic (-din′ik) relieving giddiness or vertigo.

antidiuresis (-di″u-re′sis) the suppression of secretion of urine by the kidneys.

antidiuretic (-di″u-ret′ik) 1. pertaining to or causing suppression of urine. 2. an agent that causes suppression of urine.

antidote (an′tĭ-dōt) an agent that counteracts a poison. **antido′tal,** adj. **chemical a.,** one that neutralizes the poison by changing its chemical nature. **mechanical a.,** one that prevents absorption of the poison. **physiologic a.,** one that counteracts the effects of the poison by producing opposing physiologic effects. **universal a.,** a mixture, considered by some to be useful in poisoning by acids, alkaloids, glycosides, and heavy metals, consisting of 2 parts activated charcoal, 1 part magnesium oxide, and 1 part tannic acid, given as $\frac{1}{2}$ oz. in a half glass of warm water, followed by gastric lavage or an emetic, except after ingestion of a corrosive substance.

antidromic (an″tĭ-drom′ik) conducting impulses in a direction opposite to the normal; said of neurons in the posterior roots of the spinal cord.

antidysenteric (-dis″en-ter′ik) preventing, alleviating, or curing dysentery; an agent that so acts.

antieczematic (-ek″zĕ-mat′ik) effective against eczema; an agent having such effects.

antiemetic (-e-met′ik) preventing or alleviating nausea and vomiting; also, an agent that so acts.

antienzyme (-en′zīm) an agent that prevents or retards the action of an enzyme.

antiepileptic (-ep″ĭ-lep′tik) combating epilepsy; an agent that so acts.

antiepithelial (-ep″ĭ-the′le-al) destructive to epithelial cells.

antiesterase (-es′ter-ās) an agent that inhibits or counteracts the activity of ester-hydrolyzing enzymes.

antifebrile (-feb′ril) antipyretic.

antifertilizin (-fer″tĭ-li′zin) a substance with which fertilizin reacts in agglutinating spermatozoa of certain marine vertebrates.

antifibrinolysin (-fi″brĭ-no-li′sin) an inhibitor of fibrinolysin.

antifibrinolytic (-fi″brĭ-no-lit′ik) inhibiting fibrinolysis.

antiflatulent (-flach′ŭ-lent) relieving or preventing flatulence; also, an agent that so acts.

antifungal (-fung′gal) 1. destructive to fungi; suppressing the growth or reproduction of fungi; effective against fungal infections. 2. an agent that so acts.

antigalactic (-gah-lak′tik) 1. diminishing secretion of milk. 2. an agent that tends to suppress milk secretion.

antigen (an′tĭ-jen) any substance capable of inducing antibody formation and of reacting specifically in some detectable manner with the antibodies so induced; antigens may be soluble (e.g., toxins and foreign proteins) or particulate (e.g., bacteria and tissue cells). **antigen′ic,** adj. **Au a., Australia a.,** an antigen found in the sera of patients with acute serum hepatitis and rarely in patients with infectious hepatitis; it is also found in the sera of large numbers of apparently normal people in the tropics and southeast Asia. So named because it was first detected in the serum of an Australian aborigine. **B a.,** an antigenic component of the K antigen complex. **beef heart a.,** an antigen for the Wassermann reaction made by extracting fresh normal beef heart tissue with absolute alcohol; hearts of guinea pigs, rabbits, and humans are also used. **blood group a's,** secreted soluble mucopolysaccharides possessing the H, A, and B haptenic structures characteristic of erythrocytes and some other body tissues. **capsular a.,** specific capsular substance. **carbohydrate a's,** numerous polysaccharides isolated from bacteria which function as specific haptens or as complete antigens. **carcinoembryonic a.,** a cancer-specific glycoprotein antigen of colon carcinoma, also present in many adenocarcinomas of endodermal origin and in normal gastrointestinal tissues of human embryos. **cholesterinized a.,** beef heart antigen to which has been added 0.4 per cent of cholesterol. **complete a.,** one which both stimulates an immune response and reacts with the products of that response. **conjugated a.,** one produced by coupling a hapten to a protein carrier molecule through covalent bonds; when it induces immunization, the resultant immune response is directed against both the hapten and the carrier. **D a.,** a red cell antigen of the Rh blood group system, important in the development of isoimmunization in Rh-negative persons exposed to the blood of Rh-positive persons. **E a.,** a red cell antigen of the Rh blood group system. **fetal a's,** antigens demonstrable during fetal life but not normally in adults; their reappearance in adults is attributed to reactivation of genes associated with cellular transformation to the malignant state. See also *fetoprotein*. **flagellar a.,** H antigen. **Forssman a.,** a heterogenetic antigen inducing the production of antisheep hemolysin, occurring in various unrelated species, mainly in the organs but not in the erythrocytes (guinea pig, horse), but sometimes only in the erythrocytes (sheep), and occasionally in both (chicken). **H a.** (Ger. *Hauch,* film), the antigen which occurs in the flagella of motile bacteria. **hepatitis a., hepatitis-associated a.,** Australia a. **heterogenetic a., heterologous a., heterophil a.,** an antigen common to more than one species and whose species distribution is unrelated to its phylogenetic distribution (viz., Forssman's antigen, lens protein, certain caseins, etc.). **histocompatibility a's,** genetically determined isoantigens found on the surface of nucleated cells of most tissues, which incite an immune response when grafted onto a genetically different individual and thus determine compatibility of tissues in transplantation. **HL-A a.,** histocompatibility antigens on the surface of nucleated cells determined by a single major chromosomal locus, the HL-A locus; they are important in cross-matching for transplantation procedures. **homologous a.,** isoantigen. **isogeneic a.,** an antigen carried by an individual which is capable of eliciting an immune response in genetically different individuals of the same species, but not in an individual bearing it. **isophil a.,** isoantigen. **K a's,** antigens that function as blocking antigens in that their presence interferes with agglutination with O antisera. **O a.** (Ger. *ohne Hauch,* without film), one occurring in the lipopolysaccharide layer of the wall of gram-negative bacteria. **organ-specific a.,** any antigen occurring only in a particular organ and serving to distinguish it from other organs; it may be limited to an organ of a single species or be characteristic of the same organ in many species. **partial a.,** hapten. **private a's,** antigens of the low frequency blood groups, probably differing from ordinary blood group systems only in their incidence. **public a's,** antigens of the high frequency blood groups, so called because they are found in almost all persons tested. **serum hepatitis a., SH a.,** Australia a. **somatic surface a's, K a's.** **T a.,** a nonstructural, complement-fixing viral antigen synthesized in the early stage of the infectious cycle; it persists in cells that have been modified by oncogenic adenoviruses. **tumor-specific a.,** cell-surface antigens of tumors that elicit a specific immune response in the host; abbreviated TSA. **V a., Vi a.,** an antigen contained in the capsule of a bacterium, as the typhoid bacillus, and thought to contribute to its virulence.

antigenemia (an″tĭ-jĕ-ne′me-ah) the presence of antigens in the blood.

antigenicity (-jĕ-nis′ĭ-te) ability of a substance to stimulate antibody formation.

antiglobulin (-glob′u-lin) a substance that opposes the action of a globulin.

antigoitrogenic (-goi″tro-jen′ik) inhibiting the development of goiter.

antihallucinatory (-hal-lu′sĭ-nah-to″re) counteracting hallucinogenesis; suppressing hallucinations.

antihelix (-he′liks) anthelix.

antihelmintic (-hel-min′tik) anthelmintic.

antihemolysin (-he-mol′ĭ-sin) any agent that opposes the action of a hemolysin.

antihemorrhagic (-hem″o-raj′ik) 1. exerting a hemostatic effect; counteracting hemorrhage. 2. an agent that so acts.

antihidrotic (-hi-drot′ik) anhidrotic.

antihistamine (-his′tah-min) a drug that counteracts the effect of histamine.

antihistaminic (-his″tah-min′ik) counteracting the effect of histamine; also, a drug that so acts.

antihormone (-hor′mōn) a substance which counteracts a hormone.

antihypercholesterolemic (-hi″per-ko-les′ter-ol-e″mik) 1. effective against hypercholesterolemia. 2. an agent that prevents or relieves hypercholesterolemia.

antihypertensive (-ten′siv) counteracting high blood pressure; also, an agent that reduces high blood pressure.

antihysteric (-his-ter′ik) preventing or relieving hysteria; also, agent that so acts.

anti-icteric (-ik″ter′ik) relieving icterus.

anti-immune (-ĭ-mūn′) preventing immunity.

anti-infective (-in-fek′tiv) 1. counteracting infection. 2. a substance that so acts.

anti-inflammatory (-in-flam′ah-to″re) counteracting or suppressing inflammation; also, an agent that so acts.

anti-isolysin (-i-sol′ĭ-sin) a substance that counteracts an isolysin.

antikenotoxin (-ke″no-tok′sin) a substance that inhibits the action of kenotoxin.

antiketogenesis (-ke″to-jen′ĕ-sis) inhibition of the formation of ketone bodies.

antiketogenic (-ke″to-jen′ik) preventing or inhibiting the formation of ketone bodies.

antilactase (-lak′tās) a substance that counteracts lactase.

antileukocytic (-lu″ko-sit′ik) destructive to white blood corpuscles (leukocytes).

antilewisite (-lu′ĭ-sīt) dimercaprol.

antilipemic (-li-pe′mik) counteracting high levels of lipids in the blood; also an agent that so acts.

antilithic (-lith′ik) preventing calculus formation; also, an agent that so acts.

antilysin (-li′sin) a substance that opposes the action of a lysin.

antilysis (-li′sis) inhibition of lysis.

antilytic (-lit′ik) 1. pertaining to antilysis. 2. inhibiting or preventing lysis.

antimalarial (-mah-la′re-al) 1. therapeutically effective against malaria. 2. an agent having such effects.

antimere (an′tĭ-mēr) one of the segments of the body bounded by planes at right angles to the long axis of the body.

antimetabolite (an″tĭ-mĕ-tab′o-līt) a substance bearing a close structural resemblance to one required for normal physiological functioning, and exerting its effect by interfering with the utilization of the essential metabolite.

antimetropia (-mĕ-tro′pe-ah) hyperopia of one eye, with myopia in the other.

antimongoloid (-mon′go-loid) having a feature opposite to one characteristic of Down's syndrome (mongolism), e.g., antimongoloid slant of the palpebral fissures.

antimony (an′tĭ-mo″ne) chemical element (see table), at no. 51, symbol Sb, forming various medicinal and poisonous salts; ingestion of antimony compounds, and rarely industrial exposure to them, may produce symptoms similar to acute arsenic poisoning, with vomiting a prominent symptom. **antimo′nial**, adj. **a. potassium tartrate**, a compound used in treatment of parasitic infections, e.g., schistosomiasis or leishmaniasis. **a. sodium thioglycollate**, sodium antimonyl-thioglycollate. **tartrated a.**, a. potassium tartrate.

antimorph (-morf) a mutant gene that acts to antagonize or inhibit the influence of its allele. **antimor′phic**, adj.

antimycotic (-mi-kot′ik) suppressing the growth of fungi; antifungal.

antinarcotic (-nar-kot′ik) counteracting narcotic depression.

antinauseant (-naw′ze-ant) 1. counteracting nausea. 2. an agent that so acts.

antineoplastic (-ne″o-plas′tik) 1. inhibiting or preventing development of neoplasms; checking maturation and proliferation of malignant cells. 2. an agent having such properties.

antinephritic (-nĕ-frit′ik) counteracting nephritis.

antineuralgic (-nu-ral′jik) relieving neuralgia.

antineuritic (-nu-rit′ik) relieving neuritis.

antinion (ant-in′e-on) the frontal pole of the head; the median frontal point farthest from the inion.

antiodontalgic (an″tĭ-o-don-tal′jik) relieving toothache.

antiopsonin (-op′so-nin) a substance having an inhibitory influence on opsonins.

antiovulatory (-ov′u-lah-to″re) suppressing ovulation.

antioxidant (-ok′sĭ-dant) a substance added to a product to prevent or delay its deterioration by the oxygen in air.

antioxidation (-ok″sĭ-da′shun) prevention of oxidation.

antiparalytic (-par″ah-lit′ik) relieving paralytic symptoms.

antiparasitic (-par″ah-sit′ik) 1. destroying parasites. 2. an agent that destroys parasites.

antipediculotic (-pĕ-dik″u-lot′ik) 1. effective against lice. 2. an agent effective against lice.

antipepsin (-pep′sin) an antienzyme that inhibits the action of pepsin.

antiperiodic (-pe″re-od′ik) preventing periodic recurrence of symptoms, as occurs in malaria.

antiperistalsis (-per″ĭ-stal′sis) reversed peristalsis. **antiperistal′tic**, adj.

antiplasmin (-plaz′min) a substance in the blood that inhibits plasmin.

antiplastic (-plas′tik) 1. unfavorable to healing. 2. an agent that suppresses formation of blood or other cells.

antiprotease (-pro′te-ās) a substance that checks the proteolytic action of enzymes.

antiprothrombin (-pro-throm′bin) an anticoagulant that retards the conversion of prothrombin into thrombin.

antiprotozoal (-pro″to-zo′al) lethal to protozoa, or checking their growth or reproduction; also, an agent that so acts.

antiprotozoan (-pro″to-zo′an) antiprotozoal.

antipruritic (-proo-rit′ik) 1. preventing or relieving itching. 2. an agent that counteracts itching.

antipsoriatic (-so″re-at′ik) effective againt psoriasis; an agent effective against psoriasis.

antipsychotic (-si-kot′ik) neuroleptic (1).

antipyretic (-pi-ret′ik) relieving or reducing fever; also, an agent that so acts.

antipyrine (-pi′rēn) an analgesic, $C_{11}H_{12}N_2O$.

antipyrotic (-pi-rot′ik) 1. effective in the treatment of burns. 2. an agent used in the treatment of burns.

antirachitic (-rah-kit′ik) therapeutically effective against rickets.

antiradiation (-ra″de-a′shun) capable of counteracting the effects of radiation; effective against radiation injury.

antirheumatic (-roo-mat′ik) relieving or preventing rheumatism; also, an agent that so acts.

antirickettsial (-rĭ-ket′se-al) effective against rickettsiae; also, an agent having such effects.

antiscabietic (-ska″be-et′ik) effective against scabies; also, an agent having such effects.

antiscorbutic (-skor-bu′tik) effective in the prevention or relief or scurvy.

antisepsis (-sep′sis) prevention of sepsis by the

inhibition or destruction of the causative organism.

antiseptic (-sep′tik) 1. preventing sepsis. 2. a substance that inhibits the growth and development of microorganisms but does not necessarily kill them.

antiserum (-se′rum) a serum containing antibody(ies), obtained from an animal immunized either by injection of antigen or by infection with microorganisms containing antigen.

antisialagogue (-si-al′ah-gog) counteracting saliva formation; also, an agent that inhibits flow of saliva. **antisialagog′ic,** adj.

antisialic (-si-al′ik) checking the flow of saliva; also, an agent that so acts.

antispasmodic (-spaz-mod′ik) 1. preventing or relieving spasms. 2. an agent that so acts.

Antistine (an-tis′tin) trademark for preparations of antazoline.

antistreptococcic (an″ti-strep″to-kok′sik) antagonistic to streptococci.

antisudoral, antisudorific (-soo′dor-al; -su″-dor-if′ik) inhibiting perspiration; also an agent that so acts.

antisympathetic (-sim″pah-thet′ik) 1. producing effects resembling those of interruption of the sympathetic nerve supply. 2. an agent that produces such effects.

antisyphilitic (-sif″ĭ-lit′ik) 1. effective against syphilis. 2. a remedy for syphilis.

antithenar (-the′nar) placed opposite to the palm or sole.

antithrombin (-throm′bin) any naturally occurring or therapeutically administered substance that neutralizes the action of thrombin and thus limits or restricts blood coagulation.

antithromboplastin (-throm″bo-plas′tin) any agent or substance that prevents or interferes with the interaction of blood coagulation factors as they generate prothrombinase (thromboplastin).

antithyroid (-thi′roid) counteracting thyroid functioning, especially in its synthesis of thyroid hormones.

antitoxin (-tok′sin) antibody produced in response to a toxin of bacterial (usually an exotoxin), animal (zootoxin), or plant (phytotoxin) origin, which neutralizes the effects of the toxin. **antitox′ic,** adj. **botulism a.,** a sterile solution of antitoxic substances from blood serum or plasma of healthy horses immunized against toxins of both types of *Clostridium botulinum.* **diphtheria a.,** a sterile solution of refined and concentrated antibody globulins from the blood serum or plasma of a healthy animal (usually the horse) immunized against diphtheria toxin. **gas gangrene a.,** a sterile solution of antibody globulins from the blood of horses immunized against toxins of certain species of pathogenic clostridia. **scarlet fever streptococcus a.,** a sterile solution of antitoxic substances (i.e., immunoglobulins) from the serum of healthy animals immunized against toxin from the streptococci causing scarlet fever. **tetanus a.,** a sterile solution of refined and concentrated antibody globulins from blood serum or plasma of a healthy animal (usually the horse) immunized

against tetanus toxin or toxoid. **tetanus and gas gangrene a's,** a sterile solution of antitoxic substances (immunoglobulins) from the blood of healthy animals immunized against the toxins of *Clostridium tetani, C. perfringens,* and *C. septicum.*

antitragus (-tra′gus) a projection on the ear opposite the tragus.

antitrichomonal (-trich″o-mo′nal) effective against *Trichomonas;* also, an agent having such effects.

antitrope (an′tĭ-trōp) one of two symmetrical but oppositely oriented structures. **antitrop′ic,** adj.

antitrypanosomal (an″tĭ-trĭ-pan″o-so′mal) effective against trypanosomes; also, an agent having such effects.

antitrypsin (-trip′sin) a substance that inhibits the action of trypsin. **antitryp′tic,** adj. **alpha₁-a.,** a blood plasma protein which inhibits trypsin activity; it is a glycoprotein synthesized in the liver and forming the main component of serum $alpha_1$-globulin. Deficiency of this protein, an inherited defect, is associated with pulmonary emphysema and with liver disease.

antitryptase (-trip′tās) a substance that inhibits or counteracts the action of tryptase.

antituberculin (-tu-ber′ku-lin) an antibody developed after injection of tuberculin into the body.

antituberculotic (-tu-ber″ku-lot′ik) effective in the treatment of tuberculosis; also, an agent having such properties.

antitussive (-tus′siv) 1. effective against cough. 2. an agent that suppresses coughing.

antivenereal (-vĕ-ne′re-al) counteracting venereal disease.

antivenin (-ven′in) a material used in treatment of poisoning by animal venom. **black widow spider (Latrodectus mactans) a.,** an antitoxic serum prepared by immunizing horses against venom of the black widow spider. **a. (Crotalidae) polyvalent, crotaline a.,** polyvalent, a serum containing specific venom-neutralizing globulin, produced by hyperimmunization of horses with venoms of the fer-de-lance and the Florida, Texas, and tropical rattlesnakes, used for treatment of envenomation by most pit vipers throughout the world.

antiviral (-vi′ral) destroying viruses or suppressing their replication; also, an agent that so acts.

antixerophthalmic (-ze″rof-thal′mik) counteracting xerophthalmia.

antixerotic (-ze-rot′ik) counteracting or preventing dryness.

antizymotic (-zi-mot′ik) inhibiting or suppressing the action of enzymes.

antr(o)- word element [L.], *chamber; cavity;* often used with specific reference to the maxillary antrum or sinus.

antrectomy (an-trek′to-me) excision of an antrum.

Antrenyl (an′trĕ-nil) trademark for a preparation of oxyphenonium.

antritis (an-tri′tis) inflammation of an antrum, chiefly of the maxillary antrum (sinus).

antroatticotomy (an′′tro-at′′ĭ-kot′o-me) attico-antrotomy.

antrocele (an′tro-sēl) cystic accumulation of fluid in the maxillary antrum.

antronasal (an′′tro-na′zal) pertaining to the maxillary antrum and nasal fossa.

antroscope (an′tro-skōp) an instrument for inspecting the maxillary antrum (sinus).

antrostomy (an-tros′to-me) opening of an antrum for drainage.

antrotomy (an-trot′o-me) incision of an antrum.

antrotympanic (an′′tro-tim-pan′ik) pertaining to the tympanic (mastoid) antrum and tympanum.

antrotympanitis (-tim′′pah-ni′tis) inflammation of the tympanic (mastoid) antrum and tympanum.

antrum (an′trum), pl. *an′tra* [L.] a cavity or chamber. **an′tral**, adj. **a. of Highmore,** maxillary sinus. **mastoid a., a. mastoi′deum,** an air space in the mastoid portion of the temporal bone communicating with the tympanic cavity and the mastoid cells. **a. maxilla′re, maxillary a.,** maxillary sinus. **pyloric a., a. pylor′icum,** the dilated portion of the pyloric part of the stomach, between the body of the stomach and pyloric canal. **tympanic a., a tympan′icum,** mastoid a.

Anturane (an′tu-rān) trademark for a preparation of sulfinpyrazone.

anuclear (a-nu′kle-ar) having no nucleus.

anulus (an′u-lus), pl. *an′uli* [L.] NA spelling of *annulus;* used in names of certain ringlike or encircling structures of the body.

anuresis (an′′u-re′sis) 1. retention of urine in the bladder. 2. anuria. **anuret′ic,** adj.

anuria (ah-nu′re-ah) complete suppression of urine formation by the kidney. **anu′ric,** adj.

anus (a′nus) the opening of the rectum on the body surface; the distal orifice of the alimentary canal. **imperforate a.,** congenital absence of the anal canal or persistence of the anal membrane so that the anus is closed, either completely or partially.

anvil (an′vil) incus.

anxiety (ang-zi′ĕ-te) a feeling of apprehension, uncertainty, and fear without apparent stimulus, associated with physiological changes (tachycardia, sweating, tremor, etc.). **free-floating a.,** fear in the absence of known cause for anxiety. **neurotic a.,** that in which the apprehension is objectively out of proportion to any apparent cause. **separation a.,** apprehension due to removal of significant persons or familiar surroundings, common in infants six to 10 months old.

A.O.A. American Optometric Association; American Orthopaedic Association; American Orthopsychiatric Association; American Osteopathic Association.

A.O.P.A. American Orthotics and Prosthetics Association.

aorta (a-or′tah), pl. *aor′tae, aor′tas*[Gr.] the great artery arising from the left ventricle, being the main trunk from which the systemic arterial system proceeds; see *Table of Arteries* for parts of aorta, and see Plate VIII. **overriding a.,** a congenital anomaly occurring in tetralogy of Fallot, in which the aorta is displaced to the right so that it appears to arise from both ventricles and straddles the ventricular septal defect.

aortal (a-or′tal) aortic.

aortalgia (a′′or-tal′je-ah) pain in the region of the aorta.

aortic (a-or′tik) of or pertaining to the aorta.

aorticopulmonary (a-or′′tĭ-ko-pul′mo-ner′′e) pertaining to or lying between the aorta and pulmonary artery.

aortitis (a′′or-ti′tis) inflammation of the aorta.

aortogram (a-or′to-gram) the film produced by aortography.

aortography (a′′or-tog′rah-fe) radiography of the aorta after introduction into it of a contrast material.

aortopathy (a′′or-top′ah-the) any disease of the aorta.

aortorrhaphy (a′′or-tor′ah-fe) suture of the aorta.

aortosclerosis (a-or′′to-skle-ro′sis) sclerosis of the aorta.

aortotomy (a′′or-tot′o-me) incision of the aorta.

A.O.S. American Ophthalmological Society; American Otological Society.

A.O.T.A. American Occupational Therapy Association.

A.P.A. American Pharmaceutical Association; American Physiotherapy Association; American Psychiatric Association; American Psychoanalytic Association; American Psychological Association; American Psychopathological Association.

apallesthesia (ah-pal′′es-the′ze-ah) pallanesthesia.

Apamide (ap′ah-mīd) trademark for a preparation of acetaminophen.

apancrea (ah-pan′kre-ah) absence of the pancreas.

apancreatic (ah-pan′′kre-at′ik) due to absence of the pancreas.

aparalytic (ah′′par-ah-lit′ik) without paralysis.

apathic (ah-path′ik) without sensation or feeling.

apathism (ap′ah-thizm) slowness of response to stimuli.

apathy (ap′ah-the) lack of feeling or emotion; indifference. **apathet′ic,** adj.

APC abbreviation for acetylsalicylic acid, acetophenetidin, and caffeine, used as an analgesic or antipyretic.

APE anterior pituitary extract.

apellous (ah-pel′us) 1. skinless; not covered with skin; not cicatrized (said of a wound). 2. having no prepuce.

aperient (ah-pe′re-ent) a mild laxative or gentle purgative.

aperistalsis (ah′′per-ĭ-stal′sis) absence of peristaltic action.

apertognathia (ah-per″tog-na′the-ah) open bite.

apertura (ap″er-tu′rah), pl. *apertu′rae* [L.] aperture.

aperture (ap′er-chūr) an opening or orifice. **numerical a.,** an expression of the measure of efficiency of a microscope objective.

apex (a′peks), pl. *a′pices* [L.] tip; the pointed end of a conical part; the top of a body, organ, or part. **ap′ical,** adj. **root a.,** the terminal end of the root of the tooth.

A.P.H.A. American Public Health Association.

A.Ph.A. American Pharmaceutical Association.

aphacia (ah-fa′se-ah) aphakia.

aphagia (ah-fa′je-ah) loss of the power of swallowing.

aphakia (ah-fa′ke-ah) absence of the lens of an eye, occurring congenitally or as a result of trauma or surgery. **apha′kic,** adj.

aphalangia (ah″fah-lan′je-ah) absence of fingers or toes.

aphasia (ah-fa′zhe-ah) defect or loss of the power of expression by speech, writing, or signs, or of comprehending spoken or written language, due to injury or disease of the brain centers. For types of aphasia not given below, see *agrammatism, anomia, paragrammatism,* and *paraphasia.* **apha′sic,** adj. **amnestic a.,** anomic a. **anomic a.,** amnestic or nominal aphasia; inability to name objects, qualities, or conditions. **ataxic a.,** expressive a. **auditory a.,** word deafness; loss of the ability to comprehend spoken language. **Broca's a.,** expressive a. **conduction a.,** aphasia due to lesion of the path between sensory and motor speech centers. **expressive a.,** that in which the patient understands written and spoken words and knows what he wishes to say, but cannot utter the words. **fluent a.,** that in which speech is well articulated and grammatically correct but is lacking in content. **gibberish a.,** jargon a. **global a.,** total aphasia involving all the functions which go to make up speech or communication. **jargon a.,** that with utterance of meaningless phrases. **mixed a.,** global a. **motor a.,** expressive a. **nominal a.,** anomic a. **nonfluent a.,** that in which little speech is produced and is uttered slowly, with great effort and poor articulation; due to a lesion in Broca's area. **receptive a.,** inability to understand written, spoken, or tactile speech symbols. **sensory a.,** receptive a. **total a.,** global a. **visual a.,** word blindness; loss of ability to comprehend written language.

aphasiologist (ah-fa″ze-ol′o-jist) one who specialized in aphasiology, as a neurologist or psychologist.

aphasiology (-ol′o-je) the scientific study of aphasia and the specific neurologic lesions producing it.

aphasmid (a-faz′mid) any nematode that does not possess phasmids.

aphemia (ah-fe′me-ah) loss of power of speech due to a central lesion; see *expressive aphasia.*

aphonia (a-fo′ne-ah) loss of voice; inability to produce vocal sounds. **a. clerico′rum,** see under *dysphonia.*

aphonic (a-fon′ik) 1. pertaining to aphonia. 2. without audible sound.

aphose (ah′fōz) any subjective visual sensation (phose) due to absence or interruption of light sensation.

aphotic (a-fōt′ik) without light; totally dark.

aphrasia (ah-fra′zhe-ah) inability to speak.

aphrenia (ah-fre′ne-ah) dementia.

aphrodisiac (af″ro-diz′e-ak) 1. arousing sexual desire. 2. a drug that arouses sexual desire.

aphtha (af′thah), pl. *aph′thae* [L.] (usually plural) small ulcers, especially the whitish or reddish spots in the mouth characteristic of aphthous stomatitis. **aph′thous,** adj. **Bednar's a.,** an infected traumatic ulcer on the posterior hard palate in infants. **contagious aphthae, epizootic aphthae,** foot-and-mouth disease.

aphthosis (af-tho′sis) a condition marked by the presence of aphthae.

aphylaxis (a″fi-lak′sis) absence of phylaxis or immunity. **aphylac′tic,** adj.

apical (ap′i-kal) pertaining to an apex.

apicectomy (a″pĭ-sek′to-me) excision of the apex of the petrous portion of the temporal bone.

apicitis (-si′tis) inflammation of an apex, as of the lung or the root of a tooth.

apicoectomy (-ko-ek′to-me) excision of the apical portion of the root of a tooth through an opening in overlying tissues of the jaw.

apicolysis (a″pĭ-kol′ĭ-sis) surgical collapse of the apex of the lung to obliterate the apical cavity.

A.P.L. trademark for a preparation of human chorionic gonadotropin.

aplacental (a″plah-sen′tal) having no placenta.

aplanatic (ap″lah-nat′ik) correcting spherical aberration, as an aplanatic lens.

aplasia (ah-pla′zhe-ah) lack of development of an organ or tissue, or of the cellular products from an organ or tissue. **aplas′tic,** adj. **a. axia′lis extractica′lis congen′ita,** familial centrolobar sclerosis. **a. cu′tis congen′ita,** localized failure of development of skin, most commonly of the scalp; the defects are usually covered by a thin translucent membrane or scar tissue, or may be raw, ulcerated, or covered by granulation tissue. **nuclear a.,** Möbius' syndrome.

A.P.M. Academy of Physical Medicine; Academy of Psychosomatic Medicine.

apnea (ap′ne-ah) 1. cessation of breathing. 2. asphyxia. **apne′ic,** adj.

apneumia (ap-nu′me-ah) congenital absence of the lungs.

apneusis (ap-nu′sis) sustained inspiratory effort unrelieved by expiration; it follows excision of the pneumotaxic center of the pons. **apneu′stic,** adj.

apo- word element [Gr.], *away from; separated; derived from.*

apochromat (ap″o-kro′mat) an apochromatic objective.

apochromatic (-kro-mat′ik) free from chromatic and spherical aberrations.

apocrine (ap′o-krīn) exhibiting that type of glandular secretion in which the free end of the secreting cell is cast off along with the secretory products accumulated therein (e.g., mammary and sweat glands).

apodia (ah-po′de-ah) congenital absence of one or both feet.

apoenzyme (ap″o-en′zīm) the protein component of an enzyme separable from the prosthetic group (coenzyme) but requiring the presence of the prosthetic group to form the functioning compound (holoenzyme).

apoferritin (-fer′ĭ-tin) a colorless protein in the mucosa of the small intestine, forming a compound with iron called *ferritin.*

apogee (ap′o-je) the state of greatest severity of a disease.

apolar (ah-po′lar) having neither poles nor processes; without polarity.

apomorphine (ap″o-mor′fēn) a morphine derivative, $C_{17}H_{17}NO_2$, used as a potent and prompt emetic; also used as the hydrochloride salt.

aponeurectomy (-nu-rek′to-me) excision of an aponeurosis.

aponeurorrhaphy (-nu-ror′ah-fe) suture of an aponeurosis.

aponeurosis (-nu-ro′sis), pl. *aponeuro′ses* [Gr.] a sheetlike tendinous expansion, mainly serving to connect a muscle with the parts it moves. **aponeurot′ic,** adj.

aponeurositis (-nu-ro-si′tis) inflammation of an aponeurosis.

aponeurotomy (-nu-rot′o-me) incision of an aponeurosis.

apophyseal (-fiz′e-al) pertaining to or of the nature of an apophysis.

apophysis (ah-pof′ĭ-sis), pl. *apoph′yses* [Gr.] any outgrowth or swelling, especially a bony outgrowth that has never been entirely separated from the bone of which it forms a part, such as a process, tubercle, or tuberosity.

apophysitis (ah-pof″ĭ-zi′tis) inflammation of an apophysis.

apoplectiform (ap″o-plek′tĭ-form) resembling apoplexy.

apoplexy (ap′o-plek″se) 1. sudden neurologic impairment due to a cerebrovascular disorder, limited classically to intracranial hemorrhage, but extended by some to include occlusive cerebrovascular lesions; see *stroke syndrome.* 2. copious extravasation of blood within any organ. **apoplec′tic,** adj. **adrenal a.,** sudden massive hemorrhage into the adrenal gland, occurring in Waterhouse-Friderichsen syndrome. **pancreatic a.,** extensive hemorrhage of the pancreas; seen in cardiac failure and portal hypertension.

aporepressor (ap″o-re-pres′or) in genetic theory, a product of regulator genes that combines with the corepressor to form the complete repressor.

apostasis (ah-pos′tah-sis) 1. an abscess. 2. the end or crisis of an attack or disease.

aposthia (-the-ah) congenital absence of the prepuce.

apothecary (ah-poth′ĕ-ka′re) pharmacist.

apotripsis (ap″o-trip′sis) removal of a corneal opacity.

apozymase (-zi′mās) that portion of a zymase which requires the presence of a cozymase to become a complete zymase.

apparatus (ap″ah-ra′tus) an arrangement of a number of parts acting together to perform a special function. **Abbe-Zeiss a.,** Thoma-Zeiss counting chamber. **absorption a.,** an apparatus used in gas analysis. **acoustic a., auditory a.,** the organ of hearing; see Plate XII. **Barcroft's a.,** a differential manometer for studying small samples of blood or other tissues. **Beckmann's a.,** an apparatus for determining molecular weight by lowering the freezing point or raising the boiling point of a solution. **Fell-O'Dwyer a.,** a device used in artificial respiration and for prevention of collapse of the lung in chest operations. **Golgi a.,** see under *complex.* **juxtaglomerular a.,** see under *cell.* **Kirschner's a.,** a wire and stirrup apparatus for applying skeletal traction in leg fractures. **lacrimal a., a. lacrima′lis,** the lacrimal gland and ducts and associated structures. **Sayre's a.,** an apparatus for suspending a patient during the application of a plaster of Paris jacket. **Soxhlet's a.,** an apparatus by which fatty or lipid constituents can be extracted from solid matter by repeated treatment with distilled solvent. **vasomotor a.,** the neuromuscular mechanism controlling the constriction and dilation of blood vessels, and thus the amount of blood supplied to a part.

appendage (ah-pen′dij) a subordinate portion of a structure, or an outgrowth, such as a tail. Also, a limb or limblike structure. **epiploic a's,** appendices epiploicae.

appendectomy (ap″en-dek′to-me) excision of the vermiform appendix.

appendicectomy (ah-pen″dĭ-sek′to-me) appendectomy.

appendicitis (-si′tis) inflammation of the vermiform appendix.

appendicolithiasis (-ko-lĭ-thi′ah-sis) formation of calculi in the vermiform appendix.

appendicolysis (-li′sis) surgical division of adhesions about the appendix.

appendicostomy (ah-pen″dĭ-kos′to-me) surgical creation of an opening into the vermiform appendix to irrigate or drain the large bowel.

appendicular (ap″en-dik′u-lar) 1. pertaining to an appendix or appendage. 2. pertaining to the limbs.

appendix (ah-pen′diks), pl. *appen′dices* [L.] 1. a supplementary, accessory, or dependent part attached to a main structure. 2. vermiform a. **auricular a.,** auricle (2). **appen′dices epiplo′icae,** small peritoneum-covered tabs of fat attached in rows along the teniae coli. **vermiform a., a. vermifor′mis,** a wormlike diverticulum of the cecum. **xiphoid a.,** see under *process.*

apperception (ap″er-sep′shun) the process of receiving, appreciating, and interpreting sensory impressions.

appestat (ap′pĕ-stat) the brain center (probably in the hypothalamus) concerned in controlling the appetite.

appetite (ap′ĕ-tīt) desire, chiefly desire for food.

applanometer (ap″lah-nom′ĕ-ter) a mechanical or electronic instrument for determining intraocular pressure in the detection of glaucoma; see *tonometer.*

appliance (ah-pli′ans) a device used for performing or for facilitating the performance of a particular function. **prosthetic a.,** a device affixed to or implanted in the body to substitute for or assist the function of a defective or missing body part or organ.

apposition (ap″o-zish′un) juxtaposition; the placing of things in proximity; specifically, the deposition of successive layers upon those already present, as in cell walls.

apprehension (ap″re-hen′shun) 1. perception and understanding. 2. anticipatory fear or anxiety.

approach (ah-prōch′) 1. in surgery, the specific procedures by which an organ or part is exposed. 2. in psychiatry, the manner in which personal conflicts are dealt with.

approximal (ah-prok′sĭ-mal) close together.

apraxia (ah-prak′se-ah) inability to perform purposeful movements in the absence of motor or sensory impairment, especially inability to use objects correctly. **amnestic a.,** loss of ability to carry out a movement on command due to inability to remember the command. **cortical a.,** motor a. **ideational a.,** sensory a. **innervation a., motor a.,** loss of ability to make proper use of an object, although its proper nature is recognized. **sensory a.,** loss of ability to make proper use of an object due to lack of perception of its purpose.

Apresoline (ah-pres′o-lēn) trademark for preparations of hydralazine.

aprobarbital (ap″ro-bar′bĭ-tal) a hypnotic and sedative, $C_{10}H_{14}N_2O_3$.

aproctia (ah-prok′she-ah) imperforate anus.

aprosopia (ap″ro-so′pe-ah) congenital absence, partial or complete, of facial structures.

aprosopus (ah-pros′o-pus) a fetus exhibiting aprosopia.

A.P.S. American Pediatric Society; American Physiological Society; American Proctologic Society; American Psychological Society; American Psychosomatic Society.

apsychia (ah-si′ke-ah) loss of consciousness.

A.P.T.A. American Physical Therapy Association.

aptyalism (ap-ti′ah-lizm) xerostomia; deficiency or absence of saliva.

apulmonism (ah-pul′mo-nizm) congenital absence, complete or partial, of a lung.

apus (a′pus) an individual without feet.

apyknomorphous (ah″pik-no-mor′fus) not having the stainable cell elements placed compactly; said of certain nerve cells.

apyogenous (ah″pi-oj′ĕ-nus) not caused by pus.

apyretic (a″pi-ret′ik) without fever; afebrile.

apyrexia (ah″pi-rek′se-ah) absence of fever.

apyrogenic (ah-pi″ro-jen′ik) not producing fever.

A.Q. acheivement quotient.

aq. [L.] *aq′ua* (water). **aq. dest.,** *aq′ua destilla′ta* (distilled water).

aqua (ak′wah) [L.] 1. water, H_2O. 2. a saturated solution of a volatile oil or other aromatic or volatile substance in purified water.

aquaphobia (ak″wah-fo′be-ah) morbid fear of water.

Aquatag (ak′wah-tag) trademark for a preparation of benzthiazide.

aqueduct (ak′we-dukt″) any canal or passage. **cerebral a.,** a narrow channel in the midbrain connecting the third and fourth ventricles. **a. of cochlea, cochlear a.,** cochlear canaliculus; a small canal in the petrous portion of the temporal bone that interconnects the scala tympani with the subarachnoid cavity. **sylvian a., a. of Sylvius, ventricular a.,** cerebral a.

aqueous (a′kwe-us) 1. watery; prepared with water. 2. see under *humor.*

Ar chemical symbol, *argon.*

A.R.A. American Rheumatism Association.

arachnid (ah-rak′nid) any member of the class Arachnida.

Arachnida (ah-rak′nĭ-dah) a class of the Arthropoda, including the spiders, scorpions, ticks, and mites.

arachnidism (-dizm) the systemic condition produced by the bite of a venomous spider.

arachnitis (ar″ak-ni′tis) arachnoiditis.

arachnodactyly (ah-rak″no-dak′tĭ-le) extreme length and slenderness of fingers and toes.

arachnoid (ah-rak′noid) 1. resembling a spider's web. 2. the delicate membrane interposed between the dura mater and the pia mater, and with them constituting the meninges.

arachnoiditis (ah-rak″noid-i′tis) inflammation of the arachnoid.

arachnophobia (ah-rak″no-fo′be-ah) morbid fear of spiders.

arachnopia (-pi′ah) the pia mater and arachnoid membrane together.

Aralen (ar′ah-len) trademark for a preparation of chloroquine.

Aramine (ar′ah-min) trademark for a preparation of metaraminol.

araphia (ah-ra′fe-ah) dysraphia. **ara′phic,** adj.

arbor (ar′bor), pl. *arbo′res* [L.] a treelike structure or part. **a. vi′tae,** 1. treelike outlines seen in a median section of the cerebellum. 2. palmate folds.

arborescent (ar″bo-res′ent) branching like a tree.

arborization (ar″bor-ĭ-za′shun) a collection of branches, as the branching terminus of a nerve-cell process.

arborvirus (-vi′rus) arbovirus.

arbovirus (ar″bo-vi′rus) any of a group of viruses, including the causative agents of yellow fever, viral encephalitides, and certain febrile infections, transmitted to man by various mosquitoes and ticks; those transmitted by ticks are often considered in a separate category (tickborne viruses).

A.R.C. American Red Cross; anomalous retinal correspondence.

arc (ark) a structure or projected path having a curved or bowlike outline; by extension, a visible electrical discharge generally taking the outline of an arc. In neurophysiology, the pathway of neural reactions. **reflex a.,** the neural arc utilized in a reflex action; an impulse travels centrally over afferent fibers to a nerve center, and the response outward to an effector organ or part over efferent fibers; see Plate XIV.

arch (arch) a structure of bowlike or curved outline. **abdominothoracic a.,** the lower boundary of the front of the thorax. **a. of aorta,** the curving portion between the ascending aorta and the descending aorta, giving rise to the brachiocephalic trunk, the left common carotid and the left subclavian artery. **aortic a's,** paired vessels arching from the ventral to the dorsal aorta through the branchial clefts of fishes and amniote embryos. In mammalian development, arches 1 and 2 disappear; 3 joins the common to the internal carotid artery; 4 becomes the arch of the aorta and joins the aorta and subclavian artery; 5 disappears; 6 forms the pulmonary arteries and, until birth, the ductus arteriosus. **branchial a's,** paired arched columns that bear the gills in lower aquatic vertebrates and which, in embryos of higher vertebrates, become modified into structures of the ear and neck. **a's of Corti,** series of arches made up of rods of Corti. **costal a.,** the anterior portion of the inferior thoracic aperture, consisting of the costal cartilages of ribs 7 to 10, inclusive. **dental a.,** the curving structure formed by the teeth in their normal position; the *inferior dental a.* is formed by the mandibular teeth, the *superior dental a.* by the maxillary teeth. **double aortic a.,** a congenital anomaly in which the aorta divides into two branches which embrace the trachea and esophagus and reunite to form the descending aorta. **a's of foot,** the longitudinal and transverse arches of the foot. The longitudinal arch comprises the pars medialis, formed by the calcaneus, talus, and the navicular, cuneiform and first three tarsal bones; and the pars lateralis formed by the calcaneus, the cuboid bone, and the lateral two metatarsal bones. The transverse arch comprises the navicular, cuneiform, cuboid, and five metatarsal bones. **hemal a.,** the arch formed by the body, pedicles, and transverse processes of a vertebra, a pair of ribs and their costal cartilages, and the sternum. **hyoid a.,** the second branchial arch, from which are developed the styloid process, stylohyoid ligament, and lesser cornu of the hyoid bone. **lingual a.,** a wire appliance that conforms to the lingual aspect of the dental arch, used to promote or prevent movement of the teeth in orthodontic work. **mandibular a.,** 1. the first branchial arch, from which are developed the bone of the lower jaw, malleus, and incus. 2. inferior dental a. **maxillary a.,** 1. the palatal arch. 2. superior dental a. 3. residual dental a. **nasal a.,** one formed by the nasal bones and the nasal processes of the maxilla. **neural a.,** vertebral a. **open pubic a.,** a congenital anomaly in which the pubic arch is not fused, the bodies of the pubic bones being spread apart. **oral a., palatal a.,** one formed by the roof of the mouth from the teeth (or residual dental arch) on one side to those on the other. **palatomaxillary a.,** palatal a. **palmar a's,** two arches in the palm, one (*deep palmar a.*) formed by anastomosis of the terminal part of the radial artery with the deep branch of the ulnar, and the other (*superficial palmar a.*) by anastomosis of the terminal part of the ulnar artery with the superficial palmar branch of the radial. **passive lingual a.,** an orthodontic appliance for maintaining space and preserving arch length when bilateral primary molars are prematurely lost. **pharyngeal a's,** branchial a's. **plantar a.,** the arch in the foot formed by anastomosis of the lateral plantar artery with the deep plantar branch of the dorsal artery. **postaural a's,** branchial a's. **pubic a., a. of pubis,** the arch formed by the conjoined rami of the ischial and pubic bones on two sides of the body. **pulmonary a.,** the most caudal of the aortic arches, which become the pulmonary arteries. **residual dental a.,** the curved contour of the ridge remaining after tooth removal. **right aortic a.,** a congenital anomaly in which the aorta is displaced to the right and passes behind the esophagus, thus forming a vascular ring that may cause compression of the trachea and esophagus. **stationary lingual a.,** a lingual arch soldered to the anchor bands. **supraorbital a.,** curved margin of frontal bone forming upper boundary of orbit. **tarsal a's,** two arches of the median palpebral artery, one of which supplies the upper eyelid, the other the lower. **tendinous a.,** a linear thickening of fascia over some part of a muscle. **vertebral a.,** the bony arch composed of the laminae and pedicles of a vertebra. **visceral a's,** branchial a's. **zygomatic a.,** one formed by processes of zygomatic and temporal bones.

arch(i)- word element [Gr.], *ancient; beginning; first; original.*

archamphiaster (ark-am′fe-as″ter) the primitive amphiaster associated with polar body formation.

archencephalon (ark″en-sef′ah-lon) the primitive brain from which the midbrain and forebrain develop.

archenteron (ark-en′ter-on) the primitive digestive cavity of those embryonic forms whose blastula become a gastrula by invagination.

archeocyte (ar′ke-o-sīt″) any free or wandering ameboid cell.

archeokinetic (ar″ke-o-ki-net′ik) relating to the primitive type of motor nerve mechanism as seen in the peripheral and ganglionic nervous systems.

archespore (ar′kĕ-spōr) the mass of cells giving rise to spore mother cells.

archetype (-tīp) an ideal, original, or standard type or form.

archiblast (ar′kĭ-blast) 1. the components of an ovum that actively form the embryo. 2. His′ term for the fundamental part of the blastodermic layers as distinguished from the parablast or peripheral portion of the mesoderm. **archiblas′tic,** adj.

archigaster (ar″kĭ-gas′ter) archenteron.

archil (ar′kil) the lichen *Roccella tinctoria;* also,

a violet coloring matter from this and other lichens.

archinephron (ar″kĭ-nef′ron) a unit of the pronephros.

archineuron (-nu′ron) the neuron at which an efferent impulse starts.

archipallium (-pal′e-um) that part of the pallium (cerebral cortex) which, with the paleopallium, develops in association with the olfactory system and which is phylogenetically older than the neopallium and lacks its layered structure.

arciform (ar′sĭ-form) arcuate.

arctation (ark-ta′shun) narrowing of an opening or canal.

arcualia (ar″ku-a′le-ah) nodules of cartilage in the continuous mesenchymal sheath in close apposition to the external surface of the notochord in vertebrate embryos.

arcuate (ar′ku-āt) bow-shaped; arranged in arches.

arcuation (ar″ku-a′shun) a curvature, especially an abnormal curvature.

arcus (ar′kus), pl. *ar′cus* [L.] arch; bow. **a. adipo′sus,** a. senilis. **a. juveni′lis,** a condition identical to arcus senilis, except that it occurs congenitally or before or during middle life. **a. seni′lis,** a gray opaque line surrounding the margin of the cornea, but separated from the margin by an area of clear cornea, usually occurring bilaterally in persons of 50 years or older as a result of lipoid degeneration.

area (a′re-ah), pl. *a′reae, areas* [L.] a limited space; in anatomy, a specific surface or functional region. **association a's,** areas of the cerebral cortex (excluding primary areas) connected with each other and with the neothalamus; they are responsible for higher mental and emotional processes, including memory, learning, etc. **auditory a.,** a. vestibularis. **Bamberger's a.,** an area of cardiac dullness in the left intercostal region, suggestive of pericardial effusion. **Betz cell a.,** motor a. **Broca's motor speech a.,** an area comprising parts of the opercular and triangular portions of the inferior frontal gyrus; injury to this area may result in motor aphasia. **Broca's parolfactory a.,** a. subcallosa. **Brodmann's a's,** areas of the cerebral cortex distinguished by differences in arrangement of their six cellular layers; identified by numbering each area. **embryonic a.,** see under *disk.* **excitable a.,** a motor area. **germinal a., a. germinati′va,** embryonic disk. **impression a.,** the surface of the oral structures recorded in an impression. **Kiesselbach's a.,** one on the anterior part of the nasal septum above the intermaxillary bone, richly supplied with capillaries, and a common site of nosebleed. **motor a.,** that area of the cerebral cortex which, on brief electrical stimulation, shows the lowest threshold and shortest latency for the production of muscle movement. **a. opa′ca,** the outer opaque area of the embryonic disk, as seen in the bird egg. **a. pellu′cida,** the central clear part of the embryonic disk, as seen in the bird egg. **a. perfora′ta,** perforated space. **precentral a.,** motor a. **prefrontal a.,** the cortex of the frontal lobe immediately in front of the premotor cortex, concerned chiefly with associative functions. **premotor a.,** the motor cortex of the frontal lobe immediately in front of the precentral gyrus. **primary a's,** areas of the cerebral cortex comprising the motor and sensory regions; cf. *association a's.* **psychomotor a.,** motor a. **silent a.,** any area of the brain in which pathologic conditions may occur without producing symptoms. **a. subcallo′sa, subcallosal a.,** an area of the cortex on the medial surface of each cerebral hemisphere, immediately in front of the gyrus subcallosus. **thymus-dependent a's,** those areas of the peripheral lymphoid organs populated by the thymus-dependent lymphocytes, e.g., the pericortical areas of the lymph nodes, the centers of the malpighian corpuscle of the spleen, and the internodular zone of Peyer's patches. **thymus-independent a's,** those areas of the peripheral lymphoid organs populated by thymus-independent lymphocytes, e.g., the medullary and outer cortical regions of the lymph node. **a. vasculo′sa,** part of area opaca, where the blood vessels are first seen, as in the bird egg. **a. vestibula′ris,** the lateral and median part of the floor of the fourth ventricle over which pass the striae medullares. **a. vitelli′na,** the yolk area beyond the area vasculosa in mesoblastic eggs. **vocal a.,** the part of the glottis between the vocal cords.

areflexia (ah″re-flek′se-ah) absence of the reflexes.

arenavirus (ah″re-nah-vi′rus) any of a group of morphologically similar, ether-sensitive viruses which seem to contain RNA.

areola (ah-re′o-lah), pl. *are′olae* [L.] 1. any minute space or interstice in a tissue. 2. a circular area of different color surrounding a central point, as that surrounding the nipple of the breast. **Chaussier's a.,** the indurated area encircling a malignant pustule.

areolar (-lar) pertaining to or containing areolae; containing minute spaces.

Arfonad (ar′fon-ad) trademark for a preparation of trimethaphan camsylate.

Arg arginine.

Argas (ar′gas) a genus of ticks (family Argasidae), parasitic in poultry and other birds and sometimes man. **A. per′sicus,** the fowl tick, parasitic in chickens and turkeys, the vector of fowl spirochetosis.

Argasidae (ar-gas′ĭ-de) a family of arthropods (superfamily Ixodidea) made up of the soft-bodied ticks.

argentaffin (ar-jen′tah-fin) staining readily with silver and chromium salts; see also under *cell.*

argentaffinoma (ar″jen-taf″fĭ-no′mah) carcinoid, a tumor of the gastrointestinal tract formed from the argentaffin cells of the enteric canal and producing carcinoid syndrome.

argentation (-ta′shun) staining with silver.

argentic (ar-jen′tik) containing silver.

argentum (-tum) [L.] silver (symbol Ag).

argillaceous (ar″jĭ-la′shus) composed of clay.

arginase (ar′jĭ-nās) an enzyme existing primarily in the liver, which splits arginine into urea and ornithine.

arginine (-nin) an amino acid, $C_6H_{14}N_4O_2$, one of the hexone bases produced by hydrolysis or digestion of proteins.

argininosuccinate (ar″jĭ-nĭ″no-suk′sĭ-nāt) a compound formed by the condensation of aspartic acid and citrulline; an intermediate in the urea cycle.

argininosuccinicacidemia (-suk-sin″ik-as″ĭ-de′me-ah) presence in the blood of argininosuccinic acid.

argininosuccinicaciduria (-suk-sin″ik-as″ĭ-du′re-ah) excretion in the urine of argininosuccinic acid, a feature of an inborn error of metabolism marked also by mental retardation.

argon (ar′gon) chemical element (see table), at no. 18, symbol Ar.

argyria (ar-jĭ′re-ah) poisoning by silver or its salts; chronic argyria is marked by a permanent ashen-gray discoloration of the skin, conjunctivae, and internal organs.

argyric (-rik) pertaining to or caused by silver.

argyrism (ar′jĭ-rizm) argyria.

argyrophil (ar-ji′ro-fil) capable of binding silver salts.

argyrosis (ar″jĭ-ro′sis) argyria.

arhinia (ah-rin′e-ah) congenital absence of the nose.

ariboflavinosis (a-ri″bo-fla″vĭ-no′sis) deficiency of riboflavin in the diet, marked by angular cheilosis, nasolabial lesions, optic changes, and seborrheic dermatitis.

Aristocort (ah-ris′to-cort) trademark for a preparation of triamcinolone.

Arlidin (ar′lĭ-din) trademark for preparations of nylidrin.

arm (arm) 1. brachium: the upper extremity from shoulder to elbow; popularly, the entire extremity, from shoulder to hand. 2. an armlike part, e.g., the portion of the chromatid extending in either direction from the centromere of a mitotic chromosome. **bird a.,** a wasted condition of the forearm due to muscular atrophy.

armamentarium (ar″mah-men-ta′re-um) the equipment of a practitioner or institution, including books, instruments, medicines, and surgical appliances.

A.R.M.H. Academy of Religion and Mental Health.

Armillifer (ar-mil′lĭ-fer) a genus of wormlike endoparasites of reptiles; the larvae of A. armilla′tus and A. monilifor′mis are occasionally found in man.

arnica (ar′nĭ-kah) the dried flowerheads of Arnica montana, use topically as a tincture for contusions, sprains, and superficial wounds.

A.R.N.M.D. Association for Research in Nervous and Mental Disease.

A.R.O. Association for Research in Ophthalmology.

aromatic (ar″o-mat′ik) 1. having a spicy odor. 2. in chemistry, denoting a compound characterized by the benzene ring.

arousal (ah-row′sal) a state of responsiveness to sensory stimulation.

arrector (ah-rek′tor), pl. arrecto′res [L.] raising, or that which raises; an arrector muscle.

arrest (ah-rest′) cessation or stoppage, as of a function or a disease process. **cardiac a.,** sudden cessation of cardiac function. **epiphyseal a.,** premature interruption of longitudinal growth of bone by fusion of the epiphysis and diaphysis. **maturation a.,** interruption of the process of development, as of blood cells, before the final stage is reached. **sinus a.,** a pause in cardiac rhythm due to a momentary failure of the sinus node to initiate an impulse.

arrheno- word element [Gr.], male; masculine.

arrhenoblastoma (ah-re″no-blas-to′mah) a neoplasm of the ovary, sometimes causing virilization.

arrhinia (ah-rin′e-ah) arhinia.

arrhythmia (ah-rith′me-ah) variation from the normal rhythm of the heart beat. **arrhyth′mic,** adj. **sinus a.,** the physiologic cyclic variation in heart rate related to vagal impulses to the sinoatrial node; it occurs commonly in children and in the aged.

A.R.R.S. American Roentgen Ray Society.

A.R.S. American Radium Society.

arsenate (ar′sĕ-nāt) any salt of arsenic acid.

arseniasis (ar″sĭ-ni′ah-sis) chronic arsenic poisoning; see arsenic (1).

arsenic (ar′sĕ-nik) 1. a medicinal and poisonous element (see table), at. no. 33, symbol As. Acute arsenic poisoning may result in shock and death, with skin rashes, vomiting, diarrhea, abdominal pain, muscular cramps, and swelling of eyelids, feet, and hands; the chronic form, due to ingestion of small amounts of arsenic over long periods, is marked by skin pigmentation accompanied by scaling, hyperkeratosis of palms and soles, transverse lines on the fingernails, headache, peripheral neuropathy, and confusion. 2. arsenic trioxide. 3. pertaining to or containing arsenic in a pentavalent state. **a. trioxide,** white arsenic, As_2O_3, having a sweetish taste and erythropoietic effect.

arsenical (ar-sen′ĭ-kal) 1. pertaining to or containing arsenic. 2. a compound containing arsenic.

arsenicalism, arsenism (ar-sen′ĭ-kal-izm; ar′sen-izm) chronic arsenic poisoning; see arsenic (1).

arsenoblast (ar-sen′o-blast) the male element of a zygote; a male pronucleus.

arsenolysis (ar″sen-ol′ĭ-sis) the enzyme-induced, reversible combination and separation of sugar and arsenic acid.

arsenotherapy (ar″sĕ-no-ther′ah-pe) treatment with arsenic and arsenical compounds.

arsine (ar′sēn) a very poisonous gas, AsH_3; some of its compounds have been used in warfare.

arsphenamine (ars-fen′ah-min) a yellow hygroscopic powder containing arsenic, introduced as the first specific for the treatment of syphilis, yaws, and other spirillum infections; it has been replaced by other arsenicals and by antibiotics.

arsthinol (ars′thĭ-nol) an arsenical preparation, $C_{11}H_{14}A_2NO_3S_2$, used as an amebicide.

A.R.T. Accredited Record Technicians.

Artane (ar'tān) trademark for preparations of trihexyphenidyl hydrochloride.

artefact (ar'te-fakt) artifact.

arteralgia (ar''ter-al'je-ah) pain emanating from an artery, such as headache from an inflamed temporal artery.

arteria (ar-te're-ah), pl. *arte'riae* [L.] artery. **a. luso'ria,** an abnormally situated retroesophageal vessel, usually the subclavian artery from the aortic arch.

arteriectasis (ar-te''re-ek'tah-sis) dilatation and, usually, lengthening of an artery.

arteriectomy (-ek'to-me) excision of a portion of an artery.

arterio- word element [L., Gr.], *artery.*

arteriogram (ar-te're-o-gram'') a radiograph of an artery.

arteriograph (-graf) the film produced by arteriography.

arteriography (ar-te''re-og'rah-fe) radiography of an artery or arterial system after injection of a contrast medium into the blood stream. **catheter a.,** a radiography of vessels after introduction of contrast material through a catheter inserted into an artery. **selective a.,** radiography of a specific vessel which is opacified by a medium introduced directly into it, usually via a catheter.

arteriol(o)- word element [L.], *arteriole.*

arteriola (ar-te''re-o'lah), pl. *arterio'lae*[L.] arteriole. **arterio'lae rec'tae re'nis,** branches of the arcuate arteries of the kidney that supply the pyramids.

arteriole (ar-te're-ōl) a minute arterial branch. **arterio'lar,** adj. **glomerular a., afferent,** a branch of an interlobar artery that goes to a renal artery. **glomerular a., efferent,** one arising from a renal glomerulus, breaking up into capillaries to supply renal tubules. **postglomerular a.,** efferent glomerular a. **precapillary a's,** terminal arterioles that end in capillaries. **preglomerular a.,** afferent glomerular a. **straight a's,** arteriolae rectae renis.

arteriolith (ar-te're-o-lith'') a chalky concretion in an artery.

arteriolitis (ar-tēr''ĭ-o-li'tis) inflammation of the arterioles.

arteriology (ar-te''re-ol'o-je) the sum of knowledge regarding the arteries; the science or study of the arteries.

arteriolonecrosis (ar-te''re-o''lo-nĕ-kro'sis) necrosis or destruction of arterioles.

arteriolosclerosis (-skle-ro'sis) sclerosis and thickening of the walls of arterioles. The hyaline form may be associated with nephrosclerosis, the hyperplastic with malignant hypertension, nephrosclerosis, and scleroderma. **arteriolosclerot'ic,** adj.

arteriomotor (ar-te''re-o-mo'ter) involving or causing dilation or constriction of arteries.

arteriomyomatosis (-mi''o-mah-to'sis) growth of muscular fibers in the walls of an artery, causing thickening.

arterionecrosis (-nĕ-kro'sis) necrosis of arteries.

arteriopathy (ar-te''re-op'ah-the) any disease of an artery. **hypertensive a.,** widespread involvement, chiefly of arterioles and small arteries, associated with arterial hypertension and characterized primarily by hypertrophy of the tunica media.

arterioplasty (ar-te're-o-plas''te) surgical repair or reconstruction of an artery; applied especially to Matas' operation for aneurysm.

arteriopressor (-pres'or) increasing arterial blood pressure.

arteriorrhaphy (ar-te''re-or'ah-fe) suture of an artery.

arteriorrhexis (ar-te''re-o-rek'sis) rupture of an artery.

arteriosclerosis (-skle-ro'sis) a group of diseases characterized by thickening and loss of elasticity of the arterial walls occurring in three forms, atherosclerosis, Mönckeberg's arteriosclerosis, and arteriolosclerosis. **arteriosclerot'ic,** adj. **Mönckeberg's a.,** arteriosclerosis with extensive deposits of calcium in the middle coat of the artery. **a. oblit'erans,** that in which proliferation of the intima of the small vessels has caused complete obliteration of the lumen of the artery. **peripheral a.,** arteriosclerosis of the extremities. **senile a.,** arteriosclerosis occurring in old age.

arteriospasm (ar-te're-o-spazm'') spasm of an artery.

arteriostenosis (ar-te''re-o-stĕ-no'sis) constriction of an artery.

arteriosympathectomy (-sim''pah-thek'to-me) periarterial sympathectomy.

arteriotony (ar-te''re-ot'o-ne) blood pressure.

arteriovenous (ar-te''re-o-ve'nus) both arterial and venous; pertaining to or affecting an artery and a vein.

arteritis (ar''ter-i'tis) inflammation of an artery. **brachiocephalic a., a. brachiocephal'ica,** pulseless disease. **coronary a.,** inflammation of the coronary arteries. **a. oblit'erans,** endarteritis obliterans. **rheumatic a.,** generalized inflammation of arterioles and arterial capillaries occurring in rheumatic fever. **Takayasu's a.,** pulseless disease. **temporal a.,** a chronic disease of older persons, largely involving the carotid arterial system, marked by proliferative inflammation, often with giant cells and granulomas, and by headache, constitutional symptoms, and ocular involvement.

artery (ar'ter-e) a vessel in which blood flows away from the heart, in the systemic circulation carrying oxygenated blood. **arte'rial,** adj. For named arteries of the body, *see table,* and see Plates VIII and IX. **end a.,** one which undergoes progressive branching without development of channels connecting with other arteries.

arthr(o)- word element [Gr.], *joint; articulation.*

arthragra (ar-thrag'rah) gouty pain in a joint.

arthralgia (ar-thral'je-ah) pain in a joint.

arthrectomy (ar-threk'to-me) excision of a joint.

arthritide (ar'thrĭ-tīd) a skin eruption of gouty origin.

arthritis (ar-thri'tis) inflammation of a joint. **arthrit'ic,** adj. **acute a.,** arthritis marked by pain, heat, redness, and swelling. **atrophic a.,** rheu-

COMMON NAME*	NA EQUIVALENT†	ORIGIN*	BRANCHES*	DISTRIBUTION
accompanying a. of sciatic nerve. *See* sciatic a.				
acromiothoracic a. *See* thoracoacromial a.				
alveolar a's, anterior superior	aa. alveolares superiores anteriores	infraorbital a.	dental branches	incisor and canine regions of upper jaw, maxillary sinus
alveolar a., inferior	a. alveolaris inferior	maxillary a.	dental, mylohyoid branches, mental a.	lower jaw, lower lip, chin
alveolar a., posterior superior	a. alveolaris superior posterior	maxillary a.	dental branches	molar and premolar regions of upper jaw, maxillary sinus, buccinator muscle
angular a.	a. angularis	facial a.		lacrimal sac, lower eyelid, nose
aorta	aorta	left ventricle		
abdominal aorta	aorta abdominalis	lower portion of descending aorta, from aortic hiatus of diaphragm to bifurcation into common iliac a's	inferior phrenic, lumbar, median sacral, superior and inferior mesenteric, middle suprarenal, renal, and testicular or ovarian a's, celiac trunk	
arch of aorta	arcus aortae	continuation of ascending aorta	brachiocephalic trunk, left common carotid and left subclavian a's; continues as descending (thoracic) aorta	
ascending aorta	aorta ascendens	proximal portion of aorta, arising from left ventricle	right and left coronary a's; continues as arch of aorta	
descending aorta. *See* thoracic aorta; abdominal aorta	aorta descendens	continuation of arch of aorta		
thoracic aorta	aorta thoracica	proximal portion of descending aorta, continuing from arch of aorta to aortic hiatus of diaphragm	bronchial, esophageal, pericardiac, and mediastinal branches, superior phrenic a's, posterior intercostal a's [III–XI], subcostal a's; continues as abdominal aorta	
appendicular a.	a. appendicularis	ileocolic a.		vermiform appendix

*a. = artery; a's = (pl.) arteries.
†a. = [L.] arteria; aa. = [L. (pl.)] arteriae.

59

TABLE OF ARTERIES (*Continued*)

COMMON NAME*	NA EQUIVALENT†	ORIGIN*	BRANCHES*	DISTRIBUTION
arcuate a. of foot	a. arcuata pedis	dorsalis pedis a.	deep plantar branch, dorsal metatarsal a's	foot, toes
arcuate a's of kidney	aa. arcuatae renis	interlobar a.	interlobar a's, straight arterioles of kidney	parenchyma of kidney
auditory a., internal. *See* a. of labyrinth				
auricular a., deep	a. auricularis profunda	maxillary a.		skin of auditory canal, tympanic membrane, temporomandibular joint
auricular a., posterior	a. auricularis posterior	external carotid a.	auricular and occipital branches, stylomastoid a.	middle ear, mastoid cells, auricle, parotid gland, digastric and other muscles
axillary a.	a. axillaris	continuation of subclavian a.	subscapular branches, highest thoracic, thoroacoacromial, lateral thoracic, subscapular, and anterior and posterior circumflex humeral a's	upper limb, axilla, chest, shoulder
basilar a.	a. basilaris	from junction of right and left vertebral a's	pontine branches, anterior inferior cerebellar, labyrinthine, superior cerebellar, posterior cerebral a's	brain stem, internal ear, cerebellum, posterior cerebrum
brachial a.	a. brachialis	continuation of axillary a.	superficial and deep brachial, nutrient of humerus, superior and inferior ulnar collateral, radial, ulnar a's	shoulder, arm, forearm, hand
brachial a., deep	a. profunda brachii	brachial a.	nutrient to humerus, deltoid branch, middle and radial collateral a's	humerus, muscles and skin of arm
brachial a., superficial	a. brachialis superficialis	variant brachial a., taking a more superficial course than usual	see *brachial a.*	see *brachial a.*
brachiocephalic trunk	truncus brachiocephalicus	arch of aorta	right common carotid, right subclavian a's	right side of head and neck, right arm
buccal a.	a. buccalis	maxillary a.		buccinator muscle, oral mucous membrane
a. of bulb of penis a. of bulb of urethra. *See* a. of bulb of penis	a. bulbi penis	internal pudendal a.		bulbourethral gland, bulb of penis

a. of bulb of vestibule of vagina	a. bulbi vestibuli vaginae	internal pudendal a.	bulb of vestibule of vagina, Bartholin glands
carotid a., common	a. carotis communis	brachiocephalic trunk (right), arch of aorta (left)	see *carotid a., external* and *carotid a., internal*
carotid a., external	a. carotis externa	common carotid a.	neck, face, skull
			superior thyroid, ascending pharyngeal, lingual, facial, sternocleidomastoid, occipital, posterior auricular, superficial temporal, maxillary a's	
carotid a., internal	a. carotis interna	common carotid a.	middle ear, brain, hypophysis, orbit, choroid plexus of lateral ventricle
			caroticotympanic branches, ophthalmic, posterior communicating, anterior choroid, anterior cerebral, middle cerebral a's	
caudal a. *See* sacral a., median			
celiac trunk	truncus celiacus	abdominal aorta	esophagus, stomach, duodenum, spleen, pancreas, liver, gallbladder
			left gastric, common hepatic, splenic a's	
central a. of retina	a. centralis retinae	ophthalmic a.	retina
cerebellar a., inferior, anterior	a. cerebelli inferior anterior	basilar a.	lower anterior cerebellum, inner ear
			a. of labyrinth	
cerebellar a., inferior, posterior	a. cerebelli inferior posterior	vertebral a.	lower part of cerebellum, medulla, choroid plexus of fourth ventricle
cerebellar a., superior	a. cerebelli superior	basilar a.	upper part of cerebellum, midbrain, pineal body, choroid plexus of third ventricle
cerebral a., anterior	a. cerebri anterior	internal carotid a.	orbital, frontal, and parietal cortex, corpus callosum, diencephalon, corpus striatum, internal capsule, choroid, plexus of lateral ventricle
			cortical (orbital, frontal, parietal), anterior choroidal, and central branches (including medial striate a.), and anterior communicating a.	
cerebral a., middle	a. cerebri media	internal carotid a.	orbital, frontal, parietal, and temporal cortex, corpus striatum, internal capsule
			cortical (orbital, frontal, parietal, temporal) and central (striate) branches	
cerebral a., posterior	a. cerebri posterior	terminal bifurcation of basilar a.	occipital and temporal lobes, basal ganglia, choroid plexus of lateral ventricle, thalamus, midbrain
			cortical (temporal, occipital, parieto-occipital), central, and choroid branches	

61

COMMON NAME*	NA EQUIVALENT†	ORIGIN*	BRANCHES*	DISTRIBUTION
cervical a., ascending	a. cervicalis ascendens	inferior thyroid a.	spinal branches	muscles of neck, vertebrae, vertebral canal
cervical a., deep	a. cervicalis profunda	costocervical trunk		deep neck muscles
cervical a., transverse	a. transversa colli	subclavian a.	deep and superficial branches	root of neck, muscles of scapula
choroid a., anterior	a. choroidea anterior	internal carotid or middle cerebral a.		choroid plexus of lateral ventricle and adjacent parts
ciliary a's, anterior	aa. ciliares anteriores	ophthalmic and lacrimal a's	episcleral and anterior conjunctival a's	iris, conjunctiva
ciliary a's, posterior, long	aa. ciliares posteriores longae	ophthalmic a.		iris, ciliary processes
ciliary a's, posterior, short	aa. ciliares posteriores breves	ophthalmic a.		choroid coat of eye
circumflex femoral a., lateral	a. circumflexa femoris lateralis	deep femoral a.	ascending, descending, and transverse branches	hip joint, thigh muscles
circumflex femoral a., medial	a. circumflexa femoris medialis	deep femoral a.	deep, ascending, transverse, and acetabular branches	hip joint, thigh muscles
circumflex humeral a., anterior	a. circumflexa humeri anterior	axillary a.		shoulder joint and caput humeri, long tendon of biceps, tendon of greater pectoral muscle
circumflex humeral a., posterior	a. circumflexa humeri posterior	axillary a.		deltoid, shoulder joint, teres minor, and triceps muscles
circumflex iliac a., deep	a. circumflexa ilium profunda	external iliac a.	ascending branches	iliac region, abdominal wall, groin
circumflex iliac a., superficial	a. circumflexa ilium superficialis	femoral a.		groin, abdominal wall
circumflex a. of scapula	a. circumflexa scapulae	subscapular a.		inferolateral muscles of scapula
coccygeal a. *See* sacral a., median				
colic a., left	a. colica sinistra	inferior mesenteric a.		descending colon
colic a., middle	a. colica media	superior mesenteric a.		transverse colon
colic a., right	a. colica dextra	superior mesenteric a.		ascending colon
colic a., right, inferior. *See* ileocolic a.				
colic a., superior accessory. *See* colic a., middle				
collateral a., inferior ulnar	a. collateralis ulnaris inferior	brachial a.		arm muscles at back of elbow

collateral a., middle	a. collateralis media	deep brachial a.		triceps muscle, elbow joint brachioradial and brachial muscles
collateral a., radial	a. collateralis radialis	deep brachial a.		elbow joint, triceps muscle
collateral a., superior ulnar	a. collateralis ulnaris superior	brachial a.		
communicating a., anterior	a. communicans anterior cerebri	interconnects anterior cerebral a's		
communicating a., posterior	a. communicans posterior cerebri	interconnects internal carotid and posterior cerebral a's		
conjunctival a's, anterior	aa. conjunctivales anteriores	anterior ciliary a's		conjunctiva
conjunctival a's, posterior	aa. conjunctivales posteriores	medial palpebral a.		lacrimal caruncle, conjunctiva
coronary a., left	a. coronaria sinistra	left aortic sinus	anterior interventricular and circumflex branches	left ventricle, left atrium
coronary a., right	a. coronaria dextra	right aortic sinus	posterior interventricular branch	right ventricle, right atrium
costocervical trunk	truncus costocervicalis	subclavian a.	deep cervical and highest intercostal a's	deep neck muscles, first two intercostal spaces, vertebral column, back muscles
cremasteric a.	a. cremasterica	inferior epigastric a.		cremaster muscle, coverings of spermatic cord
cystic a.	a. cystica	right branch of hepatic a., proper		gallbladder
deep brachial. *See* brachial a., deep				
deep a. of clitoris	a. profunda clitoridis	internal pudendal a.		clitoris
deep a. of penis	a. profunda penis	internal pudendal a.		corpus cavernosum penis
deep femoral a. *See* femoral a., deep				
deep lingual a. *See* profunda linguae a.				
deferential a. *See* a. of ductus deferens				
dental a's. *See* alveolar a's				
diaphragmatic a's. *See* phrenic a's				
digital a's, collateral. *See* digital a's, palmar, proper				

TABLE OF ARTERIES (*Continued*)

COMMON NAME*	NA EQUIVALENT†	ORIGIN*	BRANCHES*	DISTRIBUTION
digital a's of foot, common. *See* metatarsal a's, plantar				
digital a's of foot, dorsal	aa. digitales dorsales pedis	dorsal metatarsal a's		dorsum of toes
digital a's of hand, dorsal	aa. digitales dorsales manus	dorsal metacarpal a's		dorsum of fingers
digital a's, palmar, common	aa. digitales palmares communes	superficial palmar arch	proper palmar digital a's	fingers
digital a's, palmar, proper	aa. digitales palmares propriae	common palmar digital a's		fingers
digital a's, plantar, common	aa. digitales plantares communes	plantar metatarsal a's	proper plantar digital a's	toes
digital a's, plantar, proper	aa. digitales plantares propriae	common plantar digital a's		toes
dorsal a. of clitoris	a. dorsalis clitoridis	internal pudendal a.		clitoris
dorsal a. of foot. *See* dorsalis pedis a.				
dorsal a. of nose	a. dorsalis nasi	ophthalmic a.	lacrimal branch	dorsum of nose
dorsal a. of penis	a. dorsalis penis	internal pudendal a.		glans, corona, and prepuce of penis
dorsalis pedis a.	a. dorsalis pedis	continuation of anterior tibial a.	lateral and medial tarsal, and arcuate a's	foot, toes
a. of ductus deferens	a. ductus deferentis	umbilical a.	ureteral artery	ureter, ductus deferens, seminal vesicles, testes
duodenal a's. *See* pancreaticoduodenal a., inferior				
epigastric a., external. *See* circumflex iliac a., deep				
epigastric a., inferior	a. epigastrica inferior	external iliac a.	pubic branch, cremasteric a., a. of round ligament of uterus	abdominal wall
epigastric a., superficial	a. epigastrica superficialis	femoral a.		abdominal wall, groin
epigastric a., superior	a. epigastrica superior	internal thoracic a.		abdominal wall, diaphragm
episcleral a's	aa. episclerales	anterior ciliary a.		iris, ciliary processes
ethmoidal a., anterior	a. ethmoidalis anterior	ophthalmic a.	anterior meningeal a.	dura mater, nose, frontal sinus, anterior ethmoidal cells

	NA Term	Origin	Branches	Distribution
ethmoidal a., posterior	a. ethmoidalis posterior	ophthalmic a.		posterior ethmoidal cells, dura mater, nose
facial a.	a. facialis	external carotid a.	ascending palatine, submental, inferior and superior labial and angular a's; tonsillar and glandular branches	face, tonsil, palate, submandibular gland
facial a., deep. *See* maxillary a.				
facial a., transverse	a. transversa faciei	superficial temporal a.		parotid region
fallopian a. *See* uterine a.				
femoral a.	a. femoralis	continuation of external iliac a.	superficial epigastric, superficial circumflex iliac, external pudendal, profunda femoris, and descending genicular a's	lower abdominal wall, external genitalia, lower limb
femoral a., deep	a. profunda femoris	femoral a.	medial and lateral circumflex femoral a's, perforating a's	thigh muscles, hip joint, gluteal muscles, femur
fibular a. *See* peroneal a.				
frontal a. *See* supratrochlear a.				
funicular a. *See* testicular a.				
gastric a., left	a. gastrica sinistra	celiac trunk	esophageal branches	esophagus, lesser curvature of stomach
gastric a., right	a. gastrica dextra	common hepatic a.		lesser curvature of stomach
gastric a's, short	aa. gastricae breves	splenic a.		upper part of stomach
gastroduodenal a.	a. gastroduodenalis	common hepatic a.	superior pancreaticoduodenal and right gastroepiploic a's	stomach, duodenum, pancreas, greater omentum
gastroepiploic a., left	a. gastroepiploica sinistra	splenic a.	epiploic branches	stomach, greater omentum
gastroepiploic a., right	a. gastroepiploica dextra	gastroduodenal a.	epiploic branches	stomach, greater omentum
genicular a., descending	a. genus descendens	femoral a.	saphenous and articular branches	knee joint, upper and medial part of leg
genicular a., inferior, lateral	a. genus inferior lateralis	popliteal a.		knee joint
genicular a., inferior, medial	a. genus inferior medialis	popliteal a.		knee joint
genicular a., middle	a. genus media	popliteal a.		knee joint, cruciate ligaments, patellar synovial and alar folds
genicular a., superior, lateral	a. genus superior lateralis	popliteal a.		knee joint, femur, patella, contiguous muscles
genicular a., superior, medial	a. genus superior medialis	popliteal a.		knee joint, femur, patella, contiguous muscles

TABLE OF ARTERIES (*Continued*)

COMMON NAME*	NA EQUIVALENT†	ORIGIN*	BRANCHES*	DISTRIBUTION
gluteal a., inferior	a. glutea inferior	internal iliac a.	sciatic a.	buttock, back of thigh
gluteal a., superior	a. glutea superior	internal iliac a.	superficial and deep branches	buttocks
helicine a's of penis	aa. helicinae penis	deep and dorsal a's of penis		erectile tissue of penis
hemorrhoidal a's. *See rectal a's*				
hepatic a., common	a. hepatica communis	celiac trunk	right gastric, gastroduodenal, proper hepatic a's	stomach, pancreas, duodenum, liver, gallbladder, greater omentum
hepatic a., proper	a. hepatica propria	common hepatic a.	right and left branches	liver, gallbladder
hyaloid a.	a. hyaloidea	fetal ophthalmic a.		fetal lens (usually not present after birth)
hypogastric a. *See iliac a., internal*				
ileal a's	aa. ilei	superior mesenteric a.		ileum
ileocolic a.	a. ileocolica	superior mesenteric a.	ascending, anterior, and posterior cecal branches, appendicular a.	ileum, cecum, vermiform appendix, ascending colon
iliac a., common	a. iliaca communis	abdominal aorta	internal and external iliac a's	pelvis, abdominal wall, lower limb
iliac a., external	a. iliaca externa	common iliac a.	inferior epigastric, deep circumflex iliac a's	abdominal wall, external genitalia, lower limb
iliac a., internal	a. iliaca interna	continuation of common iliac a.	iliolumbar, obturator, superior and inferior gluteal, umbilical, inferior vesical, uterine, middle rectal, and internal pudendal a's	wall and viscera of pelvis, buttock, reproductive organs, medial aspect of thigh
iliolumbar a.	a. iliolumbalis	internal iliac a.	iliac and lumbar branches, lateral sacral a's	pelvic muscles and bones, fifth lumbar vertebra, sacrum
infraorbital a.	a. infraorbitalis	maxillary a.	anterior superior alveolar a's	maxilla, maxillary sinus, upper teeth, lower eyelid, cheek, nose
innominate a. *See brachiocephalic trunk*				
intercostal a., highest	a. intercostalis suprema	costocervical trunk	posterior intercostal a's I and II	upper thoracic wall
intercostal a's, posterior, I and II	aa. intercostales posteriores I et II	highest intercostal a.	dorsal and spinal branches	upper thoracic wall
intercostal a's, posterior, III–XI	aa. intercostales posteriores III–XI	thoracic aorta	dorsal, lateral, and lateral cutaneous branches	thoracic wall
interlobar a's of kidney	aa. interlobares renis	renal a.		lobes of kidney
interlobular a's of kidney	aa. interlobulares renis	arcuate a's of kidney	arcuate a's of kidney	renal glomeruli

66

interlobular a's of liver	aa. interlobulares hepatis	right or left branch of proper hepatic a.		between lobules of liver
interosseous a., anterior	a. interossea anterior	posterior or common interosseous a.	median a.	deep parts of front of forearm
interosseous a., common	a. interossea communis	ulnar a.	anterior and posterior interosseous a's	antecubital fossa
interosseous a., posterior	a. interossea posterior	common interosseous a.		deep parts of back of forearm
interosseous a., recurrent	a. interossea recurrens	posterior or common interosseous a.	recurrent interosseous a.	back of elbow joint
intestinal a's		vessels arising from superior mesenteric a. and supplying intestines; they include pancreaticoduodenal, jejunal, ileal, ileocolic, and colic a's		
jejunal a's	aa. jejunales	superior mesenteric a.		jejunum
labial a., inferior	a. labialis inferior	facial a.		lower lip
labial a., superior	a. labialis superior	facial a.	septal and alar branches	upper lip and nose
a. of labyrinth	a. labyrinthi	basilar or anterior inferior cerebellar a.	vestibular and cochlear branches	internal ear
lacrimal a.	a. lacrimalis	ophthalmic a.	lateral palpebral a.	lacrimal gland, eyelids, conjunctiva
laryngeal a., inferior	a. laryngea inferior	inferior thyroid a.		larynx, trachea, esophagus
laryngeal a., superior	a. laryngea superior	superior thyroid a.		larynx
lingual a.	a. lingualis	external carotid a.	suprahyoid, sublingual, dorsal lingual, profunda linguae branches	tongue, sublingual gland, tonsil, epiglottis
lingual a., deep. See profunda linguae a.				
lumbar a's	aa. lumbales	abdominal aorta	dorsal and spinal branches	posterior abdominal wall, renal capsule
lumbar a., lowest	a. lumbalis ima	median sacral a.		sacrum, greatest gluteal muscle
malleolar a., anterior, lateral	a. malleolaris anterior lateralis	anterior tibial a.		ankle joint
malleolar a., anterior, medial	a. malleolaris anterior medialis	anterior tibial a.		ankle joint
mammary a., external. See thoracic a., lateral				
mammary a., internal. See thoracic a., internal				

TABLE OF ARTERIES (*Continued*)

COMMON NAME*	NA EQUIVALENT†	ORIGIN*	BRANCHES*	DISTRIBUTION
mandibular a. *See* alveolar a., inferior				
masseteric a.	a. masseterica	maxillary a.		masseter muscle
maxillary a.	a. maxillaris	external carotid a.	pterygoid branches; deep auricular, anterior tympanic, inferior alveolar, middle meningeal, masseteric, deep temporal, buccal, posterior superior alveolar, infraorbital, descending palatine, and sphenopalatine a's, and a. of pterygoid canal	both jaws, teeth, muscles of mastication, ear, meninges, nose, paranasal sinuses, palate
maxillary a., external. *See* facial a.				
maxillary a., internal. *See* maxillary a.				
median a.	a. mediana	anterior interosseous a.		median nerve, muscles of front of forearm
meningeal a., anterior	a. meningea anterior	anterior ethmoidal a.		dura mater of anterior cranial fossa
meningeal a., middle	a. meningea media	maxillary a.	frontal, parietal, lacrimal, anastomotic, accessory meningeal, and petrous branches, and superior tympanic a.	cranial bones, dura mater
meningeal a., posterior	a. meningea posterior	ascending pharyngeal a.		bones and dura mater of posterior cranial fossa
mental a.	a. mentalis	inferior alveolar a.		chin
mesenteric a., inferior	a. mesenterica inferior	abdominal aorta	left colic, sigmoid, and superior rectal a's	descending colon, rectum
mesenteric a., superior	a. mesenterica superior	abdominal aorta	inferior pancreaticoduodenal, jejunal, ileal, ileocolic, right and middle colic a's	small intestine, proximal half of colon
metacarpal a's, dorsal	aa. metacarpeae dorsales	dorsal carpal rete and radial a.	dorsal digital a's	dorsum of fingers
metacarpal a's, palmar metatarsal a's, dorsal metatarsal a's, plantar	aa. metacarpeae palmares aa. metatarseae dorsales aa. metatarseae plantares	deep palmar arch arcuate a. of foot plantar arch	dorsal digital a's perforating branches, common and proper plantar digital a's	deep parts of metacarpus dorsum of foot, including toes plantar surface of toes
musculophrenic a.	a. musculophrenica	internal thoracic a.		diaphragm, abdominal and thoracic walls

Artery	NA Term	Origin	Branches	Distribution
nasal a's, posterior, lateral and septal	aa. nasales posteriores laterales et septi	sphenopalatine a.		nasal cavity, nasal septum, adjacent sinuses
nutrient a's of humerus	aa. nutriciae humeri	brachial and deep brachial a's		humerus
obturator a.	a. obturatoria	internal iliac a.	pubic, acetabular, anterior and posterior branches	pelvic muscles, hip joint
obturator a., accessory	a. obturatoria accessoria	variant obturator a., arising from inferior epigastric instead of internal iliac a.		
occipital a.	a. occipitalis	external carotid a.	auricular, meningeal, mastoid, descending, occipital, and sternocleidomastoid branches	muscles of neck and scalp, meninges, mastoid cells
ophthalmic a.	a. ophthalmica	internal carotid a.	lacrimal and supraorbital a's, central a. of retina, ciliary, posterior and anterior ethmoidal, palpebral, supratrochlear, and dorsal nasal a's	eye, orbit, adjacent facial structures
ovarian a.	a. ovarica	abdominal aorta	ureteral branches	ureter, ovary, uterine tube
palatine a., ascending	a. palatina ascendens	facial a.		soft palate, wall of pharynx, tonsil, auditory tube
palatine a's, descending	a. palatina descendens	maxillary a.	greater and lesser palatine a's	soft and hard palates, tonsil
palatine a., greater	a. palatina major	descending palatine a.		hard palate
palatine a's, lesser	aa. palatinae minores	descending palatine a.		soft palate, tonsil
palpebral a's, lateral	aa. palpebrales laterales	lacrimal a.		eyelids, conjunctiva
palpebral a's, medial	aa. palpebrales mediales	ophthalmic a.	posterior conjunctival a's	eyelids
pancreaticoduodenal a's, inferior	aa. pancreaticoduodenales inferiores	superior mesenteric a.		pancreas, duodenum
pancreaticoduodenal a., superior	a., pancreaticoduodenalis superior	gastroduodenal a.		pancreas, duodenum
perforating a's	aa. perforantes	deep femoral a.		adductor, hamstring, and gluteal muscles, femur
pericardiacophrenic a.	a. pericardiacophrenica	internal thoracic a.		pericardium, diaphragm, pleura
perineal a.	a. perinealis	internal pudendal a.		perineum, skin of external genitalia
peroneal a.	a. peronea	posterior tibial a.	perforating, communicating, calcaneal, and lateral and medial malleolar branches, calcaneal rete	lateral side and back of ankle, deep calf muscles
pharyngeal a., ascending	a. pharyngea ascendens	external carotid a.	posterior meningeal, pharyngeal, inferior tympanic branches	pharynx, soft palate, ear, meninges

TABLE OF ARTERIES (*Continued*)

COMMON NAME*	NA EQUIVALENT†	ORIGIN*	BRANCHES*	DISTRIBUTION
phrenic a's, great. *See* phrenic a's, inferior				
phrenic a's, inferior	aa. phrenicae inferiores	abdominal aorta	superior suprarenal a's	diaphragm, suprarenal gland
phrenic a's, superior	aa. phrenicae superiores	thoracic aorta		upper surface of vertebral portion of diaphragm
plantar a., lateral	a. plantaris lateralis	posterior tibial a.	plantar arch, plantar metatarsal a's	sole of foot, toes
plantar a., medial	a. plantaris medialis	posterior tibial a.		sole of foot, toes
popliteal a.	a. poplitea	continuation of femoral a.	deep and superficial branches lateral and medial superior genicular, middle genicular, sural, lateral and medial inferior genicular, anterior and posterior tibial a's; articular rete of knee, patellar rete	knee and calf
princeps pollicis a.	a. princeps pollicis	radial a.	radialis indicis a.	sides and palmar aspect of thumb
principal a. of thumb. *See* princeps pollicis a.				
profunda linguae a.	a. profunda linguae	lingual a.		tongue
a. of pterygoid canal	a. canalis pterygoidei	maxillary a.		roof of pharynx, auditory tube
pudendal a's, external	aa. pudendae externae	femoral a.	anterior scrotal or anterior labial branches, inguinal branches	external genitalia, upper medial thigh
pudendal a., internal	a. pudenda interna	internal iliac a.	posterior scrotal or posterior labial branches, inferior rectal, perineal, urethral a's, a. of bulb of penis or vestibule, deep a. and dorsal a. of penis or clitoris	external genitalia, anal canal, perineum
pulmonary trunk	truncus pulmonalis	right ventricle	right and left pulmonary a's	conveys unaerated blood toward lungs
pulmonary a., left	a. pulmonalis sinistra	pulmonary trunk	numerous branches named according to segments of lung to which they distribute unaerated blood	left lung
pulmonary a., right	a. pulmonalis dextra	pulmonary trunk	numerous branches named according to segments of lung to which they distribute unaerated blood	right lung
radial a.	a. radialis	brachial a.	palmar carpal, superficial palmar and dorsal carpal branches; recurrent radial a., princeps pollicis a., deep palmar arch	forearm, wrist, hand

Common Name	NA Term	Origin	Branches	Distribution
radial a., collateral. *See* collateral a., radial				
radial a. of index finger. *See* radialis indicis a.				
radialis indicis a.	a. radialis indicis	princeps pollicis a.		index finger
radiate a's of kidney. *See* interlobular a's of kidney				
ranine a. *See* profunda linguae a.				
rectal a., inferior	a. rectalis inferior	internal pudendal a.		rectum, anal canal
rectal a., middle	a. rectalis media	internal iliac a.		rectum
rectal a., superior	a. rectalis superior	inferior mesenteric a.		rectum
recurrent a., radial	a. recurrens radialis	radial a.		brachioradial and brachial muscles, elbow region
recurrent a., tibial, anterior	a. recurrens tibialis anterior	anterior tibial a.		anterior tibial muscle and long extensor muscle of toes; knee joint, contiguous fascia and skin
recurrent a., tibial, posterior	a. recurrens tibialis posterior	anterior tibial a.		knee
recurrent a., ulnar	a. recurrens ulnaris	ulnar a.		elbow region
renal a.	a. renalis	abdominal aorta	anterior and posterior branches, ureteral branches, inferior suprarenal a.	kidney, suprarenal gland, ureter
renal a's. *See* arcuate, interlobar, and interlobular a's, and straight arterioles of kidney	aa. renis			
a. of round ligament of uterus	a. ligamenti teretis uteri	inferior epigastric a.		round ligament of uterus
sacral a's, lateral	aa. sacrales laterales	iliolumbar a.	spinal branches	structures about coccyx and sacrum
sacral a., median	a. sacralis mediana	central continuation of abdominal aorta, beyond origin of common iliac a's	lowest lumbar a.	sacrum, coccyx, rectum
scapular a., transverse. *See* suprascapular a.				
sciatic a.	a. comitans nervi ischiadici	inferior gluteal a.		accompanies sciatic nerve
sigmoid a's	aa. sigmoideae	inferior mesenteric a.		sigmoid colon

COMMON NAME*	NA EQUIVALENT†	ORIGIN*	BRANCHES*	DISTRIBUTION
spermatic a., external. *See* cremasteric a.				
sphenopalatine a.	a. sphenopalatina	maxillary a.	lateral and septal posterior nasal a's	structures adjoining nasal cavity, nasopharynx
spinal a., anterior	a. spinalis anterior	vertebral a.		spinal cord
spinal a., posterior	a. spinalis posterior	vertebral a.		spinal cord
splenic a.	a. lienalis	celiac trunk	pancreatic and splenic branches, left gastroepiploic, short gastric a's	spleen, pancreas, stomach, greater omentum
straight arterioles of kidney	arteriolae rectae renis	arcuate a's of kidney		renal pyramids
stylomastoid a.	a. stylomastoidea	posterior auricular a.	mastoid and stapedial branches, posterior tympanic a.	middle ear walls, mastoid cells, stapedius
subclavian a.	a. subclavia	brachiocephalic trunk (right), arch of aorta (left)	vertebral, internal thoracic a's, thyrocervical and costocervical trunks	neck, thoracic wall, spinal cord, brain, meninges, upper limb
subcostal a.	a. subcostalis	thoracic aorta	dorsal and spinal branches	upper posterior abdominal wall
sublingual a.	a. sublingualis	lingual a.		sublingual gland
submental a.	a. submentalis	facial a.		tissues under chin
subscapular a.	a. subscapularis	axillary a.	thoracodorsal and circumflex scapular a's	scapular and shoulder region
supraorbital a.	a. supraorbitalis	ophthalmic a.		forehead, superior muscles of orbit, upper eyelid, frontal sinus
suprarenal a., inferior	a. suprarenalis inferior	renal a.		suprarenal gland
suprarenal a., middle	a. suprarenalis media	abdominal aorta		suprarenal gland
suprarenal a's, superior	aa. suprarenales superiores	inferior phrenic a.		suprarenal gland
suprascapular a.	a. suprascapularis	thyrocervical trunk	acromial branch	clavicular, deltoid, and scapular regions
supratrochlear a.	a. supratrochlearis	ophthalmic a.		anterior scalp
sural a's	aa. surales	popliteal a.		popliteal space, calf
sylvian a. *See* cerebral a., middle				
tarsal a., lateral	a. tarsea lateralis	dorsalis pedis a.		tarsus
tarsal a's, medial	aa. tarseae mediales	dorsalis pedis a.		side of foot
temporal a's, deep	aa. temporales profundae	maxillary a.		deep parts of temporal region
temporal a., middle	a. temporalis media	superficial temporal a.		temporal region

temporal a., superficial	a. temporalis superficialis	external carotid a.	parotid, anterior auricular, frontal and parietal branches; transverse facial, zygomaticoorbital, middle temporal a's	parotid and temporal regions
testicular a.	a. testicularis	abdominal aorta	ureteral branches	ureter, epididymis, testis
thoracic a., highest	a. thoracica suprema	axillary a.		axillary aspects of chest wall
thoracic a., internal	a. thoracica interna	subclavian a.	mediastinal, thymic, bronchial, sternal, perforating, lateral costal and anterior intercostal branches; pericardiacophrenic, musculophrenic, superior epigastric a's	anterior thoracic wall, mediastinal structures, diaphragm
thoracic a., lateral	a. thoracica lateralis	axillary a.	mammary branches	pectoral muscles, mammary gland
thoracoacromial a.	a. thoracoacromialis	axillary a.	clavicular, pectoral, deltoid, and acromial branches	deltoid, clavicular, thoracic regions
thoracodorsal a.	a. thoracodorsalis	subscapular a.		subscapular and teres major and minor muscles
thyrocervical trunk	truncus thyrocervicalis	subclavian a.	inferior thyroid, suprascapular and transverse cervical a's	deep neck, including thyroid gland, scapular region
thyroid a., inferior	a. thyroidea inferior	thyrocervical trunk	pharyngeal, esophageal, tracheal branches; inferior laryngeal, ascending cervical a's	thyroid gland and adjacent structures
thyroid a., lowest. *See* thyroidea ima a.				
thyroid a., superior	a. thyroidea superior	external carotid a.	hyoid, sternocleidomastoid, superior laryngeal, cricothyroid, muscular, and glandular branches	thyroid gland and adjacent structures
thyroidea ima a.	a. thyroidea ima	arch of aorta, brachiocephalic trunk or right common carotid a.		thyroid gland
tibial a., anterior	a. tibialis anterior	popliteal a.	posterior and anterior tibial recurrent a's, lateral and medial anterior malleolar a's, lateral and medial malleolar retes	leg, ankle, foot
tibial a., posterior	a. tibialis posterior	popliteal a.	fibular circumflex branch; peroneal, medial plantar, lateral plantar a's	leg, foot
transverse a. of face. *See* facial a., transverse				

TABLE OF ARTERIES (Concluded)

COMMON NAME*	NA EQUIVALENT†	ORIGIN*	BRANCHES*	DISTRIBUTION
transverse a. of neck. See cervical a., transverse; transverse a. of scapular. See suprascapular a.				
tympanic a., anterior; tympanic a., inferior; tympanic a., posterior; tympanic a., superior	a. tympanica anterior; a. tympanica inferior; a. tympanica posterior; a. tympanica superior	maxillary a.; ascending pharyngeal a.; stylomastoid a.; middle meningeal a.		tympanic cavity; tympanic cavity; tympanic cavity; tympanic cavity
ulnar a.	a. ulnaris	brachial a.	palmar carpal, dorsal carpal, and deep palmar branches; ulnar recurrent and common interosseous a's; superficial palmar arch	forearm, wrist, hand
ulnar, a., collateral. See collateral a., ulnar, inferior and collateral a., ulnar, superior				
umbilical a.	a. umbilicalis	internal iliac a.	a. of ductus deferens, superior vesical a's	ductus deferens, seminal vesicles, testes, urinary bladder, ureter
urethral a.	a. urethralis	internal pudendal a.		urethra
uterine a.	a. uterina	internal iliac a.	ovarian and tubal branches; vaginal a.	uterus, vagina, round ligament of uterus, uterine tube, ovary
vaginal a.	a. vaginalis	uterine a.		vagina, fundus of bladder
vertebral a.	a. vertebralis	subclavian a.	spinal and meningeal branches; posterior inferior cerebellar, basilar, anterior, and posterior spinal a's	muscles of neck, vertebrae, spinal cord, cerebellum, interior of cerebrum
vesical a., inferior; vesical a's, superior	a. vesicalis inferior; aa. vesicales superiores	internal iliac a.; umbilical a.		bladder, prostate, seminal vesicles; bladder, urachus, ureter
zygomaticoorbital a.	a. zygomaticoorbitalis	superficial temporal a.		lateral side of orbit

matoid a. **chronic inflammatory a.,** rheumatoid a. **cricoarytenoid a.,** inflammation of the cricoarytenoid joint in rheumatoid arthritis; causing laryngeal stridor. **a. defor′mans,** rheumatoid a. **gouty a.,** that due to gout. **hypertrophic a.,** osteoarthritis. **psoriatic a.,** that associated with severe psoriasis, classically affecting the terminal interphalangeal joints. **rheumatoid a.,** a chronic disease of the joints, usually polyarticular, in which inflammatory changes in the synovial membranes and articular structures, with atrophy and rarefaction of the bones, result in deformity and ankylosis in the late stages; postulated causes are autoimmune mechanisms and viral infection. **rheumatoid a., juvenile,** rheumatoid arthritis in children, with swelling, tenderness, and pain involving one or more joints, leading to impaired growth and development, limitation of movement, and ankylosis and flexion contractures of the joints; often accompanied by systemic manifestations. **rheumatoid a. of spine,** rheumatoid spondylitis. **suppurative a.,** a form marked by purulent joint infiltration, chiefly due to bacterial infection but also seen in Reiter's disease. **tuberculous a.,** that due to tuberculous infection, usually affecting a single joint, marked by chronic inflammation with effusion and destruction of contiguous bone.

arthritism (ar′thrĭ-tizm) gouty or rheumatic diathesis.

Arthrobacter (ar″thro-bak′ter) a genus of Schizomycetes (family Corynebacteriaceae) found in the soil.

arthrocace (ar-throk′ah-se) caries of a joint.

arthrocele (ar′thro-sēl) a joint swelling.

arthrocentesis (ar″thro-sen-te′sis) puncture of a joint cavity with aspiration of fluid.

arthrochondritis (-kon-dri′tis) inflammation of the cartilage of a joint.

arthroclasia (-kla′ze-ah) surgical breaking down of an ankylosis to permit a joint to move freely.

arthrodesis (-de′sis) surgical fusion of a joint.

arthrodia (ar-thro′de-ah) a synovial joint which allows a gliding motion.

arthrodynia (-din′e-ah) arthralgia.

arthrodysplasia (-dis-pla′ze-ah) hereditary deformity of various joints.

arthroempyesis (-em″pi-e′sis) suppuration within a joint.

arthroendoscopy (-en-dos′ko-pe) arthroscopy.

arthrography (ar-throg′rah-fe) radiography of a joint after injection of opaque contrast material. **air a.,** pneumarthrography.

arthrogryposis (ar″thro-grĭ-po′sis) 1. persistent flexure of a joint. 2. tetanoid spasm.

arthrolith (ar′thro-lith) calculous deposit within a joint.

arthrology (ar-throl′o-je) the sum of knowledge regarding the joints.

arthrolysis (-ĭ-sis) operative loosening of adhesions in an ankylosed joint.

arthrometer (ar-throm′ĕ-ter) instrument for measuring the angles of movements of joints.

arthroneuralgia (ar″thro-nu-ral′je-ah) pain in or around a joint.

arthro-ophthalmopathy (-of″thal-mop′ah-the) an association of degenerative joint disease and eye disease.

arthropathy (ar-throp′ah-the) any joint disease. **arthropath′ic,** adj. **Charcot's a., neuropathic a.,** chronic progressive degeneration of the stress-bearing portion of a joint, with hypertrophic changes at the periphery; it is associated with neurologic disorders involving loss of sensation in the joint. **osteopulmonary a.,** clubbing of fingers and toes and enlargement of ends of the long bones, in cardiac or pulmonary disease.

arthrophyma (ar″thro-fi′mah) a joint swelling.

arthrophyte (ar′thro-fīt) abnormal growth in a joint cavity.

arthroplasty (-plas″te) plastic repair of a joint.

arthropod (-pod) an individual of the phylum Arthropoda.

Arthropoda (ar-throp′o-dah) the largest phylum of animals, composed of bilaterally symmetrical organisms with hard, segmented bodies bearing jointed legs, including, among other related forms, arachnids, crustaceans, and insects, many species of which are parasites or are vectors of disease-causing organisms.

arthropyosis (ar″thro-pi-o′sis) formation of pus in a joint cavity.

arthrosclerosis (-skle-ro′sis) stiffening or hardening of the joints.

arthroscopy (ar-thros′ko-pe) examination of the interior of a joint with an endoscope.

arthrosis (ar-thro′sis) 1. a joint or articulation. 2. disease of a joint.

arthrostomy (ar-thros′to-me) surgical creation of an opening into a joint, as for drainage.

arthrosynovitis (ar″thro-sin″o-vi′tis) inflammation of the synovial membrane of a joint.

arthrotomy (ar-throt′o-me) incision of a joint.

arthroxesis (ar-throk′sĕ-sis) scraping of an articular surface.

articular (ar-tik′u-lar) pertaining to a joint.

articulare (ar-tik″u-la′re) the point of intersection of the dorsal contours of the articular process of the mandible and the temporal bone.

articulate (ar-tik′u-lāt) 1. divided into or united by joints. 2. enunciated in words and sentences. 3. to divide into or to unite so as to form a joint. 4. in dentistry, to adjust or place the teeth in their proper relation to each other in making an artificial denture.

articulatio (-la′she-o) pl. *articulatio′nes* [L.] an articulation or joint.

articulation (-la′shun) 1. a joint; the place of union or junction between two or more bones of the skeleton. 2. enunciation of words and sentences. 3. in dentistry: (a) the contact relationship of the occlusal surfaces of the teeth while in action; (b) the arrangement of artificial teeth so as to accommodate the various positions of the mouth and to serve the purpose of the natural teeth which they are to replace.

articulator (-la″tor) a device for effecting a joint-like union. **dental a.,** a device which simulates movements of the temporomandibular joints or mandible, used in dentistry.

articulo (-lo) [L.] at the moment, or crisis. **a. mor′tis,** at the point or moment of death.

artifact (ar′tĭ-fakt) any artificial (man-made) product; a structure, substance, or feature not naturally present, but introduced by some external source or action.

artificial (ar″tĭ-fish′al) made by art; not natural or pathological.

aryl- prefix, *a radical belonging to the aromatic series.*

arytenoid (ar″ĭ-te′noid) shaped like a jug or pitcher as arytenoid cartilage.

arytenoidectomy (ar″ĭ-te-noid-ek′to-me) excision of an arytenoid cartilage.

arytenoiditis (-i′tis) inflammation of arytenoid muscle or cartilage.

arytenoidopexy (ar″ĭ-te-noi′do-pek″se) surgical fixation of arytenoid cartilage or muscle.

A.S. [L.] *au′ris sinis′tra* (left ear).

As chemical symbol, *arsenic.*

As. astigmatism.

A.S.A. American Society of Anesthesiologists; American Standards Association; American Stomatological Association; American Surgical Association.

A.S.A.I.O. American Society for Artificial Internal Organs.

A.S.B. American Society of Bacteriologists.

asbestiform (as-bes′tĭ-form) fibrous in structure, like asbestos.

asbestos (as-bes′tos) a fibrous incombustible magnesium and calcium silicate.

asbestosis (as″bes-to′sis) a lung disease due to inhalation of asbestos fibers.

ascariasis (as″kah-ri′ah-sis) infection with *Ascaris.*

ascaricide (as-kar′ĭ-sīd) an agent that destroys ascarids. **ascarici′dal,** adj.

ascarid (as′kah-rid) any of the phasmid nematodes of the Ascaridoidea, which includes the genera *Ascaridia, Ascaris, Toxocara,* and *Toxascaris.*

Ascaris (-ris) a genus of large intestinal nematode parasites. **A. lumbricoi′des,** a species causing colicky pains and diarrhea, especially in children. **A. su′is,** a name given to *A. lumbricoides* found in swine.

ascaris (-ris), pl. *ascar′ides* [L.] any member of the genus *Ascaris.*

Ascarops (-rops) a genus of parasitic nematodes. **A. strongyli′na,** a blood-sucking species found in the stomach of pigs.

A.S.C.H. American Society of Clinical Hypnosis.

aschelminth (ask′hel-minth) any worm of the phylum Aschelminthes.

Aschelminthes (ask″hel-minth′ēz) a phylum of unsegmented, bilaterally symmetrical, pseudo-coelomate, mostly vermiform animals whose bodies are almost entirely covered with a cuticle, and which possess a complete digestive tract lacking definite muscular walls.

A.S.C.I. American Society for Clinical Investigation.

ascites (ah-si′tēz) effusion and accumulation of serous fluid in the abdominal cavity. **ascit′ic,** adj. **chylous a.,** the presence of chyle in the peritoneal cavity owing to anomalies, injuries, or obstruction of the thoracic duct.

A.S.C.L.T. American Society of Clinical Laboratory Technicians.

Ascomycetes (as″ko-mi-se′tēz) a class of perfect fungi which form ascospores, including yeasts, mildew, and molds.

ascomycetous (-tus) of or pertaining to the Ascomycetes.

ascorbate (as-kor′bāt) a compound or derivative of ascorbic acid.

ascospore (as′ko-spōr) a sexual spore formed in an ascus.

A.S.C.P. American Society of Clinical Pathologists.

ascus (as′kus) the sporangium or spore case of certain lichens and fungi, consisting of a single terminal cell.

-ase suffix used in forming the names of enzymes, affixed to a stem indicating the substrate (luciferase), the general nature of the substrate (proteinase), the reaction catalyzed (hydrolase), or a combination of these (transaminase).

asemasia (as″ĕ-ma′ze-ah) aphasia in which there is lack or loss of ability to communicate by words or by signals.

asemia (ah-se′me-ah) aphasia with inability to use or understand speech or signs.

asepsis (a-sep′sis) 1. freedom from infection. 2. the prevention of contact with microorganisms. **asep′tic,** adj.

asexual (a-seks′u-al) without sex; not pertaining to sex.

asexualization (a-seks″u-al-ĭ-za′shun) sterilization of an individual, as by castration or vasectomy.

A.S.G. American Society for Genetics.

A.S.H. American Society of Hematology.

A.S.H.A. American School Health Association; American Speech and Hearing Association.

A.S.H.I. Association for the Study of Human Infertility.

A.S.H.P. American Society of Hospital Pharmacists.

asialia (ah″si-a′le-ah) aptyalism.

asiderosis (ah″sid-er-o′sis) deficiency of iron reserve of the body.

A.S.I.I. American Science Information Institute.

A.S.I.M. American Society of Internal Medicine.

-asis word element, *state; condition.*

asonia (ah-so′ne-ah) sensory amusia.

A.S.P. American Society of Parasitologists.

Asp aspartic acid.

asparagine (as-par′ah-jēn) the monamide of aspartic acid, from asparagus and many kinds of seeds; used as a diuretic and as a culture medium for certain bacteria.

aspartase (as′par-tās) an enzyme that splits aspartic acid into fumaric acid and ammonia.

aspartate (ah-spahr′tāt) a salt of aspartic acid, or aspartic acid in dissociated form.

aspecific (ah″spĕ-sif′ik) nonspecific; not caused by a specific organism.

aspect (as′pekt) that part of a surface facing in any designated direction. **dorsal a.,** that surface of a body viewed from the back (human anatomy) or from above (veterinary anatomy). **ventral a.,** that surface of a body viewed from the front (human anatomy) or from below (veterinary anatomy).

aspergilloma (as″per-jil-lo′mah) a tumor-like granulomatous mass formed by colonization of *Aspergillus* in a bronchus or pulmonary cavity; the organism may disseminate through the blood stream to the brain, heart, and kidneys.

aspergillosis (-lo′sis) a disease caused by species of *Aspergillus,* marked by inflammatory granulomatous lesions in the skin, ear, orbit, nasal sinuses, lungs, and sometimes bones and meninges.

Aspergillus (as″per-jil′us) a genus of fungi (molds), several species of which are endoparasitic and opportunistic pathogens. **A. fumiga′tus,** a species growing in soil and manure, which has been found in infections of the ear, lungs, and other organs of humans and animals, and is considered a primary pathogen of birds. Its cultures produce various antibiotics, e.g., fumagillin and helvolic acid.

aspergillustoxicosis (as″per-jil″us-tok″sĭ-ko′sis) a form of mycotoxicosis caused by *Aspergillus.*

aspermia (ah-sper′me-ah) failure of formation or emission of semen.

asphalgesia (as″fal-je′ze-ah) a burning sensation felt on touching certain articles, occurring during hypnosis.

asphyxia (as-fik′se-ah) apparent or actual cessation of life due to interruption of effective gaseous exchange in the lungs. **asphyx′ial,** adj. **a. carbon′ica,** suffocation from the inhalation of coal gas, water gas, or carbon monoxide. **fetal a.,** asphyxia *in utero* due to anoxia caused by abruptio placentae, injudicious use of anesthetics, etc. **a. liv′ida,** that in which the skin is cyanotic. **local a.,** acroasphyxia. **a. neonato′rum,** respiratory failure in the newborn; see also *respiratory distress syndrome of newborn.* **traumatic a.,** that due to sudden or severe compression of the thorax or upper abdomen, or both.

asphyxiate (as-fik′se-āt) to put into a state of asphyxia.

asphyxiation (as-fik″se-a′shun) suffocation.

aspidium (as-pid′e-um) the rhizome and stipes of the male fern, the source of an oleoresin used as an anthelmintic in intestinal tapeworm infestations.

aspirate (as′pĭ-rāt) 1. to treat by aspiration. 2. the material obtained by aspiration.

aspiration (as″pĭ-ra′shun) 1. the act of inhaling. 2. removal of fluids or gases from a cavity by suction.

aspirator (-tor) an apparatus for removal by suction of fluids or gases from a cavity.

aspirin (as′pĭ-rin) acetylsalicylic acid, $C_9H_8O_4$, an analgesic, antipyretic, and antirheumatic.

aluminum a., combination of aspirin and aluminum oxide used as an analgesic.

asplenia (ah-sple′ne-ah) absence of the spleen. **functional a.,** impaired reticuloendothelial function of the spleen, as seen in children with sickle-cell anemia.

asporogenic (as″po-ro-jen′ik) not producing spores; not reproduced by spores.

asporous (ah-spo′rus) having no true spores.

A.S.R.T. American Society of Radiologic Technologists.

assay (as-sa′) determination of the amount of a particular constituent of a mixture, or of the potency of a drug. **biological a.,** bioassay. **four-point a.,** an assay based on a mixture of two doses of test material and two doses of standard material. **immune a.,** immunoassay. **microbiological a.,** the assay of nutrient or other substances by their effect on living microorganisms.

assimilation (ah-sim″ĭ-la′shun) 1. conversion of nutritive material into living tissue; anabolism. 2. psychologically, absorption of new experiences into existing psychologic make-up.

association (ah-so″se-a′shun) close relation in time or space. In neurology, correlation involving a high degree of modifiability and also consciousness; see *association center.* In genetics, the occurrence together of two characteristics (e.g., blood group O and peptic ulcers) at a frequency greater than would be predicted on the basis of chance. **clang a.,** association of words or ideas because of similarity in sound. **free a.,** oral expression of one's ideas as they arrive spontaneously; a method used in psychoanalysis.

assortment (ah-sort′ment) the random distribution of nonhomologous chromosomes to daughter cells in metaphase of the first meiotic division.

astasia (as-ta′zhe-ah) motor incoordination with inability to stand. **astat′ic,** adj. **a.-aba′sia,** inability to stand or walk although the legs are otherwise under control.

astatine (as′tah-tēn) chemical element (*see table*), at. no. 85, symbol At.

asteatosis (as″te-ah-to′sis) any disease in which persistent dry scaling of the skin suggests scantiness or absence of sebum.

aster (as′ter) the group of radiations extending from the centrosome in mitosis.

astereognosis (ah-ster″e-og-no′sis) inability to recognize or appreciate the form of objects by feeling them.

asterion (as-te′re-on) the point on the skull at the junction of occipital, parietal, and temporal bones.

asterixis (as″ter-ik′sis) a motor disturbance marked by intermittent lapses of an assumed posture as a result of intermittency of sustained contraction of groups of muscles; called *liver flap* because of its occurrence in hepatic coma, but observed also in other conditions.

asternal (a-ster′nal) 1. not joined by a sternum. 2. pertaining to asternia.

asternia (ah-ster′ne-ah) congenital absence of the sternum.

asteroid (as'ter-oid) star-shaped.

Asterol (as'ter-ol) trademark for preparations of diamthazole.

asthen(o)- word element [Gr.], *weak; weakness.*

asthenia (as-the'ne-ah) lack or loss of strength and energy; weakness. **asthen'ic,** adj. **neurocirculatory a.,** a syndrome of breathlessness, giddiness, a sense of fatigue, precordial pain, and palpitation, seen chiefly in soldiers in active war service. **tropical anhidrotic a.,** a condition due to generalized anhidrosis in conditions of high temperature, characterized by a tendency to overfatigability, irritability, anorexia, inability to concentrate, and drowsiness, with headache and vertigo.

asthenocoria (as"the-no-ko're-ah) sluggishness of the pupillary light reflex; seen in hypoadrenalism.

asthenometer (as"the-nom'e-ter) a device used in measuring the degree of muscular asthenia or of asthenopia.

asthenope (as'the-nōp) a person with asthenopia.

asthenopia (as"the-no'pe-ah) weakness or easy fatigue of the eye, with pain in the eyes, headache, dimness of vision, etc. **asthenop'ic,** adj. **accommodative a.,** asthenopia due to strain of ciliary muscle. **muscular a.,** asthenopia due to weakness of external ocular muscles.

asthenospermia (as"the-no-sper'me-ah) reduction in vitality of spermatozoa.

asthma (az'mah) a condition marked by recurrent attacks of paroxysmal dyspnea, with wheezing due to spasmodic contraction of the bronchi. In some cases, it is an allergic manifestation in sensitized persons. **asthmat'ic,** adj. **bronchial a.,** see *asthma.* **cardiac a.,** paroxysmal dyspnea associated with heart disease. **Heberden's a.,** angina pectoris. **thymic a.,** an alleged condition occurring usually in children, with thymus enlargement, asthma, and tendency to sudden death.

asthmatiform (az-mat'ĭ-form) resembling asthma.

astigmatism (ah-stig'mah-tizm) ametropia caused by differences in curvature in different meridians of the refractive surfaces of the eye so that light rays are not sharply focused on the retina. **astigmat'ic,** adj. **compound a.,** that complicated with hypermetropia in all meridians or with myopia in all meridians. **corneal a.,** that due to irregularity in the curvature or refracting power of the cornea. **hyperopic a.,** that in which the light rays are brought to a focus behind the retina. **irregular a.,** that in which the curvature varies in different parts of the same meridian or in which refraction in successive meridians differs irregularly. **lenticular a.,** that due to a defect of the lens. **mixed a.,** that in which one principal meridian is hyperopic and the other myopic. **myopic a.,** that in which the light rays are brought to a focus in front of the retina. **regular a.,** that in which refraction changes gradually in power from one principal meridian of the eye to the other, the two meridians always being at right angles; the condition is further classified as being *against*

the rule when the meridian of greatest refractive power tends toward the horizontal, *with the rule* when it tends toward the vertical, and *oblique* when it lies 45 degrees from the horizontal and vertical.

astigmatometer (as"tig-mah-tom'e-ter) an instrument used in measuring astigmatism.

astigmia (ah-stig'me-ah) astigmatism.

astigmometer (as"tig-mom'ĕ-ter) astigmatometer.

A.S.T.M.H. American Society of Tropical Medicine and Hygiene.

astomia (ah-sto'me-ah) congenital atresia of the mouth. **asto'matous,** adj.

astomus (-mus) a fetus exhibiting astomia.

astragalectomy (ah-strag"ah-lek'to-me) excision of the astragalus.

astragalus (ah-strag'ah-lus) talus (see *Table of Bones*). **astrag'alar,** adj.

astral (as'tral) of or relating to an aster.

astringent (ah-strin'jent) causing contraction, usually locally after topical application; also, an agent that so acts.

astroblast (as'tro-blast) a cell that develops into an astrocyte.

astroblastoma (as"tro-blas-to'mah) an astrocytoma of Grade II, composed of cells with abundant cytoplasm and two or three nuclei.

astrocyte (as'tro-sīt) a neuroglial cell of ectodermal origin, characterized by fibrous or protoplasmic processes; collectively called *astroglia,* or *macroglia.*

astrocytoma (as"tro-si-to'mah) a tumor composed of astrocytes; classified in order of malignancy as: *Grade I,* consisting of fibrillary or protoplasmic astrocytes; *Grade II* (see *astroblastoma*); *Grades III* and *IV* (see *glioblastoma multiforme*).

astroglia (as-trog'le-ah) the astrocytes considered as tissue.

astrosphere (as'tro-sfēr) 1. the central mass of an aster, excluding the rays. 2. aster.

asymbolia (ah"sim-bo'le-ah) loss of ability to understand symbols, as words, figures, gestures, signs, etc.

asymmetry (a-sim'ĕ-tre) lack or absence of symmetry; dissimilarity in corresponding parts or organs on opposite sides of the body which are normally alike. In chemistry, lack of symmetry in the special arrangements of the atoms and radicals within the molecule or crystal. **asymmet'rical,** adj.

asymphytous (ah-sim'fĭ-tus) separate or distinct; not grown together.

asymptomatic (a"simp-to-mat'ik) showing or causing no symptoms.

asynchronism (a-sin'kro-nizm) lack of synchronism; disturbance of coordination.

asynclitism (ah-sin'klĭ-tizm) 1. oblique presentation of the fetal head in labor, called *anterior a.* when the anterior parietal bone is designated the point of presentation, and *posterior a.* when the posterior parietal bone is so designated. 2. maturation at different times of the nucleus and cytoplasm of blood cells.

asyndesis (ah-sin'dĕ-sis) a language disorder in

which related elements of a sentence cannot be welded together as a whole.

asynechia (ah″sĭ-nek′e-ah) absence of continuity of structure.

asynergy (a″sin′er-je) lack of coordination among parts or organs normally acting in unison; in neurology, failure of cooperation among muscle groups that is necessary for execution of movement.

asynovia (ah″sĭ-no′ve-ah) deficiency of synovial secretion.

asyntaxia (a″sin-tak′se-ah) lack of proper and orderly embryonic development.

asystole (a-sis′to-le) cardiac standstill or arrest—absence of heartbeat. **asystol′ic,** adj.

At chemical symbol, *astatine.*

at. atmosphere; atomic.

Atabrine (at′ah-brin, at′ah-brēn) trademark for quinacrine.

atactic (ah-tak′tik) lacking coordination; irregular; pertaining to or characterized by ataxia.

atactiform (-tĭ-form) resembling ataxia.

ataractic (at″ah-rak′tik) 1. pertaining to or capable of producing ataraxia. 2. an agent capable of inducing ataraxia; a tranquilizer.

ataralgesia (at″ar-al-je′ze-ah) combined sedation and analgesia intended to abolish mental distress and pain attendant on surgical procedures, with the patient remaining conscious and alert.

Atarax (at′ah-raks) trademark for preparations of hydroxyzine.

ataraxia (at″ah-rak′se-ah) a state of detached serenity without depression of mental faculties or impairment of consciousness.

ataraxic (-rak′sik) ataractic.

atavism (at′ah-vizm) apparent inheritance of a characteristic from remote rather than immediate ancestors. **atavis′tic,** adj.

ataxaphasia (ah-tak″sah-fa′ze-ah) ataxiaphasia.

ataxia (ah-tak′se-ah) failure of muscular coordination; irregularity of muscular action. **atac′-tic, atax′ic,** adj. **alcoholic a.,** a condition resembling tabes dorsalis, due to loss of proprioception in chronic alcoholism. **Friedreich's a.,** hereditary sclerosis of the dorsal and lateral columns of the spine, usually beginning in childhood or youth; it is attended with ataxia, speech impairment, scoliosis, peculiar movements, and paralysis. **locomotor a.,** tabes dorsalis. **motor a.,** inability to control the coordinate movements of the muscles. **sensory a.,** ataxia due to loss of proprioception (joint position sensation) between the motor cortex and peripheral nerves, resulting in poorly judged movements, the incoordination becoming aggravated when the eyes are closed. **a.-telangiectasia,** hereditary progressive ataxia, associated with oculocutaneous telangiectasia, sinopulmonary disease with frequent respiratory infections, and abnormal eye movements.

ataxiaphasia (ah-tak″se-ah-fa′ze-ah) inability to arrange words into sentences.

ataxophemia (-so-fe′me-ah) lack of coordination of speech muscles.

atel(o)- word element [Gr.], *incomplete; imperfectly developed.*

atelectasis (at″ĕ-lek′tah-sis) incomplete expansion of the lungs at birth, or collapse of the adult lung. **atelectat′ic,** adj. **congenital a.,** that present at birth (*primary a.*) or immediately thereafter (*secondary a.*). **primary a.,** see *congenital a.* **secondary a.,** see *congenital a.*

atelia (ah-te′le-ah) imperfect or incomplete development. **ateliot′ic,** adj.

ateliosis (ah-te″le-o′sis) hypophyseal infantilism.

atelocardia (at″ĕ-lo-kar′de-ah) imperfect development of the heart.

atelocephalous (-sef′ah-lus) having an incomplete head.

atelocephaly (-sef′ah-le) imperfect development of the skull. **atelocephal′ic,** adj.

atelocheilia (-ki′le-ah) imperfect development of the lip.

ateloglossia (-glos′e-ah) imperfect development of the tongue.

atelomyelia (-mi-e′le-ah) imperfect development of the spinal cord.

atelorhachidia (-rah-kid′e-ah) imperfect development of the vertebral column.

atelostomia (-sto′me-ah) imperfect development of the mouth.

athelia (ah-the′le-ah) congenital absence of the nipples.

athermic (ah-ther′mik) without rise of temperature; afebrile; apyretic.

athermosystaltic (ah-ther″mo-sis-tal′tik) not contracting under the action of cold or heat; said of skeletal muscle.

atherogenesis (ath″er-o-jen′ĕ-sis) formation of atheromatous lesions in arterial walls. **atherogen′ic,** adj.

atheroma (ath″er-o′mah) a mass or plaque of degenerated thickened arterial intima, occurring in atherosclerosis.

atheromatosis (ath″er-o-mah-to′sis) diffuse atheromatous arterial disease.

atheromatous (ath″er-o′mah-tus) affected with or of the nature of atheroma.

atherosclerosis (ath″er-o-skle-ro′sis) a form of arteriosclerosis in which atheromas containing cholesterol, lipoid material, and lipophages are formed within the intima and inner media of large and medium-sized arteries.

athetoid (ath′ĕ-toid) resembling or affected with athetosis.

athetosis (ath″ĕ-to′sis) repetitive involuntary, slow, sinuous, writhing movements, especially severe in the hands.

athrepsia (ah-threp′se-ah) marasmus. **athrep′-tic,** adj.

athymia (ah-thi′me-ah) 1. dementia. 2. absence of functioning thymus tissue.

athymism (-mizm) the condition induced by absence or removal of the thymus.

athyreosis (ah-thi″re-o′sis) hypothyroidism. **athyreot′ic,** adj.

athyria (ah-thi′re-ah) 1. a condition resulting from absence of the thyroid gland. 2. hypothyroidism.

atlantad (at-lan'tad) toward the atlas.

atlantal (at-lan'tal) pertaining to the atlas.

atlantoaxial (at-lan"to-ak'se-al) pertaining to the atlas and the axis.

atlantodidymus (-did'ĭ-mus) a monster with one body and two heads.

atlas (at'las) the first cervical vertebra; see *Table of Bones.*

atloaxoid (at"lo-ak'soid) pertaining to the atlas and axis.

atlodidymus (-did'ĭ-mus) atlantodidymus.

atmos (at'mos) a unit of air pressure, being the pressure of 760 mm. of mercury on one square centimeter.

atmosphere (at'mos-fēr) 1. the entire gaseous envelope surrounding the earth, extending to an altitude of 10 miles and including the troposphere, tropopause, and stratosphere. 2. a unit of pressure, equivalent to that on a surface at sea level, being about 14.7 pounds per square inch, or equivalent to that of a column of mercury 760 mm. high. **atmospher'ic**, adj.

at. no. atomic number.

atocia (ah-to'se-ah) sterility in the female.

atom (at'om) the smallest particle of an element that has all the properties of the element; it consists of a positively charged nucleus (made up of protons and neutrons) and negatively charged electrons, which move in orbits about the nucleus. **atom'ic**, adj.

atomization (at"om-ĭ-za'shun) the act or process of breaking up a liquid into a fine spray.

atomizer (at'om-īz"er) a device for dispensing liquid in a fine spray.

atonia (ah-to'ne-ah) atony.

atony (at'o-ne) lack of normal tone or strength. **aton'ic**, adj.

atopen (at'o-pen) the antigen responsible for atopy.

atopic (ah-top'ik) 1. ectopic. 2. pertaining to an atopen or to atopy; allergic.

atopognosia (ah-top"og-no'ze-ah) inability to correctly locate a sensation.

atopy (at'o-pe) a clinical hypersensitivity state or allergy with a hereditary predisposition; i.e., the tendency to develop an allergy is inherited, but the specific clinical form (hay fever, asthma, etc.) is not. The antibody reagin is involved.

atoxic (ah-tok'sik) not poisonous; not due to a poison.

ATP adenosine triphosphate.

ATPase adenosinetriphosphatase.

atransferrinemia (a-trans"fer-ĭ-ne'me-ah) absence of circulating iron-binding protein (transferrin).

atraumatic (a"traw-mat'ik) not producing injury or damage.

atresia (ah-tre'zhe-ah) congenital absence or closure of a normal body opening or tubular structure. **atret'ic**, adj. **a. a'ni**, imperforate anus. **aortic a.**, congenital absence of the opening from the left ventricle of the heart into the aorta. **biliary a.**, obliteration or hypoplasia of one or more components of the bile ducts due to arrested fetal development, resulting in persis-

tent jaundice and liver damage ranging from biliary stasis to biliary cirrhosis, with splenomegaly as portal hypertension progresses. **follicular a., a. follic'uli**, degeneration and resorption of an ovarian follicle before it reaches maturity and ruptures. **mitral a.**, congenital obliteration of the mitral valve orifice; it is associated with hyperplastic left-heart syndrome or transposition of the great vessels. **prepyloric a.**, congenital membranous obstruction of the gastric outlet, characterized by vomiting of gastric contents only. **pulmonary a.**, congenital severe narrowing of the opening between the pulmonary artery and the right ventricle, with cardiomegaly, reduced pulmonary vascularity, and right ventricular atrophy. It is usually associated with tetralogy of Fallot, transposition of the great vessels, or other cardiovascular anomalies. **tricuspid a.**, congenital absence of the opening between the right atrium and right ventricle, circulation being made possible by the presence of an atrial septal defect.

atrial (a'tre-al) pertaining to an atrium.

atrichia (ah-trik'e-ah) 1. absence of hair; alopecia. 2. absence of flagella or cilia.

atrichous (ah-trik'us) 1. having no hair. 2. having no flagella.

atriomegaly (a"tre-o-meg'ah-le) abnormal enlargement of an atrium of the heart.

atrioseptopexy (-sep'to-pek"se) surgical correction of a defect in the interatrial septum.

atrioseptoplasty (-sep'to-plas"te) plastic repair of the interatrial septum.

atrioventricular (-ven-trik'u-lar) pertaining to an atrium and ventricle of the heart.

atrioventricularis communis (-ven-trik"u-la'-ris kŏ-mu'nis) a congenital cardiac anomaly in which the endocardial cushions fail to fuse, the ostium primum persists, the atrioventricular canal is undivided, a single atrioventricular valve has anterior and posterior cusps, and there is a defect of the membranous interventricular septum.

atrium (a'tre-um), pl. *a'tria* [L.] a chamber; in anatomy, a chamber affording entrance to another structure or organ, especially the upper, smaller cavity (*a. cordis*) on either side of the heart, which receives blood from the pulmonary veins (*left a.*) or venae cavae (*right a.*) and delivers it to the ventricle on the same side. **a'trial**, adj. **common a.**, the single atrium found in a form of three-chambered heart.

atrophia (ah-tro'fe-ah) [L.] atrophy (1).

atrophic (ah-trof'ik) pertaining to or characterized by atrophy.

atrophoderma (at"ro-fo-der'mah) atrophy of the skin.

atrophy (at'ro-fe) 1. a wasting away; a diminution in the size of a cell, tissue, organ, or part. 2. to undergo or cause atrophy. **acute yellow a.**, the shrunken, yellow liver which is a complication, usually fatal, of fulminant hepatitis with massive hepatic necrosis. **Aran-Duchenne a.**, spinal muscular a. **bone a.**, resorption of bone evident in both external form and internal density. **disuse a.**, wasting due to lack of normal exercise of a part. **Duchenne-Aran**

a., spinal muscular a. **eccentric a.,** atrophy of a hollow organ with increase in size of the cavity. **healed yellow a.,** postnecrotic cirrhosis. **Leber's optic a.,** hereditary bilateral progressive optic atrophy; seen in males. **lobar a.,** progressive atrophy of the cerebral convolutions in a limited area (lobe) of the brain. **myelopathic muscular a.,** muscular atrophy due to lesion of the spinal cord, as in spinal muscular atrophy. **optic a.,** atrophy of the optic disk due to degeneration of the nerve fibers of the optic nerve and optic tract. **physiologic a.,** that affecting certain organs in all individuals as part of the normal aging process. **progressive neuropathic (peroneal) muscular a.** hereditary muscular atrophy, beginning in the muscles supplied by the peroneal nerves, progressing slowly to involve the muscles of the hands and arms. **spinal muscular a.,** progressive degeneration of the motor cells of the spinal cord, beginning usually in the small muscles of the hands, but in some cases (scapulohumeral type) in the upper arm and shoulder muscles, and progressing slowly to the leg muscles. **subacute yellow a.,** submassive hepatic necrosis associated with broad zones of necrosis, due to viral, toxic, or drug-induced hepatitis; it may have an acute course with death occurring after several weeks of liver failure, or clinical recovery may be associated with regeneration of the parenchymal cells. **yellow a.,** see *acute yellow a.,* and *subacute yellow a.*

atropine (at′ro-pēn) an anticholinergic alkaloid, $C_{17}H_{23}NO_3$, derived from belladonna, hyoscyamus, or strammonium, or produced synthetically. **a. sulfate,** a soluble compound of atropine, with similar uses.

A.T.S. American Thoracic Society; American Trudeau Society.

attack (ah-tak′) an episode or onset of illness. **vagal a., vasovagal a.,** a transient vascular and neurogenic reaction marked by pallor, nausea, sweating, bradycardia, and rapid fall in arterial blood pressure, which may result in syncope.

attenuation (ah-ten″u-a′shun) 1. the act of thinning or weakening, as (*a*) the alteration of virulence of a pathogenic microorganism by passage through another host species, decreasing the virulence of the organism for the native host and increasing it for the new host, or (*b*) the process by which a beam of radiation is reduced in energy when passed through tissue or other material.

attic (at′ik) the upper portion of the tympanic cavity, extending above the level of the tympanic membrane and containing the greater part of the incus and the head of the malleus.

atticoantrotomy (at″tĭ-ko-an-trot′o-me) surgical exposure of the attic and mastoid antrum.

atticotomy (at″ĭ-kot′o-me) incision into the attic.

attitude (at′ĭ-tūd) 1. a posture or position of the body; in obstetrics, the relation of the various parts of the fetal body to one another. 2. a pattern of mental views established by cumulative prior experience.

atto- a prefix signifying one quintillionth, or 10^{-18}; symbol a.

attraction (ah-trak′shun) 1. the force, act, or process that draws one body toward another. 2. malocclusion in which the occlusal plane is closer than normal to the eye-ear plane, causing shortening of the face; cf. *abstraction* (3). **capillary a.,** the force which causes a liquid to rise in a fine-caliber tube.

at. wt. atomic weight.

atypia (a-tip′e-ah) deviation from the normal or typical state.

atypical (-ĭ-kal) irregular; not conformable to the type; in microbiology, applied specifically to strains of unusual type.

A.U. Angström unit; [L.] *aures unitas,* both ears together or *auris uterque,* each ear.

Au chemical symbol, *gold* (L. *aurum*).

Au-antigenemia (an″tĭ-jĕ-ne″me-ah) the presence of Australia antigen in the blood.

audi(o)- word element [L.], *hearing.*

audioanalgesia (aw″de-o-an″al-je′ze-ah) alleged reduction of pain by listening to recorded music to which may be added a background of so-called white sound.

audiogenic (-jen′ik) produced by sound.

audiogram (aw′de-o-gram″) a graphic record of the findings by audiometry.

audiologist (aw″de-ol′o-jist) an expert in audiology.

audiology (-ol′o-je) the science of hearing, particularly the study of impaired hearing that cannot be improved by medication or surgical therapy.

audiometer (-om′ĕ-ter) an instrument used in audiometry.

audiometrician (aw″de-o-mĕ-trish′an) a technician specializing in audiometry.

audiometry (aw″de-om′ĕ-tre) measurement of the acuity of hearing for the various frequencies of sound waves. **Békésy a.,** that in which the patient, by pressing a signal button, traces his monaural thresholds for pure tones: the intensity of the tone decreases as long as the button is depressed and increases when it is released; both continuous and interrupted tones are used. **cortical a.,** an objective method of determining auditory acuity by recording and averaging electric potentials evoked from the cortex of the brain in response to stimulation by pure tones. **electrodermal a.,** audiometry in which the subject is conditioned by harmless electric shock to pure tones; thereafter he anticipates a shock when he hears a pure tone, the anticipation resulting in a brief electrodermal response, which is recorded; the lowest intensity at which the response is elicited is taken to be his hearing threshold. **localization a.,** a technique for measuring the capacity to locate the source of a pure tone received binaurally in a sound field.

audiosurgery (aw″de-o-ser′jer-e) surgery of the ear.

audiovisual (-vizh′u-al) simultaneously stimulating, or pertaining to simultaneous stimulation of, the senses of both hearing and sight.

audition (aw-dish′un) perception of sound; hearing. **chromatic a.,** chromesthesia in which a sensation of color is produced by sound.

auditory (aw′dĭ-to″re) pertaining to the ear or the sense of hearing.

augnathus (awg-nath′us) a fetus with a double lower jaw.

aula (aw′lah) the red areola formed around a vaccination vesicle.

aura (aw′rah) a subjective sensation or motor phenomenon that precedes and marks the onset of a paroxysmal attack, as of an epileptic attack.

aural (aw′ral) 1. pertaining to or perceived by the ear. 2. pertaining to an aura.

aurantiasis (aw″ran-ti′ah-sis) carotenemia.

Aureomycin (aw″re-o-mi′sin) trademark for preparations of chlortetracycline.

auriasis (aw-ri′ah-sis) chrysiasis.

auric (aw′rik) pertaining to or containing gold.

auricle (aw′rĭ-k′l) 1. the flap of the ear. 2. the ear-shaped appendage of either atrium of the heart; formerly used to designate the entire atrium.

auricula (aw-rik′u-lah), pl. *auric′ulae* [L.] auricle.

auricular (-lar) pertaining to an auricle or to the ear.

auriculare (aw-rik″u-la′re) a point at the top of the opening of the external auditory meatus.

auricularis (-ris) [L.] pertaining to the ear; auricular.

auriculotemporal (aw-rik″u-lo-tem′po-ral) pertaining to the ear and the temporal region.

aurin (aw′rin) a triphenylmethane derivative, $C_{19}H_{14}O_3$, used as an indicator and dye intermediate.

auripuncture (aw′rĭ-pungk″chūr) surgical puncture of the tympanic membrane.

auris (aw′ris), pl. *au′res* [L.] ear.

auriscope (aw′rĭ-skōp) otoscope.

aurotherapy (aw″ro-ther′ah-pe) use of gold salts in treatment of disease.

aurothioglucose (-thi″o-gloo′kōs) a gold preparation, $C_6H_{11}Au_5S$, used in treating rheumatoid arthritis.

aurothioglycanide (-thi″o-gli′kah-nīd) a gold preparation, C_8H_8AuNOS, used in treating rheumatic arthritis.

aurothioglycolanilide (-thi″o-gli″kol-an′ĭ-līd) aurothioglycanide.

aurum (aw′rum) [L.] gold (symbol Au).

auscult (aws-kult′) auscultate.

auscultate (aws′kul-tāt) to examine by auscultation.

auscultation (aws″kul-ta′shun) listening for sounds within the body, chiefly to ascertain the condition of the thoracic or abdominal viscera and to detect pregnancy; it may be performed with the unaided ear (*direct* or *immediate a.*) or with a stethoscope (*mediate a.*).

auscultatory (aws-kul′tah-to″re) pertaining to auscultation.

aut(o)- word element [Gr.], *self.*

autacoid (aw′tah-koid) an organic substance produced in one organ and carried by the blood to other organs, on which the substance acts.

autarcesis (aw-tar′sĕ-sis) natural immunity as distinguished from immunity of the antibody type. **autarcet′ic,** adj.

autecic, autecious (aw-te′sik; aw-te′shus) parasitic always on the same host.

autism (aw′tizm) the condition of being dominated by subjective, self-centered trends of thought or behavior which are not subject to correction by external information. **autis′tic,** adj. **infantile a.,** a condition of early life, marked by failure to relate in the ordinary way to people and situations and by repetitive activities, developmental language disorders, and inability to adjust socially.

autoagglutination (aw″to-ah-gloo″tĭ-na′shun) clumping or agglutination of an individual's cells by his own serum, as in autohemagglutination.

autoagglutinin (-ah-gloo′tĭ-nin) a factor in serum capable of causing clumping together of the subject's own cellular elements.

autoamputation (-am″pu-ta′shun) spontaneous detachment from the body and elimination of an appendage or an abnormal growth, such as a polyp.

autoantibody (-an′tĭ-bod″e) an antibody formed in response to, and reacting against, an antigenic constituent of the individual's own tissues.

autoantigen (-an′tĭ-jen) a tissue constituent that is immunogenic in the organism in which it occurs, stimulating the production of autoantibodies.

autoantitoxin (-an″tĭ-tok′sin) antitoxin produced by tissues of the body to protect it from the homologous toxin.

autocatalysis (-kah-tal′ĭ-sis) catalysis in which a product of the reaction hastens or intensifies the catalysis.

autochthonous (aw-tok′tho-nus) 1. originating in the same area in which it is found. 2. denoting a tissue graft to a new site on the same individual.

autoclasis (aw-tok′lah-sis) destruction of a part by influences within itself, as by autoimmune processes.

autoclave (aw′to-klāv) a self-locking apparatus for the sterilization of materials by steam under pressure.

Autoclip (aw′to-klip″) trademark for a stainless steel surgical clip inserted by means of a mechanical applier that automatically feeds a series of clips for wound closing.

autocytolysin (aw″to-si-tol′ĭ-sin) autolysin.

autocytolysis (-si-tol′ĭ-sis) autolysis.

autodigestion (-di-jes′chun) self-digestion; autolysis; especially, digestion of the stomach wall and contiguous structures after death.

autodiploid (-dip′loid) 1. characterized by autodiploidy. 2. an individual or cell so characterized.

autodiploidy (-dip′loi-de) the state of having two sets of chromosomes as the result of redoubling of the haploid set.

autoecholalia (-ek″o-la′le-ah) repetition of one's own words.

autoecious (aw-te′shus) autecious.

autoeczematization (aw‴to-ek-zem″ah-tĭ-za′-shun) the spread, at first locally and later more generally, of lesions from an orginally circumscribed focus of eczema.

autoeroticism (-ĕ-rot′ĭ-sizm) autoerotism.

autoerotism (-er′o-tizm) erotic behavior directed toward one's self. **autoerot′ic,** adj.

autogamy (aw-tog′ah-me) 1. self-fertilization; fertilization by union of two chromatin masses derived from the same primary nucleus within a cell. 2. reproduction in which the two gametes are derived from division of a single mother cell.

autogeneic (aw″to-jĕ-ne′ik) autogenous; pertaining to an autograft.

autogenesis (-jen′ĕ-sis) self-generation; origination within the organism. **autogenet′ic, autog′enous,** adj.

autograft (aw′to-graft) a tissue graft transferred from one part of the patient's body to another part.

autohemagglutination (aw″to-hem″ah-gloo″-tĭ-na′shun) agglutination of erythrocytes by a factor produced in the subject's own body.

autohemagglutinin (-hem″ah-gloo′tĭ-nin) a substance produced in a person's body that causes agglutination of his own erythrocytes.

autohemolysin (-he-mol′ĭ-sin) a hemolysin produced in the body of an animal which lyses its own erythrocytes.

autohemolysis (-he-mol′ĭ-sis) hemolysis of an individual's blood cells by his own serum. **autohemolyt′ic,** adj.

autohemotherapy (-he″mo-ther′ah-pe) treatment by reinjection of the patient's own blood.

autohypnosis (-hip-no′sis) a self-induced hypnotic state; the act or process of hypnotizing oneself. **autohypnot′ic,** adj.

autoimmune (-im-mūn′) directed against the body's own tissue; see under *disease* and *response.*

autoimmunity (-im-mu′nĭ-te) a condition characterized by a specific humoral or cell-mediated immune response against the constituents of the body's own tissues (autoantigens); it may result in hypersensitivity reactions or, if severe, in autoimmune disease.

autoimmunization (-im‴mu-nĭ-za′shun) induction in an organism of an immune response to its own tissue constitutents.

autoinoculation (-in-ok″u-la′shun) inoculation with microorganisms from one's own body.

autointoxication (-in-tok″sĭ-ka′shun) poisoning by a toxin generated within the body.

autoisolysin (-i-sol′ĭ-sin) a substance that lyses cells (e.g., blood cells) of the individual in which it is formed, as well as those of other members of the same species.

autokeratoplasty (-ker′ah-to-plas″te) grafting of corneal tissue from one eye to the other.

autokinesis (-ki-ne′sis) voluntary motion. **autokinet′ic,** adj.

autolesion (-le′zhun) a self-inflicted injury.

autoleukoagglutinin (-lu″ko-ah-gloo′tĭ-nin) see *leukoagglutinin.*

autologous (aw-tol′o-gus) related to self; belonging to the same organism.

autolysate (aw-tol′ĭ-sāt) a specific substance produced by autolysis.

autolysin (aw-tol′ĭ-sin) a lysin originating in an organism and capable of destroying its own cells and tissues.

autolysis (aw-tol′ĭ-sis) 1. spontaneous disintegration of cells or tissues by autologous enzymes, as occurs after death and in some pathologic conditions. 2. destruction of cells of the body by its own serum. **autolyt′ic,** adj.

automatic (aw″to-mat′ik) spontaneous; done involuntarily; self-regulating.

automatism (aw-tom′ah-tizm) performance of nonreflex acts without conscious volition. **command a.,** abnormal responsiveness to commands, as in hypnosis and certain mental states.

autonomic (aw″to-nom′ik) not subject to voluntary control; functionally independent. See under *system.*

autonomotropic (-nom″o-trop′ik) having an affinity for the autonomic nervous system.

autopathy (aw-top′ah-the) idiopathic disease; one without apparent external causation.

autophagia (aw″to-fa′je-ah) 1. eating one's own flesh. 2. nutrition of the body by consumption of its own tissues.

autophilia (-fil′e-ah) pathologic self-esteem; narcissism.

autoplasmotherapy (-plaz″mo-ther′ah-pe) therapeutic injection of one's own blood plasma.

autoplasty (aw′to-plas″te) 1. replacement or reconstruction of diseased or injured parts with tissues taken from another region of the patient's own body. 2. in psychoanalysis, instinctive modification within the psychic systems in adaptation to reality. **autoplas′tic,** adj.

autoploid (-ploid) autopolyploid.

autoploidy (aw″to-ploi′de) autopolyploidy.

autopolymer (-pol′ĭ-mer) a material which polymerizes on addition of an activator and a catalyst, without the use of heat.

autopolyploid (-pol′ĭ-ploid) 1. characterized by autopolyploidy. 2. an individual or cell characterized by autopolyploidy.

autopolyploidy (-pol″ĭ-ploi′de) the state of having more than two chromosome sets as the result of redoubling of the haploid set.

autoprecipitin (-pre-sip′ĭ-tin) an autoantibody with the characteristics of a precipitin.

autoprothrombin (-pro-throm′bin) an activation product of prothrombin.

autopsy (aw′top-se) examination of a body after death; necropsy.

autopsychic (aw″to-si′kik) pertaining to one's ideas concerning his own personality.

autoradiograph (-ra′de-o-graf) the film produced by autoradiography.

autoradiography (-ra″de-og′rah-fe) the making of a radiograph of an object or tissue by recording on a photographic plate the radiation emitted by radioactive material within the object.

autoregulation (-reg″u-la′shun) control of certain phenomena by factors inherent in a situation; specifically, (1) maintenance by an organ or tissue of a constant blood flow despite changes in arterial pressure, and (2) adjustment of blood flow through an organ in accordance with its metabolic needs.

autoreinfusion (-re″in-fu′zhun) reinfusion of the patient's own blood.

autosensitization (-sen″sĭ-ti-za′shun) autoimmunization. **erythrocyte a.,** autoerythrocyte sensitization; see under *syndrome*.

autosepticemia (-sep″tĭ-se′me-ah) septicemia from poisons developed within the body.

autoserodiagnosis (-se″ro-di″ag-no′sis) diagnostic use of autoserum.

autoserum (-se′rum) serum administered to the patient from whom it was derived.

autosite (aw′to-sīt) the larger, more normal member of asymmetrical conjoined twin fetuses, to which the parasite is attached.

autosome (-sōm) any non–sex-determining chromosome; in man there are 22 pairs of autosomes. **autoso′mal,** adj.

autosplenectomy (aw″to-sple-nek′to-me) almost complete disappearance of the spleen through progressive fibrosis and shrinkage.

autostimulation (-stim″u-la′shun) stimulation of an animal with antigenic material from its own tissues.

autosuggestion (-sug-jes′chun) suggestion arising in one's self, as opposed to heterosuggestion.

autotomography (-to-mog′rah-fe) a method of body section roentgenography involving movement of the patient instead of the x-ray tube. **autotomograph′ic,** adj.

autotopagnosia (-top-ag-no′se-ah) inability to orient correctly different parts of the body.

autotoxin (-tok′sin) a toxin which acts against the body in which it is formed.

autotransfusion (-trans-fu′zhun) reinfusion of a patient's own blood.

autotransplantation (-trans″plan-ta′shun) transfer of tissue from one part of the body to another part.

autotroph (aw′to-trōf) an autotrophic organism.

autotrophic (aw″to-trof′ik) self-nourishing; able to build organic constituents from carbon dioxide and inorganic salts.

autovaccination (-vak″sĭ-na′shun) treatment with autovaccine.

autovaccine (-vak′sēn) a vaccine prepared from cultures of organisms isolated from the patient's own tissues or secretions.

autoxidation (aw″tok-sĭ-da′shun) spontaneous oxidation of a substance that is in direct contact with oxygen.

auxanography (awk″sah-nog′rah-fe) a method used for determining the most suitable medium for the cultivation of microorganisms. **auxanograph′ic,** adj.

auxesis (awk-se′sis) increase in size of an organism, especially that due to growth of its individ-

ual cells rather than an increase in their number. **auxet′ic,** adj.

auxilytic (awk″sĭ-lit′ik) increasing the lytic or destructive power.

auxin (awk′sin) a growth-promoting plant hormone that acts by causing cell elongation rather than cell multiplication.

auxiometer (awk″se-om′ĕ-ter) an apparatus for measuring the magnifying power of lenses.

auxochrome (awk′so-krōm) a chemical group which, if introduced into a chromogen, will convert it into a dye. **auxochro′mic,** adj.

auxocyte (-sīt) an oocyte, spermatocyte, or sporocyte in the early stages of development.

auxodrome (-drōm) the course of growth of a child as plotted on a Wetzel grid.

auxometry (awks-om′ĕ-tre) measurement of rate of growth. **auxomet′ric,** adj.

auxotherapy (awk″so-ther′ah-pe) substitution therapy.

auxotroph (awk′so-trōf) an auxotrophic organism.

auxotrophic (awk″so-trof′ik) 1. requiring a growth factor not required by the parental or prototype strain; said of microbial mutants. 2. requiring specific organic growth factors in addition to the carbon source present in a minimal medium.

AV, A-V atrioventricular; arteriovenous.

av., avoir. avoirdupois.

avascular (a-vas′ku-lar) not vascular; bloodless.

avascularization (a-vas″ku-lar-i-za′shun) diversion of blood from tissues, as by ligation of vessels or tight bandaging.

aversive (ah-ver′siv) characterized by or giving rise to avoidance; noxious; cf. *appetitive*.

Avertin (ah-ver′tin) trademark for tribromoethanol.

avian (a′ve-an) of or pertaining to birds.

avidin (av′ĭ-din) a protein in egg white which interacts with biotin to render the latter inactive.

avirulence (a-vir′u-lens) lack of virulence; lack of competence of an infectious agent to produce pathologic effects. **avir′ulent,** adj.

avitaminosis (a-vi″tah-mĭ-no′sis) hypovitaminosis. **avitaminot′ic,** adj.

Avlosulfon (av″lo-sul′fon) trademark for a preparation of dapsone.

avoidance (ah-void′ance) a conscious or unconscious defensive reaction intended to escape anxiety, conflict, danger, fear, or pain.

avoirdupois (av′er-dŭ-poiz″) a system of weight used in English-speaking countries; see *Table of Weights and Measures*.

avulsion (ah-vul′shun) the tearing away of a structure or part. **phrenic a.,** extraction of a portion of the phrenic nerve, producing one-sided paralysis of the diaphragm and partial collapse of the lung.

ax. axis.

axenic (a-zen′ik) not contaminated by or associated with any foreign organisms; used in reference to pure cultures of microorganisms or to germ-free animals. Cf. *gnotobiotic*.

axiation (ak″se-a′shun) establishment of an axis; development of polarity in an ovum, embryo, organ, or other body structure.

axifugal (ak-sif′u-gal) directed away from an axis or axon.

axilla (ak-sil′ah) the armpit.

axillary (ak′sĭ-ler″e) of or pertaining to the armpit.

axio- word element [L., Gr.], *axis;* in dentistry, used in special reference to the *long axis of a tooth.*

axipetal (ak-sip′ĕ-tal) directed toward an axis or axon.

axis (ak′sis) 1. a line through the center of a body, or about which a structure revolves; a line around which body parts are arranged. 2. see *Table of Bones.* **ax′ial,** adj. **basibregmatic a.,** the vertical line from the basion to the bregma. **basicranial a.,** a line from basion to gonion. **basifacial a.,** a line from gonion to subnasal point. **binauricular a.,** a line joining the two auricular points. **celiac a.,** see under *trunk.* **dorsoventral a.,** one passing from the back to the belly surface of the body. **electrical a. of heart,** the resultant of the electromotive forces within the heart at any instant. **facial a.,** basifacial a. **frontal a.,** an imaginary line running from right to left through the center of the eyeball. **a. of heart,** a line passing through the center of the base of the heart and the apex. **optic a.,** 1. visual a. 2. the hypothetical straight line passing through the centers of curvature of the front and back surfaces of a simple lens. **sagittal a. of eye,** visual a. **visual a.,** an imaginary line passing from the midpoint of the visual field to the fovea centralis.

axis cylinder (ak″sis-sil′in-der) axon.

axofugal (ak-sof′u-gal) axifugal.

axolemma (ak″so-lem′ah) the surface membrane of an axon.

axolysis (ak-sol′ĭ-sis) degeneration of an axon.

axon, axone (ak′son; -sōn) 1. that process of a nerve cell by which impulses travel away from the cell body. 2. the axis of the body. **giant a.,** an axon of certain invertebrates, e.g., the squid, whose size (500 to 700 microns) has facilitated physiological studies of cell membrane excitation.

axoneme (ak′so-nēm) a slender axial filament, such as the axial thread of a chromosome, or that forming the central core of a flagellum.

axonometer (ak″so-nom′ĕ-ter) an apparatus for determination of cylindrical axis of a lens.

axonotmesis (ak″son-ot-me′sis) damage to nerve fibers causing complete peripheral degeneration; the internal structure is fairly well preserved, so that recovery of good quality is spontaneous.

axopetal (ak-sop′ĕ-tal) axipetal.

axophage (ak′so-fāj) a glia cell occurring in excavations in the myelin in myelitis.

axoplasm (-plazm) cytoplasm of an axon.

axopodium (ak″so-po′de-um) a more or less permanent type of pseudopodium, long and needle-like, characterized by an axial rod, composed of a bundle of fibrils inserted near the center of the cell body.

axospongium (-spun′je-um) the meshwork structure of the substance of an axon.

axostyle (ak′so-stīl) 1. the central supporting structure of an axopodium. 2. a supporting rod running through the body of a trichomonad and protruding posteriorly.

azacyclonol (a″zah-si′klo-nol) an isomer of pipradol, $C_{18}H_2NO$, used in hydrochloride form as a psychotherapeutic agent.

azapetine (-pet′ēn) an adrenergic blocking agent, $C_{17}H_{20}NO_4P$, used as the phosphate salt in peripheral vascular disease.

azaserine (-ser′ēn) an antibiotic, $C_5H_7N_3O_4$, used as an immunosuppressive agent in autoimmune disease.

azathioprine (-thi′o-prēn) a mercaptopurine derivative used as a cytotoxic and immunosuppressive agent in the treatment of leukemia and autoimmune diseases and in transplantation therapy.

azeotropy (a″ze-ot′ro-pe) absence of change in composition of a mixture of substances when it is boiled under pressure. **azeotrop′ic,** adj.

azobenzene (az″o-ben′zēn) a reduction product of nitrobenzene, $C_6H_5N:N \cdot C_6H_5$.

azoic (ah-zo′ik) destitute of living organisms.

azolitmin (az″o-lit′min) a coloring principle, $C_7H_7NO_4$, used as a pH indicator.

azoospermia (a″zo-o-sper′me-ah) lack of spermatozoa in the semen.

azote (a′zōt) [Fr.] nitrogen.

azotemia (az″o-te′me-ah) an excess of urea or other nitrogenous compounds in the blood. **azote′mic,** adj.

azotenesis (-tĕ-ne′sis) any disease due to excess of nitrogenous substances in the system.

azotification (az-o″tĭ-fi-ka′shun) fixation of atmospheric nitrogen.

azotize (az′o-tīz) to combine or charge with nitrogen.

Azotobacter (ah-zo′to-bak″ter) a genus of nitrogen-fixing schizomycetes (family Azotobacteraceae).

Azotobacteraceae (ah-zo″to-bak″tĕ-ra′se-e) a family of nitrogen-fixing schizomycetes (order Eubacteriales) widely distributed in the soil.

azotometer (az″o-tom′ĕ-ter) an instrument for measuring nitrogen content of compounds in solution.

Azotomonas (a-zo″to-mo′nas) a genus of nitrogen-fixing schizomycetes (family Pseudomonadaceae) found in the soil.

azotorrhea (az″o-to-re′ah) excessive loss of nitrogenous matter in the feces.

azoturia (-tu′re-ah) excess of urea or other nitrogenous compounds in the urine. **azotu′ric,** adj.

Azulfidine (a-zul′fĭ-dēn) trademark for a preparation of salicylazosulfapyridine.

azure (azh′ūr) any of the partially methylated homologues of the series of basic dyes extending from thionine to methylene blue, or to certain mixtures thereof; used in many staining procedures.

azuresin (azh″u-rez′in) a complex combination of azure A dye and carbacrylic cationic exchange resin used as a diagnostic aid in detection of gastric secretion.

azurophil (azh-u′ro-fil) an element or cell staining well with blue aniline dyes.

azurophilia (azh″u-ro-fil′e-ah) a condition in which the blood contains cells having azurophilic granules.

azurophilic (-fil′ik) staining well with blue aniline dyes; pertaining to or characterized by azurophilia.

azygogram (az′ĭ-go-gram) the film obtained by azygography.

azygography (az″ĭ-gog′rah-fe) radiography of the azygous venous system. **azygograph′ic,** adj.

azygos (az′ĭ-gos) 1. unpaired. 2. any unpaired part, as the azygos vein.

azygous (az′ĭ-gus) having no fellow; unpaired.

azymia (a-zim′e-ah) absence of enzyme.

B

B chemical symbol, *boron;* (physics) symbol, *gauss.*

B. Baumé scale; boils at; buccal.

B.A. Bachelor of Arts.

Ba chemical symbol, *barium.*

Babesia (bah-be′ze-ah) a genus of sporozoa found in the erythrocytes of various domestic animals; it includes *B. bigem′ina,* the causative agent of a fever in cattle, and *B. ca′nis,* the causative agent of canine piroplasmosis, both transmitted by ticks.

babesiasis, babesiosis (bah-bĕ-zi′ah-sis; bah-be″ze-o′sis) infection with *Babesia;* piroplasmosis.

baby (ba′be) an infant; a child not yet able to walk. **blue b.,** an infant born with cyanosis due to a congenital heart lesion or atelectasis. **"cloud b.,"** an apparently well infant who, because of interaction of viruses and bacteria in the respiratory tract or elsewhere, is able to contaminate the surrounding atmosphere with clouds of bacteria, and is thus reponsible for nursery epidemics. **collodion b.,** an infant born completely covered by a collodion- or parchment-like membrane; see *lamellar exfoliation of the newborn,* under *exfoliation.*

bacca (bak′ah) [L.] a berry.

baccate (-āt) resembling a berry.

bacciform (-sĭ-form) berry-shaped.

Bacillaceae (bas″il-la′se-e) a family of mostly saprophytic bacteria (order Eubacteriales), commonly found in soil; a few are insect or animal parasites and may cause disease.

bacillary (bas′ĭ-la″re) pertaining to bacilli or to rodlike structures.

bacillemia (bas″ĭ-le′me-ah) presence of bacilli in the blood.

bacilli (bah-sil′i) plural of *bacillus.*

bacilliform (bah-sil′ĭ-form) having the appearance of a bacillus.

bacillin (bah-sil′in) an antibiotic substance isolated from strains of *Bacillus subtilis,* highly active on both gram-positive and gram-negative bacteria.

bacillosis (bas″ĭ-lo′sis) infection with bacilli.

bacillotherapy (bah-sil″o-ther′ah-pe) bacteriotherapy.

bacilluria (bas″ĭ-lu′re-ah) bacilli in the urine.

Bacillus (bah-sil′lus) a genus of bacteria (family Bacillaceae), including gram-positive, spore-forming bacteria, separated into 33 species, three of which are pathogenic, or potentially so, the remainder being saprophytic soil forms. **B. abor′tus,** *Brucella abortus,* which causes infectious abortion in cattle. **B. an′thracis,** the causative agent of anthrax. **B. co′li,** *Escherichia coli.* **B. dysente′riae,** *Shigella dysenteriae.* **B. enterit′idis,** *Salmonella enteritidis.* **B. lep′rae,** *Mycobacterium leprae.* **B. mal′lei,** *Pseudomonas mallei.* **B. pneumo′niae,** *Klebsiella pneumoniae.* **B. pseudomal′lei,** *Pseudomonas pseudomallei.* **B. pyocya′neus,** *Pseudomonas aeruginosa.* **B. sub′tilis,** a common saprophytic soil and water form, often occurring as a laboratory contaminant, and, rarely, in apparently causal relation to pathologic processes, such as conjunctivitis. **B. tet′ani,** *Clostridium tetani.* **B. ty′phi, B. typho′sus,** *Salmonella typhosa.* **B. welch′ii,** *Clostridium perfringens.*

bacillus (bah-sil′us), pl. *bacil′li* [L.] 1. an organism of the genus *Bacillus.* 2. a rod-shaped bacterium; any spore-forming, rod-shaped microorganism of the order Eubacteriales. **Bang's b.,** *Brucella abortus.* **Battey bacilli,** unclassified mycobacteria that may produce tuberculosis-like disease in man. **Bordet-Gengou b.,** *Bordetella pertussis.* **Calmette-Guerin b.,** *Mycobacterium bovis* rendered completely avirulent by cultivation over a long period on bile-glycerol-potato medium; see *BCG vaccine.* **colon b.,** *Escherichia coli.* **Ducrey's b.,** *Hemophilus ducreyi.* **dysentery bacilli,** see *Shigella.* **Fick's b.,** *Proteus vulgaris.* **Flexner's b.,** *Shigella flexneri.* **Friedländer's b.,** *Klebsiella pneumoniae.* **Gärtner's b.,** *Salmonella enteritidis.* **glanders b.,** *Pseudomonas mallei.* **Hansen's b.,** *Mycobacterium leprae.* **Johne's b.,** *Mycobacterium paratuberculosis.* **Klebs-Löffler b.,** *Corynebacterium diphtheriae.* **Koch-Weeks b.,** *Hemophilus aegyptius.* **Morax-Axenfeld b.,** *Hemophilus duplex.* **Morgan's b.,** *Proteus morgani.* **Nocard's b.,** *Salmonella typhimurium.* **Pfeiffer's b.,** *Hemophilus influenzae.* **Sonne-Duval b.,** *Shigella sonnei.* **tubercle b.,** *Mycobacterium tuberculosis.* **typhoid b.,** *Salmonella typhosa.*

bacitracin (bas″ĭ-tra′sin) an antibacterial polypeptide elaborated by the licheniformis group of *Bacillus subtilis*, effective against a wide range of infections; usually applied topically, but also given intramuscularly. **zinc b.,** the zinc salt of bacitracin, used in an ointment as a topical antibacterial agent.

backbone (bak′bōn) the vertebral column.

back-cross (-kros) a mating between a heterozygote and a homozygote. **double b.,** the mating between a double heterozygote and a homozygote.

backflow (-flo) abnormal backward flow of fluids; regurgitation. **pyelovenous b.,** drainage from the renal pelvis into the venous system occurring under certain conditions of back pressure.

backscatter (-skat-er) in radiology, radiation deflected by scattering processes at angles greater than 90 degrees to the original direction of the beam of radiation.

bacter(io)- word element [Gr.], *bacteria.*

bacteremia (bak″ter-e′me-ah) presence of bacteria in the blood.

bacteria (bak-te′re-ah) plural of *bacterium.* **bacte′rial,** adj.

bactericidal (bak-tēr″ĭ-si′dal) destructive to bacteria.

bactericide (bak-tēr′ĭ-sīd) an agent which destroys bacteria.

bacterid (bak′ter-id) a skin eruption caused by bacterial infection elsewhere in the body.

bacteriemia (bak-ter″e-e′me-ah) bacteremia.

bacteriochlorophyll (bak-te″re-o-klo′ro-fil) a form of chlorophyll produced by certain bacteria and capable of carrying out photosynthesis.

bacteriocidin (-si′din) a bactericidal antibody.

bacteriocin (-sin) any of a group of substances, e.g., colicin, released by certain bacteria that kill other strains of bacteria by inducing metabolic block.

bacterioclasis (bak-te″re-ok′lah-sis) bacteriolysis.

bacteriogenic (bak-te″re-o-jen′ik) 1. bacterial in origin. 2. producing bacteria.

bacterioid (bak-te′re-oid) 1. resembling bacteria. 2. a structure resembling a bacterium.

bacteriologist (bak-te″re-ol′o-jist) an expert in bacteriology.

bacteriology (-ol′o-je) the scientific study of bacteria. **bacteriolog′ic,** adj.

bacteriolysin (-ol′ĭ-sin) an antibacterial antibody that lyses bacterial cells.

bacteriolysis (-ol′ĭ-sis) destruction or dissolution of bacteria. **bacteriolyt′ic,** adj.

bacterio-opsonin (bak-te″re-o-op-so′nin) bacteriopsonin.

bacteriopexy (-pek′se) the fixation of bacteria by histiocytes.

bacteriophage (bak-te′re-o-fāj″) a virus that lyses bacteria; see *bacterial virus.* **bacteriopha′gic,** adj. **temperate b.,** one whose genetic material (prophage) becomes an intimate part of the bacterial genome, persisting and being reproduced through many cell division cycles; the affected bacterial cell is known as a *lysogenic bacterium* (q.v.).

bacteriophagia (bak-te″re-o-fa′je-ah) destruction of bacteria by a lytic agent; bacteriolysis.

bacterioprecipitin (-pre-sip′ĭ-tin) any precipitin formed in the body in response to bacterial antigens.

bacterioprotein (-pro′te-in) a toxalbumin derived from certain bacteria.

bacteriopsonin (bak-te″re-op′so-nin) an antibody that acts on bacteria.

bacteriosis (bak-te″re-o′sis) any bacterial disease.

bacteriostatic (bak-te″re-o-stat′ik) inhibiting growth or multiplication of bacteria; an agent that so acts.

bacteriotherapy (-ther′ah-pe) treatment of disease by introducing bacteria into the system.

bacteriotoxin (-tok′sin) a toxin produced by or destructive to bacteria. **bacteriotox′ic,** adj.

Bacterium (bak-te′re-um) former name for a genus of schizomycetes the species of which are now assigned to other genera, e.g., *Aerobacter, Pseudomonas, Salmonella,* etc.

bacterium (bak-te′re-um), pl. *bacte′ria* [L., Gr.] in general, any schizomycete; formerly sometimes restricted to rod-shaped or to nonsporulating rod-shaped microorganisms. **acid-fast b.,** one not readily decolorized by acids after staining. **coliform bacteria,** see *Escherichia, Aerobacter,* and *Paracolobactrum.* **lactic acid bacteria,** those producing fermentation of carbohydrate materials to form lactic acid. **lysogenic b.,** a bacterial cell that harbors in its genome the genetic material (prophage) of a temperate bacteriophage and thus reproduces the bacteriophage in cell division; occasionally the prophage develop into the mature form, replicates, lyses the bacterial cell, and is free to infect other cells.

bacteriuria (bak-te″re-u′re-ah) presence of bacteria in the urine.

bacteroid (bak′ter-oid) 1. resembling a bacterium. 2. a structurally modified bacterium.

Bacteroidaceae (bak″tĕ-roi-da′se-e) a family of schizomycetes (order Eubacteriales).

Bacteroides (-roi′dēz) a genus of schizomycetes (family Bacteroidaceae) occurring as normal flora in the mouth and large bowel, and often in necrotic tissue, probably as secondary invaders; it includes *B. fundulifor′mis,* a pathogen of animals, causing diphtheria with abscesses in cattle, gangrenous dermatitis in horses, necrotic lesions in hogs, cattle, and sheep, and abscesses and necrotic areas in rabbits; also found in chronic ulcer of the colon in man.

bacteroides (-roi′dēz) 1. any highly pleomorphic rod-shaped bacteria. 2. an organism of the genus *Bacteroides.*

bacteruria (bak″ter-u′re-ah) bacteriuria.

baculum (bak′u-lum) a bone in the fibrous septum of the penis, found in many mammals and in primates, except man.

bag (bag) a sac or pouch. **Barnes′ b.,** a water-filled rubber bag for dilating the uterine cervix. **colostomy b.,** a receptacle worn over the stoma to receive the fecal discharge after colostomy. **Douglas b.,** a receptacle for the collection of expired air, permitting measurement of respiratory gases. **ileostomy b.,** any of various plastic or latex bags attached to the body for the collection of urine or fecal material following ileostomy or the establishment of an ileal bladder. **micturition b.,** a receptacle used for urine by ambulatory patients with urinary incontinence. **Politzer b.,** a soft bag of rubber for inflating the auditory tube. **Voorhees' b.,** a rubber bag that can be inflated with water for dilating the uterine cervix. **b. of waters,** the membranes enclosing the liquor amnii and the developing fetus *in utero.*

bagassosis (bag″ah-so′sis) a lung disease due to inhalation of dust from the residue of cane after extraction of sugar (bagasse).

BAL dimercaprol (British anti-lewisite).

balance (bal′ans) 1. an instrument for weighing. 2. harmonious adjustment of parts; harmonious performance of functions. **acid-base b.,** a normal balance between production and excretion of acid or alkali by the body, resulting in a stable concentration of H^+ in body fluids. **analytical b.,** a laboratory balance sensitive to variations of the order of 0.05 to 0.1 mg. **fluid b.,** the state of the body in relation to ingestion and excretion of water and electrolytes. **microchemical b.,** a laboratory balance sensitive to variations of the order of 0.001 mg. **nitrogen b.,** the state of the body in regard to ingestion and excretion of nitrogen. In *negative nitrogen b.* the amount excreted is greater than the quantity ingested; in *positive nitrogen b.* the amount excreted is smaller than the quantity ingested. **semimicro b.,** a balance sensitive to variations of 0.01 mg. **water b.,** fluid b.

balanic (bah-lan′ik) pertaining to the glans penis or glans clitoridis.

balanitis (bah″ah-ni′tis) inflammation of the glans penis. **gangrenous b.,** erosion of the glans penis leading to rapid destruction, believed to be due to continually unhygienic conditions together with secondary spirochetal infection.

balanoplasty (bal′ah-no-plas″te) plastic repair of the glans penis.

balanoposthitis (bal″ah-no-pos-thi′tis) inflammation of the glans penis and prepuce.

balanopreputial (-pre-pu′she-al) pertaining to the glans penis and prepuce.

balanorrhagia (-ra′je-ah) balanitis with free discharge of pus.

balantidiasis (bal″an-tĭ-di′ah-sis) infection with organisms of the genus *Balantidium.*

Balantidium (bal″an-tid′e-um) a genus of ciliated protozoa, including many species found in the intestine in vertebrates and invertebrates, including *B. co′li,* a common parasite of swine, rarely in man, in whom it may cause dysentery, and *B. su′is,* found in pigs, often considered the same as *B. coli.*

Balarsen (bah-lar′sen) trademark for preparations of arsthinol.

baldness (bawld′nes) alopecia, especially absense of hair from the scalp.

ball (bawl) a more or less spherical mass. **fatty b. of Bichat,** sucking pad. **fungus b.,** aspergilloma.

ballismus (bah-liz′mus) violent flinging movements of the limbs, as in chorea, sometimes affecting only one side of the body (hemiballismus).

ballistocardiogram (bah-lis″to-kar′de-o-gram″) the tracing made by a ballistocardiograph.

ballistocardiograph (-kar′de-o-graf″) the apparatus used in ballistocardiography.

ballistocardiography (-kar″de-og′rah-fe) the graphic recording of forces imparted to the body by cardiac ejection of blood.

ballottement (bah-lot′maw) [Fr.] a palpatory maneuver to test for a floating object, especially a maneuver for detecting pregnancy by inserting two fingers into the vagina and pushing the fetal head or breech, causing the fetus to leave and quickly return to the fingers.

balm (bahm) 1. a balsam. 2. a soothing or healing medicine. **mountain b.,** eriodictyon.

balneology (bal″ne-ol′o-je) the science dealing with baths and bathing.

balneotherapeutics (bal″ne-o-ther″ah-pu′tiks) balneotherapy.

balneotherapy (-ther′ah-pe) use of baths in the treatment of disease.

balsam (bawl′sam) a semifluid, fragrant, resinous vegetable juice; balsams are resins combined with oils. **balsam′ic,** adj. **friar's b.,** compound benzoin tincture. **gurjun b.,** an oleoresin obtained from trees of the genus *Dipterocarpus,* in India. **b. of Peru, peruvian b.,** a dark brown viscid liquid from the tree *Myroxylon pereirae,* used as a local protectant and as a rubefacient. **tolu b.,** a brown or yellowish brown, plastic solid from the tree *Myroxylon balsamum,* used as an ingredient of compound benzoin tincture and as an expectorant.

bancroftosis (ban″krof-to′sis) infestation with *Wuchereria bancrofti.*

band (band) a strip which constricts or binds a part. In dentistry, a thin metal strip formed to encircle horizontally the crown of a natural tooth or its roots. **A b.,** the dark-staining zone of a sarcomere, whose center is traversed by the H band. **coronary b.,** see under *cushion.* **H b.,** a pale zone sometimes seen traversing the center of the A band of a striated muscle fibril. **I b.,** the band within a striated muscle fibril, seen as a light region under the light microscope and as a dark region under polarized light. **iliotibial b.,** see under *tract.* **M b.,** the narrow dark band in the center of the H band. **matrix b.,** a thin piece of metal fitted around a tooth to supply a missing wall of a multisurface cavity to allow adequate condensation of amalgam into the cavity. **phonatory b's,** vocal cords; or an artificial substitute for them. **retention b.,** suspensory muscle. **Z b.,** a thin membrane seen on longitudinal section as a dark line in the center of the I band; the distance between Z bands delimits the sarcomeres of striated muscle.

bandage (ban′dij) 1. a strip or roll of gauze or other material for wrapping or binding a body part. 2. to cover by wrapping with such material. **Ace b.,** trademark for a bandage of woven elastic material. **Barton's b.,** a double fig-ure-of-8 bandage for fracture of the lower jaw. **capeline b.,** one applied like a cap or hood to the head or shoulder or to an amputation stump. **cravat b.,** one made by bringing the point of a triangular bandage to the middle of the base and then folding lengthwise to desired width. **demigauntlet b.,** one that covers the hand but leaves the fingers exposed. **Desault's b.,** one binding the elbow to the side, with a pad in the axilla, for fractured clavicle. **Esmarch's b.,** an India rubber bandage applied upward around (from the distal part to the proximal) a part in order to expel blood from it; the part is often elevated as the elastic pressure is applied. **figure-of-8 b.,** one in which the turns cross each other like the figure 8. **gauntlet b.,** one which covers the hand and fingers like a glove. **Gibney b.,** strips of ½-inch adhesive overlapped along the sides and back of the foot and leg to hold the foot in slight varus position and leave the dorsum of foot and anterior aspect of leg exposed. **Hamilton's b.,** a compound bandage for the lower jaw, composed of a leather string with straps of linen webbing. **plaster b.,** one stiffened with a paste of plaster of Paris. **pres-sure b.,** one for applying pressure. **protective b.,** one for covering underlying injured tissue or dressings. **roller b.,** a tightly rolled, circular bandage of varying width and materials, often commercially prepared. **scultetus b.,** a many-tailed bandage applied with the tails overlapping each other and held in position by safety pins. **spica b.,** a figure-of-8 bandage with turns that cross one another regularly like the letter V, usually applied to anatomical areas whose dimensions vary, as the pelvis and thigh. **suspensory b.,** one for supporting the scrotum. **T b.,** one shaped like the letter T. **triangular b.,** a triangle of cloth used as a sling; it can be folded several times to form a cravat. **Velpeau b.,** one used in immobilization of certain frac-tures about the upper end of the humerus and shoulder joint, binding the arm and shoulder to the chest.

bank (bank) a stored supply of human material or tissues for future use by other individuals, as *blood b., bone b., skin b.,* etc.

Banthine (ban'thīn) trademark for preparations of methantheline.

bantingism (ban'ting-izm) Banting treatment.

bar (bahr) 1. a unit of pressure, being the pres-sure exerted by 1 megadyne per square cm. 2. a heavy wire or wrought or cast metal segment, longer than its width, used to connect parts of a removable partial denture. **median b.,** a fi-brotic formation across the neck of the prostate gland, producing obstruction of the urethra. **Mercier's b.,** interureteric ridge.

baragnosis (bar"ag-no'sis) impairment of abil-ity to perceive differences in weight or pressure.

barbital (bahr'bĭ-tahl) the first of the barbitu-rates, being a long-acting hypnotic and seda-tive.

barbiturate (bahr-bit'u-rāt) a salt or derivative of barbituric acid; barbiturates are used for their hypnotic and sedative effects.

barbotage (bahr"bo-tahzh') [Fr.] repeated alter-nate injection and withdrawal of fluid with a syringe, as in gastric lavage or administration of an anesthetic agent into the subarachnoid space by alternate injection of part of the anes-thetic and withdrawal of cerebrospinal fluid into the syringe.

baresthesia (bar"es-the'ze-ah) sensibility for weight or pressure.

baresthesiometer (bar"es-the"ze-om'ĕ-ter) in-strument for estimating sense of weight or pres-sure.

bariatrics (bar"e-at'riks) a field of medicine en-compassing the study of overweight, its causes, prevention, and treatment.

barium (ba're-um) chemical element (*see table*), at. no. 56, symbol Ba. **b. sulfate,** a water-insolu-ble salt, $BaSO_4$, used as an opaque contrast me-dium in roentgenography of the digestive tract.

bark (bahrk) the tough external layer of a woody stem or trunk. **cinchona b., Jesuit's b., peru-vian b.,** cinchona.

baroceptor (bar"o-sep'tor) baroreceptor.

barodontalgia (-don-tal'je-ah) aerodontalgia.

barognosis (bar"og-no'sis) conscious perception of weight; the faculty by which weight is recog-nized.

baro-otitis (bar"o-o-ti'tis) barotitis.

barophilic (-fil'ik) growing best under high at-mospheric pressure; said of bacteria.

baroreceptor (-re-sep'tor) a sensory nerve end-ing that is stimulated by pressure changes, as those in blood vessel walls.

barosinusitis (-si"nu-si'tis) a symptom complex due to differences in environmental atmo-spheric pressure and the air pressure in the paranasal sinuses.

barotaxis (-tak'sis) stimulation of living matter by change of atmospheric pressure.

barotitis (-ti'tis) a morbid condition of the ear due to exposure to differing atmospheric pres-sures. **b. me'dia,** a symptom complex due to difference between atmospheric pressure of the environment and air pressure in the middle ear.

barotrauma (-traw'mah) injury due to pressure, as to structures of the ear, in high-altitude fly-ers, owing to differences between atmospheric and intratympanic pressures; see *barosinusitis* and *barotitis.*

barrier (bār'e-er) an obstruction. **blood-brain b., blood-cerebral b.,** the selective barrier sep-arating the blood from the parenchyma of the central nervous system. Abbreviated *BBB.* **placental b.,** the semipermeable barrier inter-posed between the maternal and the fetal blood by the placental membrane.

bartholinitis (bar"to-lin-i'tis) inflammation of Bartholin's glands.

Bartonella (bar"to-nel'lah) a genus of the family Bartonellaceae, including *B. bacillifor'mis,* the etiologic agent of Carrión's disease.

Bartonellaceae (-nel-la'se-e) a family of the or-der Rickettsiales, occurring as pathogenic para-sites in the erythrocytes of man and other ani-mals.

bartonellemia (-nel-le'me-ah) presence in the blood of organisms of the genus *Bartonella*.

bartonelliasis, bartonellosis (-nel-li'ah-sis; -nel-lo'sis) Carrión's disease.

baryesthesia (bar"e-es-the'ze-ah) baresthesia.

baryglossia (-glos'e-ah) barylalia.

barylalia (-la'le-ah) indistinct, thick speech, due to lesion of the central nervous system.

baryphonia (-fo'ne-ah) deepness and hoarseness of the voice.

basad (ba'sad) toward a base or basal aspect.

basal (ba'sal) pertaining to or situated near a base; in physiology, pertaining to the lowest possible level.

Basaljel (ba'sal-jel) trademark for basic aluminum carbonate gel.

base (bās) 1. the lowest part or foundation of anything; see also *basis*. 2. the main ingredient of a compound. 3. the nonacid part of a salt; a substance that combines with acids to form salts. **denture b.**, the material in which the teeth of a denture are set and which rests on the supporting tissues when the denture is in place in the mouth. **hexone b's,** bases containing six atoms of carbon, including arginine, lysine, and histadine. **nitrogenous b.,** an aromatic, nitrogen-containing molecule that serves as a proton acceptor, e.g., purine or pyrimidine. **ointment b.,** a vehicle for medicinal substances intended for external application to the body. **purine b's,** a group of chemical compounds of which purine is the base, including adenine, theobromine, uric acid, and xanthine. **pyrimidine b's,** a group of chemical compounds of which pyrimidine is the base, including uracil, thymine, and cytosine, which are common constituents of nucleic acids. **record b., temporary b., trial b.,** baseplate.

baseline (bās'līn) a known value or quantity used to measure or assess an unknown, as a baseline urine sample.

baseplate (-plāt) a sheet of plastic material used in making trial plates for artificial dentures.

basial (ba'se-al) pertaining to the basion.

basic (ba'sik) 1. pertaining to or having properties of a base. 2. capable of neutralizing acids.

basicity (ba-sis'ĭ-te) 1. the quality of being a base, or basic. 2. the combining power of an acid.

Basidiobolus (bah-sid"ĭ-ob'o-lus) a genus of phycomycetous fungi (family Entomophthoraceae, order Entomophthorales), including *B. haptospo'rus*, the cause of subcutaneous phycomycosis.

basidiospore (bah-sid'e-o-spōr) a spore of certain higher fungi formed on a basidium following karyogamy and meiosis.

basidium (-um), pl. *basid'ia* [L.] the clublike organ bearing basidiospores.

basihyoid (ba"se-hi'oid) the body of the hyoid bone; in certain lower animals, either of two lateral bones that are its homologues.

basilad (bas'ĭ-lad) toward the base.

basilar (-lar) pertaining to a base or basal part.

basilateral (ba"sĭ-lat'er-al) both basilar and lateral.

basilemma (-lem'ah) basement membrane.

basiloma (bas"ĭ-lo'mah) basal cell carcinoma.

basion (ba'se-on) the midpoint of the anterior border of the foramen magnum.

basipetal (bah-sip'ĕ-tal) descending toward the base; developing in the direction of the base, as a spore.

basis (ba'sis) the lower, basic, or fundamental part of an object, organ, or substance.

basisphenoid (ba"sĕ-sfe'noid) an embryonic bone which becomes the back part of the body of the sphenoid.

basoerythrocyte (ba"so-ĕ-rith'ro-sīt) an erythrocyte containing basophil granules.

basophil (ba'so-fil) 1. any structure, cell, or histologic element staining readily with basic dyes. 2. a granular leukocyte with an irregularly shaped, relatively pale-staining nucleus that is partially constricted into two lobes, and with cytoplasm containing coarse bluish black granules of variable size.

basophile (ba'so-fīl) basophilic.

basophilia (ba"so-fil'e-ah) 1. reaction of relatively immature erythrocytes to basic dyes whereby the stained cells appear blue, gray, or grayish-blue, or bluish granules appear. 2. abnormal increase of basophilic leukocytes in the blood. 3. basophilic leukocytosis.

basophilic (-fil'ik) staining readily with basic dyes.

basophilism (ba-sof'ĭ-lizm) abnormal increase of basophilic cells. **Cushing's b., pituitary b.,** see under *syndrome* (1).

basoplasm (ba'so-plazm) cytoplasm that stains with basic dyes.

bath (bath) 1. a medium, e.g., water, vapor, sand, or mud, with which the body is washed or in which the body is wholly or partially immersed for therapeutic or cleansing purposes; application of such a medium to the body. 2. the equipment or apparatus in which a body or object may be immersed. **colloid b.,** one containing gelatin, starch, bran, or similar substances. **contrast b.,** alternate immersion of a body part in hot and cold water. **cool b.,** one in water from 65° to 75° F. **douche b.,** application of water to the body from a jet spray. **emollient b.,** one in an emollient liquid, e.g., a decoction of bran. **graduated b.,** one in which the temperature of the water is gradually lowered. **half b.,** a bath of the hips and lower part of the body. **hip b.,** sitz b. **hot b.,** one in water from 98° to 104° F. **mud b.,** application of wet sticky earth to the body, or immersion of the body in such material. **needle b.,** a shower bath in which the water is projected in a fine, needle-like spray. **sitz b.,** immersion of only the hips and buttocks. **sponge b.,** one in which the body is not immersed but is rubbed with a wet cloth or sponge. **tepid b.,** one in water 75° to 92° F. **warm b.,** one in water 92° to 97° F. **whirlpool b.,** one in which the water is kept in constant motion by mechanical means.

bathmotropism (bath-mot'ro-pizm) influence on the excitability of muscular tissue. **bathmotrop'ic,** adj.

bathochromy (bath"o-kro'me) a shift of the absorption band toward lower frequencies (longer wavelengths) with deepening of color from yellow to red to black.

bathrocephaly (bath″ro-sef′ah-le) a developmental anomaly marked by a steplike posterior projection of the skull, caused by excessive growth of the lambdoid suture.

bathy- word element [Gr.], *deep.*

bathyanesthesia (bath″e-an″es-the′ze-ah) loss of deep sensibility.

bathyesthesia (-es-the′ze-ah) deep sensibility.

bathyhyperesthesia (-hi″per-es-the′ze-ah) abnormally increased sensitiveness of deep body structures.

bathyhypesthesia (-hīp″es-the′ze-ah) abnormally diminished deep sensibility.

bathypnea (-ne′ah) deep breathing.

battery (bat′er-e) 1. a set or series of cells affording an electric current. 2. any set, series, or grouping of similar things, as a battery of tests.

Bayer 205 (ba′er) suramin sodium.

B.C. bone conduction.

BCG bacille Calmette-Guérin (see under *vaccine*).

Be chemical symbol, *beryllium.*

beaker (bēk′er) a glass cup, usually with a lip for pouring, used by chemists and pharmacists.

beat (bēt) a throb or pulsation, as of the heart or of an artery. **apex b.,** the beat felt over the apex of the heart, normally in the fifth left intercostal space. **capture b's,** occasional ventricular responses to a sinus impulse that reaches the atrioventricular node in a nonrefractory phase. **ectopic b.,** a heart beat originating at some point other than the sinus node. **escaped b's,** heart beats that follow an abnormally long pause. **forced b.,** an extrasystole produced by artificial stimulation of the heart. **premature b.,** an early appearing beat, often an extrasystole.

bechic (bek′ik) pertaining to cough.

bed (bed) 1. a supporting structure or tissue. 2. a couch or support for the body during sleep. **capillary b.,** the capillaries, collectively, and their volume capacity; see Plate IX. **fracture b.,** one for the use of patients with broken bones. **Gatch b.,** one fitted with jointed springs, which may be adjusted to various positions. **Klondike b.,** one arranged to protect the patient from drafts in outdoor sleeping. **nail b.,** matrix unguis; the area of modified epithelium beneath the nail. **Vickers hyperbaric b.,** a small portable unit for administering hyperbaric oxygen, particularly in myocardial infarction; its maximum pressure is 2 atm.

bedbug (bed′bug) a bug of the genus *Cimex.*

bedpan (bed′pan) a shallow vessel used for defecation or urination by patients confined to bed.

Bedsonia (bed-so′ne-ah) *Chlamydia.*

bedsore (bed′sōr) decubitus ulcer.

beeswax (bēz′waks) wax from the honeycomb of the bee, *Apis mellifera;* see *yellow wax.* **bleached b.,** white wax. **unbleached b.,** yellow wax.

Beggiatoa (bej″je-ah-to′ah) a genus of schizomycetes (family Beggiatoaceae).

Beggiatoaceae (-to-a′se-e) a family of schizomycetes (order Beggiatoales).

Beggiatoales (-to-a′lēz) an order of schizomycetes.

behavior (be-hāv′yer) deportment or conduct; any or all of a person's total activity, especially that which is externally observable. **automatic b.,** automatism. **invariable b.,** activity whose character is determined by innate structure, such as reflex action. **variable b.,** behavior modified by individual experience.

behaviorism (-izm) the psychologic theory based upon objectively observable, tangible, and measurable data, rather than subjective phenomena, such as ideas and emotions.

bejel (bej′el) nonvenereal syphilis.

bel (bel) a unit used to express the ratio of two powers, usually electric or acoustic powers; an increase of 1 bel in intensity approximately doubles loudness of most sounds. See also *decibel.*

belching (belch′ing) eructation.

belemnoid (be-lem′noid) 1. dart-shaped. 2. the styloid process.

belladonna (bel″ah-don′ah) 1. *Atropa belladonna* (deadly nightshade), a plant that is the source of various alkaloids, e.g., atropine, hyoscyamine, etc. 2. belladonna leaf; the dried leaves and fruiting flowering tops of *Atropa belladonna,* used as an anticholinergic.

belly (bel′e) 1. the abdomen. 2. the fleshy, contractile part of a muscle.

belonoid (bel′o-noid) needle-shaped; styloid.

bemegride (bem′ĕ-grīd) an analeptic, $C_8H_{13}NO_2$, used especially in barbiturate poisoning.

benactyzine (ben-ak′tĭ-zēn) an ataraxic, $C_{20}H_{25}NO_3$, used as the hydrochloride salt.

Benadryl (ben′ah-dril) trademark for a preparation of diphenhydramine.

benanserin (ben-an′ser-in) a serotonin antagonist, $C_{19}H_{22}N_2O$.

bend (bend) a turn or curve; a curved part. **varolian b.,** the third cerebral flexure in the developing fetus.

bendroflumethiazide (ben″dro-floo″mĕ-thi′ah-zīd) a diuretic and antihypertensive, $C_{15}H_{14}F_3N_3O_4S_2$.

bends (bendz) pain in the limbs and abdomen due to rapid reduction of air pressure; see *decompression sickness.*

Benemid (ben′ĕ-mid) trademark for probenecid.

benign (be-nīn′) not malignant; not recurrent; favorable for recovery.

Benoquin (ben′o-kwin) trademark for a preparation of monobenzone.

benoxinate (ben-ok′sĭ-nāt) a surface anesthetic for the eye, $C_{17}H_{28}N_2O_3$, used as the hydrochloride salt.

bentonite (ben′to-nīt) a native colloidal hydrated aluminum silicate that swells in water; used as a bulk laxative and in preparations for use on the skin.

benzaldehyde (ben-zal′dĕ-hīd) artificial essential oil of almond; used as a flavoring agent.

benzalkonium chloride (ben″zal-ko′ne-um) a mixture of alkylbenzyldimethylammonium chlorides; used as a topical antiseptic in 1:750 to 1:10,000 solution.

benzcurine iodide (benz'ku-rēn) gallamine triethiodide.

Benzedrex (ben'zĕ-dreks) trademark for a propylhexedrine inhaler.

Benzedrine (-drēn) trademark for a preparation of amphetamine.

benzene (ben'zēn) a liquid hydrocarbon, C_6H_6, from coal tar; used as a solvent. **b. hexachloride,** C_6Cl_6, occurring in five isomeric forms, the gamma isomer (lindane) is a powerful insecticide.

benzestrol (ben-zes'trol) an estrogenic compound, $C_{20}H_{26}O_2$, for oral administration.

benzethonium (ben''zĕ-tho'ne-um) an ammonium derivative, $C_{27}H_{42}NO_2$; the chloride salt is used as a local antiseptic.

benzhexol (benz-hek'sol) trihexyphenidyl.

benzhydramine (-hi'drah-mēn) diphenhydramine.

benzidine (ben'zĭ-dēn) a compound, $NH_2 \cdot C_6 - H_4 \cdot C_6H_4NH_2$, used as a test for blood.

benzin, benzine (ben'zin; ben'zēn) petroleum b. **petroleum b.,** a purified distillate from petroleum, a solvent for organic compounds.

benzoate (ben'zo-āt) a salt of benzoic acid.

benzoated (-āt''ed) containing or combined with benzoic acid.

benzocaine (-kān) a local anesthetic, $C_9H_{11}NO_2$, used topically.

benzodioxan (ben''zo-di-oks'an) a class of α-adrenergic blocking agents, the most important member being piperoxan.

benzoin (ben'zo-in, ben-zo'in) a balsamic resin from *Styrax benzoin* and other *Styrax* species, used as a topical protectant and antiseptic and as an expectorant.

benzol (ben'zol) benzene.

benzonatate, benzononatine (ben-zo'nah-tāt; ben-zo''no-na'tin) an antitussive, $C_{30}H_{53}NO_{11}$.

benzphetamine (benz-fet'ah-mēn) a sympathomimetic amine, $C_{17}H_{21}N$, used as an anorexiant in the form of the hydrochloride salt.

benzthiazide (-thi'ah-zīd) a diuretic and antihypertensive, $C_{15}H_{14}ClN_3O_4S_3$.

benztropine (benz'tro-pēn) a parasympatholytic, $C_{25}H_{25}NO$, used as the mesylate salt in parkinsonism.

benzyl (ben'zil) the hydrocarbon radical, C_7H_7. **b. benzoate,** a clear, oily liquid, $C_{14}H_{12}O_2$, used as a scabicide and with dimercaprol as an antidote in metal poisoning.

benzylpenicillin (ben''zil-pen''ĭ-sil'in) penicillin G.

berberine (ber'ber-ēn) an alkaloid obtained from *Hydrastis canadensis*, *Berberis* species, and related shrubs; used as an antimalarial, carminative, and febrifuge, and in external dressing for indolent ulcers.

beriberi (ber''e-ber'e) a disease due to thiamine (vitamin B_1) deficiency, marked by polyneuritis, cardiac pathology, and edema; the epidemic form occurs primarily in areas in which white (polished) rice is the staple food.

berkelium (ber-ke'le-um) chemical element (*see table*), at. no. 97, symbol Bk.

Berubigen (be-roo'bĭ-jen) trademark for preparations of cyanocobalamin.

berylliosis (bĕ-ril''e-o'sis) a morbid condition due to exposure to fumes or finely divided dust of beryllium salts, marked by formation of granulomas, usually involving the lungs and, rarely, the skin, subcutaneous tissue, lymph nodes, liver, and other organs.

beryllium (bĕ-ril'le-um) chemical element (*see table*), at. no. 4, symbol Be.

bestiality (bes''te-al'ĭ-te) sexual connection with an animal.

beta (ba'tah) second letter of the Greek alphabet, β; used in names of chemical compounds to distinguish one of two or more isomers or to indicate position of substituting atoms or groups.

betacism (-sizm) excessive use of *b* sound in speaking.

Betadine (-dēn) trademark for preparations of povidone-iodine.

betahistine (ba''tah-his'tēn) a vasodilator, $C_8 - H_{12}N_2$, having histamine-like activity.

betaine (be'tah-in) a compound, $C_5H_{11}NO_2$, which has been used in the treatment of muscular weakness and degeneration, and in hydrochloride form as a lipotropic agent and as a substitute for hydrochloric acid.

Betalin (ba'tah-lin) trademark for preparations of vitamin B complex.

betamethasone (ba''tah-meth'ah-sōn) a synthetic glucocorticoid, $C_{22}H_{29}FO_5$, the most active of the anti-inflammatory steroids; available as a cream or tablet for topical or oral use.

betanaphthol (-naf'thol) a form of naphthol, $C_{10}H_8O$, used as an antiseptic.

Betaprone (ba'tah-prōn) trademark for preparations of propiolactone.

betapropiolactone (ba''tah-pro''pe-o-lak'tōn) propiolactone.

betatron (ba'tah-tron) an apparatus for accelerating electrons to millions of electron volts by magnetic induction.

Betaxin (be-tak'sin) trademark for preparations of thiamine hydrochloride.

betazole (ba'tah-zōl) a pyrazole derivative, $C_5 - H_9N_3$; its hydrochloride salt is used in gastric function tests to stimulate gastric secretion.

bethanechol (bĕ-tha'ne-kol) a cholinergic, $C_7 - H_{17}O_2$, used as the chloride salt.

bethanidine (bĕ-than'ĭ-dēn) an adrenergic blocking agent, $C_{10}H_{15}N_3$, used in the treatment of essential hypertension, particularly the malignant phase.

Bev billion electron volts (3.82×10^{-11} gram calorie, or 1.6×10^{-3} erg).

Bevidox (bev'ĭ-doks) trademark for a solution of cyanocobalamin.

bezoar (be'zōr) a mass formed in the stomach by compaction of repeatedly ingested material that does not pass into the intestine.

BFP biological false-positive reaction; a positive finding in serologic tests for syphilis when syphilis does not exist.

Bi chemical symbol, *bismuth*.

bi- word element [L.], *two*.

biarticular (bi″ar-tik′u-lar) affecting two joints.

biarticulate (-ar-tik′u-lāt) having two joints.

bibasic (bi-ba′sik) having two hydrogen atoms that may react with bases.

bibliotherapy (bib″le-o-ther′ah-pe) use of books and the reading of them in treatment of nervous disorders.

bicameral (bi-kam′er-al) having two chambers or cavities.

bicapsular (-kap′su-lar) having two capsules.

bicarbonate (-kar′bo-nāt) any salt containing the HCO_3^- anion. **blood b., plasma b.,** the bicarbonate of the blood plasma, an index of alkali reserve. **b. of soda,** sodium bicarbonate.

bicaudal (-kaw′dal) having two tails.

bicaudate (-kaw′dāt) bicaudal.

bicellular (-sel′u-lar) made up of two cells.

bicephalus (-sef′ah-lus) dicephalus.

biceps (bi′seps) a muscle having two heads.

bichloride (bi-klo′rīd) a chloride containing two equivalents of chlorine.

Bicillin (bi′sĭ-lin) trademark for a preparation of benzathine penicillin G.

bicipital (bi-sip′ĭ-tal) having two heads; pertaining to a biceps muscle.

biconcave (-kon′kāv) having two concave surfaces.

biconvex (-kon′veks) having two convex surfaces.

bicornate, bicornuate (-kor′nāt; -kor′nu-āt) having two horns or cornua.

bicoronal (bi″kŏ-ro′ne-al) pertaining to the two coronas, one radiating from each internal capsule of the brain.

bicorporate (bi-kor′po-rāt) having two bodies.

bicuspid (-kus′pid) 1. having two cusps. 2. a bicuspid (mitral) valve. 3. a premolar tooth.

b.i.d. [L.] *bis in di′e* (twice a day).

bidermoma (bi″der-mo′mah) a teratoma composed of cells and tissues from two germ layers.

biduous (bid′u-us) lasting two days.

bifid (bi′fid) cleft into two parts or branches.

biforate (bi-fo′rāt) having two perforations or foramina.

bifurcate (-fer′kāt) divided into two branches.

bifurcation (bi″fer-ka′shun) 1. a division into two branches. 2. the point at which division into two branches occurs.

bighead (big′hed) 1. a condition of young rams characterized by edematous swelling of the head and neck, due to *Clostridium novyi*. 2. thickening of face and ears in white sheep, due to photosensitivity after ingestion of certain plants. 3. hydrocephalus in mink.

bilateral (bi-lat′er-al) having two sides; pertaining to both sides.

bile (bīl) a fluid secreted by the liver, concentrated in the gallbladder, and poured into the small intestine via the bile ducts, which helps in alkalinizing the intestinal contents and plays a role in emulsification, absorption, and digestion of fat; its chief constituents are conjugated bile salts, cholesterol, phospholipid, bilirubin, and electrolytes.

Bilharzia (bil-har′ze-ah) *Schistosoma*.

bilharziasis (bil″har-zi′ah-sis) schistosomiasis.

bili- word element [L.], *bile*.

biliary (bil′e-a-re) pertaining to bile, to the bile ducts, or to the gallbladder.

bilicyanin (bil″ĭ-si′ah-nin) a blue pigment derived by oxidation from biliverdin.

bilifuscin (-fus′in) a pigment from human bile and gallstones.

biligenesis (-jen′ĕ-sis) production of bile.

biligenic (-jen′ik) producing bile.

bilihumin (-hu′min) an insoluble ingredient of gallstones.

bilin (bi′lin) any of a group of yellow bile pigments, including stercobilin and urobilin.

bilious (bil′yus) characterized by bile, by excess of bile, or by biliousness.

biliousness (-nes) a symptom complex comprising nausea, abdominal discomfort, headache, and constipation, formerly attributed to excessive bile secretion.

biliprasin (bil″ĭ-pra′sin) a green pigment from bile.

bilirachia (-ra′ke-ah) presence of bile pigments in spinal fluid.

bilirubin (-roo′bin) a bile pigment produced by breakdown of heme and reduction of biliverdin; it normally circulates in plasma and is taken up by liver cells and conjugated to form bilirubin diglucuronide, the water-soluble pigment excreted in bile.

bilirubinemia (-roo″bĭ-ne′me-ah) presence of bilirubin in the blood.

bilirubinuria (-nu′re-ah) presence of bilirubin in the urine.

biliuria (bil″e-u′re-ah) presence of bile acids in the urine.

biliverdin (bil″ĭ-ver′din) a green bile pigment formed by catabolism of hemoglobin and converted to bilirubin in the liver; it may also arise from oxidation of bilirubin.

bilobate (bi-lo′bāt) having two lobes.

bilobular (-lob′u-lar) having two lobules.

bilocular (-lok′u-lar) having two compartments.

bimanual (-man′u-al) with both hands.

bimastoid (-mas′toid) pertaining to both mastoid processes.

binary (bi′nah-re) made up of two elements or of two equal parts; denoting a number system with a base of two.

binaural (bi-naw′ral, bin-aw′ral) pertaining to both ears.

binauricular (bin″aw-rik′u-lar) pertaining to both auricles of the ears.

binder (bīnd′er) a girdle or large bandage for support of the abdomen or breasts. **abdominal b.,** one applied to the abdomen after childbirth to support relaxed abdominal walls. **obstetric b.,** an abdominal girdle or bandage chiefly for women in labor who have pendulous abdomen.

binocular (bin-ok′u-lar) 1. pertaining to both eyes. 2. having two eyepieces, as in a microscope.

binomial (bi-no′me-al) composed of two terms,

e.g., names of organisms formed by combination of genus and species names.

binotic (bin-ot′ik) binaural.

binovular (bin-ov′u-lar) pertaining to or derived from two distinct ova.

binuclear (bi-nu′kle-ar) having two nuclei.

binucleation (bi″nu-kle-a′shun) formation of two nuclei within a cell through division of the nucleus without division of the cytoplasm.

binucleolate (bi-nu′kle-o-lāt) having two nucleoli.

bio- word element [Gr.], *life; living.*

bioacoustics (bi″o-ah-koo′stiks) the science dealing with the communicating sounds made by animals.

bioassay (-as-sa′) determination of the active power of a drug sample by comparing its effects on a live animal or an isolated organ preparation with those of a reference standard.

bioastronautics (-as″tro-naw′tiks) scientific study of effects of space and interplanetary travel on biological systems.

bioavailability (-ah-vāl″ah-bil′ĭ-te) the degree to which a drug or other substance becomes available to the target tissue after administration.

biochemistry (-kem′is-tre) the chemistry of living organisms and of vital processes.

biocidal (-si′dal) destructive to living organisms.

bioclimatologist (-kli″mah-tol′o-jist) one skilled in bioclimatology.

bioclimatology (-tol′o-je) scientific study of effects on living organisms of conditions of natural environment (rainfall, daylight, temperature, etc.) prevailing in specific regions of the earth.

biocolloid (-kol′oid) a colloid from animal, plant, or microbial tissue.

biocybernetics (-si″ber-net′iks) the science of communications and control in animals.

biodegradable (-de-grād′ah-b'l) susceptible of degradation by biological processes, as by bacterial or other enzymatic action.

biodegradation (-deg″rah-da′shun) the series of processes by which living systems render chemicals less noxious to the environment.

Bio-des (bi′o-des) trademark for a preparation of diethylstilbestrol.

biodetritus (bi″o-de-tri′tus) detritus produced by the disintegration and decomposition of once-living material.

biodynamics (-di-nam′iks) scientific study of the nature and déterminants of all organismic (including human) behavior.

bioelectricity (-e″lek-tris′ĭ-te) electrical phenomena apparent in living cells.

bioelectronics (-tron′iks) the study of the role of intermolecular transfer of electrons in biological regulation and defense.

biofeedback (-fēd′bak) the provision of visual or auditory evidence to a person of the status of an autonomic body function, as by the sounding of a tone when blood pressure is at a desirable level, so that he may exert control over the function.

bioflavonoid (-fla′vo-noid) a generic term for a group of compounds widely distributed in plants and concerned with maintenance of a normal state of the walls of small blood vessels.

biogen (bi′o-jen) one of several labile proteins supposedly representing the ultimate basis of life.

biogenesis (bi″o-jen′ĕ-sis) 1. origin of life, or of living organisms. 2. the theory that living organisms originate only from other living organisms.

biogeography (-je-og′rah-fe) the scientific study of the geographic distribution of living organisms.

biokinetics (-ki-net′iks) the science of movements within developing organisms.

biologic (-loj′ik) pertaining to biology.

biological (-loj′ĭ-kal) 1. pertaining to biology. 2. a medicinal preparation made from living organisms and their products, including serums, vaccines, etc.

biologist (bi-ol′o-jist) a specialist in biology.

biology (bi-ol′o-je) scientific study of living organisms. **molecular b.,** study of molecular structures and events underlying biological processes, including relation between genes and the functional characteristics they determine. **radiation b.,** scientific study of effects of ionizing radiation on living organisms.

bioluminescence (bi″o-lu″mĭ-nes′ens) chemoluminescence occurring in living cells.

biolysis (bi-ol′ĭ-sis) decomposition of organic matter by living organisms.

biolytic (bi″o-lit′ik) 1. pertaining to or characterized by biolysis. 2. destructive to life.

biomass (bi′o-mas) the entire assemblage of living organisms of a particular region, considered collectively.

biomathematics (bi″o-math″ĕ-mat′iks) mathematics as applied to the phenomena of living things.

biome (bi′ōm) a large, distinct, easily differentiated community of organisms arising as a result of complex interactions of climatic factors, biota, and substrate; usually designated, according to kind of vegetation present, as tundra, coniferous or deciduous forest, grassland, etc.

biomechanics (bi″o-mĕ-kan′iks) the application of mechanical laws to living structures.

biomedicine (bi″o-med′ĭ-sin) clinical medicine based on the principles of the natural sciences (biology, biochemistry, etc.). **biomed′ical,** adj.

biometeorologist (-me″te-or-ol′o-jist) one skilled in biometeorology.

biometeorology (-ol′o-je) scientific study of effects on living organisms of the extraorganic aspects (temperature, humidity, barometric pressure, rate of air flow, and air ionization) of the physical environment, whether natural or artificially created, and also their effects in closed ecological systems, as in satellites or submarines.

biometer (bi-om′ĕ-ter) instrument for measuring carbon dioxide given off by living tissue.

biometrics (bi″o-met′riks) biometry.

biometry (bi-om′ĕ-tre) the application of statistical methods to biological facts.

biomicroscope (bi"o-mi'kro-skōp) a microscope for examining living tissue in the body.

biomicroscopy (-mi-kros'ko-pe) microscopic examination of living tissue in the body.

bion (bi'on) an individual living organism.

bionecrosis (bi"o-ně-kro'sis) necrobiosis.

bionergy (bi-on'er-je) life force; the force exercised in the living organism.

bionics (-iks) scientific study of functions, characteristics, and phenomena observed in the living world, and the application of knowledge gained therefrom to nonliving systems.

bionucleonics (bi"o-nu"kle-on'iks) scientific study of biological applications of radioactive and rare stable isotopes.

biophysics (-fiz'iks) the science dealing with the application of physical methods and theories to biological problems.

biophysiology (-fiz"e-ol'o-je) that portion of biology including organogeny, morphology, and physiology.

bioplasm (bi'o-plazm) 1. protoplasm. 2. the more vital or essential part of cytoplasm. **bioplas'mic,** adj.

biopsy (bi'op-se) removal and examination, usually microscopic, of tissue from the living body, performed to establish precise diagnosis. **aspiration b.,** biopsy in which tissue is obtained by application of suction through a needle attached to a syringe. **endoscopic b.,** removal of tissue by appropriate instruments through an endoscope. **excisional b.,** biopsy of tissue removed by surgical cutting. **incisional b.,** biopsy of a selected portion of a lesion. **needle b.,** biopsy in which tissue is obtained by puncture of a tumor, the tissue within the lumen of the needle being detached by rotation, and the needle withdrawn. **punch b.,** biopsy in which tissue is obtained by a punch. **sternal b.,** biopsy of bone marrow of the sternum removed by puncture or trephining.

bios (bi'os) any of a group of growth factors for single-celled organisms such as yeast; it is probably a mixture of B vitamins and pantothenic acid. **b. I,** inositol. **b. II,** biotin.

bioscience (bi"o-si'ens) the study of biology wherein all the applicable sciences (physics, chemistry, etc.) are applied.

bioset (bi'o-set) a grouping of biological components.

biospectrometry (bi"o-spek-trom'ě-tre) spectrometry of the quantity of a substance in living tissue.

biospectroscopy (-spek-tros'ko-pe) the spectroscopy of living tissue.

biosphere (bi'o-sfēr) 1. that part of the universe in which living organisms are known to exist, comprising the atmosphere, hydrosphere, and lithosphere. 2. the sphere of action between an organism and its environment.

biostatistics (bi"o-stah-tis'tiks) vital statistics.

biosynthesis (-sin'thě-sis) creation of a compound by physiologic processes in a living organism. **biosynthet'ic,** adj.

biota (bi-o'tah) all the living organisms of a particular area; the combined flora and fauna of a region.

biotaxis (bi"o-tak'sis) the selecting and arranging powers of living cells.

biotaxy (-tak'se) 1. biotaxis. 2. taxonomy.

biotelemetry (-tel-em'ě-tre) the recording and measuring of certain vital phenomena of living organisms that are situated at a distance from the measuring device.

biotic (bi-ot'ik) 1. pertaining to life or living organisms. 2. pertaining to the biota.

biotics (bi-ot'iks) the functions and qualities peculiar to living organisms, or the sum of knowledge regarding these qualities.

biotin (bi'o-tin) a member of the vitamin B complex, $C_{10}H_{16}O_3N_2S$, required by or occurring in all forms of life tested.

biotomy (bi-ot'o-me) 1. study of animal and plant life by dissection. 2. vivisection.

biotoxication (bi"o-tok"si-ka'shun) intoxication due to a biotoxin.

biotoxicology (-tok"si-kol'o-je) scientific study of poisons produced by living organisms, and treatment of conditions produced by them.

biotoxin (-tok'sin) a poisonous substance produced by a living organism.

biotransformation (-trans"for-ma'shun) the series of chemical alterations of a compound (e.g., a drug) occurring within the body, as by enzymatic activity.

biotype (bi'o-tīp) 1. a group of individuals having the same genotype. 2. any of a number of strains of a species of microorganisms having differentiable physiologic characteristics.

biovular (bi-ov'u-lar) binovular.

biparental (bi"pah-ren'tal) derived from two parents, male and female.

biparous (bip'ah-rus) producing two ova or offspring at one time.

bipenniform (bi-pen'ĭ-form) doubly feather-shaped; said of muscles whose fibers are arranged on each side of a tendon like barbs on a feather shaft.

biperiden (-per'ĭ-den) a synthetic anticholinergic, $C_{21}H_{29}HO$, used to reduce tremors of parkinsonism.

bipolar (-po'lar) 1. having two poles. 2. pertaining to both poles.

bipotentiality (bi"po-ten"she-al'ĭ-te) ability to develop or act in either of two possible ways.

biramous (bi-ra'mus) having two branches.

birefractive (bi"re-frak'tiv) doubly refractive.

birefringence (-re-frin'jens) the quality of transmitting light unequally in different directions. **birefrin'gent,** adj. **flow b.,** that exhibited only when the substance is in solution and flowing. **form b.,** that produced by regular orientation of submicroscopic asymmetrical particles in a substance or object, differing in refractive index from the surrounding medium.

birth (berth) a coming into being; act or process of being born. **complete b.,** entire separation of the infant from the maternal body (after cutting of the umbilical cord). **multiple b.,** the birth of two or more offspring produced in the same gestation period. **premature b.,** birth of a premature infant.

birthmark (berth′mark) nevus; a circumscribed blemish or spot on the skin of congenital origin. **physiologic b.,** one so common as to be considered normal; once applied to nevus flammeus in the suboccipital region.

bisacodyl (bis-ak′o-dil) a cathartic, $C_{22}H_{19}NO_4$.

bisacromial (bis″ah-kro′me-al) pertaining to the two acromial processes.

bisalbuminemia (-al-bu″mĭ-ne′me-ah) a congenital abnormality marked by the presence of two distinct serum albumins that differ in mobility on electrophoresis.

bisection (bi-sek′shun) division into two parts by cutting.

bisexual (-seks′u-al) 1. having gonads of both sexes. 2. hermaphrodite. 3. both heterosexual and homosexual.

bisferious (bis-fe′re-us) dicrotic; having two beats.

bishydroxycoumarin (bis″hi-drok″se-koo′-mah-rin) an anticoagulant, $C_{19}H_{12}O_6$.

bisiliac (bis-il′e-ak) pertaining to the two iliac bones or to any two corresponding points on them.

bis in die (bis in de′a) [L.] twice a day.

bismuth (biz′muth) chemical element (see table), at. no. 83, symbol Bi. Its salts have been used in inflammatory diseases of the stomach and intestines and in syphilis. **b. glycolylarsanilate,** glycobiarsol. **b. subcarbonate,** a basic salt used as a topical protectant, intestinal astringent, and antacid. **b. subgallate,** bright yellow, amorphous powder, applied locally in skin diseases. **b. subnitrate, b. white,** a basic salt, used as an antacid.

bismuthosis (biz″muth-o′sis) chronic bismuth poisoning, with anuria, stomatitis, dermatitis, and diarrhea.

bistephanic (bi″stě-fan′ik) pertaining to the stephanions, especially to the shortest distance between them (bistephanic width).

bistoury (bis′too-re) a long, narrow, straight or curved, surgical knife.

bistrimin (-trĭ-min) phenyltoloxamine.

bisulfate (bi-sul′fāt) an acid sulfate.

bite (bīt) 1. seizure with the teeth. 2. a wound or puncture made by a living organism. 3. an impression made by closure of the teeth upon some plastic material, e.g., wax. 4. occlusion (2). **closed b.,** malocclusion in which the incisal edges of the mandibular anterior teeth protrude past those of the maxillary teeth. **cross b.,** crossbite. **edge-to-edge b., end-to-end b.,** occlusion in which the incisors of both jaws are closed. **open b.,** occlusion in which certain opposing teeth fail to come together when the jaws are closed; usually confined to anterior teeth. **over-b.,** overbite.

bite-block (bīt′blok) occlusion rim.

bitelock (-lok) a dental device for retaining occlusion rims in the same relation outside the mouth which they occupied in the mouth.

bitemporal (bi-tem′po-ral) pertaining to both temples or temporal bones.

biteplate (bīt′plāt) an appliance, usually plastic and wire, worn in the palate as a diagnostic or therapeutic adjunct in orthodontics or prosthodontics.

bite-wing (-wing) a wing or fin attached along the center of the tooth side of a dental x-ray film and bitten on by the patient, permitting production of images of the corona of the teeth in both dental arches and their contiguous periodontal tissues.

Bitis (bi′tis) a genus of venomous, brightly colored, thick-bodied, viperine snakes, possessing heart-shaped heads; including the puff adder (*B. arientans*), Gaboon viper (*B. gabonica*), and rhinoceros viper (*B. nasicornis*).

bitrochanteric (bi-tro″kan-ter′ik) pertaining to both trochanters on one femur or to both greater trochanters.

bitumen (bĭ-too′men) any of various natural and artificial dry petroleum products.

bituminosis (bĭ-too″mĭ-no′sis) a form of pneumoconiosis due to dust from soft coal.

biuret (bi′u-ret) a urea derivative, $C_2O_2N_3H_5$; presence is detected after addition of sodium hydroxide and copper sulfate solutions by a pinkish-violet color (protein test) or a pink and finally a bluish color (urea test).

bivalent (bi-va′lent, biv′ah-lent) 1. having a valence of two. 2. denoting homologous chromosomes associated in pairs during the first meiotic prophase.

bivalve (bi′valv) having two valves, as the shells of such mollusks as clams.

biventral (bi-ven′tral) 1. having two bellies. 2. digastric muscle.

bizygomatic (-zi″go-mat′ik) pertaining to the two most prominent points on the two zygomatic arches.

Bk chemical symbol, *berkelium.*

black (blak) reflecting no light or true color; of the darkest hue. **ivory b.,** animal charcoàl.

blackhead (blak′hed) 1. comedo. 2. histomoniasis of turkeys.

blackleg (-leg) symptomatic anthrax.

blackout (-owt) loss of vision and momentary lapse of consciousness due to diminished circulation to the brain and retina.

bladder (blad′er) a membranous sac, such as one serving as receptacle for a secretion, especially the urinary bladder. **atonic b.,** a condition marked by a dilated, poorly contracting urinary bladder without evidence of a lesion of the central nervous system. **automatic b.,** neurogenic bladder due to complete transection of the spinal cord above the sacral segments, with loss of micturition reflexes and bladder sensation, involuntary voiding, and an abnormal amount of residual urine. **autonomic b., autonomous b.,** neurogenic bladder due to a lesion in the sacral portion of the spinal cord that interrupts the reflex arc controlling the bladder, with loss of normal bladder sensation and reflexes, inability to initiate urination normally, and incontinence. **chyle b.,** cisterna chyli. **cord b.,** automatic b. **irritable b.,** a condition of the bladder marked by increased frequency of contraction with associated desire to urinate. **motor para-**

lytic b., neurogenic bladder due to impairment of the motor neurons or nerves controlling the bladder; the *acute* form is marked by painful distention and inability to initiate micturition, and the *chronic* form by difficulty in initiating micturition, straining, decreased size and force of stream, interrupted stream, and recurrent urinary tract infection. **neurogenic b.,** any condition of dysfunction of the urinary bladder due to a lesion of the central or peripheral nervous system. **neurogenic b., atonic,** neurogenic bladder due to destruction of the sensory nerve fibers from the bladder to the spinal cord, with absence of control of bladder functions and of desire to void, overdistention of the bladder, and an abnormal amount of residual urine; most frequently associated with tabes dorsalis (*tabetic b.*) and pernicious anemia. **neurogenic b., uninhibited,** neurogenic bladder due to a lesion in the region of the upper motor neurons with subtotal interruption of corticospinal pathways, with urgency, frequent involuntary voiding, and small-volume threshold of activity. **sacculated b.,** a bladder with pouches between the hypertrophied muscular fibers. **tabetic b.,** see *atonic neurogenic b.* **urinary b.,** the musculomembranous sac in the anterior part of the pelvic cavity that serves as a reservoir for urine, which it receives through the ureters and discharges through the urethra.

blanch (blanch) to become pale.

blast (blast) 1. an immature stage in cellular development before appearance of the definitive characteristics of the cell; used also as a word termination, as in adamantoblast, etc. 2. the wave of air pressure produced by the detonation of high-explosive bombs or shells or by other explosions; it causes pulmonary concussion and hemorrhage (*lung blast, blast chest*), laceration of other thoracic and abdominal viscera, ruptured ear drums, and minor effects in the central nervous system. 3. see *blasto-*.

blastema (blas-te′mah) 1. the primitive substance from which cells are formed. 2. a group of cells giving rise to a new individual (in asexual reproduction) or to an organ or part (in either normal development or in regeneration).

blasto- word element [Gr.], *a bud; budding.*

Blastocaulis (blas″to-kaw′lis) a genus of schizomycetes (family Pasteuriaceae).

blastocoele (blas′to-sēl) the fluid-filled central segmentation cavity of the blastula. **blastocoe′lic,** adj.

blastocyst (-sist) the mammalian conceptus in the post-morula stage, consisting of the trophoblast and an inner cell mass.

blastocyte (-sīt) an undifferentiated embryonic cell.

blastocytoma (blas″to-si-to′mah) blastoma.

blastoderm (blas′to-derm) the single layer of cells forming the wall of the blastula, or the cellular cap above the floor of segmented yolk in the discoblastula of telolecithal ova.

blastodisc (-disk) the convex structure formed by the blastomeres at the animal pole of an ovum undergoing incomplete cleavage.

blastogenesis (blas″to-jen′ĕ-sis) 1. development

of an individual from a blastema, i.e., by asexual reproduction. 2. transmission of inherited characters by the germ plasm. 3. morphological transformation of small lymphocytes into larger cells resembling blast cells on exposure to phytohemagglutinin or to antigens to which the donor is immunized.

blastolysis (blas-tol′ĭ-sis) destruction or splitting up of germ substance. **blastolyt′ic,** adj.

blastoma (blas-to′mah) a neoplasm composed of embryonic cells derived from the blastema of an organ or tissue. **blasto′matous,** adj.

blastomatosis (blas″to-mah-to′sis) the formation of blastomas; tumor formation.

blastomere (blas′to-mēr) one of the cells produced by cleavage of a fertilized ovum forming the blastoderm.

Blastomyces (blas″to-mi′sēz) a genus of pathogenic fungi growing as mycelial forms at room temperature and as yeastlike forms at body temperature; applied to the yeasts pathogenic for man and animals. **B. brasilien′sis,** *Paracoccidioides brasiliensis.* **B. dermatit′idis,** the agent of North American blastomycosis.

blastomycete (-mi′sēt) any organism of the genus *Blastomyces;* also, any yeastlike organism.

blastomycosis (-mi-ko′sis) 1. infection with *Blastomyces.* 2. any infection caused by a yeastlike organism. **North American b.,** a chronic infection due to *Blastomyces dermatitidis,* predominately involving the skin, lungs, and bones. **South American b.,** paracoccidioidomycosis.

blastopore (blas′to-pōr) the opening of the archenteron to the exterior of the embryo, at the gastrula stage.

blastospore (-spōr) a spore formed by budding, as in yeast.

blastula (blas′tu-lah), pl. *blas′tulae.* The usually spherical body produced by cleavage of a fertilized ovum, consisting of a single layer of cells (blastoderm) surrounding a fluid-filled cavity (blastocoele).

blastulation (blas″tu-la′shun) conversion of the morula to the blastula by development of a blastocoele.

blaze (blāz) an abnormal streak or spot of white in the scalp hair.

bleb (bleb) a large flaccid vesicle, usually at least 1 cm. in diameter.

bleeder (blēd′er) 1. one who bleeds freely; a hemophiliac. 2. any large blood vessel cut during surgery.

bleeding (-ing) 1. the escape of blood, as from an injured vessel. 2. the letting of blood. **functional b.,** bleeding from the uterus when no organic lesions are present. **implantation b.,** that occurring at the time of implantation of the fertilized ovum in the decidua. **occult b.,** escape of blood in such small quantity that it can be detected only by chemical test or by microscopic or spectroscopic examination. **placentation b.,** bleeding from the uterus during the early weeks of pregnancy, when the maternal blood vessels are being eroded.

blenn(o)- word element [Gr.], *mucus.*

blennadenitis (blen″ad-ĕ-ni′tis) inflammation of mucous glands.

blennogenic (-o-jen′ik) producing mucus.

blennoid (blen′oid) resembling mucus.

blennorrhagia (blen″o-ra′je-ah) 1. any excessive discharge of mucus; blennorrhea. 2. gonorrhea.

blennorrhea (-re′ah) any free discharge of mucus, especially a gonorrheal discharge from the urethra or vagina; gonorrhea. **blennorrhe′al,** adj. **inclusion b.,** see under *conjunctivitis.*

blennostasis (blen-nos′tah-sis) suppression of an abnormal mucous discharge, or correction of an excessive one. **blennostat′ic,** adj.

blennothorax (blen″o-tho′raks) an accumulation of mucus in the chest.

blennuria (blen-u′re-ah) mucus in the urine.

blephar(o)- word element [Gr.], *eyelid; eyelash.*

blepharadenitis (blef″ar-ad″ĕ-ni′tis) inflammation of the meibomian glands.

blepharal (blef′ar-al) pertaining to the eyelids.

blepharectomy (blef″ar-ek′to-me) partial or complete excision of an eyelid.

blepharism (blef′ah-rizm) spasm of the eyelid; continuous blinking.

blepharitis (blef″ah-ri′tis) inflammation of the eyelids. **angular b.,** inflammation involving the angles of the eyelids. **squamous b.,** blepharitis in which the edge of the eyelid is covered with small, white or gray scales. **ulcerative b.,** that marked by small ulcerated areas along the eyelid margin, multiple, suppurative lesions, and loss of lashes.

blepharoadenitis (blef″ah-ro-ad″ĕ-ni′tis) blepharadenitis.

blepharoatheroma (-ath″er-o′mah) an encysted tumor or sebaceous cyst of an eyelid.

blepharochalasis (-kal′ah-sis) hypertrophy and loss of elasticity of the skin of the upper eyelid.

blepharoconjunctivitis (-kon-junk″tĭ-vi′tis) inflammation of eyelids and conjunctiva.

blepharoncus (blef″ar-ong′kus) a tumor on the eyelid.

blepharophimosis (blef″ah-ro-fĭ-mo′sis) abnormal narrowness of the palpebral fissures.

blepharoplast (blef′ah-ro-plast″) a minute granule forming one part of the kinetoplast, and from which the axoneme arises.

blepharoplasty (-plas″te) plastic surgery of the eyelids.

blepharoplegia (blef″ah-ro-ple′je-ah) paralysis of an eyelid.

blepharoptosis (blef′ar-op-to′sis) drooping of an upper eyelid; ptosis.

blepharopyorrhea (blef″ah-ro-pi″ŏ-re′ah) purulent ophthalmia.

blepharorrhaphy (blef″ah-ror′ah-fe) 1. suture of an eyelid. 2. tarsorrhaphy.

blepharospasm (blef′ah-ro-spazm″) spasm of the orbicular muscle of the eyelids.

blepharostat (-stat″) an instrument for holdng the eyelids apart.

blepharostenosis (blef″ah-ro-stĕ-no′sis) blepharophimosis.

blepharosynechia (-sĭ-nek′e-ah) a growing together or adhesion of the eyelids.

blepharotomy (blef″ah-rot′o-me) surgical incision of an eyelid; tarsotomy.

blight (blīt) any fungal disease of plants.

blind (blīnd) not having the sense of sight.

blindness (blīnd′nes) lack or loss of ability to see; lack of perception of visual stimuli. **blue b.,** tritanopia. **blue-yellow b.,** 1. tritanopia. 2. tetartanopia. **color b.,** popular term for any deviation from normal perception of color. **day b.,** defective vision in bright light. **epidemic b.,** a form of avian leukosis with blindness and misshapen pupil or irregular depigmentation of the iris in one or both eyes. **flight b.,** amaurosis fugax due to high centrifugal forces encountered in aviation. **green b.,** deuteranopia. **letter b.,** inability to recognize individual letters. **mind b.,** psychic b. **moon b.,** periodic ophthalmia. **night b.,** failure or imperfection of vision at night or in dim light. **note b.,** inability to read musical notes because of a brain lesion. **object b.,** inability to recognize the nature and purpose of objects seen. **psychic b.,** failure of proper interpretation of visual stimuli due to a brain lesion. **red b.,** protanopia. **snow b.,** dimness of vision, usually temporary, due to glare of sun upon snow. **text b., word b.,** visual aphasia.

blister (blis′ter) a vesicle, especially a bulla. **blood b.,** a vesicle having bloody contents, as may be caused by a pinch or bruise. **fever b.,** see *herpes simplex.*

bloat (blōt) 1. tympany of the stomach. 2. enteritis in young rabbits, accompanied by gaseous distention of the abdomen.

block (blok) 1. an obstruction or stoppage. 2. regional anesthesia. **bundle-branch b.,** see under *heart block.* **caudal b.,** anesthesia produced by injection of a local anesthetic into the caudal or sacral canal. **epidural b.,** anesthesia produced by injection of the anesthetic between the vertebral spines and beneath the ligamentum flavum into the extradural space. **field b.,** regional anesthesia obtained by blocking conduction in nerves with chemical or physical agents. **heart b.,** see *heart block.* **mental b.,** obstruction to thought or memory, particularly that produced by emotional factors. **nerve b.,** regional anesthesia secured by injection of anesthetics in close proximity to the appropriate nerve. **paracervical b.,** anesthesia of the inferior hypogastric plexus and ganglia produced by injection of the local anesthetic into the lateral fornices of the vagina. **parasacral b.,** regional anesthesia produced by injection of a local anesthetic around the sacral nerves as they emerge from the sacral foramina. **paravertebral b.,** infiltration of the cervicothoracic ganglion with procaine hydrochloride. **perineural b.,** regional anesthesia produced by injection of the anesthetic agent close to the nerve. **presacral b.,** anesthesia produced by injection of the local anesthetic into the sacral nerves on the anterior aspect of the sacrum. **pudendal b.,** anesthesia produced by blocking the pudendal nerves, accomplished by injection of the local anesthetic into the tuberosity of the ischium.

sacral b., anesthesia produced by injection of the local anesthetic into the extradural space of the spinal canal. **saddle b.,** the production of anesthesia in a region corresponding roughly with the areas of the buttocks, perineum, and inner aspects of the thighs, by introducing the anesthetic agent low in the dural sac. **subarachnoid b.,** anesthesia produced by the injection of a local anesthetic into the subarachnoid space around the spinal cord. **vagal b., vagus nerve b.,** blocking of vagal impulses by injection of a solution of local anesthetic into the vagus nerve at its exit from the skull.

Blockain (blok′ān) trademark for preparations of propoxycaine.

blocking (-ing) 1. interruption of an afferent nerve pathway; see *block.* 2. inhibition of an intracellular biosynthetic process, as by injection of dactinomycin. 3. difficulty in recollection, or interruption of a train of thought or speech, due to emotional factors, usually unconscious.

blood (blud) the fluid circulating through the heart, arteries, capillaries, and veins, carrying nutriment and oxygen to body cells, and removing waste products and carbon dioxide. It consists of the liquid portion (the plasma) and the formed elements (erythrocytes, leukocytes, and platelets). **aerated b., arterial b.,** that which carries oxygen to the tissues through the systemic arteries. **central b.,** that from the pulmonary venous system; sometimes used to designate splanchnic blood, or blood obtained from chambers of the heart or from bone marrow. **citrated b.,** blood treated with sodium citrate to prevent its coagulation. **cord b.,** that contained in umbilical vessels at time of delivery of the infant. **defibrinated b.,** whole blood from which fibrin has been separated during the clotting process. **occult b.,** that present in such small quantities that it is detectible only by chemical tests or by spectroscopic or microscopic examination. **peripheral b.,** that obtained from acral areas, or from the circulation remote from the heart; the blood in the systemic circulation. **splanchnic b.,** that circulating in thoracic, abdominal, and pelvic viscera, further distinguished on the basis of specific organ, e.g., pulmonary, hepatic, splenic. **venous b.,** blood that has given up its oxygen to the tissues and is carrying carbon dioxide back through the systemic veins for gas-exchange in the lungs. **whole b.,** that from which none of the elements has been removed, especially that drawn from a selected donor under aseptic conditions, containing citrate ion or heparin.

blood group (blud′grōōp) 1. an erythrocytic allotype (or phenotype) defined by one or more cellular antigenic groupings controlled by allelic genes. A considerable number of blood group systems are now known, the most widely used in matching blood for transfusion being the ABO and the Rh blood groups. 2. any characteristic, function, or trait of a cellular or fluid component of blood, considered as the expression (phenotype or allotype) of the actions and interactions of dominant genes, and useful in medicolegal and other studies of human inheritance;

such characteristics include the antigenic groups of erythrocytes, leukocytes, platelets, and plasma proteins.

blood plasma (blud plaz′mah) the fluid portion of the blood, in which the microscopically visible formed elements (erythrocytes, leukocytes, blood platelets) are suspended.

blood pressure (blud presh′ur) see under *pressure.*

blood serum (blud se′rum) the clear liquid that separates from blood when it is allowed to clot completely, and is therefore blood plasma from which fibrogen has been removed during clotting.

blood type (blud′ tīp) see *blood group.*

blowpipe (blo′pīp) a tube through which a current of air is forced upon a flame to concentrate and intensify the heat.

B.L.R.O.A. British Laryngological, Rhinological, and Otological Association.

blue (blu) 1. one of the principal colors of the visible spectrum, lying between green and violet; the color of the clear sky. 2. a dye of blue color. **alcian b.,** a copper-containing dye for staining acid mucopolysaccharides; it may be combined with periodic acid–Schiff reagent. **alizarin b.,** a blue dyestuff derived from anthracene. **aniline b.,** a mixture of the trisulfonates of triphenyl rosaniline and of diphenyl rosaniline. **Berlin b.,** Prussian b. **brilliant cresyl b.,** an oxazin dye, usually $C_{15}H_{16}N_3OCl$, used in staining blood. **bromophenol b.,** a dye, tetrabromophenolsulfonphthalein, used as an indicator in determining hydrogen ion concentration, being yellow at pH 3 and blue at pH 4.6. **Evans b.,** a green, bluish green, or brown odorless powder, $C_{34}H_{24}N_6Na_4O_{14}S_4$, injected intravenously in determining blood volume. **indigo b.,** indigotin. **methylene b.,** dark green crystals or cystalline powder with a bronze-like luster, $C_{16}H_{18}ClN_3S·3H_2O$, used as an antidote in cyanide poisoning, in the treatment of methemoglobinemia, and as a stain and an indicator. **Prussian b.,** an amorphous blue powder, $Fe_4[Fe(CN)_6]_3$. **thymol b.,** an indicator, being red at pH 1.2 and yellow at 2.8 (for acids), and yellow at 8.0 and blue at 9.6 (for alkalis). **toluidine b., toluidine b., O,** the chloride salt or zinc chloride double salt of aminodimethylaminotoluphenazthionium chloride; useful as a stain for demonstrating basophilic and metachromatic substances. **trypan b.,** an acid, azo dye that has been used in vital staining and as a remedy in protozoal infections.

blush (blush) sudden, brief erythema of the face and neck, resulting from vascular dilatation due to emotion or heat.

B.M.A. British Medical Association.

B.M.R. basal metabolic rate.

BNA Basle Nomina Anatomica, a system of anatomic nomenclature adopted at the annual meeting of the German Anatomic Society in 1895; superseded by *Nomina Anatomica.*

B.O.A. British Orthopaedic Association.

body (bod′e) 1. the trunk, or animal frame, with its organs. 2. the largest and most important part of any organ. 3. any mass or collection of material. **acetone b's,** ketone b's. **alkapton b's,** a class of substances with an affinity for alkali, found in urine and causing alkaptonuria; the compound most commonly found, and most commonly referred to by the term, is homogentisic acid. **amygdaloid b.,** corpus amygdaloideum. **amylaceous b's,** corpora amylacea. **aortic b's,** small neurovascular structures on either side of the aorta in the region of the aortic arch, containing chemoreceptors that play a role in reflex regulation of respiration. **b's of Arantius,** small tubercles, one at the center of the free margin of each of the three cusps of the aortic and pulmonary valves. **asbestos b's,** golden yellow bodies of various shapes in sputum, lung secretions, and feces of patients with asbestosis, formed by deposition of calcium and iron salts and proteins on asbestos spicules. **Aschoff b's,** submiliary collections of cells and leukocytes in the interstitial tissues of the heart in rheumatic myocarditis. **asteroid b.,** an irregularly star-shaped inclusion body found in the giant cells in sarcoidosis and other diseases. **Auer b's,** finely granular, lamellar bodies having acid-phosphatase activity, found in the cytoplasm of myeloblasts, myelocytes, monoblasts, and granular histiocytes, rarely in plasma cells, and virtually pathognomonic of leukemia. **Babès-Ernst b's,** metachromatic granules. **Barr b.,** sex chromatin. **Cabot's ring b's,** lines in the form of loops or figures-of-8, seen in stained erythrocytes in severe anemias. **carotid b.,** a small neurovascular structure lying in the bifurcation of the right and left carotid arteries, containing chemoreceptors that monitor oxygen content in blood and help to regulate respiration. **cavernous b.,** corpus cavernosum. **cell b.,** the portion of a cell containing the nucleus independent of any such projections as an axon or dentrite that the cell may have. **chromaffin b.,** paraganglion. **ciliary b.,** the thickened part of the vascular tunic of the eye, connecting the choroid and iris. **crescent b.,** achromocyte. **cytoid b's,** globular, shiny white structures resembling cell nuclei in size and shape, appearing in degenerated retinal nerve fibers; seen histologically in cotton-wool spots. **demilune b.,** achromocyte. **Döhle's inclusion b's,** small bodies seen in the cytoplasm of neutrophils in many infectious diseases, burns, aplastic anemia, and other disorders, and after administration of toxic agents. **Donovan's b's,** *Donovania granulomatis.* **elementary b.,** 1. blood platelet. 2. inclusion b. **fimbriate b.,** corpus fimbriatum. **foreign b.,** a mass of material which is not normal to the place where it is found. **fruiting b.,** a specialized structure, as an apothecium, which produces spores. **geniculate b., lateral,** an eminence of the metathalamus, just lateral to the medial geniculate body, marking the end of the optic tract. **geniculate b., medial,** an eminence of metathalamus just lateral to the superior colliculi, concerned with hearing. **Hassall's b's,** see under *corpuscle.* **Heinz b's, Heinz-Ehrlich b's,** inclusion bodies resulting from oxidative injury to and precipitation of hemoglobin; seen in the presence of certain abnormal hemoglobins and erythrocytes with enzyme deficiencies. **b. of**

Highmore, mediastinum testis. **Howell's b's, Howell-Jolly b's,** smooth, round remnants of nuclear chromatin seen in erythrocytes in various anemias and leukemias and after splenectomy. **hyaline b's,** drusen. **hyaloid b.,** vitreous b. **immune b.,** antibody. **inclusion b's,** round, oval, or irregular shaped bodies in the cytoplasm and nuclei of cells, as in disease due to viral infection, such as rabies, smallpox, etc. **intermediary b.,** amboceptor. **ketone b's,** the substances acetone, acetoacetic acid, and β-hydroxybutyric acid; except for acetone (which may arise spontaneously from acetoacetic acid), they are normal metabolic products of lipid within the liver, and are oxidized by muscles; excessive production leads to urinary secretion of these bodies, as in diabetes mellitus. **Lafora's b's,** intracytoplasmic inclusions consisting of a complex of glycoprotein and acid mucopolysaccharide, widespread deposits are found in myoclonus epilepsy. **Leishman-Donovan b's,** round or oval bodies found in the reticuloendothelial cells, especially those of the spleen and liver, in kala-azar; they are nonflagellate intracellular forms of *Leishmania donovani.* Also used to designate similar forms of *L. tropica* found in macrophages in lesions of cutaneous leishmaniasis. **Lieutaud's b.,** vesical trigone. **malpighian b's,** renal corpuscles. **mamillary b.,** either of the pair of small spherical masses in the interpeduncular fossa of the midbrain, forming part of the hypothalamus. **metachromatic b's,** see under *granule.* **Negri b's,** round or oval inclusion bodies seen in the cytoplasm and sometimes in the processes of neurons of rabid animals after death. **Nissl b's,** large granular bodies that stain with basic dyes, forming the reticular substance of the cytoplasm of neurons, and having ribonucleoprotein as one of the main constituents. **olivary b.,** olive (2). **pacchionian b's,** arachnoid granulations. **para-aortic b's,** enclaves of chromaffin cells near the sympathetic ganglia along the abdominal aorta, serving as chemoreceptors responsive to oxygen, carbon dioxide, and hydrogen in concentration and which help control respiration. **parabasal b.,** an oval or rodlike body forming one part of the kinetoplast. **parietal b.,** the anterior eyelike structure arising from the median part of the dorsal wall of the thalamus in some lower vertebrates. **pineal b.,** a small conical structure attached by a stalk to the posterior wall of the third ventricle. **pituitary b.,** see under *gland.* **polar b's,** small cells consisting of a tiny bit of cytoplasm and a nucleus, formed during maturation divisions of the oocyte. **psammoma b's,** usually microscopic, laminated masses of calcareous material, occurring in both benign and malignant epithelial and connective-tissue tumors, and sometimes associated with chronic inflammation. **quadrigeminal b's,** corpora quadrigemina. **restiform b.,** inferior cerebellar peduncle. **Rosenmüller's b.,** epoophoron. **Russell b's,** globular plasma cell inclusions, representing aggregates of immunoglobulins synthesized by the cell. **Seidelin b's,** bodies found in the red cells in yellow fever. **b. of stomach,** that portion of the stomach between the fundus and the pyloric part. **striate b.**, corpus striatum. **suprarenal b.**, adrenal gland. **tigroid b's**, Nissl b's. **trachoma b's**, inclusion bodies found in clusters in the cytoplasm of the epithelial cells of the conjunctiva in trachoma. **vitreous b.**, the transparent gel filling the inner portion of the eyeball between the lens and retina. **wolffian b.**, mesonephros.

boil (boil) furuncle. **Aleppo b., Delhi b., Natal b., Oriental b.**, cutaneous leishmaniasis.

bolometer (bo-lom′ĕ-ter) 1. an instrument for measuring the force of the heart beat. 2. an instrument for measuring minute degrees of radiant heat.

boloscope (bo′lo-skōp) an apparatus for locating metallic foreign bodies in the tissues.

bolus (bo′lus) 1. a rounded mass of food or pharmaceutical preparation ready to swallow, or such a mass passing through the gastrointestinal tract. 2. a concentrated mass of pharmaceutical preparation, e.g., an opaque contrast medium, given intravenously. 3. a mass of scattering material, such as wax or paraffin, placed between the radiation source and the skin to achieve a precalculated isodose pattern in the tissue irradiated. **alimentary b.**, the mass of food in the oropharynx or esophagus, compising one swallow.

bond (bond) the linkage between atoms or radicals of a chemical compound, or the mark indicating the number and attachment of the valencies of an atom in constitutional formulas, represented by a pair of dots or a line between atoms, e.g., H—O—H, H—C≡C—H or H:O:H, H:C:::C:H. **covalent b.**, chemical bonds in which electrons can be shared, as the peptide bonds in proteins. **high-energy b.**, a chemical bond the hydrolysis of which yields high levels of free energy; such bonds involve phosphate (*high-energy phosphate b.*) or sulfur (*high-energy sulfur b.*) or other mixed anhydride types of chemical structure. **hydrogen b.**, a weak, primarily electrostatic, bond between a hydrogen atom bound to a highly electronegative element (such as oxygen or nitrogen) in a given molecule, or part of a molecule, and a second highly electronegative atom in another molecule or in a different part of the same molecule. **peptide b.**, a ·CO·NH· group produced in linking amino acids to form peptides.

bone (bōn) 1. the hard, rigid form of connective tissue constituting most of the skeleton of vertebrates, composed chiefly of calcium salts. 2. any distinct piece of the skeleton of the body. See *Table of Bones* for regional listing and alphabetical listing of common names of bones of the body, and see Plates II and III. **ankle b.**, talus. **basiotic b.**, a small bone in the fetus between the basilar process and the basisphenoid. **brittle b's**, osteogenesis imperfecta. **cancellated b., cancellous b.**, bone made up of thin intersecting lamellae, usually found internal to compact bone. **cartilage b.**, bone developing within cartilage, ossification taking place within a cartilage model. **cavalary b.**, rider's b. **cheek b.**, zygomatic b. **coffin b.**, the third phalanx of the horse's foot. **collar b.**, clavicle. **compact b.**, bone substance that is dense and hard. **cortical**

b., the compact bone of the shaft of a bone that surrounds the marrow cavity. **exercise b.**, a bone developed in a muscle, tendon, or fascia, due to excessive exercise. **flat b.**, one whose thickness is slight, sometimes consisting of only a thin layer of compact bone, or of two layers with intervening cancellated bone and marrow; usually curved rather than flat. **heel b.**, calcaneus. **incisive b.**, the portion of the maxilla bearing the incisors; developmentally, it is the premaxilla, which in humans later fuses with the maxilla, but in most other vertebrates persists as a separate bone. **ivory b's**, osteopetrosis. **jaw b.**, the mandible or maxilla, especially the mandible. **jugal b.**, zygomatic b. **lingual b.**, hyoid b. **long b.**, one whose length exceeds its breadth and thickness. **malar b.**, zygomatic b. **marble b's**, osteopetrosis. **mastoid b.**, see under *process*. **membrane b.**, bone developing within a connective tissue membrane. **pelvic b.**, hip b. **petrous b.**, the petrous portion of the temporal bone. **pneumatic b.**, bone that contains air-filled spaces. **premaxillary b.**, premaxilla. **pterygoid b.**, see under *process*. **pyramidal b.**, triquetal b. **rider's b.**, localized ossification of the inner aspect of the lower end of the tendon of the adductor muscle of the thigh; sometimes seen in horseback riders. **semilunar b.**, lunate b. **shin b.**, tibia. **short b.**, one of approximately equal length, width, and thickness. **solid b.**, compact b. **spongy b.**, cancellous b. **squamous b.**, the upper forepart of the temporal bone, forming an upright plate. **sutural b's**, variable and irregularly shaped bones in the sutures between the bones of the skull. **thigh b.**, femur. **triangular b.**, triquetral b. **turbinated b.**, nasal conchae. **tympanic b.**, the part of the temporal bone surrounding the middle ear. **unciform b.**, hamate b. **wormian b's**, sutural b's.

bonelet (bōn′let) an ossicle, or small bone.

Bonine (bo′nēn) trademark for preparations of meclizine.

Boophilus (bo-of′ĭ-lus) a genus of hard-bodied ticks primarily parasitic on cattle. *B. annula′tus* (*B. bo′vis*) and *B. mi′croplus* are vectors of *Babesia bigemina*, the cause of a fever in cattle; *B. decolora′tus* is a vector of *Anaplasma marginale*, the cause of gallsickness in cattle.

booster (boōst′er) see under *dose*.

boot (boot) an encasement for the foot; a protective casing or sheath. **Gibney b.**, an adhesive tape support used in treatment of sprains and other painful conditions of the ankle, the tape being applied in a basket-weave fashion with strips placed alternately under the sole of the foot and around the back of the leg. **Unna's paste b.**, a dressing for varicose ulcers, consisting of a paste made from gelatin, zinc oxide, glycerin; the entire leg is covered with paste and covered with spiral bandages, applied in alternate layers until a rigid boot is made.

borate (bo′rāt) a salt of boric acid.

borax (bo′raks) sodium borate.

borborygmus (bor″bor-ig′mus) a rumbling noise caused by propulsion of gas through the intestines.

TABLE OF BONES, LISTED BY REGIONS OF THE BODY

REGION	NAME	TOTAL NUMBER	REGION	NAME	TOTAL NUMBER
Axial skeleton			Upper limb (×2)		64
Skull		21	Shoulder	scapula	
	(eight paired – 16)			clavicle	
	inferior nasal concha		Upper arm	humerus	
	lacrimal		Lower arm	radius	
	maxilla			ulna	
	nasal		Wrist	carpal (8)	
	palatine			(capitate)	
	parietal			(hamate)	
	temporal			(lunate)	
	zygomatic			(pisiform)	
	(five unpaired – 5)			(scaphoid)	
	ethmoid			(trapezium)	
	frontal			(trapezoid)	
	occipital			(triquetral)	
	sphenoid		Hand	metacarpal (5)	
	vomer		Fingers	phalanges (14)	
Ossicles of each ear		6	Lower limb (×2)		62
	incus		Pelvis	hip bone (1)	
	malleus			(ilium)	
	stapes			(ischium)	
Lower jaw				(pubis)	
	mandible	1	Thigh	femur	
Neck			Knee	patella	
	hyoid	1	Leg	tibia	
Vertebral column		26		fibula	
	cervical vertebrae (7)		Ankle	tarsal (7)	
	(atlas)			(calcaneus)	
	(axis)			(cuboid)	
	thoracic vertebrae (12)			(cuneiform, medial)	
	lumbar vertebrae (5)			(cuneiform, intermediate)	
	sacrum (5 fused)			(cuneiform, lateral)	
	coccyx (4–5 fused)			(navicular)	
Chest				(talus)	
	sternum	1	Foot	metatarsal (5)	
	ribs (12 pairs)	24	Toes	phalanges (14)	

Table of Bones

COMMON NAME*	NA EQUIVALENT†	REGION	DESCRIPTION	ARTICULATIONS
astragalus. *See* talus				
atlas	atlas	neck	first cervical vertebra, ring of bone supporting the skull	with occipital b. and axis
axis	axis	neck	second cervical vertebra, with thick process (odontoid process) around which first cervical vertebra pivots	with atlas above and third cervical vertebra below
calcaneus	calcaneus	foot	the "heel bone," of irregularly cuboidal shape, largest of the tarsal b's	with talus and cuboid b.
capitate b.	o. capitatum	wrist	third from thumb side of 4 bones of distal row of carpal b's	with second, third, and fourth metacarpal b's, and hamate, lunate, trapezoid, and scaphoid b's
carpal b's	oss. carpi	wrist	see *capitate, hamate, lunate, pisiform b's, scaphoid, trapezium, trapezoid,* and *triquetral b's*	
clavicle	clavicula	shoulder	elongated, slender, curved bone (collar bone) lying horizontally at root of neck, in upper part of thorax	with sternum and ipsilateral scapula and cartilage of first rib
coccyx	o. coccygis	lower back	triangular bone formed usually by fusion of last 4 (sometimes 3 or 5) (coccygeal) vertebrae	with sacrum
concha, inferior nasal	concha nasalis inferior	skull	thin, rough plate of bone attached by one edge to side of each nasal cavity, the free edge curling downward	with ethmoid and ipsilateral lacrimal and palatine b's and maxilla
cuboid b.	o. cuboideum	foot	pyramidal bone, on lateral side of foot, in front of calcaneus	with calcaneus, lateral cuneiform b., fourth and fifth metatarsal b's, occasionally with navicular b.
cuneiform b., intermediate	o. cuneiforme intermedium	foot	smallest of 3 cuneiform b's, located between medial and lateral cuneiform b's	with navicular, medial, and lateral cuneiform b's, and second metatarsal b.
cuneiform b., lateral	o. cuneiforme laterale	foot	wedge-shaped bone at lateral side of foot, intermediate in size between medial and intermediate cuneiform b's	with cuboid, navicular, intermediate cuneiform b's and second, third, and fourth metatarsal b's
cuneiform b., medial	o. cuneiforme mediale	foot	largest of 3 cuneiform b's, at medial side of foot	with navicular, intermediate cuneiform, and first and second metatarsal b's
epistropheus. *See* axis				

*b. = bone; b's = (pl.) bones.
†o. = os; oss. = (L. pl.) ossa.

TABLE OF BONES (Continued)

COMMON NAME*	NA EQUIVALENT†	REGION	DESCRIPTION	ARTICULATIONS
ethmoid b.	o. ethmoidale	skull	unpaired bone in front of sphenoid b. and below frontal b., forming part of nasal septum and superior and medial conchae of nose	with sphenoid and frontal b's, vomer, and both lacrimal, nasal, and palatine b's, maxillae, and inferior nasal conchae
fabella		knee	sesamoid b. in lateral head of gastrocnemius muscle	with femur
femur	femur	thigh	longest, strongest, heaviest bone of the body (thigh b.)	proximally with hip b., distally with patella and tibia
fibula	fibula	leg	lateral and smaller of 2 bones of leg	proximally with tibia, distally with tibia and talus
frontal b.	o. frontale	skull	unpaired bone constituting anterior part of skull	with ethmoid and sphenoid b's, and both parietal, nasal, lacrimal, and zygomatic b's, and maxillae
hamate b.	o. hamatum	wrist	most medial of 4 bones of distal row of carpal b's	with fourth and fifth metacarpal b's and lunate, capitate, and triquetral b's
hip b.	o. coxae	pelvis and hip	broadest bone of skeleton, composed originally of 3 bones which become fused together in acetabulum: *ilium*, broad, flaring, uppermost portion; *ischium*, thick, three-sided part behind and below acetabulum and behind obturator foramen; *pubis*, consisting of body (expanded anterior portion), inferior ramus (extending backward and fusing with ramus of ischium) and superior ramus (extending from body to acetabulum)	with femur, anteriorly with its fellow (at symphysis pubis), posteriorly with sacrum
humerus	humerus	arm	long bone of upper arm	proximally with scapula, distally with radius and ulna
hyoid b.	o. hyoideum	neck	U-shaped bone at root of tongue, between mandible and larynx	none; attached by ligaments and muscles to skull and larynx
ilium	o. ilium	pelvis	see *hip b.*	
incus	incus	ear	middle ossicle of chain in the middle ear, so named because of its resemblance to an anvil	with malleus and stapes
innominate b. *See* hip b.				
ischium	o. ischii	pelvis	see *hip b.*	
lacrimal b.	o. lacrimale	skull	thin, uneven scale of bone near rim of medial wall of each orbit	with ethmoid and frontal b's, and ipsilateral inferior nasal concha and maxilla
lunate b.	o. lunatum	wrist	second from thumb side of 4 bones of proximal row of carpus	with radius, and capitate, hamate, scaphoid, and triquetral b's

malleus	malleus	ear	most lateral ossicle of chain in middle ear, so named because of its resemblance to a hammer	with incus; fibrous attachment to tympanic membrane
mandible	mandibula	lower jaw	horseshoe-shaped bone carrying lower teeth	with temporal b's
maxilla	maxilla	skull (upper jaw)	paired bone, below orbit and at either side of nasal cavity, carrying upper teeth	with ethmoid and frontal b's, vomer, fellow maxilla, and ipsilateral inferior nasal concha and lacrimal, nasal, palatine, and zygomatic b's
maxilla, inferior. *See* mandible				
maxilla, superior. *See* maxilla				
metacarpal b's	oss. metacarpalia	hand	five miniature long bones of hand proper, slightly concave on palmar surface	first—trapezium and proximal phalanx of thumb; second—third metacarpal b., trapezium, trapezoid, capitate, and proximal phalanx of index finger (second digit); third—second and fourth metacarpal b's, capitate and proximal phalanx of middle finger (third digit); fourth—third and fifth metacarpal b's, capitate, hamate, and proximal phalanx of ring finger (fourth digit); fifth—fourth metacarpal b., hamate b. and proximal phalanx of little finger (fifth digit)
metatarsal b's	oss. metatarsalia	foot	five miniature long bones of foot, concave on plantar and slightly convex on dorsal surface	first—medial cuneiform b., proximal phalanx of great toe, and occasionally with second metatarsal b.; second—medial, intermediate, and lateral cuneiform b's, third and occasionally with first metatarsal b., and proximal phalanx of second toe; third—lateral cuneiform b., second and fourth metatarsal b's and proximal phalanx of third toe; fourth—lateral cuneiform b., cuboid b., third and fifth metatarsal b's, and proximal phalanx of fourth toe; fifth—cuboid b., fourth metatarsal b., and proximal phalanx of fifth toe
multangulum majus. *See* trapezium; trapezoid b.				
nasal b.	o. nasale	skull	paired bone, the two uniting in median plane to form bridge of nose	with frontal and ethmoid b's, fellow of opposite side, and ipsilateral maxilla
navicular b.	o. naviculare	foot	bone at medial side of tarsus, between talus and cuneiform b's	with talus and 3 cuneiform b's, occasionally with cuboid b.

COMMON NAME*	NA EQUIVALENT†	REGION	DESCRIPTION	ARTICULATIONS
occipital b. os magnum. *See capitate b.*	o. occipitale	skull	unpaired bone constituting back and part of base of skull	with sphenoid b. and atlas and both parietal and temporal b's
palatine b.	o. palatinum	skull	paired bone, the two forming posterior portion of bony palate	with ethmoid and sphenoid b's, vomer, fellow of opposite side, and ipsilateral inferior nasal concha and maxilla
parietal b.	o. parietale	skull	paired bone between frontal and occipital b's, forming superior and lateral parts of skull	with frontal, occipital, sphenoid, fellow parietal, and ipsilateral temporal b's
patella	patella	knee	small, irregularly rectangular compressed (sesamoid) bone over anterior aspect of knee (kneecap)	with femur
phalanges (proximal middle and distal phalanges)	oss. digitorum (phalanx proximalis, phalanx media, and phalanx distalis)	fingers and toes	miniature long bones, two only in thumb and great toe, three in each of other fingers and toes	proximal phalanx of each digit with corresponding metacarpal or metatarsal b., and phalanx distal to it; other phalanges with phalanges proximal and distal (if any) to them
pisiform b.	o. pisiforme	wrist	medial and palmar of 4 bones of proximal row of carpal b's	with triquetral b.
pubic b.	o. pubis	pelvis	*see hip b.*	
radius	radius	forearm	lateral and shorter of 2 bones of forearm	proximally with humerus and ulna; distally with ulna and lunate and scaphoid b's
ribs	costae	chest	12 pairs of thin, narrow, curved long bones, forming posterior and lateral walls of chest	all posteriorly with thoracic vertebrae; upper 7 pairs (true ribs) with sternum; lower 5 pairs (false ribs), by costal cartilages, with rib above or (lowest 2—floating ribs) unattached anteriorly
sacrum	o. sacrum	lower back	wedge-shaped bone formed usually by fusion of 5 vertebrae below lumbar vertebrae, constituting posterior wall of pelvis	with fifth lumbar vertebra above, coccyx below, and with ilium at each side
scaphoid	o. scaphoideum	wrist	most lateral of 4 bones of proximal row of carpal b's	with radius, trapezium, and trapezoid, capitate and lunate b's
scapula	scapula	shoulder	wide, thin, triangular bone (shoulder blade) opposite second to seventh ribs in upper part of back	with ipsilateral clavicle and humerus
sesamoid b's	oss. sesamoidea	chiefly hands and feet	small, flat, round bones related to joints between phalanges or between digits and metacarpal or metatarsal b's; include also 2 at knee (fabella and patella)	

sphenoid b.	o. sphenoidale	base of skull	unpaired, irregularly shaped bone, constituting part of sides and base of skull and part of lateral wall of orbit	with frontal, occipital, and ethmoid b's, vomer and both parietal, temporal, palatine, and zygomatic b's
stapes	stapes	ear	most medial ossicle of chain in middle ear, so named because of its resemblance to a stirrup	with incus; ligamentous attachment to fenestra vestibuli
sternum	sternum	chest	elongated flat bone, forming anterior wall of chest, consisting of 3 segments: *manubrium* (topmost segment), *body* (in youth composed of 4 separate segments joined by cartilage), and *xiphoid process* (lowermost segment)	with both clavicles and upper 7 pairs of ribs
talus tarsal b's	talus oss. tarsi	ankle ankle and foot	the "ankle bone," second largest of tarsal b's see *calcaneus, cuboid, intermediate, lateral,* and *medial cuneiform b's, navicular b.,* and *talus*	with tibia, fibula, calcaneus, and navicular b.
temporal b.	o. temporale	skull	irregularly shaped bone, one on either side, forming part of side and base of skull, and containing middle and inner ear	with occipital, sphenoid, mandible, and ipsilateral parietal and zygomatic b's
tibia	tibia	leg	medial and larger of 2 bones of lower leg (shin b.)	proximally with femur and fibula, distally with talus and fibula
trapezium	o. trapezium	wrist	most lateral of 4 bones of distal row of carpal b's	with first and second metacarpal b's and trapezoid and scaphoid b's
trapezoid b.	o. trapezoideum	wrist	second from thumb side of 4 bones of distal row of carpal b's	with second metacarpal b. and capitate, trapezium, and scaphoid b's
triquetral b.	o. triquetrum	wrist	third from thumb side of 4 bones of proximal row of carpal b's	with hamate, lunate, and pisiform b's and articular disk
turbinate b., inferior. *See* concha, inferior nasal				
ulna	ulna	forearm	medial and longer of 2 bones of forearm	proximally with humerus and radius, distally with radius and articular disk
vertebrae (cervical, thoracic [dorsal], lumbar, sacral, and coccygeal)	vertebrae (vertebrae cervicales, vertebrae thoracicae, vertebrae lumbales, vertebrae sacrales, vertebrae coccygeae)	back	separate segments of vertebral column; about 33 in the child; uppermost 24 remain separate as true, movable vertebrae; the next 5 fuse to form the sacrum; the lowermost 3–5 fuse to form the coccyx	except first cervical (atlas) and fifth lumbar, each vertebra articulates with adjoining vertebrae above and below; the first cervical articulates with the occipital b. and second cervical vertebra (axis); the fifth lumbar with the fourth lumbar vertebra and sacrum; the thoracic vertebrae articulate also with the heads of the ribs
vomer	vomer	skull	thin bone forming posterior and posteroinferior part of nasal septum	with ethmoid and sphenoid b's and both maxillae and palatine b's
zygomatic b.	o. zygomaticum	skull	bone forming hard part of cheek and lower, lateral portion of rim of each orbit	with frontal and sphenoid b's and ipsilateral maxilla and temporal b.

border (bor′der) a bounding line, edge, or surface. **brush b.,** a specialization of the free surface of a cell, consisting of minute cylindrical processes (microvilli) that greatly increase the surface area. **vermilion b.,** the exposed red portion of the upper or lower lip.

Bordetella (bor″dĕ-tel′lah) a genus of bacteria (family Brucellaceae), including *B. bronchisep′tica,* a common cause of bronchopneumonia in guinea pigs and other rodents, in swine, and in lower primates; *B. parapertus′sis,* found occasionally in whooping cough; and *B. pertus′sis,* the cause of whooping cough in man.

borism (bo′rizm) poisoning by a boron compound.

boron (bo′ron) chemical element (*see table*), at. no. 5, symbol B.

Borrelia (bo-rel′e-ah) a genus of bacteria (family Treponemataceae), parasitic in many animals, some species causing relapsing fever in man and other mammals and in birds; it includes *B. anseri′na,* the etiologic agent of fowl spirochetosis; *B. recurren′tis,* an etiologic agent of relapsing fever; and *B. vincen′tii,* parasitic in the human mouth, occurring in large numbers with a fusiform bacillus in necrotizing ulcerative gingivitis and in necrotizing ulcerative gingivostomatitis.

boss (bos) a rounded eminence.

bosselated (bos′ĕ-lāt″ed) marked or covered with bosses.

bot (bot) the larva of botflies, which may be parasitic in the stomach of animals and sometimes man.

Bothriocephalus (both″re-o-sef′ah-lus) *Diphyllobothrium.*

botryoid (bot′re-oid) shaped like a bunch of grapes.

bottle (bot′′l) a hollow narrow-necked vessel of glass or other material. **wash b.,** 1. a flexible squeeze-bottle with delivery tube, or one with two tubes through the cork, so arranged that blowing into one forces a stream of liquid from the other; used in washing chemical materials. 2. one containing some washing fluid, through which gases are passed for the purpose of freeing them from impurities.

botuliform (bot-u′lĭ-form) sausage-shaped.

botulin (bot′u-lin) a neurotoxin produced by *Clostridium botulinum,* sometimes found in imperfectly canned or preserved foods.

botulism (bot′u-lizm) an extremely severe type of food poisoning due to a neurotoxin (botulin) produced by *Clostridium botulinum* in improperly canned or preserved foods.

bougie (boo′zhe) a slender, flexible, hollow or solid, cylindrical instrument for introduction into the urethra or other tubular organ, usually for calibrating or dilating constricted areas. **bulbous b.,** one with a bulb-shaped tip. **filiform b.,** one of very slender caliber. **soluble b.,** one that will melt or dissolve *in situ.*

bougienage (boo″zhĕ-nahzh′) passage of a bougie.

bouquet (boo-ka′) a structure resembling a cluster of flowers.

bouton (boo-taw′) [Fr.] button. **b. de Biskra, b.**

d′orient, cutaneous leishmaniasis. **b's terminaux,** end-feet.

bovine (bo′vīn) pertaining to, characteristic of, or derived from the ox (cattle).

bowel (bow′el) the intestine.

bowleg (bo′leg) genu varum; an outward curvature of one or both legs near the knee.

B.P. 1. blood pressure. 2. British Pharmacopoeia, a publication of the General Medical Council, describing and establishing standards for medicines, preparations, materials, and articles used in the practice of medicine, surgery, or midwifery.

b.p. boiling point.

B.P.A. British Paediatric Association.

Br chemical symbol, *bromine.*

brace (brās) an orthopedic appliance or apparatus (an orthosis) used to support, align, or hold parts of the body in correct position; also, usually in the plural, an orthodontic appliance for correction of malaligned teeth.

brachi(o)- word element [L., Gr.], *arm.*

brachial (bra′ke-al) pertaining to the arm.

brachialgia (bra″ke-al′je-ah) pain in the arm.

brachiation (-a′shun) locomotion in a position of suspension by means of the hands and arms, as exhibited by monkeys swinging from branch to branch.

brachiocephalic (-o-sĕ-fal′ik) pertaining to the arm and head.

brachiocrural (-kroo′ral) pertaining to the arm and leg.

brachiocubital (-ku′bĭ-tal) pertaining to the arm and elbow or forearm.

brachiocyrtosis (-ser-to′sis) crookedness of the arm.

brachium (bra′ke-um), pl. *bra′chia* [L.] 1. the arm; specifically, the arm from shoulder to elbow. 2. an armlike process or structure. **b. collic′uli inferio′ris,** fibers of the auditory pathway connecting the inferior quadrigeminal body to the medial geniculate body. **b. collic′uli superio′ris,** fibers connecting the optic tract and lateral geniculate body with the superior quadrigeminal body. **b. conjuncti′vum [cerebel′li],** superior cerebellar peduncle. **b. op′ticum,** one of the processes extending from the corpora quadrigemina to the optic thalamus. **b. pon′tis,** middle cerebellar peduncle.

brachy- word element [Gr.], *short.*

brachybasia (brak″e-ba′ze-ah) a slow, shuffling, short-stepped gait.

brachycardia (-kar′de-ah) bradycardia.

brachycephalia (-sĕ-fa′le-ah) brachycephaly.

brachycephalic (-sĕ-fal′ik) having a short wide head, with a cephalic index of 81.0 to 85.4.

brachycephaly (-sef′ah-le) the state of being brachycephalic.

brachycheilia (-ki′le-ah) shortness of the lip.

brachydactyly (-dak′tĭ-le) abnormal shortness of fingers and toes.

brachygnathia (brak″ig-na′the-ah) abnormal shortness of the lower jaw.

brachymetacarpia (brak″e-met″ah-kar′pe-ah) abnormal shortness of the metacarpal bones.

brachymetatarsia (-met″ah-tar′se-ah) abnormal shortness of the metatarsal bones.

brachymetropia (-mĕ-trop′pe-ah) myopia. **brachymetrop′ic,** adj.

brachyphalangia (-fah-lan′je-ah) abnormal shortness of one or more of the phalanges.

brachytherapy (-ther′ah-pe) treatment with ionizing radiation whose source is applied to the surface of the body or located a short distance from the area being treated.

brady- word element [Gr.], *slow.*

bradyacusia (brad″e-ah-ku′ze-ah) dullness of hearing.

bradyarrhythmia (-ah-rith′me-ah) bradycardia.

bradyarthria (-ar′thre-ah) bradylalia.

bradycardia (-kar′de-ah) slowness of the heart beat, as evidenced by slowing of the pulse rate to less than 60. **bradycar′diac,** adj.

bradycinesia (-si-ne′ze-ah) bradykinesia.

bradydiastole (-di-as′to-le) abnormal prolongation of the diastole.

bradyecoia (-e-koi′ah) partial deafness.

bradyesthesia (-es-the′ze-ah) slowness or dullness of perception.

bradygenesis (-jen′ĕ-sis) prolongation of certain stages in embryonic development.

bradyglossia (-glos′e-ah) abnormal slowness of utterance.

bradykinesia (-ki-ne′ze-ah) abnormal slowness of movement; sluggishness of physical and mental responses. **bradykinet′ic,** adj.

bradykinin (-ki′nin) a kinin composed of a chain of amino acids liberated by the action of trypsin or certain snake venoms on a globulin of blood plasma.

bradylalia (-la′le-ah) abnormally slow utterance of words due to a brain lesion.

bradylexia (-lek′se-ah) abnormal slowness in reading, due neither to defect of intelligence or of vision nor to ignorance of the alphabet.

bradylogia (-lo′je-ah) abnormal slowness of speech due to slowness of thinking, as in a mental disorder.

bradyphagia (-fa′je-ah) abnormal slowness of eating.

bradyphasia (-fa′ze-ah) bradylalia.

bradyphemia (-fe′me-ah) slowness of speech.

bradyphrasia (-fra′ze-ah) slowness of speech due to mental disorder.

bradypnea (-ne′ah) abnormal slowness of breathing.

bradyspermatism (-sper′mah-tizm) abnormally slow ejaculation of semen.

bradysphygmia (-sfig′me-ah) bradycardia.

bradystalsis (-stal′sis) abnormal slowness of peristalsis.

bradytachycardia (-tak″e-kar′de-ah) alternating attacks of bradycardia and tachycardia.

bradytocia (-to′she-ah) slow parturition.

bradyuria (-u′re-ah) abnormally slow discharge of urine.

brain (brān) encephalon; that part of the central nervous system contained within the cranium, comprising the forebrain, midbrain, and hindbrain, and developed from the anterior part of the embryonic neural tube; see also *cerebrum.*

brain stem (brān′stem) the stemlike portion of the brain connecting the cerebral hemispheres with the spinal cord, and comprising the pons, medulla oblongata, and midbrain; considered by some to include the diencephalon.

brainwashing (brān-wash′ing) mental conditioning of a captive designed to secure attitudes conformable to the captors' wishes.

branch (branch) ramus; a division or offshoot from a main stem, especially of blood vessels, nerves, or lymphatics.

branchial (brang′ke-al) pertaining to or resembling gills of a fish or derivatives of homologous parts in higher forms.

branchiogenic (brang″ke-o-jen′ik) gill-forming; forming a branchial arch.

branchiomerism (-om′er-izm) metamerism based on the serial repetition of the branchial arches.

brash (brash) a burning sensation in the stomach. **weaning b.,** diarrhea in infants occurring as a result of weaning.

breast (brest) the front of the chest, especially the modified cutaneous, glandular structure it bears, the mamma. In female mammals, the breast contains milk-secreting elements for nourishing the young. See *mammary gland.* **chicken b.,** pigeon b. **funnel b.,** see under *chest.* **pigeon b.,** prominence of the sternum due to obstruction to infantile respiration or to rickets.

breast-feeding (brest′fēd′ing) the nursing of an infant at the mother's breast.

breath (breth) the air taken in and expelled by the expansion and contraction of the thorax. **liver b.,** hepatic fetor.

breathing (brēth′ing) the alternate inspiration and expiration of air into and out of the lungs. **frog b., glossopharyngeal b.,** respiration unaided by the primary or ordinary accessory muscles of the pharynx; used by patients with chronic muscle paralysis to augment their vital capacity. **intermittent positive pressure b.,** the active inflation of the lungs during inspiration under positive pressure from a cycling valve.

breech (brēch) the buttocks.

bregma (breg′mah) the point on the surface of the skull at the junction of the coronal and sagittal sutures. **bregmat′ic,** adj.

brevicollis (brev″ĭ-kol′is) shortness of the neck.

Brevital (brev′ĭ-tal) trademark for a preparation of methohexital.

bridge (brij) 1. a dental prosthesis bearing one or more artificial teeth, attached to adjacent natural teeth. 2. pons. 3. a protoplasmic structure uniting adjacent elements of a cell, similar in plants and animals. **cantilever b.,** a fixed partial denture attached at one end to one or more natural teeth or roots, the other end not being rigidly attached. **cytoplasmic b.,** a band of protoplasm joining two adjacent blastomeres. **extension b.,** a bridge having an artificial tooth attached beyond the point of anchorage of the bridge. **Gaskell's b.,** bundle of His. **inter-**

cellular b's, processes of cell substance connecting adjoining cells; see *desmosome*. **b. of Varolius,** pons (2).

bridgework (brij′werk) a partial denture retained by attachments other than clasps. **fixed b.,** one retained with crowns or inlays cemented to the natural teeth. **removable b.,** one retained by attachments which permit its removal.

brim (brim) the edge of the superior strait of the pelvis.

brisement (brēz-maw′) [Fr.] the breaking up or tearing of anything. **b. forcé,** the breaking up or tearing of a bony ankylosis.

broach (brōch) a fine barbed instrument for dressing a tooth canal or extracting the pulp.

bromatotherapy (bro″mah-to-ther′ah-pe) dietotherapy.

bromatoxism (-tok′sizm) food poisoning.

bromelain (bro′mĕ-lān) a proteolytic and milk-clotting enzyme derived from the pineapple plant, *Ananas sativus.* In the plural, a concentrate of these enzymes, used as an anti-inflammatory agent. Also used in tenderizing meat, preparing protein hydrolysates, and chill-proofing beer.

bromethol (bro-meth′ol) tribromoethanol.

bromhidrosis (bro″mĭ-dro′sis) the secretion of foul-smelling perspiration.

bromide (bro′mīd) a binary compound of bromine.

bromidrosis (bro″mĭ-dro′sis) bromhidrosis.

brominated (bro″mĭ-nāt′ed) combined with or containing bromine.

bromine (bro′mēn) chemical element (*see table*), at. no. 35, symbol Br.

brominism (bro′min-izm) poisoning by excessive use of bromine or its compounds; symptoms include acne, headache, coldness of arms and legs, fetid breath, sleeplessness, weakness, and impotence.

bromisovalum (brōm″i-so-val′um) a urea derivative used as a sedative and mild hypnotic.

bromochlorotrifluoroethane (bro″mo-klo″ro-tri-flu″o-ro-eth′ān) halothane.

bromoderma (-der′mah) skin eruption due to use of bromides.

bromodiphenhydramine (-di″fen-hi′drah-min) an antihistaminic, $C_{17}H_{20}BrNO$, used as the hydrochloride salt.

bromomania (-ma′ne-ah) mental disorder induced by misuse of bromides.

bromomenorrhea (-men″o-re′ah) menstruation characterized by an offensive odor.

5-bromouracil (-u′rah-sil) a pyrimidine analogue with mutagenic properties.

brompheniramine (brōm″fen-ir′ah-mēn) an antihistaminic, $C_6H_9BrN_2$, used as the maleate salt.

Bromsulphalein (brōm-sul′fah-lin) trademark for a preparation of sulfobromophthalein.

Bromural (brōm-u′ral) trademark for preparations of bromisovalum.

bronchadenitis (brongk″ad-ĕ-ni′tis) inflammation of the bronchial glands.

bronchi (brong′ki) plural of *bronchus.*

bronchial (brong′ke-al) pertaining to or affecting one or more bronchi.

bronchiarctia (brong″ke-ark′she-ah) bronchostenosis.

bronchiectasis (-ek′tah-sis) chronic dilatation of one or more bronchi.

bronchiloquy (brong-kil′o-kwe) high-pitched pectoriloquy due to lung consolidation.

bronchiocele (brong′ke-o-sēl″) dilatation or swelling of a bronchiole.

bronchiocrisis (brong″ke-o-kri′sis) bronchial crisis.

bronchiogenic (-jen′ik) bronchogenic.

bronchiole (brong′ke-ōl) one of the finer subdivisions of the branched bronchial tree. **respiratory b.,** the final branch of a bronchiole; a subdivision of a terminal bronchiole, it has alveolar outcroppings and itself divides into several alveolar ducts.

bronchiolectasis (brong″ke-o-lek′tah-sis) dilatation of the bronchioles.

bronchiolitis (-li′tis) bronchopneumonia.

bronchiolus (brong-ki′o-lus), pl. *bronchi′oli* [L.] bronchiole.

bronchiospasm (brong′ke-o-spazm″) bronchospasm.

bronchiostenosis (brong″ke-o-stĕ-no′sis) bronchostenosis.

bronchitis (brong-ki′tis) inflammation of one or more bronchi. **bronchit′ic,** adj. **catarrhal b.,** acute bronchitis with profuse mucopurulent discharge. **croupous b.,** a form marked by violent cough and paroxysms of dyspnea, in which casts of the bronchial tubes are expectorated with Charcot-Leyden crystals and eosinophil cells. **fibrinous b.,** croupous b. **b. oblit′erans,** that in which the smaller bronchi become filled with nodules composed of fibrinous exudate. **plastic b.,** croupous b. **putrid b.,** chronic bronchitis with offensive sputum.

bronchocandidiasis (brong″ko-kan″dĭ-di′ah-sis) candidiasis of the respiratory tree, occurring in a mild afebrile form manifested as chronic bronchitis, and in a usually fatal form resembling tuberculosis.

bronchocavernous (-kav′er-nus) both bronchial and cavitary.

bronchocele (brong′ko-sēl) localized dilatation of a bronchus.

bronchoconstriction (brong″ko-kon-strik′-shun) bronchostenosis.

bronchoconstrictor (-kon-strik′tor) 1. narrowing the lumina of the air passages of the lungs. 2. an agent that causes such constriction.

bronchodilatation (-dil″ah-ta′shun) a dilated state of a bronchus, or the site at which a bronchus is dilated.

bronchodilator (-di-la′tor) 1. expanding the lumina of the air passages of the lungs. 2. an agent which causes dilatation of the bronchi.

bronchoegophony (-ĕ-gof′o-ne) egobronchophony.

bronchoesophageal (-ĕ-sof″ah-je′al) pertaining to or communicating with a bronchus and the esophagus.

bronchoesophagology (-ĕ-sof″ah-gol′o-je) that

branch of medicine dealing with the tracheo-bronchial tree and esophagus.

bronchoesophagoscopy (-ĕ-sof″ah-gos′ko-pe) instrumental examination of the bronchi and esophagus.

bronchogenic (-jen′ik) originating in bronchi.

bronchogram (brong′ko-gram) the film obtained by bronchography.

bronchography (bron-kog′rah-fe) radiography of the lungs after instillation of an opaque medium in the bronchi.

broncholith (brong′ko-lith) lung calculus.

broncholithiasis (brong″ko-lĭ-thi′ah-sis) a condition in which calculi are present within the lumen of the tracheobronchial tree.

bronchology (brong-kol′o-je) the study and treatment of diseases of the tracheobronchial tree. **bronchologˈic,** adj.

bronchomalacia (brong″ko-mah-la′she-ah) a deficiency in the cartilaginous wall of the trachea or a bronchus that may lead to atelectasis or obstructive emphysema.

bronchomoniliasis (-mo″nĭ-li′ah-sis) broncho-candidiasis.

bronchomotor (-mo′tor) affecting the caliber of the bronchi.

bronchopathy (brong-kop′ah-the) any disease of the bronchi.

bronchophony (brong-kof′o-ne) the sound of the voice as heard through the stethoscope applied over a healthy large bronchus.

bronchoplasty (brong′ko-plas″te) plastic surgery of a bronchus; surgical closure of a bronchial fistula.

bronchoplegia (brong″ko-ple′je-ah) paralysis of the muscles of the walls of the bronchial tubes.

bronchopleural (-ploor′al) pertaining to a bronchus and the pleura, or communicating with a bronchus and the pleural cavity.

bronchopneumonia (-nu-mo′ne-ah) inflammation of the lungs, usually beginning in the terminal bronchioles.

bronchopneumopathy (-nu-mop′ah-the) disease of the bronchi and lung tissue.

bronchopulmonary (-pul′mo-ner″e) pertaining to the bronchi and the lungs.

bronchorrhagia (-ra′je-ah) hemorrhage from the bronchi.

bronchorrhaphy (brong-kor′ah-fe) suture of a bronchus.

bronchorrhea (brong″ko-re′ah) excessive discharge of mucus from the bronchi.

bronchoscope (brong′ko-skōp) an instrument for inspecting the interior of or removing foreign bodies from the tracheobronchial tree. **bronchoscopˈic,** adj.

bronchoscopy (brong-kos′ko-pe) examination of the tracheobronchial tree through a bronchoscope.

bronchospasm (brong′ko-spazm) spasmodic contraction of the smooth muscle coating of the bronchi, as occurs in asthma.

bronchospirography (brong″ko-spi-rog′rah-fe) the recording of bronchospirometry results.

bronchospirometry (-spi-rom′ĕ-tre) determination of vital capacity, oxygen intake, and car-

bon dioxide excretion of a single lung, or simultaneous measurements of the function of each lung separately. **differential b.,** measurement of the function of each lung separately.

bronchostaxis (-stak′sis) bleeding from the bronchial wall.

bronchostenosis (-stĕ-no′sis) stricture or cicatricial diminution of the caliber of a bronchial tube.

bronchostomy (brong-kos′to-me) the surgical creation of an opening through the chest wall into the bronchus.

bronchotomy (brong-kot′o-me) incision of a bronchus.

bronchotracheal (brong″ko-tra′ke-al) pertaining to bronchi and trachea.

bronchovesicular (-vĕ-sik′u-ler) pertaining to the bronchi and alveoli.

bronchus (brong′kus), pl. *bron′chi* [L.] one of the larger passages conveying air to (right or left principal bronchus) and within the lungs (lobar and segmental bronchi).

brow (brow) the forehead, or either lateral half of it.

brown (brown) 1. a reddish yellow color. 2. a dye that is brown in color. **aniline b., Bismarck b.,** a brown aniline dye used as a stain and counterstain in histology.

B.R.S. British Roentgen Society.

Brucella (broo-sel′lah) a genus of schizomycetes (family Brucellaceae). **B. abor′tus,** the causative agent of infectious abortion in cattle and the commonest cause of brucellosis in man. **B. bronchisep′tica,** *Bordetella bronchiseptica.* **B. meliten′sis,** a causative agent of brucellosis, occurring primarily in goats. **B. o′vis,** the causative agent of an infectious disease in sheep. **B. su′is,** a species found in swine, which is capable of producing severe disease in man.

brucella (broo-sel′ah), pl. *brucel′lae.* Any member of *Brucella.* **brucel′lar,** adj.

Brucellaceae (broo″sel-la′se-e) a family of schizomycetes (order Eubacteriales), some genera of which are parasites of and pathogenic for warm-blooded animals, including man and birds.

Brucellergen (broo-sel′er-jen) trademark for a solution of nucleoproteins derived from *Brucella,* used in a skin test for brucellosis.

brucellosis (broo″sel-lo′sis) a generalized infection of man involving primarily the reticuloendothelial system, caused by species of *Brucella.*

Brugia (broo′je-ah) a genus of filarial worms, including *B. malayi,* a species similar to, and often found in association with, *Wuchereria bancrofti,* which causes human filariasis and elephantiasis throughout Southeast Asia, the China Sea, and eastern India.

bruise (brōōz) a contusion; an injury produced by impact without breakage of the skin, due to hemorrhage into tissue from ruptured vessels.

bruit (brwe, brōōt) [Fr.] a sound or murmur heard in auscultation, especially an abnormal one. **aneurysmal b.,** blowing sound heard over an aneurysm. **placental b.,** see under *souffle.*

bruxism (bruk'sizm) grinding of the teeth, especially during sleep.

B.S. Bachelor of Surgery; Bachelor of Science; breath sounds; blood sugar.

BSA body surface area.

BSP Bromsulphalein.

B.T.U., B.Th.U. British thermal unit.

buba (boo'bah) 1. mucocutaneous leishmaniasis. 2. yaws.

bubo (bu'bo) an enlarged and inflamed lymph node, particularly in the axilla or groin, due to such infections as plague, syphilis, gonorrhea, lymphogranuloma venereum, and tuberculosis. **climatic b.,** lymphogranuloma venereum. **indolent b.,** a hard, nearly painless bubo that shows no tendency to break. **pestilential b.,** that associated with plague. **sympathetic b.,** bubo due to friction and injury.

bubonalgia (bu'bo-nal'je-ah) pain in the groin.

bubonic (bu-bon'ik) characterized by or pertaining to buboes.

bubonocele (bu-bon'o-sēl) inguinal or femoral hernia forming a swelling in the groin.

bucardia (bu-kar'de-ah) cor bovinum.

bucca (buk'ah) [L.] the cheek.

buccal (buk'al) pertaining to or directed toward the cheek.

bucco- word element [L.], *cheek.*

buccoaxial (buk"o-ak'se-al) pertaining to or formed by the buccal and axial walls of a tooth cavity.

buccoclusion (-kloo'zhun) malocclusion in which the dental arch or a quadrant or group of teeth is buccal to the normal.

buccoversion (-ver'zhun) position of a tooth lying buccally to the line of occlusion.

buclizine (bu'klĭ-zēn) a minor tranquilizer having antihistaminic, antiemetic, and anticholinergic activities; used as the dihydrochloride salt.

bucnemia (buk-ne'me-ah) diffuse, tense, inflammatory swelling of the leg.

bud (bud) any small part of the embryo or adult metazoon more or less resembling the bud of a plant and presumed to have potential for growth and differentiation. **end b.,** the remnant of the primitive knot, from which arises the caudal part of the trunk. **limb b.,** a swelling on the trunk of an embryo that becomes a limb. **tail b.,** 1. the primordium of the caudal appendage. 2. end b. **taste b.,** one of the end organs of the gustatory nerve containing the receptor surfaces for the sense of taste. **ureteric b.,** an outgrowth of the mesonephric duct giving rise to all but the nephrons of the permanent kidney. **b. of urethra,** bulb of penis.

budding (bud'ing) gemmation.

buffer (buf'er) 1. a chemical system that prevents change in concentration of another chemical substance. 2. a physical or physiological system that tends to maintain constancy.

bulb (bulb) a rounded mass or enlargement. **bul'bar,** adj. **b. of aorta,** the enlargement of the aorta at its point of origin from the heart. **auditory b.,** the membranous labyrinth and cochlea. **b. of corpus cavernosum,** bulb of penis. **b. of eye,** the eyeball. **gustatory b.,** taste bud. **b. of hair,** the bulbous expansion at the proximal end of a hair in which the hair shaft is generated. **Krause's b's,** end-bulbs. **olfactory b.,** the bulblike expansion of the olfactory tract on the under surface of the frontal lobe of each cerebral hemisphere; the olfactory nerves enter it. **b. of penis,** the enlarged proximal part of the corpus spongiosum. **taste b.,** see under *bud.* **b. of urethra,** b. of penis. **b. of vestibule of vagina, vestibulovaginal b.,** a body consisting of paired masses of erectile tissue, one on either side of the vaginal opening.

bulbiform (bul'bĭ-form) bulb-shaped.

bulbitis (bul-bi'tis) inflammation of the bulb of the penis.

bulbourethral (bul"bo-u-re'thral) pertaining to the bulb of the urethra (bulb of penis).

bulbous (bul'bus) having the form or nature of a bulb; bearing or arising from a bulb.

bulbus (bul'bus), pl. *bul'bi* [L.] bulb. **b. aor'tae,** bulb of aorta. **b. carot'icus,** carotid sinus. **b. oc'uli,** the eyeball. **b. olfacto'rius,** olfactory bulb. **b. pe'nis,** bulb of penis. **b. pi'li,** bulb of hair. **b. ure'thrae,** bulb of penis. **b. vestib'uli vagi'nae,** bulb of vestibule of vagina.

bulimia (bu-lim'e-ah) abnormal increase in sensation of hunger. **bulim'ic,** adj.

bulla (bul'ah), pl. *bul'lae* [L.] a blister; a circumscribed, fluid-containing, elevated lesion of the skin, usually more than 5 mm. in diameter. **bul'late, bul'lous,** adj.

bullosis (bul-lo'sis) the production of, or a condition characterized by, bullous lesions.

BUN blood urea nitrogen; see *urea nitrogen.*

bundle (bun'd'l) a collection of fibers or strands, as of muscle fibers, or a fasciculus or band of nerve fibers. **atrioventricular b.,** b. of His. **fundamental b., ground b.,** that part of the white matter of the spinal cord bordering the gray matter and containing fibers that travel for a distance of only a few segments of the cord. **b. of His,** a band of cardiac muscle fibers connecting the atria with the ventricles of the heart. **Keith's b., sinoatrial b.,** a bundle of fibers in the wall of the right atrium between the openings of the venae cavae. **Thorel's b.,** a bundle of muscle fibers in the human heart connecting the sinoatrial and atrioventricular nodes. **b. of Vicq d'Azyr,** a band of fibers from the mamillary body to the anterior nucleus of the thalamus.

bundle branch (bun'd'l branch) a branch of the bundle of His.

bunion (bun'yun) an abnormal prominence on the inner aspect of the first metatarsal head, with bursal formation, and resulting in lateral or valgus displacement of the great toe. **tailor's b.,** bunionette.

bunionectomy (bun"yun-ek'to-me) excision of a bunion.

bunionette (-et') enlargement of the lateral aspect of the fifth metatarsal head.

Bunostomum (bu"no-sto'mum) a genus of hookworms that parasitize cattle, sheep, and other ruminants.

buphthalmos (būf-thal′mos) abnormal enlargement of the eyes; see *infantile glaucoma.*

bur, burr (ber) a form of drill used for creating openings in bone or similar hard material.

buret, burette (bu-ret′) a graduated glass tube used to deliver a measured amount of liquid.

burimamide (bu-rim′ah-mīd) an antagonist to histamine, competing for the histamine₂ receptor site on cells.

burn (bern) injury to tissues caused by the contact with heat, flame, chemicals, electricity, or radiation. First degree burns show redness; second degree burns show vesication; third degree burns show necrosis through the entire skin. Burns of the first and second degree are partial-thickness burns, those of the third are full-thickness burns.

burner (bern′er) the part of a lamp, stove, or furnace from which the flame issues. **Argand b.,** one that burns oil or gas, with an inner tube for supplying air to the flame. **Bunsen b.,** a gas burner in which the gas is mixed with air before ignition, in order to give complete oxidation.

burnishing (ber′nish-ing) a dental procedure somewhat related to polishing and abrading.

bursa (ber′sah), pl. *bur′sae, bursas* [L.] a fluid-filled sac or saclike cavity situated in places in tissues where friction would otherwise occur. **bur′sal,** adj. **b. of Achilles** (tendon), one between the calcaneal tendon and the back of the calcaneus. **b. anseri′na,** one between the tendons of the sartorius, gracilis, and semitendinosus muscles, and the tibial collateral ligments. **Boyer's b.,** one beneath hyoid bone. **Calori's b.,** one between the trachea and the arch of the aorta. **Fleischmann's b.,** one beneath the tongue. **gluteal b.,** one beneath the gluteus maximus muscle. **His' b.,** the dilatation at the end of the archenteron. **iliac b.,** one at the point of insertion of the iliopsoas muscle into the lesser trochanter. **Luschka's b.,** b. pharyngea (1). **b. muco′sa,** synovial b. **omental b., b. omenta′lis,** the lesser sac of the peritoneum. **b. pharyn′gea, pharyngeal b.,** 1. a recess in the pharynx of the fetus and newborn. 2. a cyst in the pharyngeal tonsil. **popliteal b.,** one in the popliteal space beneath the tendon of the semimembranosus and the tendon of the inner head of the gastrocnemius. **prepatellar b.,** one of the bursae in front of the patella; it may be subcutaneous, subfascial, or subtendinous in location. **subacromial b., b. subacromia′lis,** one between the acromion and the insertion of the supraspinatus muscle, extending between the deltoid and greater tubercle of the humerus. **subdeltoid b., b. subdeltoi′dea,** one between the deltoid and the shoulder joint capsule, usually connected to the subacromial bursa. **synovial b., b. synovia′lis,** a closed synovial sac interposed between surfaces that glide upon each other; it may be subcutaneous, submuscular, subfascial, or subtendinous in location.

bursectomy (ber-sek′to-me) excision of a bursa.

bursitis (ber-si′tis) inflammation of a bursa; specific types of bursitis are named according to the bursa affected, e.g., prepatellar bursitis, subacromial bursitis, etc. **Duplay's b.,** inflam-

mation of the acromial or subdeltoid bursa. **subacromial b., subdeltoid b.,** inflammation and calcification of the subacromial or subdeltoid bursa. **Thornwaldt's b.,** chronic inflammation of the pharyngeal bursa.

bursolith (ber′so-lith) a calculus in a bursa.

bursopathy (ber-sop′ah-the) any disease of a bursa.

bursotomy (ber-sot′o-me) incision of a bursa.

busulfan (bu-sul′fan) an antineoplastic, $C_6H_{14}O_6S_2$, used in treating myelocytic leukemia.

butabarbital (bu″tah-bar′bĭ-tal) a short- to intermediate-acting barbiturate, $C_{10}H_{15}N_2O_3$; its sodium salt is used as a sedative and hynotic.

butacaine (-kān) a local anesthetic, $C_{18}H_{30}N_2O_2$; the sulfate salt is used as a topical anesthetic in the eye and on mucous membranes, in solution or as ointment.

butalbital (bu-tal′bĭ-tal) a sedative, $C_{11}H_{16}N_2O_3$.

butallylonal (bu″tah-lil′o-nal) a central nervous system depressant, $C_{11}H_{15}BrN_2O_3$.

butamben (bu-tam′ben) butyl aminobenzoate.

butane (bu′tān) an aliphatic hydrocarbon from petroleum, C_4H_{10}, occurring as a colorless flammable gas.

Butazolidin (bu″tah-zol′ĭ-din) trademark for a preparation of phenylbutazone.

Butesin (bu-te′sin) trademark for a preparation of butyl aminobenzoate.

butethamine (bu-teth′ah-mēn) a local anesthetic, $C_{13}H_{20}N_2O_2$, used in dentistry in the form of the hydrochloride salt.

Butisol (bu′tĭ-sol) trademark for preparations of butabarbital.

butter (but′er) oily mass procured by churning cream, or a substance of similar consistency. **cacao b.,** theobroma oil. **b. of zinc,** zinc chloride.

buttock (but′ok) either of the two fleshy prominences formed by the gluteal muscles on the lower part of the back.

button (but′on) 1. a knoblike elevation or structure. 2. a spool- or disk-shaped device used in surgery for construction of intestinal anastomosis. **Biskra b.,** cutaneous leishmaniasis. **Jaboulay's b.,** a device used for lateral intestinal anastomosis. **mescal b's,** transverse slices of the flowering heads of a Mexian cactus, *Lophophora williamsii,* whose major active prinsiple is mescaline. **Murphy's b.,** a metallic device used for connecting the ends of a dividing intestine.

butyl (bu′til) a hydrocarbon radical, C_4H_9. **b. aminobenzoate,** an ester used as a local anesthetic in powder, ointment, suppository, and lozenge forms. **b. chloride,** an ester used as a veterinary anthelmintic for dogs and horses.

butylene (bu′tĭ-lēn) a gaseous hydrocarbon, C_4H_8.

butylparaben (bu″til-par′ah-ben) an antifungal agent, $C_{11}H_{14}O_3$, used as a pharmaceutic preservative.

butyraceous (bu″tĭ-ra′shus) of a buttery consistency.

butyrate (bu′tĭ-rāt) a salt of butyric acid.

butyrin (-rin) a triglyceride of butyric acid, C_3-$H_5(C_4H_7O_2)_3$, an acrid, bitter, liquid fat.

butyroid (bu'tĭ-roid) resembling or having the consistency of butter.

butyrometer (bu"tĭ-rom'ĕ-ter) a apparatus for estimating the butter fat of milk.

butyrophenone (bu"tĭ-ro-fe'nōn) a chemical class of major tranquilizers especially useful in the treatment of manic and moderate to severe agitated states and in the control of the vocal utterances and tics of Gilles de la Tourette's syndrome.

butyrous (bu'tĭ-rus) resembling butter.

bypass (bi'pas) an auxiliary flow; a shunt; a surgically created pathway circumventing the normal anatomical pathway, as an aortoiliac or a jejunal bypass.

byssinosis (bis"ĭ-no'sis) pneumoconiosis due to inhalation of cotton dust.

C

C 1. chemical symbol, *carbon.* 2. in the electrocardiogram, C stands for chest (precordial) lead; see *precordial lead.* 3. symbol for *complement.*

C. 'cathode (cathodal); Celsius or centigrade (scale); cervical; clearance; clonus; closure; contraction; cylinder.

c. contact; curie.

CA chronologic age.

Ca chemical symbol, *calcium;* cathode (cathodal); cancer.

cac(o)- word element [Gr.], *bad; ill.*

cacanthrax (kak-an'thraks) malignant anthrax.

cacao (kah-ka'o) 1. cocoa. 2. the seeds of the tropical American tree *Theobroma cacao.*

cacesthesia (kak"es-the'ze-ah) any morbid sensation or disorder of sensibility.

cachet (kah-sha') a disk-shaped wafer or capsule enclosing a dose of medicine.

cachexia (kah-kek'se-ah) a profound and marked state of constitutional disorder; general ill health and malnutrition. **cachec'tic,** adj. **c. hypophysiopri'va,** the train of symptoms resulting from total deprivation of pituitary function, including loss of sexual function, bradycardia, hypothermia, apathy, and coma. **malarial c.,** the physical signs resulting from antecedent attacks of severe malaria, including anemia, sallow skin, yellow sclera, splenomegaly, hepatomegaly, and, in children, retardation of growth and puberty. **pachydermic c.,** myxedema. **pituitary c.,** see *panhypopituitarism.* **c. strumipri'va, c. thyreopri'va,** myxedema resulting from deprivation of thyroid function.

cachinnation (kak"ĭ-na'shun) excessive, hysterical laughter.

cacodyl (kak'o-dil) a poisonous arsenical compound, $C_4H_{12}As_2$, which is inflammable when exposed to air.

cacodylate (-dil"āt) a salt of cacodylic acid.

cacogenics (kak"o-jen'iks) racial deterioration due to the mating and propagation of inferior individuals. **cacogen'ic,** adj.

cacogeusia (-gu'se-ah) a bad taste.

cacomelia (-me'le-ah) congenital deformity of a limb.

cacosmia (kak-oz'me-ah) 1. bad odor; stench. 2. a hallucination of unpleasant odor.

cactinomycin (kak"tĭ-no-mi'sin) actinomycin C, an antibiotic from *Streptomyces chrysomallus,* composed of a mixture of actinomycins; used as an antineoplastic.

cacumen (kah-ku'men), pl. *cacu'mina* [L.] 1. the top or apex of an organ. 2. the top of a plant. 3. culmen.

cadaver (kan-dav'er) a dead body; generally applied to a human body preserved for anatomical study. **cadav'eric, cadav'erous,** adj.

cadaverine (-in) a relatively nontoxic ptomaine, $C_5H_{14}N_2$, formed by decarboxylation of lysine; it is sometimes one of the products of *Vibrio proteus* and of *V. cholerae,* and occasionally found in the urine in cystinuria.

cadmiosis (kad"me-o'sis) pneumoconiosis due to inhalation of and tissue reaction to cadmium dust.

cadmium (kad'me-um) chemical element (*see table*), at. no. 48, symbol Cd; its salts are poisonous. Inhalation of cadmium fumes causes pulmonary edema, followed by proliferative interstitial pneumonia, and is associated with various degrees of lung damage; poisoning may also be due to ingestion of foods contaminated by cadmium-plated containers, causing violent gastrointestinal symptoms. **c. sulfide,** a salt used in 1% suspension in treatment of seborrheic dermatitis.

caduceus (kah-du'se-us) the wand of Hermes or Mercury; used as a symbol of the medical profession and as the emblem of the Medical Corps of the U.S. Army. See also *staff of Æsculapius.*

cae- for words beginning thus, see also those beginning *ce-.*

caelotherapy (se"lo-ther'ah-pe) the therapeutic use of religion and religious symbols.

caffea (kaf'e-ah) coffee.

caffeine (kah-fēn', kaf'fe-in) a central nervous system stimulant, $C_8H_{10}N_4O_2$, from coffee, tea, guarana, and maté. **citrate c., citrated c.,** a mixture of caffeine and citric acid, used as a central nervous system stimulant. **c. and sodium benzoate,** a mixture of equal parts of anhydrous caffeine and sodium benzoate, used as a central nervous system stimulant.

caffeinism (kaf'ēn-izm, kaf'e-in-izm") an agitated state induced by excessive ingestion of caffeine.

cage (kāj) a box or enclosure. **thoracic c.,** the bony structure enclosing the thorax, consisting of the ribs, vertebral column, and sternum.

Cal. large calorie (kilogram calorie).

cal. small calorie (gram calorie).

calamine (kal'ah-mīn) a preparation of zinc and ferric oxides, used topically as a protectant and astringent.

calamus (kal'ah-mus) 1. a reed or reedlike structure. 2. the peeled, dried rhizome of *Acorus calamus;* mild aromatic. **c. scripto'rius,** the pen-shaped, lowest portion of the floor of the fourth ventricle, situated between the restiform bodies.

calcaneoapophysitis (kal-ka''ne-o-ah-pof''ĭ-si'-tis) inflammation of the posterior part of the calcaneus, marked by pain and swelling.

calcaneoastragaloid (-ah-strag'ah-loid) pertaining to the calcaneus and astragalus.

calcaneodynia (-din'e-ah) pain in the heel.

calcaneotibial (-tib'e-al) pertaining to the calcaneus and tibia.

calcaneum (kal-ka'ne-um) calcaneus.

calcaneus (kal-ka'ne-us) [L.] see *Table of Bones.* **calca'neal, calca'nean,** adj.

calcar (kal'kar) a spur or spur-shaped structure. **c. a'vis,** the lower of two medial elevations in the posterior horn of the lateral cerebral ventricle, produced by the lateral extension of the calcarine sulcus.

calcareous (kal-kār'e-us) pertaining to or containing lime; chalky.

calcarine (kal'kar-in) 1. spur-shaped. 2. pertaining to the calcar.

calcariuria (kal-kār''e-u're-ah) presence of lime (calcium) salts in the urine.

calcemia (kal-se'me-ah) hypercalcemia.

calcibilia (kal''sĭ-bil'e-ah) presence of calcium in the bile.

calcic (kal'sik) of or pertaining to lime or calcium.

calcicosis (kal''sĭ-ko'sis) lung disease due to inhalation of marble dust.

calciferol (kal-sif'er-ol) 1. see *vitamin D.* 2. ergocalciferol.

calcific (kal-sif'ik) forming lime.

calcification (kal''sĭ-fĭ-ka'shun) the deposit of calcium salts in a tissue. **dystrophic c.,** the deposition of calcium in abnormal tissue, such as scar tissue or atherosclerotic plaques, without abnormalities of blood calcium. **Mönckeberg's c.,** see under *arteriosclerosis.*

calcine (kal'sīn) to reduce to a dry powder by heat.

calcinosis (kal''sĭ-no'sis) a condition characterized by abnormal deposition of calcium salts in the tissues. **c. circumscrip'ta,** localized deposition of calcium in small nodules in subcutaneous tissues or muscle. **c. universa'lis,** widespread deposition of calcium in nodules or plaques in the dermis, panniculus, and muscles.

calipenia (-pe'ne-ah) deficiency of calcium.

calcipexis, calcipexy (kal''sĭ-pek'sis; kal'sĭ-pek''se) fixation of calcium in the tissues. **calcipec'tic, calcipex'ic,** adj.

calciphilia (kal''sĭ-fil'e-ah) a tendency to calcification.

calciphylaxis (-fi-lak'sis) the formation of calcified tissue in response to administration of a challenging agent after induction of a hypersensitive state. **calciphylac'tic,** adj.

calciprivia (-priv'e-ah) deprivation or loss of calcium. **calcipri'vic,** adj.

calcitonin (-to'nin) a polypeptide hormone secreted by C cells of the thyroid gland, and sometimes of the thymus and parathyroids, which lowers calcium and phosphate concentration in plasma and inhibits bone resorption.

calcium (kal'se-um) chemical element (*see table*), at. no. 20, symbol Ca; it is found in nearly all organized tissues and is also known as *coagulation Factor IV* because of its role in multiple phases of blood coagulation. **c. aminosalicylate,** an antibacterial compound, $C_{14}H_{12}CaN_2$-O_6, used in tuberculosis. **c. benzoylpas,** $C_{28}H_{20}$-$CaN_2O_8 \cdot 5H_2O$, a tuberculostatic. **c. carbonate,** a compound occurring naturally in bone, shells, etc., and prepared artificially (precipitated) as a source of calcium. *Precipitated c. carbonate* may be prepared by reaction of a soluble calcium salt with a soluble carbonate; used as an antacid. **c. chloride,** a salt used in solution to restore electrolyte balance. **c. cyanamide,** $CaCN_2$, obtained by the interaction of nitrogen and calcium carbide in an electric furnace, which inhibits one or more of the enzymes required for oxidation of acetaldehyde formed from alcohol; used as a fertilizer, defoliant, herbicide, pesticide, and anthelmintic for swine. **c. cyclamate,** $C_{12}H_{24}CaN_2O_6S_2 \cdot 2H_2O$; a noncaloric sweetener. **c. cyclobarbital,** $C_{24}H_{30}CaN_4O_6$, a central depressant. **c. disodium edetate, c. disodium edathamil,** see *edetate.* **c. gluconate,** a calcium replenisher. **c. glycerophosphate,** a calcium and phosphorus dietary supplement. **c. hydroxide,** an alkali used in preparation of calcium hydroxide solution. **c. ipodate,** $C_{24}H_{24}$-$CaI_6N_4O_4$, a diagnostic radiopaque medium used in cholangiography and cholecystography. **c. lactate,** a calcium supplement. **c. levulinate,** a salt used infrequently as a calcium supplement. **c. mandelate,** $C_{16}H_{14}CaO_6$, a urinary antiseptic. **c. oxalate,** a compound occurring in urine as crystals and in certain calculi. **c. oxide,** lime (1). **c. oxytetracycline,** $C_{44}H_{46}CaN_4$-O_{18}, an antibacterial. **c. pantothenate,** calcium salt of the dextrorotatory isomer of pantothenic acid; used as a growth-promoting vitamin. **c. phosphate,** one of three salts containing calcium and the phosphate radical: *dibasic* and *tribasic c. phosphate* are used as sources of calcium; *monobasic c. phosphate* is used in fertilizers and as a calcium and phosphorus supplement. **c. saccharin,** $C_{14}H_8CaN_2O_6S_2 \cdot 3\frac{1}{2}H_2O$, a non-nutritive sweetener. **c. sulfate,** a compound occurring as gypsum or as plaster of Paris.

calciuria (kal''sĭ-u're-ah) calcium in the urine.

calcospherite (kal''ko-sfēr'ĭt) one of the minute globular bodies formed during calcification by chemical union of calcium particles and albuminous matter of cells.

calculifragous (kal″ku-lif′rah-gus) breaking up calculi.

calculogenesis (-lo-jen′ĕ-sis) the formation of calculi.

calculosis (-lo′sis) lithiasis.

calculus (kal′ku-lus), pl. *cal′culi* [L.] an abnormal concretion, usually composed of mineral salts, occurring within the animal body. **cal′culous,** adj. **biliary calculi,** stones of the gallbladder (cholelithiasis) composed almost entirely of the excessive blood pigment liberated by hemolysis, with calcium deposits in some. **bronchial c.,** lung c. **dental c.,** calcium phosphate and carbonate, with organic matter, deposited on tooth surfaces. **fusible c.,** a urinary calculus composed of phosphates of ammonium, calcium, and magnesium, which fuses to a black mass when tested under the blowpipe. **lacrimal c.,** one in a lacrimal gland or duct. **lung c.,** a concretion formed in the bronchi by accretion about an inorganic nucleus, or from calcified portions of lung tissue or adjacent lymph nodes. **renal c.,** one in the kidney. **salivary c.,** one in a salivary gland or duct. **urinary c.,** one in any part of the urinary tract. **vesical c.,** one in the urinary bladder.

calefacient (kal″ĕ-fa′shent) causing a sensation of warmth; an agent that so acts.

calf (kaf) sura; the fleshy back part of the leg below the knee.

caliber (kal′ĭ-ber) the diameter of the opening of a canal or tube.

calibration (kal″ĭ-bra′shun) determination of the accuracy of an instrument, usually by measurement of its variation from a standard, to ascertain necessary correction factors.

calibrator (-ter) an instrument for dilating a tubular structure or for determining the caliber of such a structure.

calicectasis (kal″ĭ-sek′tah-sis) dilatation of a calix of the kidney.

calicectomy (kal″ĭ-sek′to-me) excision of a calix of the kidney.

calicivirus (kal″ĭ-sĭ-vi′rus) any of a subgroup of picornaviruses, including the virus of vesicular exanthem.

caliculus (kah-lik′u-lus), pl. *calic′uli* [L.] a small cup or cup-shaped structure.

caliectasis (kal″e-ek′tah-sis) calicectasis.

californium (kal″ĭ-fōr′ne-um) chemical element (*see table*), at. no. 98, symbol Cf.

calipers (kal′ĭ-perz) an instrument with two bent or curved legs used for measuring thickness or diameter of a solid.

calisthenics (kal″is-then′iks) systematic exercise for attaining strength and gracefulness.

calix (ka′liks), pl. *cal′ices* [L.] a cup-shaped organ or cavity, e.g., one of the recesses of the pelvis of the kidney which enclose the pyramids. **calice′al,** adj.

Calliphora (kal-lif′o-rah) a genus of flies, the blowflies or bluebottle flies, which deposit their eggs in decaying matter, on wounds, or in body openings; the maggots are a cause of myiasis.

callosity (kah-los′ĭ-te) a callus (1).

callosum (kah-lo′sum) corpus callosum. **callo′sal,** adj.

callous (kal′us) of the nature of a callus; hard.

callus (kal′us) 1. localized hyperplasia of the horny layer of the epidermis due to pressure or friction. 2. an unorganized network of woven bone formed about the ends of a broken bone, which is absorbed as repair is completed (*provisional c.*), and ultimately replaced by true bone (*definitive c.*).

calmative (kal′mah-tiv, kah′mah-tiv) 1. sedative; allaying excitement. 2. an agent having such effects.

calomel (kal′o-mel) a heavy, white, impalpable powder, Hg_2Cl, used as a cathartic.

calor (kal′er) [L.] heat; one of the cardinal signs of inflammation.

caloric (kah-lo′rik) pertaining to heat or to calories.

calorie (kal′o-re) a unit of heat; commonly used alone to designate *small c.* **gram c.,** small c. **International Table c., I.T. c.,** a unit of heat, equivalent to 4.1868 joules. **large c.,** kilocalorie; the calorie used in metabolic studies, being the amount of heat required to raise the temperature of 1 kg. of water 1° C. **mean c.,** one one-hundredth of the amount of heat required to raise the temperature of 1 gm. of water from 0 to 100° C. **small c.,** the amount of heat required to raise the temperature of 1 gm. of water 1° C. **standard c.,** small c. **thermochemical c.,** a unit of heat, equivalent to 4.184 joules.

calorifacient (kah-lor″ĭ-fa′shent) producing heat.

calorific (kal″o-rif′ik) producing heat.

calorigenetic (kah-lor″ĭ-jĕ-net′ik) calorigenic.

calorigenic (-jen′ik) producing or increasing production of heat or energy; increasing oxygen consumption.

calorimeter (kal″o-rim′ĕ-ter) an instrument for measuring the amount of heat produced in any system or organism.

calorimetry (-rim′ĕ-tre) measurement of the heat eliminated or stored in any system.

caloripuncture (kah-lor′ĭ-punk″tūr) puncture by use of heat.

caloritropic (-trop″ik) thermotropic.

calory (kal′o-re) calorie.

calvacin (kal′vah-sin) an antineoplastic substance derived from the fungus *Calvatia gigantea.*

calvaria (kal-va′re-ah) the domelike superior portion of the cranium, comprising the superior portions of the frontal, parietal, and occipital bones.

calvarium (kal-va′re-um) calvaria.

calx (kalks) 1. lime or chalk. 2. the heel. **c. chlora′ta,** chlorinated lime. **c. sulfura′ta,** sulfurated lime.

calyculus (kah-lik′u-lus), pl. *calyc′uli* [L.] caliculus.

Calymmatobacterium (kah-lim″mah-to-bak′te′re-um) a genus of schizomycetes (family Brucellaceae), composed of pleomorphic nonmotile, gram-negative rods. **C. granulomato′sis,** *Donovania granulomatosis.*

calyx (ka′liks) calix.

camera (kam′er-ah), pl. *cam′erae* [L.] a cavity or chamber. **c. ante′rior bul′bi,** anterior chamber of the eye. **c. oc′uli,** either the anterior or the posterior chamber of the eye. **c. poste′rior bul′bi,** posterior chamber of the eye. **c. vi′trea bul′bi,** vitreous chamber.

Camoquin (kam′o-kwin) trademark for a preparation of amodiaquine.

camphor (kam′fer) 1. a ketone derived from the Asian tree *Cinnamomum camphora* or produced synthetically; used topically as an antipruritic. 2. any compound with characteristics similar to those of camphor.

camphorated (-āt″ed) containing or tinctured with camphor.

campimeter (kam-pim′ĕ-ter) an apparatus for mapping the central portion of the visual field on a flat surface.

campimetry (-tre) the determination of defects in the visual field by use of a campimeter.

camptocormia (kamp″to-kor′me-ah) a static deformity consisting of forward flexion of the trunk.

camptodactyly (-dak′tĭ-le) permanent flexion of one or more fingers.

camptospasm (kamp′to-spazm) camptocormia.

canal (kah-nal′) a relatively narrow tubular passage or channel. **adductor c.,** a fascial tunnel in the middle third of the medial part of the thigh, containing the femoral vessels and saphenous nerve. **Alcock's c.,** a tunnel formed by a splitting of the obturator fascia, which encloses the pudendal vessels and nerve. **alimentary c.,** the musculomembranous digestive tube extending from the mouth to the anus; see Plate IV. **anal c.,** the terminal portion of the alimentary canal, from the rectum to the anus. **c. of Arantius,** ductus venosus. **archinephric c.,** pronephric duct. **Arnold's c.,** a channel in the petrous portion of the temporal bone for passage of the vagus nerve. **arterial c.,** ductus arteriosus. **atrioventricular c.,** the common canal connecting the primitive atrium and ventricle; it sometimes persists as a congenital anomaly. **birth c.,** the canal through which the fetus passes in birth. **blunderbuss c.,** descriptive term for an incompletely formed tooth root in which the apical third of the root canal has a wider diameter than the coronal two thirds. **caroticotympanic c's,** tiny passages in the temporal bone connecting the carotid canal and the tympanic cavity, carrying communicating twigs between the internal carotid and tympanic plexuses. **carotid c.,** a tunnel in the petrous portion of the temporal bone that transmits the internal carotid artery to the cranial cavity. **cervical c.,** the part of the uterine cavity lying within the cervix. **Cloquet's c.,** hyaloid c. **cochlear c.,** see under *duct.* **condylar c.,** an occasional opening in the condylar fossa for transmission of the transverse sinus. **c. of Corti,** a space between the outer and inner rods of Corti. **crural c.,** femoral c. **c. of Cuvier,** ductus venosus. **dentinal c's,** dental canaliculi.

Dorello's c., an occasional opening in the temporal bone through which the abducens nerve and inferior petrosal sinus enter the cavernous sinus. **facial c.,** a canal for the facial nerve in the petrous portion of the temporal bone. **femoral c.,** the medial part of the femoral sheath lateral to the base of the lacunar ligament. **Gartner's c.,** see under *duct.* **genital c.,** any canal for the passage of ova or for copulatory use. **haversian c.,** any of the anastomosing channels of the haversian system in compact bone, containing blood and lymph vessels and nerves. **Hirschfeld's c's,** interdental c's. **c. of Huguier,** a small canal opening into the facial canal just before its termination, transmitting the chorda tympani nerve. **Hunter's c.,** adductor c. **Huschke's c.,** a canal formed by the tubercles of the tympanic ring, usually disappearing during childhood. **hyaloid c.,** a passage running from in front of the optic disk to the lens of the eye; in the fetus, it transmits the hyaloid artery. **hypoglossal c.,** an opening in the occipital bone, transmitting the hypoglossal nerve and a branch of the posterior meningeal artery. **incisive c.,** one of the small canals opening into the incisive fossa of the hard palate, transmitting the nasopalatine nerves. **infraorbital c.,** a small canal running obliquely through the floor of the orbit, transmitting the infraorbital vessels and nerve. **inguinal c.,** the oblique passage in the lower anterior abdominal wall, through which passes the round ligament of the uterus in the female, and the spermatic cord in the male. **interdental c's,** channels in the alveolar process of the mandible between the roots of the central and lateral incisors, for passage of anastomosing blood vessels between the sublingual and inferior dental arteries. **Jacobson's c.,** tympanic canaliculus. **Löwenberg's c.,** the part of the cochlear duct above the membrane of Corti. **medullary c.,** 1. vertebral c. 2. see under *cavity.* **nasolacrimal c.,** a canal formed by the maxilla laterally and the lacrimal bone and inferior nasal concha medially, transmitting the nasolacrimal duct. **neurenteric c.,** a temporary communication in the embryo between the cavities of the yolk sac and the amnion. **c. of Nuck,** a pouch of peritoneum extending into the inguinal canal, accompanying the round ligament in the female, or the testis in its descent into the scrotum in the male; usually obliterated in the female. **nutrient c. of bone,** haversian c. **optic c.,** a passage for the optic nerve and ophthalmic artery at the apex of the orbit. **parturient c.,** birth c. **perivascular c.,** a lymph space about a blood vessel. **c. of Petit,** zonular spaces. **portal c.,** a space within the capsule of Glisson and liver substance, containing branches of the portal vein, of the hepatic artery, and of the hepatic duct. **pterygoid c.,** a canal in the sphenoid bone transmitting the pterygoid vessels and nerves. **pterygopalatine c.,** a passage in the sphenoid and palatine bones for the greater palatine vessels and nerve. **pudendal c.,** Alcock's c. **pulp c.,** root c. **pyloric c.,** the short narrow part of the stomach extending from the gastroduodenal junction to the pyloric antrum. **root c.,** that part of the pulp cavity extending from the pulp chamber to the apical foramen. **sacculocochlear c.,** the canal connecting the saccule and cochlea. **sacral c.,** the continuation of the vertebral canal through the sacrum. **Schlemm's c.,** venous sinus of sclera. **semicircular c's,** three long canals (anterior, lateral, and posterior) of the bony labyrinth. **spermatic c.,** the inguinal canal in the male. **spinal c.,** vertebral c. **spiral c. of cochlea,** cochlear duct. **spiral c. of modiolus,** a canal following the course of the bony spiral lamina of the cochlea and containing the spiral ganglion. **Stilling's c.,** hyaloid c. **tarsal c.,** see under *sinus*. **tympanic c.,** see under *canaliculus*. **uterine c.,** the cavity of the uterus. **vertebral c.,** the canal formed by the series of vertebral foramina together, enclosing the spinal cord and meninges. **vidian c.,** pterygoid c. **Volkmann's c's,** canals communicating with the haversian canals, for passage of blood vessels through bone. **c. of Wirsung,** pancreatic duct. **zygomaticotemporal c.,** see under *foramen*.

canaliculus (kan″ah-lik′u-lus), pl. *canalic′uli* [L.] an extremely narrow tubular passage or channel. **canalic′ular,** adj. **bile canaliculi,** fine tubular channels forming a three-dimensional network within the parenchyma of the liver. **cochlear c.,** see under *aqueduct*. **dental canaliculi,** minute channels in dentin, extending from the pulp cavity to the overlying cement and enamel. **haversian canaliculi,** minute passages in bones connecting with the haversian canals. **lacrimal c.,** the short passage in an eyelid, beginning at the lacrimal point and draining tears from the lacrimal lake to the lacrimal sac. **mastoid c.,** a small channel in the temporal bone transmitting the tympanic branch of the vagus nerve. **tympanic c.,** a small opening on the inferior surface of the petrous portion of the temporal bone, transmitting the tympanic branch of the glossopharyngeal nerve and a small artery.

canalis (kah-nal′is), pl. *cana′les* [L.] a canal or channel.

canalization (kan″al-i-za′shun) 1. the formation of canals, natural or morbid. 2. the surgical establishment of canals for drainage.

canaloplasty (kah-nal′o-plas″te) plastic reconstruction of a passage, as of the external auditory meatus.

canavanine (kah-nav′ah-nin) a naturally occurring amino acid, isolated from soybean meal.

cancellated (kan′sel-lāt″ed) having a lattice-like structure.

cancellous (kan′sĕ-lus) of a reticular, spongy, or lattice-like structure; said mainly of bony tissue.

cancellus (kan-sel′us), pl. *cancel′li* [L.] the lattice-like structure in bone; any structure arranged like a lattice.

cancer (kan′ser) any malignant, cellular tumor; cancers are divided into two broad categories of carcinoma and sarcoma. **can′cerous,** adj. **black c.,** malignant melanoma. **chimney-sweeps' c.,** carcinoma of the scrotum due to soot poisoning. **c. en cuirasse,** carcinoma of the thorax. **epithelial c.,** carcinoma.

canceremia (kan″ser-e′me-ah) the presence of cancer cells in the blood.

cancericidal (-ĭ-si′dal) destructive to cancer cells.

cancerigenic (kan″ser-ĭ-jen′ik) giving rise to a malignant tumor.

cancerism (kan′ser-izm) a tendency to the development of malignant disease.

cancerophobia, cancerphobia (-o-fo′be-ah; -fo′be-ah) carcinophobia.

cancriform (kang′krĭ-form) resembling cancer.

cancroid (kang′kroid) 1. cancer-like. 2. a skin cancer of a low grade of malignancy.

cancrum (kang′krum) [L.] canker. **c. o′ris,** see *noma*. **c. puden′di,** see *noma*.

candicidin (kan″dĭ-si′din) an antifungal agent produced by *Streptomyces griseus*.

Candida (kan′dĭ-dah) a genus of yeastlike fungi that are commonly part of the normal flora of the mouth, skin, intestinal tract, and vagina, but can cause a variety of infections (see *candidiasis*). *C. al′bicans* is the usual pathogen.

candidal (-dal) pertaining to or caused by *Candida*.

candidemia (kan″dĭ-de′me-ah) presence in the blood of fungi of the genus *Candida*.

candidiasis (-di′ah-sis) infection by fungi of the genus *Candida*, generally *C. albicans*, most commonly involving the skin, oral mucosa (thrush), respiratory tract, and vagina; rarely there is a systemic infection or endocarditis.

candidid (kan′dĭ-did) a secondary skin eruption that is the expression of hypersensitivity to infection with *Candida* elsewhere on the body.

candidin (-din) a skin test antigen derived from *Candida albicans*, used in testing for the development of delayed-type hypersensitivity to the microorganism.

candidosis (kan″dĭ-do′sis) candidiasis.

canine (ka′nīn) 1. of pertaining to, or characteristic of a dog. 2. a canine tooth.

canities (kah-nish′e-ēz) grayness or whiteness of the scalp hair.

canker (kang′ker) an ulceration, especially of the lip or oral mucosa.

Cannabis (kan′ah-bis) a genus of plants, hemp, including *C. in′dica*, an Asiatic variety of common hemp and *C. sati′va*, the common hemp. See *cannabis*.

cannabis (kan′ah-bis) the dried flowering tops of hemp plants (*Cannabis sativa*), which have euphoric principles (tetrahydrocannabinols); classified as a hallucinogen and prepared as bhang, ganja, hashish, and marihuana.

cannabism (-bizm) a morbid state produced by misuse of cannabis.

cannula (kan′u-lah) a tube for insertion into a duct or cavity; during insertion its lumen is usually occupied by a trocar. **Bellocq's c.,** a curved cannula for plugging the posterior nares to control nosebleed.

cannulate (kan′u-lāt) to introduce a cannula, which may be left in place.

cannulation (kan″u-la′shun) introduction of a cannula into a tubelike organ or body cavity.

canthal (kan′thal) pertaining to a canthus.

canthectomy (kan-thek'to-me) excision of the canthus.

canthitis (kan-thi'tis) inflammation of the canthus.

cantholysis (kan-thol'ĭ-sis) surgical division of a canthus or a canthal ligament.

canthoplasty (kan'tho-plas"te) plastic surgery of a canthus.

canthorrhaphy (kan-thor'ah-fe) the suturing of the palpebral fissure at either canthus.

canthotomy (kan-thot'o-me) incision of a canthus.

canthus (kan'thus), pl. *can'thi* [L.] the angle at either end of the fissure between the eyelids.

Cantil (kan'til) trademark for a preparation of mepenzolate.

C.A.P. College of American Pathologists.

cap (kap) a protective covering for the head or for a similar structure; a structure resembling such a covering. **cradle c.**, crusta lactea. **duodenal c.**, the part of the duodenum adjacent to the pylorus, forming the superior flexure. **enamel c.**, the enamel organ after it covers the top of the growing tooth papilla. **knee c.**, patella; see *Table of Bones*. **skull c.**, calvaria.

capacitance (kah-pas'ĭ-tans) 1. the property of being able to store an electric charge. 2. the ratio of charge to potential in a conductor.

capacitation (kah-pas"ĭ-ta'shun) the process by which spermatozoa become capable of fertilizing an ovum after it reaches the ampullar portion of the uterine tube.

capacitor (kah-pas'ĭ-tor) a device for holding and storing charges of electricity.

capacity (kah-pas'ĭ-te) the power to hold, retain, or contain, or the ability to absorb; usually expressed numerically as the measure of such ability. **functional residual c.**, the amount of air remaining at the end of normal quiet respiration. **heat c.**, thermal c. **inspiratory c.**, the volume of gas that can be taken into the lungs in a full inspiration, starting from the resting inspiratory position; equal to the tidal volume plus the inspiratory reserve volume. **maximal breathing c.**, the greatest volume of gas that can be breathed per minute by voluntary effort. **thermal c.**, the amount of heat absorbed by a body in being raised 1° C. **total lung c.**, the amount of gas contained in the lung at the end of a maximal inspiration. **vital c.**, the volume of gas that can be expelled from the lungs from a position of full inspiration, with no limit to duration of inspiration; equal to inspiratory capacity plus expiratory reserve volume.

capelet (kap'ĕ-let) a swelling on the point of a horse's hock or on its elbow.

capillarectasia (kap"ĭ-lār"ek-ta'ze-ah) dilatation of capillaries.

Capillaria (kap"il-la're-ah) a genus of parasitic nematodes, including *C. contor'ta*, found in domestic fowl; *C. hepat'ica*, found in the liver of rats and other mammals, including man; and *C. philippinen'sis*, found in the human intestine in Luzon, causing severe diarrhea, malabsorption, and high mortality.

capillariasis (kap"ĭ-lah-ri'ah-sis) infection with nematodes of the genus *Capillaria*, especially *C. philippinensis*.

capillariomotor (kap"ĭ-lār"e-o-mo'tor) pertaining to the functional activity of the capillaries.

capillaritis (kap"ĭ-lār-i'tis) inflammation of the capillaries.

capillarity (kap"ĭ-lār'ĭ-te) the action by which the surface of a liquid where it is in contact with a solid, as in a capillary tube, is elevated or depressed.

capillary (kap'ĭ-ler"e) 1. pertaining to or resembling a hair. 2. one of the minute vessels connecting the arterioles and venules, the walls of which act as a semipermeable membrane for interchange of various substances between the blood and tissue fluid; see Plate IX. **lymph c.**, **lymphatic c.**, one of the minute vessels of the lymphatic system; see Plate IX.

capillus (kah-pil'us), pl. *capil'li* [L.] a hair; used in the plural to designate the aggregate of hair on the scalp.

capitate (kap'ĭ-tāt) head-shaped.

capitation (kap"ĭ-ta'shun) the annual fee paid to a physician or group of physicians by each participant in a health plan.

capitatum (kap"ĭ-ta'tum) the capitate bone; see *Table of Bones*.

capitellum (kap"ĭ-tel'um) capitulum.

capitonnage (kap"ĭ-to-nahzh') [Fr.] closure of a cyst by applying sutures to approximate the opposing surfaces of the cavity.

capitular (kah-pit'u-ler) pertaining to a capitulum or head of a bone.

capitulum (kah-pit'u-lum), pl. *capit'ula* [L.] a small eminence on a bone, as the eminence on the distal end of the humerus, by which it articulates with another bone.

Capla (kap'lah) trademark for a preparation of mebutamate.

capnohepatography (kap"no-hep"ah-tog'rah-fe) radiography of the liver after intravenous injection of carbon dioxide gas.

capotement (kah-pōt-maw') [Fr.] a splashing sound heard in dilatation of the stomach.

cappie (kap'e) a disease of young sheep characterized by thinning of the bones of the scalp, possibly due to phosphorus-deficient diet.

capping (cap'ing) the provision of a protective or obstructive covering. **pulp c.**, the covering of an exposed or nearly exposed dental pulp with some material to provide protection against external influences and to encourage healing.

caproate (kap'ro-āt) any salt of caproic acid.

caprylate (kap'rĭ-lāt) any salt of caprylic acid.

Capsebon (kap'se-bon) trademark for a suspension of cadmium sulfide.

capsicum (kap'sĭ-kum) the dried fruit of various species of *Capsicum* (pepper plants), used as an irritant and carminative.

capsid (kap'sid) the shell of protein that protects the nucleic acid of a virus; it is composed of structural units, or capsomers. According to the number of subunits possessed by capsomers, they are called dimers (2), trimers (3), pentamers (5), or hexamers (6).

capsitis (kap-si′tis) inflammation of the capsule of the crystalline lens.

capsomer, capsomere (kap′so-mer; kap′so-mēr) a morphological unit of the capsid of a virus.

capsotomy (kap-sot′o-me) capsulotomy.

capsula (kap′su-lah), pl. *cap′sulae* [L.] capsule.

capsulation (kap″su-la′shun) enclosure in a capsule.

capsule (kap′sūl) 1. an enclosing structure, as a soluble container enclosing a dose of medicine. 2. a cartilaginous, fatty, fibrous, membranous structure enveloping another structure, organ, or part. **cap′sular**, adj. **articular c.,** the saclike envelope enclosing the cavity of a synovial joint. **auditory c.,** the cartilaginous capsule of the embryo that becomes the bony labyrinth of the inner ear. **bacterial c.,** an envelope of gel surrounding a bacterial cell, usually polysaccharide but sometimes polypeptide in nature; it is associated with the virulence of pathogenic bacteria. **Bonnet's c.,** Tenon's c. **Bowman's c.,** glomerular c. **c's of brain,** see *external c.* and *internal c.* **cartilage c.,** a basophilic zone of cartilage matrix bordering on a lacuna and its enclosed cartilage cells. **dental c.,** periodontium. **external c.,** the layer of white fibers between the putamen and claustrum. **Gerota's c.,** the fascia surrounding the kidney. **Glisson's c.,** the connective tissue sheath accompanying the hepatic ducts and vessels through the hepatic portal. **glomerular c., c. of glomerulus,** the globular dilatation forming the beginning of a uriniferous tubule within the kidney, and surrounding the glomerulus. **c. of heart,** pericardium. **internal c.,** a fanlike mass of white fibers separating the lentiform nucleus laterally from the head of the caudate nucleus, the dorsal thalamus, and the tail of the caudate nucleus medially. **joint c.,** articular c. **c. of lens,** the elastic envelope covering the lens of the eye. **malpighian c.,** glomerular c. **optic c.,** the embryonic structure from which the sclera develops. **otic c.,** the skeletal element enclosing the inner ear mechanism. In the human embryo, it develops as cartilage at various ossification centers and becomes completely bony and unified at about the 33rd week of fetal life. **renal c., adipose,** the investment of fat surrounding the fibrous capsule of the kidney, continuous at the hilus with the fat in the renal sinus. **renal c., fibrous,** the connective tissue investment of the kidney, continuous through the hilus to line the renal sinus. **sodium iodide** ^{131}**I c's,** capsules containing radioactive iodine as sodium iodide, used in tests of thyroid disease and in suppression of thyroid function. **telemetering c.,** a small radio transmitter encased in a capsule that can be swallowed or otherwise inserted in the body to give information about conditions (pressure, temperature, pH, etc.) within an organ. **Tenon's c.,** the connective tissue enveloping the posterior eyeball.

capsulectomy (kap″su-lek′to-me) excision of a capsule, especially a joint capsule or lens capsule.

capsulitis (kap″su-li′tis) inflammation of a capsule, as that of the lens. **adhesive c.,** adhesive inflammation between the joint capsule and the peripheral articular cartilage of the shoulder, with obliteration of the subdeltoid bursa, characterized by increasing pain, stiffness, and limitation of motion.

capsulolenticular (kap″su-lo-len-tik′u-ler) pertaining to the lens of the eye and its capsule.

capsuloma (kap″su-lo′mah) a capsular or subcapsular tumor of the kidney.

capsuloplasty (kap′su-lo-plas″te) plastic repair of a joint capsule.

capsulorrhaphy (kap″su-lor′ah-fe) suturing of a capsule, especially a joint capsule.

capsulotomy (kap″su-lot′o-me) incision of a capsule, as that of the lens or of a joint.

captodiamine (kap″to-di′ah-mēn) a dimethylethylamine derivative, $C_{21}H_{29}NS_2$, used as an antihistaminic, sedative, and tranquilizer.

captodramin (-dram′in) captodiamine.

caput (kap′ut), pl. *cap′ita* [L.] the head; a general term applied to the expanded or chief extremity of an organ or part. **c. co′li,** the cecum. **c. gallinag′inis,** the verumontanum. **c. medu′sae,** dilated cutaneous veins around the umbilicus, seen mainly in the newborn and in patients suffering from cirrhosis of the liver. **c. succeda′neum,** edema occurring in and under the fetal scalp during labor.

C.A.R. Canadian Association of Radiologists.

caramel (kar′ah-mel) a concentrated solution obtained by heating sugar or glucose until it is a uniform dark brown mass, used as a coloring agent for pharmaceuticals.

caramiphen (kah-ram′ĭ-fen) an anticholinergic, $C_{18}H_{28}ClNO_2$, used as the hydrochloride salt in parkinsonism.

caraway (kar′ah-wa) dried ripe fruit of *Carum carvi;* used as a flavoring agent.

carbachol (kar′bah-kol) an ophthalmic cholinergic, $C_6H_{15}ClN_2O_2$, applied topically to the conjunctiva to constrict the pupil.

carbamate (kar′bah-māt) any ester of carbamic acid. **ethyl c.,** urethan.

carbamazepine (kar″bah-maz′ĕ-pēn) a drug, $C_{15}H_{12}N_2O$, used in the U.S. as an analgesic in the management of trigeminal neuralgia, and in other countries as an anticonvulsant.

carbamide (kar-bam′īd) urea in anhydrous, lyophilized, sterile powder form; injected intravenously in dextrose or invert sugar solution to induce diuresis.

carbaminohemoglobin (kar-bam″ĭ-no-he″moglo′bin) a combination of carbon dioxide and hemoglobin, CO_2HHb, being one of the forms in which carbon dioxide exists in the blood.

carbamoyl (kar′bah-moil) the radical NH_2—CO—; see *carbamoyltransferase.*

carbamoyltransferase (kar″bah-moil-trans′-fer-ās) an enzyme that catalyzes the transfer of carbamoyl, as from carbamoylphosphate to *L*-ornithine to form orthophosphate and citrulline in the synthesis of urea.

carbamylcholine (kar″bah-mil-ko′lēn) carbachol.

carbarsone (kar′bar-sōn) an arsenical compound, $C_7H_9AsN_2O_4$, used as an antiamebic.

carbenicillin (kar″ben-ĭ-sil′in) a semisynthetic antibiotic of the penicillin group, prepared as both the disodium and the potassium salt and used in urinary tract infections.

carbetapentane (kar-ba″tah-pen′tān) an antitussive, $C_{20}H_{31}NO_3$, used as the hydrochloride salt.

carbinol (kar′bĭ-nol) methanol.

carbinoxamine (kar″bin-ok′sah-mēn) a pyridine derivative, $C_{16}H_{19}ClN_2O$; its maleate salt is used as an antitussive.

carbo (kar′bo) [L.] charcoal. **c. anima′lis,** animal charcoal. **c. lig′ni,** wood charcoal, deodorant, absorbent, and disinfectant.

Carbocaine (-kān) trademark for preparations of mepivacaine.

carbocholine (kar″bo-ko′lēn) carbachol.

carbocyclic (-si′klik) having, or pertaining to, a closed chain or ring formation which includes only carbon atoms; said of chemical compounds.

carbohemia (-he′me-ah) the presence of carbon monoxide in the blood.

carbohemoglobin (-he″mo-glo′bin) carbaminohemoglobin.

carbohydrase (-hi′drās) any of a group of enzymes that catalyze the hydrolysis of higher carbohydrates to lower forms.

carbohydrate (-hi′drāt) a compound of carbon, hydrogen, and oxygen, the latter two usually in the proportion of water $(CH_2O)_n$; the most important carbohydrates are the starches, sugars, celluloses, and gums. They are classified into mono-, di-, tri-, poly-, and heterosaccharides.

carbohydraturia (-hi″drah-tu′re-ah) excess of carbohydrates in the urine.

carbol-fuchsin (kar″bol-fook′sin) a stain for microorganisms, containing basic fuchsin and dilute phenol; see also under *solution.*

carboligase (kar″bo-li′gās) an enzyme found in both plant and animal tissues that catalyzes the linking up of carbon atoms and thus changes pyruvic acid to acetyl-methyl-carbinol.

carbolism (kar′bo-lizm) phenol poisoning; see *phenol* (1).

carbolize (-līz) to treat with phenol.

carboluria (kar″bo-lu′re-ah) the presence of phenol in the urine.

carbomer (kar′bo-mer) a polymer of acrylic acid, cross-linked with a polyfunctional agent; a suspending agent.

carbomycin (kar″bo-mi′sin) a crystalline monobasic antibiotic isolated from the elaborated products of *Streptomyces halstedii* or produced by other means; it is bacteriostatic for gram-positive organisms.

carbon (kar′bon) chemical element (*see table*), at. no. 6, symbol C. ^{13}C, a natural isotope of carbon, of atomic mass 13, used as a tracer in chemical reactions in living tissue. ^{14}C, a radioactive isotope of carbon, of atomic mass 14, used in cancer and metabolic research. **c. dioxide,** an odorless, colorless gas, CO_2, resulting from oxidation of carbon, and formed in the tissues and eliminated by the lungs; used with oxygen to stimulate respiration, and in solid form (*carbon dioxide snow*) as an escharotic. **c. monox-**

ide, an odorless gas, CO, formed by burning carbon or organic fuels with a scanty supply of oxygen; inhalation causes central nervous system damage and asphyxiation by combining irreversibly with blood hemoglobin. **c. tetrachloride,** a clear, colorless, mobile liquid; the inhalation of its vapors can depress central nervous system activity and cause degeneration of the liver and kidneys.

carbonate (-āt) a salt of carbonic acid. **ferrous c.,** $FeCO_3$; used in iron deficiency anemia.

carbonemia (kar″bo-ne′me-ah) carbohemia.

carbonize (kar′bo-nīz) to char or to convert into charcoal.

carbonuria (kar″bo-nu′re-ah) the presence in the urine of carbon dioxide or other carbon compounds.

carbonyl (kar′bo-nil) the bivalent organic radical, C:O, characteristic of aldehydes, ketones, carboxylic acid, and esters. **c. chloride,** phosgene.

carboxyhemoglobin (kar-bok″se-he″mo-glo′bin) a compound formed from hemoglobin on exposure to carbon monoxide.

carboxyl (kar-bok′sil) the monovalent radical —COOH, occurring in those organic acids termed carboxylic acids.

carboxylase (kar-bok′sĭ-lās) an enzyme that catalyzes the removal of carbon dioxide from the carboxyl group of alpha amino keto acids. **acetyl-CoA c.,** an enzyme that catalyzes the conversion of ATP, acetyl-CoA, CO_2, and water to ADP, orthophosphate, and malonyl-CoA.

carboxylation (kar-bok″sil-a′shun) the addition of a carboxyl group, as to pyruvate to form oxaloacetate.

carboxylesterase (-es′ter-ās) an enzyme that catalyzes the hydrolysis of the esters of carboxylic acids.

carboxyltransferase (-trans′fer-ās) an enzyme that catalyzes carboxylation.

carboxy-lyase (kar-bok′se-li′ās) any of a group of lyases that catalyze the removal of a carboxyl group; it includes the carboxylases and decarboxylases.

carboxymyoglobin (-mi″o-glo′bin) a compound formed from myoglobin on exposure to carbon monoxide.

carboxypeptidase (-pep′tĭ-dās) an exopeptidase that acts only on the peptide linkage of a terminal amino acid containing a free carboxyl group.

carboxypolypeptidase (-pol″e-pep′tĭ-dās) an exopeptidase that attacks the peptide linkage of a terminal amino acid possessing a free carboxyl group, releasing a free amino acid from a polypeptide.

carbromal (kar-bro′mal) a sedative and hypnotic, $C_7H_{13}BrN_2O_2$.

carbuncle (kar′bung-k'l) a necrotizing infection of skin and subcutaneous tissues composed of a cluster of furuncles, usually due to *Staphylococcus aureus*, with multiple drainage sinuses. **carbunc′ular,** adj. **malignant c.,** anthrax.

carbunculoid (kar-bung′ku-loid) resembling a carbuncle.

carbunculosis (kar-bung″ku-lo′sis) a condition marked by formation of numerous carbuncles.

carbutamide (kar-bu′tah-mīd) a hypoglycemic agent, $C_{11}H_{17}N_3O_3S$.

carcass (kar′kas) a dead body; generally applied to other than a human body.

Carcholin (kar′ko-lin) trademark for a preparation of carbachol.

carcinectomy (kar″sĭ-nek′to-me) excision of carcinoma.

carcinoembryonic (kar″sin-o-em″bre-on′ik) relating to carcinoma and to the embryonic state; see under *antigen.*

carcinogen (kar-sin′o-jen) any substance which causes cancer. **carcinogen′ic,** adj.

carcinogenesis (kar″sĭ-no-jen′ĕ-sis) production of cancer.

carcinogenicity (-jĕ-nis′ĭ-te) the ability or tendency to produce cancer.

carcinoid (kar′sĭ-noid) argentaffinoma.

carcinolysis (kar″sĭ-nol′ĭ-sis) destruction of cancer cells. **carcinolyt′ic,** adj.

carcinoma (kar″sĭ-no′mah) a malignant new growth made up of epithelial cells tending to infiltrate surrounding tissues and to give rise to metastases. **adenocystic c., adenoid cystic c.,** cylindroma; carcinoma marked by cylinders or bands of hyaline or mucinous stroma separated or surrounded by nests or cords of small epithelial cells, occurring in the mammary and salivary glands, and mucous glands of the respiratory tract. **alveolar c.,** see under *adenocarcinoma.* **basal cell c.,** an epithelial tumor of the skin that seldom metastasizes but has potentialities for local invasion and destruction. **basosquamous cell c.,** carcinoma that histologically exhibits both basal and squamous elements. **bronchogenic c.,** carcinoma of the lung, so called because it arises from the epithelium of the bronchial tree. **chorionic c.,** choriocarcinoma. **colloid c.,** mucinous c. **cylindrical cell c.,** that in which the cells are cylindrical or nearly so. **embryonal c.,** a highly malignant, primitive form of carcinoma, probably of germinal cell or teratomatous derivation, usually arising in a gonad. **epidermoid c.,** that in which the cells tend to differentiate in the same way as those of the epidermis; i.e., they tend to form prickle cells and undergo cornification. **giant cell c.,** carcinoma containing many giant cells. **hair matrix c.,** basal cell c. **Hürthle cell c.,** see under *tumor.* **c. in si′tu,** a neoplastic entity wherein the tumor cells have not invaded the basement membrane but are still confined to the epithelium of origin; popularly applied to such cells in the uterine cervix. **medullary c.,** that composed mainly of epithelial elements with little or no stroma. **mucinous c.,** adenocarcinoma producing significant amounts of mucin. **oat cell c.,** a radiosensitive tumor composed of small, oval, undifferentiated cells that are intensely hematoxyphilic and typically bronchogenic. **papillary c.,** carcinoma in which there are papillary excrescences. **prickle cell c.,** squamous cell c. **renal cell c.,** carcinoma of the renal parenchyma, composed of tubular cells in varying arrangements. **scirrhous c.,** carcinoma with a hard structure owing to the formation of dense connective tissue in the stroma. **c. sim′plex,** an undifferentiated carcinoma. **spindle cell c.,** squamous cell carcinoma marked by fusiform development of rapidly proliferating cells. **squamous cell c.,** that arising from squamous epithelium and having cuboid cells.

carcinomatosis (kar″sĭ-no″mah-to′sis) the condition of widespread dissemination of cancer throughout the body.

carcinomatous (kar″sĭ-no′mah-tus) pertaining to or of the nature of cancer; malignant.

carcinophilia (kar″sĭ-no-fil′e-ah) special affinity for cancerous tissue. **carcinophil′ic,** adj.

carcinophobia (-fo′be-ah) morbid dread of cancer.

carcinosarcoma (-sar-ko′mah) a malignant tumor composed of carcinomatous and sarcomatous tissues. **embryonal c.,** Wilms' tumor.

carcinosis (kar″sĭ-no′sis) carcinomatosis. **miliary c.,** that marked by development of numerous nodules resembling miliary tuberculosis.

cardamom (kar′dah-mom) the fruit of *Elettaria cardamomum,* a plant of tropical Asia.

cardi(o)- word element [Gr.], *heart.*

cardia (kar′de-ah) 1. the cardiac opening. 2. the cardiac part of the stomach; that part of the stomach surrounding the esophagogastric junction, distinguished by the presence of cardiac glands.

cardiac (kar′de-ak) 1. pertaining to the heart. 2. pertaining to the cardia.

cardialgia (kar″de-al′je-ah) cardiodynia.

cardiant (kar′de-ant) a drug or agent that affects the heart.

cardiectasis (kar″de-ek′tah-sis) dilatation of the heart.

cardioaccelerator (kar″de-o-ak-sel′er-a″tor) quickening the heart action; an agent that so acts.

cardioactive (-ak′tiv) having an effect upon the heart.

cardioangiology (-an″je-ol′o-je) the medical specialty dealing with the heart and blood vessels.

cardioaortic (-a-or′tik) pertaining to the heart and aorta.

cardioarterial (-ar-te′re-al) pertaining to the heart and arteries.

cardiocele (kar′de-o-sēl″) hernial protrusion of the heart through a fissure of the diaphragm or through a wound.

cardiocentesis (kar″de-o-sen-te′sis) surgical puncture of the heart.

cardiochalasia (-kah-la′ze-ah) relaxation or incompetence of the sphincter action of the cardiac opening of the stomach.

cardiocinetic (-si-net′ik) cardiokinetic.

cardiocirrhosis (-sir-ro′sis) cirrhosis of the liver complicating heart disease, with recurrent intractable congestive heart failure.

cardiodiaphragmatic (-di″ah-frag-mat′ik) pertaining to the heart and diaphragm.

cardiodilator (-di′la-tor) an instrument for dilating the cardia.

cardiodiosis (-di-o′sis) dilatation of the cardiac opening of the stomach.

cardiodynamics (-di-nam′iks) study of the forces involved in the heart's action.

cardiodynia (-din′e-ah) pain in the heart.

cardiogenesis (-jen′ĕ-sis) development of the heart in the embryo.

cardiogenic (-jen′ik) originating in the heart.

Cardiografin (-gra′fin) trademark for preparations of meglumine diatrizoate.

cardiogram (kar′de-o-gram″) a tracing of a cardiac event produced by cardiography. **apex c.,** the record produced by apex cardiography. **precordial c.,** kinetocardiogram.

cardiograph (-graf″) an instrument used for recording some element of the heart beat. **cardiograph′ic,** adj.

cardiography (kar″de-og′rah-fe) the graphic recording of a physical or functional aspect of the heart, e.g., electrocardiography, kinetocardiography, phonocardiography, vibrocardiography. **apex c.,** the graphic recording of low-frequency pulsations at the anterior chest wall over the apex of the heart. **ultrasonic c.,** echocardiography. **vector c.,** vectorcardiography.

Cardio-Green (kar″de-o-grēn) trademark for a preparation of indocyanine green.

cardiohepatic (-hĕ-pat′ik) pertaining to the heart and liver.

cardioinhibitor (-in-hib′ĭ-ter) an agent that restrains the heart's action.

cardioinhibitory (-in-hib′ĭ-to-re) restraining or inhibiting the heart movements.

cardiokinetic (-ki-net′ik) 1. exciting or stimulating the heart. 2. an agent that so acts.

cardiolipin (-lip′in) a substance extracted from fresh beef hearts which, when combined with lecithin and cholesterol, forms an antigen for use in flocculation and precipitation tests for syphilis.

cardiologist (kar″de-ol′o-jist) a physician skilled in the diagnosis and treatment of heart disease.

cardiology (-ol′o-je) the study of the heart and its functions.

cardiolysin (-ol′ĭ-sin) a lysin which acts on the heart muscle.

cardiolysis (-ol′ĭ-sis) the operation of freeing the heart from its adhesions to the sternal periosteum in adhesive mediastinopericarditis.

cardiomalacia (kar″de-o-mah-la′she-ah) morbid softening of the muscular substance of the heart.

cardiomegaly (-meg′ah-le) hypertrophy of the heart.

cardiomelanosis (-mel″ah-no′sis) melanosis of the heart.

cardiometer (kar″de-om′ĕ-ter) an instrument for estimating the power of the heart's action.

cardiomotility (kar″de-o-mo-til′ĭ-te) the movements of the heart; motility of the heart.

cardiomyoliposis (-mi″o-lĭ-po′sis) fatty degeneration of the heart muscle.

cardiomyopathy (-mi-op′ah-the) a general diagnostic term designating primary myocardial disease.

cardiomyopexy (-mi′o-pek″se) surgical removal of the epicardium and application of a pedicled flap of adjacent muscle to the denuded myocardium and pericardium, as a means of supplying collateral circulation to the heart.

cardionector (-nek′tor) the structures regulating the heart beat, comprising the sinoatrial node, bundle of His, and atrioventricular node.

cardionephric (-nef′rik) pertaining to the heart and kidney.

cardioneural (-nu′ral) pertaining to the heart and nervous system.

cardioneurosis (-nu-ro′sis) neurocirculatory asthenia.

cardio-omentopexy (-o-men′to-pek″se) suture of a portion of the omentum to the heart.

cardiopaludism (-pal′u-dizm) heart disease due to malaria.

cardiopathy (kar″de-op′ah-the) any disorder or disease of the heart.

cardiopericardiopexy (kar″de-o-per″ĭ-kar′de-o-pek″se) surgical establishment of adhesive pericarditis, for relief of coronary disease.

cardiopericarditis (-per″ĭ-kar-di′tis) inflammation of the heart and pericardium.

cardiophobia (-fo′be-ah) morbid dread of heart disease.

cardioplasty (kar′de-o-plas″te) esophagogastroplasty.

cardioplegia (kar″de-o-ple′je-ah) interruption of myocardial contraction, as by use of chemical compounds or cold in cardiac surgery.

cardiopneumatic (-nu-mat′ik) of or pertaining to the heart and respiration.

cardiopneumograph (-nu′mo-graf) an apparatus for registering cardiopneumatic movements.

cardioptosis (kar″de-op′tŏ-sis) downward displacement of the heart.

cardiopulmonary (kar″de-o-pul′mo-ner″e) pertaining to the heart and lungs.

cardiopuncture (-punk′tūr) cardiocentesis.

cardiopyloric (-pi-lor′ik) pertaining to the cardiac opening of the stomach and the pylorus.

cardiorenal (-re′nal) pertaining to the heart and kidneys.

cardiorrhaphy (kar″de-or′ah-fe) suture of the heart muscle.

cardiorrhexis (kar″de-o-rek′sis) rupture of the heart.

cardiosclerosis (-skle-ro′sis) fibrous induration of the heart.

cardiospasm (kar′de-o-spazm″) achalasia of the esophagus.

cardiosphygmograph (kar″de-o-sfig′mo-graf) a combination of the cardiograph and sphygmograph for recording the movements of the heart and an arterial pulse.

cardiosplenopexy (-splen′o-pek″se) suture of the splenic parenchyma to the denuded surface of the heart for revascularization of the myocardium.

cardiotachometer (-tah-kom′ĕ-ter) an instrument for continuously portraying or recording the heart rate.

cardiotachometry (-tah-kom'ĕ-tre) continuous recording of the heart rate for long periods.

cardiotherapy (-ther'ah-pe) the treatment of diseases of the heart.

cardiotomy (kar"de-ot'o-me) 1. surgical incision of the heart. 2. surgical incision into the cardia.

cardiotonic (kar"de-o-ton'ik) having a tonic effect on the heart; an agent that so acts.

cardiotopometry (-to-pom'ĕ-tre) measurement of the area of cardiac dullness.

cardiotoxic (-tok'sik) having a poisonous or deleterious effect upon the heart.

cardiovalvular (-val'vu-lar) pertaining to the heart valves.

cardiovalvulotome (-val'vu-lo-tōm") an instrument for incising a heart valve.

cardiovascular (-vas'ku-lar) pertaining to the heart and blood vessels.

cardioversion (kar'de-o-ver"zhun) the restoration of sinus rhythm by electrical shock.

cardioverter (-ver"ter) an energy-storage capacitor-discharge type of condenser which is discharged with an inductance; it delivers a direct-current shock which restores sinus rhythm in atrial fibrillation.

carditis (kar-di'tis) inflammation of the heart; myocarditis.

cardivalvulitis (kar"di-val"vu-li'tis) inflammation of the heart valves.

Cardrase (kar'drās) trademark for a preparation of ethoxzolamide.

caries (ka're-ēz, kār'ez) decay, as of bone or teeth. **ca'rious,** adj. **dental c.,** a destructive process causing decalcification of the tooth enamel and leading to continued destruction of enamel and dentin, and cavitation of the tooth. **dry c.,** a form of tuberculous caries of the joints and ends of bones. **c. fungo'sa,** tuberculosis of bone. **necrotic c.,** form in which pieces of the bone lie in a suppurating cavity. **c. sic'ca,** dry c.

carina (kah-ri'nah), pl. *cari'nae* [L.] a ridgelike structure. **c. tra'cheae,** a downward and backward projection of the lowest tracheal cartilage, forming a ridge between the openings of the right and left principal bronchi. **c. urethra'lis vagi'nae,** the column of rugae in the lower anterior wall of the vagina, immediately below the urethra.

cariogenesis (kār"e-o-jen'ĕ-sis) development of caries.

cariogenic (-jen'ik) conducive to caries.

cariogenicity (-jĕ-nis'ĭ-te) the quality of being conducive to caries.

carisoprodol (kar"i-so'pro-dol) an analgesic and skeletal muscle relaxant, $C_{12}H_{24}N_2O_4$.

carminative (kar-min'ah-tive) 1. relieving flatulence. 2. an agent that relieves flatulence.

carmine (kar'min, kar'mīn) a red coloring matter used as a histologic stain. **indigo c.,** sodium indigotindisulfonate.

carminophil (kar"min'o-fil) 1. easily stainable with carmine. 2. a cell or element readily taking a stain from carmine.

carnitine (kar'nĭ-tēn) a vitamin of the B complex present in meat extracts.

carnivore (kar'nĭ-vōr) any animal that eats primarily flesh, particularly mammals of the order Carnivora, which includes cats, dogs, bears, etc. **carniv'orous,** adj.

carnosinase (kar'no-sĭ-nās) an enzyme that hydrolyzes carnosine (amino-acyl-L-histidine) and other dipeptides containing L-histidine into their constituent amino acids.

carnosine (kar'no-sin) a dipeptide, $C_9H_{14}N_4O_2$, composed of beta-alanine and histidine, found in skeletal muscle of vertebrates.

carnosinemia (kar"no-sĭ-ne'me-ah) excessive amounts of carnosine in the blood; it has been associated with a progressive neurologic disease characterized by severe mental defect and myoclonic seizures, and is probably due to a genetic deficiency of carnosinase in the serum.

carnosinuria (-nu're-ah) an aminoaciduria characterized by excess of carnosine in the urine; it occurs in carnosinemia or may be dietary in origin, especially in young children.

caro (ka'ro), pl. *car'nes* [L.] flesh, or muscular tissue.

carotenase (kar-ot'ĕ-nās) an enzyme that converts carotene into vitamin A.

carotene (kar'o-tēn) a yellow or red pigment from carrots, sweet potatoes, milk and body fat, egg yolk, etc.; it is a chromolipoid hydrocarbon existing in several forms (α-, β-, and γ-carotene), which can be converted into vitamin A in the body.

carotenemia (kar"o-tĕ-ne'me-ah) presence of excessive carotene in the blood; sometimes occurring in sufficient amounts to cause yellowing of the skin.

carotenodermia (kah-rot"ĕ-no-der'me-ah) yellowness of the skin due to carotenemia.

carotenoid (kah-rot'ĕ-noid) 1. any member of a group of red, orange, or yellow pigmented polyisoprenoid lipids found in carrots, sweet potatoes, green leaves, and some animal tissues; examples are the carotenes, lycopene, and xanthophyll. 2. marked by yellow color. 3. lipochrome.

carotenosis (kar"o-tĕ-no'sis) deposition of carotene in tissues, especially the skin.

caroticotympanic (kah-rot"ĭ-ko-tim-pan'ik) pertaining to carotid canal and tympanum.

carotid (kah-rot'id) pertaining to the carotid artery, the principal artery of the neck; see *Table of Arteries.*

carotin (kar'o-tin) carotene.

carotinase (kar-ot'ĭ-nās) carotenase.

carotodynia (kah-rot"o-din'e-ah) tenderness along the course of the carotid artery.

carp (karp) a fruiting body of a fungus.

carpal (kar'pal) pertaining to the carpus.

carpectomy (kar-pek'to-me) excision of a carpal bone.

carphenazine (kar-fen'ah-zēn) a major tranquilizer, $C_{24}H_{31}N_3O_2$, used as the maleate salt.

carphology (kar-fol'o-je) involuntary picking at the bedclothes, seen in grave fevers and in conditions of great exhaustion.

carpitis (kar-pi'tis) inflammation of the synovial membranes of the bones of the carpal joint in domestic animals, producing swelling, pain, and lameness.

carpometacarpal (kar″po-met″ah-kar′pal) pertaining to the carpus and metacarpus.

carpopedal (-pe′dal) affecting the wrist and foot.

carpophalangeal (-fah-lan′je-al) pertaining to the carpus and phalanges.

carpoptosis (-to′sis) wristdrop.

carpus (kar′pus) the joint between the arm and hand, made up of eight bones; the wrist. Also, the corresponding forelimb joint in quadrupeds.

carrageen, carragheen (kar′ah-gēn) the dried and bleached plant of the seaweed *Chondrus crispus* or *Gigartina mammillosa,* containing a valuable polysaccharide widely used as a gel, thickening agent, and emulsifier; it also has demulcent properties.

carrageenan, carragheenin (kar″ah-ge′nan) a colloidal extractive derived from carrageen.

carrier (kar′e-er) one who harbors disease organisms in his body without manifest symptoms, thus acting as a carrier or distributor of infection; also, a heterozygote, i.e., one who carries a recessive gene, autosomal or sex-linked, together with its normal allele.

carrier-free (kar′e-er-fre″) a term denoting a radioisotope of an element in pure form, i.e., essentially undiluted with a stable isotope carrier.

cart (kart) a wheeled vehicle for conveying patients or equipment and supplies in a hospital. **crash c.,** resuscitation c. **dressing c.,** one containing all supplies and equipment that may be necessary for changing dressings of surgical or injured patients. **resuscitation c.,** one containing all equipment necessary for initiating emergency resuscitation.

cartilage (kar′tĭ-lij) a specialized, fibrous connective tissue present in adults, and forming most of the temporary skeleton in the embryo, providing a model in which most of the bones develop, and constituting an important part of the organism's growth mechanism; the three most important types are hyaline cartilage, elastic cartilage, and fibrocartilage. Also, a general term for a mass of such tissue in a particular site in the body. **alar c's,** the cartilages of the wings of the nose. **aortic c.,** the second costal cartilage on the right side. **arthrodial c., articular c.,** that lining the articular surface of synovial joints. **arytenoid c's,** the two pyramid-shaped cartilages of the larynx. **connecting c.,** that connecting the surfaces of an immovable joint. **corniculate c.,** a small nodule of cartilage at the apex of each arytenoid cartilage. **costal c.,** a bar of hyaline cartilage that attaches a rib to the sternum in the case of true ribs, or to the immediately above rib in the case of the upper false ribs. **cricoid c.,** a ringlike cartilage forming the lower and back part of the larynx. **cuneiform c.,** either of the paired cartilages, one on either side in the aryepiglottic fold. **dentinal c.,** the substance remaining after the lime salts of dentin have been dissolved in an acid. **diarthrodial c.,** articular c. **elastic c.,** cartilage whose matrix contains yellow elastic fibers. **ensiform c.,** xiphoid process. **epactal**

c's, one or more small cartilages in the lateral wall of the nose. **floating c.,** a detached portion of semilunar cartilage in the knee joint. **hyaline c.,** a flexible, somewhat elastic, semitransparent substance with an opalescent bluish tint, composed of a basophilic, fibril-containing substance with cavities in which the chondrocytes occur. **interosseous c.,** connecting c. **investing c.,** articular c. **Jacobson's c.,** vomeronasal c. **mandibular c., Meckel's c.,** the embryonic cartilaginous bar into which the lower part of the mandibular arch is converted. **ossifying c.,** temporary c. **palpebral c.,** tarsal plate. **parachordal c.,** one of the two embryonic cartilages beside the occipital part of the notochord. **permanent c.,** cartilage which does not normally become ossified. **precursory c.,** temporary c. **Reichert's c.,** hyoid arch. **reticular c.,** elastic c. **Santorini's c.,** corniculate c. **semilunar c.,** one of the two interarticular cartilages of the knee joint. **sesamoid c's,** small cartilages found in the thyrohyoid ligament (*sesamoid c. of larynx*), on either side of the nose (*sesamoid c. of nose*), and occasionally in the vocal ligaments (*sesamoid c. of vocal ligament*). **slipping rib c.,** a loosened or deformed cartilage whose slipping over an adjacent rib cartilage may produce discomfort or pain. **stratified c.,** fibrocartilage. **tarsal c.,** see under *plate.* **temporary c.,** cartilage that is being replaced by bone or that is normally destined to be replaced by bone. **thyroid c.,** the shield-shaped cartilage of the larynx. **triticeous c.,** a small cartilage in the thyrohyoid ligament. **tympanomandibular c.,** Meckel's c. **vomeronasal c.,** either of the two narrow strips of cartilage, one on each side, of the nasal septum supporting the vomeronasal organ. **Weitbrecht's c.,** a pad of fibrocartilage sometimes present within the articular cavity of the acromioclavicular joint. **Wrisberg's c.,** cuneiform c. **xiphoid c.,** see under *process.* **Y c.,** Y-shaped cartilage within the acetabulum, joining the ilium, ischium, and pubes. **yellow c.,** elastic c.

cartilaginiform (kar″tĭ-lah-jin′ĭ-form) resembling cartilage.

cartilaginous (-laj′ĭ-nus) consisting of or of the nature of cartilage.

cartilago (kar″tĭ-lah′go), pl. *cartilag′ines* [L.] cartilage.

caruncle (kar′ung-k'l) a small fleshy eminence, often abnormal. **hymenal c's,** small elevations of the mucous membrane around the vaginal opening, being relics of the torn hymen. **lacrimal c.,** the red eminence at the medial angle of the eye. **myrtiform c's,** hymenal c's. **sublingual c.,** an eminence on either side of the frenulum of the tongue, on which the major sublingual duct and the submandibular duct open. **urethral c.,** a small red eminence in the mucous membrane of the female urinary meatus.

caruncula (kah-rung′ku-la), pl. *carun′culae* [L.] caruncle.

carver (kar′ver) a tool for producing and perfecting anatomic form in artificial teeth and dental restorations.

caryo- for words beginning thus, see those beginning *karyo-.*

casanthranol (kah-san'thrah-nōl) a purified mixture of the anthranol glycosides derived from *Cascara sagrada;* a cathartic.

cascade (kas-kād') a series of steps or stages (as of a physiological process) which, once initiated continues to the final step by virtue of each step being triggered by the preceding one, sometimes with cumulative effect.

cascara (kas-kār'ah) bark. **c. sagra'da,** dried bark of the shrub *Rhamnus purshiana,* used as a cathartic.

case (kās) a particular instance of a disease. **index c.,** the case of the original patient (propositus or proband) that stimulates investigation of other members of the family to discover a possible genetic factor in the condition. In epidemiology, the first case of a contagious disease. **trial c.,** a box containing convex and concave spherical and cylindrical lenses, arranged in pairs, a trial spectacle frame, and other devices used in testing vision.

casease (ka'se-ās) a protease from bacterial cultures, capable of dissolving albumin and the casein of milk and cheese.

caseation (ka"se-a'shun) 1. the precipitation of casein. 2. a form of necrosis in which tissue is changed into a dry, amorphous mass resembling cheese.

casein (ka'se-in) a phosphoprotein, the principal protein of milk, the basis of curd and of cheese. NOTE: In British nomenclature casein is called *caseinogen,* and paracasein is called *casein.* **vegetable c.,** a protein resembling casein, e.g., wheat gluten.

caseinogen (ka"se-in'o-jen) the British term for casein.

caseous (ka'se-us) resembling cheese or curd.

caseworm (kās'werm) echinococcus.

cassette (kah-set') [Fr.] a light-proof housing for x-ray film, containing front and back intensifying screens, between which the film is placed; a magazine for film or magnetic tape.

cast (kast) 1. a positive copy of an object, e.g., a mold of a hollow organ (a renal tubule, bronchiole, etc.), formed of effused plastic matter and extruded from the body, as a urinary cast; named according to constituents, as epithelial, fatty, waxy, etc. 2. a positive copy of the tissues of the jaws, made in an impression, and over which denture bases or other restorations may be fabricated. 3. to form an object in a mold. 4. a stiff dressing or casing, usually made of plaster of Paris, used to immobilize body parts. 5. strabismus. **dental c.,** see *cast* (2). **hanging c.,** one applied to the arm in fracture of the shaft of the humerus, suspended by a sling looped around the neck. **quarter c.,** a cut in the quarter of a horse's hoof. **urinary c.,** one formed from gelled protein in the renal tubules, which becomes molded to the tubular lumen.

castrate (kas'trāt) 1. to deprive of the gonads, rendering the individual incapable of reproduction. 2. a castrated individual.

castration (kas-tra'shun) excision of the gonads, or their destruction as by radiation or parasites. **female c.,** bilateral oophorectomy, or spaying. **male c.,** bilateral orchiectomy. **parasitic c.,** de-

fective sexual development due to parasitic infestation in early life.

casualty (kaz'u-al-te) 1. an accident; an accidental wound; death or disablement from an accident; also the person so injured. 2. in the armed forces, one missing from his unit as a result of death, injury, illness, capture, because his whereabouts are unknown, or other reasons.

casuistics (kaz"u-is'tiks) the recording and study of cases of disease.

cat(a)- word element [Gr.], *down; lower; under; against; along with; very.*

catabasis (kah-tab'ah-sis) the stage of decline of a disease. **catabat'ic,** adj.

catabiosis (kat"ah-bi-o'sis) the normal senescence of cells. **catabiot'ic,** adj.

catabolergy (-bol'er-je) the energy used in catabolism.

catabolin (kah-tab'o-lin) catabolite.

catabolism (-lizm) any destructive process by which complex substances are converted by living cells into more simple compounds, with release of energy. **catabol'ic,** adj.

catabolite (-līt) a compound produced in catabolism.

catacrotism (kah-tak'ro-tizm) a pulse anomaly in which a small additional wave or notch appears in the descending limb of the pulse tracing. **catacrot'ic,** adj.

catadicrotism (kat"ah-di'kro-tizm) a pulse anomaly in which two small additional waves or notches appear in the descending limb of the pulse tracing. **catadicrot'ic,** adj.

catadioptric (-di-op'trik) deflecting and reflecting light at the same time.

catagen (kat'ah-jen) the brief portion in the hair growth cycle in which growth (anagen) stops and resting (telogen) starts.

catagenesis (kat"ah-jen'ĕ-sis) involution or retrogression.

catalase (kat'ah-lās) a crystalline enzyme which specifically catalyzes the decomposition of hydrogen peroxide and is found in almost all cells except certain anaerobic bacteria. **catalat'ic,** adj.

catalepsy (-lep"se) a condition of diminished responsiveness usually characterized by a trance-like state and constantly maintained immobility, often with flexibilitas cerea. **catalep'tic,** adj.

cataleptiform (kat"ah-lep'tĭ-form) resembling catalepsy.

cataleptoid (-lep'toid) cataleptiform.

catalysis (kah-tal'ĭ-sis) increase in the velocity of a chemical reaction or process produced by the presence of a substance that is not consumed in the net chemical reaction or process; *negative catalysis* denotes the slowing down or inhibition of a reaction or process by the presence of such a substance. **catalyt'ic,** adj.

catalyst (kat'ah-list) any substance that brings about catalysis.

catalyze (-līz) to cause or produce catalysis.

catamnesis (kat"am-ne'sis) the follow-up history of a patient after he is discharged from treatment or a hospital.

cataphasia (kat″ah-fa′ze-ah) speech disorder with constant repetition of a word or phrase.

cataphora (kah-taf′ŏ-rah) lethargy with intervals of imperfect waking.

cataphoresis (kat″ah-fo-re′sis) the passage of charged particles toward the negative pole (cathode) in electrophoresis.

cataphoria (-fo′re-ah) a downward turning of the visual axis of both eyes after visual functional stimuli have been removed. **cataphor′ic,** adj.

cataphrenia (-fre′ne-ah) mental debility of the dementia type which tends to recovery. **cataphren′ic,** adj.

cataphylaxis (-fi-lak′sis) movement of leukocytes and antibodies to the site of an infection. **cataphylac′tic,** adj.

cataplasia (-pla′ze-ah) atrophy in which tissues revert to earlier, more embryonic conditions.

cataplexy (kat′ah-plek″se) a condition marked by abrupt attacks of muscular weakness and hypotonia triggered by such emotional stimulus, as mirth, anger, fear, etc., often associated with narcolepsy. **cataplec′tic,** adj.

cataract (kat′ah-rakt) an opacity of the crystalline lens of the eye or its capsule. **catarac′tous,** adj. **after-c.,** 1. any membrane in the pupillary area after extraction or absorption of the lens. 2. secondary c. (1). **atopic c.,** one occurring, usually during the third decade, in patients who have had atopic dermatitis for many years. **blue c., blue dot c.,** a condition in which small blue punctate opacities are scattered throughout the nucleus and cortex of the lens. **brown c., brunescent c.,** senile cataract appearing as a brown opacity. **capsular c.,** one consisting of an opacity in the capsule of the lens. **complicated c.,** a cataract occurring secondarily to other intraocular disease. **coronary c.,** one in which club-shaped opacities form a ring or crown around the lens, the center of the lens and the extreme periphery remaining clear. **cortical c.,** an opacity in the cortex of the lens. **cupuliform c.,** a senile cataract in the posterior cortex of the lens just under the capsule. **hypermature c.,** one in which the lens capsule is wrinkled and the contents have become solid and shrunken, or soft and liquid. **lamellar c.,** an opacity affecting only certain layers between the cortex and nucleus of the lens. **lenticular c.,** opacity of the lens not affecting the capsule. **mature c.,** one in which the lens is completely opaque. **membranous c.,** a condition in which the lens substance has shrunk, leaving remnants of the capsule and fibrous tissue formation. **morgagnian c.,** a hypermature cataract in which the cortex has become completely liquefied and the nucleus settles at the bottom of the capsule. **nuclear c.,** one in which the opacity is in the central nucleus of the eye. **polar c.,** one seated at the center of the anterior (*anterior polar c.*) or posterior (*posterior polar c.*) pole of the lens. **pyramidal c.,** a conoid anterior cataract with its apex projecting forward into the aqueous humor. **secondary c.,** 1. one that forms after most of the lens has been removed. 2. complicated c. **senile c.,** the cataract of old persons. **siliculose c., siliquose c.,** one in which there is absorption of the lens, with calcareous deposit in the capsule, so that the atrophied lens resembles a silique. **snowflake c.,** one marked by numerous grayish or bluish white flaky opacities, often seen in young diabetics. **toxic c.,** that due to exposure to a toxic drug, e.g., naphthalene. **traumatic c.,** opacification of the lens due to injury to the eye. **zonular c.,** lamellar c.

cataracta (kat″ah-rak′tah) cataract. **c. brunes′cens,** brown cataract. **c. ceru′lea,** blue dot cataract.

cataractogenic (kat″ah-rak″to-jen′ik) tending to induce the formation of cataracts.

catarrh (kah-tahr′) inflammation of a mucous membrane (particularly of the head and throat), with free discharge. **catar′rhal,** adj.

catarrhine (kat′ah-rīn) having nostrils that are close together and directed downward.

catastate (kat′ah-stāt) catabolite.

catathymic (kat″ah-thi′mik) pertaining to psychic disorders marked by perseveration.

catatonia (-to′ne-ah) catatonic schizophrenia. **cataton′ic,** adj.

catatricrotism (-tri′kro-tizm) a pulse anomaly in which three small additional waves or notches appear in the descending limb of the pulse tracing. **catatricrot′ic,** adj.

catatropia (-tro′pe-ah) a downward turning of the visual axis of both eyes in the presence of visual fusional stimuli.

catechin (kat′ĕ-kin) an astringent principle from catechu, used in tanning and dyeing.

catechol (kat′ĕ-kol) a compound, *o*-dihydroxybenzene, $C_6H_4(OH)_2$, used as a reagent and comprising the aromatic portion in the synthesis of catecholamines.

catecholamine (kat″ĕ-kol-ah-mēn″) any of a group of sympathomimetic amines (including dopamine, epinephrine, and norepinephrine), the aromatic portion of whose molecule is catechol.

catechu (kat′ĕ-ku) a powerful astringent extracted from leaves and twigs of *Ourouparia gambir.* **black c.,** an astringent from the heartwood of *Acacia catechu.*

catelectrotonus (kat″e-lek-trot′o-nus) increase of nerve or muscle irritability when near the cathode.

Catenabacterium (kah-te″nah-bak-te′re-um) a genus of anaerobic, gram-positive schizomycetes (tribe Lactobacilleae) found in the intestinal tract and occasionally associated with purulent infections.

catgut (kat′gut) a sterile strand obtained from collagen derived from healthy mammals, used as a surgical ligature.

catharsis (kah-thar′sis) 1. a cleansing or purgation. 2. the bringing into consciousness and the emotional reliving of a forgotten (repressed) painful experience as a means of releasing anxiety and tension; see also *abreaction.*

cathartic (kah-thar′tik) 1. causing bowel evacuation; an agent that so acts. 2. producing catharsis. **bulk c.,** one stimulating bowel evacuation by increasing fecal volume. **lubricant c.,** one that acts by softening the feces and reducing friction between them and the intestinal wall. **saline c.,** one that increases fluidity of intestinal contents by retention of water by osmotic forces, and indirectly increases motor activity. **stimulant c.,** one that directly increases motor activity of the intestinal tract.

cathectic (kah-thek′tik) pertaining to cathexis.

cathepsin (kah-thep′sin) a proteinase found in most cells, which takes part in cell autolysis and self-digestion of tissues.

catheter (kath′ĕ-ter) a tubular, flexible instrument passed through body channels for withdrawal of fluids from (or introduction of fluids into) a body cavity. **Bozeman's c.,** a double-current uterine catheter. **cardiac c.,** a long, fine catheter designed for passage, usually through a peripheral blood vessel, into the chambers of the heart under roentgenologic control. **de Pezzer's c.,** a self-retaining catheter with a bulbous extremity. **double-current c.,** a catheter having two channels; one for injection and one for removal of fluid. **elbowed c.,** one bent at an angle near the beak. **eustachian c.,** one for inflating the eustachian tube. **faucial c.,** a eustachian catheter for passage through the fauces. **female c.,** a short catheter for passage through the female urethra. **Foley c.,** an indwelling catheter retained in the bladder by a balloon which may be inflated with air or liquid. **Gouley's c.,** a solid, curved steel catheter grooved on its inferior surface so that it can be passed over a guide through a urethral stricture. **indwelling c.,** one held in position in the urethra. **Itard's c.,** a variety of eustachian catheter. **lobster-tail c.,** one with three joints at the tip. **Mercier's c.,** a flexible catheter elbowed at the end. **Nélaton's c.,** one of soft rubber. **Phillips' c.,** a urethral catheter with a woven filiform guide. **prostatic c.,** one with a short angular tip for passing an enlarged prostate. **railway c.,** a straight elastic catheter with an open end to be introduced with a filiform guide in cases of stricture. **Schrötter's c.,** a hard-rubber catheter of varying caliber, used for dilating laryngeal strictures. **self-retaining c.,** one so constructed as to be retained at will and to effect bladder drainage. **two-way c.,** a double-channel catheter used in irrigation. **vertebrated c.,** one made in small sections fitted together so as to be flexible. **winged c.,** one with two projections on the end to retain it in the bladder.

catheterization (kath″ĕ-ter-i-za′shun) passage of a catheter into a body channel or cavity. **cardiac c.,** passage of a small catheter through a vein in an arm or leg or the neck and into the heart, permitting the securing of blood samples, determination of intracardiac pressure, and detection of cardiac anomalies.

catheterize (kath′ĕ-ter-īz″) to introduce a catheter into a body cavity.

cathexis (kah-thek′sis) the charge or attachment of mental or emotional energy upon an idea or object.

cathode (kath′ōd) 1. the negative electrode, from which electrons are emitted and to which positive ions are attracted. 2. the electrode through which current leaves a nerve or other substance.

cathodic (kah-thod′ik) pertaining to or emanating from a cathode.

Cathomycin (kath′o-mi″sin) trademark for preparations of novobiocin.

cation (kat′i-on) a positively charged ion.

cauda (kaw′dah), pl. *cau′dae* [L.] a tail or taillike appendage. **c. cerebel′li,** vermis cerebelli. **c. equi′na,** the collection of spinal roots descending from the lower spinal cord and occupying the vertebral canal below the cord.

caudad (kaw′dad) directed toward the tail or distal end; opposite to cephalad.

caudal (kaw′dal) 1. pertaining to a cauda. 2. situated more toward the cauda, or tail, than some specified reference point; toward the inferior (in humans) or posterior (in animals) end of the body.

caudate (kaw′dāt) having a tail.

caudatum (kaw-da′tum) the caudate nucleus.

caul (kawl) a piece of amnion sometimes enveloping a child's head at birth.

caumesthesia (kaw″mes-the′ze-ah) a sensation of burning heat even though the body temperature is not elevated.

causalgia (kaw-zal′je-ah) a burning pain, often with trophic skin changes, due to peripheral nerve injury.

caustic (kaws′tik) 1. burning or corrosive; destructive to living tissues. 2. having a burning taste. 3. an escharotic or corrosive agent. **Lugol's c.,** one part each of iodine and potassium iodide, with two parts of water. **lunar c.,** toughened silver nitrate. **mitigated c.,** silver nitrate diluted with potassium nitrate.

cauterant (kaw′ter-ant) 1. any caustic material or application. 2. caustic.

cauterization (kaw″ter-i-za′shun) destruction of tissue with a cautery.

cautery (kaw′ter-e) 1. the application of a caustic agent, a hot iron, an electric current, or other agent to destroy tissue. 2. an agent used for such purpose. **actual c.,** a red-hot iron used as a cauterizing agent. 2. the application of an agent that actually burns tissue. **cold c.,** cauterization by carbon dioxide. **galvanic c.,** galvanocautery. **potential c., virtual c.,** cauterization by an escharotic.

cava (ka′vah) 1. plural of *cavum.* 2. a vena cava. **ca′val,** adj.

caverna (ka-ver′nah), pl. *caver′nae* [L.] a cavity.

caverniloquy (kav″er-nil′o-kwe) low-pitched pectoriloquy indicative of a pulmonary cavity.

cavernitis (-ni′tis) inflammation of the corpora cavernosum or corpus spongiosum of the penis.

cavernoma (-no′mah) cavernous hemangioma.

cavernositis (-no-si′tis) cavernitis.

cavernostomy (-nos′to-me) operative drainage of a pulmonary abscess cavity.

cavernous (kav′er-nus) pertaining to a hollow, or containing hollow spaces.

cavitary (kav′ĭ-ta″re) characterized by the presence of a cavity or cavities.

cavitas (kav′ĭ-tas), pl. *cavita′tes* [L.] cavity.

cavitation (kav″ĭ-ta′shun) the formation of cavities; also, a cavity.

cavitis (ka-vi′tis) inflammation of a vena cava.

cavity (kav′ĭ-te) a hollow place or space, or a potential space, within the body or one of its organs; in dentistry, the lesion produced by caries. **abdominal c.,** the cavity of the body between the diaphragm and pelvis, containing the abdominal organs. **amniotic c.,** the closed sac between the embryo and the amnion, containing the amniotic fluid. **buccal c.,** that portion of the oral cavity between the cheeks and the teeth and gingivae. **cleavage c.,** blastocoele. **complex c.,** a carious lesion involving three or more surfaces of a tooth in its prepared state. **compound c.,** a carious lesion involving two surfaces of a tooth in its prepared state. **cotyloid c.,** acetabulum. **cranial c.,** the space enclosed by the bones of the cranium. **dental c.,** the carious defect (lesion) produced by destruction of enamel and dentin in a tooth. **glenoid c.,** a depression in the lateral angle of the scapula for articulation with the humerus. **medullary (marrow) c.,** the cavity in the diaphysis of a long bone containing the marrow. **nasal c.,** the proximal part of the respiratory tract, separated by the nasal septum and extending from the nares to the pharynx. **nerve c.,** pulp c. **oral c.,** the cavity of the mouth, bounded by the jaw bones and associated structures (muscles and mucosa). **pelvic c.,** the space within the walls of the pelvis. **pericardial c.,** the potential space between the epicardium and the parietal layer of the serous pericardium. **peritoneal c.,** the potential space between the parietal and the visceral peritoneum. **pleural c.,** the potential space between the parietal and the visceral pleura. **pleuroperitoneal c.,** the temporarily continuous coelomic cavity in the embryo that is later partitioned by the developing diaphragm. **prepared c.,** a lesion from which all carious tissue has been removed, preparatory to filling of the tooth. **pulp c.,** the pulp-filled central chamber in the crown of a tooth. **Rosenmüller's c.,** a wide, slitlike lateral extension of the nasopharynx, cranial and dorsal to the pharyngeal orifice of the auditory tube. **segmentation c.,** blastocoele. **serous c.,** a celomic cavity, like that enclosed by the pericardium, peritoneum, or pleura, not communicating with the outside body, whose lining membrane secretes a serous fluid. **sigmoid c.,** either of two depressions in head of the ulna for articulation with the humerus and radius. **simple c.,** a carious lesion whose preparation involves only one tooth surface. **somatic c.,** coelom. **somite c.,** myocoele. **tension c's,** cavities of the lung in which the air pressure is greater than that of the atmosphere. **thoracic c.,** the part of the ventral body cavity between the neck and the diaphragm. **tympanic c.,** middle ear. **uterine c.,** the flattened space within the uterus communicating proximally on either side with the uterine tubes and below with the vagina. **yolk c.,** the space between the embryonic disk and the yolk of the developing ovum of some animals.

cavum (ka′vum), pl. *ca′va* [L.] cavity.

cavus (ka′vus) [L.] hollow.

c.b.c. complete blood (cell) count.

cc. cubic centimeter.

CCA chimpanzee coryza agent (respiratory syncytial virus).

c.cm. cubic centimeter.

C.D. curative dose.

C.D.₅₀ median curative dose.

Cd 1. chemical symbol, *cadmium.* 2. caudal or coccygeal.

Ce chemical symbol, *cerium.*

ceasmic (se-as′mik) characterized by persistence of embryonic fissures after birth.

cebocephalus (se″bo-sef′ah-lus) a fetus exhibiting cebocephaly.

cebocephaly (-sef′ah-le) monkey-like deformity of the head, with the eyes close together and the nose defective.

cecal (se′kal) pertaining to a cecum.

cecectomy (se-sek′to-me) excision of the cecum.

cecitis (se-si′tis) inflammation of the cecum.

ceco- word element [L.], *cecum.*

cecocele (se′ko-sēl) a hernia containing part of the cecum.

cecocolopexy (se″ko-ko′lo-pek″se) an operation for fixing the cecum and ascending colon.

cecocolostomy (-ko-los′to-me) surgical anastomosis of the cecum and colon.

cecoileostomy (-il″e-os′to-me) ileocecostomy.

Cecon (se′kon) trademark for preparations of ascorbic acid.

cecopexy (se′ko-pek″se) fixation or suspension of the cecum to correct excessive mobility.

cecoplication (se″ko-pli-ka′shun) plication of the cecal wall to correct ptosis or dilatation.

cecorrhaphy (se-kor′ah-fe) suture or repair of the cecum.

cecosigmoidostomy (se″ko-sig″moid-os′to-me) formation, usually by surgery, of an opening between the cecum and sigmoid.

cecostomy (se-kos′to-me) surgical creation of an artificial opening or fistula into the cecum.

cecotomy (se-kot′o-me) incision of the cecum.

cecum (se′kum) 1. the first part of the large intestine, forming a dilated pouch distal to the ileum and proximal to the colon, and giving off the vermiform appendix. 2. any blind pouch.

Cedilanid (se″dĭ-lan′id) trademark for a preparation of lanatoside C.

Celbenin (sel′bĕ-nin) trademark for a preparation of methicillin.

-cele word element [Gr.], *tumor; hernia; cavity.*

celi(o)- word element [Gr.], *abdomen; through the abdominal wall.*

celiac (se′le-ak) pertaining to the abdomen.

celiectomy (se″le-ek′to-me) 1. excision of the celiac branches of the vagus nerve. 2. excision of an abdominal organ.

celiocentesis (se″le-o-sen-te′sis) puncture into the abdominal cavity.

celiocolpotomy (-kol-pot′o-me) incision into the abdomen through the vagina.

celioenterotomy (-en″ter-ot′o-me) incision through the abdominal wall into the intestine.

celiogastrotomy (-gas-trot′o-me) incision through the abdominal wall into the stomach.

celioma (se″le-o′mah) a tumor of the abdomen.

celiomyomectomy (-mi″o-mek′to-me) myomectomy by an abdominal incision.

celiomyositis (se″le-o-mi″o-si′tis) inflammation of the abdominal muscles.

celioparacentesis (-par″ah-sen-te′sis) paracentesis of the abdominal cavity.

celiopathy (se″le-op′ah-the) any abdominal disease.

celiorrhaphy (se″le-or′ah-fe) suture of the abdominal wall.

celioscope (se′le-o-skōp″) an endoscope for use in celioscopy.

celioscopy (se″le-os′ko-pe) examination of an abdominal cavity through a celioscope.

celiotomy (se″le-ot′o-me) incision into the abdominal cavity. **vaginal c.**, incision into the abdominal cavity through the vagina.

celitis (se-li′tis) any abdominal inflammation.

cell (sel) 1. any of the minute protoplasmic masses making up organized tissue, consisting of a nucleus surrounded by cytoplasm enclosed in a cell membrane; in some low forms of life, e.g., bacteria, a morphological nucleus is absent, although nucleoproteins (and genes) are present. 2. a small, more or less closed space. **acid c's**, parietal c's. **adventitial c's**, macrophages that occur along the walls of blood vessels. **air c.**, one containing air, as in the lungs or auditory tube. **alpha c's**, 1. cells in the islands of Langerhans that secrete glucagon and contain large granules that are insoluble in alcohol. 2. acidophilic cells of the anterior pituitary. **alveolar c.**, any cell of the walls of the pulmonary alveoli; often restricted to the cells of the alveolar epithelium (squamous alveolar cells and great alveolar cells) and alveolar phagocytes. **Alzheimer's c's**, 1. giant astrocytes with large prominent nuclei found in the brain in hepatolenticular degeneration and hepatic coma. 2. degenerated astrocytes. **amacrine c.**, see *amacrine* (2). **ameboid c.**, any cell that can change its shape and move about. **Anichkov's (Anitschkow's) c.**, see under *myocyte*. **antipodal c's**, a group of four cells in the early embryo. **apolar c.**, a neuron with no processes or poles. **argentaffin c's**, cells of the basilar portion of the gastric glands and crypts of Lieberkühn that stain readily with silver and chromium salts; their cytoplasm contains granules capable of reducing silver compounds. **Arias-Stella c's**, columnar cells in the endometrial epithelium which have a hyperchromatic enlarged nucleus and which appear to be associated with chorionic tissue in an intrauterine or extrauterine site. **Aschoff's c's**, a type of giant cell as seen in the rheumatic nodule in the myocardium. **band c.**, a neutrophil in which the nucleus is not lobulated but in the form of a continuous band, horseshoe shaped, twisted, or coiled. **basal c.**, an early keratinocyte, present in the basal layer of the epidermis. **basket c.**, a neuron of the cerebral cortex whose fibers form a basket-like nest in which a Purkinje cell rests. **beaker c.**, goblet c. **beta c's**, 1. basophilic cells of the pancreas that secrete insulin and make up most of the bulk of the islands of Langerhans; they contain granules that are soluble in alcohol. 2. basophilic cells of the anterior pituitary. **Betz c's**, large pyramidal ganglion cells forming a layer of the gray matter of the brain. **bipolar c.**, a neuron with two processes. **blast c.**, the least differentiated blood cell. **blood c's**, see under *corpuscle*. **bone c.**, a nucleated cell in the lacunae of bone. **bristle c's**, the hair cells associated with the auditory and cochlear nerves. **burr c.**, a form of spiculed mature erythrocyte, the echinocyte, having multiple, small projections evenly spaced over the cell circumference; observed in azotemia, gastric carcinoma, and bleeding peptic ulcer. **cameloid c.**, elliptocyte. **cartilage c's**, connective tissue cells in the cartilage capsules. **central c's**, chief c's (1). **chief c's**, 1. epithelial cells, columnar or cuboidal, which line the gastric glands and secrete pepsin and extrinsic factor. 2. epithelioid cells with pale-staining cytoplasm and large nuclei with prominent nucleoli; cords of these cells form the bulk of the pineal body. 3. polyhedral cells of the parathyroid glands with pale, clear cytoplasm and a vesicular nucleus. **chromaffin c's**, cells staining readily with chromium salts, especially those of the adrenal medulla and similar cells occurring in widespread accumulations throughout the body in various organs, whose cytoplasm shows fine brown granules when stained with potassium bichromate. **chromophobe c's**, small, faintly staining cells having scanty, nongranular cytoplasm, found, often in clusters, in the anterior pituitary. **ciliated c.**, any cell having cilia. **Claudius' c's**, large cells on each side of the arches of Corti. **cleavage c.**, any of the cells derived from the fertilized ovum by mitosis; a blastomere. **columnar c.**, an elongate epithelial cell. **Corti's c's**, the cells of the organ of Corti. **crescent c's**, crescents of Giannuzzi. **Crooke's c's**, the basophils in Crooke's hyaline degeneration. **daughter c.**, one formed by division of a mother cell. **decidual c.**, a connective-tissue cell of the uterine mucous membrane, enlarged and specialized during pregnancy. **Deiters' c's**, 1. the outer phalangeal cells of the organ of Corti. 2. neuroglia c's. **demilune c's**, crescents of Giannuzzi. **Dorothy Reed c's**, Sternberg-Reed c's. **Downey c's**, atypical lymphocytes of three types invariably present in infectious mononucleosis: type I is a mature cell with a reniform, or lobulated nucleus with vacuolated, basophilic foamy cytoplasm; type II cells contain a plasmacytoid nucleus with less vacuolated and basophilic cytoplasm; type III has a finer chromatin pattern and one or two nucleoli. **elementary c's, embryonal c's**, small round cells produced by cleavage of the ovum. **enamel c.**, ameloblast. **endothelial c's**, cells composing endothelium. **enterochromaffin c's**, chromaffin cells of the intestinal mucosa that stain with chromium salts and are impregnable with silver; they are sites of synthesis and storage of serotonin. **epithelial c's**, cells composing the epithelium. **epithelioid c's**, 1. large polyhedral cells of connective tissue origin. 2. large phagocytes with prominent, pale-staining nuclei, characteristic of the granulomas of leprosy, tuberculosis, etc. **ethmoidal c's,** air-containing spaces in the ethmoid bone, collectively forming the ethmoidal sinus. **fat c's,** connective tissue cells bloated with stored fat. **Ferrata's c.,** hemohistioblast. **fiber c.,** any elongated and linear cell. **flagellate c.,** any cell having a flagellum, usually motile. **flame c's,** flagellate cells at the termination of collecting tubules of the excretory system of flatworms and nemerteans. **floor c's,** cells of the floor of the arch of Corti. **foam c's,** cells with a vacuolated appearance due to the presence of complex lipoids; seen notably in xanthoma. **follicle c's, follicular c's,** specialized epithelial cells surrounding the ovum in a primary ovarian follicle; in a vesicular ovarian follicle, they form the stratum granulosum and cumulus and secrete the follicular fluid. After ovulation they are transformed into glandular cells of the corpus luteum. **formative c.,** a cell of the inner cell mass of the conceptus, a blastomere destined to form part of the embryo. **G c's,** granular enterochromaffin cells in the mucosa of the pyloric part of the stomach, a source of gastrin. **ganglion c.,** a large nerve cell, especially one of those of the spinal ganglia. **Gaucher's c.,** a large cell characteristic of Gaucher's disease, with eccentrically placed nuclei and fine wavy fibrils parallel to the long axis of the cell. **germ c.,** an ovum or a spermatozoon. **c's of Giannuzzi,** see under *crescent.* **giant c.,** a very large, multinucleate cell; applied to megakaryocytes of bone marrow and to giant cells occurring in the lesions of tuberculosis and other infectious granulomas and about foreign bodies. **gitter c's,** microglia. **glia c's,** neuroglia c's. **goblet c.,** an epithelial cell bulged out like a goblet by contained mucin. **Golgi's c's,** see under *neuron.* **granular c.,** one containing granules, such as a keratinocyte in the stratum granulosum of the epidermis, when it contains a dense collection of darkly staining granules. **granulosa c's,** follicular c's. **gustatory c's,** taste c's. **hair c's,** epithelial cells with hairlike processes, found in the organ of Corti. **Hargraves' c.,** L.E. c. **heart failure c's, heart lesion c's,** macrophages containing granules of iron, found in the pulmonary alveoli and sputum in congestive heart failure. **HeLa c's,** cells of the first continuously cultured carcinoma strain, descended from a human cervical carcinoma. **helmet c.,** an abnormal red cell form resembling a helmet, seen in hemolytic anemia. **Hensen's c's,** the outermost supporting cells covering the organ of Corti. **Hofbauer c's,** large chromophilic cells in the chorionic villi which are probably clasmatocytes. **Hortega c's,** microglia. **Hürthle c's,** large eosinophilic cells sometimes found in the thyroid gland; see also under *tumor.* **interfollicular c's,** Hürthle c's. **interstitial c's,** the cells of the connective tissue of the ovary or of the testis (Leydig c's) which furnish the internal secretion of those structures. **islet c's,** the cells composing the islands of Langerhans. **juxtaglomerular c's,** specialized cells containing secretory granules, located in the tunica media of the afferent glomerular arterioles, thought to stimulate aldo-

sterone secretion and to play a role in renal autoregulation. **Kupffer's c's,** large, stellate or pyramidal, intensely phagocytic cells lining the walls of the hepatic sinusoids and forming part of the reticuloendothelial system. **Langerhans' c's,** 1. star-shaped cells in the germinative layer of the epidermis. 2. spindle-shaped cells in the acini of the pancreas. **L.E. c.,** a mature neutrophilic polymorphonuclear leukocyte, which has phagocytized a spherical, homogeneous-appearing inclusion, itself derived from another neutrophil; a characteristic of lupus erythematosus, but also found in analogous connective tissue disorders. **Leydig's c's,** 1. interstitial cells of the testis, which secrete testosterone. 2. mucous cells that do not pour their secretion out over the epithelial surface. **light c's,** Hürthle c's. **lutein c's,** the plump, pale-staining, polyhedral cells of the corpus luteum. **lymph c.,** lymphocyte. **lymphoid c's,** lymphocytes and plasma cells. **malpighian c.,** keratinocyte. **marrow c.,** any of the immature blood cells developing in bone marrow. **mast c.,** a connective tissue cell capable of elaborating basophilic, metachromatic cytoplasmic granules that contain histamine, heparin, and, in some species, serotonin. **mastoid c's,** air spaces of various size and shape in the mastoid process of the temporal bone. **mossy c.,** an astrocyte with protoplasmic processes. **mother c.,** one that divides to form new, or daughter, cells. **mucous c's,** cells which secrete mucus or mucin. **mulberry c.,** 1. a vacuolated plasma cell. 2. a rounded cell with centrally placed nuclei and coarse cytoplasmic vacuoles near the outer border, developing at the periphery of a retrogressing corpus luteum. **myeloid c.,** marrow c. **myeloma c.,** one found in bone marrow and sometimes in peripheral blood in multiple myeloma. **nerve c.,** neuron. **neuroglia c's, neuroglial c's,** the branching, non-neural cells of the neuroglia; they are of three types: astroglia (macroglia), oligodendroglia, and microglia. **Niemann-Pick c's,** Pick's c's. **nevus c.,** a small oval or cuboidal cell with a deeply staining nucleus and scanty pale cytoplasm, sometimes containing melanin granules, possibly derived from Schwann cells or from embryonal nevoblasts; they are clustered in rounded masses (called *theques*) in the epidermis, and reach the dermis by a kind of centripetal extrusion (*abtropfung*). **nucleated c.,** any cell having a nucleus. **olfactory c's,** a set of specialized cells of the mucous membranes of the nose, which are receptors of smell. **oxyntic c's,** parietal c's. **packed human blood c's, packed red blood c's (human),** whole blood from which plasma has been removed; used therapeutically. **Paget c's,** degenerating cells, swollen, rounded, and pigmented, found in the epidermis in Paget's disease of the nipple and in extramammary Paget's disease. **Paneth's c's,** narrow, pyramidal, or columnar epithelial cells with a round or oval nucleus close to the base of the cell, occurring in the fundus of the crypts of Lieberkühn; they contain large secretory granules that may contain peptidase. **parafollicular c's,** Hürthle c's. **parietal c's,** large spheroidal or pyramidal cells found along the walls of the gastric glands;

they are the source of hydrochloric acid in the gastric juice. **peptic c's,** chief c's (1). **pheochrome c's,** chromaffin c's. **Pick's c's,** round, oval, or polyhedral cells with foamy, lipid-containing cytoplasm, found in the bone marrow and spleen in Niemann-Pick disease. **pigment c's,** cells containing granules of pigment. **plasma c.,** a spherical or ellipsoidal cell with a single nucleus containing chromatin, an area of perinuclear clearing, and generally abundant, sometimes vacuolated cytoplasm; they are involved in the synthesis, storage, and release of antibody. **polar c's,** see under *body.* **polychromatic c's, polychromatophil c's,** immature erythrocytes staining with both acid and basic stains in a diffuse mixture of blue-gray and pink. **pregnancy c.,** an altered chromophobe cell seen in the anterior pituitary gland in pregnancy. **prickle c.,** a cell with delicate radiating processes connecting with similar cells, being a dividing keratinocyte of the prickle-cell layer of the epidermis. **primordial germ c's,** the earliest germ cells, at first located outside the gonad but migrating in early embryonic development. **pulmonary epithelial c's,** extremely thin nonphagocytic squamous cells with flattened nuclei, constituting the outer layer of the aveolar wall in the lungs. **Purkinje's c's,** large branching neurons in the middle layer of the cerebellar cortex. **red c., red blood c.,** erythrocyte. **resting c.,** one not undergoing karyokinesis. **reticular c's,** the cells forming the reticular fibers of connective tissue; those forming the framework of lymph nodes, bone marrow, and spleen form part of the reticuloendothelial system and may differentiate into macrophages. **reticuloendothelial c.,** see under *system.* **Rieder's c.,** a myeloblast seen in acute leukemia, having a nucleus with several wide and deep indentations suggesting lobulation. **Rouget c's,** contractile cells on the walls of capillaries. **Sala's c's,** star-shaped cells of connective tissue in the fibers forming the sensory nerve endings of the pericardium. **scavenger c.,** one that absorbs and removes irritant products. **Schwann's c.,** one of the large nucleated masses of protoplasm lining the inner surface of the sheath of Schwann, or neurilemma. **segmented c.,** a neutrophil with a nucleus divided into definite lobes. **Sertoli's c's,** cells in the testicular tubules to which the spermatids become attached and which support, protect, and apparently nourish the spermatids until they develop into mature spermatozoa. **Sézary c.,** a reticular lymphocyte having a large convoluted or folded nucleus with a narrow rim of cytoplasm that may contain vacuoles; seen in many proliferative states of the reticuloendothelial system and in the skin and blood in the Sézary syndrome. **sickle c.,** a crescentic or sickle-shaped erythrocyte; see also under *anemia.* **signet-ring c.,** a cell in which the nucleus has been pressed to one side by an accumulation of intracytoplasmic mucin; see *Krukenberg's tumor.* **smudge c's,** disrupted leukocytes appearing during preparation of peripheral blood smears. **somatic c's,** the cells of the somatoplasm; undifferentiated body cells. **sperm c.,** a spermatozoon. **spider c.,** 1. astrocyte. 2. one

seen in rhabdomyosarcoma, with thread-like processes radiating to the outer cell wall. **spur c.,** a form of spiculed mature erythrocyte, whose prototype is the acanthocyte of congenital abetalipoproteinemia. **squamous c.,** a flat, scalelike epithelial cell. **stab c., staff c.,** band c. **stellate c.,** any star-shaped cell, as a Kupffer cell or astrocyte, having many filaments extending in all directions. **stem c.,** a generalized mother cell whose descendants specialize, often in different directions, as an undifferentiated mesenchymal cell that may be considered to be a progenitor of the blood and fixed-tissue cells of the bone marrow. **Sternberg's giant c's, Sternberg-Reed c's,** enlarged, atypical histiocytes with multiple or hyperlobulated nucleoli; a characteristic feature of Hodgkin's disease. **stipple c.,** an erythrocyte containing granules that take a basic or bluish stain with Wright's stain. **target c.,** an abnormally thin erythrocyte showing, when stained, a dark center and a peripheral ring of hemoglobin, separated by a pale, unstained zone containing less hemoglobin; seen in various anemias and other disorders. **tart c.,** a macrophage or monocytoid reticuloendothelial cell containing a phagocytized nucleus with well preserved nuclear structure. **taste c's,** cells in taste buds associated with the nerves of taste. **tendon c's,** flattened cells of connective tissue occurring in rows between the primary bundles of the tendons. **totipotential c.,** an embryonic cell capable of developing into any variety of body cell. **Touton c's,** large cells containing lipoid material found in the lesions of xanthoma and histiocytosis X. **Türk c.,** a nongranular, mononuclear cell having features of both an atypical lymphocyte and a plasma cell, seen in the peripheral blood in severe anemias, chronic infections, and leukemoid reactions. **Tzanck c.,** a degenerated epithelial cell caused by acantholysis, found especially in pemphigus. **vasofactive c., vasoformative c.,** one that joins with other cells to form blood vessels. **visual c's,** the neuroepithelial elements of the retina. **wandering c's,** cells capable of ameboid movement, e.g., macrophages, lymphocytes, etc. **white c., white blood c.,** leukocyte. **zymogenic c's,** chief c's (1).

cella (sel′ah), pl. *cel′lae* [L.] cell.

cellobiase (sel″lo-bi′ās) β-glucosidase; see *glucosidase.*

cellobiose (-bi′ōs) a disaccharide, $C_{12}H_{22}O_{11}$, formed from cellulose by the action of cellulase.

celloidin (sĕ-loi′din) a concentrated preparation of pyroxylin, used in microscopy for embedding specimens for section cutting.

cellula (sel′u-lah), pl. *cel′lulae* [L.] cell.

cellular (-ler) pertaining to or composed of cells.

cellularity (sel″u-lar′ĭ-te) the state of a tissue or other mass as regards the number of constituent cells.

cellulase (sel′u-lās) an enzyme that hydrolyzes cellulose to cellobiose, secreted by bacteria and by fungi that destroy wood; a concentrate of such enzymes derived from *Aspergillus niger* is used as a digestive aid.

cellule (-ūl) a small cell.

cellulicidal (sel″u-lĭ-si′dal) destroying cells.

cellulifugal (-lif′u-gal) directed away from a cell body.

cellulipetal (-lip′ĕ-tal) directed toward a cell body.

cellulitis (-li′tis) inflammation of cellular tissue, especially purulent inflammation of loose connective tissue. **anaerobic c.,** inflammation of the subcutaneous tissue in which the infecting bacteria, most commonly *Clostridium perfringens,* proliferate and produce gas in the tissue (but not in muscle); the onset is gradual, pain is absent, and systemic symptoms are not severe. **dissecting c.,** inflammation with suppuration spreading between layers of the involved tissue. **gangrenous c.,** that leading to death of the tissue followed by bacterial invasion and putrefaction. **gaseous c.,** inflammation due to a gas-producing organism and presence of gas in the tissues. **pelvic c.,** parametritis.

cellulofibrous (-lo-fi′brus) partly cellular and partly fibrous.

celluloid (sel′u-loid) a plastic compound of pyroxylin and camphor.

celluloneuritis (sel″u-lo-nu-ri′tis) inflammation of neurons.

cellulose (sel′u-lōs) a carbohydrate, $(C_6H_{10}O_5)_n$, forming the skeleton of most plant structures and plant cells. **absorbable c., oxidized c.,** an absorbable oxidation product of cellulose, used as a local hemostatic. **tetranitrate c.,** $(C_{12}H_{16}N_4O_{18})_n$, the principal constituent of pyroxylin.

celom (sel′lom) coelom.

Celontin (se-lon′tin) trademark for a preparation of methsuximide.

celoschisis (se-los′kĭ-sis) congenital fissure of the abdominal wall.

celoscope (se′lo-skōp) celioscope.

celosomia (se″lo-so′me-ah) congenital fissure or absence of the sternum, with hernial protrusion of the viscera.

celosomus (-so′mus) a fetus exhibiting celosomia.

celothelioma (-the″le-o′mah) mesothelioma.

celotomy (se-lot′o-me) herniotomy.

celovirus (sel″o-vi′rus) CELO virus.

celozoic (-zo′ik) inhabiting the intestinal canal of the body; said of parasites.

cement (se-ment′) 1. a substance that produces a solid union between two surfaces. 2. in dentistry, a filling material used to aid the retention of gold castings and to insulate the tooth pulp. 3. cementum. **dental c.,** cementum. **intercellular c.,** a mucilaginous substance that holds cells, especially epithelial cells, together. **muscle c.,** the myoglia. **nerve c.,** the neuroglia.

cementicle (se-men′tĭ-k'l) a small, discrete globular mass of cementum in the region of a tooth root.

cementoblast (se-men′to-blast) a large cuboidal cell, found between the fibers on the surface of the cementum, which is active in cementum formation.

cementoblastoma (se-men″to-blas-to′mah) an odontogenic fibroma whose cells are developing into cementoblasts and in which there is only a small proportion of calcified tissue.

cementoclasia (-kla′se-ah) disintegration of the cementum of a tooth.

cementocyte (se-men′to-sīt) a cell in the lacunae of cellular cementum, frequently having long processes radiating from the cell body toward the periodontal surface of the cementum.

cementogenesis (se-men″to-jen′ĕ-sis) development of cementum on the root dentin of a tooth.

cementoma (se″men-to′mah) a mass of cementum lying free at the apex of a tooth, probably a reaction to injury.

cementosis (-to′sis) proliferation of cementum.

cementum (se-men′tum) the bonelike connective tissue covering the root of a tooth and assisting in tooth support.

cenesthesia (sen″es-the′ze-ah) the general feeling or sense of conscious existence; the sense of normal functioning of body organs. **cenesthe′sic, cenesthet′ic,** adj.

ceno- word element [Gr.], *new; empty;* or denoting relationship to a common feature or characteristic.

cenopsychic (se″no-si′kik) of recent appearance in mental development.

cenosis (se-no′sis) a morbid discharge. **cenot′ic,** adj.

cenosite (se′no-sīt) coinsite.

cenotype (sen′o-tīp) the original from which other types have arisen.

censor (sen′sor) 1. a member of a committee on ethics or for critical examination of a medical or other society. 2. the psychic influence which prevents unconscious thoughts and wishes coming into consciousness.

center (sen′ter) 1. the middle point of a body. 2. a collection of neurons concerned with performance of a particular function. **accelerating c.,** one in the brain stem involved in acceleration of the heart. **apneustic c.,** a nerve center in the brain stem controlling normal respiration. **auditory c.,** the center for hearing, in the more anterior of the transverse temporal gyri. **Broca's c.,** speech c. **cardioinhibitory c.,** one in the medulla oblongata that exerts an inhibitory influence on the heart. **ciliospinal c.,** one in the lower cervical and upper dorsal portions of the spinal cord involved in dilatation of the pupil. **coughing c.,** one in the medulla oblongata above the respiratory center, which controls the act of coughing. **deglutition c.,** swallowing c. **epiotic c.,** the center of ossification forming the mastoid process. **facial c.,** one in the lower part of the ascending frontal convolution, controlling facial movements. **germinal c.,** the area in lymphoid tissue where mitotic figures are observed, differentiation and formation of lymphocytes occur, and elements related to antibody synthesis are found. **gustatory c.,** one supposed to control taste, located in the cortex of the uncinate convolution. **health c.,** 1. a community health organization for creating health work and coordinating the efforts of all health agencies. 2. an educational complex consisting of a medical school and various allied health professional schools. **Kronecker's c.,** cardioinhibitory c. **medullary respiratory c.,** one in the medulla oblongata that coordinates respiratory movements. **motor c.,** any center that originates, controls, inhibits, or maintains motor impulses. **nerve c.,** an aggregation, in brain or spinal cord, of cell bodies of neurons. **ossification c.,** any point at which ossification begins in a bone. **pneumotaxic c.,** one in the upper pons that rhythmically inhibits inspiration. **reflex c.,** any center in the brain or cord in which a sensory impression is changed into a motor impulse. **respiratory c's,** a series of the centers (the apneustic, pneumotaxic, and medullary respiratory c's) in the medulla and pons that coordinate respiratory movements. **Setschenow's c's,** reflex inhibitory centers in the medulla oblongata and spinal cord. **speech c.,** one in the left (or right) inferior frontal gyrus concerned with aspects of speech. **swallowing c.,** one on the floor of the fourth ventricle concerned with deglutition. **thermoregulatory c's,** hypothalamic centers regulating the conservation and dissipation of heat. **vasomotor c's,** centers in the tuber cinereum, medulla oblongata, and spinal cord, believed to regulate the contraction and dilatation of blood vessels. **Wernicke's c.,** the speech center in the cortex of the left temporooccipital convolution. **word c.,** one concerned with the recognition of words, different areas being involved for recognition of written and of spoken words.

centesimal (sen-tes′ĭ-mal) divided into hundredths.

-centesis word element [Gr.], *puncture and aspiration of.*

centi- word element [L.], *hundred;* used in naming units of measurement to indicate one hundredth (10^{-2}) of the unit designated by the root with which it is combined; symbol c.

centigrade (sen′tĭ-grād) having 100 gradations (steps or degrees), as the Celsius (centigrade) scale; abbreviated C.

centigram (-gram) one hundredth of a gram; abbreviated cg.

centiliter (-le″ter) one hundredth of a liter; abbreviated cl.

centimeter (-me″ter) one hundredth of a meter, or approximately 0.3937 inch; abbreviated cm. **cubic c.,** a unit of capacity, being that of a cube each side of which measures 1 cm.; abbreviated cc., cm.^{3}, or cu. cm.

centinormal (sen″tĭ-nor′mal) one hundredth of normal strength.

centipoise (-poiz) one hundredth of a poise.

centrad (sen′trad) toward a center.

central (sen′tral) pertaining to a center; located at the midpoint.

centraphose (sen′trah-fōz) a subjective sensation of darkness.

centrencephalic (sen″tren-sĕ-fal′ik) pertaining to the center of the encephalon.

centric (sen′trik) pertaining to a center.

centriciput (sen-tris′ĭ-put) the central part of the upper surface of the head, located between the occiput and sinciput.

centrifugal (sen-trif′u-gal) moving away from a center.

centrifugate (sen-trif′u-gāt) material subjected to centrifugation.

centrifugation (sen-trif″u-ga′shun) the process of separating lighter portions of a solution, mixture, or suspension from the heavier portions by centrifugal force.

centrifuge (sen′trĭ-fūj) 1. a machine by which centrifugation is effected. 2. to subject to centrifugation. **microscope c.,** a high-speed centrifuge with a built-in microscope permitting a specimen to be viewed under centrifugal force.

centrilobular (sen″trĭ-lob′u-lar) pertaining to the central portion of a lobule.

centriole (sen′tre-ōl) either of two minute organelles that migrate to opposite poles of a cell during cell division and serve to organize the alignment of the spindles.

centripetal (sen-trip′ĕ-tal) moving toward a center.

centro- word element [L., Gr.], *center; a central location.*

centrokinesia (sen″tro-ki-ne′se-ah) movement originating from central stimulation. **centrokinet′ic,** adj.

centrolecithal (-les′ĭ-thal) having the yolk in the center.

centromere (sen′tro-mēr) the clear constricted portion of the chromosome at which the chromatids are joined and by which the chromosome is attached to the spindle during cell division. **centromer′ic,** adj.

centrosclerosis (sen″tro-skle-ro′sis) osteosclerosis of the marrow cavity of a bone.

centrosome (sen′tro-sōm) a specialized area of condensed cytoplasm containing the centrioles and playing an important part in mitosis.

centrosphere (-sfēr) centrosome.

centrostaltic (sen″tro-stal′tik) pertaining to a center of motion.

centrum (sen′trum), pl. *cen′tra* [L.] 1. a center. 2. the body of a vertebra.

cephal(o)- word element [Gr.], *head.*

cephalad (sef′ah-lad) toward the head.

cephalalgia (sef″al-al′je-ah) headache.

cephaledema (-ĕ-de′mah) edema of the head.

cephalexin (sef″ah-lek′sin) an oral cephalosporin used in the treatment of pneumococcal and Group-A streptococcal respiratory infections and infections of the urinary tract, skin, and soft tissue.

cephalhematocele (sef″al-he-mat′o-sēl) a hematocele under the pericranium, communicating with one or more dural sinuses.

cephalhematoma (-he″mah-to′mah) a tumor or swelling filled with blood beneath the pericranium.

cephalhydrocele (-hi′dro-sēl) a serous or watery accumulation under the pericranium.

cephalic (sĕ-fal′ik) pertaining to the head, or to the head end of the body.

cephalin (sef′ah-lin) 1. a monaminomonophosphatide in brain tissue, nerve tissue, and yolk of egg. 2. a crude phospholipid usually extracted from brain tissue, used as a clotting agent in blood coagulation work.

cephalitis (sef″ah-li′tis) encephalitis.

cephalocele (sĕ-fal′o-sēl) protrusion of a part of the cranial contents.

cephalocentesis (sef″ah-lo-sen-te′sis) surgical puncture of the head.

cephalodynia (-din′e-ah) pain in the head.

cephalogaster (-gas′ter) the anterior portion of the enteric canal of the embryo.

cephaloglycin (-gli′sin) an analogue of cephalosporin C used in urinary tract infections.

cephalogram (-gram) an x-ray image of the structures of the head; cephalometric radiograph.

cephalogyric (-ji′rik) pertaining to turning motions of the head.

cephalohematoma (-he″mah-to′mah) cephalhematoma.

cephalomelus (sef″ah-lom′e-lus) a monster with an accessory limb growing from the head.

cephalometer (sef″ah-lom′ĕ-ter) an instrument for measuring the head; an orienting device for positioning the head for radiographic examination and measurement.

cephalometrics (sef″ah-lo-met′riks) cephalometry.

cephalometry (sef″ah-lom′ĕ-tre) scientific measurement of the dimensions of the head.

cephalomotor (sef″ah-lo-mo′tor) moving the head; pertaining to motions of the head.

Cephalomyia (-mi′yah) Oestrus.

cephalonia (sef″ah-lo′ne-ah) a condition in which the head is abnormally enlarged, with sclerotic hyperplasia of the brain.

cephalopathy (sef″ah-lop′ah-the) any disease of the head.

cephalopelvic (sef″ah-lo-pel′vik) pertaining to the relationship of the fetal head to the maternal pelvis.

cephaloridine (sef″ah-lor′ĭ-dēn) a broad-spectrum antibiotic of the cephalosporin group.

cephalosporin (sef″ah-lo-spōr′in) any of a group of broad-spectrum, penicillinase-resistant antibiotics from Cephalosporium, including cephalexia, cephaloridine, cephaloglycin, and cephalothin, which share the nucleus 7-aminocephalosporanic acid. **c. C,** a component of cephalosporin, $C_{16}H_{21}N_3O_8S$, used as an antimicrobial. **c. P,** an antibacterial steroid, $C_{33}H_{50}O_8$; the crude form contains at least five components $(P_1, P_2, P_3, P_4, P_5,)$, P_1 being the major active substance.

Cephalosporium (-spo′re-um) a genus of soil-inhabiting fungi (family Moniliaceae); some species are the source of the cephalosporins.

cephalostat (sef′ah-lo-stat″) a head-positioning device which assures reproducibility of the relations between an x-ray beam, a patient's head, and an x-ray film.

cephalothin (-thin) a semisynthetic analogue of the natural antibiotic cephalosporin C, $C_{16}H_{15}$-$N_2NaO_6S_2$, used against various bacteria, including many penicillin-resistant staphylococci.

cephalothoracic (sef″ah-lo-tho-ras′ik) pertaining to the head and thorax.

cephalothoracopagus (-tho″rah-kop′ah-gus) a double monster united in the frontal plane, the fusion extending from the crown of the head to the middle abdominal region.

cephalotomy (sef″ah-lot′o-me) 1. the cutting up of the fetal head to facilitate delivery. 2. dissection of the fetal head.

cephalotropic (sef″ah-lo-trop′ik) having an affinity for brain tissue.

cephalotrypesis (-tri-pe′sis) trephination of the skull.

ceptor (sep′tor) 1. in Ehrlich's side-chain theory, receptors that have been thrown off into the blood stream. 2. any apparatus that receives external stimuli or impressions and transfers them to nerve centers.

cera (se′rah) [L.] wax. **c. al′ba,** white wax. **c. fla′va,** yellow wax.

ceramics (sĕ-ram′iks) the modeling and processing of objects made of clay or similar materials. **dental c.,** the use of porcelain and similar materials in restorative dentistry.

ceramidase (ser-am′ĭ-dās) an enzyme occurring in most mammalian tissue that catalyzes the reversible acylation-deacylation of ceramides.

ceramide (ser′ah-mīd) any of a group of naturally occurring sphingolipids in which the NH_2 group of sphingosine is acylated with a fatty acyl CoA derivative to form an N-acylsphingosine. **galactosyl c.,** cerebroside. **c. glucoside,** the major sphingolipid accumulated in Gaucher's disease. **c. trihexoside,** the major sphingolipid accumulated in Fabry's disease.

cerasin (ser′ah-sin) a class of gums from cherry, plum, and other trees, containing carbohydrate.

cerasine (ser′ah-sīn) a red azo dye, used as a cytoplasmic stain.

cerate (sēr′āt) a medicinal preparation for external use, compounded of fat or wax, or both, intermediate in consistency between an ointment and a plaster.

ceratin (ser′ah-tin) keratin.

ceratitis (ser″ah-ti′tis) keratitis.

cerato- for words beginning thus, see also those beginning kerato-.

ceratonosus (ser″ah-ton′o-sus) any disease of the cornea.

Ceratophyllus (ser-ah-tof′ĭ-lus) a genus of fleas.

ceratum (se-ra′tum) [L.] cerate.

cercaria (ser-ka′re-ah), pl. cerca′riae [Gr.] the final, free-swimming larval stage of a trematode parasite.

cerclage (ser-klahzh′) [Fr.] encircling of a part with a ring or loop, as for correction of an incompetent cervix uteri or fixation of adjacent ends of a fractured bone.

cercus (ser′kus) a bristle-like structure.

cerea flexibilitas (sēr′e-ah flek″sĭ-bil′ĭ-tas) waxy flexibility.

cerebellar (ser″ĕ-bel′ar) pertaining to the cerebellum.

cerebellifugal (ser″ĕ-bel-lif′u-gal) conducting away from the cerebellum.

cerebellipetal (-lip′ĕ-tal) conducting toward the cerebellum.

cerebellitis (-li′tis) inflammation of the cerebellum.

cerebellospinal (ser″ĕ-bel″o-spi′nal) proceeding from the cerebellum to the spinal cord.

cerebellum (ser″ĕ-bel′um) the part of the metencephalon situated on the back of the brain stem, to which it is attached by three cerebellar peduncles on each side; it consists of a median lobe (vermis) and two lateral lobes (the hemispheres).

cerebral (ser′ĕ-bral, sĕ-re′bral) pertaining to the cerebrum.

cerebration (ser″ĕ-bra′shun) functional activity of the brain.

cerebrifugal (-brif′u-gal) conducting or proceeding away from the cerebrum.

cerebripetal (-brip′ĕ-tal) conducting or proceeding toward the cerebrum.

cerebritis (-bri′tis) inflammation of the cerebrum.

cerebrocuprein (-bro-ku′pre-in) a copper protein isolated from the human and bovine brain.

cerebroid (ser′ĕ-broid) resembling brain substance.

cerebroma (ser″ĕ-bro′mah) any abnormal mass of brain substance.

cerebromalacia (-bro-mah-la′she-ah) abnormal softening of the substance of the cerebrum.

cerebromeningitis (-men″in-ji′tis) meningoencephalitis.

cerebropathia (-path′e-ah) [L.] cerebropathy. **c. psy′chica toxe′mica,** Korsakoff's psychosis.

cerebropathy (ser″ĕ-brop′ah-the) any disorder of the brain.

cerebrophysiology (ser″ĕ-bro-fiz″e-ol′o-je) the physiology of the cerebrum.

cerebropontile (-pon′til) pertaining to cerebrum and pons.

cerebrosclerosis (-skle-ro′sis) morbid hardening of the substance of the cerebrum.

cerebrose (ser′ĕ-brōs) galactose (of cerebrosides).

cerebroside (sĕ-re′bro-sīd) a general designation for sphingolipids in which sphingosine is combined with galactose or glucose; found chiefly in nervous tissue.

cerebrosis (ser″ĕ-bro′sis) any disease of the cerebrum.

cerebrospinal (ser″ĕ-bro-spi′nal) pertaining to the brain and spinal cord.

cerebrospinant (-spi′nant) an agent which affects the brain and spinal cord.

cerebrotomy (ser″ĕ-brot′o-me) anatomy or dissection of the brain.

cerebrum (ser′ĕ-brum, sĕ-re′brum) the main portion of the brain, occupying the upper part of the cranial cavity; its two hemispheres, united by the corpus callosum, form the largest part of the central nervous system in man. The term is sometimes applied to the postembryonic forebrain and midbrain together or to the entire brain.

cerium (se′re-um) chemical element (*see table*), at. no. 58, symbol Ce.

cerolysin (se-rol′ĭ-sin) a lysin which decomposes wax or cerumen.

ceroma (se-ro′ma) a tumor that has undergone waxy degeneration.

ceroplasty (se′ro-plas″te) the making of anatomical models in wax.

cerulein (sĕ-roo′le-in) a peptide analogue of cholecystokinin and gastrin isolated from the skin of frogs; in mammals it is a powerful stimulant of gallbladder contraction.

ceruloplasmin (sĕ-roo″lo-plaz′min) an alpha$_2$-globulin of plasma, being a glycoprotein in which most of the plasma copper is transported.

cerumen (sĕ-roo′men) earwax; the waxlike substance found within the external meatus of the ear. **ceru′minal, ceru′minous,** adj.

ceruminolysis (sĕ-roo″mĭ-nol′ĭ-sis) dissolution or disintegration of cerumen in the external auditory meatus. **ceruminolyt′ic,** adj.

ceruminosis (-no′sis) excessive or disordered secretion of cerumen.

cervic(o)- word element [L.], *neck; cervix.*

cervical (ser′vĭ-kal) pertaining to the neck or to the cervix.

cervicectomy (ser″vĭ-sek′to-me) excision of the cervix uteri.

cervicitis (-si′tis) inflammation of the cervix uteri.

cervicobrachialgia (ser″vĭ-ko-brak″e-al′je-ah) pain in the neck radiating to the arm, due to compression of nerve roots of the cervical spinal cord.

cervicocolpitis (-kol-pi′tis) inflammation of the cervix uteri and vagina.

cervicofacial (-fa′shal) pertaining to the neck and face.

cervicoplasty (ser′vĭ-ko-plas″te) plastic surgery on the neck.

cervicovesical (ser″vĭ-ko-ves′ĭ-kal) relating to the cervix uteri and urinary bladder.

Cervilaxin (ser″vĭ-lak′sin) trademark for a preparation of relaxin.

cervix (ser′viks), pl. *cer′vices* [L.] neck; the front portion of the neck (collum), or a constricted part of an organ (e.g., cervix uteri). **incompetent c.,** one that is abnormally prone to dilate in the second trimester of pregnancy, resulting in premature expulsion of the fetus. **c. u′teri,** the narrow lower end of the uterus, between the isthmus and the opening of the uterus into the vagina. **c. vesi′cae,** the lower, constricted part of the urinary bladder, proximal to the opening of the urethra.

cesium (se′ze-um) chemical element (*see table*), at. no. 55, symbol Cs.

cesticidal (ses″tĭ-si′dal) destructive to cestodes.

Cestoda (ses-to′dah) a subclass of Cestoidea comprising the true tapeworms, which have a head (scolex) and segments (proglottides). The adults are endoparasitic in the alimentary tract and associated ducts of various vertebrate hosts; their larvae may be found in various organs and tissues.

Cestodaria (ses″to-da′re-ah) a subclass of tapeworms, the unsegmented tapeworms of the class Cestoidea, which are endoparasitic in the intestines and coelom of various primitive fishes and rarely in reptiles.

cestode (ses'tōd) 1. any individual of the class Cestoidea, especially any member of the subclass Cestoda. 2. cestoid.

cestodology (ses"to-dol'o-je) the scientific study of cestodes.

cestoid (ses'toid) resembling a tapeworm.

Cestoidea (ses-toi'de-ah) a class of tapeworms (phylum Platyhelminthes), characterized by the absence of a mouth and digestive tract and by the presence of a noncuticular layer covering their bodies.

cetylpyridinium (se"til-pi"ri-din'e-um) a local anti-infective, $C_{21}H_{38}ClN \cdot H_2O$, used as the chloride salt.

Cevalin (se'vah-lin) trademark for preparations of ascorbic acid (vitamin C).

Cevex (se'veks) trademark for a liquid preparation of ascorbic acid (vitamin C).

Ce-Vi-Sol (se'vi-sol) trademark for a preparation of ascorbic acid (vitamin C).

C.F. carbolfuchsin; citrovorum factor.

Cf chemical symbol, *californium.*

C.F.T. complement fixation test.

cg. centigram.

C.G.S., c.g.s. centimeter-gram-second (system), a system of measurements based on the centimeter as the unit of length, the gram as the unit of mass, and the second as the unit of time.

Ch¹ Christchurch chromosome.

C.H.A. Catholic Hospital Association.

chafe (chāf) irritation of the skin, as by rubbing together of opposing skin folds.

chagoma (chă-go'mah) a skin tumor occurring in Chagas' disease.

chain (chān) a collection of objects linked together in a linear fashion, or end to end. **branched c.,** an open chain of atoms, usually carbon, with one or more side chains attached to it. **closed c.,** several atoms linked together to form a ring, which may be saturated, as in cyclopentane, or aromatic, as in benzene. **heavy c.,** any of the large polypeptide chains of five classes that, paired with the light chains, make up the antibody molecule. Heavy chains bear the antigenic determinants that differentiate the immunoglobulin classes. **light c.,** either of the two small polypeptide chains (molecular weight 22,000) that, when linked to heavy chains by disulfide bonds, make up the antibody molecule; they are of two types, kappa and lambda, which are unrelated to immunoglobulin class differences. **open c.,** several atoms linked together to form an open chain; compounds of this series are called *acrylic, aliphatic, fatty,* or *paraffin* compounds. **side c.,** a chain of atoms attached to a larger chain or to a ring.

chalasia (kah-la'ze-ah) relaxation of a bodily opening, such as the cardiac sphincter (a cause of vomiting in infants).

chalazion (kah-la'ze-on) a small eyelid mass resulting from chronic inflammation of a meibomian gland.

chalcosis (kal-ko'sis) copper deposits in tissue.

chalicosis (kal"ĭ-ko'sis) pneumoconiosis due to inhalation of fine particles of stone.

chalk (chawk) amorphous calcium carbonate, a white, lusterless, slightly alkaline, insoluble earth. **prepared c.,** a native form of calcium carbonate freed from its impurities by elutriation; used as an antacid.

chalone (kal'ōn) a postulated group of tissue-specific substances said to inhibit cell proliferation and whose action is reversible.

chalybeate (kah-lib'e-āt) containing or charged with iron.

chamaecephaly (kam"e-sef'ah-le) the condition of having a low flat head, i.e., a cephalic index of 70 or less. **chamaecephal'ic,** adj.

chamber (chām'ber) an enclosed space. **air c.,** relief c. **anterior c.,** the part of the aqueous-containing space of the eyeball between the cornea and iris. **aqueous c.,** the part of the eyeball filled with aqueous humor; see *anterior c.* and *posterior c.* **counting c.,** a shallow glass chamber specially ruled to facilitate the counting of discrete particles in the sample under study. **diffusion c.,** an apparatus for separating a substance by means of a semipermeable membrane. **Haldane c.,** an air-tight chamber in which animals are confined for metabolic studies. **hyperbaric c.,** an enclosed space in which gas (oxygen) can be raised to greater than atmospheric pressure. **ionization c.,** an enclosure containing two or more electrodes between which an electric current may be passed when the enclosed gas is ionized by radiation; used for determining the intensity of roentgen and other rays. **posterior c.,** that part of the aqueous-containing space of the eyeball between the iris and the lens. **pulp c.,** the natural cavity in the central portion of the tooth crown that is occupied by the dental pulp. **relief c.,** the recess in a denture surface that rests on the oral structures, to reduce or eliminate pressure. **Thoma-Zeiss counting c.,** a device for counting blood or other cells. **vitreous c.,** the vitreous-containing space in the eyeball, bounded anteriorly by the lens and ciliary body and posteriorly by the posterior wall of the eyeball.

chancre (shang'ker) 1. the primary sore of syphilis, also known as *hard, hunterian,* or *true chancre,* occurring at the site of entry of the infection. 2. a papular lesion occurring at the site of entry of infection in skin tuberculosis or sporotrichosis. **hard c., hunterian c.,** see *chancre.* **c. re'dux,** chancre developing on the scar of a healed primary chancre. **simple c., soft c.,** chancroid. **true c.,** see *chancre.*

chancroid (shang'kroid) a soft, nonsyphilitic venereal sore caused by *Hemophilus ducreyi.* **phagedenic c.,** chancroid with a tendency to slough. **serpiginous c.,** a variety tending to spread in curved lines.

chancrous (shang'krus) of the nature of chancre.

character (kar'ak-ter) a quality or attribute indicative of the nature of an object or an organism; in genetics, the expression of a gene or group of genes as seen in a phenotype. **acquired c.,** a noninheritable modification produced in an animal as a result of its own activities or of environmental influences. **dominant c.,** a mendelian character that is expressed when it is transmitted by a single gene. **mendelian c's,** in genetics, the separate and distinct traits exhibited by an animal or plant and dependent on the genetic constitution of the organism. **primary sex c's,** those characters of the male and female concerned directly in reproduction. **recessive c.,** a mendelian character that is expressed only when transmitted by both genes (one from each parent) determining the trait. **secondary sex c's,** those characters specific to the male and female but not directly concerned in reproduction. **sex-conditioned c., sex-influenced c.,** an autosomal trait whose full expression is conditioned by the sex of the individual, e.g., human baldness. **sex-linked c.,** one transmitted consistently to individuals of one sex only, being carried in the sex chromosome.

charcoal (char'kōl) carbon prepared by charring other organic material. **activated c.,** residue of destructive distillation of various organic materials, treated to increase its adsorptive power; used as a general purpose antidote. **animal c.,** charcoal prepared from bone, which is purified (*purified animal c.*) by removal of materials dissolved in hot hydrochloric acid and water; adsorbent and decolorizer.

charlatan (shar'lah-tan) a pretender to knowledge or skills not possessed; a quack.

charleyhorse (char'le-hors) soreness and stiffness in a muscle, especially the quadriceps, due to overstrain or contusion.

chart (chart) a record of data in graphic or tabular form. **reading c.,** a chart with material printed in gradually increasing type sizes, used in testing acuity of near vision. **Reuss' c's,** charts with colored letters printed on colored backgrounds, used in testing color vision. **Snellen's c.,** a chart printed with block letters in gradually decreasing sizes, used in testing visual acuity.

chauffage (sho-fahzh') [Fr.] treatment with a low-heated cautery that is passed to and fro close to the tissue.

Ch.B. [L.] *Chirur'giae Baccalau'reus* (Bachelor of Surgery).

ChE cholinesterase.

check-bite (chek'bīt) a sheet of hard wax or modeling compound placed between the teeth, used to check occlusion of the teeth.

cheek (chēk) bucca; a fleshy protuberance, especially the fleshy portion of either side of the face. Also, the mucous membrane-covered inner surface of the cheeks. **cleft c.,** a congenital fissure of the cheek.

cheil(o)- word element [Gr.], *lip*.

cheilectropion (ki"lek-tro'pe-on) eversion of the lip.

cheilitis (ki-li'tis) inflammation of the lips. **actinic c., c. actin'ica,** pain and swelling of the lips and development of a scaly crust on the vermilion border after exposure to actinic rays. **solar c.,** involvement of the lips after exposure to actinic rays; such involvement may be acute (*actinic c.*), or chronic, with alteration of the epithelium and sometimes fissuring or ulceration.

cheilognathoprosoposchisis (ki"lo-na"tho-pros"o-pos'kĭ-sis) congenital oblique facial cleft continuing into the lip and upper jaw.

cheiloplasty (ki'lo-plas"te) surgical repair of a defect of the lip.

cheilorrhaphy (ki-lor'ah-fe) suture of the lip; surgical repair of harelip.

cheiloschisis (ki-los'kĭ-sis) harelip.

cheilosis (ki-lo'sis) fissuring and dry scaling of the vermilion surface of the lips and angles of the mouth, a characteristic of riboflavin deficiency.

cheilostomatoplasty (ki"lo-sto-mat'o-plas"te) surgical restoration of the lips and mouth.

cheilotomy (ki-lot'o-me) incision of the lip.

cheir(o)- word element [Gr.], *hand.* See also words beginning *chir(o)-*.

cheiralgia (ki-ral'je-ah) pain in the hand.

cheirarthritis (ki"rar-thri'tis) inflammation of the joints of the hands and fingers.

cheirognostic (ki"rog-nos'tik) pertaining to or characterized by the ability to distinguish stimuli as originating on the right or left side of the body.

cheirokinesthesia (ki"ro-kin"es-the'ze-ah) the subjective perception of movements of the hand, especially in writing.

cheiromegaly (-meg'ah-le) abnormal enlargement of the hands and fingers.

cheiroplasty (ki'ro-plas"te) plastic surgery on the hand.

cheiropodalgia (ki"ro-po-dal'je-ah) pain in the hands and feet.

cheiropompholyx (-pom'fo-liks) pompholyx.

cheiroscope (ki'ro-skōp) an instrument used in the training of binocular vision.

cheirospasm (-spazm) spasm of the muscles of the hand.

chelate (ke'lāt) to combine with a metal in complexes in which the metal is part of a ring. By extension, a chemical compound in which a metallic ion is sequestered and firmly bound into a ring within the chelating molecules. Chelates are used in chemotherapy of metal poisoning.

Chel-Iron (kēl'i-ron) trademark for preparations of ferrocholinate.

cheloid (ke'loid) keloid.

chem(o)- word element [Gr.], *chemical; chemistry.*

chemabrasion (kēm-ah-bra'shun) superficial destruction of the epidermis and the upper layer of the dermis by application of a cauterant to the skin; done to remove scars, tattoos, etc.

chemexfoliation (kēm'eks-fo'le-a"shun) chemabrasion.

chemical (kem'ĭ-kal) 1. pertaining to chemistry. 2. a substance composed of chemical elements, or obtained by chemical processes.

chemicogenesis (kem"ĭ-ko-jen'ĕ-sis) initiation of segmentation of an ovum by chemical means.

chemiluminescence (kem"ĭ-lu"mĭ-nes'ens) chemoluminescence.

cheminosis (-no′sis) any disease due to chemical agents.

chemism (kem′izm) chemical activity; chemical property or relationship.

chemist (kem′ist) 1. an expert in chemistry. 2. (British) pharmacist.

chemistry (kem′is-tre) the science dealing with the elements and atomic relations of matter, and of various compounds of the elements. **colloid c.,** chemistry dealing with the nature and composition of colloids. **inorganic c.,** that branch of chemistry dealing with compounds not occurring in the plant or animal worlds. **organic c.,** that branch of chemistry dealing with carbon-containing compounds.

chemoautotroph (ke″mo-aw′to-trōf) a chemoautotrophic microorganism.

chemoautotrophic (-aw″to-trof′ik) capable of synthesizing cell constituents from carbon dioxide by means of energy derived from inorganic reactions.

chemobiotic (-bi-ot′ik) a compound of a chemotherapeutic agent and an antibiotic.

chemocautery (-kaw′ter-e) cauterization by application of a caustic substance.

chemodectoma (-dek-to′mah) any tumor of the chemoreceptor system, e.g., a carotid body tumor.

chemokinesis (-ki-ne′sis) increased activity of an organism caused by a chemical substance.

chemoluminescence (-loo″mĭ-nes′ens) luminescence produced by direct transformation of chemical energy into light energy.

chemolysis (ke-mol′ĭ-sis) chemical decomposition.

chemomorphosis (ke″mo-mor-fo′sis) change of form from chemical action.

chemonucleolysis (-nu″kle-ol′ĭ-sis) dissolution of a portion of the nucleus pulposus by injection of a chemolytic agent (e.g., chymopapain) for treatment of a herniated intervertebral disk.

chemopallidectomy (-pal″ĭ-dek′to-me) destruction of tissue of the globus pallidus by a chemical agent.

chemoprophylaxis (-pro″fĭ-lak′sis) prevention of disease by chemical means.

chemopsychiatry (-si-ki′ah-tre) the treatment of mental and emotional disorders by the use of drugs.

chemoreceptor (-re-sep′tor) a receptor sensitive to stimulation by chemical substances.

chemosensitive (-sen′sĭ-tiv) sensitive to changes in chemical composition.

chemosensory (-sen′so-re) relating to the perception of chemical substances, as in odor detection.

chemoserotherapy (-se″ro-ther′ah-pe) treatment of infection by drugs and serum.

chemosis (ke-mo′sis) edema of the conjunctiva of the eye.

chemosterilant (ke″mo-ster′ĭ-lant) a chemical compound which upon ingestion causes sterility of an organism.

chemosurgery (-ser′jer-e) destruction of tissue by chemical means for therapeutic purposes.

chemosynthesis (-sin′thĕ-sis) the building up of chemical compounds under the influence of chemical stimulation, specifically the formation of carbohydrates from carbon dioxide and water as a result of energy derived from chemical reactions. **chemosynthet′ic,** adj.

chemotaxis (-tak′sis) taxis in response to the influence of chemical stimulation. **chemotac′-tic,** adj. **leukocyte c.,** the response of leukocytes to products formed in immunologic reactions, wherein leukocytes are attracted to and accumulate at the site of the reaction; a part of the inflammatory response.

chemotherapy (-ther′ah-pe) treatment of disease by chemical agents.

chemotic (ke-mot′ik) 1. pertaining to or affected with chemosis. 2. an agent that increases lymph production in the ocular conjunctiva.

chemotropism (ke-mot′ro-pizm) tropism in response to the influence of chemical stimulation. **chemotrop′ic,** adj.

chemurgy (kem′er-je) chemistry applied to the industrial use of raw organic products.

cherubism (cher′u-bizm) hereditary and progressive bilateral swelling at the angle of the mandible, sometimes involving the entire jaw, imparting a cherubic look to the face, in some cases enhanced by upturning of the eyes.

chest (chest) the thorax, especially its anterior aspect. **flail c.,** one whose wall moves paradoxically with respiration, owing to multiple fractures of the ribs. **funnel c.,** a congenital abnormality of the anterior chest wall in which the sternum is depressed. **pigeon c.,** see under *breast.*

chiasm (ki′azm) a decussation or X-shaped crossing. **optic c.,** the structure in the forebrain formed by the decussation of the fibers of the optic nerve from each half of each retina.

chiasma (ki-az′mah) chiasm; in genetics, the points at which members of a chromosome pair are in contact during the prophase of meiosis and because of which recombination, or crossing over, occurs on separation.

chickenpox (chik′en-poks) varicella; a highly contagious disease caused by the herpes zoster virus, characterized by crops of vesicular eruptions appearing over a period of a few days to a week after an incubation period of 17–21 days; usually benign in children, but in infants and adults may be accompanied by severe symptoms.

chigger (chig′er) the six-legged red larva of mites of the family Trombiculidae (e.g., *Eutrombicula alfreddugèsi, E. splendens, Trombicula autumnalis),* which attach to their host's skin, and whose bite produces a wheal, usually with intense itching and severe dermatitis. Some species are vectors of the rickettsiae of scrub typhus.

chigoe (chig′o) the flea, *Tunga penetrans,* of subtropical and tropical America and Africa; the pregnant female burrows into the skin of the feet, legs, or other part of the body, causing intense irritation and ulceration, sometimes leading to spontaneous amputation of a digit.

chilblain (chil′blān) a recurrent localized itching, swelling, and painful erythema of the fingers, toes, or ears, caused by mild frostbite.

child (chīld) the human young, from infancy to puberty.

childbed (chīld'bed) the puerperal state or period.

childbirth (-berth'') the act or process of giving birth to a child; see *labor.*

chill (chil) a sensation of cold, with convulsive shaking of the body.

Chilomastix (ki''lo-mas'tiks) a genus of parasitic protozoa found in the intestines of vertebrates, including *C. mesnil'i,* a very common, widely distributed species found as a commensal in the human cecum and colon.

Chilopoda (ki-lop'o-dah) a class of the phylum Arthropoda, including the centipedes.

chimera (ki-me'rah) an organism whose body contains different cell populations derived from different zygotes of the same or different species, occurring spontaneously or produced artificially. **heterologous c.,** one in which the foreign cells are derived from an organism of a different species. **homologous c.,** one in which the foreign cells are derived from an organism of the same species, but of a different genotype. **isologous c.,** one in which the foreign cells are derived from a different organism having the identical genotype, as from an identical twin. **radiation c.,** an organism with immunologic characteristics of host and donor after a bone marrow graft from an antigenically different donor, the host having first been subjected to irradiation to inhibit his immune response.

chimerism (ki'mer-izm) the state of being a chimera; the presence in an individual of cells of different origin.

chin (chin) the anterior prominence of the lower jaw; the mentum.

chionablepsia (ki''o-nah-blep'se-ah) snow blindness.

chir(o)- word element [Gr.], *hand.* See also words beginning *cheir(o)-.*

chiropodist (ki-rop'ŏ-dist) podiatrist.

chiropody (ki-rop'ŏ-de) podiatry.

chiropractic (ki''ro-prak'tik) a system of therapeutics that attributes disease to dysfunction of the nervous system, and attempts to restore normal function by manipulation and treatment of the body structures, especially those of the vertebral column.

chiropractor (-prak'tor) a practitioner of chiropractic.

chi-square (ki'skwār) see under *test.*

chitin (ki'tin) a horny polysaccharide, the principal constituent of the shells of arthropods and shards of beetles, and found in certain fungi.

chitobiose (ki''to-bi'ōs) a disaccharide composed of two glucosamine units, obtained by hydrolysis of de-acetylated chitin (chitosan).

chlamydemia (klah-mĭ-de'me-ah) the presence of chlamydiae in the blood.

Chlamydia (klah-mid'e-ah) a genus of the family Chlamydiaceae. **C. psitta'ci,** a species, strains of which cause psittacosis, ornithosis, and a variety of diseases in animals. **C. tra-**

cho'matis, a species, various strains of which cause trachoma, inclusion conjunctivitis, urethritis, bronchopneumonia of laboratory mice, proctitis, and lymphogranuloma venereum.

chlamydia (klah-mid'e-ah), pl. *chlamyd'iae.* Any member of *Chlamydia.*

Chlamydiaceae (klah-mid''e-a'se-e) a family of bacteria (order Chlamydiales), containing a single genus, *Chlamydia.*

Chlamydiales (klah-mid'e-al-ēz) an order of coccoid, gram-negative, parasitic microorganisms that multiply only within the cytoplasm of vertebrate host cells by a unique development cycle.

chlamydiosis (klah-mid''e-o'sis) any infection or disease caused by *Chlamydia.*

Chlamydobacteriaceae (klah-mi''do-bak-te''re-a'se-e) a family of schizomycetes (order Chlamydobacteriales).

Chlamydobacteriales (-bak-te''re-a''lēz) an order of schizomycetes.

chlamydospore (klam'ĭ-do-spor'') a thick-walled intercalary or terminal asexual spore formed by the rounding-up of a cell; it is not shed.

chloasma (klo-az'mah) melasma. **c. gravida'-rum,** see under *melasma.* **c. hepat'icum,** discoloration of the skin allegedly due to disorder of the liver. **c. uteri'num,** melasma gravidarum.

chlophedianol (klo''fĕ-di'ah-nol) an antitussive agent, $C_{17}H_{20}NO$, used as the hydrochloride salt.

chloracne (klor-ak'ne) an acneiform eruption due to exposure to chlorine compounds.

chloral (klo'ral) 1. an oily liquid, $Cl_3C \cdot CHO$, with a pungent, irritating odor, prepared by the mutual action of alcohol and chlorine; used in manufacture of chloral hydrate and DDT. 2. c. hydrate. **c. betaine,** an adduct formed by the reaction of chloral hydrate with betaine; used as a sedative. **c. hydrate,** a crystalline substance used as a hypnotic.

chloralism (-izm) a morbid condition due to excessive use of chloral.

chlorambucil (klor-am'bu-sil) an antineoplastic, $C_{14}H_{19}Cl_2NO_2$, derived from nitrogen mustard.

chloramphenicol (klor''am-fen'ĭ-kol) an antibacterial and antirickettsial, $C_{11}H_{12}Cl_2N_2O_5$.

chlorate (klo'rāt) a salt of chloric acid.

chlorbutol (klor'bu-tol) chlorobutanol.

chlorcyclizine (klor-si'klĭ-zēn) an antihistaminic, $C_{18}H_{21}ClN_2$, used as the hydrochloride salt.

chlordane (klor'dān) a poisonous substance of the chlorinated hydrocarbon group, used as an insecticide.

chlordantoin (klor-dan'to-in) a topical antifungal agent, $C_{11}H_{17}Cl_3N_2O_2S$.

chlordiazepoxide (klor''di-a''ze-pok'sīd) a minor tranquilizer, $C_{16}H_{14}ClN_3O$.

chlorellin (klo-rel'in) a bacteriostatic substance derived from the fresh water algae *Chlorella.*

chloremia (klo-re'me-ah) hyperchloremia.

chloretic (klo-ret′ik) an agent which accelerates the flow of bile.

Chloretone (klo′re-tōn) trademark for a preparation of chlorobutanol.

chlorguanide (klor-gwan′īd) proguanil.

chlorhydria (-hi′dre-ah) an excess of hydrochloric acid in the stomach.

chloride (klo′rīd) a salt of hydrochloric acid; any binary compound of chlorine in which the latter is the negative element. **ferric c.,** $FeCl_3 \cdot 6H_2O$; used as a reagent and topically as an astringent and styptic.

chloridimeter (klo″rĭ-dim′ĕ-ter) an instrument used in chloridimetry.

chloridimetry (-dim′ĕ-tre) measurement of the chloride content of a fluid.

chloriduria (-du′re-ah) excess of chlorides in the urine.

chlorinated (klo′rĭ-nat″ed) charged with chlorine.

chlorine (klo′rēn) chemical element (*see table*), at. no. 17, symbol Cl.

chlorisondamine (klor″i-son′dah-mēn) an isoindoline derivative, $C_{14}H_{20}Cl_6N_2$, used to produce ganglionic blockade and to reduce blood pressure.

chlorite (klo′rīt) a salt of chlorous acid; disinfectant and bleaching agent.

chlormadinone (klor-mah′dĭ-nōn) a progestin, $C_{23}H_{29}ClO_4$.

chlormerodrin (-mer′o-drin) a mercurial diuretic, $C_5H_{11}ClHgN_2O_2$.

chlormezanone (-mez′ah-nōn) a muscle relaxant and tranquilizer, $C_{11}H_{12}ClNO_3S$.

Chlorobium (klo-ro′be-um) a genus of schizomycetes (family Chlorobacteriaceae).

chlorobutanol (klo″ro-bu′tah-nol) an antibacterial and dental analgesic, $C_4H_7Cl_3O_5$.

chloroform (klo′ro-form) a colorless, mobile liquid, $CHCl_3$, with ethereal odor and sweet taste, used as a solvent; once widely used as an inhalation anesthetic and analgesic, and as an antitussive, carminative, and counterirritant.

chloroformism (-form″izm) 1. the habitual use of chloroform for its narcotic effect. 2. the anesthetic effect of the vapor of chloroform.

chlorolabe (klor′o-lāb) the pigment in retinal cones that is more sensitive to the green portion of the spectrum than are the other pigments (cyanolabe and erythrolabe).

chloroleukemia (klo″ro-lu-ke′me-ah) myelogenous leukemia in which no specific tumor masses are observed at autopsy, but the body organs and fluids show a definite green color.

chlorolymphosarcoma (-lim″fo-sar-ko′mah) chloroma.

chloroma (klo-ro′mah) a malignant, green-colored tumor arising from myeloid tissue.

Chloromycetin (klo″ro-mi-se′tin) trademark for preparations of chloramphenicol.

chloromyeloma (-mi″ĕ-lo′mah) chloroma with multiple growths in bone marrow.

chloropexia (-pek″se-ah) the fixation of chlorine in body tissues.

chlorophane (klo′ro-fān) a green-yellow pigment from the retina.

chlorophenol (klo″ro-fe′nol) a topical antiseptic, $C_6H_4Cl \cdot OH$, prepared by the action of chlorine on phenol.

chlorophenothane (-fe′no-thān) DDT; an insecticide, $C_{14}H_9Cl_5$, used as a pediculicide.

chlorophyll (klo′ro-fil) the green coloring matter of plants by which photosynthesis is accomplished.

chlorophyllin (-fil″in) any of the water-soluble salts obtained by alkaline hydrolysis of chlorophyll with replacement of the methyl and phytyl ester groups by sodium or potassium.

chloroplast (-plast) any of the chlorophyll-bearing bodies of plant cells.

chloroprivic (klo″ro-pri′vik) deprived of chlorides; due to loss of chlorides.

chloroprocaine (-pro′kān) a local anesthetic, $C_{13}H_{19}ClN_2O_2$, used as the hydrochloride salt.

chloropsia (klo-rop′se-ah) defect of vision in which objects appear to have a greenish tinge.

chloroquine (klo′ro-kwin) an antimalarial and lupus erythematosus suppressant, $C_{18}H_{26}ClN_3$.

chlorosis (klo-ro′sis) a disorder, generally of pubescent females, characterized by greenish yellow discoloration of the skin and hypochromic erythrocytes. **chlorot′ic,** adj.

chlorothen (klo′ro-then) an antihistaminic, $C_{14}H_{18}ClN_3S$, used as the citrate salt.

chlorothiazide (klo″ro-thi′ah-zīd) a diuretic and antihypertensive, $C_7H_6ClN_3O_4S_2$.

chlorothymol (-thi′mol) an antibacterial, $C_{10}H_{13}ClO$.

chlorotrianisene (-tri-an′ĭ-sēn) an estrogenic compound, $C_{23}H_{21}ClO_3$, used especially in relieving menopausal symptoms.

chlorpheniramine (klor″fen-ir′ah-mēn) an antihistaminic, $C_{16}H_{19}ClN_2$, used as the maleate salt.

chlorphenoxamine (-ok′sah-mēn) a compound, $C_{18}H_{22}ClNO$, used as the hydrochloride salt to reduce muscular rigidity in parkinsonism.

chlorpromazine (klor-pro′mah-zēn) a major tranquilizer, $C_{17}H_{19}ClN_2S$, used in rectal suppositories; the hydrochloride salt is administered orally, muscularly, or intravenously.

chlorpropamide (-pro′pah-mīd) an oral hypoglycemic, $C_{10}H_{13}ClN_2O_3S$.

chlorprophenpyridamine (klor″pro-fen-pi-rid′ah-mēn) chlorpheniramine.

chlorprothixene (-pro-thiks′ēn) a major tranquilizer, $C_{18}H_{18}ClNS$.

chlorquinaldol (klor-kwin′al-dol) a keratoplastic, bactericidal, and fungicidal agent, $C_{10}H_7Cl_2NO$, used topically in dermatoses.

chlortetracycline (klor″tet-rah-si′klēn) an antibiotic obtained from *Streptomyces aureofaciens;* the hydrochloride salt is used as an antibacterial and antiprotozoal.

chlorthalidone (klor-thal′ĭ-dōn) a diuretic, $C_{14}H_{11}ClN_2O_4S$.

Chlor-Trimeton (-tri′mĕ-ton) trademark for preparations of chlorpheniramine.

chloruresis (klor″u-re′sis) excretion of chlorides in the urine. **chloruret′ic,** adj.

chloruria (klo-ru′re-ah) excess chlorides in the urine.

chlorzoxazone (klor-zok′sah-zōn) a skeletal muscle relaxant, $C_7H_4ClNO_2$.

Ch.M. [L.] *Chirur′giae Ma′gister* (Master of Surgery).

choana (ko-a′nah), pl. *choa′nae* [L.] 1. any funnel-shaped cavity or infundibulum. 2. [pl.] the paired openings between the nasal cavity and the nasopharynx.

Choanotaenia (ko-a″no-te′ne-ah) a genus of tapeworms, including *C. infundib′ulum,* an important parasite of chickens and turkeys.

choke (chōk) 1. to interrupt respiration by obstruction or compression, or the condition resulting from such interruption. 2. [pl.] a burning sensation in the substernal region, with uncontrollable coughing, occurring during decompression.

chol(o)- word element [Gr.], *bile.*

cholagogue (ko′lah-gog) an agent that stimulates gallbladder contraction to promote bile flow. **cholagog′ic,** adj.

Cholan-DH (ko′lan) trademark for preparations of dehydrocholic acid.

cholangeitis (ko-lan″je-i′tis) cholangitis.

cholangiectasis (-ek′tah-sis) dilatation of a bile duct.

cholangiocarcinoma (ko-lan″je-o-kar″sĭ-no′-mah) adenocarcinoma of the bile ducts.

cholangioenterostomy (-en″ter-os′to-me) surgical anastomosis of a bile duct to the intestine.

cholangiogastrostomy (-gas-tros′to-me) anastomosis of a bile duct to the stomach.

cholangiogram (ko-lan′je-o-gram″) the film obtained by cholangiography.

cholangiography (ko-lan″je-og′rah-fe) radiography of the bile ducts.

cholangiole (ko-lan′je-ōl) one of the fine terminal elements of the bile duct system. **cholangi′olar,** adj.

cholangiolitis (ko-lan″je-o-li′tis) inflammation of the cholangioles. **cholangiolit′ic,** adj.

cholangioma (-o′mah) a tumor of the bile ducts.

cholangiostomy (ko″lan-je-os′to-me) fistulization of a bile duct.

cholangiotomy (-ot′o-me) incision into a bile duct.

cholangitis (ko″lan-ji′tis) inflammation of a bile duct. **cholangit′ic,** adj.

cholanopoiesis (ko″lah-no-poi-e′sis) the synthesis of bile acids or of their conjugates and salts by the liver.

cholanopoietic (-poi-et′ik) 1. promoting cholanopoiesis. 2. an agent that promotes cholanopoiesis.

cholate (ko′lāt) a salt or ester of cholic acid.

chole- word element [Gr.], *bile.*

cholebilirubin (ko″le-bil″e-ru′bin) a pigment, $C_{32}H_{50}O_{11}N_2$, differing from bilirubin, occurring in gallbladder bile; it gives a direct reaction to the van den Bergh test.

cholecalciferol (-kal-sif′er-ol) vitamin D_3, an oil-soluble antirachitic vitamin.

cholecyanin (-si′ah-nin) bilicyanin.

cholecyst (ko′le-sist) the gallbladder.

cholecystagogue (ko″le-sis′tah-gog) an agent that promotes evacuation of the gallbladder.

cholecystalgia (-sis-tal′je-ah) biliary colic.

cholecystectasia (-sis″tek-ta′ze-ah) distention of the gallbladder.

cholecystectomy (-sis-tek′to-me) excision of the gallbladder.

cholecystenterostomy (-sis″ten-ter-os′to-me) formation of a new communication between the gallbladder and the intestine.

cholecystic (-sis′tik) pertaining to the gallbladder.

cholecystis (-sis′tis) the gallbladder.

cholecystitis (-sis-ti′tis) inflammation of the gallbladder. **emphysematous c.,** that due to gas-producing organisms, marked by gas in the gallbladder lumen, often infiltrating into the gallbladder wall and surrounding tissues.

cholecystocolostomy (-sis″to-ko-los′to-me) surgical anastomosis of the gallbladder and the colon.

cholecystoduodenostomy (-du″o-dĕ-nos′to-me) surgical anastomosis of the gallbladder and the duodenum.

cholecystogastrostomy (-gas-tros′to-me) surgical anastomosis between the gallbladder and the stomach.

cholecystogram (-sis′to-gram) a roentgenogram of the gallbladder.

cholecystography (-sis-tog′rah-fe) roentgenography of the gallbladder. **cholecystograph′ic,** adj.

cholecystojejunostomy (-sis″to-je-ju-nos′to-me) surgical anastomosis of the gallbladder and the jejunum.

cholecystokinetic (-ki-net′ik) stimulating contraction of the gallbladder.

cholecystokinin (-kin′in) a hormone secreted in the small intestine that stimulates gallbladder contraction and secretion of pancreatic enzymes.

cholecystolithiasis (-lĭ-thi′ah-sis) cholelithiasis.

cholecystopexy (-sis′to-pek″se) surgical suspension or fixation of the gallbladder.

cholecystorrhaphy (-sis-tor′ah-fe) suture or repair of the gallbladder.

cholecystostomy (-sis-tos′to-me) the creation of an opening into the gallbladder for drainage.

cholecystotomy (-sis-tot′o-me) incision of the gallbladder.

choledochal (kol′ĕ-dok-al) pertaining to the common bile duct.

choledochectomy (kol″ĕ-do-kek′to-me) excision of part of the common bile duct.

choledochitis (-ki′tis) inflammation of the common bile duct.

choledocho- word element [Gr.], *common bile duct.*

choledochoduodenostomy (ko-led″ŏ-ko-du″o-dĕ-nos′to-me) surgical anastomosis of the common bile duct to the duodenum.

choledochoenterostomy (-en″ter-os′to-me) surgical anastomosis of the common bile duct to the intestine.

choledochogastrostomy (-gas-tros′to-me) surgical anastomosis of the common bile duct to the stomach.

choledochojejunostomy (-je-ju-nos′to-me) surgical anastomosis of the common bile duct to the jejunum.

choledocholithiasis (-lĭ-thi′ah-sis) calculi in the common bile duct.

choledocholithotomy (-lĭ-thot′o-me) incision into common bile duct for removal of stone.

choledochoplasty (ko-led′o-ko-plas″te) plastic repair of the common bile duct.

choledochorrhaphy (ko-led″o-kor′ah-fe) suture or repair of the common bile duct.

choledochostomy (-kos′to-me) creation of an opening into the common bile duct for drainage.

choledochotomy (-kot′o-me) incision into the common bile duct.

choledochus (ko-led′o-kus) the common bile duct.

Choledyl (kōl′ĕ-dil) trademark for a preparation of oxtriphylline.

choleic (ko-le′ik) pertaining to the bile.

cholelith (ko′lĕ-lith) gallstone.

cholelithiasis (ko″le-lĭ-thi′ah-sis) the presence or formation of gallstones.

cholelithotomy (-lĭ-thot′o-me) incision of the biliary tract for removal of gallstones.

cholelithotripsy (-lith′o-trip″se) crushing of a gallstone.

cholelithotrity (-lĭ-thot′rĭ-te) cholelithotripsy.

cholemesis (ko-lem′ĕ-sis) vomiting of bile.

cholemia (ko-le′me-ah) bile or bile pigment in the blood. **chole′mic,** adj.

choleperitoneum (ko″le-per″ĭ-to-ne′um) the presence of bile in the peritoneum.

cholepoiesis (-poi-e′sis) the formation of bile in the liver. **cholepoiet′ic,** adj.

choleprasin (-pra′sin) one of the bile pigments isolated from gallstones.

cholera (kol′er-ah) Asiatic cholera; an acute infectious disease endemic and epidemic in Asia, caused by *Vibrio cholerae,* marked by severe diarrhea with extreme fluid and electrolyte depletion, and by vomiting, muscle cramps, and prostration. **Asiatic c.,** see *cholera.* **chicken c.,** see *fowl c.* **dry c.,** c. sicca. **fowl c.,** hemorrhagic septicemia due to *Pasteurella multocida,* affecting all domestic fowl and various other fowl all over the world. **c. ful′minans,** c. sicca. **hog c.,** an acute, highly infectious and highly fatal viral disease of swine. **c. infan′tum,** a noncontagious diarrhea occurring in infants; formerly common in the summer months. **c. sic′ca, c. sid′erans,** cholera in which death occurs before diarrhea has appeared.

choleragen (kol′er-ah-jen) the exotoxin produced by the cholera vibrio, which is thought to stimulate electrolyte and water secretion into the small intestine.

choleraic (kol″ĕ-ra′ik) of, pertaining to, or of the nature of cholera.

choleresis (ko-ler′ĕ-sis) the secretion of bile by the liver.

choleretic (ko″ler-et′ik) stimulating bile production by the liver; an agent that so acts.

cholerine (kol′er-ēn) 1. the earliest stage of cholera. 2. a relatively mild form of cholera.

choleroid (-oid) resembling cholera.

cholestasis (ko″lĕ-sta′sis) stoppage or suppression of bile flow, having intrahepatic or extrahepatic causes. **cholestat′ic,** adj.

cholesteatoma (-ste″ah-to′mah) a cystlike mass with a lining of stratified squamous epithelium filled with desquamating debris frequently including cholesterol, which occurs in the meninges, central nervous system, and bones of the skull, but most commonly in the middle ear and mastoid region.

cholesteatosis (-ste-ah-to′sis) fatty degeneration due to cholesterol esters.

cholesteremia (ko-les″ter-e′me-ah) hypercholesterolemia.

cholesterin (ko-les′ter-in) cholesterol.

cholesterinemia (ko-les″ter-in-e′me-ah) cholesterolemia.

cholesterinuria (-u′re-ah) cholesteroluria.

cholesterol (ko-les′ter-ol) 1. a monatomic alcohol, $C_{27}H_{45}O$, found in animal fats and oils, bile, blood, brain tissue, milk, egg yolk, myelin sheaths of nerve fibers, liver, kidneys, and adrenal glands. 2. a preparation of cholesterol used as a pharmaceutic aid.

cholesterolemia (ko-les″ter-ol-e′me-ah) hypercholesterolemia.

cholesterolosis (-o′sis) cholesterosis.

cholesteroluria (-u′re-ah) the presence of cholesterol in the urine.

cholesterosis (ko-les″ter-o′sis) a condition in which cholesterol is deposited in tissues in abnormal amounts.

choletherapy (ko″le-ther′ah-pe) treatment by administration of bile salts.

choleuria (-u′re-ah) choluria.

choleverdin (-ver′din) biliverdin.

choline (ko′lēn) an amine, $C_5H_{15}O_2N$, sometimes classed as a vitamin, from many animal and vegetable tissues and produced synthetically; the basic constituent of lecithin and the precursor of acetylcholine, it prevents fat deposition in the liver. **c. acetylase, c. acetyltransferase,** an enzyme that brings about the synthesis of acetylcholine.

cholinergic (ko″lin-er′jik) parasympathomimetic: activated or transmitted by choline (acetylcholine); said of nerve fibers that liberate acetylcholine at a synapse when a nerve impulse passes, i.e., the parasympathetic fibers. Also, an agent that produces such an effect.

cholinesterase (-es′ter-ās) 1. an enzyme that catalyzes the hydrolysis of acylcholine to choline and an anion. 2. acetylcholinesterase.

cholinolytic (ko″lin-o-lit′ik) 1. blocking the action of acetylcholine, or of cholinergic agents. 2. an agent that blocks the action of acetylcholine in cholinergic areas, i.e., organs supplied by parasympathetic nerves, and voluntary muscles.

cholinomimetic (-mi-met′ik) having an action similar to that of choline.

cholochrome (ko′lo-krōm) a biliary pigment.

Cholografin (ko″lo-gra′fin) trademark for preparations of iodipamide.

cholohemothorax (-he″mo-tho′raks) the presence of bile and blood in the thorax.

chololithiasis (-lĭ-thi′ah-sis) cholelithiasis.

cholothorax (-tho′raks) cholohemothorax.

choluria (ko-lu′re-ah) the presence of bile in the urine; discoloration of the urine with bile pigments. **cholu′ric,** adj.

chondr(o)- word element [Gr.], *cartilage.*

chondral (kon′dral) pertaining to cartilage.

chondralgia (kon-dral′je-ah) pain in a cartilage.

chondrectomy (kon-drek′to-me) surgical removal of a cartilage.

chondrification (kon″drĭ-fi-ka′shun) conversion into cartilage.

chondrin (kon′drin) a protein from cartilage.

chondrio- word element [Gr.], *cartilage; granule.*

chondriome (kon′dre-ōm) the total mitochondrial content of a cell.

chondriosome (kon′dre-o-sōm″) mitochondrion.

chondritis (kon-dri′tis) inflammation of a cartilage.

chondroadenoma (kon″dro-ad″ĕ-no′mah) adenochondroma.

chondroangioma (-an″je-o′mah) a benign mesenchymoma containing chondromatous and angiomatous elements.

chondroblast (kon′dro-blast) an immature cartilage-producing cell.

chondroblastoma (kon″dro-blas-to′mah) a benign tumor arising from young chondroblasts in the epiphysis of a bone.

chondrocalcinosis (-kal″sĭ-no′sis) 1. deposition of calcium in cartilage. 2. pseudogout.

chondroclast (kon′dro-klast) a giant cell believed to be concerned in absorption of cartilage.

Chondrococcus (kon″dro-kok′kus) a genus of schizomycetes (family Myxococcaceae) found in animal dung.

chondroconia (-ko′ne-ah) Schridde's granules.

chondrocostal (-kos′tal) pertaining to the ribs and costal cartilages.

chondrocranium (-kra′ne-um) the cartilaginous cranial structure of the embryo.

chondrocyte (kon′dro-sīt) a cartilage cell. **chondrocyt′ic,** adj.

chondrodermatitis (kon″dro-der″mah-ti′tis) an inflammatory process that involves cartilage and skin; used almost exclusively to mean *c. nodula′ris chron′ica hel′icis,* a condition marked by a painful nodule on the helix of the ear.

chondrodynia (-din′e-ah) pain in a cartilage.

chondrodysplasia (-dis-pla′ze-ah) enchondromatosis.

chondrodystrophia (-dis-tro′fe-ah) chondrodystrophy. **c. feta′lis,** achondroplasia.

chondrodystrophy (-dis′tro-fe) a disorder of cartilage formation.

chondroendothelioma (-en″do-the″le-o′mah) an endothelioma containing cartilage tissue.

chondroepiphysitis (-ep″ĭ-fiz-i′tis) inflammation involving the epiphyseal cartilages.

chondrofibroma (-fi-bro′mah) a fibroma with cartilaginous elements.

chondrogen (kon′dro-jen) a substance regarded as the basis of cartilage and of corneal tissue.

chondrogenesis (kon″dro-jen′ĕ-sis) formation of cartilage.

chondrogenic (-jen′ik) giving rise to or forming cartilage.

chondroid (kon′droid) resembling cartilage.

chondroitin (kon-dro′ĭ-tin) a mucopolysaccharide, $C_{18}H_{27}NO_{14}$; its sulfate ester is widespread in connective tissue, particularly cartilage, and in the cornea.

chondroitinuria (kon″dro-ĭ-tin-u′re-ah) the presence of chondroitic acid in the urine.

chondrolipoma (-lĭ-po′mah) a benign tumor containing cartilaginous and fatty tissue.

chondroma (kon-dro′mah) a tumor or tumor-like growth of cartilage cells. **joint c.,** a mass of cartilage in the synovial membrane of a joint. **c. sarcomato′sum,** chondrosarcoma. **synovial c.,** a cartilaginous body formed in a synovial membrane.

chondromalacia (kon″dro-mah-la′she-ah) abnormal softening of cartilage.

chondromatosis (-mah-to′sis) formation of multiple chondromas. **synovial c.,** a rare condition in which cartilage is formed in the synovial membrane of joints, tendon sheaths, or bursae, sometimes becoming detached and producing a number of loose bodies.

chondromere (kon′dro-mēr) a cartilaginous vertebra of the fetal vertebral column.

chondrometaplasia (kon″dro-met″ah-pla′ze-ah) a condition characterized by metaplastic activity of the chondroblasts.

chondromucin (-mu′sin) a compound of chondroitic acid and mucin forming the intercellular substance of cartilage.

chondromucoid (-mu′koid) chondromucin.

chondromucoprotein (-mu″ko-pro′te-in) the principal constituent of the ground substance of cartilage, a copolymer of a mucoprotein, chondroitin-4-sulfate (chondroitin sulfate A), and chondroitin-6-sulfate (chondroitin sulfate C).

Chondromyces (-mi′sēz) a genus of schizomycetes (family Polyangiaceae), found in animal manure and decaying fungi.

chondromyoma (-mi-o′mah) a benign tumor containing myomatous and cartilaginous elements.

chondromyxoma (-mik-so′mah) myxoma with cartilaginous elements.

chondromyxosarcoma (-mik″so-sar-ko′mah) a sarcoma containing cartilaginous and mucous tissue.

chondro-osseous (-os′e-us) composed of cartilage and bone.

chondro-osteodystrophy (-os″te-o-dis′tro-fe) Morquio's syndrome.

chondropathy (kon-drop′ah-the) disease of cartilage.

chondrophyte (kon′dro-fīt) a cartilaginous growth at the articular extremity of a bone.

chondroplasia (kon″dro-pla′ze-ah) the formation of cartilage by specialized cells (chondrocytes).

chondroplast (kon′dro-plast) chondroblast.

chondroplasty (-plas″te) plastic repair of cartilage.

chondroporosis (kon″dro-po-ro′sis) the formation of sinuses or spaces in cartilage.

chondroprotein (-pro′te-in) any of a series of glycoproteins occurring in cartilage.

chondrosamine (kon-dro′sam-in) a galactosamine which results from hydrolysis of chondrosin.

chondrosarcoma (kon″dro-sar-ko′ma) a malignant tumor derived from cartilage cells or their precursors. **central c.,** one within the interior of a bone.

chondrosin (kon′dro-sin) a disaccharide, the most common aldohexuronic acid in nature occurring as a structural unit; obtained by hydrolysis of chondroitins and chondroitin sulfates.

chondrosis (kon-dro′sis) the formation of cartilage.

chondrosteoma (kon″dros-te-o′mah) osteochondroma.

chondrosternal (kon″dro-ster′nal) pertaining to the costal cartilages and sternum.

chondrosternoplasty (-ster′no-plas″te) surgical correction of funnel chest.

chondrotomy (kon-drot′o-me) the dissection or surgical division of cartilage.

chondroxiphoid (kon″dro-zi′foid) pertaining to the xiphoid process.

chondrus (kon′drus) the dried, sun-bleached plant of the seaweed *Chondrus crispus;* used as a protective agent for the skin.

chonechondrosternon (ko″ne-kon″dro-ster′-non) funnel chest.

chord (kord) cord.

chorda (kor′dah), pl. *chor′dae* [L.] a cord or sinew. **chor′dal,** adj. **c. dorsa′lis,** notochord. **c. gubernac′ulum,** a portion of the gubernaculum testis or of the round ligament of the uterus that develops in the inguinal crest and adjoining body wall. **c. mag′na,** Achilles tendon. **chor′dae tendin′eae,** tendinous cords connecting the two atrioventricular valves to the appropriate papillary muscles in the heart ventricles. **c. tym′pani,** a nerve originating from the intermediate nerve, distributed to the submandibular, sublingual, and lingual glands and anterior two-thirds of the tongue; it is a parasympathetic and special senory nerve. **c. umbilica′lis,** umbilical cord. **c. voca′lis,** see *vocal cords.* **chor′dae willis′ii,** Willis' cords.

Chordata (kor-da′tah) a phylum of the animal kingdom comprising all animals having a notochord during some developmental stage.

chordate (kor′dāt) 1. an animal of the Chordata. 2. having a notochord.

chordee (kor′de) downward deflection of the penis, due to a congenital anomaly or to urethral infection.

chorditis (kor-di′tis) inflammation of the vocal or the spermatic cords.

chordoma (kor-do′mah) a malignant tumor arising from the embryonic remains of the notochord.

chordoskeleton (kor″do-skel′ĕ-ton) the part of the skeleton formed about the notochord.

chordotomy (kor-dot′o-me) surgical division of the anterolateral tracts of the spinal cord.

chorea (ko-re′ah) the ceaseless occurrence of rapid, jerky involuntary movements. **chore′ic,** adj. **acute c.,** Sydenham's c. **Bergeron's c.,** electric chorea of childhood, characterized by violent rhythmic spasms, but running a benign course; see also *c. major.* **chronic c.,** Huntington's c. **Dubini's c.,** an acute, fatal form of electric chorea due to acute infection of the central nervous system. **electric c.,** a variety with violent and sudden movements. See *Bergeron's c., Dubini's c.,* and *Henoch's c.* **c. gravida′rum,** Sydenham's chorea occurring in early pregnancy, with or without a previous history of rheumatic fever. **Henoch's c.,** chronic progressive electric chorea; see also *c. major.* **hereditary c., Huntington's c.,** a hereditary disease marked by chronic progressive chorea and mental deterioration. **c. insa′niens,** a grave form of chorea associated with mania, and usually ending fatally. **limp c.,** chorea accompanied by extreme muscular weakness. **maniacal c.,** c. insaniens. **mimetic c.,** chorea caused by imitation. **Sydenham's c.,** an acute, usually self-limited disorder, chiefly occurring between the ages of 5 and 15, or during pregnancy, closely linked with rheumatic fever, and marked by involuntary movements that gradually become severe, affecting all motor activities.

choreiform (ko-re′ĭ-form) resembling chorea.

choreoathetosis (ko″re-o-ath″ĕ-to′sis) a condition characterized by choreic and athetoid movements. **choreoath′etoid,** adj.

choreophrasia (-fra′ze-ah) meaningless repetition of words or phrases.

chorioadenoma (-ad″ĕ-no′mah) adenoma of the chorion. **c. destru′ens,** a form of hydatidiform mole in which molar chorionic villi penetrate into the myometrium and/or parametrium or are transported to distant sites, most often the lungs.

chorioallantois (-ah-lan′to-is) an extraembryonic structure formed by union of the chorion and allantois which by means of vessels in the associated mesoderm serves in gas exchange. In reptiles and birds, it is a membrane apposed to the shell; in many mammals, it forms the placenta. **chorioallanto′ic,** adj.

chorioamnionitis (-am″ne-o-ni′tis) bacterial infection of the fetal membranes.

chorioangioma (-an″je-o′mah) an angioma of the chorion.

choriocapillaris (-kap″ĭ-la′ris) the capillary layer of the choroid.

choriocarcinoma (-kar″sĭ-no′mah) a malignant neoplasm of trophoblastic cells, formed by abnormal proliferation of the placental epithelium, without production of chorionic villi.

choriocele (ko′re-o-sēl″) protrusion of the chorion through an aperture.

chorioepithelioma (ko″re-o-ep″ĭ-the″le-o′mah) choriocarcinoma.

choriogenesis (-jen′ĕ-sis) the development of the chorion.

chorioid (ko′re-oid) choroid.

chorioma (ko″re-o′mah) any trophoblastic proliferation, benign or malignant.

choriomeningitis (ko″re-o-men″in-ji′tis) cerebral meningitis with lymphocytic infiltration of the choroid plexus. **lymphocytic c.,** a form of viral meningitis, usually occurring in adults between the ages of 20 and 40, during the fall and winter months.

chorion (ko′re-on) the outermost of the fetal membranes, composed of trophoblast lined with mesoderm; it develops villi, becomes vascularized by allantoic vessels, and forms the fetal part of the placenta. **chorion′ic,** adj. **c. frondo′sum,** the part of chorion covered by villi. **c. lae′ve,** the smooth, membranous part of the chorion. **shaggy c.,** c. frondosum.

Chorioptes (ko″re-op′tēz) a genus of parasitic mites infesting domestic animals and causing a kind of mange.

chorioretinal (ko″re-o-ret′ĭ-nal) pertaining to the choroid and retina.

chorioretinitis (-ret″ĭ-ni′tis) inflammation of the choroid and retina.

chorioretinopathy (-ret″ĭ-nop′ah-the) a noninflammatory process involving both the choroid and retina.

chorista (ko-ris′tah) defective development due to, or marked by, displacement of the primordium.

choristoma (ko″ris-to′mah) a mass of histologically normal tissue in an abnormal location.

choroid (ko′roid) the middle, vascular coat of the eye, between the sclera and the retina. **choroid′al,** adj.

choroidea (ko-roi′de-ah) choroid.

choroideremia (ko-roi″der-e′me-ah) hereditary (X-linked) primary choroidal degeneration which, in males, eventually leads to blindness as degeneration of the retinal pigment epithelium progresses to complete atrophy; in females, it is nonprogressive and vision is usually normal.

choroiditis (ko″roi-di′tis) inflammation of the choroid.

choroidocyclitis (ko-roi″do-sik-li′tis) inflammation of the choroid and ciliary processes.

choroidoiritis (-i-ri′tis) inflammation of the choroid and iris.

choroidoretinitis (-ret″ĭ-ni′tis) inflammation of the choroid and retina.

chrom(o)- word element [Gr.], *color.*

chromaffin (kro-maf′in) staining strongly with chromium salts, as certain cells of the adrenal glands, along sympathetic nerves, etc.

chromaffinity (kro″mah-fin′ĭ-te) the property of staining strongly with chrome salts.

chromaffinoma (kro-maf″ĭ-no′mah) 1. any tumor containing chromaffin cells. 2. pheochromocytoma.

chromaffinopathy (-nop′ah-the) disease of the chromaffin system.

chromaphil (kro′mah-fil) chromaffin.

chromat(o)- word element [Gr.], *color; chromatin.*

chromate (kro′māt) any salt of chromic acid.

chromatelopsia (kro″mat-el-op′se-ah) imperfect perception of colors.

chromatic (kro-mat′ik) 1. pertaining to color; stainable with dyes. 2. pertaining to chromatin.

chromatid (kro′mah-tid) either of two parallel, spiral filaments joined at the centromere which make up a chromosome, and which divide in cell division, each going to a different pole of the dividing cell and each becoming a chromosome of one of the two daughter cells.

chromatin (kro′mah-tin) the more readily stainable portion of the cell nucleus, composed of DNA attached to a protein base; it is the carrier of the genes. **sex c.,** Barr body; the persistent mass of the material of the inactivated X chromosome in cells of normal females.

chromatin-negative (-neg′ah-tiv) lacking sex chromatin, a characteristic of the nuclei of cells in a normal male.

chromatin-positive (-poz′ĭ-tiv) containing sex chromatin, a characteristic of the nuclei of cells in a normal female.

chromatism (kro′mah-tizm) 1. hallucinatory perception of color. 2. abnormal pigmentation.

chromatogenous (kro″mah-toj′ĕ-nus) producing color or coloring matter.

chromatogram (kro-mat′o-gram) the record produced by chromatography.

chromatograph (-graf) 1. to analyze by chromatography. 2. the apparatus used in chromatography.

chromatography (kro″mah-tog′rah-fe) the separation of closely related compounds in a mixture by introducing the mixture (mobile phase) into an adsorbent medium (stationary phase), the constituent compounds forming bands at different levels along the medium according to their velocity through it. **chromatograph′ic,** adj. **electric c.,** electrochromatography. **gas c.,** that in which an inert gas is used to move the vapors of the materials to be separated through a column of inert material. **gas-liquid c.,** that in which the substances to be separated are moved by an inert gas along a long tube filled with a finely divided inert solid coated with a nonvolatile oil; each component migrates at a rate determined by its solubility in oil and its vapor pressure. **paper c.,** that in which a sheet of blotting paper, usually filter paper, is substituted for the adsorption column. **partition c.,** a method of separation of solutes utilizing the partition of the solutes between two liquid phases, namely, the original solvent and the film of solvent on the adsorption column. **thin-layer c.,** chromatography through a thin layer of inert material, such as cellulose.

chromatokinesis (kro″mah-to-ki-ne′sis) movement of chromatin during the life and division of a cell.

chromatolysis (kro″mah-tol′ĭ-sis) 1. the solution and disintegration of the chromatin of cell nuclei. 2. disintegration of Nissl bodies of a neuron as a result of injury, fatigue, or exhaustion.

chromatometer (-tom′ĕ-ter) an instrument for measuring color or color perception.

chromatophil (kro-mat′o-fil) a cell or structure which stains easily. **chromatophil′ic,** adj.

chromatophore (-fōr) any pigmentary cell or color-producing plastid.

chromatopsia (kro″mah-top′se-ah) a visual defect in which (a) colorless objects appear to be tinged with color, or (b) colors are imperfectly perceived.

chromatoptometer (kro″mop-tom′ĕ-ter) a device for measuring color perception.

chromatoptometry (-top-tom′ĕ-tre) measurement of color perception.

chromaturia (kro″mah-tu′re-ah) abnormal coloration of the urine.

chromesthesia (kro″mes-the′ze-ah) association of imaginary color sensations with actual sensations of taste, hearing, or smell.

chromhidrosis (kro″mĭ-dro′sis) secretion of colored sweat.

chromicize (kro′mĭ-sīz) to treat with chromium.

chromidiosis (kro-mid″e-o′sis) outflow of chromatin and nuclear substance from the nucleus to the cytoplasm of a cell.

chromidium (kro-mid′e-um), pl. *chromid′ia.* A granule of extranuclear chromatin in the cytoplasm of a cell.

chromidrosis (kro″mĭ-dro′sis) chromhidrosis.

chromium (kro′me-um) chemical element (*see table*), at. no. 24, symbol Cr. **c. oxide,** a substance used in dentistry as a polishing agent, especially for stainless steel. **c. trioxide,** chromic acid (2).

Chromobacterium (kro″mo-bak-te′re-um) a genus of schizomycetes (family Rhizobiaceae) that characteristically produce a violet pigment.

chromoblast (kro′mo-blast) an embryonic cell which develops into a pigment cell.

chromoblastomycosis (kro″mo-blas″to-mi-ko′-sis) chromomycosis.

chromocyte (kro′mo-sīt) any colored cell or pigmented corpuscle.

chromocystoscopy (kro″mo-sis-tos′ko-pe) cystoscopy of the ureteral orifices after oral administration of a dye which is excreted in the urine.

chromodacryorrhea (-dak″re-o-re′ah) the shedding of bloody tears.

chromogen (kro′mo-jen) any substance giving origin to a coloring matter.

chromogenesis (kro″mo-jen′ĕ-sis) the formation of color or pigment.

chromogenic (-jen′ik) producing color or pigment.

chromolipoid (-lip′oid) lipochrome.

chromolysis (kro-mol′ĭ-sis) chromatolysis.

chromomere (kro′mo-mēr) 1. any of the beadlike granules occurring in series along a chromonema. 2. granulomere.

chromomycosis (kro″mo-mi-ko′sis) a chronic fungal infection of the skin, producing wartlike nodules or papillomas that may ulcerate.

chromonema (-ne′mah) any of the coiled threads in anaphase and telophase chromo-somes, later giving rise to the spireme. **chromone′mal,** adj.

chromoparic (-par′ik) producing color.

chromopectic (-pek′tik) pertaining to, characterized by, or promoting chromopexy.

chromopexic (-pek′sik) chromopectic.

chromopexy (kro′mo-pek″se) the fixation of pigment, especially by the liver in the formation of bilirubin.

chromophage (-fāj) pigmentophage.

chromophane (-fān) a retinal pigment.

chromophil (-fil) any easily stainable cell or tissue. **chromophil′ic,** adj.

chromophobe (-fōb) any cell, structure, or tissue not readily stainable, applied especially to the chromophobe cells of the anterior pituitary gland.

chromophobia (kro″mo-fo′be-ah) the quality of staining poorly with dyes. **chromopho′bic,** adj.

chromophore (kro′mo-fōr) any chemical group whose presence gives a decided color to a compound and which unites with certain other groups (auxochromes) to form dyes.

chromophoric (kro″mo-fōr′ik) 1. bearing color. 2. pertaining to a chromophore.

chromophose (kro′mo-fōs) a subjective sensation of color.

chromoplasm (-plazm) chromatin.

chromoplastid (kro″mo-plas′tid) any pigment-producing cell other than a chloroplast.

chromoprotein (-pro′te-in) a colored conjugated protein, e.g., the red hemoglobin of higher animals, which has a respiratory function and is closely related to the chlorophyll of higher plants.

chromopsia (kro-mop′se-ah) chromatopsia.

chromoscopy (kro-mos′ko-pe) diagnosis of renal function by color of the urine after administration of dyes. **gastric c.,** diagnosis of gastric function by the color of the gastric contents; a test for achylia gastrica.

chromosome (kro′mo-sōm) in animal cells, a structure in the nucleus containing a linear thread of DNA which transmits genetic information and is associated with RNA and histones; during cell division the material composing the chromosome is compactly coiled, making it visible with appropriate staining and permitting its movement in the cell with minimal entanglement; each organism of a species is normally characterized by the same number of chromosomes in its somatic cells, 46 being the number normally present in man, including the two (XX or XY) which determine the sex of the organism. In bacterial genetics, a closed circle of double-stranded DNA which contains the genetic material of the cell and is attached to the cell membrane; the bulk of this material forms a compact bacterial nucleus. **chromoso′mal,** adj. **bivalent c.,** see *bivalent* (2). **Christchurch c.,** an autosome of Group G, with deletion of the short arms, first found in two siblings with chronic lymphocytic leukemia; now considered to be a variant found incidentally in patients with different defects. Symbol Ch[1]. **gametic c.,** one in a haploid cell (gamete) consisting of a double strand of DNA. **homologous c's,** the chromosomes of a matching pair in the diploid complement that contain alleles of specific genes. **Ph¹ c., Philadelphia c.,** an abnormality of chromosome 21, characterized by shortening of its long arms, seen in the leukocytes of most patients with chronic leukemia. **ring c.,** a chromosome in which both ends have been lost (deletion) and the two broken ends have reunited to form a ring-shaped figure. **sex c's,** chromosomes associated with sex determination, in mammals constituting an unequal pair, the X and the Y chromosome. **somatic c.,** autosome. **W c's,** the sex chromosomes of certain insects, birds, and fishes, in which the female is heterogametic (i.e., has a W and a Z chromosome) and the males are homogametic (having only Z chromosomes). **X c.,** the female sex chromosome, being carried by half the male gametes and all female gametes; female diploid cells have two X chromosomes. **Y c.,** the male sex chromosome, being carried by half the male gametes and none of the female gametes; male diploid cells have an X and a Y chromosomes. **Z c's,** see *W c's.*

chromotoxic (kro″mo-tok′sik) destructive to hemoglobin or due to destruction of hemoglobin.

chromotropic (-trop′ik) turning to or attracting color or pigment.

chron(o)- word element [Gr.], *time.*

chronaxie, chronaxy (kro′nak-se) the minimum time an electric current must flow at a voltage twice the rheobase to cause a muscle to contract.

chronic (kron′ik) persisting for a long time.

chronobiology (kron″o-bi-ol′o-je) the scientific study of the effect of time on living systems.

chronognosis (kron″og-no′sis) perception of the lapse of time.

chronograph (kron′o-graf) an instrument for recording small intervals of time.

chronoscope (-skōp) an instrument for measuring small intervals of time.

chronotaraxis (kron″o-tar-ak′sis) disorientation in relation to time.

chronotropic (-trop′ik) affecting the time or rate.

chronotropism (kro-not′ro-pizm) interference with regularity of a periodical movement, such as the heart's action.

chrys(o)- word element [Gr.], *gold.*

chrysarobin (kris″ah-ro′bin) a mixture of neutral principles derived from goa powder; used in treatment of psoriasis and other chronic skin diseases.

chrysiasis (krĭ-si′ah-sis) deposition of gold in living tissue.

chrysoderma (kris″o-der′mah) permanent pigmentation of the skin due to gold deposit.

Chrysomyia (-mi′yah) a genus of flies whose larvae may be secondary invaders of wounds or internal parasites of man.

Chrysops (kris′ops) a genus of bloodsucking tropical flies, the grove flies, including *C. disca′- lis,* a vector of tularemia in the western United States, and *C. sila′cea,* an intermediate host of *Loa loa.*

chrysotherapy (kris″o-ther′ah-pe) treatment with gold salts.

chthonophagia (thon″o-fa′je-ah) geophagia.

chylangioma (ki-lan″je-o′mah) a tumor of intestinal lymph vessels filled with chyle.

chyle (kīl) the milky fluid taken up by the lacteals from food in the intestine during digestion, consisting of lymph and triglyceride fat (chylomicrons) in a stable emulsion, and passed into the veins by the thoracic duct, becoming mixed with blood.

chylectasia (ki″lek-ta′ze-ah) dilatation of a chylous vessel, e.g., a lacteal.

chylemia (ki-le′me-ah) the presence of chyle in the blood.

chylifacient (ki″lĭ-fa′shent) forming chyle.

chylifaction (-fak′shun) chylification. **chylifac′tive,** adj.

chyliferous (ki-lif′er-us) 1. forming chyle. 2. conveying chyle.

chylification (ki″lĭ-fĭ-ka′shun) the formation of chyle.

chyliform (ki′lĭ-form) resembling chyle.

chylocele (ki′lo-sēl) elephantiasis scroti.

chylocyst (-sist) cisterna chyli.

chyloderma (ki″lo-der′mah) elephantiasis filariensis.

chylology (ki-lol′o-je) the study of chyle.

chylomediastinum (ki″lo-me″de-as-ti′num) the presence of chyle in the mediastinum.

chylomicron (-mi′kron) a stable droplet containing triglyceride fat, cholesterol, phospholipids, and protein, found in intestinal lymphatics (lacteals) and blood during and after meals.

chylomicronemia (-mi″kro-ne′me-ah) an excess of chylomicrons in the blood.

chylopericardium (-per″ĭ-kar′de-um) the presence of effused chyle in the pericardium.

chyloperitoneum (-per″ĭ-to-ne′um) the presence of effused chyle in the peritoneal cavity.

chylophoric (-for′ik) conveying chyle.

chylopneumothorax (-nu″mo-tho′raks) the presence of chyle and air in the pleural cavity.

chylopoiesis (-poi-e′sis) chylification. **chylopoiet′ic,** adj.

chylothorax (-tho′raks) the presence of effused chyle in the pleural cavity.

chylous (ki′lus) pertaining, mingled with, or of the nature of chyle.

chyluria (ki-lu′re-ah) the presence of chyle in the urine, giving it a milky appearance.

Chymar (ki′mar) trademark for preparations of chymotrypsin.

chymase (ki′mās) an enzyme of the gastric juice which hastens the action of the pancreatic juice.

chyme (kīm) the semifluid, homogeneous, creamy or gruel-like material produced by gastric digestion of food.

chymification (ki″mĭ-fĭ-ka′shun) conversion of food into chyme; gastric digestion.

chymosin (ki-mo′sin) rennin.

chymotrypsin (ki″mo-trip′sin) an endopeptidase with action similar to that of trypsin, produced in the intestine by activation of chymotrypsinogen by trypsin; a product crystallized from an extract of the pancreas of the ox is used clinically.

chymotrypsinogen (-trip-sin′o-jen) the inactive precursor of chymotrypsin, the form in which it is secreted by the pancreas.

C.I. color index.

Ci abbreviation for *curie* recommended by the International Commission on Radiological Units and Measurements.

cib. [L.] *ci′bus* (food).

cicatrectomy (sik″ah-trek′to-me) excision of a cicatrix.

cicatricial (sik″ah-trish′al) pertaining to or of the nature of a cicatrix.

cicatrix (sĭ-ka′triks, sik′ah-triks), pl. *cica′trices* [L.] a scar; the fibrous tissue left after the healing of a wound. **vicious c.,** one causing deformity or impairing the function of an extremity.

cicatrization (sik″ah-tri-za′shun) the formation of a cicatrix or scar.

cicutoxin (sik″u-toks′in) a very poisonous principle from plants of the genus *Cicuta,* including the water hemlocks *C. maculata* and *C. virosa.*

-cide word element [L.], *destruction or killing* (homicide); *an agent which kills or destroys* (germicide). **-ci′dal,** adj.

cili(o)- word element [L.], *cilia; ciliary* (*body*).

cilia (sil′e-ah), sing. *cil′ium* [L.] 1. the eyelashes. 2. minute, motile, hairlike processes attached to the free surface of a cell.

ciliariscope (sil″e-ar′ĭ-skōp) an instrument for examining ciliary region of eye.

ciliarotomy (-ar-ot′o-me) surgical division of the ciliary zone.

ciliary (sil′e-er″e) pertaining to or resembling cilia; used particularly in reference to certain eye structures, as the ciliary body or muscle.

Ciliata (sil″e-a′tah) a class of protozoa (subphylum Ciliophora) whose members possess cilia throughout the life cycle; a few species are parasitic.

ciliate (sil′e-āt) 1. having cilia. 2. any individual of the Ciliophora.

ciliated (sil′e-āt″ed) provided with cilia.

ciliectomy (sil″e-ek′to-me) 1. excision of a portion of the ciliary body. 2. excision of the portion of the eyelid containing the roots of the lashes.

Ciliophora (sil″e-of′o-rah) a subphylum of protozoa whose members possess cilia during some developmental stage and usually have two kinds of nuclei (a micro- and a macronucleus); it includes the Ciliata and Suctoria.

cilioretinal (sil″e-o-ret′ĭ-nal) pertaining to the ciliary body and retina.

cilioscleral (-skle′ral) pertaining to the ciliary body and sclera.

ciliospinal (-spi′nal) pertaining to the ciliary body and spinal cord.

cilium (sil′e-um) singular of *cilia.*

Cillobacterium (sil″lo-bak-te′re-um) a genus of schizomycetes (tribe Lactobacilleae) found in the intestinal tract and occasionally associated with purulent infections.

cillosis (sil-lo′sis) spasmodic quivering of the eyelid.

cimbia (sim′be-ah) a white band running across the ventral surface of the crus cerebri.

Cimex (si′meks) a genus of blood-sucking insects (order Hemiptera), the bedbugs; it includes *C. boue′ti* of West Africa and South America, *C. lectula′rius* the common bedbug of temperate regions, and *C. rotunda′tus* of the tropics.

cinchona (sin-ko′nah) the dried bark of the stem or root of various South American trees of the genus *Cinchona;* it is the source of quinine, cinchonine, and other alkaloids.

cinchonine (sin′ko-nēn) an alkaloid, $C_{19}H_{22}N_2O$, from cinchona, used like quinine as an antimalarial.

cinchonism (sin′ko-nizm) the morbid or injurious effects of the injudicious use of cinchona or its alkaloids.

cine- word element [Gr.], *movement;* see also words beginning *kine-.*

cineangiocardiography (sin″e-an″je-o-kar″-de-og′rah-fe) the photographic recording of fluoroscopic images of the heart and great vessels by motion picture techniques.

cineangiography (-an″je-og′rah-fe) the photographic recording of fluoroscopic images of the blood vessels by motion picture techniques.

cinedensigraphy (sin″ĕ-den-sig′rah-fe) graphic recording of movements of interal body structures by means of roentgen rays and radiosensitive cells.

cinefluorography (-floo″or-og′rah-fe) cineradiography.

cinematics (-mat′iks) kinematics.

cinematography (-mah-tog′rah-fe) the taking of motion pictures.

cinematoradiography (-mah-to-ra″de-og′rah-fe) the recording of x-ray images by motion picture techniques; cinefluorography.

cinemicrography (-mi-krog′rah-fe) the making of motion pictures of a small object through the lens system of a microscope.

cinephlebography (-flĕ-bog′rah-fe) cineradiography of the veins after administration of a contrast medium. In *ascending functional c.,* the contrast medium is introduced into a vein in the foot and its progress is observed as it courses through the tibial, popiteal, femoral, and iliac veins.

cineplasty (sin′ĕ-plas″te) kineplasty.

cineradiography (sin″ĕ-ra″de-og′rah-fe) the making of a motion picture record of successive images appearing on a fluoroscopic screen.

cinerea (sĭ-ne′ra-ah) the gray matter of the nervous system. **cine′real,** adj.

cineroentgenofluorography (sin″e-rent″gen-o-floo″or-og′rah-fe) cineradiography.

cinesi- for words beginning thus, see those beginning *kinesi-.*

cineto- for words beginning thus, see those beginning *kineto-.*

cingulectomy (sing″gu-lek′to-me) bilateral extirpation of the anterior half of the gyrus cinguli.

cingulotomy (sing″gu-lot′o-me) the creation of lesions in the cingulum of the frontal lobe for relief of intractable pain.

cingulum (sing'gu-lum), pl. *cin'gula* [L.] 1. an encircling structure or part; a girdle. 2. a bundle of association fibers partly encircling the corpus callosum not far from the median plane, interrelating the cingulate and hippocampal gyri. 3. the lingual lobe of an anterior tooth. **cing'ulate,** adj.

cinnamon (sin'ah-mun) the dried bark of *Cinnamomum loureirii;* cordial, carminative, and flavoring agent.

C.I.O.M.S. Council for International Organization of Medical Sciences.

circadian (ser''kah-de'an, ser-ka'de-an) denoting a period of about 24 hours; see under *rhythm.*

circinate (ser'sĭ-nāt) resembling a ring, or circle.

circle (ser'k'l) a round figure, structure, or part. **Berry's c's,** charts with circles on them for testing stereoscopic vision. **defensive c.,** the coexistence of two conditions which tend to have an antagonistic or inhibiting effect on each other. **diffusion c.,** a confused image formed on the retina when the retina is not at the focus of the eye. **c. of Haller,** a circle of arteries in the sclera around the site of the entrance of the optic nerve. **Minsky's c.,** a device for the graphic recording of eye lesions. **sensory c.,** a body area within which it is impossible to distinguish separately the impressions arising from two sites of stimulation. **Weber's c's,** circles on the skin delineating the distance at which two simultaneously applied points can be separately distinguished. **c. of Willis,** the anastomotic loop of vessels near the base of the brain.

circling (ser'kling) movement in a circle; a name applied to listeriosis in sheep, because of the tendency of affected animals to move in a circle.

circulation (ser''ku-la'shun) movement in regular or circuitous course, as the movement of blood through the heart and blood vessels. **allantoic c.,** circulation in the fetus through the umbilical vessels. **collateral c.,** that carried on through secondary channels after obstruction of the principal channel supplying the part. **coronary c.,** that within the coronary vessels. **extracorporeal c.,** circulation of blood outside the body, as through an artificial kidney or a heart-lung apparatus. **fetal c.,** that propelled by the fetal heart through the fetus, umbilical cord, and placental villi. **first c.,** primitive c. **hypophyseoportal c.,** that passing from the capillaries of the median eminence of the hypothalamus into the portal vessels to the sinusoids of the adenohypophysis. **intervillous c.,** the flow of maternal blood through the intervillous space of the placenta. **lesser c.,** pulmonary c. **omphalomesenteric c.,** vitelline c. **placental c.,** the fetal circulation; also, the maternal circulation through the intervillous space. **portal c.,** a general term denoting the circulation of blood through larger vessels from the capillaries of one organ to those of another; applied especially to the passage of blood from the gastrointestinal tract and spleen through the portal vein to the liver. **primitive c.,** that by which the earliest nutriment and oxygen are conveyed to the developing embryo. **pulmo-**

nary c., the flow of blood from the right ventricle through the pulmonary artery to the lungs, where carbon dioxide is exchanged for oxygen, and back through the pulmonary vein to the left atrium. **sinusoidal c.,** that occurring through the sinusoids of an organ. **systemic c.,** the general circulation, carrying oxygenated blood from the left ventricle to the body tissues, and returning venous blood to the right atrium. **umbilical c.,** allantoic c. **vitelline c.,** the circulation through the blood vessels of the yolk sac.

circulatory (ser'ku-lah-tor''e) pertaining to circulation.

circulus (ser'ku-lus), pl. *cir'culi* [L.] a circle.

circum- word element [L.], *around.*

circumcision (ser''kum-sizh'un) removal of all or part of the foreskin, or prepuce. **female c.,** incision of the fold of skin over the glans clitoridis; clitoridotomy.

circumcorneal (-kōr'ne-al) surrounding the cornea.

circumduction (-duk'shun) circular movement of a limb or of the eye.

circumflex (ser'kum-fleks) curved like a bow.

circuminsular (ser''kum-in'su-lar) surrounding, situated, or occurring about the insula.

circumlental (-len'tal) situated or occurring around the lens.

circumnuclear (-nu'kle-ar) surrounding or occurring around the nucleus.

circumocular (-ok'u-ler) surrounding or occurring around the eye.

circumrenal (-re'nal) around the kidney.

circumscribed (ser'kum-skrībd) bounded or limited; confined to a limited space.

circumstantiality (ser''kum-stan''she-al'ĭ-te) thinking or conversation characterized by unnecessary elaboration of trivial details.

circumvallate (-val'āt) surrounded by a ridge or trench, as the vallate papillae.

cirrhosis (sĭ-ro'sis) interstitial inflammation of an organ, particularly the liver; see *c. of liver.* **cirrhot'ic,** adj. **atrophic c.,** cirrhosis in which the liver is decreased in size. **biliary c.,** cirrhosis of the liver from chronic bile retention, due to obstruction or infection of the major extra- or intrahepatic bile ducts (*secondary biliary c.*), or of unknown etiology (*primary biliary c.*), and sometimes occurring after administration of certain drugs. **Cruveilhier-Baumgarten c.,** see under *syndrome.* **fatty c.,** a form in which liver cells become infiltrated with fat. **hypertrophic c.,** primary biliary c. **Laennec's c.,** cirrhosis of the liver associated with alcohol abuse. **c. of liver,** a group of liver diseases marked by loss of normal hepatic architecture, with fibrosis and nodular regeneration. **metabolic c.,** cirrhosis of the liver associated with metabolic diseases, such as hemochromatosis, Wilson's disease, glycogen storage disease, galactosemia, and disorders of amino acid metabolism. **portal c.,** Laennec's c. **posthepatitic c.,** that (usually macronodular) resulting as a sequel to acute hepatitis. **postnecrotic c.,** that which follows submassive necrosis of the liver (subacute yellow atrophy) due to toxic or viral hepatitis; the reticulin framework of normal lobules collapses and may be replaced by broad bands of fibrous tissue separating regeneration nodules (multilobular liver) of varying size. **Todd's c.,** primary biliary c.

cirrus (sir'us), pl. *cir'ri* [L.] a slender, usually flexible, appendage, as the muscular retractile copulatory organ of certain trematodes, or one of the organs of locomotion of ciliate protozoa, which are composed of fused cilia.

cirsectomy (ser-sek'to-me) excision of a portion of a varicose vein.

cirsoid (ser'soid) resembling a varix.

cirsomphalos (ser-som'fah-los) caput medusae.

cis (sis) [L.] in organic chemistry, having certain atoms or radicals on the same side; in genetics, having the two mutant genes of a pseudoallele on the same chromosome.

11-*cis* retinal see *retinal* (2).

cistern (sis'tern) a closed space serving as a reservoir for fluid, e.g., one of the enlarged spaces of the body containing lymph or other fluid. **cister'nal,** adj. **c. of Pecquet,** receptaculum chyli.

cisterna (sis-ter'nah), pl. *cister'nae* [L.] cistern. **c. cerebellomedulla'ris,** the enlarged subarachnoid space between the undersurface of the cerebellum and the posterior surface of the medulla oblongata. **c. chy'li,** the dilated part of the thoracic duct at its origin in the lumbar region.

cistron (sis'tron) the smallest unit of genetic material that must be intact to function as a transmitter of genetic information; as traditionally construed, approximately synonymous with gene.

citrate (sit'rāt, si'trāt) a salt of citric acid.

citrated (sit'rāt-ed) containing a citrate, especially potassium citrate.

citreoviridin (si''tre-o-vir'ĭ-din) a toxic compound isolated from the fungus *Penicillium citreoviride,* said to have the empirical formula of $C_{23}H_{30}O_6$.

citrinin (sit'rĭ-nin) a toxic antibiotic, $C_{13}H_{14}O_5$, produced by *Penicillium citrinum* and some species of *Aspergillus;* active against gram-positive bacteria.

citronella (sit''ron-el'ah) a fragrant grass, the source of a volatile oil (citronella oil) used in perfumes and insect repellents.

citrulline (sit-rul'lēn) an alpha-amino acid involved in urea production.

citrullinuria (sit-rul''lĭ-nu're-ah) presence in the urine of large amounts of citrulline, with increased levels also in both plasma and cerebrospinal fluid.

cittosis (sit-to'sis) pica.

Cl chemical symbol, *chlorine.*

cladosporiosis (klad''o-spo''re-o'sis) any infection with *Cladosporium,* including black degeneration of the brain, chromomycosis, and tinea nigra.

Cladosporium (-spo're-um) a genus of imperfect fungi (order Moniliales). *C. herbarum* produces "black spot" on meat in cold storage, growing at a temperature of 18° F. (–8° C.); *C. carrioni* is an agent of chromomycosis; *C. wernecki* and *C.*

mansoni are agents of tinea nigra; *C. trichoides* and other species cause black degeneration of the brain.

clairvoyance (klār-voi'ans) [Fr.] a form of extrasensory perception in which knowledge of objective events is acquired without the use of the senses.

clamp (klamp) a surgical device for compressing a part or structure. **rubber dam c's,** metallic devices used to retain the dam on a tooth.

clap (klap) gonorrhea.

clapotement (klah-pōt-maw') [Fr.] a splashing sound, as in succussion.

clarificant (klah-rif'ĭ-kant) a substance which clears a liquid of turbidity.

clasmatocyte (klaz-mat'o-sīt) a macrophage.

clasmatosis (klaz''mah-to'sis) the breaking off of parts of a cell; the process of cytoplasmic fragmentation by which plasmacytes are said to release synthesized immunoglobulins.

clasmocytoma (klaz''mo-si-to'mah) reticulum cell sarcoma.

clasp (klasp) a device by which something is held.

class (klas) 1. a taxonomic category subordinate to a phylum and superior to an order. 2. a group of variables all of which show a value falling between certain limits.

classification (klas''sĭ-fĭ-ka'shun) the systematic arrangement of similar entities on the basis of certain differing characteristics. **Angle's c.,** a classification of dental malocclusion based on the mesiodistal (anteroposterior) position of the mandibular dental arch and teeth relative to the maxillary dental arch and teeth; see under *malocclusion.* **Caldwell-Moloy c.,** classification of female pelves as gynecoid, android, anthropoid, and platypelloid; see under *pelvis.* **Denver c.,** the classification of human chromosomes on the basis of size and centromere position; the 23 pairs of chromosomes are arranged individually and numbered, or in seven groups (A to G) in order of decreasing length. **Keith-Wagener-Barker c.,** a classification of hypertension and arteriolosclerosis based on retinal changes. **Kraepelin's c.,** a classification of manic-depressive and schizophrenic groups of mental disease. **Lancefield c.,** the classification of hemolytic streptococci into groups on the basis of serologic action.

clastic (klas'tik) 1. undergoing or causing division. 2. separable into parts.

clastothrix (klas'to-thriks) trichorrhexis nodosa.

clathrate (klath'rāt) 1. having the shape or appearance of a lattice; pertaining to clathrate compounds. 2. [pl.] inclusion complexes in which molecules of one type are trapped within cavities of the crystalline lattice of another substance.

claudication (klaw''dĭ-ka'shun) limping; lameness. **intermittent c.,** pain, tension, and weakness in the legs on walking, which intensifies to produce lameness and is relieved by rest; it is seen in occlusive arterial disease. **venous c.,** intermittent claudication due to venous stasis.

claustrophilia (klaws"tro-fil'e-ah) an abnormal desire to be in a closed room or space.

claustrophobia (-fo'be-ah) morbid fear of closed places.

claustrum (klaws'trum), pl. *claus'tra* [L.] the thin layer of gray matter lateral to the external capsule, separating it from the white matter of the insula.

clava (kla'vah) gracile tubercle.

clavacin (klav'ah-sin) patulin.

Claviceps (klav'ĭ-seps) a genus of parasitic fungi that infest various plant seeds. *C. purpu'rea* is the source of ergot.

clavicle (klav'ĭ-k'l) see *Table of Bones.* **clavic'u-lar,** adj.

clavicotomy (klav"ĭ-kot'o-me) surgical division of the clavicle.

clavicula (klah-vik'u-lah) [L.] clavicle.

claviformin (klav"ĭ-for'min) patulin.

clavus (kla'vus), pl. *cla'vi* [L.] a corn. **c. hys-ter'icus,** a sensation as if a nail were being driven into the head.

clawfoot (klaw'foot) a high-arched foot with the toes hyperextended at the metatarsophalangeal joint and flexed at the distal joints.

clawhand (-hand) flexion and atrophy of the hand and fingers.

clearance (klēr'ans) the act of clearing; specifically, complete removal by the kidneys of a solute or solution from a specific volume of blood per unit of time. **blood-urea c.,** the volume of blood cleared of urea per minute by renal elimination. **creatinine c.,** the volume of plasma cleared of creatinine after parenteral administration of a specified amount of the substance. **inulin c.,** an expression of the renal efficiency in eliminating inulin from the blood. **urea c.,** blood-urea c.

cleavage (klēv'ij) division into distinct parts; the early successive splitting of a fertilized ovum into smaller cells (blastomeres) by mitosis. **complete c.,** holoblastic c. **determinate c.,** that in which definite blastomeres give rise to specific embryonic parts. **equatorial c.,** that which occurs in a plane passing through the equator of the egg. **holoblastic c.,** that involving the entire egg. **incomplete c.,** meroblastic c. **indeterminate c.,** that in which the fate of the blastomeres is not fixed, each blastomere, when isolated, being capable of altering its destiny and developing into a whole embryo. **latitudinal c.,** that which occurs in planes passing at right angles to the egg axis. **meridional c.,** that which occurs in planes passing through the egg axis. **meroblastic c., partial c.,** that involving only the protoplasmic portions of the egg.

cleft (kleft) a fissure or longitudinal opening, especially one occurring during the embryonic development. **branchial c's,** a series of openings in the early embryo, separating the branchial arches. **visceral c's,** branchial c's.

cleid(o)- word element [Gr.], *clavicle.*

cleidocranial (kli"do-kra'ne-al) pertaining to the clavicle and the head.

cleidomastoid (-mas'toid) pertaining to the clavicle and mastoid process.

cleidotomy (kli-dot'o-me) surgical division of the clavicle of the fetus in difficult labor to facilitate delivery.

clemizole (klem'ĭ-zōl) an antihistaminic, C_{19}-$H_{20}ClN_3$.

click (klik) a brief, sharp sound, especially any of the short, dry clicking heart sounds during systole, indicative of various heart conditions.

clidinium bromide (klĭ-din'e-um) an anticholinergic, $C_{22}H_{26}BrNO_3$.

climacteric (kli-mak'ter-ik, kli"mak-ter'ik) the syndrome of endocrine, somatic, and psychic changes occurring at the end of the female reproductive period (menopause); it may also accompany normal diminution of sexual activity in the male.

climatology (kli"mah-tol'o-je) the scientific study of natural environmental conditions (e.g., rainfall, temperature) prevailing in specific regions of the earth.

climatotherapy (kli"mah-to-ther'ah-pe) treatment of disease by means of a favorable climate.

climax (kli'maks) the period of greatest intensity, as in the course of a disease.

clindamycin (klin"dah-mi'sin) a semisynthetic antibiotic derivative of lincomycin, $C_{18}H_{33}Cl$-N_2O_5S; used as an antibacterial and antiparasitic agent.

clinic (klin'ik) 1. a clinical lecture; examination of patients before a class of students; instruction at the bedside. 2. an establishment where patients are admitted for special study and treatment by a group of physicians practicing medicine together. **ambulant c.,** one for patients not confined to the bed. **dry c.,** a clinical lecture with case histories, but without patients present.

clinical (klin'ĭ-k'l) pertaining to a clinic or to the bedside; pertaining to or founded on actual observation and treatment of patients, as distinguished from theoretical or basic sciences.

clinician (klĭ-nish'an) an expert clinical physician and teacher.

clinicopathologic (klin"ĭ-ko-path'o-loj-ik) pertaining both to symptoms of disease and to its pathology.

Clinistix (klin'ĭ-stiks) trademark for an enzyme-impregnated plastic strip used to test for glucose in the urine.

Clinitest (-test) trademark for reagent tablets containing copper sulfate, used in testing for urine.

clinocephaly (kli"no-sef'ah-le) congenital flatness or concavity of the vertex of the head.

clinodactyly (-dak'til-e) permanent deviation or deflection of one or more fingers.

clinoid (kli'noid) bed-shaped.

clinoscope (kli'no-skōp) an instrument for measuring the paralysis of the ocular muscles as shown by torsion of the eyeballs.

clip (klip) a metallic device for approximating the edges of a wound or for the prevention of bleeding from small individual blood vessels.

cliseometer (klis"e-om'ĕ-ter) an instrument for measuring the angles between the axis of the body and that of the pelvis.

Clistin (klis'tin) trademark for preparations of carbinoxamine.

clition (klit'e-on) the midpoint of the anterior border of the clivus.

clitoridectomy (klit″o-rĭ-dek'to-me) excision of the clitoris.

clitoriditis (-di'tis) clitoritis.

clitoridotomy (-dot'o-me) incision of the clitoris; female circumcision.

clitoris (klit'o-ris) the small, elongated, erectile body in the female, situated at the anterior angle of the rima pudendi and homologous with the penis in the male.

clitorism (klit'o-rizm) 1. hypertrophy of the clitoris. 2. persistent erection of the clitoris.

clitoritis (klit″o-ri'tis) inflammation of the clitoris.

clivus (kli'vus), pl. *cli'vi*[L.] a bony surface in the posterior cranial fossa sloping upward from the foramen magnum to the dorsum sellae.

cloaca (klo-a'kah), pl. *cloa'cae* [L.] 1. a common passage for fecal, urinary, and reproductive discharge in most lower vertebrates. 2. the terminal end of the hindgut before division into rectum, bladder, and genital primordia in mammalian embryos. 3. an opening in the involucrum of a necrosed bone. **cloa'cal,** adj.

cloacogenic (klo″ah-ko-jen'ik) originating from the cloaca or from persisting cloacal remnants; said of a group of rare transitional-cell nonkeratinizing epidermoid anal cancers.

clock (klok) a device for measuring time. **biological c.,** the physiologic mechanism which governs the rhythmic occurrence of certain biochemical, physiologic, and behavioral phenomena in living organisms.

clofibrate (klo-fi'brāt) an anticholesterolemic, $C_{12}H_{15}ClO_3$.

clomiphene (klo'mĭ-fēn) a nonsteroid estrogen analogue, $C_{26}H_{28}ClNO$, used as the citrate salt to stimulate ovulation.

clonazepam (klo-naz'ĕ-pam) a benzodiazepine derivative, $C_{15}H_{10}ClN_3O_3$, used as an oral anticonvulsant.

clone (klōn) 1. the asexual progeny of a single cell. 2. a strain of cells descended in culture from a single cell; the establishment or initiation of such a strain. 3. to establish or initiate such a strain. **clo'nal,** adj.

clonic (klon'ik) pertaining to or characterized by clonus.

clonicity (klo-nis'ĭ-te) the condition of being clonic.

clonicotonic (klon″ĭ-ko-ton'ik) both clonic and tonic.

clonidine (klo'nĭ-dēn) a centrally acting antihypertensive agent, $C_9H_9Cl_2N_3$.

clonism (klon'izm) a succession of clonic spasms.

clonograph (klon'o-graf) an instrument for recording spasmodic movements of parts and tendon reflexes.

Clonorchis (klo-nor'kis) a genus of Asiatic liver flukes.

clonospasm (klon'o-spazm) clonic spasm.

clonus (klo'nus) alternate involuntary muscular contraction and relaxation in rapid succession.

ankle c., foot c., a series of abnormal reflex movements of the foot, induced by sudden dorsiflexion, causing alternate contraction and relaxation of the triceps surae muscle. **toe c.,** abnormal rhythmic movement of the big toe, induced by suddenly extending the first phalanx. **wrist c.,** spasmodic movement of the hand, induced by forcibly extending the hand at the wrist.

Clopane (klo'pān) trademark for preparations of cyclopentamine.

Clostridium (klo-strid'e-um) a genus of anaerobic spore-forming bacteria (family Bacillaceae). **C. bifermen'tans,** a species common in feces, sewage, and soil and associated with gas gangrene. **C. botuli'num,** the agent causing botulism in man. **C. histolyt'icum,** a species found in feces and soil. **C. kluy'veri,** a species used in the study of both microbial synthesis and microbial oxidation of fatty acids. **C. no'vyi,** an important cause of gas gangrene. **C. oedemat'iens,** *C. novyi.* **C. perfrin'gens,** the most common etiologic agent of gas gangrene, differentiable into several different types: type A (classic gangrene in man), B (lamb dysentery), C (struck in sheep), D (enterotoxemia in sheep), E (enterotoxemia in lambs and calves), F (enteritis necroticans in man). **C. sporog'enes,** a species widespread in nature, reportedly associated with pathogenic anaerobes in gangrenous infections. **C. ter'tium,** a species found in feces, sewage, and soil and present in some gangrenous infections. **C. tet'ani,** a common inhabitant of soil and human and horse intestines, and the cause of tetanus in man and domestic animals. **C. welch'ii,** British name for *C. perfringens.*

clostridium (klo-strid'ĭ-um), pl. *clostrid'ia* [Gr.] an individual of the genus *Clostridium.*

clot (klot) 1. a semisolidified mass of coagulum, as of blood or lymph. 2. to form such a mass. **agonal c., agony c.,** one formed in the heart during the death agony. **antemortem c.,** one formed in the heart or in a large vessel before death. **blood c.,** one formed of blood, either in or out of the body. **chicken fat c.,** a yellow-appearing blood clot, due to settling out of erythrocytes before clotting. **currant jelly c.,** a reddish clot, due to the presence of erythrocytes enmeshed in it. **distal c.,** one formed in a vessel on the distal side of a ligature. **external c.,** one formed outside a blood vessel. **heart c.,** one formed within the heart after death. **internal c.,** a blood clot formed within a blood vessel. **laminated c.,** a blood clot formed by successive deposits, giving it a layered appearance. **marantic c.,** a blood clot due to enfeebled circulation and general malnutrition. **muscle c.,** one formed by coagulation of muscle plasm. **passive c.,** one formed in the sac of an aneurysm through which the blood has stopped circulating. **plastic c.,** one formed from the intima of an artery at the point of ligation, forming a permanent obstruction of the artery. **postmortem c.,** one formed in the heart or in a large blood vessel after death. **proximal c.,** one formed in a vessel on the proximal side of a ligature. **stratified c.,** laminated c.

clotrimazole (klo-trim′ah-zōl) a topical antifungal agent, $C_{22}H_{17}ClN_2$.

cloxacillin (kloks″ah-sil′in) a semisynthetic penicillin; its sodium salt is used in treating staphylococcal infections due to penicillinase-positive organisms.

clubbing (klub′ing) proliferation of soft tissue about the terminal phalanges of fingers or toes, without osseous change.

clubfoot (-foot) a congenitally deformed foot; see *talipes.*

clubhand (-hand) a hand deformity analogous to clubfoot; talipomanus.

clumping (klump′ing) the aggregation of particles, such as bacteria, into irregular masses.

cluneal (kloo′ne-al) pertaining to the buttocks.

clunis (kloo′nis), pl. *clu′nes* [L.] buttock.

clysis (kli′sis) the administration other than orally of any of several solutions to replace lost body fluid, supply nutriment, or raise blood pressure; also, the solution so administered.

clyster (klis′ter) an enema.

C.M. [L.] *Chirur′giae Ma′gister* (Master in Surgery).

Cm chemical symbol, *curium.*

cm. centimeter.

cm.² square centimeter.

cm.³ cubic centimeter.

C.M.A. Canadian Medical Association.

c./min. cycles per minute.

c.mm. cubic millimeter.

C.N.A. Canadian Nurses' Association.

cnemial (ne′me-al) pertaining to the shin.

C.N.M. Certified Nurse-Midwife.

C.N.S. central nervous system.

Co chemical symbol, *cobalt.*

C.O.A. Canadian Orthopaedic Association.

CoA coenzyme A.

coacervate (ko-as′er-vāt) a collection of less fully hydrated particles of a colloid system, with less solvent bound to them than they had before.

coacervation (ko-as″er-va′shun) the formation of coacervates in a colloid system.

coadaptation (ko″ad-ap-ta′shun) the mutual, correlated, adaptive changes in two interdependent organs.

coagglutination (ko″ah-gloo″tĭ-na′shun) the aggregation of particulate antigens combined with agglutinins of more than one specificity.

coagglutinin (ko″ah-gloo′tĭ-nin) partial agglutinin.

coagulability (ko-ag″u-lah-bil′ĭ-te) the state of being capable of forming or of being formed into clots.

coagulant (ko-ag′u-lant) promoting, accelerating, or making possible coagulation of blood; an agent that so acts.

coagulase (-lās) an antigenic substance of bacterial origin, produced chiefly by staphylococci, which may be causally related to thrombus formation.

coagulate (-lāt) 1. to cause to clot. 2. to become clotted.

coagulation (ko-ag″u-la′shun) 1. formation of a clot. 2. in surgery, the disruption of tissue by physical means to form an amorphous residuum, as in electrocoagulation and photocoagulation. **blood c.,** the sequential process by which the multiple coagulation factors of blood interact, ultimately resulting in formation of an insoluble clot, divisible into three stages: (1) formation of intrinsic and extrinsic prothrombin converting principle; (2) formation of thrombin; (3) formation of stable fibrin polymers. **electric c.,** destruction of tissue by application of a bipolar current delivered by a needle point.

coagulative (ko-ag′u-la″tiv) associated with or promoting coagulation; of the nature of coagulation.

coagulopathy (ko-ag″u-lop′ah-the) any disorder of blood coagulation. **consumption c.,** a disorder characterized by reduction in elements involved in blood coagulation due to their utilization in excessive blood clotting, usually in disseminated intravascular coagulation.

coagulum (ko-ag′u-lum), pl. *coag′ula* [L.] a clot. **closing c.,** the clot that closes the gap made in the uterine lining by the implanting blastocyst.

coalescence (ko″ah-les′ens) the fusion or blending of parts.

coapt (ko′apt) to approximate, as the edges of a wound.

coarctate (ko-ark′tāt) 1. to press close together; contract. 2. pressed together; restrained.

coarctation (ko″ark-ta′shun) stricture or narrowing. **c. of aorta,** a localized malformation marked by deformity of the aortic media, causing narrowing, usually severe, of the lumen of the vessel. **reversed c.,** pulseless disease.

coat (kōt) tunica; a membrane or other tissue covering or lining an organ. **buffy c.,** the thin yellowish layer of leukocytes overlying the packed erythrocytes in centrifuged blood.

cobalamin (ko-bal′ah-min) a cobalt-containing complex common to all members of the vitamin B_{12} group.

cobalt (ko′bawlt) chemical element (*see table*), at. no. 27, symbol Co. Its radioactive isotope, cobalt 60 (^{60}Co), is used in the treatment of malignancies.

coca (ko′kah) the leaves of the South American plant *Erythroxylon coca,* a source of cocaine.

cocaine (ko-kān′, ko′kān) an alkaloid, $C_{17}H_{21}NO_4$, obtained from leaves of various species of *Erythroxylon* (coca plants) or produced synthetically; used as a local anesthetic.

cocainism (ko′kān-izm) the morbid condition caused by misuse of cocaine.

cocainize (ko-kān′īz) to put under the influence of cocaine.

cocarboxylase (ko″kar-bok′sĭ-lās) phosphorylated thiamine.

cocarcinogen (ko″kar-sin′o-jen) an agent that increases the effect of a carcinogen by direct concurrent local effect on the tissue.

cocarcinogenesis (ko-kar″sĭ-no-jen′ĕ-sis) the development, according to one theory, of cancer only in preconditioned cells as a result of conditions favorable to its growth.

cocci (kok′si) plural of *coccus*.

Coccidia (kok-sid′e-ah) an order of sporozoa, including two genera, *Eimeria* and *Isospora*, commonly parasitic in epithelial cells of the intestinal tract, but also found in the liver and other organs.

coccidia (kok-sid′e-ah) plural of *coccidium*.

coccidial (-al) of, pertaining to, or caused by Coccidia.

coccidian (-an) 1. pertaining to Coccidia. 2. any individual of the Coccidia.

Coccidioides (kok-sid″e-oi′dēz) a genus of pathogenic fungi, including *C. im′mitis*, the cause of coccidioidomycosis.

coccidioidin (-din) a sterile preparation containing by-products of growth products of *Coccidioides immitis*, injected intracutaneously as a test for coccidioidomycosis.

coccidioidoma (-do′mah) residual pulmonary granulomatous nodules seen roentgenographically as solid round foci in coccidioidomycosis.

coccidioidomycosis (-oi″do-mi-ko′sis) infection with *Coccidioides immitis*, occurring as a respiratory infection, due to spore inhalation, varying in severity from that of a common cold to symptoms resembling those of influenza (*primary c.*), or as a virulent and severe, chronic, progressive, granulomatous disease resulting in involvement of cutaneous and subcutaneous tissues, viscera, central nervous system, and lungs (*secondary c.*).

coccidioidosis (-oi-do′sis) coccidioidomycosis.

coccidiosis (-o′sis) infection by coccidia. In man, applied to the presence of *Isospora hominis* or *I. belli* in stools; such infection is often asymptomatic, rarely causing a severe watery mucous diarrhea.

coccidium (kok-sid′e-um), pl. *coccid′ia* [L.] any member of the order Coccidia.

coccigenic (kok″sĭ-jen′ik) produced by cocci.

coccinella (-nel′ah) [L.] cochineal.

coccobacillus (kok″o-bah-sil′us) an oval bacterial cell intermediate between the coccus and bacillus forms. **coccobac′illary,** adj.

coccobacteria (-bak-te′re-ah) a common name for spheroid bacteria, or for various bacterial cocci.

coccoid (kok′oid) resembling a coccus.

cocculin (kok′u-lin) picrotoxin.

coccus (kok′us), pl. *coc′ci* [L.] a spherical bacterium, usually slightly less than 1 μ in diameter. **coc′cal,** adj.

coccyalgia (kok″se-al′je-ah) coccygodynia.

coccycephalus (-sef′ah-lus) a monster whose head is beak-shaped.

coccydynia (kok″sĭ-din′e-ah) coccygodynia.

coccygeal (kok-sij′e-al) pertaining to or located in the region of the coccyx.

coccygectomy (kok″sĭ-jek′to-me) excision of the coccyx.

coccygodynia (-go-din′e-ah) pain in the coccyx and neighboring region.

coccygotomy (-got′o-me) incision of the coccyx.

coccyx (kok′siks) see *Table of Bones.*

cochineal (koch′ĭ-nēl) dried female insects of

Coccus cacti, enclosing young larvae; used as a coloring agent for pharmaceuticals and as a biological stain.

cochlea (kok′le-ah) a spiral tube forming part of the inner ear, which is the essential organ of hearing. See Plate XII. **coch′lear,** adj.

cochleariform (kok″le-ar′ĭ-form) spoon-shaped.

cochleitis (-i′tis) inflammation of the cochlea.

cochleovestibular (kok″le-o-ves-tib′u-ler) pertaining to the cochlea and vestibule of the ear.

Cochliomyia (-mi′yah) a genus of flies, including *C. hominivo′rax,* the screw-worm fly, which deposits its eggs on animal wounds; after hatching, the larvae burrow into the wound and feed on living tissue.

cocillana (ko″sil-yah′nah) the bark of the South American tree *Guarea rusbyi,* used as an emetic, expectorant, and cathartic.

cocoa (ko′ko) powder prepared from roasted, cured kernels of ripe seeds of *Theobroma cacao,* used as a flavoring agent.

coconscious (ko-kon′shus) not in the field of the conscious, yet capable of being remembered.

coconsciousness (-nes) consciousness secondary to the main stream of consciousness.

cocontraction (ko″kon-trak′shun) coordination of antagonist muscles.

coctolabile (kok″to-la′bil) capable of being altered or destroyed by heating.

coctoprecipitin (-pre-sip′ĭ-tin) a precipitin produced by injecting a heated serum or other antigen.

coctostabile (-sta′bil) not altered by heating to the boiling point of water.

code (kōd) 1. a set of rules for regulating conduct. 2. a system by which information can be communicated. **genetic c.,** the arrangement of nucleotides in the polynucleotide chain of a chromosome governing transmission of genetic information to proteins, i.e., determining the sequence of amino acids in the polypeptide chain making up each protein synthesized by the cell. **triplet c.,** the three-base sequence (nucleotide) in the DNA molecule which codes for one amino acid.

codeine (ko′dēn) an alkaloid, $C_{18}H_{21}NO_3 \cdot H_2O$, obtained from opium or prepared from morphine by methylation; used as a narcotic analgesic and as an antitussive. The phosphate and sulfate salts are soluble in water.

codominance (ko-dom′ĭ-nans) the full expression in a heterozygote of both alleles of a pair without either being influenced by the other, as in a person with blood group AB. **codom′inant,** adj.

codon (ko′don) a series of three adjacent bases in one polynucleotide chain of a DNA or RNA molecule, which codes for a specific amino acid.

coe- for words beginning thus, see also those beginning *ce-*.

coefficient (ko″ĕ-fish′ent) 1. an expression of the change or effect produced by variation in certain factors, or of the ratio between two different quantities. 2. a number or figure put before a chemical formula to indicate how many times the formula is to be multiplied. **c. of absorp-**

tion, the volume of a gas absorbed by a unit volume of a liquid at 0° C. and a pressure of 760 mm. Hg. **Baumann's c.,** ratio of the ethereal to the total sulfates in the urine. **biological c.,** the amount of potential energy consumed by the body at rest. **Bouchard's c.,** the ratio between the amount of urine and the total solids of the urine. **Falta's c.,** the percentage of ingested sugar eliminated from the system. **c. of partage,** the ratio between the amount of an acid absorbed by ether from an aqueous solution of the acid and the amount that remains in solution. **phenol c.,** a measure of the bactericidal activity of a chemical compound in relation to phenol; expressed as a ratio of the activity of a dilution of the unknown to that of phenol when both dilutions kill in 10 mins. but not in 5 mins. under the specified conditions. **sedimentation c.,** the rate in centimeters per second per unit centrifugal field at which a particle (e.g., protein) in solution travels in the analytical ultracentrifuge. A rate of 1×10^{-13} cm./second/unit centrifugal field is defined as one Svedberg unit (S). **c. of thermal conductivity,** a number indicating the quantity of heat passing in a unit of time through a unit thickness of a substance when the difference in temperature is 1° C. **c. of thermal expansion,** the change in volume per unit volume of a substance produced by a 1° C. temperature increase. **urotoxic c.,** the quantity of urotoxic units produced per unit weight and eliminated in the urine per unit time. **Yvon's c.,** the ratio between the quantity of urea and the phosphates of the urine.

-coele word element [Gr.], *cavity; space.*

Coelenterata (se-len″ter-a′tah) a phylum of invertebrates which includes the hydras, jellyfish, sea anemones, and corals.

coelenterate (se-len′ter-āt) 1. pertaining or belonging to the Coelenterata. 2. any member of the Coelenterata.

coeloblastula (se″lo-blas′tu-lah) the common type of blastula, consisting of a hollow sphere composed of blastomeres.

coelom (se′lom) body cavity, especially the cavity in the mammalian embryo between the somatopleure and splanchnopleure, which is both intra- and extraembryonic; the principal cavities of the trunk arise from the intraembryonic portion. **coelom′ic,** adj.

coelomate (sēl′o-māt) 1. having a coelom. 2. an individual of the Eucoelomata; eucoelomate.

coelosomy (se″lo-so′me) a developmental anomaly characterized by protrusion of the viscera from and their presence outside the body cavity.

coenurosis (se″nu-ro′sis) gid.

Coenurus (se-nu′rus) a genus of certain tapeworm larva, including *C. cerebra′lis,* the larva of *Multiceps multiceps,* which causes gid.

coenurus (se-nu′rus) the larval stage of tapeworms of the genus *Multiceps,* a semitransparent, fluid-filled, bladder-like organism that contains multiple scoleces attached to the inner surface of its wall and that does not form brood capsules. It develops in various parts of the host body, especially in the central nervous system.

coenzyme (ko-en′zīm) an organic molecule, usually containing phosphorus and some vitamins, sometimes separable from the enzyme protein; a coenzyme and an apoenzyme must unite in order to function (as a holoenzyme). **c. A,** a coenzyme essential for carbohydrate and fat metabolism; among its constituents are pantothenic acid and a terminal SH group, which forms thioester linkages with various acids, e.g., acetic acid (acetyl CoA). **c. I,** nicotinamide-adenine dinucleotide. **c. II,** nicotinamide-adenine dinucleotide phosphate. **c. Q,** any of a group of related quinones with isoprenoid units in the side chains (the ubiquinones), occurring in the lipid fraction of mitochondria and serving, along with the cytochromes, as an intermediate in electron transport; they are similar in structure and function to vitamin K_1.

coeur (ker) [Fr.] heart. **c. en sabot** (on să-bo′) a heart whose shape on a radiograph vaguely resembles that of a wooden shoe; noted in tetralogy of Fallot.

cofactor (ko′fak-tor) an element or principle, e.g., a coenzyme, with which another must unite in order to function.

coffee (kof′e) the dried seeds of the tropical trees *Coffea arabica* and *C. liberica;* its active principles include caffeine, coffee oil, sugars, proteins, and many volatile flavor oils. Also, a drink made by decoction or infusion of these seeds.

Cogentin (ko-jen′tin) trademark for preparations of benztropine.

cognition (kog-nish′un) that operation of the mind process by which we become aware of objects of thought and perception, including all aspects of perceiving, thinking, and remembering. **cog′nitive,** adj.

cohesion (ko-he′zhun) the force causing various particles to unite. **cohe′sive,** adj.

coil (koil) a winding structure or spiral.

coinosite (koi′no-sīt) a free commensal organism.

coition (ko-ish′un) coitus.

coitophobia (ko″ĭ-to-fo′be-ah) morbid fear of coitus.

coitus (ko′ĭ-tus) sexual connection per vaginam between male and female. **c. incomple′tus, c. interrup′tus,** coitus in which the penis is withdrawn from the vagina before ejaculation. **c. reserva′tus,** coitus in which ejaculation of semen is intentionally suppressed.

colation (ko-la′shun) the process of straining or filtration, or the product of such a process.

colchicine (kol′chĭ-sēn) an alkaloid, $C_{22}H_{25}NO_6$, from the tree *Colchicum autumnale* (meadow saffron), used as a suppressant for gout.

cold (kōld) 1. privation, or relatively low degree, of heat. 2. common cold; a catarrhal disorder of the upper respiratory tract, which may be viral, a mixed infection, or an allergic reaction, and marked by acute coryza, slight temperature rise, chilly sensations, and general indisposition. **common c.,** see *cold* (2). **rose c.,** a form of seasonal hay fever caused by the pollen of roses.

coldsore (kold′sor) see *herpes simplex.*

colectomy (ko-lek′to-me) excision of the colon or of a portion of it.

Colesiota (ko-le″se-o′tah) a genus of microorganisms of uncertain classification, including *C. conjuncti′vae*, the agent causing infectious ophthalmia of sheep.

Colettsia (ko-let′se-ah) a genus of microorganisms of uncertain classification, including *C. pe′coris*, a parasitic species found in the conjunctiva of domestic animals.

colibacillemia (ko″li-bas″i-le′me-ah) the presence of *Escherichia coli* in the blood.

colibacillosis (-lo′sis) infection with *Escherichia coli.*

colibacilluria (-lu′re-ah) the presence of *Escherichia coli* in the urine.

colibacillus (ko″li-bah-sil′us) *Escherichia coli.*

colic (kol′ik) 1. acute paroxysmal abdominal pain. 2. pertaining to the colon. **appendicular c.**, vermicular c. **biliary c.**, colic due to passage of gallstones along the bile duct. **Devonshire c.**, lead c. **gallstone c.**, biliary c. **gastric c.**, pain in the stomach. **hepatic c.**, biliary c. **lead c.**, colic due to lead poisoning. **menstrual c.**, dysmenorrhea. **ovarian c.**, ovarian pain. **painter's c.**, lead c. **renal c.**, pain due to thrombosis of the renal vein or artery, dissection of the renal artery, renal infarction, intrarenal mass lesions, or passage of a stone within the collecting system. **salivary c.**, pain in the region of the salivary gland in cases of salivary calculus. **sand c.**, chronic indigestion. **uterine c.**, severe colic arising in the uterus, usually at the menstrual period. **vermicular c.**, pain in the vermiform appendix caused by catarrhal inflammation resulting from blockage of the outlet of the appendix.

colica (kol′i-kah) [L.] colic.

colicin (kol′i-sin) a protein secreted by certain strains of *Escherichia coli* and lethal to other strains of the same species.

colicky (kol′ik-e) pertaining to or affected by colic.

colicoplegia (ko″li-ko-ple′je-ah) combined lead colic and lead paralysis.

colicystitis (-sis-ti′tis) cystitis due to *Escherichia coli.*

colicystopyelitis (-sis″to-pi″ĕ-li′tis) inflammation of the bladder and renal pelvis due to *Escherichia coli.*

coliform (kol′i-form) resembling or being *Escherichia coli.*

colinephritis (ko″li-ne-fri′tis) nephritis due to *Escherichia coli.*

coliphage (kol′i-fāj) any bacteriophage that infects *Escherichia coli.*

coliplication (ko″li-pli-ka′shun) coloplication.

colipuncture (-punk″tūr) colocentesis.

colipyelitis (-pi″ĕ-li′tis) pyelitis caused by *Escherichia coli.*

colisepsis (-sep′sis) infection with *Escherichia coli.*

colistimethate (ko-lis″ti-meth′āt) a colistin derivative; the sodium salt, $C_{49}H_{89}N_{13}NaO_{22}S_4$, is used as an antibacterial.

colistin (ko-lis′tin) an antibiotic produced by *Bacillus polymyxa* var. *colistinus,* or the same substance produced by other means, related to polymyxin, and used in the treatment of urinary tract infections; the water-soluble sulfate salt, effective against several gram-negative bacilli but not against *Proteus,* is used as an intestinal antibacterial.

colitides (ko-lit′i-dēz) plural of *colitis;* inflammatory disorders of the colon considered collectively.

colitis (ko-li′tis) inflammation of the colon. **amebic c.**, colitis due to *Entamoeba histolytica;* amebic dysentery. **granulomatous c.**, transmural colitis with the formation of noncaseating granulomas. **mucous c.**, a chronic noninflammatory disease marked by excessive secretion of mucus and disordered colonic motility, with colic, constipation, and/or diarrhea with passage of mucus. **regional c., segmental c.**, transmural or granulomatous inflammatory disease of the colon; regional enteritis involving the colon. It may be associated with ulceration, strictures, or fistulas. **transmural c.**, inflammation of the full thickness of the bowel, rather than mucosal and submucosal disease, usually with the formation of noncaseating granulomas. It may be confined to the colon, segmentally or diffusely, or may be associated with small bowel disease (regional enteritis). Clinically, it may resemble ulcerative colitis, but the ulceration is often longitudinal or deep, the disease is often segmental, stricture formation is common, and fistulas, particularly in the perineum, are a frequent complication. **ulcerative c.**, chronic ulceration in the colon, chiefly of the mucosa and submucosa, clinically manifested by cramping abdominal pain, rectal bleeding, and loose discharges of blood, pus, and mucus with scanty fecal particles.

colitoxemia (ko″li-tok-se′me-ah) toxemia due to infection with *Escherichia coli.*

colitoxicosis (-tok″si-ko′sis) intoxication caused by *Escherichia coli.*

colitoxin (-tok′sin) a toxin from *Escherichia coli.*

coliuria (-u′re-ah) the presence of *Escherichia coli* in the urine.

collagen (kol′ah-jen) an albuminoid, a main supportive protein of skin, tendon, bone, cartilage, and connective tissue. **collag′enous**, adj.

collagenase (kol-laj′ĕ-nās) an enzyme that hydrolyzes peptides containing proline, including collagen and gelatin.

collagenation (kol-laj″ĕ-na′shun) the appearance of collagen in developing cartilage.

collagenic (kol″ah-jen′ik) 1. producing collagen. 2. pertaining to collagen.

collagenoblast (kol-laj′ĕ-no-blast″) a cell arising from a fibroblast and which, as it matures, is associated with collagen production; it may also form cartilage and bone by metaplasia.

collagenocyte (-sīt″) a mature collagen-producing cell.

collagenogenic (kol-laj″ĕ-no-jen′ik) pertaining to or characterized by collagen production; forming collagen or collagen fibers.

collagenolysis (kol″ah-jen-ol′ĭ-sis) dissolution or digestion of collagen. **collagenolyt′ic**, adj.

collagenosis (kol″ah-jĕ-no′sis) collagen disease.

collapse (kŏ-laps′) 1. a state of extreme prostration and depression, with failure of circulation. 2. abnormal falling in of the walls of a part or organ. **circulatory c.,** shock; circulatory insufficiency without congestive heart failure.

collateral (kŏ-lat′er-al) 1. secondary or accessory; not direct or immediate. 2. a small side branch, as of a blood vessel or nerve.

colliculectomy (kŏ-lik″u-lek′to-me) excision of the colliculus seminalis.

colliculitis (-li′tis) inflammation about the colliculus seminalis.

colliculus (kŏ-lik′u-lus), pl. *collic′uli* [L.] a small elevation. **c. semina′lis,** a prominent portion of the male urethral crest on which are the opening of the prostatic utricle and, on either side, the orifices of the ejaculatory ducts.

collimation (kol″ĭ-ma′shun) in microscopy, the process of making light rays parallel; the adjustment of two or more optical axes with respect to each other. In radiology, the elimination of the more divergent portion of an x-ray beam.

colliquation (-kwa′shun) liquefactive degeneration of tissue.

colliquative (kŏ-lik′wah-tiv) characterized by excessive liquid discharge, or by liquefaction of tissue.

collodiaphyseal (kol″o-di″ah-fiz′e-al) pertaining to the neck and shaft of a long bone, especially the femur.

collodion (kŏ-lo′de-on) a syrupy liquid compounded of pyroxylin, ether, and alcohol, which dries to a clear, tenacious film; used as a topical protectant. **flexible c.,** a preparation of collodion, camphor, and castor oil; used as a topical protectant. **salicylic acid c.,** flexible collodion containing salicylic acid; used topically as a keratolytic.

colloid (kǫl′oid) 1. resembling glue. 2. a state of matter composed of single large molecules or aggregations of smaller molecules (disperse particles, 0.1 μ to 1 $\mu\mu$) of solid, liquid, or gas, in a continuous medium (disperse medium), which may be solid, liquid, or gas.

colloidal (kŏ-loi′dal) of the nature of a colloid.

colloidin (-din) a jelly-like principle produced in colloid degeneration.

colloidoclasia (kŏ-loi″do-kla′ze-ah) breaking up of the physical equilibrium of the colloid of the body, producing anaphylactic shock.

collum (kol′um), pl. *col′la* [L.] the neck, or a necklike part. **c. distor′tum,** torticollis. **c. val′gum,** coxa valga.

collutory (kol′u-to″re) mouthwash or gargle.

collyrium (kŏ-lir′e-um), pl. *collyr′ia* [L.] a lotion for the eyes; an eye wash.

colo- word element [Gr.], *colon.*

coloboma (kol″o-bo′mah) an apparent absence or defect of some ocular tissue, usually due to failure of a part of the fetal fissure to close; it may affect the choroid, ciliary body, eyelid, iris, lens, optic nerve, or retina. **bridge c.,** coloboma of the iris in which a strip of iris tissue bridges over the fissure. **Fuchs'** **c.,** a small, crescent-shaped defect of the choroid at the lower edge of the optic disk. **c. lob′uli,** fissure of the ear lobe.

colocecostomy (-se-kos′to-me) cecocolostomy.

colocentesis (-sen-te′sis) surgical puncture of the colon.

colocholecystostomy (-ko″le-sis-tos′to-me) cholecystocolostomy.

coloclysis (ko-lok′lĭ-sis) irrigation of the colon.

coloclyster (ko″lo-klis′ter) an enema injected into the colon through the rectum.

colocolostomy (-ko-los′to-me) surgical formation of an anastomosis between two portions of the colon.

colocutaneous (-ku-ta′ne-us) pertaining to the colon and skin, or communicating with the colon and the cutaneous surface of the body.

colocynth (kol′o-sinth) dried pulp of unripe but full-grown fruit of *Citrullus colocynthis;* used as a drastic cathartic.

colocynthin (kol″o-sin′thin) a strongly purgative principle fom colocynth.

coloenteritis (ko″lo-en″ter-i′tis) enterocolitis.

colofixation (-fik-sa′shun) the fixation or suspension of the colon in cases of ptosis.

Cologel (kol′o-jel) trademark for a preparation of methylcellulose.

coloileal (ko″lo-il′e-al) ileocolic.

colon (ko′lon) the part of the large intestine extending from the cecum to the rectum. See Plate IV. **colon′ic,** adj. **ascending c.,** the portion of the colon which passes cephalad from the cecum to the right colic flexure. **descending c.,** the portion of the colon which passes caudad from the left colic flexure to the sigmoid colon. **irritable c.,** mucous colitis. **left c.,** the distal portion of the large intestine, developed embryonically from the hindgut and functioning in the storage and elimination from the body of nonabsorbed residue of ingested material. **right c.,** the proximal portion of the large intestine, developed embryonically from the terminal portion of the midgut and functioning in absorption of ingested material. **sigmoid c.,** that portion of the left colon situated in the pelvis and extending from the descending colon to the rectum. **spastic c.,** mucous colitis. **transverse c.,** that portion of the large intestine passing transversely across the upper part of the abdomen, between the right and left colic flexures.

colonalgia (ko″lon-al′je-ah) pain in the colon.

colonitis (-i′tis) colitis.

colonopathy (-op′ah-the) any disease or disorder of the colon.

colonorrhagia (ko″lon-o-ra′je-ah) hemorrhage from the colon.

colonorrhea (-re′ah) mucous colitis.

colonoscope (ko-lon′o-skōp) an elongated flexible fiberoptic endoscope which permits visual examination of the entire colon.

colonoscopy (ko″lon-os′ko-pe) endoscopic examination of the colon, either transabdominally during laparotomy, or transanally by means of a colonoscope.

colony (kol′o-ne) a discrete group of organisms, as a collection of bacteria in a culture.

colopexy (ko′lo-pek″se) surgical fixation or suspension of the colon.

coloplication (ko″lo-pli-ka′shun) the operation of taking a reef in the colon.

coloproctectomy (-prok-tek′to-me) surgical removal of the colon and rectum.

coloproctitis (-prok-ti′tis) inflammation of colon and rectum.

coloproctostomy (-prok-tos′to-me) colorectostomy.

coloptosis (ko″lop-to′sis) downward displacement of the colon.

colopuncture (ko′lo-punk″tūr) colocentesis.

color (kul′er) 1. a property of a surface or substance due to absorption of certain light rays and reflection of others within the range of wavelengths (roughly 370–760 mμ) adequate to excite the retinal receptors. 2. radiant energy within the range of adequate chromatic stimuli of the retina, i.e., between the infrared and ultraviolet. 3. a sensory impression of one of the rainbow hues. **complementary c's,** a pair of colors the sensory mechanisms for which are so linked that when they are mixed on the color wheel they cancel each other out, leaving neutral gray. **confusion c's,** different colors which are liable to be mistakenly matched by persons with defective color vision, and hence are used for detecting different types of color vision defects. **primary c's,** (a) according to the Newton theory, the seven rainbow hues: violet, indigo, blue, green, yellow, orange, red; (b) in painting and printing, blue, yellow, red; (c) according to the Helmholz theory, red, green, blue. **pure c.,** one whose stimulus consists of homogeneous wavelengths, with little or no admixture of wavelengths of other hues.

coloration (kul″er-a′shun) the state of being colored. **protective c.,** coloration of the body blending with the environmental background, to make the organism less visible to predators. **warning c.,** brilliant, conspicuous coloration of poisonous or unpalatable animals, as a warning to potential predators.

colorectitis (ko″lo-rek-ti′tis) coloproctitis.

colorectostomy (-rek-tos′to-me) formation of an artificial opening between the colon and rectum.

colorectum (-rek′tum) the distal 10 inches (25 cm.) of the bowel, including the distal portion of the colon and the rectum, regarded as a unit. **colorec′tal,** adj.

colorimeter (kul″er-im′ĕ-ter) an instrument for measuring color differences, especially one for measuring the color of blood in order to determine the proportion of hemoglobin.

colorrhaphy (ko-lor′ah-fe) suture of the colon.

colosigmoidostomy (ko″lo-sig″moid-os′to-me) surgical anastomosis of a formerly remote portion of the colon to the sigmoid.

colostomy (ko-los′to-me) the surgical creation of an opening between the colon and the body surface; also, the opening (stoma) so created. **dry c.,** that performed in the left colon, the discharge from the stoma consisting of soft or formed fecal matter. **ileotransverse c.,** surgical anastomosis between the ileum and the transverse colon. **wet c.,** colostomy in (a) the right colon, the drainage from which is liquid, or (b) the left colon following anastomosis of the ureters to the sigmoid or descending colon so that urine is also expelled through the same stoma.

colostrorrhea (ko-los″tro-re′ah) spontaneous discharge of colostrum.

colostrum (ko-los′trum) the thin, yellow, milky fluid secreted by the mammary gland a few days before or after parturition.

colotomy (ko-lot′o-me) incision of the colon.

colotyphoid (ko″lo-ti′foid) typhoid fever in which there is follicular ulceration of the colon, with extensive lesions in the small intestine.

colovaginal (-vaj′ĭ-nal) pertaining to or communicating with the colon and vagina.

colovesical (-ves′ĭ-kal) pertaining to or communicating with the colon and bladder.

colp(o)- word element [Gr.], *vagina.*

colpalgia (kol-pal′je-ah) pain in the vagina.

colpatresia (kol″pah-tre′ze-ah) atresia or occlusion of the vagina.

colpectasia (kol″pek-ta′ze-ah) distention or dilatation of the vagina.

colpectomy (kol-pek′to-me) excision of the vagina.

colpeurysis (kol-pu′rĭ-sis) dilatation of the vagina.

colpitis (kol-pi′tis) inflammation of the vagina; vaginitis.

colpocele (kol′po-sēl) vaginal hernia.

colpocleisis (kol″po-kli′sis) surgical closure of the vaginal canal.

colpocystitis (-sis-ti′tis) inflammation of the vagina and bladder.

colpocystocele (-sis′to-sēl) hernia of the bladder into the vagina.

colpocytogram (-si′to-gram) differential listing of cells observed in vaginal smears.

colpocytology (-si-tol′o-je) the quantitative and differential study of cells exfoliated from the epithelium of the vagina.

colpodynia (-din′e-ah) pain in the vagina.

colpohyperplasia (-hi″per-pla′ze-ah) excessive growth of the mucous membrane and wall of the vagina.

colpomicroscope (-mi′kro-skōp) an instrument for microscopic examination of the tissues of the cervix *in situ.*

colpomicroscopy (-mi-kros′ko-pe) examination by means of the colpomicroscope.

colpoperineoplasty (-per″ĭ-ne′o-plas″te) plastic repair of the vagina and perineum.

colpoperineorrhaphy (-per″ĭ-ne-or′ah-fe) suture of the ruptured vagina and perineum.

colpopexy (kol′po-pek″se) suture of a relaxed vagina to the abdominal wall.

colpoplasty (-plas″te) plastic surgery involving the vagina.

colpoptosis (kol″pop-to′sis) prolapse of the vagina.

colporrhagia (kol″po-ra′je-ah) hemorrhage from the vagina.

colporrhaphy (kol-por′ah-fe) 1. suture of the vagina. 2. the operation of denuding and suturing the vaginal wall to narrow the vagina.

colporrhexis (kol″po-rek′sis) laceration of the vagina.

colposcope (kol′po-skōp) a speculum for examining the vagina and cervix by means of a magnifying lens.

colposcopy (kol-pos′ko-pe) examination by means of a colposcope.

colpospasm (kol′po-spazm) vaginal spasm.

colpostenosis (kol″po-stĕ-no′sis) contraction or narrowing of the vagina.

colpostenotomy (-stĕ-not′o-me) a cutting operation for stricture of the vagina.

colpotomy (kol-pot′o-me) incision of the vagina with entry into the cul-de-sac.

colpoxerosis (kol″po-ze-ro′sis) abnormal dryness of the vulva and vagina.

colt-ill (kōlt′il) see under *ill.*

columella (kol″u-mel′ah), pl. *columel′lae* [L.] a little column. **c. coch′leae,** modiolus. **c. na′si,** the fleshy external termination of the septum of the nose.

column (kol′um) an anatomical part in the form of a pillar-like structure; anything resembling a pillar. **anal c's,** vertical folds of mucous membrane at the upper half of the anal canal. **anterior c.,** the anterior portion of the gray substance of the spinal cord, in transverse section seen as a horn. **c's of Bertini,** renal c's. **c. of Burdach,** fasciculus cuneatus of the spinal cord. **Clarke's c.,** nucleus thoracicus. **enamel c's,** adamantine prisms. **fat c's,** columns of adipose tissue extending from subcutaneous tissue to hair follicles and sweat glands. **c. of Goll,** fasciculus gracilis of spinal cord. **gray c's,** the longitudinally oriented parts of the spinal cord in which the nerve cell bodies are found, comprising the gray substance of the spinal cord. **lateral c.,** the lateral portion of the spinal cord, in transverse section seen as a horn; present only in the thoracic and upper lumbar regions. **c's of Morgagni,** anal c's. **posterior c.,** the posterior portion of gray substance of the spinal cord, in transverse section seen as a horn. **posteroexternal c.,** the outer wider portion of the posterior column of the cord. **rectal c's,** anal c's. **renal c's,** inward extensions of the cortical substance of the kidney between contiguous renal pyramids. **c. of Sertoli,** an elongated Sertoli cell in the parietal layer of the seminiferous tubules. **spinal c.,** vertebral c. **vertebral c.,** the rigid structure in the midline of the back, composed of the vertebrae.

columna (ko-lum′nah), pl. *colum′nae* [L.] column.

columnization (kol″um-nĭ-za′shun) the supporting of the prolapsed uterus by means of tampons.

Coly-Mycin (kol′e-mi″sin) trademark for preparations of colistimethate.

colypeptic (ko″le-pep′tik) kolypeptic.

coma (ko′mah) 1. a state of profound unconsciousness from which the patient cannot be aroused, even by powerful stimuli. 2. a comet-shaped image caused by light passing obliquely through a lens. **alcoholic c.,** stupor accompanying severe alcoholic intoxication. **apoplectic c.,** the stupor accompanying stroke.

diabetic c., the coma of severe diabetic acidosis. **Kussmaul's c.,** the coma and air hunger of diabetic acidosis. **metabolic c.,** the coma accompanying metabolic encephalopathy. **trance c.,** lethargy produced by hypnosis. **uremic c.,** lethargic state due to uremia. **c. vigil,** apparent wakefulness with absent or grossly diminished response to outside stimuli.

comatose (ko′mah-tōs) pertaining to or affected with coma.

combustion (kom-bust′yun) rapid oxidation with emission of heat.

comedo (kom′ĕ-do), pl. *comedo′nes.* A plug of keratin and sebum within the dilated orifice of a hair follicle.

comedomastitis (kom″ĕ-do-mas-ti′tis) mammary duct ectasia.

comes (ko′mēz), pl. *com′ites*[L.] an artery or vein accompanying a nerve trunk.

comfortization (kum″for-tĭ-za′shun) the scientific application of physiologic principles to promote comfort in potentially stressful situations, as in aircraft design.

commensal (kŏ-men′sal) 1. living on or within another organism, and deriving benefit without harming or benefiting the host individual. 2. a parasitic organism that causes no harm to the host.

commensalism (-izm) symbiosis in which one population (or individual) is benefited and the other is neither benefited nor harmed.

comminuted (kom′ĭ-nūt″ed) broken or crushed into small pieces, as a comminuted fracture.

comminution (kom″ĭ-nu′shun) the act of breaking, or condition of being broken, into small fragments.

commissura (kom″ĭ-su′rah), pl. *commissu′rae* [L.] commissure. **c. cerebel′li,** pons (2). **c. mag′na,** corpus callosum.

commissure (kom′ĭ-shūr) a site of union of corresponding parts; used also with specific reference to the sites of junction between adjacent cusps of the heart valves. **anterior c. of cerebrum,** the band of fibers connecting the parts of the two cerebral hemispheres. **Gudden's c.,** see *supraoptic c's.* **Meynert's c.,** see *supraoptic c's.* **middle c. of cerebrum,** band of gray matter joining the optic thalami; it develops as a secondary adhesion and may be absent. **posterior c. of cerebrum,** a large fiber bundle crossing from one side of the cerebrum to the other dorsal to where the aqueduct opens into the third ventricle. **supraoptic c's,** commissural fibers crossing the midline of the human brain dorsal to the caudal border of the optic chiasm, representing the combined commissures of Gudden and Meynert.

commissurorrhaphy (kom″ĭ-shūr-or′ah-fe) suture of the components of a commissure, to lessen the size of the orifice.

commissurotomy (-ot′o-me) surgical incision or digital disruption of the components of a commissure to increase the size of the orifice; commonly done to separate adherent, thickened leaflets of a stenotic mitral valve.

communicable (kŏ-mu′nĭ-kah-b′l) capable of being transmitted from one person to another.

communicans (kŏ-mu′nĭ-kans) [L.] communicating.

community (kŏ-mu′nĭ-te) a body of individuals living in a defined area or having a common interest or organization. **biotic c.,** an assemblage of populations living in a defined area.

compaction (kom-pak′shun) a complication of labor in twin births in which there is simultaneous full engagement of the leading fetal poles of both twins, so that the true pelvic cavity is filled and further descent is prevented.

Compazine (kom′pah-zēn) trademark for preparations of prochlorperazine.

compensation (kom″pen-sa′shun) the counterbalancing of any defect of structure or function. In psychoanalysis, the mechanism by which an approved character trait is put forward to hide from the ego the existence of an opposite trait. In cardiology, the maintenance of an adequate blood flow without distressing symptoms. **compen′satory,** adj. **dosage c.,** in genetics, the mechanism by which the effect of the two X chromosomes of the normal female is rendered identical to that of the one X chromosome of the normal male.

complaint (kom-plānt′) a disease, symptom, or disorder. **chief c.,** the symptom or group of symptoms about which the patient first consults the doctor; the presenting symptom.

complement (kom′plĕ-ment) a complex series of enzymatic proteins in normal serum that combine with antigen-antibody complex; complement comprises nine functioning components symbolized as C1 through C9, which cause lysis of cells and destruction of bacteria, and are involved in various immunological and biological activities.

complementation (kom″plĕ-men-ta′shun) in genetics, the restoration of wild-type function as a result of two distinct mutations on the same chromosome. In virology, the interaction of two defective bateriophages resulting in replication of both. **interallelic c.,** intragenic c. **intercistronic c., intergenic c.,** the essentially full restoration of wild-type function in a *cis-trans* test when two mutations, in transposition, are located in different cistrons (genes). **intracistronic c., intragenic c.,** the partial restoration of function sometimes seen in the *cis-trans* test when the two mutations are located at different sites within the same cistron.

complex (kom′pleks) 1. the sum or combination of various things, like or unlike, as a complex of symptoms; see *syndrome.* 2. a group of associated, partially or wholly repressed ideas, usually outside of awareness, which can evoke emotional forces that influence an individual's behavior. 3. that portion of an electrocardiogram representing the systole of an atrium or ventricle. **anomalous c.,** a complex varying from the normal type, as an electrocardiographic complex. **atrial c.,** the portion (P wave) of the electrocardiogram produced by excitation of the atrium. **avian leukosis c.,** see *avian leukosis.* **Cain c.,** the rivalry, competition, or destructive impulses between brothers. **calcarine c.,** calcar avis. **castration c.,** the fear (usually fantasied) of damage to or loss of sexual organs as punishment for forbidden sexual desires. **Clérambault-Kandinsky c.,** a mental state in which the patient thinks his mind is controlled by some outside influence or by another person. **Eisenmenger c.,** a defect of the interventricular septum with severe pulmonary hypertension, hypertrophy of the right ventricle, and latent or overt cyanosis. **Electra c.,** libidinous fixation of a daughter toward her father. **father c.,** Electra c. **Golgi c.,** Golgi apparatus; a complex structure within cells, made up of several elements, each consisting of a number of saccules; it plays a role in internal and external secretion. **inferiority c.,** unconscious feelings of inferiority, producing timidity or, as a compensation, exaggerated aggressiveness and expression of superiority (*superiority c.*). **Jocasta c.,** libidinous fixation of a mother toward a son. **Lear c.,** libidinous fixation of a father toward a daughter. **Lutembacher's c.,** see under *syndrome.* **mother c., Oedipus c.,** libidinous fixation of a son toward his mother. **sex c.,** the correlation between the internal secretions and the sex function. **superiority c.,** see *inferiority c.* **symptom c.,** syndrome. **ventricular c.,** the portion (Q, R, S, and T waves) of the electrocardiogram produced by excitation of the ventricles.

complexion (kom-plek′shun) the color and appearance of the skin of the face.

compliance (kom-pli′ans) the quality of yielding to pressure or force without disruption, or an expression of the measure of ability to do so, as an expression of the distensibility of an air- or fluid-filled organ, e.g., lung or urinary bladder, in terms of unit of volume change per unit of pressure change.

complication (kom″plĭ-ka′shun) 1. a disease(s) concurrent with another disease. 2. the occurrence of two or more diseases in the same patient.

compos mentis (kom′pos men′tis) [L.] sound of mind; sane.

compound (kom′pownd) 1. made up of two or more parts or ingredients. 2. a substance made up of two or more materials. 3. in chemistry, a substance consisting of two or more elements in union. **acyclic c.,** an open-chain compound; see under *chain.* **aliphatic c.,** an open-chain compound containing no multiple bonds; see under *chain.* **clathrate c's,** inclusion complexes in which molecules of one type are trapped within cavities of the crystalline lattice of another substance. **cyclic c.,** a closed-chain compound; see under *chain.* **heterocyclic c.,** a closed-chain compound in which the ring is made up of dissimilar atoms. **inorganic c.,** a compound of chemical elements containing no carbon atoms. **organic c.,** a compound of chemical elements containing carbon atoms. **organometallic c.,** one in which carbon is linked to a metal. **quaternary ammonium c.,** see *tetraethylammonium.* **saturated c.,** a chemical compound in which all the valences of the elements composing it are satisfied. **unsaturated c.,** a chemical compound in which not all the valences of the elements composing it are satisfied.

compress (kom′pres) a pad or bolster of folded

linen or other material, applied with pressure; sometimes medicated, it may be wet or dry, or hot or cold. **cribriform c.,** one perforated with holes. **fenestrated c.,** one with an opening for discharge of secretions. **graduated c.,** one consisting of layers of gradually decreasing size. **Priessnitz c.,** a cold wet compress.

compression (kom-presh′un) 1. act of pressing upon or together; the state of being pressed together. 2. in embryology, the shortening or omission of certain developmental stages.

compressor (kom-pres′er) any agent by which compression may be achieved.

compulsion (kom-pul′shun) an overwhelming urge to perform an irrational act or ritual. **compul′sive,** adj.

conarium (ko-na′re-um) the pineal body.

conation (ko-na′shun) in psychology, the power that impels effort of any kind; the conscious tendency to act.

conative (kon′ah-tiv) pertaining to the basic strivings of a person, as expressed in his behavior and actions.

concanavalin (kon″kah-nav′ah-lin) either of two phytohemagglutinins isolated along with canavalin from the meal of the Jack bean (*Canavalia ensiformis* and other species of *Canavalia*), which agglutinate the blood of mammals as a result of reaction with polyglucosans. *Concanavalin A* has been shown to inhibit the growth of ascites tumors.

concave (kon′kāv) rounded and somewhat depressed or hollowed out.

concavity (kon-kav′ĭ-te) a depression or hollowed surface.

concavoconcave (kon-ka″vo-kon′kāv) concave on each of two opposite surfaces.

concavoconvex (-kon′veks) having one concave and one convex surface.

concentrate (kon′sen-trāt) 1. to bring to a common center; to gather at one point. 2. to increase the strength by diminishing the bulk of, as of a liquid; to condense. 3. a drug or other preparation that has been strengthened by evaporation of its nonactive parts.

concentration (kon″sen-tra′shun) 1. increase in strength by evaporation. 2. the ratio of the mass or volume of a solute to the mass or volume of the solution or solvent. **hydrogen ion c.,** the degree of concentration of hydrogen ions in a solution; related approximately to the pH of the solution by the equation $(H^+) = 10^{-pH}$.

concept (kon′sept) the image of a thing held in the mind.

conception (kon-sep′shun) 1. fertilization of the ovum by the spermatozoon. 2. concept.

conceptus (kon-sep′tus) the sum of derivatives of a fertilized ovum at any developmental stage from fertilization until birth, including extraembryonic membranes as well as the embryo or fetus.

concha (kong′kah), pl. *con′chae* [L.] a shell-shaped structure. **c. of auricle,** the hollow of the auricle of the external ear, bounded anteriorly by the tragus and posteriorly by the anthelix. **c. bullo′sa,** a cystic distention of the middle nasal concha. **ethmoidal c., inferior,** nasal c., middle. **ethmoidal c., superior,** nasal c., superior. **ethmoidal c., supreme,** nasal c., supreme. **nasal c., inferior,** a bone forming the lower part of the lateral wall of the nasal cavity. **nasal c., middle,** the lower of two bony plates projecting from the inner wall of the ethmoid labyrinth and separating the superior from the middle meatus of the nose. **nasal c., superior,** the upper of two bony plates projecting from the inner wall of the ethmoid labyrinth and forming the upper boundary of the superior meatus of the nose. **nasal c., supreme,** a third thin bony plate occasionally found projecting from the inner wall of the ethmoid labyrinth, above the two usually found. **c. santori′ni,** nasal c., supreme. **sphenoidal c.,** a thin curved plate of bone at the anterior and lower part of the body of the sphenoid bone, on either side, forming part of the roof of the nasal cavity.

conchitis (kong-ki′tis) inflammation of a concha.

conchotomy (kong-kot′o-me) incision of a nasal concha.

conclination (kon″klĭ-na′shun) inward rotation of the upper pole of the vertical meridian of each eye.

concordance (kon-kor′dans) in genetics, the occurrence of a given trait in both members of a twin pair. **concor′dant,** adj.

concrescence (kon-kres′ens) a growing together of parts originally separate.

concretio (kon-kre′she-o) concretion. **c. cor′dis,** adhesive pericarditis in which the pericardial cavity is obliterated.

concretion (kon-kre′shun) 1. a calculus or inorganic mass in a natural cavity or in tissue. 2. abnormal union of adjacent parts. 3. a process of becoming harder or more solid.

concussion (kon-kush′un) a violent shock or jar, or the condition resulting from such an injury. **c. of the brain,** loss of consciousness, transient or prolonged, due to a blow to the head; there may be transient amnesia, vertigo, nausea, weak pulse, and slow respiration. **c. of the labyrinth,** deafness with tinnitus due to a blow on or explosion near the ear.

condensation (kon″den-sa′shun) 1. the act of rendering, or the process of becoming, more compact; in dentistry, the packing of filling materials into a tooth cavity. 2. the fusion of events, thoughts, or concepts to produce a new and simpler concept. 3. the process of passing from a gaseous to a liquid or solid phase.

condenser (kon-den′ser) 1. a vessel or apparatus for condensing gases or vapors. 2. a device for illuminating microscopic objects. 3. an apparatus for concentrating energy or matter. 4. a dental instrument used to pack plastic filling material into the prepared cavity of a tooth. **Abbe's c.,** as originally designed, a two-lens condenser combination placed below the stage of a microscope.

condition (kon-dish′un) to train; to subject to conditioning.

conditioning (-ing) learning in which a response is elicited by a neutral stimulus which previously has been repeatedly presented in conjunction with the stimulus that originally elicited the response.

condom (kon′dum) a sheath or cover to be worn over the penis in coitus to prevent impregnation or infection.

conductance (kon-duk′tans) ability to conduct or transmit, as electricity or other energy or material; in studies of respiration, an expression of the amount of air reaching the alveoli per unit of time per unit of pressure, the reciprocal of resistance.

conduction (kon-duk′shun) conveyance of energy, as of heat, sound, or electricity. **aerial c.,** conduction of sound waves to the organ of hearing through the air. **aerotympanal c.,** conduction of sound waves to the ear through the air and the tympanum. **air c.,** aerial c. **bone c.,** conduction of sound waves to the inner ear through the bones of the skull. **saltatory c.,** the passage of a potential from node to node of a nerve fiber, rather than along the membrane.

conductivity (kon″duk-tiv′ĭ-te) capacity for conduction.

condylarthrosis (kon″dil-ar-thro′sis) a modification of the spheroidal form of synovial joint in which the articular surfaces are ellipsoidal rather than spheroid.

condyle (kon′dīl) a rounded projection on a bone, usually for articulation with another bone. **con′dylar,** adj.

condylectomy (kon″dil-ek′to-me) excision of a condyle.

condylion (kon-dil′e-on) the most lateral point on the surface of the head of the mandible.

condyloid (kon′dĭ-loid) resembling a condyle.

condyloma (kon″dĭ-lo′mah) an elevated lesion of the skin. **condylo′matous,** adj. **c. acumina′-tum,** a small, pointed papilloma of viral origin, usually occurring on the mucous membrane or skin of the external genitals or in the perianal region. **flat c., c. la′tum,** a broad, flat syphilitic condyloma occurring on the folds of moist skin, especially about the genitals and anus.

condylotomy (-lot′o-me) transection of a condyle.

condylus (kon′dĭ-lus), pl. *con′dyli* [L.] condyle.

cone (kōn) 1. a solid figure or body having a circular base and tapering to a point, especially one of the conelike bodies of the retina. 2. in radiology, a conical or open-ended cylindrical structure used as an aid in centering the radiation beam and as a guide to source-to-film distance. **ether c.,** a cone-shaped device used over the face in administration of inhalation anesthesia. **c. of light,** the triangular light reflex on the membrana tympani. **pressure c.,** the area of compression exerted by a mass in the brain, as in uncal or transtentorial herniation. **retinal c's,** highly specialized conical or flask-shaped outer segments of the visual cells, which, with the retinal rods, form the light-sensitive elements of the retina. **sarcoplasmic c.,** the conical mass of sarcoplasm at each end of the nucleus of a smooth or cardiac muscle fiber. **twin c's,** retinal cone cells in which two cells are blended.

conexus (kŏ-nek′sus) a connecting structure.

confabulation (kon-fab″u-la′shun) the recitation of imaginary experiences to fill gaps in memory.

confection (kon-fek′shun) a medicated sweetmeat or electuary. **c. of senna,** a mild laxative containing powdered senna leaf, with other ingredients.

configuration (kon-fig″u-ra′shun) 1. the general form of a body. 2. see *gestalt.*

confinement (kon-fīn′ment) restraint within a specific area, especially at childbirth.

conflict (kon′flikt) a painful state of consciousness due to clash between opposing emotional forces, found to a certain extent in every person.

confluence (kon′floo-ens) a running together; a meeting of streams. **con′fluent,** adj. **c. of sinuses,** the dilated point of confluence of the superior sagittal, straight, occipital, and two transverse sinuses of the dura mater.

conformator (kon′for-ma″tor) an instrument for determining outlines of skull.

confusion (kon-fu′zhun) disturbed orientation in regard to time, place, or person, sometimes accompanied by disordered consciousness.

congeneic (kon″jĕ-ne′ik) of or relating to a strain of animals developed from an inbred (isogenic) strain by repeated matings with animals from another stock that have a foreign gene, the final congeneic strain then presumably differing from the original inbred strain by the presence of this gene.

congener (kon′jĕ-ner) something closely related to another thing, as a chemical compound closely related to another in composition and exerting similar or antagonistic effects. **congen′erous,** adj.

congenital (kon-jen′ĭ-tal) present at and existing from the time of birth.

congestin (kon-jes′tin) a toxic substance from tentacles of sea anemones that, when injected into dogs, causes intense congestion of the splanchnic vessels, and hemorrhage.

congestion (kon-jes′chun) abnormal accumulation of blood in a part. **hypostatic c.,** congestion of a dependent part of the body or an organ due to gravitational forces, as in venous insufficiency. **passive c.,** that due to lack of vital power or to obstruction to escape of blood from the part. **pulmonary c.,** engorgement of the pulmonary vessels, with transudation of fluid into the alveolar and interstitial spaces; it occurs in cardiac disease, infections, and certain injuries. **venous c.,** passive c.

congestive (kon-jes′tiv) pertaining to or associated with congestion.

conglobate (kon-glo′bāt) aggregated in a rounded mass or clump.

conglobation (kon″glo-ba′shun) the act of forming, or the state of being formed, into a rounded mass.

conglutin (kon-gloo′tin) a proteid from almonds and from seeds of various legumes.

conglutinant (kon-gloo′tĭ-nant) promoting union, as of the lips of a wound.

conglutination (-gloo″tĭ-na′shun) 1. the adherence of tissues to each other. 2. agglutination of erythrocytes that is dependent upon both complement and antibodies.

coniofibrosis (ko″ne-o-fi-bro′sis) pneumoconiosis with exuberant growth of connective tissue in the lungs.

coniosis (ko″ne-o′sis) a diseased state due to inhalation of dust.

coniosporosis (ko″ne-o-spo-ro′sis) a condition characterized by asthmatic symptoms and acute pneumonitis, caused by inhalation of spores of *Coniosporium corticale,* a fungus growing under the bark of certain trees; observed in workers engaged in peeling logs.

coniotoxicosis (-tok″sĭ-ko′sis) pneumoconiosis in which the irritant affects the tissues directly.

conization (ko″ni-za′shun) the removal of a cone of tissue, as in partial excision of the cervix uteri.

conjugata (kon″ju-ga′tah) the conjugate diameter of the pelvis. **c. ve′ra,** the true conjugate diameter of the pelvis.

conjugate (kon′ju-gāt) 1. paired, or equally coupled; working in unison. 2. a conjugate diameter of the pelvic inlet; used alone usually to denote the true conjugate diameter; see under *diameter.*

conjugation (kon″ju-ga′shun) a joining. In unicellular organisms, a form of sexual reproduction in which two individuals join in temporary union to transfer genetic material. In biochemistry, the joining of a toxic substance with some natural substance of the body to form a detoxified product for elimination.

conjunctiva (kon″junk-ti′vah), pl. *conjuncti′vae* [L.] the delicate membrane lining the eyelids and covering the eyeball. **conjuncti′val,** adj.

conjunctivitis (kon-junk″tĭ-vi′tis) inflammation of the conjunctiva. **acute contagious c.,** pinkeye; a highly contagious form of conjunctivitis caused by *Hemophilus aegyptius.* **allergic c., anaphylactic c.,** hay fever. **atopic c.,** allergic conjunctivitis of the immediate type, due to such airborne allergens as pollens, dusts, spores, and animal hair. **gonorrheal c.,** a severe form due to infection with gonococci. **granular c.,** trachoma. **inclusion c.,** conjunctivitis primarily affecting newborn infants, caused by a strain of *Chlamydia trachomatis,* beginning as acute purulent conjunctivitis and leading to papillary hypertrophy of the palpebral conjunctiva. **phlyctenular c.,** that marked by small vesicles surrounded by a reddened zone. **spring c., vernal c.,** a form characteristically occurring in the spring.

conjunctivoma (kon-junk″tĭ-vo′mah) a tumor of the eyelid composed of conjunctival tissue.

conjunctivoplasty (kon″junk-ti′vo-plas″te) plastic repair of the conjunctiva.

connector (kun-nek′tor) a device which joins together two separate parts or units, e.g., the bilateral parts of a removable partial denture.

conoid (ko′noid) cone-shaped.

consanguinity (kon″sang-gwin′ĭ-te) blood relationship; kinship.

conscious (kon′shus) capable of responding to sensory stimuli and having subjective experiences; awake; aware.

consciousness (-nes) the state of being conscious; responsiveness of the mind to impressions made by the senses. **double c.,** see *multiple personality.*

conservative (kon-ser′vah-tiv) designed to preserve health, restore function, and repair structures by nonradical methods.

consolidation (kon-sol″ĭ-da′shun) solidification; the process of becoming or the condition of being solid; said especially of the lung as it fills with exudate in pneumonia.

constant (kon′stant) 1. not failing; remaining unaltered. 2. a quantity that is not subject to change. **Avogadro's c.,** the number of particles of the type specified by the chemical formula in 1 (gram) mole of any substance having a chemical formula; the numerical value of the constant is 6.0232×10^{23}. **Michaelis c.,** a constant representing the substrate concentration at which the velocity of an enzyme reaction is half the maximal velocity; symbol K_m. **sedimentation c.,** a measure, commonly expressed in Svedberg units, of the relative sedimentation rate of molecules under an induced gravitational field, as in a centrifuge; symbol S.

constipated (kon′stĭ-pāt″ed) affected with constipation.

constipation (kon″stĭ-pa′shun) infrequent or difficult evacuation of feces.

constitution (kon″stĭ-tu′shun) 1. the make-up or functional habit of the body. 2. the arrangement of atoms in a molecule.

constitutional (-al) 1. affecting the whole constitution of the body; not local. 2. pertaining to the constitution.

constriction (kon-strik′shun) 1. a narrowing or compression of a part; a stricture. 2. a diminution in range of thinking or feeling, associated with diminished spontaneity.

constrictor (kon-strik′tor) that which causes constriction.

consultant (-sul′tant) a physician called in for advice and counsel.

consultation (kon″sul-ta′shun) a deliberation by two or more physicians about diagnosis or treatment in a particular case.

consumption (kon-sump′shun) 1. the act of consuming, or the process of being consumed. 2. wasting of the body; formerly, tuberculosis of the lungs. **luxus c.,** ingestion of excess protein which does not form part of the tissues but remains in the body as a reserve supply.

contact (kon′takt) 1. a mutual touching of two bodies or persons. 2. an individual known to have been sufficiently near an infected person to have been exposed to the transfer of infectious material. **balancing c.,** the contact between the upper and lower occlusal surfaces of the teeth on the side opposite the working contact. **complete c.,** contact of the entire adjoining surfaces of two teeth. **direct c., immediate c.,** the contact of a healthy person with a person having a communicable disease, the disease being transmitted as a result. **indirect c., mediate c.,** that achieved through some intervening medium, as propagation of a communicable disease through the air or by means of fomites. **occlusal c.,** contact between the upper and lower teeth when the jaws are closed. **proximal c., proximate c.,** touching of the proximal surfaces of two adjoining teeth. **weak c.,** contact in which adjoining surfaces of two teeth barely touch. **working c.,** that between the upper and lower teeth on the side toward which the mandible has been moved in mastication.

contactant (kon-tak′tant) an allergen capable of inducing delayed contact-type hypersensitivity of the epidermis after one or more episodes of contact.

contactology (kon″tak-tol′o-je) the specialized field of knowledge related to the prescription and use of contact lenses.

contagion (kon-ta′jun) 1. the spread of disease from person-to-person. 2. a contagious disease. **direct c., immediate c.,** communication of disease by direct contact with a sick person. **mediate c.,** communication of disease from a sick to a well person through an intervening object or person. **psychic c.,** communication of psychological symptoms through mental influence.

contagiosity (kon-ta″je-os′ĭ-te) the quality of being contagious.

contagious (kon-ta′jus) capable of being transmitted from one person to another.

contaminant (kon-tam′ĭ-nant) something that causes contamination.

contamination (kon-tam″ĭ-na-shun) 1. the soiling or making inferior by contact or mixture. 2. the deposition of radioactive material in any place where it is not desired.

content (kon′tent) that which is contained within a thing. **latent c.,** the part of a dream which is hidden in the unconsciousness. **manifest c.,** the part of a dream which is remembered after awakening.

continence (kon′tĭ-nens) ability to exercise voluntary control over natural impulses. **con′tinent,** adj.

contra- word element [L.], *against; opposed.*

contra-angle (kon″trah-ang′g'l) an angulation by which the working point of a surgical instrument is brought close to the long axis of its shaft.

contra-aperture (-ap′er-tūr) a second opening made in an abscess to facilitate the discharge of its contents.

contraception (-sep′shun) the prevention of conception or impregnation.

contraceptive (-sep′tiv) 1. diminishing the likelihood of or preventing conception. 2. an agent that so acts. **intrauterine c.,** see *contraceptive device.* **oral c.,** a hormonal compound taken orally in order to block ovulation and prevent the occurrence of pregnancy.

contractile (kon-trak′til) having the power or tendency to contract in response to a suitable stimulus.

contractility (kon″trak-til′ĭ-te) capacity for becoming short in response to a suitable stimulus.

contraction (kon-trak′shun) a drawing together; a shortening or shrinkage. **carpopedal c.,** the condition resulting from chronic short-

ening of the muscles of the fingers, toes, arms, and legs in tetany. **cicatricial c.,** the contraction occurring in the tissues of a healing wound as a cicatrix forms. **clonic c.,** muscular contraction alternating with relaxation. **closing c.,** contraction occuring at the point of application of the stimulus when the electrical circuit is closed. **Dupuytren's c.,** see under *contracture.* **Hicks' c's,** light, usually painless, irregular uterine contractions during pregnancy, gradually increasing in intensity and frequency and becoming more rhythmic during the third trimester. **hourglass c.,** contraction of an organ, as the stomach or uterus, at or near the middle. **idiomuscular c.,** contraction produced by direct electrical stimulation of a wasted muscle. **isometric c.,** muscle contraction without appreciable shortening or change in distance between its origin and insertion. **isotonic c.,** muscle contraction without appreciable change in the force of contraction; the distance between the muscle's origin and insertion becomes lessened. **opening c.,** contraction occurring at the point of application of the stimulus when the electrical circuit is opened. **paradoxical c.,** contraction of a muscle caused by the passive approximation of its extremities. **postural c.,** the state of muscular tension and contraction which just suffices to maintain the posture of the body. **rheumatic c.,** tetany. **tetanic c.,** sustained muscular contraction without intervals of relaxation. **tonic c.,** tetanic c. **Volkmann's c.,** see under *contracture.*

contracture (kon-trak′tūr) abnormal shortening of muscle tissue, rendering the muscle highly resistant to passive stretching. **Dupuytren's c.,** flexion deformity of the fingers or toes, due to shortening, thickening, and fibrosis of the palmar or plantar fascia. **ischemic c.,** muscular contracture and degeneration due to interference with the circulation from pressure, or from injury or cold. **organic c.,** permanent and continuous contracture. **Volkmann's c.,** contraction of the fingers and sometimes of the wrist, or of analogous parts of the foot, with loss of power, after severe injury or improper use of a tourniquet.

contrafissure (kon″trah-fish′er) a fracture in a part opposite the site of the blow.

contraincision (-in-sizh′un) counterincision to promote drainage.

contraindication (-in″dĭ-ka′shun) any condition which renders a particular line of treatment improper or undesirable.

contralateral (-lat′er-al) pertaining to, situated on, or affecting the opposite side.

contrecoup (kon″truh-koo′) [Fr.] denoting an injury, as to the brain, occurring at a site opposite to the point of impact.

control (kon-trōl′) 1. the governing or limitation of certain objects or events. 2. a standard against which experimental observations may be evaluated, as a procedure identical to the experimental procedure except for absence of the one factor being studied; also any individual of the group exhibiting the standard characteristics. **birth c.,** regulation of childbearing by measures designed to prevent conception.

contuse (kon-tūz′) to bruise; to wound by beating.

contusion (kon-too′zhun) injury to a part without a break in the skin; a bruise.

conus (ko′nus), pl. *co′ni* [L.] 1. a cone or cone-shaped structure. 2. posterior staphyloma of the myopic eye. **c. arterio′sus,** the anterosuperior portion of the right ventricle of the heart, at the entrance to the pulmonary trunk. **c. medulla′ris,** the cone-shaped lower end of the spinal cord, at the level of the upper lumbar vertebrae. **c. termina′lis,** c. medullaris. **co′ni vasculo′si,** lobules of epididymis.

convalescence (kon″vah-les′ens) the stage of recovery from an illness, operation, or injury.

convalescent (kon″vah-les′ent) 1. pertaining to or characterized by convalescence. 2. a patient who is recovering from a disease, operation, or injury.

convection (kon-vek′shun) the act of conveying or transmission, specifically transmission of heat in a liquid or gas by circulation of heated particles.

convergence (kon-ver′jens) 1. inclination toward a common point; the coordinated movement of the two eyes toward fixation of the same near point. 2. the point of meeting of convergent lines. **conver′gent,** adj. **negative c.,** outward deviation of the visual axes. **positive c.,** inward deviation of the visual axes.

conversion (kon-ver′zhun) 1. the transformation of emotions into physical manifestations. 2. manipulative correction of malposition of a fetal part during labor.

convertin (kon-ver′tin) coagulation Factor VII.

convex (kon′veks) having a rounded, somewhat elevated surface.

convexoconcave (kon-vek″so-kon′kāv) having one convex and one concave surface.

convexoconvex (-kon′veks) convex on two surfaces.

convolution (kon″vo-lu′shun) a tortuous irregularity or elevation caused by the infolding of a structure upon itself. **Broca's c.,** inferior frontal gyrus. **Heschl's c.,** anterior transverse temporal gyrus.

convulsion (kon-vul′shun) an involuntary contraction or series of contractions of the voluntary muscles. **epileptiform c.,** convulsion marked by loss of consciousness. **mimetic c., mimic c.,** facial spasm or tic. **puerperal c.,** involuntary spasms in women just before, during, or just after childbirth. **salaam c.,** nodding spasm. **tetanic c.,** tonic spasm with loss of consciousness. **uremic c.,** convulsion due to uremia, or retention in the blood of material that should have been eliminated by the kidneys.

convulsive (kon-vul′siv) pertaining to, characterized by, or of the nature of convulsion.

Cooperia (koo-pe′re-ah) a genus of parasitic nematodes sometimes found in the small intestine of ruminants.

cooperid (koo′per-id) an individual of the genus *Cooperia.*

coordination (ko-or″dĭ-na′shun) the harmonious functioning of interrelated organs and parts.

cope (kōp) in dentistry, the upper or cavity side of a denture flask.

coping (kōp′ing) a thin, metal covering or cap, such as the plate of metal applied over the prepared crown or root of a tooth prior to attaching an artificial crown.

copiopia (ko″pe-o′pe-ah) eyestrain.

copolymer (ko-pol′ĭ-mer) a polymer containing monomers of more than one kind.

copper (kop′er) chemical element (*see table*), at. no. 29, symbol Cu. **c. sulfate,** cupric sulfate.

copperhead (-hed) 1. a venomous snake (a pit viper), *Agkistrodon contortrix,* of the United States, having a brown to copper-colored body with dark bands. 2. a very venomous elapid snake, *Denisonia superba,* of Australia, Tasmania, and the Solomon Islands.

coprecipitin (ko″pre-sip′ĭ-tin) any of two or more precipitins in serum.

copremesis (kop-rem′ĕ-sis) the vomiting of fecal matter.

coproantibody (kop″ro-an′tĭ-bod-e) an antibody (chiefly IgA) present in the intestinal tract, associated with immunity to enteric infection.

coprolalia (-la′le-ah) the utterance of obscene words, especially words relating to feces.

coprolith (kop′ro-lith) hard fecal concretion in the intestine.

coprology (kop-rol′o-je) the study of the feces.

coproma (kop-ro′mah) stercoroma.

coprophagia (kop″ro-fa′je-ah) the ingestion of dung, or feces.

coprophilia (-fil′e-ah) a psychopathologic interest in filth, especially in feces and defecation.

coprophilic (-fil′ik) 1. pertaining to or characterized by coprophilia. 2. inhabiting dung or feces; said of bacteria.

coprophobia (-fo′be-ah) abnormal repugnance to defecation and to feces.

coproporphyria (-por-fir′e-ah) hereditary porphyria marked by excessive excretion of coproporphyrin, chiefly in the feces.

coproporphyrin (-por′fĭ-rin) a porphyrin formed in the blood-forming organs and intestine and found in the urine and feces in coproporphyrinuria.

coproporphyrinogen (-por″fĭ-rin′o-jen) the fully reduced, colorless compound giving rise to coproporphyrin by oxidation.

coproporphyrinuria (-por″fĭ-rin-u′re-ah) the presence of coproporphyrin in the urine.

coprostasis (kop-ros′tah-sis) fecal impaction.

coprozoa (kop″ro-zo′ah) protozoa found in feces outside the body, but not in the intestines.

coprozoic (-zo′ik) living in fecal matter.

copula (kop′u-lah) any connecting part or structure.

copulation (kop″u-la′shun) sexual congress or coitus; usually applied to the mating process in animals lower than man.

cor (kor) [L.] heart. **c. adipo′sum,** fatty heart. **c. bilocula′re,** a two-chambered heart with one atrium and one ventricle, and a common atrioventricular valve. **c. bovi′num,** a greatly enlarged heart due to a hypertrophied left ventricle. **c. hirsu′tum,** c. villosum. **c. pseudo-**

trilocula′re biatria′tum, a congenital anomaly in which the heart functions as a three-chambered heart, the blood passing from the right to the left atrium and thence to the left ventricle and aorta. **c. pulmona′le,** heart disease due to pulmonary hypertension secondary to disease of the blood vessels of the lung. **c. triatria′tum,** a heart with three atrial chambers, the pulmonary veins emptying into an accessory chamber above the true left atrium and communicating with it by a small opening. **c. trilocula′re,** three-chambered heart. **c. trilocula′re biatria′tum,** a three-chambered heart with two atria communicating, by the tricuspid and mitral valves, with a single ventricle. **c. trilocula′re biventricula′re,** a three-chambered heart with one atrium and two ventricles. **c. villo′sum,** a roughened state of the pericardium, due to an exudate on its surface, occurring in pericarditis.

coracidium (kor″ah-sid′e-um), pl. *coracid′ia* [L.] the individual free-swimming or free-crawling, spherical, ciliated embryo of certain tapeworms, e.g., *Diphyllobothrium latum.*

coracoacromial (kor″ah-ko-ah-kro′me-al) pertaining to the coracoid and acromion processes.

coracoid (kor′ah-koid) 1. like a crow's beak. 2. the coracoid process.

Coramine (ko′rah-min) trademark for preparations of nikethamide.

cord (kord) any long, cylindrical, flexible structure. **Braun's c′s,** strings of cells which have been observed in the kidney of the early embryo. **dental c.,** a cordlike mass of cells from which the enamel organ develops. **Ferrein's c′s,** the lower, or true, vocal cords. **genital c.,** in the embryo, the midline fused caudal part of the two urogenital ridges, each containing a mesonephric and paramesonephric duct. **gubernacular c.,** chorda gubernaculum. **nerve c.,** any nerve trunk or bundle of nerve fibers. **sexual c's,** the seminiferous tubules during the early fetal stage. **spermatic c.,** the structure extending from the abdominal inguinal ring to the testis, comprising the pampiniform plexus, nerves, ductus deferens, testicular artery, and other vessels. **spinal c.,** that part of the central nervous system lodged in the vertebral canal, extending from the foramen magnum to the upper part of the lumbar region; see Plates XI and XIV. **umbilical c.,** the structure connecting the fetus and placenta, and containing the vessels through which fetal blood passes to and from the placenta. **vocal c's,** folds of mucous membrane in the larynx; the superior pair being called the *false,* and the inferior pair the *true,* vocal cords. **Willis' c's,** fibrous bands traversing the inferior angle of the superior sagittal sinus.

cordal (kor′dal) pertaining to a cord; used specifically in referring to the vocal cords.

cordate (kor′dāt) heart-shaped.

cordectomy (kor-dek′to-me) excision of a cord, as of a vocal cord.

cordiform (kor′dĭ-form) heart-shaped.

corditis (kor-di′tis) inflammation of the spermatic cord.

cordopexy (kor′do-pek″se) surgical fixation of a vocal cord.

cordotomy (kor-dot′o-me) 1. section of a vocal cord. 2. chordotomy.

Cordran (kor′dran) trademark for a preparation of flurandrenolide.

core(o)- word element [Gr.], *pupil of eye.*

coreclisis (kor″ĕ-kli′sis) iridencleisis.

corectasis (kor-ek′tah-sis) dilatation of the pupil.

corectome (ko-rek′tōm) cutting instrument for iridectomy.

corectomedialysis (ko-rek″to-me″de-al′ĭ-sis) surgical creation of an artificial pupil by detaching the iris from the ciliary ligament.

corectomy (ko-rek′to-me) iridectomy.

corectopia (kor″ek-to′pe-ah) abnormal location of the pupil of the eye.

coredialysis (ko″re-di-al′ĭ-sis) surgical separation of the external margin of the iris from the ciliary body.

corediastasis (-di-as′tah-sis) dilatation of the pupil.

corelysis (ko-rel′ĭ-sis) operative destruction of the pupil; especially detachment of adhesions of the pupillary margin of the iris from the lens.

coremorphosis (ko″re-mor-fo′sis) surgical formation of an artificial pupil.

corenclisis (ko″ren-kli′sis) iridencleisis.

coreometer (ko″re-om′ĕ-ter) pupillometer.

coréometry (-om′ĕ-tre) pupillometry.

coreoplasty (ko′re-o-plas″te) any plastic operation on the pupil.

corepressor (ko″re-pres′sor) in genetic theory, a small molecule that combines with an aporepressor to form the complete repressor.

coretomy (ko-ret′o-me) iridotomy.

corium (ko′re-um) the dermis; the layer of the skin deep to the epidermis, consisting of a dense bed of vascular connective tissue, and containing the nerves and terminal organs of sensation, the hair roots, and sebaceous and sweat glands.

corn (korn) a horny induration and thickening of the stratum corneum, caused by friction and pressure and forming a conical mass pointing down into the corium, producing pain and irritation. **soft c.,** one between the toes, kept softened by moisture, often leading to painful inflammation under the corn.

cornea (kor′ne-ah) the transparent anterior part of the eye. See Plate XIII. **cor′neal,** adj. **conical c.,** keratoconus.

corneitis (kor″ne-i′tis) keratitis.

corneoiritis (kor″ne-o-i-ri′tis) inflammation of the cornea and iris.

corneosclera (-skle′rah) the cornea and sclera regarded as one organ.

corneous (kor′ne-us) hornlike or horny; consisting of keratin.

corniculum (kor-nik′u-lum) [L.] corniculate cartilage.

cornification (kor″nĭ-fi-ka′shun) 1. conversion into keratin, or horn. 2. conversion of epithelium to the stratified squamous type.

cornified (kor′nĭ-fīd) converted into horny tissue (keratin); keratinized.

cornu (kor′nu), pl. *cor′nua* [L.] horn; a hornlike excrescence or projection; in anatomical nomenclature, a structure that appears horn-shaped, especially in section. **c. ammo′nis,** hippocampus. **c. cuta′neum,** a horny excrescence on human skin. **c. sacra′le,** either of two hook-shaped processes extending down from the arch of the last sacral vertebra.

cornual, cornuate (kor′nu-al; kor′nu-āt) pertaining to a horn, especially to the horns of the spinal cord.

corona (kŏ-ro′nah), pl. *coro′nae* [L.] a crown; in anatomical nomenclature, a crownlike eminence or encircling structure. **coro′nal,** adj. **dental c., c. den′tis,** the crown of a tooth; anatomical crown. **c. glan′dis pe′nis,** rim around proximal part of glans penis. **c. radia′ta,** 1. the radiating crown of projection fibers passing from the internal capsule to every part of the cerebral cortex. 2. an investing layer of radially elongated follicle cells surrounding the zona pellucida. **c. ven′eris,** a ring of syphilitic sores around the forehead.

coronad (kor′o-nad) toward the crown of the head or any corona.

coronaritis (kor″o-nar-i′tis) coronary arteritis.

coronary (kor′ŏ-ner″e) encircling in the manner of a crown; a term applied to vessels, ligaments, etc., especially to the arteries of the heart, and, by extension, to pathologic involvement of them.

coronavirus (kor″o-nah-vi′rus) any of a group of morphologically similar, ether-sensitive viruses, probably RNA, causing infectious bronchitis of birds, hepatitis in mice, gastroenteritis in swine, and respiratory infections in humans.

coroner (kor′o-ner) an officer who holds inquests in regard to violent, sudden, or unexplained deaths.

coronoidectomy (kor″o-noi-dek′to-me) surgical removal of the coronoid process of the mandible.

coroscopy (ko-ros′ko-pe) retinoscopy.

corotomy (ko-rot′o-me) iridotomy.

corpulency (kor′pu-len-se) undue fatness; obesity.

corpus (kor′pus), pl. *cor′pora* [L.] body. **c. adipo′sum buc′cae,** sucking pad. **c. al′bicans,** white fibrous tissue that replaces the regressing corpus luteum in the human ovary in the latter half of pregnancy, or soon after ovulation when pregnancy does not supervene. **cor′pora amyla′cea,** small hyaline masses of degenerate cells found in the prostate, neuroglia, etc. **c. amygdaloi′deum,** a small mass of subcortical gray matter within the tip of the temporal lobe, anterior to the inferior horn of the lateral ventricle of the brain. **cor′pora aran′tii,** bodies of Arantius. **cor′pora bigem′ina,** corpora quadrigemina. **c. callo′sum,** an arched mass of white matter in the depths of the longitudinal fissure, composed of transverse fibers connecting the cerebral hemispheres. **c. caverno′sum,** either of the columns of erectile tissue forming the body of the clitoris (*c. cavernosum clitoridis*)

or penis (*c. cavernosum penis*). **c. cilia′re,** ciliary body. **c. denta′tum,** dentate nucleus. **c. fimbria′tum,** band of white matter bordering the lateral edge of the lower cornu of the lateral ventricle of the cerebrum. **cor′pora fla′va,** waxy bodies in the central nervous system and elsewhere. **c. genicula′tum,** see *lateral geniculate body* and *medial geniculate body.* **c. hemorrhag′icum,** 1. an ovarian follicle containing blood. 2. a corpus luteum containing a blood clot. **c. highmoria′num,** mediastinum testis. **c. interpeduncula′re,** nucleus interpeduncu-lare. **c. lu′teum,** a yellow glandular mass in the ovary formed by an ovarian follicle that has matured and discharged its ovum. **c. pyrami-da′le,** pyramid of the medulla oblongata. **cor′-pora quadrigem′ina,** four rounded eminences on the posterior mesencephalon. **cor′pora restifor′mia,** inferior cerebellar peduncle. **c. spongio′sum pe′nis,** a column of erectile tissue forming the urethral surface of the penis, in which the urethra is found. **c. ster′ni,** the body of the sternum, located between the manubrium and the xiphoid process. **c. stria′tum,** a subcortical mass of gray and white substance in front of and lateral to the thalamus in each cerebral hemisphere. **c. subthalam′icum,** nucleus subthalamicus. **c. vit′reum,** the vitreous body of the eye. **c. wolffia′num,** mesonephros.

corpuscle (kor′pus′l) any small mass or body. **corpus′cular,** adj. **amylaceous c's,** corpora amylacea. **basal c.,** a small thickening at the base of each cilium in ciliated cells. **Bizzozero's c's,** platelets. **blood c's,** formed elements of the blood, i.e., erythrocytes and leukocytes. **Burck-hardt's c's,** yellowish bodies found in trachoma secretion. **cartilage c's,** see under *cell.* **cement c.,** cementocyte. **chorea c's,** round hyaline bodies in the sheaths of the vessels of the corpora striata and internal capsule in chorea. **chro-mophil c's,** Nissl bodies. **chyle c.,** a lymphocyte found in chyle. **colloid c's,** corpora amylacea. **colostrum c's,** large rounded bodies in colostrum, containing droplets of fat and sometimes a nucleus. **concentric c's,** Hassall's c's. **cor-neal c's,** star-shaped corpuscles within the corneal spaces. **Donné's c's,** colostrum c's. **Drys-dale's c's,** transparent microscopic cells in the fluid of ovarian cysts. **genital c's,** small encapsulated nerve endings in the mucous membranes in the genital region. **ghost c.,** phantom c. **Gluge's c's,** granular corpuscles in diseased nerve tissue. **Golgi's c's,** encapsulated end-organs found in a tendon at its junction with muscular fibers. **Grandry's c's,** Merkel's c's. **Has-sall's c's,** small concentrically striated bodies in the thymus. **Hayem's elementary c's,** platelets. **Krause's c's,** end-bulbs. **lamellated c's,** large encapsulated nerve endings found throughout the body, concerned with perception of different sensations. **Leber's c's,** Has-sall's c's. **Lostorfer's c's,** granular bodies in the blood in syphilis. **lymph c's,** lymphocytes in lymph. **lymphoid c's,** lymphocytes in tissues. **malpighian c's,** renal c's. **Meissner's c's,** tactile c's. **Merkel's c's,** tactile corpuscles in the submucosa of the tongue and mouth. **Mie-scher's c's,** sarcosporidian cysts. **nerve c's,**

sheath cells between the neurilemma and medullary sheath. **Norris' c's,** colorless transparent disks in the blood serum. **Nunn's c's,** epithelial cells in ovarian cysts that have undergone fatty degeneration. **Pacini's c's, pacinian c's,** lamellated corpuscles concerned in perception of pressure. **phantom c.,** an artifactual red blood cell from which the hemoglobin has been dissolved. **Purkinje's c's,** large, branched nerve cells composing the middle layer of the cortex of the cerebellum. **pus c.,** one of the cells of pus, chiefly neutrophilic leukocytes. **Rainey's c's,** sarcosporidian cysts. **red blood c.,** erythrocyte. **renal c's,** bodies forming the beginning of nephrons, each consisting of the glomerulus and glomerular capsule. **shadow c.,** phantom c. **tactile c's,** medium-sized nerve endings in the skin, chiefly in the palms and soles. **thymus c's,** Hassall's c's. **Traube's c.,** phantom c. **Vater's c's,** lamellated c's. **Virchow's c's,** corneal c's. **Wagner's c's,** tactile c's. **white blood c.,** leukocyte.

corpusculum (kor-pus'ku-lum), pl. *corpus'cula* [L.] corpuscle.

correction (kŏ-rek'shun) a setting right, e.g., the provision of specific lenses for improvement of vision, or an arbitrary adjustment made in values or devices in performance of experimental procedures.

correlation (kor″ĕ-la'shun) in neurology, the union of afferent impulses within a nerve center to bring about an appropriate response. In statistics, the degree of association of variable phenomena, as intelligence and birth order.

correspondence (kor″ĕ-spon'dens) the condition of being in agreement or conformity. **anomalous retinal c.,** a condition in which disparate points on the retinas of the two eyes come to be associated sensorially. **harmonious retinal c.,** the condition in which the corresponding points on the retinas of the two eyes are associated sensorially. **retinal c.,** the state concerned with the impingement of image-producing stimuli on the retinas of the two eyes.

corrosive (kŏ-ro'siv) destructive to the texture or substance of the tissues; an agent that so acts.

Cortate (kor'tāt) trademark for preparations of desoxycorticosterone.

Cort-Dome (kort'dōm) trademark for preparations of hydrocortisone.

Cortef (kor'tef) trademark for preparations of hydrocortisone.

cortex (kor'teks), pl. *cor'tices* [L.] an outer layer, as the bark of the trunk or the rind of a fruit, or the outer layer of an organ or other structure, as distinguished from its inner substance. **cor'tical,** adj. **adrenal c.,** the outer, firm layer comprising the larger part of the adrenal gland; it secretes various hormones. **cerebellar c.,** the superficial gray matter of the cerebellum. **cerebral c., c. cer'ebri,** the convoluted layer of gray substance covering each cerebral hemisphere; see *archipallium, paleopallium,* and *neopallium.* **c. len'tis,** the softer, external part of the lens of the eye. **provisional c.,** the cortex of the fetal adrenal gland that undergoes involution in early fetal life. **renal c.,** the outer part

of the substance of the kidney, composed mainly of glomeruli and convoluted tubules.

cortexone (kor-tek'sōn) desoxycorticosterone.

corticate (kor'tĭ-kāt) having a cortex or bark.

corticectomy (kor″tĭ-sek'to-me) excision of an area of cerebral cortex (scar or microgyrus) in treatment of focal epilepsy.

corticifugal (-sif'u-gal) proceeding, conducting, or moving away from the cortex.

corticipetal (-sip'ĕ-tal) proceeding, conducting, or moving toward the cortex.

corticoadrenal (kor″tĭ-ko-ah-dre'nal) pertaining to the adrenal cortex.

corticobulbar (-bul'bar) pertaining to or connecting the cerebral cortex and the medulla oblongata.

corticoid (kor'tĭ-koid) a hormone of the adrenal cortex, or other natural or synthetic compound with similar activity.

corticopontine (kor″tĭ-ko-pon'tīn) pertaining to or connecting the cerebral cortex and the pons.

corticospinal (-spi'nal) pertaining to or connecting the cerebral cortex and the spinal cord.

corticosteroid (-ste'roid) any of the steroids produced by the adrenal cortex, e.g., cortisol, corticosterone, etc. Also, their synthetic equivalents.

corticosterone (-stēr'on) a steroid found in the adrenal cortex that maintains life in adrenalectomized animals, having several other activities attributed to the adrenal cortex.

corticotrophic (-trof'ik) corticotropic.

corticotrophin (-tro'fin) corticotropin.

corticotropic (-trop'ik) having a stimulating effect on the adrenal cortex; pertaining to corticotropin.

corticotropin (-tro'pin) a hormone secreted by the anterior pituitary gland, having a stimulating effect on the adrenal cortex; a preparation from the anterior pituitary gland of mammals is used to stimulate adrenal cortex activity and to test its function.

Cortifoam (kor'tĭ-fōm) trademark for an aerosol foam containing 10% hydrocortisone acetate; used as an intrarectal anti-inflammatory.

cortisol (kor'tĭ-sol) see *hydrocortisone.*

cortisone (kor'tĭ-sōn) a glucocorticoid with significant mineralocorticoid activity, isolated from the adrenal cortex, largely inactive in man until converted to hydrocortisone (cortisol); the acetate is used as an anti-inflammatory agent.

Cortogen (kor'to-jen) trademark for preparations of cortisone.

Cortone (kor'tōn) trademark for preparations of cortisone.

Cortrophin (kor-tro'fin) trademark for preparations of corticotropin.

corundum (kŏ-run'dum) native aluminum oxide, Al_2O_3, used in dentistry as an abrasive and polishing agent.

coruscation (kor″us-ka'shun) the sensation as of a flash of light before the eyes.

corybantism (kor″ĭ-ban'tism) wild, frenzied, and sleepless delirium.

corymbiform (ko-rim'bĭ-form) clustered; said of

lesions grouped around a single, usually larger, lesion.

Corynebacteriaceae (ko-ri″ne-bak-te″re-a′-se-e) a family of schizomycetes (order Eubacteriales).

Corynebacterium (-bak-te′re-um) a genus of bacteria (family Corynebacteriaceae), including *C. diphthe′riae*, the etiologic agent of diphtheria, *C. minutis′simum*, the etiologic agent of erythrasma, *C. pseudodiphtherit′icum*, a nonpathogenic species present in the respiratory tract, and *C. pseudotuberculo′sis*, which sometimes causes pseudotuberculosis in domestic animals.

coryza (ko-ri′zah) profuse discharge from the mucous membrane of the nose.

coryzavirus (ko-ri″zah-vi′rus) rhinovirus.

C.O.S. Canadian Ophthalmological Society; Clinical Orthopaedic Society.

cosmetic (koz-met′ik) 1. beautifying; tending to preserve, restore, or confer comeliness. 2. a beautifying substance or preparation.

cost(o)- word element [L.], *rib.*

costa (kos′tah), pl. *cos′tae* [L.] 1. a rib. 2. a thin, firm, rodlike structure running along the base of the undulating membrane of certain flagellates. **cos′tal**, adj.

costalgia (kos-tal′je-ah) pain in the ribs.

costalis (kos-ta′lis) [L.] costal.

costectomy (kos-tek′to-me) excision of a rib.

costive (kos′tiv) 1. pertaining to, characterized by, or producing constipation. 2. an agent that depresses intestinal motility.

costiveness (-nes) constipation.

costocervical (kos″to-ser′vĭ-kal) pertaining to ribs and neck.

costochondral (-kon′dral) pertaining to a rib and its cartilage.

costoclavicular (-klah-vik′u-ler) pertaining to the ribs and clavicle.

costocoracoid (-kor′ah-koid) pertaining to the ribs and coracoid process.

costogenic (-jen′ik) arising from a rib, especially from a defect of the marrow of the ribs.

costoscapularis (-skap″u-la′ris) the serratus anterior muscle.

costosternal (-ster′nal) pertaining to the ribs and sternum.

costosternoplasty (-ster″no-plas′′te) surgical repair of funnel chest, a segment of rib being used to support the sternum.

costotomy (kos-tot′o-me) incision or division of a rib or costal cartilage.

costotransverse (kos″to-trans-vers′) lying between the ribs and the transverse processes of the vertebrae.

costotransversectomy (-trans″ver-sek′to-me) excision of a part of a rib along with the transverse process of a vertebra.

costovertebral (-ver′tĕ-bral) pertaining to a rib and a vertebra.

costoxiphoid (-zi′foid) connecting the ribs and xiphoid cartilage.

cosyntropin (ko-sin-tro′pin) a synthetic corticotropin used in the screening of adrenal insufficiency on the basis of plasma cortisol response after intramuscular or intravenous injection.

Cothera (ko-ther′ah) trademark for a preparation of dimethoxanate.

cothromboplastin (ko-throm″bo-plas′tin) coagulation Factor VII.

cotton (kot′un) a textile material derived from the seeds of cultivated varieties of *Gossypium;* used as a dressing. **absorbent c.**, purified cotton from which the natural wax has been removed. **collodion c.**, pyroxylin. **purified c.**, cotton freed from impurities, deprived of fatty matter, bleached and sterilized; used as a surgical aid.

co-twin (ko′twin) one of a pair of twins.

cotyledon (kot″ĭ-le′don) any subdivision of the uterine surface of the placenta.

cotyloid (kot′ĭ-loid) cup-shaped.

couching (kowch′ing) surgical displacement of the lens in cataract.

cough (kof) 1. sudden noisy expulsion of air from lungs. 2. to produce such an expulsion of air. **dry c.**, cough without expectoration. **ear c.**, reflex cough produced by disease of the ear. **hacking c.**, a short, frequent, shallow and feeble cough. **productive c.**, cough attended with expectoration of material from the bronchi. **reflex c.**, cough due to irritation of some remote organ. **stomach c.**, cough caused by reflex irritation from stomach disorder. **wet c.**, productive cough. **whooping c.**, see under W.

coulomb (koo′lom) the unit of electrical charge, defined as the quantity of electrical charge transferred by 1 ampere in 1 second.

Coumadin (koo′mah-din) trademark for a preparation of warfarin.

count (kownt) a numerical computation or indication. **Addis c.**, the determination of the number of erythrocytes, leukocytes, epithelial cells, casts, and protein content in an aliquot of a 12-hour urine specimen. **blood c.**, determination of the number of formed elements in a measured volume of blood, usually a cubic millimeter (as of red blood cells, white blood cells, or platelet count). **differential c.**, a count on a stained blood smear, of the proportion of different types of leukocytes (or other cells), expressed in percentages. **direct platelet c.**, estimation of the number of platelets per cubic millimeter of blood. **filament-nonfilament c.**, determination of the number of juvenile and mature leukocytes, as in the differential blood count. **indirect platelet c.**, the count of the total number of platelets per cubic millimeter of blood by counting the platelets on a stained blood film. **platelet c.**, the count of the total number of platelets per cubic millimeter of blood by counting the platelets on a stained blood film. **Schilling's c.**, a differential blood cell count in which the leukocytes are divided into four groups.

counter (kown′ter) an instrument or apparatus by which numerical value in computed; in radiology, a device for enumerating ionizing events. **Coulter c.**, an automatic photoelectric instrument used in enumeration of formed elements in the peripheral blood. **Geiger c., Geiger-**

Müller c., an amplifying device that indicates the presence of ionizing particles. **scintillation c.,** a device for indicating the emission of ionizing particles, permitting determination of the concentration of radioactive isotopes in the body or other substance.

counterextension   (kown″ter-eks-ten′shun) traction in a proximal direction coincident with traction in opposition to it.

counterincision (-in-sizh′un) a second incision made to promote drainage or to relieve tension on the edges of a wound.

counterirritant (-ir′ĭ-tant) 1. producing counterirritation. 2. an agent which produces counterirritation.

counterirritation (-ir″ĭ-ta′shun) superficial irritation intended to relieve some other irritation.

counteropening (-o″pen-ing) a second incision made across an earlier one to promote drainage.

counterpoison (kown′ter-poi″zon) a poison given to counteract another poison.

counterpulsation (kown″ter-pul-sa′shun) a technique for assisting the circulation and decreasing the work of the heart, by synchronizing the force of an external pumping device with cardiac systole and diastole.

counterpuncture (kown′ter-punk″tūr) a second opening made opposite another.

counterstain (-stān) a stain applied to render the effects of another stain more discernible.

countertraction (-trak″shun) traction opposed to another traction; used in reduction of fractures.

countertransference (kown″ter-trans-fer′ens) in psychoanalysis, the emotional reaction aroused in the physician by the patient.

coup (koo) [Fr.] stroke. **c. de fouet** (koo duh fwa) ["stroke of the whip"] rupture of the plantaris muscle accompanied by a sharp disabling pain. **c. de sabre** (koo-duh sahb) ["saber stroke"] resembling the scar of a saber wound; used to designate such a lesion of linear scleroderma on the forehead and scalp. **c. de sang** (koo duh sang) congestion of the brain. **c. sur coup** (koo sur koo) ["blow on blow"] administration of a drug in small doses at short intervals to secure rapid, complete, or continuous action.

coupling (kup′ling) in genetics, occurrence in a double heterozygote on the same chromosome of the two mutant alleles of interest; in cardiology, serial occurrence of a normal heart beat followed closely by a premature beat.

covalence (ko-va′lens) a chemical bond between two atoms in which electrons are shared between the two nuclei. **cova′lent,** adj.

covariance (ko-va′re-ans) the expected value of the product of the deviations of corresponding values of two random variables from their respective means.

coverglass (kuv′er-glas) a thin glass plate that covers a mounted microscopical object or a culture.

coverslip (-slip) coverglass.

cowage (kow′aj) 1. a perennial herb, *Mucuna pruriens,* of the East Indies. 2. the hairs of the cowage pods, which cause severe itching, are used medicinally as a vermifuge, anthelmintic, and counterirritant in admixture with such vehicles as honey. Also used as "itching powders" of joke-shop fame.

Cowdria (kow′dre-ah) a genus of rickettsiae (tribe Ehrlichieae), comprising organisms pathogenic for certain vertebrates but not for man.

cowperitis (kow″per-i′tis) inflammation of Cowper's (bulbourethral) glands.

cowpox (kow′poks) a mild eruptive disease of milk cows, usually confined to the udder and teats, due to vaccinia virus, and transmissible to man.

coxa (kok′sah), pl. *cox′ae*[L.] the hip; loosely, the hip joint. **c. mag′na,** broadening of the head and neck of the femur. **c. pla′na,** osteochondrosis of the capitular epiphysis of the femur. **c. val′ga,** deformity of the hip joint with increase in the angle of inclination between the neck and shaft of the femur. **c. va′ra,** deformity of the hip joint with decrease in the angle of inclination between the neck and shaft of the femur.

coxalgia (kok-sal′je-ah) 1. hip-joint disease. 2. pain in the hip.

coxarthropathy (koks″ar-throp′ah-the) hip-joint disease.

Coxiella (kok″se-el′ah) a genus of rickettsiae, including *C. burnet′ii,* the etiologic agent of Q fever.

coxitis (kok-si′tis) inflammation of the hip joint.

coxodynia (kok″so-din′e-ah) pain in the hip.

coxofemoral (-fem′o-ral) pertaining to the hip and thigh.

coxotomy (kok-sot′o-me) the operation of opening the hip joint.

coxotuberculosis (kok″so-tu-ber″ku-lo′sis) tuberculosis of the hip joint.

coxsackievirus (kok-sak′e-vi″rus) one of a heterogeneous group of viruses producing, in man, a disease resembling poliomyelitis, but without paralysis.

cozymase (ko-zi′mās) nicotinamide-adenine dinucleotide.

C.P. candle power.

CPC clinicopathological conference.

CPK creatine phosphokinase.

c.p.m. counts per minute, an expression of the particles emitted after administration of a radioactive material such as ^{131}I.

c.p.s. cycles per second.

CR conditioned reflex (response).

Cr chemical symbol, *chromium.*

cradle (kra′d'l) a frame placed over the body of a bed patient for application of heat or cold or for protecting injured parts from contact with bed covers. **electric c., heat c.,** a tunnel- or hood-shaped cradle equipped with light bulbs, for application of heat to the body.

Craigia (kra′ge-ah) a genus of flagellate protozoa; its flagellate stages are thought by some to be *Chilomastix mesnili,* and its ameboid stages *Entamoeba coli.*

cramp (kramp) a painful spasmodic muscular contraction. **heat c.,** spasm accompanied by pain, weak pulse, and dilated pupils; seen in workers in intense heat. **intermittent c.,** intermittent abnormal muscular contractions. **recumbency c's,** cramping in muscles of legs and feet occurring while resting or during light sleep. **writers' c.,** an occupational neurosis marked by spasmodic contraction of the muscles of the fingers, hand, and forearm, with neuralgic pain.

crani(o)- word element [L.], *skull.*

craniad (kra′ne-ad) in a cranial direction; toward the anterior (in animals) or superior (in humans) end of the body.

cranial (kra′ne-al) pertaining to the cranium, or to the anterior (in animals) or superior (in humans) end of the body.

craniectomy (kra″ne-ek′to-me) excision of a segment of the skull.

craniocele (kra′ne-o-sēl″) protrusion of part of the brain through the skull.

craniocerebral (kra″ne-o-ser′ĕ-bral) pertaining to the cranium and cerebrum.

cranioclasis (kra″ne-ok′lah-sis) craniotomy (2).

cranioclast (kra′ne-o-klast″) an instrument for performing craniotomy (2).

cranioclasty (-klas″te) craniotomy (2).

craniocleidodysostosis (kra″ne-o-kli″do-dis″-os-to′sis) cleidocranial dysostosis.

craniodidymus (-did′ĭ-mus) a monster with two heads.

craniofacial (-fa′shal) of or pertaining to the cranium and face.

craniofenestria (-fĕ-nes′tre-ah) defective development of the fetal skull, with areas in which no bone is formed.

craniograph (kra′ne-o-graf″) an instrument for outlining the skull.

craniolacunia (kra″ne-o-lah-ku′ne-ah) defective development of the fetal skull, with depressed areas on the inner surface.

craniomalacia (-mah-la′she-ah) abnormal softness of the bones of the skull.

craniometer (kra″ne-om′ĕ-ter) an instrument for use in craniometry.

craniometry (-om′ĕ-tre) measurement of the skull and facial bones.

craniopagus (-op′ah-gus) a double monster joined at the head.

craniopathy (-op′ah-the) any disease of the skull. **metabolic c.,** a condition characterized by lesions of the calvaria with multiple metabolic changes, and by headache, obesity, and visual disorders.

craniopharyngeal (kra″ne-o-fah-rin′je-al) pertaining to the cranium and pharynx.

craniopharyngioma (-fah-rin″je-o′mah) a tumor arising from cell rests derived from the infundibulum of the hypophysis or Rathke's pouch.

cranioplasty (kra′ne-o-plas″te) any plastic operation on the skull.

craniopuncture (-punk″tūr) exploratory puncture of the skull.

craniorachischisis (kra″ne-o-rah-kis′kĭ-sis) congenital fissure of skull and spinal column.

craniosacral (-sa′kral) pertaining to the skull and sacrum.

cranioschisis (kra″ne-os′kĭ-sis) congenital fissure of the skull.

craniosclerosis (kra″ne-o-skle-ro′sis) thickening of the bones of the skull.

cranioscopy (kra″ne-os′ko-pe) diagnostic examination of the head.

craniospinal (kra″ne-o-spi′nal) pertaining to the skull and the spine.

craniostenosis (-ste-no′sis) deformity of the skull due to premature closure of the cranial sutures.

craniostosis (kra″ne-os-to′sis) congenital ossification of the cranial sutures.

craniosynostosis (kra″ne-o-sin″os-to′sis) premature closure of the sutures of the skull.

craniotabes (-ta′bēz) reduction in mineralization of the skull, with abnormal softness of the bone, usually affecting the occipital and parietal bones along the lambdoidal sutures.

craniotome (kra′ne-o-tōm″) a cutting instrument used in craniotomy.

craniotomy (kra″ne-ot′o-me) 1. any operation on the cranium. 2. puncture of the skull and removal of its contents to decrease the size of the head of a dead fetus and aid delivery.

craniotympanic (kra″ne-o-tim-pan′ik) pertaining to the skull and tympanum.

cranium (kra′ne-um), pl. *cra′nia* [L.] the skeleton of the head, variously construed as including all of the bones of the head, all except the mandible, or the eight bones forming the vault lodging the brain.

craquelé (krak-la′) [Fr.] profusely cracked.

crater (kra′ter) an excavated area surrounded by an elevated margin.

craterization (kra″ter-i-za′shun) excision of bone tissue to create a crater-like depression.

cravat (krah-vat′) a triangular bandage.

cream (krēm) the oily or fatty part of milk from which butter is prepared, or a fluid mixture of similar consistency. **cold c.,** a preparation of spermaceti, white wax, mineral oil, sodium borate, and purified water, applied topically to skin; also used as a vehicle for medications. **leukocytic c.,** buffy coat. **c. of tartar,** potassium bitartrate.

Creamalin (krēm′ah-lin) trademark for preparations of aluminum hydroxide gel.

crease (krēs) a line or slight linear depression. **flexion c., palmar c.,** any of the normal grooves across the palm which accommodate flexion of the hand by separating folds of tissue. **simian c.,** a single transverse palmar crease formed by fusion of the proximal and distal palmar creases; seen in congenital disorders such as Down's syndrome. **Sydney c.,** a proximal transverse palmar crease that extends to the ulnar border of the hands.

creatinase (kre-at′ĭ-nās) an enzyme that catalyzes the decomposition of creatine into urea and ammonia.

creatine (kre′ah-tin) a crystallizable nitrogenous compound synthesized in the body; phosphorylated creatine is an important storage form of high-energy phosphate. **c. phosphate,** phosphocreatine.

creatinemia (kre″ah-tĭ-ne′me-ah) excessive creatine in the blood.

creatinine (kre-at′ĭ-nin) a basic substance procurable from creatine and from urine.

creatinuria (kre-at″ĭ-nu′re-ah) increased concentration of creatine in the urine.

cremasteric (kre″mas-ter′ik) pertaining to the cremaster muscle.

crena (kre′nah), pl. *cre′nae* [L.] a notch or cleft.

crenate, crenated (kre′nāt; kre′nāt-ed) scalloped or notched.

crenation (kre-na′shun) the formation of abnormal notching around the edge of an erythrocyte; the notched appearance of an erythrocyte due to its shrinkage after suspension in a hypertonic solution.

crenocyte (kre′no-sīt) a crenated erythrocyte.

crenocytosis (kre″no-si-to′sis) the presence of crenated erythrocytes in the blood.

Crenothrix (kre′no-thriks) a genus of schizomycetes (family Crenotrichaceae).

creosol (kre′o-sol) one of the active constituents of creosote, $C_8H_{10}O_2$.

creosote (kre′o-sōt) a mixture of phenols from wood tar; used externally as an antiseptic and internally in chronic bronchitis as an expectorant. A mixture of carbonates of various constituents of creosote (*c. carbonate*) is used the same as the base.

crepitant (krep′ĭ-tant) having a dry, crackling sound.

crepitation (krep″ĭ-ta′shun) a dry, crackling sound or sensation, such as that produced by the grating of the ends of a fractured bone.

crepitus (krep′ĭ-tus) 1. the discharge of flatus from the bowels. 2. crepitation. 3. a crepitant rale. **c. re′dux,** crepitus heard in the resolving stage of pneumonia.

crescent (kres′ent) 1. shaped like a new moon. 2. a crescent-shaped structure. **crescen′tic,** adj. **c's of Giannuzzi,** crescent-shaped patches of serous cells surrounding the mucous tubercles in mixed glands. **myopic c.,** a crescentic staphyloma in the fundus of the eye in myopia. **sublingual c.,** the crescent-shaped area on the floor of the mouth, bounded by the lingual wall of the mandible and the base of the tongue.

cresol (kre′sol) a mixture of isomeric cresols from coal tar, containing not more than 5% phenol; used as a disinfectant.

crest (krest) a projection, or projecting structure or ridge, especially one surmounting a bone or its border. **ampullar c.,** the most prominent part of a localized thickening of the membrane lining the ampullae of the semicircular ducts. **cross c.,** a ridge of enamel extending across the face of a tooth. **dental c.,** the maxillary ridge passing along the alveolar processes of the fetal maxillary bones. **frontal c.,** a median ridge on the internal surface of the frontal bone. **iliac c.,** the thickened, expanded upper border of the ilium. **intertrochanteric c.,** a ridge on the posterior femur connecting the greater with the lesser trochanter. **lacrimal c., anterior,** the lateral margin of the groove on the posterior border of the frontal process of the maxilla. **lacrimal c., posterior,** a vertical ridge dividing the lateral or orbital surface of the lacrimal bone into two parts. **nasal c.,** a ridge on the internal border of the nasal bone. **neural c.,** a cellular band dorsolateral to the embryonic neural tube that gives origin to the cerebrospinal ganglia. **obturator c.,** a strong ridge forming the inferior border of the superior ramus of the pubic bone. **occipital c., external,** a ridge sometimes extending on the external surface of the occipital bone from the external protuberance toward the foramen magnum. **occipital c., internal,** a median ridge on the internal surface of the occipital bone, extending from the midpoint of the cruciform eminence toward the foramen magnum. **palatine c.,** a transverse ridge sometimes seen on the inferior surface of the horizontal plate of the palatine bone. **pubic c.,** the thick, rough anterior border of the body of the pubic bone. **sacral c., intermediate,** either of two indefinite ridges just medial to the dorsal sacral foramina. **sacral c., lateral,** either of two series of tubercles lateral to the dorsal sacral foramina. **sacral c., median,** a median ridge on the dorsal surface of the sacrum. **sphenoidal c.,** a median ridge on the anterior surface of the body of the sphenoid bone. **supramastoid c.,** the superior border of the posterior root of the zygomatic process of the temporal bone. **supraventricular c.,** a ridge on the inner wall of the right ventricle, marking off the conus arteriosus. **temporal c.,** a ridge extending upward and backward from the zygomatic process of the frontal bone. **c. of tibia,** the prominent ridge on the front of the tibia. **turbinated c.,** a horizontal ridge on the internal surface of the palate bone. **urethral c.,** a prominent longitudinal mucosal fold along the posterior wall of the female urethra, or a median elevation along the posterior wall of the male urethra, lying between the prostatic sinuses. **c. of vestibule,** a ridge between the spherical and elliptical recesses of the vestibule, dividing posteriorly to bound the cochlear recess.

cretin (kre′tin) a patient exhibiting cretinism.

cretinism (kre′tĭ-nizm) arrested physical and mental development with dystrophy of bones and soft tissues, due to congenital lack of thyroid secretion. **athyreotic c.,** cretinism due to thyroid aplasia or destruction of the thyroid of the fetus in utero. **sporadic goitrous c.,** a genetically determined condition in which enlargement of the thyroid gland is associated with deficiency in the supply of circulating thyroid hormone.

cretinoid (kre′tĭ-noid) resembling a cretin, or suggestive of cretinism.

cretinous (kre′tĭ-nus) affected with cretinism.

crevice (krev′is) a fissure. **gingival c.,** the space between the cervical enamel of a tooth and the overlying unattached gingiva.

crevicular (krĕ-vik′u-lar) pertaining to a crevice, especially the gingival crevice.

cribrate (krib′rāt) perforated, as a sieve.

cribration (krĭ-bra′shun) 1. the quality of being

cribriform. 2. the process or act of sifting or passing through a sieve.

cribriform (krib′rĭ-form) perforated like a sieve.

cribrum (kri′brum), pl. *cri′bra* [L.] lamina cribrosa of the ethmoid bone.

cricoarytenoid (kri″ko-ar″ĭ-te′noid) pertaining to the cricoid and arytenoid cartilages.

cricoid (kri′koid) 1. ring-shaped. 2. the cricoid cartilage.

cricoidectomy (kri″koi-dek′to-me) excision of the cricoid cartilage.

cricopharyngeal (kri″ko-fah-rin′je-al) pertaining to the cricoid cartilage and pharynx.

cricothyreotomy (-thi″re-ot′o-me) incision through the cricoid and thyroid cartilages.

cricothyroid (-thi′roid) pertaining to the cricoid and thyroid cartilages.

cricotomy (kri-kot′o-me) incision of the cricoid cartilage.

cricotracheotomy (kri″ko-tra″ke-ot′o-me) incision of the trachea through the cricoid cartilage.

cri du chat (kre-du-shah) [Fr.] see under *syndrome.*

crinogenic (kri″no-jen′ik, krin″o-jen′ik) causing secretion in a gland.

crisis (kri′sis), pl. *cri′ses* [L.] 1. the turning point of a disease for better or worse; especially a sudden change, usually for the better, in the course of an acute disease. 2. a sudden paroxysmal intensification of symptoms in the course of a disease. **addisonian c.,** fatigue, nausea, vomiting, and weight loss accompanying an acute attack of Addison's disease. **aplastic c.,** sudden temporary disappearance of erythroblasts from bone marrow, seen under various circumstances, including certain hemolytic states and infections. **asthmatic c.,** status asthmaticus. **bronchial c.,** paroxysms of dyspnea in tabes dorsalis. **clitoris c.,** attacks of sexual excitement in women with tabes dorsalis. **deglobulinization c.,** a condition occurring in congenital spherocytic anemia, with sudden onset of fever, abdominal pain, and vomiting, associated with reticulocytopenia, leukopenia, thrombocytopenia, and erythroblastopenia. **Dietl's c.,** a sudden severe attack of nephralgia or gastric pain, chills, fever, nausea, vomiting, and general collapse; said to be due to partial turning of the kidney upon its pedicle. **gastric c.,** paroxysms of intense pain in abdomen in tabes dorsalis. **genital c. of newborn,** estrinization of the vaginal mucosa and hyperplasia of the breast, influenced by transplacentally acquired estrogens. **hemoclastic c.,** temporary leukopenia, with relative lymphocytosis, lowered blood pressure, and changes in blood coagulability, due to toxic protein-split products in the blood, and occurring in anaphylactic shock after a meal of albuminoids in persons with disordered liver function. **nephralgic c.,** paroxysmal pain in the ureter in tabes dorsalis. **nitritoid c.,** redness of the face, dyspnea, feeling of distress, cough, and precordial pain sometimes following the injection of arsphenamine. **rectal c.,** severe pain in rectum in tabes dorsalis. **salt-losing c.,** see under *syndrome.* **tabetic c.,** a painful paroxysm occurring in tabes dorsalis. **thyroid c., thyrotoxic c.,** sudden and dangerous increase of symptoms of thyrotoxicosis. **vesical c.,** paroxysms of pain in bladder in tabes dorsalis.

crista (kris′tah), pl. *cris′tae* [L.] crest. **cris′tae cu′tis,** dermal ridges; ridges of the skin produced by the projecting papillae of the corium on the palm of the hand or sole of the foot, producing a fingerprint or footprint characteristic of the individual. **c. gal′li,** a thick, triangular process projecting upward from the cribriform plate of the ethmoid bone.

Crithidia (krĭ-thid′e-ah) a genus of parasitic protozoa found in the digestive tract of arthropods and other invertebrates.

C.R.N.A. Certified Registed Nurse Anesthetist.

cromolyn (kro′mŏ-lin) a bronchodilator, $C_{23}H_{14}O_{11}$, used as the sodium salt.

cross (kros) 1. a cross-shaped figure or structure. 2. any organism produced by crossbreeding; a method of crossbreeding.

crossbite (kros′bīt) malocclusion in which the mandibular teeth are in buccal version (or complete lingual version in posterior segments) to the maxillary teeth.

crossbreeding (-brēd-ing) hybridization; the mating of organisms of different strains or species.

cross-eye (-i) esotropia.

crossing over (kros′ing o′ver) the exchanging of material between homologous chromosomes during the first meiotic division, resulting in new combinations of genes.

crossmatching (kros-mach′ing) see under *matching.*

crotalid (krot′ah-lid) 1. any smake of the family Crotalidae; a pit viper. 2. of or pertaining to the family Crotalidae.

Crotalidae (kro-tal′ĭ-de) a family of venomous snakes, the pit vipers.

crotalin (krot′ah-lin) a protein in rattlesnake venom.

Crotalus (krot′ah-lus) a genus of rattlesnakes.

crotamiton (kro″tah-mi′ton) an acaricide, $C_{13}H_{17}NO$, used in the treatment of scabies and as an antipruritic.

crotaphion (kro-taf′e-on) the cranial point at the tip of great wing of sphenoid bone.

crotonism (kro′ton-izm) poisoning by croton oil, with burning of the mouth and sometimes emesis, followed by severe watery diarrhea and colic; sometimes accompanied by headache, somnolence, vertigo, prostration, and collapse. Death from circulatory or respiratory failure may occur.

crotoxin (kro-tok′sin) a neurotoxin from rattlesnake venom.

croup (krōōp) a condition seen chiefly in infants and children, due to acute obstruction of the larynx caused by allergy, foreign body, infection, or new growth, marked by a resonant barking cough, hoarseness, and persisitent stridor. **croup′ous,** adj. **catarrhal c.,** that accompanied by catarrhal discharge. **false c., spasmodic c.,** spasm of laryngeal muscles with slight inflammation.

crown (krown) 1. the topmost part of an organ or structure, e.g., the top of the head. 2. artificial c. **anatomical c.,** the upper, enamel-covered part of a tooth. **artificial c.,** a metal, porcelain, or plastic reproduction of a crown affixed to the remaining natural structure of a tooth. **clinical c.,** the portion of a tooth exposed beyond the gingiva. **physiological c.,** the portion of a tooth distal to the gingival crevice or to the gum margin.

crowning (krown′ing) the appearance of a large segment of the fetal scalp at the vaginal orifice in childbirth.

crucial (kroo′shal) severe and decisive.

cruciate (kroo′she-āt) shaped like a cross.

crucible (kroo′sĭ-b'l) a vessel for melting refractory substances.

cruciform (kroo′sĭ-form) cross-shaped.

crura (kroo′rah) plural of *crus*.

crural (kroor′al) pertaining to the leg or to any crus.

cruror (kroo′or) a blood clot.

crus (krus), pl. *cru′ra* [L.] 1. the leg, from knee to foot. 2. a leglike part. **cru′ral,** adj. **c. cer′ebri,** a structure comprising fiber tracts descending from the cerebral cortex to form the longitudinal fascicles of the pons. **c. of clitoris,** the continuation of the corpus cavernosum of the clitoris, diverging posteriorly to be attached to the pubic arch. **crura of diaphragm,** two fibromuscular bands that arise from the lumbar vertebrae and insert into the central tendon of the diaphragm. **crura of fornix,** two flattened bands of white substance that unite to form the body of the fornix. **c. of penis,** the continuation of each corpus cavernosum of the penis, diverging posteriorly to be attached to the pubic arch.

crust (krust) a formed outer layer, especially an outer layer of solid matter formed by drying of a bodily exudate or secretion. **milk c.,** crusta lactea.

crusta (krus′tah), pl. *crus′tae* [L.] 1. a crust. 2. crus cerebri. **c. lac′tea,** seborrhea of the scalp of nursing infants. **c. petro′sa,** cementum.

Crustacea (krus-ta′she-ah) a class of arthropods including the lobsters, crabs, shrimps, wood lice, water fleas, and barnacles.

crutch (kruch) a staff extending from the armpit to the ground, with a crosspiece at the top fitting under the arm and a crossbar for the hand, used to support the weight of the body in walking.

crux (kruks), pl. *cru′ces* [L.] cross. **c. of heart,** the intersection of the walls separating the right and left sides and the atrial and ventricular heart chambers. **cru′ces pilo′rum,** crosslike figures formed by the pattern of hair growth, the hairs lying in opposite directions.

cry(o)- word element [Gr.], *cold.*

cryalgesia (kri″al-je′ze-ah) pain on application of cold.

cryanesthesia (-an-es-the′ze-ah) loss of power of perceiving cold.

cryesthesia (-es-the′ze-ah) abnormal sensitiveness to cold.

crymoanesthesia (kri″mo-an″es-the′ze-ah) anesthesia produced by refrigeration.

crymodynia (-din′e-ah) rheumatic pain occurring in cold or damp weather.

cryobank (kri′o-bank″) a facility for freezing and preserving semen at low temperatures (usually −196.5° C.) for future use.

cryobiology (kri″o-bi-ol′o-je) the science dealing with the effect of low temperatures on biological systems.

cryocautery (-kaw′ter-e) cold cautery.

cryocrit (kri′o-krit) the percentage of the total volume of blood serum or plasma occupied by cryoprecipitates after centrifugation.

cryoextraction (kri″o-eks-trak′shun) application of extremely low temperature for the removal of a cataractous lens.

cryofibrinogen (-fi-brin′o-jen) an abnormal fibrinogen that precipitates at low temperatures and redissolves at 37° C.

cryofibrinogenemia (-fi-brin″o-jen-e′me-ah) the presence of cryofibrinogen in the blood.

cryogenic (-jen′ik) producing low temperatures.

cryoglobulin (-glob′u-lin) an abnormal globulin that precipitates at low temperatures and redissolves at 37° C.

cryoglobulinemia (-glob″u-lin-e′me-ah) the presence in the blood of cryoglobulin.

cryohypophysectomy (-hi″po-fiz-ek′to-me) destruction of the pituitary gland by the application of cold.

cryometer (kri-om′ĕ-ter) a thermometer for measuring very low temperature.

cryopathy (kri-op′ah-the) a morbid condition caused by cold.

cryophilic (kri″o-fil′ik) psychrophilic.

cryophylactic (-fi-lak′tik) resistant to very low temperatures; said of bacteria.

cryoprecipitate (-pre-sip′ĭ-tāt) any precipitate that results from cooling.

cryoprobe (kri′o-prōb) an instrument for applying extreme cold to tissue.

cryoprotein (kri″o-pro′te-in) a blood protein that precipitates on cooling.

cryoscope (kri′o-skōp) an instrument for performing cryoscopy.

cryoscopy (kri-os′ko-pe) examination of fluids based on the principle that the freezing point of a solution varies according to the amount and nature of the solute. **cryoscop′ic,** adj.

cryostat (kri′o-stat) 1. a device by which temperature can be maintained at a very low level. 2. in pathology and histology, a chamber containing a microtome for sectioning frozen tissue.

cryosurgery (kri″o-ser′jer-e) the destruction of tissue by application of extreme cold.

cryothalamectomy (-thal″ah-mek′to-me) destruction of a portion of the thalamus by application of extreme cold.

cryotherapy (-ther′ah-pe) the therapeutic use of cold.

cryotolerant (-tol′er-ant) able to withstand very low temperatures.

crypt (kript) a blind pit or tube on a free surface. **alveolar c.,** the bony compartment surrounding a developing tooth. **anal c's,** see under *sinus.* **dental c.,** the space occupied by a developing tooth. **enamel c.,** a space bounded by dental ledges on either side and usually by the enamel organ, and filled with mesenchyma. **c's of Fuchs, c's of iris,** pitlike depressions in the iris. **c's of Lieberkühn,** intestinal glands. **Luschka's c's,** deep indentations of the gallbladder mucosa which penetrate into the muscular layer of the organ. **c's of Morgagni,** anal sinuses. **synovial c.,** a pouch in the synovial membrane of a joint. **c's of tongue,** deep, irregular invaginations from the surface of the lingual tonsil. **tonsillar c's,** epithelium-lined clefts in the palatine tonsils.

crypt(o)- word element [Gr.], *concealed; crypt.*

crypta (krip'tah), pl. *cryp'tae* [L.] crypt.

cryptectomy (krip-tek'to-me) excision or obliteration of a crypt.

cryptenamine (krip-ten'ah-mīn) a mixture of alkaloids from an extract of *Veratrum viride,* used to lower blood pressure.

cryptesthesia (krip"tes-the'ze-ah) subconscious perception of occurrences not ordinarily perceptible to the senses.

cryptitis (krip-ti'tis) inflammation of a crypt, especially the anal crypts.

cryptocephalus (krip"to-sef'ah-lus) a fetus with an inconspicuous head.

cryptococcosis (-kok-o'sis) infection by *Cryptococcus neoformans,* having a predilection for the brain and meninges but also invading the skin, lungs, and other parts.

Cryptococcus (-kok'us) a genus of yeastlike fungi, including *C. neofor'mans,* the cause of cryptococcosis in man.

cryptodidymus (-did'ĭ-mus) a twin monster, one fetus being enclosed within the body of the other.

cryptogam (krip'to-gam) one of the lower plants that have no true flowers, but propagate by spores.

cryptogenic (krip"to-jen'ik) of obscure or doubtful origin.

cryptoglioma (-gli-o'mah) a stage of retinal glioma in which the eyeball shrinks, masking the presence of the growth.

cryptolith (krip'to-lith) a concretion in a crypt.

cryptomenorrhea (krip"to-men"o-re'ah) the occurrence of menstrual symptoms without external bleeding, as in imperforate hymen.

cryptomerorachischisis (-me"ro-rah-kis'kĭ-sis) spina bifida occulta.

cryptomnesia (krip"tom-ne'ze-ah) subconscious memory. **cryptomne'sic,** adj.

cryptophthalmia, cryptophthalmos, cryptophthalmus (krip"tof-thal'me-ah; -thal'mos; -thal'mus) congenital absence of the palpebral fissure, the skin extending from the forehead to the cheek, and the eye malformed or rudimentary.

cryptopodia (krip"to-po'de-ah) swelling of the lower leg and foot, covering all but the sole.

cryptopyic (-pi'ik) attended by concealed suppuration.

cryptorchid (krip-tor'kid) a person with undescended testes.

cryptorchidectomy (krip"tor-kĭ-dek'to-me) excision of an undescended testis.

cryptorchidism (krip-tor'kĭ-dizm) cryptorchism.

cryptorchidopexy (krip-tor'kĭ-do-pek"se) orchiopexy.

cryptorchism (krip-tor'kizm) failure of one or both testes to descend into the scrotum.

cryptoxanthin (krip"to-zan'thin) a yellow carotenoid widely distributed in nature (egg yolk, green grass, yellow corn, etc.), which can be converted into vitamin A in the body.

cryptozygous (-zi'gus) having the calvaria wider than the face, so that the zygomatic arches are concealed when the head is viewed from above.

crystal (kris'tal) a naturally produced angular solid of definite form. **blood c's,** hematoidin crystals in the blood. **Böttcher's c's,** microscopic crystals seen on adding a drop of solution of ammonium phosphate to a drop of prostatic fluid. **Charcot-Leyden c's,** crystalline structures found in secretions from sites where eosinophils are abundant, as in the sputum in bronchial asthma. **Charcot-Neumann c's,** minute crystals of spermine phosphate found in semen and various animal tissues. **coffin-lid c's,** peculiar indented crystals of ammoniomagnesium phosphate from alkaline urine. **dumbbell c's,** crystals of calcium oxalate occurring in urine. **hedgehog c's,** wedge-shaped spiny crystals of uric acid. **knife-rest c's,** coffin lid c's. **rock c.,** quartz; a transparent form of silica used in making lenses. **Teichmann's c's,** crystals of hemin.

crystalbumin (kris"tal-bu'min) 1. albumin found in water extract of the crystalline lens. 2. a general term for crystallizable albumins.

crystallin (kris'tah-lin) a globulin in the crystalline lens.

crystalline (kris'tah-līn) 1. resembling a crystal in nature or clearness. 2. pertaining to crystals.

crystallization (kris"tah-li-za'shun) conversion into crystalline form.

crystallography (kris"tah-log'rah-fe) the science dealing with the study of crystals. **x-ray c.,** the determination of the three-dimensional structure of molecules by means of diffraction patterns produced by x-rays.

crystalloid (kris'tah-loid) 1. resembling a crystal. 2. a noncolloid substance.

crystalluria (kris"tah-lu're-ah) the excretion of crystals in the urine, causing renal irritation.

Crysticillin (kris"tĭ-sil'in) trademark for preparations of procaine penicillin G.

Crystodigin (kris"to-dij'in) trademark for preparations of digitoxin.

Crystoids (kris'toidz) trademark for a preparation of hexylresorcinol.

C.S. current strength.

Cs chemical symbol, *cesium.*

C.S.A.A. Child Study Association of America.

C.S.F. cerebrospinal fluid.

C.S.G.B.I. Cardiac Society of Great Britain and Ireland.

C.S.M. cerebrospinal meningitis.

C.T.A. Canadian Tuberculosis Association.

Ctenocephalides (te″no-se-fal′ĭ-dēz) a genus of fleas, including *C. ca′nis,* frequently found on dogs, which may transmit the dog tapeworm to man, and *C. fe′lis,* commonly parasitic on cats.

C-terminal (ter′min-al) the end of the peptide chain carrying the free alpha carboxyl group of the last amino acid, conventionally written to the right.

Cu chemical symbol, *copper* (L. *cuprum*).

cu. cubic.

cubitus (ku′bĭ-tus) 1. elbow. 2. the upper limb distal to the humerus: the elbow, forearm, and hand. 3. ulna. **cu′bital,** adj. **c. val′gus,** deformity of the elbow in which it deviates away from the midline of the body when extended. **c. va′rus,** deformity of the elbow in which it deviates toward the midline of the body when extended.

cuboid (ku′boid) resembling a cube.

cu. cm. cubic centimeter.

cuff (kuf) a small, bandlike structure encircling a part or object. **musculotendinous c.,** one formed by intermingled muscle and tendon fibers. **rotator c.,** a musculotendinous structure encircling and giving strength to the shoulder joint.

cuffing (kuf′ing) formation of a cufflike surrounding border, as of leukocytes about a blood vessel, observed in certain infections.

cuirass (kwe-ras′) a covering for the chest. **tabetic c.,** an area of diminished sense of touch encircling the chest in tabes dorsalis.

cul-de-sac (kul-dĕ-sak′) [Fr.] a blind pouch. **Douglas' c.,** rectouterine excavation.

culdocentesis (kul″do-sen-te′sis) transvaginal puncture of Douglas' cul-de-sac for aspiration of fluid.

culdoscope (kul′do-skōp) an endoscope used in culdoscopy.

culdoscopy (kul-dos′ko-pe) visual examination of the female viscera through an endoscope introduced into the pelvic cavity through the posterior vaginal fornix.

Culex (ku′leks) a genus of mosquitoes found throughout the world, many species of which are vectors of disease-producing organisms.

culicide (ku′lĭ-sīd) an agent which destroys mosquitoes.

culicifuge (ku-lis′ĭ-fūj) an agent which repels mosquitoes.

culicine (ku-lĭ-sin, ku′lĭ-sīn) 1. a member of the genus *Culex* or related genera. 2. pertaining to, involving, or affecting mosquitoes of the genus *Culex* or related species.

culmen (kul′men), pl. *cul′mina* [L.] the anterior and upper part of the monticulus cerebelli.

cultivation (kul″tĭ-va′shun) the propagation of living organisms, especially the growing of cells in artificial media.

culture (kul′tūr) 1. the propagation of microorganisms or of living tissue cells in media conducive to their growth. 2. to induce such propaga-

tion. 3. the product of such propagation. **cul′-tural,** adj. **cell c.,** a growth of cells *in vitro;* although the cells proliferate they do not organize into tissue. **continuous flow c.,** the cultivation of bacteria in a continuous flow of fresh medium to maintain bacterial growth in logarithmic phase. **fractional c.,** obtaining of a single species of microorganism from a culture containing more than one. **hanging-drop c.,** a culture in which the material to be cultivated is inoculated into a drop of fluid attached to a coverglass inverted over a hollow slide. **plate c.,** one grown on a medium, usually agar or gelatin, on a Petri dish. **pure c.,** a culture of a single cell species, without presence of any contaminants. **slant c.,** one made on the surface of solidified medium in a tube which has been tilted to provide a greater surface area for growth. **stab c.,** one in which the medium is inoculated by thrusting a needle deep into its substance. **streak c.,** one in which the medium is inoculated by drawing an infected wire across it. **tissue c.,** the cultivation of tissue cells *in vitro.* **type c.,** a culture of a species of microorganism usually maintained in a central collection of type or standard cultures.

culture medium (kul′tūr me′de-um) any substance or preparation used for the cultivation of living cells.

cu. mm. cubic millimeter.

cumulus (ku′mu-lus), pl. *cu′muli* [L.] a small elevation. **c. ooph′orus,** a mass of follicular cells surrounding the ovum in the vesicular ovarian follicle.

cuneate, cuneiform (ku′ne-āt; ku-ne′ĭ-form) wedge-shaped.

cuneocuboid (ku″ne-o-ku′boid) pertaining to the cuneiform and cuboid bones.

cuneus (ku′ne-us), pl. *cu′nei* [L.] a wedge-shaped lobule on the medial aspect of the occipital lobe of the cerebrum.

cuniculus (ku-nik′u-lus), pl. *cunic′uli* [L.] a burrow in the skin made by the itch mite.

cunnilingus (kun″ĭ-ling′gus) [L.] oral stimulation of the female genitals.

cup (kup) 1. a depression or hollow. 2. a cupping glass. **glaucomatous c.,** a form of optic disk depression peculiar to glaucoma. **optic c.,** physiologic c. **physiologic c.,** a slight depression sometimes observed in the optic disk.

cupola (ku′pŏ-lah) cupula.

cupping (kup′ing) 1. the application of a cupping glass. 2. the formation of a cup-shaped depression.

cupric (ku′prik) pertaining to or containing divalent copper.

cuprous (ku′prus) pertaining to or containing monovalent copper.

cupruresis (ku″proo-re′sis) the urinary excretion of copper.

cupruretic (ku″proo-ret′ik) pertaining to or promoting the urinary excretion of copper.

cupula (ku′pu-lah), pl. *cu′pulae* [L.] a small, inverted cup or dome-shaped cap over a structure.

curare (koo-rah′re) any of a wide variety of highly toxic extracts from various botanical sources, including various species of *Strychnos,* a genus of tropical trees; used originally as arrow poisons in South America. An extract of the shrub, *Chondodendron tomentosum,* has been used as a skeletal muscle relaxant.

curarization (ku″rar-i-za′shun) administration of curare (usually tubocurarine) to induce muscle relaxation by its blocking activity at the myoneural junction.

curarimimetic (koo-rah″re-mi-met′ik) producing effects similar to those of curare.

cure (kūr) 1. the course of treatment of any disease, or of a special case. 2. the successful treatment of a disease or wound. 3. a system of treating diseases. 4. a medicine effective in treating a disease. **grape c.,** treatment by a diet consisting of grapes. **hunger c.,** treatment of disease by severe fasting. **Karell c.,** see under *treatment.* **starvation c.,** hunger cure. **water c.,** hydrotherapy.

curet (ku-ret′) 1. a spoon-shaped instrument for cleansing a diseased surface. 2. to use a curet.

curettage (ku″rĕ-tahzh′) [Fr.] the cleansing of a diseased surface, as with a curet. **medical c.,** induction of bleeding from the endometrium by administration and withdrawal of a progestational agent. **periapical c.,** removal with a curet of diseased periapical tissue without excision of the root tip.

curette (ku-ret′) curet.

curettement (-ment) curettage. **physiologic c.,** enzymatic débridement.

curie (ku′re) a unit of radioactivity, defined as the quantity of any radioactive nuclide in which the number of disintegrations per second is 3.700×10^{10}.

curiegram (-gram) a photographic print made by radium emanation.

curie-hour (-our″) a unit of dose equivalent to that obtained by exposure for one hour to radioactive material disintegrating at the rate of 3.7×10^{10} atoms per second.

curietherapy (ku″re-ther′ah-pe) originally, radium or radon therapy; now applied to therapy given by emanations from any radioactive source.

curium (ku′re-um) a chemical element (*see table*), at. no. 96, symbol Cm.

current (kur′ent) that which flows; electric transmission in a circuit. **action c.,** the current generated in the cell membrane of a nerve or muscle by the action potential. **alternating c.,** a current which periodically flows in opposite directions. **direct c.,** a current flowing in one direction only.

curvatura (ker″vah-tu′rah), pl. *curvatu′rae* [L.] curvature.

curvature (ker′vah-tūr) a nonangular deviation from a normally straight course. **greater c. of stomach,** the left or lateral and inferior border of the stomach, marking the inferior junction of the anterior and posterior surfaces. **lesser c. of stomach,** the right or medial border of the stomach, marking the superior junction of the anterior and posterior surfaces. **Pott's c.,** abnormal posterior curvature of the spine due to tuberculous caries. **spinal c.,** abnormal deviation of the vertebral column.

curve (kerv) a line which is not straight, or which describes part of a circle, especially a line that represents varying values in a graph. **Barnes' c.,** the segment of a circle the center of which is the sacral promontory, its concavity being directed dorsally. **c. of Carus,** the normal axis of the pelvic outlet. **dental c.,** c. of occlusion. **dissociation c. of oxyhemoglobin,** a graphic curve representing the normal variation in the amount of oxygen which combines with hemoglobin as a function of the tension of oxygen and carbon dioxide. The dissociation curve is said to shift to the right when less than a normal amount of oxygen is taken up by the blood at a given P_{O_2}, and to shift to the left when more than a normal amount is taken up. **dye-dilution c.,** a graph representing the concentration of a fixed dose of a dye (as in the systemic circulation) at specific time intervals; used in studies of cardiac output. **frequency c.,** a curve representing graphically the probabilities of different numbers of recurrences of an event. **growth c.,** the curve obtained by plotting increase in size or numbers against the elapsed time. **isodose c's,** lines delimiting body areas receiving the same quantity of radiation in radiotherapy. **muscle c.,** myogram. **c. of occlusion,** a curved line determined by the occlusal surfaces and incisal edges of existing teeth, when viewed from the side. **Price-Jones c.,** a graphic curve representing the variation in the size of the red blood corpuscles. **probability c.,** frequency c. **Spee's c.,** c. of occlusion. **temperature c.,** a graphic tracing showing the variations in body temperature. **tension c's,** lines observed in cancellous tissue of bones, determined by the exertion of stress during development. **Wunderlich's c.,** the typical temperature curve of typhoid fever.

cushingoid (koosh′ing-oid) resembling Cushing's syndrome, said of signs and symptoms.

cushion (koosh′un) a soft or padlike part. **endocardial c's,** elevations on the atrioventricular canal of the embryonic heart which later help form the interatrial septum.

cusp (kusp) a pointed or rounded projection, such as on the crown of a tooth, or a segment of a cardiac valve. **semilunar c.,** any of the semilunar segments of the aortic valve (having posterior, right, and left cusps) or the pulmonary valve (having anterior, right, and left cusps).

cuspid (kus′pid) 1. having one cusp or point. 2. a canine tooth.

cuspidate (kur′pĭ-dāt) provided with cusps.

cuspis (kus′pis), pl. *cus′pides* [L.] a cusp.

cutaneous (ku-ta′ne-us) pertaining to the skin.

cutdown (kut′down) creation of a small incised opening, especially over a vein (*venous c.*), to facilitate venipuncture and permit passage of a needle or cannula for withdrawal of blood or administration of fluids.

cuticle (ku′tĭ-k'l) 1. a layer of more or less solid substance covering the free surface of an epithelial cell. 2. eponychium (1). **dental c., enamel c.,** the calcified epithelial remnants on the tooth enamel after complete formation of the enamel.

cuticula (ku-tik′u-lah), pl. *cutic′ulae*[L.] cuticle.

cutin (ku′tin) 1. a waxy constituent of the cuticle of plants. 2. a preparation of ox gut used as suture material and as a wound dressing.

cutireaction (ku″tĭ-re-ak′shun) an inflammatory or irritative reaction on the skin, occurring in certain infectious diseases, or on application or injection of a preparation of the organism causing the disease. **von Pirquet's c.,** Pirquet reaction.

cutis (ku′tis) the skin. **c. anseri′na,** transitory elevation of the hair follicles due to contraction of the arrectores pilorum muscles; a reflection of sympathetic nerve discharge. **c. elas′tica, c. hyperelas′tica,** Ehlers-Danlos syndrome. **c. lax′a,** a hereditary disorder in which the skin and subcutaneous tissues hypertrophy, so that the skin hangs in folds. **c. marmora′ta,** transitory mottling of the skin sometimes due to exposure to cold. **c. pen′dula,** c. laxa. **c. rhomboida′lis nu′chae,** thickening of the skin of the neck with striking accentuation of its markings, giving an appearance of diamond-shaped plaques. **c. ve′ra,** corium. **c. ver′ticis gyra′ta,** enlargement and thickening of the skin of the scalp, which lies in folds resembling gyri and sulci of the brain.

cuvette (ku-vet′) [Fr.] a glass container generally having well defined characteristics (dimensions, optical properties), to contain solutions or suspensions for study.

CV cardiovascular.

CVS cardiovascular system.

cwt. hundredweight.

Cy cyanogen.

cyan(o)- word element [Gr.], *blue.*

cyanamide (si-an′ah-mīd) 1. deliquescent crystals, HN:C:NH, from calcium cyanamide or sulfuric acid. 2. calcium cyanamide.

cyanemia (si″ah-ne′me-ah) blueness of the blood.

cyanhemoglobin (si″an-he″mo-glo′bin) a compound formed by action of hydrocyanic acid on hemoglobin, giving the bright red color to blood.

cyanide (si′ah-nīd) a binary compound of cyanogen.

cyanmethemoglobin (si″an-met-he″mo-glo′-bin) a crystalline substance formed by the action of hydrocyanic acid on methemoglobin in the cold, or on oxyhemoglobin at body temperature; the pigment most widely used in hemoglobinometry.

cyanmetmyoglobin (-mi″o-glo′bin) a compound formed from metmyoglobin by addition of the cyanide ion to yield reduction to the ferrous state.

cyanocobalamin (si″ah-no-ko-bal′ah-min) vitamin B_{12}; a hematopoietic vitamin found in liver, fish meal, eggs, and other natural sources, or produced from cultures of *Streptomyces griseus,* which combines with intrinsic factor for absorption and is needed for erythrocyte maturation. Absence of intrinsic factor leads to malabsorption of cyanocobalamin and results in pernicious anemia. **radio active c.,** cyanocobalamin containing radio active cobalt of mass number 57 or 60, used in diagnosis of pernicious anemia.

cyanogen (si-an′o-jen) the radical CN—; also NCCN, the latter a very poisonous gas.

cyanogenesis (si″ah-no-jen′ĕ-sis) the formation of cyanogen or hydrocyanic acid.

cyanogenetic (-jĕ-net′ik) pertaining to or characterized by the formation of hydrocyanic acid.

cyanolabe (si′ah-no-lāb″) the pigment in retinal cones that is more sensitive to the blue range of the spectrum than are chlorolabe and erythrolabe.

cyanophil (si-an′o-fil) 1. cyanophilous. 2. a cell or other histologic element readily stainable with blue dyes.

cyanophilous (si″ah-nof′ĭ-lus) stainable with blue dyes.

cyanopia (si″ah-no′pe-ah) cyanopsia.

cyanopsia (si″ah-nop′se-ah) defect of vision in which objects appear tinged with blue.

cyanopsin (si″an-op′sin) a bluish visual pigment present in the retinal cones of some animals.

cyanosed (si′ah-nōsd) cyanotic.

cyanosis (si″ah-no′sis) a bluish discoloration of skin and mucous membranes due to excessive concentration of reduced hemoglobin in the blood. **cyanot′ic,** adj. **autotoxic c.,** enterogenous c. **central c.,** that due to arterial unsaturation, the aortic blood carrying reduced hemoglobin. **enterogenous c.,** a syndrome due to absorption of nitrites and sulfides from the intestine, principally marked by methemoglobinemia and/or sulfhemoglobinemia associated with cyanosis, and accompanied by severe enteritis, abdominal pain, constipation or diarrhea, headache, dyspnea, dizziness, syncope, anemia, and, occasionally, digital clubbing and indicanuria. **peripheral c.,** that due to an excessive amount of reduced hemoglobin in the venous blood as a result of extensive oxygen extraction at the capillary level. **pulmonary c.,** central cyanosis due to poor oxygenation of the blood in the lungs. **c. ret′inae,** cyanosis of the retina, observable in certain congenital cardiac defects. **shunt c.,** central cyanosis due to the mixing of unoxygenated blood with arterial blood in the heart or great vessels.

cybernetics (si″ber-net′iks) the science of the processes of communication and control in the animal and in the machine.

cycl(o)- word element [Gr.], *round; recurring; ciliary body of the eye.*

Cyclaine (si′klān) trademark for preparations of hexylcaine.

cyclamate (si′klah-māt) any salt of cyclamic acid; the sodium and calcium salts have been widely used as non-nutritive sugar substitutes.

Cyclamycin (si′klah-mi″sin) trademark for a preparation of troleandomycin.

cyclandelate (si-klan′dĕ-lāt) a vasodilator, C_{17}-$H_{24}O$, for peripheral vascular disease.

cyclarthrosis (si″klar-thro′sis) a pivot joint.

cyclase (si′klās) an enzyme that catalyzes the formation of a cyclic phosphodiester. **adenyl c., adenylate c.,** an enzyme found in the liver and muscle cell membranes, which catalyzes the conversion of adenosine triphosphate (ATP) to cyclic adenosine monophosphate (AMP) plus pyrophosphate, and is activated by many hormones.

cyclazocine (si″klah-zo′sēn) a benzomorphine compound that acts as a narcotic antagonist.

cycle (si′k'l) a succession or recurring series or events. **carbon c.**, the steps by which carbon (in the form of carbon dioxide) is extracted from the atmosphere by living organisms and ultimately returned to the atmosphere. It comprises a series of interconversions of carbon compounds beginning with the production of carbohydrates by plants during photosynthesis, proceeding through animal consumption, and ending and beginning again in the decomposition of the animal or plant or in the exhalation of carbon dioxide by animals. **cardiac c.**, a complete cardiac movement, or heart beat, including systole, diastole, and intervening pause. **citric acid c.**, tricarboxylic acid c. **estrous c.**, the recurring periods of heat (estrus) in adult females of most mammals and the correlated changes in the reproductive tract from one period to another. **hair c.**, the successive phases of hair growth, from initiation to loss from the follicle, consisting of anagen, catagen, and telogen. **Krebs c.**, tricarboxylic acid c. **Krebs-Henseleit c.**, urea c. **menstrual c.**, the period of regularly recurring physiologic changes in the endometrium that culminate in its shedding (menstruation). **mosquito c.**, that period in the life of a malarial parasite that is spent in the body of the mosquito host. **nitrogen c.**, the steps by which nitrogen is extracted from the nitrates of soil and water, incorporated as amino acids and proteins in living organisms, and ultimately reconverted to nitrates: (1) conversion of nitrogen to nitrates by bacteria; (2) the extraction of the nitrates by plants and the building of amino acids and proteins by adding an amino group to the carbon compounds produced in photosynthesis; (3) the ingestion of plants by animals, and (4) the return of nitrogen to the soil in animal excretions or on the death and decomposition of plants and animals. **ornithine c.**, urea c. **ovarian c.**, the sequence of physiologic changes in the ovary involved in ovulation. **reproductive c.**, the cycle of physiologic changes in the reproductive organs, from the time of fertilization of the ovum through gestation and parturition. **sex c., sexual c.**, 1. the physiologic changes recurring regularly in the genital organs of female mammals when pregnancy does not supervene. 2. the period of sexual reproduction in an organism which also reproduces asexually. **tricarboxylic acid c.**, the cyclic metabolic mechanism by which the complete oxidation of the acetyl moiety of acetyl-coenzyme A is effected; the process is the chief source of mammalian energy, during which carbon chains of sugars, fatty acids, and amino acid are metabolized to yield carbon dioxide, water, and high-energy phosphate bonds. **urea c.**, a cyclic series of reactions that produce urea, a major route for removal of the ammonia produced in the metabolism of amino acids in the liver and kidney. **uterine c.**, the phenom-

ena occurring in the endometrium during the estrous or menstrual cycle, preparing it for implantation of the blastocyst. **vaginal c.**, the rhythmic alteration in the epithelial lining of the vagina in conjunction with the ovarian cycle.

cyclectomy (sĭ-klek′to-me) 1. excision of a piece of the ciliary body. 2. excision of a portion of the ciliary border of the eyelid.

cyclencephalus (si″klen-sef′ah-lus) a monster with the cerebral hemispheres blended into one.

cyclic (sik′lik) pertaining to or occurring in a cycle or cycles; applied to chemical compounds containing a ring of atoms in the nucleus.

cyclicotomy (si″klĭ-kot′o-me) cyclotomy.

cyclitis (si-kli′tis) inflammation of the ciliary body.

cyclizine (si′klĭ-zēn) an antihistamine, $C_{18}H_{22}N_2$; the hydrochloride salt is used as an antinauseant to prevent motion sickness.

cyclobarbital (si″klo-bar′bĭ-tal) a barbiturate, $C_{12}H_{16}N_2O_3$, used as an intravenous anesthetic and hypnotic.

cyclocephalus (-sef′ah-lus) a cyclops.

cyclochoroiditis (-ko″roi-di′tis) inflammation of ciliary body and choroid.

cyclocryotherapy (-kri″o-ther′ah-pe) freezing of the ciliary body; done in the treatment of glaucoma.

cyclocumarol (-koo′mah-rōl) an anticoagulant, $C_{20}H_{18}O_4$.

cyclodialysis (-di-al′ĭ-sis) creation of a communication between the anterior chamber of the eye and the suprachoroidal space, in glaucoma.

cyclodiathermy (-di″ah-ther′me) destruction of a portion of the ciliary body by diathermy.

cyclogram (si′klo-gram) a tracing of the visual field made with a cycloscope.

cycloguanil (si″klo-gwan′il) an antimalarial, $C_{11}H_{14}ClN_5$, used as the pamoate salt.

Cyclogyl (si′klo-jil) trademark for a preparation of cyclopentolate.

cycloid (si′kloid) 1. containing a ring of atoms; said of organic chemical compounds. 2. cyclothymic (2).

cycloisomerase (si″klo-i-som′er-ās) an enzyme that catalyzes intramolecular lyase reactions.

cyclokeratitis (-ker″ah-ti′tis) inflammation of cornea and ciliary body.

cyclo-ligase (-li′gas) an enzyme that catalyzes the formation of carbon-nitrogen, C—N bonds, and the breakdown of a pyrophosphate bond, as of ATP.

cyclomethycaine (-meth′ĭ-kān) a local anesthetic, $C_{22}H_{33}NO_3$.

cyclopentamine (-pen′tah-mēn) a sympathomimetic amine, $C_9H_{19}N$; used as a nasal decongestant in the form of the hydrochloride salt.

cyclopenthiazide (-pen-thi′ah-zīd) an antihypertensive and diuretic, $C_{13}H_{18}ClN_3O_4S_2$.

cyclopentolate (-pen′to-lāt) an anticholinergic, $C_{17}H_{25}NO_3$; used as a topical cycloplegic and mydriatic in the form of the hydrochloride salt.

cyclophoria (-fo′re-ah) heterophoria in which there is deviation of the eye from the anteroposterior axis in the absence of visual fusional stimuli. **negative c.,** incyclophoria. **positive c.,** excyclophoria.

cyclophosphamide (-fos'fah-mīd) a neoplastic suppressant, $C_7H_{15}Cl_2NO_2P\cdot H_2O$, used in the treatment of lymphomas and leukemias.

cyclopia (si-klo'pe-ah) a developmental anomaly characterized by a single orbital fossa, with the globe absent or rudimentary, apparently normal, or duplicated, or the nose absent or present as a tubular appendix located above the orbit.

cycloplegia (si''klo-ple'je-ah) paralysis of the ciliary muscle; paralysis of accommodation.

cycloplegic (-ple'jik) 1. pertaining to, characterized by, or causing cycloplegia. 2. an agent which produces cycloplegia.

cyclopropane (-pro'pān) a colorless, highly inflammable and explosive gas, C_3H_6, used as an inhalation anesthetic.

Cyclops (si'klops) a genus of minute crustaceans, species of which are hosts of *Diphyllobothrium* and *Dracunculus.*

cyclops (si'klops) a monster exhibiting cyclopia.

cycloscope (si'klo-skōp) a form of perimeter for mapping the visual fields.

cycloserine (si''klo-ser'ēn) an antibiotic, C_3H_6-N_2O_2, produced by *Streptomyces orchidaceus* or obtained synthetically; used as a tuberculostatic and in treatment of urinary tract infections.

cyclosis (si-klo'sis) movement of the cytoplasm within a cell, without deformation of the cell wall.

Cyclospasmol (si''klo-spaz'mol) trademark for preparations of cyclandelate.

cyclothiazide (-thi'ah-zīd) a diuretic and antihypertensive, $C_{14}H_{16}ClN_3O_4S_2$.

cyclothymia (-thi'me-ah) a condition characterized by alternating moods of elation and dejection.

cyclothymic (-thi'mik) 1. pertaining to or characterized by cyclothymia. 2. a cyclothymic personality.

cyclotomy (si-klot'o-me) incision of the ciliary muscle.

cyclotron (si'klo-tron) an apparatus for accelerating protons or deutrons to high energies by means of a constant magnet and an oscillating electric field.

cyclotropia (si''klo-tro'pe-ah) permanent deviation of an eye around the anteroposterior axis in the presence of visional fusional stimuli, resulting in diplopia. **negative c.,** incyclotropia. **positive c.,** excyclotropia.

cycrimine (si'krĭ-mēn) an anticholinergic, C_{19}-$H_{29}NO$, used as the hydrochloride salt in the treatment of parkinsonism.

cyesis (si-e'sis) pregnancy. **cyet'ic,** adj.

cylindrodendrite (sil''in-dro-den'drīt) a collateral branch of an axon.

cylindroid (sil'in-droid) 1. shaped like a cylinder. 2. a urinary cast of various origins, which tapers to a slender tail that is often twisted or curled upon itself.

cylindroma (sil''in-dro'mah) 1. adenoid cystic carcinoma. 2. a benign skin tumor, usually on the face and scalp, in which the stroma has the form of elongated, twisted cords of hyaline material. **cylindrom'atous,** adj.

cylindruria (sil''in-droo're-ah) presence of cylindroids in the urine.

cymbocephaly (sim''bo-sef'ah-le) scaphocephaly.

cynanche (sĭ-nan'ke) severe sore throat with threatened suffocation. **c. malig'na,** a gangrenous or putrid sore throat, often diphtheritic or scarlatinal. **c. tonsilla'ris,** peritonsillar abscess.

cynanthropy (sin-an'thro-pe) delusion in which the patient believes himself a dog.

cynophobia (sin''o-fo'be-ah) morbid fear of dogs.

cyotrophy (si-ot'ro-fe) nutrition of the fetus.

cyproheptadine (si''pro-hep'tah-dēn) a histamine and serotonin antagonist, $C_{21}H_{21}N$; its hydrochloride salt is used as an antipruritic.

cyrtometer (sir-tom'ĕ-ter) a device for measuring curved surfaces of the body.

cyrtosis (sir-to'sis) 1. kyphosis. 2. distortion of the bones.

Cys cysteine.

cyst (sist) 1. any closed epithelium-lined cavity or sac, normal or abnormal, usually containing liquid or semisolid material. 2. a stage in the life cycle of certain parasites, during which they are enveloped in a protective wall. **adventitious c.,** one formed about a foreign body or exudate. **alveolar c's,** dilatations of pulmonary alveoli, which may fuse by breakdown of their septa to form large air cysts (pneumatoceles). **Baker's c.,** a swelling behind the knee due to escape of synovial fluid that has become enclosed in a sac or membrane. **Bartholin c.,** a retention cyst of Bartholin's gland, usually occurring as a result of earlier infection of the gland. **Blessig's c's,** cystic spaces formed at the periphery of the retina. **blood c.,** one containing extravasated blood. **blue dome c.,** a benign retention cyst of the breast which shows a blue color. **bone c., aneurysmal,** a solitary lesion of bone which causes a bulging of the overlying cortex, resembling somewhat the saccular protrusion of the aortic wall in aortic aneurysm. **Boyer's c.,** an enlargement of the subhyoid bursa. **bronchogenic c.,** a spherical cyst of bronchial origin lined with bronchial epithelium which may contain secretory elements, generally found in the mediastinum or the lung. **chocolate c.,** one filled with hemosiderin following local hemorrhage, such as may occur in the ovary in ovarian endometriosis. **choledochal c.,** a congenital cystic dilatation of the common bile duct which may cause pain in the right upper quadrant, jaundice, fever, or vomiting, or be asymptomatic. **colloid c.,** one with jelly-like contents. **daughter c.,** a small parasitic cyst developed from the wall of a larger one. **dentigerous c.,** an odontogenic cyst surrounding the crown of a tooth, originating after the crown is completely formed. **dermoid c.,** a tumor lined by stratified epithelium, containing hair follicles, sweat and sebaceous glands, nerve elements, and teeth. **dermoid c. of**

ovary, a benign cystic teratoma of the ovary, consisting of a grayish white mass with a fibrous wall, containing sebum, hair, and sometimes bone, teeth, and some histologically well differentiated components. **echinococcus c.,** hydatid c. **epidermal c., epidermal inclusion c., epidermoid c.,** one containing keratinized material and lined by keratinizing squamous epithelium, usually found in the skin. **exudation c.,** one formed by an exudate in a closed cavity. **fissural c.,** one arising along a line of fusion of various embryonic processes. **follicular c.,** one due to occlusion of the duct of a follicle or small gland, especially one formed by enlargement of a graafian follicle as a result of accumulated transudate. **globulomaxillary c.,** one within the maxilla at the junction of the globular portion of the medial nasal process and the maxillary process. **hydatid c.,** the larval cyst stage of the tapeworms *Echinococcus granulosus* and *E. multilocularis,* containing daughter cysts with many scoleces. **incisive canal c.,** median anterior maxillary c. **Iwanoff's c's,** Blessig's c's. **keratin c.,** one arising in the pilosebaceous apparatus lined by stratified squamous epithelium, and containing largely macerated keratin, and often sufficient sebum to render the contents greasy and often rancid. **median anterior maxillary c.,** one in or near the incisive canal, arising from proliferation of epithelial remnants of the nasopalatine duct. **median palatal c.,** one in the midline of the hard palate, between the lateral palatal processes. **meibomian c.,** a cyst of the meibomian gland, sometimes applied to a chalazion. **mother c.,** a parasitic cyst enclosing other cysts. **myxoid c.,** a nodular lesion usually overlying a distal interphalangeal finger joint in the dorsolateral or dorsomesial position, consisting of focal mucinous degeneration of the collagen of the dermis; not a true cyst, lacking an epithelial wall, it does not communicate with the underlying synovial space. **Naboth's c's, nabothian c's,** see under *follicle.* **nasoalveolar c., nasolabial c.,** a fissural cyst arising outside the bones at the junction of the globular portion of the medial nasal process, the lateral nasal process, and the maxillary process, sometimes secondarily involving the maxilla. **nasopalatine duct c.,** median anterior maxillary c. **odontogenic c.,** any cyst derived from odontogenic epithelium and therefore found exclusively in the jaws. **osseous hydatid c's,** hydatid cysts formed by the larvae of *Echinococcus granulosus* in bone, which may become weakened and eroded by the exuberant growth. **parasitic c.,** one formed by a larval parasite. **periodontal c., apical,** radicular c. **pilonidal c.,** a hair-containing sacrococcygeal dermoid cyst or sinus, often opening at a postanal dimple. **preauricular c., congenital,** one due to imperfect fusion of the first and second branchial arches in formation of the auricle, communicating with a pitlike depression in front of the helix and above the tragus (ear pit). **radicular c.,** an epithelium-lined sac, which may contain cholesterol, at the apex of a tooth. **retention c.,** one due to retention of glandular secretion. **sarcosporidian c's,** cylindrical cysts containing parasitic spores, found in muscles of those infected with *Sarcocystis.* **sebaceous c.,** a retention cyst of a sebaceous gland, containing cheesy, yellow, fatty material, usually occurring on the face, neck, scalp, or trunk. **seminal c.,** one containing semen. **solitary bone c.,** a pathologic bone space in the metaphyses of long bones of growing children; of disputed origin, it may be either empty or filled with fluid and have a delicate connective tissue lining. **sterile c.,** a true hydatid cyst that fails to produce brood capsules. **sublingual c.,** ranula. **tarry c.,** 1. one resulting from hemorrhage into a corpus luteum. 2. a bloody cyst resulting from endometriosis. **tarsal c.,** chalazion. **theca-lutein c.,** a cyst of the ovary in which the cystic cavity is lined with theca interna cells. **trichilemmal c.,** keratin c. **unicameral bone c.,** solitary bone c. **unilocular c.,** one with a single cavity. **vitelline c.,** a congenital cyst lined with ciliated epithelium occurring along the gastrointestinal canal; the remains of the omphalomesenteric duct. **wolffian c.,** a cyst of the broad ligament developed from vestiges of the wolffian body, or mesonephros.

cyst(o)- word element [Gr.], *cyst; bladder.*

cystadenocarcinoma (sis-tad″ĕ-no-kar″sĭ-no′-mah) adenocarcinoma with extensive cyst formation.

cystadenoma (sis-tad″ĕ-no′mah) cystoma blended with adenoma. **mucinous c.,** a multilocular tumor produced by ovarian epithelial cells and having mucin-filled cavities. **papillary c.,** any tumor producing patterns that are both papillary and cystic. **serous c.,** a cystic tumor of the ovary containing thin, clear yellow serum and some solid tissue.

cystalgia (sis-tal′je-ah) pain in the bladder.

cystathionine (sis″tah-thi′o-nēn) a thio-ester of homocysteine and serine, occurring as an intermediate in cystine synthesis.

cystathioninuria (-thi″o-nin-u′re-ah) abnormal increase in excretion of cystathionine in the urine.

cystectasia (sis″tek-ta′ze-ah) dilatation of the bladder.

cystectomy (sis-tek′to-me) 1. excision of a cyst. 2. excision or resection of the bladder.

cysteine (sis′te-in) a sulfur-containing amino acid produced by enzymatic or acid hydrolysis of proteins, readily oxidized to cystine; sometimes found in urine.

cystencephalus (sis″ten-sef′ah-lus) a monster with a membranous sac in place of a brain.

cystic (sis′tik) 1. pertaining to or containing cysts. 2. pertaining to the urinary bladder or to the gallbladder.

cysticercosis (sis″tĭ-ser-ko′sis) infection with cysticerci.

cysticercus (-ser′kus) pl. *cysticer′ci* [Gr.] a larval form of tapeworm.

cystiform (sis′tĭ-form) resembling a cyst.

cystigerous (sis-tij′er-us) containing cysts.

cystine (sis′tēn, sis′tin) a sulfur-containing amino acid produced by digestion or acid hydrolysis of proteins, sometimes found in the urine and kidneys, and readily reduced to two molecules of cysteine.

cystinemia (sis″tĭ-ne′me-ah) the presence of cystine in the blood.

cystinosis (-no′sis) Fanconi's syndrome (2).

cystinuria (-nu′re-ah) the occurrence of cystine in the urine.

cystistaxis (-stak′sis) oozing of blood from the mucous membrane into the bladder.

cystitis (sis-ti′tis) inflammation of the urinary bladder. **catarrhal c., acute,** that resulting from injury, irritation of foreign bodies, gonorrhea, etc., and marked by burning in the bladder, pain in the urethra, and painful micturition. **cystic c., c. cys′tica,** that marked by formation of submucosal cysts in the bladder neck. **c. follicula′ris,** that in which the bladder mucosa is studded with nodules containing lymph follicles. **c. glandula′ris,** that in which the mucosa contains mucin-secreting glands. **interstitial c., chronic,** a bladder condition with an inflammatory lesion, usually in the vertex, and involving the entire thickness of the wall. **panmural c.,** interstitial c., chronic. **c. papillomato′sa,** that with papillomatous growths on the inflamed mucous membrane.

cystitome (sis′tĭ-tōm) an instrument for opening the lens capsule.

cystitomy (sis-tit′o-me) surgical division of the lens capsule.

cystoadenoma (sis″to-ad″ĕ-no′mah) cystadenoma.

cystocarcinoma (-kar″sĭ-no′mah) carcinoma associated with cysts.

cystocele (sis′to-sēl) herniation of the urinary bladder into the vagina.

cystodynia (sis″to-din′e-ah) pain in the bladder.

cystoelytroplasty (-el′ĭ-tro-plas″te) surgical repair of a vesicovaginal injuries.

cystoepithelioma (-ep″ĭ-the″le-o′mah) a tumor with cystic and epitheliomatous elements.

cystofibroma (-fi-bro′mah) fibroma containing cysts.

cystogastrostomy (-gas-tros′to-me) surgical anastomosis of a cyst to the stomach for drainage.

cystogram (sis′to-gram) the film obtained by cystography.

cystography (sis-tog′rah-fe) radiography of the urinary bladder. **voiding c.,** radiography of the bladder while the patient is urinating.

cystoid (sis′toid) 1. resembling a cyst. 2. a cystlike, circumscribed collection of softened material, having no enclosing capsule.

cystojejunostomy (sis″to-je-ju-nos′to-me) surgical anastomosis of a cyst to the jejunum.

cystolith (sis′to-lith) a vesical calculus.

cystolithectomy (sis″to-lĭ-thek′to-me) surgical removal of a vesical calculus.

cystolithiasis (-lĭ-thi′ah-sis) formation of vesical calculi.

cystolithic (-lith′ik) pertaining to a vesical calculus.

cystolithotomy (-lĭ-thot′o-me) cystolithectomy.

cystoma (sis-to′mah) a tumor containing cysts of neoplastic origin; a cystic tumor.

cystometer (sis-tom′ĕ-ter) an instrument for studying the neuromuscular mechanism of the bladder by means of measurements of pressure and capacity.

cystometrogram (sis″to-met′ro-gram) the record obtained by cystometrography.

cystometrography (-mĕ-trog′rah-fe) the graphic recording of intravesical volumes and pressures.

cystomorphous (-mor′fus) resembling a cyst or bladder.

cystoparalysis (-pah-ral′ĭ-sis) cystoplegia.

cystopexy (sis′to-pek″se) fixation of the bladder to the abdominal wall.

cystoplasty (-plas″te) plastic repair of the bladder.

cystoplegia (sis″to-ple′je-ah) paralysis of the bladder.

cystoproctostomy (-prok-tos′to-me) surgical creation of a communication between the urinary bladder and the rectum.

cystoptosis (sis″top-to′sis) prolapse of part of the inner bladder into the urethra.

cystopyelitis (sis″to-pi″ĕ-li′tis) inflammation of the bladder and renal pelvis.

cystopyelonephritis (-pi″ĕ-lo-ne-fri′tis) combined cystitis and pyelonephritis.

cystorrhaphy (sis-tor′ah-fe) suture of the bladder.

cystorrhea (sis″to-re′ah) mucous discharge from the bladder.

cystosarcoma (-sar-ko′mah) an unusually large fibroadenoma of the mammary gland, with a cellular, sarcoma-like stoma; it is locally aggressive and sometimes metastasizes.

cystoscope (sis′to-skōp) an endoscope for visual examination of the bladder.

cystoscopy (sis-tos′ko-pe) visual examination of the urinary tract with a cystoscope.

cystostomy (sis-tos′to-me) surgical formation of an opening into the bladder.

cystotomy (sis-tot′o-me) incision of the bladder.

cystoureteritis (sis″to-u-re″ter-i′tis) inflammation of the urinary bladder and ureters.

cystoureterogram (-u-re′ter-o-gram″) a roentgenogram of the bladder and ureter.

cystourethrography (-u″re-throg′rah-fe) roentgenography of the urinary bladder and urethra.

cystourethroscope (-u-re′thro-skōp″) an instrument for examining the posterior urethra and bladder.

cyt(o)- word element [Gr.], *a cell.*

cytarabine (si-tār′ah-bēn) an antimetabolite, $C_9H_{13}N_3O_5$, which inhibits DNA synthesis, and hence has antineoplastic and antiviral properties.

cytase (si′tās) 1. Metchnikoff's name for complement. 2. an enzyme in various plant seeds capable of solubilizing the cell wall.

-cyte word element [Gr.], *a cell.*

cytidine (si′tĭ-dēn) a nucleoside consisting of cytosine and ribose, a constituent of RNA.

cytoanalyzer (si″to-an″ah-li′zer) an electronic

optical apparatus for the detection of malignant cells in smears.

cytoarchitectonic (-ar″kĭ-tek-ton′ik) pertaining to cellular structure or the arrangement of cells in tissue.

cytobiology (-bi-ol′o-je) the biology of cells.

cytocentrum (-sen′trum) centrosome.

cytochalasin (-kal′ah-sin) any of a group of fungal metabolites that affect the motility of polymorphonuclear leukocytes.

cytochemistry (-kem′is-tre) the identification and localization of the different chemical compounds and their activities within the cell.

cytochrome (si′to-krōm) any of a class of hemoproteins, widely distributed in animal and plant tissues, whose main function is electron transport; distinguished according to their prosthetic group as *a, b, c,* and *d.*

cytochylema (si″to-ki-le′mah) hyaloplasm (1).

cytocide (si′to-sīd) an agent which destroys cells. **cytoci′dal,** adj.

cytocinesis (si″to-si-ne′sis) cytokinesis.

cytoclasis (si-tok′lah-sis) the destruction of cells. **cytoclas′tic,** adj.

cytode (si′tōd) a non-nucleated cell or cell element.

cytodendrite (si″to-den′drīt) dendrite.

cytodiagnosis (-di″ag-no′sis) diagnosis based on examination of cells.

cytodieresis (-di-er′ĕ-sis) cell division, i.e., meiosis or mitosis.

cytodistal (-dis′tal) denoting that part of an axon remote from the cell body.

cytogene (si′to-jēn) a self-perpetuating cytoplasmic particle that traces its origin to the genes of the nucleus.

cytogenesis (si″to-jen′ĕ-sis) the origin and development of the cell.

cytogeneticist (-jĕ-net′ĭ-sist) a specialist in cytogenetics.

cytogenetics (-jĕ-net′iks) that branch of genetics devoted to the cellular constituents concerned in heredity, i.e., the chromosomes. **cytogenet′ical,** adj. **clinical c.,** the branch of cytogenetics concerned with relations between chromosomal abnormalities and pathologic conditions.

cytogenic (-jen′ik) 1. pertaining to cytogenesis. 2. forming or producing cells.

cytogenous (si-toj′ĕ-nus) producing cells.

cytoglycopenia (si″to-gli″ko-pe′ne-ah) deficient glucose content of body or blood cells.

cytohistogenesis (-his″to-jen′ĕ-sis) the development of the structure of cells.

cytoid (si′toid) resembling a cell.

cytokinesis (-ki-ne′sis) the changes that occur in the cytoplasm during meiosis, mitosis, and fertilization.

cytokinin (-ki′nin) any of a class of phytohormones (N^6-substituted adenines) whose principal functions are the induction of cell division (cytokinesis) and the regulation of differentiation of tissue (organogenesis).

cytologist (si-tol′o-jist) a specialist in cytology.

cytology (si-tol′o-je) the study of cells, their origin, structure, function, and pathology. **cytolog′ic,** adj. **exfoliative c.,** microscopic examination of cells desquamated from a body surface as a means of detecting malignant change.

cytolysin (si-tol′ĭ-sin) a substance or antibody that produces cytolysis.

cytolysis (si-tol′ĭ-sis) the dissolution of cells.

cytolysosome (si″to-li′so-sōm) a lysosome fused with mitochondria and other cell organelles and associated with cell autolysis.

cytomegalovirus (-meg″ah-lo-vi′rus) any of a group of highly host-specific herpesviruses, infecting man, monkeys, or rodents, producing unique large cells with intranuclear inclusions; the virus specific for man causes cytomegalic inclusion disease.

Cytomel (si′to-mel) trademark for a preparation of liothyronine.

cytometaplasia (si″to-met″ah-pla′ze-ah) alteration in the function or form of cells.

cytometer (si-tom′ĕ-ter) a device for counting blood cells.

cytometry (si-tom′ĕ-tre) the counting of blood cells.

cytomitome (si″to-mi′tōm) a fibril or fibrillary structure in the cytoplasm.

cytomorphology (-mor-fol′o-je) the morphology of body cells.

cytomorphosis (-mor-fo′sis) the changes through which cells pass in development.

cyton (si′ton) the cell body of a neuron.

cytopathic (si″to-path′ik) pertaining to or characterized by pathologic changes in cells.

cytopathogenesis (-path″o-jen′ĕ-sis) production of pathologic changes in cells. **cytopathogenet′ic,** adj.

cytopathogenic (-path″o-jen′ik) capable of producing pathologic changes in cells.

cytopathogenicity (-path″o-je-nis′ĭ-te) the ability to cause pathologic changes in cells.

cytopathology (-pah-thol′o-je) the study of cells in disease; cellular pathology.

cytopenia (-pe′ne-ah) deficiency in the cells of the blood.

Cytophaga (si-tof′ah-gah) a genus of schizomycetes (family Cytophagaceae), species of which dissolve vegetable fiber and hydrolyze cellulose.

Cytophagaceae (si″to-fah-ga′se-e) a family of schizomycetes (order Myxobacterales) which are saprophytic soil microorganisms.

cytophagocytosis (-fag″o-si-to′sis) cytophagy.

cytophagous (si-tof′ah-gus) devouring or consuming cells; said of phagocytes.

cytophagy (si-tof′ah-je) the ingestion of cells by phagocytes.

cytophilic (si″to-fil′ik) having an affinity for cells.

cytophotometer (-fo-tom′ĕ-ter) a photometer for measuring localization of organic compounds within cells by measuring the light intensity through selected stained areas of cytoplasm.

cytophylaxis (-fi-lak′sis) 1. the protection of cells against cytolysis. 2. increase in cellular activity.

cytophyletic (-fi-let′ik) pertaining to the genealogy of cells.

cytophysics (-fiz′iks) the physics of cell activity.

cytophysiology (-fiz″e-ol′o-je) the physiology of cells.

cytopipette (-pi-pet′) a pipette for taking cytological smears.

cytoplasm (si′to-plazm) the protoplasm of a cell exclusive of that of the nucleus (nucleoplasm). **cytoplas′mic,** adj.

cytoplastin (si′to-plas″tin) the plastin of cytoplasm.

cytoproximal (si″to-prok′si-mal) denoting that part of an axon nearer to the cell body.

cytoscopy (si-tos′ko-pe) examination of cells.

cytosine (si′to-sēn) the base oxyaminopyrimidine, $C_4H_5N_3O$, a component of nucleic acid. **c. arabinoside,** cytarabine.

cytoskeleton (si″to-skel′ĕ-ton) a conspicuous internal reinforcement in the cytoplasm of a cell, containing minute filaments aggregated in bundles.

cytosol (si′to-sol) the liquid medium of the cytoplasm, i.e., cytoplasm minus organelles and nonmembranous insoluble components.

cytosome (-sōm) the body of a cell apart from its nucleus.

cytospongium (si″to-spun′je-um) spongioplasm.

cytost (si′tost) a specific toxin given off from a cell as a result of injury to it.

cytostatic (si″to-stat′ik) 1. suppressing the growth and multiplication of cells. 2. an agent that so acts.

cytostome (si′to-stōm) the cell mouth; the aperture through which food enters certain protozoa.

cytotaxis (si″to-tak′sis) the movement and arrangement of cells with respect to a specific source of stimulation. **cytotac′tic,** adj.

cytothesis (si-toth′ĕ-sis) restitution of cells to their normal condition.

cytotoxic (si″to-tok′sik) having a deleterious effect upon cells.

cytotoxin (-tok′sin) a toxin or antibody having a specific toxic action upon cells of special organs.

cytotrophoblast (-trof′o-blast) the cellular (inner) layer of the trophoblast.

cytotropism (si-tot′ro-pizm) 1. cell movement in response to external stimulation. 2. the tendency of viruses, bacteria, drugs, etc., to exert their effect upon certain cells of the body. **cytotrop′ic,** adj.

Cytoxan (si-tok′san) trademark for preparations of cyclophosphamide.

cytozoic (si″to-zo′ik) living within or attached to cells; said of parasites.

cytula (sit′u-lah) the impregnated ovum.

cyturia (si-tu′re-ah) the presence of cells of any sort in the urine.

D

D chemical symbol, *deuterium.*

D. 1. deciduous; density; [L.] *dex′ter* (right); diopter; dose; duration. 2. symbol for the unit of vitamin D potency.

D- chemical prefix (small capital) specifying that the substance corresponds in chemical configuration to the standard substance D-glyceraldehyde. Opposed to L-. For carbohydrates, the configuration of the highest numbered asymmetric carbon atoms determines whether the substance is D- or L-; for amino acids, the lowest numbered asymmetric carbon atom is the key.

d- chemical abbreviation, *dextrorotatory.*

dacry(o)- word element [Gr.], *tears* or *the lacrimal apparatus of the eye.*

dacryagogic (dak″re-ah-goj′ik) 1. inducing a flow of tears. 2. serving as a channel for discharge of secretion of the lacrimal glands.

dacryagogue (dak′re-ah-gog) 1. an agent that induces a flow of tears. 2. a lacrimal duct.

dacryoadenalgia (dak″re-o-ad″ĕ-nal′je-ah) pain in a lacrimal gland.

dacryoadenectomy (-ad″ĕ-nek′to-me) excision of a lacrimal gland.

dacryoadenitis (-ad″ĕ-ni′tis) inflammation of a lacrimal gland.

dacryoblennorrhea (-blen″o-re′ah) mucous flow from the lacrimal apparatus.

dacryocele (dak′re-o-sēl″) dacryocystocele.

dacryocyst (-sist″) the lacrimal sac.

dacryocystalgia (dak″re-o-sis-tal′je-ah) pain in the lacrimal sac.

dacryocystectomy (-sis-tek′to-me) excision of the wall of the lacrimal sac.

dacryocystitis (-sis-ti′tis) inflammation of the lacrimal sac.

dacryocystoblennorrhea (-sis″to-blen″o-re′ah) chronic catarrhal inflammation of the lacrimal sac, with constriction of the lacrimal gland.

dacryocystocele (-sis′to-sēl) hernial protrusion of the lacrimal sac.

dacryocystoptosis (-sis″top-to′sis) prolapse of the lacrimal sac.

dacryocystorhinostenosis (-sis″to-ri″no-stĕ-no′sis) narrowing of the duct leading from the lacrimal sac to the nasal cavity.

dacryocystorhinostomy (-ri-nos′to-me) surgical creation of an opening between the lacrimal sac and nasal cavity.

dacryocystorhinotomy (-ri-not′o-me) passage of a probe through the lacrimal sac into the nasal cavity.

dacryocystostenosis (-stĕ-no'sis) narrowing of the lacrimal sac.

dacryocystostomy (-sis-tos'to-me) creation of a new opening into the lacrimal sac.

dacryocystotomy (-sis-tot'o-me) incision of the lacrimal sac and duct.

dacryohemorrhea (-he''mo-re'ah) the discharge of tears mixed with blood.

dacryolith (dak're-o-lith'') a lacrimal calculus.

dacryolithiasis (dak''re-o-lĭ-thi'ah-sis) the presence of dacryoliths.

dacryoma (dak''re-o'mah) a tumor-like swelling due to obstruction of the lacrimal duct.

dacryon (dak're-on) the point where the lacrimal, frontal, and upper maxillary bones meet.

dacryops (dak're-ops) 1. a watery state of the eye. 2. distention of a lacrimal duct by contained fluid.

dacryopyorrhea (dak''re-o-pi''o-re'ah) the discharge of tears mixed with pus.

dacryopyosis (-pi-o'sis) suppuration of the lacrimal apparatus.

dacryorrhea (-re'ah) excessive flow of tears.

dacryosolenitis (-so-lĕ-ni'tis) inflammation of a lacrimal duct.

dacryostenosis (-stĕ-no'sis) stricture or narrowing of a lacrimal duct.

dacryosyrinx (-sir'inks) 1. a lacrimal duct. 2. a lacrimal fistula. 3. a syringe for irrigating the lacrimal ducts.

Dactil (dak'til) trademark for a preparation of piperidolate.

dactinomycin (dak''tĭ-no-mi'sin) actinomycin D, an antibiotic derived from several species of *Streptomyces*, $C_{62}H_{86}N_{12}O_{16}$; used as an antineoplastic.

dactyl (dak'til) a digit.

dactyl(o)- word element [Gr.], *a digit; a finger or toe.*

dactylitis (dak''tĭ-li'tis) inflammation of a finger or toe.

dactylography (dak''tĭ-log'rah-fe) the study of fingerprints.

dactylogryposis (dak''tĭ-lo-grĭ-po'sis) permanent flexion of the fingers.

dactylology (dak''tĭ-lol'o-je) communication between individuals by signs made with the hands and fingers.

dactylolysis (dak''tĭ-lol'ĭ-sis) 1. surgical correction of syndactyly. 2. loss or amputation of a digit. **d. sponta'nea,** spontaneous loss of digits, as in ainhum or in leprosy.

dactylomegaly (dak''tĭ-lo-meg'ah-le) abnormally large fingers or toes.

dactyloscopy (dak''tĭ-los'ko-pe) examination of fingerprints for identification.

dactylus (dak'tĭ-lus), pl. *dac'tyli* [L.] a digit.

daltonism (dawl'ton-izm) red-green blindness.

dam (dam) rubber dam; a thin sheet of latex rubber used to isolate teeth from mouth fluids during dental therapy.

damp (damp) foul air or noxious gas(es) in a mine. **after-d.,** a gaseous mixture of nitrogen, carbon dioxide, and usually carbon monoxide, formed in a mine by explosion of fire damp or dust. **black d., choke d.,** a gaseous mixture formed in a mine by the gradual absorption of the oxygen and the giving off of carbon dioxide by the coal. **cold d.,** foggy vapor charged with carbon dioxide. **fire d.,** light explosive hydrocarbon gases, chiefly methane, CH_4, found in coal mines. **white d.,** carbon monoxide.

damping (damp'ing) steady diminution of the amplitude of successive vibrations of a specific form of energy, as of electricity.

D and C dilatation (of cervix) and curettage (of uterus).

dander (dan'der) small scales from the hair or feathers of animals, which may be a cause of allergy in sensitive persons.

dandruff (dan'druf) 1. dry scaly material shed from the scalp; applied to that normally shed from the scalp epidermis as well as to the excessive scaly material associated with disease. 2. seborrheic dermatitis of the scalp.

Danilone (dan'ĭ-lōn) trademark for a preparation of phenindione.

danthron (dan'thron) a cathartic, $C_{14}H_8O_4$.

dantrolene (dan'tro-lēn) a skeletal muscle relaxant, $C_{14}H_{10}N_4O_5$.

dapsone (dap'sōn) an antibacterial, $C_{12}H_{12}N_2$-O_2S, used as a leprostatic and a dermatitis herpetiformis suppressant.

Daranide (dar'ah-nīd) trademark for a preparation of dichlorphenamide.

Daraprim (dar'ah-prim) trademark for a preparation of pyrimethamine.

Darbid (dar'bid) trademark for a preparation of isopropamide.

Daricon (dar'ĭ-kon) trademark for a preparation of oxyphencyclimine.

darnel (dar'nel) a rye grass, *Lolium temulentum*, the seeds of which contain a narcotic poison; ingestion of contaminated flour may produce vertigo, staggering, vomiting, visual disturbances, burning pain in the mouth, and prostration.

Dartal (dar'tal) trademark for a preparation of thiopropazate.

dartoid (dar'toid) resembling the dartos.

dartos (dar'tos) the contractile tissue under the skin of the scrotum.

Darvon (dar'von) trademark for a preparation of propoxyphene.

darwinism (dar'wĭ-nizm) the theory of evolution according to which higher organisms have been developed from lower ones through the influence of natural selection.

daughter (daw'ter) 1. decay product. 2. arising from cell division, as a daughter cell.

db decibel.

DBI trademark for a preparation of phenformin.

D.C. Dental Corps; direct current; Doctor of Chiropractic.

D & C dilatation (of cervix) and curettage (of uterus).

D.D.S. Doctor of Dental Surgery.

DDT dichloro-diphenyl-trichloroethane, a powerful insect poison; used in dilution as a powder or in an oily solution as a spray.

de- word element [L.], *down; from;* sometimes negative or privative, and often intensive.

deacidification (de″ah-sid″ĭ-fĭ-ka′shun) neutralization of acidity.

deactivation (de-ak″tĭ-va′shun) the process of making or becoming inactive.

deacylase (de-as′il-ās) any hydrolase that catalyzes the removal of an acyl group.

deaf (def) lacking the sense of hearing or not having the full power of hearing.

deafferentation (de-af″er-en-ta′shun) the elimination or interruption of afferent (sensory) nerve fibers.

deaf-mute (def′mūt) a person unable to hear or speak.

deaf-mutism (def-mu′tizm) inability to hear or speak.

deafness (def′nes) lack or loss, complete or partial, of the sense of hearing. **acoustic trauma d.,** that due to continuous exposure to excessively loud noises. **apoplectiform d.,** Meniere's disease in which the hearing impairment is sudden in onset and fluctuates. **bass d.,** deafness to certain low tones. **boilermakers′ d.,** that due to working where the noise level is extremely high. **cerebral d.,** that due to a brain lesion. **conduction d.,** that due to defect of the sound-conducting apparatus. **cortical d.,** that due to disease of the cortical centers. **functional d.,** that due to defective functioning of the auditory apparatus without organic lesions. **hysterical d.,** that which may appear or disappear in a hysterical patient without discoverable cause. **labyrinthine d.,** that due to disease of the labyrinth. **nerve d., neural d.,** that due to a lesion of the auditory nerve on the central neural pathways. **perceptive d., sensorineural d.,** that due to a lesion in the sensory mechanism (cochlea) of the ear or to a lesion of the acoustic nerve or central neural pathways or to a combination of such lesions. **tone d.,** sensory amusia. **transmission d.,** conduction d. **word d.,** auditory aphasia; receptive aphasia in which sounds are heard but convey no meaning to the mind.

dealcoholization (de-al″ko-hol-i-za′shun) removal of alcohol from an object.

deamidase (de-am′ĭ-dās) an enzyme that splits amides to form carboxylic acid and ammonia.

deamidation (de-am″ĭ-da′shun) deamidization.

deamidization (de-am″ĭ-di-za′shun) liberation of the ammonia from an amide.

deaminase (de-am′ĭ-nās) an enzyme causing deamination, or removal of the amino group from organic compounds, named according to its substrate as *adenosine d., cytidine d., guanine d.,* etc.

deamination (de-am″ĭ-na′shun) removal of the amino group, —NH_2, from a compound.

Deaner (de′ner) trademark for a preparation of deanol acetamidobenzoate.

deanol acetamidobenzoate (de′ah-nol as″et-am″ĭ-do-ben′zo-āt) a central stimulant with parasympathomimetic activity, $C_{13}H_{20}N_2O_4$.

death (deth) the cessation of life; permanent cessation of all vital bodily functions. **black d.,** bubonic plague. **brain d.,** irreversible coma.

cell d., complete degeneration or necrosis of cells. **cot d., crib d.,** sudden infant death syndrome. **somatic d.,** cessation of all vital cellular activity.

debanding (de-band′ing) the removal of fixed orthodontic appliances.

debility (de-bil′ĭ-te) lack or loss of strength; weakness.

débride (da-brēd′) [Fr.] to remove by débridement.

débridement (da-brēd-maw′) [Fr.] the removal of foreign material and contaminated or devitalized tissue from or adjacent to a traumatic or infected lesion until surrounding healthy tissue is exposed.

debris (dĕ-bre′) [Fr.] devitalized tissue or foreign matter. In dentistry, soft foreign material loosely attached to a tooth surface.

debrisoquin (deb-ris′o-kwin) an antihypertensive agent, $C_{10}H_{13}N_3$, used as the sulfate salt.

deca- word element [Gr.], *ten;* used in naming units of measurement to indicate a quantity 10 times the unit designated by the root with which it is combined.

Decadron (dek′ah-dron) trademark for preparations of dexamethasone.

Deca-Durabolin (de″ka-dur-ab′o-lin) trademark for a preparation of nandrolone decanoate.

decagram (dek′ah-gram) ten grams.

decalcification (de-kal″sĭ-fĭ-ka′shun) 1. loss of calcium salts from a bone or tooth. 2. the processs of removing calcareous matter.

decalcify (de-kal′sĭ-fi) to deprive of calcium or its salts.

decaliter (dek′ah-le″ter) ten liters.

decameter (-me″ter) ten meters.

decamethonium (-mĕ-tho′ne-um) a muscle relaxant, $C_{16}H_{38}N_2$, used in surgical anesthesia and in electroshock treatment, in the form of its bromide or iodide salt.

decannulation (de-kan″u-la′shun) the removal of a cannula.

decanormal (dek″ah-nor′mal) having ten times the strength of normal.

decantation (de″kan-ta′shun) the pouring of a clear supernatant liquid from a sediment.

decapeptide (dek″ah-pep′tĭd) a peptide containing 10 amino acids.

decapitation (de-kap″ĭ-ta′shun) the removal of the head, as of an animal, fetus, or bone.

decapsulation (de-kap″su-la′shun) removal of a capsule, especially the renal capsule.

decarboxylase (de″kar-bok′sĭ-lās) any of the lyase class of enzymes that catalyze the removal of a carbon dioxide molecule from a compound.

decarboxylation (de″kar-bok″sĭ-la′shun) removal of the carboxyl group from a compound.

decavitamin (dek″ah-vi′tah-min) a combination of vitamins in capsular or tablet form, each of which contains vitamins A and D, ascorbic acid, calcium pantothenate, cyanocobalamin, folic acid, niacinamide, pyridoxine hydrochloride, riboflavin, thiamine hydrochloride, and a suitable form of alpha tocopherol.

decay (de-ka′) 1. the gradual decomposition of

dead organic matter. 2. the process or stage of decline, as in aging. **beta d.,** disintegration of the nucleus of an unstable radionuclide in which the mass number is unchanged, but atomic number is increased or decreased by 1, as a result of emission of a negatively or positively charged (beta) particle.

decerebrate (de-ser′ĕ-brāt) to eliminate cerebral function by transecting the brain stem or by ligating the common carotid arteries and basilar artery at the center of the pons; an animal so prepared, or a brain-damaged person with similar neurologic signs.

decerebration (de-ser″ĕ-bra′shun) the act of decerebrating.

dechloridation (de-klo″rĭ-da′shun) the removal of chloride, or salt.

decholesterolization (de-ko-les″ter-ol-i-za′-shun) reduction of cholesterol levels in the blood.

Decholin (de′ko-lin) trademark for preparations of dehydrocholic acid.

deci- word element [L.], *one-tenth;* used in naming units of measurement to indicate one-tenth of the unit designated by the root with which it is combined (10^{-1}); symbol d.

decibel (des′ĭ-bel) a unit used to express the ratio of two powers, usually electric or acoustic powers, equal to one-tenth of a bel; one decibel equals approximately the smallest difference in acoustic power the human ear can detect.

decidua (de-sid′u-ah) a name applied to the endometrium during pregnancy, which is shed after childbirth. **decid′ual,** adj. **basal d., d. basa′lis,** that portion on which the implanted ovum rests. **capsular d., d. capsula′ris,** that portion directly overlying the implanted ovum and facing the uterine cavity. **menstrual d., d. menstrua′lis,** the hyperemic uterine mucosa shed during menstruation. **parietal d., d. parieta′lis,** the decidua exclusive of the area occupied by the implanted ovum. **d. reflex′a,** capsular decidua. **d. seroti′na,** basal d. **d. subchoria′lis,** the maternal component of the tissue comprising the closing ring of Winkler-Waldeyer. **true d., d. ve′ra,** parietal d.

deciduate (de-sid′u-āt) characterized by shedding.

deciduation (de-sid″u-a′shun) the shedding of the decidua.

deciduitis (-i′tis) a bacterial disease leading to changes in the decidua.

deciduoma (-o′mah) an intrauterine mass containing decidual cells.

deciduosis (-o′sis) the presence of decidual tissue or of tissue resembling the endometrium of pregnancy in an ectopic site.

deciduous (de-sid′u-us) falling off; subject to being shed, as deciduous teeth.

decigram (des′ĭ-gram) one tenth of a gram.

deciliter (-le″ter) one tenth of a liter.

decimeter (-me″ter) one tenth of a meter.

decinormal (des″ĭ-nor′mal) of one tenth normal strength.

decipara (des″ĭ-pah′rah) a woman who has had ten pregnancies which resulted in viable offspring; para X.

declination (dek″lĭ-na′shun) cyclophoria.

declive (de-klīv′) a slope or a slanting surface. In anatomy, the part of the vermis of the cerebellum just caudal to the primary fissure.

declivis (de-kli′vis) [L.] declive.

Declomycin (dek′lo-mi″sin) trademark for preparations of demeclocycline.

decoction (de-kok′shun) 1. the process of boiling. 2. a preparation made by boiling.

decoloration (de-kul″er-a′shun) 1. removal of color; bleaching. 2. lack or loss of color.

decompensation (de″kom-pen-sa′shun) inability of the heart to maintain adequate circulation, marked by dyspnea, venous engorgement, and edema.

decomposition (de-kom″po-zish′un) the separation of compound bodies into their constituent principles.

decompression (de″kom-presh′un) removal of pressure, especially the slow lessening of pressure on deep-sea divers and caisson workers to prevent bends, and the reduction of pressure on persons as they ascend to great heights. **cardiac d.,** d. of heart. **cerebral d.,** relief of intracranial pressure by removal of a skull flap and incision of the dura mater. **d. of heart,** pericardiotomy with evacuation of a hematoma. **nerve d.,** relief of pressure on a nerve by surgical removal of the constricting fibrous or bony tissue. **d. of pericardium,** d. of heart. **d. of rectum,** proctostomy for imperforate anus. **d. of spinal cord,** surgical relief of pressure on the spinal cord, which may be due to hematoma, bone fragments, etc.

decongestant (de″kon-jes′tant) 1. tending to reduce congestion or swelling. 2. an agent that reduces congestion or swelling.

decongestive (de″kon-jes′tiv) reducing congestion.

decontamination (de″kon-tam-ĭ-na′shun) the freeing of a person or object of some contaminating substance, e.g., war gas, radioactive material, etc.

decortication (de-kor″tĭ-ka′shun) 1. removal of the outer covering from a plant, seed, or root. 2. removal of portions of the cortical substance of a structure or organ.

decrepitation (de-krep″ĭ-ta′shun) the explosion or crackling of certain substances (salt, crystals, etc.) upon heating.

decrudescence (de″kroo-des′ens) diminution or abatement of the intensity of symptoms.

decubitus (de-ku′bĭ-tus) 1. an act of lying down; the position assumed in lying down. 2. decubitus ulcer. **decu′bital,** adj. **Andral's d.,** lying on the unaffected side in the early stages of pleurisy. **dorsal d.,** lying on the back. **lateral d.,** lying on one side, designated *right lateral decubitus* when the subject lies on the right side and *left lateral decubitus* when he lies on the left side. **ventral d.,** lying on the stomach.

decussate (de-kus′āt) 1. to cross in the form of an X. 2. crossed like the letter X.

decussatio (de″kus-sa′she-o), pl. *decussatio′nes* [L.] decussation.

decussation (de″kus-sa′shun) a crossing over; the intercrossing of fellow parts or structures in the form of an X. **Forel's d.,** the ventral tegmental decussation of the rubrospinal and rubroreticular tracts in the mesencephalon. **fountain d. of Meynert,** the dorsal tegmental decussation of the tectospinal tract in the mesencephalon. **d. of the pyramids,** the anterior part of the lower medulla oblongata in which most of the fibers of the pyramids intersect.

dedifferentiation (de-dif″er-en″she-a′shun) regression from a more specialized or complex form to a simpler state.

de-epicardialization (de″ep-ĭ-kar″dĭ-al-i-za′-shun) a surgical procedure for the relief of intractable angina pectoris, in which epicardial tissue is destroyed by application of a caustic agent to promote development of collateral circulation.

def (de′e-ef) an expression of dental caries experience in deciduous teeth, *d* representing the number of teeth indicated for filling; *e* the number indicated for extraction; *f* the number of filled teeth.

defatted (de-fat′ed) deprived of fat.

defecation (def″ĕ-ka′shun) 1. the evacuation of fecal matter from the rectum. 2. the removal of impurities, as chemical defecation.

defect (de′fekt) an imperfection, failure, or absence. **aortic septal d.,** a congenital anomaly in which there is abnormal communication between the ascending aorta and pulmonary artery just above the semilunar valves. **atrial septal d., atrioseptal d.,** a congenital anomaly in which there is persistent patency of the atrial septum, owing to failure of closure of the ostium primum or ostium secundum. **ectodermal d., congenital,** a hereditary condition affecting chiefly males, marked by smooth glossy skin, absence of sweat glands, abnormality of teeth, defective hair formation, saddle nose, prominent frontal bones, large chin, and thick lips. **endocardial cushion d's,** a spectrum of septal defects resulting from imperfect fusion of the endocardial cushions, and ranging from persistent ostium primum to persistent common atrioventricular canal; see *atrial septal d.* and *atrioventricularis communis.* **filling d.,** any localized defect in the contour of the stomach, duodenum, or intestine, as seen in the roentgenogram after barium enema. **retention d.,** a defect in the power of recalling or remembering names, numbers, or events. **septal d.,** a defect in a cardiac septum resulting in an abnormal communication between the opposite chambers of the heart. **ventricular septal d.,** a congenital cardiac anomaly in which there is persistent patency of the ventricular septum in either the muscular or fibrous portions, most often due to failure of the bulbar septum to completely close the interventricular foramen.

defective (de-fek′tiv) 1. imperfect. 2. a person lacking in some physical, mental, or moral quality.

defeminization (de-fem″ĭ-ni-za′shun) loss of female sexual characteristics.

defense (de-fens′) behavior directed to protection of the individual from injury.

deferens (def′er-ens) [L.] deferent.

deferent (def′er-ent) conveying away, as from a center.

deferentectomy (def″er-en-tek′to-me) excision of a ductus deferens.

deferential (def″er-en′shal) pertaining to the ductus deferens.

deferentitis (def″er-en-ti′tis) inflammation of the ductus deferens.

deferoxamine (de″fer-oks′ah-mēn) an iron-chelating agent, $C_{25}H_{48}N_2O_8$, isolated from *Streptomyces pilosus.*

defervescence (def″er-ves′ens) the period of abatement of fever.

defibrillation (de-fib″rĭ-la′shun) 1. termination of atrial or ventricular fibrillation, usually by electroshock. 2. separation of tissue fibers by blunt dissection.

defibrillator (de-fib″rĭ-la′tor) an electronic apparatus used to produce defibrillation by application of brief electroshock to the heart, directly or through electrodes placed on the chest wall.

defibrination (de-fi″brĭ-na′shun) deprival of fibrin.

deficiency (de-fish′en-se) a lack or shortage; a condition characterized by presence of less than normal or necessary supply or competence.

deficit (def′ĭ-sit) a lack or deficiency. **oxygen d.,** see *anoxemia, anoxia,* and *hypoxia.*

deflection (de-flek′shun) a turning aside; in psychoanalysis, an unconscious diversion of ideas from conscious attention.

defluvium (de-floo′ve-um) [L.] a falling out, as of the hair.

defluxion (de-fluk′shun) 1. a sudden disappearance. 2. a copious discharge, as of catarrh. 3. a falling out, as of hair.

deformability (de-form″ah-bil′ĭ-te) the ability of cells, such as erythrocytes, to change shape as they pass through narrow spaces, such as the microvasculature.

deformation (de″for-ma′shun) 1. deformity. 2. the process of adapting in shape or form.

deformity (de-for′mĭ-te) distortion of any part or general disfigurement of the body; malformation. **Åkerlund d.,** an indentation (in addition to the niche) in the duodenal cap in the radiograph in duodenal ulcer. **Arnold-Chiari d.,** protrusion of the cerebellum and medulla oblongata down into the spinal canal through the foramen magnum. **gun stock d.,** cubitus varus. **Madelung's d.,** radial deviation of the hand secondary to overgrowth of the distal ulna or shortening of the radius. **reduction d.,** congenital absence of a portion or all of a body part, especially of the limbs. **silver-fork d.,** see under *fracture.* **Sprengel's d.,** congenital elevation of the scapula, due to failure of descent in fetal life. **Volkmann's d.,** see under *disease.*

defundation (de″fun-da′shun) excision of the fundus of the uterus.

Deg. degeneration; degree.

degenerate 1. (de-jen′er-āt) to change from a higher to a lower form. 2. (de-jen′er-it) characterized by degeneration. **3.** a person whose moral or physical state is below the normal.

degeneration (de-jen″er-a′shun) deterioration; change from a higher to a lower form, especially change of tissue to a lower or less functionally active form. **degen′erative**, adj. **Abercrombie's d.**, amyloid d. **adipose d.**, fatty d. **albuminoid d., albuminous d.**, cloudy swelling. **amyloid d.**, that with deposit of lardacein in the tissues; indicates impaired nutritive function, and is seen in wasting diseases. **ascending d.**, wallerian degeneration affecting centripetal nerve fibers and progressing toward the brain or spinal cord. **atheromatous d.**, atheroma. **calcareous d.**, degeneration of tissue with deposit of calcareous material. **caseous d.**, caseation (2). **cellulose d.**, amyloid d. **colloid d.**, assumption by the tissues of a gumlike or gelatinous material. **congenital macular d.**, hereditary macular degeneration, marked by the presence of a cystlike lesion that in the early stages resembles egg yolk. **Crooke's hyaline d.**, degeneration of basophils of the pituitary gland, in which they lose their specific granulations and the cytoplasm becomes progressively hyalinized; a constant finding in Cushing's syndrome, but also occurring in Addison's disease. **cystic d.**, that with formation of cysts. **descending d.**, wallerian degeneration extending peripherally along nerve fibers. **disciform macular d.**, a form of macular degeneration occurring in persons over 40 years of age, in which sclerosis involving the macula and retina is produced by hemorrhages between Bruch's membrane and the pigment epithelium. **fatty d.**, deposit of fat globules in a tissue. **fibrinous d.**, necrosis with deposit of fibrin within the cells of the tissue. **fibroid d.**, degeneration into fibrous tissue. **fibrous d.**, fibrosis. **gray d.**, degeneration of the white substance of the spinal cord, in which it loses myelin and assumes a gray color. **hepatolenticular d.**, a hereditary disorder of copper metabolism, marked by a pigmented ring at the outer margin of the cornea, degenerative changes in the brain, cirrhosis of the liver, splenomegaly, tremor, rigidity, contractures, psychic disturbances, dysphagia, and increasing weakness and emaciation. **hyaline d.**, a regressive change in cells in which the cytoplasm takes on a homogeneous, glassy appearance; also used loosely to describe the histologic appearance of tissues. **hyaloid d.**, amyloid d. **hydropic d.**, a form in which the epithelial cells absorb much water. **lattice d. of retina**, a frequently bilateral, usually benign asymptomatic condition, characterized by patches of fine gray or white lines that intersect at irregular intervals in the peripheral retina, usually associated with numerous, round, punched-out areas of retinal thinning or retinal holes. **lipoidal d.**, a form somewhat resembling fatty degeneration but in which the extraneous material is lipoid. **mucoid d.**, that with deposit of myelin and lecithin in the cells. **mucous d.**, that with accumulation of mucus in epithelial tissues. **myxomatous d.**, that with accumulation of mucus in connective tissues. **parenchymatous d.**, cloudy swelling. **polypoid d.**, development of polypoid growths on a mucous membrane. **secondary d.**, wallerian d. **spongy d. of central nervous system, spongy d. of white matter**, a rare hereditary form of leukodystrophy marked by early onset, widespread demyelination and vacuolation of the cerebral white matter giving rise to a spongy appearance, and by severe mental retardation, megalocephaly, atony of the neck muscles, spasticity of the arms and legs, and blindness; death usually occurs at about 18 months of age. **subacute combined d. of spinal cord**, degeneration of both the posterior and lateral columns of the spinal cord, producing various motor and sensory disturbances; it is due to vitamin B_{12} deficiency and usually associated with pernicious anemia. **vitreous d.**, hyaline d. **wallerian d.**, fatty degeneration of nerve fiber that has been severed from its nutritive source. **waxy d.**, amyloid d. **Zenker's d.**, hyaline degeneration and necrosis of striated muscle.

degloving (de-gluv′ing) intra-oral surgical exposure of the bony mandibular chin; it can be performed in the posterior region if necessary.

deglutition (deg″loo-tish′un) the act of swallowing.

degradation (deg″rah-da′shun) conversion of a chemical compound to one less complex as by splitting off one or more groups of atoms.

degree (de-gre′) **1.** a grade or rank awarded scholars by a college or university. **2.** a unit of measure of temperature. **3.** a unit of measure of arcs and angles, one degree being $\frac{1}{360}$ of a circle.

degustation (de″gus-ta′shun) the act or function of tasting.

dehiscence (de-his′ens) a splitting open. **wound d.**, separation of the layers of a surgical wound.

dehumidifier (de″hu-mid′ĭ-fi″er) an apparatus for reducing the moisture content of the air.

dehydrase (de-hi′drās) a term once applied to both the dehydrogenases and the dehydratases.

dehydratase (de-hi′drah-tās) any lyase (hydro-lyase) that catalyzes the removal of H_2O, leaving double bonds (or adding groups to double bonds).

dehydration (de″hi-dra′shun) **1.** removal of water from a substance. **2.** the condition resulting from excessive loss of body water.

dehydrocholesterol (de-hi″dro-ko-les′ter-ol) a sterol present in skin which, on ultraviolet irradiation, produces vitamin D. **7-d., activated**, cholecalciferol.

11-dehydrocorticosterone (-kor″tĭ-ko′stēr-ōn) a steriod, $C_{21}H_{28}O_4$, from the adrenal cortex and produced synthetically, having a slight effect on protein and carbohydrate metabolism; used like cortisone.

dehydroepiandrosterone (-ep″ĭ-an-dros′ter-ōn) an androgen, $C_{19}H_{28}O_2$, occurring in normal human urine and synthesized from cholesterol; abbreviated DHA.

dehydrogenase (de-hi′dro-jen-ās″) an enzyme that mobilizes the hydrogen of a substrate so that it can pass to a hydrogen acceptor.

dehydrogenate (-jen-āt″) to remove hydrogen from.

dehydroretinal (de-hi″dro-ret′ĭ-nal) the aldehyde of dehydroretinol, derived·from the visual pigment porphyropsin, found in fresh-water fishes and certain vertebrates and amphibians; its metabolic role is analogous to that of rhodopsin in other animals.

dehydroretinol (-ret′ĭ-nol) vitamin A_2; the form, $C_{20}H_{28}O$, of vitamin A found in the retina and liver of fresh-water fishes and certain invertebrates and amphibians; it differs from retinol (vitamin A_1) in having one more conjugated double bond and has approximately one-third the biological activity of retinol.

deionization (de-i″on-i-za′shun) the production of a mineral-free state by the removal of ions.

déjà vu (da′zhah voo′) [Fr.] an illusion that a new situation is a repetition of a previous experience.

dejecta (de-jek′tah) excrement.

dejection (de-jek′shun) 1. a mental state marked by depression and melancholy. 2. discharge of feces; defecation. 3. excrement; feces.

delacrimation (de-lak″rĭ-ma′shun) excessive flow of tears.

delactation (de″lak-ta′shun) 1. weaning. 2. cessation of lactation.

Delalutin (del″ah-lu′tin) trademark for a preparation of hydroxyprogesterone.

delamination (de-lam″ĭ-na′shun) separation into layers, as of the blastoderm.

Delatestryl (del″ah-tes′tril) trademark for a preparation of testosterone.

de-lead (de-led′) to induce the removal of lead from tissues and its excretion in the urine by the administration of chelating agents.

deleterious (del″ĕ-te′re-us) injurious; harmful.

deletion (de-le′shun) in genetics, loss of genetic material from a chromosome.

delinquent (de-lin′kwent) characterized by antisocial, illegal, or criminal conduct; a person exhibiting such conduct, especially a minor (*juvenile d.*).

deliquescence (del″ĭ-kwes′ens) the condition of becoming moist or liquified as a result of absorption on water from the air. **deliques′cent,** adj.

delirium (dĕ-lēr′e-um) a mental disturbance of relatively short duration usually reflecting a toxic state, marked by illusions, hallucinations, delusions, excitement, restlessness, and incoherence. **chronic alcoholic d.,** Korsakoff's psychosis. **d. tre′mens,** an acute mental disturbance marked by delirium with trembling and great excitement, attended by anxiety, mental distress, sweating, gastrointestinal symptoms, and precordial pain; a form of alcoholic psychosis ordinarily seen after withdrawal from heavy alcohol intake.

deliver (de-liv′er) 1. to aid in childbirth. 2. to remove, as a fetus, placenta, or lens of the eye.

delivery (de-liv′er-e) expulsion or extraction of the child and fetal membranes at birth. **abdominal d.,** delivery of an infant through an incision made into the intact uterus through the abdominal wall. **breech d.,** delivery in which the fetal buttocks present first. **forceps d.,** extraction of the child from the maternal passages by application of forceps to the fetal

head; designated *low* or *midforceps delivery* according to the degree of engagement of the fetal head and *high* when engagement has not occurred. **postmortem d.,** delivery of a child after death of the mother. **spontaneous d.,** birth of an infant without any aid from an attendant.

delle (del′eh) the clear area in the center of a stained erythrocyte.

dellen (del′en) saucer-shaped excavations at the periphery of the cornea, usually on the temporal side.

delomorphous (del″o-mor′fus) having definitely formed and well-defined limits, as a cell or tissue.

delta (del′tah) 1. the fourth letter of the Greek alphabet, Δ or δ; used in chemical names to denote the fourth of a series of isomeric compounds or the carbon atom fourth from the carboxyl group, or to denote the fourth of any series. 2. a triangular area.

Delta-Cortef (del′tah kor″tef) trademark for a preparation of prednisolone.

Deltalin (del′tah-lin) trademark for a preparation of synthetic vitamin D_2.

Deltasone (-sōn) trademark for a preparation of prednisone.

deltoid (del′toid) 1. triangular. 2. the deltoid muscle.

Deltra (del′trah) trademark for a preparation of prednisone.

delusion (de-lu′zhun) a false belief inconsistent with an individual's own knowledge and experience. **delu′sional,** adj. **depressive d.,** a delusion of unworthiness or futility. **expansive d.,** abnormal belief in one's own greatness, goodness, or power. **d. of grandeur,** delusional conviction of one's own importance, power, wealth, etc., as in megalomania, dementia paralytica, and paranoid schizophrenia. **d. of negation,** a morbid belief that some part of the body is missing or that the world has ceased to exist. **nihilistic d.,** belief that the self and external reality no longer exist. **d. of persecution,** a morbid belief on the part of a patient that he is being persecuted, slandered, and injured. **systematized d.,** a delusion formulated in a logical manner; a delusion having a logical structure. **unsystematized d.,** a delusion made up of disconnected parts.

Delvinal (del″vĭ-nal) trademark for preparations of vinbarbital.

deme (dēm) a population of very similar organisms interbreeding in nature and occupying a circumscribed area.

demecarium (dem″ĕ-ka′re-um) a cholinesterase inhibitor, $C_{32}H_{52}N_4O_4$, used as the bromide salt in the treatment of glaucoma and esotropia.

demeclocycline (dem″ĕ-klo-si′klēn) a broad-spectrum antibiotic produced by a mutant strain of *Streptomyces aureofaciens*, closely related to the other tetracyclines; the base and the hydrochloride salt are used as antibacterials.

demecycline (-si′klēn) an antibacterial, $C_{21}H_{22}N_2O_8$.

dementia (de-men′she-ah) organic loss of intellectual function. **Binswanger's d.,** dementia due to demyelination of the subcortical white matter of the brain with sclerotic changes in the blood vessels supplying it. **paralytic d., d. paralyt'ica,** a chronic meningoencephalitis marked by degeneration of the cortical neurons, progressive dementia, and generalized paralysis, which, if untreated, is ultimately fatal. **d. prae'cox,** in the U.S., a former name for schizophrenia; commonly used in Europe to denote process schizophrenia. **d. praeseni'lis, presenile d.,** dementia of unknown cause beginning at middle age and marked by cortical atrophy and secondary ventricular dilatation. **secondary d.,** that following and due to another form of psychosis. **senile d.,** see under *psychosis.* **terminal d.,** that occurring as a final result of nervous or mental disease.

Demerol (dem'er-ol) trademark for preparations of meperidine.

demethylchlortetracycline (de-meth''il-klor''-tet-rah-si'klēn) demeclocycline.

demilune (dem'ĭ-lūn) a crescent-shaped structure or cell. **Heidenhain's d's,** crescents of Giannuzzi.

demineralization (de-min''er-al-i-za'shun) excessive elimination of mineral or organic salts from tissues of the body.

demodectic (dem''o-dek'tik) pertaining to or caused by *Demodex.*

Demodex (dem'o-deks) a genus of mites parasitic within the hair follicles of the host, including the species *D. folliculo'rum* in man, and *D. ca'nis* and *D. e'qui,* which cause mange in dogs and horses, respectively.

demogram (de'mo-gram) a graphic representation of the population of a given area according to the time period and the age and sex of the individuals composing it.

demography (de-mog'rah-fe) the statistical science dealing with populations, including matters of health, disease, births, and mortality.

demorphinization (de-mor''fĭ-nĭ-za'shun) gradual withdrawal of morphine from one addicted to its use.

demucosation (de''mu-ko-za'shun) removal of the mucous membrane from a part.

demulcent (de-mul'sent) 1. soothing; bland. 2. a soothing mucilaginous or oily medicine or application.

demyelinate (de-mi'ĕ-lin-āt) to destroy or remove the myelin sheath from a nerve or nerves.

demyelination (-a'shun) destruction or loss of the myelin sheath of a nerve or nerves.

denarcotize (de-nar'ko-tīz) to deprive of narcotics or of narcotic properties.

denaturant (de-na'tūr-ant) a denaturing agent.

denaturation (de-na''chur-a'shun) a change in the usual nature of a substance, as by the addition of methanol or acetone to alcohol to render it unfit for drinking, or the change in molecular structure of proteins due to splitting of hydrogen bonds caused by heat or certain chemicals.

denatured (de-na'churd) changed by denaturation.

dendraxon (den-drak'son) a nerve cell whose axon splits up into terminal filaments immediately after leaving the cell.

dendriform (den'drĭ-form) tree-shaped.

dendrite (den'drīt) one of the threadlike extensions of the cytoplasm of a neuron; dendrites, which typically branch into treelike processes, compose most of the receptive surface of a neuron.

dendritic (den-drit'ik) 1. branched like a tree. 2. pertaining to or possessing dendrites.

dendroid (den'droid) branching like a tree.

dendron (den'dron) dendrite.

dendrophagocytosis (den''dro-fag''o-si-to'sis) the absorption by microglial cells of broken portions of astrocytes.

denervation (de''ner-va'shun) interruption of the nerve connection to an organ or part.

dengue (den'ge) an infectious, eruptive, febrile, viral disease of tropical areas, transmitted by *Aedes* mosquitoes, and marked by severe pains in the head, eyes, muscles, and joints, sore throat, catarrhal symptoms, and sometimes a skin eruption and painful swellings of parts.

denial (dě-ni'al) a defense mechanism in which the existence of intolerable actions, ideas, etc., are unconsciously denied.

denidation (de''ni-da'shun) degeneration and expulsion of the endometrium during the menstrual cycle.

dens (dens), pl. *den'tes* [L.] a tooth or toothlike structure. **d. in den'te,** a malformed tooth caused by invagination of the crown before it is calcified, giving the appearance of a "tooth within a tooth."

densimeter (den-sim'ĕ-ter) densitometer.

densitometer (den''sĭ-tom'ĕ-ter) an instrument for determining the density of a liquid.

densitometry (-tom'ĕ-tre) determination of variations in density by comparison with that of another material or with a certain standard.

density (den'sĭ-te) 1. the ratio of the mass of a substance to its volume. 2. the quality of being compact or dense. 3. the quantity of matter in a given space. 4. the quantity of electricity in a given area, volume, or time.

densography (den-sog'rah-fe) the exact determination of the contrast densities in a roentgenogram by a photoelectric cell.

dent(o)- word element [L.], *tooth; toothlike.*

dental (den'tal) pertaining to the teeth.

dentalgia (den-tal'je-ah) toothache.

dentate (den'tāt) notched; tooth-shaped.

dentes (den'tēz) [L.] plural of *dens.*

dentia (den'she-ah) a condition relating to development or eruption of the teeth. **d. prae'cox,** premature eruption of the teeth; presence of teeth in the mouth at birth. **d. tar'da,** delayed eruption of the teeth, beyond the usual time for their appearance.

dentibuccal (den''tĭ-buk'al) pertaining to the cheek and teeth.

denticle (den'tĭ-k'l) 1. a small toothlike process. 2. a distinct calcified mass within the pulp chamber of a tooth.

dentification (den''tĭ-fi-ka'shun) formation of tooth substance.

dentifrice (den'tĭ-fris) a preparation for cleansing and polishing the teeth.

dentigerous (den-tij′er-us) bearing teeth.

dentilabial (den″tĭ-la′be-al) pertaining to the teeth and lips.

dentilingual (-ling′gwal) pertaining to the teeth and tongue.

dentin (den′tin) the chief substance of the teeth, surrounding the tooth pulp and covered by enamel on the crown and by cementum on the roots. **den′tinal**, adj. **adventitious d.**, secondary d. **circumpulpar d.**, the inner portion of dentin, adjacent to the pulp, consisting of thinner fibrils. **cover d.**, the peripheral portion of dentin, adjacent to the enamel or cementum, consisting of coarser fibers than the circumpulpar dentin. **interglobular d.**, imperfectly calcified dentinal matrix situated between calcified globules. **intermediate d.**, the soft matrix of the predentin. **irregular d.**, secondary d. **mantle d.**, cover d. **opalescent d.**, dentin giving an unusual translucent or opalescent appearance to the teeth, as occurs in dentinogenesis imperfecta. **primary d.**, dentin formed before the eruption of a tooth. **sclerotic d.**, transparent d. **secondary d.**, new dentin formed in response to stimuli associated with the normal aging process or with pathological conditions, such as caries or injury, or cavity preparation; it is highly irregular in nature. **transparent d.**, dentin in which some dentinal tubules have become sclerotic or calcified, producing the appearance of translucency.

dentinoblastoma (den″tĭ-no-blas-to′mah) dentinoma.

dentinogenesis (-jen′ĕ-sis) the formation of dentin. **d. imperfec′ta**, a hereditary condition marked by imperfect formation and calcification of dentin, giving the teeth a brown or blue opalescent appearance.

dentinogenic (-jen′ik) forming or producing dentin.

dentinoid (den′tĭ-noid) 1. resembling dentin. 2. predentin.

dentinoma (den″tĭ-no′mah) a tumor of odontogenic origin, consisting mainly of dentin.

dentinosteoid (den″tin-os′te-oid) a tumor composed of or containing dentin and bone.

dentinum (den-ti′num) dentin.

dentist (den′tist) a person who has received a degree in dentistry and is authorized to practice dentistry.

dentistry (den′tis-tre) 1. that branch of the healing arts concerned with the teeth, oral cavity, and associated structures, including prevention, diagnosis, and treatment of disease and restoration of defective or missing tissue. 2. the work done by dentists, e.g., the creation of restorations, crowns and bridges, and surgical procedures performed in and about the oral cavity. 3. the practice of the dental profession collectively. **cosmetic d., esthetic d.**, dentistry concerned with the repair and restoration of carious, broken, or defective teeth in such manner as to improve on their original appearance. **geriatric d.**, gerodontics. **operative d.**, dentistry concerned with restoration of parts of the teeth that are defective as a result of disease, trauma, or abnormal development to a state of normal function, health, and esthetics. **pediatric d.**, pedodontics. **preventive d.**, dentistry concerned with maintenance of a normal masticating mechanism by fortifying the structures of the oral cavity against damage and disease. **prosthetic d.**, prosthodontics.

dentition (den-tish′un) the teeth in the dental arch; ordinarily used to designate the natural teeth in position in their alveoli. **deciduous d.**, the teeth that erupt first and are later replaced by the permanent dentition. **delayed d.**, retarded d. **mixed d.**, the complement of teeth in the jaws after eruption of some of the permanent teeth, but before all the deciduous teeth are shed. **permanent d.**, the teeth that erupt and take their places after the deciduous teeth are lost. **precocious d.**, abnormally accelerated appearance of the deciduous or permanent teeth. **predeciduous d.**, cornified epithelial structures found in the mouth before eruption of the true deciduous teeth. **primary d.**, deciduous d. **retarded d.**, abnormally delayed appearance of the deciduous or permanent teeth. **secondary d.**, permanent d. **transitional d.**, mixed d.

dentoalveolar (den″to-al-ve′o-ler) pertaining to a tooth and its alveolus.

dentoalveolitis (-al″ve-o-li′tis) peridontal disease.

dentofacial (-fa′shal) of or pertaining to the teeth and alveolar process and the face.

dentotropic (-trop′ik) turning toward or having an affinity for tissues composing the teeth.

dentulous (den′tu-lus) having natural teeth.

denture (den′chur) a complement of teeth, either natural or artificial; ordinarily used to designate an artificial replacement for the natural teeth and adjacent tissues. **clasp d.**, a removable partial denture retained and stabilized by means of clasps. **complete d.**, an appliance replacing all the teeth of one jaw, as well as associated structures of the jaw. **full d.**, complete d. **immediate d.**, one inserted immediately after extraction of the teeth. **implant d.**, one constructed with a metal substructure embedded within the underlying soft structures of the jaws. **interim d.**, a denture to be used for a short interval of time for reasons of esthetics, mastication, occlusal support, convenience, or to condition the patient to the acceptance of an artificial substitute for missing natural teeth until more definite prosthetic dental treatment can be provided. **partial d.**, a removable (*removable partial d.*) or permanently attached (*fixed partial d.*) appliance replacing one or more missing teeth in one jaw and receiving support and retention from underlying tissues and some or all of the remaining teeth. **permanent d.**, a denture inserted after oral tissues have healed and the condition of the alveolar ridges has become fairly stabilized. **provisional d.**, an interim denture used for the purpose of conditioning the patient to the acceptance of an artificial substitute for missing natural teeth. **temporary d.**, interim d. **transitional d.**, a partial denture which is to serve as a temporary prosthesis and to which teeth will be added as more teeth are lost and which will be replaced after postextraction tissue changes have occurred. **trial d.,** one made for verification of its esthetic qualities, the making of records, or other procedures before the final denture is completed.

denucleated (de-nu′kle-āt″ed) deprived of the nucleus.

denudation (de″nu-da′shun) the stripping or laying bare of any part.

deodorant (de-o′dor-ant) an agent that masks offensive odors.

deodorize (-īz) to neutralize or absorb odor.

deodorizer (-īz″er) a deodorizing agent.

deorsumduction (de-or″sum-duk′shun) deorsumversion.

deorsumvergence (-ver′jens) deorsumversion.

deorsumversion (-ver′zhun) the turning downward of a part, especially of the eyes.

deossification (de-os″ĭ-fĭ-ka′shun) loss or removal of the mineral elements of bone.

deoxidation (de-ok″sĭ-da′shun) the removal of oxygen from a chemical compound.

deoxy- chemical prefix designating a compound containing one less oxygen atom than the reference substance; see also words beginning *desoxy-*.

deoxycorticosterone (de - ok″sĭ - kor″tĭ - ko - stēr′ōn) desoxycorticosterone.

deoxygenation (-jĕ-na′shun) the act of depriving of oxygen.

deoxyribonuclease (-ri″bo-nu′kle-ās) an enzyme that catalyzes the hydrolysis (depolymerization) of deoxyribonucleic acid (DNA).

deoxyribonucleoprotein (-nu′kle-o-pro″te-in) a nucleoprotein in which the sugar is D-2-deoxyribose.

deoxyribonucleoside (-nu′kle-o-sīd) a nucleoside having a purine or pyrimidine base bonded to deoxyribose.

deoxyribonucleotide (-nu′kle-o-tīd) a nucleotide having a purine or pyrimidine base bonded to deoxyribose, which in turn is bonded to a phosphate group.

deoxyribose (-ri′bōs) an aldopentose, $CH_2 \cdot OH \cdot \cdot (CHOH)_2 \cdot CH_2 \cdot CHO$, found in deoxyribonucleic acids, deoxyribonucleotides, and deoxyribonucleosides.

dependence (de-pend′ens) the psychophysical state of a drug user in which the usual or increasing doses of the drug are required to prevent the onset of withdrawal symptoms.

depersonalization (de-per″sun-al-i-za′shun) feelings of unreality or strangeness concerning either the environment or the self or both.

dephosphorylation (de-fos″for-ĭ-la′shun) removal of the trivalent PO_3 group from organic molecules.

depilate (dep′ĭ-lāt) to remove hair.

depilation (dep″ĭ-la′shun) removal of hair.

depilatory (dĕ-pil′ah-tor″e) 1. having the power to remove hair. 2. an agent for removing or destroying hair.

depolarization (de-po″lar-i-za′shun) the process or act of neutralizing polarity.

depolymerization (de-pol″ĭ-mer-i-za′shun) the conversion of a compound into one of smaller

molecular weight and different physical properties without changing the percentage relations of the elements composing it.

depolymerize (de-pol′ĭ-mĕ-rīz″) to cause to undergo depolymerization.

deposit (de-poz′it) 1. sediment or dregs. 2. extraneous inorganic matter collected in the tissues or in an organ of the body.

depot (de′po, dep′o) a body area in which a substance, e.g., a drug, can be accumulated, deposited, or stored and from which it can be distributed. **fat d.,** a site in the body in which large quantities of fat are stored, as in adipose tissue.

Depo-Testosterone (de″po-tes-tos′ter-ōn) trademark for a sustained-action preparation of testosterone.

depressant (de-pres′ant) diminishing any functional activity; an agent that so acts. **cardiac d.,** an agent that depresses the rate or force of contraction of the heart.

depressed (de-prest′) carried below the normal level; associated with depression.

depression (de-presh′un) 1. a hollow or depressed area; downward or inward displacement. 2. a lowering or decrease of functional activity. 3. in psychiatry, a morbid sadness, dejection, or melancholy. **agitated d.,** psychotic depression accompanied by continuous restlessness. **anaclitic d.,** impairment of an infant's physical, social, and intellectual development which sometimes follows a sudden separation from the mothering person. **congenital chondrosternal d.,** congenital deformity with a deep, funnel-shaped depression in the anterior chest wall. **involutional d.,** see under *melancholia*. **pacchionian d's,** small pits on the internal cranium on either side of the groove for the superior sagittal sinus, occupied by the arachnoid granulations. **reactive d.,** depression due to some external situation, and relieved when that situation is removed. **situational d.,** reactive d.

depressomotor (de-pres″o-mo′tor) 1. retarding or abating motor activity. 2. an agent that so acts.

depressor (de-pres′or) anything that depresses, as a muscle, agent, or instrument, or an afferent nerve whose stimulation causes a fall in blood pressure.

depth (depth) distance measured perpendicularly downward from a surface. **focal d.,** the measure of the power of a lens to yield clear images of objects at different distances.

deradelphus (der″ah-del′fus) a twin monster fused at or near the navel, and having one head.

derangement (de-rānj′ment) 1. mental disorder. 2. disarrangement of a part or organ.

dereism (de′re-izm) mental activity in which fantasy runs unhampered by logic and experience. **dereis′tic,** adj.

derencephalus (der″en-sef′ah-lus) a monster with a rudimentary skull and bifid cervical vertebrae, the brain resting in the bifurcation.

derepression (de″re-presh′un) 1. elevation of the level of an enzyme above the normal, either by lowering of the corepressor concentration or by a mutation that decreases the formation of aporepressor or the response to the complete repressor. 2. the inhibition of the repressor substance produced by the regulator genes with the result that the operator gene is free to initiate the process of polypeptide formation.

derivative (de-riv′ah-tiv) a chemical substance derived from another substance either directly or by modification or partial substitution.

derma (der′mah) corium.

dermabrasion (der″mah-bra′shun) planing of the skin done by mechanical means, e.g., sandpaper, wire brushes, etc.; see *planing.*

Dermacentor (-sen′tor) a genus of ticks that are important transmitters of disease. **D. albipic′tus,** a species found in Canada and northern and western United States, parasitic on cattle, horses, moose, and elk. **D. anderso′ni,** a species parasitic on various wild mammals, responsible for transmitting Rocky Mountain spotted fever, Colorado tick fever, and tularemia to man and for causing tick paralysis. **D. varia′bilis,** the chief vector of Rocky Mountain spotted fever in the central and eastern United States, the dog being the principal host of the adults, but also parasitic on cattle, horses, rabbits, and man. **D. venus′tus,** *D. andersoni.*

dermal (der′mal) pertaining to the true skin.

Dermanyssus (der″mah-nis′us) a genus of mites, including *D. galli′nae,* the bird mite, poultry (chicken or fowl) mite, or chicken louse, which sometimes infests man.

dermato(o)- word element [Gr.], *skin.*

dermatic (der-mat′ik) dermal.

dermatitis (der″mah-ti′tis), pl. *dermatit′ides.* Inflammation of the skin. **actinic d., d. actin′ica,** that due to exposure to actinic radiation, such as that from the sun, ultraviolet waves, or x- or gamma radiation. **d. artefac′ta,** a skin condition marked by lesions that are self-inflicted by the patient, whether by chemical or physical means. **atopic d.,** a chronic pruritic eruption of unknown etiology; allergic, hereditary, and psychogenic factors appear to be involved. **berlock d.,** dermatitis, typically of the neck, face, and breast, with drop-shaped or guadrilateral patches or streaks, induced by sequential exposure to perfume or other toilet articles and then to sunlight. **contact d.,** 1. acute dermatitis due to contact with a substance to which the person is allergic or sensitive; when severe, called *d. veneata.* 2. primary-irritant (nonallergic) d. **d. dysmenorrhe′ica,** a rosacea-like eruption on the cheeks of women, recurring during or just before painful menstrual periods. **exfoliative d.,** virtually universal erythema, desquamation, scaling, and itching of the skin, and loss of hair. **d. exfoliati′va neonato′rum,** exfoliative dermatitis supervening in bullous impetigo of the newborn. **d. gestatio′nis,** herpes gestationis. **d. herpetifor′mis,** dermatitis occurring in successive crops of grouped erythematous papular, vesicular, eczematous, or bullous lesions, accompanied by burning and itching. **d. hypostat′ica,** stasis d. **industrial d.,** contact dermatitis, usually of the allergic type, caused by material used in the patient's occupation. **infectious eczematoid d.,** a pustular eczematoid eruption frequently following or oc-

curring coincidentally with some pyogenic process. **meadow d., meadow-grass d.,** phototoxic dermatitis marked by an eruption of vesicles and bullae arranged in streaks and bizarre configurations, caused by exposure to sunlight after contact with meadow grass, usually *Agrimonia eupatoria.* **d. medicamento′sa,** drug eruption. **d. papilla′ris capillit′ii,** folliculitis keloidalis. **d. pediculoi′des ventrico′sus,** grain itch. **photocontact d.,** allergic contact dermatitis caused by the action of sunlight on skin sensitized by contact with a substance capable of causing this reaction, such as a halogenated salicylanilide, sandalwood oil, or hexachlorophene. **phototoxic d.,** erythema followed by hyperpigmentation of sun-exposed areas of the skin, resulting from sequential exposure to agents containing photosensitizing substances, such as coal tar and certain perfumes, drugs, or plants containing psoralens, and then to sunlight. **primary-irritant d.,** dermatitis induced by a substance acting as an irritant rather than as a sensitizer or allergen. **radiation d.,** radiodermatitis. **rat-mite d.,** inflammation of the skin due to a bite of the rat-mite, *Ornithonyssus bacoti.* **d. re′pens,** acrodermatitis continua. **roentgen-ray d.,** radiodermatitis. **schistosome d.,** swimmer's itch. **seborrheic d., d. seborrhe′ica,** a chronic, usually pruritic, dermatitis with erythema, dry, moist, or greasy scaling, and yellow crusted patches on various areas, especially the scalp, with exfoliation of an excessive amount of dry scales (dandruff). **stasis d.,** an eczematous eruption of the lower legs, usually due to impeded circulation, with edema, pigmentation, and often chronic ulceration. **uncinarial d.,** ground itch. **d. venena′ta,** see *contact d.* (1). **x-ray d.,** radiodermatitis.

dermatoautoplasty (der″mah-to-aw′to-plas″te) autotransplantation of skin.

Dermatobia (der″mah-to′be-ah) a genus of botflies, including *D. hominis,* whose larvae are parasitic in the skin of man, mammals, and birds.

dermatocele (der′mah-to-sēl″) cutis laxa.

dermatofibroma (der″mah-to-fi-bro′mah) a fibrous tumor-like nodule of the dermis.

dermatofibrosarcoma (-fi″bro-sar-ko′mah) a fibrosarcoma of the skin.

dermatogen (der-mat′o-jen) a skin antigen that may be associated with any skin disorder.

dermatoglyphics (der″mah-to-glif′iks) the study of the patterns of ridges of the skin of the fingers, palms, toes, and soles; of interest in anthropology and law enforcement as a means of establishing identity and in medicine, both clinically and as a genetic indicator, particularly of chromosomal abnormalities.

dermatographia (-graf′e-ah) urticaria due to physical allergy in which a pale, raised welt or wheal with a red flare on each side is elicited by stroking or scratching the skin with a dull instrument.

dermatographism (der″mah-tog′rah-fizm) dermographia.

dermatoheteroplasty (der″mah-to-het′er-o-plas″te) the grafting of skin derived from an individual of another species.

dermatologic, dermatological (-loj′ik; -loj′ĭ-kal) pertaining to dermatology; of or affecting the skin.

dermatologist (der″mah-tol′o-jist) a physician who specializes in dermatology.

dermatology (-tol′o-je) the medical specialty concerned with the diagnosis and treatment of skin diseases.

dermatolysis (-tol′ĭ-sis) cutis laxa.

dermatome (der′mah-tōm) 1. an instrument for cutting thin skin slices for grafting. 2. the area of skin supplied with afferent nerve fibers by a single posterior spinal root. 3. the lateral part of an embryonic somite.

dermatomegaly (der″mah-to-meg′ah-le) cutis laxa.

dermatomere (der′mah-to-mēr″) any segment or metamere of the embryonic integument.

dermatomycosis (der″mah-to-mi-ko′sis) a superficial fungal infection of the skin or its appendages.

dermatomyoma (-mi-o′mah) a dermal leiomyoma.

dermatomyositis (-mi″o-si′tis) a collagen disease marked by nonsuppurative inflammation of the skin, subcutaneous tissue, and muscles, with necrosis of muscle fibers.

dermatopathic (-path′ik) pertaining or attributable to disease of the skin, as dermatopathic lymphadenopathy.

dermatopathology (-pah-thol′o-je) pathology concerned with lesions of the skin.

dermatopathy (der″mah-top′ah-the) dermopathy.

dermatophilosis (der′mah-to-fi-lo′sis) an actinomyotic disease caused by *Dermatophilus congolensis,* affecting cattle, sheep, horses, goats, deer, and sometimes man. In man, it is marked by nonpainful pustules on the hands and arms; the lesions break down and form shallow red ulcers which regress spontaneously, leaving some scarring. In sheep, it is marked by exudative red scaling lesions that form pyramidal masses.

Dermatophilus (der″mah-tof′ĭ-lus) 1. *Tunga.* 2. a genus of pathogenic actinomycetes. **D. con-golen′sis,** the etiologic agent of dermatophilosis. **D. pen′etrans,** *Tunga penetrans* (chigoe).

dermatophyte (der′mah-to-fīt″) a fungus parasitic upon the skin, including *Microsporum, Epidermophyton,* and *Trichophyton.*

dermatophytid (der″mah-tof′ĭ-tid) a secondary skin eruption which is an expression of hypersensitivity to a dermatophyte, especially *Epidermophyton,* infection, occurring on an area remote from the site of infection.

dermatophytosis (der″mah-to-fi-to′sis) a fungous infection of the skin; often used to refer to tinea pedis (athlete's foot).

dermatoplasty (der′mah-to-plas″te) a plastic operation on the skin; operative replacement of destroyed or lost skin. **dermatoplas′tic,** adj.

dermatopolyneuritis (der″mah-to-pol″ĭ-nu-ri′tis) acrodynia.

dermatosclerosis (-skle-ro′sis) scleroderma.

dermatosis (der″mah-to′sis) any skin disease, especially one not characterized by inflammation. **Bowen's precancerous d.,** Bowen's disease. **chick nutritional d.,** a disease of chicks marked by eruptions on head and feet, due to lack of pantothenic acid. **industrial d.,** see under *dermatitis.* **d. papulo′sa ni′gra,** a form of seborrheic keratosis seen chiefly in Negroes, with multiple miliary pigmented papules usually on the cheek bones, but sometimes occurring more widely on the face and neck. **precancerous d.,** any skin condition in which the lesions—warts, moles, or other excrescences—are likely to undergo malignant degeneration. **progressive pigmentary d.,** a slowly progressive purpuric and pigmentary disease of the skin affecting chiefly the shins, ankles, and dorsum of the feet. **Schamberg's d.,** progressive pigmentary d. **stasis d.,** a chronic, usually eczematous dermatitis, almost always of the anteromesial aspect of the lower leg, and often complicated by ulceration; probably due to deficient venous return. **subcorneal pustular d.,** a bullous dermatosis resembling dermatitis herpetiformis, with single and grouped vesicles and pustules beneath the horny layer of the skin.

dermatosome (der′mah-to-sōm″) a thickening on each spindle fiber in the equatorial region in mitosis.

dermatotherapy (der″mah-to-ther′ah-pe) treatment of skin diseases.

dermatotropic (-trop′ik) having a specific affinity for the skin.

dermatozoon (-zo′on) any animal parasite on the skin; an ectoparasite.

dermis (der′mis) the true skin, or corium. **der′-mal, der′mic,** adj.

dermoblast (der′mo-blast) that part of the mesoblast, developing into the true skin.

dermographia (der″mo-graf′e-ah) dermatographia.

dermographism (der-mog′rah-fizm) dermatographia.

dermoid (der′moid) 1. skinlike. 2. dermoid cyst.

dermoidectomy (der″moi-dek′to-me) excision of a dermoid cyst.

dermomycosis (der″mo-mi-ko′sis) dermatophytosis.

dermomyotome (-mi′o-tōm) all but the sclerotome of a mesodermal somite; the primordium of skeletal muscle and, perhaps, of corium.

dermopathy (der-mop′ah-the) any skin disorder. **diabetic d.,** any of several cutaneous manifestations of diabetes.

dermophyte (der′mo-fīt) dermatophyte.

dermoplasty (-plas″te) dermatoplasty.

dermoskeleton (der″mo-skel′ĕ-ton) exoskeleton.

dermosynovitis (-sin″o-vi′tis) inflammation of skin overlying an inflamed bursa or tendon sheath.

dermotropic (-trop′ik) dermatotropic.

dermovascular (-vas′ku-ler) pertaining to the blood vessels of the skin.

derodidymus (der″o-did′ĭ-mus) dicephalus.

Deronil (der′o-nil) trademark for a preparation of dexamethasone.

descemetitis (des″ĕ-mĕ-ti′tis) inflammation of Descemet's membrane.

descemetocele (des″ĕ-met′o-sēl) hernia of Descemet's membrane.

descensus (de-sen′sus), pl. *descen′sus* [L.] downward displacement or prolapse. **d. tes′tis,** normal migration of the testis from its fetal position in the abdominal cavity to its location within the scrotum, usually during the last three months of gestation. **d. u′teri,** prolapse of the uterus.

desensitization (de-sen″sĭ-tĭ-za′shun) 1. the reduction or abolition of sensitivity to a particular antigen; also, the condition of having undergone desensitization. 2. in psychiatry, the removal of a mental complex.

desensitize (de-sen′sĭ-tīz) 1. to deprive of sensation. 2. to subject to desensitization.

deserpidine (de-ser′pĭ-dēn) an antihypertensive and tranquilizer, $C_{32}H_{38}N_2O$, isolated from *Rauwolfia.*

desexualize (de-seks′u-al-īz) to deprive of sexual characters; to castrate.

desiccant (des′ĭ-kant) 1. promoting dryness. 2. an agent that promotes dryness.

desiccate (des′ĭ-kāt) to render thoroughly dry.

desiccation (des″ĭ-ka′shun) the act of drying.

desiccative (des′ĭ-ka″tiv) causing to dry up.

desipramine (des-ip′rah-mēn) an antidepressant, $C_{18}H_{22}N_2$, used as the hydrochloride salt.

deslanoside (des-lan′o-sīd) a cardiotonic glycoside, $C_{47}H_{74}O_{19}$, obtained from lanatoside C; used where digitalis is recommended.

desm(o)- word element [Gr.], *ligament.*

desmitis (des-mi′tis) inflammation of a ligament.

desmocranium (des″mo-kra′ne-um) the mass of mesoderm at the cranial end of the notochord in the early embryo, forming the earliest stage of the skull.

desmocyte (des′mo-sīt) fibroblast.

desmogenous (des-moj′ĕ-nus) of ligamentous origin.

desmography (des-mog′rah-fe) a description of ligaments.

desmoid (des′moid) 1. fibrous or fibroid. 2. a lesion produced by progressive fibroblastic proliferation in striated muscle and sometimes in periosteum.

desmolase (des′mo-lās) any enzyme that catalyzes the addition or removal of some chemical group to or from a substrate without hydrolysis.

desmology (des-mol′o-je) science of ligaments.

desmoma (des-mo′mah) desmoid tumor.

desmopathy (des-mop′ah-the) any disease of the ligaments.

desmoplasia (des″mo-pla′ze-ah) the formation and development of fibrous tissue. **desmoplas′tic,** adj.

desmosome (des′mo-sōm) a small thickening at the middle of an intercellular bridge, which is the site of attachment of adjoining cells.

desmosterol (des-mos′ter-ol) the immediate precursor in the biosynthesis of cholesterol.

desmotomy (des-mot′o-me) incision or division of a ligament.

desoxy- for words beginning thus, see also those beginning *deoxy-.*

desoxycorticosterone (des-ok″sĭ-kor″tĭ-ko-stēr′ōn) a mineralocorticoid precursor of corticosterone concerned in water and electrolyte metabolism, but having no effect on carbohydrate metabolism; used in the form of the acetate and pivalate esters in adrenal insufficiency.

Desoxyn (des-ok′sin) trademark for a preparation of methamphetamine.

desoxyribonuclease (des-ok″sĭ-ri″bo-nu′kle-ās) deoxyribonuclease.

desoxyribose (-ri′bōs) deoxyribose.

desquamation (des″kwah-ma′shun) the shedding of epithelial elements, chiefly of the skin, in scales or sheets. **desquam′ative,** adj.

dest. [L.] *destilla′ta* (distilled).

desulfhydrase (de″sulf-hi′drās) an enzyme that removes hydrogen sulfide from a compound.

desulfurase (de-sul′fu-rās) desulfhydrase.

DET diethyltryptamine.

detachment (de-tach′ment) the condition of being separated or disconnected. **d. of retina, retinal d.,** separation of the inner layers of the retina from the pigment epithelium.

detector (de-tek′tor) an instrument or apparatus for revealing the presence of something. **lie d.,** polygraph.

detergent (de-ter′jent) 1. purifying, cleansing. 2. an agent that purifies or cleanses.

determinant (de-ter′mĭ-nant) a factor that establishes the nature of an entity or event. **antigenic d.,** the structural component of an antigen molecule responsible for its specific interaction with antibody molecules elicited by the same or related antigen.

determination (de-ter″mĭ-na′shun) the establishment of the exact nature of an entity or event. **sex d.,** the process by which the sex of an organism is fixed; associated, in man, with the presence or absence of the Y chromosome. **embryonic d.,** the loss of pluripotentiality in any embryonic part and its start on the way to an unalterable fate.

determinism (de-ter′mĭ-nizm) the theory that all phenomena are the result of antecedent conditions and that nothing occurs by chance.

detoxicate (de-tok′sĭ-kāt) detoxify.

detoxication (de-tok″sĭ-ka′shun) detoxification.

detoxification (-fĭ-ka′shun) 1. reduction of the toxic properties of a substance. 2. treatment designed to assist in recovery from the toxic effects of a drug. **metabolic d.,** reduction of the toxic properties of a substance by chemical changes induced in the body, producing a compound which is less poisonous or more readily eliminated.

detoxify (de-tok′sĭ-fi) to subject to detoxification.

detrition (de-trish′un) the wearing away, as of teeth, by friction.

detritus (de-tri′tus) particulate matter produced by or remaining after the wearing away or disintegration of a substance or tissue.

detruncation (de″trung-ka′shun) decollation; decapitation, especially of a fetus.

detrusor (de-tru′sor) a general term for a body part, e.g., a muscle, that pushes down.

detumescence (de″tu-mes′ens) the subsidence of congestion and swelling.

deutan (du′tan) a person exhibiting deuteranomalopia or deuteranopia.

deuteranomalopia (du″ter-ah-nom″ah-lo′pe-ah) a variant of normal color vision with imperfect perception of the green hues.

deuteranomalopsia (-lop′se-ah) deuteranomalopia.

deuteranomaly (du″ter-ah-nom′ah-le) deuteranomalopia. **deuteranom′alous**, adj.

deuteranope (du′ter-ah-nōp″) a person exhibiting deuteranopia.

deuteranopia, deuteranopsia (du″ter-ah-no′-pe-ah; -ah-nop′se-ah) defective color vision, with confusion of greens and reds, and retention of the sensory mechanism for two hues only—blue and yellow. **deuteranop′ic**, adj.

deuterate (du′ter-āt) to treat (combine) with deuterium (^{2}H).

deuterium (du-te′re-um) see *hydrogen*. **d. oxide,** heavy water.

deuterohemophilia (du″ter-o-he″mo-fil′e-ah) a group of hemorrhagic disorders resembling classical hemophilia, due to coagulation factor deficiencies or to the action of certain anticoagulants.

deuteron (du′ter-on) the nucleus of deuterium atoms; deuterons are used as bombing particles for nuclear disintegration.

deuteropathy (du″ter-op′ah-the) a disease that is secondary to another disease.

deutoplasm (du′to-plazm) the inactive materials in protoplasm, especially reserve foodstuffs, as yolk.

devascularization (de-vas″ku-ler-ĭ-za′shun) interruption of circulation of blood to a part due to obstruction or destruction of blood vessels supplying it.

Devegan (dev′e-gan) trademark for a preparation of acetarsone.

development (de-vel′up-ment) the process of growth and differentiation. **developmen′tal**, adj. **mosaic d.,** embryonic development in a fixed, unalterable way, local regions being independent portions of a mosaic whole. **psychosexual d.,** development of the psychological aspect of sexuality from birth to maturity. **regulative d.,** embryonic development in which the determination of various organs and parts is gradually attained through the action of inductors.

deviant (de′ve-ant) 1. varying from a determinable standard. 2. a person with characteristics varying from what is considered standard or normal. **color d.,** a person whose color perception varies from the norm. **sex d.,** a person whose sexual behavior varies from that normally considered biologically or socially accepted.

deviation (de″ve-a′shun) variation from the regular standard or course. In ophthalmology, a tendency for the visual axes of the eyes to fall out of alignment due to muscular imbalance. **conjugate d.,** deflection of the eyes in the same direction at the same time. **minimum d.,** the smallest deviation of a ray that a given prism can produce. **standard d.,** the measure of variability of any frequency curve.

device (de-vīs′) something contrived for a specific purpose. **contraceptive d.,** one used to prevent conception, as a diaphragm or condom to prevent entrance of spermatozoa into the uterine cervix, or one inserted into the uterus (*intrauterine d.*) to prevent implantation of a fertilized ovum. **intrauterine d. (IUD),** a plastic or metallic device inserted in the uterus to prevent implantation of the fertilized ovum; available in various shapes, including loops, coils, bows, rings, shields, springs, M's, and T's.

deviometer (de″ve-om′ĕ-ter) an instrument for measuring the deviation in strabismus.

devitalization (de-vi″tal-i-za′shun) deprivation of vitality or life, as of a tissue.

devitalize (de-vi′tal-īz) to deprive of life or vitality.

devitalized (-īzed) devoid of vitality or life.

devolution (dev″o-lu′shun) the reverse of evolution; catabolic change.

dexamethasone (dek″sah-meth′ah-sōn) an anti-inflammatory adrenocortical steriod, $C_{22}H_{29}FO_5$.

dexbrompheniramine (deks″brōm-fen-ir′ah-mēn) the dextrorotatory isomer of brompheniramine, $C_{18}H_{19}BrN_2$, used as an antihistaminic in the form of the maleate salt.

dexchlorpheniramine (-klōr-fen-ir′ah-mēn) the dextrorotatory isomer of chlorpheniramine, $C_{18}H_{19}ClN_2$, used as an antihistaminic in the form of the maleate salt.

Dexedrine (dek′sĕ-drēn) trademark for preparations of dextroamphetamine.

Dexoval (dek′so-val) trademark for a preparation of methamphetamine.

Dexon (dek′son) trademark for a synthetic suture material, polyglycolic acid, a polymer that is completely absorbable and nonirritating.

dexter (dek′ster) [L.] right; on the right side.

dextr(o)- word element [L.], *right*.

dextrad (dek′strad) to or toward the right side.

dextral (dek′stral) pertaining to the right side.

dextrality (dek-stral′ĭ-te) the preferential use of the right member of the major paired organs of the body.

dextran (dek′stran) a water-soluble polysaccharide of glucose (dextrose) produced by the action of *Leuconostoc mesenteroides* on sucrose; used as a plasma volume extender.

dextraural (dek-straw′ral) hearing better with the right ear.

dextriferron (deks″tri-fer′on) a complex of ferric hydroxide and partially hydrolyzed dextrin used in the treatment of iron-deficiency anemia.

dextrin (dek′strin) a carbohydrate formed during the hydrolysis of starch to sugar.

dextrin-1,6-glucosidase (deks″trin-glu-ko′sĭ-dās) dextrin 6-glucanohydrolase: an enzyme that catalyzes the hydrolysis of α-1-6-glucan links in dextrins containing short 1,6-linked side chains.

dextrinosis (dek″strĭ-no′sis) accumulation in the tissues of an abnormal polysaccharide. **limit d.,** Forbes' disease.

dextrinuria (dek″strin-u′re-ah) presence of dextrin in the urine.

dextroamphetamine (dek″stro-am-fet′ah-mēn) the dextrorotatory isomer of amphetamine, having substantially more central nervous system stimulating effect than the levorotatory (levamfetamine) or racemic forms of amphetamine; abuse of this drug may lead to dependence.

dextrocardia (-kar′de-ah) location of the heart in the right side of the thorax, the apex pointing to the right. **mirror-image d.,** location of the heart in the right side of the chest, the atria being transposed and the right ventricle lying anteriorly and left of the left ventricle.

dextroclination (-klĭ-na′shun) rotation of the upper poles of the vertical meridians of the eyes to the right.

dextrocularity (dek″strok-u-lar′ĭ-te) having greater visual power in the right eye, therefore using it more than the left.

dextroduction (dek″stro-duk′shun) movement of an eye to the right.

dextrogastria (-gas′tre-ah) displacement of the stomach to the right.

dextrogram (dek′stro-gram) an electrocardiographic tracing showing right axis deviation, indicative of right ventricular hypertrophy.

dextrogyration (dek″stro-ji-ra′shun) rotation to the right.

dextromanual (-man′u-al) right-handed.

dextromethorphan (-meth′or-fan) a synthetic morphine derivative, $C_{18}H_{25}NO$, used as an antitussive in the form of the hydrobromide salt.

dextropedal (dek-strop′ĕ-dal) right-footed.

dextroposition (dek″stro-po-zish′un) displacement to the right.

dextropropoxyphene (-pro-pok′sĭ-fēn) propoxyphene.

dextrorotatory (-ro′tah-tor″e) turning the plane of polarization to the right.

dextrose (dek′strōs) a monosaccharide, $C_6H_{12}O_6 \cdot H_2O$, usually obtained by hydrolysis of starch; used intravenously as a fluid and nutrient replenisher.

dextrosinistral (dek″stro-sin′is-tral) extending from right to left; also applied to a left-handed person trained to use the right hand in certain performances.

dextrosuria (-su′re-ah) dextrose in the urine.

dextrotorsion (-tor′shun) dextroclination.

dextrotropic (-trop′ik) turning to the right.

dextroversion (-ver′zhun) 1. version to the right, especially movement of the eyes to the right. 2. location of the heart in the right chest, the left ventricle remaining in the normal position on the left, but lying anterior to the right ventricle.

DFP diisopropyl fluorophosphate; see *isoflurophate.*

dg. decigram.

di- word element [Gr., L.], *two.*

dia- word element [Gr.], *through; between; apart; across; completely.*

diabetes (di″ah-be′tēz) any disorder characterized by excessive urine excretion. **adult-onset d.,** maturity-onset d. **brittle d.,** diabetes that is difficult to control, characterized by unexplained oscillation between hypoglycemia and acidosis. **bronze d., bronzed d.,** hemochromatosis. **chemical d.,** a mild abnormality of carbohydrate tolerance manifested by hyperinsulinemia or hyperglycemia only when the patient is subjected to stress loads of glucose. **d. insip′idus,** a metabolic disorder due to deficiency of antidiuretic hormone, resulting in failure of tubular reabsorption of water in the kidney and the consequent passage of a large amount of urine and great thirst. **d. insip′idus, nephrogenic,** a congenital and familial form of diabetes insipidus due to failure of the renal tubules to reabsorb water; there is excessive production of antidiuretic hormone but the tubules fail to respond to it. **juvenile d.,** severe diabetes mellitus of the brittle type, occurring abruptly during the first two decades of life. **latent d.,** chemical d. **maturity-onset d.,** a mild form of diabetes mellitus with onset after about 40 years of age; although pancreatic insulin reserve is diminished, it is almost always sufficient to prevent ketoacidosis, and dietary control is usually effective. **d. melli′tus,** a metabolic disorder in which there is inability to oxidize carbohydrates, due to disturbance of the normal insulin mechanism, producing hyperglycemia, glycosuria, polyuria, thirst, hunger, emaciation, weakness, acidosis, sometimes leading to dypsnea, lipemia, ketonuria, and finally coma. **phlorizin d.,** that produced by administration of phlorizin. **phosphate d.,** a genetically determined failure of renal tubular reabsorption of phosphates, resulting in osteomalacia; believed to be due to impaired ability to utilize vitamin D. **puncture d.,** that produced by puncture of the medulla oblongata. **renal d.,** see under *glycosuria.* **subclinical d.,** a state characterized by an abnormal glucose tolerance test result, but without clinical signs of diabetes.

diabetic (di″ah-bet′ik) 1. pertaining to or characterized by diabetes. 2. a person exhibiting diabetes.

diabetid (di″ah-be′tid) a cutaneous manifestation of diabetes; diabetic dermopathy.

diabetogenic (di″ah-bet″o-jen′ik) producing diabetes.

diabetogenous (di″ah-be-toj′ĕ-nus) caused by diabetes.

diabetometer (di″ah-be-tom′ĕ-ter) a polariscope for use in estimating the percentage of sugar in urine.

Diabinese (di-ab′ĭ-nēs) trademark for preparations of chlorpropamide.

diabrotic (di″ah-brot′ik) 1. ulcerative; caustic. 2. a corrosive or escharotic substance.

diacetate (di-as′ĕ-tāt) any salt of acetoacetic acid.

diacetemia (di-as″ĕ-te′me-ah) the presence of acetoacetic acid in the blood.

diaceturia (-tu′re-ah) diacetic acid in the urine.

diacetyl (di-as′ĕ-til) a yellow liquid, CH₃-COCOCH₃, having the odor of butter. **d. peroxide,** a compound, CH₃CO·O·O·CO·CH₃, used in solution as an antiseptic.

diacetylmorphine (di″ah-se″til-mor′fēn) heroin.

diacid (di-as′id) having two replaceable hydrogen atoms; a dibasic acid having the acid activity of two molecules of a monobasic acid.

diaclasis (di″ak′lah-sis) osteoclasis.

diaclast (di′ah-klast) an instrument for perforating the fetal skull in craniotomy.

diacrisis (di-ak′rĭ-sis) 1. diagnosis. 2. a disease marked by a morbid state of the secretions. 3. a critical discharge or excretion.

diacritic (di″ah-krit′ik) distinguishing; diagnostic.

diad (di′ad) dyad.

diaderm (di′ah-derm) the blastoderm during that stage in which it consists of an ectoderm and an entoderm.

diadochokinesia (di″ah-do″ko-ki-ne′ze-ah) the function of arresting one motor impulse and substituting one that is diametrically opposite.

diadochokinesis (-ki-ne′sis) diadochokinesia.

Diadol (di′ah-dol) trademark for a preparation of allobarbital.

Diafen (di′ah-fen) trademark for a preparation of diphenylpyraline.

diagnose (di′ag-nōs) to identify or recognize a disease.

diagnosis (di″ag-no′sis) determination of the nature of a case of a disease. **diagnos′tic,** adj. **clinical d.,** diagnosis based on signs, symptoms, and laboratory findings during life. **differential d.,** the determination of which one of several diseases may be producing the symptoms. **d. by exclusion,** the determination of a disease by excluding all other conditions. **physical d.,** diagnosis based on information obtained by inspection, palpation, percussion, and auscultation. **serum d.,** serodiagnosis.

diagnostician (di″ag-nos-tish′an) an expert in diagnosis.

diagnostics (di″ag-nos′tiks) the science and practice of diagnosis of disease.

diagram (di′ah-gram) a graphic representation, in simplest form, of an object or concept, made up of lines and lacking pictorial elements. **vector d.,** a diagram representing the direction and magnitude of electromotive forces of the heart for one entire cycle, based on analysis of the scalar electrocardiogram.

diagraph (-graf) an instrument for recording outlines, as in craniometry.

diakinesis (di″ah-ki-ne′sis) the stage of first meiotic prophase in which the nucleolus and nuclear envelope disappear and the spindle fibers form.

dialysance (-li′sans) the minute rate of net exchange of solute molecules passing through a membrane in dialysis.

dialysate (di-al′ĭ-sāt) the material passing through the membrane in dialysis.

dialysis (di-al′ĭ-sis) the process of separating crystalloids and colloids in solution by the difference in their rates of diffusion through a semipermeable membrane: crystalloids pass through readily, colloids very slowly or not at all. See also *hemodialysis.* **lymph d.,** removal of urea and other elements from lymph collected from the thoracic duct, treated outside the body, and later reinfused. **peritoneal d.,** dialysis through the peritoneum, the dialyzing solution being introduced into and removed from the peritoneal cavity, as either a continuous or an intermittent procedure.

dialyzer (di′ah-līz″er) a hemodialyzer.

diameter (di-am′ĕ-ter) the length of a straight line passing through the center of a circle and connecting opposite points on its circumference. **anteroposterior d.,** the distance between two points located on the anterior and posterior aspects, respectively, of the structure being measured, such as the true conjugate diameter of the pelvis or occipitofrontal diameter of the skull. **Baudelocque's d.,** external conjugate d. **conjugate d.,** see *pelvic d.* **cranial d's,** distances measured between certain landmarks of the skull, such as *biparietal,* that between the two parietal eminences; *bitemporal,* that between the two extremities of the coronal suture; *cervicobregmatic,* that between the center of the anterior fontanel and the junction of the neck with the floor of the mouth; *frontomental,* that between the forehead and chin; *occipitofrontal,* that between the external occipital protuberance and most prominent midpoint of the frontal bone; *occipitomental,* that between the external occipital protuberance and the most prominent midpoint of the chin; *suboccipitobregmatic,* that between the lowest posterior point of the occiput and the center of the anterior fontanel. **extracanthic d.,** the distance between the lateral points of junction of the upper and lower eyelids. **intercanthic d.,** the distance between the medial points of junction of the upper and lower eyelids. **pelvic d.,** any diameter of the pelvis, such as *diagonal conjugate,* joining the posterior surface of the pubis to the tip of the sacral promontory; *external conjugate* joining the depression under the last lumbar spine to the upper margin of the pubis; *true* (*internal*) *conjugate,* the anteroposterior diameter of the pelvic inlet, measured from the upper margin of the pubic symphysis to the sacrovertebral angle; *oblique,* joining the one sacroiliac articulation to the iliopubic eminence of the other side; *transverse* (of inlet), joining the two most widely separated points of the pelvic inlet; *transverse* (of outlet) joining the medial surfaces of the ischial tuberosities.

diamide (di-am′id) a double amide.

diamidine (di-am′ĭ-dēn) a compound that contains two amidine groups.

diamine (di-am′in, di′ah-min) a double amine.

diaminodiphenylsulfone (di-am″ĭ-no-di-fen″-il-sul′fōn) dapsone.

diaminuria (di-am″ĭ-nu′re-ah) the presence of diamines in the urine.

Diamox (di′ah-moks) trademark for preparations of acetazolamide.

diamthazole (di-am′thah-zōl) an antifungal agent, $C_{15}H_{23}N_3OS$, used as the dihydrochloride salt.

Dianabol (di-an′ah-bol) trademark for preparations of methandrostenolone.

Diaparene (di-ap″ah-rēn) trademark for a preparation of methylbenzothonium.

diapause (di′ah-pawz) a state of inactivity and arrested development accompanied by greatly decreased metabolism, as in many eggs, insect pupae, and plant seeds; it is a mechanism for surviving adverse winter conditions.

diapedesis (di″ah-pĕ-de′sis) the outward passage of blood cells through intact vessel walls.

diaphanometry (-fah-nom′ĕ-tre) measurement of the transparency of a liquid.

diaphanoscope (-fan′o-skōp) an instrument for transilluminating a body cavity.

diaphanoscopy (-fah-nos′ko-pe) examination by the diaphanoscope.

diaphemetric (-fĕ-met′rik) pertaining to measurement of tactile sensibility.

diaphorase (di-af′o-rās) a flavoprotein that catalyzes the oxidation of nicotinamide-adenine dinucleotide (NAD) or nicotinamide-adenine dinucleotide phosphate (NADP).

diaphoresis (di″ah-fo-re′sis) perspiration, especially profuse prespiration.

diaphoretic (-fo-ret′ik) 1. pertaining to, characterized by, or promoting diaphoresis. 2. an agent that promotes diaphoresis.

diaphragm (di′ah-fram) 1. the musculomembranous partition separating the abdominal and thoracic cavities. 2. any separating membrane or structure. 3. a disk with one or more openings or with an adjustable opening, mounted in relation to a lens or source of radiation, by which part of the light or radiation may be excluded from the area. **diaphragmat′ic,** adj. **Bucky d., Bucky-Potter d.,** a device used in radiography to prevent scattered radiation from reaching the film, thereby securing better contrast and definition. **contraceptive d.,** a device of molded rubber or other soft plastic material, fitted over the cervix uteri to prevent entrance of spermatozoa. **pelvic d.,** the portion of the floor of the pelvis formed by the coccygeus muscles and the levator muscles of the anus, and their fascia. **polyarcuate d.,** one showing abnormal scalloping of the margins on radiographic visualization. **urogenital d.,** the musculomembranous layer superficial to the pelvic diaphragm, extending between the ischiopubic rami and surrounding the urogenital ducts.

diaphragma (di″ah-frag′mah), pl. *diaphragmata* [Gr.] diaphragm (1).

diaphragmatocele (-frag-mat′o-sēl) diaphragmatic hernia.

diaphragmitis (-frag-mi′tis) inflammation of the diaphragm.

diaphyseal, diaphysial (di″ah-fiz′e-al) pertaining to or affecting the shaft of a long bone (diaphysis).

diaphysectomy (-fĭ-zek′to-me) excision of part of a diaphysis.

diaphysis (di-af′ĭ-sis), pl. *diaph′ysis* [Gr.] the shaft of a long bone, between the epiphyses.

diaphysitis (di″ah-fĭ-zi′tis) inflammation of a diaphysis.

diaplasis (di-ap′lah-sis) the setting of a fracture or reduction of a dislocation.

diapophysis (di″ah-pof′ĭ-sis) an upper transverse process of a vertebra.

diapyesis (-pi-e′sis) suppuration. **diapyet′ic,** adj.

diarrhea (-re′ah) abnormally frequent evacuation of watery stools. **diarrhe′al, diarrhe′ic,** adj. **choleraic d.,** acute diarrhea with serous stools, accompanied by circulatory collapse, thus resembling cholera. **fermental d., fermentative d.,** that caused by fermentation due to microorganisms. **lienteric d.,** diarrhea marked by stools containing undigested food. **mucous d.,** diarrhea with mucus in the stools. **osmotic d.,** that due to the presence of osmotically active nonabsorbable solutes, e.g., magnesium sulfate, in the intestine. **parenteral d.,** diarrhea due to infections outside the gastrointestinal tract. **summer d.,** acute diarrhea in children during the intense heat of summer. **traveler's d.,** diarrhea occurring among travelers, particularly in those visiting tropical or subtropical areas where sanitation is suboptimal; it is currently considered to be due to infection with enteropathogenic *Escherichia coli.* **tropical d.,** see under *sprue.*

diarthric (di-ar′thrik) pertaining to or affecting two different joints; biarticular.

diarthrodial (di″ar-thro′dĭ-al) of the nature of a diarthrosis.

diarthrosis (di″ar-thro′sis), pl. *diarthro′ses* [Gr.] a synovial joint.

diarticular (di″ar-tik′u-ler) diarthric.

diaschisis (di-as′kĭ-sis) loss of functional connection between various centers or neuron tracts forming one of the cerebral mechanisms.

diascope (di′ah-skōp) a glass or clear plastic plate pressed against the skin for observing changes produced in the underlying skin after the blood vessels are emptied and the skin is blanched.

diascopy (di-as′ko-pe) 1. examination by means of a diascope. 2. transillumination.

Diasone (di′ah-sōn) trademark for a preparation of sodium sulfoxone.

diastase (di′ah-stās) a combination of enzymes produced during germination of seeds, and contained in malt; it converts starch into maltose and then into dextrose. **d. ve′ra,** pancreatin.

diastasis (di-as′tah-sis) 1. dislocation or separation of two normally attached bones between which there is no true joint. 2. diastasis cordis; the rest period of the cardiac cycle, occurring just before systole.

diastema (di″ah-ste′mah) a space or cleft.

diastematocrania (-stem″ah-to-kra′ne-ah) longitudinal congenital fissure of the cranium.

diastematomyelia (-mi-e′le-ah) abnormal congenital division of the spinal cord by a bony spicule or fibrous band protruding from a vertebra or two, each of the halves surrounded by a dural sac.

diastematopyelia (-pi-e′le-ah) congenital median fissure of the pelvis.

diaster (di-as′ter) amphiaster.

diastole (di-as′to-le) the dilatation, or the period of dilatation, of the heart, especially of the ventricles. **diastol′ic,** adj.

diataxia (di″ah-tak′se-ah) ataxia affecting both sides of the body. **cerebral infantile d., d. cerebra′lis infanti′lis,** cerebral infantile ataxic paralysis.

diathermal, diathermic (-ther′mal; -ther′mik) pertaining to diathermy; permeable by heat waves.

diathermy (-ther′me) the heating of body tissues due to their resistance to the passage of high-frequency electromagnetic radiation. In *medical d.* the tissues are warmed, in *surgical d.* tissue is destroyed. **short-wave d.,** diathermy with high-frequency current of wavelength less than 30 meters.

diathesis (di-ath′ĕ-sis) an unusual constitutional susceptibility or predisposition to a particular disease. **diathet′ic,** adj.

diatom (di′ah-tom) a unicellular microscopic form of alga having a cell wall of silica.

diatomic (di″ah-tom′ik) 1. containing two atoms. 2. dibasic. 3. composed of diatoms.

diatrizoate (-tri-zo′āt) a salt of diatrizoic acid used in combination with sodium hydroxide or meglumine as a radiopaque medium.

diaxon (di-ak′son) a nerve cell with two axons.

diazepam (di-az′ĕ-pam) a minor tranquilizer and skeletal muscle relaxant, $C_{16}H_{13}ClN_2O$.

diazo- (di-az′o) the group, —N_2—.

diazotize (di-az′o-tīz) to introduce the diazo group into a compound.

dibasic (di-ba′sik) containing two replaceable hydrogen atoms, or furnishing two hydrogen ions.

dibenzylchlorethamine (di″ben-zil-klōr-eth′ah-mēn) an alpha-adrenergic blocking agent, $C_{16}H_{18}ClN$, used in the treatment of peripheral vascular disorders and in the diagnosis of pheochromocytoma.

Dibenzyline (di-ben′zĭ-lēn) trademark for a preparation of phenoxybenzamine.

dibothriocephaliasis (di-both″re-o-sef″ah-li′ah-sis) diphyllobothriasis.

Dibothriocephalus (-sef′ah-lus) *Diphyllobothrium.*

dibucaine (di-bu′kān) a local anesthetic, $C_{20}H_{29}$-N_3O_2, used topically and intraspinally in the form of the base and as the hydrochloride salt; the latter is also used intramuscularly for infiltration anesthesia.

Dibuline (di′bu-lēn) trademark for a preparation of dibutoline.

dibutoline (di-bu′to-lēn) an anticholinergic, C_{30}-$H_{66}N_4O_8$; the sulfate salt is used as a mydriatic, cycloplegic, and gastrointestinal antispasmodic.

dicentric (di-sen′trik) 1. pertaining to, developing from, or having two centers. 2. having two centromeres.

dicephalous (di-sef′ah-lus) having two heads.

dicephalus (-ah-lus) a two-headed monster.

dicephaly (-ah-le) a developmental anomaly characterized by the presence of two heads.

dichlorisone (di-klor′ĭ-sōn) a steroid, $C_{21}H_{26}Cl_2$-O_4, used as a topical antipruritic.

dichloroisoproterenol (di-klo″ro-i″so-pro-ter′-ĕ-nol) a beta-adrenergic blocking agent, $C_{11}H_{15}$-Cl_2NO, used in the treatment of various cardiac disorders.

dichlorphenamide (di″klor-fen′ah-mīd) a carbonic anhydrase inhibitor, $C_6H_6Cl_2O_4S_2$, used to reduce intraocular pressure in glaucoma.

dichorial (di-ko′re-al) dichorionic.

dichorionic (di-ko″re-on′ik) having two distinct chorions.

dichroic (di-kro′ik) characterized by dichroism.

dichroism (di′kro-izm) the quality or condition of showing one color in reflected and another in transmitted light.

dichromasy (di-kro′mah-se) dichromatism.

dichromat (di′kro-mat) a person exhibiting dichromatopsia.

dichromate (di-kro′māt) a salt containing the bivalent Cr_2O_7 radical.

dichromatic (di″kro-mat′ik) pertaining to or characterized by dichromatism.

dichromatism (di-kro′mah-tizm) 1. the quality of existing in or exhibiting two different colors. 2. dichromatopsia.

dichromatopsia (di″kro-mah-top′se-ah) a condition characterized by ability to perceive only two of the 160 colors discriminated by the normal eye.

dichromic (di-kro′mik) 1. showing only two colors. 2. containing two atoms of chromium.

dichromophil (di-kro′mo-fil) amphophilic; amphophil.

dichromophilism (di″kro-mof′ĭ-lizm) capacity for double staining, i.e., with both acid and basic dyes.

dicloxacillin (di-kloks″ah-sil′in) a semisynthetic penicillin used in infections with penicillin-resistant gram-positive organisms.

Dicodid (di-ko′did) trademark for preparations of hydrocodone.

dicoelous (di-se′lus) 1. hollowed on each of two sides. 2. having two cavities.

dicophane (di′ko-fān) chlorophenothane.

dicoria (di-ko′re-ah) double pupil.

dicoumarin (di-koo′mah-rin) bishydroxycoumarin.

Dicrocoelium (dik″ro-se′le-um) a genus of flukes, including *D. dentrit′icum,* which has been found in human biliary passages.

dicrotism (di′krŏ-tizm) the occurrence of two sphygmographic waves or elevations to one beat of the pulse. **dicrot′ic,** adj.

Dictyocaulus (dik″te-o-kaw′lus) a genus of nematode parasites of the bronchial.tree of horses, sheep, goats, cattle, and deer.

dictyoma (dik″te-o′mah) diktyoma.

dictyotene (-o-tēn″) the protracted stage resembling suspended prophase in which the primary oocyte persists from late fetal life until discharged from the ovary at or after puberty.

dicumarol (di-koo′mah-rol) bishydroxycoumarin.

Dicurin (di-kur′in) trademark for a preparation of merethoxylline.

dicyclic (di-si′klik) pertaining to or having two cycles; in chemistry, having two rings in the molecular structure.

dicyclomine (di-si′klo-mēn) an anticholinergic, $C_{19}H_{35}NO_2$, used as a gastrointestinal antispasmodic.

didactylism (di-dak′tĭ-lizm) the presence of only two digits on a hand or foot.

didactylous (di-dak′tĭ-lus) having only two digits on a hand or foot.

didelphia (di-del′fe-ah) the condition of having a double uterus.

didymalgia (did″ĭ-mal′je-ah) pain in a testis.

didymitis (did″ĭ-mi′tis) inflammation of a testis.

didymous (did′ĭ-mus) occurring in pairs.

didymus (did′ĭ-mus) a testis; also used as a word termination designating a fetus with duplication of parts or one consisting of conjoined symmetrical twins.

die (di) a form used in the construction of something, as a positive reproduction of the form of a prepared tooth in a suitable hard substance.

diecious (di-e′shus) sexually distinct; denoting species in which male and female genitals do not occur in the same individual. In botany, having staminate and pistillate flowers on separate plants.

dieldrin (di-el′drin) an insecticide, $C_{12}H_8Cl_6O$.

dielectric (di″e-lek′trik) transmitting electricity by induction, but not by conduction; the term is applied to an insulating substance through or across which electric force may act by induction without conduction.

diembryony (di-em′bre-on″e) the production of two embryos from a single egg.

diencephalon (di″en-sef′ah-lon) 1. the posterior part of the forebrain, consisting of the hypothalamus, thalamus, metathalamus, and epithalamus. 2. the posterior of the two brain vesicles formed by specialization in embryonic development. See also *brain stem.*

dienestrol (di″en-es′trol) an estrogen, $C_{18}H_{18}O_2$, used in the treatment of menopausal symptoms and atrophic vaginitis and to suppress lactation.

Dientamoeba (di-en″tah-me′bah) a genus of amebas commonly found in the colon and appendix of man, including *D. frag′ilis,* a species that has been associated with diarrhea.

dieresis (di-er′ĕ-sis) 1. the division or separation of parts normally united. 2. the surgical separation of parts.

diet (di′et) the customary amount and kind of food and drink taken by a person from day to day; more narrowly, a diet planned to meet specific requirements of the individual, including or excluding certain foods. **absolute d.,** fasting. **acid-ash d.,** one of meat, fish, eggs, and cereals with little fruit or vegetables and no cheese or milk. **alkali-ash d.,** one of fruit, vegetables, and milk with as little as possible of meat, fish, eggs and cereals. **balanced d.,** one containing foods which furnish all the nutritive factors in proper proportion for adequate nutrition. **Banting d.,** one designed to reduce obesity. **bland d.,** one that is free of irritating or stimulating foods. **diabetic d.,** one prescribed in diabetes mellitus, usually limited in the amount of sugar or readily available carbohydrate. **elimination d.,** one for diagnosis of food allergy, based on sequential omission of foods that might cause the symptoms. **gouty d.,** one for mitigation of gout, restricting nitrogenous, especially high-purine foods, and substituting dairy products, with prohibition of wines and liquors. **high calorie d.,** one furnishing more calories than needed to maintain weight, often more than 3500–4000 calories per day. **high fat d.,** ketogenic d. **high protein d.,** one containing large amounts of protein, consisting largely of meat, fish, milk, legumes, and nuts. **Karell d.,** a milk diet for nephritis and heart disease. **ketogenic d.,** one containing large amounts of fat, with minimal amounts of protein and carbohydrate. **low calorie d.,** one containing fewer calories than needed to maintain weight, e.g., less than 1200 calories per day for an adult. **low fat d.,** one containing limited amounts of fat. **low fiber d.,** low residue d. **low purine d.,** one for mitigation of gout, omitting meat, fowl, and fish and substituting milk, eggs, cheese, and vegetable protein. **low residue d.,** one giving the least possible fecal residue. **low salt d., low sodium d.,** one containing very little sodium chloride; often prescribed for hypertension and edematous states. **Minot-Murphy d.,** one containing large amounts of liver; given for pernicious anemia. **purine-free d.,** see *low purine d.* **salt-free d.,** low salt d. **Sippy d.,** one for peptic ulcer and conditions requiring a smooth diet, at first consisting of only milk and cream, with gradual addition of other foods, the amounts increasing until on day 28 the patient is placed on the regular ward diet. **smooth d.,** one that avoids the use of roughage foods. **subsistence d.,** one that provides the minimal requirements for life. **Taylor's d.,** a preparation of white of egg, olive oil, and sugar given when the urine is to be tested for chlorides.

dietary (di′ĕ-ter″e) 1. pertaining to diet. 2. a course or system of diet.

dietetic (di″ĕ-tet′ik) pertaining to diet or proper food.

dietetics (-iks) the science of diet and nutrition.

diethazine (di-eth′ah-zēn) an anticholinergic, $C_{18}H_{22}N_2S$; the hydrochloride salt is used as an antiparkisonian agent.

diethylcarbamazine (di-eth″il-kar-bam′ah-zēn) an antifilarial agent, $C_{10}H_{21}N_3O$, used as the citrate salt.

diethylpropion (-pro′pe-on) an appetite suppressant, $C_{13}H_{19}NO$, used as the hydrochloride salt.

diethylstilbestrol (-stil-bes′trol) a synthetic estrogenic compound, $C_{18}H_{20}O_2$, used to treat menopausal symptoms, vaginitis, and suppressed lactation.

diethyltoluamide (-tol-u′ah-mīd) an arthropod repellent, $C_{12}H_{17}NO$.

diethyltryptamine (-trip′tah-mēn) a synthetic hallucinogenic substance closely related to dimethyltryptamine; abbreviated DET.

dietitian (di″ĕ-tish′an) one skilled in the use of diet in health and disease.

dietotherapy (di″ĕ-to-ther′ah-pe) the regulation of diet in treating disease.

differential (dif″er-en′shal) pertaining to a difference or differences.

differentiation (dif″er-en″she-a′shun) 1. the distinguishing of one thing from another. 2. the act or process of acquiring completely individual characters, as occurs in progressive diversification of embryonic cells and tissues. 3. increase in morphological or chemical heterogeneity.

diffraction (dĭ-frakt′shun) the bending or breaking up of a ray of light into its component parts.

diffusate (dĭ-fu′zāt) material that has diffused through a membrane.

diffuse 1. (dĭ-fūs′) not definitely limited or localized. 2. (dĭ-fūz′) to pass through or to spread widely through a tissue or substance.

diffusible (dĭ-fu′zĭ-b'l) capable of rapid diffusion.

diffusion (dĭ-fu′zhun) 1. the state or process of being widely spread. 2. the spontaneous mixing of the molecules of two or more substances resulting from random thermal motion; its rate is proportional to the concentrations of the substances and increases with the temperature. **double d.,** an immunodiffusion test in which both antigen and antibody diffuse into a common area so that, if the antigen and antibody are interacting, they combine to form bands of precipitate. **gel d.,** a test in which antigen and antibody diffuse toward one another through a gel medium to form a precipitate.

digastric (di-gas′trik) 1. having two bellies. 2. digastric muscle.

digenetic (di″jĕ-net′ik) having two stages of multiplication, one sexual in the mature forms, the other asexual in the larval stages.

digestant (di-jes′tant) assisting or stimulating digestion; an agent that so acts.

digestion (di-jes′chun) 1. the act or process of converting food into chemical substances that can be absorbed and assimilated. 2. the subjection of a substance to prolonged heat and moisture, so as to disintegrate and soften it. **diges′tive,** adj. **artificial d.,** digestion carried on outside the body. **gastric d.,** digestion by the action of gastric juice. **gastrointestinal d.,** the gastric and intestinal digestions together. **intestinal d.,** digestion by the action of intestinal juices. **pancreatic d.,** digestion by the action of pancreatic juice. **peptic d.,** gastric d. **primary d.,** gastrointestinal d. **salivary d.,** the change of starch into maltose by the saliva.

digit (dij′it) a finger or toe. **dig′ital,** adj.

Digitaline Nativelle (dij″ĭ-tal′ēn na″tĭ-vel′) trademark for preparations of digitoxin.

Digitalis (dij″ĭ-tal′is) a genus of herbs; *D. lana′ta,* a Balkan species, yields digoxin and lanatoside, and the leaves of *D. purpu′rea,* the purple foxglove, furnish digitalis.

digitalis (dij″ĭ-tal′is) the dried leaf of *Digitalis purpurea;* used as a cardiotonic agent.

digitalization (dij″ĭ-tal-i-za′shun) the administration of digitalis in a dosage schedule designed to produce and then maintain optimal therapeutic concentrations of its cardiotonic glycosides.

digitate (dij′ĭ-tāt) having digit-like branches.

digitation (dij″ĭ-ta′shun) 1. a finger-like process. 2. surgical creation of a functioning digit by making a cleft between two adjacent metacarpal bones, after amputation of some or all of the fingers.

digitiform (dij′ĭ-tĭ-form″) finger-like.

digitigrade (-grād″) characterized by walking or running on the toes; applied to animals whose digits only touch the ground, the posterior part of the foot being more or less raised, as horses and cattle.

digitonin (dij″ĭ-to′nin) a saponin, $C_{55}H_{90}O_{29}$, from *Digitalis purpurea;* used as a reagent to precipitate cholesterol.

digitoxin (dij″ĭ-tok′sin) a cardiotonic glycoside, $C_{41}H_{64}O_{13}$, from *Digitalis purpurea* and other *Digitalis* species; used in the treatment of congestive heart failure.

digitus (dij′ĭ-tus), pl. *dig′iti* [L.] a digit.

diglossia (di-glos′e-ah) bifid tongue.

diglyceride (di-glis′er-īd) a glyceride containing two fatty acid molecules in ester linkage.

dignathus (dig-na′thus) a fetus with two lower jaws.

digoxin (dĭ-jok′sin) a cardiotonic glycoside, $C_{41}H_{64}O_{14}$, from the leaves of *Digitalis lanata;* used in the treatment of congestive heart failure.

dihydric (di-hi′drik) having two hydrogen atoms in each molecule.

dihydrocodeinon (di-hi″dro-ko′de-ĭ-nōn) hydrocodone.

dihydroergotamine (-er-got′ah-mēn) a product of catalytic hydrogenation of ergotamine; used in treatment of migraine.

dihydromorphinone (-mor′fĭ-nōn) hydromorphone.

dihydrotachysterol (-tah-kis′ter-ol) a synthetic steroid, $C_{28}H_{46}O$, from ergosterol; used as a blood-calcium regulator.

dihydroxyaluminum (di″hi-drok″se-ah-lu′mĭ-num) an aluminum compound having two hydroxyl groups in a molecule; available as *d. aminoacetate* and *d. sodium carbonate,* which are used as antacids.

dihydroxycholecalciferol (-ko″le-kal-sif′er-ol) a group of active metabolites of cholecalciferol (vitamin D_3) numbered according to the carbon atom(s) on which a hydroxyl group is substituted; 1,25-dihydroxycholecalciferol is the most active form known.

3,4-dihydroxyphenylalanine (-fen″il-al′ah-nēn) dopa.

diiodohydroxyquin (di″i-o″do-hi-drok′se-kwin) an antiamebic, $C_9H_5I_2NO$.

3,5-diiodothyronine (-thi′ro-nēn) an organic iodine-containing compound, $C_{15}H_{13}I_2NO_4$, obtained in the manufacture of synthetic thyroxine.

diiodotyrosine (-ti′ro-sēn) an organic iodine-containing precursor of thyroxine, liberated from thyroglobulin by hydrolysis.

diktyoma (dik″te-o′mah) a tumor of the ciliary epithelium resembling embryonic retinal tissue in structure.

dilaceration (di-las″er-a′shun) a tearing apart, as of a cataract. In dentistry, an abnormal angulation or curve in the root or crown of a formed tooth.

Dilantin (di-lan′tin) trademark for diphenylhydantoin.

dilatation (dil″ah-ta′shun) 1. the condition, as of an orifice or tubular structure, of being dilated or stretched beyond normal dimensions. 2. the act of dilating or stretching. **d. of heart,** compensatory enlargement of the cavities of the heart, with thinning of its walls.

dilatator (dil″ah-ta′tor) dilator.

dilation (di-la′shun) 1. the act of dilating or stretching. 2. dilatation.

dilator (di-la′tor) a structure (muscle) that dilates, or an instrument used to dilate.

Dilaudid (di-law′did) trademark for preparations of hydromorphone.

Diloderm (di′lo-derm) trademark for a preparation of dichlorisone.

diluent (dil′u-ent) 1. diluting. 2. an agent that dilutes or renders less potent or irritant.

dilution (di-lu′shun) 1. reduction of concentration of an active substance by admixture of a neutral agent. 2. a substance that has undergone dilution. **serial d.,** 1. the progressive dilution of a substance in a series of tubes in predetermined ratios. 2. a method of obtaining a pure bacterial culture by rapid transfer of an exceedingly small amount of material from one nutrient medium to a succeeding one of the same volume.

dimenhydrinate (di″men-hi′drĭ-nāt) an antihistaminic, $C_{17}H_{21}NO\cdot C_7H_7ClN_4O_2$, used as an antinauseant.

dimer (di′mer) 1. a compound formed by combination of two identical molecules. 2. a capsomer having two structural subunits.

dimercaprol (di″mer-kap′rol) antilewisite or British antilewiste (BAL); a compound, C_3H_8-OS_2, used as an antidote against poisoning with arsenic, gold, mercury, and other metals.

Dimetane (di′mĕ-tān) trademark for preparations of brompheniramine.

dimethicone (di-meth′ĭ-kōn) a silicone oil used as a skin protective; available as ointment, spray, and cream.

dimethindene (di″meth-in′dēn) an antihistaminic, $C_{20}H_{24}N_2$, used as the maleate salt.

dimethisoquin (di″mĕ-thi′so-kwin) a local anesthetic, $C_{17}H_{24}N_2O$, used as the hydrochloride salt.

dimethisterone (di″meth-is′ter-ōn) a synthetic progestin, $C_{23}H_{32}O_2$, used as an oral contraceptive, either alone or in combination with ethinyl estradiol.

dimethoxanate (di″mĕ-thok′sĭ-nāt) an antitussive, $C_{19}H_{22}N_2O_3S$, used as the hydrochloride salt.

dimethyl- having two methyl groups in the molecule.

dimethylamine (di-meth″il-am′in) a ptomaine, $(CH_3)_2NH$, from decaying gelatin, decomposing yeast, rotten fish, etc.

***p*-dimethylaminoazobenzene** (-am″ĭ-no-az″o-ben′zēn) a carcinogenic dye, $C_6H_5N_2C_6H_4\cdot N$-$(CH_3)_2$, used as a pH indicator.

Dimethylane (di-meth′ĭ-lān) trademark for preparations of promoxolane.

dimethyl phthalate (di-meth′il thal′āt) an insect repellent, $C_{10}H_{10}O_4$.

dimethyl sulfoxide (di-meth′il sul-fok′sīd) DMSO; a powerful solvent, C_2H_6OS, which has the ability to penetrate plant and animal tissues and to preserve living cells during freezing; it has been proposed as a topical analgesic and anti-inflammatory agent and to increase penetrability of other substances.

dimethyltryptamine (di-meth″il-trip′tah-mēn) a hallucinogenic substance, $C_{12}H_{16}N_2$, derived from the plant *Prestonia amazonica;* abbreviated DMT.

dimetria (di-me′tre-ah) a condition characterized by double uterus.

Dimocillin (di″mo-sil′in) trademark for preparations of sodium methicillin.

dimorphism (di-mor′fizm) the quality of existing in two distinct forms. **dimor′phic, dimor′phous,** adj. **sexual d.,** 1. physical or behavioral differences associated with sex. 2. having some properties of both sexes, as in the early embryo and in some hermaphrodites.

dineuric (di-nu′rik) having two neurons or axons.

Dinoflagellata (di″no-flaj″ĕ-la′tah) an order of minute, chiefly marine, plantlike protozoa; certain members sometimes flourish in numbers so vast as to cover and discolor the seawater (red tide), causing the death of many fish and invertebrates. Included are the genera *Gonyaulax* and *Gymnodinium.*

dinoflagellate (-flaj′ĕ-lāt) 1. of or pertaining to the order Dinoflagellata. 2. any individual of the order Dinoflagellata.

dinucleotide (di-nu′kle-o-tīd″) one of the cleavage products into which a polynucleotide may be split, itself composed of two mononucleotides. **flavin-adenine d.,** a coenzyme that is a condensation product of riboflavin phosphate and adenylic acid; it forms the prosthetic group of certain enzymes, including D-amino acid oxidase and xanthine oxidase, and is important in electron transport in mitochondria. **nicotinamide-adenine d.,** NAD: a coenzyme widely distributed in nature and involved in electron transfer in mitochondria; the products of its hydrolysis are 1 molecule each of adenine and nicotinamide and 2 each of *d*-ribose and phosphoric acid. **nicotinamide-adenine d. phosphate,** NADP: a coenzyme required for a limited number of reactions, similar to nicotinamide-adenine dinucleotide, except for inclusion of 3 phosphate units.

Dioctophyma (di-ok″to-fi′mah) a genus of nematodes, including *D. rena′le*, the kidney worm, found in dogs, cattle, horses, and other animals, and rarely in man; it is highly destructive to kidney tissue.

dioctyl calcium sulfosuccinate (di-ok′til kal′se-um sul″fo-suk′sĭ-nāt) a wetting agent and nonlaxative fecal softener, $C_{40}H_{74}CaO_{14}S_2$.

dioctyl sodium sulfosuccinate (so′de-um sul″fo-suk′sĭ-nāt) a cathartic, wetting agent, and fecal softener, $C_{20}H_{37}Na_7S$.

Diodoquin (di″o-do′kwin) trademark for a preparation of diiodohydroxyquin.

Diodrast (di′o-drast) trademark for a preparation of iodopyracet.

dioecious (di-e′shus) diecious.

diopter (di-op′ter) a unit adopted for refractive power of lenses, being the reciprocal of the focal length expressed in meters; symbol D. **prism d.**, a unit of prismatic deviation, being the deflection of 1 cm. at a distance of one meter; symbol Δ.

dioptometer (di″op-tom′ĕ-ter) an instrument for testing ocular refraction.

dioptometry (-tom′ĕ-tre) the measurement of ocular accommodation and refraction.

dioptre (di′op-ter) diopter.

dioptric (di-op′trik) pertaining to refraction or to transmitted and refracted light; refracting.

dioptrics (di-op′triks) the science of refracted light.

diosgenin (di-os′jen-in) an aglycone of the saponin dioscin, obtained from yams of the genus *Dioscorea*, and used as a precursor in the synthesis of pregnenolone, progesterone, and other steroids.

diovulatory (di-ov′u-lah-to″re) ordinarily discharging two ova in one ovarian cycle.

dioxide (di-ok′sīd) an oxide with two oxygen atoms.

dioxyline (di-ok′sĭ-lēn) a coronary and peripheral vasodilator, $C_{22}H_{25}NO_4$, used as the phosphate salt.

Dipaxin (di-pak′sin) trademark for preparations of diphenadione.

dipeptidase (di-pep′tĭ-dās) an enzyme that catalyzes the hydrolysis of the peptide linkage in a dipeptide.

dipeptide (di-pep′tīd) a peptide which, on hydrolysis, yields two amino acids.

diperodon (di-per′o-don) a surface anesthetic and analgesic, $C_{22}H_{27}N_3O_4$, used as the hydrochloride salt.

Dipetalonema (di-pet″ah-lo-ne′mah) a genus of nematode parasites (superfamily Filarioidea), including *D. per′stans* and *D. strepto′ca*, species primarily parasitic in man, other primates serving as reservoir hosts.

diphallus (di-fal′lus) double penis.

diphasic (di-fa′zik) having two phases.

diphebuzol (di-feb′u-zol) phenylbutazone.

diphemanil (di-fe′mah-nil) an anticholinergic, $C_{21}H_{27}NO_4S$, used to inhibit gastric secretion

and motility, relieve pylorospasm, control sweating, and relieve pruritus.

diphenadione (di-fen″ah-di′ōn) an anticoagulant, $C_{23}H_{16}O_3$.

diphenhydramine (di″fen-hi′drah-min) an antihistaminic, $C_{17}H_{21}NO$, used as the hydrochloride salt.

diphenicillin (-ĭ-sil′in) an acid- and penicillinase-resistant semisynthetic penicillin available as the sodium salt for oral and intramuscular use.

diphenoxylate (-ok′sĭ-lāt) an antidiarrheal, $C_{30}H_{32}N_2O_2$, used as the hydrochloride salt.

diphenylhydantoin (di-fen″il-hi-dan′to-in) an anticonvulsant, $C_{15}H_{12}N_2O_2$, used in the treatment of all forms of epilepsy except petit mal.

diphenylpyraline (-pi′rah-lēn) an antihistaminic, $C_{18}H_{23}NO$, used as the hydrochloride salt.

diphonia (di-fo′ne-ah) the production of two different voice tones in speaking.

diphosphothiamin (di-fos″fo-thi′ah-min) the coenzyme that is involved in the decarboxylation of α-keto acids.

diphtheria (dif-the′re-ah) an acute infectious disease caused by *Corynebacterium diphtheriae* and its toxin, primarily affecting the membranes of the nose, throat, or larynx, and marked by formation of a gray-white pseudomembrane, with fever, pain, and, in the laryngeal form, aphonia and respiratory obstruction. The toxin may also cause myocarditis and neuritis. **diphthe′rial, diphther′ic, diphtherit′ic**, adj.

diphtheroid (dif′thĕ-roid) 1. resembling diphtheria or the diphtheria bacillus. 2. any member of *Corynebacterium* other than *C. diphtheriae*. 3. pseudodiphtheria.

diphthongia (dif-thon′je-ah) the production of double vocal sounds.

diphyllobothriasis (di-fil″o-both-ri′ah-sis) infection with *Diphyllobothrium*.

Diphyllobothrium (-both′re-um) a genus of large tapeworms, including *D. la′tum* (broad or fish tapeworm), found in the intestine of man, cats, dogs, and other fish-eating mammals; its first intermediate host is a crustacean and the second a fish, the infection in man being acquired by eating inadequately cooked fish.

diphyodont (dif′e-o-dont″) having two dentitions, a deciduous and a permanent.

diplacusis (dip″lah-koo′sis) the perception of a single auditory stimulus as two separate sounds. **binaural d.**, different perception by the two ears of a single auditory stimulus. **disharmonic d.**, binaural diplacusis in which a pure tone is heard differently in the two ears. **echo d.**, binaural diplacusis in which a sound of brief duration is heard at different times in the two ears. **monaural d.**, diplacusis in which a pure tone is heard in the same ear as a split tone of two frequencies.

diplegia (di-ple′je-ah) paralysis of like parts on either side of the body. **diple′gic**, adj.

diplobacillus (dip″lo-bah-sil′us) a short, rod-shaped organism occurring in pairs.

diplobacterium (-bak-te′re-um) diplobacillus.

diploblastic (-blas′tik) having two germ layers.

diplocardia (-kar′de-ah) separation of the two halves of the heart.

Diplococcus (-kok′us) a genus of bacteria (tribe Streptococceae), including *D. pneumo′niae*, the commonest cause of lobar pneumonia, including some 80 serotypes distinguishable by the polysaccharide hapten of the capsular substance.

diplococcus (-kok′us), pl. *diplococ′ci.* 1. any of the spherical, lanceolate, or coffee-bean-shaped bacteria occurring usually in pairs as a result of incomplete separation after cell division in a single plane. 2. any organism of the genus *Diplococcus.*

diplocoria (-ko′re-ah) double pupil.

diploë (dip′lo-e) the spongy layer between the inner and outer compact layers of the flat bones of the skull. **diploet′ic, diplo′ic,** adj.

diplogenesis (dip″lo-jen′ĕ-sis) the production of a double monster.

diploid (dip′loid) 1. having two sets of chromosomes, as normally found in the somatic cells; in man, the diploid number is 46. 2. an individual or cell having two full sets of homologous chromosomes.

diploidy (dip′loi-de) the state of being diploid.

diplomyelia (dip″lo-mi-e′le-ah) lengthwise fissure and seeming doubleness of the spinal cord.

diplonema (-ne′mah) the double chromosomes in the diplotene stage.

diplopia (dĭ-plo′pe-ah) the perception of two images of a single object. **binocular d.,** perception of a separate image of a single object by each of the two eyes. **crossed d.,** diplopia in which the image belonging to the right eye is displaced to the left of the image belonging to the left eye. **direct d.,** that in which the image belonging to the right eye appears to the right of the image belonging to the left eye. **heteronymous d.,** crossed d. **homonymous d.,** direct d. **horizontal d.,** that in which the images lie in the same horizontal plane, being either direct or crossed. **monocular d.,** perception by one eye of two images of a single object. **paradoxical d.,** crossed d. **torsional d.,** that in which the upper pole of the verticle axis of one image is inclined toward or away from that of the other. **vertical d.,** that in which one image appears above the other in the same vertical plane.

diplopiometer (dĭ-plo″pe-om′ĕ-ter) an instrument for measuring diplopia.

diploscope (dip′lo-skōp) an instrument for studying double vision.

diplosome (-sōm) the two centrioles of a mammalian cell.

diplosomia (dip″lo-so′me-ah) a condition in which complete twins are joined at some of their body parts.

diplotene (dip′lo-tēn) that stage of the first prophase of meiosis during which the paired bivalent chromosomes begin to repel one another.

dipole (di′pōl) 1. a molecule having charges of equal and opposite sign. 2. a pair of electric charges or magnetic poles separated by a short distance.

diprosopus (di-pros′o-pus) a monster with varying degrees of duplication of the face.

diprotrizoate (di″pro-tri′zo-āt) a compound used as a contrast medium in roentgenography of the urinary tract.

dipsesis (dip-se′sis) excessive thirst. **dipset′ic,** adj.

dipsogen (dip′so-jen) an agent or measure that induces thirst and promotes ingestion of fluids.

dipsogenic (dip″so-jen′ik) engendering thirst.

dipsomania (-ma′ne-ah) alcoholism.

dipsosis (dip-so′sis) excessive thirst.

dipsotherapy (dip″so-ther′ah-pe) the therapeutic limitaion of amount of fluids ingested.

Diptera (dip′ter-ah) an order of insects, including flies, gnats, and mosquitoes.

dipterous (dip′ter-us) 1. having two wings. 2. pertaining to insects of the order Diptera.

dipygus (di-pi′gus) a fetus with a double pelvis.

dipylidiasis (dip″ĭ-lĭ-di′ah-sis) infection with *Dipylidium caninum.*

Dipylidium (dip″ĭ-lid′e-um) a genus of tapeworms. *D. cani′num,* the dog tapeworm, is parasitic in dogs and cats and is occasionally found in man.

dipyridamole (di″pi-rid′ah-mōl) a coronary vasodilator, $C_{24}H_{40}N_8O_4$.

dipyrone (di′pi-rōn) an analgesic and antipyretic, $C_{13}H_{16}N_3NaO_4S \cdot H_2O$.

director (di-rek′tor) a grooved instrument for guiding a surgical instrument.

Dirofilaria (di″ro-fĭ-la′re-ah) a genus of filarial nematodes (superfamily Filarioidea), including *D. immit′is,* the heartworm, found in the right heart and veins of the dog, wolf, and fox.

dirofilariasis (-fil″ah-ri′ah-sis) infection with organisms of the genus *Dirofilaria.*

dis- word element [L.], *reversal* or *separation;* [Gr.], *duplication.*

disaccharidase (di-sak′ah-rĭ-dās″) an enzyme that catalyzes the hydrolysis of disaccharides.

disaccharide (di-sak′ah-rid, -sak′ah-rīd) any of a class of sugars yielding two monosaccharides on hydrolysis.

disarticulation (dis″ar-tik″u-la′shun) amputation or separation at a joint.

disassimilation (-ah-sim″ĭ-la′shun) catabolism.

disc (disk) disk.

discharge (dis-charj′) 1. a setting free, or liberation. 2. matter or force set free. 3. an excretion or substance evacuated.

discission (dĭ-sizh′un) incision, or cutting into, as of a soft cataract.

discitis (dis-ki′tis) diskitis.

disclination (dis″klĭ-na′shun) outward rotation of both eyes.

discoblastula (dis″ko-blas′tu-lah) the specialized blastula formed by cleavage of a fertilized telolecithal ovum, consisting of a cellular cap (blastoderm) separated by the blastocele from a floor of uncleaved yolk.

discogenic (-jen′ik) caused by derangement of an intervertebral disk.

discogram (dis′ko-gram) diskogram.

discography (dis-kog′rah-fe) diskography.

discoid (dis′koid) 1. disk-shaped. 2. a disklike medicated tablet. 3. a dental instrument with a disklike or circular blade.

discopathy (dis-kop′ah-the) any disease of an intervertebral disk.

discoplacenta (dis″ko-plah-sen′tah) a discoid placenta.

discordance (dis-kor′dans) the occurrence of a given trait in only one member of a twin pair. **discor′dant,** adj.

discrete (dis-krēt′) made up of separated parts or characterized by lesions which do not become blended.

discus (dis′kus), pl. *dis′ci*[L.] disk. **d. ooph′orus, d. ovig′erus, d. prolig′erus,** cumulus oophorus.

discutient (dis-ku′shent) scattering, or causing a disappearance; a remedy that so acts.

disdiaclast (-di′ah-klast) any of the doubly refracting elements of the contractile substance of a muscle.

disease (dĭ-zēz′) a definite morbid process, often with a characteristic train of symptoms. **Acosta's d.,** mountain sickness. **Adams' d., Adams-Stokes d.,** sudden attacks of unconsciousness, with or without convulsions, due to heart block. **Addison's d.,** bronzelike pigmentation of the skin, severe prostration, progressive anemia, low blood pressure, diarrhea, and digestive disturbance, due to adrenal hypofunction. **akamushi d.,** scrub typhus. **Albers-Schönberg d.,** osteopetrosis. **Almeida's d.,** paracoccidioidomycosis. **Alper's d.,** poliodystrophy cerebri. **Alzheimer's d.,** presenile dementia. **Andersen's d.,** amylopectinosis. **Aran-Duchenne d.,** spinal muscular atrophy. **arc-welder's d.,** pulmonary siderosis. **Aujeszky's d.,** pseudorabies. **Australian X d.,** an acute epidemic encephalitis of viral origin observed in Australia during the summer months between 1917 and 1926, resembling Japanese B encephalitis symptomatically and pathologically. **autoimmune d.,** any of a group of disorders in which tissue injury is associated with humoral or cell-mediated responses to body constituents; they may be systemic or organ-specific. **Ayerza's d.,** a form of polycythemia vera marked by chronic cyanosis, chronic dyspnea, chronic bronchitis, bronchiectasis, hepatosplenomegaly, hyperplasia of bone marrow, and associated with sclerosis of the pulmonary artery. **Bamberger-Marie d.,** hypertrophic pulmonary osteoarthropathy. **Bang's d.,** infectious abortion in cattle. **Banti's d.,** congestive splenomegaly; originally, a primary disease of the spleen with splenomegaly and pancytopenia, now considered secondary to portal hypertension. **Barlow's d.,** scurvy in infants. **Barraquer's d.,** progressive lipodystrophy. **Basedow's d.,** Graves' d. **Bayle's d.,** paralytic dementia. **Bazin's d.,** erythema induratum. **Bechterew's d.,** rheumatoid spondylitis. **Behçet's d.,** see under *syndrome*. **Benson's d.,** asteroid hyalitis. **Bernhardt's d.,** meralgia paresthetica. **Besnier-Boeck d.,** sarcoidosis. **Best's d.,** congenital macular degeneration. **Bielschowsky's d., Bielschowsky-Jansky d.,** late infantile amaurotic familial idiocy, differing from the infantile form (*Tay-Sachs d.*) in that it occurs between 3 and 4 years of age, progresses more slowly, and the cherry-red retinal spot is frequently absent, but there are pigmentary changes of the retinas. **Biermer's d.,** pernicious anemia. **black d.,** a fatal disease of sheep, and sometimes of man, in the United States and Australia, due to *Clostridium novyi,* marked by necrotic areas in the liver. **bleeder's d.,** hemophilia. **Blocq's d.,** astasia-abasia. **Bloodgood's d.,** cystic d. of breast. **Blount's d.,** osteochondrosis deformans tibiae. **Boeck's d.,** sarcoidosis. **Borna d.,** a fatal enzootic encephalitis of viral origin, affecting horses, cattle, and sheep. **Bornholm d.,** epidemic pleurodynia. **Bourneville's d.,** tuberous sclerosis. **Bowen's d.,** intraepidermal squamous cell carcinoma, often occurring in multiple primary sites. **Breda's d.,** yaws. **Bright's d.,** a descriptive term once used for kidney disease with proteinuria, usually glomerulonephritis. **Brill's d.,** a recrudescence of typhus occurring as long as 70 years after the initial acute episode of epidemic typhus; it is milder than the primary infection. **Brill-Symmers d.,** giant follicular lymphoma. **Brill-Zinsser d.,** Brill's d. **Buerger's d.,** thromboangiitis obliterans. **Busse-Buschke d.,** cryptococcosis. **Caffey's d.,** infantile cortical hyperostosis. **caisson d.,** decompression sickness. **California d.,** coccidioidomycosis. **Calvé-Perthes d.,** osteochondrosis of capitular epiphysis of femur. **Camurati-Engelmann d.,** diaphyseal dysplasia. **Canavan's d.,** spongy degeneration of the central nervous system. **Carrión's d.,** an infectious disease in South America due to *Bartonella bacilliformis,* transmitted by the sandfly *Phlebotomus verrucarum,* appearing in an acute febrile anemic stage (*Oroya fever*) followed by a nodular skin eruption (*verruga peruana*). **cat-scratch d.,** see under *fever*. **celiac d.,** nontropical sprue. **Chagas' d., Chagas-Cruz d.,** trypanosomiasis due to *Trypanosoma cruzi;* it runs an acute course in children and a chronic course in adults. **Charcot's d.,** see under *arthropathy*. **Charcot-Marie-Tooth d.,** progressive neuropathic (peroneal) muscular atrophy. **Christian-Weber d.,** nodular nonsuppurative panniculitis. **Christmas d.,** hemophilia B. **chronic granulomatous d.,** chronic suppurative lymphadenitis, eczematoid dermatitis, hepatosplenomegaly, and chronic pulmonary disease associated with a genetically determined defect in the intracellular bactericidal function of leukocytes. **circling d.,** see *circling*. **Coats' d.,** chronic progressive retinopathy usually affecting male children, in which the fundus reveals an exudative retinal detachment associated with telangiectatic blood vessels and multiple hemorrhages; it may lead to total retinal detachment, iritis, glaucoma, and cataract. **collagen d.,** any of a group of diseases characterized by widespread pathologic changes in connective tissue; they include lupus erythematosus, dermatomyositis, scleroderma, polyarteritis nodosa, thrombotic purpura, rheumatic fever, and rheumatoid arthritis. **communicable d.,** a disease the causative agents of which may pass or be carried from one person to another directly or indirectly. **complicating d.,** one occurring in the course of some other disease as a complication. **Concato's d.,** progressive malignant polyserositis with large effusions into the pericardium, pleura, and peritoneum. **constitutional d.,** one involving a system of organs or one with widespread symptoms. **contagious d.,** communicable d. **Cori's d.,** Forbes' d. **coxsackievirus A d.,** herpangina. **Crigler-Najjar d.,** see under *syndrome.* **Crohn's d.,** regional ileitis. **Crouzon's d.,** craniofacial dysostosis. **Cruveilhier's d.,** 1. simple ulcer of the stomach. 2. spinal muscular atrophy. **Cushing's d.,** Cushing's syndrome in which the hyperadrenocorticism is secondary to excessive pituitary secretion of adrenocorticotropic hormone. **cystic d. of breast,** a form of productive mastitis marked by the formation of many small cysts. **cystine storage d.,** Fanconi syndrome (2). **cytomegalic inclusion d.,** a disease, especially of newborns, due to infection with a cytomegalovirus, and characterized by hepatosplenomegaly and often by microcephaly and mental or motor retardation. **Darier's d.,** keratosis follicularis. **Darling's d.,** histoplasmosis. **deficiency d.,** a condition caused by dietary or metabolic deficiency, including all diseases due to an insufficient supply of essential nutrients. **degenerative joint d.,** osteoarthritis. **Dejerine's d., Dejerine-Sottas d.,** progressive hypertrophic interstitial neuropathy. **demyelinating d.,** any condition characterized by destruction of myelin. **de Quervain's d.,** painful tenosynovitis due to relative narrowness of the common tendon sheath of the abductor pollicis longus and extensor pollicis brevis. **Dercum's d.,** adiposis dolorosa. **Devic's d.,** neuromyelitis optica. **Duchenne's d.,** 1. spinal muscular atrophy. 2. progressive bulbar paralysis. 3. tabes dorsalis. **Duchenne-Aran d.,** spinal muscular atrophy. **Duhring's d.,** dermatitis herpetiformis. **Duke's d.,** a febrile disease of childhood marked by an exanthematous eruption, probably a mild form of scarlet fever. **Duplay's d.,** see under *bursitis.* **Durand-Nicolas-Favre d.,** lymphogranuloma venereum. **Duroziez's d.,** congenital mitral stenosis. **Ebstein's d.,** see under *anomaly.* **Economo's d.,** lethargic encephalitis. **Engelmann's d.,** diaphyseal dysplasia. **epizootic d.,** one affecting a large number of animals in some particular region within a short period of time. **Erb's d.,** idiopathic muscular atrophy. **Erb-Goldflam d.,** myasthenia gravis. **Eulenburg's d.,** myotonia congenita. **extrapyramidal d.,** any of a group of clinical disorders marked by abnormal involuntary movements, alterations in muscle tone, and postural disturbances; they include parkinsonism, chorea, athetosis, etc. **Fabry's d.,** angiokeratoma corporis diffusum. **Fahr-Volhard d.,** the malignant form of arteriolar nephrosclerosis. **Fanconi's d.,** see under *syndrome.* **Feer's d.,** acrodynia. **fibrocystic d. of pancreas,** cystic fibrosis. **fifth d.,** erythema infectiosum. **fifth venereal d.,** lymphogranuloma venereum. **flint d.,** chalicosis. **focal d.,** a localized disease. **foot-and-mouth d.,** an acute, contagious viral disease of wild and domestic cloven-footed animals, very rarely of man, marked by a vesicular eruption on the lips, buccal cavity, pharynx,

legs, and feet, sometimes involving the udder or teats. **Forbes' d.,** glycogenosis (type III) in which a deficiency of the debrancher enzyme dextrin-1,6-glucosidase affects the heart and liver, with hepatomegaly, hypoglycemia, acidosis, stunted growth, and doll facies. **Fordyce's d.,** a developmental anomaly marked by enlarged and ectopic sebaceous glands that appear as minute yellowish papules on the oral mucosa. **Fothergill's d.,** 1. scarlatina anginosa. 2. trigeminal neuralgia. **fourth d.,** Duke's d. **fourth venereal d.,** 1. gangrenous balanitis. 2. granuloma inguinale. **Fox-Fordyce d.,** a persistent and recalcitrant, itchy, papular eruption, chiefly of the axillae and pubes, due to inflammation of apocrine sweat glands. **Frei's d.,** lymphogranuloma venereum. **Freiberg's d.,** osteochondrosis of the head of the second metatarsal bone. **Friedländer's d.,** endarteritis obliterans. **Friedreich's d.,** paramyoclonus multiplex. **functional d.,** one involving functions without detectable tissue damage. **Gamna's d.,** splenomegaly with thickening of the splenic capsule and the presence of small brownish areas (Gamna nodules), ferruginous pigment being deposited in the splenic pulp. **Garrés d.,** sclerosing nonsuppurative osteomyelitis. **Gaucher's d.,** a hereditary disorder of glucocerebroside metabolism, marked by the presence of Gaucher's cells in the marrow, and by hepatosplenomegaly and erosion of the cortices of long bones and pelvis. The adult form is associated with moderate anemia and thrombocytopenia, and yellowish pigmentation of the skin; in the infantile form there is, in addition, marked central nervous system impairment; in the juvenile form there are rapidly progressive systemic manifestations but moderate central nervous system involvement. **Gee's d., Gee-Herter d., Gee-Herter-Heubner d.,** nontropical sprue of children. **Gee-Thaysen d.,** nontropical sprue of adults. **Gierke's d.,** glycogenosis (type I) in which deficiency of the hepatic enzyme glucose-6-phosphatase results in liver and kidney involvement, with hepatomegaly, hypoglycemia, hyperuricemia, and gout. **Gilbert's d.,** benign hereditary hyperbilirubinemia marked by mild intermittent jaundice and often by fatigue, weakness, and abdominal pain. **Gilles de la Tourette's d.,** see under *syndrome.* **Glanzmann's d.,** see *thrombasthenia.* **Glisson's d.,** rickets. **glycogen storage d.,** glycogenosis. **Goldflam's d., Goldflam-Erb d.,** myasthenia gravis. **Graves' d.,** an association of hyperthyroidism, goiter, and exophthalmos, with accelerated pulse rate, profuse sweating, nervous symptoms, psychic disturbances, emaciation, and elevated basal metabolism. **Greenfield's d.,** infantile metachromatic leukodystrophy. **Gull's d.,** atrophy of the thyroid gland with myxedema. **Günther's d.,** congenital erythropoietic porphyria. **H d.,** Hartnup d. **Hailey-Hailey d.,** benign familial pemphigus. **Hamman's d.,** spontaneous interstitial emphysema of the lungs. **Hand's d.,** Hand-Schüller-Christian d. **hand-foot-and-mouth d.,** a mild, highly infectious viral disease of children, with vesicular lesions in the mouth and on the hands and feet. **Hand-Schüller-Christian d.,** chronic idiopathic histiocytosis, with multifocal histiocytic lipogranulomas of bone and of the skin and viscera; the histiocytes contain abundant cholesterol. **Hanot's d.,** biliary cirrhosis. **Hansen's d.,** leprosy. **Hartnup's d.,** a genetically determined disorder of intestinal and renal transport of neutral alpha-amino acids, marked by a pellagra-like skin rash, with transient cerebellar ataxia, constant renal aminoaciduria, and other biochemical abnormalities. **Hashimoto's d.,** struma lymphomatosa. **heavy-chain d.,** a monoclonal gammopathy in which there is elaboration of IgG that lacks certain antigenic determinants. The resultant globulin fragment (molecular weight, 53,000), resembling the Fc fragment, is found in both serum and urine. Symptoms include recurring bacterial infections, anemia, enlargment of lymphoid organs, and edema of the palate. Histologically there is lymphoma, ranging from Hodgkin's disease to reticulum cell sarcoma. Heavy-chain disease involving the IgA and IgM systems has also been reported. **Heerfordt's d.,** uveoparotid fever. **Heine-Medin d.,** the major form of poliomyelitis. **hemolytic d. of newborn,** erythroblastosis fetalis. **hemorrhagic d. of newborn,** a self-limited hemorrhagic disorder of the first few days of life, due to deficiency of vitamin K–dependent coagulation Factors II, VII, IX, and X. **Hers' d.,** glycogenosis (type VI), in which a deficiency of liver phosphorylase affects the liver and leukocytes, with hepatomegaly, moderate hypoglycemia, mild acidosis, and growth retardation. **Heubner-Herter d.,** nontropical sprue of children. **hip-joint d.,** tuberculosis of the hip joint. **Hippel's d.,** von Hippel's d. **Hirschsprung's d.,** congenital megacolon. **His' d.,** His-Werner d., trench fever. **Hodgkin's d.,** a malignant condition marked clinically by painless, progressive enlargement of lymph nodés, spleen, and general lymphoid tissue; other symptoms may include anorexia, lassitude, weight loss, fever, pruritus, night sweats, and anemia. Sternberg-Reed cells are characteristically present. **Hodgson's d.,** aneurysmal dilatation of the proximal part of the aorta. **hoof-and-mouth d.,** foot-and-mouth d. **hookworm d.,** infection with the hookworm *Ancylostoma duodenale* or *Necator americanus,* the larvae of which enter the body through the skin or are ingested with contaminated food or water, and migrate to the small intestine where, as adults, they attach to the intestinal mucosa and ingest blood; symptoms may include abdominal pain, diarrhea, colic or nausea, and anemia. In dogs, it is caused by *Uncinaria stenocephala.* **Hutchinson-Gilford d.,** progeria. **hyaline membrane d.,** a disorder of newborn infants, usually premature, characterized by the formation of a hyaline-like membrane lining the terminal respiratory passages. Extensive atelectasis is attributed to lack of surfactant. See *respiratory distress syndrome of newborn.* **hydatid d.,** an infection, usually of the liver, due to larval forms of tapeworms of the genus *Echinococcus,* marked by development of expanding cysts. **Iceland d.,** benign myalgic encephalomyelitis. **immune-complex d.,** a state in which circulating antigen-anti-

body complexes, formed by coexisting immune reactions, induce vascular injury. **infectious d.,** one due to organisms ranging in size from viruses to parasitic worms; it may be contagious in origin, result from nosocomial organisms, or be due to endogenous microflora from the nose and throat, skin, or bowel. **intercurrent d.,** one occurring during the course of another disease with which it has no connection. **iron-storage d.,** hemochromatosis. **Jensen's d.,** retinochoroiditis juxtapapillaris. **Johne's d.,** a usually fatal, chronic enteritis of cattle, but also affecting sheep, goats, and deer, caused by *Mycobacterium paratuberculosis.* **Kahler's d.,** multiple myeloma. **Kashin-Beck d.,** a disabling degenerative disease of the peripheral joints and spine, endemic in eastern Siberia, northern China, and Korea; believed to be caused by ingestion of cereal grains infected with the fungus *Fusarium sporotrichiella.* **Katayama d.,** schistosomiasis japonica. **Kedani d.,** scrub typhus. **Kienböck's d.,** 1. slowly progressive osteochondrosis of the lunate bone; it may affect other wrist bones. 2. traumatic cavitation of the spinal cord. **Klippel's d.,** arthritic general pseudo-paralysis. **Köhler's bone d.,** 1. osteochondrosis of the tarsal navicular bone in children. 2. thickening of the shaft of the second metatarsal bone and changes about its articular head, with pain in the second metatarsophalangeal joint on walking or standing. **Krabbe's d.,** a familial form of leukoencephalopathy beginning in infancy, marked pathologically by cerebral demyelination and by the presence of large globoid bodies in the white substance. **Kufs' d.,** late juvenile, or adult, amaurotic familial idiocy, occurring between 15 and 26 years of age, differing from the infantile form (*Tay-Sachs d.*) in that it shows no racial predilection, and from the infantile, late infantile (*Bielschowsky's d.*), and juvenile (*Spielmeyer-Vogt d.*) forms in that ocular lesions are absent; clinical findings are those of cerebellar or basal ganglia disorders. **Kugelberg-Welander d.,** a hereditary juvenile form of muscular atrophy, due to lesions of the anterior horns of the spinal cord, with onset principally between 2 and 17 years of age; it is marked by atrophy and weakness of the proximal muscles of the lower extremities and pelvic girdle, followed by involvement of the distal muscles and muscular twitchings. **Kümmell's d.,** compression fracture of vertebra, with symptoms occurring a few weeks after injury, including spinal pain, intercostal neuralgia, motor disturbances of the legs, and kyphosis which is painful on pressure and easily reduced by extension. **Kussmaul's d.,** periarteritis nodosa. **Kyasanur Forest d.,** a highly fatal viral disease of monkeys in the Kyasanur Forest of India, communicable to man, in whom it produces hemorrhagic symptoms. **Lafora's d.,** myoclonus epilepsy. **leaf-curl d.,** a viral disease of plants characterized by curling or crinkling of the leaves. **Leber's d.,** see under *atrophy.* **Legg's d., Legg-Calvé d., Legg-Calvé-Perthes d., Legg-Calvé-Waldenström d.,** osteochondrosis of the capitular head of the femoral epiphysis. **Leiner's d.,** erythroderma desquamativum. **Leriche's d.,** Sudeck's atrophy.

Letterer-Siwe d., a nonlipid reticuloendotheliosis of early childhood, marked by a hemorrhagic tendency, eczematoid skin eruption, hepatosplenomegaly with lymph node involvement, and progressive anemia. **Libman-Sacks d.,** verrucous endocarditis associated with systemic lupus erythematosus. **Lignac-Fanconi d.,** Fanconi's syndrome (2). **Lindau's d., Lindau-von Hippel d.,** von Hippel-Lindau d. **Little's d.,** congenital spastic stiffness of the limbs, a form of cerebral spastic paralysis due to lack of development of the pyramidal tracts. **Lobstein's d.,** see *osteogenesis imperfecta.* **Lowe's d.,** oculocerebrorenal syndrome. **lumpy skin d.,** a highly infectious viral disease of cattle in Africa, which may result in permanent sterility or death, marked by the formation of nodules on the skin and sometimes on the mucous membranes. **Lutz-Splendore-Almeida d.,** paracoccidioidomycosis. **McArdle's d.,** glycogenosis (type V) in which a deficiency of muscle phosphorylase affects the skeletal muscles, with muscle cramps and a depressed blood lactate level during exercise. **Madelung's d.,** 1. see under *deformity.* 2. see under *neck.* **Majocchi's d.,** purpura annularis telangiectodes. **maple bark d.,** a granulomatous interstitial pneumonitis due to inhalation of spores from *Cryptostroma corticale,* a mold found beneath the bark of maple logs. **maple syrup urine d.,** a hereditary disease involving an enzyme defect in the metabolism of the branched chain amino acids, marked clinically by mental and physical retardation, feeding difficulties, and a characteristic odor of the urine. **Marchiafava-Micheli d.,** paroxysmal noctural hemoglobinuria; see *intermittent hemoglobinuria.* **Marie's d.,** acromegaly. **Marie-Bamberger d.,** hypertrophic pulmonary osteoarthropathy. **Marie-Strümpell d.,** rheumatoid spondylitis. **Marie-Tooth d.,** progressive neuropathic (peroneal) muscular atrophy. **mast cell d.,** urticaria pigmentosa. **Mediterranean d.,** see *β-thalassemia.* **Menetrier's d.,** giant hypertrophic gastritis. **Meniere's d.,** deafness, tinnitus, and dizziness, in association with nonsuppurative disease of the labyrinth. **Merzbacher-Pelizaeus d.,** familial centrolobar sclerosis. **Meyer's d.,** adenoid vegetations of the pharynx. **Mikulicz's d.,** benign, self-limited lymphocytic infiltration and enlargement of the lacrimal and salivary glands of uncertain etiology. **Milroy's d.,** hereditary permanent lymphedema of the legs due to lymphatic obstruction. **Minamata d.,** a severe neurologic disorder due to alkyl mercury poisoning, leading to severe permanent neurologic and mental disabilities or death; once prevalent among those who ate contaminated seafood from Minamata Bay, Japan. **Mitchell's d.,** erythromelalgia. **Möbius' d.,** periodic migraine with paralysis of the oculomotor muscles. **Mondor's d.,** phlebitis affecting the large subcutaneous veins normally crossing the lateral chest wall and breast from the epigastric or hypochondriac region to the axilla. **Morquio's d.,** see under *syndrome.* **Morquio-Ullrich d.,** Morquio's syndrome. **Morton's d.,** tenderness or pain in the metatarsophalangeal joint of the third or fourth toe. **Morvan's d.,** a form of sy-

ringomyelia, with painless ulceration of the fingertips and analgesic paralysis and atrophy of the forearms and hands. **mosaic d's,** infectious viral diseases of plants, marked by mottling of the foliage. **motor neuron d.,** any disease of a motor neuron, including spinal muscular atrophy, progressive bulbar paralysis, amyotrophic lateral sclerosis, and lateral sclerosis. **Newcastle d.,** a viral disease of birds, including domestic fowl, characterized by respiratory and gastrointestinal or pneumonic and encephalitic symptoms; also transmissible to man. **Nicolas-Favre d.,** lymphogranuloma venereum. **Niemann's d., Niemann-Pick d.,** a hereditary disease with massive hepatosplenomegaly, brownish yellow discoloration of skin, nervous system involvement, and the presence in the liver, spleen, lungs, lymph nodes, and bone marrow of foamy reticular cells containing phospholipids. **Norrie's d.,** a hereditary disorder consisting of bilateral blindness from retinal malformation, mental retardation, and deafness. **oasthouse urine d.,** Smith-Strang d. **occupational d.,** disease due to various factors involved in one's employment. **Oguchi's d.,** a form of hereditary night blindness occurring in Japan. **Ollier's d.,** enchondromatosis. **Oppenheim's d.,** amyotonia congenita. **organic d.,** one due to or accompanied by structural changes. **Ormond's d.,** retroperitoneal fibrosis. **Osgood-Schlatter d.,** osteochondrosis of the tuberosity of the tibia. **Osler's d.,** 1. polycythemia vera. 2. hereditary hemorrhagic telangiectasia. **Osler-Vaquez d.,** polycythemia vera. **Owren's d.,** parahemophilia. **Paget's d.,** 1. (of bone) osteitis deformans. 2. (of breast) an inflammatory cancerous affection of the areola and nipple. 3. an extramammary counterpart of Paget's disease (2), usually involving the vulva, and sometimes other sites, as the perianal and axillary regions. **Parkinson's d.,** paralysis agitans. **parrot d.,** psittacosis. **Parrot's d.,** see under *pseudoparalysis.* **Parry's d.,** Graves' d. **pearl d.,** tuberculosis of the peritoneum and mesentery of cattle. **Pel-Ebstein d.,** Hodgkin's d. **Pelizaeus-Merzbacher d.,** familial centrolobar sclerosis. **Pellegrini's d., Pellegrini-Stieda d.,** calcification of medial collateral ligament of knee due to trauma. **periodontal d.,** any disease or disorder of the periodontium. **Perthes' d.,** osteochondrosis of capitular femoral epiphysis. **Peyronie's d.,** induration of the corpora cavernosa of the penis, producing a fibrous chordee. **Pfeiffer's d.,** infectious mononucleosis. **Pick's d.,** 1. lobar atrophy. 2. ascites and fibrotic liver disease associated with constrictive pericarditis. **pink d.,** acrodynia. **Pompe's d.,** glycogenosis (type II) in which deficiency of the enzyme α-1,4-glucosidase results in generalized glycogen accumulation, with cardiomegaly, cardiorespiratory failure, and death; affected children appear imbecilic and are hypotonic. **Poncet's d.,** tuberculous arthritis. **Pott's d.,** tuberculosis of the spine, with osteitis or caries of the vertebrae, marked by stiffness of the spine, pain on motion, tenderness on pressure, and prominence of certain vertebral spines. **pulseless d.,** progressive obliteration of the brachiocephalic trunk and left subclavian and left common carotid arteries above their origin in the aortic arch, leading to loss of the pulse in both arms and carotids and to symptoms associated with ischemia of the brain, eyes, face, and arms. **Quincke's d.,** angioneurotic edema. **Raynaud's d.,** a primary or idiopathic vascular disorder, most often affecting women, marked by bilateral attacks of Raynaud's phenomenon. **Recklinghausen's d.,** 1. neurofibromatosis. 2. (of bone) osteitis fibrosa cystica generalisata. **Rendu-Osler-Weber d.,** hereditary hemorrhagic telangiectasia. **rheumatic heart d.,** the most important manifestation and sequel to rheumatic fever, consisting chiefly of valvular deformities. **Riggs' d.,** compound periodontitis. **Ritter's d.,** dermatitis exfoliativa neonatorum. **Roger's d.,** a ventricular septal defect; the term is usually restricted to small, asymptomatic defects. **Rokitansky's d.,** acute yellow atrophy of the liver. **runt d.,** a syndrome produced by immunologically competent cells in a foreign host that is unable to reject them, resulting in gross retardation of host development and in death. **Sandhoff's d.,** a variant of Tay-Sach's disease marked by a progressively more rapid course, due to a defect in the enzymes hexosaminidase A and B. **San Joaquin Valley d.,** coccidioidomycosis. **Schamberg's d.,** progressive pigmentary dermatosis. **Scheuermann's d.,** osteochondrosis of vertebral epiphyses in juveniles. **Schilder's d.,** a subacute or chronic leukoencephalopathy of children and adolescents, with massive destruction of the white substance of the cerebral hemispheres; clinical symptoms include blindness, deafness, bilateral spasticity, and mental deterioration. **Schimmelbusch's d.,** cystic d. of breast. **Schlatter-Osgood d.,** Osgood-Schlatter d. **Schönlein's d.,** see under *purpura.* **Schönlein-Henoch d.,** see under *purpura.* **Schüller's d.,** Hand-Schüller-Christian d. **Schüller-Christian d.,** Hand-Schüller-Christian d. **secondary d.,** 1. a morbid condition subsequent to or a consequence of another disease. 2. one due to introduction of incompatible, immunologically competent cells into a host rendered incapable of rejecting them by heavy exposure to ionizing radiation. **self-limited d.,** one which by its very nature runs a limited and definite course. **serum d.,** see under *sickness.* **silo-filler's d.,** pulmonary inflammation, often with acute pulmonary edema, due to inhalation of the irritant gases (especially oxides of nitrogen) which collect in recently filled silos. **Simmonds' d.,** see *panhypopituitarism.* **sixth d.,** exanthema subitum. **sixth venereal d.,** lymphogranuloma venereum. **Smith-Strang d.,** a hereditary defect in methionine absorption, in which the urine has a characteristic odor resembling that of the interior of an oasthouse due to alpha-hydroxybutyric acid formed by bacterial action on the unabsorbed methionine; it is marked by white hair, mental retardation, convulsions, and attacks of hyperpnea. **Spielmeyer-Vogt d.,** juvenile amaurotic familial idiocy, occurring between 5 and 10 years of age, and marked by "salt and pepper" pigmentation of the retinas; it shows no racial predilection as does the infantile form (*Tay-Sachs d.*). **Stan-**

ton's d., melioidosis. **Steinert's d.,** myotonic dystrophy. **stiff lamb d.,** stiffness and lameness of lambs, due to infection with *Erysipelothrix insidiosa.* **Still's d.,** juvenile rheumatoid arthritis. **Stokes' d.,** Graves' d. **Stokes-Adams d.,** Adams-Stokes d. **storage d.,** a metabolic disorder in which a specific substance (a lipid, a protein, etc.) accumulates in certain cells in unusually large amounts. **Strümpell's d.,** 1. hereditary lateral sclerosis with the spasticity mainly limited to the legs. 2. polioencephalomyelitis. **Strümpell-Leichtenstein d.,** hemorrhagic encephalitis. **Strümpell-Marie d.,** rheumatoid spondylitis. **Sturge-Weber d.,** see under *syndrome.* **Stuttgart d.,** leptospirosis affecting dogs. **Sudeck's d.,** post-traumatic osteoporosis. **Sutton's d.,** 1. halo nevus. 2. periadenitis mucosa necrotica recurrens. **sweet clover d.,** a hemorrhagic disease of cattle due to ingestion of spoiled sweet clover. **Swift's d.,** acrodynia. **Takayasu's d.,** pulseless d. **Tangier d.,** a familial disorder characterized by a deficiency of high-density lipoproteins in the blood serum, with storage of cholesterol esters in the tonsils and other tissues. **Tay-Sachs d.,** the infantile form of amaurotic idiocy, a hereditary disorder of lipid metabolism affecting chiefly Jewish infants, in which sphingolipids accumulate in the brain; it is marked by cerebromacular degeneration, progressive dementia, progressive loss of vision, paralysis, and death. It is distinguished by a cherry-red spot with a gray border on both retinas. **Teschen d.,** infectious porcine encephalomyelitis. **Thomsen's d.,** myotonia congenita. **thyrocardiac d.,** thyrotoxic heart d. **thyrotoxic heart d.,** heart disease associated with hyperthyroidism, marked by atrial fibrillation, cardiac enlargement, and congestive heart failure. **tsutsugamushi d.,** scrub typhus. **tunnel d.,** decompression sickness. **vagabonds' d.,** discoloration of the skin in persons subjected to louse bites over long periods. **Vaquez's d.,** polycythemia vera. **venereal d.,** a contagious disease usually acquired in sexual intercourse or other genital contact, including syphilis, gonorrhea, chancroid, granuloma inguinale, lymphogranuloma venereum, and balanitis gangrenosa. **veno-occlusive d. of liver,** acute or chronic, partial or complete occlusion of the branches of the hepatic veins by endophlebitis and thrombosis, leading to centrilobular necrosis, fibrosis, and ascites; most often seen in children. **Vincent's d.,** necrotizing ulcerative gingivostomatitis. **Volkmann's d.,** congenital deformity of the foot due to tibiotarsal dislocation. **von Hippel's d.,** angiomatosis confined principally to the retina. **von Hippel-Lindau d.,** a hereditary condition marked by angiomatosis of the retina and cerebellum, which may be associated with similar lesions of the spinal cord and cysts of the viscera; neurologic symptoms, including seizures and mental retardation, may be present. **von Jaksch's d.,** anemia pseudoleukemica infantum. **von Willebrand's d.,** angiohemophilia. **Waldenström's d.,** osteochondrosis of the capitular femoral epiphysis. **Weber-Christian d.,** nodular nonsuppurative panniculitis. **Weil's d.,** leptospiral jaundice. **Werlhof's d.,** idiopathic thrombocytopenia purpura. **Wernicke's d.,** see under *encephalopathy.* **Westphal-Strümpell d.,** hepatolenticular degeneration. **Whipple's d.,** intestinal lipodystrophy, a malabsorption syndrome marked by diarrhea, steatorrhea, skin pigmentation, arthralgia and arthritis, lymphadenopathy, central nervous system lesions, and infiltration of the intestinal muscosa with marcrophages containing PAS-positive material. **white muscle d.,** 1. muscular dystrophy in calves, due to vitamin E deficiency. 2. stiff lamb d. **Whitmore's d.,** melioidosis. **Wilson's d.,** hepatolenticular degeneration. **Winckel's d.,** a fatal disease of the newborn, with jaundice, hemoglobinuria, bloody urine, hemorrhage, cyanosis, collapse, and convulsions. **Wolman's d.,** primary familial xanthomatosis in infants, associated with involvement and calcification of the adrenal glands, failure to thrive, vomiting, diarrhea, hepatomegaly, splenomegaly, foam cells in the bone marrow and other tissues, and early death. **woolsorter's d.,** pulmonary anthrax. **x d.,** 1. hyperkeratosis (3). 2. aflatoxicosis.

disengagement (dis″en-gāj′ment) emergence of the fetus, or part thereof, from the vaginal canal.

disequilibrium (-e-kwĭ-lib′re-um) unstable equilibrium.

disgerminoma (dis-jer″mĭ-no′mah) dysgerminoma.

dish (dish) a shallow vessel of glass or other material for laboratory work. **evaporating d.,** a laboratory vessel, usually wide and shallow, in which material is evaporated by exposure to heat. **Petri d.,** a shallow glass dish for growing bacterial cultures. **Stender d.,** one of various forms and sizes, used in preparing and staining histologic specimens.

disinfect (dis″in-fekt′) to free from pathogenic organisms, or to render them inert.

disinfectant (-in-fek′tant) 1. freeing from infection. 2. an agent that disinfects, particularly one used on inanimate objects.

disinfection (-in-fek′shun) the act of disinfecting. **concomitant d., concurrent d.,** immediate disinfection and disposal of discharges and infective matter all through the course of a disease. **terminal d.,** disinfection of a sick room and its contents at the termination of a disease.

disinfestation (-in-fes-ta′shun) destruction of insects, rodents, or other animal forms present on the person or his clothes or in his surroundings, and which may transmit disease.

disinsectization (-in-sek″tĭ-za′shun) removal from or extermination of insects.

disintegrant (dis-in′tĕ-grant) an agent used in pharmaceutical preparation of tablets, which causes them to disintegrate and release their medicinal substances on contact with moisture.

Disipal (dis′ĭ-pal) trademark for a preparation of orphenadrine.

disjunction (dis-junk′shun) the act or state of being disjoined. In genetics, the moving apart of bivalent chromosomes at the first anaphase of meiosis. **craniofacial d.,** Le Fort III fracture.

disk (disk) a circular or rounded flat plate.

articular d., a pad of fibrocartilage or dense fibrous tissue present in some synovial joints. **Bowman's d's,** flat, disklike plates making up striated muscle fibers. **choked d.,** papilledema. **cupped d.,** a pathologically depressed optic disk. **dental d.,** a thin, round piece of paper or other material for carrying polishing powders or specially treated for use in various procedures on the teeth. **embryonic d.,** a flattish area in a cleaved ovum in which the first traces of the embryo are seen. **gelatin d.,** a disk or lamina of gelatin variously medicated, used chiefly in eye diseases. **germ d., germinal d.,** embryonic d. **Hensen's d.,** H band. **intervertebral d's,** layers of fibrocartilage between the bodies of adjacent vertebrae. **intra-articular d's,** fibrous structures within the capsules of diarthrodial joints. **optic d.,** the intraocular part of the optic nerve formed by fibers converging from the retina and appearing as a pink to white disk. **Placido's d.,** a disk marked with concentric circles, used in examining the cornea. **slipped d.,** popular term for herniation of an intervertebral disk.

diskectomy (dis-kek′to-me) excision of an intervertebral disk.

diskiform (dis′kĭ-form) in the shape of a disk.

diskitis (dis-ki′tis) inflammation of a disk, especially of an intervertebral disk.

diskogram (dis′ko-gram) a film produced by diskography.

diskography (dis-kog′rah-fe) radiography of the vertebral column after injection of radiopaque material into an intervertebral disk.

dislocation (dis″lo-ka′shun) displacement of a part. **complete d.,** one completely separating the surfaces of a joint. **compound d.,** one in which the joint communicates with the air through a wound. **consecutive d.,** one in which the displaced bone is not in the same position as when dislocated. **incomplete d.,** a slight displacement. **old d.,** one in which inflammatory or fibrotic changes have occurred. **partial d.,** incomplete d. **pathologic d.,** one due to paralysis, synovitis, infection, or other disease. **primitive d.,** one in which the bones remain as originally displaced. **recent d.,** one in which no inflammatory changes have occurred. **simple d.,** one in which there is no communication with the air through a wound. **subspinous d.,** dislocation of the head of the humerus into the space below the spine of the scapula.

dismemberment (dis-mem′ber-ment) amputation of a limb or a portion of it.

disocclude (dis″ŏ-klood′) to grind a tooth so that it does not touch its antagonist in the other jaw in any masticatory movements.

Disomer (di′so-mer) trademark for a preparation of dexbrompheniramine.

disomus (di-so′mus) a double-bodied monster.

disorder (dis-or′der) a derangement or abnormality of function; a morbid physical or mental state. **affective d's,** the group of psychoses characterized chiefly by a predominant mood (extreme depression or elation) or by alternations between such moods, including involutional melancholia and manic-depressive psychosis. **character d.,** a mental disorder characterized by maladaptive behavior, emotional responses that are socially unacceptable, and minimal feelings of anxiety or other symptoms that usually accompany neuroses. **functional d.,** a disorder not associated with any clearly defined physical or structural change. **mental d.,** any psychiatric illness or disease, whether functional or of organic origin. **personality d.,** a mental disorder which stems from the personality of the individual and in which there is minimal feeling of subjective anxiety and little or no feeling of distress. **psychophysiologic d.,** a mental disorder in which physical symptoms are presumed to be of psychogenic origin. **psychosomatic d.,** psychophysiologic d.

disorganization (dis-or″gan-i-za′shun) the process of destruction of any organic tissue; any profound change in the tissues of an organ or structure which causes the loss of most or all of its proper characters.

disorientation (-o″re-en-ta′shun) the loss of proper bearings, or a state of mental confusion as to time, place, or identity.

dispensary (-pen′ser-e) 1. a place for dispensation of free or low cost medical treatment. 2. any place where drugs and medicines are actually dispensed.

dispensatory (-pen′sah-tor″e) a book which describes medicines and their preparation and uses. **D. of the United States of America,** a collection of monographs on unofficial drugs and drugs recognized by the Pharmacopeia of the United States, the Pharmacopoeia of Great Britain, and the National Formulary, also on general tests, processes, reagents, and solutions of the U.S.P. and N.F., as well as drugs used in veterinary medicine.

dispersate (dis′per-sāt) a suspension of finely divided particles of a substance.

disperse (dis-pers′) to scatter the component parts, as of a tumor or the fine particles in a colloid system; also, the particles so dispersed.

dispersion (dis-per′zhun) 1. the act of scattering or separating; the condition of being scattered. 2. the incorporation of one substance into another. 3. a colloid solution.

dispersoid (-per′soid) a colloid in which the dispersity is relatively great.

dispireme (di-spi′rēm) the stage of cell division following the diaster.

displacement (dis-plās′ment) removal to an abnormal location or position; in psychology, unconscious transference of an emotion from its original object onto a more acceptable substitute.

disproportion (dis″pro-por′shun) a lack of the proper relationship between two elements or factors. **cephalopelvic d.,** a condition in which the fetal head is too large for the mother's pelvis.

disruption (dis-rup′shun) the act of separating forcibly, or the state of being abnormally separated.

dissect (dĭ-sekt′, di-sekt′) to cut apart, or separate; especially, the exposure of structures of a cadaver for anatomical study.

dissection (dĭ-sek′shun) 1. the act of dissecting. 2. a part or whole of an organism prepared by dissecting. **blunt d.,** dissection accomplished by separating tissues along natural cleavage lines, without cutting. **sharp d.,** dissection accomplished by incising tissues with a sharp edge.

dissector (dĭ-sek′tor) 1. one who dissects. 2. a handbook used as a guide for dissecting.

disseminated (dis-sem′ĭ-nāt″ed) scattered; distributed over a considerable area.

dissimilation (dĭ-sim″ĭ-la′shun) catabolism.

dissociation (dĭ-so″se-a′shun) 1. the act of separating or the state of being separated. 2. an intrapsychic defense process in which one or more groups of mental processes become separated off from normal consciousness and then function as a unitary whole. **atrial d.,** independent beating of the left and right atria, each with normal rhythm or with various combinations of normal rhythm, atrial flutter, or atrial fibrillation. **atrioventricular d.,** control of the atria by one pacemaker and of the ventricles by another, independent pacemaker.

dissogeny (dĭ-soj′ĕ-ne) the state of having sexual maturity in both a larval and an adult stage.

dissolution (dis″o-lu′shun) 1. the process in which one substance is dissolved in another. 2. separation of a compound into its components by chemical action. 3. liquefaction. 4. death.

dissolve (dĭ-zolv′) 1. to cause a substance to pass into solution. 2. to pass into solution.

distad (dis′tad) in a distal direction.

distal (dis′tal) remote; farther from any point of reference.

distalis (dis-ta′lis) [L.] distal.

distance (dis′tans) the measure of space intervening between two objects or two points of reference. **focal d.,** see under *length.* **hearing d.,** the maximum distance at which sound-producing stimuli can be perceived by the ear. **infinite d.,** in optics, a distance of 20 ft. or more; rays entering the eye from an object at that distance are practically as parallel as if they came from an infinite point. **interarch d.,** the vertical distance between the maxillary and mandibular arches under certain specified conditions of vertical dimension. **interocclusal d.,** the distance between the occluding surfaces of the maxillary and mandibular teeth with the mandible in physiologic rest position. **interocular d.,** the distance between the eyes, usually used in reference to the interpupillary distance. **target-skin d.,** the distance between the anode from which roentgen rays are reflected and the skin of the body surface interposed in their path. **working d.,** the distance between the front lens of a microscope and the object when the instrument is correctly focused.

distemper (dis-tem′per) a name for several infectious diseases of animals, especially *canine distemper,* a highly fatal viral disease of dogs, marked by fever, loss of appetite, and a discharge from the nose and eyes.

distichia (-tik′e-ah) distichiasis.

distichiasis (dis″tĭ-ki′ah-sis) the presence of a double row of eyelashes, one or both of which are turned in against the eyeball.

distillate (dis′tĭ-lāt) a product of distillation.

distillation (dis″tĭ-la′shun) conversion of a liquid into vapors which are reconverted to liquid form, as a means of eliminating contaminants from the original solution. **destructive d., dry d.,** decomposition of a solid by heating in the absence of air, resulting in volatile liquid products. **fractional d.,** that attended by the successive separation of volatilizable substances in order of their respective volatility.

distobuccal (dis″to-buk′al) pertaining to or formed by the distal and buccal surfaces of a tooth, or by the distal and buccal walls of a tooth cavity.

distobucco-occlusal (-buk″o-ŏ-kloo′zal) pertaining to or formed by the distal, buccal, and occlusal surfaces of a tooth.

distobuccopulpal (-pul′pal) pertaining to or formed by the distal, buccal, and pulpal walls of a tooth cavity.

distocervical (dis″to-ser′vĭ-kal) 1. pertaining to the distal surface of the neck of a tooth. 2. distogingival.

distoclusion (-kloo′zhun) malrelation of the dental arches with the lower jaw in a distal or posterior position in relation to the upper.

distogingival (-jin-ji′val) pertaining to or formed by the distal and gingival walls of a tooth cavity.

distomia (di-sto′me-ah) the presence of two mouths.

distomiasis (dis″to-mi′ah-sis) infection due to trematodes or flukes.

distomolar (-mo′lar) a supernumerary molar; any tooth distal to a third molar.

distortion (dĭ-stor′shun) the state of being twisted out of normal shape or position; in psychiatry, the conversion of material offensive to the superego into acceptable form. **parataxic d.,** distortions in judgment and perception, particularly in interpersonal relations, based upon the need to perceive objects and relationships in accord with a pattern from earlier experience.

distraction (dĭ-strak′shun) 1. diversion of attention. 2. separation of joint surfaces without rupture of their binding ligaments and without displacement.

distress (dĭ-stres′) physical or mental anguish or suffering. **idiopathic respiratory d. of newborn,** see *respiratory distress syndrome of newborn.*

distrix (dis′triks) the splitting of hairs at their distal ends.

disulfiram (di-sul′fĭ-ram) a disulfide compound, $C_{10}H_{20}N_2S_4$, used to treat alcoholics.

dithiazanine iodide (di″thi-az′ah-nēn) an anthelmintic, $C_{23}H_{23}IN_2S_2$, used against strongylids and whipworms.

diurese (di″u-rēs′) the act of effecting diuresis.

diuresis (di″u-re′sis) increased excretion of urine.

diuretic (di″u-ret′ik) 1. increasing urine excretion or the amount of urine. 2. an agent that promotes urine secretion.

Diuril (di′u-ril) trademark for preparations of chlorothiazide.

diurnal (di-er′nal) pertaining to or occurring during the daytime, or period of light.

divagation (di″vah-ga′shun) incoherent or wandering speech.

divalent (di-va-lent) 1. bivalent. 2. carrying an electronic charge of two units.

divergence (di-ver′jens) a moving apart, or inclination away from a common point. **diver′gent,** adj.

diverticular (di″ver-tik′u-lar) pertaining to or resembling a diverticulum.

diverticulectomy (di″ver-tik″u-lek′to-me) excision of a diverticulum.

diverticulitis (di″ver-tik″u-li′tis) inflammation of a diverticulum.

diverticulogram (di″ver-tik′u-lo-gram) a roentgenogram of a diverticulum.

diverticulosis (di″ver-tik″u-lo′sis) the presence of diverticula.

diverticulum (di″ver-tik′u-lum), pl. *divertic′ula* [L.] a circumscribed pouch or sac occurring normally or created by herniation of the lining mucous membrane through a defect in the muscular coat of a tubular organ. **false d.,** an intestinal diverticulum due to the protrusion of the mucous membrane through a tear in the muscular coat. **intestinal d.,** one formed by hernial protrusion of the mucous membrane through a defect in the muscular coat of the intestine. **Meckel's d.,** an occasional sacculation or appendage of the ileum, derived from an unobliterated yolk stalk. **Nuck's d.,** see under *canal.* **pharyngoesophageal d.,** a diverticulum at the pharyngoesophageal junction. **pituitary d.,** Rathke's pouch. **pressure d., pulsion d.,** one formed by hernial protrusion of the mucous membrane through the muscular coat of the esophagus as a result of pressure from within. **Rokitansky's d.,** a traction diverticulum of the esophagus. **traction d.,** a localized distortion, angulation, or funnel-shaped bulging of the esophageal wall, due to adhesions resulting from external lesion. **Zenker's d.,** pharyngoesophageal d.

division (dĭ-vizh′un) the act of separating into parts. **cell d.,** fission of a cell. **direct cell d.,** see *amitosis.* **indirect cell d.,** see *meiosis* and *mitosis.* **maturation d.,** meiosis.

divulsion (dĭ-vul′shun) the act of separating or pulling apart.

divulsor (dĭ-vul′ser) an instrument for dilating the urethra.

dizygotic (di″zi-got′ik) pertaining to or derived from two separate zygotes (fertilized ova).

dizziness (diz′ĭ-nes) a disturbed sense of relationship to space; a sensation of unsteadiness and a feeling of movement within the head; vertigo is sometimes used erroneously as a synonym.

DL chemical prefix (small capitals) denoting that the substance is an equimolecular mixture of two enantiomorphs, one of which corresponds in configuration to D-glyceraldehyde, the other to L-glyceraldehyde.

D.M.D. Doctor of Dental Medicine.

D.M.F. *d*ecayed, *m*issing, *f*illed (teeth): an index used in dental surveys.

D.M.R.D. Diploma in Medical Radio-Diagnosis (Brit.).

D.M.R.T. Diploma in Medical Radio-Therapy (Brit.).

DMSO dimethyl sulfoxide.

DNA deoxyribonucleic acid.

DNase deoxyribonuclease.

D.N.B. dinitrobenzene.

D.O. Doctor of Osteopathy.

D.O.A. dead on admission (arrival).

Doca (do′kah) trademark for desoxycorticosterone acetate.

Docibin (do′si-bin) trademark for a crystalline preparation of vitamin B_{12}.

dock (dok) to remove part or all of the tail of an animal.

doctor (dok′tor) a practitioner of the healing arts, as one graduated from a college of medicine, osteopathy, dentistry, or veterinary medicine, and licensed to practice.

dol (dōl) a unit of pain intensity.

dolich(o)- word element [Gr.], *long*.

dolichocephalic (dol″ĭ-ko-sĕ-fal′ik) long headed; having a cephalic index of 75.9 or less.

dolichoderus (-dēr′us) an individual with a long neck.

dolichofacial (-fa′shal) having a long face.

dolichomorphic (-mor′fik) having a long, thin, asthenic body type.

dolichopellic (-pel′ik) having a pelvic index of 95 or above.

Dolophine (do′lo-fēn) trademark for a preparation of methadone.

dolor (do′lor) [L.] pain; one of the cardinal signs of inflammation. **d. cap′itis,** headache.

dolorific (do″lor-if′ik) producing pain.

dolorimeter (-im′ĕ-ter) an instrument for measuring pain in dols.

dolorogenic (do-lor″o-jen′ik) dolorific.

DOM 2,5-dimethoxy-4-methylamphetamine.

dominance (dom′ĭ-nans) 1. the supremacy, or superior manifestation, in a specific situation of one of two or more competitive or mutually antagonist factors. 2. the appearance, in a heterozygote, of one of two alternative parental characters. **incomplete d.,** failure of one gene to be completely dominant, heterozygotes showing a phenotype intermediate between the two parents.

dominant (dom′ĭ-nant) 1. exerting a ruling or controlling influence; in genetics, capable of expression when carried by only one of a pair of homologous chromosomes. 2. a dominant allele or trait.

donor (do′ner) 1. an organism that supplies living tissue to be used in another body, as a person who furnishes blood for transfusion, or an organ for transplantation. 2. a substance or compound that contributes part of itself to another substance (acceptor). **hydrogen d.,** a substance or compound that gives up hydrogen to another substance. **universal d.,** a person with group O blood; such blood is sometimes used in emergency transfusion.

Donovania (don″o-va′ne-ah) a genus of schizomycetes, inluding *D. granulomatis,* the etiologic agent of granuloma inguinale.

dopa (do′pah) 3,4-dihydroxyphenylalanine, produced by oxidation of tyrosine by tyrosinase; it is the precursor of dopamine and an intermediate product in the biosynthesis of norepinephrine, epinephrine, and melanin. L-dopa, the naturally occurring form, and levodopa, the synthetic form, are used in parkinsonism and manganese poisoning.

dopamine (-mēn) a compound, hydroxytyramine, produced by the decarboxylation of dopa, an intermediate product in the synthesis of norepinephrine.

dopaminergic (-mēn-er′jik) activated or transmitted by dopamine; pertaining to tissues or organs affected by dopamine.

dopa-oxidase (-ok′sĭ-dās) an enzyme that oxidizes dopa to melanin in the skin, producing pigmentation.

Dorbane (dor′bān) trademark for a preparation of danthron.

Doriden (dor′ĭ-den) trademark for preparations of glutethimide.

Dormison (dor′mĭ-son) trademark for a preparation of methylparafynol.

dornase (dor′nās) a shortened term for *deoxyribonuclease;* also a word termination, as in strepto*dornase.* **pancreatic d.,** a stabilized preparation of deoxyribonuclease, prepared from beef pancreas; used as an aerosol to reduce the tenacity of pulmonary secretions.

Dornavac (dor′nah-vak) trademark for a preparation of pancreatic dornase.

dors(o)- word element [L.], *the back; the dorsal aspect.*

Dorsacaine (dor′sah-kān) trademark for a preparation of benoxinate.

dorsad (dor′sad) toward the back.

dorsal (dor′sal) directed toward or situated on the back surface; opposite of ventral.

dorsalgia (dor-sal′je-ah) pain in the back.

dorsalis (dor-sa′lis) [L.] dorsal.

dorsiflexion (dor″sĭ-flek′shun) backward flexion or bending, as of the hand or foot.

dorsocephalad (dor″so-sef′ah-lad) toward the back of the head.

dorsolateral (-lat′er-al) pertaining to the back and the side.

dorsoventral (-ven′tral) 1. pertaining to the back and belly surfaces of a body. 2. passing from the back to the belly surface.

dorsum (dor′sum), pl. *dor′sa* [L.] 1. the back; the posterior or superior surface of a body or body part, as of the foot or hand. 2. the aspect of an anatomical structure or part corresponding in position to the back; posterior in the human.

dosage (do′sij) the determination and regulation of the size, frequency, and number of doses.

dose (dōs) the quantity to be administered at one time, as a specified amount of medication or a given quantity of radiation. **absorbed d.,** that amount of energy from ionizing radiations absorbed per unit mass of matter, expressed in rads. **air d.,** the intensity of a roentgen-ray or gamma-ray beam in air, expressed in roentgens. **booster d.,** an amount of immunogen (vaccine, toxoid, or other antigen preparation), usually smaller than the original amount, injected at an appropriate interval after primary immunization to sustain the immune response to that immunogen. **curative d.,** that which is sufficient to restore normal health. **curative d., median,** a dose that abolishes symptoms in 50% of test subjects; abbrev. C.D.$_{50}$. **divided d.,** a fraction of the total quantity of a drug prescribed to be given at intervals, usually during a 24-hour period. **effective d.,** that quantity of a drug that will produce the effects for which it is given. **effective d., median,** that quantity of an agent that produces its effects in 50% of test subjects. **erythema d.,** the amount of radiation which, when applied to the skin, causes temporary reddening. **fatal d.,** lethal d. **infective d.,** that amount of pathogenic organisms that will cause infection in susceptible subjects. **infective d., median,** the amount of pathogenic microorganisms that will cause infection in 50% of the test subjects. **lethal d.,** that quantity of an agent that will or may be sufficient to cause death. **lethal d., median,** the quantity of an agent that will kill 50% of the test subjects; in radiology, the amount of radiation that will kill, within a specified period, 50% of individuals in a large group or population. **lethal d., minimum,** 1. the amount of toxin that will just kill an experimental animal. 2. the smallest quantity of diphtheria toxin that will kill a guinea pig of 250-gm. weight in 4 to 5 days when injected subcutaneously. **maximum d.,** the largest dose consistent with safety. **maximum permissible d.,** the largest amount of ionizing radiation that one may safely receive according to recommended limits in radiation protection guides. **minimum d.,** the smallest dose that will produce an appreciable effect. **permissible d.,** that amount of ionizing radiation which is not expected to lead to appreciable bodily injury. **skin d.,** 1. the air dose of radiation at the skin surface, comprising the primary radiation plus backscatter. 2. the absorbed dose in the skin. **threshold erythema d.,** the single skin dose that will produce in 80% of those tested, a faint but definite erythema within 30 days, and in the other 20%, no visible reaction. Abbreviated T.E.D. **tolerance d.,** the largest quantity of an agent that may be administered without harm.

dosimeter (do-sim'ĕ-ter) an instrument used to detect and measure exposure to radiation.

dosimetry (do-sim'ĕ-tre) scientific determination of amount, rate, and distribution of radiation emitted from a source of ionizing radiation.

dot (dot) a small spot or speck. **Gunn's d's,** white dots seen about the macula lutea on oblique illumination. **Maurer's d's,** irregular dots, staining red with Leishman's stain, seen in erythrocytes infected with *Plasmodium falciparum*. **Mittendorf's d.,** a congenital anomaly manifested as a small gray or white opacity just inferior and nasal to the posterior pole of the lens, representing the remains of the lenticular attachment of the hyaloid artery; it does not affect vision. **Schüffner's d's,** small granules seen in erythrocytes infected with *Plasmodium*

vivax when stained by certain methods. **Trantas' d's,** small, white calcareous-looking dots in the limbus of the conjunctiva in vernal conjunctivitis.

double-blind (dŭ'b'l-blīnd') denoting a study of the effects of a specific agent in which neither the administrator nor the recipient, at the time of administration, knows whether the active or an inert substance is given.

doublet (dub'let) a combination of two similar or complementary entities.

douche (dōōsh) [Fr.] a stream of water directed against a part of the body or into a cavity. **air d.,** a current of air blown into a cavity, particularly into the tympanum to open the eustachian tube.

douglasitis (dug"lah-si'tis) inflammation of the rectouterine excavation (Douglas' cul-de-sac).

dourine (doo-rēn') a contagious venereal disease of equine species, due to *Trypanosoma equiperdum*.

dowel (dow'el) a peg or pin for fastening an artificial crown or core to a natural tooth root, or affixing a die to a working model for construction of a crown, inlay, or partial denture.

doxapram (dok'sah-pram) a respiratory stimulant, $C_{24}H_{30}N_2O_2$, used as the hydrochloride salt.

Doxinate (dok'si-nāt) trademark for a preparation of dioctyl sodium sulfosuccinate.

doxycycline (dok"se-si'klēn) a broad-spectrum antibiotic, $C_{22}H_{24}N_2O$, synthetically derived from oxytetracycline, active against a wide range of gram-positive and gram-negative organisms.

doxylamine (dok"sil-am'ēn) an antihistaminic, $C_{17}H_{22}N_2O$, used as the bisuccinate salt.

D.P. Doctor of Pharmacy; Doctor of Podiatry.

D.P.H. Department of Public Health; Diplomate in Public Health; Doctor of Public Health.

DPT diptheria-pertussis-tetanus; see under *vaccine.*

DR reaction of degeneration.

Dr. Doctor.

dr. dram.

drachm (dram) dram.

dracunculiasis, dracunculosis (drah-kung"-ku-li'ah-sis; -lo'sis) infection by nematodes of the genus *Dracunculus.*

Dracunculus (drah-kung'ku-lus) a genus of nematode parasites, including *D. medinen'sis* (guinea worm), a threadlike worm, 30–120 cm. long, which is widely distributed in India, Africa, and Arabia, inhabiting subcutaneous and intermuscular tissues of man and certain other animals.

draft (draft) potion or dose.

drain (drān) any device by which a channel or open area may be established for exit of fluids or purulent material from a cavity, wound, or infected area. **cigarette d.,** one made by drawing a strip of gauze or surgical sponge into a tube of gutta-percha. **controlled d.,** a square of gauze, filled with gauze strips, pressed into a wound, the corners of the square and ends of the strips left protruding. **Mikulicz's d.,** a single layer of gauze, packed with several thick wicks of gauze, pushed into a wound cavity. **Penrose d.,** cigarette d. **quarantine d.,** one left in place after laparotomy to drain the peritoneal cavity. **stab wound d.,** one brought out through a small puncture wound at some distance from the operative incision, to prevent infection of the operation wound. **Wylie d.,** a hard rubber pessary with a grooved stem.

drainage (drān'ij) systematic withdrawal of fluids and discharges from a wound, sore, or cavity. **capillary d.,** that effected by strands of hair, catgut, spun glass, or other material of small caliber which acts by capillary attraction. **closed d.,** drainage of an empyema cavity carried out with protection against the entrance of outside air into the pleural cavity. **open d.,** drainage of an empyema cavity through an opening in the chest wall into which one or more rubber drainage tubes are inserted, the opening not being sealed against the entrance of outside air. **postural d.,** therapeutic drainage in bronchiectasis and lung abscess by placing the patient head downward so that the trachea will be inclined below the affected area. **through d.,** that effected by passing a perforated tube through the cavity, so that irrigation may be effected by injecting fluid into one aperture and letting it escape out of another. **tidal d.,** drainage of the urinary bladder by an apparatus which alternately fills the bladder to a predetermined pressure and empties it by a combination of siphonage and gravity flow.

dram (dram) a unit of measure in the avoirdupois (27.34 grains, $\frac{1}{16}$ ounce) or apothecaries' (60 grains, $\frac{1}{8}$ ounce) system. **fluid d.,** a unit of liquid measure of the apothecaries' system, containing 60 minims; equivalent to 3.697 ml.

Dramamine (dram'ah-mēn) trademark for preparations of dimenhydrinate.

dramatism (dram'ah-tizm) pompous and dramatic speech and behavior in mental disorder.

dream (drēm) a conscious series of images, emotions, or thoughts occurring during sleep.

drepanocyte (drep'ah-no-sīt″) a sickle cell. **drepanocyt'ic,** adj.

drepanocytosis (drep″ah-no-si-to'sis) the presence of sickle cells in the blood.

dressing (dres'ing) any of various materials used for covering and protecting a wound. **antiseptic d.,** gauze impregnated with antiseptic material. **occlusive d.,** one that seals a wound from contact with air or bacteria. **pressure d.,** one by which pressure is exerted on the covered area to prevent collection of fluids in underlying tissues.

drift (drift) a chance variation, as in gene frequency from one generation to another; the smaller the population, the greater are the random variations.

Drinalfa (drin-al'fah) trademark for preparations of methamphetamine.

drip (drip) the slow, drop-by-drop infusion of a liquid. **Murphy d.,** the continuous drop by drop administration per rectum of saline solution. **postnasal d.,** drainage of excessive mucous or

mucopurulent discharge from the postnasal region into the pharynx.

Drisdol (driz'dol) trademark for preparations of ergocalciferol (vitamin D).

drive (drīv) the force that activates human impulses.

drocarbil (dro-kar'bil) a veterinary anthelmintic, $C_{16}H_{23}AsN_2O_7$.

Drolban (drol'ban) trademark for a preparation of dromostanolone.

dromograph (drom'o-graf) a recording flowmeter for measuring blood flow.

dromostanolone (dro″mo-stan'o-lōn) an androgenic, anabolic steroid, $C_{23}H_{36}O_3$; used in the form of the propionate ester as an antineoplastic agent in the treatment of breast carcinoma.

dromotropic (-trop'ik) affecting conductivity of a nerve fiber.

drop (drop) 1. a minute sphere of liquid as it hangs or falls. 2. a descent or falling below the usual position.

droperidol (dro-per'ĭ-dol) a tranquilizer of the butyrophenone series, $C_{22}H_{22}FN_3O_2$, used as a narcoleptic preanesthetic, and, in combination with fentanyl citrate (known as *Innovar*), as a neuroleptanalgesic.

dropper (drop'er) a pipet or tube for dispensing liquid in drops.

dropsical (drop'sĭ-kal) affected with or pertaining to dropsy.

dropsy (drop'se) the abnormal accumulation of serous fluid in cellular tissues or in a body cavity.

drowning (drown'ing) suffocation and death resulting from filling of the lungs with water or other substance or fluid.

Dr.P.H. Doctor of Public Health.

drug (drug) 1. any medicinal substance. 2. a narcotic. 3. to administer a drug to.

druggist (drug'ist) pharmacist.

drum (drum) 1. the middle ear. 2. the tympanic membrane.

drumhead (drum'head) the tympanic membrane.

drumstick (-stik) a nuclear lobule attached by a slender strand to the nucleus of some polymorphonuclear leukocytes of normal females but not of normal males.

drusen (droo'sen) 1. hyaline excrescences in Bruch's membrane of the eye, usually due to aging. 2. rosettes of granules occurring in the lesions of actinomycosis.

dualism (du'al-izm) 1. the theory that there are two distinct stem cells for blood cell formation: one for the lymphatic cells and the other for the myeloid cells. 2. the doctrine that body and mind are independent units.

duazomycin (du-az″o-mi'sin) an antibiotic substance with antineoplastic properties, produced by *Streptomyces ambofaciens*.

Ducobee (doo'ko-be) trademark for preparations of vitamin B_{12}; see *cyanocobalamin*.

duct (dukt) a passage with well-defined walls, especially a tubular structure for the passage of excretions or secretions. **duc'tal,** adj. **aberrant d.,** any duct that is not usually present or that takes an unusual course or direction. **alveolar d's,** small passages connecting the respiratory bronchioles and alveolar sacs. **Bartholin's d.,** the larger of the sublingual ducts, which opens into the submandibular duct. **Bellini's d's,** the excretory or collecting portions of the renal tubules. **bile d's, biliary d's,** the passages for the conveyance of bile in and from the liver. **Botallo's d.,** ductus arteriosus. **branchial d's,** the drawn-out branchial grooves which open into the temporary cervical sinus of the embryo. **cochlear d.,** a spiral tube in the bony canal of the cochlea, divided into the scala tympani and scala vestibuli by the lamina spiralis. **common bile d.,** the duct formed by the union of the cystic and hepatic ducts. **d's of Cuvier,** two short venous trunks in the fetus opening into the atrium of the heart; the right one becomes the superior vena cava. **cystic d.,** the passage connecting the gallbladder neck and the common bile duct. **deferent d.,** ductus deferens. **efferent d.,** any duct which gives outlet to a glandular secretion. **ejaculatory d.,** the duct formed by union of the ductus deferens and the duct of the seminal vesicle, opening into the prostatic urethra on the colliculus seminalis. **endolymphatic d.,** a canal connecting the membranous labyrinth of the ear with the endolymphatic sac. **excretory d.,** one that is merely conductive and not secretory. **galactophorous d's,** lactiferous d's. **gall d's,** bile d's. **Gartner's d.,** a closed rudimentary duct lying parallel to the uterine tube, into which transverse ducts of the epoophoron open; it is the remains of the part of the mesonephros that participates in formation of the reproductive organs. **genital d.,** see under *canal.* **hepatic d.,** the excretory duct of the liver, or one of its branches in the lobes of the liver. **interlobular d's,** channels between different lobules of a gland. **lacrimal d.,** see under *canaliculus.* **lacrimonasal d.,** nasolacrimal d. **lactiferous d's,** ducts conveying the milk secreted by the mammary lobes to and through the nipples. **Luschka's d's,** tubular structures in the wall of the gallbladder; some are connected with bile ducts, but none with the lumen of the gallbladder. **lymphatic d's,** channels for conducting lymph. **lymphatic d., left,** thoracic d. **lymphatic d., right,** a vessel draining lymph from the upper right side of the body, receiving lymph from the right subclavian, jugular, and mediastinal trunks when those vessels do not open independently into the right brachiocephalic vein. **mammary d's,** lactiferous d's. **mesonephric d.,** an embryonic duct of the mesonephros, which in the male becomes the ductus deferens and in the female is largely obliterated. **metanephric d.,** ureter. **milk d's,** lactiferous d's. **d. of Müller, müllerian d.,** paramesonephric d. **nasolacrimal d.,** the canal conveying the tears from the lacrimal sac to the inferior meatus of the nose. **omphalomesenteric d.,** yolk stalk. **pancreatic d.,** the main excretory duct of the pancreas, which usually unites with the common bile duct before entering the duodenum. **papillary d's,** the straight excretory or collecting portions of the renal tubules, which descend through the renal medulla to a renal papilla. **paramesonephric d.,** either of the paired embryonic ducts developing into the uterine tubes, uterus, and vagina in the female and becoming largely obliterated in the male. **paraurethral d's,** ducts inconstantly present in the female, which drain a group of the urethral glands into the vestibule. **parotid d.,** the duct by which the parotid gland empties into the mouth. **perilymphatic d.,** a small canal connecting the scala tympani of the cochlea with the subarachnoid space. **pronephric d.,** the duct of the pronephros, which later serves as the mesonephric duct. **prostatic d's,** ducts from the prostate, opening into or near the prostatic sinuses on the posterior urethra. **d's of Rivinus,** the small sublingual ducts which open into the mouth on the sublingual fold. **salivary d's,** the ducts of the salivary glands. **Santorini's d.,** a small inconstant duct draining a part of the head of the pancreas into the minor duodenal papilla. **secretory d.,** a smaller duct that is tributary to an excretory duct of a gland and that also has a secretory function. **semicircular d's,** the long ducts of the membranous labyrinth of the ear. **seminal d's,** the passages for conveyance of spermatozoa and semen. **spermatic d.,** ductus deferens. **d. of Steno, d. of Stensen,** parotid d. **sublingual d's,** the excretory ducts of the sublingual gland. **submandibular d., submaxillary d.,** the duct that drains the submandibular gland and opens at the sublingual caruncle. **tear d.,** lacrimal canaliculus. **thoracic d.,** the canal that ascends from the cisterna chyli to the junction of the left subclavian and left internal jugular vein. **thyroglossal d.,** an embryonic duct extending between the thyroid primordium and the posterior tongue. **urogenital d's,** the paramesonephric and mesonephric ducts. **Wharton's d.,** submandibular d. **d. of Wirsung,** pancreatic d. **wolffian d.,** mesonephric d.

ductile (duk′til) susceptible of being drawn out without breaking.

ductless (dukt′les) having no excretory duct.

ductule (duk′tūl) a minute duct.

ductulus (duk′tu-lus), pl. *duc′tuli* [L.] ductule.

ductus (duk′tus), pl. *duc′tus* [L.] duct. **d. arterio′sus,** fetal blood vessel which joins the aorta and pulmonary artery. **d. arterio′sus, patent,** abnormal persistence of an open lumen in the ductus arteriosus after birth. **d. choledo′chus,** common bile duct. **d. def′erens,** the excretory duct of the testis which joins the excretory duct of the seminal vesicle to form the ejaculatory duct. **d. veno′sus,** a major blood channel that develops through the embryonic liver from the left umbilical vein to the inferior vena cava.

Dulcolax (dul′ko-laks) trademark for preparations of bisacodyl.

dull (dul) not resonant on percussion.

dullness (dul′nes) diminished resonance on percussion; also a peculiar percussion sound that lacks the normal resonance.

dumb (dum) unable to speak; mute.

dumbness (dum′nes) mutism, or aphasia.

dumping (dump′ing) see under *syndrome.*

duodenal (du″o-de′nal) of or pertaining to the duodenum.

duodenectomy (du″o-dĕ-nek′to-me) excision of the duodenum, total or partial.

duodenitis (du″o-dĕ-ni′tis) inflammation of the duodenum.

duodenocholedochotomy (du″o-de″no-ko-led″o-kot′o-me) incision of the duodenum and common bile duct.

duodenoenterostomy (-en″ter-os′to-me) anastomosis of the duodenum to some other part of the small intestine.

duodenography (du″o-dĕ-nog′rah-fe) radiography of the duodenum.

duodenohepatic (du″o-dĕ-no-hĕ-pat′ik) pertaining to the duodenum and liver.

duodenoileostomy (-il″e-os′to-me) anastomosis of the duodenum to the ileum.

duodenojejunostomy (-je″ju-nos′to-me) anastomosis of the duodenum to the jejunum.

duodenorrhaphy (du″o-dĕ-nor′ah-fe) suture of the duodenum.

duodenoscope (du″o-de′no-skōp) an endoscope for examining the duodenum.

duodenoscopy (du″o-dĕ-nos′ko-pe) examination of the duodenum by an endoscope.

duodenostomy (-nos′to-me) surgical formation of a permanent opening into the duodenum.

duodenotomy (-not′o-me) incision of the duodenum.

duodenum (du″o-de′num) the first or proximal portion of the small intestine, extending from the pylorus to the jejunum.

Duphaston (du-fas′ton) trademark for preparations of dydrogesterone.

duplication (du-plĭ-ka′shun) a doubling; in genetics, the presence of an extra segment of chromosome.

dupp (dup) a syllable used to represent the second heart sound in auscultation.

Durabolin (du-rab′o-lin) trademark for a preparation of nandrolone.

Duracillin (du″rah-sil-in) trademark for preparations of crystalline procaine penicillin G.

dural (du′ral) pertaining to the dura mater.

dura mater (du′rah ma′ter) the outermost, toughest of the three meninges (membranes) of the brain and spinal cord.

duroarachnitis (du″ro-ar″ak-ni′tis) inflammation of the dura mater and arachnoid.

dust (dust) a finely powdered substance. **blood d.,** hemoconia. **ear d.,** statoconia.

D.V.M. Doctor of Veterinary Medicine.

dwarf (dwarf) an abnormally undersized person. **achondroplastic d.,** a dwarf having a relatively large head with saddle nose and brachycephaly, short extremities, and usually lordosis. **Amsterdam d.,** a dwarf affected with de Lange's syndrome. **asexual d.,** an adult dwarf with deficient sexual development. **ateliotic d.,** a dwarf with infantile skeleton, with persistent nonunion between epiphyses and diaphyses. **infantile d.,** a person with retardation of mental and physical development. **micromelic d.,** a dwarf with very small limbs. **normal d.,** an abnormally undersized but perfectly formed person. **phocomelic d.,** a dwarf in whom the diaphyses of the long bones are abnormally short. **pituitary d.,** a dwarf whose condition is due to hypofunction of the anterior pituitary. **pure d.,** normal d. **rachitic d.,** a person dwarfed by rickets, having a high forehead with prominent bosses, bent long bones, and Harrison's groove. **renal d.,** a dwarf whose failure to achieve normal bone maturation is due to renal failure. **sexual d.,** a dwarf with normal sexual development.

dwarfism (dwarf′fizm) the state of being a dwarf; underdevelopment of body.

Dy chemical symbol, *dysprosium.*

dyad (di′ad) a double chromosome resulting from the halving of a tetrad.

Dyclone (di′klōn) trademark for a preparation of dyclonine.

dyclonine (di′klo-nēn) a topical anesthetic, C_{18}-$H_{27}O_2$, used as the hydrochloride salt.

dydrogesterone (di″dro-jes′ter-ōn) a synthetic progestin, $C_{21}H_{28}O_2$, used orally in treatment of amenorrhea and of abnormal uterine bleeding due to hormonal imbalance.

dye (di) any of various colored substances containing auxochromes and thus capable of coloring substances to which they are applied; used for staining and coloring, as test reagents, and as therapeutic agents. **acid d., acidic d.,** one which is acidic in reaction and usually unites with positively charged ions of the material acted upon. **amphoteric d.,** one containing both reactive basic and reactive acidic groups, and staining both acidic and basic elements. **anionic d.,** acid d. **basic d.,** one which is basic in reaction and unites with negatively charged ions of the material acted upon. **cationic d.,** basic d.

dynamic (di-nam′ik) pertaining to or manifesting force.

dynamics (di-nam′iks) the scientific study of forces in action; a phase of mechanics.

dynamogenesis (di″nah-mo-jen′ĕ-sis) the development of energy or force. **dynamogen′ic,** adj.

dynamograph (di-nam′o-graf) a self-registering dynamometer.

dynamometer (di″nah-mom′ĕ-ter) an instrument for measuring the force of muscular contraction.

dynamoneure (di-nam′o-nūr) a spinal neuron connected with the muscles.

dynamoscope (-skōp) a device for performing dynamoscopy.

dynamoscopy (di″nah-mos′ko-pe) the observation of function of an organ or structure, as of muscle action, or of kidney function by ureteral catheterization.

dyne (dīn) the metric unit of force, being that amount which would, during each second, produce an acceleration of 1 cm. per second in a particle of 1 gram mass.

dyphilline (di-fil′in) a theophylline compound, $C_{10}H_{14}N_4O_4$, used as a diuretic and as a bronchodilator and peripheral vasodilator.

dys- prefix [Gr.], *bad; difficult; disordered.*

dysacousia, dysacousis (dis″ah-koo′se-ah; -ah-koo′sis) dysacusis.

dysacusis (-ak-koo-sis) 1. a hearing impairment in which the loss is not measurable in decibels, as in disturbances in discrimination of speech or tone quality, pitch, or loudness, etc. 2. a condition in which certain sounds produce discomfort.

dysadrenalism (dis″ad-re′nal-izm) any disorder of adrenal function, whether of decreased or heightened function.

dysadrenia (dis″ah-dre′ne-ah) dysadrenalism.

dysaphia (dis-a′fe-ah) impairment of the sense of touch.

dysarteriotony (dis″ar-tēr″e-ot′o-ne) abnormality of blood pressure.

dysarthria (dis-ar′thre-ah) imperfect articulation of speech due to disturbances of muscular control resulting from central or peripheral nervous system damage.

dysarthrosis (dis″ar-thro′sis) 1. deformity or malformation of a joint. 2. dysarthria.

dysaudia (dis-aw′de-ah) impaired hearing.

dysautonomia (dis″aw-to-no′me-ah) a hereditary condition marked by defective lacrimation, skin blotching, emotional instability, motor incoordination, and hyporeflexia.

dysbarism (dis′bar-izm) any clinical syndrome due to difference between the surrounding atmospheric pressure and the total gas pressure in the tissues, fluids, and cavities of the body.

dysbasia (dis-ba′ze-ah) difficulty in walking, especially that due to nervous lesion.

dysbulia (dis-bu′le-ah) weakness or perversion of will. **dysbu′lic,** adj.

dyscephaly (dis-sef′ah-le) malformation of the cranium and bones of the face. **dyscephal′ic,** adj.

dyschezia (dis-ke′ze-ah) difficult or painful defecation.

dyschiria (dis-ki′re-ah) loss of power to tell which side of the body has been touched.

dyscholia (dis-ko′le-ah) a disordered condition of the bile.

dyschondroplasia (dis″kon-dro-pla′ze-ah) enchondromatosis.

dyschromatopsia (dis″kro-mah-top′se-ah) disorder of color vision.

dyschromia (dis-kro′me-ah) any disorder of pigmentation of skin or hair.

dyschronism (dis-kro′nizm) separate in time; disturbance of any time relation.

dyscinesia (dis″si-ne′ze-ah) dyskinesia.

dyscoria (dis-ko′re-ah) abnormality in the form or shape of the pupil or in the reaction of the two pupils.

dyscorticism (dis-kor′ti-sizm) disordered functioning of the adrenal cortex.

dyscrasia (dis-kra′ze-ah) a morbid condition. **dyscrat′ic,** adj. **blood d.,** any abnormal or pathologic condition of the blood.

dysdiadochokinesia (dis″di-ah-do″ko-ki-ne′ze-ah) derangement of the function of diadochokinesia. **dysdiadochokinet′ic,** adj.

dysembryoma (dis″em-bre-o′mah) teratoma.

dysentery (dis′en-ter″e) any of a number of disorders marked by inflammation of the intestine, especially of the colon, with abdominal pain, tenesmus, and frequent stools containing blood and mucus. **dysenter′ic,** adj. **amebic d.,** dysentery caused by *Entamoeba histolytica;* amebic colitis. **bacillary d.,** dysentery caused by *Shigella.* **viral d.,** dysentery caused by a virus, occurring in epidemics and marked by acute watery diarrhea.

dyserethesia (dis″er-ĕ-the′ze-ah) impairment of sensibility.

dysergasia (-ga′ze-ah) a behavior disorder due to organic changes in the nervous system, with disorientation, hallucination, and delirious reactions.

dysergia (dis-er′je-ah) motor incoordination due to defect of efferent nerve impulse.

dysesthesia (dis″es-the′ze-ah) 1. impairment of any sense, especially of the sense of touch. 2. a painful, persistent sensation induced by a gentle touch of the skin. **auditory d.,** dysacusis (2).

dysfunction (dis-funk′shun) disturbance, impairment, or abnormality of functioning of an organ.

dysgalactia (dis″gah-lak′te-ah) disordered milk secretion.

dysgammaglobulinemia (dis-gam″mah-glob″-u-lin-e′me-ah) an immunological deficiency state marked by selective deficiencies of one or more, but not all, classes of immunoglobulins, resulting in heightened susceptibility to those infectious diseases vulnerable to immunoglobulin-associated defense mechanisms. **dysgammaglobuline′mic,** adj.

dysgenesis (dis-jen′ĕ-sis) defective development; malformation. **gonadal d.,** any of a variety of gonadal developmental anomalies, including gonadal aplasia, Turner's syndrome, etc.

dysgenics (dis-jen′iks) the study of racial deterioration.

dysgerminoma (dis-jer″mĭ-no′mah) a solid, often radiosensitive, malignant ovarian neoplasm derived from undifferentiated germinal cells; the counterpart of seminoma of the testis.

dysgeusia (dis-gu′ze-ah) impairment of the sense of taste.

dysglobulinemia (dis-glob″u-lin-e′me-ah) any disorder of the blood globulins.

dysglycemia (dis″gli-se′me-ah) any disorder of blood sugar metabolism.

dysgnathia (dis-na′the-ah) any oral abnormality extending beyond the teeth to involve the maxilla or mandible, or both. **dysgnath′ic,** adj.

dysgnosia (dis-no′ze-ah) any abnormality of the intellect.

dysgonic (dis-gon′ik) seeding badly; said of bacterial cultures that grow poorly.

dysgraphia (dis-gra′fe-ah) inability to write properly; it may be part of a language disorder due to disturbance of the parietal lobe or of the motor system.

dyshematopoiesis (dis-hem″ah-to-poi-e′sis) defective blood formation. **dyshematopoiet′ic,** adj.

dyshemopoiesis (dis-he″mo-poi-e′sis) dyshematopoiesis.

dyshidrosis (dis″hĭ-dro′sis) 1. pompholyx. 2. any disorder of eccrine sweat glands.

dysjunction (dis-junk′shun) see *disjunction*.

dyskaryosis (dis″kar-e-o′sis) abnormality of the nucleus of a cell. **dyskaryot′ic,** adj.

dyskeratoma (dis″ker-ah-to′mah) a dyskeratotic tumor. **warty d.,** a solitary brownish red nodule with a soft, yellowish, central keratotic plug, most commonly occurring on the face, neck, scalp, or axilla, or in the mouth; histologically it resembles an individual lesion of keratosis follicularis.

dyskeratosis (dis″ker-ah-to′sis) abnormal, premature, or imperfect keratinization of the keratinocytes. **dyskeratot′ic,** adj.

dyskinesia (dis″ki-ne′ze-ah) impairment of the power of voluntary movement. **dyskinet′ic,** adj. **d. al′gera,** a condition in which movement is painful. **biliary d.,** derangement of the filling and emptying mechanism of the gallbladder. **d. intermit′tens,** intermittent disability of the limbs due to impaired circulation.

dyslalia (dis-la′le-ah) impairment of ability to speak associated with abnormality of external speech organs.

dyslexia (dis-lek′se-ah) impairment of ability to comprehend written language, due to a central lesion. **dyslex′ic,** adj.

dyslochia (dis-lo′ke-ah) disordered lochial discharge.

dyslogia (dis-lo′je-ah) impairment of the reasoning power; also, impairment of speech, due to mental disorders.

dysmaturity (dis″mah-tūr′ĭ-te) the condition of being small or immature for gestational age; said of fetuses that are the product of a pregnancy involving placental dysfunction. **pulmonary d.,** Wilson-Mikity syndrome.

dysmelia (dis-me′le-ah) malformation of a limb or limbs due to disturbance in embryonic development.

dysmenorrhea (dis″men-or-re′ah) painful menstruation. **dysmenorrhe′al,** adj. **congestive d.,** that accompanied by great congestion of the uterus. **essential d.,** that for which there is no demonstrable cause. **inflammatory d.,** that due to inflammation. **membranous d.,** that marked by membranous exfoliations derived from the uterus. **obstructive d.,** that due to mechanical obstruction to the discharge of menstrual fluid. **primary d.,** essential d. **secondary d.,** that due to a pelvic lesion. **spasmodic d.,** that due to spasmodic uterine contraction.

dysmetria (dis-me′tre-ah) inability to properly direct or limit motions.

dysmimia (dis-mim′e-ah) impairment of the power to express thought by gestures.

dysmnesia (dis-ne′ze-ah) disordered memory.

dysmyotonia (dis″mi-o-to′ne-ah) muscular dystonia; abnormal tonicity.

dysodontiasis (dis″o-don-ti′ah-sis) defective, delayed, or difficult eruption of the teeth.

dysontogenesis (dis″on-to-jen′ĕ-sis) defective embryonic development. **dysontogenet′ic,** adj.

dysopia (dis-o′pe-ah) defective vision.

dysorexia (dis″o-rek′se-ah) impaired or deranged appetite.

dysosmia (dis-oz′me-ah) impairment of the sense of smell.

dysosteogenesis (dis-os″te-o-jen′ĕ-sis) defective bone formation; dysostosis.

dysostosis (dis″os-to′sis) defective ossification; defect in the normal ossification of fetal cartilages. **cleidocranial d.,** a hereditary condition marked by defective ossification of the cranial bones, complete or partial absence of the clavicles, and dental and vertebral anomalies. **craniofacial d.,** a hereditary condition marked by acrocephaly, exophthalmos, hypertelorism, strabismus, parrot-beaked nose, and hypoplastic maxilla with relative mandibular prognathism. **mandibulofacial d.,** a hereditary disorder occurring in a complete form (*Franceschetti's syndrome*) with antimongoloid slant of the palpebral fissures, coloboma of the lower lid, micrognathia and hypoplasia of the zygomatic arches, and microtia, and in an incomplete form (*Treacher Collins syndrome*) with the same anomalies in lesser degree. **metaphyseal d.,** a skeletal abnormality in which the epiphyses are normal or nearly so, and the metaphyseal tissues are replaced by masses of cartilage, producing interference with enchondral bone formation and expansion and thinning of the metaphyseal cortices. **d. mul′tiplex,** Hurler's syndrome. **orodigitofacial d.,** orofaciodigital syndrome.

dysoxidizable (dis-ok′sĭ-dīz″ah-b'l) not easily oxidizable.

dyspancreatism (dis-pan′kre-ah-tizm″) disorder of function of the pancreas.

dyspareunia (dis″pah-ru′ne-ah) difficult or painful coitus in women.

dyspepsia (dis-pep′se-ah) impairment of the power or function of digestion; usually applied to epigastric discomfort after meals. **dyspep′tic,** adj. **acid d.,** that associated with excessive acidity of the stomach. **intestinal d.,** that arising in the intestines. **nervous d.,** that which is functional in origin.

dysphagia (dis-fa′je-ah) difficulty in swallowing.

dysphasia (dis-fa′ze-ah) impairment of speech, consisting in lack of coordination and failure to arrange words in their proper order; due to a central lesion.

dysphemia (dis-fe′me-ah) stuttering or other speech disorder due to psychoneurosis.

dysphonia (dis-fo′ne-ah) any voice impairment; difficulty in speaking. **dysphon′ic,** adj. **d. clerico′rum,** loss of the voice from overuse, as by clergymen.

dysphoria (dis-fo′re-ah) disquiet; restlessness; malaise.

dysphrasia (dis-fra′ze-ah) imperfection of speech due to a central or cerebral defect.

dyspigmentation (dis″pig-men-ta′shun) a disorder of pigmentation of skin or hair.

dyspituitarism (dis″pĭ-tu′ĭ-tar-izm″) a condition due to disordered activity of the pituitary gland.

dysplasia (dis-pla′ze-ah) abnormality of development; in pathology, alteration in size, shape, and organization of adult cells. **dysplas′tic,** adj. **anhidrotic ectodermal d.,** congenital ectodermal defect. **anteroposterior facial d.,** defective development resulting in abnormal anteroposterior relations of the maxilla and mandible to each other or to the cranial base. **chondroectodermal d.,** achondroplasia with defective development of skin, hair, and teeth, polydactyly, and defect of cardiac septum. **congenital alveolar d.,** respiratory distress syndrome of newborn. **cretinoid d.,** a developmental abnormality characteristic of cretinism, consisting of retarded ossification and smallness of the internal and sexual organs. **dental d.,** developmental abnormality producing abnormal relationship of a varying number of teeth with their opposing members. **diaphyseal d.,** thickening of the cortex of the midshaft area of the long bones, progressing toward the epiphyses, and sometimes also in the flat bones. **epiphyseal d.,** faulty growth and ossification of the epiphyses with roentgenographically apparent stippling and decreased stature, not associated with thyroid disease. **fibrous d. (of bone),** thinning of the cortex of bone and replacement of bone marrow by gritty fibrous tissue containing bony spicules, causing pain, disability, and gradually increasing deformity; only one bone may be involved (*monostotic fibrous d.*), with the process later affecting several or many bones (*polyostotic fibrous d.*). **fibrous d. of jaw,** cherubism. **hereditary ectodermal d.,** congenital ectodermal defect. **hidrotic ectodermal d.,** a hereditary condition marked by generalized hypotrichosis, dystrophy of the nails, and hyperpigmentation; hyperkeratosis of the palms and soles and mental deficiency may also occur. **metaphyseal d.,** a disturbance in enchondral bone growth, failure of modeling causing the ends of the shafts to remain larger than normal in circumference. **thymic d.,** any of a group of hereditary disorders characterized by faulty development of the thymus, which may be associated with (*a*) normal serum immunoglobulin levels and impaired cell-mediated immunity (*Nezelof's syndrome*), (*b*) Swiss type agammaglobulinemia and impairment of both cell-mediated and humoral immunity, or (*c*) variable deficiencies of immunoglobulins, the severity being dependent on the degree of the deficiency.

dyspnea (disp-ne′ah) labored or difficult breathing. **dyspne′ic,** adj. **functional d.,** respiratory distress not caused by organic disease and unrelated to exertion but associated with anxiety states. **paroxysmal nocturnal d.,** respiratory distress related to posture (especially reclining at night), usually attributed to congestive heart failure with pulmonary edema.

dyspragia (dis-pra′je-ah) painful performance of any function.

dyspraxia (dis-prak′se-ah) partial loss of ability to perform coordinated acts.

dysprosium (dis-pro′ze-um) chemical element (*see table*), at. no. 66, symbol Dy.

dysproteinemia (dis-pro″te-in-e′me-ah) disorder of the protein content of the blood.

dysraphia (dis-ra′fe-ah) incomplete closure of the embryonic neural tube.

dysrhythmia (dis-rith′me-ah) a disturbance of rhythm. **cerebral d., electroencephalographic d.,** a disturbance or irregularity in the rhythm of the brain waves as recorded by electroencephalography.

dyssebacea (dis″se-ba′she-ah) disorder of sebaceous follicles; specifically, a condition seen (but not exclusively) in riboflavin deficiency, marked by greasy, branny seborrhea on the midface, with erythema in the nasal folds, canthi, or other skin folds.

dyssomnia (dis-som′ne-ah) a disorder of sleep.

dysspermia (dis-sper′me-ah) impairment of the spermatozoa, or of the semen.

dysstasia (dis-sta′ze-ah) difficulty in standing. **dysstat′ic,** adj.

dyssynergia (dis″sin-er′je-ah) muscular incoordination. **d. cerebella′ris myoclon′ica,** a condition characterized by cerebellar dyssynergia, myoclonus, and epilepsy. **d. cerebella′ris progressi′va,** a condition marked by generalized tremors associated with disturbance of muscle tone and of muscular coordination; due to disorder of cerebellar function.

dystaxia (dis-tak′se-ah) difficulty in controlling voluntary movements.

dystectia (dis-tek′she-ah) defective closure of the neural tube.

dysthymia (dis-thi′me-ah) mental depression; also, any intellectual anomaly.

dysthyroidism (dis-thi′roi-dizm) imperfect development and function of the thyroid.

dystocia (dis-to′se-ah) abnormal labor or childbirth. **fetal d.,** that due to the shape, size, or position of the fetus. **maternal d.,** that due to some condition inherent in the mother. **placental d.,** difficult delivery of the placenta.

dystonia (dis-to′ne-ah) impairment of muscular tonus. **dyston′ic,** adj. **d. musculo′rum defor′mans,** a hereditary disorder marked by involuntary, irregular, clonic contortions of the muscles of the trunk and extremities, which twist the body forward and sideways in a grotesque fashion.

dystopia (dis-to′pe-ah) malposition; displacement. **dystop′ic,** adj.

dystrophia (dis-tro′fe-ah) [Gr.] dystrophy. **d. adiposogenita′lis,** adiposogenital dystrophy. **d. epithelia′lis cor′neae,** dystrophy of the corneal epithelium, with erosions. **d. myoton′ica,** myotonic dystrophy. **d. un′guium,** changes in the texture, structure, and/or color of the nails due to no demonstrable cause, but presumed to be attributable to some disturbance of nutrition. **d. un′guis media′na canalifor′mis,** a fissure or groove near the middle of a nail, starting at the cuticle and extending (with nail growth) to the free edge.

dystrophoneurosis (dis-trof″o-nu-ro′sis) 1. any nervous order due to poor nutrition. 2. impairment of nutrition due to nervous disorder.

dystrophy (dis′tro-fe) any disorder due to defective or faulty nutrition. **dystroph′ic,** adj. **adiposogenital d.,** a condition marked by adiposity of the feminine type, genital hypoplasia, changes in secondary sex characters, and metabolic disturbances; seen with lesions of the hypothalamus. **Duchenne's muscular d.,** pseudohypertrophic muscular d. **Landouzy-Déjerine d.,** a relatively benign form of muscular dystrophy, with marked atrophy of the muscles of the face, shoulder girdle, and arm. **Leyden-Möbius d.,** limb-girdle muscular d. **limb-girdle muscular d.,** slowly progressive muscular dystrophy, usually beginning in childhood, marked by weakness and wasting in the shoulder or pelvic girdle. **median canaliform d. of the nail,** dystrophia unguis mediana canaliformis. **muscular d.,** a group of genetically determined, painless, degenerative myopathies marked by muscular weakness and atrophy without nervous system involvement; see *pseudohypertrophic muscular d., Landouzy-Déjerine d.,* and *limb-girdle muscular d.* **myotonic d.,** a rare, slowly progressive, hereditary disease, marked by myotonia followed by muscular atrophy (especially of the face and neck), cataracts, hypogonadism, frontal balding, and cardiac disorders. **progressive muscular d.,** muscular d. **pseudohypertrophic muscular d.,** muscular dystrophy affecting the shoulder and pelvic girdles, beginning in childhood and marked by increasing weakness, pseudohypertrophy of the muscles, followed by atrophy, and a peculiar swaying gait with the legs kept wide apart. **Salzmann's nodular corneal d.,** a progressive hypertrophic degeneration of the epithelial layer of the cornea, Bowman's membrane, and the outer portion of the corneal stroma.

dystrypsia (dis-trip′se-ah) derangement of intestinal or pancreatic digestion due to lack of trypsin.

dysuria (dis-u′re-ah) painful or difficult urination. **dysu′ric,** adj.

E

E. electromotive force; emmetropia; eye.

ear (ēr) the organ of hearing; see Plate XII. **Blainville's e.,** congenital difference in size or shape of the ears. **Cagot e.,** one without a lower lobe. **cauliflower e.,** a partially deformed auricle due to injury and subsequent perichondritis. **diabetic e.,** mastoiditis complicating diabetes. **external e.,** the auricle and external meatus together. **inner e., internal e.,** the vestibule, cochlea, and semicircular canals together. **middle e.,** an air space in the temporal bone containing the auditory ossicles; see Plate XII.

earache (ēr′āk) pain in the ear; otalgia.

earwax (ēr′waks) cerumen.

eburnation (e″ber-na′shun) conversion of bone into a hard, ivory-like mass.

EBV Epstein-Barr virus.

ecaudate (e-kaw′dāt) tail-less.

ecbolic (ek-bol′ik) oxytocic.

ecbovirus (ek″bo-vi′rus) an enteric orphan virus isolated from cattle.

eccentric (ek-sen′trik) 1. situated or occurring away from a center. 2. proceeding from a center.

eccentrochondroplasia (ek-sen″tro-kon″dro-pla′ze-ah) Morquio's syndrome.

eccentro-osteochondrodysplasia (-os″te-o-kon″dro-dis-pla′ze-ah) Morquio's syndrome.

ecchondroma (ek″kon-dro′mah) a hyperplastic growth of cartilaginous tissue on the surface of a cartilage or projecting under the periosteum of a bone.

ecchondrosis (ek″kon-dro′sis) ecchondroma.

ecchymoma (ek″ĭ-mo′mah) swelling due to blood extravasation.

ecchymosis (ek″ĭ-mo′sis), pl. *ecchymo′ses* [Gr.] a small hemorrhagic spot, larger than a petechia, in the skin or mucous membrane, forming a nonelevated, rounded or irregular, blue or purplish patch. **ecchymot′ic,** adj.

eccrine (ek′rin) exocrine, with special reference to ordinary sweat glands.

eccrisis (ek′rĭ-sis) excretion of waste products.

eccritic (ek-krit′ik) 1. promoting excretion. 2. an agent which promotes excretion.

eccyesis (ek″si-e′sis) ectopic pregnancy.

ecdovirus (ek″do-vi′rus) an enteric orphan virus isolated from dogs.

ecdysis (ek′dĭ-sis) desquamation or sloughing, especially the molting of an outer covering and development of a new one as occurs in certain arthropods, crustaceans, snakes, and lizards.

ecdysone (ek′dĭ-sōn) the hormone produced in the prothoracic glands of arthropods that induces molting (ecdysis) and metamorphosis.

ECG electrocardiogram.

ecgonine (ek′go-nin) the final basic product, $C_9H_{15}NO_3$, obtained by hydrolysis of cocaine and several related alkaloids.

echinococcosis (e-ki″no-kok-o′sis) hydatid disease.

Echinococcus (-kok′us) a genus of small tapeworms, including *E. granulo′sus,* usually parasitic in dogs and wolves, whose larvae (hydatids) may develop in mammals, forming hydatid tumors or cysts chiefly in the liver; and *E. multilocula′ris,* whose larvae form alveolar or multilocular rather than unilocular cysts and whose adult forms usually parasitize the fox and wild rodents, although man is sporadically infected.

echo (ek′o) a repeated sound, produced by reverberation of sound waves; also, the reflection of ultrasonic, radio, and radar waves. **amphoric e.,** a resonant repetition of a sound heard on auscultation of the chest, occurring at an appreciable interval after the vocal sound. **metallic e.,** a ringing repetition of the heart sounds sometimes heard in patients with pneumopericardium and pneumothorax.

echoacousia (ek″o-ah-koo′ze-ah) the subjective experience of hearing echoes after normally heard sounds.

echocardiogram (-kar′de-o-gram″) the record produced by echocardiography.

echocardiography (-kar″de-og′rah-fe) recording of the position and motion of the heart walls or internal structures of the heart and neighboring tissue by the echo obtained from beams of ultrasonic waves directed through the chest wall.

echoencephalogram (-en-sef′ah-lo-gram″) the record produced by echoencephalography.

echoencephalography (-en-sef″ah-log′rah-fe) a diagnostic technique in which pulses of ultrasonic waves are beamed through the head from both sides, and echoes from the midline structures of the brain are recorded graphically; shifts from the midline may indicate a centrally placed mass.

echogram (ek′o-gram) the record made by echography.

echography (ĕ-kog′rah-fe) the use of ultrasound as a diagnostic aid. Ultrasound waves are directed at the tissues, and a record is made, as on an oscilloscope, of the waves reflected back through the tissues, which indicate interfaces of different acoustic densities and thus differentiate between solid and cystic structures.

echolalia (ek″o-la′le-ah) automatic repetition by a patient of what is said to him.

echomimia (-mim′e-ah) echopraxia.

echomotism (-mo′tizm) echopraxia.

echopathy (ek-op′ah-the) automatic repetition by a patient of words or movements of others.

echopraxia (ek″o-prak′se-ah) the spasmodic and involuntary imitation of the movements of others.

echothiophate iodide (-thi′o-fāt) a cholinesterase inhibitor, $C_9H_{23}INO_3PS$, used in the treatment of glaucoma.

echovirus (-vi′rus) an enterovirus isolated from man, separable into many serotypes, certain of which are associated with human disease, especially aseptic meningitis.

eclabium (ek-la′be-um) eversion of a lip.

eclampsia (e-klamp′se-ah) convulsions and coma, rarely coma alone, occurring in a pregnant or puerperal woman, and associated with hypertension, edema, and/or proteinuria. **eclamp′tic,** adj. **puerperal e.,** that occurring after childbirth. **uremic e.,** that due to uremia.

eclampsism (e-klamp′sizm) preeclampsia.

eclamptogenic (e-klamp″to-jen′ik) causing convulsions.

ecmnesia (ek-ne′ze-ah) forgetfulness of recent events with remembrance of more remote ones.

ecmovirus (ek″mo-vi′rus) an enteric orphan virus isolated from monkeys.

Ecolid (e′ko-lid) trademark for a preparation of chlorisondamine.

ecologist (e-kol′o-jist) a person skilled in ecology.

ecology (e-kol′o-je) the science of organisms as affected by environmental factors; study of the environment and life history of organisms. **ecolog′ic, ecolog′ical,** adj.

ecomania (e″ko-ma′ne-ah) an attitude of mind that is dominating toward family members but humble toward those in authority.

ecosystem (ek′o-sis″tem) the fundamental unit in ecology, comprising the living organisms and the nonliving elements interacting in a certain defined area.

ecphylaxis (ek″fi-lak′sis) a condition of impotency of the antibodies in the blood. **ecphylac′tic,** adj.

écraseur (a″krah-zer′) [Fr.] an instrument with a loop of chain or wire for removing parts.

ecsovirus (ek″si-vi′rus) an enteric orphan virus isolated from swine.

E.C.T. electroconvulsive therapy.

ect(o)- word element [Gr.], *external; outside.*

ectad (ek′tad) directed outward.

ectal (ek′tal) external.

ectasia (ek-ta′ze-ah) dilatation, expansion, or distention. **ectat′ic,** adj. **mammary duct e.,** dilatation of the collecting ducts of the mammary gland, with inspissation of gland secretion and inflammatory changes in the tissues.

ectental (ek-ten′tal) pertaining to the ectoderm and entoderm, and to their line of junction.

ectethmoid (ek-teth′moid) one of the paired lateral masses of the ethmoid bone.

ecthyma (ek-thi′mah) a shallowly ulcerative form of impetigo, chiefly on the shins or forearms. **e. syphilit′icum,** an eruption of pustules in tertiary syphilis.

ectoantigen (ek″to-an′tĭ-jen) 1. an antigen that seems to be loosely attached to the outside of bacteria. 2. an antigen formed in the ectoplasm (cell membrane) of a bacterium.

ectoblast (ek′to-blast) the ectoderm.

ectocardia (ek″to-kar′de-ah) congenital displacement of the heart.

ectocervix (-ser′viks) portio vaginalis. **ectocer′vical,** adj.

ectocinerea (-sĭ-ne′re-ah) the cortical gray matter of the brain.

ectoderm (ek′to-derm) the outermost of the three primitive germ layers of the embryo; from it are derived the epidermis and epidermic tissues, such as the nails, hair, and glands of the skin, the nervous system, external sense organs (eye, ear, etc.) and mucous membrane of the mouth and anus. **ectoder′mal, ectoder′mic,** adj. **amniotic e.,** the inner layer of the amnion (and covering of the umbilical cord) that is continuous with body ectoderm. **basal e.,** trophoblast covering the eroded uterine tissue that faces the placental sinuses. **extraembryonic e.,** the epithelial covering of the chorion and lining of the amnion. **neural e.,** the region of the ectoderm destined to become the neural tube.

ectodermosis (ek″to-der-mo′sis) a disorder based on congenital maldevelopment of organs derived from the ectoderm. **e. erosi′va pluri-orificia′lis,** Stevens-Johnson syndrome.

ectoentad (-en′tad) from without inward.

ectoenzyme (-en′zīm) an extracellular enzyme.

ectogenous (ek-toj′ĕ-nus) introduced from without; arising from causes outside the organism.

ectoglobular (ek″to-glob′u-lar) formed outside the blood cells.

ectogony (ek-tog′o-ne) the influence exerted on the mother by the developing embryo.

ectohormone (ek″to-hor′mōn) a hormone secreted to the outside of the body, as a pheromone.

ectomere (ek′to-mēr) one of the blastomeres taking part in formation of the ectoderm.

ectomorph (ek′to-morf) an individual exhibiting ectomorphy.

ectomorphy (-mor″fe) a type of body build in which tissues derived from the ectoderm predominate; a somatotype in which both visceral and body structures are relatively slightly developed, the body being linear and delicate. **ectomor′phic,** adj.

-ectomy word element [Gr.], *excision; surgical removal.*

ectopagus (ek-top′ah-gus) a double monster connected along the side of the body.

ectoparasite (ek″to-par′ah-sīt) a parasite living on the outside of the host's body. **ectoparasit′ic,** adj.

ectophyte (ek′to-fīt) a vegetable parasite living on the outside of the host's body.

ectopia (ek-to′pe-ah) [Gr.] displacement or malposition, especially if congenital. **e. cor′dis,** congenital displacement of the heart outside the thoracic cavity. **e. i′ridis,** displacement of the iris, with abnormal smallness of the pupil. **e. len′tis,** abnormal position of the lens of the eye. **e. pupil′lae congen′ita,** congenital displacement of the pupil.

ectopic (ek-top′ik) 1. pertaining to or characterized by ectopia. 2. located away from normal position.

ectoplasm (ek′to-plazm) cell membrane.

ectoplastic (-plas″tik) having formative power on the surface, as ectoplastic cells.

ectopy (ek′to-pe) ectopia.

ectosteal (ek-tos′te-al) pertaining to or situated outside of a bone.

ectostosis (ek″to-sto′sis) ossification beneath the perichondrium of a cartilage or the periosteum of a bone.

ectothrix (ek′to-thriks) a fungus that grows inside the shaft of a hair, but produces a conspicuous external sheath of spores.

ectozoon (ek″to-zo′on) ectoparasite.

ectro- word element [Gr.], *miscarriage; congenital absence.*

ectrodactyly (ek″tro-dak′tĭ-le) congenital absence of all or part of a digit (*partial e.*).

ectrogeny (ek-troj′ĕ-ne) congenital absence or defect of a part. **ectrojen′ic,** adj.

ectromelia (-me′le-ah) gross hypoplasia or aplasia of one or more long bones of one or more limbs. **ectromel′ic,** adj.

ectromelus (ek-trom′ĕ-lus) an individual with rudimentary arms and legs.

ectropion (ek-tro′pe-on) eversion or turning outward, as of the margin of an eyelid. **e. u′veae,** eversion of the margin of the pupil.

ectrosyndactyly (ek″tro-sin-dak′tĭ-le) a condition in which some digits are absent and those that remain are webbed.

ectylurea (ek″til-u-re′ah) a urea compound, $C_7H_{12}N_2O_2$, used as a sedative.

eczema (ek′zĕ-mah) 1. a superficial inflammatory process involving primarily the epidermis, marked early by redness, itching, minute papules and vesicles, weeping, oozing, and crusting, and later by scaling, lichenification, and often pigmentation. 2. atopic dermatitis. **contact e.,** see under *dermatitis* (1). **facial e. of ruminants,** a photosensitive disease of ruminants, particularly in New Zealand, due to ingestion of the spores of the mold *Pithomyces chartarum,* which contain sporidesmin. **e. herpet′icum,** disseminated herpes simplex; see *Kaposi's varicelliform eruption.* **e. margina′tum,** tinea cruris. **nummular e., e. nummula′re,** that in which the patches are coin shaped; it may be a form of neurodermatitis. **stasis e.,** see under *dermatitis.* **e. vaccina′tum,** disseminated vaccinia; see *Kaposi's varicelliform eruption.*

eczematoid (ek-zem′ah-toid) resembling eczema.

eczematous (ek-zem′ah-tus) characterized by or of the nature of eczema.

E.D. effective dose; erythema dose.

E.D.$_{50}$ median effective dose; a dose that produces its effects in 50% of a population.

edema (ĕ-de′mah) an abnormal accumulation of fluid in intercellular spaces of the body. **angioneurotic e.,** recurring attacks of transient edema suddenly appearing in areas of the skin or mucous membranes and occasionally of the viscera, often associated with dermographia, urticaria, erythema, and purpura. In the hereditary form, associated with failure of inhibition of complement component C1, there tends to be more visceral involvement. **brain e.,** an excessive accumulation of fluid in the brain substance (*wet brain*). **cardiac e.,** a manifestation of congestive heart failure, due to increased venous and capillary pressures and often associated with renal sodium retention. **dependent e.,** edema affecting most severely the lowermost or dependent parts of the body. **malignant e.,** that marked by rapid extension, quick destruction of tissue, and the formation of gas. **e. neonato′rum,** a disease of premature and feeble infants resembling sclerema, marked by spreading edema with cold, livid skin. **nonpitting e.,** that in which the tissues cannot be pitted by pressure. **pitting e.,** that in which pressure leaves a persistent depression in the tissues. **pulmonary e.,** diffuse extravascular accumulation of fluid in the pulmonary tissues and air spaces due to changes in hydrostatic forces in the capillaries or to increased capillary permeability; it is marked by intense dyspnea. **Quincke's e.,** angioneurotic e.

edematogenic (ĕ-dem″ah-to-jen′ik) producing or causing edema.

edematous (ĕ-dem′ah-tus) characterized by or pertaining to edema.

edentia (e-den′she-ah) absence of the teeth.

edentulate (-tu-lāt) edentulous.

edentulous (-tu-lus) without teeth.

edetate (ed′ĕ-tāt) any salt of edetic acid, including *e. disodium calcium,* used in the diagnosis and treatment of lead poisoning, and *e. disodium,* used in the treatment of poisoning with lead and other heavy metals and, because of its affinity for calcium, in treatment of hypercalcemia.

edrophonium (ed″ro-fo′ne-um) a cholinergic, $C_{10}H_{16}NO$, used in the form of the chloride salt as a curare antagonist and as a diagnostic agent in myasthenia gravis.

EDTA edetic acid.

EEE eastern equine encephalomyelitis.

EEG electroencephalogram.

E.E.N.T. eye-ear-nose-throat.

effacement (ĕ-fās′ment) the obliteration of form or features; said of the cervix during labor when it is so changed that only the external os remains.

effect (ĕ-fekt′) the result produced by an action. **additive e.,** the combined effect produced by the action of two or more agents, being equal to the sum of their separate effects. **anachoretic e.,** anachoresis. **Bohr e.,** displacement of the oxyhemoglobin dissociation curve by a change in carbon dioxide tension. **Crabtree e.,** the inhibition of oxygen consumption on the addition of glucose to tissues or microorganisms having a high rate of aerobic glycolysis; the converse of the Pasteur effect. **cumulative e.,** see under *action.* **Doppler e.,** the relationship of the apparent frequency of waves, as of sound, light, and radio waves, to the relative motion of the source of the waves and the observer, the frequency increasing as the two approach each other and decreasing as they move apart. **Pasteur e.,** the decrease in the rate of glucose utilization glycolysis and the suppression of lactate accumulation by tissues or microorganisms in the presence of oxygen. Cf. *Crabtree e.* **photechic e.,** Russell e. **position e.,** in genetics, the changed effect produced by alteration of the relative positions of various genes on the chromosomes. **pressure e.,** the sum of the changes that are due to obstruction of tissue drainage by pressure. **Russell e.,** making a photographic plate developable by substances other than light. **side e.,** see under S.

effectiveness (ĕ-fek′tiv-nes) the ability to produce a specific result or to exert a specific measurable influence. **relative biological e.,** an expression of the effectiveness of other types of radiation in comparison with that of gamma or roentgen rays; abbreviated RBE.

effector (ĕ-fek′tor) a muscle or gland that contracts or secretes, respectively, in direct response to nerve impulses.

effemination (ĕ-fem″ĭ-na′shun) feminization.

efferent (ef′er-ent) conveying away from a center, as an efferent nerve.

effleurage (ef″lu-rahzh′) [Fr.] a stroking movement in massage.

efflorescence (ef″lo-res′ens) 1. quality of being efflorescent. 2. a rash or eruption.

efflorescent (ef″lo-res′ent) becoming powdery by losing the water of crystallization.

effluvium (ĕ-floo′ve-um), pl. *efflu′via* [L.] 1. an outflowing or shedding, as of the hair. 2. an exhalation or emanation, especially one of noxious nature.

effusion (ĕ-fu′zhun) 1. escape of a fluid into a part. 2. effused material.

egesta (e-jes′tah) undigested material thrown out from the body.

egestion (e-jes′chun) the casting out of undigestible material.

egg (eg) an animal ovum or female reproductive cell, especially one extruded from the maternal body before development of the embryo, either before or after fertilization.

ego (e′go) that part of the psyche that has consciousness, maintains its identity, and recognizes and tests reality; the conscious sense of the self.

ego-alien (e″go-āl′yen) ego-dystonic.

egobronchophony (-brong-kof′o-ne) increased vocal resonance with high-pitched bleating quality of the voice, heard on auscultation of the lungs, especially in pleural effusion.

egocentric (-sen′trik) having all one's ideas centered on one's self.

ego-dystonic (-dis-ton′ik) denoting any impulse, idea, or the like, that is repugnant to and inconsistent with an individual's conception of himself.

egoism (e′go-izm) a self-seeking for advantage at the expense of others; overevaluation of the self.

egomania (e″go-ma′ne-ah) morbid self-esteem.

egophony (e-gof′o-ne) egobronchophony.

ego-syntonic (e″go-sin-ton′ik) denoting any impulse, idea, or the like, that is in harmony with an individual's conception of himself.

egotism (e′go-tizm) overevaluation of one's self.

egotropic (e″go-trop′ik) egocentric.

Ehrlichia (ār-li′ke-ah) a genus of the tribe Ehrlichieae causing disease in dogs, cattle, and sheep.

Ehrlichieae (ār″lĭ-ki′e-e) a tribe of rickettsiae made up of organisms adapted for existence in invertebrates, chiefly arthropods, and pathogenic for certain vertebrates but not for man.

eiconometer (i″ko-nom′ĕ-ter) eikonometer.

eidetic (i-det′ik) denoting exact visualization of events or objects previously seen; a person having such an ability.

eidogen (i′do-jen) a substance elaborated by a second-grade inductor, which is capable of modifying the form of an embryonic organ already in the process of formation.

eidoptometry (i″dop-tom′ĕ-tre) measurement of the acuteness of visual perception.

eikonometer (i″ko-nom′ĕ-ter) an instrument for measuring the degree of aniseikonia.

Eimeria (i-me′re-ah) a genus of sporozoa (order Coccidia) found in the epithelial cells of man and animals, including pathogens of many economically important diseases of domestic animals.

einsteinium (īn-sti′ne-um) chemical element (*see table*), at. no. 99, symbol Es.

ejaculatio (e-jak″u-la′she-o) [L.] ejaculation. **e. prae′cox,** premature ejaculation in coitus.

ejaculation (e-jak″u-la′shun) forcible, sudden expulsion; especially expulsion of semen from the male urethra. **ejac′ulatory,** adj.

ejecta (e-jek′tah) refuse cast off from the body.

ejector (e-jek′tor) an apparatus for effecting the forcible expulsion or removal of a material or body. **saliva e.,** an apparatus for removal of saliva and water from the mouth during operations on the teeth.

EKG electrocardiogram.

EKY electrokymogram.

elaborate (e-lab′o-rāt) to produce complex substances out of simpler materials.

elapid (el′ah-pid) 1. any snake of the family Elapidae. 2. of or pertaining to the family Elapidae.

Elapidae (e-lap′ĭ-de) a family of usually terrestrial, venomous snakes, which have cylindrical tails and front fangs that are short, stout, immovable, and grooved. It includes cobras, kraits, coral snakes, copperheads, blacksnakes, brown snakes, tiger snakes, death adders, and mambas.

elastance (e-las′tans) the quality of recoiling on removal of pressure without disruption, or an expression of the measure of the ability to do so in terms of unit of volume change per unit of pressure change. It is the reciprocal of compliance.

elastase (e-las′tās) an enzyme capable of catalyzing the digestion of elastic tissue.

elastic (e-las′tik) capable of resuming normal shape after distortion.

elasticin (e-las′tĭ-sin) elastin.

elasticity (e″las-tis′ĭ-te) the quality of being elastic.

elastin (e-las′tin) a yellow scleroprotein, the essential constituent of elastic connective tissue; it is brittle when dry, but when moist is flexible and elastic.

elastofibroma (e-las″to-fi-bro′mah) a tumor consisting of both elastin and fibrous elements. **e. dor′si,** a tumor-like nodule of subscapular tissue occurring in old age.

elastoidosis, nodular (e-las″toi-do′sis) a condition characterized by comedones and yellowish, circumscribed, thickened plaques around the orbits or nose, or the nape.

elastoma (e″las-to′mah) a tumor or focal excess of elastic tissue fibers or abnormal collagen fibers of the skin. **Miescher's e.,** elastosis perforans serpiginosa.

elastometer (e″las-tom′ĕ-ter) an instrument for measuring elasticity of tissues.

elastometry (e″las-tom′ĕ-tre) the measurement of elasticity.

elastomucin (e-las″to-mu′sin) a polysaccharide component of elastic tissue.

elastorrhexis (-rek′sis) rupture of fibers composing elastic tissue.

elastosis (e″las-to′sis) degeneration of elastic tissue. **elastot′ic,** adj. **actinic e.,** degeneration of the elastic tissue of the dermis due to constant exposure to sunlight. **e. perfo′rans serpigino′sa, perforating e.,** an elastic tissue defect, occurring alone or in association with other disorders, including Down's syndrome and Ehlers-Danlos syndrome, in which elastomas are extruded through small keratotic papules in the epidermis; the lesions are usually arranged in arcuate serpiginous clusters on the sides of the nape, face, or arms.

elation (e-la′shun) emotional excitement marked by acceleration of mental and bodily activity.

Elavil (el′ah-vil) trademark for a preparation of amitriptyline.

elbow (el′bo) 1. the bend of the arm; the joint connecting the arm and forearm. 2. any angular bend. **capped e.,** a hygroma on the point of the elbow in horses or cattle. **little leaguer's e.,** medial epicondylitis of the elbow due to repeated stress on the flexor muscles of the forearm, often seen in adolescent ballplayers. **miner's e.,** enlargement of the bursa over the point of the elbow, due to resting the body weight on the elbow, as in mining. **pulled e.,** subluxation of the head of the radius distally under the round ligament. **tennis e.,** a painful condition of the outer aspect of the elbow, due to inflammation or irritation of the extensor tendon attachment of the lateral humeral epicondyle.

elcosis (el-ko′sis) fetid ulceration.

eldrin (el′drin) rutin.

electroaffinity (e-lek″tro-ah-fin′ĭ-te) the degree of tenacity with which a substance attracts electrons.

electroanalysis (-ah-nal′ĭ-sis) chemical analysis by means of electric current.

electrobiology (-bi-ol′o-je) the study of electric phenomena in living tissue.

electrobioscopy (-bi-os′ko-pe) the determination of the presence or absence of life by means of an electric current.

electrocardiogram (-kar′de-o-gram″) the record produced by electrocardiography. **scalar e.,** the conventional tracing showing only changes in magnitude of voltage and polarity (positive or negative) with time.

electrocardiograph (-kar′de-o-graf″) the apparatus used in electrocardiography.

electrocardiography (-kar″de-og′rah-fe) the graphic recording from the body surface of electric currents generated by the heart, as a means of studying the action of the heart muscle. **electrocardiograph′ic,** adj.

electrocatalysis (-kah-tal′ĭ-sis) catalysis produced by electricity.

electrocautery (-kaw′ter-e) an apparatus for cauterizing tissue by means of a platinum wire heated by electric current.

electrochemistry (-kem′is-tre) study of chemical changes produced by electric action.

electrochromatography (-kro″mah-tog′rah-fe) electrophoresis.

electrocoagulation (-ko-ag″u-la′shun) coagulation of tissue by means of an electric current.

electrocontractility (-kon″trak-til′ĭ-te) contractility in response to electrical stimulation.

electroconvulsive (-con-vul′siv) inducing convulsions by means of electricity.

electrocorticogram (-kor′tĭ-ko-gram″) the record produced by electrocorticography.

electrocorticography (-kor″tĭ-kog′rah-fe) electroencephalography with the electrodes applied directly to the cerebral cortex.

electrode (e-lek′trōd) either of the two terminals of an electrically conducting system or cell. **active e.**, one smaller than an indifferent electrode, producing electrical stimulation in a concentrated area. **calomel e.**, one capable of both collecting and giving up chloride ions in neutral or acidic aqueous media, consisting of mercury in contact with mercurous chloride; used as a reference electrode in pH measurements. **depolarizing e.**, one having a resistance greater than that of the portion of the body enclosed in the circuit. **exciting e.**, active e. **hydrogen e.**, one made by depositing platinum black on platinum and then allowing it to absorb hydrogen gas to saturation; used in determination of hydrogen ion concentration. **impregnated e.**, one with an absorbent tip impregnated with prescribed medicament. **indifferent e.**, one larger than an active electrode, dispersing electrical stimulation over a larger area. **negative e.**, cathode. **point e.**, an electrode having on one end a metallic point; used in applying current. **positive e.**, anode. **silent e.**, indifferent e. **therapeutic e.**, active e.

electrodermal (e-lek″tro-der′mal) pertaining to the electrical properties of the skin, especially to changes in its resistance.

electrodesiccation (-des″ĭ-ka′shun) destruction of tissue by dehydration, done by means of a high-frequency electric current.

electrodiagnosis (-di″ag-no′sis) diagnosis by means of electric devices.

electrodiagnostics (-di″ag-nos′tiks) the science and practice of electrodiagnosis.

electrodialyzer (-di″ah-li′zer) a blood dialyzer utilizing an applied electric field and semipermeable membranes for separating the colloids from the solution.

electroencephalogram (-en-sef′ah-lo-gram″) the record produced by electroencephalography.

electroencephalograph (-en-sef′ah-lo-graf″) the instrument used in electroencephalography.

electroencephalography (-en-sef″ah-log′rah-fe) the recording of changes in electric potential in various areas of the brain by means of electrodes placed on the scalp or on or in the brain itself. **electroencephalograph′ic**, adj.

electrogastrogram (-gas′tro-gram) the graphic record obtained by electrogastrography.

electrogastrograph (-gas′tro-graf) an instrument for recording the electrical activity of the stomach by means of swallowed gastric electrodes.

electrogastrography (-gas-trog′rah-fe) the recording of the electrical activity of the stomach as measured between its lumen and the body surface. **electrogastrograph′ic**, adj.

electrogram (e-lek′tro-gram) any record produced by changes in electric potential. **His bundle e.**, an intracardiac electrocardiogram of potentials in the bundle of His, done through a cardiac catheter.

electrohemostasis (e-lek″tro-he″mo-sta′sis) arrest of hemorrhage by electrocautery.

electrohysterography (-his″ter-og′rah-fe) recording of changes in electric potential associated with uterine contractions.

electrokymogram (-ki′mo-gram) the record produced by electrokymography.

electrokymograph (-ki′mo-graf) the instrument used in electrokymography.

electrokymography (-ki-mog′rah-fe) the photography on x-ray film of the motion of the heart or of other moving structures which can be visualized radiographically.

electrolysis (e″lek-trol′ĭ-sis) destruction by passage of a galvanic current, as in disintegration of a chemical compound in solution or removal of excessive hair from the body.

electrolyte (e-lek′tro-līt) a substance that dissociates into ions fused in solution, thus becoming capable of conducting electricity.

electrolytic (e-lek″tro-lit′ik) pertaining to electrolysis or to an electrolyte.

electromagnet (-mag′net) a temporary magnet made by passing electric current through a coil of wire surrounding a core of soft iron.

electromagnetism (-mag′nĕ-tizm) magnetism developed by an electric current.

electromyogram (-mi′o-gram) the record obtained by electromyography.

electromyograph (-mi′o-graf) the instrument used in electromyography.

electromyography (-mi-og′rah-fe) the recording and study of the intrinsic electrical properties of skeletal muscle. **electromyograph′ic**, adj.

electron (e-lek′tron) any of the negatively charged particles arranged in orbits around the nucleus of an atom and determining all of the atom's physical and chemical properties except mass and radioactivity.

electronarcosis (e-lek″tro-nar-ko′sis) anesthesia produced by passage of an electric current through electrodes placed on the temples.

electron-dense (e-lek′tron-dens″) in electron microscopy, having a density that prevents electrons from penetrating.

electronegative (e-lek″tro-neg′ah-tiv) bearing a negative electric charge.

electronegativity (-neg″ah-tiv′ĭ-te) electroaffinity.

electroneuromyography (-nu′ro-mi-og′rah-fe) electromyography in which the nerve of the muscle under study is stimulated by application of an electric current.

electronic (e″lek-tron′ik) pertaining to or carrying electrons.

electronystagmography (e-lek″tro-nis″tag-mog′rah-fe) electroencephalographic recordings of eye movements that provide objective documentation of induced and spontaneous nystagmus.

electro-oculogram (-ok′u-lo-gram″) the electroencephalographic tracings made while moving the eyes a constant distance between two fixation points, inducing a deflection of fairly constant amplitude; abbreviated EOG.

electropherogram (-fer′o-gram) electrophoretogram.

electrophoresis (-fo-re′sis) the movement of charged particles suspended in a liquid on various media (e.g., paper, starch, agar), under the influence of an applied electric field. **electrophoret′ic**, adj.

electrophoretogram (-fo-ret′o-gram) the record produced on or in a supporting medium by bands of material which have been separated by the process of electrophoresis.

electrophysiology (-fiz″e-ol′o-je) the study of the effects of electric reactions of the body in health.

electropositive (-poz′ĭ-tiv) having a positive charge.

electroresection (-re-sek′shun) resection by electrosurgical means.

electroretinograph (-ret′in-o-graf) an instrument for measuring the electrical response of the retina to light stimulation; abbreviated ERG.

electroscission (-sish′un) cutting of tissue by means of the electric cautery.

electroscope (e-lek′tro-skōp) an instrument for measuring radiation intensity.

electroshock (-shok) shock produced by applying electric current to the brain.

electrostimulation (e-lek″tro-stim-u-la′shun) electric stimulation of tissues.

electrostriatogram (-stri-a′to-gram) an electroencephalogram showing differences in electric potential recorded at various levels of the corpus striatum.

electrosurgery (-ser′jer-e) surgery performed by electrical methods; the active electrode may be a needle, bulb, or disk. **electrosur′gical**, adj.

electrosynthesis (-sin′thĕ-sis) chemical reactions effected by means of electricity.

electrotaxis (-tak′sis) taxis in response to electric stimuli.

electrotherapeutics, electrotherapy (-therah-pu′tiks; -ther′ah-pe) treatment of disease by means of electricity.

electrotropism (e″lek-trot′ro-pizm) tropism in response to electric stimuli.

electrovalence (e-lek″tro-va′lens) the number of charges an atom acquires in a chemical reaction by gain or loss of electrons.

electroversion (-ver′zhun) the act of electrically terminating a cardiac dysrhythmia.

electrovert (e-lek′tro-vert) to apply electricity to the heart or precordium to depolarize the heart and terminate a cardiac dysrhythmia.

electuary (e-lek′tu-er″e) a medicinal preparation consisting of a powdered drug made into a paste with honey or syrup.

eledoisin (el-ĕ-doi′sin) an endecapeptide, C_{54}-$H_{85}N_{13}O_{15}S$, from the posterior salivary gland of a species of small octopus (*Eledone*), which is a precursor of a large group of biologically active peptides; it has vasodilator, hypotensive, and extravascular smooth muscle stimulant properties.

eleidin (el-e′ĭ-din) a substance, allied to keratin, found in the stratum lucidum of the skin.

element (el′ĕ-ment) 1. any of the primary parts or constituents of a thing. 2. in chemistry, a simple substance which cannot be decomposed by chemical means and which is made up of atoms which are alike in their peripheral electronic configurations and so in their chemical properties, but which may differ in their nuclei and so in their atomic weight and in their radioactive properties. See *Table of Elements*. **formed e's (of the blood)**, erythrocytes, leukocytes, and platelets. **radioactive e.,** a chemical element which spontaneously transmutes into another element, with emission of corpuscular or electromagnetic radiations. **stable e.,** 1. a chemical element that does not spontaneously transmute into another element with emission of corpuscular or electromagnetic radiations. 2. a tissue cell of mature tissues that does not alter by mitosis. **trace e's,** chemical elements distributed throughout the tissues in very small amounts and that are either essential in nutrition, as cobalt, copper, etc., or harmful, as selenium.

eleo- word element [Gr.], *oil*.

eleoma (el″e-o′mah) a tumor or swelling caused by injection of oil into the tissues.

eleometer (el″e-om′ĕ-ter) an instrument for determining the percentage of oil in a mixture or the specific gravity of oils.

eleopten (-op′ten) the more volatile constituent of a volatile oil.

eleotherapy (el″e-o-ther′ah-pe) oleotherapy.

elephantiasis (el″ĕ-fan-ti′ah-sis) elephantiasis filariensis; a chronic filarial disease, usually seen in the tropics, due to infection with *Brugia malayi* or *Wuchereria bancrofti*, marked by inflammation and obstruction of the lymphatics and hypertrophy of the skin and subcutaneous tissues, chiefly affecting the legs and external genitals. The term is often applied to hypertrophy and thickening of the tissues from any cause. **e. filarien′sis**, true elephantiasis (see above). **e. neuromato′sa**, neurofibroma. **e. nos′tras**, that due to either chronic streptococcal erysipelas or chronic recurrent cellulitis. **e. scro′ti**, that in which the scrotum is the main seat of the disease.

elevator (el′ĕ-va″tor) an instrument for elevating tissues for removing osseous fragments or roots of teeth.

elimination (e-lim″ĭ-na′shun) 1. the act of expulsion or extrusion, especially expulsion from the body. 2. omission or exclusion.

Elipten (e-lip′ten) trademark for a preparation of aminoglutethimide.

elixir (e-lik′ser) a clear, sweetened, usually hydroalcoholic liquid containing flavoring substances and sometimes active medicinal agents, for oral use. **aromatic e.,** a preparation containing compound orange spirit, sugar, talc, and alcohol; used as a vehicle for various drugs. **aromatic e., red,** aromatic elixir colored by addition of amaranth solution. **benzaldehyde e., compound,** a preparation of benzaldehyde, vanillin, orange flower water, alcohol, simple syrup, and water; used as a vehicle for drugs. **diphenhydramine hydrochloride e.,** diphenhydramine hydrochloride 2.5 gm., orange oil 0.24 ml., cinnamon oil 0.11 ml., clove oil 0.08 ml., coriander oil 0.03 ml., anethole 0.03 ml., amaranth solution 1.6 ml., alcohol 150.0 ml., syrup 350.0 ml., and sufficient purified water to make a total of 1000 ml.; used as an antihistaminic. **high-alcoholic e.,** compound orange spirit 4 ml., saccharin 3 gm., glycerin 200 ml., and sufficient alcohol to make a total of 1000 ml. **iso-alcoholic e.,** a mixture of low- and high-alcoholic elixirs whose strength is suitable for the medicament for which it serves as a vehicle. **low-alcoholic e.,** compound orange spirit 10 ml., alcohol 100 ml., glycerin 200 ml., sucrose 320 gm., and sufficient purified water to make 1000 ml. **phenobarbital e.,** phenobarbital 4.0 gm., orange oil 0.75 ml., amaranth solution 10.0 ml., alcohol 150.0 ml., glycerin 450.0 ml., syrup 150.0 ml., and sufficient purified water to make a total of 1000 ml.; used as an anticonvulsant, hypnotic, and sedative. **sodium pentobarbital e.,** sodium pentobarbital 4.0 gm., glycerin 450.0 ml., alcohol 150.0 ml., orange oil 0.75 ml., caramel 2 gm., syrup 150.0 ml., diluted hydrochloric acid 6.0 ml., and sufficient purified water to make a total of 1000 ml.; used as a hypnotic. **terpin hydrate e.,** a preparation of terpin hydrate, sweet orange peel tincture, benzaldehyde, glycerin, alcohol, and syrup in purified water; used as an expectorant. **three bromides e.,** a mixture of ammonium, potassium, and sodium bromides, amaranth solution, and compound benzaldehyde elixir; used as a central nervous system depressant.

Elkosin (el′ko-sin) trademark for preparations of sulfisomidine.

elliptocyte (e-lip′to-sīt) an elliptical red blood cell.

elliptocytosis (e-lip″to-si-to′sis) a hereditary disorder in which the erythrocytes are largely elliptical and which is characterized by increased red cell destruction and anemia.

Elorine (el′o-rēn) trademark for a preparation of tricyclamol.

eluate (el′u-āt) the substance separated out by, or the product of, elution or elutriation.

eluent (e-lu′ent) the solution used in elution.

elution (e-loo′shun) in chemistry, separation of material by washing; the process of pulverizing substances and mixing them with water in order to separate the heavier constituents, which settle out in solution, from the lighter.

elutriation (e-loo″tre-a′shun) purification of a substance by dissolving it in a solvent and pouring off the solution, thus separating it from the undissolved foreign material.

Em. emmetropia.

emaciation (e-ma″se-a′shun) excessive leanness; a wasted condition of the body.

emailloblast (e-ma′lo-blast) ameloblast.

emanation (em″ah-na′shun) that which is given off, such as a gaseous disintegration product given off from radioactive substances or an effluvium.

emasculation (e-mas″ku-la′shun) removal of the penis or testes.

embalming (em-bahm′ing) treatment of a dead body to retard decomposition.

embarrass (em-bar′as) to impede the function of; to obstruct.

embedding (em-bed′ing) fixation of tissue in a firm medium, in order to keep it intact during cutting of thin sections.

embole (em′bo-le) 1. the reducing of a dislocated limb. 2. emboly.

embolectomy (em″bo-lek′to-me) surgical removal of an embolus from a blood vessel.

emboli (em′bo-li) plural of *embolus.*

embolic (em-bol′ik) pertaining to embolism or an embolus.

embolism (em′bo-lizm) the sudden blocking of an artery by a clot or foreign material which has been brought to its site of lodgment by the blood current. **air e.,** that due to air bubbles entering the veins after trauma or surgical procedures. **cerebral e.,** embolism of a cerebral artery. **coronary e.,** embolism of a coronary artery. **fat e.,** obstruction by a fat embolus, occurring especially after fractures of large bones. **infective e.,** obstruction by an embolus containing bacteria or septic poison. **miliary e.,** embolism affecting many small blood vessels. **paradoxical e.,** blockage of a systemic artery by a thrombus originating in a systemic vein that has passed through a defect in the interatrial or interventricular septum. **pulmonary e.,** obstruction of the pulmonary artery or one of its branches by an embolus.

embolalia (em″bo-lo-la′le-ah) interpolation of meaningless words or phrases in a spoken sentence.

embolophrasia (-fra′ze-ah) embolalia.

embolus (em′bo-lus), pl. *em′boli* [L.] a clot or other plug brought by the blood from another vessel and forced into a smaller one, thus obstructing the circulation. **fat e.,** one composed of oil or fat. **saddle e.,** one at the bifurcation of an artery, blocking both branches.

emboly (em′bo-le) invagination of the blastula to form the gastrula.

embrasure (em-bra′zhur) the interproximal space occlusal to the area of contact of adjacent teeth in the same dental arch.

embryectomy (em″bre-ek′to-me) excision of an extrauterine embryo or fetus.

embryo (em′bre-o) 1. in animals, those derivatives of the fertilized ovum that eventually become the offspring, during their period of most rapid growth, i.e., after the long axis appears until all major structures are represented. In man, the developing organism from about two weeks after fertilization to the end of the sev-

TABLE OF CHEMICAL ELEMENTS

ELEMENT (DATE OF DISCOVERY)	SYMBOL	ATOMIC NUMBER	ATOMIC WEIGHT*	VALENCE	SP. GR. OR DENSITY (GRAMS/LITER)	DESCRIPTIVE COMMENT
Actinium (1899)	Ac	89	[227]	....	10.07	radioactive element associated with uranium
Aluminum (1827)	Al	13	26.9815	3	2.6989	silvery-white metal, abundant in earth's crust, but not in free form
Americium (1944)	Am	95	[243]	3, 4, 5, 6	11.7	fourth transuranium element discovered
Antimony (prehistoric)	Sb	51	121.75	3, 5	6.691	exists in 4 allotropic forms
Argon (1894)	Ar	18	39.948	0?	1.7837 g./l.	colorless, odorless gas
Arsenic (1250)	As	33	74.9216	3, 5	5.73 / 4.73 / 1.97	(gray) semimetallic solid / (black) / (yellow)
Astatine (1940)	At	85	[210]	1, 3, 5, 7		radioactive halogen
Barium (1808)	Ba	56	137.34	2	3.5	silvery-white, alkaline earth metal
Berkelium (1949)	Bk	97	[247]	3, 4		fifth transuranium element discovered
Beryllium (1798)	Be	4	9.0122	2	1.848	light, steel-gray metal
Bismuth (1753)	Bi	83	208.980	3, 5	9.747	pinkish-white, crystalline, brittle metal
Boron (1808)	B	5	10.811	3	2.34, 2.37	crystalline or amorphous element, not occurring free in nature
Bromine (1826)	Br	35	79.909	1, 3, 5, 7	3.12 / 7.59 g./l.	mobile, reddish-brown liquid, volatilizing readily / red vapor with disagreeable odor
Cadmium (1817)	Cd	48	112.40	2	8.65	soft, bluish-white metal
Calcium (1808)	Ca	20	40.08	2	1.55	metallic element, forming more than 3 per cent of earth's crust
Californium (1950)	Cf	98	[249]	....	1.8–2.1	sixth transuranium element discovered
Carbon (prehistoric)	C	6	12.01115	2, 3, 4	1.9–2.3 / 3.15–3.53	(amorphous) element widely distributed in nature / (graphite) / (diamond)
Cerium (1803)	Ce	58	140.12	3, 4	6.67–8.23	most abundant rare earth metal
Cesium (1860)	Cs	55	132.905	1	1.873	silvery-white, soft, alkaline metal
Chlorine (1774)	Cl	17	35.453	1, 3, 5, 7	3.214 g./l.	greenish-yellow gas of the halogen group
Chromium (1797)	Cr	24	51.996	2, 3, 6	7.18–7.20	steel-gray, lustrous, hard metal
Cobalt (1735)	Co	27	58.9332	2, 3	8.9	brittle, hard metal
Copper (prehistoric)	Cu	29	63.54	1, 2	8.96	reddish, lustrous, malleable metal
Curium (1944)	Cm	96	[247]	3	7	third transuranium element discovered
Dysprosium (1886)	Dy	66	162.50	3	8.536	rare earth metal with metallic bright silver luster
Einsteinium (1952)	Es	99	[254]	....		seventh transuranium element discovered
Erbium (1843)	Er	68	167.26	3	9.051	soft, malleable rare earth metal

Element (year)	Symbol	At. no.	At. weight	Valences	Density	Description
Europium (1896)	Eu	63	151.96	2, 3	5.259	lustrous, silvery-white rare earth metal
Fermium (1953)	Fm	100	[253]	. . . .		eighth transuranium element discovered
Fluorine (1771)	F	9	18.9984	1	1.696 g./l.	pale yellow, corrosive gas of the halogen group
Francium (1939)	Fr	87	[223]	1		product of alpha disintegration of actinium
Gadolinium (1880)	Gd	64	157.25	3	7.8, 7.895	lustrous, silvery-white rare earth metal
Gallium (1875)	Ga	31	69.72	2, 3	5.907	beautiful, silvery-appearing metal
Germanium (1886)	Ge	32	72.59	2, 4	5.323	grayish-white, brittle metal
Gold (prehistoric)	Au	79	196.967	1, 3	19.32	malleable yellow metal
Hafnium (1923)	Hf	72	178.49	4	13.29	gray metal associated with zirconium
Hahnium (1970)	Ha	105	[260]			twelfth transuranium element discovered
Helium (1895)	He	2	4.0026	0	0.177 g./l.	inert gas
Holmium (1879)	Ho	67	164.930	3	8.803	relatively soft and malleable rare earth metal
Hydrogen (1766)	H	1	1.00797	1	0.08988 g./l. 0.070	(gas) most abundant element in the universe (liquid)
Indium (1863)	In	49	114.82	1, 2?, 3	7.31	soft, silvery-white metal
Iodine (1811)	I	53	126.9044	1, 3, 5, 7	4.93, 11.27 g./l.	grayish-black, lustrous solid or violet-blue gas
Iridium (1803)	Ir	77	192.2	3, 4	22.42	white, brittle metal of platinum family
Iron (prehistoric)	Fe	26	55.847	2, 3, 4, 6	7.874	fourth most abundant element in earth's crust
Krypton (1898)	Kr	36	83.80	0	3.733 g./l.	inert gas
Lanthanum (1839)	La	57	138.91	3	5.98-6.186	silvery-white, ductile, rare earth metal
Lawrencium (1961)	Lw	103	[257]	. . . .		tenth transuranium element discovered
Lead (prehistoric)	Pb	82	207.19	2, 4	11.35	bluish-white, lustrous, malleable metal
Lithium (1817)	Li	3	6.939	1	0.534	lightest of all metals
Lutetium (1907)	Lu	71	174.97	3	9.872	rare earth metal
Magnesium (1808)	Mg	12	24.312	2	1.738	silvery-white metallic element, eighth in abundance in earth's crust
Manganese (1774)	Mn	25	54.9380	1, 2, 3, 4, 6, 7	7.21-7.44	exists in 4 allotropic forms
Mendelevium (1955)	Md	101	[256]	. . . .		ninth transuranium element discovered
Mercury (prehistoric)	Hg	80	200.59	1, 2	13.546	heavy, silvery-white metal, liquid at ordinary temperatures
Molybdenum (1782)	Mo	42	95.94	2, 3, 4?, 5?, 6	10.22	silvery-white, very hard metal
Neodymium (1885)	Nd	60	144.24	3	6.80, 7.004	exists in 2 allotropic forms
Neon (1898)	Ne	10	20.183	0?	0.89990 g./l.	inert gas
Neptunium (1940)	Np	93	[237]	3, 4, 5, 6	18.0-20.45	first transuranium element discovered
Nickel (1751)	Ni	28	58.71	0, 1, 2, 3	8.902	silvery-white, malleable metal
Niobium (1801)	Nb	41	92.906	2, 3, 4?, 5	8.57	shiny white, soft, ductile metal
Nitrogen (1772)	N	7	14.0067	3, 5	1.2506 g./l.	colorless, odorless, inert element, making up 78 per cent of the air
Nobelium (?) (1958)	No	102	[253]	. . . .		acceptance of this element considered premature
Osmium (1803)	Os	76	190.2	2, 3, 4, 8	22.57	bluish-white, hard metal of platinum family
Oxygen (1774)	O	8	15.9994	2	1.429 g./l.	colorless, odorless gas, third most abundant element in the universe

Table of Chemical Elements (Continued)

ELEMENT (DATE OF DISCOVERY)	SYMBOL	ATOMIC NUMBER	ATOMIC WEIGHT*	VALENCE	SP. GR. OR DENSITY (GRAMS/LITER)	DESCRIPTIVE COMMENT
Palladium (1803)	Pd	46	106.4	2, 3, 4	12.02	steel-white metal of the platinum family
Phosphorus (1669)	P	15	30.9738	3, 5	1.82 / 2.20 / 2.25–2.69	(white) waxy solid, transparent when pure / (red) / (black)
Platinum (1735)	Pt	78	195.09	1?, 2, 3, 4	21.45	silvery-white, malleable metal
Plutonium (1940)	Pu	94	[242]	3, 4, 5, 6	19.84	second transuranium element discovered
Polonium (1898)	Po	84	[210]	2, 4, 6	9.32	very rare natural element
Potassium (1807)	K	19	39.102	1	0.862	soft, silvery, alkali metal, seventh in abundance in earth's crust
Praseodymium (1885)	Pr	59	140.907	3, 4	6.782, 6.64	soft, silvery rare earth metal
Promethium (1941)	Pm	61	[147]	3		produced by irradiation of neodymium and praseodymium; identity established in 1945
Protactinium (1917)	Pa	91	[231]	4 or 5	15.37	bright lustrous metal
Radium (1898)	Ra	88	[226]	2	5(?)	brilliant white, radioactive metal
Radon (1900)	Rn	86	[222]	0	9.73 g./l.	heaviest known gas
Rhenium (1925)	Re	75	186.2	−1, 2, 3, 4, 5, 6, 7	21.02	silvery-white lustrous metal
Rhodium (1803)	Rh	45	102.905	−2, 3, 4, 5, 6, 7	12.41	silvery-white metal of platinum family
Rubidium (1861)	Rb	37	85.47	1, 2, 3, 4	1.532	soft, silvery-white, alkali metal
Ruthenium (1844)	Ru	44	101.07	0, 1, 2, 3, 4, 5, 6, 7, 8	12.41	hard white metal of platinum family
Rutherfordium (1969)	Rf	104	[261]			eleventh transuranium element discovered
Samarium (1879)	Sm	62	150.35	2, 3	7.536–7.40	bright silver lustrous metal
Scandium (1879)	Sc	21	44.956	3	2.992	soft, silvery-white metal
Selenium (1817)	Se	34	78.96	2, 4, 6	4.79, 4.28	exists in several allotropic forms
Silicon (1823)	Si	14	28.086	4	2.33	a relatively inert element, second in abundance in earth's crust
Silver (prehistoric)	Ag	47	107.870	1, 2	10.50	malleable, ductile metal with brilliant white luster
Sodium (1807)	Na	11	22.9898	1	0.971	most abundant of alkali metals, sixth in abundance in earth's crust
Strontium (1808)	Sr	38	87.62	2	2.54	exists in 3 allotropic forms
Sulfur (prehistoric)	S	16	32.064	2, 4, 6	1.957, 2.07	exists in several isotopic and many allotropic forms
Tantalum (1802)	Ta	73	180.948	2?, 3, 4?, 5	16.6	gray, heavy, very hard metal
Technetium (1937)	Tc	43	[99]	3?, 4, 6, 7	11.50	first element produced artificially
Tellurium (1782)	Te	52	127.60	2, 4, 6	6.24	silvery-white, lustrous element

Element	Symbol	At. No.	At. Mass	Valence	Density	Description
Terbium (1843)	Tb	65	158.924	3, 4	8.272	silvery-gray, malleable, ductile rare earth metal
Thallium (1861)	Tl	81	204.37	1, 3	11.85	very soft, malleable metal
Thorium (1828)	Th	90	232.038	4	11.66	silvery-white, lustrous metal
Thulium (1879)	Tm	69	168.934	2, 3		least abundant rare earth metal
Tin (prehistoric)	Sn	50	118.69	2, 4	5.75, 7.31	(gray) malleable metal existing in 2 or 3 allotropic forms, changing from white to gray on cooling and back to white on warming (white)
Titanium (1791)	Ti	22	47.90	2, 3, 4	4.54	lustrous white metal
Tungsten (1783)	W	74	183.85	2, 3, 4, 5, 6	19.3	steel-gray to tin-white metal
Uranium (1789)	U	92	238.03	3, 4, 5, 6	18.95	heavy, silvery-white metal
Vanadium (1801)	V	23	50.942	2, 3, 4, 5	6.11	bright, white metal
Xenon (1898)	Xe	54	131.30	0?	5.887 g./l.	one of the so-called rare or inert gases
Ytterbium (1878)	Yb	70	173.04	2, 3	6.977, 6.54	exists in 2 allotropic forms
Yttrium (1794)	Y	39	88.905	3	4.45	rare earth metal with silvery metallic luster
Zinc (1746)	Zn	30	65.37	2	7.133	bluish-white, lustrous metal, malleable at 100–150° C.
Zirconium (1789)	Zr	40	91.22	4	6.4	grayish-white, lustrous metal

*Figures in brackets represent mass number of most stable isotope.

TABLE OF ELEMENTS BY ATOMIC NUMBERS

1 hydrogen	16 sulfur	31 gallium	46 palladium	61 promethium	76 osmium	91 protactinium
2 helium	17 chlorine	32 germanium	47 silver	62 samarium	77 iridium	92 uranium
3 lithium	18 argon	33 arsenic	48 cadmium	63 europium	78 platinum	93 neptunium
4 beryllium	19 potassium	34 selenium	49 indium	64 gadolinium	79 gold	94 plutonium
5 boron	20 calcium	35 bromine	50 tin	65 terbium	80 mercury	95 americium
6 carbon	21 scandium	36 krypton	51 antimony	66 dysprosium	81 thallium	96 curium
7 nitrogen	22 titanium	37 rubidium	52 tellurium	67 holmium	82 lead	97 berkelium
8 oxygen	23 vanadium	38 strontium	53 iodine	68 erbium	83 bismuth	98 californium
9 fluorine	24 chromium	39 yttrium	54 xenon	69 thulium	84 polonium	99 einsteinium
10 neon	25 manganese	40 zirconium	55 cesium	70 ytterbium	85 astatine	100 fermium
11 sodium	26 iron	41 niobium	56 barium	71 lutetium	86 radon	101 mendelevium
12 magnesium	27 cobalt	42 molybdenum	57 lanthanum	72 hafnium	87 francium	102 [see nobelium]
13 aluminum	28 nickel	43 technetium	58 cerium	73 tantalum	88 radium	103 lawrencium
14 silicon	29 copper	44 ruthenium	59 praseodymium	74 tungsten	89 actinium	104 rutherfordium
15 phosphorus	30 zinc	45 rhodium	60 neodymium	75 rhenium	90 thorium	105 hahnium

enth or eighth week. 2. in plants, the element of the seed that develops into a new individual. **em′bryonal, embryon′ic,** adj. **presomite e.,** the embryo at any stage before the appearance of the first somite. **previllous e.,** the embryo at any stage before the appearance of the chorionic villi. **somite e.,** the embryo at any stage between the appearance of the first and the last somites.

embryocardia (em″bre-o-kar′de-ah) a symptom in which the heart sounds resemble those of the fetus, there being very little difference in the quality of the first and second sounds.

embryoctony (em″bre-ok′to-ne) destruction of the living embryo or fetus.

embryogeny (em″bre-oj′ĕ-ne) the origin or development of the embryo. **embryogenet′ic, embryogen′ic,** adj.

embryologist (em″bre-ol′o-jist) an expert in embryology.

embryology (em″bre-ol′o-je) the science of the development of the individual during the embryonic stage and, by extension, in several or even all preceding and subsequent stages of the life cycle. **embryolog′ic,** adj.

embryoma (em″bre-o′mah) a general term applied to neoplasms thought to be derived from embryonic cells or tissues, including dermoid cysts, teratomas, embryonal carcinomas, etc. **e. of kidney,** Wilms' tumor.

embryonization (em-bre″o-nĭ-za′shun) reversion of a tissue or cell to the embryonic form.

embryonoid (em′bre-ŏ-noid″) resembling an embryo.

embryopathy (em″bre-op′ah-the) a morbid condition resulting from interference with normal embryonic development. **rubella e.,** rubella syndrome.

embryoplastic (em′bre-o-plas″tik) pertaining to or concerned in formation of an embryo.

embryotomy (em″bre-ot′o-me) dissection of the fetus in difficult labor.

embryotoxon (em″bre-o-tok′son) a ringlike opacity at the margin of the cornea. **anterior e.,** embryotoxon. **posterior e.,** a developmental anomaly in which there is a ringlike opacity at Schwalbe's ring, with thickening and anterior displacement of the latter; it is seen in Axenfeld's syndrome and Rieger's syndrome.

embryotroph (em′bre-o-trōf″) the total nutriment (histotroph and hemotroph) made available to the embryo.

embryotrophy (em″bre-ot′ro-fe) the nutrition of the early embryo.

embryulcus (-ul′kus) a blunt hook for removal of the fetus from the uterus.

emedullate (e-med′u-lāt) to remove bone marrow.

emergent (e-mer′jent) 1. coming out from a cavity or other part. 2. coming on suddenly.

emery (em′er-e) an abrasive substance consisting of corundum and various impurities, such as iron oxide.

emesis (em′ĕ-sis) the act of vomiting. Also used as a word termination, as in *hematemesis.*

emetic (e-met′ik) 1. causing vomiting. 2. an agent that causes vomiting.

emetine (em′ĕ-tēn) an alkaloid, $C_{29}H_{40}N_2O_4$, derived from ipecac or produced synthetically; its hydrochloride salt is used as an antiamebic.

emetocathartic (em″ĕ-to-kah-thar′tik) both emetic and cathartic; an emetocathartic agent.

E.M.F. electromotive force.

-emia word element [Gr.], *condition of the blood.*

emigration (em″ĭ-gra′shun) the escape of leukocytes through the walls of small blood vessels; diapedesis.

eminence (em′ĭ-nens) a projection or boss.

eminentia (em″ĭ-nen′she-ah), pl. *eminen′tiae* [L.] eminence.

emiocytosis (e″me-o-si-to′sis) the ejection of material, e.g., insulin granules, from a cell.

emissary (em′ĭ-sār″e) affording an outlet, referring especially to the venous outlets from the dural sinuses through the skull.

emission (e-mish′un) a discharge; specifically an involuntary discharge of semen. **nocturnal e.,** reflex emission of semen during sleep.

Emivan (em′ĭ-van) trademark for preparations of ethamivan.

emmenagogue (ĕ-men′ah-gog) an agent or measure that promotes menstruation.

emmenia (ĕ-me′ne-ah) the menses. **emmen′ic,** adj.

emmenology (em″ĕ-nol′o-je) the sum of knowledge about menstruation and its disorders.

emmetrope (em′ĕ-trōp) a person who has no refractive error of vision.

emmetropia (em″ĕ-tro′pe-ah) the ideal optical condition, parallel rays coming to a focus on the retina. **emmetrop′ic,** adj.

Emmonsia (ĕ-mon′se-ah) a genus of imperfect, saprophytic, soil fungi; two species, *E. cres′cens* and *E. par′va,* cause adiospiromycosis in rodents and man.

emollient (e-mol′yent) 1. softening or soothing. 2. an agent that softens or soothes the skin, or soothes an irritated internal surface.

emotion (e-mo′shun) a state of mental excitement characterized by alteration of feeling tone and by physiological changes.

emotivity (e″mo-tiv′ĭ-te) capacity for emotion.

empathize (em′pah-thīz) to experience or feel empathy; to enter into another's feelings.

empathy (em′pah-the) the recognition of and entering into another's feelings. **empath′ic,** adj.

emperipolesis (em-per″ĭ-po-le′sis) lymphocytic penetration of and movement within another cell.

emphysema (em″fĭ-se′mah) 1. a pathologic accumulation of air in tissues or organs. 2. pulmonary e. **atrophic e.,** overdistention and stretching of lung tissues due to atrophic changes. **bullous e.,** single or multiple large cystic alveolar dilatations of lung tissue. **centriacinar e., centrilobular e.,** focal dilatations of the respiratory bronchioles rather than alveoli, distributed throughout the lung in the midst of grossly normal lung tissue. **interlobular e.,** accumulation of air in the septa between lobules of the lungs. **interstitial e.,** presence of air in the peribronchial and interstitial tissues of the lungs. **intestinal e.,** a condition marked by accumulation of gas under the serous tunic of the intestine. **lobar e.,** emphysema involving less than all the lobes of the affected lung. **lobar e., congenital, lobar e., infantile,** a condition characterized by overinflation, commonly affecting one of the upper lobes and causing respiratory distress in early life. **e. of lungs,** pulmonary e. **mediastinal e.,** pneumomediastinum. **obstructive e.,** overinflation of the lungs associated with partial bronchial obstruction which interferes with exhalation. **panacinar e., panlobular e.,** generalized obstructive emphysema affecting all lung segments, with atrophy and dilatation of the alveoli and destruction of the vascular bed. **pulmonary e.,** increase beyond normal in the size of the air space in the lungs distal to the terminal bronchioles. **subcutaneous e.,** the presence of air or gas in subcutaneous tissues. **surgical e.,** subcutaneous emphysema following an operation. **unilateral e.,** that affecting only one lung, frequently due to congenital defects in circulation. **vesicular e.,** panacinar e.

emphysematous (em″fĭ-sem′ah-tus) of the nature of or affected with emphysema.

empiricism (em-pir′ĭ-sizm) skill or knowledge based entirely on experience. **empir′ic, empir′ical,** adj.

Empirin (em′pĭ-rin) trademark for tablets containing acetylsalicylic acid, phenacetin, and caffeine.

emprosthotonos (em″pros-thot′ŏ-nos) tetanic forward flexure of the body.

empyema (em″pi-e′mah) accumulation of pus in a body cavity. **empye′mic,** adj. **thoracic e.,** pyothorax; suppurative inflammation of the pleural space.

empyesis (em″pi-e′sis) a pustular eruption.

emulgent (e-mul′jent) 1. effecting a straining or purifying process. 2. a renal artery or vein. 3. a medicine that stimulates bile or urine flow.

emulsifier (e-mul″sĭ-fi′er) a substance used to make an emulsion.

emulsion (e-mul′shun) a mixture of two immiscible liquids, one being dispersed throughout the other in small droplets; a colloid system in which both the dispersed phase and the dispersion medium are liquids.

emulsoid (e-mul′soid) a colloid system in which the dispersion medium is liquid, usually water, and the disperse phase consists of highly complex organic substances, such as starch or glue, which absorb much water, swell, and become distributed throughout the dispersion medium.

emunctory (e-mungk′to-re) 1. excretory or cleansing. 2. an excretory organ or duct.

emylcamate (e-mil′kah-māt) a tranquilizer, $C_7H_{15}NO_2$.

enamel (e-nam′el) the white, compact, and very hard substance covering and protecting the dentin of a tooth crown. **brown e., hereditary,** amelogenesis imperfecta. **curled e.,** enamel in which the columns are bent. **dwarfed e.,** that which is less thick than normal. **mottled e.,** defective enamel, with a chalky white appearance or brownish stain, caused by excessive amounts of fluoride in drinking water and food preparations during period of enamel calcification. **nanoid e.,** dwarfed e.

enameloma (en-am″el-o′mah) a small spherical nodule of enamel attached to a tooth at the cervical line or on the root.

enamelum (e-nam′el-um) [L.] enamel.

enanthema (en″an-the′ma) an eruption upon a mucous surface. **enanthem′atous,** adj.

enantiobiosis (en-an″te-o-bio′sis) commensalism in which the associated organisms are mutually antagonistic.

enantiomorph (en-an′te-o-morf″) one of a pair of isomeric substances, the structures of which are mirror opposites of each other.

enarthrosis (en″ar-thro′sis) a joint in which the rounded head of one bone is received into a socket in another, as in the hip bone.

encapsulation (en-kap″su-la′shun) enclosure within a capsule.

encarditis (en″kar-di′tis) endocarditis.

encephal(o)- word element [Gr.], *brain.*

encephalalgia (en″sef-ah-lal′je-ah) pain within the head.

encephalatrophy (en″sef-ah-lat′ro-fe) atrophy of the brain.

encephalic (en″sĕ-fal′ik) 1. pertaining to the encephalon. 2. within the skull.

encephalitis (en″sef-ah-li′tis) inflammation of the brain. **encephalit′ic,** adj. **acute disseminated e.,** postinfection e. **Australian X e.,** an acute encephalitis of viral origin observed in Australia during the summer months between 1917 and 1926. **cortical e.,** inflammation involving only the cortex of the brain. **Economo's e.,** lethargic e. **epidemic e.,** a viral encephalitis occurring epidemically. **equine e.,** 1. see under *encephalomyelitis.* 2. Borna disease. **hemorrhagic e.,** herpes encephalitis in which there is inflammation of the brain with hemorrhagic foci and perivascular exudate. **herpes e.,** that caused by herpesvirus, resembling equine encephalomyelitis. **e. hyperplas′tica,** acute nonsuppurating e. **infantile e.,** encephalitis in children from infectious disease. **influenzal e.,** that occurring as a complication of influenza. **Japanese B e.,** a form of epidemic encephalitis of varying severity occurring in Japan and other Pacific islands, China, U.S.S.R., and probably much of the Far East. **lead e.,** encephalitis with cerebral edema due to lead poisoning. **lethargic e.,** a form of epidemic encephalitis characterized by increasing languor, apathy, and drowsiness. **Murray Valley e.,** a viral encephalitis occurring epidemically in 1950 and 1951 in the Murray Valley, Victoria, Australia, believed to be a recrudescence of Australian X disease; a few cases occurred in 1956 and it has been reported in New Guinea. **e. neonato′rum,** encephalitis of the newborn. **e. periaxia′lis diffu′sa,** Schilder's disease. **postinfection e.,** an acute disease of the central nervous system seen in patients convalescing from infectious, usual viral, diseases. **postvaccinal e.,** acute encephalitis sometimes occurring after vaccination. **purulent e., pyogenic e.,** suppurative e. **Russian autumnal e.,** Japanese B e. **Russian endemic e., Russian forest-spring e., Russian spring-summer e., Russian tick-borne e., Russian vernal e.,** a form of epidemic encephalitis acquired in forests from infected ticks and transmitted in other ways, as by ingestion of the flesh or milk of infected animals. **St. Louis e.,** a viral disease first observed in Illinois in 1932, closely resembling western equine encephalomyelitis clinically; it is usually transmitted by certain mosquitoes. **Schilder's e.,** see under *disease.* **e. subcortica'lis chron'ica,** Binswanger's dementia. **suppurative e.,** encephalitis accompanied by suppuration and abscess formation. **vaccinal e.,** postvaccinal e. **vernal e.,** Russian spring-summer e.

encephalitogenic (en"sef-ah-lĭ-to-jen'ik) causing encephalitis.

encephalocele (en-sef'ah-lo-sēl") hernial protrusion of brain substance through a congenital or traumatic opening of the skull.

encephalocystocele (en-sef"ah-lo-sis'to-sēl) hernial protrusion of the brain distended by fluid.

encephalogram (en-sef'ah-lo-gram") the film obtained by encephalography.

encephalography (en-sef"ah-log'rah-fe) radiography of the brain.

encephaloid (en-sef'ah-loid) 1. resembling the brain or brain substance. 2. medullary carcinoma.

encephalolith (en-sef'ah-lo-lith") a brain calculus.

encephalology (en-sef"ah-lol'o-je) the sum of knowledge regarding the brain, its functions, and its diseases.

encephaloma (en-sef"ah-lo'mah) 1. any swelling or tumor of the brain. 2. medullary carcinoma. '

encephalomalacia (en-sef"ah-lo-mah-la'she-ah) softening of the brain.

encephalomeningitis (-men"in-ji'tis) meningoencephalitis.

encephalomeningocele (-mĕ-ning'go-sēl) protrusion of the brain and meninges through a defect in the skull.

encephalomeningopathy (-men"in-gop'ah-the) disease involving the brain and meninges.

encephalomere (en-sef'ah-lo-mēr") one of the segments making up the embryonic brain.

encephalometer (en"sef-ah-lom'ĕ-ter) an instrument used in locating certain of the brain regions.

encephalomyelitis (en-sef"ah-lo-mi"ĕ-li'tis) inflammation of the brain and spinal cord. **acute disseminated e.,** postinfection encephalitis. **benign myalgic e.,** a disease, usually occurring in epidemics, characterized by headache, fever, myalgia, muscular weakness, and emotional lability. **equine e.,** see *equine e., eastern, Venezuelan,* and *western.* **equine e., eastern,** a viral disease similar to western equine encephalomyelitis, but occurring in a region extending from New Hampshire to Texas and as far west as Wisconsin, and in Canada, Mexico, the Carribean, and parts of Central and South Amer-

ica. **equine e., Venezuelan,** a viral disease of horses and mules; the infection in man resembles influenza, with little or no indication of nervous system involvement; the causative agent was first isolated in Venezuela. **equine e., western,** a viral disease of horses and mules, communicable to man, occurring chiefly as a meningoencephalitis, with little involvement of the medulla or spinal cord; observed in the United States chiefly west of the Mississippi River. **granulomatous e.,** a disease marked by granulomas and necrosis of the walls of the cerebral and spinal ventricles. **infectious porcine e.,** a highly fatal disease of swine, due to a picornavirus, marked by flaccid ascending paralysis. **mouse e., murine e.,** Theiler's disease. **postvaccinal e.,** inflammation of the brain and spinal cord following vaccination or infection with vaccinia virus.

encephalomyeloneuropathy (-mi"ĕ-lo-nu-rop'ah-the) a disease involving the brain, spinal cord, and peripheral nerves.

encephalomyelopathy (-mi"ĕ-lop'ah-the) a disease involving the brain and spinal cord.

encephalomyeloradiculitis (-mi"ĕ-lo-rah-dik"u-li'tis) inflammation of the brain, spinal cord, and spinal nerve roots.

encephalomyeloradiculopathy (-mi"ĕ-lo-rah-dik"u-lop'ah-the) a disease involving the brain, spinal cord, and spinal nerve roots.

encephalomyocarditis (-mi"o-kar-di'tis) a viral disease marked by degenerative and inflammatory changes in skeletal and cardiac muscle and by central lesions resembling those of poliomyelitis.

encephalon (en-sef'ah-lon) the brain.

encephalopathy (en-sef"ah-lop'ah-the) any degenerative brain disease. **biliary e., bilirubin e.,** kernicterus. **boxer's e.,** traumatic e. **hepatic e.,** a condition, usually occurring secondarily to advanced liver disease, marked by disturbances of consciousness that may progress to deep coma (hepatic coma), psychiatric changes of varying degree, flapping tremor, and fetor hepaticus. **hypernatremic e.,** a severe hemorrhagic encephalopathy induced by the hyperosmolarity accompanying hypernatremia and dehydration. **lead e.,** brain disease caused by lead poisoning. **portal-systemic e.,** hepatic e. **progressive subcortical e.,** Schilder's disease. **traumatic e.,** general slowing of mental functions, occasional confusion, and scattered memory loss, due to cumulative punishment absorbed in the boxing ring. **Wernicke's e.,** an inflammatory hemorrhagic form due to thiamine deficiency associated with chronic alcoholism, but also occurring as a complication of certain other diseases, with paralysis of the eye muscles, diplopia, nystagmus, ataxia, and mental changes ranging from deterioration and forgetfulness to delirium tremens and Korsakoff's psychosis.

encephalopuncture (en-sef"ah-lo-punk'tūr) surgical puncture of the brain.

encephalopyosis (-pi-o'sis) suppuration or abscess of the brain.

encephalorachidian (-rah-kid′e-an) cerebrospinal.

encephalorrhagia (-ra′je-ah) hemorrhage within or from the brain.

encephalosclerosis (-skle-ro′sis) hardening of the brain.

encephalosis (en″sef-ah-lo′sis) any organic brain disease.

encephalotomy (-lot′o-me) 1. craniotomy (2). 2. dissection or anatomy of the brain.

enchondroma (en″kon-dro′mah) a benign growth of cartilage arising in the metaphysis of a bone. **enchondro′matous,** adj.

enchondromatosis (en-kon″dro-mah-to′sis) a condition characterized by hamartomatous proliferation of cartilage cells within the metaphysis of several bones, causing thinning of the overlying cortex and distortion of the growth in length.

enchondrosarcoma (-sar-ko′mah) central chondroma.

enclave (en′klāv) tissue detached from its normal connection and enclosed within another organ.

enclitic (en-klit′ik) having the planes of the fetal head inclined to those of the maternal pelvis.

encopresis (en″ko-pre′sis) incontinence of feces not due to organic defect or illness.

encysted (en-sist′ed) enclosed in a sac, bladder, or cyst.

end(o)- word element [Gr.], *within; inward.*

endadelphos (end″ah-del′fos) a monster in which a parasitic twin is enclosed within the body of the other twin (the autosite).

Endamoeba (en″dah-me′bah) a genus of amebas parasitic in the intestines of invertebrates.

endangiitis (en″dan-je-i′tis) inflammation of the endangium.

endangium (en-dan′je-um) tunica intima (inner coat) of a blood vessel.

endaortitis (en″da-or-ti′tis) inflammation of the membrane lining the aorta.

endarterectomy (en″dar-ter-ek′to-me) excision of thickened atheromatous areas of the innermost coat of an artery.

endarterial (end″ar-te′re-al) within an artery.

endarteritis (en″dar-ter-i′tis) inflammation of the innermost coat (tunica intima) of an artery. **e. oblit′erans,** a form in which the lumen of the smaller vessels become narrowed or obliterated as a result of proliferation of the tissue of the intimal layer.

end-artery (end-ar′ter-e) an artery that does not anastomose with other arteries.

end-body (end′bod-e) end-piece.

endbrain (-brān) telencephalon.

end-bulb (-bulb) one of the small encapsulated bodies at the end of sensory nerve fibers in skin, mucous membranes, muscles, and other areas.

endemic (en-dem′ik) 1. present in a community at all times. 2. a disease of low morbidity that is constantly present in a human community, but clinically recognizable in only a few.

endemiology (en-de″me-ol′o-je) the science dealing with all the factors relating to occurrence of endemic disease.

endemoepidemic (en″de-mo-ep″ĭ-dem′ik) endemic, but occasionally becoming epidemic.

endergonic (en″der-gon′ik) characterized or accompanied by the absorption of energy; requiring the input of free energy.

end-feet (end′fēt) botton- or knoblike terminal enlargements of naked nerve fibers which end in relation to dendrites of another cell.

ending (-ing) a termination, especially the peripheral termination of a nerve or nerve fiber.

endoaneurysmorrhaphy (en″do-an″u-riz-mor′ah-fe) opening of an aneurysmal sac and suture of the orifices.

endoangiitis (-an″je-i′tis) endangiitis.

endoappendicitis (-ah-pen″dĭ-si′tis) inflammation of the mucous membrane of the vermiform appendix.

endoarteritis (-ar″ter-i′tis) endarteritis.

endoblast (en′do-blast) entoderm.

endobronchitis (en″di-brong-ki′tis) inflammation of the epithelial lining of the bronchi.

endocardial (-kar′de-al) 1. situated or occurring within the heart. 2. pertaining to the endocardium.

endocarditis (-kar-di′tis) inflammation of the endocardium. **endocardit′ic,** adj. **atypical verrucous e.,** see *verrucous e.* **bacterial e.,** a febrile systemic disease marked by bacterial or fungal infection of the heart valves, with formation of pathogen-laden vegetations: the *acute* form has an abrupt onset and a rapidly progressive course, and is caused by virulent organisms—e.g., *Staphylococcus aureus,* gram-negative bacteria, and fungi—capable of invading other tissues; the *subacute* form has an insidious onset and protracted course, and is due to various bacteria, usually α-hemolytic streptococci. **constrictive e.,** Löffler′s e. **Libman-Sacks e.,** see *verrucous e.* **Löffler′s e., Löffler′s parietal fibroplastic e.,** endocarditis associated with eosinophilia, marked by fibroplastic thickening of the endocardium, resulting in congestive heart failure, persistent tachycardia, hepatomegaly, splenomegaly, serous effusions into the pleural cavity, and edema of the limbs. **marantic e.,** nonbacterial thrombotic e. **mural e.,** that affecting the lining of the walls of the heart chambers only. **nonbacterial verrucous e.,** see *verrucous e.* **parietal e.,** mural e. **rheumatic e.,** that associated with rheumatic fever. **rickettsial e.,** endocarditis caused by invasion of the heart valves with *Coxiella burnetii;* it is a sequela of Q fever, usually occurring in persons who have had rheumatic fever. **syphilitic e.,** that resulting from extension of syphilitic infection from the aorta. **tuberculous e.,** that resulting from extension of a tuberculous infection from the pericardium and myocardium. **valvular e.,** that affecting the membrane over the heart valves only. **vegetative e.,** verrucous e. **verrucous e.,** nonbacterial endocarditis with formation of shreds of fibrin on the ulcerated valves, often found in association with systemic lupus erythematosus, in which case it is known as *Libman-Sacks disease* or *atypical verrucous endocarditis.*

endocardium (en″do-kar′de-um) the endothelial lining membrane of the heart and the connective tissue bed on which it lies.

endocervicitis (-ser″vĭ-si′tis) inflammation of the endocervix.

endocervix (-ser′viks) 1. the mucous membrane lining the canal of the cervix uteri. 2. the region of the opening of the cervix into the uterine cavity. **endocer′vical,** adj.

endochondral (-kon′dral) situated, formed, or occurring within cartilage.

endocolitis (-ko-li′tis) inflammation of the mucous membrane of the colon.

endocranial (-kra′ne-al) within the cranium.

endocranitis (-kra-ni′tis) inflammation of the endocranium.

endocranium (-kra′ne-um) the endosteal layer of the dura mater of the brain.

endocrinasthenia (-krin″es-the′ne-ah) a hormonal imbalance resulting in psychosis or psychoneurosis.

endocrine (en′do-krin) 1. secreting internally. 2. pertaining to internal secretions; hormonal. See also under *system*.

endocrinism (en-dok′rĭ-nizm) endocrinopathy.

endocrinologist (en″do-krĭ-nol′o-jist) an individual skilled in endocrinology, and in the diagnosis and treatment of disorders of the glands of internal secretion, i.e., the endocrine glands.

endocrinology (en″do-krĭ-nol′o-je) the study of the endocrine system.

endocrinopathy (en″do-krĭ-nop′ah-the) any disease due to disorder of the endocrine system. **endocrinopath′ic,** adj.

endocrinotherapy (-kri″no-ther′ah-pe) treatment of disease by the administration of endocrine preparations; hormonotherapy.

endocrinous (en-dok′rĭ-nus) of or pertaining to an internal secretion (hormone) or to a gland producing such a secretion, i.e., to an endocrine gland.

endocystitis (en″do-sis-ti′tis) inflammation of the bladder mucosa.

endocytosis (-si-to′sis) the uptake by a cell of particles that are too large to diffuse through its wall; it includes both phagocytosis and pinocytosis.

endoderm (en′do-derm) entoderm.

Endodermophyton (en″do-der-mof′ĭ-ton) *Trichophyton.*

endodontia (-don′she-ah) endodontics.

endodontics (-don′tiks) the branch of dentistry concerned with the etiology, prevention, diagnosis, and treatment of conditions that affect the tooth pulp, root, and periapical tissues.

endodontist (-don′tist) a dentist who specializes in endodontics.

endodontitis (-don-ti′tis) pulpitis.

endodontium (-don′she-um) dental pulp.

endodontology (-don-tol′o-je) endodontics.

endoenteritis (-en″ter-i′tis) inflammation of the intestinal mucosa.

endoenzyme (-en′zīm) an intracellular enzyme.

endogamy (en-dog′ah-me) 1. fertilization by union of separate cells having the same chromatin ancestry. 2. restriction of marriage to persons within the same community. **endog′amous,** adj.

endogenic (en″do-jen′ik) endogenous.

endogenous (en-doj′ĕ-nus) produced within or caused by factors within the organism.

endointoxication (en″do-in-tok″sĭ-ka′shun) poisoning by an endogenous toxin.

endolaryngeal (-lah-rin′je-al) situated or occurring within the larynx.

Endolimax (-li′maks) a genus of amebas found in the colon of man, other mammals, birds, amphibians, and cockroaches.

endolymph (en′do-limf) the fluid within the membranous labyrinth. **endolymphat′ic,** adj.

endolympha (en″do-lim′fah) endolymph.

endolysin (en-dol′ĭ-sin) a bactericidal substance in cells, acting directly on bacteria.

endomesoderm (en″do-mes′o-derm) mesoderm originating from the entoderm of the two-layered blastodisk.

endometrectomy (-me-trek′to-me) excision of the uterine mucosa.

endometrial (-me′tre-al) pertaining to the endometrium.

endometrioid (-me′tre-oid) resembling endometrium.

endometrioma (-me″tre-o′mah) a solitary non-neoplastic mass containing endometrial tissue.

endometriosis (-me″tre-o′sis) the aberrant occurrence of tissue which more or less perfectly resembles the endometrium, in various locations in the pelvic cavity. **endometriot′ic,** adj. **e. exter′na, external e.,** endometriosis. **e. inter′na, internal e.,** adenomyosis. **ovarian e.,** that involving the ovary, either in the form of small superficial islands or in the form of epithelial ("chocolate") cysts of various sizes. **stromal e.,** adenomyosis in which all or nearly all of the tissue infiltrating the myometrium consists of stroma.

endometritis (-me-tri′tis) inflammation of the endometrium. **puerperal e.,** that following childbirth. **syncytial e.,** a benign tumor-like lesion with infiltration of the uterine wall by large syncytial trophoblastic cells.

endometrium (-me′tre-um) the mucous membrane lining the uterus.

endomitosis (-mi-to′sis) reproduction of nuclear elements not followed by chromosome movements and cytoplasmic division. **endomitot′ic,** adj.

endomorph (en′do-morf) an individual having the type of body build in which entodermal tissues predominate: there is relative preponderance of soft roundness throughout the body, with large digestive viscera and fat accumulations, and with large trunk and thighs and tapering extremities.

endomorphy (-mor″fe) the condition of being an endomorph. **endomor′phic,** adj.

endomyocarditis (en″do-mi″o-kar-di′tis) inflammation of endocardium and myocardium.

endomysium (-mis′e-um) the sheath of delicate reticular fibrils surrounding each muscle fiber.

endoneuritis (-nu-ri′tis) inflammation of the endoneurium.

endoneurium (-nu′re-um) the interstitial connective tissue in a peripheral nerve, separating individual nerve fibers. **endoneu′rial,** adj.

endonuclease (-nu′kle-ās) a nuclease that cleaves internal bonds of polynucleotides.

endoparasite (-par′ah-sīt) a parasite that lives within the host's body. **endoparasit′ic,** adj.

endopelvic (-pel′vik) within the pelvis.

endopeptidase (-pep′tĭ-dās) a peptidase capable of acting on any peptide linkage in a peptide chain.

endopericarditis (-per″ĭ-kar-di′tis) inflammation of the endocardium and pericardium.

endoperimyocarditis (-per″ĭ-mi″o-kar-di′tis) inflammation of the endocardium, pericardium, and myocardium.

endoperitonitis (-per″ĭ-to-ni′tis) inflammation of the serous lining of peritoneal cavity.

endophlebitis (-fle-bi′tis) inflammation of the intima of a vein.

endophthalmitis (en″dof-thal-mi′tis) inflammation of the ocular cavities and their adjacent structures.

endophyte (en′do-fīt) a parasitic plant organism living within its host's body.

endophytic (en″do-fit′ik) 1. pertaining to an endophyte. 2. growing inward; proliferating on the interior of an organ or structure.

endoplasm (en′do-plazm) the more centrally located cytoplasm of a cell. **endoplas′mic,** adj.

endopolyploid (en″do-pol′ĭ-ploid) having reduplicated chromatin within an intact nucleus, with or without an increase in the number of chromosomes (applied only to cells and tissues).

endopolyploidy (-pol″ĭ-ploi′de) 1. endomitosis. 2. polysomaty. 3. autopolyploidy due to a previous endomitotic cycle.

endoreduplication (-re-du″plĭ-ka′shun) replication of chromosomes without subsequent cell division.

end organ (end″or′gan) one of the larger, encapsulated endings of sensory nerves.

endosalpingitis (en″do-sal″pin-ji′tis) inflammation of the endosalpinx.

endosalpingoma (-sal″ping-go′mah) adenomyoma of the uterine tube.

endosalpingosis (-sal″ping-go′sis) 1. endometriosis involving the uterine tube. 2. ovarian endometriosis in which the abnormal mucosa resembles tubal mucosa rather than endometrium.

endoscope (en′do-skōp) an instrument for examining the interior of a hollow viscus.

endoscopy (en-dos′ko-pe) visual examination by means of an endoscope. **endoscop′ic,** adj. **peroral e.,** examination of organs accessible to observation through an endoscope passed through the mouth.

endosepsis (en″do-sep′sis) septicemia originating from causes inside the body.

endoskeleton (-skel′ĕ-ton) the cartilaginous and bony skeleton of the body, exclusive of that part of the skeleton of dermal origin.

endosmometer (en″dos-mom′ĕ-ter) an instrument for measurement of endosmosis.

endosmosis (en″dos-mo′sis) inward osmosis; inward passage of liquid through a membrane of a cell or cavity. **endosmot′ic,** adj.

endosome (en′do-sōm) a body thought to consist of deoxyribonucleic acid, observed in the vesicular nucleus of certain protozoa.

endospore (-spōr) 1. a spore produced in the hypha or cell. 2. the inner wall of a spore.

endosteal (en-dos′te-al) 1. pertaining to the endosteum. 2. occurring or located within a bone.

endosteitis (en-dos″te-i′tis) inflammation of the endosteum.

endosteoma (en-dos″te-o′mah) a tumor in the medullary cavity of a bone.

endosteum (en-dos′te-um) the tissue lining the medullary cavity of a bone.

endostoma (en″dos-to′mah) endosteoma.

endotendineum (en″do-ten-din′e-um) the delicate connective tissue separating the secondry bundles (fascicles) of a tendon.

endothelia (-the′le-ah) [Gr.] plural of *endothelium.*

endothelial (-the′le-al) pertaining to or made up of endothelium.

endotheliochorial (-the″le-o-ko′re-al) denoting a type of placenta in which syncytial trophoblast embeds maternal vessels bared to their endothelial lining.

endotheliocyte (-the′le-o-sīt″) endothelial leukocyte.

endothelioid (-the′le-oid) resembling endothelium.

endotheliolysin (-the″le-ol′ĭ-sin) an antibody which causes the dissolution of endothelial cells. **endotheliolyt′ic,** adj.

endothelioma (-the″le-o′mah) a tumor arising from the endothelial lining of blood vessels.

endotheliomatosis (-the″le-o″mah-to′sis) formation of multiple, diffuse endotheliomas.

endotheliosis (-the″le-o′sis) proliferation of endothelial elements.

endotheliotoxin (-the″le-o-tok′sin) a specific toxin that acts on endothelium of capillaries and small veins, producing hemorrhage.

endothelium (-the′le-um), pl. *endothe′lia* [Gr.] the layer of epithelial cells that lines the cavities of the heart and of the blood and lymph vessels, and the serous cavities of the body.

endothermal, endothermic (-ther′mal; -ther′mik) 1. characterized by the absorption of heat. 2. pertaining to endothermy.

endothermy (en′do-ther″me) production of heat in the tissues by the resistance they offer to the passage of high-frequency current.

endothrix (-thriks) a dermatophyte whose growth and spore production are confined chiefly within the hair shaft.

endotoxemia (en″do-toks-e′me-ah) the presence of endotoxins in the blood, which may result in shock.

endotoxin (-tok′sin) a heat-stable toxin present in the intact bacterial cell but not in cell-free filtrates of cultures of intact bacteria. Endotoxins are lipopolysaccharide complexes that occur in the cell wall; they are pyrogenic and increase capillary permeability. **endotox′ic**, adj.

endotracheal (-tra′ke-al) within the trachea.

endotrachelitis (-tra″kel-i′tis) endocervicitis.

endovasculitis (-vas″ku-li′tis) endangiitis.

Endoxan (en-dok′san) trademark for a preparation of cyclophosphamide.

end piece (end′pēs) in early immunological theory, the pseudoglobulin fraction of guinea pig serum, which corresponds to the C2 component of complement.

end plate (-plāt) a flattened discoid expansion at the myoneural junction, where a myelinated motor nerve fiber joins a skeletal muscle fiber.

endrin (en′drin) a highly toxic insecticide of the chlorinated hydrocarbon group.

enema (en′ĕ-mah) 1. introduction of fluid into the rectum. 2. a solution introduced into the rectum to promote evacuation of feces or as a means of introducing nutrient or medicinal substances, or opaque material in roentgen examination of the lower intestinal tract. **analeptic e.**, an enema consisting of a pint of tepid water containing ½ teaspoonful of salt. **barium e., contrast e.**, a suspension of barium injected into and retained in the intestines during roentgenographic examination; intestinal deformities are demonstrated by filling defects revealed by the column of radiopaque barium. **double contrast e.**, injection and evacuation of a barium suspension, followed by inflation of the intestines with air, to facilitate roentgen visualization of the intestinal mucosa. **Fleet e.**, trademark for an enema containing, in each 100 ml., 16 gm. sodium biphosphate and 6 gm. sodium phosphate, packaged in a plastic squeeze bottle fitted with a 2-inch, prelubricated rectal tube.

energometer (en″er-gom′ĕ-ter) an instrument for studying the pulse.

energy (en′er-je) power which may be translated into motion, overcoming resistance, or effecting physical change; the ability to do work. **free e.**, the energy equal to the maximum amount of work that can be obtained from a process occurring under conditions of fixed temperature and pressure. **kinetic e.**, the energy of motion. **nuclear e.**, energy that can be liberated by changes in the nucleus of an atom (as by fission of a heavy nucleus or fusion of light nuclei into heavier ones with accompanying loss of mass). **potential e.**, energy at rest or not manifested in actual work.

enervation (en″er-va′shun) 1. lack of nervous energy. 2. removal of a nerve or a section of a nerve.

enflagellation (en-flaj″ĕ-la′shun) the formation of flagella; flagellation.

ENG electronystagmography.

engagement (en-gāj′ment) the entrance of the fetal head or presenting part into the superior pelvic strait.

engastrius (en-gas′tre-us) a double monster in which one fetus is contained within the abdomen of the other.

engorgement (en-gorj′ment) local congestion; distention with fluids; hyperemia.

engram (en′gram) the traces allegedly left in the nervous system by any experience.

engraphia (en-gra′fe-ah) the theory that stimuli leave definite traces (engrams) on the protoplasm, which, with repetition, induce a habit that persists after the stimuli have ceased.

enhexymal (en-hek′sĭ-mal) hexobarbital.

enkatarrhaphy (en″kah-tar′ah-fe) the operation of burying a structure by suturing together the sides of tissues adjacent to it.

enol (e′nol) one of two tautomeric forms of a substance, the other being the keto form; the enol is formed from the keto by migration of hydrogen from the adjacent carbon atom to the carbonyl group.

enolase (e′no-lās) an enzyme in glycolytic systems that changes phosphoglyceric acid into phosphopyruvic acid.

enophthalmos (en″of-thal′mos) a backward displacement of the eyeball into the orbit.

enostosis (en″os-to′sis) a bony growth within a bone cavity or on the internal surface of the bone cortex.

Enovid (en-o′vid) trademark for preparations of mestranol and norethynodrel, used to inhibit ovulation.

ensiform (en′sĭ-form) sword-shaped; xiphoid.

ensomphalus (en-som′fah-lus) a double monster with blended bodies, two separate navels, and two umbilical cords.

enstrophe (en′stro-fe) inversion, especially of the margin of the eyelids.

E.N.T. ear, nose, and throat.

entad (en′tad) toward a center; inwardly.

ental (en′tal) inner; central.

entamebiasis (en″tah-me-bi′ah-sis) infection by *Entamoeba*.

Entamoeba (en″tah-me′bah) a genus of amebas parasitic in the intestines of vertebrates, including three species commonly parasitic in man: *E. co′li*, found in the intestinal tract; *E. gingiva′lis* (*E. bucca′lis*), found in the mouth; and *E. histolyt′ica*, the cause of amebic dysentery and tropical abscess of the liver.

entasia (en-ta′ze-ah) a constrictive spasm; tonic spasm.

enter(o)- word element [Gr.], *intestines*.

enteral (en′ter-al) within, by way of, or pertaining to the small intestine.

enteralgia (en″ter-al′je-ah) pain in the intestine.

enterectomy (-ek′to-me) excision of a portion of the intestine.

enterelcosis (-el-ko′sis) ulceration of the intestine.

enterepiplocele (-e-pip′lo-sēl) enteroepiplocele.

enteric (en-ter′ik) pertaining to the small intestine.

enteric-coated (en-ter″ik-kōt′ed) designating a special coating applied to tablets or capsules that prevents release and absorption of active ingredients until they reach the intestine.

enteritis (en″ter-i′tis) inflammation of the intestine, especially of the small intestine. **e. anaphylac'tica,** hemorrhagic inflammation of both the large and the small intestine following a second dose of anaphylactogen in sensitized dogs. **choleriform e.,** an acute cholera-like diarrheal disease with a high fatality rate prevalent in epidemic and endemic forms in the Western Pacific area since 1938. **e. cys'tica chron'ica,** a form marked by cystic dilatations of the intestinal glands, due to closure of their openings. **diphtheritic e.,** enteritis marked by the presence of a false membrane and severe ulceration of the mucosa beneath the membrane. **e. gra'vis,** an often fatal disease characterized by severe abdominal pain, nausea, vomiting, and bloody diarrhea, with mucosal necrosis and hemorrhage and edema of the submucosa, most prominent in the jejunum and proximal ileum. **e. membrana'cea, membranous e., mucomembranous e., mucous e., myxomembranous e.,** mucous colitis. **e. necrot'icans,** intestinal inflammation due to *Clostridium perfringens* type F, marked by necrosis. **e. nodula'ris,** enteritis with enlargement of the lymph nodes. **pellicular e.,** mucous colitis. **phlegmonous e.,** a condition with symptoms resembling those of peritonitis; it may be secondary to other intestinal diseases, e.g., chronic obstruction, strangulated hernia, carcinoma. **e. polypo'sa,** that marked by polypoid growths in the intestine, due to proliferation of the connective tissue. **protozoan e.,** that in which the intestine is infested with protozoan organisms of various species. **pseudomembranous e.,** see under *enterocolitis.* **regional e.,** see under *ileitis.* **streptococcal e.,** primary phlegmonous enteritis due to *Streptococcus pyogenes.* **terminal e.,** regional ileitis.

enteroanastomosis (en″ter-o-ah-nas″to-mo′sis) enteroenterostomy.

Enterobacteriaceae (-bak-te″re-a′se-e) a family of gram-negative, rod-shaped bacteria (order Eubacteriales) occurring as plant or animal parasites or as saprophytes.

enterobiasis (-bi′ah-sis) infection with nematodes of the genus *Enterobius,* especially *E. vermicularis.*

Enterobius (en″ter-o′be-us) a genus of intestinal nematodes (superfamily Oxyuroidea), including *E. vermicula'ris,* the seatworm or pinworm, parasitic in the upper large intestine, and occasionally in the female genitals and bladder; infection is frequent in children, sometimes causing itching.

enterocele (en′ter-o-sēl″) intestinal hernia.

enterocentesis (en″ter-o-sen-te′sis) surgical puncture of the intestine.

enteroclysis (en″ter-ok′lĭ-sis) the injection of liquids into the intestine.

enterococcus (en″ter-o-kok′kus), pl. *enterococ'ci* [Gr.] any streptococcus of the human intestine.

enterocoele (en′ter-o-sēl″) the body cavity formed by outpouchings from the archenteron.

enterocolectomy (en″ter-o-ko-lek′to-me) resection of the intestine, including the ileum, cecum, and colon.

enterocolitis (-ko-li′tis) inflammation of the small intestine and colon. **hemorrhagic e.,** enterocolitis characterized by hemorrhagic breakdown of the intestinal mucosa, with inflammatory cell infiltration. **necrotizing e., pseudomembranous e.,** an acute, superficial necrosis of the mucosa of the small intestine and colon, with shock and dehydration, and passage per rectum of seromucus, often mixed with blood, and shreds or casts of the bowel wall.

enterocolostomy (-ko-los′to-me) surgical anastomosis of the small intestine to the colon.

enterocrinin (en″ter-ok′rĭ-nin) an extract of the mucosa of the small intestine, said to be a physiological hormone, which stimulates the intestine to secretory activity.

enterocutaneous (en″ter-o-ku-ta′ne-us) pertaining to or communicating with the intestine and the skin, or surface of the body.

enterocyst (en′ter-o-sist″) a cyst proceeding from subperitoneal tissue.

enterocystocele (en″ter-o-sis′to-sēl) hernia of the bladder and intestine.

enterocystoma (-sis-to′mah) vitelline cyst.

enterodynia (-din′e-ah) pain in the intestine.

enteroenterostomy (-en″ter-os′to-me) surgical anastomosis between two segments of the intestine.

enteroepiplocele (en″ter-o-e-pip′lo-sēl) hernia of the small intestine and omentum.

enterogastritis (-gas-tri′tis) gastroenteritis.

enterogastrone (-gas′trōn) anthelone E; a hormone of the duodenum which mediates the humoral inhibition of gastric secretion and motility produced by ingestion of fat.

enterogenous (en″ter-oj′ĕ-nus) 1. arising from the primitive foregut. 2. originating within the small intestine.

enterogram (en′ter-o-gram″) an instrumental tracing of the movements of the intestine.

enterography (en″ter-og′rah-fe) a description of the intestine.

enterohepatitis (en″ter-o-hep″ah-ti′tis) 1. inflammation of the intestine and liver. 2. histomoniasis of turkeys.

enterohepatocele (-hep′ah-to-sēl″) an umbilical hernia containing intestine and liver.

enterohydrocele (-hi′dro-sēl) hernia with hydrocele.

enterokinase (-ki′nās) enteropeptidase.

enterokinesia (-ki″ne′se-ah) peristalsis.

enterokinetic (-ki-net′ik) pertaining to or stimulating peristalsis.

enterokinin (-ki′nin) an extract of the mucosa of the small intestine, said to be a physiological hormone, which stimulates intestinal motility.

enterolith (en′ter-o-lith″) a calculus in the intestine.

enterolithiasis (en″ter-o-lĭ-thi′ah-sis) the presence of intestinal calculi.

enterology (en″ter-ol′o-je) scientific study of the intestine.

enterolysis (en″ter-ol′ĭ-sis) surgical separation of intestinal adhesions.

enteromegaly (en″ter-o-meg′ah-le) enlargement of the intestine.

enteromerocele (-me′ro-sēl) femoral hernia.

enteromycosis (-mi-ko′sis) fungal disease of the intestine.

enteron (en′ter-on) the gut or alimentary canal; usually used in medicine with specific reference to the small intestine.

enteroparesis (en″ter-o-pah-re′sis) relaxation of the intestine resulting in dilatation.

enteropathogen (-path′o-jen) a microorganism which causes a disease of the intestine. **enteropathogen′ic,** adj.

enteropathogenesis (-path″o-jen′ĕ-sis) the production of disease or disorder of the intestine.

enteropathy (en″ter-op′ah-the) any disease of the intestine. **gluten e.,** nontropical sprue. **protein-losing e.,** a nonspecific term referring to conditions, e.g., adult celiac disease, associated with excessive loss of enteric plasma proteins.

enteropeptidase (en″ter-o-pep′tĭ-dās) an enzyme of the intestinal juice which activates the proteolytic enzyme of the pancreatic juice by converting trypsinogen into trypsin.

enteropexy (en′ter-o-pek″se) surgical fixation of the intestine to the abdominal wall.

enteroplasty (-plas″te) plastic repair of the intestine.

enteroplegia (en″ter-o-ple′je-ah) adynamic ileus.

enteroptosis (en″ter-op-to′sis) abnormal downward displacement of the intestine. **enteroptot′ic,** adj.

enterorrhagia (en″ter-o-ra′je-ah) intestinal hemorrhage.

enterorrhaphy (en″ter-or′ah-fe) suture of the intestine.

enterorrhexis (en″ter-o-rek′sis) rupture of the intestine.

enteroscope (en′ter-o-skōp″) an instrument for inspecting the inside of the intestine.

enterosepsis (en″ter-o-sep′sis) sepsis developed from the intestinal contents.

enterospasm (en′ter-o-spazm″) intestinal spasm.

enterostasis (en″ter-o-sta′sis) intestinal stasis.

enterostaxis (-stak′sis) slow hemorrhage through the intestinal mucosa.

enterostenosis (-stě-no′sis) narrowing or stricture of the intestine.

enterostomy (en″ter-os′to-me) formation of a permanent opening into the intestine through the abdominal wall. **enterosto′mal,** adj.

enterotomy (en″ter-ot′o-me) incision of the intestine.

enterotoxemia (en″ter-o-tok-se′me-ah) a condition characterized by the presence in the blood of toxins produced in the intestines.

enterotoxigenic (-tok″sĭ-jen′ik) producing, produced by, or pertaining to production of enterotoxin.

enterotoxin (-tok′sin) 1. a toxin specific for the cells of the intestinal mucosa. 2. a toxin arising in the intestine. 3. an exotoxin that is protein in nature and relatively heat-stable, produced by staphylococci.

enterotoxism (-tok′sizm) autointoxication of enteric origin.

enterotropic (-trop′ik) affecting the intestine.

enterovaginal (-vaj′ĭ-nal) pertaining to or communicating with the intestine and the vagina.

enterovesical (-ves′ĭ-kal) pertaining to or communicating with the intestine and urinary bladder.

Entero-Vioform (-vi′o-form) trademark for a preparation of iodochlorhydroxyguin.

enterovirus (-vi′rus) one of a subgroup of the picornaviruses infecting the gastrointestinal tract and discharged in the excreta, including coxsackieviruses, echoviruses, and polioviruses.

enterozoon (-zo′on) an animal parasite in the intestine. **enterozo′ic,** adj.

enthalpy (en′thal-pe) the heat content of a physical system.

enthesis (en′the-sis) the use of artificial material in the repair of a defect or deformity of the body.

enthetic (en-thet′ik) 1. pertaining to enthesis. 2. brought in from outside.

ento- word element [Gr.], *within; inner.*

entoblast (en′to-blast) the entoderm.

entocele (-sēl) internal hernia.

entochoroidea (en″to-ko-roi′de-ah) the inner layer of the choroid.

entocone (en′to-kōn) the medial posterior cusp of an upper molar tooth.

entocornea (en″to-kor′ne-ah) Descemet's membrane.

entoderm (en′to-derm) the innermost of the three primitive germ layers of the embryo; from it are derived the epithelium of the pharynx, respiratory tract (except the nose), digestive tract, bladder, and urethra. **entoder′mal, entoder′mic,** adj.

entoectad (en″to-ek′tad) from within outward.

entomere (en′to-mēr) a blastomere normally destined to become entoderm.

entomion (en-to′me-on) the tip of mastoid angle of parietal bone.

entomology (en″to-mol′o-je) that branch of biology concerned with the study of insects. **medical e.,** that concerned with insects which cause disease or serve as vectors of pathogens.

entomophilous (-mof′ĭ-lus) fertilized by insect-borne pollen; said of certain flowers.

entophyte (en′to-fīt) endophyte.

entopic (en-top′ik) occurring in the proper place.

entoptic (en-top′tik) originating within the eye.

entoptoscopy (en″top-tos′ko-pe) inspection of the interior of the eye.

entoretina (en″to-ret′ĭ-nah) the nervous or inner layer of the retina.

entotic (en-tot′ik) situated in or arising within the ear.

entozoon (en″to-zo′on) an internal animal parasite. **entozo′ic,** adj.

entropion (en-tro′pe-on) inversion, or the turning inward, as of the margin of an eyelid. **e. u′veae,** inversion of the margin of the pupil.

entropionize (-pe-ŏ-nīz″) to put into a state of inversion.

entypy (en′tĭ-pe) a method of gastrulation in which the entoderm lies external to the amniotic ectoderm.

enucleate (e-nu′kle-āt) to remove whole and clean, as the eye from its socket.

enucleation (e-nu″kle-a′shun) removal of an organ or other mass intact from its supporting tissues, as of the eyeball from the orbit.

enuresis (en″u-re′sis) involuntary discharge of urine; usually referring to involuntary discharge of urine during sleep at night. **enuret′ic**, adj.

envenomation (en-ven″o-ma′shun) the poisonous effects caused by the bites, stings, or effluvia of insects and other arthropods, or the bites of snakes.

environment (en-vi′ron-ment) the sum total of all the conditions and elements that make up the surroundings and influence the development of an individual.

Enzactin (en-zak′tin) trademark for preparations of triacetin.

enzootic (en″zo-ot′ik) 1. present in an animal community at all times, but occurring in only small numbers of cases. 2. a disease of low morbidity which is constantly present in an animal community.

enzygotic (en″zi-got′ik) developed from one zygote.

enzymatic (en″zi-mat′ik) of, relating to, caused by, or of the nature of an enzyme.

enzyme (en′zīm) a protein capable of accelerating or producing by catalytic action some change in a substrate for which it is often specific. **activating e.,** one which activates a given amino acid by attaching it to the corresponding transfer ribonucleic acid. **adaptive e.,** induced e. **allosteric e.,** one containing· an allosteric site; see under *site.* **autolytic e.,** one that produces autolysis of the cell in which it exists. **brancher e., branching e.,** α-glucan-branching glycosyltransferase: an enzyme involved in conversion of amylose to amylopectin; deficiency causes amylopectinosis (glycogenosis, type IV). **clotting e., coagulating e.,** one that catalyzes the conversion of soluble into insoluble proteins. **constitutive e.,** one produced by a microorganism regardless of the presence or absence of the specific substrate. **curdling e.,** clotting e. **debrancher e., debranching e.,** dextrin-1,6-glucosidase: one acting on glucose residues of the glycogen molecule, it is important in glycogenolysis. Deficiency cause Forbes disease (glycogenosis, type III). **digestive e.,** a substance that catalyzes the process of digestion. **extracellular e.,** one existing outside the cell secreting it. **glycolytic e.,** one that catalyzes the conversion of sugar to pyruvic acid. **induced e., inducible e.,** one whose production requires or is stimulated by a specific small molecule, the *inducer,* which is the substrate of the enzyme or a compound structurally related to it. **inhibitory e.,** one whose action blocks another reaction or a reaction sequence. **lipolytic e.,** one that catalyzes the hydrolysis of fat. **mucolytic e.,** one that catalyzes the hydrolytic depolymerization of mucopolysaccharides.

oxidation e., oxidase. **proteolytic e.,** one that catalyzes the hydrolysis of proteins and various split products of proteins, the final product being small peptides and amino acids. **Q e.,** α-glucan-branching glycosyltransferase; see under *glycosyltransferase.* **redox e.,** one that catalyzes oxidation-reduction reactions. **reducing e.,** reductase. **repressible e.,** one whose rate of production is decreased as the concentration of certain metabolites is increased. **respiratory e's,** enzymes of the mitochondria, e.g., cytochrome oxidase, which serve as catalysts for cellular oxidations. **splitting e.,** one that catalyzes the splitting of a fragment from a molecule, e.g., the splitting out of CO_2 from a carboxyl group (decarboxylation). **steatolytic e.,** lipolytic e. **transferring e.,** a transferase; an enzyme that catalyzes the transference of various radicals between molecules. **uricolytic e.,** one that catalyzes the conversion of uric acid to urea. **yellow e's,** flavoproteins isolated from several sources, which take part in oxidations and reductions.

enzymic (en-zi′mik) enzymatic.

enzymology (en″zi-mol′o-je) the study of enzymes and enzymatic action.

enzymolysis (en″zi-mol′ĭ-sis) disintegration induced by an enzyme.

enzymopathy (en″zi-mop′ah-the) an inborn error of metabolism consisting of defective or absent enzymes, as in the glycogenoses or the mucopolysaccharidoses.

enzymopenia (en-zi″mo-pe′ne-ah) deficiency of an enzyme in the blood. **enzymope′nic,** adj.

enzymuria (en″zi-mu′re-ah) presence of enzymes in the urine.

eonism (e′o-nizm) transvestism in the male.

eosin (e′o-sin) any of a class of rose-colored stains or dyes, all being bromine derivatives of fluorescein; *eosin Y,* the sodium salt of tetrabromfluorescein, is much used in histologic and laboratory procedures.

eosinopenia (e″o-sin″o-pe′ne-ah) abnormal deficiency of eosinophils in the blood.

eosinophil (e″o-sin′o-fil) a granular leukocyte having a nucleus with two lobes connected by a thread of chromatin, and cytoplasm containing coarse, round granules of uniform size.

eosinophilia (e″o-sin″o-fil′e-ah) 1. the formation and accumulation of an abnormally large number of eosinophils in the blood. 2. the condition of being readily stained with eosin. **tropical e.,** a disease characterized by anorexia, malaise, cough, leukocytosis, and an increase in eosinophils.

eosinophilic (-fil′ik) staining readily with eosin; pertaining to eosinophils or to eosinophilia.

eosinophilous (e″o-sĭ-nof′ĭ-lus) eosinophilic.

eosinotactic (e″o-sin″o-tak′tik) attracting or repelling eosinophilic cells.

epactal (e-pak′tal) 1. supernumerary. 2. any wormian bone.

epaxial (ep-ak′se-al) situated upon or above an axis.

epencephalon (ep″en-sef′ah-lon) 1. cerebellum. 2. metencephalon.

ependyma (ĕ-pen'dĭ-mah) the membrane lining the cerebral ventricles and the central canal of the spine. **epen'dymal,** adj.

ependymitis (ep"en-dĭ-mi'tis) inflammation of the ependyma.

ependymoblast (ep"en-di'mo-blast) an embryonic ependymal cell.

ependymocyte (ĕ-pen'dĭ-mo-sīt) an ependymal cell.

ependymoma (ĕ-pen"dĭ-mo'mah) a neoplasm, usually slow growing and benign, composed of differentiated ependymal cells.

ependymopathy (ĕ-pen"dĭ-mop'ah-the) any disease of the ependyma.

Eperythrozoon (ep"ĕ-rith"ro-zo'on) a genus of the family Bartonellaceae; its members are of limited pathogenicity, infecting rodents, cattle, sheep, and swine.

ephapse (e-faps') a point of lateral contact (other than a synapse) between nerve fibers across which impulses are conducted directly through the nerve membranes. **ephap'tic,** adj.

ephebiatrics (ĕ-fe"be-at'riks) the branch of medicine which deals especially with the diagnosis and treatment of diseases and problems peculiar to youth.

ephebic (ĕ-fe'bik) pertaining to youth or the period of puberty and adolescence.

ephebogenesis (ef"ĕ-bo-jen'ĕ-sis) the bodily changes occurring at puberty. **ephebogenet'ic,** adj.

ephebology (ef"ĕ-bol'o-je) the study of puberty.

Ephedra (ef'ĕ-drah) a genus of low, branching shrubs indigenous to China and India; certain species furnish ephedrine.

ephedrine (ĕ-fed'rin, ef'ĕ-drin) an adrenergic, $C_{10}H_{15}NO$, extracted from several species of *Ephedra* or produced synthetically; used as a bronchodilator in the form of the hydrochloride or sulfate salt.

ephelis (ĕ-fe'lis), pl. *ephel'ides* [Gr.] a freckle.

Ephynal (ef'ĭ-nal) trademark for a preparation of vitamin E.

epi- word element [Gr.], *upon; over.*

epiandrosterone (ep"ĭ-an-dros'ter-ōn) an androgenic steroid less active than androsterone and excreted in small amounts in normal human urine.

epiblast (ep'ĭ-blast) 1. ectoderm. 2. ectoderm, except for the neural plate. **epiblas'tic,** adj.

epiblepharon (ep"ĭ-blef'ah-ron) a developmental anomaly in which a horizontal fold of skin stretches across the border of the eyelid; on the lower lid it may press the lashes against the eyeball.

epiboly (e-pib'o-le) gastrulation in which smaller blastomeres at the animal pole of the fertilized ovum grow over and enclose the cells of the vegetal hemisphere.

epibulbar (ep"ĭ-bul'bar) situated upon the eyeball.

epicanthus (-kan'thus) a vertical fold of skin on either side of the nose, sometimes covering the inner canthus; a normal characteristic in persons of certain races, but anomalous in others. **epican'thal, epican'thic,** adj.

epicardia (-kar'de-ah) the portion of the esophagus below the diaphragm.

epicardium (-kar'de-um) the visceral pericardium.

epichorion (-ko're-on) the portion of the uterine mucosa enclosing the implanted conceptus.

epicomus (-ko'mus) a monster with a parasitic twin joined at the summit of the head.

epicondylalgia (-kon"dĭ-lal'je-ah) pain in the muscles or tendons attached to the epicondyle of the humerus.

epicondyle (-kon'dīl) an eminence upon a bone, above its condyle.

epicondylitis (-kon"dĭ-li'tis) inflammation of an epicondyle or of tissues adjoining the humeral epicondyle.

epicondylus (-kon'dĭ-lus), pl. *epicon'dyli* [L.] epicondyle.

epicranium (-kra'ne-um) structures collectively which cover the skull.

epicrisis (-kri'sis) a secondary crisis.

epicritic (-krit'ik) determining accurately; said of cutaneous nerve fibers sensitive to fine variations of touch or temperature.

epicystitis (-sis-ti'tis) inflammation of the structures above the bladder.

epicystotomy (-sis-tot'o-me) cystotomy by the suprapubic method.

epicyte (ep'ĭ-sīt) cell membrane.

epidemic (ep"ĭ-dem'ik) 1. attacking many people in a region at the same time; widely diffused and rapidly spreading. 2. a disease of high morbidity which is only occasionally present in the human community.

epidemicity (-dĕ-mis'ĭ-te) the quality of being widely diffused and rapidly spreading throughout a community.

epidemiogenesis (-de"me-o-jen'ĕ-sis) the spread of a communicable disease to epidemic proportions.

epidemiography (-de"me-og'rah-fe) a treatise upon or an account of epidemics.

epidemiology (-de"me-ol'o-je) 1. the study of the relationships of various factors determining the frequency and distribution of diseases in the human community. 2. the field of medicine dealing with the determination of specific causes of localized outbreaks of infection, toxic poisoning, or other disease of recognized etiology.

epidermidalization (-der"mid-ah-li-za'shun) development of epidermal cells (stratified epithelium) from mucous cells (columnar epithelium).

epidermidosis (ep"i-der"mĭ-do'sis) any disease of the epidermis.

epidermis (-der'mis) the outermost, nonvascular layer of the skin, derived from the embryonic ectoderm, varying in thickness from $\frac{1}{200}$ to $\frac{1}{20}$ inch, and made up of, from within outward, of five layers: basal layer, prickle-cell layer, granular layer, clear layer, and horny layer. **epider'mal, epider'mic,** adj.

epidermitis (-der-mi'tis) inflammation of the epidermis.

epidermodysplasia (-der"mo-dis-pla'ze-ah)

faulty development of the epidermis. **e. ver-rucifor'mis,** a condition due to a virus identical with or closely related to the virus of common warts, in which the lesions are red or red-violet and widespread, and tend to become malignant.

epidermoid (-der'moid) 1. resembling the epidermis. 2. an intracranial cystlike mass formed by inclusion of epidermal elements.

epidermoidoma (-der"moi-do'mah) a cerebral or meningeal tumor formed by inclusion of ectodermal elements at the time of closure of the neural groove.

epidermolysis (-der-mol'ĭ-sis) a loosened state of the epidermis with formation of blebs and bullae either spontaneously or at the site of trauma. **e. bullo'sa,** a variety with development of bullae and vesicles, often at the site of trauma; in the hereditary forms, there may be severe scarring after healing, or extensive denuded areas after rupture of the lesions.

epidermomycosis (-der"mo-mi-ko'sis) dermatophytosis.

epidermophytid (-der-mof'ĭ-tid) dermatophytid.

epidermophytin (-der-mof'ĭ-tin) a filtrate of *Epidermophyton* cultures that induces a hypersensitivity reaction of the tuberculin type; used in treatment of epidermophytosis.

Epidermophyton (-der-mof'ĭ-ton) a genus of fungi, including *E. flocco'sum,* which attacks both skin and nails but not hair, and is one of the causative agents of tinea cruris, tinea pedis (athlete's foot), and onychomycosis.

epidermophytosis (-der"mo-fi-to'sis) a fungal skin infection, especially one due to *Epidermophyton;* dermatophytosis.

epididymectomy (ep"ĭ-did"ĭ-mek'to-me) excision of the epididymis.

epididymis (-did'ĭ-mis) an elongated, cordlike structure along the posterior border of the testis, in the ducts of which the spermatozoa are stored. **epidid'ymal,** adj.

epididymitis (-did"ĭ-mi'tis) inflammation of the epididymis.

epididymo-orchitis (-did"ĭ-mo-or-ki'tis) inflammation of the epididymis and testis.

epididymotomy (-did"ĭ-mot'o-me) incision of the epididymis.

epididymovasostomy (-did"ĭ-mo-vas-os'to-me) surgical anastomosis of the epididymis to the ductus deferens.

epidural (ep"ĭ-du'ral) situated upon or outside the dura mater.

epidurography (-du-rog'rah-fe) radiography of the spine after a radiopaque medium has been injected into the epidural space.

epiestriol (-es'tre-ol) an estrogenic steroid found in pregnant women.

epigastralgia (-gas-tral'je-ah) pain in the epigastrium.

epigastrium (-gas'tre-um) the upper and middle region of the abdomen, located within the sternal angle. **epigas'tric,** adj.

epigastrius (-gas'tre-us) a double monster in which the parasite forms a tumor on the epigastrium of the autosite.

epigastrocele (-gas'tro-sēl) epigastric hernia.

epigenesis (-jen'ĕ-sis) the development of an organism from an undifferentiated cell, consisting in the successive formation and development of organs and parts that do not preexist in the fertilized egg. **epigenet'ic,** adj.

epiglottidean (-glŏ-tid'e-an) pertaining to the epiglottis.

epiglottidectomy (-glot"ĭ-dek'to-me) excision of the epiglottis.

epiglottiditis (-glot"ĭ-di'tis) inflammation of the epiglottis.

epiglottis (-glot'is) the lidlike cartilaginous structure overhanging the entrance to the larynx, guarding it during swallowing; see Plate IV. **epiglot'tic,** adj.

epiglottitis (-glŏ-ti'tis) epiglottiditis.

epilation (-la'shun) the removal of hair by the roots.

epilemma (-lem'ah) endoneurium.

epilepsia (ep"ĭ-lep'se-ah) epilepsy. **e. partia'lis contin'ua,** continuous clonic movements of a limited part of the body, due to an abnormal neuronal discharge.

epilepsy (ep'ĭ-lep"se) paroxysmal transient disturbances of brain function that may be manifested as episodic impairment or loss of consciousness, abnormal motor phenomena, psychic or sensory disturbances, or perturbation of the autonomic nervous system; symptoms are due to disturbance of the electrical activity of the brain. **abdominal e.,** paroxysmal abdominal pain as an expression of neuronal discharge from the brain. **cortical e.,** seizure phenomena originating in the cerebral cortex. **cursive e.,** psychomotor epilepsy manifested by running. **focal e.,** minor epileptic seizures in which the seizures are predominantly one-sided or local, or present localized features. **generalized e.,** epilepsy in which the seizures are generalized; they may have a focal onset or be generalized from the beginning. **grand mal e.,** epilepsy, often preceded by an aura, in which a sudden loss of conciousness is immediately followed by generalized convulsions. **idiopathic e.,** epilepsy of unknown etiology. **jacksonian e.,** epilepsy marked by unilateral clonic movements that start in one muscle group and spread systematically to adjacent groups, reflecting the march of epileptic activity through the motor cortex. **myoclonus e.,** slowly progressive hereditary epilepsy beginning in childhood, with intermittent or continuous clonus of muscle groups, resulting in difficulties in voluntary movements; there is mental deterioration and the presence of Lafora bodies in various cells. **nocturnal e.,** that in which the attack occurs at night or during sleep. **petit mal e.,** epilepsy seen especially in children, in which there is sudden momentary unconsciousness with only minor myoclonic jerks. **photogenic e.,** epilepsy in which seizures are induced by a flickering light. **post-traumatic e.,** recurring convulsions due to head injury. **procursive e.,** cursive e. **psychomotor e.,** that associated with disease of the temporal lobe, with impaired consciousness of variable degree, the patient carrying out a series of coordinated acts that are out of place, bizarre, and serve no useful purpose and for which he is amnesic. **reflex e.**, an epileptic seizure occurring in response to a sensory stimulus. **sensory e.**, seizures manifested by hallucinations of sight, smell, or taste. **sleep e.**, narcolepsy. **spinal e.**, succession of clonic and tonic spasms in spastic paraplegia. **temporal lobe e.**, psychomotor e. **thalamic e.**, that ascribed to disease of the thalamus. **tonic e.**, seizure characterized by generalized rigidity.

epileptic (ep″ĭ-lep′tik) 1. pertaining to or affected with epilepsy. 2. a person affected with epilepsy.

epileptiform (-lep′tĭ-form) 1. resembling epilepsy or its manifestations. 2. occurring in severe or sudden paroxysms.

epileptogenic (-lep″to-jen′ik) causing an epileptic seizure.

epileptoid (-lep′toid) epileptiform.

epileptology (-lep-tol′o-je) the study of epilepsy.

epiloia (ep″ĭ-loi′ah) tuberous sclerosis.

epimandibular (-man-dib′u-lar) situated on the lower jaw.

epimenorrhagia (-men″o-ra′je-ah) too frequent and excessive menstruation.

epimenorrhea (-men″o-re′ah) abnormally frequent menstruation.

epimer (ep′ĭ-měr) either of two optical isomers that differ in the configuration around one asymmetrical carbon atom.

epimerase (ĕ-pim′er-āse″) an isomerase that catalyzes the inversion of asymmetric groups in substrates (epimers) having more than one center of asymmetry.

epimere (ep′ĭ-mēr) the dorsal portion of a somite, from which is formed muscles innervated by the dorsal ramus of a spinal nerve.

epimerite (ep″ĭ-mer′īt) an organelle of certain protozoa by which they attach themselves to epithelial cells.

epimerization (ĕ-pim″er-i-za′shun) the changing of one epimeric form of a compound into another, as by enzymatic action.

epimorphosis (ep″ĭ-mor-fo′sis) the regeneration of a part of an organism by proliferation at the cut surface. **epimor′phic**, adj.

epimysium (-mis′e-um) the fibrous sheath around an entire skeletal muscle. See Plate XIV.

epinephrine (-nef′rin) a hormone secreted by the adrenal medulla, and released predominantly in response to hypoglycemia. It is a potent stimulator of the sympathetic nervous system (adrenergic receptors), being a powerful vasopressor, increasing blood pressure, and stimulating the heart muscle. It also relaxes bronchial smooth muscle. Also produced synthetically and used pharmaceutically for these properties.

epinephrinemia (-nef″rĭ-ne′me-ah) the presence of epinephrine in the blood.

epinephros (-nef′ros) adrenal gland.

epineural (-nu′ral) situated upon a neural arch.

epineurium (-nu′re-um) the sheath of a peripheral nerve. **epineu′rial**, adj.

epinosis (-no′sis) a psychic or imaginary state of illness secondary to an original illness.

epiotic (-ot′ik) situated on above the ear.

epipharynx (-far′inks) nasopharynx. **epipharyn′geal**, adj.

epiphenomenon (-fĕ-nom′ĕ-non) an accessory, exceptional, or accidental occurrence in the course of any disease.

epiphora (e-pif′o-rah) overflow of tears due to obstruction of lacrimal duct.

epiphysiolysis (ep″ĭ-fiz″e-ol′ĭ-sis) separation of the epiphysis from the bone shaft.

epiphysis (e-pif′ĭ-sis), pl. _epiph′yses_ [Gr.] 1. the end of a long bone, usually wider than the shaft, and either entirely cartilaginous or separated from the shaft by a cartilaginous disk. 2. part of a bone formed from a secondary center of ossification, commonly found at the ends of long bones on the margins of flat bones, and at tubercles and processes; during the period of growth, epiphyses are separated from the main portion of the bone by cartilage. **epiphys′eal**, adj. **capital e.**, the epiphysis at the head of a long bone. **e. cer′ebri**, pineal body. **slipped e.**, dislocation of the epiphysis of a bone, as of the epiphysis of the head of the femur. **stippled epiphyses**, epiphyseal dysplasia.

epiphysitis (e-pif″ĭ-si′tis) inflammation of an epiphyses or of the cartilage joining the epiphysis to a bone shaft.

epiphyte (ep′ĭ-fīt) an external plant parasite.

epiphytic (ep″ĭ-fit′ik) 1. pertaining to or caused by epiphytes. 2. a widely diffused outbreak of an infectious disease in plants.

epipial (-pi′al) situated upon the pia mater.

epiplocele (e-pip′lo-sēl) omental hernia.

epiploectomy (ep″ĭ-plo-ek′to-me) omentectomy.

epiploenterocele (-en′ter-o-sēl″) a hernia containing intestine and omentum.

epiplomerocele (-me′ro-sēl) a femoral hernia containing omentum.

epiplomphalocele (ep″ĭ-plom-fal′o-sēl) an umbilical hernia containing omentum.

epiploon (e-pip′lo-on), pl. _epip′loa_ [Gr.] the omentum. **epiplo′ic**, adj.

epiplopexy (-pek″se) omentopexy.

epiplorrhaphy (e″pip-lor′ah-fe) omentorrhaphy.

epiploscheocele (e″pip-los′ke-o-sēl″) a scrotal hernia containing omentum.

epipygus (ep″ĭ-pi′gus) pygomelus.

episclera (-skle′rah) the loose connective tissue between the sclera and the conjunctiva.

episcleral (-skle′ral) 1. overlying the sclera. 2. pertaining to the episclera.

episcleritis (-skle-ri′tis) inflammation of the episcleral and adjacent tissues.

episioperineoplasty (e-piz″e-o-per″ĭ-ne′o-plas″te) plastic repair of the vulva and perineum.

episioperineorrhaphy (-per″ĭ-ne-or′ah-fe) suture of the vulva and perineum.

episioplasty (ep-iz′e-o-plas″te) plastic repair of the vulva.

episiorrhaphy (e-piz″e-or′ah-fe) 1. suture of the

labia majora. 2. suture of a lacerated perineum.

episiostenosis (e-piz″e-o-stĕ-no′sis) narrowing of the vulvar orifice.

episiotomy (e-piz″e-ot′o-me) incision of the vulva for obstetric purposes.

episome (ep′ĭ-sōm) in bacterial genetics, any accessory extrachromosomal replicating genetic element that can exist either autonomously or integrated with the chromosome.

epispadias (ep″ĭ-spa′de-as) congenital absence of the upper wall of the urethra, occurring in both sexes, but more commonly in the male, the urethral opening being located anywhere on the dorsum of the penis. **epispa′diac, epispa′dial,** adj.

episplenitis (-sple-ni′tis) inflammation of the capsule of the spleen.

epistaxis (-stak′sis) nosebleed; hemorrhage from the nose, usually due to rupture of small vessels overlying the anterior part of the cartilaginous nasal septum.

episternal (-ster′nal) 1. situated on or over the sternum. 2. pertaining to the episternum.

episternum (-ster′num) a bone present in reptiles and monotremes that may be represented as part of the manubrium, or first piece of the sternum.

epistropheus (-stro′fe-us) axis (see *Table of Bones*).

epitendineum (-ten-din′e-um) the fibrous sheath covering a tendon.

epithalamus (-thal′ah-mus) the part of the thalamencephalon just superior and posterior to the thalamus, comprising the pineal body and adjacent structures; considered by some to include the stria medullaris.

epithalaxia (-thah-lak′se-ah) desquamation of epithelium, especially that of the intestine.

epithelial (-the′le-al) pertaining to or composed of epithelium.

epithelialization (-the″le-al-i-za′shun) healing by the growth of epithelium over a denuded surface.

epithelialize (-the′le-al-īz″) to cover with epithelium.

epitheliitis (-the″le-i′tis) inflammation of epithelium.

epitheliochorial (ep″ĭ-the″le-o-ko′re-al) denoting a type of placenta in which the chorion is apposed to the uterine epithelium but does not erode it.

epitheliofibril (-fi′bril) a fibril running through the cytoplasm of epithelial cells.

epitheliogenetic (-jĕ-net′ik) due to epithelial proliferation.

epithelioid (ep″ĭ-the′le-oid) resembling epithelium.

epitheliolysin (-the″le-ol′ĭ-sin) a cytolysin formed in the serum in response to injection of epithelial cells from a different species; it is capable of destroying epithelial cells of animals of the donor species.

epitheliolysis (-the″le-ol′ĭ-sis) destruction of epithelial tissue. **epitheliolyt′ic,** adj.

epithelioma (-the″le-o′mah) any tumor derived from epithelium. **epithelio′matous,** adj. **e.**

adenoi′des cys′ticum, trichoepithelioma. **basal cell e.,** basal cell carcinoma. **Malherbe's e., Malherbe's calcifying e.,** pilomatricoma.

epithelium (-the′le-um), pl. *epithe′lia* [Gr.] the cellular covering of internal and external body surfaces, including the lining of vessels and small cavities. It consists of cells joined by small amounts of cementing substances and is classified according to the number of layers and the shape of the cells. **ciliated e.,** that bearing vibratile cilia on the free surface. **columnar e.,** epithelium whose cells are of much greater height than width. **cuboidal e.,** that composed of cube-shaped cells. **germinal e.,** thickened peritoneal epithelium covering the gonad from earliest development; formerly thought to give rise to germ cells. **glandular e.,** that composed of secreting cells. **laminated e.,** stratified e. **pigmentary e., pigmented e.,** that made up of cells containing granules of pigment. **pseudostratified e.,** that in which the cells are so arranged that the nuclei occur at different levels, giving the appearance of being stratified. **pyramidal e.,** columnar epithelium whose cells have been modified by pressure into truncated pyramids. **rod e.,** that composed of rod-shaped cells. **sense e., sensory e.,** neuroepithelium (1). **simple e.,** that composed of a single layer of cells. **squamous e.,** that composed of flattened platelike cells. **stratified e.,** that composed of cells arranged in layers. **tessellated e.,** simple squamous e. **transitional e.,** that characteristically found lining hollow organs that are subject to great mechanical change due to contraction and distention, originally thought to represent a transition between stratified squamous and columnar epithelium.

epithelization (ep″ĭ-the″li-za′shun) epithelialization.

epithiazide (-thi′ah-zīd) an antihypertensive and diuretic, $C_{10}H_{11}ClF_3N_3O_4S_3$.

epitonic (ep″ĭ-ton′ik) abnormally tense or tonic.

epitope (ep′ĭ-tōp) an antigenic determinant (see under *determinant*) of known structure.

epitrichium (ep″ĭ-trik′e-um) periderm.

epitrochlea (-trok′le-ah) the inner condyle of the humerus.

epitympanum (-tim′pah-num) the upper part of the tympanum. **epitympan′ic,** adj.

epizoic (-zo′ik) pertaining to or caused by epizoa.

epizoicide (-zo′ĭ-sīd) an agent that destroys epizoa.

epizoon (-zo′on), pl. *epizo′a* [Gr.] an external animal parasite. **epizo′ic,** adj.

epizootic (-zo-ot′ik) 1. attacking many animals in any region at the same time; widely diffused and rapidly spreading. 2. a disease of high morbidity which is only occasionally present in an animal community.

epizootiology (-zo-ot″e-ol′o-je) the scientific study of factors in the frequency and distribution of infectious diseases among animals.

eponychium (ep″o-nik′e-um) 1. the narrow band of epidermis extending from the nail wall onto the nail surface. 2. the horny fetal epidermis at the site of the future nail.

eponym (ep′o-nim) a name or phrase formed

from or including a person's name, as Hodgkin's disease. **eponym'ic, epon'ymous,** adj.

epoophorectomy (ep″o-of″o-rek′to-me) excision of the epoophoron.

epoophoron (-of′o-ron) a vestigial structure associated with the ovary.

epoxy (ĕ-pok′se) 1. containing one atom of oxygen bound to two different carbon atoms. 2. a resin composed of epoxy polymers and characterized by adhesiveness, flexibility, and resistance to chemical actions.

Eprolin (ep′ro-lin) trademark for a preparation of vitamin E.

epulis (ep-u′lis), pl. *epu'lides* [Gr.] any tumor of the gingiva.

epulosis (ep″u-lo′sis) cicatrization. **epulot′ic,** adj.

Equanil (ek′wah-nil) trademark for preparations of meprobamate.

equation (e-kwa′zhun) an expression of equality between two parts. **Henderson-Hasselbalch e.,** a formula for calculating the pH of a buffer solution such as blood plasma,

$$pH = pK' + \log \frac{(BA)}{(HA)};$$ (HA) is the concentration

of a weak acid; (BA) the concentration of a weak salt of this acid; pK′ the buffer system. **personal e.,** the variation introduced into any study or relationship because of differences in individuals.

equator (e-kwa′tor) an imaginary line encircling a globe or globular body midway between its poles. **equato′rial,** adj.

equiaxial (e″kwe-ak′se-al) having axes of the same length.

equilibration (e″kwĭ-lĭ-bra′shun) the achievement of a balance between opposing elements or forces. **occlusal e.,** modification of the occlusal stress, to produce simultaneous occlusal contacts, or to achieve hormonious occlusion.

equilibrium (e″kwĭ-lib′re-um) a state of balance between opposing forces or influences. **dynamic e.,** the condition of balance between varying, shifting, and opposing forces that is characteristic of living processes.

equilin (ek′wil-in) a conjugated estrogen, C_{18}-$H_{20}O_2$, isolated from urine of pregnant horses.

equine (e′kwīn) pertaining to, characteristic of, or derived from the horse.

equinovarus (e-kwi″no-va′rus) talipes equinovarus.

equipotential (e″kwĭ-po-ten′shal) having similar and equal power or capability.

equivalent (e-kwiv′ah-lent) 1. of equal force, power, value, etc. 2. something that has equivalent properties. **chemical e.,** that weight in grams of a substance that will produce or react with 1 mole of hydrogen ion or 1 mole of electrons. **epilepsy e.,** any disturbance, mental or physical, which may take the place of an epileptic seizure. **gram e.,** chemical e. **Joule's e.,** the mechanical equivalent of heat or the amount of work expended in raising the temperature of a pound of water through 1° F.; 772 foot-pounds. Symbol J. **neutralization e.,** the equivalent

weight of an acid as determined by neutralization with a standard base.

E.R. external resistance.

Er chemical symbol, *erbium*.

E.R.A. Electroshock Research Association.

erasion (e-ra′zhun) removal by scraping, or curettage.

erbium (er′be-um) chemical element (*see table*), at. no. 68, symbol Er.

erectile (ĕ-rek′tīl) capable of erection.

erection (e-rek′shun) the condition of being rigid and elevated, as erectile tissue when filled with blood.

erector (e-rek′tor) [L.] a structure that erects, as a muscle which raises or holds up a part.

eremacausis (er″ĕ-mah-kaw′sis) the slow oxidation, combustion, or decay of organic matter.

erethism (er′ĕ-thizm) excessive irritability or sensibility to stimulation. **erethis′mic, erethis′tic,** adj.

erethisophrenia (er″ĕ-thiz″o-fre′ne-ah) exaggerated mental excitability.

erg (erg) a unit of work or energy, equivalent to 2.4×10^{-8} gram calories, or to 0.624×10^{12} electron volts.

ergasia (er-ga′ze-ah) 1. a hypothetical substance which stimulates the activity of body cells. 2. any mentally integrated function, activity, reaction, or attitude of the individual.

ergastic (er-gas′tik) 1. having potential energy. 2. pertaining to ergasia.

ergastoplasm (er-gas′to-plazm) granular endoplasmic reticulum.

ergocalciferol (er″go-kal-sif′er-ol) calciferol; vitamin D_2: an activation product, $C_{28}H_{44}O$, of ergosterol, produced by ultraviolet radiation of ergosterol; used as an antirachitic vitamin.

ergocornine (-kor′nēn) an alkaloid, $C_{31}H_{39}N_5$-O_5, from ergot, once used in peripheral vascular disorders.

ergocristine (-kris′tēn) an alkaloid, $C_{35}H_{39}N_5$-O_5, from ergot, once used in peripheral vascular disorders.

ergocryptine (-krip′tēn) an alkaloid, $C_{32}H_{41}N_5$-O_5, from ergot, once used in peripheral vascular disorders.

ergograph (er′go-graf) an instrument for measuring work done in muscular action.

ergonomics (er″go-nom′iks) the science relating to man and his work, including the factors affecting the efficient use of human energy.

ergonovine (-no′vin) an alkaloid, $C_{19}H_{23}N_3O_2$, from ergot or produced synthetically, used as an oxytocic and to relieve migraine.

ergophore (er′go-fōr) in Ehrlich's side-chain theory, the group of atoms in a molecule that brings about the specific activity of the substance.

ergoplasm (-plazm) ergastoplasm.

ergosome (-sōm) polyribosome.

ergostat (-stat) a machine to be worked for muscular exercise.

ergosterol (er-gos′ter-ol) a sterol, $C_{28}H_{43}\cdot OH$, occurring in animal and plant tissues which, on ultraviolet irradiation becomes a potent antirachitic substance, ergocalciferol.

ergot (er′got) the dried sclerotium of the fungus *Claviceps purpurea*, which is developed on rye plants; ergot alkaloids are used as oxytocics and in treatment of migraine. See also *ergotism*.

ergotamine (er-got′ah-min) an alkaloid of ergot, $C_{33}H_{35}N_5O_5$; the tartrate salt is used for relief of migraine.

ergotaminine (er″go-tam′ĭ-nēn) an isomer of ergotamine.

ergotherapy (-ther′ah-pe) treatment of disease by physical effort.

ergotism (er′go-tizm) chronic poisoning produced by ingestion of ergot, marked by cerebrospinal symptoms, spasms, cramps, or by a kind of dry gangrene.

ergotoxine (er″go-tok′sēn) a toxic crystalline alkaloid originally isolated from ergot (*Claviceps purpurea*), consisting of a mixture of ergocornine, ergocristine, and ergocryptine, which exert both oxytocic and adrenergic blocking effects. Because of the variability of these effects, neither ergotoxine nor any of its constituents is currently used in medicine.

Ergotrate (er′go-trāt) trademark for preparations of ergonovine.

eriodictyon (er″e-o-dik′te-on) the dried leaf of *Eriodictyon californicum*, used in pharmaceutical preparations.

erogenous (ĕ-roj′ĕ-nus) arousing erotic feelings.

erosio (e-ro′ze-o) [L.] erosion. **e. intergita′lis blastomycet′ica,** an eroded lesion occurring between the fingers, almost always between the third and fourth fingers, due to *Candida albicans*.

erosion (e-ro′zhun) an eating or gnawing away; a shallow or superficial ulceration; in dentistry, the wasting away or loss of substance of a tooth by a chemical process that does not involve known bacterial action. **ero′sive,** adj. **cervical e.,** destruction of the squamous epithelium of the vaginal portion of the cervix, due to irritation; the eroded area is covered by columnar epithelium.

erotic (ĕ-rot′ik) pertaining to sexual love or to lust.

erotism (er′o-tizm) a sexual instinct or desire; expression of one's instinctual energy or drive, especially the sex drive. **anal e.,** fixation of libido at (or regression to) the anal phase of infantile development, producing egotistic, dogmatic, stubborn, miserly character. **genital e.,** achievement and maintenance of libido at genital phase of psychosexual development, permitting acceptance of normal adult relationships and responsibilities. **oral e.,** fixation of libido at (or regression to) the oral phase of infantile development, producing passive, insecure, sensitive character.

erotize (er′o-tīz) to endow with erotic meaning or significance.

erotogenic (ĕ-ro″to-jen′ik) producing erotic feelings.

erotomania (-ma′ne-ah) morbidly exaggerated sexual behavior or reaction; preoccupation with sexuality.

erotopathy (er″o-top′ah-the) any perversion of the sexual impulse.

erotophobia (ĕ-ro″to-fo′be-ah) morbid dread of sexual love.

errhine (er′īn) promoting a nasal discharge; an agent that so acts.

Ertron (er′tron) trademark for preparations of ergocalciferol (vitamin D_2).

eructation (e″ruk-ta′shun) belching; casting up wind from the stomach through the mouth.

eruption (e-rup′shun) 1. the act of breaking out, appearing, or becoming visible, as eruption of the teeth. 2. visible efflorescent lesions of the skin due to disease, with redness, prominence, or both; a rash. **creeping e.,** larva migrans. **drug e.,** an eruption or a solitary lesion caused by a drug taken internally. **fixed e.,** a circumscribed inflammatory skin lesion(s) recurring at the same site(s) over a period of months or years; each attack lasts only a few days but leaves residual pigmentation which is cumulative. **Kaposi's varicelliform e.,** a generalized and serious vesiculopustular eruption of viral origin, superimposed on preexisting atopic dermatitis; it may be due to the herpes simplex virus (*eczema herpeticum*) or vaccinia (*eczema vaccinatum*).

eruptive (e-rup′tiv) pertaining to or characterized by eruption.

ERV expiratory reserve volume.

erysipelas (er″ĭ-sip′ĕ-las) a contagious disease of the skin and subcutaneous tissues due to infection with *Streptococcus pyogenes*, with redness and swelling of affected areas, constitional symptoms, and sometimes vesicular and bullous lesions. **swine e.,** a contagious and highly fatal disease of pigs, caused by *Erysipelothrix insidiosa*.

erysipelatous (er″ĭ-sĭ-pel′ah-tus) pertaining to or of the nature of erysipelas.

erysipeloid (er″ĭ-sip′ĕ-loid) a dermatitis or cellulitis of the hand chiefly affecting fish handlers and caused by *Erysipelothrix insidiosa*.

Erysipelothrix (er″ĭ-sip′ĕ-lo-thriks″) a genus of gram-positive bacteria (family Corynebacteriaceae), containing the single species *E. insidio′sa* (*E. rhusiopath′iae*), the causative agent of swine erysipelas and erysipeloid.

erysiphake (er-is′ĭ-fāk) an instrument for removing the lens in cataract by suction.

erythema (er″ĭ-the′mah) redness of the skin due to congestion of the capillaries. **e. ab ig′ne,** that due to exposure to radiant heat. **e. annula′re,** a type of erythema multiforme with ring-shaped lesions. **e. annula′re centrif′ugum,** a chronic variant of erythema multiforme usually affecting the thighs and lower legs, with single or multiple erythematous-edematous papules that enlarge peripherally and clear in the center to produce annular lesions, which may coalesce. **epidemic arthritic e.,** Haverhill fever. **e. indura′tum,** chronic necrotizing vasculitis, usually occurring on the calves of young women; its association with tuberculosis is in dispute. **e. infectio′sum,** a mildly contagious, sometimes epidemic, disease of children between the ages of four and twelve, marked by a rose-colored, coarsely lacelike macular rash. **e. i′ris,** a type of erythema multiforme in which the lesions form concentric rings, producing a target-like appearance. **e. margina′tum,** a type of erythema multiforme in which the reddened areas are disk-shaped with elevated edges. **e. mi′grans,** geographic tongue. **e. multifor′me,** a symptom complex with highly polymorphic skin lesions, including macular papules, vesicles, and bullae; attacks are usually self-limited but recurrences are the rule. **e. nodo′sum,** an acute inflammatory skin disease marked by tender red nodules, usually on the shins, due to exudation of blood and serum. **toxic e., e. tox′icum,** a generalized erythematous or erythematomacular eruption due to administration of a drug or to bacterial toxins or other toxic substances. **e. tox′icum neonato′rum,** a self-limited urticarial condition affecting infants in the first few days of life. **e. venena′tum,** toxic e.

erythematous (er″ĭ-them′ah-tus) characterized by erythema.

erythr(o)- word element [Gr.], *red; erythrocyte.*

erythralgia (er″ĭ-thral′je-ah) erythromelalgia.

erythrasma (er″ĭ-thraz′mah) a chronic bacterial infection of the major skin folds due to *Corynebacterium minutissimum,* marked by red or brownish patches on the skin.

erythredema polyneuropathy (ĕ-rith″rĕ-de′mah pol″ĭ-nu-rop′ah-the) acrodynia.

erythremia (er″ĭ-thre′me-ah) polycythemia vera.

erythrin (er′ĭ-thrin) an antibacterial peptide isolated from erythrocytes.

erythrism (ĕ-rith′rizm) redness of the hair and beard with a ruddy complexion. **erythris′tic,** adj.

erythritol (ĕ-rith′rĭ-tol) a polyhydric alcohol, $C_4H_{10}O_4$, which is about twice as sweet as sucrose, found in algae, lichens, grasses, and several fungi.

erythrityl (ĕ-rith′rĭ-til) the univalent radical, C_4H_9, from erythritol. **e. tetranitrate,** a vasodilator used in angina pectoris and coronary insufficiency; because of its explosiveness it must be diluted, as with lactose.

erythroblast (ĕ-rith′ro-blast) originally, any nucleated erythrocyte, but now more generally used to designate the nucleated precursor from which an erythrocyte develops. **basophilic e.,** see under *normoblast.* **early e.,** basophilic normoblast. **late e.,** orthochromatic normoblast. **orthochromatic e.,** see under *normoblast.* **polychromatic e.,** polychromatic normoblast.

erythroblastemia (ĕ-rith″ro-blas-te′me-ah) the presence in the peripheral blood of abnormally large numbers of nucleated red cells; erythroblastosis.

erythroblastoma (-blas-to′mah) a tumor-like mass composed of nucleated red blood cells.

erythroblastopenia (-blas″to-pe′ne-ah) abnormal deficiency of erythroblasts.

erythroblastosis (-blas-to′sis) 1. the presence of erythroblasts in the circulating blood. 2. avian leukosis marked by increased numbers of immature erythrocytes in the circulating blood.

erythroblastot′ic, adj. **e. feta′lis, e. neonato′rum,** hemolytic anemia of the fetus or newborn due to transplacental transmission of maternally formed antibody against the fetus' erythrocytes, usually secondary to an incompatibility between the mother's Rh blood group and that of her offspring.

erythrochloropia (-klo-ro′pe-ah) ability to distinguish red and green, but not blue or yellow.

erythrochromia (-kro′me-ah) hemorrhagic, red pigmentation of the spinal fluid.

erythroclasis (er″ĭ-throk′lah-sis) fragmentation of the red blood cells. **erythroclas′tic,** adj.

erythrocuprein (ĕ-rith″ro-koo′prin) a copperprotein compound contained in erythrocytes.

erythrocyanosis (-si″ah-no′sis) coarsely mottled bluish red discoloraion on the legs and thighs, especially of girls; thought to be a circulatory reaction to exposure to cold.

erythrocyte (ĕ-rith′ro-sīt) a red blood cell or corpuscle; one of the formed elements in peripheral blood. Normally, in the human, the mature form is a non-nucleated, yellowish, biconcave disk, containing hemoglobin and transporting oxygen. For immature forms, see *normoblast.* **achromic e.,** a colorless erythrocyte. **basophilic e.,** one that takes the basic stain. **"Mexican hat" e.,** leptocyte. **orthochromatic e.,** one that takes only the acid stain. **polychromatic e., polychromatophilic e.,** one that, on staining, shows shades of blue combined with tinges of pink. **target e.,** leptocyte.

erythrocythemia (ĕ-rith″ro-si-the′me-ah) an increase in the number of erythrocytes in the blood, as in erythrocytosis.

erythrocytic (-sit′ik) of or pertaining to erythrocytes.

erythrocytin (-si′tin) a substance in red cells thought to function in the first stage of blood coagulation.

erythrocytolysin (-si-tol′ĭ-sin) a substance that produces erythrocytolysis.

erythrocytolysis (-si-tol′ĭ-sis) dissolution of erythrocytes and escape of the hemoglobin.

erythrocytometer (-si-tom′ĕ-ter) a device for measuring or counting erythrocytes.

erythrocyto-opsonin (-si″to-op-so′nin) hemopsonin.

erythrocytorrhexis (-si″to-rek′sis) the escape from erythrocytes of round, shiny granules and the splitting off of particles.

erythrocytoschisis (-si-tos′kĭ-sis) degeneration of erythrocytes into platelet-like bodies.

erythrocytosis (-si-to′sis) increase in the total red cell mass secondary to any of a number of nonhematogenic systemic disorders in response to a known stimulus (*secondary polycythemia*), in contrast to primary polycythemia (*polycythemia vera*). **leukemic e., e. megalosplen′ica,** polycythemia vera. **stress e.,** an apparent polycythemia seen in active, anxiety-prone persons, resulting from diminished plasma volume.

erythrodegenerative (-de-jen′er-a″tiv) characterized by degeneration of erythrocytes.

erythroderma (-der′mah) abnormal redness of the skin over widespread areas of the body. **congenital ichthyosiform e.,** a generalized hereditary dermatitis with scaling, which occurs in bullous and nonbullous forms. **e. de-squamati′vum,** a condition resembling and probably identical with severe seborrheic dermatitis, affecting newborn breast-fed infants, characterized by generalized exfoliative dermatitis and marked erythroderma. **e. ichthyosifor′me congen′itum,** congenital ichthyosiform e. **lymphomatous e.,** widespread redness of the skin associated with lymphoma. **maculopapular e.,** a reddish eruption composed of macules and papules. **psoriatic e., e. psoriat′icum,** a generalized psoriasis vulgaris, showing the chemical characteristics of exfoliative dermatitis.

erythrodermia (-der′me-ah) erythroderma.

erythrodextrin (-dek′strin) a dextrin stained red by iodine.

erythrodontia (-don′she-ah) reddish brown pigmentation of the teeth.

erythrogenesis (-jen′ĕ-sis) the production of erythrocytes. **e. imperfec′ta,** congenital hypoplastic anemia (1).

erythrogenic (-jen′ik) 1. producing erythrocytes. 2. producing a sensation of red. 3. producing or causing erythema.

erythrogonium (-go′ne-um) promegaloblast.

erythroid (er′ĭ-throid) 1. of a red color; reddish. 2. pertaining to the developmental series of cells ending in erythrocytes.

erythrokeratodermia (ĕ - rith″ ro - ker″ ah - to - der′me-ah) a reddening and hyperkeratosis of the skin. **e. figura′ta varia′bilis, e. varia′bilis,** a rare hereditary disorder marked by circumscribed erythematous and hyperkeratotic plaques on the skin which vary in size and shape within hours or days; they appear shortly after birth and persist into adolescence or adulthood.

erythrokinetics (-ki-net′iks) the quantitative, dynamic study of in vivo production and destruction of erythrocytes.

erythrolabe (ĕ-rith′ro-lāb) the pigment in retinal cones that is more sensitive to the red range of the spectrum than are the other pigments (chlorolabe and cyanolabe).

erythroleukemia (ĕ-rith″ro-lu-ke′me-ah) a malignant blood dyscrasia, one of the myeloproliferative disorders, with atypical erythroblasts and myeloblasts in the peripheral blood.

erythroleukosis (-lu-ko′sis) erythroblastosis (2).

erythrolysin (er″ĭ-throl′ĭ-sin) erythrocytolysin.

erythrolysis (er″ĭ-throl′ĭ-sis) erythrocytolysis.

erythromania (ĕ-rith″ro-ma′ne-ah) uncontrollable blushing.

erythromelalgia (-mel-al′je-ah) paroxysmal, bilateral vasodilation, particularly of the extremities, with burning pain and increased skin temperature and redness.

erythrometer (er″ĭ-throm′ĕ-ter) 1. an instrument or color scale for measuring degrees of redness. 2. erythrocytometer.

erythromycin (ĕ-rith″ro-mi′sin) a broad-spectrum antibiotic, $C_{37}H_{67}NO_{13}$, produced by a strain of *Streptomyces erythreus;* used against gram-positive bacteria.

erythron (er′ĭ-thron) the circulating erythrocytes in the blood, their precursors, and all the body elements concerned in their production.

erythroneocytosis (ĕ-rith″ro-ne″o-si-to′sis) presence of immature erythrocytes in the blood.

erythronoclastic (er″ĭ-thron′o-klas″tik) destroying erythron.

erythropenia (ĕ-rith″ro-pe′ne-ah) deficiency in the number of erythrocytes.

erythrophage (ĕ-rith′ro-fāj) a phagocyte that ingests erythrocytes.

erythrophagia, erythrophagocytosis (-fa′je-ah; -fag″o-si-to′sis) phagocytosis of erythrocytes.

erythropheresis (ĕ-rith″ro-fĕ-re′sis) the reduction of the red cell volume by removal of whole blood and replacement with plasma or albumin.

erythrophil (ĕ-rith′ro-fil) 1. a cell or other element that stains easily with red. 2. erythrophilous.

erythrophilous (er″ĭ-throf′ĭ-lus) easily staining red.

erythrophobia (ĕ-rith″ro-fo′be-ah) 1. a neurotic manifestation marked by blushing at the slightest provocation. 2. morbid aversion to red.

erythrophose (ĕ-rith′ro-fōz) any red phose.

erythrophthisis (ĕ-rith″ro-thi′sis) a condition characterized by severe impairment of the restorative power of the erythrocyte-forming tissues.

erythroplasia (-pla′ze-ah) a condition of the mucous membranes characterized by erythematous papular lesions. **e. of Queyrat,** squamous cell carcinoma *in situ,* manifested as a circumscribed, velvety, erythematous papular lesion on the glans penis, coronal sulcus, or prepuce, leading to scaling and superficial ulceration.

erythropoiesis (-poi-e′sis) the formation of erythrocytes. **erythropoiet′ic,** adj.

erythropoietin (-poi′ĕ-tin) the term applied to the substance(s) serving as the humoral regulator of erythropoiesis.

erythroprosopalgia (-pros″o-pal′je-ah) a nervous disorder marked by redness and pain in the face.

erythropsia (er″ĭ-throp′se-ah) a defect of vision in which objects appear tinged with red.

erythropsin (er″ĭ-throp′sin) rhodopsin.

erythrorrhexis (ĕ-rith″ro-rek′sis) erythrocytorrhexis.

erythrosedimentation (-sed″ĭ-men-ta′shun) the sedimentation of erythrocytes.

erythrosis (er″ĭ-thro′sis) 1. reddish or purplish discoloration of the skin and mucous membranes, as in polycythemia vera. 2. hyperplasia of the hematopoietic tissue.

erythrostasis (ĕ-rith″ro-sta′sis) the stoppage of erythrocytes in the capillaries, as in sickle cell anemia.

erythruria (er″ĭ-throo′re-ah) excretion of red urine.

Es chemical symbol, *einsteinium.*

escape (es-kāp′) the act of becoming free. **nodal e.,** extrasystole in which the atrioventricular node is the pacemaker. **vagal e.,** the exhaustion of or adaptation to neural chemical mediators in the regulation of systemic arterial pressure. **ventricular e.,** extrasystole in which a ventricular pacemaker becomes effective before the sinoatrial pacemaker; it usually occurs with slow sinus rates and often, but not necessarily, with increased vagal tone.

eschar (es′kar) 1. a slough produced by a thermal burn, by a corrosive application, or by gangrene. 2. tache noire. **escharot′ic,** adj.

Escherichia (esh″ĕ-rik′e-ah) a genus of widely distributed, gram-negative bacteria (family Enterbacteriaceae), occasionally pathogenic for man. **E. co′li,** a species constituting the greater part of the normal intestinal flora of man and other animals; it is a frequent cause of urinary tract infections and epidemic diarrheal disease, especially in children.

Escherichieae (esh″er-ĭ-ki′e-e) a tribe of bacteria (family Enterobacteriaceae), comprising the coliform bacteria.

eschrolalia (es″kro-la′le-ah) coprolalia.

escorcin (es-kor′sin) a brown powder, $C_9H_8O_4$, prepared from a substance extracted from the horse chestnut; used in detecting corneal and conjunctival lesions.

escutcheon (es-kuch′an) the pattern of distribution of the pubic hair.

eserine (es′er-ēn) physostigmine.

Esidrix (es′ĭ-driks) trademark for a preparation of hydrochlorothiazide.

-esis word element, *state; condition.*

Eskabarb (es′kah-barb) trademark for a preparation of phenobarbital.

Eskadiazine (es″kah-di′ah-zēn) trademark for a preparation of sulfadiazine.

esmarch (es′mark) an Esmarch bandage.

eso- word element [Gr.], *within.*

esodic (e-sod′ik) afferent.

esoethmoiditis (es″o-eth″moid-i′tis) inflammation of the ethmoid sinuses.

esogastritis (-gas-tri′tis) inflammation of the gastric mucosa.

esophageal (ĕ-sof″ah-je′al, ĕ-so-fa′je-al) of or pertaining to the esophagus.

esophagectasia (ĕ-sof″ah-jek-ta′se-ah) dilatation of the esophagus.

esophagectomy (ĕ-sof″ah-jek′to-me) excision of a portion of the esophagus.

esophagism (ĕ-sof′ah-jizm) spasm of the esophagus.

esophagitis (ĕ-sof″ah-ji′tis) inflammation of the esophagus. **peptic e.,** that due to a reflux of acid and pepsin from the stomach.

esophagobronchial (ĕ-sof″ah-go-brong′ke-al) pertaining to or communicating with the esophagus and a bronchus.

esophagocele (ĕ-sof′ah-go-sēl″) abnormal distention of the esophagus; protrusion of the esophageal mucosa through a rupture in the muscular coat.

esophagoduodenostomy (ĕ-sof″ah-go-du″o-de-nos′to-me) anastomosis of the esophagus to the duodenum.

esophagodynia (-din′e-ah) pain in the esophagus.

esophagoenterostomy (-en″ter-os′to-me) surgi-cal formation of an anastomosis between the esophagus and small intestine.

esophagoesophagostomy (-ĕ-sof″ah-gos′to-me) anastomosis between two formerly remote parts of the esophagus.

esophagogastrectomy (-gas-trek′to-me) excision of the esophagus and stomach.

esophagogastric (-gas′trik) pertaining to the esophagus and the stomach.

esophagogastroanastomosis (-gas″tro-ah-nas″to-mo′sis) esophagogastrostomy.

esophagogastroplasty (-gas′tro-plas″te) plastic repair of the esophagus and stomach.

esophagogastroscopy (-gas-tros′ko-pe) endoscopic inspection of the esophagus and stomach.

esophagogastrostomy (-gas-tros′to-me) anastomosis of the esophagus to the stomach.

esophagography (ĕ-sof″ah-gog′rah-fe) roentgenography of the esophagus.

esophagojejunostomy (ĕ-sof″ah-go-je″ju-nos′-to-me) anastomosis of the esophagus to the jejunum.

esophagomalacia (-mah-la′she-ah) softening of the walls of the esophagus.

esophagometer (ĕ-sof″ah-gom′ĕ-ter) an instrument for measuring the esophagus.

esophagomyotomy (ĕ-sof″ah-go-mi-ot′o-me) incision through the muscular coat of the esophagus.

esophagoplasty (ĕ-sof′ah-go-plas″te) plastic repair of the esophagus.

esophagoplication (ĕ-sof″ah-go-pli-ka′shun) infolding of the wall of an esophageal pouch.

esophagoptosis (ĕ-sof″ah-gop-to′sis) prolapse of the esophagus.

esophagorespiratory (ĕ-sof″ah-go-rĕ-spīr′ah-to″re) pertaining to or communicating with the esophagus and respiratory tract (trachea or a bronchus).

esophagoscope (ĕ-sof′ah-go-skōp″) an endoscope for examination of the esophagus.

esophagoscopy (ĕ-sof″ah-gos′ko-pe) endoscopic examination of the esophagus.

esophagospasm (ĕ-sof′ah-go-spazm) spasm of the esophagus.

esophagostenosis (-stĕ-no′sis) stricture of the esophagus.

esophagostomy (ĕ-sof″ah-gos′to-me) creation of an artificial opening into the esophagus.

esophagotomy (ĕ-sof″ah-got′o-me) incision of the esophagus.

esophagotracheal (ĕ-sof″ah-go-tra′ke-al) pertaining to or communicating with the esophagus and trachea.

esophagus (ĕ-sof′ah-gus) the musculomembranous passage extending from the pharynx to the stomach. See Plate IV.

esophoria (es″o-fo′re-ah) deviation of the visual axis toward that of the other eye in the absence of visual fusional stimuli.

esosphenoiditis (-sfe″noid-i′tis) osteomyelitis of the sphenoid bone.

esotropia (-tro′pe-ah) cross-eye; deviation of the visual axis of one eye toward that of the other eye. **esotrop′ic,** adj.

E.S.P. extrasensory perception.

E.S.R. erythrocyte sedimentation rate.

essence (es′ens) 1. the distinctive or individual principle of anything. 2. mixture of alcohol with a volatile oil.

essential (ĕ-sen′shal) 1. constituting the inherent part of a thing; giving a substance its peculiar and necessary qualities. 2. indispensable; required in the diet, as essential fatty acids. 3. idiopathic; having no obvious external cause.

E.S.T. electric shock therapy.

ester (es′ter) a compound formed from an alcohol and an acid by removal of water.

esterase (es′ter-ās) any enzyme which catalyzes the hydrolysis of an ester into its alcohol and acid.

esterification (es-ter″ĭ-fi-ka′shun) conversion of an acid into an ester.

esterify (es-ter′ĭ-fi) to combine with an alcohol with elimination of a molecule of water, forming an ester.

esterolysis (es″ter-ol′ĭ-sis) the hydrolysis of an ester into its alcohol and acid. **esterolyt′ic,** adj.

esthematology (es″them-ah-tol′o-je) esthesiology.

esthesiogenic (es-the″ze-o-jen′ik) producing sensation.

esthesiology (es-the″ze-ol′o-je) the scientific study or description of the sense organs and sensations.

esthesiometer (es-the″ze-om′ĕ-ter) tactometer.

esthesioneurosis (es-the″ze-o-nu-ro′sis) any disorder of the sensory nerves.

esthesiophysiology (-fiz″e-ol′o-je) the physiology of sensation and sense organs.

esthesodic (es″the-zod′ik) conducting or pertaining to conduction of sensory impulses.

esthetics (es-thet′iks) the branch of philosophy dealing with beauty; in dentistry, a philosophy concerned especially with the appearance of a dental restoration, as achieved through its color or form.

Estinyl (es′tĭ-nil) trademark for a preparation of ethinyl estradiol.

estival (es′tĭ-val, ĕ-sti′val) pertaining to or occurring in summer.

estivation (es″tĭ-va′shun) the dormant state in which certain animals pass the summer.

estivoautumnal (es″tĭ-vo-aw-tum′nal) occurring in summer and autumn.

estradiol (es″trah-di′ol, es-tra′de-ol) the most potent naturally occurring estrogen in humans; pharmacologically, it is usually used in the form of its esters (e.g., *e. benzoate, e. cypionate, e. valerate*), or as a semisynthetic derivative (*ethinyl e.*). For properties and uses, see *estrogen.*

estrin (es′trin) estrogen.

estrinization (es″trin-ĭ-za′shun) production of the cellular changes in the vaginal epithelium characteristic of estrus.

estriol (es′tre-ol) a relatively weak human estrogen, being a metabolic product of estradiol and estrone found in high concentrations in urine; see *estrogen.*

estrogen (es′tro-jen) a generic term for es-

trus-producing compounds; the female sex hormones, including estradiol, estriol, and estrone. In humans, the estrogens are formed in the ovary, adrenal cortex, testis, and fetoplacental unit, and are responsible for female secondary sex characteristic development, and during the menstrual cycle, act on the female genitalia to produce an environment suitable for fertilization, implantation, and nutrition of the early embryo. Estrogen is used as a palliative in postmenopausal cancer of the breast and in prostatic cancer, as oral contraceptives, for relief of menopausal discomforts, etc.

estrogenic (es″tro-jen′ik) estrus-producing; having the properties of, or similar to, an estrogen.

estrone (es′trōn) an estrogen isolated from pregnancy urine, the human placenta, and palm kernel oil, and also prepared synthetically; for properties, see *estrogen.*

estrous (es′trus) pertaining to estrus.

estruation (es″troo-a′shun) estrus.

Estrugenone (es″troo-jen′ōn) trademark for a preparation of estrone.

estrum (es′trum) estrus.

estrus (es′trus) the recurrent, restricted period of sexual receptivity in female mammals other than human females, marked by intense sexual urge. **es′trual,** adj.

e.s.u. electrostatic unit.

Etamon (et′ah-mon) trademark for a preparation of tetraethylammonium.

ethambutol (ĕ-tham′bu-tōl) a tuberculostatic agent, $C_{10}H_{24}N_2O_2$.

ethamivan (ĕ-tham′ĭ-van) a respiratory stimulant, $C_{12}H_{17}NO_3$.

ethanol (eth′ah-nol) alcohol (1).

ethanolamine (eth″ah-nol-ah′mēn) a colorless, moderately viscous liquid with an ammonical odor, $NH_2 \cdot CH_2 \cdot CH_2OH$, contained in cephalins and phospholipids, and derived metabolically by decarboxylation of serine. The oleate is used as a sclerosing agent in the treatment of varicose veins.

ethchlorvynol (eth-klor′vĭ-nol) a sedative, C_7H_9ClO.

ethene (eth′ēn) ethylene.

ether (e′ther) 1. diethyl ether: a colorless, transparent, mobile, very volatile, highly inflammable liquid, $C_2H_5 \cdot O \cdot C_2H_5$, with a characteristic odor; given by inhalation to produce general anesthesia. 2. any of various volatile liquids, mostly containing diethyl ether or resembling it. **acetic e.,** ethyl acetate. **diethyl e.,** see *ether* (1). **formic e.,** ethyl formate. **hydriodic e.,** ethyl iodide. **hydrobromic e.,** ethyl bromide. **hydrochloric e.,** ethyl chloride. **nitrofurfuryl methyl e.,** a compound used as a topical fungicide and sporicide for skin infections. **vinyl e.,** a clear colorless liquid used as an inhalation anesthetic to produce general anesthesia.

ethereal (e-the′re-al) 1. pertaining to, prepared with, containing, or resembling ether. 2. evanescent; delicate.

etherization (e″ther-i-za′shun) induction of anesthesia by means of ether.

ethinamate (ĕ-thin′ah-māt) a short-acting, non-barbiturate sedative, $C_{19}H_{13}NO_2$.

ethinyl trichloride (eth′ĭ-nil tri-klo′rīd) trichloroethylene.

ethionamide (ĕ-thi″on-am′īd) a tuberculostatic, $C_8H_{10}N_2S$.

ethionine (ĕ-thi′o-nin) the ethyl homologue of methionine.

ethisterone (ĕ-this′ter-ōn) a synthetic progestational steroid, $C_{21}H_{28}O_2$.

ethmocarditis (eth″mo-kar-di′tis) inflammation of the connective tissue of the heart.

ethmocephalus (-sef′ah-lus) a monster with an imperfect head, more or less union of the eyes, and a rudimentary nose.

ethmofrontal (-fron′tal) pertaining to the ethmoid and frontal bones.

ethmoid (eth′moid) 1. sievelike; cribriform. 2. the ethmoid bone.

ethmoidal (eth-moi′dal) pertaining to the ethmoid bone.

ethmoidectomy (eth″moi-dek′to-me) excision of ethmoidal cells or of a portion of the ethmoid bone.

ethmoiditis (eth″moi-di′tis) inflammation of the ethmoid bone or ethmoid sinuses.

ethmoidotomy (eth″moi-dot′o-me) incision into the ethmoid sinus.

ethmolacrimal (eth″mo-lak′rĭ-mal) pertaining to the ethmoid and the lacrimal bones.

ethmomaxillary (-mak′sĭ-lār-e) pertaining to the ethmoid and maxillary bones.

ethmosphenoid (-sfe′noid) pertaining to the ethmoid and sphenoid bones.

ethmoturbinal (-tur′bĭ-nal) pertaining to the superior and middle nasal conchae.

ethnic (eth′nik) pertaining to a social group who share cultural bonds or physical (racial) characteristics.

ethnobiology (eth″no-bi-ol′o-je) the scientific study of physical characteristics of different races of mankind.

ethnology (eth-nol′o-je) the science dealing with the races of men, their descent, relationship, etc.

ethoheptazine (eth″o-hep′tah-zēn) an analgesic, $C_{16}H_{23}NO_2$.

ethohexadiol (-heks-a′de-ol) an insect repellant, $C_8H_{18}O_2$.

ethologist (e-thol′o-jist) a person skilled in ethology.

ethology (e-thol′o-je) the scientific study of animal behavior, particularly in the natural state. **etholog′ical,** adj.

ethopropazine (eth″o-pro′pah-zēn) a homologue of promethazine, $C_{19}H_{24}N_2S$, used as the hydrochloride salt in the treatment of parkinsonism.

ethosuximide (-suk′sĭ-mīd) an anticonvulsant, $C_7H_{11}NO_2$.

ethotoin (e-tho′to-in) a phenylhydantoin derivative, $C_{11}H_{12}N_2O_2$, used as an anticonvulsant in grand mal epilepsy.

ethoxazene (eth-ok′sah-zēn) an azo dye, $C_{14}H_{16}$-N_4O; its hydrochloride salt is used for its local analgesic action to relieve pain associated with urinary tract infections.

ethoxzolamide (eth″ok-zol′ah-mīd) a carbonic anhydrase inhibitor, $C_9H_{10}N_2O_3S_2$, used as a diuretic and to reduce intraocular pressure in glaucoma.

ethyl (eth′il) the monovalent radical, C_2H_5. **e. acetate,** a flavoring agent and antispasmodic, $CH_3COOC_2H_5$. **e. aminobenzoate,** benzocaine. **e. biscoumacetate,** an anticoagulant, $C_{22}H_{16}O_8$. **e. bromide,** an inhalation anesthetic, C_2H_5Br. **e. carbamate,** urethan. **e. chaulmoograte,** a mixture of the ethyl esters of the unsaturated fatty acids—chaulmoogric and hydnocarpic—of chaulmoogra oil, used in leprosy and sarcoidosis. **e. chloride,** a local anesthetic, C_2H_5Cl, applied topically to intact skin. **e. formate,** a volatile liquid used as a solvent and flavoring agent. **e. iodide,** a colorless liquid used as a reagent. **e. oxide,** a pharmaceutical solvent. **e. phenylephrine,** ethylphenylephrine. **e. vanillin,** a flavoring agent, $C_9H_{10}O_3$.

ethylcellulose (eth″il-sel′u-lōs) an ethyl ether of cellulose; used as a pharmaceutical tablet binder.

ethylene (eth′ĭ-lēn) a colorless flammable gas, $CH_2:CH_2$, with a slightly sweet odor and taste; used as an inhalation anesthetic.

ethylenediamine (eth″ĭ-lēn-di′ah-mēn) a solvent, $C_2H_8N_2$, used in pharmaceutical preparations.

ethylmorphine (eth″il-mor′fēn) the ethyl ester of morphine, $C_{19}H_{23}NO_3$; its hydrochloride salt is used as an antitussive and narcotic, and topically as a chemotic.

ethylnoradrenaline (-nor-ah-dren′ah-lin) ethylnorepinephrine.

ethylnorepinephrine (-nor-ep″ĭ-nef′rin) a sympathomimetic, $C_{10}H_{15}NO_3$, used as the hydrochloride salt in treatment of bronchial asthma.

ethylparaben (-par′ah-ben) an antifungal agent, $C_9H_{10}O_3$.

ethylphenylephrine (-fen″il-ef′rin) a sympathomimetic circulatory stimulant, $C_{10}H_{15}NO_2$, used as the hydrochloride salt.

ethynodiol (ĕ-thi″no-di′ōl) a semisynthetic steroid, $C_{24}H_{32}O_4$; the diacetate ester is used as an anovulatory progesterone.

ethynyl (eth″ĭ-nil) the group —C≡CH, when it occurs in organic compounds; present in various oral contraceptives.

etiolation (e″te-o-la′shun) 1. blanching or paleness of a plant grown in the dark due to lack of chlorophyll. 2. the process by which the skin becomes pale when deprived of sunlight.

etiology (e″te-ol′o-je) the science dealing with causes of disease. **etiolog′ic, etiolog′ical,** adj.

etioporphyrin (e″te-o-por′fir-in) a porphyrin obtained from hematoporphyrin.

Eu chemical symbol, *europium.*

eu- word element [Gr.], *normal; good; well; easy.*

Eubacteriales (u″bak-te″re-a′lēz) an order of schizomycetes comprising the true bacteria.

Eubacterium (u″bak-te′re-um) a genus of schizomycetes (tribe Lactobacilleae) found in the intestinal tract as parasites and as saprophytes in soil and water.

eubiotics (u″bi-ot′iks) the science of healthy living.

eucalyptol (u″kah-lip′tol) the chief constituent of eucalyptus oil, also obtained from other oils, and used as a flavoring agent, expectorant, and local anesthetic.

eucatropine (u-kat′ro-pēn) a mydriatic, $C_{17}H_{25}$-NO_3, used as the hydrochloride salt.

euchlorhydria (u″klor-hi′dre-ah) the presence of the normal amount of hydrochloric acid in the gastric juice.

eucholia (u-ko′le-ah) normal condition of the bile.

euchromatin (u-kro′mah-tin) that state of chromatin in which it stains lightly, is genetically active, and is considered to be partially or fully uncoiled.

euchromatopsy (u-kro′mah-top″se) normal color vision.

eucrasia (u-kra′ze-ah) 1. a state of health; proper balance of different factors constituting a healthy state. 2. a state in which the body reacts normally to ingested or injected drugs, proteins, etc.

eudiemorrhysis (u″di-ĕ-mor′ĭ-sis) the normal flow of blood through the capillaries.

eudiometer (u″de-om′ĕ-ter) an instrument for measuring and analyzing gases.

eudipsia (u-dip′se-ah) ordinary, normal thirst.

euergasia (u″er-ga′ze-ah) normal psychobiologic functioning.

euesthesia (u″es-the′ze-ah) a normal state of the senses.

eugenics (u-jen′iks) the study and control of procreation as a means of improving hereditary characteristics of future generations. **eugen′ic,** adj. **negative e.,** that concerned with prevention of reproduction by individuals having inferior or undesirable traits. **positive e.,** that concerned with promotion of optimal mating and reproduction by individuals having desirable or superior traits.

eugenol (u′jĕ-nol) the chief constituent of clove oil, $C_{10}H_{12}O_2$; also obtained from other sources and used as a dental topical analgesic and antiseptic.

euglobulin (u-glob′u-lin) one of a class of globulins characterized by being insoluble in water but soluble in saline solutions.

euglycemia (u″gli-se′me-ah) a normal level of glucose in the blood. **euglyce′mic,** adj.

eugnathic (u-nath′ik) characterized by a normal state of the maxilla and mandible.

eugonic (u-gon′ik) growing luxuriantly; said of bacterial cultures.

eukaryon (u-kar′e-on) 1. a highly organized nucleus bounded by a nuclear membrane, a characteristic of cells of higher organisms; cf. *prokaryon.* 2. eukaryote.

eukaryosis (u″kar-e-o′sis) the state of having a true nucleus.

eukaryote (u-kar′e-ōt) an organism whose cells have a true nucleus bounded by a nuclear membrane, and exhibit mitosis; cf. *prokaryote.*

eukaryotic (u″kar-e-ot′ik) pertaining to a eukaryon or to a eukaryote.

eukinesia (u″ki-ne′ze-ah) normal or proper motor function or activity. **eukinet′ic,** adj.

eulaminate (u-lam′ĭ-nāt) having the normal number of laminae, as certain areas of the cerebral cortex.

eumetria (u-me′tre-ah) a normal condition of nerve impulse, so that a voluntary movement just reaches the intended goal; the proper range of movement.

eunuch (u′nuk) a male deprived of the testes or external genitals, especially one castrated before puberty (so that male secondary sex characteristics fail to develop).

eunuchoid (u′nu-koid) 1. resembling a eunuch. 2. a person who resembles a eunuch.

eunuchoidism (u′nŭ-koi-dizm″) deficiency of the testes or of their secretion, with impaired sexual power and eunuchoid symptoms. **female e.,** hypogonadism in which the ovaries fail to function at puberty, resulting in infertility, absence of development of secondary sex characteristics, infantile sexual organs, and excessive growth of the long bones. **hypergonadotropic e.,** that associated with high levels of gonadotropins, as in Klinefelter's syndrome. **hypogonadotropic e.,** that due to lack of gonadotropin secretion.

eupancreatism (u-pan′kre-ah-tizm″) normal functioning of the pancreas.

eupepsia (u-pep′se-ah) good digestion; the presence of a normal amount of pepsin in the gastric juice. **eupep′tic,** adj.

euphoretic (u″fo-ret′ik) 1. pertaining to, characterized by, or producing euphoria. 2. an agent that produces euphoria.

euphoria (u-fo′re-ah) bodily comfort; well-being; absence of pain or distress. In psychiatry, abnormal or exaggerated sense of well-being. **euphor′ic,** adj.

euphoriant (u-for′e-ant) euphoretic.

euplastic (u-plas′tik) readily becoming organized; adapted to tissue formation.

euploid (u′ploid) 1. having a balanced set or sets of chromosomes, in any number. 2. a euploid individual or cell.

euploidy (u′ploi-de) the state of being euploid.

eupnea (ūp-ne′ah) normal respiration. **eupne′ic,** adj.

eupraxia (u-prak′se-ah) intactness of reproduction of coordinated movements. **euprac′tic,** adj.

Eurax (u′raks) trademark for preparations of crotamiton.

eurhythmia (u-rith′me-ah) regularity of the pulse.

europium (u-ro′pe-um) chemical element (*see table*), at. no. 63, symbol Eu.

Eurotium (u-ro′she-um) a genus of fungi or molds.

eury- word element [Gr.], *wide; broad.*

eurycephalic (u″rĭ-sĕ-fal′ik) having a wide head.

euryon (u″re-on) a point on either parietal bone

marking either end of the greatest transverse diameter of the skull.

eusystole (u-sis'to-le) a normal state of systole of the heart.

euthanasia (u''thah-na'zhe-ah) 1. an easy or painless death. 2. mercy killing; the deliberate ending of life of a person suffering from an incurable disease.

euthenics (u-then'iks) the science of race improvement by regulation of environment.

euthermic (u-ther'mik) characterized by the proper temperature; promoting warmth.

euthyroid (u-thi'roid) having a normally functioning thyroid gland.

eutocia (u-to'she-ah) normal labor, or childbirth.

Eutrombicula (u''trom-bik'u-lah) a subgenus of *Trombicula;* see *chigger.*

eutrophia (u-tro'fe-ah) a state of normal (good) nutrition. **eutroph'ic,** adj.

eutrophication (u''tro-fi-ka'shun) the accidental or deliberate promotion of excessive growth (multiplication) of an organism to the disadvantage of other organisms in the same ecosystem by oversupplying it with nutrients.

ev, Ev electron volt.

evacuant (e-vak'u-ant) 1. promoting evacuation. 2. an agent which promotes evacuation.

evacuation (e-vak''u-a'shun) 1. an emptying, as of the bowels. 2. a dejection or stool; material discharged from the bowels.

evagination (e-vaj''i-na'shun) an outpouching of a layer or part.

evanescent (ev''ah-nes'ent) vanishing; passing away quickly; unstable; unfixed.

eventration (e''ven-tra'shun) 1. protrusion of the bowels through the abdomen. 2. removal of the abdominal viscera. **diaphragmatic e.,** elevation of the dome of the diaphragm, usually due to phrenic nerve paralysis.

eversion (e-ver'zhun) a turning inside out; a turning outward.

evert (e-vert') to turn inside out; to turn outward.

Evipal (ev'i-pal) trademark for a preparation of hexobarbital.

evisceration (e-vis''er-a'shun) 1. extrusion of the viscera, or internal organs; disembowelment. 2. removal of the contents of the eyeball, leaving the sclera.

evocation (ev''o-ka'shun) the calling forth of morphogenetic potentialities through contact with organizer material.

evocator (ev'o-ka''tor) a chemical substance emitted by an organizer that evokes a specific morphogenetic response from the embryonic tissue in contact with it.

evolution (ev''o-lu'shun) a developmental process in which an organ or organism becomes more and more complex by differentiation of its parts; a continuous and progressive change according to certain laws and by means of resident forces. **convergent e.,** the appearance of similar forms and/or functions in two or more lines not sufficiently related phylogenetically to account for the similarity. **organic e.,** the

origin and development of species; the theory that existing organisms are the result of descent with modification from those of past times.

evulsion (e-vul'shun) extraction by force.

ex- word element [L.], *away from; without; outside; sometimes; completely.*

exacerbation (eg-zas''er-ba'shun) increase in severity of a disease or any of its symptoms.

examination (eg-zam''i-na'shun) inspection or investigation, especially as a means of diagnosing disease, qualified according to the methods used, as physical, cystoscopic, etc.

exanthem (eg-zan'them) 1. any eruptive disease or fever. 2. an eruption characterizing an eruptive fever. **e. sub'itum,** a disease of children, with continuous or remittent fever lasting about 3 days, falling by crisis, and followed by a rash on the trunk.

exanthema (eg''zan-the'mah), pl. *exanthem'ata* [Gr.] exanthem.

exanthematous (eg''zan-them'ah-tus) characterized by or of the nature of an eruption or rash.

exarticulation (eks''ar-tik-u-la'shun) amputation at a joint; partial removal of a joint.

excalation (eks''kah-la'shun) absence or exclusion of one member of a normal series, such as a vertebra.

excavatio (eks''kah-va'she-o), pl. *excavatio'nes* [L.] excavation.

excavation (-va'shun) 1. the act of hollowing out. 2. a hollowed-out space, or pouchlike cavity. **atrophic e.,** cupping of the optic disk, due to atrophy of the optic nerve fibers. **dental e.,** removal of carious material from a tooth in preparation for filling. **e. of optic disk, physiologic e.,** a depression in the center of the optic disk. **rectouterine e.,** a sac formed by a fold of peritoneum dipping down between the uterus and rectum. **rectovesical e.,** the space between the rectum and bladder in the peritoneal cavity of the male. **vesicouterine e.,** the space between the bladder and uterus in the peritoneal cavity of the female.

excavator (eks'kah-va''tor) a scoop or gouge for surgical use. **dental e.,** an instrument for removing carious material from a tooth.

excementosis (ek-se''men-to'sis) hyperplasia of the cementum of the root of a tooth.

excerebration (ek''ser-ĕ-bra'shun) removal of the brain.

excernent (ek-ser'nent) causing an evacuation or discharge.

exchanger (eks-chānj'er) an apparatus by which something may be exchanged. **heat e.,** a device placed in the circuit of extracorporeal circulation to induce rapid cooling and rewarming of blood.

excipient (ek-sip'e-ent) any more or less inert substance added to a drug to give suitable consistency or form to the drug; a vehicle.

excise (ek-sīz') to remove by cutting.

excision (ek-sizh'un) removal, as of an organ, by cutting.

excitability (ek-sīt″ah-bil′ĭ-te) readiness to respond to a stimulus; irritability.

excitant (ek-sīt′ant) an agent producing excitation of the vital functions, or of those of the brain.

excitation (ek″si-ta′shun) an act of irritation or stimulation; a condition of being excited; the addition of energy, as the excitation of a molecule by absorption of photons. **direct e.,** electrostimulation of a muscle by placing the electrode on the muscle itself. **indirect e.,** electrostimulation of a muscle by placing the electrode on its nerve.

excitomotor (ek-si″to-mo′tor) tending to produce motion or motor function; an agent that so acts.

excitor (ek-si′tor) a nerve which stimulates a part to greater activity.

excitosecretory (ek-si″to-se-kre′to-re) producing increased secretion.

excitovascular (-vas′ku-ler) causing vascular changes.

exclave (eks′klāv) a detached part of an organ.

exclusion (ek-skloo′zhun) a shutting out or elimination; surgical isolation of a part, as of a segment of intestine, without removal from the body.

excochleation (eks″kok-le-a′shun) curettement of a cavity.

excoriation (eks-ko″re-a′shun) any superficial loss of substance, as that produced on the skin by scratching.

excrement (eks′krĕ-ment) fecal matter; matter cast out as waste from the body.

excrementitious (eks″krĕ-men-tish′us) pertaining to or of the nature of excrement.

excrescence (eks-kres′ens) an abnormal outgrowth; a projection of morbid origin. **excres′cent,** adj.

excreta (eks-kre′tah) excretion products; waste material excreted from the body.

excrete (eks-krēt′) to throw off or eliminate, as waste matter, by a normal discharge.

excretion (eks-kre′shun) 1. the act, process, or function of excreting. 2. material that is excreted. **ex′cretory,** adj.

excursion (eks-kur′zhun) a range of movement regularly repeated in performance of a function, e.g., excursion of the jaws in mastication. **excur′sive,** adj.

excyclophoria (ek″si-klo-fo′re-ah) cyclophoria in which the upper pole of the visual axis deviates toward the temple.

excyclotropia (-tro′pe-ah) cyclotropia in which the upper pole of the visual axis deviates toward the temple.

excystation (ek″sis-ta′shun) escape from a cyst or envelope, as in that stage in the life cycle of parasites occurring after the cystic form has been swallowed by the host.

exemia (ek-se′me-ah) loss of fluid from the blood vessels, the red blood cells being left behind.

exencephalus (eks″en-sef′ah-lus) a monster with an imperfect cranium, the brain lying outside the skull.

exenteration (eks-en″ter-a′shun) surgical removal of the inner organs; evisceration. **pelvic e.,** excision of the organs and adjacent structures of the pelvis.

exenterative (eks-en′ter-ah-tiv) pertaining to or requiring exenteration, as exenterative surgery.

exercise (ek′ser-sīz) performance of physical exertion for improvement of health or correction of physical deformity. **active e.,** motion imparted to a part by voluntary contraction and relaxation of its controlling muscles. **active resistive e.,** motion voluntarily imparted to a part against resistance. **isometric e.,** active exercise performed against stable resistance, without change in the length of the muscle. **isotonic e.,** active exercise without appreciable change in the force of muscular contraction, with shortening of the muscle. **passive e.,** motion imparted to a part by another person or outside force, or produced by voluntary effort of another segment of the patient's own body.

exeresis (eks-er′ĕ-sis) surgical removal or excision.

exergonic (ek″ser-gon′ik) accompanied by the release of free energy.

exfetation (eks″fe-ta′shun) ectopic or extrauterine pregnancy.

exflagellation (eks-flaj″ĕ-la′shun) the protrusion or formation of flagelliform microgametes from a microgametocyte in malarial parasites and some related sporozoa.

exfoliation (eks-fo″le-a′shun) a falling off in scales or layers. **exfo′liative,** adj. **lamellar e. of newborn,** a congenital hereditary disorder in which the infant (collodion baby) is born entirely covered with a collodion- or parchment-like membrane that peels off within 24 hours, after which there may be complete healing, or the scales may re-form and the process repeated; in the more severe form, the infant (harlequin fetus) is entirely covered with thick, horny, armor-like scales, and is usually stillborn or dies soon after birth.

exhalation (eks″hah-la′shun) 1. the giving off of watery or other vapor, or of an effluvium. 2. a vapor or other substance exhaled or given off. 3. the act of breathing out.

exhaustion (eg-zawst′yun) 1. privation of energy with consequent inability to respond to stimuli; lassitude. 2. withdrawal. 3. a condition of emptiness caused by withdrawal. 4. emptying by a process of withdrawal. **heat e.,** an effect of excessive exposure to heat, marked by subnormal body temperature with dizziness, headache, nausea, and sometimes delirium and/or collapse. **heat e., anhidrotic,** tropical anhidrotic asthenia.

exhibitionism (ek″sĭ-bish′uh-nizm) a sexual deviation in which pleasure is gained by exposure of the genitals to persons of the opposite sex in socially unacceptable circumstances.

exhibitionist (ek″sĭ-bish′ĕ-nist) a person who indulges in exhibitionism.

exo- word element [Gr.], *outside; outward.*

exobiology (ek″so-bi-ol′o-je) the science concerned with study of life on planets other than the earth.

exocardia (-kar'de-ah) ectocardia.

exocardial (-kar'de-al) situated, occurring, or developed outside the heart.

exocoelom (-se'lum) the portion of the coelom external to the embryo.

exocolitis (-ko-li'tis) inflammation of the outer coat of the colon.

exocrine (ek'so-krin) 1. secreting externally via a duct. 2. denoting such a gland or its secretion.

exocytosis (ek''so-si-to'sis) 1. the discharge from a cell of particles that are too large to diffuse through the wall; the opposite of endocytosis. 2. the aggregation of migrating leukocytes in the epidermis as part of the inflammatory response.

exodeviation (-de''ve-a'shun) a turning outward; in ophthalmology, exotropia.

exodic (ek-sod'ik) efferent; centrifugal.

exodontia (ek''so-don'she-ah) exodontics.

exodontics (-don'tiks) that branch of dentistry dealing with extraction of teeth.

exodontist (-don'tist) a dentist who practices exodontics.

exoenzyme (-en'zīm) an enzyme which acts outside the cell which secretes it.

exoerythrocytic (-ĕ-rith''ro-sit'ik) occurring outside the erythrocyte; applied to developmental stages of malarial parasites taking place in cells other than erythrocytes.

exogamy (ek-sog'ah-me) 1. protozoan fertilization by union of elements that are not derived from the same cell. 2. marriage outside a particular group.

exogastrula (ek''so-gas'troo-lah) an abnormal gastrula in which invagination is hindered and the mesentoderm bulges outward.

exogenous (ek-soj'ĕ-nus) originating outside or caused by factors outside the organism.

exomphalos (eks-om'fah-los) 1. hernia of the abdominal viscera into the umbilical cord. 2. congenital umbilical hernia.

exonuclease (ek''so-nu'kle-ās) a nuclease that cleaves single mononucleotides from the end of a polynucleotide chain.

exopeptidase (-pep'tĭ-dās) a proteolytic enzyme whose action is limited to terminal peptide linkages.

exophoria (-fo're-ah) deviation of the visual axis of one eye away from that of the other eye in the absence of visual fusional stimuli. **exopho'ric,** adj.

exophthalmometry (ek''sof-thal-mom'ĕ-tre) measurement of the extent of protrusion of the eyeball in exophthalmos. **exophthalmomet'ric,** adj.

exophthalmos (ek''sof-thal'mus) abnormal protrusion of the eye. **exophthal'mic,** adj.

exophytic (ek''so-fit'ik) growing outward; in oncology, proliferating on the exterior or surface epithelium of an organ or other structure in which the growth originated.

exoplasm (ek'so-plazm) cell membrane.

exoserosis (ek''so-se-ro'sis) an oozing of serum or exudate.

exoskeleton (-skel'ĕ-ton) a hard structure formed on the outside of the body, as a crustacean's shell; in vertebrates, applied to structures produced by the epidermis, as hair, nails, hoofs, teeth, etc.

exosmosis (ek''sos-mo'sis) osmosis or diffusion from within outward.

exostosis (ek''sos-to'sis), pl. *exosto'ses* [Gr.] a benign growth projecting from a bone surface characteristically capped by cartilage. **exostot'ic,** adj. **e. cartilagin'ea,** a variety of osteoma consisting of a layer of cartilage developing beneath the periosteum of a bone. **hereditary multiple exostoses,** a hereditary condition in which multiple bony excrescences grow out from the cortical surfaces of long bones.

exothermal, exothermic (ek''so-ther'mal; -ther'mik) marked or accompanied by evolution of heat; liberating heat or energy.

exotoxin (-tok'sin) a potent toxin formed and excreted by the bacterial cell, and free in the surrounding medium. **exotox'ic,** adj.

exotropia (-tro'pe-ah) strabismus in which there is permanent deviation of the visual axis of one eye away from that of the other, resulting in diplopia. **exotro'pic,** adj.

expander (ek-span'der) extender. **plasma volume e.,** artificial plasma extender.

expectorant (ek-spek'to-rant) 1. promoting expectoration. 2. an agent that promotes expectoration. **liquefying e.,** an expectorant that promotes the ejection of mucus from the respiratory tract by decreasing its viscosity.

expectoration (ek-spek''to-ra'shun) 1. the coughing up and spitting out of material from the lungs, bronchi, and trachea. 2. sputum.

experiment (ek-sper'ĭ-ment) a procedure done in order to discover or demonstrate some fact or general truth. **experimen'tal,** adj. **control e.,** one made under standard conditions, to test the correctness of other observations.

expiration (eks''pĭ-ra'shun) 1. the act of breathing out, or expelling air from the lungs. 2. termination, or death. **expi'ratory,** adj.

expire (ek-spīr') 1. to breathe out. 2. to die.

explant 1. (eks-plant') to take from the body and place in an artificial medium for growth. 2. (eks'plant) tissue taken from the body and grown in an artificial medium.

exploration (eks''plo-ra'shun) investigation or examination for diagnostic purposes. **explo'ratory,** adj.

exposure (eks-po'zhur) 1. the act of laying open, as surgical exposure. 2. the condition of being subjected to something, as to infectious agents, extremes of weather or radiation, which may have a harmful effect. 3. in radiology, a measure of the amount of ionizing radiation at the surface of the irradiated object, e.g., the body.

expression (eks-presh'un) 1. the aspect or appearance of the face as determined by the physical or emotional state. 2. the act of squeezing out or evacuating by pressure.

expressivity (eks''pres-siv'ĭ-te) the extent to which a heritable trait is manifested by an individual carrying the principal gene or genes that determine it.

expulsive (ek-spul'siv) driving or forcing out; tending to expel.

exsanguination (eks-sang″wĭ-na′shun) extensive loss of blood due to internal or external hemorrhage.

exsection (ek-sek′shun) excision.

exsiccation (ek″sĭ-ka′shun) the act of drying out; in chemistry, the deprival of a crystalline substance of its water of crystallization.

exsorption (ek-sorp′shun) the movement of substances out of cells, especially the movement of substances out of the blood into the intestinal lumen.

exstrophy (ek′stro-fe) the turning inside out of an organ. **e. of bladder,** congenital deficiency of the abdominal wall and bladder, the latter organ appearing to be turned inside out, with the internal surface of the posterior wall showing through the opening in the anterior wall.

ext. external; extract.

extender (ek-sten′der) something that enlarges or prolongs. **artificial plasma e.,** a substance that can be transfused to maintain fluid volume of the blood in event of great necessity, supplemental to the use of whole blood and plasma.

extension (ek-sten′shun) 1. the movement by which the two ends of any jointed part are drawn away from each other. 2. a movement bringing the members of a limb into or toward a straight condition. **Buck's e.,** extension of fractured leg by weights, the foot of the bed being raised so that the body makes counterextension. **Codivilla's e.,** extension for fractures made by a weight pulling on calipers or a nail passed through the lower end of the bone. **nail e.,** extension exerted on the distal fragment of a fractured bone by means of a nail or pin (Steinmann pin) driven into the fragment. **Steinmann e.,** nail e.

extensor (eks-ten′sor) [L.] any muscle that extends a joint.

exteriorize (eks-te′re-or-īz) 1. to form a correct mental reference of the image of an object seen. 2. in psychiatry, to turn one's interest outward. 3. to transpose an internal organ to the exterior of the body.

extern (eks′tern) a medical student or graduate in medicine who assists in patient care in the hospital but does not reside there.

external (eks-ter′nal) situated or occurring on the outside. In anatomy, situated toward or near the outside; lateral.

externalize (eks-ter′nah-līz) to direct outwardly an internal conflict.

externus (eks-ter′nus) external; in anatomy, denoting a structure farther from the center of the part or cavity.

exteroceptor (ek″ster-o-sep′tor) a sensory nerve ending stimulated by the immediate external environment, such as those in the skin and mucous membranes. **exterocep′tive,** adj.

exterofective (-fek′tiv) responding to external stimuli; a term applied to the cerebrospinal nervous system.

extima (eks′tĭ-mah) outermost; the outermost coat of a blood vessel.

extinction (eks-ting′shun) in psychology, the disappearance of a conditioned response as a result of nonreinforcement; also, the process by which the disappearance is accomplished.

extirpation (eks″ter-pa′shun) complete removal or eradication of an organ or tissue.

extorsion (eks-tor′shun) tilting of the upper part of the vertical meridian of the eye away from the midline of the face.

extra- word element [L.], *outside; beyond the scope of; in addition.*

extra-articular (eks″trah-ar-tik′u-ler) situated or occurring outside a joint.

extracapsular (-kap′su-ler) situated or occurring outside a capsule.

extracellular (-sel′u-lar) outside a cell or cells.

extracorporeal (-kor-po′re-al) situated or occurring outside the body.

extracorticospinal (-kor″tĭ-ko-spi′nal) outside the corticospinal tract.

extract (eks′trakt) a concentrated preparation of a vegetable or animal drug. **allergenic e.,** an extract of the protein of any substance to which a person may be sensitive. **beef e.,** a concentrate from beef broth. **cell-free e.,** the solution obtained by rupturing cells and removing all particulate matter. **chondodendron tomentosum e.,** an alcoholic extract from curare obtained from the South American shrub *Chondodendron tomentosum;* used as a skeletal muscle relaxant. **dry e.,** powdered e. **Goulard's e.,** lead subacetate solution. **liver e.,** one prepared from mammalian livers; used as a hematopoietic. **malt e.,** a product containing dextrin, maltose, a small amount of glucose, and amylolytic enzymes; used as a nutritive and emulsifying agent. **ox bile e.,** one prepared from the fresh bile of the ox; used as a choleretic. **parathyroid e.,** see under *injection.* **pilular e.,** one whose solvent has been partially evaporated, leaving a plastic mass. **powdered e.,** one whose solvent has been entirely evaporated, leaving a fine, dry powder. **semiliquid e.,** one evaporated to a syrupy consistency. **solid e.,** pilular e. **trichinella e.,** an aqueous extract of specially treated larvae of *Trichinella spiralis,* usually obtained from inoculated rodents; used as a skin test for trichinella infection.

extraction (eks-trak′shun) 1. the process or act of pulling or drawing out. 2. the preparation of an extract. **breech e.,** extraction of an infant from the uterus in breech presentation. **flap e.,** extraction of a cataract by an incision which makes a flap of cornea. **serial e.,** the selective extraction of deciduous teeth during an extended period of time to allow autonomous adjustment. **vacuum e.,** delivery of a fetus by application of a vacuum.

extractive (eks-trak′tiv) any substance present in an organized tissue, or in a mixture in a small quantity, and requiring extraction by a special method.

extractor (eks-trak′tor) an instrument for removing a calculus or foreign body.

extracystic (eks″trah-sis′tik) outside a cyst or the bladder.

extradural (-du′ral) situated or occurring outside the dura mater.

extraembryonic (-em″bre-on′ik) not occurring

as part of the embryo proper; applied specifically to the fetal membranes.

extragenital (-jen′ĭ-tal) unrelated to, not originating in, or remote from the genital organs.

extrahepatic (-hĕ-pat′ik) situated or occurring outside the liver.

extraligamentous (-lig″ah-men′tus) occurring outside a ligament.

extramalleolus (-mal-e′o-lus) the external malleolus.

extramarginal (-mar′jĭ-nal) below the limit of consciousness.

extramastoiditis (-mas″toi-di′tis) inflammation of tissues adjoining the mastoid process.

extramedullary (-med′u-ler″e) situated or occurring outside a medulla, especially the medulla oblongata.

extramural (-mu′ral) situated or occurring outside the wall of an organ or structure.

extranuclear (-nu′kle-ar) situated or occurring outside a cell nucleus.

extraocular (-ok′u-lar) outside the eyeball.

extraperitoneal (-per″ĭ-to-ne′al) outside the peritoneum.

extraplacental (-plah-sen′tal) independent of the placenta.

extrapleural (-ploo′ral) outside the pleura.

extrapulmonary (-pul′mo-na″re) not connected with the lungs.

extrapyramidal (-pĭ-ram′ĭ-dal) outside the pyramidal tracts; see under *system.*

extrasystole (-sis′to-le) a premature cardiac contraction that is independent of the normal rhythm and arises in response to an impulse outside the sinoatrial node. **atrial e.,** one in which the stimulus is thought to arise in the atrium elsewhere than at the sinus. **atrioventricular e.,** one in which the stimulus is thought to arise in the atrioventricular node. **infranodal e.,** ventricular e. **interpolated e.,** a contraction taking place between two normal heart beats. **nodal e.,** atrioventricular e. **retrograde e.,** a premature ventricular contraction, followed by a premature atrial contraction, due to transmission of the stimulus backward, usually over the bundle of His. **ventricular e.,** one in which either a pacemaker or re-entry site is in the ventricular structure.

extratubal (-tu′bal) outside a tube.

extrauterine (-u′ter-īn) situated or occurring outside the uterus.

extravaginal (-vaj′ĭ-nal) outside the vagina.

extravasation (eks-trav″ah-za′shun) 1. a discharge or escape, as of blood, from a vessel into the tissues; blood or other substance so discharged. 2. the process of being extravasated.

extravascular (eks″trah-vas′ku-lar) situated or occurring outside a vessel or the vessels.

extraventricular (-ven-trik′u-lar) situated or occurring outside a ventricle.

extraversion (-ver′zhun) extroversion.

extravert (eks′trah-vert) extrovert.

extremitas (eks′trem′ĭ-tas), pl. *extremita′tes* [L.] extremity.

extremity (eks-trem′ĭ-te) 1. the distal or termi-

nal portion of elongated or pointed structures. 2. the arm or leg.

extrinsic (eks-trin′sik) of external origin.

extroversion (eks″tro-ver′zhun) 1. a turning inside out; exstrophy. 2. direction of one's energies and attention outward from the self.

extrovert (eks′tro-vert) a person whose interest is turned outward.

extrude (ek-strood′) 1. to force out, or to occupy a position distal to that normally occupied. 2. in dentistry, to occupy a position occlusal to that normally occupied.

extrudoclusion (eks-troo″do-kloo′zhun) extrusion (2).

extrusion (eks-troo′zhun) 1. a pushing out. 2. in dentistry, the condition of a tooth pushed too far forward from the line of occlusion.

extubation (eks″tu-ba′shun) removal of a tube used in intubation.

exuberant (eg-zu′ber-ant) copious or excessive in production; showing excessive proliferation.

exudate (eks′u-dāt) a fluid with a high content of protein and cellular debris which has escaped from blood vessels and has been deposited in tissues or on tissue surfaces, usually as a result of inflammation.

exudation (eks″u-da′shun) 1. the escape of fluid, cells, or cellular debris from blood vessels and deposition in or on the tissue. 2. exudate.

exudative (eks-oo′dah-tiv) of or pertaining to a process of exudation.

exumbilication (eks″um-bil″ĭ-ka′shun) 1. marked protrusion of the navel. 2. umbilical hernia.

eye (i) the organ of vision; see Plate XIII. **black e.,** a bruise of the tissue around the eye, marked by discoloration, swelling, and pain. **compound e.,** the multifaceted eye of insects. **cross e.,** esotropia. **exciting e.,** the eye that is primarily injured and from which the influences start which involve the other eye in sympathetic ophthalmia. **Klieg e.,** conjunctivitis, edema of the eyelids, lacrimation, and photophobia due to exposure to intense lights (Klieg lights). **pink e.,** acute contagious conjunctivitis. **reduced e., schematic e.,** 1. an apparatus with two refracting elements, one representing the cornea and the other the lens. 2. a diagrammatic illustration of the eye structure. **shipyard e.,** epidemic keratoconjunctivitis. **wall e.,** 1. leukoma of the cornea. 2. exophoria.

eyeball (i′bawl) the ball or globe of the eye.

eyebrow (i′brow) 1. supercilium; the transverse elevation at the junction of the forehead and the upper eyelid. 2. supercilia; the hairs growing on this elevation.

eyecup (i′kup) 1. a small vessel for application of cleansing or medicated solution to the exposed area of the eyeball. 2. physiologic cup.

eyeglass (i′glas) a lens for aiding the sight.

eyeground (i′grownd) the fundus of the eye as seen with the ophthalmoscope.

eyelash (i′lash) cilium; one of the hairs growing on the edge of an eyelid.

eyelid (i′lid) either of two movable folds (upper

and lower) protecting the anterior surface of the eyeball. **third e.,** nictitating membrane.

eyepiece (i'pēs) the lens or system of lenses of a microscope (or telescope) nearest the user's eye, serving to further magnify the image produced by the objective.

eyespot (i'spot) the light-sensitive pigmented spot of certain invertebrates.

eyestrain (i'strān) fatigue of the eye from overuse or from uncorrected defect in focus of the eye.

F

F chemical symbol, *fluorine.*

F. Fahrenheit; field of vision; formula; French.

F₁ first filial generation.

F₂ second filial generation.

fabella (fah-bel'ah), pl. *fabel'lae* [L.] see *Table of Bones.*

fabism (fa'bizm) favism.

F.A.C.D. Fellow of American College of Dentists.

face (fās) 1. the anterior, or ventral, aspect of the head from the forehead to the chin, inclusive. 2. any presenting aspect or surface. **fa'cial,** adj. **frog f.,** flatness of the face due to intranasal disease. **hippocratic f.,** facies hippocratica. **moon f.,** the peculiar rounded face seen in various conditions, as in Cushing's syndrome, or after administration of adrenal corticoids.

face-bow (fās'bo) a device used in dentistry to record the positional relations of the maxillary arch to the temporomandibular joints (or opening axis of the jaw) and to orient dental casts in this same relationship to the opening axis of the articulator.

facet (fas'et) a small plane surface on a hard body, as on a bone.

facetectomy (fas″ĕ-tek'to-me) excision of the articular facet of a vertebra.

faci(o)- word element [L.], *face.*

facial (fa'shal) of or pertaining to the face.

facies (fa'she-ēz), pl. *fa'cies* [L.] 1. the face. 2. a specific surface of a body structure, part, or organ. 3. the expression or appearance of the face. **adenoid f.,** the dull expression, with open mouth, sometimes seen in children with adenoid growths. **f. hepat'ica,** a thin face with sunken eyeballs, sallow complexion, and yellow conjunctivae, characteristic of certain chronic liver disorders. **f. hippocrat'ica,** a drawn, pinched, and pale appearance of the face indicative of approaching death. **f. leonti'na,** a peculiar, deeply furrowed, lion-like appearance of the face seen in certain cases of advanced lepromatous leprosy.

facilitation (fah-sil″ĭ-ta'shun) hastening or assistance of a natural process; the increased excitability of a neuron after stimulation by a subthreshold presynaptic impulse.

facing (fās'ing) a piece of porcelain cut to represent the outer surface of a tooth.

faciobrachial (fa″she-o-bra'ke-al) pertaining to the face and the arm.

faciocervical (-ser'vĭ-kal) pertaining to the face and neck.

faciolingual (-ling'gwal) pertaining to the face and tongue.

facioplasty (fa'she-o-plas″te) restorative or plastic surgery of the face.

facioplegia (fa″she-o-ple'je-ah) facial paralysis. **faciople'gic,** adj.

facioscapulohumeral (-skap″u-lo-hu'mer-al) pertaining to the face, scapula, and arm.

F.A.C.O.G. Fellow of the American College of Obstetricians and Gynecologists.

F.A.C.P. Fellow of American College of Physicians.

F.A.C.S. Fellow of American College of Surgeons.

F.A.C.S.M. Fellow of the American College of Sports Medicine.

factitial (fak-tish'al) artificially produced; unintentionally produced.

factitious (fak-tish'us) artificial.

factor (fak'tor) an agent or element that contributes to the production of a result. **accelerator f.,** coagulation Factor V. **animal protein f.,** a substance found in animal protein essential to maximal growth of animals. **antianemia f.,** cyanocobalamin. **antihemophilic f.,** coagulation Factor VIII. **antihemorrhagic f.,** vitamin K. **antinuclear f. (ANF),** an autoantibody against constituents of cell nuclei, present in the sera in systemic lupus erythematosus and occasionally in rheumatoid arthritis and other collagen diseases. **antipernicious anemia f.,** cyanocobalamin. **antirachitic f.,** vitamin D. **antiscorbutic f.,** ascorbic acid. **antisterility f.,** vitamin E. **Bittner milk f.,** mouse mammary tumor agent. **Castle's f.,** intrinsic f. **citrovorum f.,** folinic acid. **clotting f's,** coagulation f's. **coagulation f's,** factors essential to normal blood clotting, whose absence, diminution, or excess may lead to abnormality of the clotting mechanism. Twelve factors, commonly designated by Roman numerals (I to V and VII to XIII) have been described (factor VI is no longer considered to have a clotting function). Platelet factors, designated by Arabic numerals, also play a role in coagulation. *Factor I,* fibrinogen; it is converted to fibrin by the action of thrombin. Deficiency results in afibrinogemia or hypofibrinogenemia. *Factor II,* prothrombin; it is converted to thrombin by extrinsic prothrombin converting principle. Deficiency leads to hypoprothrombinemia. *Factor III,* tissue thromboplastin; important in formation of extrinsic prothrombin converting principle. *Factor IV,* calcium. *Factor*

V, proaccelerin; it functions in both intrinsic and extrinsic pathways of blood coagulation. Deficiency leads to parahemophilia. *Factor VII,* proconvertin; it functions in the extrinsic pathway of blood coagulation. Deficiency, either hereditary or acquired (vitamin K deficiency), leads to hemorrhagic tendency. *Factor VIII,* antihemophilic factor. Deficiency, a sex-linked recessive trait, results in classical hemophilia. *Factor IX,* plasma thromboplastin component; Christmas factor. Deficiency results in hemophilia B. *Factor X,* Stuart factor. Deficiency may result in a systemic coagulation disorder. *Factor XI,* plasma thromboplastin antecedent. Deficiency results in hemophilia C. *Factor XII,* Hageman factor; it initiates the intrinsic process of blood clotting *in vitro. Factor XIII,* fibrin stabilizing factor; it polymerizes fibrin monomers. Deficiency causes a clinical hemorrhagic diathesis. **Curling f.,** griseofulvin. **Duran Reynals' f.,** hyaluronidase. **extrinsic f.,** cyanocobalamin. **F f., fertility f.,** the episome that determines the mating type of conjugating bacteria, being present in the donor (male) bacterium and absent in the recipient (female). **Hageman f.,** coagulation Factor XII. **intrinsic f.,** a glycoprotein secreted by gastric glands, necessary for absorption of cyanocobalamin (*extrinsic f.*). **LE f.,** an immunoglobulin (a 7S antibody) that reacts with leukocyte nuclei, found in the serum in systemic lupus erythematosus. **modifying f's,** multiple factors which affect the degree of expressivity of another gene. **multiple f's,** two or more genes which cooperate, blend, or cumulate to produce a certain character. **platelet f's,** factors important in hemostasis which are contained in or attached to the platelets: *platelet factor 1* is adsorbed coagulation Factor V from the plasma; *platelet factor 2* is an accelerator of the thrombin-fibrinogen reaction; *platelet factor 3* plays a role in the generation of intrinsic prothrombin converting principle; *platelet factor 4* is capable of inhibiting the activity of heparin. **R f., resistance f.,** the bacterial plasmid (R plasmid) responsible for resistance to antibiotics; it is transmitted to other bacterial cells by conjugation, as well as to the progeny of any cell containing it. **Rh f., Rhesus f.,** genetically determined antigens present on the surface of erythrocytes; incompatibility for these antigens between mother and offspring is responsible for erythroblastosis fetalis. **rheumatoid f.,** a protein of high molecular weight in the serum of most patients with rheumatoid arthritis, detectable by serologic tests. **spreading f.,** hyaluronidase. **Stuart f., Stuart-Prower f.,** coagulation Factor X.

facultative (fak′ul-ta″tiv) not obligatory; pertaining to or characterized by the ability to adjust to particular circumstances or to assume a particular role.

faculty (fak′ul-te) 1. a normal power or function, especially of the mind. 2. the teaching staff of an institution of learning.

FAD flavin adenine dinucleotide.

fae- for words beginning thus, see those beginning *fe-.*

failure (fāl′yer) inability to perform or to func-

tion properly. **heart f.,** see under *H.* **kidney f., renal f.,** inability of the kidney to excrete metabolites at normal plasma levels under normal loading, or inability to retain electrolytes when intake is normal; in the acute form, marked by uremia and usually by oliguria, with hyperkalemia and pulmonary edema.

faint (fānt) syncope.

falcate (fal′kāt) falciform.

falcial (-shal) pertaining to a falx.

falciform (-sĭ-form) sickle-shaped.

falcular (-ku-ler) falciform.

fallout (fawl′owt) the settling to the earth's surface of radioactive fission products from the atmosphere after a nuclear explosion.

falx (falks), pl. *fal′ces* [L.] a sickle-shaped structure. **f. cerebel′li,** a fold of dura mater separating the cerebellar hemispheres. **f. cer′ebri,** the fold of dura mater in the longitudinal fissure, separating the cerebral hemispheres.

F.A.M.A. Fellow of American Medical Association.

familial (fah-mil′e-al) occurring in or affecting more members of a family than would be expected by chance.

family (fam′ĭ-le) 1. a group descended from a common ancestor. 2. a taxonomic subdivision subordinate to an order (or suborder) and superior to a tribe (or subfamily).

fang (fang) 1. the root of a tooth. 2. one of the teeth of a carnivore with which it seizes and tears its prey, or the envenomed tooth of a serpent.

fango (fan′go) volcanic mud.

fangotherapy (fan″go-ther′ah-pe) the therapeutic use of fango in packs or baths.

Fannia (fan′e-ah) a genus of flies whose larvae have caused both intestinal and urinary myiasis in man.

fantasy (fan′tah-se) an imaged sequence of events or mental images that serves to satisfy unconscious wishes or to express unconcious conflicts.

farad (far′ad) the unit of electric capacity; capacity to hold 1 coulomb with a potential of 1 volt.

faraday (far′ah-da) the quantity of electrical charge associated with one gram equivalent of an electrochemical reaction, equal to about 96,510 coulombs.

faradism (far′ah-dizm) 1. faradization. 2. induced current.

faradization (far″ah-dĭ-za′shun) therapeutic use of interrupted current.

farcy (far′se) see *glanders.*

fardel-bound (far′del-bownd) having an inflamed abomasum and a distended omasum, making chewing of the cud impossible; a condition affecting cattle and sheep.

farinaceous (far″ĭ-na′shus) 1. of the nature of flour or meal. 2. starchy; containing starch.

farsightedness (far-sīt′ed-nes) hyperopia.

fascia (fash′e-ah), pl. *fas′ciae* [L.] a sheet or band of fibrous tissue such as lies deep to the skin or invests muscles and various body organs. **fas′cial,** adj. **aponeurotic f.,** a dense, firm, fibrous, membrane investing the trunk and limbs and giving off sheaths to the various muscles. **f. cribro'sa,** the superficial fascia of the thigh covering the saphenous opening. **crural f.,** the investing fascia of the leg. **deep f.,** aponeurotic f. **endothoracic f.,** that beneath the serous lining of the thoracic cavity. **extrapleural f.,** a prolongation of the endothoracic fascia sometimes found at the root of the neck, important as possibly modifying the auscultatory sounds at the apex of the lung. **f. la'ta,** the external investing fascia of the thigh. **Scarpa's f.,** the deep, membranous layer of the subcutaneous abdominal fascia. **superficial f.,** 1. a fascial sheet lying directly beneath the skin. 2. subcutaneous tissue. **Tenon's f.,** see under *capsule*. **thyrolaryngeal f.,** that covering the thyroid body and attached to the cricoid cartilage. **transverse f.,** that between the transversalis muscle and the peritoneum. **Tyrrell's f.,** that between the bladder and rectum.

fascicle (fas'ĭ-k'l) a small bundle or cluster, especially of nerve or muscle fibers.

fascicular (fah-sik'u-lar) clustered together; pertaining to or arranged in bundles or clusters; pertaining to a fascicle.

fasciculated (fah-sik'u-lāt-ed) clustered together or occurring in bundles, or fasciculi.

fasciculation (fah-sik''u-la'shun) 1. the formation of fascicles. 2. a small local involuntary muscular contraction visible under the skin, representing spontaneous discharge of a number of fibers innervated by a single motor nerve filament.

fasciculus (fah-sik'u-lus), pl. *fascic'uli* [L.] fascicle. **f. cuneatus of medulla oblongata,** the continuation into the medulla oblongata of the fasciculus cuneatus of the spinal cord. **f. cuneatus of spinal cord,** the lateral portion of the posterior funiculus of the spinal cord, composed of ascending fibers that end in the nucleus cuneatus. **f. gracilis of medulla oblongata,** the continuation into the medulla oblongata of the fasciculus gracilis of the spinal cord. **f. gracilis of spinal cord,** the median portion of the posterior funiculus of the spinal cord, composed of ascending fibers that end in the nucleus gracilis.

fasciectomy (fas''e-ek'to-me) excision of fascia.

fasciitis (-i'tis) inflammation of a fascia. **nodular f., proliferative f.,** a benign, reactive proliferation of fibroblasts in the subcutaneous tissues, commonly affecting the deep fascia. **pseudosarcomatous f.,** a benign soft tissue tumor occurring subcutaneously and sometimes arising from deep muscle and fascia.

fasciodesis (-od'ĕ-sis) suture of a fascia to skeletal attachment.

Fasciola (fah-si'o-lah) a genus of flukes, including *F. hepat'ica,* the common liver fluke of herbivores, occasionally found in the human liver.

fasciola (fah-si'o-lah), pl. *fasci'olae* [L.] 1. a small band of striplike structure. 2. a small bandage. **fasi'olar,** adj.

fascioliasis (fas''e-o-li'ah-sis) infection with *Fasciola*.

fasciolopsiasis (-lop-si'ah-sis) infection with *Fasciolopsis*.

Fasciolopsis (-lop'sis) a genus of trematodes, including *F. bus'ki,* the largest of the intestinal flukes, found in the small intestines of residents throughout Asia.

fascioplasty (fas'e-o-plas''te) plastic repair of a fascia.

fasciorrhaphy (fas''e-or'ah-fe) repair of a lacerated fascia.

fasciotomy (fas''e-ot'o-me) incision of a fascia.

fast (fast) 1. immovable, or unchangeable; resistant to the action of a specific drug, stain, or destaining agent. 2. abstention from food.

fastigium (fas-tij'e-um) [L.] 1. the highest point in the roof of the fourth ventricle of the brain. 2. the acme, or highest point. **fastig'ial,** adj.

fat (fat) 1. adipose tissue. 2. an ester of glycerol with fatty acids, usually palmitic, oleic, or stearic acid. **brown f.,** brown adipose tissue. **wool f.,** anhydrous lanolin. **wool f., hydrous,** lanolin. **wool f., refined,** anhydrous lanolin.

fatal (fa'tal) causing death; deadly; mortal; lethal.

fatigability (fat''ĭ-gah-bil'ĭ-te) easy suseptibility to fatigue.

fatigue (fah-tēg') a state of increased discomfort and decreased efficiency due to prolonged or excessive exertion; loss of power or capacity to respond to stimulation.

fatty (fat'e) pertaining to or characterized by fat.

fauces (faw'sēz) the passage between the throat and pharynx. **fau'cial,** adj.

faucitis (faw-si'tis) inflammation of the fauces.

fauna (faw'nah) the collective animal organisms of a given locality.

faveolate (fah-ve'o-lāt) honeycombed; alveolate.

faveolus (fah-ve'o-lus) foveola.

favid (fa'vid) a secondary skin eruption due to allergy in favus.

favism (fa'vizm) an acute hemolytic anemia precipitated by fava beans (ingestion, or inhalation of pollen), usually caused by deficiency of glucose-6-phosphate dehydrogenase in the erythrocytes.

favus (fa'vus) a type of tinea capitis, with formation of prominent honeycomb-like masses, due to *Trichophyton schoenleini.* **f. of fowl,** a chronic dermatomycosis affecting the comb of fowl, caused by *Trichophyton megnini.*

F-Cortef (ef-kor'tef) trademark for a preparation of fludrocortisone.

F.D. focal distance; fatal dose (now called *lethal dose*).

F.D.A. Food and Drug Administration.

F.D.I. Fédération Dentaire Internationale (International Dental Association).

Fe chemical symbol, *iron* (L. *ferrum*).

fear (fēr) a normal emotional response, in contrast to anxiety and phobia, to consciously recognized external sources of danger, which is manifested by alarm, apprehension, or disquiet.

febricide (feb'rĭ-sīd) lowering bodily temperature in fever; an agent that so acts.

febrifacient (feb''rĭ-fa'shent) producing fever.

febrific (fĕ-brik'ik) producing fever.

febrifugal (fĕ-brif'u-gal) dispelling fever.

febrifuge (feb′rĭ-fūj) an agent that reduces body temperature in fever; antipyretic.

febrile (feb′ril) pertaining to fever; feverish.

febris (feb′ris) [L.] fever. **f. meliten′sis, f. un′dulans,** brucellosis.

fecalith (fe′kah-lith) an intestinal concretion formed around a center of fecal matter.

fecaloid (fe′kal-oid) resembling feces.

fecaloma (fe″kal-o′mah) stercoroma.

fecaluria (-u′re-ah) presence of fecal matter in the urine.

feces (fe′sēz), pl. of *faex* [L.] excrement discharged from the bowels. **fe′cal,** adj.

fecula (fek′u-lah) 1. lees or sediment. 2. starch.

feculent (fek′u-lent) 1. having dregs or sediment. 2. excrementitious.

fecundation (fe″kun-da′shun) fertilization; impregnation.

fecundity (fe-kun′dĭ-te) the ability to produce offspring frequently and in large numbers. In demography, the physiological ability to reproduce, as opposed to fertility.

feeblemindedness (fe″b′l-mīnd′ed-nes) former name for mental retardation.

feedback (fēd′bak) the return of some of the output of a system as input so as to exert some control in the process; feedback is *negative* when the return exerts an inhibitory control; *positive* when it exerts a stimulatory effect.

feeding (-ing) the taking or giving of food. **artificial f.,** feeding of a baby with food other than mother's milk. **breast f.,** see under B. **forced f.,** administration of food by force to those who cannot or will not receive it. **sham f.,** feeding in which the food is chewed and swallowed but does not enter the stomach, because of diversion to the exterior by an esophageal fistula or other device.

fellatio (fĕ-la′she-o) oral stimulation or manipulation of the penis.

felon (fel′on) a purulent infection involving the pulp of the distal phalanx of a finger.

feltwork (felt′werk) a complex of closely interwoven fibers, as of nerve fibers.

female (fe′māl) 1. an individual of the sex that produces ova or bears young. 2. feminine.

feminine (fem′ĭ-nin) pertaining to the female sex, or having qualities normally characteristic of the female.

feminism (fem′ĭ-nizm) the appearance or existence of female secondary sex characters in the male.

feminization (fem″ĭ-ni-za′shun) 1. the normal induction or development of female sex characters. 2. the induction or development of female secondary sex characters in the male. **testicular f.,** a condition in which the subject is phenotypically female, but lacks nuclear sex chromatin and is of XY chromosomal sex.

femoral (fem′o-ral) pertaining to the femur or to the thigh.

femorocele (fem′o-ro-sēl″) femoral hernia.

femorotibial (fem″o-ro-tib′e-al) pertaining to the femur and tibia.

femto- (fem′to) a combining form used in naming units of measurement to indicate one-quadrillionth (10^{-15}) of the unit designated by the root with which it is combined.

femur (fe′mur), pl. *fem′ora* [L.] 1. see *Table of Bones.* 2. the thigh.

fenestra (fĕ-nes′trah), pl. *fenes′trae* [L.] a window-like opening. **f. coch′leae,** a round opening in the inner wall of the middle ear covered by the secondary tympanic membrane. **f. ova′lis,** vestibuli. **f. rotun′da,** f. cochleae. **f. vestib′uli,** an oval opening in the inner wall of the middle ear, which is closed by the base of the stapes.

fenestrate (fen′es-trāt) to pierce with one or more openings.

fenestration (fen″es-tra′shun) 1. the act of perforating or condition of being perforated. 2. the surgical creation of a new opening in the labyrinth of the ear for restoration of hearing in otosclerosis. **aortopulmonary f.,** aortic septal defect.

fenfluramine (fen-floor′ah-mēn) an amphetamine derivative, $C_{12}H_{16}F_3N$, used as an anorexic in the form of the hydrochloride salt.

fentanyl (fen′tah-nil) a piperidine derivative $C_{22}H_{22}N_2O$; the citrate salt is used as a narcotic analgesic and, in combination with droperidol (known as *Innovar*), as a neuroleptanalgesic.

Feosol (fe′o-sol) trademark for preparations of ferrous sulfate.

Fergon (fer′gon) trademark for preparations of ferrous gluconate.

ferment 1. (fer-ment′) to undergo fermentation. 2. (fer′ment) any substance that causes fermentation.

fermentation (fer″men-ta′shun) enzymatic decomposition, especially of carbohydrates; the anaerobic conversion of foodstuffs to particular products, as opposed to aerobic conversion (oxidation). **acetic f.,** conversion of alcoholic solution into acetic acid or vinegar. **alcoholic f.,** formation of alcohol from carbohydrates. **ammoniacal f.,** formation of ammonia and carbon dioxide from urea by urease. **butyric f.,** change of carbohydrates, milk, etc., into butyric acid. **caseous f.,** the coagulation of soluble casein by rennin. **diastatic f.,** the change of starch into glucose by ptyalin or certain other enzymes. **lactic f.,** the conversion of sugars to lactic acid by various bacteria; the souring of milk. **viscous f.,** production of gummy substances, as in wine, milk, or urine, under the influence of various bacilli.

fermium (fer′me-um) chemical element (*see table*), at. no. 100, symbol Fm.

ferning (fern′ing) the appearance of a fernlike pattern in a dried specimen of cervical mucus, an indication of the presence of estrogen.

-ferous word element [L.], *bearing; producing.*

ferredoxin (fer″ĕ-dok′sin) a nonheme iron-containing protein, also having a high sulfide content, which serves as an acceptor molecule in electron transport from chlorophyll during the formation of NADPH in photosynthesis.

ferric (fer′ik) containing iron in its plus-three oxidation state, Fe(III) (sometimes designated Fe^{3+}).

ferritin (fer′ĭ-tin) the iron-apoferritin complex,

which is one of the chief forms in which iron is stored in the body.

Ferrobacillus (fer″o-bah-sil′lus) a genus of schizomycetes (family Siderocepsaceae) which oxidize ferrous iron in the ferric state.

ferrocholinate (-ko′lin-āt) a compound of ferric hydroxide and choline dihydrogen citrate; used orally in iron-deficiency anemia.

ferrokinetics (-ki-net′iks) the turnover or rate of change of iron in the body.

Ferrolip (fer′o-lip) trademark for preparations of ferrocholinate.

ferroprotein (fer″o-pro′te-in) a protein combined with an iron-containing radical; ferroproteins are respiratory carriers.

ferrotherapy (-ther′ah-pe) therapeutic use of iron and iron compounds.

ferrous (fer′us) containing iron in its plus-two oxidation state, Fe(II) (sometimes designated Fe^{2+}); for ferrous compounds see under the salt, e.g., sulfate.

ferruginous (fĕ-roo′jĭ-nus) 1. containing iron or iron rust. 2. of the color of iron rust.

ferrule (fer′ool) a band of metal applied to a tooth to strengthen it.

ferrum (fer′um) [L.] iron (symbol Fe).

fertility (fer-til′ĭ-te) the capacity to conceive or induce conception. **fer′tile**, adj.

fertilization (fer″tĭ-lĭ-za′shun) union of male and female elements, leading to development of a new individual. **external f.**, union of the gametes outside the bodies of the originating organisms, as in most fish. **internal f.**, union of the gametes inside the body of the female, the sperm having been transferred from the body of the male by an accessory sex organ or other means.

fertilizin (fer″tĭ-li′zin) a substance of the plasma membrane and gelatinous coat of the ovum of some species; considered to have the specific receptor groups that bind the spermatozoon to the ovum.

fervescence (fer-ves′ens) increase of fever or body temperature.

fester (fes′ter) to suppurate superficially.

festinant (fes′tĭ-nant) accelerating.

festination (fes″tĭ-na′shun) an involuntary tendency to take short accelerating steps in walking.

festoon (fes-toon′) a carving in the base material of a denture that simulates the contours of the natural tissues being replaced.

fetal (fe′tal) of or pertaining to a fetus or the period of its development.

fetalization (fe″tal-i-za′shun) retention in the adult of characters that at an earlier stage of evolution were only infantile and were rapidly lost as the organism attained maturity.

fetation (fe-ta′shun) 1. development of the fetus. 2. pregnancy.

feticide (fēt′ĭ-sīd) the destruction of the fetus.

fetid (fet′id) having a rank, disagreeable smell.

fetish (fet′ish, fe′tish) an object symbolically endowed with special meaning; an object or body part charged with special erotic interest.

fetoglobulin (fe′to-glob′u-lin) fetoprotein.

fetography (fe-tog′rah-fe) radiography of the fetus *in utero*.

fetology (fe-tol′o-je) that branch of medicine dealing with the fetus *in utero*.

fetometry (fe-tom′ĕ-tre) measurement of the fetus, especially of its head.

fetoplacental (fe″to-plah-sen′tal) pertaining to the fetus and placenta.

fetoprotein (-pro′tēn) a fetal antigen that also occurs in adults in certain diseases; α-fetoprotein appears in the serum of patients with hepatoma and embryonal adenocarcinoma; γ-fetoprotein in that of patients with a variety of neoplasms, including sarcomas and leukemias; and β-fetoprotein (found to be identical with normal liver ferritin) in fetal liver and in adults with a variety of liver diseases.

fetor (fe′tor) stench or offensive odors. **f. o′ris**, halitosis. **hepatic f., f. hepat′icus**, the peculiar odor of the breath characteristic of hepatic disease.

fetus (fe′tus) [L.] the developing young in the uterus, specifically the unborn offspring in the postembryonic period, in man from seven or eight weeks after fertilization until birth. **f. acardi′acus**, acardius. **calcified f., lithopedion. f. compres′sus**, f. papyraceus. **f. in fe′tu**, a small, imperfect fetus, incapable of independent life, contained within the body of another fetus. **harlequin f.**, a newborn infant with the severest form of lamellar exfoliation of the newborn. **mummified f.**, a dried-up and shriveled fetus. **f. papyra′ceus**, a dead fetus pressed flat by the growth of a living twin. **parasitic f.**, an incomplete minor fetus attached to a larger, more completely developed fetus, or autosite.

fever (fe′ver) 1. pyrexia; elevation of body temperature above the normal (98.6° F. or 37° C.). 2. any disease characterized by elevation of body temperature. **African tick f.**, relapsing fever caused by *Borrelia duttonii*. **American mountain f.**, Colorado tick f. **aphthous f.**, foot-and-mouth disease. **Assam f.**, kala-azar. **biliary f. of dogs**, canine piroplasmosis. **blackwater f.**, a dangerous complication of falciparum malaria, with passage of dark red to black urine, severe toxicity, and high mortality. **boutonneuse f.**, a tickborne disease endemic in the Mediterranean area, Crimea, Africa, and India, due to infection with *Rickettsia conorii*, with chills, fever, primary skin lesion (tache noire), and rash appearing on the second to fourth day. **breakbone f.**, dengue. **carbuncular f.**, a kind of anthrax in horses and cattle, with gangrenous swellings in the skin. **cat-bite f.**, an infectious disease due to *Pasteurella multocida*, transmitted by a cat bite, marked by formation of an abscess at the site of inoculation. **cat-scratch f.**, a benign, subacute, regional lymphadenitis due to a cat bite or scratch or a scratch from a surface contaminated by a cat, marked by a primary papular eruption at the site of inoculation. **Chagres f.**, a severe type of malarial fever. **childbed f.**, puerperal septicemia. **Colorado tick f.**, a tickborne, nonexanthematous, febrile, viral disease occurring in the Rocky Mountain regions of the United States. **continued f.**, one not varying more than 1.0° to 1.5° F. in 24 hours. **dandy f.,** dengue. **deer fly f.,** tularemia. **desert f.,** primary coccidioidomycosis. **drug f.,** febrile reaction to a therapeutic agent, including vaccines, antineoplastics, antimicrobials, etc. **elephantoid f.,** a recurrent acute febrile condition occurring with filariasis; it may be associated with elephantiasis or lymphangitis. **enteric f.,** 1. typhoid f. 2. paratyphoid. **epidemic hemorrhagic f.,** an acute infectious disease characterized by fever, purpura, peripheral vascular collapse, and acute renal failure, caused by a filterable agent thought to be transmitted to man by mites or chiggers. **eruptive f., exanthematous f.,** any fever accompanied by eruption on the skin. **exanthematic f. of Marseille,** boutonneuse f. **familial Mediterranean f.,** a hereditary disease usually occurring in Armenians and Sephardic Jews, and marked by short recurrent attacks of fever with pain in the abdomen, chest, or joints and erythema resembling that seen in erysipelas; it is sometimes complicated by amyloidosis. **famine f.,** 1. relapsing f. 2. typhus. **Far East hemorrhagic f.,** epidemic hemorrhagic f. **Gibraltar f.,** brucellosis. **glandular f.,** infectious mononucleosis. **harvest f.,** spirochetosis affecting harvest workers, due to *Leptospira grippotyphosa,* with fever, diarrhea, conjunctivitis, stupor, vomiting, and diarrhea. **Hasami f.,** a mild fever of Japan caused by *Leptospira autumnalis.* **Haverhill f.,** an acute form of rat-bite fever due to *Streptobacillus moniliformis,* transmitted by the bite of an infected rat, with an erythematous eruption, severe generalized arthritis, adenitis, headache, and vomiting. **hay f.,** a seasonal form of allergic rhinitis, with acute conjunctivitis, lacrimation, itching, swelling of the nasal mucosa, nasal catarrh, sudden attacks of sneezing, and often asthmatic symptoms; regarded as an anaphylactic or allergic condition excited by a specific allergen (e.g., pollen) to which the person is sensitized. **hay f., nonseasonal, hay f. perennial,** nonseasonal allergic rhinitis. **hectic f.,** a fever recurring daily. **hemoglobinuric f.,** malaria attended with hemoglobinuria. **hemorrhagic f's,** a group of viral diseases of diverse etiology but having many similar clinical characteristics: increased capillary permeability, leukopenia, and thrombocytopenia are common to all. They are manifested by sudden onset, fever, headache, generalized myalgia, backache, conjunctivitis, and severe prostration, followed by various hemorrhagic symptoms, which result in focal inflammatory reaction and necrosis, with mild leukocytosis. **hospital f.,** epidemic typhus. **icterohemorrhagic f.,** leptospiral jaundice. **Ikwa f.,** trench f. **intermittent f.,** an attack of malaria or other fever, with recurring paroxysms of elevated temperature separated by intervals during which the temperature is normal. **jail f.,** epidemic typhus. **Japanese river f.,** scrub typhus. **jungle f.,** falciparum malaria occurring in the East Indies. **Kagami f.,** infectious mononucleosis. **Kedani f.,** scrub typhus. **Kenya f.,** Kenya typhus. **Kew Gardens spotted f.,** rickettsialpox. **Lassa f.,** a highly fatal, acute, febrile disease caused by an extremely virulent virus, oc-

curring in West Africa, and characterized by progressively increasing prostration, sore throat, ulcerations of the mouth or throat, rash, and general aches and pains. **Malta f.,** brucellosis. **marsh f.,** 1. leptospiral jaundice. 2. malaria. **Mediterranean f.,** brucellosis. See also *familial Mediterranean f.* **metal fume f.,** an occupational disorder with malaria-like symptoms, due to inhalation of volatilized metals. **milk f.,** 1. a fever said to attend establishment of lactation after delivery. 2. an endemic fever said to be due to the use of unwholesome cow's milk. 3. a form of paralysis due to a metabolic disorder, affecting cows near delivery, and usually accompanied by hypocalcemia. **mountain f.,** 1. Colorado tick f. 2. Rocky Mountain spotted f. 3. brucellosis. **mountain tick f.,** Colorado tick f. **mud f.,** leptospiral jaundice. **Murchison-Pel-Ebstein f.,** a type typical of Hodgkin's disease, characterized by irregular episodes of pyrexia of several days' duration, with intervening periods in which the temperature is normal. **Neapolitan f.,** brucellosis. **Oroya f.,** the acute febrile anemic stage of Carrión's disease. **paludal f.,** malaria. **Panama f.,** Chagres f. **pappataci f.,** phlebotomus f. **paratyphoid f.,** paratyphoid. **parenteric f.,** a disease clinically resembling typhoid fever and paratyphoid, but not caused by *Salmonella.* **parrot f.,** psittacosis. **periodic f.,** a hereditary condition characterized by repetitive febrile episodes and anatomic disturbances, occurring in precise or irregular cycles of days, weeks, or months. **petechial f.,** cerebrospinal meningitis. **pharyngoconjunctival f.,** an epidemic disease due to an adenovirus, occurring chiefly in school children, with fever, pharyngitis, conjunctivitis, rhinitis, and enlarged cervical lymph nodes. **Philippine hemorrhagic f.,** dengue. **phlebotomus f.,** a febrile viral disease of short duration, transmitted by the sandfly *Phlebotomus papatasii,* with dengue-like symptoms, occurring in Mediterranean and Middle East countries. **pinta f.,** a disease observed in northern Mexico, identical with Rocky Mountain spotted fever. **pretibial f.,** an infection due to *Leptospira autumnalis,* marked by a rash on the pretibial region, with lumbar and postorbital pain, malaise, coryza, and fever. **puerperal f.,** septicemia accompanied by fever, in which the focus of infection is a lesion of the mucous membrane of the parturient canal due to trauma during childbirth; usually due to a streptococcus. **Q f.,** a febrile rickettsial infection, usually respiratory, first described in Australia, caused by *Coxiella burnetii.* **quartan f.,** see under *malaria.* **quintan f.,** trench f. **rabbit f.,** tularemia. **rat-bite f.,** an infectious disease following the bite of a rat or other rodent, occurring in two forms: *Haverhill fever* and *sodoku.* **recurrent f., relapsing f.,** any of a group of infectious diseases due to various species of *Borrelia,* marked by alternating periods of fever and apyrexia, each lasting from five to seven days. **remittent f.,** one varying 2° F. or more in 24 hours, but without return to normal temperature. **rheumatic f.,** a febrile disease occurring as a sequela to Group A hemolytic streptococcal infections, characterized by multiple focal inflammatory lesions of the connective tissue structures, especially of the heart, blood vessels, and joints, and by the presence of Aschoff bodies in the myocardium and skin. **Rift Valley f.,** a febrile disease with dengue-like symptoms, due to an arbovirus, transmitted by mosquitoes or by contact with diseased animals; first observed in the Rift Valley, Kenya. **rock f.,** brucellosis. **Rocky Mountain spotted f.,** infection with *Rickettsia rickettsii,* transmitted by ticks, marked by fever, muscle pain, and weakness followed by a macular petechial eruption that begins on the hands and feet and spreads to the trunk and face, by central nervous system symptoms, etc. **sandfly f.,** phlebotomus f. **San Joaquin f.,** the primary stage of coccidioidomycosis. **scarlet f.,** an acute disease caused by Group A hemolytic streptococci, marked by pharyngotonsillitis and a skin rash caused by an erythrogenic toxin produced by the organism; the rash is a diffuse, bright scarlet erythema with many points of deeper red. Desquamation of the skin begins as a fine scaling with eventual peeling of the palms and soles. **septic f.,** fever due to septicemia. **seven-day f.,** 1. a fever with dengue-like symptoms affecting Europeans in India. 2. nanukayami. **shin bone f.,** trench f. **ship f.,** epidemic typhus. **slime f.,** leptospiral jaundice. **slow f.,** brucellosis. **solar f.,** dengue. **Songo f.,** epidemic hemorrhagic f. **South African tick-bite f.,** a tickborne infection in South Africa, due to *Rickettsia conorii,* the etiologic agent of boutonneuse fever. **spirillum f.,** sodoku. **spotted f.,** a febrile disease characterized by a skin eruption, such as Rocky Mountain spotted fever, boutonneuse fever, and other infections due to tickborne rickettsiae, and typhus fever and epidemic cerebrospinal meningitis. **sun f.,** dengue. **swamp f.,** 1. leptospiral jaundice. 2. equine infectious anemia. 3. malaria. **tertian f.,** see under *malaria.* **thermic f.,** sunstroke. **three-day f.,** phlebotomus f. **tick f.,** any infectious disease transmitted by the bite of a tick. **trench f.,** a louseborne rickettsial disease due to *Rickettsia quintana,* with febrile paroxysms, leg pains, chills, sweating, rash, splenomegaly, and a tendency to relapse. **tsutsugamushi f.,** scrub typhus. **typhoid f.,** infection by *Salmonella typhosa* chiefly involving the lymphoid follicles of the ileum, with chills, fever, headache, cough, prostration, abdominal distention, splenomegaly, and a maculopapular rash; perforation of the bowel occurs in about 5% of untreated cases. **typhomalarial f.,** a fever with typhoid symptoms, but believed to be malarial in origin. **typhus f.,** typhus. **undulant f.,** brucellosis. **uveoparotid f.,** a manifestation of sarcoidosis, marked by chronic inflammation of the parotid gland and uvea, with chronic iridocyclitis, unilateral facial paralysis, lassitude, and a subfebrile temperature. **valley f.,** primary coccidioidomycosis. **Volhynia f.,** trench f. **yellow f.,** an acute, infectious, mosquito-borne viral disease, endemic primarily in tropical South America and Africa, marked by fever, jaundice due to necrosis of the liver, and albuminuria.

FFA free fatty acids.

fiber (fi′ber) an elongated threadlike structure.

A f's, myelinated fibers of the somatic nervous system having a diameter of 1μ–22μ and a conduction velocity of 5–120 meters per second. **accelerating f's, accelerator f's,** adrenergic fibers that transmit the impulses which accelerate the heart beat. **adrenergic f's,** nerve fibers that liberate epinephrine-like substances at the time of passage of nerve impulses across a synapse. **alpha f's,** motor and proprioceptive fibers of the A type having conduction velocities of 70–120 meters per second and ranging from 13μ to 22μ in diameter. **alveolar f's,** fibers of the periodontal membrane extending from the cementum of the tooth root to the walls of the alveolus. **apical f's,** fibers of the periodontal membrane extending from the cementum of the apical portion of the tooth root to the deepest portion of the alveolus. **arcuate f.,** any of the bow-shaped fibers in the brain, such as those connecting adjacent gyri in the cerebral cortex, or the external or internal arcuate fibers of the medulla oblongata. **association f's,** nerve fibers that interconnect portions of the cerebral cortex within a hemisphere. Short association fibers interconnect neighboring gyri; long fibers interconnect more widely separated gyri and are arranged into bundles or fasciculi. **B f's,** myelinated preganglionic autonomic axons having a fiber diameter of $\leq 3\mu$ and a conduction velocity of 3–15 meters per second. **basilar f's,** those that form the middle layer of the zona arcuata and the zona pectinata of the organ of Corti. **beta f's,** touch and temperature fibers of the A type having conduction velocities of 30–70 meters per second and ranging from 8μ to 13μ in diameter. **C f's,** unmyelinated postganglionic fibers of the autonomic nervous system, also the unmyelinated fibers at the dorsal roots, having a conduction velocity of 0.6–2.3 meters per second and a diameter of 0.3μ–1.3μ. **cholinergic f's,** nerve fibers that liberate acetylcholine at the synapse. **chromosomal f's,** traction f's. **collagenous f.,** a soft, flexible, white fiber, the most characteristic constituent of all types of connective tissues. **Corti's f's,** see under *rod.* **dark f's,** muscle fibers rich in sarcoplasm and having a dark appearance. **dendritic f's,** those which pass in a treelike form from the cortex to the white substance of the brain. **depressor f's,** 1. nerve fibers which, when stimulated reflexly, cause a diminished vasomotor tone and thereby a decrease in arterial pressure. **elastic f's,** yellowish fibers of elastic quality traversing the intercellular substance of connective tissue. **gamma f's,** A fibers that conduct touch and pressure impulses and innervate the intrafusal fibers of the muscle spindle; they conduct at velocities of 15–40 meters per second and range from 3μ to 7μ in diameter. **Gerdy's f's,** fibers of the superficial ligament bridging the clefts between the fingers on the palm of the hand. **Gottstein's f's,** the external cells and the nerve fibers associated with them, forming part of the expansion of the auditory nerve in the cochlea. **gray f's,** unmyelinated nerve fibers found largely in the sympathetic nerves. **Herxheimer's f's,** spiral fibers in the stratum mucosum of the skin. **internuncial f's,** fibers connecting nerve cells.

intrafusal f's, modified muscle fibers which, surrounded by fluid and enclosed in a connective tissue envelope, compose the muscle spindle. **lattice f's,** reticular f's. **light f's,** muscle fibers poor in sarcoplasm and more transparent than dark fibers. **medullated f's,** myelinated f's. **motor f's,** nerve fibers transmitting impulses to a muscle fiber. **Müller's f's,** elongated neuroglial cells traversing all the layers of the retina, forming its principal supporting element. **muscle f.,** any of the cells comprising the contractile elements of muscular tissue, see Plate XIV. **myelinated f's,** grayish white nerve fibers encased in a myelin sheath. **nerve f.,** a slender process of a neuron, especially the prolonged axon which conducts nerve impulses; see Plate XI. **nonmedullated f's,** unmyelinated f's. **osteogenetic f's, osteogenic f's,** precollagenous fibers formed by osteoclasts and becoming the fibrous component of bone matrix. **oxytalan f.,** a connective tissue fiber resistant to acid hydrolysis, found in structures subjected to mechanical stress, such as tendons, ligaments, etc. **perforating f's,** Sharpey's f's. **postganglionic f's,** fibers constituting a postganglionic neuron. **precollagenous f.,** a reticular fiber, so called on the supposition that it is an immature collagenous fiber. **preganglionic f's,** fibers constituting a preganglionic neuron. **pressor f's,** 1. nerve fibers which, when stimulated reflexly, cause or increase vasomotor tone. 2. cardiac pressor f's. **projection f's,** bundles of axons connecting the cerebral cortex with the subcortical centers, brain stem, and spinal cord. **Purkinje's f's,** modified cardiac muscle fibers in the subendothelial tissue concerned with conducting impulses in the heart. **radicular f's,** fibers in the roots of the spinal nerves. **f's of Remak,** gray f's. **reticular f.,** immature connective tissue fibers staining with silver, forming the reticular framework of lymphoid and myeloid tissue, and occurring in interstitial tissue of glandular organs, papillary layer of the skin, and elsewhere. **Sharpey's f's,** those that pass from the periosteum and embed in the periosteal lamellae. **spindle f's,** achromatic filaments extending between the poles of a dividing cell and making a spindle-shaped configuration. **T f.,** a fiber given off at right angles from the axon of a nerve cell. **Tomes' f's,** branching processes of odontoblasts in the dentinal canals. **traction f's,** those of the spindle in mitosis along which the daughter chromosomes move apart. **unmyelinated f's,** nerve fibers that lack the myelin sheath. **white f's,** collagenous f's.

fibercolonoscope (fi″ber-ko-lōn′o-skōp) a fiberscope for viewing the colon.

fibergastroscope (-gas′tro-skōp) a fiberscope for viewing the stomach.

fiber-illuminated (fi′ ber - il - loo″ min - a′ ted) transmitting light by means of bundles of glass or plastic fibers, utilizing a lens system to transmit the image; said of endoscopes of such design.

fiberoptic (fi″ber-op′tik) pertaining to fiberoptics; coated with glass or plastic fibers having special optical properties.

fiberoptics (-op′tiks) the transmission of an image along flexible bundles of glass or plastic fibers having special optical properties and orientation.

fiberscope (fi′ber-skōp) a flexible endoscope whose lumen is coated with glass or plastic fibers having special optical properties.

fibr(o)- word element [L.], *fiber; fibrous.*

fibra (fi′brah), pl. *fi′brae* [L.] fiber.

fibril (fi′bril) a minute fiber or filament. **fibril′lar, fib′rillary,** adj. **dentinal f's,** component fibrils of the dentinal matrix.

fibrilla (fi-bril′ah), pl. *fibril′lae* [L.] a fibril.

fibrillation (fi″brĭ-la′shun) 1. a small, local, involuntary, muscular contraction, due to spontaneous activation of single muscle cells or muscle fibers. 2. the quality of being made up of fibrils. 3. the initial degenerative changes in osteoarthritis, marked by softening of the articular cartilage and development of vertical clefts between groups of cartilage cells. **atrial f.,** atrial arrhythmia marked by rapid randomized contractions of the atrial myocardium, causing a totally irregular, and often rapid, ventricular rate. **ventricular f.,** cardiac arrhythmia marked by fibrillary contractions of the ventricular muscle due to rapid repetitive excitation of myocardial fibers without coordinated ventricular contraction.

fibrillogenesis (fi-bril″o-jen′ĕ-sis) the formation and development of fibrils.

fibrin (fi′brin) an insoluble protein that is essential to clotting of blood, formed from fibrinogen by action of thrombin.

fibrinase (-ās) coagulation Factor XIII.

fibrinocellular (fi″brĭ-no-sel′u-ler) made up of fibrin and cells.

fibrinogen (fi-brin′o-jen) 1. coagulation Factor I. 2. a sterile compound derived from normal human plasma and dried from the frozen state; used to promote blood clotting.

fibrinogenemia (fi-brin″o-jĕ-ne′me-ah) hyperfibrinogenemia.

fibrinogenesis (fi″brĭ-no-jen′ĕ-sis) the production of fibrin.

fibrinogenic (fi-brin″o-jen′ik) producing or causing the formation of fibrin.

fibrinogenolysis (fi″brin-o-jĕ-nol′ĭ-sis) the proteolytic destruction of fibrinogen in circulating blood. **fibrinogenolyt′ic,** adj.

fibrinogenopenia (fi-brin″o-jen″o-pe′ne-ah) deficiency of fibrinogen in the blood. **fibrinogenope′nic,** adj.

fibrinoid (fi′brĭ-noid) 1. resembling fibrin. 2. a homogeneous, eosinophilic, relatively acellular refractile substance with some of the staining properties of fibrin.

fibrinokinase (fi″brĭ-no-ki′nās) a non–water-soluble plasminogen activator derived from animal tissues.

fibrinolysin (fi″brĭ-nol′ĭ-sin) 1. plasmin. 2. a preparation of proteolytic enzyme formed from profibrinolysin (plasminogen) by action of physical agents or by specific bacterial kinases; used to promote dissolution of thrombi.

fibrinolysis (fi″brĭ-nol′ĭ-sis) the dissolution of fibrin by enzymatic action. **fibrinolyt′ic,** adj.

fibrinopenia (fi″brĭ-no-pe′ne-ah) deficiency of fibrinogen in the blood.

fibrinopeptide (-pep′tīd) either of two peptides (A and B) split off from fibrinogen during coagulation by the action of thrombin.

fibrinoplastin (-plas′tin) paraglobulin.

fibrinopurulent (-pu′roo-lent) characterized by the presence of both fibrin and pus.

fibrinoscopy (fi″brĭ-nos′ko-pe) inoscopy.

fibrinous (fi′brĭ-nus) pertaining to or of the nature of fibrin.

fibrinuria (fi″brĭ-nu′re-ah) the presence of fibrin in the urine.

fibroadenoma (fi″bro-ad″ĕ-no′mah) adenoma containing fibrous elements.

fibroadipose (-ad′ĭ-pōs) both fibrous and fatty.

fibroangioma (-an″je-o′mah) an angioma containing much fibrous tissue.

fibroareolar (-ah-re′o-lar) both fibrous and areolar.

fibroblast (fi′bro-blast) an immature fiber-producing cell of connective tissue capable of differentiating into chondroblast, collagenoblast, or osteoblast. **fibroblas′tic,** adj.

fibroblastoma (fi″bro-blas-to′mah) any tumor arising from fibroblasts, now classified as fibromas or fibrosarcomas.

fibrobronchitis (-brong-ki′tis) croupous bronchitis.

fibrocalcific (-kal-sif′ik) pertaining to or characterized by partially calcified fibrous tissue.

fibrocarcinoma (-kar″sĭ-no′mah) scirrhous carcinoma.

fibrocartilage (-kar′tĭ-lij) cartilage made up of parallel, thick, compact collagenous bundles, separated by narrow clefts containing the typical cartilage cells (chondrocytes). **fibrocartilag′inous,** adj. **elastic f.,** that containing elastic fibers. **interarticular f.,** any articular disk.

fibrocartilago (-kar″tĭ-lah′go), pl. *fibrocartilag′ines* [L.] fibrocartilage.

fibrocellular (-sel′u-ler) both fibrous and cellular.

fibrochondritis (-kon-dri′tis) inflammation of fibrocartilage.

fibrochondroma (-kon-dro′mah) chondroma that contains areas of fibrosis.

fibrocyst (fi′bro-sist) cystic fibroma.

fibrocystic (fi″bro-sis′tik) characterized by an overgrowth of fibrous tissue and development of cystic spaces, especially in a gland.

fibrocystoma (-sis-to′mah) cystic fibroma.

fibrocyte (fi′bro-sīt) fibroblast.

fibrodysplasia (fi″bro-dis-pla′ze-ah) fibrous dysplasia.

fibroelastic (-e-las′tik) both fibrous and elastic.

fibroelastosis (-e″las-to′sis) overgrowth of fibroelastic elements. **endocardial f.,** a condition characterized by left ventricular hypertrophy, conversion of the endocardium into a thick fibroelastic coat, with ventricular capacity sometimes reduced, but often increased.

fibroenchondroma (-en″kon-dro′mah) enchondroma containing fibrous elements.

fibroepithelioma (-ep″ĭ-the″le-o′mah) a tumor composed of both fibrous and epithelial elements.

fibroglia (fi-brog′le-ah) border fibrils in close relation to the surface of fibroblasts.

fibroglioma (fi″bro-gli-o′mah) a glioma containing excessive fibrous tissue.

fibroid (fi′broid) 1. having a fibrous structure; resembling a fibroma. 2. fibroma. 3. leiomyoma; *fibroids* is a colloquial clinical term for leiomyoma of the uterus.

fibroidectomy (fi″broid-ek′to-me) excision of a uterine fibroma.

fibrolipoma (fi″bro-lĭ-po′mah) a lipoma containing excessive fibrous tissue. **fibrolipo′matous,** adj.

fibroma (fi-bro′mah) a tumor composed mainly of fibrous or fully developed connective tissue. **ameloblastic f.,** an odontogenic fibroma, marked by simultaneous proliferation of both epithelial and mesenchymal tissue, without formation of enamel or dentin. **cementifying f.,** cementoblastoma; a tumor usually occurring in the mandible of older persons and consisting of fibroblastic tissue containing masses of cementum-like tissue. **chondromyxoid f. of bone,** a benign neoplasm apparently derived from cartilage-forming connective tissue. **cystic f.,** one that has undergone cystic degeneration. **f. myxomato′des,** myxofibroma. **nonosteogenic f.,** a degenerative and proliferative lesion of the medullary and cortical tissues of bone. **odontogenic f.,** a benign tumor of the jaw arising from the embryonic portion of the tooth germ, the dental papilla, or dental follicle, or later from the periodontal membrane. **ossifying f., ossifying f. of bone,** a benign, relatively slow-growing, central bone tumor, usually of the jaws, especially the mandible, which is composed of fibrous connective tissue within which bone is formed.

fibromatogenic (fi-bro″mah-to-jen′ik) producing or causing fibroma.

fibromatoid (fi-bro′mah-toid) resembling fibroma; fibroma-like.

fibromatosis (fi″bro-mah-to′sis) 1. the presence of multiple fibromas. 2. the formation of a fibrous, tumor-like nodule arising from the deep fascia, with a tendency to local recurrence. **f. gingi′vae,** a diffuse fibroma of the gingivae and palate, manifested as a dense, smooth or nodular overgrowth of the tissues. **palmar f.,** fibromatosis involving the palmar fascia, and resulting in Dupuytren's contracture. **plantar f.,** fibromatosis involving the plantar fascia manifested as single or multiple nodular swellings, sometimes accompanied by pain but usually unassociated with contractures.

fibromatous (fi-bro′mah-tus) pertaining to or of the nature of fibroma.

fibromuscular (fi″bro-mus′ku-ler) both fibrous and muscular.

fibromyitis (-mi-i′tis) inflammation of muscle with fibrous degeneration.

fibromyoma (-mi-o′mah) a myoma containing fibrous elements.

fibromyomectomy (-mi″o-mek′to-me) excision of a fibromyoma (leiomyoma).

fibromyositis (-mi″o-si′tis) inflammation of fibromuscular tissue.

fibromyxoma (-mik-so′mah) myxofibroma.

fibromyxosarcoma (-mik″so-sar-ko′mah) a sarcoma containing fibrous and mucous elements.

fibroneuroma (-nu-ro′mah) neurofibroma.

fibropapilloma (-pap″ĭ-lo′mah) a papilloma containing much fibrous tissue.

fibroplasia (-pla′ze-ah) the formation of fibrous tissue. **fibroplas′tic,** adj. **retrolental f.,** a condition characterized by retinal vascular proliferation and tortuosity and by the presence of fibrous tissue behind the lens, leading to detachment of the retina and arrest of growth of the eye, generally attributed to use of excessively high concentrations of oxygen in the care of premature infants.

fibropurulent (-pu′roo-lent) containing both fibers and pus.

fibrosarcoma (-sar-ko′mah) a sarcoma derived from collagen-producing fibroblasts. **odontogenic f.,** a malignant tumor of the jaws, originating from one of the mesenchymal components of the tooth or tooth germ.

fibroserous (-se′rus) composed of both fibrous and serous elements.

fibrosis (fi-bro′sis) formation of fibrous tissue; fibroid degeneration. **fibrot′ic,** adj. **cystic f., cystic f. of pancreas,** a generalized hereditary disorder of infants, children, and young adults, associated with widespread dysfunction of the exocrine glands, marked by signs of chronic pulmonary disease, obstruction of pancreatic ducts by amorphous eosinophilic concretions with consequent pancreatic enzyme deficiency, by abnormally high electrolyte levels in sweat, and occasionally by biliary cirrhosis. **diffuse interstitial pulmonary f.,** progressive fibrosis of the pulmonary alveolar walls, with steadily progressive dypsnea, resulting in death from oxygen lack or right heart failure. **endomyocardial f.,** idiopathic myocardiopathy occurring endemically in various regions of Africa and rarely in other areas, characterized by cardiomegaly, marked thickening of the endocardium with dense, white fibrous tissue that frequently extends to involve the inner third or half of the myocardium, and congestive heart failure. **mediastinal f.,** development of whitish, hard fibrous tissue in the upper portion of the mediastinum, sometimes obstructing the air passages and large blood vessels. **neoplastic f.,** proliferative f. **panmural f. of bladder,** chronic interstitial cystitis. **periureteric f.,** progressive development of fibrous tissue spreading from the great midline vessels and causing strangulation of one or both ureters. **postfibrinous f.,** that occurring in tissues in which fibrin has been deposited. **proliferative f.,** that in which the fibrous elements continue to proliferate after the original causative factor has ceased to operate. **pulmonary f.,** diffuse interstitial pulmonary f. **f. u′teri,** a morbid condition characterized by overgrowth of the smooth muscle and increase in the collagenous

fibrous tissue, producing a thickened, coarse, tough myometrium.

fibrositis (fi″bro-si′tis) inflammatory hyperplasia of the white fibrous tissue, especially of the muscle sheaths and facial layers of the locomotor system.

fibrothorax (-tho′raks) adhesion of the two pleural layers, the lung being covered by thick nonexpansible fibrous tissue.

fibrous (fi′brus) composed of or containing fibers.

fibula (fib′u-lah), pl. *fib′ulae* [L.] see *Table of Bones.* **fib′ular,** adj.

fibulocalcaneal (fib″u-lo″kal-ka′ne-al) pertaining to fibula and calcaneus.

F.I.C.D. Fellow of the International College of Dentists.

ficin (fi′sin) a highly active, crystallizable proteinase from the sap of fig trees, which catalyzes the hydrolysis of many proteins at acid (4.1) pH, the clotting of milk, and "digestion" of some living worms, e.g., whipworms. It also shows esterase activity. It has been used in dogs as a trichuricide.

F.I.C.S. Fellow of the International College of Surgeons.

field (fēld) 1. an area or open space, as an operative field or visual field. 2. a range of specialization in knowledge, study, or occupation. 3. in embryology, the developing region within a range of modifying factors. **auditory f.,** the space or range within which stimuli may be perceived as sound. **high-power f.,** the area of a slide visible under the high magnification system of a microscope. **individuation f.,** a region in which an organizer influences adjacent tissue to become a part of a total embryo. **low-power f.,** the area of a slide visible under the low magnification system of a microscope. **morphogenetic f.,** an embryonic region out of which definite structures normally develop. **visual f.,** the area within which stimuli will produce the sensation of sight with the eye in a straight-ahead position.

FIGLU formiminoglutamic acid.

figure (fig′ūr) 1. an object of particular form. 2. a number, or numeral. **mitotic f′s,** stages of chromosome aggregation exhibiting a pattern characteristic of mitosis.

fila (fi′lah) [L.] plural of *filum.*

filaceous (fi-la′shus) composed of filaments.

filament (fil′ah-ment) a delicate fiber or thread.

filamentous (fil″ah-men′tus) composed of long, threadlike structures.

filamentum (fil″ah-men′tum), pl. *filamen′ta* [L.] filament.

Filaria (fĭ-la′re-ah) a former generic name for members of the superfamily Filarioidea. **F. bancrof′ti,** *Wuchereria bancrofti.* **F. medinen′sis,** *Dracunculus medinensis.* **F. san′guinis-hom′inis,** *Wuchereria bancrofti.*

filaria (fĭ-la′re-ah), pl. *fila′riae* [L.] a nematode worm of the superfamily Filarioidea. **fila′rial,** adj.

filariasis (fil″ah-ri′ah-sis) infection with filariae.

filaricide (fĭ-lăr′ĭ-sīd) an agent which destroys filariae. **filaricid′al,** adj.

filariform (-form) resembling filariae; threadlike.

Filarioidea (fĭ-la″re-oi′de-ah) a superfamily or order of parasitic nematodes, the adults being threadlike worms that invade the tissues and body cavities where the female deposits microfilariae (prelarvae).

filiform (fil′ĭ-form, fi′lĭ-form) 1. threadlike. 2. an extremely slender bougie.

filipin (fil′ĭ-pin) an antifungal antibiotic, $C_{35}H_{58}O_{11}$.

fillet (fil′et) 1. a loop, as of cord or tape, for making traction. 2. in the nervous system, a long band of nerve fibers.

filling (fil′ing) 1. material inserted in a prepared tooth cavity. 2. restoration of the crown with appropriate material after removal of carious tissue from a tooth. **complex f.,** one for a complex cavity. **composite f.,** one consisting of a composite resin. **compound f.,** one for a cavity that involves two surfaces of a tooth. **permanent f.,** one intended to provide complete function while the tooth remains in the oral cavity. **temporary f.,** one designed to be removed after a short period of insertion.

film (film) 1. a thin layer or coating. 2. a thin sheet of material (e.g., gelatin, cellulose acetate) specially treated for use in photography or radiography; used also to designate the sheet after exposure to the energy to which it is sensitive. **bite-wing f.,** an x-ray film for radiography of oral structures, with a protruding tab to be held between the upper and lower teeth. **gelatin f., absorbable,** sterile, nonantigenic, absorbable, water-insoluble film used as an aid in surgical closure and repair of defects in dura and pleura. **spot f.,** a radiograph of a small anatomic area obtained (*a*) by rapid exposure during fluoroscopy to provide a permanent record of a transiently observed abnormality, or (*b*) by limitation of radiation passing through the area to improve definition and detail of the image produced. **x-ray f.,** film sensitized to roentgen (x-) rays, either before or after exposure.

film badge (film baj) a pack of radiographic film or films, used for the detection and approximate measurement of radiation exposure of personnel.

filopodium (fi″lo-po′de-um), pl. *filopo′dia* [L.] a filamentous pseudopodium composed of ectoplasm.

filopressure (-presh′ūr) compression of a blood vessel by a thread.

filter (fil′ter) a device for eliminating certain elements, as (1) particles of certain size from a solution, or (2) rays of certain wavelength from a stream of radiant energy. **Berkefeld's f.,** one composed of diatomaceous earth, impermeable to ordinary bacteria. **Millipore f.,** trademark for a device used to filter nutrient solutions as they are administered intravenously. **Pasteur-Chamberland f.,** a hollow column of unglazed porcelain through which liquids are forced by pressure or by vacuum exhaustion. **Wood's f.,** see under *light*.

filterable (-ah-b′l) capable of passing through the pores of a filter.

filtrable (fil′trah-b′l) filterable.

filtrate (fil′trāt) a liquid that has passed through a filter.

filtration (fil-tra′shun) passage through a filter or through a material that prevents passage of certain molecules.

filum (fi′lum), pl. *fi′la* [L.] a threadlike structure or part. **f. termina′le,** a slender, threadlike prolongation of the spinal cord from the conus medullaris to the back of the coccyx.

fimbria (fim′bre-ah), pl. *fim′briae* [L.] 1. a fringe, border, or edge; a fringelike structure. 2. one of the minute filamentous appendages of certain bacteria, associated with antigenic properties of the cell surface. **f. hippocam′pi,** the band of white matter along the median edge of the ventricular surface of the hippocampus. **fimbriae of uterine tube,** the numerous divergent fringelike processes on the distal part of the infundibulum of the uterine tube.

fimbriate (fim′bre-āt) fringed.

fimbriocele (fim′bre-o-sēl″) hernia containing the fimbriae of the uterine tube.

finger (fing′ger) one of the five digits of the hand. **baseball f.,** partial permanent flexion of the terminal phalanx of a finger caused by a ball or other object striking the end or back of the finger, resulting in rupture of the attachment of the extensor tendon. **clubbed f.,** one with enlargement of the terminal phalanx without constant osseous changes. **hammer f.,** mallet f. **index f.,** the second digit of the hand; the forefinger. **mallet f.,** permanent flexion of the distal phalanx of a finger. **ring f.,** the fourth digit of the hand. **webbed f's,** syndactyly; fingers more or less united by strands of tissue.

fingerprint (-print) 1. an impression of the cutaneous ridges of the fleshy distal portion of a finger. 2. in biochemistry, the characteristic pattern of a peptide after subjection to an analytical technique.

first aid (ferst ād) emergency care and treatment of an injured or ill person before complete medical and surgical treatment can be secured.

fission (fish′un) 1. the act of splitting. 2. asexual reproduction in which the cell divides into two (*binary f.*) or more (*multiple f.*) daughter parts, each of which becomes an individual organism. 3. nuclear fission; the splitting of the atomic nucleus, with release of energy.

fissiparous (fi-sip′ah-rus) propagated by fission.

fissula (fis′u-lah), pl. *fis′sulae* [L.] a small cleft.

fissura (fis-su′rah), pl. *fissu′rae* [L.] fissure. **f. in a′no,** anal fissure.

fissure (fish′er) 1. any cleft or groove, normal or otherwise, especially a deep fold in the cerebral cortex involving its entire thickness. 2. a fault in the enamel surface of a tooth. **abdominal f.,** a congenital cleft in the abdominal wall. **anal f., f. in a′no,** painful lineal ulcer at the margin of the anus. **anterior median f.,** a longitudinal furrow along the midline of the anterior aspect of the spinal cord and medulla oblongata. **auricular f.,** an external fissure of the skull between the tympanic portion and the mastoid process of the temporal bone, transmitting the auricular branch of the vagus nerve. **basisylvian f.,** the part of the sylvian fissure between the temporal lobe and the orbital surface of the frontal bone. **f. of Bichat,** transverse f. (2). **branchial f.,** see under *cleft.* **calcarine f.,** see under *sulcus.* **central f.,** see under *sulcus.* **collateral f.,** see under *sulcus.* **enamel f.,** fissure (2). **glaserian f.,** a fissure between the tympanic and squamous parts of the temporal bone. **Henle's f's,** spaces filled with connective tissue between the muscular fibers of the heart. **hippocampal f.,** see under *sulcus.* **longitudinal f.,** the deep fissure between the cerebral hemispheres. **palpebral f.,** the longitudinal opening between the eyelids. **parieto-occipital f.,** see under *sulcus.* **portal f.,** porta hepatis. **posterior median f.,** see under *sulcus.* **presylvian f.,** the anterior branch of the fissure of Sylvius. **Rolando's f.,** central sulcus. **f. of round ligament,** one on the visceral surface of the liver lodging the round ligament in the adult. **spheno-occipital f.,** the fissure between the basilar part of the occipital bone and the sphenoid bone. **sylvian f., f. of Sylvius,** one extending laterally between the temporal and frontal lobes, and turning posteriorly between the temporal and parietal lobes. **transverse f.,** 1. porta hepatis. 2. the transverse cerebral fissure between the diencephalon and the cerebral hemispheres. **zygal f.,** a cerebral fissure consisting of two branches connected by a stem.

fistula (fis'tu-lah) an abnormal passage or communication, usually between two internal organs, or leading from an internal organ to the body surface. **anal f.,** one near the anus which may or may not communicate with the rectum. **arteriovenous f.,** one between an artery and a vein. **blind f.,** one open at one end only, opening on the skin (*external blind f.*) or on an internal mucous surface (*internal blind f.*). **branchial f.,** a persisting branchial cleft. **complete f.,** one extending from the skin to an internal body cavity. **craniosinus f.,** one between the cerebral space and one of the sinuses, permitting escape of cerebrospinal fluid into the nose. **Eck's f.,** an artificial communication made between the portal vein and the vena cava. **fecal f.,** a colonic fistula opening on the external body surface, discharging feces. **gastric f.,** an abnormal passage communicating with the stomach; often applied to a surgically created opening from the stomach through the abdominal wall. **horseshoe f.,** a semicircular fistulous tract near the anus, with both openings on the skin. **incomplete f.,** blind f. **pulmonary arteriovenous f., congenital,** a congenital anomalous communication between the pulmonary arterial and venous systems, allowing unoxygenated blood to enter the systemic circulation. **rectovaginal f.,** one between the rectum and vagina. **rectovesical f.,** one between the rectum and bladder. **salivary f.,** an abnormal passage communicating with a salivary duct. **Thiry's f.,** an opening created into the intestine to obtain specimens of intestinal juice. **umbilical f.,** one communicating with the gut or the urachus at the umbilicus. **vesical f.,** one communicating with the urinary bladder. **vesicovaginal f.,** an opening from the bladder to the vagina.

fistulatome (-tōm") an instrument for cutting a fistula.

fistulectomy (fis"tu-lek'to-me) excision of a fistula.

fistulization (fis"tu-li-za'shun) 1. the process of becoming fistulous. 2. the surgical creation of fistula.

fistulotomy (fis"tu-lot'o-me) incision of a fistula.

fistulous (fis'tu-lus) pertaining to or of the nature of a fistula.

fit (fit) a convulsion, paroxysm, or sudden attack. **running f.,** 1. an episode marked by hysteria and uncontrolled running. 2. cursive epilepsy.

fixation (fik-sa'shun) 1. the process of making or the state of being immovable. 2. in psychiatry, the cessation of the development of personality at a stage short of complete maturity. 3. in microscopy, the preservation of tissue so that its structure may be examined in detail with minimal alteration of the normal state. 4. in chemistry, the process whereby a substance is removed from the gaseous or solution phase and localized. 5. in ophthalmology, direction of the gaze so that the visual image of the object falls on the fovea centralis. 6. in film processing, the chemical removal of all undeveloped salts of the film emulsion, as on x-ray films. **complement f., f. of complement,** addition of another serum containing an antibody and the corresponding antigen to a hemolytic serum, making the complement incapable of producing hemolysis. **parent f.,** inordinate attachment of an individual for a parent, persisting into adult life.

fixative (fik'sah-tiv) an agent used in preserving a histologic or pathologic specimen so as to maintain the normal structure of its constituent elements.

flaccid (flak'sid) weak, lax, and soft.

flagellar (flah-jel'ar) of or pertaining to a flagellum.

flagellate (flaj'ĕ-lāt) 1. any microorganism having flagella. 2. any protozoon of the subphylum Mastigophora. 3. having flagella.

flagellation (flaj"el-la'shun) 1. massage by tapping the part with the fingers. 2. whipping or being whipped to achieve erotic pleasure. 3. exflagellation.

flagelliform (flah-jel'ĭ-form) shaped like a flagellum or lash.

flagellosis (flaj"ĕ-lo'sis) infestation with flagellate protozoa.

flagellospore (flah-jel'o-spōr) zoospore.

flagellum (flah-jel'um), pl. *flagel'la* [L.] a mobile, whiplike process, such as the coiled, filamentous appendage, originating in the cell wall or outer layers of cytoplasm of rod-shaped bacteria, certain protozoa, etc., and serving as an organ of locomotion.

flail (flāl) exhibiting abnormal or pathologic mobility, as flail chest or flail joint.

flame (flām) 1. the luminous, irregular appearance usually accompanying combustion, or an appearance resembling it. 2. to render an object sterile by exposure to a flame.

flange (flanj) a projecting border or edge; in dentistry, that part of the denture base which extends from around the embedded teeth to the border of the denture.

flank (flank) the side of the body between ribs and ilium.

flap (flap) 1. a mass of tissue for grafting, usually including skin, only partially removed from one part of the body so that it retains its own blood supply during transfer to another site. 2. an uncontrolled movement. **circular f.,** a flap of somewhat circular outline. **island f.,** a flap consisting of skin and subcutaneous tissue, with a pedicle made up of only the nutrient vessels. **jump f.,** one cut from the abdomen and attached to a flap of the same size on the forearm; the forearm flap is transferred later to some other part of the body to fill a defect there. **liver f.,** asterixis. **pedicle f.,** one consisting of the full thickness of the skin and the subcutaneous tissue, attached by a pedicle. **rope f.,** one made by elevating a long strip of tissue from its bed except at its two ends, the cut edges then being sutured together to form a tube. **skin f.,** a full-thickness mass or flap of tissue containing epidermis, dermis, and subcutaneous tissue. **sliding f.,** a flap carried to its new position by a sliding technique. **tube f., tunnel f.,** rope f.

flare (flār) a diffuse area of redness on the skin around the point of application of an irritant, due to a vasomotor reaction.

flask (flask) 1. a laboratory vessel, usually of glass and with a constricted neck. 2. a metal case in which materials used in making artificial dentures are placed for processing. **Erlenmeyer f.,** a conical glass flask with a broad base and narrow neck. **volumetric f.,** a narrow-necked vessel of glass calibrated to contain or deliver an exact volume at a given temperature.

flatfoot (flat′foot) a condition in which one or more arches of the foot have flattened out.

flatness (-nes) a peculiar sound lacking resonance, heard on percussing an abnormally solid part.

flatulence (flat′u-lens) excessive formation of gases in the stomach or intestine.

flatulent (flat′u-lent) characterized by flatulence; distended with gas.

flatus (fla′tus) 1. gas or air in the gastrointestinal tract. 2. gas or air expelled through the anus.

flatworm (flat′werm) an individual organism of the phylum Platyhelminthes.

flav(o)- word element [L.], *yellow.*

flavanone (fla′vah-nōn) flavonoid compounds formed by reduction of the 2:3 double bond of a flavone.

flavin (fla′vin) any of a group of water-soluble yellow pigments widely distributed in animals and plants, including riboflavin and yellow enzymes.

flavivirus (fla″ve-vi′rus) a subcategory of togaviruses; the type species is the yellow fever virus.

Flavobacterium (fla″vo-bak-te′re-um) a genus of schizomycetes (family Achromobacteraceae), characteristically producing yellow, orange, red, or yellow-brown pigmentation, found in soil and water; some species are said to be pathogenic.

flavone (fla′vōn) a crystalline substance, the 4-keto series of flavonoids, able to reverse increased capillary fragility; numerous yellow dyes having similar properties are derived from it.

flavonoid (fla′vo-noid) a generic term for a group of compounds widely distributed in higher plants; one subgroup (anthocyanins) accounts for most of the yellow, red, and blue pigmentation, while another (bioflavonoids) are concerned in maintenance of a normal state of capillary walls.

flavonol (-nol) a yellow crystalline flavonoid, formed by introduction of an OH group at C-3 of a flavone.

flavoprotein (fla″vo-pro′te-in) a conjugated protein containing flavin.

flavoxate (fla-voks′āt) a smooth muscle relaxant, $C_{24}H_{25}NO_4$; the hydrochloride salt is used in treatment of spasms of the urinary tract.

flaxseed (flak′sēd) linseed.

fl.dr. fluid dram.

flea (fle) a small, wingless, bloodsucking insect; many fleas are parasitic and may act as disease carriers.

fleece (flēs) a mass of interlacing fibrils. **f. of Stilling,** the lacework of white fibers surrounding the dentate nucleus.

flesh (flesh) the soft, muscular tissue of the animal body. **goose f.,** cutis anserina. **proud f.,** exuberant amounts of soft, edematous, granulation tissue developing during healing of large surface wounds.

flex (fleks) to bend or put in a state of flexion.

flexibilitas (flek″sĭ-bil′ĭ-tas) [L.] flexibility. **f. ce′rea,** waxy flexibility.

flexibility (flek″sĭ-bil′ĭ-te) the state of being unusually pliant. **waxy f.,** a cataleptic state in which the limbs retain any position in which they are placed.

flexion (flek′shun) the act of bending or the condition of being bent.

flexor (flek′ser) any muscle that flexes a joint; see *Table of Muscles.*

flexura (flek-shu′rah), pl. *flexu′rae* [L.] flexure.

flexure (flek′sher) a bend or fold; a curvation. **caudal f.,** the bend at the aboral end of the embryo. **cephalic f.,** the curve in the midbrain of the embryo. **cervical f.,** a bend in the neural tube of the embryo at the junction of the brain and spinal cord. **colic f., left,** the angular junction of the transverse and descending colon. **colic f., right,** the angular junction of the ascending and transverse colon. **cranial f.,** cephalic f. **dorsal f.,** one of the flexures in the mid-dorsal region of the embryo. **duodenojejunal f.,** the bend at the junction of duodenum and jejunum. **hepatic f.,** right colic f. **lumbar f.,** the ventral curvature in the lumbar region of the back. **mesencephalic f.,** a bend in the neural tube of the embryo at the level of the mesencephalon. **nuchal f.,** cervical f. **pontine f.,** a flexure of the hindbrain in the embryo. **sacral f.,** caudal f. **sigmoid f.,** see under *colon.* **splenic f.,** left colic f.

floccillation (flok″sĭ-la′shun) carphology.

floccose (flok′ōs) woolly; said of bacterial growth composed of short, curved chains variously oriented.

flocculation (flok″u-la′shun) a colloid phenomena in which the disperse phase separates in discrete, usually visible, particles rather than in a continuous mass, as in coagulation.

flocculent (flok′u-lent) containing downy or flaky shreds.

flocculus (flok′u-lus), pl. *floc′culi* [L.] 1. a small tuft or mass, as of wool or other fibrous material. 2. a small mass on the lower side of each cerebral hemisphere, continuous with the nodule of the vermis. **floc′cular,** adj.

flora (flo′rah) the collective plant organisms of a given locality. **intestinal f.,** the bacteria normally residing within the lumen of the intestine.

Floraquin (flor′ah-kwin) trademark for a preparation of diiodohydroxyquin.

Florinef (flor′ĭ-nef) trademark for preparations of fludrocortisone.

Floropryl (flor′o-pril) trademark for preparations of isoflurophate.

flowmeter (flo′me-ter) an apparatus for measuring the rate of flow of liquids or gases.

floxuridine (floks-ūr′ĭ-dēn) a derivative of fluouracil, $C_9H_{11}FN_2O_5$, used as an antiviral and antineoplastic agent. Abbreviated FUDR.

fl.oz. fluid ounce.

flu (floo) popular name for *influenza.*

fluctuation (fluk″tu-a′shun) a variation, as about a fixed value or mass; a wavelike motion.

fludrocortisone (floo″dro-kor′tĭ-sōn) a synthetic adrenal corticoid with effects similar to those of hydrocortisone and desoxycorticosterone.

fluid (floo′id) 1. a liquid or gas; any liquid of the body. 2. composed of molecules which freely change their relative positions without separation of the mass. **allantoic f.,** the fluid contained in the allantois. **amniotic f.,** the liquid within the amnion that bathes the developing fetus and protects it from mechanical injury. **cerebrospinal f.,** the fluid contained within the ventricles of the brain, the subarachnoid space, and the central canal of the spinal cord. **extracellular f.,** a general term for all the body fluids outside the cells, including the interstitial fluid, plasma, lymph, cerebrospinal fluid, etc. **interstitial f.,** the extracellular fluid bathing most tissues, excluding the fluid within the lymph and blood vessels. **intracellular f.,** the portion of the total body water with its dissolved solutes which are within the cell membranes. **labyrinthine f.,** perilymph. **Müller's f.,** a fluid for preserving anatomic specimens. **Scarpa's f.,** endolymph. **seminal f.,** semen. **serous f.,** normal lymph of a serous cavity. **synovial f.,** synovia.

fluidextract (floo″id-ek′strakt) a liquid preparation of a vegetable drug, containing alcohol as a solvent or preservative, or both, of such strength that each milliliter contains the extraction of 1 gm. of the standard drug it represents.

fluidrachm (floo′ĭ-dram) fluid dram.

fluke (flook) any trematode.

flumen (floo′men), pl. *flu′mina* [L.] a stream. **flu′mina pilo′rum,** the lines along which the hairs of the body are arranged.

flumethasone (floo-meth′ah-sōn) an anti-inflammatory glucocorticoid, $C_{22}H_{28}F_2O_5$, used topically in the treatment of certain dermatoses.

flumethiazide (floo″mĕ-thi′ah-zīd) a diuretic and antihypertensive, $C_8H_6F_3N_3O_4S$.

fluocinolone acetonide (floo″o-sin′o-lōn) an anti-inflammatory glucocorticoid, $C_{24}H_{30}F_2O_6$, used topically in eczematous dermatoses.

fluocortolone (-kor′to-lōn) an anti-inflammatory glucocorticoid, $C_{22}H_{29}FO_4$.

fluorescein (-res′e-in) a fluorescing dye, $C_{20}H_{10}$-O_5; its sodium salt is used in solution to reveal corneal lesions and as a test of circulation in the retina and extremities.

fluorescence (-res′ens) the property of emitting light while exposed to light, the wavelength of the emitted light being longer than that of the absorbed light. **fluores′cent,** adj.

fluoridation (floo″or-ĭ-da′shun) treatment with fluorides; the addition of fluorides to a public water supply as a public health measure to reduce the incidence of dental caries.

fluoride (floo′o-rīd) any binary compound of fluorine.

fluoridization (floo″or-ĭ-di-za′shun) 1. application of fluoride solution to the teeth. 2. fluoridation.

fluorine (floo′or-ēn) chemical element (*see table*), at. no. 9, symbol F.

fluorochrome (floo′or-o-krōm) a fluorescent compound, as a dye, used to mark protein with a fluorescent label.

fluorography (floo″or-og′rah-fe) photofluorography.

Fluoromar (floor′o-mar) trademark for a preparation of fluroxene.

fluorometholone (floor″o-meth′o-lōn) an anti-inflammatory glucocorticoid, $C_{22}H_{29}FO_4$, used topically in dermatoses having an allergic or inflammatory basis and associated with pruritus.

fluoroscope (floo′or-o-skōp) an instrument for visual observation of the form and motion of the deep structures of the body by means of x-ray shadows projected on a fluorescent screen.

fluoroscopy (floo″or-os′ko-pe) examination by means of the fluoroscope.

fluorosis (floo″o-ro′sis) a condition due to ingestion of excessive amounts of fluorine. **dental f.,** a mottled discoloration of the enamel of the teeth occurring in chronic endemic fluorosis. **endemic f., chronic,** that due to unusually high concentrations of fluorine in the natural drinking water supply, typically causing dental fluorosis but also combined osteosclerosis and osteomalacia.

fluorouracil (floo″or-o-ūr′ah-sil) an antimetabolite, $C_4H_3FN_2O_2$, used as an antineoplastic agent.

Fluothane (floo′o-thān) trademark for a preparation of halothane.

fluoxymesterone (floo-ok″se-mes′ter-ōn) an anabolic androgenic steroid, $C_{20}H_{29}FO_3$, used in the palliative treatment of certain cancers.

fluphenazine (floo-fen′ah-zēn) a major tranquilizer, $C_{22}H_{26}F_3N_3OS$, used as the enanthate and hydrochloride salts.

fluprednisolone (floo″pred-nis′o-lōn) an antiinflammatory glucocorticoid, $C_{21}H_{27}FO_5$, used in treating joint diseases and allergic disorders.

flurandrenolide (floor″an-dren′o-līd) a glucocorticoid, $C_{27}H_{33}FO$, used topically in certain dermatoses.

flurazepam (floor-az′ĕ-pam) a hypnotic, $C_{21}H_{23}$-$ClFN_3O$, used as the hydrochloride salt.

flurogestone (floor″o-jes′tōn) a progestin, C_{23}-$H_{31}FO_5$, used as the acetate ester.

flurothyl (floor′o-thil) a volatile liquid, C_4H_4-F_6O, used as a convulsant administered by inhalation for therapy of psychiatric disorders for which electroconvulsive therapy is usually employed.

fluroxene (floor-oks′ēn) a volatile liquid, C_4H_5-F_3O, administered by inhalation to produce general anesthesia.

flush (flush) redness, usually transient, of the face and neck. **hectic f.,** a persistent or chronic flush associated with chronic debilitating disease, usually febrile. **malar f.,** hectic flush at the malar eminence.

flutter (flut′er) a rapid vibration or pulsation. **atrial f.,** cardiac arrhythmia in which the atrial contractions are rapid (200–320 per minute), but regular. **diaphragmatic f.,** peculiar wavelike fibrillations of the diaphragm of unknown cause. **impure f.,** atrial flutter in which the atrial rhythm is irregular. **mediastinal f.,** abnormal motility of the mediastinum during respiration. **pure f.,** atrial flutter in which the atrial rhythm is regular. **ventricular f.,** a possible transition stage between ventricular tachycardia and ventricular fibrillation, the electrocardiogram showing rapid, uniform and virtually regular oscillations, 250 or more per minute.

flutter-fibrillation (-fi-brĭ-la′shun) impure flutters that vary from moment to moment in their resemblance to flutter or fibrillation, respectively.

flux (fluks) 1. an excessive flow or discharge. 2. matter discharged.

fly (fli) a dipterous, or two-winged, insect which is often the vector of organisms causing disease. **deer f.,** *Chrysops discalis*. **tsetse f.,** see *Glossina*.

Fm chemical symbol, *fermium*.

FMN flavin mononucleotide.

focus (fo′kus), pl. *fo′ci* [L.] 1. the point of convergence of light rays or sound waves. 2. the chief center of a morbid process. **fo′cal,** adj.

foe- for words beginning thus, see those beginning *fe-*.

fog (fog) a colloid system in which the dispersion medium is a gas and the disperse particles are liquid.

fogging (fog′ing) in ophthalmology, a method of determining refractive error in astigmatism, the patient being first made artificially myopic in order to relax accommodation.

foil (foil) metal in the form of an extremely thin, pliable sheet.

folate (fo′lāt) any of a group of substances whose molecules are made up of a form of pteroic acid conjugated with L-glutamic acid. Folates act as coenzymes that promote one-carbon transfer, and are present in natural foods, including mammalian cells.

fold (fold) plica; a thin, recurved margin, or doubling. **amniotic f.,** the folded edge of the amnion where it rises over and finally encloses the embryo. **aryepiglottic f.,** a fold of mucous membrane extending on each side between the lateral border of the epiglottis and the summit of the arytenoid cartilage. **circular f's,** the permanent transverse folds of the luminal surface of the small intestine. **costocolic f.,** phrenicocolic ligament. **Douglas' f.,** a crescentic line marking the termination of the posterior layer of the sheath of the rectus abdominis muscle, just below the level of the iliac crest. **gastric f's,** the series of folds in the mucous membrane of the stomach. **gluteal f.,** the crease separating the buttocks from the thigh. **head f.,** a fold of blastoderm at the cephalic end of the developing embryo. **Kohlrausch's f's,** transverse f's. **lacrimal f.,** a fold of mucous membrane at the lower opening of the nasolacrimal duct. **Marshall's f.,** vestigial f. **medullary f.,** neural f. **mesonephric f.,** see under *ridge*. **mucosal f., mucous f.,** a fold of mucous membrane. **nail f.,** the fold of palmar skin around the base and sides of the nail. **neural f.,** one of the paired folds lying on either side of the neural plate that form the neural tube. **palmate f's,** folds on the anterior and posterior walls of the cervical canal. **semilunar f. of conjunctiva,** a mucous fold at the medial angle of the eye. **spiral f.,** a spirally arranged elevation in the mucosa of the first part of the cystic duct. **tail f.,** a fold of blastoderm at the caudal end of the developing embryo. **transverse f's,** three permanent transverse folds in the rectum. **urogenital f.,** see under *ridge*. **ventricular f., vestibular f.,** a false vocal cord. **vestigial f.,** a pericardial fold enclosing the remnant of the embryonic left anterior cardinal vein. **vocal f.,** the true vocal cord.

folie (fo-le′) [Fr.] psychosis; insanity. **f. à deux** (ah duh′) occurrence of identical psychosis simultaneously in two closely associated persons. **f. circulaire** (ser-ku-lair′) circular psychosis. **f. du doute** (du doot) pathologic inability to make even the most trifling decisions. **f. du pourquoi** (du poor-kwah′) psychopathologic constant questioning. **f. gémellaire** (zha-mĕ-lair′) psychosis occurring simultaneously in twins. **f. musculaire** (mus″ku-lār′) severe chorea. **f. raisonnante** (rez-un-nahnt′) the delusional form of any psychosis.

folium (fo′le-um), pl. *fo′lia* [L.] a leaflike structure, especially one of the leaflike subdivisions of the cerebellar cortex.

follicle (fol′lĭ-k'l) a sac or pouchlike depression or cavity. **follic′ular,** adj. **atretic f.,** an involuted vesicular ovarian follicle. **dental f.,** the structure within the substance of the jaws enclosing a tooth before its eruption; the dental sac and its contents. **Fleischmann's f.,** an occasional follicle in the mucosa of the floor of the mouth. **gastric f's,** lymphoid masses in the gastric mucosa. **graafian f's,** vesicular ovarian f's. **hair f.,** one of the tubular invaginations of the epidermis enclosing the hairs, and from which the hairs grow. **intestinal f's,** see under *gland*. **Lieberkühn's f's,** the intestinal glands. **lingual f's,** nodular masses of lymphoid tissue at the root of the tongue, constituting the lingual tonsil. **lymph f., lymphatic f.,** 1. a small collection of actively proliferating lymphocytes in the cortex of a lymph node. 2. a small collection of lymphoid tissue in the mucous membrane of the gastrointestinal tract, where they occur singly (*solitary lymphatic f.*) or closely packed together (*aggregated lymphatic f's*). **Montgomery's f's,** nabothian f's. **Naboth's f's, nabothian f's,** cystlike formations due to occlusion of the lumina of glands in the mucosa of the uterine cervix, causing them to be distended with retained secretion. **ovarian f.,** the ovum and its encasing cells, at any stage in its development. **ovarian f's, primary,** immature ovarian follicles, each comprising an immature ovum and the few specialized epithelial cells surrounding it. **ovarian f's, primordial,** an ovarian follicle consisting of an egg enclosed by a single layer of cells. **ovarian f's, vesicular,** graafian follicles; maturing ovarian follicles among whose cells fluid has begun to accumulate, leading to the formation of a single cavity and leaving the ovum located in the cumulus oophorous. **sebaceous f.,** a hair follicle with a relatively large sebaceous gland, producing a relatively insignificant hair. **solitary f's,** 1. areas of concentrated lymphatic tissue in the mucosa of the colon. 2. small lymph follicles scattered throughout the mucosa and submucosa of the small intestine. **thyroid f's,** discrete cystlike units filled with a colloid substance, constituting the lobules of the thyroid gland.

folliculi (fo-lik′u-li) plural of *folliculus*.

folliculitis (fŏ-lik″u-li′tis) inflammation of a follicle. **f. bar′bae,** sycosis vulgaris. **f. decal′vans,** suppurative folliculitis leading to scarring, with permanent hair loss on the involved area. **keloid f., f. keloida′lis,** infection of the hair follicles on the back of the neck, with formation of persistent hard follicular papules, leading to development of typical keloidal plaques. **f. ulerythemato′sa reticula′ta,** a condition in which numerous, closely crowded, small atrophic areas separated by narrow ridges appear on the face, the affected area being erythematous and the skin stretched and hard. **f. variolifor′mis,** see under *acne*.

folliculoma (fŏ-lik″u-lo′mah) granulosa-theca cell tumor.

folliculosis (fŏ-lik″u-lo′sis) excessive development of lymph follicles.

folliculus (fŏ-lik′u-lus), pl. *follic′uli* [L.] follicle.

Follutein (fol-lu′te-in) trademark for a preparation of chorionic gonadotropin.

Folvite (fōl′vīt) trademark for preparations of folic acid.

fomentation (fo″men-ta′shun) treatment by warm moist applications; also, the substance thus applied.

fomes (fo′mēz), pl. *fo′mites* [L.] an inanimate object or material on which disease-producing agents may be conveyed.

fomite (fo′mīt) fomes.

fontanel, fontanelle (fon″tah-nel′) a soft spot; one of the membrane-covered spaces remaining at the junction of the sutures in the incompletely ossified skull of the fetus or infant.

fonticulus (fon-tik′u-lus), pl. *fontic′uli* [L.] a fontanel.

food (food) anything which, when taken into the body, serves to nourish or build up tissues or supply body heat.

foot (foot) the distal portion of the primate leg, upon which the individual stands and walks. **athlete's f.,** tinea pedis. **club f.,** see *talipes*. **dangle f., drop f.,** a condition in which the foot hangs in a plantar-flexed position, due to lesion of the peroneal nerve. **flat f.,** flatfoot. **fungus f.,** maduromycosis. **immersion f.,** a condition resembling trench foot occurring in persons who have spent long periods in water. **Madura f.,** maduromycosis. **march f.,** painful swelling of the foot, usually with fracture of a metatarsal bone, after excessive foot strain. **sucker f.,** an expansion of a process of an astrocyte, by which the latter is attached to a small blood vessel. **trench f.,** a condition of the feet resembling frostbite, due to the prolonged action of water on the skin combined with circulatory disturbance due to cold and inaction.

footdrop (foot′drop) dropping of the foot from paralysis of the anterior muscles of the leg.

foot-pound (-pownd) the amount of energy necessary to raise 1 pound of mass a distance of 1 foot.

foramen (fo-ra′men), pl. *foram′ina* [L.] a natural opening or passage, especially one into or through a bone. **aortic f.,** hiatus aorticus. **apical f.,** an opening at or near the apex of the root of a tooth. **auditory f., external,** external acoustic meatus. **auditory f., internal,** a passage for the auditory and facial nerves in petrous bone. **Botallo's f.,** f. ovale (1). **cecal f., f. ce′cum,** 1. a blind opening between the frontal crest and the crista galli. 2. a depression on the dorsum of the tongue at the median sulcus. **condyloid f., anterior,** hypoglossal canal. **condyloid f., posterior,** condylar canal. **cotyloid f.,** a passage between the margin of the acetabulum and the transverse ligament. **epiploic f.,** an opening connecting the two sacs of the peritoneum, below and behind the porta hepatis. **esophageal f.,** see under *hiatus*. **ethmoidal foramina, foram′ina ethmoida′lia,** small openings in the ethmoid bone at the junction of the medial wall with the roof of the orbit, the *anterior* transmitting the nasal branch of the ophthalmic nerve and the anterior ethmoid vessels, the *posterior* transmitting the posterior ethmoid vessels. **great f.,** f. magnum. **incisive f.,** one of the openings of the incisive canals into the incisive fossa of the hard palate. **infraorbital f.,** a passage for the infraorbital nerve and artery. **interventricular f.,** a communication between the lateral and third ventricle. **inter-vertebral f.,** a passage for a spinal nerve and vessels formed by notches on pedicles of adjacent vertebrae. **jugular f.,** an opening formed by the jugular notches on the temporal and occipital bones. **f. of Key and Retzius,** an opening at the end of each lateral recess of the fourth ventricle by which the ventricular cavity communicates with the subarachnoid space. **f. la′cerum, f. la′cerum me′dium,** a gap formed at the junction of the great wing of the sphenoid bone, tip of the petrous part of the temporal bone, and basilar part of the occipital bone. **f. la′cerum poste′rius,** jugular f. **f. of Magendie,** a deficiency in the lower part of the roof of the fourth ventricle through which the ventricular cavity communicates with the subarachnoid space. **f. mag′num,** a large opening in the anterior inferior part of the occipital bone, between the cranial cavity and vertebral canal. **mastoid f.,** an opening in the temporal bone behind the mastoid process. **medullary f.,** vertebral f. (1). **mental f.,** an opening on the lateral part of the mandible, for passage of the mental nerve and vessels. **f. of Monro,** interventricular f. **nutrient f.,** any of the passages admitting nutrient vessels to the medullary cavity of bone. **obturator f.,** the large opening between the os pubis and ischium. **olfactory f.,** any of the many openings of the cribriform plate of the ethmoid bone. **optic f.,** see under *canal.* **f. ova′le,** 1. a fetal opening between the heart's atria. 2. an aperture in the great wing of the sphenoid for vessels and nerves. **palatine f., anterior** incisive f. **palatine f., greater,** the lower opening of the greater palatine canal, found laterally on the horizontal plate of each palatine bone, transmitting a palatine nerve and artery. **parietal f.,** a passage in the parietal bone for vessels. **pterygopalatine f.,** greater palatine f. **quadrate f.,** vena cava f. **f. rotun′-dum,** a round opening in the great wing of sphenoid for the maxillary branch of the trigeminal nerve. **sacral f., anterior,** eight openings (four on each side) for anterior branches of sacral nerves. **sacral f., posterior,** eight openings (four on each side) for posterior branches of sacral nerves. **Scarpa's f.,** an opening behind the upper medial incisor, for the nasopalatine nerve. **sciatic f.,** either of two foramina, the greater and the smaller sciatic foramina, formed by the sacrotuberal and sacrospinal ligaments in the sciatic notch of the hip bone. **sphenopalatine f.,** 1. a space between the orbital and sphenoidal processes of the palatine bone, opening into the nasal cavity, and transmitting the sphenopalatine artery and nasal nerves. 2. greater palatine f. **spinous f.,** a hole in the great wing of the sphenoid for the middle meningeal artery. **f. of Stensen,** incisive canal. **stylomastoid f.,** an opening between the styloid and mastoid processes, for the facial nerve and the stylomastoid artery. **supraorbital f.,** a passage in the frontal bone for the supraorbital artery and nerve; often present as a notch bridged only by fibrous tissue. **thebesian foramina,** minute openings in the walls of the right atrium through which the smallest cardiac veins empty into the heart. **thyroid f.,** 1.

an inconstant opening in the thyroid cartilage, due to incomplete union of the fourth and fifth branchial cartilages. 2. obturator f. **transverse f.,** the passage in either transverse process of a cervical vertebra that, in the upper six vertebrae, transmits the vertebral vessels. **vena cava f.,** an opening in the diaphragm for the inferior vena cava and some branches of the right vagus nerve. **vertebral f.,** 1. the large opening in a vertebra formed by its body and arch. 2. transverse f. **vertebroarterial f.,** transverse f. **f. of Vesalius,** an occasional opening medial to the foramen ovale of the sphenoid, for passage of a vein from the cavernous sinus. **Weitbrecht's f.,** a foramen in the capsule of the shoulder joint. **f. of Winslow,** epiploic f. **zygomaticotemporal f.,** an opening on the temporal surface of the zygomatic bone.

foramina (fo-ram′ĭ-nah) plural of *foramen.*

force (fōrs) energy or power; that which originates or arrests motion or other activity. **catabolic f.,** energy derived from the metabolism of food. **electromotive f.,** that which gives rise to an electric current. **occlusal f.,** the force exerted on opposing teeth when the jaws are brought into approximation. **reserve f.,** energy above that required for normal functioning; in the heart, the power that will take care of the additional circulatory burden imposed by exertion. **Van der Waals f's,** the relatively weak, short-range forces of attraction existing between atoms and molecules, which results in the attraction of nonpolar organic compounds to each other (hydrophobic bonding).

forceps (fōr′seps), pl. *for′cipes* [L.] 1. a two-bladed instrument with a handle for compressing or grasping tissues in surgical operations, and for handling sterile dressings, etc. 2. any forcipate organ or part. **alligator f.,** strong toothed forceps having a double clamp. **f. ante′rior,** f. minor. **artery f.,** one for grasping and compressing an artery. **aural f.,** one for operations on the ear. **axis-traction f.,** specially jointed obstetrical forceps so made that traction can be applied in the line of the pelvic axis. **bayonet f.,** a forceps whose blades are offset from the axis of the handle. **capsule f.,** one for removing the lens capsule in cataract. **Chamberlen f.,** the original form of obstetrical forceps. **clamp f.,** a forceps-like clamp with an automatic lock, for compressing arteries, etc. **dental f.,** one for the extraction of teeth. **dressing f.,** one with scissor-like handles for grasping lint, drainage tubes, etc., in dressing wounds. **epilating f.,** one for pulling out hairs. **extraction f.,** dental f. **fixation f.,** one for holding a part steady during operation. **Hodge's f.,** a form of obstetrical forceps. **Kocher's f.,** a strong forceps for holding tissues during operation or for compressing bleeding tissue. **Laborde's f.,** a flat forceps for making traction on the tongue to stimulate the respiratory center in asphyxiation. **Levret's f.,** an obstetrical forceps curved to correspond with the curve of the parturient canal. **Liston's f.,** a bone-cutting forceps. **lithotomy f.,** one for removing stones from the bladder. **Löwenberg's f.,** one for removing adenoid growth. **f. ma′jor,** the terminal fibers of the corpus callosum that pass from the splenium into the occipital lobes. **f. mi′nor,** the terminal fibers of the corpus callosum that pass from the genu to the frontal lobes. **mouse-tooth f.,** one with one or more fine teeth at the tip of each blade. **obstetrical f.,** one for extracting the fetal head from the maternal passages. **Péan's f.,** a clamp for hemostasis. **f. poste′rior,** forceps major. **rongeur f.,** one for use in cutting bone. **sequestrum f.,** one with small but strong serrated jaws for removing pieces of bone forming a sequestrum. **Simpson's f.,** a form of obstetrical forceps. **speculum f.,** a long, slender forceps for use through a speculum. **Tarnier's f.,** a form of obstetrical forceps. **tenaculum f.,** one having a sharp hook at the end of each jaw. **torsion f.,** one for making torsion on an artery to arrest hemorrhage. **tracheal f.,** a long, slender forceps for removing foreign bodies from the trachea. **volsella f., vulsellum f.,** one with teeth for grasping and applying traction. **Willett f.,** a vulsellum for applying scalp traction to control hemorrhage in placenta previa.

forcipate (fōr′sĭ-pāt) shaped like a forceps.

forcipressure (fōr′sĭ-presh″ūr) pressure with forceps, chiefly for arresting hemorrhage.

forearm (fōr′arm) antebrachium; the part of the arm between elbow and wrist.

forebrain (-brān) prosencephalon: 1. the part of the brain developed from the anterior of the three primary brain vesicles, comprising the diencephalon and telencephalon. 2. the most anterior of the primary brain vesicles.

foreconscious (-kon-shus) preconscious.

forefinger (-fing-ger) index finger.

forefoot (-fut) 1. one of the front feet of a quadruped. 2. the fore part of the foot.

foregut (-gut) the endodermal canal of the embryo cephalic to the junction of the yolk stalk, giving rise to the pharynx, lung, esophagus, stomach, liver, and most of the small intestine.

forehead (-ed) frons; the part of the face above the eyes. **bony f.,** the skeleton of the forehead, formed by the anterior part of the skull (frontal bone).

foreskin (-skin) the prepuce.

forewaters (-wat-erz) the part of the amniotic sac that pouches into the uterine cervix in front of the presenting part of the fetus.

fork (fork) a pronged instrument. **tuning f.,** a device that produces harmonic vibration when its two prongs are struck; used to test hearing and bone conduction.

formaldehyde (fōr-mal′dĕ-hīd) a powerful disinfectant gas, HCHO, usually used in solution.

formalin (fōr′mah-lin) a 37% aqueous solution of gaseous formaldehyde used as a fixative.

formamidase (form-am′ĭ-dās) an enzyme that catalyzes the hydrolysis of formylkynurenine to kynurenine and formate in tryptophan metabolism.

formate (fōr′māt) a salt of formic acid.

formatio (fōr-ma′she-o), pl. *formatio′nes* [L.] formation.

formation (fōr-ma′shun) 1. the process of giving shape or form; the creation of an entity, or of a structure of definite shape. 2. a structure of def-

inite shape. **reaction f.,** the development of mental mechanisms which hold in check and repress the components of forbidden wishes. **reticular f.,** areas of diffuse neurons collectively resembling a network in the spinal cord, brain stem, and thalamus; it controls many of the unconscious motor activities of the body.

forme (fōrm), pl. *formes* [Fr.] form. **f. fruste** (fōrm froost) (pl. *formes frustes*) an atypical, especially a mild or incomplete, form, as of a disease. **f. tardive** (fōrm tahr-dēv′) a late-occurring form of a disease that usually appears at an earlier age.

formication (fōr″mĭ-ka′shun) a sensation as if small insects were crawling on the skin.

formiciasis (-si′ah-sis) morbid condition caused by ant bites.

formilase (fōr′mĭ-lās) an enzyme which changes acetic acid into unstable formic acid.

formol (fōr′mol) formaldehyde solution.

formula (fōr′mu-lah), pl. *for′mulae, for′mulas* [L.] an expression, using numbers or symbols, of the composition of, or of directions for preparing, a compound, such as a medicine, or of a procedure to follow to obtain a desired result, or of a single concept. **chemical f.,** a combination of symbols used to express the chemical composition of a substance. **configurational f.,** spatial f. **constitutional f.,** empirical f. **dental f.,** an expression in symbols of the number and arrangement of teeth in the jaws. Letters represent the various types of teeth: I, *incisor;* C, *canine;* P, *premolar,* M, *molar.* Each letter is followed by a horizontal line. Numbers above the line represent maxillary teeth; those below, mandibular teeth. The human dental formula is $I_2^2C_1^1M_2^2 = 10$ (one side only) for deciduous teeth, and $I_2^2C_1^1P_2^2M_3^3 = 16$ (one side only) for permanent teeth. **empirical f.,** a chemical formula which expresses the proportions of the elements present in a substance. **molecular f.,** a chemical formula expressing the number of atoms of each element present in a molecule of a substance, without indicating how they are linked. **official f.,** one officially established by a pharmacopeia or other recognized authority. **rational f.,** structural f. **spatial f., stereochemical f.,** a chemical formula giving the numbers of atoms of each element present in a molecule of a substance, which atom is linked to which, the types of linkages involved and the relative positions of the atoms in space. **structural f.,** a chemical formula showing the spatial arrangement of the atoms and the linkage of every atom. **vertebral f.,** an expression of the number of vertebrae in each region of the spinal column; the human vertebral formula is $C_7T_{12}L_5S_5Cd_4 = 33$.

formulary (fōr′mu-ler″e) a collection of formulae. **National F.,** see under *N.*

formyl (fōr′mil) the radical, HCO or H·C:O—, of formic acid.

formylase (form′ĭ-lās) formamidase.

fornix (fōr′niks), pl. *for′nices* [L.] 1. an archlike structure or the vaultlike space created by such a structure. 2. fornix of cerebrum; either of a pair of arched fiber tracts that unite under the corpus callosum, so that together they comprise two columns, a body, and two crura.

Foroblique (fōr-o-blēk′) trademark for an obliquely forward visual telescopic system used in certain cystoscopes.

Forthane (fōr′thān) trademark for a preparation of methylhexaneamine.

fossa (fos′ah), pl. *fos′sae*[L.] a trench or channel; in anatomy, a hollow or depressed area. **acetabular f.**, a nonarticular area in the floor of the acetabulum. **adipose fossae**, spaces in the female breast which contain fat. **amygdaloid f.**, the depression in which the tonsil is lodged. **canine f.**, a depression on the external surface of the maxilla. **cerebral f.**, any of the depressions on the floor of the cranial cavity. **condylar f., condyloid f.**, either of two pits on the lateral part of the occipital bone. **coronoid f.**, a depression in the humerus for the coronoid process of the ulna. **cranial f.**, any one of three hollows (anterior, middle, and posterior) in the base of the cranium for the lobes of the brain. **digastric f.**, a depression on the inner surface of the mandible, giving attachment to the anterior belly of the digastric muscle. **digital f.**, trochanteric f. **duodenojejunal f.**, either of two peritoneal pockets, one behind the inferior and the other behind the superior duodenal fold. **epigastric f.**, 1. one in the epigastric region. 2. urachal f. **ethmoid f.**, the groove in the cribriform plate of the ethmoid bones, for the olfactory bulb. **glenoid f.**, mandibular f. **hyaloid f.**, a depression in the front of the vitreous body, lodging the lens. **hypophyseal f.**, a depression in the sphenoid, lodging the pituitary gland. **iliac f.**, a concave area occupying much of the inner surface of the ala of the ilium, especially anteriorly; from it arises the iliacus muscle. **incisive f.**, a slight depression on the anterior surface of the maxilla above the incisor teeth. **infratemporal f.**, an irregularly shaped cavity medial or deep to the zygomatic arch. **interpeduncular f.**, a depression between the two cerebral peduncles, the floor of which is the posterior perforated substance. **ischiorectal f.**, a potential space between the pelvic diaphragm and the skin below it; an anterior recess extends a variable distance between the pelvic and urogenital diaphragms. **Jobert's f.**, a fossa in the popliteal region bounded by the adductor magnus and the gracilis and sartorius. **jugular f.**, the depression at the base of the neck just above the sternum. **lacrimal f.**, a shallow depression in the roof of the orbit, lodging the lacrimal gland. **mandibular f.**, a depression in the temporal bone in which the condyle of the mandible rests. **mastoid f.**, a small triangular area between the posterior wall of the external acoustic meatus and the posterior root of the zygomatic process of the temporal bone. **nasal f.**, the portion of the nasal cavity anterior to the middle meatus. **navicular f.**, 1. the vaginal vestibule between the vaginal orifice and the frenulum of the pudendal labia. 2. the lateral expansion of the urethra of the glans penis. 3. a depression on the internal pterygoid process of the sphenoid, giving attachment to the tensor veli palatini muscle. **olfactory f.**, ethmoid f.

oral f., stomodeum. **f. ova′lis cor′dis**, a fossa in the right atrium of the heart; remains of fetal foramen ovale. **ovarian f.**, a shallow pouch on the posterior surface of the broad ligament in which the ovary is located. **patellar f.**, hyaloid f. **pituitary f.**, hypophyseal f. **rhomboid f.**, the floor of the fourth ventricle, made up of the dorsal surfaces of the medulla oblongata and pons. **Rosenmüller's f.**, see under *cavity*. **subarcuate f.**, a depression in the posterior inner surface of the petrous portion of the temporal bone. **subpyramidal f.**, a depression on the internal wall of the middle ear. **subsigmoid f.**, a fossa between the mesentery of the sigmoid flexure and that of the descending colon. **supraspinous f.**, a depression above the spine of the scapula. **sylvian f.**, fissure of Sylvius. **temporal f.**, an area on the side of the cranium bounded by the temporal lines, the frontal process of the zygomatic bone, and the zygomatic arch, lodging the temporal muscle. **tibiofemoral f.**, a space between the articular surfaces of the tibia and femur mesial or lateral to the inferior pole of the patella. **trochanteric f.**, a depression on the medial surface of the greater trochanter, receiving the tendon of the obturator externus muscle. **urachal f.**, one on the inner abdominal wall, between the urachus and the hypogastric artery. **Waldeyer's f.**, the two duodenal fossae regarded as one. **zygomatic f.**, infratemporal f.

fossette (fŏ-set′) 1. a small depression. 2. a small, deep corneal ulcer.

fossula (fos′u-lah), pl. *fos′sulae*[L.] a small fossa.

foulage (foo-lahzh′) [Fr.] kneading and pressing of the muscles in massage.

foul brood (fowl brood) a contagious disease of honeybees due to *Bacillus alvei*.

foundation (fown-da′shun) the structure or basis on which something is built. **denture f.**, the portion of the structures and tissues of the mouth available to support a denture.

fourchette (foor-shet′) [Fr.] the posterior union of the labia minora.

fovea (fo′ve-ah), pl. *fo′veae* [L.] a small pit or depression. **f. centra′lis**, a small pit in the center of the macula lutea, the area of clearest vision, where the retinal layers are spread aside, and light falls directly on the cones. **sublingual f.**, a depression on the inside of the mandible, lodging part of the lingual gland. **submandibular f.**, a depression on the medial aspect of the mandible, lodging part of the submandibular gland.

foveate (fo′ve-āt) pitted.

foveation (fo″ve-a′shun) formation of pits on a surface as on the skin; a pitted condition.

foveola (fo-ve′o-lah), pl. *fove′olae* [L.] a minute pit or depression.

foxglove (foks′gluv) see *digitalis*.

Fr chemical symbol, *francium*.

fractionation (frak″shun-a′shun) 1. in radiology, division of the total dose of radiation into small doses administered at intervals. 2. in chemistry, separation of a substance into components, as by distillation or crystallization.

fracture (frak′tūr) 1. the breaking of a part, especially a bone. 2. a break or rupture in a bone. **avulsion f.**, separation of a small fragment of bone cortex at the site of attachment of a ligament or tendon. **Barton's f.**, fracture of the distal end of the radius into the wrist joint. **Bennett's f.**, fracture of the base of the first metacarpal bone running into the carpometacarpal joint, complicated by subluxation. **blow-out f.**, fracture of the orbital floor caused by a sudden increase of intraorbital pressure due to traumatic force; the orbital contents herniate into the maxillary sinus so that the inferior rectus or inferior oblique muscle may become incarcerated in the fracture site, producing diplopia on looking up. **capillary f.**, one that appears on a radiogram as a fine, hairlike line, the segments of bone not being separated; sometimes seen in fractures of the skull. **closed f.**, one that does not produce an open wound in the skin. **Colles' f.**, fracture of the lower end of the radius, the lower fragment being displaced backward; if the lower fragment is displaced forward, it is a *reversed Colles' fracture*. **comminuted f.**, one in which the bone is splintered or crushed. **complete f.**, one involving the entire cross section of the bone. **compound f.**, open f. **compression f.**, one produced by compression. **depressed f.**, fracture of the skull in which a fragment is depressed. **direct f.**, one at the site of injury. **dislocation f.**, fracture of a bone near an articulation with concomitant dislocation of that joint. **double f.**, fracture of a bone in two places. **Dupuytren's f.**, Pott's f. **Duverney's f.**, fracture of the ilium just below the anterior inferior spine. **fissure f.**, a crack extending from a surface into, but not through, a long bone. **greenstick f.**, one in which one side of a bone is broken, the other being bent. **horizontal maxillary f.**, Le Fort I f. **impacted f.**, one in which one fragment is firmly driven into the other. **incomplete f.**, one which does not involve the complete cross section of the bone. **indirect f.**, one at a point distant from the site of injury. **interperiosteal f.**, incomplete or greenstick fracture. **intrauterine f.**, fracture of a fetal bone incurred *in utero*. **lead pipe f.**, one in which the bone cortex is slightly compressed and bulged on one side with a slight crack on the other side of the bone. **Le Fort's f.**, bilateral horizontal fracture of the maxilla. Le Fort fractures are classified as follows: *Le Fort I f.*, a horizontal segmented fracture of the alveolar process of the maxilla, in which the teeth are usually contained in the detached portion of the bone. *Le Fort II f.*, unilateral or bilateral fracture of the maxilla, in which the body of the maxilla is separated from the facial skeleton and the separated portion is pyramidal in shape; the fracture may extend through the body of the maxilla down the midline of the hard palate, through the floor of the orbit, and into the nasal cavity. *Le Fort III f.*, a fracture in which the entire maxilla and one or more facial bones are completely separated from the craniofacial skelton; such fractures are almost always accompanied by multiple fractures of the facial bones. **Monteggia's f.**, one in the proximal half of the shaft of the ulna, with dislocation of the head of the radius. **open f.**, one in

which a wound through the adjacent or overlying soft tissues communicates with the site of the break. **parry f.**, Monteggia's f. **pathologic f.**, one occurring from mild injury, due to preexisting bone involvement with tumor, cyst, infection, or the like. **pertrochanteric f.**, one passing through the greater trochanter of the femur. **ping-pong f.**, an indented fracture of the skull, resembling the indentation that can be produced with the finger in a ping-pong ball; when elevated it resumes and retains its normal position. **Pott's f.**, fracture of the lower part of the fibula with serious injury of the lower tibial articulation. **pyramidal f. (of maxilla)**, Le Fort II f. **silver-fork f.**, Colles' f. **simple f.**, closed f. **Smith's f.**, reversed Colles' f. **spiral f.**, one in which the bone has been twisted apart. **spontaneous f.**, pathologic f. **sprain f.**, the separation of a tendon from its insertion, taking with it a piece of bone. **Stieda's f.**, fracture of the internal condyle of the femur. **transcervical f.**, one through the neck of the femur. **transverse facial f.**, Le Fort III f. **transverse maxillary f.**, a term sometimes used for horizontal maxillary fracture (Le Fort I f.). **trophic f.**, one due to nutritional (trophic) disturbance. **Wagstaffe's f.**, separation of the internal malleolus.

fracture-dislocation (frak′tūr dis″lo-ka′shun) fracture of a bone near a joint, also involving dislocation.

frae- for words beginning thus, see those beginning *fre-*.

fragilitas (frah-jil′ĭ-tas) [L.] fragility. **f. crin′ium**, a brittleness of the hair. **f. os′sium**, osteogenesis imperfecta. **f. un′guium**, abnormal brittleness of the nails.

fragility (frah-jil′ĭ-te) susceptibility, or lack of resistance, to influences capable of causing disruption of continuity or integrity. **f. of blood**, erythrocyte f. **capillary f.**, abnormal susceptibility of capillary walls to rupture. **erythrocyte f.**, susceptibility of erythrocytes to hemolysis when exposed to increasingly hypotonic saline solutions (*osmotic f.*) or when subjected to mechanical trauma (*mechanical f.*).

fragmentation (frag″men-ta′shun) division into small pieces.

frambesia (fram-be′ze-ah) yaws. **f. trop′ica**, yaws.

frambesioma (fram-be″ze-o′mah) mother yaw.

frame (frām) a rigid structure for giving support to or for immobilizing a part. **Balkan f.**, an apparatus for continuous extension in treatment of fractures of the femur, consisting of an overhead bar, with pulleys attached, by which the leg is supported in a sling. **Bradford f.**, a canvas-covered, rectangular frame of pipe; used as a bed frame in disease of the spine or thigh. **quadriplegic standing f.**, a device for supporting in the upright position a patient whose four limbs are paralyzed. **Stryker f.**, one consisting of canvas stretched on anterior and posterior frames, on which the patient can be rotated around his longitudinal axis. **trial f.**, an eyeglass frame designed to permit insertion of different lenses used in correcting refractive errors of vision.

Francisella (fran″sĭ-sel′ah) a genus of microorganisms, including *F.* (*Pasteurella*) *tularen′sis,* the etiologic agent of tularemia.

francium (fran′se-um) chemical element (*see table*), at. no. 87, symbol Fr.

F.R.C.P. Fellow of the Royal College of Physicians.

F.R.C.S. Fellow of the Royal College of Surgeons.

freckle (frek″l) a pigmented spot on the skin due to accumulation of melanin resulting from exposure to sunlight. **melanotic f. of Hutchinson,** a noninvasive malignant melanoma occurring most often on the face of women during the fourth decade.

freemartin (fre′mar-tin) a sexually maldeveloped female calf born as a twin to a normal male calf; it is usually sterile and intersexual as a result of male hormone reaching it through anastomosed placental vessels.

freeze-drying (frēz-dri′ing) a method of tissue preparation in which the tissue specimen is frozen and then dehydrated at low temperature in a high vacuum.

freeze-etching (-ech′ing) a method used to study unfixed cells by electron microscopy, in which the object to be studied is placed in 20% glycerol, frozen at −100° C., and then mounted on a chilled holder.

fremitus (frem′ĭ-tus) a vibration perceptible on palpation. **friction f.,** the vibration caused by the rubbing together of two dry body surfaces. **hydatid f.,** see under *thrill.* **rhonchal f.,** palpable vibrations produced by passage of air through a mucus-filled, large bronchial tube. **tactile f.,** vibration, as in the chest wall, felt on the thorax while the patient is speaking. **tussive f.,** one felt on the chest when the patient coughs. **vocal f.,** one caused by speaking, perceived on auscultation.

frenectomy (fre-nek′to-me) excision of a frenum (frenulum).

frenoplasty (fre′no-plas″te) the correction of an abnormally attached frenum by surgically repositioning it.

frenotomy (fre-not′o-me) the cutting of a frenum (frenulum).

frenulum (fren′u-lum), pl. *fren′ula* [L.] a small fold of integument or mucous membrane that limits the movements of an organ or part. **f. of clitoris,** a fold formed by union of the labia minora with the clitoris. **f. of ileocecal valve,** a fold formed by the joined extremities of the ileocecal valve, partially encircling the lumen of the colon. **f. labio′rum puden′di,** fourchette. **f. lin′guae,** f. of tongue. **f. of lip,** a median fold of mucous membrane connecting the inside of each lip to the corresponding gum. **f. of Morgagni,** f. of ileocecal valve. **f. of prepuce of penis,** the fold under the penis connecting it with the prepuce. **f. of superior medullary velum,** a band lying in the superior medullary velum at its attachment to the inferior colliculi. **f. of tongue,** the vertical fold of mucous membrane under the tongue, attaching it to the floor of the mouth. **f. val′vulae co′li,** f. of ileocecal valve. **f. ve′li,** f. of superior medullary velum.

frenum (fre′num), pl. *fre′na* [L.] a restraining structure or part; see *frenulum.* **fre′nal,** adj.

frequency (fre′kwen-se) the number of occurrences of a determinable entity per unit of population or of time, e.g., cases of a disease per 100,000 population.

freudian (froi′de-an) pertaining to Sigmund Freud, the founder of psychoanalysis, and to his doctrines regarding the causes and treatment of neuroses and psychoses.

friable (fri′ah-b′l) easily pulverized or crumbled.

friction (frik′shun) the act of rubbing.

frigidity (frĭ-jid′ĭ-te) coldness; especially, sexual unresponsiveness of the female to physical stimulation.

frigolabile (frig″o-la′bĭl) easily affected or destroyed by cold.

frigorific (-rif′ik) producing coldness.

frigostable (-sta′b′l) resistant to cold or low temperatures.

frigotherapy (-ther′ah-pe) cryotherapy.

frit (frit) imperfectly fused material used as a basis for making glass and in the formation of porcelain teeth.

frog (frog) 1. a smooth-skinned, fully web-footed, tailless, leaping amphibian, commonly used as a laboratory animal. 2. the band of horny substance in the middle of the sole of a horse's foot.

frolement (frōl-maw′) [Fr.] 1. a rustling sound heard on auscultation in pericardial disease. 2. a brushing movement in massage.

frons (fronz) [L.] the forehead.

frontad (frun′tad) toward a front, or frontal aspect.

frontal (frun′tal) 1. pertaining to the forehead. 2. denoting a longitudinal plane of the body.

frontalis (fron-ta′lis) [L.] frontal.

frontomalar (frun″to-ma′lar) pertaining to the frontal and malar bones.

frontomaxillary (-mak′sĭ-ler″e) pertaining to the frontal bone and maxilla.

frontonasal (-na′zal) pertaining to the frontal sinus and the nose.

fronto-occipital (-ok-sip′ĭ-tal) pertaining to the forehead and the occiput.

frontoparietal (-pah-ri′ĕ-tal) pertaining to the frontal and parietal bones.

frontotemporal (-tem′po-ral) pertaining to the frontal and temporal bones.

frost (frost) a deposit resembling frozen dew or vapor. **urea f.,** the appearance on the skin of salt crystals left by evaporation of the sweat in urhidrosis.

frostbite (frost′bīt) injury to tissues due to exposure to cold.

frottage (fro-tahzh′) [Fr.] 1. rubbing movement in massage. 2. sexual gratification by rubbing against a person of the opposite sex.

frotteur (fro-tur′) one who practices frottage (2).

fructivorous (fruk-tiv′o-rus) subsisting on or eating fruit.

fructofuranose (fruk″to-fu′rah-nōs) the combining and more reactive form of fructose.

β-fructofuranosidase (-fu″rah-no′sĭ-dās) an enzyme occurring in yeasts and other organisms that catalyzes the hydrolysis of sugars with a terminal unsubstituted β-D-fructofuranosyl residue.

fructokinase (-ki′nās) an enzyme that catalyzes the transfer of a high-energy phosphate group to D-fructose.

fructose (fruk′tōs) a sugar, $C_6H_{12}O_6$, found in honey and many sweet fruits; used as a fluid and nutrient replenisher.

fructosemia (fruk″to-se′me-ah) the presence of fructose in the blood, as in fructose intolerance.

fructoside (fruk′to-sīd) a compound that bears the same relation to fructose as a glucoside does to glucose.

fructosuria (fruk″to-su′re-ah) the presence of fructose in the urine. **essential f.,** a benign hereditary disorder of carbohydrate metabolism due to a defect in fructokinase and manifested only by fructose in the blood and urine.

fructosyl (fruk′to-sil) a radical of fructose.

fruit (frōot) the matured ovary of a plant, including the seed and its envelopes.

frustration (frus-tra′shun) increased emotional tension due to failure to achieve sought gratifications or satisfactions.

FSH follicle-stimulating hormone.

Fuadin (fu′ah-din) trademark for a preparation of stibophen.

fuchsin (fook′sin) any of several red to purple dyes. **acid f.,** a mixture of sulfonated fuchsins; used in various complex stains. **basic f.,** a histologic stain, a mixture of pararosaniline, rosaniline, and magenta II. Also, a mixture of rosaniline and pararosaniline hydrochlorides used as a local anti-infective.

fuchsinophilia (fook″sin-o-fil′e-ah) the property of staining readily with fuchsin dyes. **fuchsinophil′ic,** adj.

fucose (fu′kōs) a monosaccharide occurring as L-fucose in a number of mucopolysaccharides and mucoproteins.

fucosidase (fu-ko′sĭ-dās) an enzyme occurring in two forms that catalyzes the hydrolysis of fucoside to an alcohol and fucose.

fucosidosis (fu″ko-sĭ-do′sis) a hereditary neurovisceral disease due to deficient enzymatic activity of fucosidase and resulting in accumulation of fucose in all tissues; it is marked by progressive cerebral degeneration, muscle weakness with eventual spasticity, emaciation, cardiomegaly, thick skin, and excessive sweating.

fugacity (fu-gas′ĭ-te) a measure of the escaping tendency of a substance from one phase to another phase, or from one part of a phase to another part of the same phase.

-fugal word element [L.], *driving away; fleeing from; repelling.*

fugue (fūg) a dissociative reaction in which amnesia is accompanied by physical flight from customary surroundings.

fulgurate (ful′gu-rāt) 1. to come and go like a flash of lightning. 2. to destroy by contact with electric sparks generated by a high-frequency current.

fulguration (ful″gu-ra′shun) destruction of living tissue by electric sparks generated by a high-frequency current.

fulminate (ful′mĭ-nāt) to occur suddenly with great intensity. **ful′minant,** adj.

Fulvicin (ful′vĭ-sin) trademark for a preparation of griseofulvin.

fumagillin (fu″mah-jil′in) an antibiotic, $C_{26}H_{34}$-O_7, elaborated by strains of *Aspergillus fumigatus.*

fumarase (fu′mah-rās) an enzyme that catalyzes the interconversion of fumarate and malate.

fumarate (fu′mar-āt) a salt of fumaric acid. **ferrous f.,** the anhydrous salt of a combination of ferrous iron and fumaric acid; used as a hematinic.

fumigation (fu″mĭ-ga′shun) exposure to disinfecting fumes.

fuming (fūm′ing) emitting a visible vapor.

Fumiron (fum′i-ron) trademark for a preparation of ferrous fumarate.

functio (fungk′she-o) [L.] function. **f. lae′sa,** loss of function; one of the cardinal signs of inflammation.

function (fungk′shun) the special, normal, or proper action of any part or organ.

functional (fungk′shun-al) of pertaining to a function; affecting the function but not the structure.

fundament (fun′dah-ment) 1. a base or foundation, as the breech or rump. 2. the anus and parts adjacent to it.

fundectomy (fun-dek′to-me) excision of the fundus of an organ, as of the stomach.

fundiform (fun′dĭ-form) shaped like a loop or sling.

fundoplication (fun″do-pli-ka′shun) mobilization of the lower end of the esophagus and plication of the fundus of the stomach up around it.

fundus (fun′dus), pl. *fun′di* [L.] the bottom or base of anything; the bottom or base of an organ, or the part of a hollow organ farthest from its mouth. **fun′dal, fun′dic,** adj. **f. of eye,** the back portion of the interior of the eyeball, visible through the pupil by use of the ophthalmoscope. **f. of gallbladder,** the inferior, dilated portion of the gallbladder. **f. of stomach,** the part of the stomach to the left and above the level of the opening of the esophagus. **f. tym′pani,** the floor of the tympanic cavity. **f. of urinary bladder,** the base or posterior surface of the urinary bladder. **f. of uterus,** the part of the uterus above the orifices of the uterine tubes.

fundusectomy (fun″du-sek′to-me) excision of the fundus of the stomach.

funduscope (fun′dus-skōp) ophthalmoscope. **funduscop′ic,** adj.

fungal (fung′al) pertaining to or caused by a fungus.

fungate (fun′gāt) to produce fungus-like growths; to grow rapidly, like a fungus.

fungemia (fun-je′me-ah) the presence of fungi in the blood stream.

fungi (fun′ji) plural of *fungus.*

fungicide (fun′jĭ-sīd) an agent that destroys fungi. **fungici′dal,** adj.

fungicidin (fun″jĭ-si′din) nystatin.

fungiform (fun′jĭ-form) shaped like a fungus, or mushroom.

fungistasis (fun″jĭ-sta′sis) inhibition of the growth of fungi. **fungistat′ic,** adj.

fungistat (fun′jĭ-stat) a substance that inhibits the growth of fungi.

fungitoxic (fun″jĭ-tok′sik) exerting a toxic effect upon fungi.

Fungizone (fun′jĭ-zōn) trademark for a preparation of amphotericin B.

fungoid (fun′goid) resembling a fungus. **chignon f.,** a nodular growth on the hair.

fungosity (fun-gos′ĭ-te) a fungoid growth or excrescence.

fungous (fun′gus) of the nature of, caused by, or resembling a fungus.

fungus (fun′gus), pl. *fun′gi* [L.] a general term for a group of eukaryotic protists (mushrooms, yeasts, molds, etc.) marked by the absence of chlorophyll and the presence of a rigid cell wall. **cerebral f.,** hernia cerebri. **club f.,** Basidiomycetes. **fission f.,** schizomycete. **imperfect f.,** a fungus whose perfect (sexual) stage is unknown. **mycelial f.,** any fungus that forms mycelia, in contrast to a yeast fungus. **perfect f.,** a fungus for which both sexual and asexual types of spore formation are known. **ray f.,** *Actinomyces.* **sac f.,** Ascomycetes. **slime f.,** Mycetozoa.

funicle (fu′nĭ-k′l) funiculus.

funiculitis (fu-nik″u-li′tis) 1. inflammation of the spermatic cord. 2. inflammation of that portion of a spinal nerve root lying within the intervertebral canal.

funiculus (fu-nik′u-lus), pl. *funic′uli* [L.] a cord; a cordlike structure or part. **funic′ular,** adj. **anterior f.,** the white substance of the spinal cord lying on either side between the anterior median fissure and the ventral root. **cuneate f.,** see under *fasciculus.* **lateral f.,** 1. the white substance of the spinal cord lying on either side between the dorsal and ventral roots. 2. the continuation into the medulla oblongata of all the fiber tracts of the lateral funiculus of the spinal cord with exception of the lateral pyramidal tract. **posterior f.,** the white substance of the spinal cord lying on either side between the posterior median sulcus and the dorsal root. **f. spermat′icus,** the spermatic cord.

funiform (fu′nĭ-form) resembling a rope or cord.

funis (fu′nis) any cordlike structure, particularly the umbilical cord. **fu′nic,** adj.

Furacin (fu′rah-sin) trademark for preparations of nitrofurazone.

Furadantin (fūr″ah-dan′tin) trademark for preparations of nitrofurantoin.

Furaspor (fūr″ah-spōr) trademark for a preparation of nitrofurfuryl methyl ether.

furazolidone (fu″rah-zol′ĭ-dōn) an antibacterial and antiprotozoal, $C_8H_7N_3O_5$.

furcal (fer′kal) forked.

furcation (fur-ka′shun) the anatomical area of a multirooted tooth where the roots divide.

furfuraceous (fer″fu-ra′shus) fine and loose; said of scales resembling bran or dandruff.

furfural, furfurol (fur′fu-ral; -rol) an aromatic compound from the distillation of bran, sawdust, etc., which causes convulsions in animals.

furor (fu′ror) fury; rage. **f. epilep′ticus,** an attack of intense anger occurring in epilepsy.

furosemide (fu-ro′sĕ-mīd) a thiazide diuretic, $C_{12}H_{11}ClN_2O_5S$.

Furoxone (fer-ok′sōn) trademark for preparations of furazolidone.

furrow (fur′o) a groove or trench. **atrioventricular f.,** the transverse groove marking off the atria of the heart from the ventricles. **digital f.,** any one of the transverse folds across the joints on the palmar surface of a finger. **genital f.,** a groove that appears on the genital tubercle of the fetus at the end of the second month. **gluteal f.,** the furrow which separates the buttocks. **Liebermeister's f's,** depressions sometimes seen on the upper surface of the liver from pressure of the ribs, generally due to tight lacing or tight garments. **mentolabial f.,** the hollow just above the chin. **nympholabial f.,** a groove separating the labium majus and labium minus on each side. **primitive f.,** see under *groove.* **scleral f.,** see under *sulcus.* **Sibson's f.,** the lower border of the pectoralis major muscle.

furuncle (fu′rung-k′l) a boil; a painful nodule formed in the skin by circumscribed inflammation of the corium and subcutaneous tissue, enclosing a central slough or "core"; due to staphylococci entering the skin through hair follicles. **furun′cular,** adj.

furunculoid (fu-rung′ku-loid) resembling a furuncle or boil.

furunculosis (fu-rung″ku-lo′sis) 1. the persistent sequential occurrence of furuncles over a period of weeks or months. 2. the simultaneous occurrence of a number of furuncles.

furunculus (fu-rung′ku-lus) [L.] furuncle.

Fusarium (fu-sa′re-um) a genus of fungi; some species are plant pathogens and some are opportunistic infectious agents of man and animals.

fuscin (fu′sin) a brown pigment of the retinal epithelium.

fusible (fu′zĭ-b′l) capable of being melted.

fusiform (fu′zĭ-form) spindle-shaped.

fusimotor (fu″sĭ-mo′tor) denoting motor nerve fibers (of gamma motoneurons) that innervate intrafusal fibers of the muscle spindle.

fusion (fu′zhun) 1. the act or process of melting. 2. the abnormal coherence of adjacent parts or bodies. 3. the coordination of separate images of the same object in the two eyes into one. 4. the operative formation of an ankylosis or arthrosis. **diaphyseal-epiphyseal f.,** operative establishment of bony union between the epiphysis and diaphysis of a bone. **nerve f.,** nerve anastomosis done to induce regeneration for resupplying empty tracts of a nerve with new growth of fibers. **nuclear f.,** the fusion of two atomic nuclei to form a single heavier nucleus, resulting in the release of enormous amounts of energy. **spinal f.,** spondylosyndesis.

fusional (-al) marked by fusion.

Fusobacterium (fu″zo-bak-te′re-um) a genus of anaerobic gram-negative bacteria found as normal flora in the mouth and large bowel, and often in necrotic tissue, probably as secondary invaders. *F. plautivincen'ti* is found in necrotizing ulcerative gingivitis (trench mouth) and necrotizing ulcerative stomatitis.

fusocellular (-sel'u-ler) having spindle-shaped cells.

fusospirillosis (-spi"rĭ-lo'sis) necrotizing ulcerative gingivitis.

fusospirochetal (-spi"ro-ke'tal) of or caused by fusiform bacilli and spirochetes.

fusospirochetosis (-ke-to'sis) infection with fusiform bacilli and spirochetes.

G

G gram; gingival; glucose; gonidial.

g gravity; the unit of force exerted upon a body during acceleration and deceleration.

g. gram (or grams).

Ga chemical symbol, *gallium.*

gadolinium (gad"o-lin'e-um) chemical element (*see table*), at. no. 64, symbol Gd.

gag (gag) 1. a surgical device for holding the mouth open. 2. to retch, or to strive to vomit.

gait (gāt) the manner or style of walking. **antalgic g.,** the limp characteristic of coxalgia, with avoidance of weight-bearing on the affected side. **ataxic g.,** an unsteady, uncoordinated walk, employing a wide base. **cerebellar g.,** a staggering walk indicative of cerebellar disease. **festinating g.,** a gait in which the patient involuntarily moves with short, accelerating steps, often on tiptoe, as in paralysis agitans; festination. **helicopod g.,** a gait in which the feet describe half circles, as in some hysterical disorders. **spastic g.,** a gait in which the legs are held together and move in a stiff manner, the toes seeming to drag and catch. **steppage g.,** the gait in drop foot in which the advancing leg is lifted high so that the toes can clear the ground. **tabetic g.,** an ataxic gait in which the feet slap the ground. **waddling g.,** a gait suggesting that of a duck, characteristic of progressive muscular dystrophy.

galact(o)- word element [Gr.], *milk.*

galactacrasia (gah-lak"tah-kra'ze-ah) abnormal condition of the breast milk.

galactagogue (gah-lak'tah-gog) promoting milk flow; an agent that so acts.

galactan (gah-lak'tan) a carbohydrate which yields galactose upon hydrolysis.

galactemia (gal"ak-te'me-ah) the presence of milk in the blood.

galactic (gah-lak'tik) 1. pertaining to milk. 2. galactagogue.

galactin (gah-lak'tin) prolactin.

galactischia (gal"ak-tisk'e-ah) suppression of milk secretion.

galactoblast (gah-lak'to-blast) a colostrum corpuscle in the acini of the mammary gland.

galactobolic (gah-lak"to-bol'ik) of or relating to the action of neurohypophyseal peptides which contract the mammary myoepithelium and cause ejection of milk.

galactocele (gah-lak'to-sēl) 1. a milk-containing, cystic enlargement of the mammary gland. 2. hydrocele filled with milky fluid.

galactokinase (gah-lak"to-ki'nās) an enzyme that catalyzes the transfer of a high-energy phosphate group from a donor to D-galactose, producing D-galactose-1-phosphate.

galactolipid, galactolipin (-lip'id; -lip'in) a cerebroside which yields galactose on hydrolysis.

galactoma (gal"ak-to'mah) galactocele (1).

galactometer (gal"ak-tom'ĕ-ter) an instrument for measuring the specific gravity of milk.

galactophagous (gal"ak-tof'ah-gus) subsisting upon milk.

galactophlysis (gal"ak-tof'lĭ-sis) a vesicular eruption containing milky fluid.

galactophore (gah-lak'to-fōr) 1. galactophorous. 2. a milk duct.

galactophoritis (gah-lak"to-fo-ri'tis) inflammation of the milk ducts.

galactophorous (gal"ak-tof'o-rus) conveying milk.

galactophygous (gal"ak-tof'ĭ-gus) arresting the flow of milk.

galactoplania (gah-lak"to-pla'ne-ah) secretion of milk in some abnormal part.

galactopoiesis (-poi-e'sis) the production of milk by the mammary glands.

galactopoietic (-poi-et'ik) 1. pertaining to, marked by, or promoting milk production. 2. an agent that promotes milk flow.

galactopyra (-pi'rah) milk fever.

galactorrhea (-re'ah) excessive or spontaneous milk flow; persistent secretion of milk irrespective of nursing.

galactosamine (-sam'in) an amino derivative of galactose.

galactoscope (gah-lak'to-skōp) a device for showing the proportion of cream in milk.

galactose (gah-lak'tōs) a monosaccharide, $C_6H_{12}O_6$. D-galactose is found in lactose, cerebrosides of the brain, raffinose of the sugar beet, and in many gums and seaweeds; L-galactose in flaxseed mucilage.

galactosemia (gah-lak"to-se'me-ah) a hereditary disorder of carbohydrate metabolism, characterized by hepatomegaly, cataracts, mental retardation, vomiting, diarrhea, jaundice, poor weight gain, and malnutrition in early infancy.

galactosidase (-si'dās) an enzyme that catalyzes the conversion of galactoside to galactose; it occurs in two forms: α-galactosidase (melibiase) and β-galactosidase (lactase).

galactoside (gah-lak'to-sīd) a glycoside containing galactose.

galactosis (gal″ak-to'sis) the formation of milk by the lacteal glands.

galactostasis (gal″ak-tos'tah-sis) 1. cessation of milk secretion. 2. abnormal collection of milk in the mammary glands.

galactosuria (gah-lak″to-su're-ah) the presence of galactose in the urine.

galactotherapy (-ther'ah-pe) treatment of a nursing infant by medication given the mother or wet nurse.

galactotoxin (-tok'sin) a basic substance formed in milk.

galactotoxism, galactoxism (-tok'sizm; gal″-ak-tok'sizm) poisoning by milk.

galactozymase (gah-lak″to-zi'mās) a starch-liquefying enzyme.

galacturia (gal″ak-tu're-ah) chyluria.

galea (ga'le-ah), pl. *ga'leae* [L.] a helmet-shaped structure. **g. aponeurot'ica,** the aponeurosis connecting the two bellies of the occipitofrontalis muscle.

galenicals, galenics (gah-len'ĭ-kals; -iks) medicines prepared according to Galen's formulas; now used to denote standard preparations containing one or several organic ingredients, as contrasted with pure chemical substances.

gall (gawl) the bile.

gallamine triethiodide (gal'ah-mīn tri″eth-i'o-dīd) a skeletal muscle relaxant, $C_{30}H_{60}I_3N_3$-O_3.

gallate (gal'āt) a salt of gallic acid.

gallbladder (gawl'blad-er) the pear-shaped reservoir for bile on the posteroinferior surface of the liver.

gallium (gal'le-um) chemical element (*see table*), at. no. 31, symbol Ga.

gallon (gal'on) a unit of liquid measure (4 quarts, 3.785 liters, or 3785 ml.).

gallop (gal'op) a disordered rhythm of the heart; see under *rhythm.*

gallsickness (gawl-sik'nes) a disease of cattle caused by *Anaplasma marginale,* marked by high fever, anemia, and icterus.

gallstone (gawl'stōn) a calculus formed in the gallbladder or bile duct.

galvanism (gal'vah-nizm) 1. unidirectional electric current derived from a chemical battery. 2. galvanotherapy.

galvanization (gal″vah-ni-za'shun) galvanotherapy.

galvanocautery (gal″vah-no-kaw'ter-e) cautery by a wire heated by galvanic current.

galvanocontractility (-kon″trak-til'ĭ-te) contractility in response to a galvanic stimulus.

galvanometer (gal″vah-nom'ĕ-ter) an instrument for measuring current by electromagnetic action.

galvanonervous (gal″vah-no-ner'vus) produced by application of galvanic current to a nerve.

galvanopalpation (-pal-pa'shun) testing of nerves of the skin by galvanic current.

galvanosurgery (-ser'jer-e) the use of galvanocautery in surgery.

galvanotaxis (-tak'sis) the tendency of an organism to arrange itself in a medium so that its axis bears a certain relation to direction of the current in the medium.

galvanotherapy (-ther'ah-pe) the therapeutic use of galvanic current.

galvanotropism (gal″vah-not'ro-pizm) the tendency of an organism to turn or move under the action of electric current.

gamete (gam'ēt) 1. one of two cells, male (*spermatozoon*) and female (*ovum*), whose union is necessary in sexual reproduction to initiate the development of a new individual. 2. the malarial parasite in its sexual form in a mosquito's stomach, either male (*microgamete*) or female (*macrogamete*); the latter is fertilized by the former to develop into an ookinete. **gamet'ic,** adj.

gametocide (gam'ĕ-to-sīd″) an agent that destroys gametes or gametocytes. **gametoci'dal,** adj.

gametocyte (gah-met'o-sīt) that sexual stage of the malarial parasite in the blood which may produce gametes when taken into the mosquito host; it may be male (*microgametocyte*) or female (*macrogametocyte*).

gametogenesis (gam″ĕ-to-jen'ĕ-sis) the development of the male and female sex cells (gametes). **gametogen'ic,** adj.

gametogony (gam″ĕ-tog'o-ne) the development of merozoites into male and female gametes, which later fuse to form a zygote.

gamma (gam'ah) third letter of the Greek alphabet, γ; used in names of chemical compounds to distinguish one of three or more isomers or to indicate position of substituting atoms or groups.

gamma benzene hexachloride (gam'ah ben'-zēn hek″sah-klor'īd) a pediculicide and scabicide, $C_6H_6Cl_6$.

gammacism (-sizm) imperfect utterance of *g* and *k* sounds.

gamma globulin see under *globulin.*

gammaglobulinopathy (gam″ah-glob″u-lin-op'ah-the) gammopathy.

gammopathy (gam-mop'ah-the) abnormal proliferation of the lymphoid cells producing immunoglobulins; the gammopathies include multiple myeloma, macroglobulinemia, and Hodgkin's disease.

gamogenesis (gam″o-jen'ĕ-sis) sexual reproduction. **gamogenet'ic,** adj.

gangli(o)- word element [Gr.], *ganglion.*

ganglia (gang'gle-ah) plural of *ganglion.*

gangliated (gang'gle-āt″ed) ganglionated.

gangliectomy (gang″gle-ek'to-me) ganglionectomy.

gangliform (gang'glĭ-form) having the form of a ganglion.

gangliitis (gang'gle-i'tis) ganglionitis.

ganglioblast (gang'gle-o-blast″) an embryonic cell of the cerebrospinal ganglia.

gangliocyte (-sīt″) a ganglion cell.

gangliocytoma (gang″gle-o-si-to'mah) ganglioneuroma.

ganglioform (gang'gle-o-form″) gangliform.

ganglioglioma (gang"gle-o-gli-o′mah) a glioma rich in mature neurons or ganglion cells.

ganglioglioneuroma (-gli"o-nu-ro′mah) ganglioneuroma.

ganglioma (gang"gle-o′mah) ganglioneuroma.

ganglion (gang′gle-on), pl. *gan′glia, ganglions* [Gr.] 1. a knot, or knotlike mass; in anatomy, a group of nerve cell bodies, located outside the central nervous system; occasionally applied to certain nuclear groups within the brain or spinal cord, e.g., basal ganglia. 2. a form of cystic tumor on an aponeurosis or a tendon. **gan′-glial, ganglion′ic,** adj. **Acrel's g.,** a cystic tumor on an extensor tendon of the wrist. **Andersch's g.,** inferior g. (1). **Arnold's g.,** otic g. **Auerbach's g.,** myenteric plexus. **autonomic ganglia,** aggregations of cell bodies of neurons of the autonomic nervous system. **basal ganglia,** masses of gray matter in the cerebral hemisphere, comprising the corpus striatum, amygdaloid body, and claustrum; sometimes including the thalamus, tuber cinereum, geniculate bodies, and quadrigeminal bodies. **Bidder's ganglia,** ganglia on the cardiac nerves, situated at the lower end of the atrial septum. **Bochdalek's g.,** superior dental plexus. **cardiac ganglia,** ganglia of the cardiac plexus near the arterial ligament. **carotid g.,** an occasional small enlargement in the internal carotid plexus. **celiac ganglia,** two irregularly shaped ganglia, one on each crus of the diaphragm within the celiac plexus. **cephalic ganglia,** parasympathetic ganglia in the head, consisting of the ciliary, otic, pterygopalatine, and submandibular ganglia. **cerebrospinal ganglia,** those associated with the cranial and spinal nerves. **cervical g.,** 1. any of the three ganglia (inferior, middle, and superior) of the sympathetic trunk in the neck region. 2. one near the cervix uteri. **cervicothoracic g.,** one formed by fusion of the inferior cervical and the first thoracic ganglia. **cervicouterine g.,** cervical g. (2). **ciliary g.,** a parasympathetic ganglion in the posterior part of the orbit. **Cloquet's g.,** a swelling of nasopalatine nerve in anterior palatine canal. **coccygeal g.,** glomus coccygeum. **Corti's g.,** spiral g. **dorsal root g.,** spinal g. **Ehrenritter's g.,** superior g. (1). **false g.,** an enlargement on a nerve that does not have a true ganglionic structure. **Frankenhäuser's g.,** cervical g. (2). **gasserian g.,** trigeminal g. **geniculate g.,** the sensory ganglion of the facial nerve, on the geniculum of the facial nerve. **hepatic g.,** one near the hepatic artery. **g. im′-par,** the ganglion commonly found in front of the coccyx, where the sympathetic trunks of the two sides unite. **inferior g.,** 1. the lower of two ganglia of the glossopharyngeal nerve as it passes through the jugular foramen. 2. the lower of two ganglia of the vagus nerve as it passes through the jugular foramen. **jugular g.,** superior g. (1 and 2). **Lee's g.,** cervical g. (2). **Ludwig's g.,** one near the right atrium of the heart, connected with the cardiac plexus. **lumbar ganglia,** the ganglia on the sympathetic trunk, usually four or five on either side. **lymphatic g.,** a lymph node. **Meckel's g.,** pterygopalatine g. **Meissner's g.,** one of the small groups of nerve cells in Meissner's plexus. **mesenteric g., inferior,** a sympathetic ganglion near the origin of the inferior mesenteric artery. **mesenteric g., superior,** one or more sympathetic ganglia at the sides of, or just below, the superior mesenteric artery. **otic g.,** a parasympathetic ganglion immediately below the foramen ovale; its postganglionic fibers supply the parotid gland. **parasympathetic ganglia,** aggregations of cell bodies of neurons of the parasympathetic nervous system. **petrous g.,** inferior g. (1). **phrenic g.,** a sympathetic ganglion often found within the phrenic plexus at its junction with the cardiac plexus. **pterygopalatine g.,** a parasympathetic ganglion in the parasympathetic fossa. **Remak's g.,** a sympathetic ganglion in the heart wall near the superior vena cava. **renal ganglia,** sympathetic ganglia within the renal plexus. **Ribes' g.,** the alleged ganglion in the termination of the internal carotid plexus around the anterior communicating artery of the brain. **sacral ganglia,** those of the sacral part of the sympathetic trunk, usually three or four on either side. **Scarpa's g.,** vestibular g. **Schacher's g.,** ciliary g. **semilunar g.,** 1. trigeminal g. 2. [pl.] celiac ganglia. **sensory g.,** any of the ganglia of the peripheral nervous system that transmit sensory impulses; also, the collective masses of nerve cell bodies in the brain subserving sensory functions. **simple g.,** a cystic tumor in a tendon sheath. **sphenopalatine g.,** pterygopalatine g. **spinal g.,** one on the dorsal root of each spinal nerve. **spiral g.,** the ganglion on the cochlear nerve, located within the modiolus, sending fibers peripherally to the organ of Corti and centrally to the cochlear nuclei of the brain stem. **splanchnic g.,** 1. one on the greater splanchnic nerve near the twelfth thoracic vertebra. 2. celiac plexus. **stellate g.,** cervicothoracic g. **submandibular g., submaxillary g.,** a parasympathetic ganglion located superior to the deep part of the submandibular gland, on the lateral surface of the hyoglossal muscle. **superior g.,** 1. the upper of two ganglia on the glossopharyngeal nerve as it passes through the jugular foramen. 2. the upper of two ganglia of the vagus nerve just as it passes through the jugular foramen. **sympathetic ganglia,** aggregations of cell bodies of neurons of the sympathetic nervous system. **thoracic ganglia,** those on the thoracic portion of the sympathetic trunk, 11 or 12 on either side. **trigeminal g.,** one on the sensory root of the fifth cranial nerve in a cleft in the dura mater on the anterior surface of the petrous part of the temporal bone, giving off the ophthalmic and maxillary and part of the mandibular nerve. **tympanic g.,** an enlargement on the tympanic branch of the glossopharyngeal nerve. **vagal g.,** 1. inferior g. (2). 2. superior g. (2). **Valentin's g.,** one on a superior dental nerve. **ventricular ganglia,** Bidder's ganglia. **vestibular g.,** the sensory ganglion of the vestibular part of the eighth cranial nerve, located in the upper part of the lateral end of the internal acoustic meatus. **Walther's g.,** glomus coccygeum. **Wrisberg's g.,** cardiac g. **wrist g.,** cystic enlargement of a tendon sheath on the back of the wrist.

ganglionated (gang′gle-o-nāt″ed) provided with ganglia.

ganglionectomy (gang″gle-o-nek′to-me) excision of a ganglion.

ganglioneuroma (-nu-ro′mah) a benign neoplasm composed of nerve fibers and mature ganglion cells.

ganglionitis (-ni′tis) inflammation of a ganglion.

ganglionostomy (-nos′to-me) surgical creation of an opening into a cystic tumor on a tendon sheath or aponeurosis.

ganglioplegic (-ple′jik) blocking transmission of impulses through the sympathetic and parasympathetic ganglia; an agent that so acts.

ganglioside (gang′gle-o-sīd) a class of galactose-containing cerebrosides found in central nervous system tissues; they are glycolipids of the basic composition ceramide-glucose-galactose-N-acetyl neuraminic acid. The form GM_1 accumulates in tissues in generalized gangliosidosis, the form GM_2 in Tay-Sachs disease.

gangliosidosis (gang″gle-o-si-do′sis) a lipid storage disorder marked by accumulation of gangliosides in tissues due to an enzyme defect. In generalized gangliosidosis, a hereditary defect in β-galactosidase causes accumulation of galactoside GM_1, resulting in mental retardation, hepatomegaly, skeletal deformities, and, often, cherry red spot. See also *Tay-Sachs disease.*

gangosa (gang-go′sah) one of the late lesions of yaws, manifested as a destructive ulceration of the nose, nasopharynx, and hard palate.

gangrene (gang′grēn) death of tissue, usually in considerable mass, generally with loss of vascular (nutritive) supply and followed by bacterial invasion and putrefaction. **diabetic g.,** moist gangrene associated with diabetes. **dry g.,** that occurring without subsequent bacterial decomposition, the tissues becoming dry and shriveled. **embolic g.,** a condition following cutting off of blood supply by embolism. **gas g.,** an acute, severe, painful condition in which the muscles and subcutaneous tissues become filled with gas and a serosanguineous exudate; due to infection of wounds by anaerobic bacteria, among which are various species of *Clostridium*. **moist g.,** that associated with proteolytic decomposition resulting from bacterial action. **symmetric g.,** gangrene of corresponding digits on both sides, due to vasomotor disturbances.

gangrenosis (gang″grě-no′sis) the development of gangrene.

gangrenous (gang′grě-nus) pertaining to, marked by, or of the nature of gangrene.

ganoblast (gan′o-blast) ameloblast.

Gantrisin (gan′trĭ-sin) trademark for preparations of sulfisoxazole.

gap (gap) an unoccupied interval in time; an opening or hiatus. **air-bone g.,** the lag between the audiographic curves for air- and bone-conducted stimuli, as an indication of loss of bone conduction of the ear. **auscultatory g.,** a period in which sound is not heard in the auscultatory method of sphygmomanometry. **interocclusal g.,** see under *distance.* **isochromatid g.,** a non-staining region at the same level in two sister chromatids. **silent g.,** auscultatory.

Garamycin (gar″ah-mi′sin) trademark for a preparation of gentamicin.

gargle (gar′g′l) 1. a solution for rinsing mouth and throat. 2. to rinse the mouth and throat by holding a solution in the open mouth and agitating it by expulsion of air from the lungs.

gargoylism (gar′goil-izm) Hurler's syndrome.

gas (gas) any elastic aeriform fluid in which the molecules are separated from one another and so have free paths. **gas′eous,** adj. **coal g.,** a gas, poisonous because it contains carbon monoxide, produced by destructive distillation of coal; much used for domestic cooking. **laughing g.,** nitrous oxide. **marsh g.,** methane. **olefiant g.,** ethylene. **tear g.,** one which produces severe lacrimation by irritating the conjunctivae.

gaskin (gas′kin) the thigh of a horse.

gasometry (gas-om′ĕ-tre) measurement of the amount of gas present in a mixture.

gaster (gas′ter) [Gr.] stomach.

Gasterophilus (-of′ĭ-lus) a genus of botflies the larvae of which develop in the gastrointestinal tract of horses and may sometimes infect man.

gastr(o)- word element [Gr.], *stomach.*

gastradenitis (gas″trad-ĕ-ni′tis) inflammation of the stomach glands.

gastralgia (gas-tral′je-ah) gastric colic.

gastrectomy (gas-trek′to-me) excision of the stomach (*total g.*) or of a portion of it (*partial* or *subtotal g.*).

gastric (gas′trik) pertaining to, affecting, or originating in the stomach.

gastricsin (gas-trik′sin) a proteolytic enzyme isolated from gastric juice; its precursor is pepsinogen but it differs from pepsin in molecular weight and in the amino acids at the N terminal.

gastrin (gas′trin) a polypeptide hormone secreted by certain cells of the pyloric glands, which strongly stimulates secretion of gastric acid and pepsin, and weakly stimulates secretion of pancreatic enzymes and gallbladder contraction.

gastrinoma (gas″trin-o′mah) a gastrin-secreting, non-beta islet cell tumor of the pancreas, associated with Zollinger-Ellison syndrome.

gastritis (gas-tri′tis) inflammation of the stomach. **atrophic g.,** chronic gastritis with atrophy of the mucous membrane and glands. **catarrhal g.,** inflammation and hypertrophy of the gastric mucosa, with excessive secretion of mucus. **erosive g., exfoliative g.,** that in which the gastric surface epithelium is eroded. **giant hypertrophic g.,** excessive proliferation of the gastric mucosa, producing diffuse thickening of the stomach wall. **hypertrophic g.,** gastritis with infiltration and enlargment of the glands. **phlegmonous g.,** a variety with abscesses in the stomach walls. **polypous g.,** hypertrophic gastritis with polypoid projections of the mucosa. **pseudomembranous g.,** that in which a false membrane occurs in patches within the stomach. **toxic g.,** that due to action of a poison or corrosive agent.

gastroacephalus (gas″tro-a-sef′ah-lus) a twin monster, the autosite bearing a headless parasite on its abdomen.

gastroanastomosis (-ah-nas″to-mo′sis) gastrogastrostomy.

gastrocamera (-kam′er-ah) a small camera which can be passed down the esophagus to photograph the inside of the stomach.

gastrocardiac (-kar′de-ak) pertaining to the stomach and the heart.

gastrocele (gas′tro-sēl) hernial protrusion of the stomach or of a gastric pouch.

gastrocnemius (gas″trok-ne′me-us) see *Table of Muscles.*

gastrocoele (gas′tro-sēl) archenteron.

gastrocolic (gas″tro-kol′ik) pertaining to or communicating with the stomach and colon.

gastrocolitis (-ko-li′tis) inflammation of the stomach and colon.

gastrocolostomy (-ko-los′to-me) surgical anastomosis of the stomach to the colon.

gastrocolotomy (-ko-lot′o-me) incision into the stomach and colon.

gastrocutaneous (-ku-ta′ne-us) pertaining to the stomach and skin, or communicating with the stomach and the cutaneous surface of the body, as a gastrocutaneous fistula.

gastrodiaphane (-di′ah-fān) a small electric lamp for use in gastrodiaphany.

gastrodiaphany (-di-af′ah-ne) examination of the stomach by transillumination of its walls with a gastrodiaphane.

gastrodidymus (-did′ĭ-mus) symmetrical twins fused in the abdominal region.

Gastrodiscoides (-dis-koi′dēz) a genus of trematodes parasitic in the intestinal tract.

gastroduodenal (-du″o-de′nal) pertaining to the stomach and duodenum.

gastroduodenitis (-du-od″ĕ-ni′tis) inflammation of the stomach and duodenum.

gastroduodenoscopy (-du″o-dĕ-nos′ko-pe) endoscopic examination of the stomach and duodenum.

gastroduodenostomy (-du″o-de-nos′to-me) surgical anastomosis of the stomach to a formerly remote part of the duodenum.

gastrodynia (-din′e-ah) pain in the stomach.

gastroenteralgia (-en″ter-al′je-ah) pain in the stomach and intestine.

gastroenteric (-en-ter′ik) pertaining to the stomach and intestine.

gastroenteritis (-en″ter-i′tis) inflammation of the stomach and intestine.

gastroenteroanastomosis (-en″ter-o-ah-nas″-to-mo′sis) anastomosis between the stomach and small intestine.

gastroenterocolitis (-en″ter-o-ko-li′tis) inflammation of the stomach, small intestine, and colon.

gastroenterologist (-en″ter-ol′o-jist) a physician specializing in gastroenterology.

gastroenterology (-en″ter-ol′o-je) the study of the stomach and intestine and their diseases.

gastroenteropathy (-en″ter-op′ah-the) any disease of the stomach and intestine.

gastroenteroptosis (-en″ter-op-to′sis) downward displacement or prolapse of the stomach and intestine.

gastroenterostomy (-en″ter-os′to-me) surgical anastomosis of the stomach to the intestine.

gastroenterotomy (-en″ter-ot′o-me) incision into the stomach and intestine.

gastroepiploic (-ep″ĭ-plo′ik) pertaining to the stomach and epiploon (omentum).

gastroesophageal (-ĕ-sof″ah-je′al) pertaining to the stomach and esophagus.

gastroesophagitis (-e-sof″ah-ji′tis) inflammation of the stomach and esophagus.

gastroesophagostomy (-e-sof″ah-gos′to-me) surgical anastomosis between the stomach and esophagus.

gastrofiberscope (-fi′ber-skōp) a fiberscope for viewing the stomach.

gastrogastrostomy (-gas-tros′to-me) surgical anastomosis of two previously remote portions of the stomach.

gastrogavage (-gah-vahzh′) artificial feeding through a tube passed into the stomach.

gastrogenic (-jen′ik) originating in the stomach.

Gastrografin (-gra′fin) trademark for a preparation of meglumine diatrizoate.

gastrograph (gas′tro-graf) an instrument for registering motions of stomach.

gastrohepatic (gas″tro-hĕ-pat′ik) pertaining to the stomach and liver.

gastrohepatitis (-hep″ah-ti′tis) inflammation of the stomach and liver.

gastroileac (-il′e-ak) pertaining to the stomach and ileum.

gastroileitis (-il″e-i′tis) inflammation of the stomach and ileum.

gastroileostomy (-il″e-os′to-me) surgical anastomosis of the stomach to the ileum.

gastrointestinal (-in-tes′tĭ-nal) pertaining to the stomach and intestine.

gastrojejunocolic (-je-ju″no-kol′ik) pertaining to the stomach, jejunum, and colon.

gastrojejunostomy (-je-ju-nos′to-me) surgical anastomosis of the stomach to the jejunum.

gastrolienal (-li′ĕ-nal) gastrosplenic.

gastrolith (gas′tro-lith) a calculus in the stomach.

gastrolithiasis (gas″tro-lĭ-thi′ah-sis) the presence or formation of gastroliths.

gastrology (gas-trol′o-je) study of the stomach and its diseases.

gastrolysis (gas-trol′ĭ-sis) surgical division of perigastric adhesions to mobilize the stomach.

gastromalacia (gas″tro-mah-la′she-ah) softening of the wall of the stomach.

gastromegaly (-meg′ah-le) enlargement of the stomach.

gastromelus (gas-trom′ĕ-lus) a fetus with a supernumerary leg on the abdomen.

gastromycosis (gas″tro-mi-ko′sis) fungal infection of the stomach.

gastromyotomy (-mi-ot′o-me) incision through the muscular coats of the stomach.

gastromyxorrhea (-mik″so-re′ah) excessive secretion of mucus by the stomach.

gastrone (gas'trōn) a reputed hormonal inhibitor of gastric acid secretion, extracted from gastric mucus.

gastroparalysis (gas"tro-pah-ral'ĭ-sis) paralysis of the stomach.

gastroparesis (-par'ĕ-sis) gastroparalysis.

gastropathy (gas-trop'ah-the) any disease of the stomach.

gastropexy (gas'tro-pek"se) surgical fixation of the stomach.

Gastrophilus (gas-trof'ĭ-lus) *Gasterophilus.*

gastrophrenic (gas"tro-fren'ik) pertaining to the stomach and diaphragm.

gastroplasty (gas'tro-plas"te) plastic repair of the stomach.

gastroplegia (gas"tro-ple'je-ah) gastroparalysis.

gastroplication (-pli-ka'shun) treatment of gastric dilatation by stitching a fold in the stomach wall.

gastroptosis (gas"trop-to'sis) downward displacement of the stomach.

gastropulmonary (gas"tro-pul'mo-ner"e) pertaining to the stomach and lungs.

gastropylorectomy (-pi"lo-rek'to-me) excision of the pyloric part of the stomach.

gastropyloric (-pi-lor'ik) pertaining to the entire stomach and to the pylorus.

gastrorrhagia (-ra'je-ah) hemorrhage from the stomach.

gastrorrhaphy (gas-tror'ah-fe) suture of the stomach.

gastrorrhea (gas"tro-re'ah) excessive secretion by the glands of the stomach.

gastroschisis (gas-tros'kĭ-sis) congenital fissure of the abdominal wall.

gastroscope (gas'tro-skōp) an endoscope for inspecting the interior of the stomach. **gastroscop'ic,** adj.

gastroscopy (gas-tros'ko-pe) inspection of the interior of the stomach with a gastroscope.

gastrospasm (gas'tro-spazm) spasm of the stomach.

gastrosplenic (gas"tro-splen'ik) pertaining to the stomach and spleen.

gastrostaxis (-stak'sis) the oozing of blood from the stomach mucosa.

gastrostenosis (-stĕ-no'sis) contraction or shrinkage of the stomach.

gastrostogavage (gas-tros"to-gah-vahzh') feeding through a gastric fistula.

gasgrostolavage (-lah-vahzh') irrigation of the stomach through a gastric fistula.

gastrostomy (gas-tros'to-me) creation of an artificial opening into the stomach.

gastrothoracopagus (gas"tro-thor"ah-kop'ah-gus) symmetrical conjoined twins joined at the abdomen and thorax.

gastrotomy (gas-trot'o-me) incision into the stomach.

gastrotonometer (gas"tro-to-nom'ĕ-ter) an instrument for measuring intragastric pressure.

gastrotropic (-trop'ik) having an affinity for or exerting a special effect on the stomach.

gastrotympanities (-tim"pah-ni'tēz) tympanitic distention of the stomach.

gastrula (gas'troo-lah) the embryonic state following the blastula; the simplest type consists of two layers (ectoderm and endoderm) which have invaginated to form the archenteron and an opening, the blastopore.

gastrulation (gas"troo-la'shun) the formation of a gastrula.

gauntlet (gawnt'let) a bandage covering the hand and fingers like a glove.

gauss (gows) the unit of magnetic flux density.

gauze (gawz) a light, open-meshed fabric of muslin or similar material. **absorbent g.,** white cotton cloth of various thread counts and weights, supplied in various lengths and widths and in different forms (rolls or folds). **petrolatum g.,** a sterile material produced by saturation of sterile absorbent gauze with sterile white petrolatum.

gavage (gah-vahzh') [Fr.] 1. forced feeding, especially through a tube passed into the stomach. 2. superalimentation.

g-cal. gram calorie (small calorie).

Gd chemical symbol, *gadolinium.*

Ge chemical symbol, *germanium.*

gegenhalten (ga"gen-halt'en) [Ger.] an involuntary resistance to passive movement, as may occur in cerebral cortical disorders.

gel (gel) a colloid that is firm in consistency, although containing much liquid; a colloid in gelatinous form. **aluminum hydroxide g.,** a suspension of aluminum oxide in the form of aluminum hydroxide and hydrated oxide, used to reduce gastric acidity, as a demulcent and protective for gastric mucosa, as a vehicle to increase absorption of orally administered penicillin, and in conjunction with a low phosphorus diet in the treatment of renal disease. **aluminum phosphate g.,** a water suspension of aluminum phosphate and some flavoring agents; used as a gastric antacid, astringent, and demulcent. **basic aluminum carbonate g.,** an aluminum hydroxide-aluminum carbonate gel, used as a phosphorus-binding agent in prevention of recurrent phosphatic calculi and as a gastric antacid.

gelasmus (jĕ-las'mus) hysterical laughter.

gelastic (jĕ-las'tik) pertaining to laughter.

gelatin (jel'ah-tin) a substance obtained by partial hydrolysis of collagen derived from skin, white connective tissue, and bones of animals; used as a suspending agent and in the manufacture of capsules and suppositories; suggested for use as a plasma substitute, and has been used as an adjuvant protein food. **zinc g.,** a preparation of zinc oxide, gelatin, glycerin, and purified water, applied topically as a protective.

gelatinase (jĕ-lat'ĭ-nās) an enzyme that liquefies gelatin, but does not affect fibrin and egg albumin; occurs among bacteria, molds, and yeasts.

gelatiniferous (jel"ah-tin-if'er-us) producing gelatin.

gelatinize (jĕ-lat'ĭ-nīz) to convert into, or become converted into, gelatin.

gelatinoid (jĕ-lat'ĭ-noid) resembling gelatin.

gelatinolytic (jĕ-lat"ĭ-no-lit'ik) dissolving or splitting up gelatin.

gelatinosa (jel″ah-tĭ-no′sah) [L.] gelatinous.

gelatinous (jĕ-lat′ĭ-nus) like jelly or softened gelatin.

gelation (jĕ-la′shun) conversion of a sol into a gel.

geld (geld) to remove the testes, especially of the horse.

Gelfilm (jel′film) trademark for absorbable gelatin film.

Gelfoam (-fōm) trademark for preparations of absorbable gelatin sponge.

gelose (jel′ōs) agar.

gelosis (je-lo′sis) a hard lump in a tissue, especially in muscle.

gemellology (jem″el-ol′o-je) the scientific study of twins and twinning.

geminate (jem′ĭ-nāt) paired; occurring in twos.

gemistocyte (jem-is′to-sīt) an astrocyte in which the cell body swells considerably, the nucleus is in an eccentric position, and the cytoplasm is clearly visible. **gemistocyt′ic**, adj.

gemmation (jĕ-ma′shun) budding; asexual reproduction in which a portion of the cell body is thrust out and then becomes separated, forming a new individual.

gemmule (jem′ūl) 1. a reproductive bud; the immediate product of gemmation. 2. one of the many little excrescences upon the protoplasmic process of a nerve cell.

Gemonil (jem′o-nil) trademark for a preparation of metharbital.

-gen word element [Gr.], *an agent that produces.*

genal (je′nal) pertaining to the cheek; buccal.

gender (jen′der) sex; the category to which an individual is assigned on the basis of sex.

gene (jēn) the biologic unit of heredity, self-reproducing and located at a definite position (locus) on a particular chromosome. **allelic g's,** genes situated at corresponding loci in a pair of chromosomes. **complementary g's,** two independent pairs of nonallelic genes, neither of which will produce its effect in the absence of the other. **dominant g.,** one that produces an effect (the phenotype) in the organism regardless of the state of the corresponding allele. **histocompatibility g.,** one that determines the specificity of tissue antigenicity and thus the compatibility of donor and recipient in tissue transplantation and blood transfusion. **holandric g's,** genes located on the Y chromosome and appearing only in male offspring. **leaky g.,** one in which a switch in the sequence of bases in a nucleotide results in the production of a mutant protein that, because of a single amino acid replacement, has only partial enzymatic activity; a hypomorph. **lethal g.,** one whose presence brings about the death of the organism or permits survival only under certain conditions. **mutant g.,** one that has undergone a detectable mutation. **operator g.,** one serving as a starting point for reading the genetic code, and which, through interaction with a repressor, controls the activity of structural genes associated with it in the operon. **recessive g.,** one that produces an effect in the organism only when it is transmitted by both parents. **regulator g., repressor g.,** one that synthesizes re-

pressor, a substance which, through interaction with the operator gene, switches off the activity of the structural genes associated with it in the operon. **sex-linked g.,** one carried on a sex chromosome, especially on an X chromosome. **structural g.,** one that specifies the amino acid sequence of a polypeptide chain. **supplementary g's,** two independent pairs of genes which interact in such a way that one dominant will produce its effect even in the absence of the other, but the second requires the presence of the first to be effective.

genera (jen′er-ah) plural of *genus.*

generation (jen″ĕ-ra′shun) 1. the process of reproduction. 2. a class composed of all individuals removed by the same number of successive ancestors from a common predecessor, or occupying positions on the same level in a genealogical (pedigree) chart. **alternate g.,** the alternate generation by asexual and sexual means in an animal or plant species. **asexual g.,** production of a new organism not originating from union of gametes. **filial g., first,** the first-generation offspring of two parents; symbol F_1. **filial g., second,** all of the offspring produced by two individuals of the first filial generation; symbol F_2. **parental g.,** the generation with which a particular genetic study is begun; symbol P_1. **sexual g.,** production of a new organism from the zygote formed by the union of gametes. **spontaneous g.,** the discredited concept of continuous generation of living organisms from nonliving matter.

generative (jen′ĕ-ra″tiv) pertaining to reproduction.

generic (jĕ-ner′ik) 1. pertaining to a genus. 2. nonproprietary; denoting a drug name not protected by a trademark, usually descriptive of the drug's chemical structure.

genesiology (jĕ-ne″ze-ol′o-je) the sum of what is known concerning reproduction.

genesis (jen′ĕ-sis) creation; origination; used as a word termination joined to an element indicating the thing created, e.g., carcinogenesis.

genetic (jĕ-net′ik) 1. pertaining to reproduction or to birth or origin. 2. inherited.

geneticist (jĕ-net′ĭ-sist) a specialist in genetics.

genetics (jĕ-net′iks) the study of heredity. **biochemical g.,** the science concerned with the chemical and physical nature of genes and the mechanism by which they control the development and maintenance of the organism. **clinical g.,** the study of the possible genetic factors influencing the occurrence of a pathologic condition.

genetotrophic (jĕ-net″o-trof′ik) pertaining to genetics and nutrition; relating to problems of nutrition that are hereditary in nature, or transmitted through the genes.

genetous (jen′ĕ-tus) dating from fetal life.

Geneva Convention (jĕ-ne′vah) an international agreement of 1864, whereby, among other pledges, the signatory nations pledged themselves to treat the wounded and the army medical and nursing staff as neutrals on the field of battle.

genial (je′ne-al) pertaining to the chin.

genic (jen′ik) pertaining to or caused by the genes.

-genic word element [Gr.], *giving rise to; causing.*

genicular (jĕ-nik′u-lar) pertaining to the knee.

geniculate (jĕ-nik′u-lāt) bent, like a knee.

geniculum (jĕ-nik′u-lum), pl. *genic′ula* [L.] a little knee; used in anatomic nomenclature to designate a sharp kneelike bend in a small structure or organ.

genion (je′ne-on) apex of lower genial tubercle.

genioplasty (je′ne-o-plas″te) plastic surgery of the chin.

genital (jen′ĭ-tal) 1. pertaining to reproduction, or to the reproductive organs. 2. [pl.] the reproductive organs.

genitalia (jen″ĭ-ta′le-ah) the reproductive organs. **external g.,** the reproductive organs external to the body, including pudendum, clitoris, and female urethra in the female, and scrotum, penis, and male urethra in the male. **indifferent g.,** the reproductive organs of the embryo prior to the establishment of definitive sex.

genitaloid (jen′ĭ-tal-oid″) pertaining to the primordial sex cells, before future sexuality is distinguishable.

genito- word element [L.], *the organs of reproduction.*

genitocrural (jen″ĭ-to-kroo′ral) pertaining to the genitalia and the thigh.

genitofemoral (-fem′o-ral) genitocrural.

genitoplasty (jen′ĭ-to-plas″te) plastic surgery on the genital organs.

genitourinary (jen″ĭ-to-u′rĭ-ner″e) urogenital.

genoblast (jen′o-blast) 1. the nucleus of the impregnated ovum. 2. a mature germ cell.

genocopy (-kop″e) an individual whose phenotype mimics that of another genotype but whose character is determined by a distinct assortment of genes.

genodermatosis (je″no-der″mah-to′sis) a genetic disorder of the skin, usually generalized.

genome (je′nōm) the complete set of hereditary factors contained in the haploid set of chromosomes. **genom′ic,** adj.

genotype (jen″o-tīp) 1. the entire genetic constitution of an individual; also, the alleles present at one or more specific loci. 2. the type species of a genus. **genotyp′ic,** adj.

-genous word element [Gr.], *arising or resulting from; produced by.*

gentamicin (jen″tah-mi′sin) an antibiotic elaborated by fungi of the genus *Micromonospora*, effective against *Pseudomonas* and certain other gram-negative bacilli; the sulfate salt is prepared as a cream and ointment for topical application.

gentian (jen′shan) the dried rhizome and roots of *Gentiana lutea;* has been used as a bitter tonic.

gentianophilic (jen″shan-o-fil′ik) staining readily with gentian violet.

gentianophobic (-fo′bik) not staining with gentian violet.

genu (je′nu), pl. *gen′ua* [L.] the knee; any kneelike structure. **g. extror′sum,** bowleg. **g. in-**

tror′sum, knock-knee. **g. recurva′tum,** hyperextensibility of the knee joint. **g. val′gum,** knock-knee. **g. va′rum,** bowleg.

genus (je′nus), pl. *gen′era* [L.] a taxonomic category (taxon) subordinate to a tribe (or subtribe) and superior to a species (or subgenus).

geo- word element [Gr.], *the earth; the soil.*

geobiology (je″o-bi-ol′o-je) the biology of terrestrial life.

geode (je′ōd) a dilated lymph space.

geomedicine (je″o-med′ĭ-sin) the branch of medicine dealing with the influence of climatic and environmental conditions on health.

geophagia, geophagism (je″o-fa′je-ah; je-of′ah-jizm) the eating of earth (soil) or clay.

geotaxis (je″o-tak′sis) geotropism.

geotragia (-tra′je-ah) geophagia.

geotrichosis (-trĭ-ko′sis) a candidiasis-like infection due to *Geotrichum candidum*, which may attack the bronchi, lungs, mouth, or intestinal tract.

Geotrichum (je-ot′rĭ-kum) a genus of yeastlike fungi, including *G. can′didum*, found in the feces and in dairy products.

geotropism (je-ot′ro-pizm) a tendency of growth or movement toward or away from the earth; the influence of gravity on growth.

ger-, gero-, geronto- word element [Gr.], *old age; the aged.*

geratic (jĕ-rat′ik) pertaining to old age.

geratology (jer″ah-tol′o-je) gereology.

gereology (jer″e-ol′o-je) the science dealing with old age.

geriatrics (-at′riks) the department of medicine dealing especially with the problems of aging and diseases of the elderly. **dental g.,** gerodontics. **geriat′ric,** adj.

geriodontics (-o-don′tiks) gerodontics.

germ (jerm) 1. a pathogenic microorganism. 2. a living substance capable of developing into an organ, part, or organism as a whole; a primordium. **dental g.,** collective tissues from which a tooth is formed. **enamel g.,** the epithelial rudiment of the enamel organ. **wheat g.,** the embryo of wheat which contains tocopherol, thiamine, riboflavin, and other vitamins.

germanin (jer′mah-nin) sodium suramin.

germanium (jer-ma′ne-um) chemical element (*see table*), at. no. 32, symbol Ge.

germicidal (jer″mĭ-si′dal) lethal to pathogenic microorganisms.

germicide (jer′mĭ-sīd) an agent that kills pathogenic microorganisms.

germinal (jer′mĭ-nal) pertaining to or of the nature of a germ cell or the primitive stage of development.

germination (jer″mĭ-na′shun) the sprouting of a seed or spore or of a plant embryo.

germinative (jer′mĭ-na″tiv) pertaining to germination or to a germ cell.

germinoma (jer″mĭ-no′mah) a neoplasm of germ tissue (testis or ovum), e.g., a seminoma.

gerocomia (jer″o-ko′me-ah) the care of old men; the hygiene of old age.

geroderma, gerodermia (-der′mah; -der′me-ah) dystrophy of the skin and genitals, giving the appearance of old age.

gerodontics (-don′tiks) dentistry dealing with the dental problems of older people. **gerodon′tic,** adj.

gerodontist (-don′tist) a dentist specializing in gerodontics.

gerodontology (-don-tol′o-je) study of the dentition and dental problems in the aged and aging.

geromarasmus (-mah-raz′mus) the emaciation sometimes characteristic of old age.

geromorphism (-mor′fizm) premature senility.

gerontal (jĕ-ron′tal) pertaining to old age.

gerontologist (jer″on-tol′o-jist) a physician specializing in gerontology.

gerontology (jer″on-tol′o-je) the scientific study of the problems of aging in all its aspects.

gerontopia (-to′pe-ah) senopia.

gerontotherapeutics (je-ron″to-ther″ah-pu′-tiks) the science of retarding and preventing the development of many of the aspects of senescence.

gerontoxon (jer″on-tok′son) arcus senilis.

gestagen (jes′tah-jen) any hormone with progestational activity.

gestalt (ges-tawlt′) a whole perceptual configuration.

gestaltism (gĕ-stawl′tizm) the theory in psychology that the objects of mind, as immediately presented to direct experience, come as complete unanalyzable wholes or forms (Gestalten) which cannot be split up into parts.

gestation (jes-ta′shun) the period of development of the young in viviparous animals, from the time of fertilization of the ovum; see also *pregnancy.*

gestosis (jes-to′sis) any toxemic manifestation in pregnancy.

GFR glomerular filtration rate.

ghost (gōst) a faint or shadowy figure lacking the customary substance of reality. **blood g.,** phantom corpuscle.

G.I. gastrointestinal; globin insulin.

giantism (ji′an-tizm) 1. gigantism. 2. excessive size, as of cells or nuclei.

Giardia (je-ar′de-ah) a genus of flagellate protozoa parasitic in the intestinal tract of man and animals, which may cause protracted, intermittent diarrhea with symptoms suggesting malabsorption; *G.* lam′blia (*G. intestina′lis*) is the species found in man.

giardiasis (je″ar-di′ah-sis) infection with *Giardia.*

gibberellin (gib″ber-el′in) any of a class of phytohormones whose most striking activity is the promotion of lateral bud development in decapitated plant stems; first isolated from fungi of the genus *Gibberella.*

gibbosity (gĭ-bos′ĭ-te) the condition of being humped; kyphosis.

gibbous (gib′us) humped; protuberant.

gibbus (gib′us) a hump.

gid (gid) a disease of the brain and spinal cord of domestic animals, especially sheep, due to *Coe-*

nurus cerebralis, and marked by unsteadiness of gait.

giga- word element [Gr.], *huge;* used in naming units of measurement to designate an amount 10^9 (one billion) times the size of the unit to which it is joined, e.g., gigameter (10^9 meters); symbol G.

gigantism (ji-gan′tizm) abnormal overgrowth; excessive size and stature. **cerebral g.,** gigantism in the absence of increased levels of growth hormone, attributed to a cerebral defect; infants are large, and accelerated growth continues for the first 4 or 5 years, the rate being normal thereafter. The hands and feet are large, the head large and dolichocephalic, the eyes have an antimongoloid slant, with hypertelorism. The child is clumsy, and mental retardation of varying degree is usually present. **eunuchoid g.,** gigantism in which the body shows the proportions of a eunuch and sexual deficiency. **pituitary g.,** Launois' syndrome.

gigantomastia (ji-gan′to-mas′te-ah) extreme hypertrophy of the breast.

ginger (jin′jer) the dried rhizome of the tropical plant *Zingiber officinale;* used as a flavoring agent.

gingiva (jin-ji′vah, jin′jĭ-vah), pl. *gingi′vae* [L.] the gum; the mucous membrane, with supporting fibrous tissue, covering the tooth-bearing border of the jaw. **gingi′val,** adj. **alveolar g.,** the portion covering the alveolar process. **areolar g.,** the portion attached to the alveolar process by loose areolar connective tissue. **free g.,** the portion covering part of the crowns of the teeth, but not attached to them. **marginal g.,** gingival margin.

gingivalgia (jin″jĭ-val′je-ah) pain in the gingivae.

gingivally (jin-ji′val-e) toward the gingiva.

gingivectomy (jin″jĭ-vek′to-me) surgical excision of all loose infected and diseased gingival tissue.

gingivitis (jin″jĭ-vi′tis) inflammation of the gingiva. **atrophic g., senile,** a condition characterized by hyperkeratinization and areas of desquamation in the gingiva. **fusospirochetal g.,** necrotizing ulcerative g. **herpetic g.,** infection of the gingivae by the herpes simplex virus. **necrotizing ulcerative g., ulceromembranous g., Vincent's g.,** trench mouth; a gingival infection marked by redness and swelling, necrosis, pain, hemorrhage, a necrotic odor, and often a pseudomembrane; see also under *gingivostomatitis.*

gingivo- word element [L.], *gingival.*

gingivoglossitis (jin″jĭ-vo-glos-si′tis) inflammation of the gingivae and tongue.

gingivolabial (-la′be-al) pertaining to the gingivae and lips.

gingivoplasty (jin′jĭ-vo-plas″te) surgical remodeling of the gingiva.

gingivosis (jin″jĭ-vo′sis) a chronic, diffuse inflammation of the gingivae, with desquamation of papillary epithelium and mucous membrane.

gingivostomatitis (jin″jĭ-vo-sto″mah-ti′tis) inflammation of the gingivae and oral mucosa. **herpetic g.,** that due to infection with herpes simplex virus, with redness of the oral tissues, formation of multiple vesicles and painful ulcers, and fever. **necrotizing ulcerative g.,** that due to extension of necrotizing ulcerative gingivitis to other areas of the oral mucosa.

ginglymoarthrodial (jing″glĭ-mo-ar-thro′de-al) partly ginglymoid and partly arthrodial.

ginglymoid (jing′glĭ-moid) resembling a hinge; pertaining to a ginglymus.

ginglymus (jing′glĭ-mus) a joint that allows movement in but one plane, forward and backward, as does a door hinge.

girdle (ger′d'l) cingulum; an encircling structure or part; anything encircling the body. **pectoral g.,** shoulder g. **pelvic g.,** the encircling bony structure supporting the lower limbs. **shoulder g., thoracic g.,** the encircling bony structure supporting the upper limbs.

Gitaligin (jĭ-tal′ĭ-jin) trademark for a preparation of gitalin.

gitalin (jit′ah-lin) amorphous gitalin; a mixture of digitalis glycosides used as a cardiotonic in congestive heart failure and cardiac arrhythmias.

githagism (gith′ah-jizm) poisoning by seeds of the corn cockle *Agrostemma githago.*

gizzard (giz′ard) the muscular second stomach of a bird.

glabella (glah-bel′ah) the area on the frontal bone above the nasion and between the eyebrows.

glabrous (gla′brus) smooth and bare.

gladiolus (glah-di′o-lus) corpus sterni.

glairy (glār′e) resembling egg white.

gland (gland) an aggregation of cells specialized to secrete or excrete materials not related to their ordinary metabolic needs. **accessory g.,** a minor mass of glandular tissue near or at some distance from a gland of similar structure. **acinous g.,** one made up of one or more acini. **adrenal g.,** a flattened body above either kidney, consisting of a cortex and a medulla, the former elaborating steroid hormones, and the latter epinephrine and norepinephrine. **aggregate g's, agminated g's,** Peyer's patches. **alveolar g.,** acinous g. **apocrine g.,** one whose discharged secretion contains part of the secreting cells. **areolar g's,** sebaceous glands in the mammary areola. **axillary g's,** lymph nodes situated in the axilla. **Bartholin's g.,** one of two small bodies on either side of the vaginal orifice. **Blandin's g's,** anterior lingual g's. **Bowman's g's,** olfactory g's. **bronchial g's,** seromucous glands in the mucosa and submucosa of bronchial walls. **Bruch's g's,** lymph follicles in the conjunctiva of lower lid. **Brunner's g's,** duodenal g's. **buccal g's,** seromucous glands on the inner surface of the cheeks. **bulbocavernous g., bulbourethral g.,** one of two glands embedded in the substance of the sphincter of the urethra, posterior to the membranous part of the urethra. **cardiac g's,** mucin-secreting glands of the cardiac part (cardia) of the stomach. **celiac g's,** lymph nodes anterior to the abdominal aorta. **ceruminous g's,** cerumen-secreting glands in the skin of the external auditory canal. **cervical g's,** 1. the lymph nodes of the

neck. 2. compound clefts in the wall of the uterine cervix. **ciliary g's,** sweat glands that have become arrested in their development, situated at the edges of the eyelids. **circumanal g's,** specialized sweat and sebaceous glands around the anus. **closed g.,** endocrine g. **Cobelli's g's,** mucous glands in the esophageal mucosa just above the cardia. **coccygeal g.,** glomus coccygeum. **compound g.,** one made up of a number of smaller units whose excretory ducts combine to form ducts of progressively higher order. **conglobate g.,** a lymph node. **Cowper's g.,** bulbourethral g. **ductless g's,** endrocrine g's. **duodenal g's,** glands in the submucosa of the duodenum, opening into the glands of the small intestine. **Duverney's g.,** bulbourethral g. **Ebner's g's,** serous glands at the back of the tongue near the taste buds. **eccrine g.,** one of the ordinary, or simple, sweat glands, which is of the merocrine type. **endocrine g's,** organs whose secretions (hormones) are released directly into the circulatory system; they include the pituitary, thyroid, parathyroid, and adrenal glands, the pineal body, and the gonads. **excretory g.,** one that excretes waste products from the system. **exocrine g.,** one whose secretion is discharged through a duct opening on an internal or external surface of the body. **fundic g's, fundus g's,** tubular glands in the mucosa of the fundus and body of the stomach, containing acid- and pepsin-secreting cells. **Galeati's g's,** duodenal g's. **gastric g's,** the secreting glands of the stomach, including the fundic, cardiac, and pyloric glands. **gastric g's, proper,** fundic g's. **Gay's g's,** circumanal g's. **genal g's,** buccal g's. **glossopalatine g's,** mucous glands at the posterior end of the smaller sublingual glands. **gustatory g's,** Ebner's g's. **guttural g.,** one of the mucous glands of the pharynx. **Harder's g's, harderian g's,** accessory lacrimal glands at the inner corner of the eye in animals that have nictitating membranes. **haversian g's,** synovial villi. **hematopoietic g's,** glandlike bodies that take part in blood formation, e.g., the spleen. **hemolymph g's,** see under *node.* **holocrine g.,** one whose discharged secretion contains the entire secreting cells. **intestinal g's,** straight tubular glands in the mucous membrane of the instestine, opening, in the small intestine, between the bases of the villi, and containing argentaffin cells. **jugular g.,** accessory lacrimal glands deep in the conjunctival connective tissue, mainly near the upper fornix. **Krause's g's,** mucous glands in the middle portion of the conjunctiva. **lacrimal g's,** the glands which secrete tears. **g's of Lieberkühn,** intestinal g's. **lingual g's,** the seromucous glands on the surface of the tongue. **lingual g's, anterior,** the seromucous glands near the apex of the tongue. **Littre's g's,** 1. preputial g's. 2. urethral g's (male). **Luschka's g.,** glomus coccygeum. **lymph g.,** see under *node.* **mammary g.,** the specialized gland of the skin of female mammals, which secretes milk for nourishment of the young. **meibomian g's,** sebaceous follicles between the cartilage and conjunctiva of eyelids. **merocrine g.,** one in which the secretory cells maintain their integrity throughout the secretory cycle. **mixed g's,** 1. seromucous g's. 2. glands that have both exocrine and endocrine portions. **Moll's g's,** ciliary g's. **monoptychic g.,** one in which the tubules or alveoli are lined with a single layer of secreting cells. **Montgomery's g's,** areolar g's. **Morgagni's g's,** urethral g's (male). **mucous g's,** glands which secrete mucus. **nabothian g's,** see under *follicle.* **Nuhn's g's,** anterior lingual g's. **oil g.,** sebaceous g. **olfactory g's,** small mucous glands in the olfactory mucosa. **parathyroid g's,** small bodies in the region of the thyroid gland, developed from the entoderm of the branchial clefts, occurring in a variable number of pairs, commonly two; they secrete parathyroid hormone and are concerned chiefly with the metabolism of calcium and phosphorus. **paraurethral g's,** see under *duct.* **parotid g.,** the largest of the three, paired salivary glands, located in front of the ear. **peptic g's,** fundic g's. **Peyer's g's,** see under *patch.* **pineal g.,** see under *body.* **pituitary g.,** the hypophysis; the epithelial body of dual origin at the base of the brain in the sella turcica, attached by a stalk to the hypothalamus; it consists of two main lobes, the *anterior lobe,* secreting several important hormones which regulate the proper functioning of the thyroids, gonads, adrenal cortex, and other endocrine organs, and the *posterior lobe,* whose cells serve as a reservoir for hormones having antidiuretic and oxytocic action, releasing them as needed. **preen g.,** a large, compound alveolar structure on the back of birds, above the base of the tail, which secretes an oily "water-proofing" material that the bird applies to its feathers and skin by preening. **preputial g's,** small sebaceous glands of the corona of the penis and the inner surface of the prepuce, which secrete smegma. **prostate g.,** see *prostate.* **pyloric g's,** the mucin-secreting glands of the pyloric part of the stomach. **racemose g's,** glands composed of acini arranged like grapes on a stem. **Rivinus g.,** sublingual g. **saccular g.,** one consisting of a sac or sacs, lined with glandular epithelium. **salivary g's,** glands of the oral cavity whose combined secretion constitutes the saliva, including the parotid, sublingual, and submandibular glands and numerous small glands in the tongue, lips, cheeks, and palate. **sebaceous g's,** holocrine glands in the corium that secrete an oily substance and sebum. **sentinel g.,** an enlarged lymph node, considered to be pathognomonic of some pathologic condition elsewhere. **seromucous g's,** glands that are both mucous and serous. **serous g.,** a gland that secretes a watery albuminous material, commonly but not always containing enzymes. **sex g's, sexual g's,** see *testis* and *ovary.* **simple g.,** one with a nonbranching duct. **Skene's g's,** paraurethral ducts. **solitary g's,** see under *follicle.* **sublingual g.,** a salivary gland on either side under the tongue. **submandibular g., submaxillary g.,** a salivary gland on the inner side of each ramus of the lower jaw. **sudoriferous g's,** sweat g's. **suprarenal g.,** adrenal g. **Susanne's g.,** a mucous gland of the mouth, beneath the alveolingual groove. **sweat g's,** glands that secrete sweat, situated in the corium or subcutaneous tissue, opening by a duct on the body surface. The ordinary or *eccrine sweat g's* are distributed over most of the body surface, and promote cooling by evaporation of the secretion; the *apocrine sweat g's* empty into the upper portion of a hair follicle instead of directly onto the skin, and are found only in certain body areas, as around the anus and in the axilla. **target g.,** one specifically affected by a pituitary hormone. **tarsal g's,** meibomian g's. **thymus g.,** see *thymus.* **thyroid g.,** an endocrine gland consisting of two lobes, one on each side of the trachea, joined by a narrow isthmus, producing hormones (thyroxine and triiodothyronine), which require iodine for their elaboration and which are concerned in regulating metabolic rate; it also secretes calcitonin. **tubular g.,** any gland made up of or containing a tubule or tubules. **tubuloacinar g.,** one that is both tubular and acinous. **Tyson's g's,** preputial g's. **urethral g's,** mucous glands in the wall of the urethra. **vaginal g.,** any gland of the vaginal mucosa. **Virchow's g.,** sentinel node. **vulvovaginal g.,** Bartholin g. **Waldeyer's g's,** glands in the attached edge of the eyelid. **Weber's g's,** the tubular mucous glands of the tongue. **Zeis' g's,** modified rudimentary sebaceous glands attached directly to the eyelash follicles. **Zuckerkandl's g's,** para-aortic bodies.

glanders (glan′derz) a contagious disease of horses, communicable to man, due to *Pseudomonas mallei,* and marked by purulent inflammation of the mucous membranes and cutaneous eruption of nodules that coalesce and break down, forming deep ulcers, which may end in necrosis of cartilage and bone; the more chronic and constitutional form is known as *farcy.*

glandilemma (glan″dĭ-lem′ah) the capsule or outer envelope of a gland.

glandula (glan′du-lah), pl. *glan′dulae* [L.] a gland.

glandular (glan′du-lar) 1. pertaining to or of the nature of a gland. 2. pertaining to the glans penis.

glandule (glan′dūl) a small gland.

glans (glanz), pl. *glan′des* [L.] a small, rounded mass or glandlike body. **g. clitor′idis,** erectile tissue on the free end of the clitoris. **g. pe′nis,** the cap-shaped expansion of the corpus spongiosum at the end of the penis.

glass (glas) 1. a hard, brittle, often transparent material, usually consisting of the fused amorphous silicates of potassium or sodium, and of calcium, with silica in excess. 2. a container, usually cylindrical, made from glass. 3. (pl.) lenses worn to aid or improve vision; see also *glasses* and *lens.* **cupping g.,** a vessel from which the air has been exhausted, applied to the skin in order to draw blood to the surface. **soluble g., water g.,** a potassium or sodium silicate sometimes used in preparing immovable bandages. **Wood's g.,** see under *light.*

glasses (glas′ez) spectacles; lenses arranged in a frame holding them in the proper position before the eyes, as an aid to vision. **bifocal g., Franklin g.,** those with lenses having two different refracting powers, one for distant and one for near vision. **trifocal g.,** glasses with lenses having three different refractive powers, one for distant, one for intermediate, and one for near vision.

glaucarubin (glaw″kah-ru′bin) a crystalline glycoside obtained from the fruit of *Simaruba glauca;* used as an amebicide.

glaucoma (glaw-ko′mah) a group of eye diseases characterized by an increase in intraocular pressure, causing pathological changes in the optic disk and typical visual field defects. **congenital g.,** that due to defective development of the structures in and around the anterior chamber of the eye and resulting in impairment of aqueous humor; see *infantile g.* and *juvenile g.* **Donders′ g.,** g. simplex. **infantile g.,** buphthalmos; hydrophthalmos; congenital glaucoma that may be fully developed at birth with enlarged eyes and hazy corneas, or may develop at any time up to two or three years of age. **juvenile g.,** congenital glaucoma differing from the infantile form in that it occurs in older children and young adults, and there is no gross enlargement of the eyeball. **narrow-angle g.,** a form of primary glaucoma in an eye characterized by a shallow anterior chamber and a narrow angle, in which filtration is compromised as a result of the iris blocking the angle. **open-angle g.,** a form of primary glaucoma in an eye in which the angle of the anterior chamber remains open, but filtration is gradually diminished because of the tissues of the angle. **primary g.,** increased intraocular pressure occurring in an eye without previous disease. **secondary g.,** increased intraocular pressure due to disease or injury to the eye. **g. sim′plex,** glaucoma without pronounced symptoms, but attended with progressive loss of vision.

glaucomatous (-tus) pertaining to or of the nature of glaucoma.

glaze (glāz) in dentistry, a ceramic veneer added to a procelain restoration, to simulate enamel.

gleet (glēt) 1. chronic gonorrheal urethritis. 2. a urethral discharge, especially one that is mucous or purulent.

glenoid (gle′noid) resembling a pit or socket.

glia (gli′ah) neuroglia.

gliacyte (-sīt) a cell of the neuroglia.

gliadin (-din) an alcohol-soluble protein from wheat.

glial (gli′al) of or pertaining to the neuroglia.

gliobacteria (gli″o-bac-te′re-ah) rod-shaped schizomycetes surrounded by a zooglea.

glioblastoma (-blas-to′mah) any malignant astrocytoma. **g. multifor′me,** astrocytoma Grade III or IV; a rapidly growing tumor, usually of the cerebral hemispheres, composed of spongioblasts, astroblasts, and astrocytes.

gliococcus (-kok′us) a micrococcus that forms gelatinous matter.

gliocyte (gli′o-sīt) gliacyte.

gliocytoma (gli″o-si-to′mah) glioma.

gliogenous (gli-oj′ĕ-nus) produced or formed by neuroglia.

glioma (gli-o′mah) a tumor composed of neuroglia in any of its states of development; sometimes extended to include all intrinsic neoplasms of the brain and spinal cord, as astrocy-

tomas, ependymomas, etc. **g. ret′inae,** retinoblastoma.

gliomatosis (gli″o-mah-to′sis) excessive development of the neuroglia, especially of the spinal cord, in certain cases of syringomylia.

gliomatous (gli-o′mah-tus) pertaining to or of the nature of glioma.

glioneuroma (gli″o-nu-ro′mah) glioma combined with neuroma.

gliosarcoma (-sar-ko′mah) glioma combined with sarcoma.

gliosis (gli-o′sis) an excess of astroglia in damaged areas of the central nervous system.

gliosome (gli′o-sōm) one of the small cytoplasmic processes of neuroglial cells.

gliotoxin (gli″o-tok′sin) an antibiotic substance obtained from several unrelated species of fungi, including *Trichoderma* (*Gliocladium*).

glissonitis (glis″o-ni′tis) inflammation of Glisson's capsule.

globi (glo′bi) 1. plural of *globus.* 2. encapsulated globular masses containing bacilli; seen in smears of lepromatous leprosy lesions.

globin (glo′bin) the protein constituent of hemoglobin; also, any member of a group of proteins similar to the typical globin.

globinometer (glo″bĭ-nom′ĕ-ter) an instrument for determining the proportion of oxyhemoglobin in the blood.

globoside (glob′o-sīd) a sphingoglycolipid containing acetylated amino sugars and simple hexoses, occurring in human serum, spleen, liver, and erythrocytes, and accumulating in tissues in Sandhoff's disease.

globule (glob′ūl) a small spherical mass; a little globe or pellet, as of medicine. **glob′ular,** adj.

globulin (glob′u-lin) a class of proteins which are insoluble in water, but soluble in saline solutions (euglobulins), or water-soluble proteins (pseudoglobulins) whose other physical properties resemble true globulins; see *serum g.* **accelerator g.,** coagulation Factor V. **alpha g's,** globulins in plasma which, in neutral or alkaline solutions, have the greatest electrophoretic mobility, in this respect most nearly resembling the albumins. **antihemophilic g.,** coagulation Factor VIII. **beta g's,** globulins in plasma which, in neutral or alkaline solutions, have an electrophoretic mobility between that of the alpha and that of the gamma globulins. **gamma g's,** a group of plasma globulins which, in neutral or alkaline solutions, have the slowest electrophoretic mobility and which have sites of antibody activity; see *immunoglobulin.* **immune g.,** 1. immunoglobulin. 2. a serum globulin that has been modified in response to infection or to injection of certain materials and contains antibodies to the antigens eliciting their production; used as a passive immunizing agent against measles or tetanus and in prophylaxis or treatment of pertussis. **serum g.,** the fraction of proteins precipitated from blood serum by half saturation with ammonium sulfate; the principal groups include the α-, β-, and γ-globulins.

globulinuria (glob″u-lin-u′re-ah) the presence of globulins in the urine.

globus (glo'bus), pl. *glo'bi* [L.] 1. a sphere or ball; a spherical structure. 2. a subjective sensation as of a lump or mass. **g. hyster'icus,** subjective sensation of a lump in the throat. **g. pal'lidus,** the smaller and more medial part of the lentiform nucleus of the brain.

glomangioma (glo-man″je-o'mah) a benign, often painful tumor derived from a glomus, usually occurring on the distal portion of the fingers or toes, in the skin, or in deeper structures.

glomectomy (glo-mek'to-me) excision of a glomus.

glomera (glom'er-ah) plural of *glomus.*

glomerular (glo-mer'u-lar) pertaining to or of the nature of a glomerulus, especially a renal glomerulus.

glomeruli (glo-mer'u-li) plural of *glomerulus.*

glomerulitis (glo-mer″u-li'tis) inflammation of the renal glomeruli.

glomerulonephritis (glo-mer″u-lo-ně-fri'tis) nephritis with inflammation of the capillary loops in the renal glomeruli. **lobular g.,** a form in which all glomeruli are affected, with accentuation of the lobulation of the glomerular tufts; it is marked by constant proteinuria and microscopic hematuria.

glomerulopathy (glo-mer″u-lop'ah-the) any disease of the renal glomeruli. **diabetic g.,** intercapillary glomerulosclerosis.

glomerulosclerosis (glo-mer″u-lo-skle-ro'sis) fibrosis and scarring resulting in senescence of the renal glomeruli. **intercapillary g.,** a degenerative complication of diabetes, manifested as albuminuria, nephrotic edema, hypertension, renal insufficiency, and retinopathy.

glomerulus (glo-mer'u-lus), pl. *glomer'uli* [L.] a small tuft or cluster, as of blood vessels or nerve fibers; often used alone to designate one of the renal glomeruli. **olfactory g.,** one of the small globular masses of dense neuropil in the olfactory bulb containing the first synapse in the olfactory pathway. **renal glomeruli,** coils of blood vessels, one projecting into the expanded end or capsule of each of the uriniferous tubules.

glomoid (glo'moid) resembling a glomus.

glomus (glo'mus), pl. *glom'era* [L.] a small histologically recognizable body composed primarily of fine arterioles connecting directly with veins, and having a rich nerve supply. **glom'era aor'tica,** aortic bodies. **g. carot'icum,** carotid body. **g. choroi'deum,** an enlargement of the choroid plexus of the lateral ventricle. **g. coccyg'eum,** a collection of arteriovenous anastomoses close to the tip of the coccyx formed by the middle sacral artery. **g. jugula're,** an aggregation of chemoreceptors in the bulb of the jugular vein.

gloss(o)- word element [Gr.], *tongue.*

glossal (glos'al) pertaining to the tongue.

glossalgia (glŏ-sal'je-ah) pain in the tongue.

glossectomy (glŏ-sek'to-me) excision of all or a portion of the tongue.

Glossina (glŏ-si'nah) a genus of biting flies, the tsetse flies, which serve as vectors of trypanosomes causing various forms of trypanosomiasis in man and animals.

glossitis (glŏ-si'tis) inflammation of the tongue. **g. area'ta exfoliati'va,** geographic tongue. **rhomboid g., median,** a congenital anomaly of the tongue, with a flat or slightly raised reddish patch or plaque on the midline of the dorsal surface.

glossocele (glos'o-sēl) swelling and protrusion of the tongue.

glossodynia (glos″o-din'e-ah) pain in the tongue.

glossoepiglottidean (-ep″ĭ-glŏ-tid'e-an) pertaining to the tongue and epiglottis.

glossograph (glos'o-graf) an apparatus for registering tongue movements in speech.

glossohyal (glos″o-hi'al) pertaining to the tongue and hyoid bone.

glossolalia (-la'le-ah) unintelligible speech.

glossology (glŏ-sol'o-je) 1. sum of knowledge regarding the tongue. 2. treatise on nomenclature.

glossopathy (glŏ-sop'ah-the) any disease of the tongue.

glossopharyngeal (glos″o-fah-rin'je-al) pertaining to the tongue and pharynx.

glossoplasty (glos'o-plas″te) plastic surgery of the tongue.

glossorrhaphy (glŏ-sōr'ah-fe) suture of the tongue.

glossospasm (glos'o-spazm) spasm of the tongue.

glossotomy (glŏ-sot'o-me) incision of the tongue.

glossotrichia (glos″o-trik'e-ah) hairy tongue.

glottic (glo'ik) pertaining to the glottis or to the tongue.

glottis (glot'tis), pl. *glot'tides* [Gr.] the vocal apparatus of the larynx, consisting of the true vocal cords and the opening between them.

Glu glutamic acid or glutamyl.

glucagon (gloo'kah-gon) a polypeptide hormone secreted by the pancreatic alpha cells that increases blood glucose concentration; its hydrochloride salt is used parenterally as a hyperglycemic.

glucagonoma (gloo″kah-gon-o'mah) a malignant glucagon-secreting tumor of the alpha cells of the pancreas.

glucinium (gloo-sin'e-um) beryllium.

glucocerebroside (gloo″ko-ser'ě-bro-sīd) a cerebroside with a glucose sugar.

glucocorticoid (-kor'tĭ-koid) any corticoid substance that increases gluconeogenesis, raising the concentration of liver glycogen and blood sugar.

Gluco-Ferrum (-fer'rum) trademark for preparations of ferrous gluconate.

glucofuranose (-fu'rah-nōs) a form of glucose in which carbon atoms 1 and 4 are bridged by an oxygen atom.

glucogenic (-jen'ik) giving rise to or producing glucose.

glucokinase (-ki'nās) an enzyme that in the presence of ATP catalyzes glucose to glucose 6-phosphate.

glucokinetic (-ki-net'ik) activating sugar so as to maintain the sugar level of the body.

glucokinin (-kin′in) a substance obtained from vegetable tissues and yeast; when injected into animals, it produces hyperglycemia, and in depancreatized dogs has an insulin-like effect.

gluconate (gloo′ko-nāt) a salt of gluconic acid, containing the $HOCH_2(CHOH)_5COO—$ radical. **ferrous g.,** a compound used in the treatment of iron deficiency anemia.

gluconeogenesis (gloo″ko-ne″o-jen′ĕ-sis) the synthesis of glucose by the liver and kidney from noncarbohydrate sources, such as amino and fatty acids.

glucophore (gloo′ko-fōr) the group of atoms in a molecule which gives the compound a sweet taste.

glucoprotein (gloo″ko-pro′te-in) glycoprotein.

glucopyranose (-pi′rah-nōs) a form of glucose in which carbon atoms 1 and 5 are bridged by an oxygen atom.

glucosamine (-sam′in) an α-amino derivative of dextrose (δ-glucose), obtained from mucin and chitin.

glucosan (gloo′ko-san) an anhydro-polymer yielding a hexose on hydrolysis.

glucosazone (gloo″ko-sa′sōn) a crystalline substance produced by treating dextrose with phenylhydrazine and acetic acid.

glucose (gloo′kōs) 1. D-glucose; a monosaccharide, $C_6H_{12}O_6$, in certain foodstuffs, especially fruit, and in normal blood; the chief source of energy for living organisms. 2. liquid g. **liquid g.,** a thick syrupy, sweet liquid, consisting chiefly of dextrose, with dextrins, maltose, and water, obtained by incomplete hydrolysis of starch; used as a flavoring agent, as a food, and in the treatment of dehydration. **g. 1-phosphate,** an intermediate in carbohydrate metabolism. **g. 6-phosphate,** an intermediate in carbohydrate metabolism.

glucosidase (gloo-ko′sĭ-dās) an enzyme of the hydrolase class that splits a glucoside, occurring as α-, β-, and α-1,3-glucosidase; α-g. (maltase) occurs in the intestinal juice, and β-g. (cellobiase) in the kidney, liver, and intestinal mucosa.

glucoside (gloo′ko-sīd) a glycoside in which the sugar constituent is glucose.

glucosin (-sin) any of a group of bases derived from glucose by the action of ammonia; some are highly toxic.

glucosulfone (gloo″ko-sul′fōn) a dapsone derivative; the sodium salt, $C_{24}H_{34}N_2Na_2O_{18}S_3$, is used as a leprostatic and tuberculostatic.

glucosuria (-su′re-ah) 1. the presence of dextrose in the urine. 2. dextrosuria.

β-glucuronidase (gloo″ku-ron′ĭ-dās) an enzyme that attacks glycosidic linkages in natural and synthetic glucuronides and has been implicated in estrogen metabolism and cell division; occurs in the spleen, liver, and endocrine glands.

glucuronide (gloo-ku′ron-īd) any compound with glucuronic acid.

glutamate (gloo′tah-māt) a salt of glutamic acid; in biochemistry, the term is often used interchangeably with glutamic acid.

glutaminase (gloo-tam′ĭ-nās) an enzyme that catalyzes the splitting of glutamine into glutamic acid and ammonia.

glutamine (gloo′tah-min) an amide of glutamic acid, occurring in the juices of many plants and in some animal tissues; it is an important carrier of urinary ammonia and is broken down in the kidney by glutaminase.

glutamyl (gloo′tah-mil) the univalent radical of glutamic acid.

Glutan H-C-L (gloo′tan) trademark for capsules containing glutamic acid hydrochloride.

glutaraldehyde (gloo″tahr-al′dĕ-hīd) a compound, $CHO \cdot (CH_2)_3 \cdot CHO$, used as a tissue fixative for light and electron microscopy because of its preservation of fine structural detail and localization of enzyme activity.

glutathione (gloo″tah-thi′ōn) a tripeptide in animal and plant tissues composed of glutamic acid, cysteine, and aminoacetic acid, it acts as a respiratory carrier of oxygen. **oxidized g.,** the precursor of reduced glutathione. **reduced g.,** a tripeptide present in red cells, deficiency of which probably predisposes erythrocytes to the oxidant and hemolytic effects of certain drugs.

gluteal (gloo′te-al) pertaining to the buttocks.

glutelin (gloo′tĕ-lin) a simple protein from the seeds of cereals.

gluten (gloo′ten) the protein of wheat and other grains that gives to the dough its tough elastic character.

glutethimide (gloo-teth′ĭ-mīd) a hypnotic and sedative, $C_{13}H_{15}NO_2$.

glutin (gloo′tin) 1. a viscid substance from the glutelin of wheat. 2. gelatin in its soft or dissolved state.

glutinous (gloo′tĭ-nus) adhesive; sticky.

glutitis (gloo-ti′tis) inflammation of the glutei muscles.

Gly glycine.

glycemia (gli-se′me-ah) the presence of glucose in the blood.

glyceraldehyde (glis″er-al′dĕ-hīd) a compound, glyceric aldehyde, $CH_2OHCHOHCHO$, formed by the oxidation of glycerol.

glyceride (glis′er-īd) an organic acid ester of glycerol, designated, according to the number of ester linkages, as mono-, di-, or triglyceride.

glycerin (glis′er-in) glycerol; a clear, colorless, syrupy liquid, $C_3H_8O_3$, used as a humectant and solvent for drugs; it is a trihydric sugar alcohol, being the alcoholic component of fats.

glycerite (glis′er-īt) a preparation of a medicinal substance in glycerin.

glycerol (glis′er-ol) glycerin.

glycerophosphate (glis″er-o-fos′fāt) a combination of a base with glycerin and phosphoric acid.

glycerose (glis′er-ōs) a sugar formed by oxidizing glycerol; there are two glyceroses, glyceraldehyde and dihydroxyacetone.

glyceryl (glis′er-il) the trivalent radical, C_3H_5O, of glycerin. **g. monostearate,** an emulsifying agent. **g. triacetate,** triacetin. **g. trinitrate,** nitroglycerin.

glycine (gli′sēn) aminoacetic acid.

glycobiarsol (gli″ko-bi-ar′sol) an amebicide, C_8-$H_9A_2BiNO_6$, used in intestinal amebiasis.

glycocalyx (-kal′iks) the glycoprotein-polysaccharide covering that surrounds many cells.

glycocholate (-ko′lāt) a salt of glycocholic acid.

glycocoll (gli′ko-kol) aminoacetic acid.

glycogen (-jen) a polysaccharide, the chief carbohydrate storage material in animals, formed by and largely stored in the liver and to a lesser extent in muscles; it is depolymerized to glucose and liberated as needed. **glycogen′ic,** adj.

glycogenase (-jĕ-nās″) an enzyme which splits glycogen into dextrin and maltose.

glycogenesis (gli″ko-jen′ĕ-sis) the conversion of glucose to glycogen for storage in the liver. **glycogenet′ic,** adj.

glycogenic (-jen′ik) pertaining to, characterized by, or promoting glycogenesis; pertaining to glycogen.

glycogenolysis (-jĕ-nol′ĭ-sis) the splitting up of glycogen in the liver, yielding glucose. **glycogenolyt′ic,** adj.

glycogenosis (-jĕ-no′sis), pl. *glycogeno′ses.* A group of genetically determined disorders of glycogen metabolism, marked by abnormal storage of glycogen in the body tissues. See *Gierke's disease* (glycogenosis, type I), *Pompe's disease* (type II), *Forbes' disease* (type III), *amylopectinosis* (type IV), *McArdle's disease* (type V), and *Hers' disease* (type VI). **generalized g.,** Pompe's disease. **hepatorenal g.,** Gierke's disease. **myophosphorylase deficiency g.,** McArdle's disease.

glycogenous (gli-koj′ĕ-nus) glycogenic.

glycogeusia (gli″ko-gu′se-ah) a sweet taste in the mouth.

glycol (gli′kol) any of a group of aliphatic dihydric alcohols, having marked hygroscopic properties and useful as solvents and plasticizers.

glycolipid (gli″ko-lip′id) a lipid containing carbohydrate groups, usually galactose but also glucose, inositol, or others; the glycolipids include the cerebrosides.

glycolysis (gli-kol′ĭ-sis) the breaking down of sugars into simpler compounds chiefly pyruvate or lactate. **glycolyt′ic,** adj.

glycometabolic (gli″ko-met″ah-bol′ik) pertaining to the metabolism of sugar.

glyconeogenesis (-ne″o-jen′ĕ-sis) gluconeogenesis.

glyconucleoprotein (-nu″kle-o-pro′te-in) a nucleoprotein bearing carbohydrate groups.

glycopenia (-pe′ne-ah) a deficiency of sugar in the tissues.

glycopexis (-pek′sis) fixation or storing of sugar or glycogen. **glycopec′tic,** adj.

glycophilia (-fil′e-ah) a condition in which a small amount of glucose produces hyperglycemia.

glycoprotein (-pro′te-in) any of a class of conjugated proteins consisting of a compound of protein with a carbohydrate group.

glycoptyalism (-ti′ah-lizm) glycosialia.

glycopyrrolate (-pir′o-lāt) an anticholinergic, $C_{19}H_{28}BrNO_3$, used in gastrointestinal disorders.

glycorrhachia (-ra′ke-ah) the presence of glucose in the cerebrospinal fluid.

glycorrhea (-re′ah) any sugary discharge from the body.

glycosamine (-sam′in) glucosamine.

glycosecretory (-se-kre′to-re) concerned in secretion of glycogen.

glycosemia (-se′me-ah) glycemia.

glycosialia (-si-a′le-ah) sugar in the saliva.

glycosialorrhea (-si″ah-lo-re′ah) excessive flow of saliva containing glucose.

glycosidase (gli″ko-sĭ-dās) any of a large group of hydrolytic enzymes acting on glycosyl compounds.

glycoside (gli′ko-sīd) any compound containing a carbohydrate molecule (sugar), particularly any such natural product in plants, convertible, by hydrolytic cleavage, into a sugar and a nonsugar component (aglycone), and named specifically for the sugar contained, as glucoside (glucose), pentoside (pentose), fructoside (fructose), etc. **cardiac g.,** any of a group of glycosides in certain plants (*Digitalis*, etc.), having a characteristic action on the heart.

glycosometer (gli″ko-som′ĕ-ter) an instrument for determining proportion of glucose in urine.

glycosphingolipid (-sfing″o-lip′id) a sphingolipid containing the sugar glucose or galactose.

glycostatic (-stak′ik) tending to maintain a constant sugar level.

glycosuria (-su′re-ah) abnormally high sugar content in the urine. **renal g.,** that due to inherited inability of the renal tubules to reabsorb glucose completely.

glycosyl (gli′ko-sil) a radical derived from a carbohydrate.

glycotropic (gli″ko-trop′ik) having an affinity for sugar; causing hyperglycemia.

glycuresis (gli″ku-re′sis) the normal increase in glucose content of the urine which follows an ordinary carbohydrate meal.

glycyrrhiza (glis″ĭ-ri′zah) licorice; the dried rhizome and roots of the legume *Glycyrrhiza glabra,* used as a flavored vehicle for drugs.

glycyrrhizin (glis″ĭ-ri′zin) a sweet substance, $C_{42}H_{62}O_{16}$, from glycyrrhiza.

Glytheonate (gli-the′o-nāt) trademark for a preparation of theophylline sodium glycinate.

gm gram.

gnat (nat) a small dipterous insect. In Great Britain the term is applied to mosquitoes; in America to insects smaller than mosquitoes.

gnath(o)- word element [Gr.], *jaw.*

gnathic (nath′ik) pertaining to the jaw or cheeks.

gnathion (na′the-on) the most outward and everted point on the profile curvature of the chin.

gnathitis (na-thi′tis) inflammation of the jaw.

gnathocephalus (na″tho-sef′ah-lus) a headless monster with jaws.

gnathodynamometer (-di″nah-mom′ĕ-ter) an instrument for measuring the force exerted in closing the jaws.

gnathology (nah-thol′o-je) a science dealing

with the masticatory apparatus as a whole, including morphology, anatomy, histology, physiology, pathology, and therapeutics.

gnathoplasty (na'tho-plas"te) plastic surgery of the jaw or cheek.

gnathoschisis (nah-thos'kĭ-sis) congenital cleft of the upper jaw, as in cleft palate.

Gnathostoma (nah-thos'to-mah) a genus of nematodes parasitic in cats, swine, cattle, and sometimes man.

gnathostomiasis (nah-thos"to-mi'ah-sis) infection with *Gnathostoma*.

gnosia (no'se-ah) the faculty of perceiving and recognizing. **gnos'tic**, adj.

gnotobiology (no"to-bi-ol'o-je) gnotobiotics.

gnotobiota (-bi-o'tah) the specifically and entirely known microfauna and microflora of a specially reared laboratory animal.

gnotobiote (-bi'ōt) a specially reared laboratory animal whose microflora and microfauna are specifically known in their entirety. **gnotobiot'ic**, adj.

gnotobiotics (-bi-ot'iks) the science of rearing gnotobiotes.

goiter (goi'ter) enlargement of the thyroid gland, causing a swelling in the front part of the neck. **aberrant g.**, goiter of a supernumerary thyroid gland. **adenomatous g.**, that caused by adenoma or multiple colloid nodules of the thyroid gland. **Basedow's g.**, a colloid goiter which has become hyperfunctioning after administration of iodine. **colloid g.**, a large, soft thyroid gland with distended spaces filled with colloid. **cystic g.**, one with cysts formed by mucoid or colloid degeneration. **diving g.**, a movable goiter, located sometimes above and sometimes below the sternal notch. **exophthalmic g.**, goiter characterized by exophthalmos; see *Graves' disease*. **fibrous g.**, goiter in which the capsule and the stroma of the thyroid gland are hyperplastic. **follicular g.**, parenchymatous g. **intrathoracic g.**, one in which a portion of the enlarged gland is in the thoracic cavity. **lingual g.**, enlargement of the upper end of the thyroglossal duct, forming a tumor at the posterior part of the dorsum of the tongue. **lymphadenoid g.**, struma lymphomatosa. **nodular g.**, goiter with circumscribed nodules within the gland. **parenchymatous g.**, one marked by increase in follicles and proliferation of epithelium. **perivascular g.**, one that surrounds a large blood vessel. **plunging g.**, diving g. **retrovascular g.**, one with a process or processes behind an important blood vessel. **simple g.**, simple hyperplasia of the thyroid gland. **substernal g.**, one in which a portion of the enlarged gland is beneath the sternum. **suffocative g.**, one which causes dyspnea by pressure. **toxic g.**, Graves' disease. **vascular g.**, one due chiefly to dilatation of the blood vessels. **wandering g.**, diving g.

goitre (goi'ter) goiter.

goitrin (goi'trin) a goitrogenic substance isolated from rutabagas and turnips.

goitrogen (goi'tro-jen) a goiter-producing agent.

goitrogenic (goi"tro-jen'ik) producing goiter.

goitrogenicity (-jĕ-nis'ĭ-te) the tendency to produce goiter.

goitrous (goi'trus) pertaining to goiter.

gold (gōld) chemical element (*see table*), at. no. 79, symbol Au; gold compounds (all of which are poisonous) are used in medicine, chiefly in treating arthritis. **annealed g.**, gold which has been heated in a flame to increase its cohesive properties. **g. aurothiosulfate**, gold sodium thiosulfate. **cohesive g.**, chemically pure gold that forms a solid mass when properly condensed into a tooth cavity. **crystal g., crystalline g., fibrous g., mat g.**, pure gold composed of flakelike crystals formed by electrodeposition. **g. sodium thiomalate**, $C_4H_3AuNa_2O_4S\cdot H_2O$; used in treatment of rheumatoid arthritis and nondisseminated lupus erythematosus. **g. sodium thiosulfate**, $Na_3Au(S_2O_3)_2\cdot 2H_2O$; used in treatment of rheumatoid arthritis. **g. thioglucose**, aurothioglucose.

gomitoli (go-mit'o-li) a network of capillaries in the upper infundibular stem (of the hypothalamus) that surround terminal arterioles of the superior hypophyseal arteries and that lead into portal veins to the adenohypophysis.

gomphosis (gom-fo'sis) a type of fibrous joint in which a conical process is inserted into a socket-like portion.

gon- word element [Gr.], 1. *seed; semen*. 2. *knee*.

gonad (go'nad, gon'ad) a gamete-producing gland; an ovary or testis. **gonad'al, gonad'ial**, adj. **indifferent g.**, the sexually undifferentiated gonad of the early embryo. **third g.**, the adrenal gland, so called because of its interrelations with the sex glands.

gonadectomy (go"nah-dek'to-me) removal of a gonad.

gonadopathy (gon"ah-dop'ah-the) any disease of the gonads.

gonadotherapy (gon"ah-do-ther'ah-pe) treatment with gonadal hormones.

gonadotrophic (-trōf'ik) gonadotropic.

gonadotrophin (-trōf'in) gonadotropin.

gonadotropic (-trop'ik) stimulating the gonads; applied to hormones of the anterior pituitary which influence the gonads.

gonadotropin (-trōp'in) a substance which has a stimulating effect upon the gonads, especially the hormone secreted by the anterior pituitary. **chorionic g.**, a gonad-stimulating principle from human pregnancy urine or from the serum of pregnant mares; also, a dry sterile preparation of this principle from human pregnancy urine, used in the treatment of underdevelopment of the sex glands.

gonaduct (gon'ah-dukt) the duct of a gonad; an oviduct or seminal duct.

gonagra (go-nag'rah) gout in the knee.

gonalgia (go-nal'je-ah) pain in the knee.

gonangiectomy (go-nan"je-ek'to-me) vasectomy.

gonarthritis (gon"ar-thri'tis) inflammation of the knee joint.

gonarthrocace (-ar-throk'ah-se) tuberculous arthritis of the knee.

gonarthrotomy (-throt'o-me) incision into the knee joint.

gonecystis (gon"e-sis'tis) a seminal vesicle.

gonecystitis (-sis-ti'tis) inflammation of a seminal vesicle.

gonecystolith (-sis'to-lith) a concretion in a seminal vesicle.

gonecystopyosis (-sis"to-pi-o'sis) suppuration in a seminal vesicle.

gonidium (go-nid'e-um), pl. *gonid'ia* [Gr.] 1. the algal component of the thallus of a lichen. 2. a motile reproductive unit of certain nitrogen-fixing bacteria.

goniometer (go"ne-om'ĕ-ter) an instrument for measuring angles. **finger g.,** one for measuring the limits of flexion and extension of the interphalangeal joints of the fingers.

gonion (go'ne-on), pl. *go'nia* [Gr.] the most inferior, posterior, and lateral point on the external angle of the mandible. **go'nial,** adj.

goniopuncture (go"ne-o-punk'chur) insertion of a knife blade through the clear cornea, just within the limbus, across the anterior chamber of the eye and through the opposite corneoscleral wall, in treatment of glaucoma.

gonioscope (go'ne-o-skōp") an optical instrument for examining the anterior chamber of the eye and for demonstrating ocular motility and rotation.

gonioscopy (go"ne-os'ko-pe) examination of the angle of the anterior chamber with a gonioscope.

goniotomy (-ot'o-me) an operation for glaucoma; it consists in opening Schlemm's canal under direct vision.

gono- word element [Gr.], *seed; semen.*

gonocele (gon'o-sēl) spermatocele.

gonococcemia (gon"o-kok-se'me-ah) the presence of gonococci in the blood.

gonococcide (-kok'sīd) an agent destructive to gonococci.

gonococcus (-kok'us), pl. *gonococ'ci* [L.] an individual of the species *Neisseria gonorrhoeae,* the etiologic agent of gonorrhea. **gonococ'cal, gonococ'cic,** adj.

gonocyte (gon'o-sīt) the primitive reproductive cell of the embryo.

gonophore (-fōr) an accessory generative organ, such as the oviduct.

gonorrhea (gon"o-re'ah) infection with *Neisseria gonorrhoeae,* most often transmitted venereally, marked in males by urethritis with pain and purulent discharge; commonly asymptomatic in females, but may extend to produce salpingitis, oophoritis, tubo-ovarian abscess, and peritonitis. Bacteremia may occur in both sexes, causing skin lesions, arthritis, and rarely meningitis or endocarditis. **gonorrhe'al,** adj.

Gonyaulax (gon"e-aw'laks) a genus of dinoflagellates found in fresh, salt, or brackish waters, having yellow to brown chromatophores; it includes *G. catanel'la,* a poisonous species, which helps to form the destructive red tide in the ocean; see also under *poison.*

gonycampsis (gon"ĭ-kamp'sis) abnormal curvature of the knee.

gonyocele (gon'e-o-sēl") synovitis or tuberculous arthritis of the knee.

gonyoncus (gon"e-ong'kus) tumor of the knee.

gorget (gor'jet) a wide-grooved lithotome director.

GOT glutamic-oxalacetic transaminase.

gouge (gowj) a hollow chisel for cutting and removing bone.

goundou (gōōn'doo) a sequel of yaws, seen in natives of Central and South America, with headache, purulent nasal discharge, and formation of bony exostoses at the side of the nose.

gout (gowt) a hereditary form of arthritis marked by hyperuricemia and by recurrent paroxysmal attacks of acute arthritis usually involving a single peripheral joint, followed by complete remission; the attacks result from deposition of crystals of monosodium urate in and around affected joints. **gout'y,** adj. **latent g., masked g.,** lithemia without the typical features of gout. **misplaced g., retrocedent g.,** gout in which the arthritic symptoms have disappeared and are followed by severe constitutional disturbances. **rheumatic g.,** rheumatoid arthritis.

G.P. general practitioner; general paresis (see *dementia paralytica*).

G6PD glucose-6-phosphate dehydrogenase.

GPT glutamic-pyruvic transaminase.

gr. grain.

gracile (gras'il) slender; delicate.

gradient (gra'de-ent) rate of increase or decrease of a variable value, or its representative curve.

graduate (grad'u-āt) 1. a person who has received a degree from a university or college. 2. a measuring vessel marked by a series of lines.

graduated (grad'u-āt"ed) marked by a succession of lines, steps, or degrees.

graft (graft) any tissue or organ for implantation or transplantation; to implant or transplant such tissue. See also *flap.* **accordion g.,** a full-thickness graft in which slits have been made to that it may be stretched to cover a larger area. **autodermic g., autoepidermic g.,** a skin graft taken from the patient's own body. **autologous g., autoplastic g.,** autograft. **avascular g.,** a graft of tissue in which not even transient vascularization is achieved. **Blair-Brown g.,** a split-skin graft of intermediate thickness. **bone g.,** a piece of bone used to take the place of a removed bone or bony defect. **cable g.,** a nerve graft made up of several sections of nerve in the manner of a cable. **cutis g.,** dermal g. **Davis g.,** pinch g. **delayed g.,** a skin graft sutured back into its bed and subsequently shifted to a new recipient site. **dermal g., dermic g.,** skin from which epidermis and subcutaneous fat have been removed; used instead of fascia in various plastic procedures. **epidermic g.,** a piece of epidermis implanted on a raw surface. **Esser g.,** a full-thickness graft spread over a mold of Stent preparation and sutured in position along with the mold. **fascia g.,** one taken from the fascia lata or the lumbar fascia. **fascicular g.,** a nerve graft in which bundles of nerve fibers are approximated and sutured separately. **free g.,** one completely freed from its bed, in contrast to a flap. **full-thickness g.,** a skin graft consisting of the full thickness of the skin, with little or none of the subcutaneous tissue. **heterodermic g.,** a skin graft taken from a donor of another species. **heterologous g., heteroplastic g.,** xenograft. **homologous g., homoplastic g.,** allograft. **isologous g., isoplastic g.,** isograft. **Krause-Wolfe g.,** full-thickness g. **lamellar g.,** replacement of the superficial layers of an opaque cornea by a thin layer of clear cornea from a donor eye. **nerve g.,** replacement of an area of defective nerve with a segment from a sound one. **Ollier-Thiersch g.,** a very thin skin graft in which long, broad strips of skin, consisting of the epidermis, rete, and part of the corium, are used. **omental g's,** free or attached segments of omentum used to cover suture lines following gastrointestinal or colonic surgery. **pedicle g.,** see under *flap.* **penetrating g.,** a full-thickness corneal transplant. **periosteal g.,** a piece of periosteum to cover a denuded bone. **pinch g.,** a piece of skin graft about ¼ inch in diameter, obtained by elevating the skin with a needle and slicing it off with a knife. **Reverdin g.,** epidermic g. **rope g.,** see under *flap.* **sieve g.,** a skin graft from which tiny circular islands of skin are removed so that a larger denuded area can be covered, the sieve-like portion being placed over one area, and the individual islands over surrounding or other denuded areas. **skin g.,** a piece of skin transplanted to replace a lost portion of the skin. **split-skin g.,** a skin graft consisting of only a portion of the skin thickness. **sponge g.,** a bit of sponge inserted into a wound to promote the formation of granulations. **thick-split g.,** a skin graft cut in pieces, often including about two thirds of the full thickness of the skin. **Thiersch's g.,** Ollier-Thiersch g. **white g.,** avascular g.

grafting (graf'ting) the implanting or transplanting of any tissue or organ.

grain (grān) 1. a seed, especially of a cereal plant. 2. the twentieth part of a scruple: 0.065 gm.; abbreviated gr.

gram (gram) the basic unit of mass (weight) of the metric system, being the equivalent of 15.432 grains; abbreviated g. or gm.

-gram word element [Gr.], *written; recorded.*

gram-equivalent (gram''e-kwiv'ah-lent) see *chemical equivalent.*

gramicidin (gram''ĭ-si'din) gramicidin D; an antibacterial polypeptide produced by *Bacillus brevis* and one of the two main components of tyrothricin. *Gramicidin S* is a closely related substance produced by a thermophilic strain of *B. brevis.*

graminivorous (-niv'o-rus) eating or subsisting on cereal grains.

gram-molecule (gram-mol'ĕ-kūl) a quantity in grams numerically equal to the molecular weight of the substance.

gram-negative (-neg'ah-tiv) see *Gram's stain.*

gram-positive (-poz'ĭ-tiv) see *Gram's stain.*

grana (gra'nah) dense green, chlorophyll-containing bodies in chloroplasts of plant cells.

grand mal (grahn mal) [Fr.] see under *epilepsy.*

granular (gran'u-lar) made up of or marked by the presence of granules or grains.

granulatio (gran''u-la'she-o), pl. *granulatio'nes* [L.] a granule, or granular mass.

granulation (-la'shun) 1. the division of a hard substance into small particles. 2. the formation in wounds of small, rounded masses of tissue during healing; also the mass so formed. **arachnoid g's,** enlarged arachnoid villi projecting into the venous sinuses and creating slight depressions on the inner surface of the cranium. **exuberant g's,** excessive proliferation of granulation tissue in healing wounds.

granule (gran'ūl) 1. a small particle or grain. 2. a small pill made from sucrose. **acidophil g's,** granules staining with acid dyes. **acrosomal g.,** the enlarged granule inside the vacuole-like structure which comprises the acrosome or spermatozoon cap. **albuminous g's,** granules seen in the cytoplasm of many normal cells, which disappear on the addition of acetic acid, but are not affected by ether or chloroform. **aleuronoid g's,** colorless myeloid colloidal bodies found in the base of pigment cells. **alpha g's,** 1. the coarse, highly refractive, eosinophil granules of leukocytes, composed of albuminous matter. 2. the acidophil granules in the cells of the pituitary gland. **Altmann's g's,** mitochondria. **amphophil g's,** beta g's. **azure g's, azurophil g's,** those staining easily with azure dyes; they are coarse reddish granules seen in many lymphocytes. **Babès-Ernst g's,** metachromatic g's. **Balfour's infective g.,** a small refractive granule seen in the erythrocytes in spirochtosis of fowls. **basal g.,** blepharoplast. **basophil g's,** granules staining with basic dyes. **beta g's,** presecretion granules found in the hypophysis and pancreatic islands. **Bettelheim's g's,** small mobile granules seen in the blood. **Bütschli's g's,** swellings on the bipolar rays of the amphiaster in the ovum. **carbohydrate g's,** particles of carbohydrate matter in body fluids in the course of being assimilated. **chromatic g's, chromophilic g's,** Nissl bodies. **cone g's,** nuclei of visual cells in outer nuclear layer of the retina which are connected with the cones. **cytoplasmic g's,** albuminous g's. **delta g's,** fine basophilic granules in the lymphocytes. **elementary g's,** hemoconia. **eosinophil g's,** those staining with eosin; see *alpha g's* (1). **epsilon g's,** neutrophil granules from protoplasm of polymorphonuclear leukocytes. **Fauvel's g's,** peribronchitic abscesses. **fuchsinophil g's,** those staining with fuchsin. **gamma g's,** basophilic granules found in the blood, marrow, and tissues. **Grawitz's g's,** minute granules seen in the erythrocytes in the basophilia of lead poisoning. **hyperchromatin g's,** azure g's. **iodophil g's,** granules staining brown with iodine, seen in polymorphonuclear leukocytes in various acute infectious diseases. **juxtaglomerular g's,** osmophilic secretory granules present in the juxtaglomerular cells, closely resembling zymogen granules. **kappa g's,** azure g's. **Kölliker's interstitial g's,** granules seen in the sarcoplasm of muscle fibers. **metachromatic g's,** granules present in many bacterial cells, having an avidity for basic dyes and causing irregular staining of the cell. **Much's g's,** granules and rods found in tuberculous sputum which do not stain by the usual processes for acid-fast bacilli, but do stain with Gram stain. **Neusser's g's,** basophil granules seen about the nuclei of leukocytes. **neutrophil g's,** epsilon g's. **Nissl g's,** see under *body.* **oxyphil g's,** alpha g's (1). **pigment g's,** small masses of coloring matter in pigment cells. **proacrosomal g.,** a small, dense granular body found in one of the vacuoles of Golgi bodies, which develops into the acrosomal granule. **protein g's,** minute particles of various proteins, some anabolic and others catabolic. **rod g's,** nuclei of visual cells in outer nuclear layer of the retina which are connected with the rods. **Schridde's g's,** granules similar to mitochondria, but smaller, found in plasma cells and lymphocytes. **Schrön's g.,** a small body, of doubtful origin, seen in the germinal spot of the ovum. **Schrön-Much g's,** Much's g's. **Schüffner's g's,** see under *dot.* **seminal g's,** the small granular bodies in the spermatic fluid. **thread g's,** mitochondria. **zymogen g's,** secretory granules in certain cells, containing enzyme precursors that become active after they have left the cell.

granuloadipose (gran″u-lo-ad′ĭ-pōs) showing fatty degeneration containing granules of fat.

granuloblast (gran′u-lo-blast″) an immature granulocyte.

granuloblastosis (gran″u-lo-blas-to′sis) a form of avian leukosis with increase in immature, granular blood cells in the circulating blood; there may be infiltration of the liver and spleen.

granulocyte (gran′u-lo-sīt″) any cell containing granules, especially a granular leukocyte. **band-form g.,** band cell.

granulocytopenia (gran″u-lo-si″to-pe′ne-ah) agranulocytosis.

granulocytopoiesis (-si″to-poi-e′sis) the production of granulocytes. **granulocytopoiet′ic,** adj.

granulocytosis (-si-to′sis) an excess of granulocytes in the blood.

granuloma (gran″u-lo′mah) a tumor-like mass or nodule of granulation tissue, with actively growing fibroblasts and capillary buds, due to a chronic inflammatory process associated with an infectious disease or invasion by nonliving foreign body. **apical g.,** modified granulation tissue containing elements of chronic inflammation located adjacent to the root apex of a tooth with infected necrotic pulp. **benign g. of thyroid,** chronic inflammation of the thyroid gland, converting it into a bulky tumor which later becomes extremely hard. **coccidioidal g.,** coccidioidomycosis. **dental g.,** one usually surrounded by a fibrous sac continuous with the periodontal ligament and attached to the root apex of a tooth. **eosinophilic g.,** a form of xanthomatosis marked by the presence of rarefactions of cysts in one or more bones, sometimes associated with eosinophilia. **g. fissura′tum,** a

firm, reddish, fissured, fibrotic granuloma of the gum and buccal mucosa, occurring on an edentulous alveolar ridge between the ridge and cheek. **foreign body g.,** a localized histiocytic reaction to a foreign body in the tissue. **Hodgkin's g.,** see under *disease.* **infectious g.,** one due to a specific microorganism, as the tubercle bacilli. **g. inguina′le,** a granulomatous venereal disease, usually seen in dark-skinned people, marked by purulent ulceration of the external genitals, caused by *Donovania granulomatis.* **lethal midline g.,** a rare, destructive necrotizing granuloma that results in destruction of the midface and invariably in death. It is nearly always preceded by longstanding nonspecific inflammation of the nose or nasal sinuses, with purulent, often bloody discharge. **lipoid g.,** one containing lipoid cells; xanthoma. **lipophagic g.,** a granuloma attended by the loss of subcutaneous fat. **Majocchi's g.,** trichophytic g. **midline g.,** lethal midline g. **paracoccidioidal g.,** paracoccidioidomycosis. **peripheral giant cell reparative g.,** a pedunculated or sessile lesion of the gingivae or alveolar ridge, apparently rising from the periodontal ligament or mucoperiosteum, and usually due to trauma. **pyogenic g.,** a fungating pedunculated growth in which the granulations consist of masses of pyogenic organisms. **septic g.,** pyogenic g. **swimming pool g.,** a granulomatous lesion that complicates injuries sustained in swimming pools, attributed to *Mycobacterium balnei;* it tends to heal spontaneously in a few months or years. **g. telangiecta′icum,** a form characterized by numerous dilated blood vessels. **trichophytic g.,** a form of tinea corporis, occurring chiefly on the lower legs, due to *Trichophyton* infecting hairs at the site of involvement, marked by raised, circumscribed, rather boggy granulomas, disseminated or arranged in chains; the lesions are slowly absorbed, or undergo necrosis, leaving depressed scars. **g. trop′icum,** yaws. **ulcerating g. of pudenda, venereal g., g. vene′reum,** g. inguinale.

granulomatosis (gran″u-lo″mah-to′sis) the formation of multiple granulomas. **g. siderot′ica,** a condition in which brownish nodules are seen in the enlarged spleen. **Wegener's g.,** a progressive disease, with granulomatous lesions of the respiratory tract, focal necrotizing arteriolitis and, finally, widespread inflammation of all organs of the body.

granulomatous (gran″u-lo′mah-tus) composed of granulomas.

granulomere (gran′u-lo-mēr″) the center portion of a platelet in a dry, stained blood smear, apparently filled with fine, purplish red granules.

granulopenia (gran″u-lo-pe′ne-ah) agranulocytosis.

granuloplastic (gran′u-lo-plas″tik) forming granules.

granulopoiesis (gran″u-lo-poi-e′sis) the formation of granulocytes. **granulopoiet′ic,** adj.

granulosa (gran″u-lo′sah) pertaining to cells of the cumulus oophorus.

granulose (gran′u-lōs) amylose (2).

granulosis (gran″u-lo′sis) the formation of granules. **g. ru′bra na′si,** redness and marked sweating confined to the nose and surrounding area of the face, with red papules and sometimes many small vesicles, seen most often in children, and usually clearing up at puberty.

granum (gra′num) [L.] grain.

graph (graf) a diagram or curve representing varying relationships between sets of data. Often used as a word ending denoting a recording instrument.

graphorrhea (graf″o-re′ah) in psychiatry, the writing of a meaningless flow of words.

graphospasm (graf′o-spazm) writers' cramp.

-graphy word element [Gr.], *writing or recording; a method of recording.* **-graph′ic,** adj.

grattage (grah-tahzh′) [Fr.] removal of granulations by scraping.

gravedo (grah-ve′do) head cold; nasal catarrh.

gravel (grav′el) calculi occurring in small particles.

gravid (grav′id) pregnant.

gravida (grav′ĭ-dah) a pregnant woman; called *g. I* (*primigravida*) during the first pregnancy, *g. II* (*secundigravida*) during the second, and so on.

gravidic (grah-vid′ik) occurring in pregnancy.

gravidocardiac (grav″ĭ-do-kar′de-ak) pertaining to heart disease in pregnancy.

gravimetric (grav″ĭ-met′rik) pertaining to measurement by weight; performed by weight, as the gravimetric method of drug assay.

gravity (grav′ĭ-te) weight; tendency toward the center of the earth. **specific g.,** the weight of a substance compared with that of another taken as a standard.

grease (gres) an inflammatory swelling in a horse's leg, with formation of cracks in the skin and excretion of oily matter.

green (grēn) 1. the color of grass or of an emerald. 2. a green dye. **benzaldehyde g.,** malachite g. **brilliant g.,** a basic dye having powerful bacteriostatic properties for gram-positive organisms; used topically as an anesthetic. **indocyanine g.,** a tricarbocyanine dye used intravenously in determination of blood volume, cardiac output, and hepatic function. **malachite g.,** a triphenylmethane dye used as a stain for bacteria and as an antiseptic for wounds. **Paris g., Schweinfurt g.,** a double salt of copper acetate and copper meta-arsenite, used as an insecticide.

Gregarina (greg″ah-ri′nah) a genus of sporozoa, species of which are parasitic in insects.

grid (grid) 1. a grating; in radiology, a device consisting essentially of a series of narrow lead strips closely spaced on their edges and separated by spacers of low density material; used to reduce the amount of scattered radiation reaching the x-ray film. 2. a chart with horizontal and perpendicular lines for plotting curves. **baby g.,** a direct-reading chart on infant growth. **Wetzel g.,** a direct-reading chart for evaluating physical fitness in terms of body build, developmental level, and basal metabolism.

grip (grip) 1. influenza. 2. a grasping or clasping. **devil's g.,** epidemic pleurodynia.

grippe (grip) influenza.

griseofulvin (gris″e-o-ful′vin) an antibiotic, $C_{17}H_{17}ClO_6$, isolated from *Penicillium griseofulvum* and other *Penicillium* species; used as a fungistatic in dermatophytoses.

groin (groin) inguen; the junctional region between the thigh and abdomen.

groove (grōōv) a narrow, linear hollow or depression. **branchial g.,** an external furrow lined with ectoderm, occurring in the embryo between two branchial arches. **Harrison's g.,** a horizontal groove along the lower border of the thorax corresponding to the costal insertion of the diaphragm. **labial g.,** an embryonic groove produced by degeneration of the central cells of the labial lamina, which later becomes the vestibule of the oral cavity. **medullary g., neural g.,** that formed by beginning invagination of the neural plate of the embryo to form the neural tube. **primitive g.,** a longitudinal furrow on the outer surface of the primitive streak.

gross (grōs) coarse or large; visible to the naked eye.

group (grōōp) 1. an assemblage of objects having certain things in common. 2. a number of atoms forming a recognizable and usually transferable portion of a molecule. **alcohol g.,** a combination of carbon, hydrogen, and oxygen atoms in a molecule, characteristic of the chemical compound alcohol; there are three: the primary, the secondary, and the tertiary alcohol group. **azo g.,** a bivalent chemical group composed of two nitrogen atoms, —N:N—. **blood g.,** see under B. **coli-aerogenes g.,** coliform bacilli or coliform bacteria; a group of microorganisms including *Escherichia coli, Aerobacter aerogenes,* and a variety of intermediate forms. **colon-thyphoid-dysentery g.,** collectively, bacteria of the genera *Escherichia, Salmonella,* and *Shigella.* **peptide g.,** the bivalent radical, —CO·NH—, formed by reaction between the NH_2 and COOH groups of adjacent amino acids. **prosthetic g.,** the non–amino acid portion of a conjugated protein. **saccharide g.,** a combination of carbon, hydrogen, and oxygen atoms in a hypothetical molecule, $C_6H_{10}O_5$, the number of which in the compound determines the specific name of the polysaccharide.

group-transfer (grōōp″trans′fer) denoting a chemical reaction (excluding oxidation and reduction) in which molecules exchange functional groups, a process catalyzed by enzymes called transferases.

growth (grōth) 1. a normal process of increase in size of an organism as a result of accretion of tissue similar to that originally present. 2. an abnormal formation, such as a tumor. 3. the proliferation of cells, as in a bacterial culture. **absolute g.,** an expression of the absolute increase in size of an organism or of a particular organ or part. **allometric g.,** the growth of different organs or parts of an organism at different rates. **appositional g.,** growth by addition at the periphery of a particular structure or part. **interstitial g.,** that occurring in the interior of parts or structures already formed. **new g.,** neoplasm.

grumous (groo′mus) lumpy or clotted.

gryposis (grĭ-po′sis) abnormal curvature, as of the nails.

G.S. Gerontological Society.

GSH reduced glutathione.

GSSG oxidized glutathione.

gt. [L.] *gutta* (drop).

GTP guanosine triphosphate.

gtt. [L.] *guttae* (drops).

GU genitourinary.

guaiac (gwi′ak) a resin from the wood of trees of the genus *Guajacum,* used as a reagent and formerly in treatment of rheumatism.

guanase (gwan′ās) guanine deaminase.

guanethidine (gwan-eth′ĭ-dēn) an adrenergic blocking agent, $C_{10}H_{22}N_4$; the sulfate salt is used as an antihypertensive.

guanidine (gwan′ĭ-dēn) a base, $NH:C(NH_2)_2$, the amidine of aminocarbamic acid.

guanine (gwan′ēn) a purine base, $C_5H_5N_5O$, one of the fundamental components of nucleic acids (DNA and RNA).

guanosine (gwan′o-sēn) a nucleoside, guanine riboside, one of the major constituents of RNA. **g. triphosphate,** an energy-rich compound involved in several metabolic reactions.

guaranine (gwah-rah′nin) caffeine.

gubernaculum (goo″ber-nak′u-lum), pl. *gubernac′ula* [L.] a guiding structure. **g. tes′tis,** the fetal ligament attaching the epididymis to the scrotum, present during descent of the testis.

guide (gīd) a device by which another object is led in its proper course, e.g., a grooved sound.

guillotine (gil′o-tēn) an instrument with a sliding blade for excising a tonsil or the uvula.

gullet (gul′et) the passage to the stomach, including both the esophagus and pharynx.

gum (gum) 1. mucilaginous excretion of various plants. 2. gingiva. **g. arabic,** acacia. **British g.,** dextrin. **g. camphor,** camphor. **g. karaya,** sterculia g. **g. opium,** opium. **sterculia g.,** dried gummy exudation from *Sterculia urens* or other *Sterculia* species; used as a bulk cathartic. **g. tragacanth,** tragacanth.

gumboil (gum′boil) gingival abscess.

gumma (gum′ah) a soft, gummy tumor, such as that occurring in tertiary syphilis.

gummatous (-tus) of the nature of gumma.

gummy (gum′e) resembling gum or gumma.

gurney (ger′ne) a wheeled cot used in hospitals.

gustation (gus-ta′shun) the act of tasting or the sense of taste. **gus′tatory,** adj.

gut (gut) 1. the intestine or bowel. 2. the primitive digestive tube, consisting of the fore-, mid-, and hindgut. 3. catgut. **blind g.,** cecum. **head g.,** foregut. **postanal g.,** an extension of the embryonic gut caudal to the cloaca. **preoral g.,** Seessel's pouch. **primitive g.,** archenteron. **tail g.,** postanal g.

gutta (gut′ah), pl. *gut′tae* [L.] a drop.

gutta-percha (gut″ah-per′chah) the coagulated latex of a number of tropical trees of the family Sapotaceae; used as a dental cement and in splints.

guttat. [L.] *guttatim* (drop by drop).

guttate (gut′āt) resembling a drop.

guttatim (gŭ-ta′tim) [L.] drop by drop.

guttering (gut′er-ing) the cutting of a gutter-like excision in bone.

guttural (gut′er-al) pertaining to the throat.

gymnastics (jim-nas′tiks) systematic muscular exercise. **Swedish g.,** a system of exercise following a rigid pattern of movement, utilizing little equipment and stressing correct body posture.

gymnocyte (jim′no-sīt) a cell with no cell wall.

Gymnodinium (jim″no-din′e-um) a genus of dinoflagellates, most species of which have many colored chromatophores, found in fresh, salt, and brackish waters; when present in great numbers, they help to form the destructive red tide in the ocean.

gymnospore (jim′no-spōr) a spore without a protective envelope.

gyn-, gyne-, gyneco-, gyno- word element [Gr.], *woman.*

gynaeco- for words beginning thus, see those beginning *gyneco-.*

gynandrism (jin-an′drizm) 1. hermaphroditism. 2. female pseudohermaphroditism.

gynandroblastoma (jĭ-nan″dro-blas-to′mah) an ovarian tumor containing elements of both arrhenoblastoma and granulosa cell tumor.

gynandroid (jĭ-nan′droid) a hermaphrodite or a female pseudohermaphrodite.

gynandromorph (jĭ-nan′dro-morf) an organism exhibiting gynandromorphism.

gynandromorphism (jĭ-nan″dro-mor′fizm) the presence of chromosomes of both sexes in different tissues of the body, producing a mosaic of male and female sex characteristics. **gynandromorph′ous,** adj.

gynecic (jĭ-ne′sik) pertaining to women.

gynecogenic (jin″ĕ-ko-jen′ik) producing female characteristics.

gynecography (jin″ĕ-kog′rah-fe) radiography of the female reproductive tract.

gynecoid (jin′ĕ-koid) woman-like.

gynecologist (jin″ĕ-kol′o-jist, gi″nĕ-) a specialist in gynecology.

gynecology (jin″ĕ-kol′o-je, gi″nĕ-) the branch of medicine dealing with diseases of the genital tract in women. **gynecolog′ic,** adj.

gynecomania (jin″ĕ-ko-ma′ne-ah) satyriasis.

gynecomastia (-mas′te-ah) excessive development of the male mammary glands, even to the functional state.

gynecopathy (jin″ĕ-kop′ah-the) any disease peculiar to women.

gynephobia (jin″ĕ-fo′be-ah) morbid aversion to women.

Gynergen (jin′er-jen) trademark for a preparation of ergotamine.

gynogenesis (jin″o-jen′ĕ-sis) development of an egg that is stimulated by a sperm in the absence of any participation of the sperm nucleus.

gynomerogon (-mer′o-gon) an organism produced by gynomerogony and containing only the maternal set of chromosomes.

gynomerogony (-mer-og′o-ne) development of a portion of a fertilized ovum containing only the female pronucleus.

gynopathic (-path′ik) pertaining to disease of women.

gynoplastics (jin′o-plas″tiks) the plastic or reconstructive surgery of female reproductive organs. **gynoplas′tic**, adj.

gypsum (jip′sum) native calcium sulfate, which, when calcined, becomes plaster of Paris.

gyrate (ji′rāt) convoluted; ring or spiral shaped.

gyration (ji-ra′shun) revolution about a fixed center.

gyre (jīr) gyrus.

gyrectomy (ji-rek′to-me) excision or resection of a cerebral gyrus, or a portion of the cerebral cortex.

Gyrencephala (ji″ren-sef′ah-lah) a group of higher mammals, including man, having a brain marked by convolutions.

gyrencephalic (ji″ren-sĕ-fal′ik) pertaining to the Gyrencephala; having a brain marked by convolutions.

gyri (ji′ri) plural of *gyrus*.

gyrose (ji′rōs) marked by curved lines or circles.

gyrospasm (ji′ro-spazm) rotatory spasm of the head.

gyrous (ji′rus) gyrose.

gyrus (ji′rus), pl. *gy′ri* [L.] one of the many well developed folds in the white medullary layer of the cerebral cortex, separated by fissures or sulci. **angular g.,** one continuous anteriorly with the supramarginal gyrus. **annectant gyri,** gyri transitivi. **gy′ri bre′ves in′sulae,** the short, rostrally placed gyri on the surface of the insula. **Broca's g.,** inferior frontal gyrus. **callosal g.,** cingulate g. **central g., anterior,** precentral g. **central g., posterior,** postcentral g. **cerebral gyri,** the tortuous elevations (convolutions) on the surface of the cerebral hemisphere, caused by infolding of the cortex and separated by fissures or sulci. **cingulate g.,** an arch-shaped convolution situated just above the corpus callosum. **dentate g.,** a serrated strip of gray matter under the medial border of the hippocampus and in its depths. **g. fornica′tus,** the marginal portion of the cerebral cortex on the medial aspect of the hemisphere, including the cingulate gyrus, parahippocampal gyrus, and others. **frontal g.,** any of the three (inferior, middle, and superior) gyri of the frontal lobe. **fusiform g.,** one on the inferior surface of the hemisphere between the inferior temporal and parahippocampal gyri, consisting of a lateral (*lateral occipitotemporal g.*) and a medial (*medial occipitotemporal g.*) part. **g. genic′uli,** a vestigial gyrus at the anterior end of the corpus callosum. **Heschl's gyri,** transverse temporal gyri. **hippocampal g.,** parahippocampal g. **infracalcarine g.,** lingual g. **lingual g.,** one on the occipital lobe forming the inferior lip of the calcarine sulcus and, with the cuneus, the visual cortex. **g. lon′gus in′sulae,** the long, occipitally directed gyrus on the surface of the insula. **marginal g.,** the middle frontal gyrus. **occipital g.,** any of the three (superior, middle, and inferior) gyri of the occipital lobe. **occipitotemporal g., lateral,** the lateral portion of the fusiform gyrus. **occipitotemporal g., medial,** the medial portion of the fusiform gyrus. **g. olfacto′rius media′lis of Retzius,** area subcallosa. **orbital gyri,** irregular gyri on the orbital surface of the frontal lobe. **parahippocampal g.,** one between the hippocampal and collateral sulci. **paraterminal g.,** a thin sheet of gray matter in front of and ventral to the genu of the corpus callosum. **postcentral g.,** the convolution of the frontal lobe immediately behind the central sulcus; the primary sensory area of the cerebral cortex. **precentral g.,** the convolution of the frontal lobe immdiately in front of the central sulcus; the primary motor area of the cerebral cortex. **preinsular gyri,** gyri breves insulae. **gy′ri profun′di cer′ebri,** the deeply placed cerebral gyri. **g. rec′tus,** one on the orbital surface of the frontal lobe. **subcallosal g.,** paraterminal g. **supracallosal g.,** indusium griseum. **supramarginal g.,** that part of the inferior parietal convolution which curves around the upper end of the sylvian fissure. **temporal g.,** any of the gyri of the temporal lobe, including the inferior, middle, superior, and transverse temporal gyri; the more prominent of the latter (*anterior transverse temporal g.*) represents the cortical center for hearing. **gyri transiti′vi,** various small folds on the cerebral surface that are too inconstant to bear special names. **uncinate g.,** the uncus.

H

H chemical symbol, *hydrogen*.

H. [L.] *ho′ra* (hour); horizontal; hyperopia.

H⁺ symbol, *hydrogen ion*.

habena (hah-be′nah) habenula (2). **habe′nal, habe′nar,** adj.

habenula (hah-ben′u-lah), pl. *haben′ulae* [L.] 1. a frenulum, or reinlike structure, such as one of a set of structures in the cochlea. 2. a small eminence on the dorsomesial eminence of the thalamus, just in front of the posterior commissure. **haben′ular,** adj.

habit (hab′it) 1. an action which has become automatic or characteristic by repetition. 2. predisposition; bodily temperament. **drug h.,** addiction to drugs. **full h.,** a full, thick, heavy-set body build indicating a possible tendency to apoplexy.

habitat (hab′ĭ-tat) the natural abode of an animal or plant species.

habituation (hah-bich″u-a′shun) 1. the gradual adaptation to a stimulus or to the environment. 2. a condition due to repeated consumption of a drug, with a desire to continue its use, but with little or no tendency to increase the dose.

habitus (hab′ĭ-tus) [L.] 1. attitude (2). 2. physique. **h. apoplec′ticus,** full habit. **h. enterop′toticus,** the body conformation seen in enteroptosis, marked by a long, narrow abdomen. **h. phthis′icus,** a body conformation predisposing to pulmonary tuberculosis, marked by pallor, emaciation, poor muscular development, and small bones.

Habronema (hab″ro-ne′mah) a genus of nematodes parasitic in the stomach of horses; their larvae may be transmitted to the horse's skin, where they may cause dermatitis and a type of granuloma; in the conjunctiva, they cause worm-containing granulomas.

habronemiasis (hab″ro-ne-mi′ah-sis) infection with *Habronema*.

hachement (ahsh-maw′) [Fr.] hacking or chopping stroke in massage.

hae- for words beginning thus, see also those beginning *he-*.

Haemadipsa (he″mah-dip′sah) a genus of leeches.

Haemaphysalis (hem″ah-fis′ah-lis) a genus of hard-bodied ticks, species of which are important vectors of disease.

Haemobartonella (he″mo-bar″to-nel′ah) a genus of microorganisms of the family Bartonellaceae, species of which are parasitic in various lower animals.

Haemophilus (he-mof′ĭ-lus) *Hemophilus*.

hafnium (haf′ne-um) chemical element (*see table*), at. no. 72, symbol Hf.

hair (hār) pilus; a threadlike structure, especially the specialized epidermal structure composed of keratin and developing from a papilla sunk in the corium, produced only by mammals and characteristic of that group of animals. Also, the aggregate of such hairs. **auditory h's,** hairlike attachments of the epithelial cells of the inner ear. **bamboo h.,** trichorrhexis nodosa. **beaded h.,** hair marked with alternate swellings and consrictions, as in monilethrix. **burrowing h.,** one that grows horizontally beneath the surface of the skin. **club h.,** one whose root is surrounded by a bulbous enlargment composed of keratinized cells, preliminary to normal loss of the hair from the follicle. **Frey's h's,** stiff hairs mounted in a handle; used for testing the sensitiveness of pressure points of the skin. **ingrown h.,** one that emerges from the skin but curves and reenters it. **lanugo h.,** the fine hair on the body of the fetus, constituting the lanugo. **moniliform h.,** beaded h. **resting h.,** see *telogen*. **sensory h's,** hairlike projections on the surface of sensory epithelial cells. **stellate h.,** one split at the end in a starlike form. **tactile h's,** hairs sensitive to touch. **taste h's,** short hairlike processes projecting freely into the lumen of the pit of a taste bud from the peripheral ends of the taste cells. **terminal h.,** the coarse hair on various areas of the body during adult years. **twisted h.,** one which at spaced intervals is twisted through an axis of 180 degrees, being abnormally flattened at the site of twisting. **wooly h.,** lanugo.

hairball (hār′bawl) trichobezoar.

halation (hah-la′shun) indistinctness of the visual image caused by strong illumination coming from the same direction as the object being viewed.

halazone (hal′ah-zōn) a disinfectant for water supplies, $C_7H_5Cl_2NO_4S$.

Haldol (hal′dol) trademark for a preparation of haloperidol.

Haldrone (hal′drōn) trademark for a preparation of paramethasone.

half-life (haf′līf) the time in which the radioactivity originally associated with a particular isotope is reduced by half through radioactive decay. **biological h.,** the time required for a living tissue, organ, or organism to eliminate one-half of a radioactive substance which has been introduced into it.

half-value (haf-val′u) see under *layer*.

halide (hal′īd) a binary compound of one of the halogens.

halisteresis (hah-lis″ter-e′sis) osteomalacia. **halisteret′ic,** adj.

halitosis (hal″ĭ-to′sis) offensive odor of the breath.

halitus (hal′ĭ-tus) an exhalation of vapor; an expired breath.

hallucination (hah-lu″sĭ-na′shun) a sense perception (sight, touch, sound, smell, or taste) that has no basis in external stimulation. **hallucinator′y,** adj. **auditory h.,** a hallucination of hearing. **gustatory h.,** a hallucination of taste. **haptic h.,** tactile h. **hypnagogic h.,** one occurring between sleeping and awakening. **olfactory h.,** a hallucination of smell. **tactile**

308

h., a hallucination of touch. **visual h.,** a hallucination of sight.

hallucinogen (hah-lu′sĭ-no-jen″) an agent that is capable of producing hallucinations. **hallucinogen′ic,** adj.

hallucinosis (hah-lu″sĭ-no′sis) a psychosis marked by hallucinations. **acute h., alcoholic h.,** alcoholic psychosis marked by auditory hallucinations and delusions of persecution.

hallux (hal′uks) the great toe. **h. doloro′sa,** a painful disease of the great toe, usually associated with flatfoot. **h. flex′us,** h. rigidus. **h. mal′leus,** hammer toe affecting the great toe. **h. rig′idus,** painful flexion deformity of the great toe with limitation of motion at the metarsophalangeal joint. **h. val′gus,** angulation of the great toe toward the other toes of the foot. **h. va′rus,** angulation of the great toe away from the other toes of the foot.

halmatogenesis (hal″mah-to-jen′ĕ-sis) a sudden alteration of type from one generation to another.

halo (ha′lo) 1. a luminous or colored circle, as the colored circle seen around a light in glaucoma. 2. a ring seen around the macula lutea in ophthalmoscopic examinations. 3. the imprint of the ciliary processes on the vitreous body. **Fick's, h.,** a colored circle appearing around a light, due to the wearing of contact lenses. **h. glaucomato′sus, glaucomatous h.,** peripapillary atrophy seen in severe or chronic glaucoma. **senile h.,** a zone of variable width around the optic papilla, due to exposure of various elements of the choroid as a result of senile atrophy of the pigmented epithelium.

haloduric (hal″o-du′rik) capable of existing in a medium containing a high concentration of salt.

halogen (hal′o-jen) a nonmetallic element of the seventh group of the periodic system: chlorine, iodine, bromine, and fluorine.

halometer (hah-lom′ĕ-ter) 1. an instrument for measuring ocular halos. 2. an instrument for estimating the size of erythrocytes by measuring the diffraction halos which they produce.

haloperidol (hal″o-per′ĭ-dol) a major tranquilizer of the butyrophenone series, $C_{21}H_{23}Cl$-FNO_2.

halophil (hal′o-fil) a microorganism that requires a high concentration of salt for optimal growth.

halophilic (hal″o-fil′ik) pertaining to or characterized by an affinity for salt; requiring a high concentration of salt for optimal growth.

Halotestin (-tes′tin) trademark for a preparation of fluoxymesterone.

halothane (hal′o-thān) an inhalation anesthetic, $C_2HBrClF_3$.

hamartia (ham-ar′she-ah) defect in tissue combination during development.

hamartoblastoma (ham-ar″to-blas-to′mah) a tumor developing from a hamartoma.

hamartoma (ham″ar-to′mah) a benign tumor-like nodule composed of an overgrowth of mature cells and tissues normally present in the affected part, but often with one element predominating.

hamartomatous (-tus) pertaining to a disturbance in growth of a tissue in which the cells of a circumscribed area outstrip those of the surrounding areas.

hamate (ham′āt) hooked, as the hamate bone.

hammer (ham′er) 1. an instrument with a head designed for striking blows. 2. malleus (1).

hamster (ham′ster) a small rodent, used extensively in laboratory experiments.

hamstring (ham′string) one of the tendons bounding the popliteal space laterally and medially. **inner h's,** tendons of gracilis, sartorius, and two other muscles of leg. **outer h.,** tendon of biceps flexor femoris.

hamulus (ham′u-lus), pl. *ham′uli* [L.] any hook-shaped process. **ham′ular,** adj.

hand (hand) the part of the upper limb distal to the forearm; the carpus, metacarpus, and fingers together. **ape h.,** one with the thumb permanently extended. **claw h.,** see *clawhand.* **cleft h.,** a malformation in which the division between the fingers extends into the metacarpus; also, a hand with the middle digits absent. **club h.,** see *clubhand.* **drop h.,** wristdrop. **Krukenberg's h.,** a forklike stump created by separating the distal ends of the radius and ulna and covering them with skin, after amputation proximal to the carpus. **lobster-claw h.,** cleft h. **writing h.,** in paralysis agitans, assumption of the position by which a pen is commonly held.

H and E hematoxylin and eosin (stain).

handedness (hand′ed-nes) the preferential use of the hand of one side in voluntary motor acts.

handpiece (-pēs) that part of a dental engine held in the operator's hand and engaging the bur or working point while it is being revolved.

hangnail (hang′nāl) a shred of eponychium on a proximal or lateral nail fold.

haphalgesia (haf″al-je′ze-ah) pain on touching objects.

haploid (hap′loid) having half the number of chromosomes characteristically found in the somatic (diploid) cells of an organism; typical of the gametes of a species whose union restores the diploid number.

haploidy (hap′loi-de) the state of being haploid.

haploscope (hap′lo-skōp) a stereoscope for testing the visual axis.

haplotype (-tīp) the group of alleles of linked genes contributed by either parent; the haploid genetic constitution contributed by either parent.

hapten (hap′ten) partial antigen; a specific nonprotein substance which does not itself elicit antibody formation, but does elicit the immune response when coupled with a carrier protein. **hapten′ic,** adj.

haptene (hap′tēn) hapten.

haptic (hap′tik) tactile.

haptics (hap′tiks) the science of the sense of touch.

haptoglobin (hap″to-glo′bin) a group of serum α_2-globulin glycoproteins that bind free hemoglobin; different types, genetically determined, are distinguished electrophoretically.

haptophore (hap′to-fōr) in Ehrlichs' side-chain theory, the specific group of the molecule of toxins, agglutinins, precipitins, opsonins, and lysins by which they become attached to their antibodies, antigens, or the receptors of cells, thus making possible their specific activity.

harelip (hār′lip) a congenital cleft of the upper lip.

Harmonyl (har′mo-nil) trademark for preparations of deserpidine.

Harrison antinarcotic act (har′ĭ-sun) a federal law enacted March 1, 1915, regulating the possession, sale, purchase, and prescription of habit-forming drugs.

hashish (hash-ēsh′) a preparation of the unadulterated resin scraped from the flowering tops of female hemp plants (*Cannabis sativa*), smoked or chewed for its intoxicating effects. It is far more potent than marihuana.

haustration (hos-tra′shun) 1. the formation of a haustrum. 2. a haustrum.

haustrum (hos′trum), pl. *haus′tra* [L.] a recess. **haus′tral,** adj. **haus′tra co′li,** sacculations in the wall of the colon produced by adaptation of its length to the tenia coli, or by the arrangement of the circular muscle fibers.

Hb hemoglobin.

HB_C hepatitis B core (antigen); an antigen in the core of the Dane particle.

H.C. Hospital Corps.

HCl hydrochloric acid.

He chemical symbol, *helium.*

head (hed) caput; the upper, anterior, or proximal extremity of a structure, especially the part of an organism containing the brain and organs of special sense. **articular h.,** an eminence on a bone by which it articulates with another bone. **big h.,** see *bighead.* **hourglass h.,** one in which the coronal suture is depressed. **nerve h.,** the optic disk. **saddle h.,** one with a sunken crown. **steeple h.,** oxycephaly. **swelled h.,** bighead (1). **tower h.,** oxycephaly.

headache (hed′āk) pain in the head. **cluster h.,** a migraine-like disorder marked by attacks of unilateral intense pain over the eye and forehead, with flushing and watering of the eyes and nose; attacks last about an hour and occur in clusters. **cough h.,** stabbing pain produced by traction on pain-sensitive structures on coughing or straining. **histamine h.,** cluster h. **migraine h.,** see *migraine.* **sick h.,** migraine. **tension h.,** a type due to prolonged overwork, emotional strain or both, affecting especially the occipital region.

headgrit (-grit) yellows (2).

healing (hēl′ing) a process of cure; the restoration of integrity to injured tissue. **h. by first intention,** that in which union or restoration of continuity occurs directly without intervention of granulations. **h. by second intention,** union by closure of a wound with granulations.

health (helth) a state of physical, mental, and social well-being. **public h.,** the field of medicine concerned with safeguarding and improving the health of the community as a whole.

healthy (helth′e) pertaining to, characterized by, or promoting health.

hearing (hēr′ing) the sense by which sounds are perceived; capacity to perceive sound.

heart (hart) cor; the viscus of cardiac muscle that maintains the circulation of the blood; see Plate VI. **athletic h.,** hypertrophy of the heart without valvular disease, sometimes seen in athletes. **bovine h.,** cor bovinum. **cervical h.,** one situated in the neck. **chaotic h.,** a heart which exhibits frequent premature systoles. **fatty h.,** 1. one that has undergone fatty degeneration. 2. a condition in which fat has accumulated about and in the heart muscle. **fibroid h.,** one affected with chronic myocarditis, in which fibrous tissue replaces portions of the myocardium. **horizontal h.,** a counterclockwise rotation of the electrical axis (deviation to the left) of the heart. **irritable h.,** neurocirculatory asthenia. **left h.,** the left atrium and ventricle, which propel the blood through the systemic circulation. **Quain's fatty h.,** fatty degeneration of the myocardium. **right h.,** the right atrium and ventricle, which propel the venous blood into the pulmonary circulation. **soldier's h.,** neurocirculatory asthenia. **three-chambered h.,** congenital absence of the ventricular or atrial septum so that the heart has a single ventricle with two atria or a single atrium with two ventricles. **tobacco h.,** one showing irregularity of action attributed to excessive use of tobacco. **triatrial h.,** cor triatriatum. **trilocular h.,** three-chambered h.

heart beat (hart′bēt) see *beat.*

heart block (-blok) impairment of conduction in heart excitation; often applied specifically to atrioventricular heart block. **atrioventricular (A-V) h.b.,** a form in which the blocking is at the atrioventricular junction. It is *first degree* when A-V conduction time is prolonged; *second degree* (*partial h.b.*) when some but not all atrial impulses reach the ventricle; *third degree* (*complete h.b.*) when no atrial impulses at all reach the ventricle, and the atria and ventricles act independently of each other. **bundle-branch h.b.,** a form in which one ventricle is excited before the other because of absence of conduction in one of the branches of the bundle of His. **complete h.b.,** see *atrioventricular h.b.* **interventricular h.b.,** bundle-branch h.b. **Mobitz type I h.b.,** second degree A-V heart block in which the P-R interval increases progressively until an atrial impulse is blocked. **Mobitz type II h.b.,** second degree A-V heart block in which the P-R interval is fixed, with periodic blocking of an atrial impulse. **sinoatrial h.b.,** partial or complete impairment of conduction from the sinoatrial node to the atria, resulting in delay or absence of an atrial beat.

heartburn (-bern) pyrosis; a retrosternal burning sensation usually due to reflux of acid into the esophagus.

heart failure (-fāl-ūr) inability of the heart to maintain a circulation sufficient to meet the body's needs; most often applied to myocardial failure affecting the right or left ventricle. **backward h.f.,** a concept of heart failure emphasizing the contribution of passive engorgement of the systemic venous system as a cause. **congestive h.f.,** that marked by breathlessness and abnormal retention of sodium and water, resulting in edema, with congestion of the lungs or peripheral circulation, or both. **forward h.f.,** a concept of heart failure emphasizing the inadequacy of cardiac output as the primary cause and considering venous distention to be secondary. **high output h.f.,** that in which cardiac output remains high, associated with hyperthyroidism, anemia, emphysema, etc. **left-sided h.f., left ventricular h.f.,** failure of adequate output by the left ventricle, marked by pulmonary congestion and edema. **low output h.f.,** that in which cardiac output is diminished, associated with cardiovascular diseases. **right-sided h.f., right ventricular h.f.,** failure of adequate output by the right ventricle, marked by venous engorgement, hepatic enlargement, and pitting edema.

heartwater (-wot-er) a fatal rickettsial disease of cattle, sheep, and goats marked by fluid accumulation in the pericardium and pleural cavity.

heartworm (-werm) an individual of the species *Dirofilaria immitis.*

heat (hēt) 1. the sensation of an increase in temperature; the energy producing such a sensation. 2. energy transferred as a result of a gradient in temperature. 3. estrus. **conductive h.,** heat transmitted by direct contact, as with a hot water bottle. **convective h.,** heat conveyed by currents of a warm medium, such as air or water. **conversive h.,** heat developed in tissues by resistance to passage of high-energy radiations. **prickly h.,** miliaria rubra.

heaves (hēvz) chronic pulmonary emphysema of horses.

hebephrenia (he″bĕ-fre′ne-ah) hebephrenic schizophrenia. **hebephren′ic,** adj.

hebetic (hĕ-bet′ik) pertaining to puberty.

hebetude (heb′ĕ-tūd) dullness; apathy.

hebiatrics (he″be-at′riks) ephebiatrics.

hebosteotomy, hebotomy (he-bos″te-ot′o-me; he-bot′o-me) pubiotomy.

hecateromeric, hecatomeric (hek″ah-ter″o-; hek″ah-to-mer′ik) having processes which divide in two, one going to each side of the spinal cord, said of certain neurons.

hecto- word element [Fr.], *hundred;* used in naming units of measurements to designate an amount 100 times (10²) the size of the unit to which it joined; symbol h.

hectogram (hek′to-gram) 100 grams; 3.527 oz. avoirdupois, or 3.215 oz. apothecaries' weight.

hectoliter (-le″ter) 100 liters; 26.4 United States, or 22 Imperial gallons.

hectometer (-me″ter) 100 meters; roughly, 328 feet, 1 inch.

hedonism (he′do-nizm) excessive devotion to pleasure.

Hedulin (hed′u-lin) trademark for a preparation of phenindione.

heel (hēl) calx; the hindmost part of the foot. **cracked h.,** pitted keratolysis.

height (hīt) the vertical measurement of an object or body. **h. of contour,** 1. a line encircling a tooth representing its greatest circumference. 2. the line encircling a tooth in a more or less horizontal plane and passing through the sur-

face point of greatest radius. 3. the line encircling a tooth at its greatest bulge or diameter with respect to a selected path of insertion.

helcoid (hel′koid) like an ulcer.

heli(o)- word element [Gr.], *sun.*

helianthin (he″le-an′thin) methyl orange.

helical (hel′ĭ-kal) shaped like a helix.

helicine (hel′ĭ-sin) 1. of spiral form. 2. of or pertaining to a helix.

helicoid (hel′ĭ-koid) resembling a coil or helix.

helicopodia (hel″ĭ-ko-po′de-ah) helicopod gait.

helicotrema (hel″ĭ-ko-tre′mah) a foramen between the scala tympani and scala vestibuli.

heliencephalitis (he″le-en-sef″ah-li′tis) encephalitis from exposure to the sun (sunstroke).

heliotaxis (he″le-o-tak′sis) phototaxis.

heliotherapy (-ther′ah-pe) therapeutic use of the sun bath.

heliotropism (he″le-ot′ro-pizm) phototropism (1).

helium (he′le-um) chemical element (*see table*), at. no. 2, symbol He.

helix (he′liks) 1. a coiled structure. 2. the superior and posterior free margin of the pinna of the ear. α-**helix, alpha h.,** the helical secondary structure of many proteins. **double h., Watson-Crick h.,** a representation of the structure of DNA, consisting of two coiled chains, each of which contains information completely specifying the other chain.

helminth (hel′minth) a parasitic worm.

helminthagogue (hel-min′thah-gog) anthelmintic.

helminthemesis (hel″min-them′ĕ-sis) the vomiting of worms.

helminthiasis (-thi′ah-sis) an infection with worms.

helminthic (hel-min′thik) pertaining to or caused by helminths.

helminthology (hel″min-thol′o-je) the scientific study of parasitic worms.

helminthoma (-tho′mah) a tumor caused by a parasitic worm.

heloma (he-lo′mah) a corn. **h. du′rum,** hard corn. **h. mol′le,** soft corn.

helotomy (he-lot′o-me) the excision or the paring of corns or calluses.

hemabarometer (hem″ah-bah-rom′ĕ-ter) an instrument for ascertaining the specific gravity of blood.

hemachrome (he′mah-krōm, hem′ah-krōm) hemochrome.

hemachrosis (hem″ah-kro′sis) excessive redness of the blood.

hemacytometer (he″mah-si-tom′ĕ-ter) hemocytometer.

hemadsorption (hem″ad-sorp′shun) the adherence of red cells to other cells. **hemadsor′bent,** adj.

hemagglutination (he″mah-gloo″tĭ-na′shun) agglutination of erythrocytes.

hemagglutinin (-gloo′tĭ-nin) an antibody that causes agglutination of erythrocytes. **cold h.,** one which acts only at temperatures near 4° C.

warm h., one which acts only at temperatures near 37° C.

hemal (he′mal) pertaining to the blood.

hemalum (hem-al′um) a mixture of hematoxylin and alum used as a nuclear stain.

hemanalysis (he″mah-nal′ĭ-sis) analysis of the blood.

hemangiectasia (he-man″je-ek′tah-sis) angiectasis.

hemangioameloblastoma (he-man″je-o-ah-mel″o-blas-to′mah) a highly vascular ameloblastoma.

hemangioblast (he-man′je-o-blast) a mesodermal cell which gives rise to both vascular endothelium and hemocytoblasts.

hemangioblastoma (he-man″je-o-blas-to′mah) a capillary hemangioma of the brain consisting of proliferated blood vessel cells or angioblasts.

hemangioendothelioblastoma (-en″do-the″le-o-blas-to′mah) a tumor of mesenchymal origin of which the cells tend to form endothelial cells and line blood vessels.

hemangioendothelioma (-en″do-the″le-o′mah) a hemangioma in which endothelial cells are the most prominent component.

hemangioendotheliosarcoma (-en″do-the″le-o-sar-ko′mah) hemangiosarcoma.

hemangiofibroma (-fi-bro′mah) a hemangioma containing fibrous tissue.

hemangioma (he-man″je-o′mah) a benign tumor made up of newly formed blood vessels. **ameloblastic h.,** a highly vascular ameloblastoma. **cavernous h.,** a red-blue spongy tumor made up of a connective tissue framework enclosing large, cavernous, vascular spaces containing blood. **sclerosing h.,** a solidly cellular lesion purportedly developing from a hemangioma by proliferation of endothelial cells and connective tissue stroma.

hemangiomatosis (he-man″je-o-mah-to′sis) the presence of multiple hemangiomas.

hemangiopericytoma (-per″ĭ-si-to′mah) a tumor composed of spindle cells with a rich vascular network, which apparently arises from pericytes.

hemangiosarcoma (-sar-ko′mah) a malignant tumor formed of endothelial and fibroblastic tissue.

hemaphein (hem″ah-fe′in) a brown coloring matter of the blood and urine. **hemaphe′ic,** adj.

hemarthrosis (hem″ar-thro′sis) extravasation of blood into a joint or its synovial cavity.

hemat(o)- word element [Gr.], *blood.* See also words beginning *hem-* and *hemo-*.

hematein (hem″ah-te′in) a brownish-red substance, $C_{16}H_{12}O_6$, derived from hematoxylin; used as an indicator and stain.

hematemesis (hem″ah-tem′ĕ-sis) the vomiting of blood.

hematencephalon (hem″at-en-sef′ah-lon) effusion of blood into the brain.

hemathermous (hem″ah-ther′mus) warmblooded.

hematic (he-mat′ik) 1. pertaining to or containing blood. 2. hematinic.

hematidrosis (hem″ah-tĭ-dro′sis) excretion of bloody sweat.

hematimeter (hem″ah-tim′ĕ-ter) hemocytometer.

hematin (hem′ah-tin) 1. heme. 2. the hydroxide of heme, $C_{34}H_{33}FeN_4O_5$; used as a reagent.

hematinemia (hem″ah-tĭ-ne′me-ah) presence of hematin (heme) in the blood.

hematinic (hem″ah-tin′ik) 1. pertaining to hematin (heme). 2. an agent that improves the quality of blood, increasing the hemoglobin level and the number of erythrocytes.

hematinometer (hem″ah-tĭ-nom′ĕ-ter) an instrument for measuring the hemoglobin of the blood.

hematinuria (hem″ah-tin-u′re-ah) the presence of hematin (heme) in the urine.

hematobilia (hem″ah-to-bil′ĭ-ah) bleeding into the biliary passages.

hematoblast (hem′ah-to-blast″) hemocytoblast.

hematocele (-sēl″) an effusion of blood into a cavity, especially into the tunica vaginalis testis. **parametric h., pelvic h., retrouterine h.,** a tumor formed by effusion of blood into the pouch of Douglas.

hematochezia (hem″ah-to-ke′ze-ah) the passage of bloody stools.

hematochromatosis (-kro″mah-to′sis) hemochromatosis.

hematochyluria (-ki-lu′re-ah) the discharge of blood and chyle with the urine, due to *Wuchereria bancrofti.*

hematocoelia (-se′le-ah) effusion of blood into the peritoneal cavity.

hematocolpometra (-kol″po-me′trah) accumulation of menstrual blood in the vagina and uterus.

hematocolpos (-kol′pos) accumulation of blood in the vagina.

hematocrit (he-mat′o-krit) the volume percentage of erythrocytes in whole blood; also, the apparatus or procedure used in its determination.

hematocryal (hem″ah-to-kri′al) poikilothermic.

hematocrystallin (-kris′tah-lin) hemoglobin.

hematocyanin (-si′ah-nin) a blue respiratory pigment occurring in the blood of mollusks and arthropods, containing 0.17–0.38% copper.

hematocyst (hem′ah-to-sist″) effusion of blood into the bladder or a cyst.

hematocyturia (hem″ah-to-si-tu′re-ah) the presence of erythrocytes in the urine.

hematogenesis (-jen′ĕ-sis) hematopoiesis.

hematogenic (-jen′ik) 1. hematopoietic. 2. hematogenous.

hematogenous (hem″ah-toj′ĕ-nus) produced by or derived from the blood; disseminated through the blood stream.

hematoid (hem′ah-toid) resembling blood.

hematoidin (hem″ah-toi′din) a substance apparently chemically identical with bilirubin but formed in the tissues from hemoglobin, particularly under conditions of reduced oxygen tension.

hematologist (he″mah-tol′o-jist) a specialist in hematology.

hematology (-tol′o-je) the science dealing with the morphology of blood and blood-forming tissues, and with their physiology and pathology.

hematolymphangioma (hem″ah-to-lim-fan″-je-o′mah) a tumor that is composed of blood and lymph vessels.

hematolysis (hem″ah-tol′ĭ-sis) hemolysis. **hematolyt′ic,** adj.

hematoma (he″mah-to′mah) a localized collection of extravasated blood, usually clotted, in an organ, space, or tissue. **subdural h.,** a massive blood clot beneath the dura mater that causes neurologic symptoms by pressure on the brain.

hematomediastinum (hem″ah-to-me″de-as-ti′-num) hemomediastinum.

hematometra (-me′trah) an accumulation of blood in the uterus.

hematometry (he″mah-tom′ĕ-tre) measurement of hemoglobin and estimation of the percentage of various cells in the blood.

hematomphalocele (hem″at-om-fal′o-sēl) an umbilical hernia containing blood.

hematomyelia (hem″ah-to-mi-e′le-ah) hemorrhage into the substance of the spinal cord.

hematomyelitis (-mi″ĕ-li′tis) acute myelitis with bloody effusion into the spinal cord.

hematomyelopore (-mi′ĕ-lo-pōr) formation of canals in the spinal cord due to hemorrhage.

hematonosis (hem″ah-ton′o-sis) any disease of the blood.

hematopathology (hem″ah-to-pah-thol′o-je) the study of diseases of the blood.

hematophagia (-fa′je-ah) 1. blood drinking. 2. subsisting on blood. 3. hemocytophagia. **hematoph′agous,** adj.

hematophilia (-fil′e-ah) hemophilia.

hematoplastic (-plas′tik) concerned in the elaboration of blood.

hematopoiesis (-poi-e′sis) the formation and development of blood cells. **extramedullary h.,** that occurring outside the bone marrow, as in the spleen, liver, and lymph nodes.

hematopoietic (-poi-et′ik) 1. pertaining to or affecting the formation of blood cells. 2. an agent that promotes the formation of blood cells.

hematoporphyrin (-por′fĭ-rin) an iron-free derivative of heme, a product of the decomposition of hemoglobin.

hematoporphyrinemia (-por″fĭ-rĭ-ne′me-ah) hematoporphyrin in the blood.

hematoporphyrinuria (-por″fĭ-rĭ-nu′re-ah) hematoporphyrin in the urine.

hematorrhachis (hem″at-o′rah-kis) hemorrhage into the vertebral canal.

hematorrhea (hem″ah-to-re′ah) copious hemorrhage.

hematosalpinx (-sal′pinks) an accumulation of blood in the uterine tube.

hematoscheocele (hem″ah-tos′ke-o-sēl″) an accumulation of blood within the scrotum.

hematoscope (hem′ah-to-skōp″) an instrument for the optical or spectroscopic examination of blood.

hematoscopy (hem″ah-tos′ko-pe) analysis of blood with the hematoscope.

hematospectroscopy (hem″ah-to-spek-tros′-ko-pe) spectroscopic examination of blood.

hematospermatocele (-sper-mat′o-sēl) a spermatocele containing blood.

hematospermia (-sper′me-ah) hemospermia.

hematosteon (hem″ah-tos′te-on) hemorrhage into the medullary cavity of a bone.

hematothermal (hem″ah-to-ther′mal) warm-blooded.

hemtotoxic (-tok′sik) 1. pertaining to blood poisoning. 2. poisonous to the blood and hematopoietic system.

hematotrachelos (-trah-ke′los) distention of the cervix uteri with blood.

hematotropic (-trop′ik) having a specific affinity for or exerting a specific effect on the blood or blood cells.

hematotympanum (-tim′pah-num) hemorrhage into the middle ear.

hematoxylin (hem″ah-tok′sĭ-lin) an acid coloring matter from the heartwood of *Haematoxylon campechianum;* used as a histologic stain and also as an indicator.

hematuria (hem″ah-tu′re-ah) the presence of blood in the urine. **endemic h.,** urinary schistosomiasis. **enzootic bovine h.,** a disease of cattle marked by blood in the urine, anemia, and debilitation. **essential h.,** that for which no cause has been determined. **false h.,** redness of the urine due to ingestion of food or drugs containing pigment. **renal h.,** that in which the blood comes from the kidney. **urethral h.,** that in which the blood comes from the urethra. **vesical h.,** that in which the blood comes from the bladder.

heme (hēm) an iron compound of protoporphyrin which constitutes the pigment portion or protein-free part of the hemoglobin molecule and is responsible for its oxygen-carrying properties.

hemeralopia (hem″er-ah-lo′pe-ah) day blindness.

hemi- word element [Gr.], *half.*

hemiacardius (hem″e-ah-kar′de-us) an unequal twin in which the heart is rudimentary, its circulation being assisted by the other twin.

hemiachromatopsia (-a″kro-mah-top′se-ah) color blindness in half, or in corresponding halves, of the visual field.

hemialbumose (-al′bu-mōs) a digestion product of certain proteins; normally found in bone marrow, and occurring in the urine in osteomalacia and diphtheria.

hemialbumosuria (-al″bu-mo-su′re-ah) hemialbumose in the urine.

hemiamyosthenia (-ah-mi″os-the′ne-ah) lack of muscular power on one side of the body.

hemianacusia (-an″ah-ku′ze-ah) loss of hearing in one ear.

hemianalgesia (-an″al-je′ze-ah) analgesia on one side of the body.

hemianencephaly (-an″en-sef′ah-le) congenital absence of one side of the brain.

hemianesthesia (-an″es-the′ze-ah) anesthesia of

one side of the body. **crossed h., h. crucia′ta,** loss of sensation on one side of the face and loss of pain and temperature sense on the opposite side of the body.

hemianopia (-ah-no′pe-ah) defective vision or blindness in half of the visual field. **hemiano′pic,** adj. **absolute h.,** blindness to light, color, and form in half of the visual field. **altitudinal h.,** that affecting a horizontal half of the visual field. **binasal h.,** that in which the defect is in the nasal half of the visual field in each eye. **binocular h.,** true h. **bitemporal h.,** that in which the defect is in the temporal half of the visual field in each eye. **complete h.,** that affecting an entire half of the visual field in each eye. **congruous h.,** that in which the defect is approximately the same in each eye. **crossed h.,** heteronymous h. **equilateral h.,** homonymous h. **heteronymous h.,** that affecting both nasal or both temporal halves of the field of vision. **homonymous h.,** that affecting the nasal half of the field of vision of one eye and the temporal half of the other. **horizontal h.,** altitudinal h. **lateral h.,** vertical h. **lower h.,** that affecting the lower half of the visual field. **nasal h.,** that affecting the medial half of the visual field, i.e., the half nearest the nose. **quadrant h., quadrantic h.,** quadrantanopia. **temporal h.,** that affecting the lateral vertical half of the visual field, i.e., the half nearest the temple. **true h.,** that affecting one vertical half of each eye, usually due to a single lesion of the optic tract, at or above the level of the chiasm. **unilateral h., uniocular h.,** that affecting half of the visual field of one eye only. **upper h.,** that affecting the upper half of the visual field. **vertical h.,** that in a lateral half of the visual field.

hemianopsia (-ah-nop′se-ah) hemianopia. **hemianop′tic,** adj.

hemianosmia (-an-oz′me-ah) absence of the sense of smell in one nostril.

hemiapraxia (-ah-prak′se-ah) apraxia on one side of the body only.

hemiataxia (-ah-tak′se-ah) ataxia on one side of the body.

hemiathetosis (-ath″ĕ-to′sis) athetosis of one side of the body.

hemiatrophy (-at′ro-fe) atrophy of one side of the body or one half of an organ or part.

hemiballism, hemiballismus (-bal′izm; -bă-liz′mus) ballismus involving one side of the body, most marked in the upper limb.

hemic (he′mik, hem′ik) pertaining to blood.

hemicardia (hem″e-kar′de-ah) the presence of only one side of a four-chambered heart.

hemicellulose (-sel′u-lōs) general name for a group of high molecular weight carbohydrates resembling cellulose but more soluble and more easily decomposed.

hemicentrum (-sen′trum) either lateral half of a vertebral centrum.

hemicephalia (-sĕ-fa′le-ah) congenital abscence of the cerebrum.

hemicephalus (-sef′ah-lus) a fetus exhibiting hemicephalia.

hemichorea (-ko-re′ah) chorea affecting only one side of the body.

hemichromatopsia (-kro″mah-top′se-ah) color blindness in half of the visual field.

hemicolectomy (-ko-lek′to-me) excision of approximately half of the colon.

hemicrania (-kra′ne-ah) 1. unilateral headache. 2. incomplete anencephaly.

hemicraniosis (-kra″ne-o′sis) hyperostosis of one side of the cranium and face.

hemidiaphoresis (-di″ah-fo-re′sis) hemihyperhidrosis.

hemidysesthesia (-dis″es-the′ze-ah) disorder of sensation on one side of the body.

hemidystrophy (-dis′tro-fe) unequal development of the two sides of the body.

hemiectromelia (-ek″tro-me′le-ah) developmental anomaly with imperfect limbs on one side of the body.

hemielastin (-e-las′tin) a substance formed by the digestion or hydrolysis of elastin.

hemiepilepsy (-ep″ĭ-lep″se) epilepsy affecting one side of the body.

hemifacial (-fa′shal) pertaining to or affecting half of the face.

hemigastrectomy (-gas-trek′to-me) excision of half of the stomach.

hemigeusia (-gu′ze-ah) absence of the sense of taste on one side of the tongue.

hemiglossectomy (-glŏ-sek′to-me) excision of one side of the tongue.

hemiglossitis (-glŏ-si′tis) inflammation of one half of the tongue.

hemignathia (-na′the-ah) a developmental anomaly characterized by partial or complete lack of the lower jaw on one side.

hemihidrosis (-hĭ-dro′sis) sweating on one side of the body only.

hemihypalgesia (-hīp″al-je′ze-ah) diminished sensitivity to pain on one side of the body.

hemihyperesthesia (-hi″per-es-the′ze-ah) increased sensitiveness of one side of the body.

hemihyperhidrosis (-hĭ-dro′sis) excessive perspiration on one side of the body.

hemihypertonia (-to′ne-ah) increased muscle tone on one side of the body.

hemihypertrophy (hem″e-hi-per′tro-fe) overgrowth of one side of the body or of a part.

hemihypesthesia (-hīp″es-the′ze-ah) diminished sensitiveness on one side of the body.

hemihypotonia (-hi″po-to′ne-ah) diminished muscle tone of one side of the body.

hemilaminectomy (-lam″ĭ-nek′to-me) removal of the vertebral laminae on one side.

hemilaryngectomy (-lar″in-jek′to-me) excision of part of the larynx.

hemilateral (-lat′er-al) affecting one lateral half of the body only.

hemilesion (-le′zhun) a lesion on one side of the spinal cord.

hemimelia (-me′le-ah) congenital absence of all or part of the distal half of a limb.

hemimelus (hem-im′ĕ-lus) an individual exhibiting hemimelia.

hemin (he′min) the crystalline chloride of heme.

heminephrectomy (hem″e-nĕ-frek′to-me) excision of part (half) of a kidney.

hemiopia (-o′pe-ah) hemianopia. **hemiop′ic,** adj.

hemipagus (hem-ip′ah-gus) twin fetuses joined laterally at the thorax.

hemiparanesthesia (hem″e-par″an-es-the′ze-ah) anesthesia of the lower half of one side.

hemiparaplegia (-par″ah-ple′je-ah) paralysis of the lower half of one side.

hemiparesis (-pah-re′sis) paresis affecting one side of the body.

hemiplacenta (-plah-sen′tah) an organ composed of the chorion, yolk sac, and, usually, allantois, which puts marsupial embryos into temporary relation with the maternal uterus.

hemiplegia (-ple′je-ah) paralysis of one side of the body. **hemiple′gic,** adj. **alternate h.,** paralysis of one side of the face and the opposite side of the body. **cerebral h.,** that due to a brain lesion. **crossed h.,** alternate h. **facial h.,** paralysis of one side of face. **spastic h.,** hemiplegia with spasticity of the affected muscles and increased tendon reflexes. **spinal h.,** that due to lesion of spinal cord.

Hemiptera (hem-ip′ter-ah) an order of insects, winged or wingless, including ordinary bugs and lice, having mouth parts adapted to piercing and sucking.

hemipterous (he-mip′ter-us) of or pertaining to insects of the order Hemiptera.

hemirachischisis (hem″e-rah-kis′kĭ-sis) rachischisis without prolapse of the spinal cord.

hemisection (-sek′shun) 1. bisection. 2. division into two equal parts.

hemispasm (hem′e-spazm) spasm affecting one side only.

hemisphere (hem′ĭ-sfēr) half of a spherical or roughly spherical structure or organ. **cerebellar h.,** either of two lobes of the cerebellum lateral to the vermis. **cerebral h.,** one of the paired structures forming the bulk of the human brain, which together comprise the cerebral cortex, centrum semiovale, basal ganglia, and rhinencephalon, and contain the lateral ventricles. **dominant h.,** that cerebral hemisphere which is more concerned than the other in the integration of sensations and the control of voluntary functions.

hemispherium (hem″ĭ-sfe′re-um), pl. *hemisphe′ria* [L.] either cerebral hemisphere.

hemithorax (hem″e-tho′raks) one side of the chest.

hemithyroidectomy (-thi″roi-dek′to-me) excision of one lobe of the thyroid gland.

hemivertebra (-ver′tĕ-brah) a developmental anomaly in which one side of a vertebra is incompletely developed.

hemizygosity (-zi-gos′ĭ-te) the state of having only one of a pair of alleles transmitting a specific character. **hemizy′gous,** adj.

hemizygote (-zi′gōt) an individual or cell exhibiting hemizygosity.

hemo- word element [Gr.], *blood.* See also words beginning *hem-* and *hemato-*.

hemoalkalimeter (he″mo-al″kah-lim′ĕ-ter) an apparatus for estimating alkalinity of the blood.

hemobilia (-bil′e-ah) hematobilia.

hemoblast (he′mo-blast) hemocytoblast. **lymphoid h. of Pappenheim,** pronormoblast.

hemoblastosis (he″mo-blas-to′sis) general term for proliferative disorders of the blood-forming tissues.

hemocatheresis (-kah-ther′ĕ-sis) the destruction of red blood cells. **hemocatheret′ic,** adj.

hemochorial (-ko′re-al) denoting a type of placenta in which maternal blood comes in direct contact with the chorion.

hemochromatosis (-kro″mah-to′sis) a disorder of iron metabolism with excess deposition of iron in the tissues, bronze skin pigmentation, hepatic cirrhosis, and diabetes mellitus. **hemochromatot′ic,** adj.

hemochrome (he′mo-krōm) an oxygen-carrying pigment of the blood.

hemochromogen (he″mo-kro′mo-jen) any compound formed by the combination of heme with a nitrogenous compound.

hemochromometer (-kro-mom′ĕ-ter) an instrument for making color tests of the blood to determine the proportion of hemoglobin.

hemoclasis (he-mok′lah-sis) hemolysis. **hemoclas′tic,** adj.

hemoconcentration (he″mo-kon″sen-tra′shun) decrease of the fluid content of the blood, with resulting increase in concentration of its formed elements.

hemoconia (-ko′ne-ah), pl. *hemoco′niae* [L.] small, round or dumbbell-shaped bodies exhibiting brownian movement, observed in blood platelets in darkfield microscopy of a wet film of blood.

hemoconiosis (-ko″ne-o′sis) presence in blood of excessive amounts of hemoconia.

hemocryoscopy (-kri-os′ko-pe) the ascertaining of the freezing point of blood.

hemocrystallin (-kris′tah-lin) hemoglobin.

hemocuprein (-ku′pre-in) a copper and protein compound isolated from erythrocytes.

hemocyanin (-si′ah-nin) hematocyanin.

hemocyte (he′mo-sīt) a blood cell.

hemocytoblast (he″mo-si′to-blast) the free stem cell from which, according to some theorists, all other blood cells are derived.

hemocytoblastoma (-si″to-blas-to′mah) a tumor containing all the cells typical of bone marrow.

hemocytocatheresis (-kah-ther′ĕ-sis) hemolysis.

hemocytogenesis (-jen′ĕ-sis) hematopoiesis.

hemocytology (-si-tol′o-je) the study of blood cells.

hemocytolysis (-si-tol′ĭ-sis) hemolysis.

hemocytometer (-si-tom′ĕ-ter) an instrument used in counting blood cells.

hemocytotripsis (-si″to-trip′sis) disintegration of blood cells by pressure.

hemodiagnosis (-di″ag-no′sis) diagnosis by examination of the blood.

hemodialysis (-di-al′ĭ-sis) removal of certain elements from the blood by virtue of difference in rates of their diffusion through a semipermeable membrane while being circulated outside the body.

hemodialyzer (-di′ah-līz″er) an apparatus for performing hemodialysis.

hemodiastase (-di′as-tās) an amylolytic enzyme in the blood.

hemodilution (-di-lu′shun) increase in fluid content of blood, resulting in diminution in the concentration of formed elements.

hemodynamics (-di-nam′iks) the study of the movements of the blood and of the forces concerned therein. **hemodynam′ic**, adj.

hemoendothelial (-en-do-the′le-al) denoting a type of placenta in which maternal blood comes in contact with the endothelium of chorionic vessels.

hemoferrum (-fer′um) oxyhemoglobin.

hemoflagellate (-flaj′ĕ-lāt) any flagellate protozoan parasite of the blood; the term includes the genera *Trypanosoma* and *Leishmania*.

hemofuscin (-fūs′in) a brownish-yellow pigment resulting from hemoglobin decomposition; it gives urine a deep ruddy color.

hemogenesis (-jen′ĕ-sis) hematopoiesis. **hemogen′ic**, adj.

hemoglobin (-glo′bin) the oxygen-carrying pigment of the erythrocytes, formed by the developing erythrocyte in the bone marrow, made up of four different globin polypeptide chains, each composed of several hundred amino acids. Hemoglobin A is normal adult hemoglobin. Many abnormal hemoglobins have been reported, including hemoglobin E, H, M, and S; homozygosity for hemoglobin S results in sickle cell anemia, heterozygosity in sickle cell trait. Symbol Hb. **fetal h.**, that forming more than half of the hemoglobin of the fetus, present in minimal amounts in adults and abnormally elevated in certain blood disorders. **muscle h.**, myoglobin. **reduced h.**, that not combined with oxygen.

hemoglobinemia (-glo″bĭ-ne′me-ah) the presence of excessive hemoglobin in the blood plasma.

hemoglobinolysis (-glo″bĭ-nol′ĭ-sis) the splitting up of hemoglobin.

hemoglobinometer (-glo″bĭ-nom′ĕ-ter) a laboratory instrument for colorimetric determination of the hemoglobin content of the blood.

hemoglobinopathy (-glo″bĭ-nop′ah-the) a hematologic disorder due to alteration in the genetically determined molecular structure of hemoglobin, with characteristic clinical and laboratory abnormalities and often overt anemia.

hemoglobinophilia (-glo″bĭ-no-fil′e-ah) the property of growing well in culture media containing hemoglobin. **hemoglobinophil′ic**, adj.

hemoglobinous (-glo′bĭ-nus) containing hemoglobin.

hemoglobinuria (-glo″bĭ-nu′re-ah) the presence of free hemoglobin in the urine. **hemoglobinu′ric**, adj. **epidemic h.**, Winckel's disease. **intermittent h.**, that occurring in isolated episodes, e.g., after exposure to cold (*paroxysmal cold h.*), or idiopathically, usually during the night, with hemosiderinuria, increased

amounts of plasma hemoglobin, a positive acid-serum or sucrose-hemolysis test, and often leukopenia or thrombocytopenia (*paroxysmal noctural h.*). **march h.**, that occurring after prolonged exercise. **toxic h.**, that which is consequent upon the ingestion of various poisons.

hemogram (he′mo-gram) a written record or graphic representation of the differential blood count.

hemohistioblast (he″mo-his′te-o-blast″) the hypothetical stem cell from which all blood cells are derived.

hemoid (he′moid) resembling blood.

hemokinesis (he″mo-ki-ne′sis) the flow of blood in the body. **hemokinet′ic**, adj.

hemokonia (-ko′ne-ah) hemoconia.

hemokoniosis (-ko″ne-o′sis) hemoconiosis.

hemolymph (he′mo-limf) 1. blood and lymph. 2. the blood of those invertebrates having open blood-vascular systems.

hemolymphangioma (he″mo-lim-fan″je-o′mah) hematolymphangioma.

hemolysate (he-mol′ĭ-sāt) the product resulting from hemolysis.

hemolysin (he-mol′ĭ-sin) a substance that liberates hemoglobin from erythrocytes by interrupting their structural integrity.

hemolysis (he-mol′ĭ-sis) the liberation of hemoglobin, consisting in separation of the hemoglobin from the red cells and its appearance in the plasma. **hemolyt′ic**, adj. **immune h.**, lysis by complement of erythrocytes sensitized as a consequence of interaction with specific antibody to the erythrocytes.

hemolysoid (he-mol′ĭ-soid) a hemolysin so altered that it still combines with erythrocytes but does not cause hemolysis.

hemolyze (he′mo-līz) to subject to or to undergo hemolysis.

hemomediastinum (he″mo-me″de-as-ti′num) an effusion of blood into the mediastinum.

hemometer (he-mom′ĕ-ter) hemoglobinometer.

hemometra (he″mo-me′trah) hematometra.

hemonephrosis (-nĕ-fro′sis) hematonephrosis.

hemopathology (-pah-thol′o-je) the study of diseases of the blood.

hemopathy (he-mop′ah-the) any disease of the blood. **hemopath′ic**, adj.

hemopericardium (he″mo-per″ĭ-kar′de-um) an effusion of blood within the pericardium.

hemoperitoneum (-per″ĭ-to-ne′um) an effusion of blood in the peritonal cavity.

hemopexin (-pek′sin) a heme-binding serum protein.

hemopexis (-pek′sis) coagulation of blood.

hemophagocyte (-fag′o-sīt) a phagocyte that destroys blood cells.

hemophil (he′mo-fil) 1. thriving on blood. 2. a microorganism which grows best in media containing hemoglobin.

hemophilia (he″mo-fil′e-ah) a hereditary hemorrhagic diathesis due to deficiency of a blood coagulation factor. **h. A**, classical hemophilia; an X-linked recessive form affecting males, due to deficiency of coagulation Factor VIII. **h. B**, a form similar to classical hemophilia but due to a lack of coagulation Factor IX. **h. C,** an autosomal dominant form due to lack of coagulation Factor XI. **classical h.,** h. A. **vascular h.,** angiohemophilia.

hemophiliac (-fil′e-ak) a person affected with hemophilia.

hemophilic (-fil′ik) 1. having an affinity for blood; in bacteriology, growing well in culture media containing blood. 2. pertaining to or characterized by hemophilia.

hemophilioid (-fil′e-oid) resembling classical hemophilia clinically; applied to a number of hereditary or acquired hemorrhagic disorders not due solely to coagulation Factor VIII deficiency.

Hemophilus (he-mof′ĭ-lus) a genus of gram-negative bacteria (family Brucellaceae), most species of which have a nutritional requirement for the constituents of fresh blood, including *H. aegyp′ticus,* the cause of acute contagious conjunctivitis; *H. ducrey′i,* the cause of chancroid; *H. du′plex,* the cause of an acute or chronic blepharoconjunctivitis; *H. influen′zae,* a species once thought to cause epidemic influenza, causes a highly fatal form of meningitis affecting mostly infants; and *H. vagina′lis,* associated, possibly causally, with human vaginitis.

hemophoric (he″mo-for′ik) conveying blood.

hemophthalmia (he″mof-thal′me-ah) extravasation of blood inside the eye.

hemoplastic (he′mo-plas″tik) hematoplastic.

hemopleura (he″mo-ploo′rah) hemothorax.

hemopneumopericardium (-nu″mo-per″ĭ-kar′de-um) effused blood and air in the pericardium.

hemopneumothorax (-nu″mo-tho′raks) pneumothorax with hemorrhagic effusion.

hemopoiesis (-poi-e′sis) hematopoiesis. **hemopoiet′ic,** adj.

hemoposia (-po′ze-ah) the drinking of blood.

hemoprecipitin (-pre-sip′ĭ-tin) a blood precipitin.

hemoprotein (-pro′tēn) a conjugated protein containing heme as the prosthetic group.

hemopsonin (he″mop-so′nin) an opsonin that renders erythrocytes more liable to phagocytosis.

hemoptysis (he-mop′tĭ-sis) the spitting of blood or of blood-stained sputum. **parasitic h.,** a disease due to infection of the lungs with lung flukes of the genus *Paragonimus,* with cough and spitting of blood and gradual deterioration of health.

hemorrhage (hem′ŏ-rij) the escape of blood from the vessels; bleeding. **hemorrhag′ic,** adj. **capillary h.,** the oozing of blood from the minute vessels. **cerebral h.,** hemorrhage into the cerebrum; see *stroke syndrome.* **concealed h.,** internal h. **fibrinolytic h.,** that due to abnormalities in the fibrinolytic system. **internal h.,** that in which the extravasated blood remains within the body. **nasal h.,** epistaxis. **petechial h.,** subcutaneous hemorrhage occurring in minute spots. **postpartum h.,** that which follows soon after labor or childbirth. **primary h.,** that occurring immediately after injury. **secondary h.,** bleeding which follows an injury after a lapse of time. **unavoidable h.,** that caused by detachment of a placenta previa. **uterine h., essential,** hemorrhage from the uterus, usually with hypertrophy of the uterine mucosa and cystic disease of the ovary.

hemorrhagenic (hem″o-rah-jen′ik) causing hemorrhage.

hemorrhagin (-ra′jin) a cytolysin in certain venoms and poisons which is destructive to endothelial cells and blood vessels.

hemorrhea (-re′ah) hematorrhea.

hemorrheology (he″mo-re-ol′o-je) the scientific study of the deformation and flow properties of cellular and plasmatic components of blood in macroscopic, microscopic, and submicroscopic dimensions, and the rheological properties of vessel structure with which the blood comes in direct contact.

hemorrhoid (hem′ŏ-roid) a varicose dilatation of a vein of the superior or inferior hemorrhoidal plexus. **hemorrhoi′dal,** adj. **external h.,** varicose dilatation of a vein of the inferior hemorrhoidal plexus, distal to the pectinate line and covered with modified anal skin. **internal h.,** a varicose dilatation of a vein of the superior hemorrhoidal plexus, originating above the pectinate line and covered by mucous membrane. **lingual h.,** varicose dilatation of the veins of the tongue, usually on the ventral surface. **prolapsed h.,** an internal hemorrhoid which has descended below the pectinate line and protruded outside the anal sphincter. **strangulated h.,** an internal hemorrhoid which has been prolapsed sufficiently and for long enough time for its blood supply to become occluded by the constricting action of the anal sphincter. **thrombosed h.,** one containing clotted blood.

hemorrhoidectomy (hem″o-roi-dek′to-me) excision of hemorrhoids.

hemosiderin (he″mo-sid′er-in) an insoluble form of tissue storage iron, visible microscopically both with and without the use of special stains.

hemosiderinuria (-sid″er-in-u′re-ah) the presence of hemosiderin in the urine.

hemosiderosis (-sid″ĕ-ro-sis) a focal or general increase in tissue iron stores without associated tissue damage.

hemospermia (-sper′me-ah) the presence of blood in the semen.

hemostasis (he″mo-sta′sis, he-mos′tah-sis) 1. the arrest of bleeding, either by the physiological properties of vasoconstriction and coagulation or by surgical means. 2. interruption of blood flow through any vessel or to any anatomical area.

hemostat (he′mo-stat) 1. a small surgical clamp for constricting blood vessels. 2. an antihemorrhagic agent.

hemostatic (he″mo-stat′ik) checking blood flow; an agent that so acts.

hemostyptic (-stip′tik) hemostatic.

hemotherapy (-ther′ah-pe) the use of blood or its products in treating disease.

hemothorax (-tho′raks) collection of blood in the pleural cavity.

hemotoxic (-tok′sik) hematotoxic.

hemotoxin (-tok′sin) an exotoxin characterized by hemolytic activity.

hemotroph (he′mo-trŏf) the sum total of nutritive substances supplied to the embryo from the maternal blood. **hemotroph′ic,** adj.

hemotympanum (he″mo-tim′pah-num) hematotympanum.

henbane (hen′bān) hyoscyamus.

henry (hen′re) the unit of electrical inductance.

hepar (he′par) [L.] the liver.

heparin (hep′ah-rin) an anticoagulant mucopolysaccharide acid found in tissues, most abundantly in the liver and lungs, or a mixture of active principles from the livers or lungs of domestic animals (sodium h.) which renders the blood incoagulable; used in the prevention and treatment of thrombosis, in bacterial endocarditis, postoperative pulmonary embolism, and frostbite, and in repair of vascular injury.

heparinize (hep′ĕr-ĭ-nīz″) to render blood incoagulable with heparin.

hepat(o)- word element [Gr.], *liver.*

hepatalgia (hep″ah-tal′je-ah) pain in the liver.

hepatatrophia (hep″ah-tah-tro′fe-ah) atrophy of the liver.

hepatectomy (hep″ah-tek′to-me) surgical excision of liver tissue.

hepatic (hĕ-pat′ik) pertaining to the liver.

hepatic(o)- word element [Gr.], *hepatic duct.*

hepaticoduodenostomy (hĕ-pat″ĭ-ko-du″o-dĕ-nos′to-me) anastomosis of the hepatic duct to the duodenum.

hepaticoenterostomy (-en″ter-os′to-me) anastomosis of the hepatic duct to the intestine (duodenum or jejunum).

hepaticogastrostomy (-gas-tros′to-me) anastomosis of the hepatic duct to the stomach.

hepaticojejunostomy (-je″ju-nos′to-me) anastomosis of the hepatic duct to the jejunum.

hepaticolithotomy (-lĭ-thot′o-me) incision of the hepatic duct, with removal of calculi.

hepaticolithotripsy (-lith′o-trip″se) the crushing of a stone in the hepatic duct.

hepaticostomy (hĕ-pat″ĭ-kos′to-me) fistulization of the hepatic duct.

hepaticotomy (hĕ-pat″ĭ-kot′o-me) incision of the hepatic duct.

hepatitis (hep″ah-ti′tis) inflammation of the liver. **anicteric h.,** a mild viral hepatitis without jaundice. **cholangiolitic h.,** inflammation of the bile ducts of the liver associated with obstructive jaundice. **infectious h.,** an acute viral (hepatitis virus A) illness, usually transmitted by oral ingestion of infected material, but also by blood transfusion (see *serum h.*), usually beginning with fever, malaise, and nonspecific gastrointestinal symptoms, followed by jaundice, pruritus, dark urine, pale stools, and hepatomegaly with tenderness. **infectious necrotic h. of sheep,** black disease. **lupoid h.,** chronic active hepatitis characterized by the presence of LE cells in the peripheral blood. **neonatal h.,** hepatitis of uncertain etiology occurring soon after birth and marked by prolonged persistent jaundice, which may progress to cirrhosis.

serum h., transfusion h., an acute viral (hepatitis virus B) illness transmitted by parenteral exposure (contaminated needles and transfusion of blood and its products) and by oral ingestion of contaminated material; its course tends to be more prolonged than that of infectious hepatitis. **viral h.,** see *infectious h.* and *serum h.*

hepatization (hep″ah-tĭ-za′shun) transformation into a liver-like mass, especially the solidified state of the lung in lobar pneumonia. The early stage, in which the pulmonary exudate is blood stained, is called *red h.* The later stage, in which the red cells disintegrate and a fibrinosuppurative exudate persists, is called *gray h.*

hepatoblastoma (hep″ah-to-blas-to′mah) a malignant intrahepatic tumor consisting chiefly of embryonic tissue, occurring in infants and young children.

hepatocele (hep′ah-to-sēl) hernia of the liver.

hepatocellular (hep″ah-to-sel′u-lar) pertaining to or affecting liver cells.

hepatocholangitis (-ko″lan-ji′tis) inflammation of the liver and bile ducts.

hepatocirrhosis (-sĭ-ro′sis) cirrhosis of the liver.

hepatocuprein (-ku′prin) a copper protein present in liver tissue.

hepatocystic (-sis′tik) pertaining to the liver and gallbladder.

hepatocyte (hep′ah-to-sīt″) a parenchymal liver cell.

hepatodynia (hep″ah-to-din′e-ah) pain in the liver.

hepatoflavin (-fla′vin) a riboflavin obtained from liver tissue.

hepatogastric (-gas′trik) pertaining to the liver and stomach.

hepatogenic (-jen′ik) 1. giving rise to or forming liver tissue. 2. hepatogenous.

hepatogenous (hep″ah-toj′ĕ-nus) 1. produced in or originating in the liver. 2. hepatogenic.

hepatogram (hep′ah-to-gram″) 1. a tracing of the liver pulse in the sphygmogram. 2. a roentgenogram of the liver.

hepatography (hep″ah-tog′rah-fe) 1. a treatise on the liver. 2. radiography of the liver. 3. the recording of the liver pulse.

hepatoid (hep′ah-toid) resembling the liver.

hepatojugular (hep″ah-to-jug′u-lar) pertaining to the liver and jugular vein; see under *reflux.*

hepatolienography (-li″ĕ-nog′rah-fe) radiography of the liver and spleen.

hepatolith (hep′ah-to-lith″) a biliary calculus in the liver.

hepatolithectomy (hep″ah-to-lĭ-thek′to-me) removal of a calculus from the liver.

hepatolithiasis (-lĭ-thi′ah-sis) the presence of calculi in the biliary ducts of the liver.

hepatology (hep″ah-tol′o-je) the scientific study of the liver and its diseases.

hepatolysin (-tol′ĭ-sin) a cytolysin destructive to liver cells.

hepatolysis (hep″ah-tol′ĭ-sis) destruction of the liver cells. **hepatolyt′ic,** adj.

hepatoma (hep″ah-to′mah) 1. any tumor of the

liver. 2. a malignant hepatic tumor whose cells resemble parenchymal liver cells.

hepatomalacia (hep″ah-to-mah-la′she-ah) softening of the liver.

hepatomegaly (-meg′ah-le) enlargement of the liver.

hepatomelanosis (-mel″ah-no′sis) melanosis of the liver.

hepatomphalocele (hep″ah-tom′fah-lo-sēl″) umbilical hernia with liver involvement in the hernial sac.

hepatonephric (hep″ah-to-nef′rik) pertaining to the liver and kidney.

hepatopathy (hep″ah-top′ah-the) any disease of the liver.

hepatopexy (hep′ah-to-pek″se) surgical fixation of a displaced liver.

hepatopleural (hep″ah-to-ploo′ral) pertaining to the liver and pleura or pleural cavity.

hepatopneumonic (-nu-mon′ik) pertaining to, affecting, or communicating with the liver and lungs.

hepatoportal (-por′tal) pertaining to the portal system of the liver.

hepatopulmonary (-pul′mo-ner″e) hepatopneumonic.

hepatorenal (-re′nal) pertaining to the liver and kidneys.

hepatorrhaphy (hep″ah-tor′ah-fe) suture of the liver.

hepatorrhexis (hep″ah-to-rek′sis) rupture of the liver.

hepatoscan (hep′ah-to-skan″) a surface scintiscan of the liver.

hepatoscopy (hep″ah-tos′ko-pe) examination of the liver.

hepatosis (hep″ah-to′sis) any functional disorder of the liver. **serous h.,** veno-occlusive disease of the liver.

hepatosplenitis (hep″ah-to-sple-ni′tis) inflammation of the liver and spleen.

hepatosplenography (-sple-nog′rah-fe) roentgenography of the liver and spleen.

hepatosplenomegaly (-sple″no-meg′ah-le) enlargement of the liver and spleen.

hepatotherapy (-ther′ah-pe) therapeutic administration of liver or liver extract.

hepatotomy (hep″ah-tot′o-me) incision of the liver.

hepatotoxemia (hep″ah-to-tok-se′me-ah) blood poisoning originating in the liver.

hepatotoxin (-tok′sin) a toxin that destroys liver cells. **hepatotox′ic,** adj.

hepta- word element [Gr.], *seven.*

heptabarbital (hep″tah-bar′bĭ-tal) a hypnotic and sedative, $C_{13}H_{18}N_2O_3$.

heptachromic (-kro′mik) 1. pertaining to or exhibiting seven colors. 2. able to distinguish all seven colors of the spectrum.

heptose (hep′tōs) a sugar whose molecule contains seven carbon atoms.

herb (erb, herb) any leafy plant without a woody stem, especially one used as a household remedy or as a flavor. **death's h.,** belladonna (2).

herbivorous (her-biv′o-rus) subsisting upon plants.

hereditary (hĕ-red′ĭ-tār″e) genetically transmitted from parent to offspring.

heredity (hĕ-red′ĭ-te) 1. the genetic transmission of a particular quality or trait from parent to offspring. 2. the genetic constitution of an individual. **autosomal h.,** transmission of a quality or trait by a gene located on an autosome. **sex-linked h., X-linked h.,** transmission of a quality or trait by a gene located on a sex chromosome; generally limited to transmission of a trait by an X-linked gene.

heredofamilial (her″ĕ-do-fah-mil′e-al) occurring in certain families under circumstances that implicate a hereditary basis.

heritability (her″ĭ-tah-bil′ĭ-te) the quality of being heritable; a measure of the extent to which a phenotype is influenced by the genotype.

heritable (her′ĭ-tah-b′l) capable of being inherited, as a genetic trait.

hermaphrodism (her-maf′ro-dizm) hermaphroditism.

hermaphrodite (her-maf′ro-dīt) an individual who exhibits hermaphroditism.

hermaphroditism (her-maf′ro-di-tizm″) a state characterized by the presence of both ovarian and testicular tissues and of ambiguous morphologic criteria of sex; see also *pseudohermaphroditism.* **bilateral h.,** that in which gonadal tissue typical of both sexes occurs on each side of the body. **false h.,** pseudohermaphroditism. **lateral h.,** presence of gonadal tissue typical of one sex on one side of the body and tissue typical of the other sex on the opposite side. **transverse h.,** that in which the external genital organs are typical of one sex and the gonads typical of the other sex. **true h.,** see *hermaphroditism.*

hermetic (her-met′ik) impervious to air.

hernia (her′ne-ah) protrusion of a portion of an organ or tissue through an abnormal opening. **her′nial,** adj. **abdominal h.,** one through the abdominal wall. **h. adipo′sa,** fat h. **Barth's h.,** one between the serosa of the abdominal wall and that of a persistent vitelline duct. **Béclard's h.,** femoral hernia at the saphenous opening. **h. cer′ebri,** protrusion of brain substance through the skull. **Cloquet's h.,** crural h., pectineal. **complete h.,** one in which the sac and its contents have passed through the hernial orifice. **crural h.,** femoral h. **crural h., pectineal,** hernia within and behind the femoral vessels, the tumor resting upon the pectineus muscle. **diaphragmatic h.,** hernia through the diaphragm. **diverticular h.,** protrusion of a congenital diverticulum of the gut. **epigastric h.,** a hernia through the linea alba above the navel. **extrasaccular h.,** sliding h. **fat h.,** hernial protrusion of peritoneal fat through the abdominal wall. **femoral h.,** protrusion of a loop of intestine into the femoral canal. **gastroesophageal h.,** hiatal hernia in which the distal esophagus and part of the stomach protrude into the thorax. **Hesselbach's h.,** femoral hernia with a pouch through the cribriform fascia. **hiatal h., hiatus h.,** protrusion of any structure through the esophageal hiatus of the diaphragm. **Holthouse's h.,** an inguinal hernia that has turned outward into the groin. **incarcerated h.,** an irreducible hernia with intestinal obstruction but no strangulation. **incisional h.,** one occurring through an old abdominal incision. **inguinal h.,** hernia into the inguinal canal. **intermuscular h., interparietal h.,** an interstitial hernia lying between one or another of the fascial or muscular planes of the abdomen. **interstitial h.,** one in which a knuckle of intestine lies between two layers of the abdominal wall. **irreducible h.,** one that cannot be restored by manipulation. **ischiatic h.,** hernia through the sacrosciatic foramen. **labial h.,** one into a labium majus. **Littre's h.,** diverticular h. **lumbar h.,** hernia in the loin. **mesocolic h.,** hernia into a pouch of the mesocolon. **obturator h.,** a protrusion through obturator foramen. **pectineal h.,** hernia beneath the pectineal fascia. **properitoneal h.,** an interstitial hernia lying between the parietal peritoneum and the transverse fascia. **reducible h.,** one that can be returned by manipulation. **retrograde h.,** herniation of two loops of intestine, the portion between the loops lying within the abdominal wall. **Richter's h.,** hernia involving only part of the lumen of the gut. **scrotal h.,** inguinal hernia which has passed into the scrotum. **sliding h., slip h., slipped h.,** hernia of the colon in which a portion of the part is drawn into or slips into a hernial sac by the inclusion in the sac of the parietal peritoneum to which it is attached. **strangulated h.,** one which is tightly constricted and in which the blood supply is cut off, and may become gangrenous. **synovial h.,** protrusion of the inner lining membrane through the stratum fibrosum of a joint capsule. **umbilical h.,** herniation of part of the umbilicus, the defect in the abdominal wall and protruding bowel being covered with skin and subcutaneous tissue. **vaginal h.,** hernia into the vagina. **ventral h.,** hernia through the abdominal wall.

herniated (her'ne-āt"ed) protruding like a hernia.

herniation (her"ne-a'shun) abnormal protrusion of an organ or other body structure through a defect or natural opening in a covering membrane, muscle, or bone. **h. of nucleus pulposus,** rupture or prolapse of the nucleus pulposus into the spinal cord.

hernioid (her'ne-oid) resembling hernia.

herniology (her"ne-ol'o-je) the study of hernia.

hernioplasty (her'ne-o-plas"te) operation for the repair of hernia.

herniorrhaphy (her"ne-or'ah-fe) surgical repair of hernia, with suturing.

herniotomy (her"ne-ot'o-me) a cutting operation for the repair of hernia.

heroin (her'o-in) diacetylmorphine; a highly addictive morphine derivative, $C_{21}H_{23}NO_5$; the importation of heroin and its salts into the United States, as well as its use in medicine, is illegal.

heroinism (-izm") addiction to heroin.

herpangina (her"pan-ji'nah) an infectious febrile disease due to a coxsackievirus, marked by vesicular or ulcerated lesions on the fauces or soft palate.

herpes (her'pēz) any inflammatory skin disease marked by the formation of small vesicles in clusters; the term is usually restricted to such diseases caused by herpesviruses and is used alone to refer to *herpes simplex* or to *herpes zoster.* **herpet'ic,** adj. **h. catarrha'lis,** h. simplex. **h. febri'lis,** see *h. simplex.* **h. genita'lis,** h. progenitalis. **h. gestatio'nis,** a variant of dermatitis herpetiformis peculiar to pregnant women, and clearing upon termination of pregnancy. **h. i'ris,** erythema multiforme in which the lesions are vesicular. **h. progenita'lis,** herpes simplex of the genitals. **h. sim'plex,** an acute viral disease marked by groups of vesicles on the skin, often on the borders of the lips or nares (*cold sores*), or on the genitals (*h. progenitalis*); it often accompanies fever (*fever blisters, h. febrilis*). **h. zos'ter,** shingles; an acute, unilateral, self-limited inflammatory disease of cerebral ganglia and the ganglia of posterior nerve roots and peripheral nerves in a segmented distribution, caused by the chickenpox virus, and characterized by groups of small vesicles in the cutaneous areas along the course of affected nerves, and associated with neuralgic pain. **h. zos'ter ophthal'micus,** herpes zoster involving the ophthalmic nerve, with a vesicular erythematous rash along the nerve path (forehead, eyelid, and cornea) preceded by lancinating pain; there is iridocyclitis, and corneal involvement that may lead to keratitis and corneal anesthesia. **h. zos'ter o'ticus,** herpes zoster of the geniculate ganglion, with motor impairment, pain, and herpetic lesions of the auricle, auditory canal, and tympanic membrane.

herpesvirus (her"pēz-vi'rus) any of a group of DNA viruses which includes the etiologic agents of herpes simplex, herpes zoster, chickenpox, cytomegalic inclusion disease, etc.

herpetiform (her-pet'ĭ-form) resembling herpes; having grouped vesicles.

hersage (ār-sahzh') [Fr.] surgical separation of the fibers of a peripheral nerve.

hertz (herts) a unit of frequency, equal to one cycle per second. Symbol, Hz.

hesperidin (hes-per'ĭ-din) a flavone glycoside, $C_{28}H_{34}O_{15}$, isolated from the rind of certain citrus fruits; used to reduce capillary permeability.

heter(o)- word element [Gr.], *other; dissimilar.*

heteradelphus (het"er-ah-del'fus) a twin monster with one fetus much more developed than the other.

heterauxesis (-awk-ze'sis) disproportionate growth of body parts.

heterecious (-e'shus) parasitic on different hosts in various stages of its existence.

heteresthesia (-es-the'ze-ah) variation of cutaneous sensibility on adjoining areas.

heteroagglutination (het"er-o-ah-glu"tĭ-na'-shun) agglutination of particulate antigens of one species by agglutinins derived from another species.

heteroagglutinin (-ah-gloo′tin-in) an agglutinin that is capable of heteroagglutination.

heteroalbumose (-al′bu-mōs) hemialbumose insoluble in water.

heteroantibody (-an″tĭ-bod′e) an antibody combining with antigens originating from a species foreign to the antibody producer.

heteroantigen (-an′tĭ-jen) an antigen originating from a species foreign to the antibody producer.

heteroauxin (-awk′sin) a plant growth hormone.

heteroblastic (-blas′tik) originating in a different kind of tissue.

heterocellular (-sel′u-lar) composed of cells of different kinds.

heterocephalus (-sef′ah-lus) a monster with two unequal heads.

heterochromatin (-kro′mah-tin) that state of chromatin in which it is dark-staining, genetically inactive, and tightly coiled.

heterochromia (-kro′me-ah) diversity of color in a part normally of one color. **h. i′ridis,** difference of color in the two irides, or in different areas in the same iris.

heterochronia (-kro′ne-ah) irregularity in time, as the formation of parts or tissues in unusual sequence, or a difference in chronaxie of a muscle and that of its nerve. **heteroch′ronous,** adj.

heterochronic (-kron′ik) 1. pertaining to heterochronia. 2. denoting different ages or stages of development.

heterochthonous (het″er-ok′tho-nus) originating in an area other than that in which it is found.

heterocrine (het′er-o-krin) secreting more than one kind of matter.

heterocyclic (het″er-o-si′klik) having a closed chain or ring formation including atoms of different elements.

heterocytotropic (-si″to-trop′ik) having an affinity for cells from different species.

heterodermic (-der′mik) denoting a skin graft from an individual of another species.

heterodont (het′er-o-dont″) having teeth of different shapes, as molars, incisors, etc.

heterodromous (het″er-od′ro-mus) moving, acting, or arranged in the opposite direction.

heterodymus (het″er-od′ĭ-mus) a fetus with a second head, neck, and thorax attached to the thorax.

heteroecious (het″er-e′shus) heterecious.

heteroerotism (het″er-o-er′o-tizm) sexual feeling directed toward another person.

heterogamety (-gam′ĕ-te) production by an individual of one sex (as the human male) of unlike gametes with respect to the sex chromosomes. **heterogamet′ic,** adj.

heterogamy (het″er-og′ah-me) reproduction resulting from the union of gametes differing in size and structure. **heterog′amous,** adj.

heterogeneity (het″er-o-jĕ-ne′ĭ-te) the state of being heterogeneous.

heterogeneous (-je′ne-us) not of uniform composition, quality, or structure.

heterogenesis (-jen′ĕ-sis) 1. alternation of generations; reproduction differing in character in successive generations. 2. asexual generation. 3. spontaneous generation. **heterogenet′ic,** adj.

heterogenous (het″er-oj′ĕ-nus) derived from a different source or species.

heterogony (het″er-og′o-ne) heterogenesis.

heterograft (het′er-o-graft″) xenograft.

heterography (het″er-og′rah-fe) writing of other than intended words.

heterohemagglutination (het″er-o-hem″ah-glu″tĭ-na′shun) agglutination of erythrocytes of one species by a hemagglutinin derived from an individual of a different species.

heterohemagglutinin (-hem″ah-glu′tĭ-nin) a hemagglutinin that agglutinates erythrocytes of organisms of other species.

heterohemolysin (-he-mol′ĭ-sin) a hemolysin which destroys red blood cells of animals of species other than that of the animal in which it is formed; it may occur naturally or be induced by immunization.

heteroimmunity (-im-mu′nĭ-te) 1. an immune state induced in an individual by immunization with cells of an animal of another species. 2. a state in which an immune response to exogenous antigen (e.g., drugs or pathogens) results in immunopathological changes. **heteroimmune′,** adj.

heterokaryon (-kar′e-on) a cell or hypha containing two or more nuclei of different genetic constitution.

heterokeratoplasty (-ker′ah-to-plas″te) grafting of corneal tissue taken from an individual of another species.

heterokinesis (-ki-ne′sis) differential distribution of sex chromosomes in the developing gametes of a heterogametic organism.

heterolalia (-la′le-ah) heterophasia.

heterolateral (-lat′er-al) contralateral.

heterologous (het″er-ol′o-gus) 1. made up of tissue not normal to the part. 2. xenogeneic.

heterolysin (het″er-ol′ĭ-sin) a lysin that lyzes cells of species other than the one in which it is formed.

heterolysis (het″er-ol′ĭ-sis) lysis of the cells of one species by lysin from a different species. **heterolyt′ic,** adj.

heteromeric (het″er-o-mer′ik) sending processes through one of the commissures to the white matter of the opposite side of the spinal cord; said of neurons.

heterometaplasia (-met″ah-pla′ze-ah) formation of tissue foreign to the part where it is formed.

heterometropia (-mĕ-tro′pe-ah) the state in which the refraction in the two eyes differs.

heteromorphosis (-mor-fo′sis) the development, in regeneration, of an organ or structure different from the one that was lost.

heteromorphous (-mor′fus) of abnormal shape or structure.

heteronomous (het″er-on′ŏ-mus) 1. in biology, subject to different laws of growth; specialized along different lines. 2. in psychology, subject to another's will.

heteronymous (het″er-on′ĭ-mus) standing in opposite relations.

hetero-osteoplasty (het″er-o-os′te-o-plas″te) osteoplasty with bone taken from an individual of another species.

heteropagus (het″er-op′ah-gus) a conjoined twin monster consisting of unequally developed components.

heteropathy (het″er-op′ah-the) abnormal or morbid sensibility to stimuli.

heterophasia (het″er-o-fa′ze-ah) the utterance of words other than those intended.

heterophemia (-fe′me-ah) heterophasia.

heterophil (het′er-o-fil″) 1. a granular leukocyte represented by neutrophils in man, but characterized in other mammals by granules which have variable sizes and staining characteristics. 2. heterophilic.

heterophilic (het″er-o-fil′ik) 1. having affinity for antigens or antibodies other than the one for which it is specific. 2. staining with a type of stain other than the usual one.

heterophonia (-fo′ne-ah) any abnormality of the voice or phonation.

heterophoria (-fo′re-ah) failure of the visual axes to remain parallel after visual fusional stimuli have been eliminated. **heterophor′ic,** adj.

heterophthalmia (het″er-of-thal′me-ah) difference in the direction of the visual axes, or in the color, of the two eyes.

Heterophyes (het″er-of′ĭ-ēz) a genus of minute trematode worms parasitic in the intestine of fish-eating mammals.

heterophyiasis (-fi-i′ah-sis) infection with *Heterophyes.*

heteroplasia (-pla′ze-ah) replacement of normal by abnormal tissue; malposition of normal cells. **heteroplas′tic,** adj.

heteroplasty (het′er-o-plas″te) heterotransplantation.

heteroploid (-ploid″) 1. characterized by heteroploidy. 2. an individual or cell with an abnormal number of chromosomes.

heteroploidy (-ploi″de) the state of having an abnormal number of chromosomes.

heteropsia (het″er-op′se-ah) unequal vision in the two eyes.

heteropyknosis (het″er-o-pik-no′sis) 1. the quality of showing variations in density throughout. 2. a state of differential condensation observed in different chromosomes, or in different regions of the same chromosome; it may be attenuated (*negative h.*) or accentuated (*positive h.*). **heteropyknot′ic,** adj.

heterosexual (-seks′u-al) 1. pertaining to, characteristic of, or directed toward the opposite sex. 2. a person with erotic interests directed toward the opposite sex.

heterosexuality (-seks″u-al′ĭ-te) sexual attraction to persons of the opposite sex.

heterosis (het″er-o′sis) the existence, in the first generation hybrid, of greater vigor than is shown by either parent strain.

heterosporous (het″er-os′po-rus) having two kinds of spores, which reproduce asexually.

heterostimulation (het″er-o-stim″u-la′shun) stimulation of an animal with antigenic material originating in another species.

heterosuggestion (-sug-jes′chun) suggestion received from another person, as opposed to autosuggestion.

heterotaxia (-tak′se-ah) abnormal position of viscera or parts. **heterotax′ic,** adj.

heterotherm (het′er-o-therm″) an animal exhibiting heterothermy.

heterothermy (-ther′me) exhibition of widely different body temperatures at different times or under different conditions. **heterother′mic,** adj.

heterotonia (het″er-o-to′ne-ah) a state characterized by variations in tension or tone. **heteroton′ic,** adj.

heterotopia (-to′pe-ah) displacement or misplacement of parts; the presence of a tissue in an abnormal location. **heterotop′ic,** adj.

heterotransplant (-trans′plant) xenograft.

heterotransplantation (-trans″plan-ta′shun) transplantation of tissues or cells from one individual to another of a different species (a xenograft).

heterotrichosis (-trĭ-ko′sis) growth of hairs of different colors on the body.

heterotroph (het′er-o-trōf″) a heterotrophic organism.

heterotrophic (het″er-o-trōf′ik) not self-sustaining; said of microorganisms requiring a reduced form of carbon for energy and synthesis.

heterotropia (-tro′pe-ah) failure of the visual axes to remain parallel when fusion is possible.

heterotypic (-tip′ik) pertaining to, characteristic of, or belonging to a different type. **heterotyp′ical,** adj.

heteroxenous (het″er-ok′sĕ-nus) requiring more than one host to complete the life cycle.

heterozygosity (het″er-o-zi-gos′ĭ-te) the state of having different alleles in regard to a given character. **heterozy′gous,** adj.

heterozygote (-zi′gōt) an individual exhibiting heterozygosity.

HETP hexaethyltetraphosphate.

Hetrazan (het′rah-zan) trademark for a preparation of diethylcarbamazine.

heuristic (hu-ris′tik) encouraging or promoting investigation; conducive to discovery.

hex(a)- word element [Gr.], *six.*

Hexa-Betalin (hek″sah-be′tah-lin) trademark for a preparation of pyridoxine.

hexachlorophene (-klo′ro-fēn) a local antiseptic and detergent for application to the skin, $C_{13}H_6Cl_6O_2$; also used to combat flukes in ruminants.

hexachromic (-kro′mik) 1. pertaining to or exhibiting six colors. 2. able to distinguish only six of the seven colors of the spectrum.

hexad (hek′sad) 1. a group or combination of six similar or related entities. 2. an element with a valence of six.

hexadactyly (hek″sah-dak′tĭ-le) the occurrence of six digits on one limb.

hexadimethrine (-di-meth′rēn) a compound

used to neutralize the anticoagulant action of heparin.

hexaethyltetraphosphate (-eth''il-tet''rah-fos'fāt) a powerful anticholinesterase, $(C_6H_5-O)_6P_4O_7$, used as an insecticide.

hexamer (heks'ah-mer) 1. a polymer composed of six monomers. 2. a capsomer having six structural subunits.

hexamethonium (hek''sah-mĕ-tho'ne-um) a ganglionic blocking agent, $C_{12}H_{30}N_2$, used in the form of salts to produce hypotension.

hexamine (hek'sah-min) methenamine.

hexane (hek'sān) a saturated hydrogen obtained by distillation from petroleum.

hexaploid (hek'sah-ploid) 1. pertaining to or characterized by hexaploidy. 2. an individual or cell having six sets of chromosomes.

hexaploidy (-ploi''de) the state of having six sets of chromosomes (6n).

hexavalent (hek''sah-va'lent) having a valence of six.

Hexavibex (-vi'beks) trademark for a preparation of pyridoxine.

hexavitamin (-vi'tah-min) a preparation of vitamins A and D, ascorbic acid, thiamine hydrochloride, riboflavin, and niacinamide.

hexestrol (hek-ses'trol) a synthetic estrogen, $C_{18}H_{22}O_2$.

hexethal (hek'sĕ-thal) a short- to intermediate-acting barbiturate, $C_{12}H_{19}N_2O_3$ used as the sodium salt.

hexetidine (hek-set'ĭ-dēn) a drug, $C_{21}H_{45}N_3$, used in the treatment of bacterial vaginitis.

hexobarbital (hek''so-bar'bĭ-tal) an ultra-short-acting sedative and hypnotic, $C_{12}H_{16}N_2O_3$; also used as the sodium salt to induce general anesthesia.

hexabarbitone (-bar'bĭ-tōn) hexobarbital.

hexocyclium methylsulfate (-si'kle-um) an anticholinergic, $C_{21}H_{36}N_2O_5S$, having antisecretory and antispasmodic activities; used in the management of peptic ulcer and other gastrointestinal disorders accompanied by hyperacidity, hypermotility, and spasm.

hexokinase (-ki'nās) an enzyme that catalyzes the transfer of a high-energy phosphate group of a donor to D-glucose, producing D-glucose-6-phosphate.

hexosamine (hek'sōs-am''in) a nitrogenous sugar in which an amino group replaces a hydroxyl group.

hexose (hek'sōs) a monosaccharide containing six carbon atoms in a molecule.

hexosephosphate (hek''sōs-fos'fāt) an ester of glucose with phosphoric acid, which aids in the absorption of sugar and is important in carbohydrate metabolism.

hexylcaine (hek'sil-kān) a local anesthetic, $C_{18}H_{23}NO_2$, used as the hydrochloride salt.

hexylresorcinol (hek''sil-rĕ-zor'sĭ-nol) an anthelmintic for intestinal roundworms and trematodes, $C_{12}H_{18}O_2$.

HF Hageman factor (coagulation Factor XII).

Hf chemical symbol, *hafnium.*

Hg chemical symbol, *mercury* (L., *hydrargyrum*).

Hgb hemoglobin.

HGF hyperglycemic-glycogenolytic factor (glucagon).

HGH human growth hormone.

hiatus (hi-a'tus), pl. *hia'tus* [L.] a gap, cleft, or opening. **hia'tal,** adj. **aortic h.,** the opening in the diaphragm through which the aorta and thoracic duct pass. **esophageal h.,** the opening in the diaphragm for the passage of the esophagus and the vagus nerves. **saphenous h.,** the depression in the fascia lata bridged by the cribriform fascia and perforated by the great saphenous vein. **semilunar h.,** the groove in the ethmoid bone through which the anterior ethmoidal air cells, the maxillary sinus, and sometimes the frontonasal duct drain via the ethmoid infundibulum.

hibernation (hi''ber-na'shun) the dormant state in which certain animals pass the winter, marked by narcosis and by sharp reduction in body temperature and metabolism. **artificial h.,** a state of reduced metabolism, muscle relaxation, and a twilight sleep resembling narcosis, produced by controlled inhibition of the sympathetic nervous system and causing attenuation of the homeostatic reactions of the organism.

hibernoma (hi''ber-no'mah) a rare benign tumor made up of large polyhedral cells with a coarsely granular cytoplasm, occurring on the back or around the hips; so called because it resembles the dorsal fat pads of hibernating animals.

hiccough, hiccup (hik'up) sharp inspiratory sound with spasm of the glottis and diaphragm.

hidr(o)- word element [Gr.], *sweat.*

hidradenitis (hi''drad-ĕ-ni'tis) inflammation of the sweat glands. **h. suppurati'va,** a severe, chronic, recurrent suppurative infection of the apocrine sweat glands.

hidradenoma (-no'mah) a general term for tumors of the skin the components of which resemble epithelial elements of sweat glands; they may be nodular (solid) or papillary.

hidrocystoma (hi''dro-sis-to'mah) a retention cyst of a sweat gland.

hidropoiesis (-poi-e'sis) the formation of sweat. **hidropoiet'ic,** adj.

hidrorrhea (-re'ah) hyperhidrosis.

hidroschesis (hi-dros'kĕ-sis) anhidrosis.

hidrotic (hĭ-drot'ik, hi-drot'ik) pertaining to, characterized by, or causing sweating.

hidrous (hi'drus) containing water.

hieralgia (hi''er-al'je-ah) pain in the sacrum.

hierolisthesis (hi''er-o-lis-the'sis) displacement of the sacrum.

hilitis (hi-li'tis) inflammation of a hilus.

hillock (hil'ok) a small prominence or elevation.

hilum (hi'lum) hilus.

hilus (hi'lus), pl. *hi'li* [L.] a depression or pit on an organ, giving entrance and exit to vessels and nerves. **hi'lar,** adj.

hindbrain (hīnd'brān) rhombencephalon: 1. the part of the brain developed from the posterior of the three primary brain vesicles, comprising the metencephalon and myelencephalon. 2. the most caudal of the three primary brain vesicles.

hindfoot (-foot) the posterior portion of the foot,

comprising the region of the talus and calcaneus.

hindgut (-gut) the embryonic structure from which the caudal intestine, chiefly the colon, is formed.

hip (hip) coxa; the area lateral to and including the hip joint; loosely, the hip joint. **snapping h.,** slipping of the hip joint, sometimes with an audible snap, due to slipping of a tendinous band over the greater trochanter.

hippo (hip′o) ipecac.

hippocampus (hip″o-kam′pus), pl. *hippocam′pi* [L.] a curved elevation in the floor of the inferior horn of the lateral ventricle; an important functional component of the limbic system, its efferent projections form the fornix. **hippocam′pal,** adj. **h. ma′jor,** hippocampus. **h. mi′nor,** calcar avis.

Hippocrates (hip-pok′rah-tēz) the famous Greek physician (5th century B.C.) generally regarded as the "Father of Medicine." Many of his writings and those of his school have survived, among which appears the Hippocratic oath, the ethical guide of the medical profession. **hippocrat′ic,** adj.

hippuria (hǐ-pu′re-ah) an excess of hippuric acid in the urine.

hippus (hip′us) abnormal exaggeration of the rhythmic contraction and dilation of the pupil, independent of changes in illumination or in fixation of the eyes.

hirci (hir′si), sing. *hir′cus* [L.] the hairs growing in the axilla.

hircus (her′kus) see *hirci.*

hirsute (her′sūt) shaggy; hairy.

hirsutism (-izm) abnormal hairiness, especially in women.

hirudicide (hǐ-roo′dǐ-sīd) an agent that is destructive to leeches. **hirudici′dal,** adj.

hirudin (hǐ-roo′din) the active principle of the buccal secretion of leeches; it prevents coagulation by acting as an antithrombin.

Hirudinea (hir″u-din′e-ah) a class of annelids, the leeches.

Hirudo (hǐ-roo′do) a genus of leeches, including *H. medicina′lis,* formerly used extensively for drawing blood.

hist(io)(o)- word element [Gr.], *tissue.*

Histadyl (his′tah-dil) trademark for preparations of methapyrilene.

Histalog (his′tah-log) trademark for a preparation of betazole.

histaminase (his-tam′ǐ-nās) an enzyme which inactivates histamine.

histamine (his′tah-min) an amine formed by decarboxylation of histadine, found in many animal and plant tissues, or produced synthetically; it causes (1) dilatation of capillaries, which increases capillary permeability, (2) constriction of bronchial smooth muscle of the lungs, and (3) increased gastric secretion, and is implicated as a mediator of immediate hypersensitivity. Used, in the form of the phosphate salt, to reduce sensitivity to allergens and as a diagnostic aid in testing gastric acid formation. **histamin′ic,** adj.

histaminemia (his″tah-min-e′me-ah) histamine in the blood.

histidase (his′tǐ-dās) an enzyme of the liver that converts histidine to urocanic acid.

histidine (his′tǐ-din) an amino acid obtainable from many proteins by the action of sulfuric acid and water; it is essential for optimal growth in infants. Its decarboxylation results in formation of histamine.

histidinemia (his″tǐ-dǐ-ne′me-ah) a hereditary metabolic defect marked by excessive histidine in the blood and urine due to deficient histidase activity; many affected persons show mild mental retardation and disordered speech development.

histidinuria (his″tǐ-dǐ-nu′re-ah) an excess of histidine in the urine; see *histidinemia.*

histiocyte (his′te-o-sīt″) a large phagocytic interstitial cell of the reticuloendothelial system; macrophage. **histiocyt′ic,** adj.

histiocytoma (his″te-o-si-to′mah) a tumor containing histiocytes.

histiocytosis (-si-to′sis) a condition marked by an abnormal appearance of histiocytes in the blood. **lipid h.,** Niemann-Pick disease. **h. X,** a generic term that embraces eosinophilic granuloma, Letterer-Siwe disease, and Hand-Schüller-Christian disease.

histiogenic (-jen′ik) histogenous.

histioid (his′te-oid) histoid.

histoblast (his′to-blast) a tissue-forming cell.

histochemistry (his″to-kem′is-tre) that branch of histology dealing with the identification of chemical components in cells and tissues.

histocompatibility (-kom-pat″ǐ-bil′ǐ-te) that quality of being accepted and remaining functional; said of that relationship between the genotypes of donor and host in which a graft generally will not be rejected. **histocompat′ible,** adj.

histodialysis (-di-al′ǐ-sis) disintegration or breaking down of tissue.

histodifferentiation (-dif″er-en″she-a′shun) the acquisition of tissue characteristics by cell groups.

histofluorescence (-floo′o-res′ens) fluorescence produced in tissues by administration of fluorescing drugs prior to exposure to x-rays.

histogenesis (-jen′ě-sis) the formation or development of tissues from the undifferentiated cells of the germ layer of the embryo. **histogenet′ic,** adj.

histogenous (his-toj′ě-nous) formed by the tissues.

histogram (his′to-gram) a graph in which values found in a statistical study are represented by vertical bars or rectangles.

histoid (his′toid) 1. developed from but one kind of tissue. 2. like one of the tissues of the body.

histoincompatibility (his″to-in″kom-pat″ǐ-bil′ǐ-te) the quality of not being accepted or not remaining functional; said of that relationship between the genotypes of donor and host in which a graft generally will be rejected. **histoincompat′ible,** adj.

histokinesis (-ki-ne′sis) movement in the tissues of the body.

histologist (his-tol′o-jist) one who specializes in histology.

histology (his-tol′o-je) that department of anatomy dealing with the minute structure, composition, and function of tissues. **histolog′ic, histolog′ical,** adj. **pathologic h.,** the science of diseased tissues.

histolysis (his-tol′ĭ-sis) dissolution or breaking down of tissues. **histolyt′ic,** adj.

histoma (his-to′mah) any tissue tumor.

histometaplastic (his″to-met″ah-plas′tik) stimulating metaplasia of tissue.

Histomonas (his-tom′o-nas) a genus of protozoa parasitic in the cecum, liver, and other tissues of various fowl.

histomoniasis (his″to-mo-ni′ah-sis) infection with *Histomonas.* **h. of turkeys,** blackhead; an infectious disease of turkeys due to *Histomonas meleagridis,* with intestinal and hepatic lesions and dark discoloration of the comb.

histone (his′tōn) a simple protein, soluble in water and insoluble in dilute ammonia, found combined as salts with acidic substances, e.g., the protein combined with nucleic acid or the globin of hemoglobin.

histonomy (his-ton′o-me) the scientific study of tissues based on the translation into biological terms of quantitative laws derived from histologic measurement.

histonuria (his″to-nu′re-ah) the presence of histone in the urine.

histopathology (-pah-thol′o-je) pathologic histology.

histophysiology (-fiz″e-ol′o-je) the correlation of function with the microscopic structure of cells and tissues.

Histoplasma (-plaz′mah) a genus of fungi, including *H. capsula′tum,* the cause of histoplasmosis in man.

histoplasmin (-plaz′min) a preparation of growth products of *Histoplasma capsulatum,* injected intracutaneously as a test for histoplasmosis.

histoplasmosis (-plaz-mo′sis) infection with *Histoplasma capsulatum;* it is usually asymptomatic but may cause acute pneumonia, or disseminated reticuloendothelial hyperplasia with hepatosplenomegaly and anemia, or an influenza-like illness with joint effusion and erythema nodosum. Reactivated infection involves the lungs, meninges, heart, peritoneum, and adrenals.

historrhexis (-rek′sis) the breaking up of tissue.

histotherapy (-ther′ah-pe) therapeutic administration of animal tissues.

histothrombin (-throm′bin) thrombin derived from connective tissue.

histotome (his′to-tōm) microtome.

histotomy (his-tot′o-me) dissection of tissues; microtomy.

histotoxic (his″to-tok′sik) poisonous to tissue.

histotroph (his′to-trōf) the sum total of nutritive substances supplied to the embryo in vivip-

arous animals from sources other than the maternal blood.

histotrophic (his″to-trōf′ik) 1. encouraging formation of tissue. 2. pertaining to histotroph.

histotropic (-trop′ik) having affinity for tissue cells.

histrionism (his′tre-o-nizm″) a morbid or hysterical adoption of an exaggerated manner and gestures. **histrion′ic,** adj.

hives (hīvz) urticaria.

Hl latent hyperopia.

Hm manifest hyperopia.

HMO health maintenance organization.

Ho chemical symbol, *holmium.*

hoarse (hōrs) having a rough quality of voice.

hoarseness (hōrs′nes) trachyphonia.

hock (hok) the tarsal joint or region of the hind leg of the horse and ox.

hodoneuromere (ho″do-nu′ro-mēr) a segment of the embryonic trunk with its pair of nerves and their branches.

hol(o)- word element [Gr.], *entire; whole.*

holandric (hol-an′drik) inherited exclusively through the male descent; transmitted through genes located on the Y chromosome.

holarthritis (hol″ar-thri′tis) hamarthritis.

holergasia (-er-ga′ze-ah) a psychiatric disorder involving the entire personality; a major psychosis. **holergas′tic,** adj.

holism (hol′izm) the conception of man as a functioning whole. **holis′tic,** adj.

holmium (hol′me-um) chemical element (*see table*), at. no. 67, symbol Ho.

holoacardius (hol″o-ah-kar′de-us) an unequal twin fetus in which the heart is absent, its circulation being accomplished by the heart of the more perfect twin. **h. aceph′alus,** one which has no head. **h. acor′mus,** one without the caudal part of the body. **h. amor′phus,** one which has no recognizable organs, being only a shapeless mass.

holoblastic (-blas′tik) undergoing cleavage in which the entire ovum participates; dividing completely.

Holocaine (ho′lo-kān) trademark for a preparation of phenacaine.

holocrine (-krin) exhibiting glandular secretion in which the entire secretory cell laden with its secretory products is cast off.

holodiastolic (hol″o-di″ah-stol′ik) pertaining to the entire diastole.

holoendemic (-en-dem′ik) affecting practically all the residents of a particular region.

holoenzyme (-en′zīm) the active compound formed by combination of a coenzyme and an apoenzyme.

holography (hol-og′rah-fe) the lensless recording of three-dimensional images on film by means of laser beams.

hologynic (hol″o-jin′ik) inherited exclusively through the female descent; transmitted through genes located on X chromosomes.

holophytic (-fit′ik) obtaining food like a plant; said of certain protozoa.

holoprosencephaly (-pros″en-sef′ah-le) developmental failure of cleavage of the prosencephalon with a deficit in midline facial development and with cyclopia in the severe form; sometimes due to trisomy 13–15.

holorachischisis (-rah-kis′kĭ-sis) fissure of the entire vertebral column with prolapse of the entire spinal cord.

holosystolic (-sis-tol′ik) pertaining to the entire systole.

holozoic (-zo′ik) having the nutritional characters of an animal, i.e., digesting protein.

homaluria (hom″ah-lu′re-ah) production and excretion of urine at a normal, even rate.

homatropine (ho-mat′ro-pin) an anticholinergic alkaloid obtained by the condensation of tropine and mandelic acid; used as a mydriatic and cycloplegic (*h. hydrobromide*) and as an inhibitor of gastric spasm and secretion (*h. methylbromide*).

homaxial (ho-mak′se-al) having axes of the same length.

homeo- word element [Gr.], *similar; same; unchanging.*

homeochrome (ho′me-o-krōm″) staining with mucin stains after formol-bichromate fixation.

homeomorphous (ho″me-o-mor′fus) of like form and structure.

homeopathy (ho″me-op′ah-the) a system of therapeutics based on the administration of minute doses of drugs which are capable of producing in healthy persons symptoms like those of the disease treated. **homeopath′ic,** adj.

homeoplasia (ho″me-o-pla′ze-ah) formation of new tissue like that normal to the part. **homeoplas′tic,** adj.

homeostasis (-sta′sis) a tendency to stability in the normal physiological states of the organism. **homeostat′ic,** adj.

homeotherapy (-ther′ah-pe) treatment or prevention of disease with a substance similar to the causative agent of the disease.

homeothermal (-ther′mal) homoiothermic.

homeotypic, homeotypical (-tip′ik; -tip′ĭ-kal) resembling the normal or usual type.

homo- 1. word element [Gr.], *same.* 2. chemical prefix indicating addition of one CH_2 group to the main compound.

homobiotin (ho″mo-bi′o-tin) a homologue of biotin having an additional CH_2 group in the side chain and acting as a biotin antagonist.

homocarnosine (-kar′no-sēn) a dipeptide consisting of γ-aminobutyric acid and histidine; it is a normal constituent of the human brain.

homocysteine (-sis-te′in) a transmethylation product of methionine; it is an intermediate in the synthesis of cystine.

homocystine (-sis-tēn) a homologue of cystine which results from demethylation of methionine.

homocystinuria (-sis″tin-u′re-ah) an inborn error of sulfur amino acid metabolism due to lack of the enzyme cystathionine synthase; it is characterized by homocystine in the urine and by mental retardation, hepatomegaly, ectopia lentis, and cardiovascular and skeletal disorders.

homocytotropic (-si″to-trop′ik) having an affinity for cells of the same species.

homodromous (ho-mod′ro-mus) moving or acting in the same or in the usual direction.

homogametic (ho″mo-gah-met′ik) having only one kind of gametes with respect to the sex chromosomes, as in the human female.

homogamy (ho-mog′ah-me) imbreeding.

homogenate (ho-moj′ě-nāt) material obtained by homogenization.

homogeneity (ho″mo-jě-ne′ĭ-te) the state of being homogeneous.

homogeneous (-je′ne-us) of uniform quality, composition, or structure throughout.

homogenesis (-jen′ě-sis) reproduction by the same process in each generation. **homogenet′ic,** adj.

homogenic (-jen′ik) homozygous.

homogenize (ho-moj′ě-nīz) to render homogeneous.

homograft (ho′mo-graft) allograft.

homoiotherm (ho-moi′o-therm) an animal exhibiting homoiothermy; a so-called warm-blooded animal.

homoiothermic (ho-moi″o-ther′mik) pertaining to or characterized by homoiothermy.

homoiothermy (ho-moi′o-ther″me) maintenance of a constant body temperature despite variation in environmental temperature, as in mammals and birds.

homolateral (ho″mo-lat′er-al) ipsilateral.

homologous (ho-mol′ŏ-gus) 1. corresponding in structure, position, origin, etc. 2. allogeneic.

homologue (hom′o-log) 1. any homologous organ or part. 2. in chemistry, one of a series of compounds distinguished by addition of a CH_2 group in successive members.

homology (ho-mol′o-je) the state of being homologous.

homolysin (ho-mol′ĭ-sin) a lysin produced by injection into the body of an antigen derived from an individual of the same species.

homonomous (ho-mon′ŏ-mus) designating homologous serial parts, such as somites.

homonymous (ho-mon′ĭ-mus) standing in the same relation.

homophilic (ho″mo-fil′ik) reacting only with a specific antigen.

homoplasty (ho′mo-plas″te) plastic surgery using an allograft. **homoplas′tic,** adj.

homorganic (hom″or-gan′ik) produced by the same or by homologous organs.

homosexual (ho″mo-seks′u-al) 1. sexually attracted by persons of the same sex. 2. a homosexual individual.

homosexuality (-seks″u-al′ĭ-te) sexual attraction toward persons of the same sex.

homosporous (ho-mos′po-rus) having spores of only one kind.

homotherm (ho′mo-therm) homoiotherm.

homotopic (ho″mo-top′ik) occurring at the same place upon the body.

homotype (ho′mo-tīp) a part having reversed symmetry with its mate, as the hand. **homotyp′ic,** adj.

homozygosis (ho″mo-zi-go′sis) the formation of a zygote by the union of gametes that have one or more identical alleles.

homozygosity (-zi-gos′ĭ-te) the state of having identical alleles in regard to a given character. **homozy′gous**, adj.

homozygote (-zi′gōt) an individual exhibiting homozygosity.

homunculus (ho-mung′ku-lus) 1. a dwarf without deformity or disproportion of parts. 2. the miniature human form once thought to be performed in the sperm or ovum.

honey (hon′e) a sweet-tasting substance produced by the honeybee, containing chiefly levulose and fructose; used as an excipient.

hoof-bound (hoof′bownd) dryness and contraction of a horse's hoof, causing lameness.

hook (hook) a curved instrument for traction or holding. **Braun's h.**, an instrument used in fetal decapitation. **Malgaigne's h's**, two pairs of hooks connected by a screw for approximating the pieces of a broken patella. **palate h., posterior h.**, one for raising the palate in rhinoscopy. **Tyrrell's h.**, a slender hook used in eye surgery.

hookworm (hook′werm) a nematode parasitic in the intestines of man and other vertebrates; two important species are *Necator americanus* (American, or New World, h.) and *Ancylostoma duodenale* (Old World h.). Infection may cause serious illness; see under *disease*, and see *ground itch.*

hoose (hooz) a bronchopulmonary disease of cattle, sheep, goats, and swine caused by nematodes.

hordeolum (hŏr-de′o-lum) stye; a localized, purulent, inflammatory infection of one or more sebaceous glands (meibomian or zeisian) of the eyelid; *external h.* occurs on the skin surface at the edge of the lid, *internal h.* on the conjunctival surface.

horizon (ho-ri′zon) a specific anatomic stage of embryonic development, of which 23 have been defined, beginning with fertilization and ending with the fetal stage.

hormesis (hŏr-me′sis) stimulation by a subinhibitory concentration of a toxic substance.

hormion (hŏr′me-on) point of union of the sphenoid bone with the posterior border of vomer.

hormonagogue (hŏr-mōn′ah-gog) an agent that stimulates hormone production.

hormone (hŏr′mōn) a chemical substance produced in the body which has a specific regulatory effect on the activity of certain cells or a certain organ or organs. **hormo′nal**, adj. **adaptive h.**, one secreted during adaptation to unusual circumstances. **adrenocortical h.**, one of the steroids produced by the adrenal cortex, of which there are four main types: (1) estrogen, (2) androgens, (3) progesterone, and (4) corticoids. **adrenocorticotropic h. (ACTH)**, corticotropin. **adrenomedullary h's**, substances secreted by the adrenal medulla, including epinephrine and norepinephrine. **androgenic h's**, the masculinizing hormones: androsterone and testosterone. **antidiuretic h.**, vasopressin. **corpus luteum h.**, progesterone. **cortical h.**, adrenocortical h. **follicle-stimulating h.**

(FSH), a gonadotropic hormone of the anterior pituitary which stimulates follicular growth and maturation in the ovary and spermatogenesis in the testis. **gonadotropic h.**, one which has an influence on the gonads. **growth h.**, a substance that stimulates growth, especially a secretion of the anterior pituitary, that directly influences protein, carbohydrate, and lipid metabolism and controls the rate of skeletal and visceral growth. **interstitial cell-stimulating h.**, luteinizing h. **lactation h., lactogenic h.**, prolactin. **luteinizing h.**, a gonadotropic hormone of the anterior pituitary gland, acting with follicle-stimulating hormone, to cause ovulation of mature follicles and secretion of estrogen by thecal and granulosa cells of the ovary; it is also concerned with corpus luteum formation. In the male, it stimulates development of the interstitial cells of the testes and their secretion of testosterone. **luteotropic h.**, luteotropin. **melanocyte-stimulating h. (MSH)**, a peptide secreted by the adenohypophysis in man and in the rhomboid fossa in lower vertebrates, influencing melanin formation and deposition in the body, and causing color changes in the skin of amphibians, fishes, and reptiles. **ovarian h's**, those secreted by the ovary, including the estrogens and gestagens. **parathyroid h.**, a polypeptide hormone secreted by the parathyroid glands, which influences calcium and phosphorus metabolism and bone formation. **placental h.**, one secreted by the placenta, including chorionic gonadotropin, relaxin, and other substances having estrogenic, progestational, or adrenocorticoid activity. **plant h.**, phytohormone. **progestational h.**, 1. progesterone. 2. [pl.] see under *agent.* **sex h's**, hormones having estrogenic (*female sex h's*) or androgenic (*male sex h's*) activity. **somatotrophic h., somatotropic h.**, growth h. **thyroid h's**, thyroxine, calcitonin, and triiodothyronine; in the singular, thyroxine and/or triiodothyronine. **thyrotropic h.**, thyrotropin.

hormonopoiesis (hŏr-mo″no-poi-e′sis) the production of hormones. **hormonopoiet′ic**, adj.

hormonotherapy (-ther′ah-pe) treatment by the use of hormones; endocrinotherapy.

horn (hŏrn) cornu; a pointed projection such as the paired processes on the head of various animals; any horn-shaped structure. **cicatricial h.**, a hard, dry outgrowth from a cicatrix, commonly scaly and rarely osseus. **cutaneous h.**, a horny excrescence on the skin, commonly on the face or scalp. **h. of pulp**, an extension of the pulp into an accentuation of the roof of the pulp chamber directly under a cusp or a developmental lobe of the tooth. **h. of spinal cord**, either of the horn-shaped structures, anterior or posterior, seen in transverse section of the spinal cord; the anterior horn is formed by the anterior column of the cord, the posterior by the posterior column.

horopter (hŏr-op′ter) the sum of all points seen in binocular vision with the eyes fixed.

horror (hor′er) dread; terror. **h. autotox′icus**, self-tolerance.

horsepox (hors′poks) a mild form of smallpox affecting horses.

hospital (hos′pit-'l) an institute for the treatment of the sick. **lying-in h., maternity h.,** one for the care of obstetric patients.

hospitalization (hos″pit-'l-i-za′shun) 1. the placing of a patient in a hospital for treatment. 2. the term of confinement in a hospital.

host (hōst) 1. an organism that harbors or nourishes another organism (the parasite). 2. the recipient of an organ or other tissue derived from another organism (the donor). **accidental h.,** one that accidentally harbors an organism that is not ordinarily parasitic in the particular species. **definitive h., final h.,** the organism in which a parasite passes its adult and sexual existence. **intermediate h.,** the organism in which a parasite passes its larval or nonsexual existence. **paratenic h.,** an animal acting as a substitute intermediate host of a parasite, usually having acquired the parasite by ingestion of the original host. **primary h.,** definitive h. **reservoir h.,** one that becomes infected by a pathogenic parasite and may serve as the source from which the parasite is transmitted to other animals. **secondary h.,** intermediate h.

5-HT serotonin (5-hydroxytryptamine).

hum (hum) a low, steady, prolonged sound. **venous h.,** a continuous blowing or singing sound heard on ausculation at the base of the neck with the patient in upright position; due to increased venous flow, it is exaggerated in anemia and fever.

Humatin (hu′mah-tin) trademark for preparations of paromomycin.

humectant (hu-mek′tant) 1. moistening. 2. a moistening or diluent medicine.

humeral (hu′mer-al) of or pertaining to the humerus.

humeroradial (hu″mer-o-ra′de-al) pertaining to the humerus and radius.

humeroscapular (-skap′u-lar) pertaining to the humerus and scapula.

humeroulnar (-ul′nar) pertaining to the humerus and ulna.

humerus (hu′mer-us), pl. *hu′meri* [L.] see *Table of Bones.*

humidity (hu-mid′ĭ-te) the degree of moisture, especially of that in the air.

humor (hu′mor), pl. *humo′res, humors* [L.] any fluid or semifluid of the body. **hu′moral,** adj. **aqueous h.,** the fluid produced in the eye and filling the spaces (anterior and posterior chambers) in front of the lens and its attachments. **ocular h.,** either of the humors (aqueous or vitreous) of the eye. **vitreous h.,** 1. the fluid portion of the vitreous body. 2. vitreous body.

Humorsol (hu′mor-sol) trademark for a solution of demecarium bromide.

humpback (hump′bak) kyphosis.

hunchback (hunch′bak) 1. kyphosis. 2. a person with kyphosis.

hunger (hung′ger) a craving, as for food. **air h.,** a distressing dyspnea occurring in paroxysms.

HVL half-value layer.

hyal(o)- word element [Gr.], *glassy.*

hyalin (hi′ah-lin) a translucent albuminoid product of amyloid degeneration.

hyaline (hi′ah-līn) glassy and transparent or nearly so.

hyalinization (hi″ah-lin″i-za′shun) conversion into a glasslike substance.

hyalinosis (hi″ah-lĭ-no′sis) hyaline degeneration.

hyalinuria (hi″ah-lĭ-nu′re-ah) hyalin in the urine.

hyalitis (hi″ah-li′tis) inflammation of the vitreous body or the vitreous (hyaloid) membrane. **asteroid h.,** asteroid hyalosis. **suppurative h.,** purulent inflammation of the vitreous body.

hyalogen (hi-al′o-jen) an albuminous substance occurring in cartilage, vitreous body, etc., and convertible into hyalin.

hyaloid (hi′ah-loid) resembling glass.

hyalomere (hi′ah-lo-mēr″) the pale, homogeneous portion of a blood platelet.

Hyalomma (hi″ah-lom′ah) a genus of ticks of Africa, Asia, and Europe; ectoparasites of animals and man, they may transmit disease and cause serious injury by their bite.

hyalomucoid (hi″ah-lo-mu′koid) the mucoid of the vitreous body.

hyalonyxis (-nik′sis) puncturing of the vitreous body.

hyalophagia (-fa′je-ah) the eating of glass.

hyaloplasm (hi′ah-lo-plazm″) 1. the more fluid, finely granular substance of the cytoplasm of a cell. 2. axoplasm. **nuclear h.,** karyolymph.

hyaloserositis (hi″ah-lo-se″ro-si′tis) inflammation serous membranes, with hyalinization of the serous exudate into a pearly investment of the affected organ. **progressive multiple h.,** Concato's disease.

hyalosis (hi″ah-lo′sis) degenerative changes in the vitreous humor. **asteroid h.,** the presence of spherical or star-shaped opacities in the vitreous humor.

hyalosome (hi-al′o-sōm) a structure resembling the nucleolus of a cell, but staining only slightly.

hyaluronate (hi″ah-lu′ro-nāt) a salt or ester of hyaluronic acid.

hyaluronidase (hi″ah-lu-ron′ĭ-dās) an enzyme that catalyzes the hydrolysis of hyaluronic acid, found in leeches, snake and spider venom, and in testes, and produced by various pathogenic bacteria, enabling them to spread through tissues; a preparation from mammalian testes is used to promote absorption and diffusion of solutions injected subcutaneously.

Hyazyme (hi′ah-zīm) trademark for a preparation of hyaluronidase.

hybrid (hi′brid) an offspring of parents of different species.

hybridism (-izm) the state of being a hybrid; the production of hybrids.

hybridization (hi″brid-ĭ-za′shun) the production of hybrids.

hydantoin (hi-dan′to-in) a crystalline base, glycolyl urea, derivable from allantoin.

hydatid (hi′dah-tid) 1. hydatid cyst. 2. any cystlike structure. **h. of Morgagni,** a cystlike remnant of the müllerian duct attached to a testis or to the oviduct. **sessile h.,** the hydatid of Morgagni connected with a testis.

hydatidiform (hi″dah-tid′ĭ-form) resembling a hydatid cyst; see under *mole*.

hydatidosis (hi″dah-tĭ-do′sis) hydatid disease.

hydatidostomy (hi″dah-tĭ-dos′to-me) incision and drainage of a hydatid cyst.

Hydeltra (hi-del′trah) trademark for preparations of prednisolone.

hydr(o)- word element [Gr.], *hydrogen; water.*

hydracetin (hi-dras′ĕ-tin) acetylphenylhydrazine.

hydragogue (hi′drah-gog) 1. producing watery discharge, especially from the bowels. 2. a cathartic that causes watery purgation.

hydralazine (hi-dral′ah-zēn) an antihypertensive, $C_8H_8N_4$, used as the hydrochloride salt.

hydramnios (hi-dram′ne-os) excess of amniotic fluid.

hydranencephaly (hi″dran-en-sef′ah-le) absence of the cerebral hemispheres, their normal site being occupied by cerebrospinal fluid. **hydranencephal′ic,** adj.

hydrargyria, hydrargyrism (hi″drar-jir′e-ah; hi-drar-jĭ-rizm) mercury poisoning; see *mercury*.

hydrargyrum (hi-drar′jĭ-rum) [L.] mercury.

hydrarthrosis (hi″drar-thro′sis) an accumulation of effused watery fluid in a joint cavity. **hydrarthro′dial,** adj.

hydrase (hi′drās) hydratase.

hydratase (hi′drah-tās) any enzyme that catalyzes the hydration or dehydration of C—O linkages.

hydrate (hi′drāt) 1. any compound of a radical with water. 2. any salt or other compound containing water of crystallization.

hydration (hi-dra′shun) the absorption of or combination with water.

hydraulics (hi-draw′liks) the science dealing with the mechanics of liquids.

hydrazine (hi′drah-zin) a gaseous diamine, H_4-N_2, or any of its substitution derivatives.

hydremia (hi-dre′me-ah) excess of water in the blood.

hydrencephalomeningocele (hi″dren-sef″ah-lo-mĕ-ning′go-sēl) hernial protrusion through a cranial defect of meninges containing cerebrospinal fluid and brain substance.

hydroa (hi-dro′ah) a vesicular eruption, with intense itching and burning, occurring on skin surfaces exposed to sunlight.

hydrobilirubin (hi″dro-bil″ĭ-roo′bin) a brownish-red pigment derived from bilirubin.

Hydrocal (hi′dro-kal) trademark for an artificial stone used in dentistry.

hydrocalycosis (hi″dro-kal″ĭ-ko′sis) distention of a renal calyx with accumulated urine.

hydrocarbon (-kar′bon) an organic compound that contains carbon and hydrogen only. **alicyclic h.,** one that has cyclic structure and aliphatic properties. **aliphatic h.,** one in which carbon atoms do not form a ring. **aromatic h.,** one that has cyclic structure and a closed conjugated system of double bonds. **cyclic h.,** one of

a series of hydrocarbons having the general formula C_nH_{2n}, the carbon atoms being thought of as having a closed ring structure. **saturated h.,** one that has the maximum number of hydrogen atoms for a given carbon structure. **unsaturated h.,** an aliphatic or alicyclic hydrocarbon that has less than the maximum number of hydrogen atoms for a given carbon structure.

hydrocele (hi′dro-sēl) a circumscribed collection of fluid, especially in the tunica vaginalis of the testis or along the spermatic cord.

hydrocelectomy (hi″dro-se-lek′to-me) excision of a hydrocele.

hydrocephalocele (-sef′ah-lo-sēl″) encephalocystocele.

hydrocephaloid (-sef′ah-loid) resembling hydrocephalus.

hydrocephalus (-sef′ah-lus) a condition characterized by abnormal accumulation of cerebrospinal fluid within the skull, with enlargement of the head, atrophy of the brain, mental deterioration, and convulsions. **hydrocephal′ic,** adj. **communicating h.,** that in which there is free access of fluid between the ventricles of the brain and the spinal canal. **h. ex vac′uo,** compensatory replacement by cerebrospinal fluid of the volume of tissue lost in atrophy of the brain. **noncommunicating h., obstructive h.,** that due to obstruction of the flow of cerebrospinal fluid within the brain ventricles or through their exit foramina. **otitic h.,** that caused by spread of inflammation of otitis media to the cranial cavity.

hydrocephaly (-sef′ah-le) hydrocephalus.

hydrochloride (-kol′rīd) a salt of hydrochloric acid.

hydrochlorothiazide (-klo″ro-thi′ah-zīd) a diuretic, $C_7H_8ClN_3O_4S_2$.

hydrocholecystis (-ko″le-sis′tis) distention of gallbladder with watery fluid.

hydrocholeresis (-ko″lĕ-re′sis) choleresis marked by increased water output, or induction of excretion of bile relatively low in specific gravity, viscosity, and total solid content.

hydrocholeretic (-ko″ler-et′ik) 1. pertaining to an increased output by the liver of bile of low specific gravity. 2. an agent that stimulates hydrocholeresis.

hydrocirsocele (-sir′so-sēl) hydrocele combined with varicocele.

hydrocodone (-ko′dōn) a synthetic analgesic, $C_{18}H_{21}NO_3$, essentially similar to codeine in its actions but more active and more prone to cause addiction; used as the bitartrate salt, mainly as an antitussive.

hydrocolloid (-kol′loid) a colloid system in which water is the dispersion medium.

hydrocolpos (-kol′pos) collection of watery fluid in the vagina.

hydrocortamate (-kor′tah-māt) a synthetic glucocorticoid, $C_{27}H_{41}NO_6$, used as the hydrochloride salt in the topical treatment of dermatoses.

hydrocortisone (-kor′tĭ-sōn) the main glucocorticoid secreted by the adrenal glands, usually referred to as cortisol in biochemistry and pharmacology; a synthetic preparation is used for its anti-inflammatory actions in the form of the alcohol and as the acetate, sodium phosphate, and sodium succinate esters.

Hydrocortone (-kor′tōn) trademark for preparations of hydrocortisone.

hydrocyst (hi′dro-sist) a cyst with watery contents.

Hydrodiuril (hi″dro-di′u-ril) trademark for a preparation of hydrochlorothiazide.

hydroencephalocele (-en-sef′ah-lo-sēl) encephalocystocele.

hydroflumethiazide (-floo″mĕ-thi′ah-zīd) an antihypertensive and diuretic, $C_8H_8F_3N_3O_4S_2$.

hydrogel (hi′dro-jel) a gel that contains water.

hydrogen (hi′dro-jen) chemical element (*see table*), at. no. 1, symbol H; it exists as the mass 1 isotope (*protium, light,* or *ordinary, h.*), mass 2 isotope (*deuterium, heavy h.*), and mass 3 isotope (*tritium*). **h. cyanide,** an extremely poisonous liquid or gas, HCN, used as a rodenticide and insecticide. **h. disulfide,** an ill-smelling gas, H_2S. **h. monoxide,** water, H_2O. **h. peroxide,** a strongly disinfectant cleansing and bleaching liquid, H_2O_2, used in dilute solution in water. **h sulfide,** an ill-smelling, colorless, poisonous gas, H_2S.

hydrogenase (-ās″) an enzyme that catalyzes the reduction of various substances by combining them with molecular hydrogen.

hydrogenate (-āt″) to cause to combine with hydrogen; to reduce with hydrogen.

hydrogenlyase (hi″dro-jen-li′ās) an adaptive enzyme formed by *Escherichia coli* which catalyzes the breakdown of formic acid to carbon dioxide and hydrogen.

hydrogymnastics (-jim-nas′tiks) therapeutic exercise performed in water.

hydrokinetic (-ki-net′ik) relating to movement of water or other fluid, as in a whirlpool bath.

hydrokinetics (-ki-net′iks) the science treating of fluids in motion.

hydrolase (hi′dro-lās) one of the six main classes of enzymes, comprising those that catalyze the hydrolytic cleavage of a compound.

Hydrolose (-lōs) trademark for a preparation of methylcellulose.

hydro-lyase (hi″dro-li′ās) any lyase that removes water from a compound in the form of the water molecule.

hydrolymph (hi′dro-limf) the thin, watery nutritive fluid of certain lower animals.

hydrolysate (hi-drol′ĭ-sāt) any compound produced by hydrolysis.

hydrolysis (hi-drol′ĭ-sis) the cleavage of a compound by the addition of water, the hydroxyl group being incorporated in one fragment and the hydrogen atom in the other. **hydrolyt′ic,** adj.

hydroma (hi-dro′mah) hygroma.

hydromeningocele (hi″dro-mĕ-ning′go-sēl) protrusion of the meninges, containing fluid, through a defect in the skull or vertebral column.

hydrometer (hi-drom′ĕ-ter) an instrument for determining the specific gravity of a fluid.

hydrometra (hi″dro-me′trah) a collection of watery fluid in the uterus.

hydrometrocolpos (-me″tro-kol′pos) a collection of watery fluid in the uterus and vagina.

hydrometry (hi-drom′ĕ-tre) measurement of specific gravity with a hydrometer.

hydromicrocephaly (hi″dro-mi″kro-sef′ah-le) smallness of the head with an abnormal amount of cerebrospinal fluid.

hydromorphone (-mor′fon) a hydrogenated ketone of morphine, $C_{17}H_{19}NO_3$; the hydrochloride salt is used as a narcotic analgesic.

hydromphalus (hi-drom′fah-lus) a cystic accumulation of watery fluid at the umbilicus.

hydromyelia (hi″dro-mi-e′le-ah) dilatation of the central canal of the spinal cord with an abnormal accumulation of fluid.

hydromyelomeningocele (-mi″ĕ-lo-mĕ-ning′-go-sēl) a defect of the spine marked by protrusion of the membranes and tissue of the spinal cord, forming a fluid-filled sac.

hydromyoma (-mi-o′mah) uterine leiomyoma with cystic degeneration.

hydronephrosis (-nĕ-fro′sis) distention of the renal pelvis and calices with urine, due to obstruction of the ureter, with atrophy of the kidney parenchyma. **hydronephrot′ic,** adj.

hydropericarditis (-per″ĭ-kar-di′tis) pericarditis with watery effusion.

hydropericardium (-per″ĭ-kar′de-um) excess of transudate in the pericardial cavity.

hydroperitoneum (-per″ĭ-to-ne′um) ascites.

hydrophilia (-fil′e-ah) the property of absorbing water. **hydrophil′ic, hydroph′ilous,** adj.

hydrophobia (-fo′be-ah) rabies.

hydrophobic (-fo′bik) 1. pertaining to hydrophobia (rabies). 2. repelling water; insoluble in water.

hydrophthalmos (hi″drof-thal′mos) distention of eyeball in infantile glaucoma.

hydrophysometra (hi″dro-fi″so-me′trah) collection of fluid and gas in the uterus.

hydropic (hi-drop′ik) pertaining to or affected with dropsy.

hydropneumatosis (hi″dro-nu″mah-to′sis) a collection of fluid and gas in the tissues.

hydropneumogony (-nu-mo′go-ne) injection of air into a joint to detect the presence of effusion.

hydropneumopericardium (-nu″mo-per″ĭ-kar′de-um) a collection of fluid and gas within the pericardium.

hydropneumoperitoneum (-per″ĭ-to-ne′um) a collection of fluid and gas in the peritoneal cavity.

hydropneumothorax (-tho′raks) a collection of fluid and gas within the pleural cavity.

hydrops (hi′drops) [L.] abnormal accumulation of serous fluid in the tissues or in a body cavity; dropsy. **fetal h., h. feta′lis,** accumulation of fluid in the entire body of the newborn infant, in erythroblastosis fetalis.

hydropyonephrosis (hi″dro-pi″o-nĕ-fro′sis) urine and pus in the renal pelvis.

hydroquinone (-kwin′ōn) a skin depigmenting agent, $C_6H_6O_2$.

hydrorrhea (-re′ah) a copious watery discharge. **h. gravida′rum,** watery discharge from the vagina during pregnancy.

hydrosalpinx (-sal′pinks) accumulation of watery fluid in the uterine tube.

hydrosarcocele (-sar′ko-sēl) hydrocele and sarcocele together.

hydroscheocele (hi-dros′ke-o-sēl″) scrotal hernia containing fluid.

hydrosol (hi′dro-sol) a sol in which the dispersion medium is water.

hydrospirometer (hi″dro-spi-rom′ĕ-ter) a spirometer in which a column of water serves as an index.

hydrostat (hi′dro-stat) a device for regulating the height of a fluid in a column or reservoir.

hydrostatics (hi″dro-stat′iks) science of equilibrium of fluids. **hydrostat′ic,** adj.

hydrosyringomyelia (-sĭ-ring″go-mi-e′le-ah) coexistence of hydromyelia and syringomyelia.

hydrotaxis (-tak′sis) taxis in response to the influence of water or moisture.

hydrotherapy (-ther′ah-pe) use of water in any form, either externally or internally, in treatment of disease.

hydrothermal (-ther′mal) of or relating to hot water.

hydrothionemia (thi″o-ne′me-ah) hydrogen sulfide in the blood.

hydrothionuria (-thi″o-nu′re-ah) hydrogen sulfide in the urine.

hydrothorax (-tho′raks) a collection of serous fluid within the pleural cavity.

hydrotropism (hi-drot′ro-pizm) a growth response of a nonmotile organism to the presence of water or moisture.

hydrotympanum (hi″dro-tim′pah-num) a collection of serous fluid in the middle ear.

hydroureter (-u-re′ter) distention of the ureter with urine or watery fluid.

hydrovarium (-va′re-um) a collection of serous fluid in an ovary.

hydroxide (hi-drok′sīd) any compound containing hydroxyl.

hydroxocobalamin (hi-drok″so-ko-bal′ah-min) an analogue of cyanocobalamin having exceptionally long-acting hematopoietic activity.

hydroxy- chemical prefix indicating the presence of the univalent radical OH.

hydroxyamphetamine (hi-drok″se-am-fet′ah-min) a sympathomimetic amine, $C_9H_{13}NO$; its hydrobromide salt is used as a nasal decongestant, pressor, and mydriatic.

hydroxyapatite (-ap′ah-tīt) an inorganic constituent of bone matrix and teeth, imparting rigidity to these structures.

hydroxybenzene (-ben′zēn) phenol.

hydroxychloroquine (-klo′ro-kwin) a drug, $C_{18}H_{26}ClN_3O$, used as the sulfate salt in the treatment of malaria, lupus erythematosus, rheumatoid arthritis, and symptomatic giardiasis.

25-hydroxycholecalciferol (-ko″le-kal-sif′er-ol) a metabolically activated form of cholecalciferol synthesized in the liver.

hydroxycorticosterone (-kor″tĭ-ko′stēr-ōn) hydrocortisone.

hydroxydione (-di′ōn) a steroid preparation, $C_{25}H_{35}O_6$; its sodium salt is used as a basal anesthetic.

hydroxyl (hi-drok′sil) the univalent radical OH.

hydroxylase (hi-drok′sĭ-lās) any enzyme that brings about the coupled oxidation of two donors, with incorporation of oxygen into one of them.

hydroxyphenamate (hi-drok″se-fen′ah-māt) a minor tranquilizer, $C_{11}H_{15}NO_3$.

hydroxyprogesterone (-pro-jes′ter-ōn) a long-acting progestational steriod, $C_{27}H_{40}O_4$, used as the caproate ester in corpus luteum deficiencies.

hydroxyproline (-pro′lēn) an amino acid produced in the digestion of hydrolytic decomposition of proteins, especially of collagens.

hydroxystilbamidine (-stil-bam′ĭ-dēn) an antileishmanial agent, $C_{16}H_{16}N_4O$, used as the isethionate salt.

5-hydroxytryptamine (-trip′tah-mēn) serotonin.

hydroxyzine (hi-drok′sĭ-zēn) a central nervous system depressant, $C_{21}H_{27}ClN_2O_2$, having antispasmodic, antihistaminic, and antifibrillatory actions; used as the hydrochloride or pamoate salt.

hydruria (hi-droo′re-ah) excretion of urine of low osmolality or low specific gravity.

hygiene (hi′jēn) science of health and its preservation. **hygien′ic,** adj. **mental h.,** the science dealing with development of healthy mental and emotional reactions and habits. **oral h.,** proper care of the mouth and teeth.

hygienist (hi′je-en″ist) a specialist in hygiene. **dental h.,** an auxiliary member of the dental profession, trained in the art of removing calcareous deposits and stains from surfaces of teeth and in providing additional services and information on prevention of oral disease.

hygienization (hi″je-en″i-za′shun) establishment of hygienic conditions.

hygro- word element [Gr.], *moisture.*

hygroma (hi-gro′mah) an accumulation of fluid in a sac, cyst, or bursa. **hygrom′atous,** adj. **h. col′li,** a watery tumor of the neck. **cystic h., h. cys′ticum,** see under *lymphangioma.* **Fleischmann's h.,** enlargement of a bursa in the floor of the mouth, to the outer side of the genioglossus muscle.

hygrometer (hi-grom′ĕ-ter) an instrument for measuring atmospheric moisture.

hygrometry (hi-grom′ĕ-tre) measurement of moisture in atmosphere.

hygroscopic (hi″gro-skop′ik) readily absorbing moisture.

Hygroton (hi′gro-ton) trademark for a preparation of chlorthalidone.

hymen (hi′men) the membranous fold partially or wholly occluding the external vaginal orifice. **hy′menal,** adj.

hymenectomy (hi″men-ek′to-me) excision of the hymen.

hymenitis (-i′tis) inflammation of the hymen.

hymenolepiasis (-o-lep-i′ah-sis) infection with *Hymenolepis.*

Hymenolepis (-ol′ĕ-pis) a genus of tapeworms,

including *H. na'na,* found in rodents, rats, and man, especially children.

hymenology (-ol'o-je) the science dealing with the membranes of the body.

hymenotomy (-ot'o-me) division of the hymen.

hyoepiglottic, hyoepiglottidean (hi″o-ep″ĭ-glot'ik; -ep″ĭ-glo-tid'e-an) pertaining to the hyoid bone and epiglottis.

hyoglossal (-glos'al) pertaining to the hyoid bone and tongue or to the hyoglossus muscle.

hyoid (hi'oid) shaped like Greek letter upsilon (υ); pertaining to the hyoid bone.

hyoscine (hi'o-sīn) scopolamine.

hyoscyamine (hi″o-si'ah-mēn) an anticholinergic alkaloid, $C_{17}H_{23}NO_3$, usually obtained from species of *Hyoscyamus* and other solanaceous plants; the hydrobromide and sulfate salts are used to produce parasympathetic blockade; the latter is used as a vagal blocking agent.

hyoscyamus (-si'ah-mus) the dried leaf of *Hyoscyamus niger,* which contains hyoscyamine and scopolamine.

hyp- see *hypo-*.

hypacusia (hi″pah-ku'ze-ah) hypoacusis.

hypalbuminosis (hi″pal-bu″mi-no'sis) hypoalbuminosis.

hypalgesia (hi″pal-je'ze-ah) diminished sensibility to pain. **hypalge'sic,** adj.

hypamnios (hi-pam'ne-os) deficiency of amniotic fluid.

hypanakinesis (hi″pan-ah-ki-ne'sis) hypokinesia.

hyparterial (hi″par-te're-al) beneath an artery.

hypaxial (hi-pak'se-al) ventral to the long axis of the body.

hyper- word element [Gr.], *abnormally increased; excessive.*

hyperacid (hi″per-as'id) abnormally or excessively acid.

hyperacidity (-ah-sid'ĭ-te) excessive acidity.

hyperactive (-ak'tiv) characterized by hyperactivity.

hyperactivity (-ak-tiv'ĭ-te) excessive activity; hyperkinetic syndrome.

hyperacusis (-ah-ku'sis) an exceptionally acute sense of hearing.

hyperadenosis (-ad″ĕ-no'sis) enlargement of glands.

hyperadiposis (-ad″ĭ-po'sis) extreme fatness.

hyperadrenalism (-ah-dre'nal-izm) overactivity of the adrenal glands.

hyperadrenia (-ah-dre'ne-ah) hyperadrenalism.

hyperadrenocorticism (-ah-dre″no-kor'tĭ-sizm) hypersecretion of the adrenal cortex.

hyperaffectivity (-af″fek-tiv'ĭ-te) abnormally increased sensibility to mild stimuli; the quality of abnormally heightened emotional reactivity. **hyperaffec'tive,** adj.

hyperaldosteronism (-al″do-stēr'ōn-izm) an abnormality of electrolyte metabolism due to excessive secretion of aldosterone; it may be primary or occur secondarily in response to extra-adrenal disease. There may be hyperten-

sion, hypokalemia, alkalosis, muscular weakness, polyuria, and polydipsia.

hyperalgesia (-al-je'ze-ah) excessive sensitiveness to pain. **hyperalge'sic,** adj.

hyperalimentation (-al″ĭ-men-ta'shun) the ingestion or administration of a greater than optimal amount of nutrients. **parenteral h.,** intravenous infusion of such nutrients as amino acids, glucose, fructose, etc.

hyperammonemia (-ah″mo-ne'me-ah) an excess of ammonia in the blood.

hyperamylasemia (-am″il-a-se'me-ah) abnormally high levels of amylase in the blood serum.

hyperanakinesia (-an″ah-ki-ne'ze-ah) excessive motor activity.

hyperaphia (-a'fe-ah) tactile hyperesthesia. **hyperaph'ic,** adj.

hyperazotemia (-az″o-te'me-ah) an excess of nitrogenous matter in the blood.

hyperazoturia (-az″o-tu're-ah) an excess of nitrogenous matter in the urine.

hyperbaric (-bār'ik) characterized by greater than normal weight; applied to gases under greater than atmospheric pressure, or to a solution of greater specific gravity than another taken as a reference standard.

hyperbarism (-bar'izm) a condition due to exposure to ambient gas pressure or atmospheric pressures exceeding the pressure within the body.

hyperbetalipoproteinemia (-ba″tah-lip″o-pro″te-in-e'me-ah) hyperlipoproteinemia (type II).

hyperbilirubinemia (-bil″i-roo″bĭ-ne'me-ah) excess of bilirubin in the blood.

hyperbrachycephalic (-brak″e-sĕ-fal'ik) having a cephalic index of 85.5 or more.

hyperbulia (-bu'le-ah) excessive wilfulness.

hypercalcemia (-kal-se'me-ah) an excess of calcium in the blood. **idiopathic h.,** a condition of infants, associated with vitamin D intoxication, characterized by elevated serum calcium levels, increased density of the skeleton, mental deterioration, and nephrocalcinosis.

hypercalciuria (-kal″se-u're-ah) an excess of calcium in the urine.

hypercapnia (-kap'ne-ah) an excess of carbon dioxide in the blood. **hypercap'nic,** adj.

hypercarbia (-kar'be-ah) hypercapnia.

hypercatharsis (-kah-thar'sis) excessive purgation. **hypercathar'tic,** adj.

hypercellularity (-sel″u-lar'ĭ-te) abnormal increase in the number of cells present, as in bone marrow. **hypercell'ular,** adj.

hypercementosis (-se″men-to'sis) excessive growth of cementum on tooth roots.

hyperchloremia (-klo-re'me-ah) an excess of chlorides in the blood. **hyperchlore'mic,** adj.

hyperchlorhydria (-klōr-hi'dre-ah) an excess of hydrochloric acid in the gastric juice.

hypercholesteremia (-ko-les″ter-e'me-ah) hypercholesterolemia.

hypercholesterolemia (-ko-les″ter-ol-e'me-ah) an excess of cholesterol in the blood. **hypercholesterole'mic,** adj. **familial h.,** hyperlipoproteinemia (type II).

hypercholia (-ko'le-ah) excessive secretion of bile.

hyperchromasia (-kro-ma'ze-ah) hyperchromatism.

hyperchromatism (-kro'mah-tizm) 1. excessive pigmentation. 2. degeneration of cell nuclei, which become filled with particles of pigment (chromatin). 3. increased staining capacity. **hyperchromat'ic**, adj.

hyperchromatosis (-kro"mah-to'sis) hyperchromatism.

hyperchromemia (-kro-me'me-ah) a high color index of the blood.

hyperchromia (-kro'me-ah) 1. hyperchromatism. 2. abnormal increase in the hemoglobin content of erythrocytes.

hyperchylia (-ki'le-ah) excessive secretion of gastric juice.

hyperchylomicronemia (-ki"lo-mi"kro-ne'me-ah) presence in the blood of an excessive number of particles of fat (chylomicrons).

hypercoagulability (-ko-ag"u-lah-bil'ĭ-te) abnormally increased coagulability of the blood.

hypercorticism (-kor"tĭ-sizm) hyperadrenocorticism.

hypercryalgesia (-kri"al-je'ze-ah) excessive sensitiveness to cold.

hypercryesthesia (-kri"es-the'ze-ah) hypercryalgesia.

hypercupremia (-ku-pre'me-ah) an excess of copper in the blood.

hypercupriuria (-ku"pre-u're-ah) an excess of copper in the urine.

hypercyanotic (-si"ah-not'ik) extremely cyanotic.

hypercythemia (-si-the'me-ah) an excess of red blood cells in the blood.

hypercytosis (-si-to'sis) abnormally increased number of cells, especially of leukocytes.

hyperdactyly (-dak'tĭ-le) the presence of supernumerary digits on hand or foot.

hyperdicrotic (-di-krot'ik) markedly dicrotic.

hyperdistention (-dis-ten'shun) excessive distention.

hyperdiuresis (-di"u-re'sis) excessive excretion of urine.

hyperdynamia (-di-na'me-ah) excessive muscular activity. **hyperdynam'ic**, adj.

hyperechema (-e-ke'mah) exaggeration of auditory sensations.

hyperemesis (-em'ĕ-sis) excessive vomiting. **hyperemet'ic**, adj. **h. gravida'rum**, the pernicious vomiting of pregnancy. **h. lacten'tium**, excessive vomiting in nursing babies.

hyperemia (-e'me-ah) an excess of blood in a part. **hypere'mic**, adj. **active h., arterial h.,** that due to local or general relaxation of arterioles. **Bier's passive h., constriction h.,** induction of venous congestion by applying a thin rubber band. **fluxionary h.,** active h. **leptomeningeal h.,** congestion of the pia-arachnoid. **passive h.,** that due to obstruction to flow of blood from the area. **reactive h.,** that due to increase in blood flow after its temporary interruption. **venous h.,** passive h.

hyperencephalus (-en-sef'ah-lus) a monster with the cranial vault absent and brain exposed.

hypereosinophilia (-e"o-sin"o-fil'e-ah) eosinophilia (2).

hyperequilibrium (-e"kwĭ-lib're-um) excessive tendency to vertigo.

hyperergasia (-er-ga'ze-ah) excessive functional activity.

hyperergia (-er'je-ah) 1. hyperergasia. 2. hyperergy.

hyperergy (-er'je) hypersensitivity to allergens; extreme allergy. **hyperer'gic**, adj.

hypererythrocythemia (-ĕ-rith"ro-si-the'me-ah) hypercythemia.

hyperesophoria (-es"o-fo're-ah) deviation of the visual axes upward and inward.

hyperesthesia (-es-the'ze-ah) abnormally increased sensitivity of the skin or of an organ of special sense. **hyperesthet'ic**, adj. **acoustic h., auditory h.,** hyperacusia. **cerebral h.,** that which is due to a cerebral lesion. **gustatory h.,** hypergeusesthesia. **muscular h.,** muscular oversensitivity to pain or fatigue. **olfactory h.,** hyperosmia. **oneiric h.,** increased sensitivity or pain during sleep and dreams. **optic h.,** abnormal sensitivity of the eye to light. **tactile h.,** excessive tactile sensibility.

hyperexophoria (-ek"so-fo're-ah) deviation of the visual axes upward and outward.

hyperextension (-ek-sten'shun) extreme or excessive extension of a limb or part.

hyperferremia (-fē-re'me-ah) an excess of iron in the blood. **hyperferre'mic**, adj.

hyperfibrinogenemia (-fi-brin"o-jĕ-ne'me-ah) excessive fibrinogen in the blood.

hyperflexion (-flek'shun) forcible overflexion of a limb or part.

hyperfunction (-funk'shun) excessive functioning of a part or organ.

hypergalactia, hypergalactosis (-gah-lak'she-ah; gal"ak-to'sis) excessive secretion of milk. **hypergalac'tous**, adj.

hypergammaglobulinemia (-gam"ah-glob"u-lĭ-ne'me-ah) increased gamma globulins in the blood. **hypergammaglobuline'mic**, adj.

hypergenesis (-jen'ĕ-sis) excessive development. **hypergenet'ic**, adj.

hypergenitalism (-jen'ĭ-tal-izm) hypergonadism.

hypergeusesthesia, hypergeusia (-gūs"es-the'ze-ah; -gu'ze-ah) abnormal acuteness of the sense of taste.

hypergia (hi-per'je-ah) 1. hypoergasia. 2. diminished sensitivity in allergy.

hyperglandular (hi"per-glan'du-ler) marked by excessive glandular activity.

hyperglobulia (-glo-bu'le-ah) polycythemia.

hyperglobulinemia (-glob"u-lĭ-ne'me-ah) excess of globulin in the blood.

hyperglycemia (-gli-se'me-ah) an excess of glucose in the blood.

hyperglycemic (-gli-se'mik) 1. pertaining to, characterized by, or causing hyperglycemia. 2. an agent that increases the glucose level of the blood.

hyperglyceridemia (-glis″er-ĭ-de′me-ah) excess of glycerides in the blood.

hyperglycinemia (-gli″sĭ-ne′me-ah) a hereditary metabolic disorder involving excessive glycine in the blood and urine. One form is characterized by episodic vomiting, lethargy, dehydration, ketosis, and increased susceptibility to infection; a second form by generalized hypotonia, lethargy, absence of reflexes, and periodic myoclonic jerks.

hyperglycinuria (-gli′sĭ-nu′re-ah) an excess of glycine in the urine; see *hyperglycinemia.*

hyperglycogenolysis (-gli″ko-jĕ-nol′ĭ-sis) excessive glycogenolysis, resulting in excessive dextrose in the body.

hyperglycorrhachia (-ra′ke-ah) excessive sugar in the cerebrospinal fluid.

hyperglycosuria (-su′re-ah) extreme glycosuria.

hypergonadism (hi″per-go′nad-izm) abnormally increased functional activity of the gonads, with excessive growth and precocious sexual development.

hyperhedonia (-he-do′ne-ah) morbid increase of the feeling of pleasure in agreeable acts.

hyperhemoglobinemia (-he″mo-glo″bĭ-ne′me-ah) an excess of hemoglobin in the blood.

hyperhidrosis (-hĭ-dro′sis) excessive perspiration. **hyperhidrot′ic,** adj.

hyperhydration (-hi-dra′shun) abnormally increased water content of the body.

hyperidrosis (-ĭ-dro′sis) hyperhidrosis.

hyperimmune (-im-mūn′) possessing very large quantities of specific antibodies in the serum.

hyperinflation (-in-fla′shun) excessive inflation or expansion, as of the lungs; overinflation.

hyperinsulinism (-in′su-lin-izm″) 1. excessive secretion of insulin. 2. insulin shock.

hyperinvolution (-in″vo-lu′shun) superinvolution.

hyperirritability (-ir″ĭ-tah-bil′ĭ-te) pathological responsiveness to slight stimuli.

hyperisotonic (-i″so-ton′ik) denoting a solution containing more than 0.45% salt, in which erythrocytes become crenated as a result of exosmosis.

hyperkalemia (-kah-le′me-ah) an excess of potassium in the blood, characterized clinically by electrocardiographic abnormalities; in severe cases, weakness and flaccid paralysis may occur. **hyperkale′mic,** adj.

hyperkeratinization (-ker″ah-tin-i-za′shun) excessive development or retention of keratin in the epidermis.

hyperkeratosis (-ker″ah-to′sis) 1. hypertrophy of the horny layer of the skin, or any disease characterized by it. 2. hypertrophy of the cornea. 3. thickening of the horny layer of the skin in cattle, due to ingestion of grease containing high levels of chlorinated hydrocarbons. **hyperkeratot′ic,** adj. **epidermolytic h.,** a hereditary disease, with hyperkeratosis, blisters, and erythema; at birth, the skin is entirely covered with thick, horny, armor-like plates that are soon shed, leaving a raw surface on which the scales re-form. **h. follicula′ris in cu′tem**

pen′etrans, a disease marked by keratotic pegs that develop in hair follicles and eccrine ducts, penetrating the epidermis and extending down into the corium, causing foreign-body reaction and pain.

hyperketonemia (-ke″to-ne′me-ah) abnormally increased concentration of ketone bodies in the blood.

hyperketonuria (-ke″to-nu′re-ah) excessive ketone in the urine.

hyperkinemia (-ki-ne′me-ah) abnormally high cardiac output. **hyperkine′mic,** adj.

hyperkinesia (-ki-ne′ze-ah) abnormally increased motor function or activity; see *hyperkinetic syndrome.* **hyperkinet′ic,** adj.

hyperlactation (-lak-ta′shun) lactation in greater than normal amount or for a longer than normal period.

hyperleukocytosis (-lu″ko-si-to′sis) an excess of leukocytes in blood.

hyperlipemia (-li-pe′me-ah) an excess of lipids in the blood. **carbohydrate-induced h.,** hyperlipoproteinemia (type IV). **fat-induced h.,** hyperlipoproteinemia (type I).

hyperlipoproteinemia (-lip″o-pro″te-in-e′me-ah) an excess of lipoproteins in the blood. The familial type occurs in five forms, distinguished chemically by the ratio of plasma levels of cholesterol and triglycerides, characterized clinically as follows. *Type I:* repeated bouts of abdominal colic, xanthoma of the skin and eyes, and hepatosplenomegaly. *Type II:* tendinous xanthoma, tuberous xanthoma, and accelerated atherosclerosis. *Type III:* planar xanthoma and, less often, tendinous xanthoma and atherosclerosis. *Type IV:* early coronary atherosclerosis and sometimes the symptoms of type I. *Type V:* the symptoms of type I.

hyperliposis (-lĭ-po′sis) excess of fat in the blood serum or tissues.

hyperlithuria (-lĭ-thu′re-ah) excess of lithic (uric) acid in the urine.

hyperlucency (-lu′sen-se) excessive radiolucency.

hypermastia (-mas′te-ah) 1. the presence of one or more supernumery mammary glands. 2. hypertrophy of the mammary gland.

hypermature (-mah-tūr′) past the stage of maturity.

hypermenorrhea (-men″ŏ-re′ah) excessive menstrual bleeding, but occurring at regular intervals and being of usual duration.

hypermetabolism (-mě-tab′o-lizm) increased metabolism. **extrathyroidal m.,** abnormally elevated basal metabolism unassociated with thyroid disease.

hypermetria (-me′tre-ah) ataxia in which movements overreach the intended goal.

hypermetrope (-mě′trōp) hyperope.

hypermetropia (-mě-tro′pe-ah) hyperopia.

hypermnesia (hi″perm-ne′ze-ah) extreme retentiveness of memory. **hypermne′sic,** adj.

hypermorph (hi′per-morf) 1. a person who is tall but of low sitting height. 2. in genetics, a mutant gene that shows an increase in the activity it influences. **hypermor′phic,** adj.

hypermotility (hi″per-mo-til′ĭ-te) abnormally increased motility, as of the gastrointestinal tract.

hypermyotonia (-mi″o-to′ne-ah) excessive muscular tonicity.

hypermyotrophy (-mi-ot′ro-fe) excessive development of muscular tissue.

hypernatremia (-na-tre′me-ah) an excess of sodium in the blood. **hypernatre′mic,** adj.

hyperneocytosis (-ne″o-si-to′sis) leukocytosis with an excessive number of immature forms of leukocytes.

hypernephroma (-nĕ-fro′mah) renal cell carcinoma whose structure resembles that of adrenocortical tissue.

hypernoia (-noi′ah) excessive mental activity.

hypernutrition (-nu-trish′un) overfeeding and its ill effects.

hyperonychia (-o-nik′e-ah) onychauxis.

hyperope (hi′per-ōp) a person with hyperopia.

hyperopia (hi″per-o′pe-ah) farsightedness; a visual defect in which parallel light rays reaching the eye come to a focus behind the retina, vision being better for far objects than for near. **hypero′pic,** adj. **absolute h.,** that which cannot be corrected by accommodation. **axial h.,** that due to shortness of the anteroposterior diameter of the eye. **facultative h.,** that which can be entirely corrected by accommodation. **latent h.,** that degree of the total hyperopia corrected by the physiologic tone of the ciliary muscle, revealed by cycloplegic examination. **manifest h.,** that degree of the total hyperopia not corrected by the physiologic tone of the ciliary muscle, revealed by cycloplegic examination. **relative h.,** facultative h. **total h.,** manifest and latent hyperopia combined.

hyperorchidism (-or′kĭ-dizm) excessive functional activity of the testes.

hyperorexia (-o-rek′se-ah) excessive appetite.

hyperorthocytosis (-or″tho-si-to′sis) leukocytosis with a normal proportion of the various forms of leukocytes.

hyperosmia (-oz′me-ah) abnormal acuteness of the sense of smell. **hyperos′mic,** adj.

hyperosmolarity (-oz″mo-lar′ĭ-te) abnormally increased osmolar concentration.

hyperostosis (-os-to′sis) hypertrophy of bone. **hyperostot′ic,** adj. **h. cra′nii,** hyperostosis involving the cranial bones. **frontal internal h.,** a new formation of bone tissue in patches on the inner surface of the cranial bone in the frontal region. **infantile cortical h.,** a disease of young infants, with soft tissue swelling over affected bones, fever, irritability, and periods of remission and exacerbation. **Morgagni's h.,** frontal internal h.

hyperoxaluria (-ok″sah-lu′re-ah) an excess of oxalate in the urine. **primary h.,** an inborn error of metabolism, with excessive urinary excretion of oxalate, nephrolithiasis, nephrocalcinosis, early onset of renal failure, and often a generalized deposit of calcium oxalate.

hyperoxemia (-ok-se′me-ah) excessive acidity of the blood.

hyperoxia (-ok′se-ah) an excess of oxygen in the system. **hyperox′ic,** adj.

hyperparasite (-par′ah-sīt) a parasite that preys on a parasite. **hyperparasit′ic,** adj.

hyperparathyroidism (-par″ah-thi′roid-izm) excessive activity of the parathyroid glands. *Primary h.* is associated with neoplasia or hyperplasia; the excess of parathyroid hormone leads to alteration in function of bone cells, renal tubules, and gastrointestinal mucosa. *Secondary h.* occurs when the serum calcium tends to fall below normal, as in chronic renal disease, etc.

hyperpepsinia (-pep-sin′e-ah) excessive secretion of pepsin.

hyperperistalsis (-per″ĭ-stal′sis) excessively active peristalsis.

hyperphalangism (-fal′an-jizm) the presence of a supernumerary phalanx on a digit.

hyperphasia (-fa′ze-ah) excessive talkativeness.

hyperphenylalaninemia (-fen″il-al″ah-nĭ-ne′-me-ah) an excess of phenylalanine in the blood, as in phenylketonuria.

hyperphonesis (-fo-ne′sis) intensification of the sound in auscultation or percussion.

hyperphoria (-fo′re-ah) upward deviation of the visual axis of one eye in the absence of visual fusional stimuli.

hyperphosphatemia (-fos″fah-te′me-ah) an excess of phosphates in the blood.

hyperphosphaturia (-fos″fah-tu′re-ah) an excess of phosphates in the urine.

hyperphrenia (-fre′ne-ah) 1. extreme mental excitement. 2. accelerated mental activity.

hyperpigmentation (-pig″men-ta′shun) abnormally increased pigmentation.

hyperpituitarism (-pĭ-tu′ĭ-tar-izm″) a condition due to pathologically increased activity of the pituitary gland, either of the basophilic cells, resulting in basophil adenoma causing compression of the pituitary gland, or of the eosinophilic cells, producing overgrowth, acromegaly, and gigantism (*true h.*).

hyperplasia (-pla′ze-ah) abnormal increase in the number of normal cells in normal arrangement in an organ or tissue, which increases its volume. **hyperplas′tic,** adj. **chronic perforating h. of pulp,** internal resorption of a tooth. **lipoid h.,** increased formation of lipoid-containing cells.

hyperplasmia (-plaz′me-ah) 1. excess in the proportion of blood plasma to corpuscles. 2. increase in size of erythrocytes due to absorption of plasma.

hyperploid (hi′per-ploid) 1. characterized by hyperploidy. 2. a hyperploid individual or cell.

hyperploidy (hi′per-ploi″de) the state of having more than the typical number of chromosomes in unbalanced sets, as in Down's syndrome.

hyperpnea (hi″perp-ne′ah) abnormal increase in depth and rate of respiration. **hyperpne′ic,** adj.

hyperpolarization (hi″per-po″lar-i-za′shun) any increase in the amount of electrical charge separated by the cell membrane, and hence in the strength of the transmembrane potential.

hyperponesis (-po-ne′sis) excessive action-potential output from the motor and premotor areas of the cortex. **hyperponet′ic,** adj.

hyperposia (-po′ze-ah) abnormally increased ingestion of fluids for relatively brief periods.

hyperpotassemia (-pot″ah-se′me-ah) hyperkalemia.

hyperpragic (-praj′ik) characterized by excessive mental activity.

hyperpraxia (-prak′se-ah) abnormal mental activity; restlessness.

hyperprolinemia (-pro″lĭ-ne′me-ah) a disorder of amino acid metabolism marked by an excess of proline in the body fluids.

hyperprosexia (-pro-sek′se-ah) preoccupation with one idea to the exclusion of all others.

hyperproteinemia (-pro″te-in-e′me-ah) an excess of protein in the blood.

hyperproteosis (-pro″te-o′sis) a condition due to an excess of protein in the diet.

hyperpsychosis (-si-ko′sis) exaggeration of mental activity with abnormal rapidity of the flow of thought.

hyperpyrexia (-pi-rek′se-ah) excessively high body temperature. **hyperpyrex′ial, hyperpyret′ic,** adj. **malignant h.,** malignant hyperthermia.

hyperreactive (-re-ak′tiv) showing a greater than normal response to stimuli.

hyperreflexia (-re-flek′se-ah) exaggeration of reflexes.

hyperresonance (-rez′o-nans) exaggerated resonance on percussion.

hypersalemia (-sah-le′me-ah) abnormally increased content of salt in the blood.

hypersalivation (-sal″ĭ-va′shun) ptyalism.

hypersecretion (-se-kre′shun) excessive secretion.

hypersensitivity (-sen″sĭ-tiv′ĭ-te) a state of altered reactivity in which the body reacts with an exaggerated immune response to a foreign agent. **hypersen′sitive,** adj. **delayed h.,** a slowly developing increase in cell-mediated immune response to a specific antigen, as occurs in graft rejection, autoimmune disease, etc. **immediate h.,** antibody-mediated hypersensitivity characterized by lesions resulting from release of histamine and other vasoactive substances, as occurs in anaphylaxis.

hypersensitization (-sen″sĭ-ti-za′shun) the process of rendering, or the condition of being, abnormally sensitive.

hypersialosis (-si″ah-lo′sis) ptyalism.

hypersomnia (-som′ne-ah) pathologically excessive sleep or drowsiness.

hypersplenism (-splen′izm) a condition characterized by exaggeration of the hemolytic function of the spleen, resulting in deficiency of peripheral blood elements, and by hypercellularity of the bone marrow and splenomegaly.

hypersthenia (-sthe′ne-ah) great strength or tonicity. **hypersthen′ic,** adj.

hypertelorism (-te′lo-rizm) abnormally increased distance between two organs or parts. **ocular h., orbital h.,** increase in the interorbital distance, often associated with cleidocranial

or craniofacial dysostosis and sometimes with mental deficiency.

Hypertensin (-ten′sin) trademark for a preparation of angiotensin amide.

hypertension (-ten′shun) persistently high arterial blood pressure; it may have no known cause (*essential, idiopathic,* or *primary h.*) or be associated with other diseases (*secondary h.*). **accelereated h.,** malignant h. **adrenal h.,** that associated with an adrenal tumor which secretes mineral corticosteroids. **benign h.,** chronic hypertension of relatively mild degree. **essential h.,** that without known cause. **Goldblatt h.,** see under *kidney.* **malignant h.,** an accelerated severe hypertensive state with papilledema of the ocular fundus and vascular hemorrhagic lesions, thickening of the small arteries and arterioles, left ventricular hypertrophy, and poor prognosis. **pale h.,** malignant h. **portal h.,** abnormally increased pressure in the portal circulation. **pulmonary h.,** abnormally increased pressure in the pulmonary circulation. **red h.,** benign h. **renal h.,** that associated with or due to renal disease with a factor of parenchymatous ischemia. **renovascular h.,** that due to occlusive disease of the renal arteries.

hypertensive (-ten′siv) 1. marked by increased blood pressure. 2. an individual with abnormally increased blood pressure.

hypertensor (-ten′sor) a pressor agent.

hyperthecosis (-the-ko′sis) hyperplasia and excessive luteinization of the cells of the inner stromal layer of the ovary.

hyperthelia (-the′le-ah) the presence of supernumerary nipples.

hyperthermalgesia (-ther″mal-je′ze-ah) abnormal sensitivity to heat.

hyperthermesthesia (-ther″mes-the′ze-ah) increased sensibility for heat.

hyperthermia (-ther′me-ah) greatly increased body temperature. **hyperther′mal, hyperther′mic,** adj. **malignant h.,** a syndrome affecting patients undergoing general anesthesia, marked by rapid rise in body temperature, signs of increased muscle metabolism, and, usually, rigidity.

hyperthrombinemia (-throm″bĭ-ne′me-ah) an excess of thrombin in the blood.

hyperthymia (-thi′me-ah) excessive emotionalism.

hyperthymic (-thi′mĭk) pertaining to hyperthymia or to hyperthymism.

hyperthymism (-thi′mizm) excessive activity of the thymus gland.

hyperthyroidism (-thi′roid-izm) excessive thyroid gland activity, marked by increased metabolic rate, goiter, and disturbances in the autonomic nervous system and in creatine metabolism; sometimes used to refer to *Graves' disease.* **hyperthy′roid,** adj.

hyperthyroxinemia (-thi-rok″sin-e′me-ah) an excess of thyroxine in the blood.

hypertonia (-to′ne-ah) a condition of excessive tone of the skeletal muscles; increased resistance of muscle to passive stretching. **h. oc′uli,** glaucoma.

hypertonic (-ton′ik) 1. denoting increased tone or tension. 2. denoting a solution having greater osmotic pressure than the solution with which it is compared.

hypertonicity (-to-nis′ĭ-te) the state or quality of being hypertonic.

hypertrichosis (-trĭ-ko′sis) excessive growth of hair.

hypertriglyceridemia (-tri-glis″er-i-de′me-ah) an excess of triglycerides in the blood; a familial form occurs in hyperlipoproteinemia types I and IV.

hypertrophy (hi-per′tro-fe) enlargement or overgrowth of an organ or part due to increase in size of its constituent cells. **hypertroph′ic,** adj. **ventricular h.,** hypertrophy of the myocardium of a ventricle.

hypertropia (hi″per-tro′pe-ah) strabismus in which there is permanent upward deviation of the visual axis of an eye.

hyperuricemia (-u″rĭ-se′me-ah) an excess of uric acid in the blood. **hyperurice′mic,** adj.

hypervalinemia (-val″ĭ-ne′me-ah) an inborn error of metabolism characterized by elevated levels of serum valine, valinuria, and failure to thrive.

hypervascular (-vas′ku-ler) extremely vascular.

hyperventilation (-ven″tĭ-la′shun) abnormally increased pulmonary ventilation, resulting in reduction of carbon dioxide tension, which, if prolonged, may lead to alkalosis.

hyperviscosity (-vis-kos′ĭ-te) excessive viscosity.

hypervitaminosis (-vi″tah-mĭ-no′sis) a condition due to ingestion of an excess of one or more vitamins; symptom complexes are associated with excessive intake of vitamins A and D. **hypervitaminot′ic,** adj.

hypervolemia (-vo-le′me-ah) abnormal increase in the plasma volume in the body.

hypesthesia (hi″pes-the′ze-ah) hypoesthesia.

hypha (hi′fah), pl. *hy′phae* [L.] one of the filaments composing the mycelium of a fungus. **hy′phal,** adj.

hyphedonia (hīp″he-do′ne-ah) diminution of power of enjoyment.

hyphema (hi-fe′mah) hemorrhage within the anterior chamber of the eye.

hyphemia (hi-fe′me-ah) 1. oligemia, or deficiency of blood. 2. hyphema.

hyphidrosis (hip″hĭ-dro′sis) too scanty perspiration.

Hyphomyces (hi″fo-mi′sēz) a genus of phycomycetous fungi. *H. des′truens* causes hyphomycosis destruens equi.

Hyphomycetes (-mi-se′tēz) the mycelial (hyphal) fungi, i.e., the molds.

hyphomycosis (-mi-ko′sis) infections with *Hyphomyces.* **h. des′truens e′qui,** a disease of horses and mules caused by *Hyphomyces destruens,* marked by subcutaneous abscesses that eventually break through the skin, leaving large raw surfaces.

hypn(o)- word element [Gr.], *sleep; hypnosis.*

hypnagogic (hip″nah-goj′ik) 1. producing sleep. 2. occurring just before sleep; said of dreams.

hypnagogue (hip′nah-gog) 1. hypnotic; pertaining to drowsiness. 2. an agent that induces sleep or drowsiness.

hypnalgia (hip-nal′je-ah) pain during sleep.

hypnoanalysis (hip″no-ah-nal′ĭ-sis) a method of psychotherapy combining psychoanalysis with hypnosis.

hypnodontics (-don′tiks) the application of hypnosis and controlled suggestion in the practice of dentistry.

hypnogenic (-jen′ik) inducing sleep or a hypnotic state.

hypnoid (hip′noid) resembling hypnosis.

hypnolepsy (hip′no-lep″se) narcolepsy.

hypnology (hip-nol′o-je) scientific study of sleep or of hypnotism.

hypnosis (hip-no′sis) an artificially induced passive state in which there is increased amenability and responsiveness to suggestions and commands. **hypnot′ic,** adj.

hypnotherapy (hip″no-ther′ah-pe) the therapeutic use of hypnosis.

hypnotic (hip-not′ik) 1. inducing sleep; also, an agent that so acts. 2. pertaining to or of the nature of hypnotism.

hypnotism (hip′no-tizm) 1. the method or practice of inducing hypnosis. 2. hypnosis.

hypnotize (-tīz) to put into a condition of hypnosis.

hypnotoxin (hip″no-tok′sin) 1. a hypothetical toxin said to accumulate during the waking hours until it is sufficient to inhibit the activity of the cortical cells and induce sleep. 2. a toxic substance derived from the tentacles of the Portuguese man-of-war, causing central nervous system depression, affecting both motor and sensory elements.

hypo (hi′po) 1. popular term for a hypodermic inoculation or syringe. 2. sodium thiosulfite.

hypo-, hyp- word element [Gr.], *beneath; under; deficient.*

hypoacidity (hi″po-ah-sid′ĭ-te) deficiency of acid; lack of normal acid.

hypoacusia, hypoacusis (-ah-ku′ze-ah; -ah-ku′sis) slightly diminished auditory sensitivity.

hypoadrenalism (-ah-dre′nal-izm) deficiency of adrenal activity, as in Addison's disease.

hypoadrenocorticism (-ah-dre″no-kor′tĭ-sizm) deficient activity of the adrenal cortex.

hypoaffectivity (-af″fek-tiv′ĭ-te) abnormally diminished sensitivity to superficial stimuli; abnormally decreased emotional reactivity.

hypoalbuminemia (-al-bu″mĭ-ne′me-ah) abnormally low blood levels of albumin.

hypoalbuminosis (-al-bu-mĭ-no′sis) abnormally low level of albumin.

hypoaldosteronism (-al″do-stēr′ōn-izm) a deficiency of aldosterone in the body.

hypoalimentation (-al″ĭ-men-ta′shun) insufficient nourishment.

hypoazoturia (-az″o-tu′re-ah) diminished nitrogenous material in the urine.

hypobaric (-bār′ik) characterized by less than

normal pressure or weight; applied to gases under less than atmospheric pressure, or to solutions of lower specific gravity than another taken as a standard of reference.

hypobarism (-bar′izm) the condition resulting when ambient gas or atmospheric pressure is below that within the body tissues.

hypobaropathy (-bār-op′ah-the) the disturbances experienced at high altitudes due to reduced air pressure.

hypoblast (hi′po-blast) the entoderm. **hypoblas′tic,** adj.

hypocalcemia (hi″po-kal-se′me-ah) reduction of blood calcium below normal.

hypocalciuria (-kal″se-u′re-ah) abnormally diminished urinary calcium levels.

hypocapnia (-kap′ne-ah) deficiency of carbon dioxide in the blood. **hypocap′nic,** adj.

hypocarbia (-kar″be-ah) hypocapnia.

hypochloremia (-klo-re′me-ah) abnormally diminished levels of chloride in the blood. **hypochlore′mic,** adj.

hypochlorhydria (-klōr-hi′dre-ah) lack of hydrochloric acid in the gastric juice.

hypochlorization (-klōr″ĭ-za′shun) reduction of sodium chloride salt in the diet.

hypochloruria (-klōr-u′re-ah) diminished chloride content in the urine.

hypocholesteremia (-ko-les″ter-e′me-ah) hypocholesterolemia.

hypocholesterolemia (-ko-les″ter-ol-e′me-ah) abnormally low levels of cholesterol in the blood. **hypocholesterole′mic,** adj.

hypochondria (-kon′dre-ah) 1. plural of *hypochondrium.* 2. hypochondriasis.

hypochondriac (-kon′dre-ak) 1. pertaining to the hypochondrium or to hypochondriasis. 2. a person affected with hypochondriasis.

hypochondriasis (-kon-dri′ah-sis) morbid anxiety about one's health, with numerous and varying symptoms that cannot be attributed to organic disease. **hypochondri′acal,** adj.

hypochondrium (-kon′dre-um), pl. *hypochon′dria.* The upper lateral abdominal region, overlying the costal cartilages, on either side of the epigastrium. **hypochon′drial,** adj.

hypochromasia (-kro-ma′ze-ah) 1. staining less intensely than normal. 2. decrease of hemoglobin in erythrocytes so that they are abnormally pale. **hypochromat′ic,** adj.

hypochromatism (-kro′mah-tizm) abnormally deficient pigmentation, especially deficiency of chromatin in a cell nucleus.

hypochromatosis (-kro″mah-to′sis) the gradual fading and disappearance of the cell nucleus (chromatin).

hypochromemia (-kro-me′me-ah) abnormally low color index of the blood.

hypochromia (-kro′me-ah) 1. hypochromasia (2). 2. hypochromatism. **hypochro′mic,** adj.

hypochylia (-ki′le-ah) deficiency of chyle.

hypocomplementemia (-kom′plĕ-men-te′me-ah) diminution of complement levels in the blood.

hypocorticism (-kor′tĭ-sizm) hypoadrenocorticism.

hypocrinism (-kri′nizm) a state due to deficient secretion of an endocrine gland.

hypocupremia (-ku-pre′me-ah) abnormally diminished levels of copper in the blood.

hypocyclosis (-si-klo′sis) insufficient accommodation in the eye.

hypocythemia (-si-the′me-ah) deficiency in the number of erythrocytes in the blood.

hypodactyly (-dak′tĭ-le) the presence of less than the normal number of fingers or toes.

Hypoderma (-der′mah) a genus of ox-warble or heel flies whose larvae cause warbles in cattle and a form of larva migrans in man.

hypodermatic (-der-mat′ik) hypodermic.

hypodermiasis (-der-mi′ah-sis) a creeping eruption of the skin in man and cattle caused by the larvae of *Hypoderma.*

hypodermic (-der′mik) applied or administered beneath the skin.

hypodermis (-der′mis) 1. the panniculus adiposus. 2. the outer cellular layer of invertebrates that secretes the cuticular exoskeleton.

hypodermoclysis (-der-mok′lĭ-sis) subcutaneous injection of fluids, e.g., saline solution.

hypodipsia (-dip′se-ah) abnormally diminished thirst.

hypodontia (-don′she-ah) partial anodontia.

hypodynamia (-di-na′me-ah) abnormally diminished power. **hypodynam′ic,** adj.

hypoeccrisia (-e-kriz′e-ah) abnormally diminished excretion. **hypoeccrit′ic,** adj.

hypoendocrinism (-en-dok′rĭ-nizm) insufficiency of endocrine gland activity.

hypoergia, hypoergy (-er′je-ah; -er′je) hyposensitivity. **hypoer′gic,** adj.

hypoesophoria (-es″o-fo′re-ah) deviation of the visual axes downward and inward.

hypoesthesia (-es-the′ze-ah) a state of abnormally decreased sensitivity to stimuli. **hypoesthet′ic,** adj.

hypoexophoria (-ek″so-fo′re-ah) deviation of the visual axes downward and laterally.

hypoferremia (-fĕ-re′me-ah) deficiency of iron in the blood.

hypofibrinogenemia (-fi-brin″o-jĕ-ne′me-ah) deficiency of fibrinogen in the blood.

hypofunction (-funk′shun) diminished function.

hypogalactia (-gah-lak′she-ah) deficiency of milk secretion. **hypogalac′tous,** adj.

hypogammaglobulinemia (-gam″ah-glob″u-lin-e′me-ah) an immunological deficiency state marked by abnormally low levels of generally all classes of serum gamma globulins, with heightened susceptibility to infectious diseases. It may be congenital or secondary, or it may be physiological, which occurs in normal infants and which, when prolonged, is called *transient h.* **hypogammaglobuline′mic,** adj.

hypogastric (-gas′trik) pertaining to the hypogastrium.

hypogastrium (-gas′tre-um) the pubic region, the lowest middle abdominal region.

hypogastropagus (-gas-trop′ah-gus) conjoined twins united at the hypogastrium.

hypogastroschisis (-gas-tros′kĭ-sis) congenital fissure of the hypogastrium.

hypogenesis (-jen′ĕ-sis) defective embryonic development. **hypogenet′ic**, adj.

hypogenitalism (-jen′ĭ-tal-izm″) hypogonadism.

hypogeusesthesia, hypogeusia (-gūs″es-the′-ze-ah; -gu′ze-ah) abnormally diminished sense of taste.

hypoglossal (-glos′al) beneath the tongue.

hypoglottis (-glot′is) 1. the underside of the tongue. 2. ranula.

hypoglycemia (-gli-se′me-ah) deficiency of glucose concentration in the blood, which may lead to nervousness, hypothermia, headache, confusion, and sometimes convulsions and coma.

hypoglycemic (-gli-se′mik) 1. pertaining to, characterized by, or causing hypoglycemia. 2. an agent that lowers blood glucose levels.

hypoglycogenolysis (-gli″ko-gĕ-nol′ĭ-sis) depressed glycogenolysis.

hypoglycorrhachia (-ra′ke-ah) abnormally low sugar content in the cerebrospinal fluid.

hypognathous (hi-pog′nah-thus) 1. having a protruding lower jaw. 2. pertaining to a hypognathus.

hypognathus (hi-pog′nah-thus) a rudimentary twin attached to the lower jaw of the autosite.

hypogonadism (hi″po-go′nad-izm) decreased functional activity of the gonads, with retardation of growth and sexual development.

hypogonadotropic (-gon″ah-do-trōp′ik) relating to or caused by deficiency of gonadotropin.

hypohidrosis (-hĭ-dro′sis) abnormally diminished secretion of sweat. **hypohidrot′ic**, adj.

hypokalemia (-kah-le′me-ah) abnormally low potassium levels in the blood, which may lead to neuromuscular and renal disorders and to electrocardiographic abnormalities.

hypokalemic (-kah-le′mik) 1. pertaining to or characterized by hypokalemia. 2. an agent that lowers blood potassium levels.

hypokinesia (-ki-ne′ze-ah) abnormally diminished motor activity. **hypokinet′ic**, adj.

hypoleydigism (-li′dig-izm) abnormally diminished secretion of androgens by Leydig's cells.

hypomagnesemia (-mag″nĕ-se′me-ah) abnormally low magnesium content of the blood, manifested chiefly by neuromuscular hyperirritability.

hypomania (-ma′ne-ah) mania of a moderate type. **hypoman′ic**, adj.

hypomastia (-mas′te-ah) abnormal smallness of the mammary glands.

hypomenorrhea (-men″ŏ-re′ah) diminution of menstral flow or duration.

hypomere (hi′po-mēr) 1. the ventrolateral portion of a myotome, innervated by an anterior ramus of a spinal nerve. 2. the lateral plate of mesoderm that develops into the walls of the body cavities.

hypometabolism (hi″po-mĕ-tab′o-lizm) decreased metabolism; low metabolic rate.

hypometria (-me′tre-ah) ataxia in which movements fall short of reaching the intended goal.

hypomnesia (hi″pom-ne′ze-ah) defective memory.

hypomorph (hi″po-morf) 1. a person who is short in standing height as compared with his sitting height. 2. in genetics, a mutant gene that shows only a partial reduction in the activity it influences. **hypomor′phic**, adj.

hypomotility (hi″po-mo-til′ĭ-te) decreased motility.

hypomyotonia (-mi″o-to′ne-ah) deficient muscular tonicity.

hypomyxia (-mik′se-ah) decreased secretion of mucus.

hyponatremia (-na-tre′me-ah) deficiency of sodium in the blood; salt depletion.

hyponeocytosis (-ne″o-si-to′sis) leukopenia with the presence of immature leukocytes in the blood.

hyponoia (-noi′ah) sluggish mental activity.

hyponychium (-nik′e-um) the thickened epidermis beneath the free distal end of the nail. **hyponych′ial**, adj.

hypo-orthocytosis (-or″tho-si-to′sis) leukopenia with a normal proportion of the various forms of leukocytes.

hypopancreatism (-pan′kre-ah-tizm″) diminished activity of the pancreas.

hypoparathyroidism (-par″ah-thi′roid-izm) the condition produced by greatly reduced function of or removal of the parathyroid glands, with hypocalcemia, which may lead to the tetany; hyperphosphatemia, with decreased bone resorption; and other symptoms.

hypophalangism (-fah-lan′jizm) absence of a phalanx on a finger or toe.

hypopharynx (hi″po-far′inks) laryngopharynx.

hypophonesis (-fo-ne′sis) diminution of the sound in auscultation or percussion.

hypophonia (-fo′ne-ah) a weak voice due to incoordination of the vocal muscles.

hypophoria (-fo′re-ah) downward deviation of the visual axis of one eye in the absence of visual fusional stimuli.

hypophosphatasia (-fos″fah-ta′ze-ah) an inborn error of metabolism marked by abnormally low serum alkaline phosphatase activity and excretion of phosphoethanolamine in the urine. It is manifested by rickets in infants and children and by osteomalcia in adults. It is most severe in babies under six months of age.

hypophosphatemia (-fos″fah-te′me-ah) deficiency of phosphates in the blood, as may occur in rickets and osteomalacia. See also *hypophosphatasia*. **hypophosphate′mic**, adj.

hypophosphaturia (-fos″fah-tu′re-ah) abnormally decreased levels of urinary phosphate.

hypophrenia (-fre′ne-ah) mental retardation. **hypophren′ic**, adj.

hypophysectomy (hi-pof″ĭ-sek′to-me) excision of the pituitary gland (hypophysis).

hypophyseoportal (hi″po-fiz″e-o-por′tal) denoting the portal system of the pituitary gland, in which hypothalamic venules connect with capillaries of the anterior pituitary.

hypophyseoprivic, hypophysioprivic (-priv′ik) deficient in hormonal secretion of the pituitary gland (hypophysis).

hypophysis (hi-pof′ĭ-sis), pl. *hypoph′yses* [Gr.]

pituitary gland. **hypophys′eal,** adj. **h. cer′e-bri,** pituitary gland. **pharyngeal h.,** a mass in the pharyngeal wall with structure similar to that of the pituitary gland. **h. sic′ca,** posterior pituitary.

hypopiesis (hi″po-pi-e′sis) abnormally low pressure, as low blood pressure. **hypopiet′ic,** adj.

hypopigmentation (-pig″men-ta′shun) abnormally diminished pigmentation.

hypopituitarism (-pĭ-tu′ĭ-tar-izm″) the condition resulting from diminution or cessation of hormal secretion by the pituitary gland, especially the anterior pituitary.

hypoplasia (-pla′ze-ah) incomplete development of an organ or tissue. **hypoplas′tic,** adj. **enamel h.,** incomplete or defective development of the enamel of the teeth. **enamel h., hereditary,** amelogenesis imperfecta. **h. of mesenchyme,** osteogenesis imperfecta.

hypopnea (hi-pop′ne-ah) abnormal decrease in depth and rate of respiration. **hypopne′ic,** adj.

hypoporosis (hi″po-po-ro′sis) deficient callus formation after bone fracture.

hypoposia (-po′ze-ah) abnormally diminished ingestion of fluids.

hypopotassemia (-pot″ah-se′me-ah) hypokalemia.

hypopraxia (-prak′se-ah) abnormally diminished activity.

hypoprosody (-pros′o-de) diminution of the normal variation of stress, pitch, and rhythm of speech.

hypoproteinemia (-pro″te-ĕ-ne′me-ah) deficiency of protein in the blood.

hypoprothrombinemia (-pro-throm″bĭ-ne′me-ah) deficiency of prothrombin in the blood.

hypopselaphesia (hi″pop-sel″ah-fe′ze-ah) dullness of the tactile sense.

hypopsychosis (hi″po-si-ko′sis) diminution of the function of thought.

hypoptyalism (-ti′ah-lizm) abnormally decreased secretion of saliva.

hypopyon (hi-po′pe-on) an accumulation of pus in the anterior chamber of the eye.

hyporeactive (hi″po-re-ak′tiv) showing less than normal response to a stimuli.

hyporeflexia (-re-flek′se-ah) diminution or weakening of reflexes.

hyposalemia (-sah-le′me-ah) abnormally decreased salt levels in the blood.

hyposalivation (-sal″ĭ-va′shun) hypoptyalism.

hyposcleral (-skle′ral) beneath the sclera.

hyposecretion (-se-kre′shun) diminished secretion, as by a gland.

hyposensitive (-sen′sĭ-tiv) 1. exhibiting abnormally decreased sensitivity. 2. being less sensitive to a specific allergen after repeated and gradually increasing doses of the offending substance.

hyposensitivity (-sen″sĭ-tiv′ĭ-te) the condition of being hyposensitive.

hyposensitization (-sen″sĭ-ti-za′shun) the act or process of rendering hyposensitive.

hyposmia (hi-poz′me-ah) diminished acuteness of the sense of smell.

hyposmolarity (hi-poz″mo-lar′ĭ-te) abnormally decreased osmolar concentration.

hyposomnia (hi″po-som′ne-ah) insomnia.

hypospadiac (-spa′de-ak) 1. pertaining to hypospadias. 2. a person affected with hypospadias.

hypospadias (-spa′de-as) a developmental anomaly in which the male urethra opens on the underside of the penis or on the perineum. **female h.,** a developmental anomaly in the female in which the urethra opens into the vagina.

hypostasis (hi-pos′tah-sis) poor or stagnant circulation in a dependent part of the body or an organ.

hypostatic (hi″po-stat′ik) 1. pertaining to, due to, or associated with hypostasis. 2. abnormally static; said of certain inherited traits that are liable to be suppressed by other traits.

hyposthenia (hi″pos-the′ne-ah) an enfeebled state; weakness. **hyposthen′ic,** adj.

hyposthenuria (hi″pos-thĕ-nu′re-ah) inability to form urine of high specific gravity.

hypostomia (hi″po-sto′me-ah) a developmental anomaly in which the mouth is a small vertical slit.

hypostypsis (-stip′sis) moderate astringency. **hypostyp′tic,** adj.

hyposynergia (-sĭ-ner′je-ah) defective coordination.

hypotelorism (-te′lo-rizm) abnormally decreased distance between two organs or parts. **ocular h., orbital h.,** abnormal decrease in the intraorbital distance.

hypotension (-ten′shun) abnormally low blood pressure. **orthostatic h., postural h.,** low blood pressure that occurs on rising to the erect position.

hypotensive (-ten′siv) marked by low blood pressure or serving to reduce blood pressure.

hypotensor (-ten′sor) a hypotensive agent.

hypothalamus (-thal′ah-mus) the part of the diencephalon forming the floor and part of the lateral wall of the third ventricle; anatomically, it includes the optic chiasm, mamillary bodies, tuber cinereum, infundibulum, and pituitary gland, but for physiological purposes the pituitary gland is considered a distinct structure. The hypothalamic nuclei serve to activate, control, and integrate the peripheral autonomic mechanisms, endocrine activities, and many somatic functions. **hypothalam′ic,** adj.

hypothenar (hi-poth′ĕ-nar) 1. the fleshy eminence on the palm along the ulnar margin. 2. relating to this eminence.

hypothermia (hi″po-ther′me-ah) low body temperature, especially such a state induced as a means of decreasing metabolism and thereby the need for oxygen, as used in various surgical procedures. **hypother′mal, hypother′mic,** adj.

hypothesis (hi-poth′ĕ-sis) a supposition that appears to explain a group of phenomena and is assumed as a basis of reasoning and experimentation. **lattice h.,** a theory of the nature of the antigen-antibody reaction which postulates reaction between multivalent antigen and divalent antibody to give an antigen-antibody complex of a lattice-like structure. **Lyon h.,** the random and fixed inactivation (in the form of sex chromatin) of one X chromosome in mammalian cells at an early stage of embryogenesis, leading to mosaicism of paternal and maternal X chromosomes in the female. **Makeham's h.,** death results from two coexisting factors: (1) chance, which is constant; (2) inability to withstand destruction, which progresses geometrically. **unitarian h.,** antibody is a single species of modified serum globulin regardless of the overt consequences of its reaction with homologous antigen, e.g., agglutination, precipitation, complement fixation, etc.

hypothrombinemia (hi″po-throm″bĭ-ne′me-ah) deficiency of thrombin in the blood.

hypothymia (-thi′me-ah) abnormally diminished emotionalism.

hypothymism (-thi′mizm) diminished thymus activity.

hypothyroidism (-thi′roi-dizm) deficiency of thyroid activity. In adults, it is marked by decreased metabolic rate, tiredness, and lethargy. See also *cretinism* and *myxedema.* **hypothy′roid,** adj.

hypotonia (-to′ne-ah) diminished tone of the skeletal muscles.

hypotonic (-ton′ik) 1. denoting decreased tone or tension. 2. denoting a solution having less osmotic pressure than one with which it is compared.

hypotonicity (-to-nis′ĭ-te) the state or quality of being hypotonic.

hypotoxicity (-tok-sis′ĭ-te) abnormally reduced toxic quality.

hypotransferrinemia (-trans-fer″ĭ-ne′me-ah) deficiency of transferrin in the blood.

hypotrichosis (-trĭ-ko′sis) presence of less than the normal amount of hair.

hypotrophy (hi-pot′ro-fe) abiotrophy.

hypotropia (hi″po-tro′pe-ah) permanent downward deviation of the visual axis of one eye.

hypotympanotomy (-tim″pah-not′o-me) surgical opening of the hypotympanum.

hypotympanum (-tim′pah-num) the lower part of the cavity of the middle ear, in the temporal bone.

hypoventilation (-ven″tĭ-la′shun) reduction in the amount of air entering the pulmonary alveoli.

hypovitaminosis (-vi″tah-mĭ-no′sis) a condition produced by lack of an essential vitamin.

hypovolemia (-vo-le′me-ah) abnormally decreased volume of circulating fluid (plasma) in the body. **hypovole′mic,** adj.

hypovolia (-vo′le-ah) diminished water content or volume, as of extracellular fluid.

hypoxanthine (-zan′thēn) an intermediate product of uric acid synthesis, formed from adenylic acid and itself a precursor of xanthine.

hypoxemia (hi″pok-se′me-ah) deficient oxygenation of the blood.

hypoxia (hi-pok′se-ah) reduction of oxygen in body tissues below physiologic levels. **hypox′ic,** adj.

hypsarrhythmia (hip″sah-rith′me-ah) an elec-troencephalographic abnormality commonly associated with infantile spasms, with random, high-voltage slow waves and spikes spreading to all cortical areas.

hypsochrome (hip′so-krōm) an atom or group whose introduction into a compound shifts the compound's maximum absorption frequency to a shorter wavelength. **hypsochro′mic,** adj.

hypsokinesis (hip″so-ki-ne′sis) a backward swaying or falling when in erect posture; seen in paralysis agitans and other forms of the amyostatic syndrome.

hyster(o)- word element [Gr.], *uterus; hysteria.*

hysteralgia (his″tĕ-ral′je-ah) pain in the uterus.

hysteratresia (his″ter-ah-tre′ze-ah) atresia of the uterus.

hysterectomy (his″tĕ-rek′to-me) excision of the uterus. **abdominal h.,** that performed through the abdominal wall. **cesarean h.,** cesarean section followed by removal of the uterus. **complete h.,** total h. **partial h.,** subtotal h. **radical h.,** excision of the uterus, upper vagina, and parametrium. **subtotal h., supracervical h.,** that in which the cervix is left in place. **total h.,** that in which the uterus and cervix are completely excised. **vaginal h.,** that performed through the vagina.

hysteresis (his″tĕ-re′sis) a time lag in the occurrence of two associated phenomena, as between cause and effect.

hystereurynter (his″ter-u-rin′ter) an instrument for dilating the os uteri.

hystereurysis (-u′rĭ-sis) dilation of the os uteri.

hysteria (his-te′re-ah) a neurosis with symptoms based on conversion, characterized by lack of control over acts and emotions, by morbid self-consciousness, by anxiety, by exaggeration of the effect of sensory impressions, and by simulation of various disorders. **hyster′ical,** adj. **anxiety h.,** that with recurring attacks of anxiety. **conversion h.,** see under *reaction.* **fixation h.,** that with symptoms based on those of an organic disease. **h. ma′jor,** that with sudden onset of dream states, stupors, and paralyses. **h. mi′nor,** that with mild convulsions in which consciousness is not lost.

hysteriac (his-te′re-ak) a person affected with hysteria.

hysterics (his-ter′iks) popular term for an uncontrollable emotional outburst.

hysterocatalepsy (his″ter-o-kat′ah-lep″se) hysteria with cataleptic symptoms.

hysterocele (his′ter-o-sēl″) metrocele.

hysterocleisis (his″ter-o-kli′sis) surgical closure of the os uteri.

hysterodynia (-din′e-ah) pain in the uterus.

hysteroepilepsy (-ep″ĭ-lep′se) severe hysteria with epileptiform convulsions.

hysterogenic (-jen′ik) causing hysterical phenomena or symptoms.

hysterography (his″tĕ-rog′rah-fe) 1. the graphic recording of the strength of uterine contractions in labor. 2. radiography of the uterus after instillation of a contrast medium.

hysteroid (his′ter-oid) resembling hysteria.

hysterolaparotomy (his″ter-o-lap″ah-rot′o-me)

incision of the uterus through the abdominal wall.

hysterolith (his'ter-o-lith'') a uterine calculus.

hysterolysis (his''tě-rol'ĭ-sis) freeing of the uterus from adhesions.

hysterometer (his''tě-rom'ě-ter) an instrument for measuring the uterus.

hysteromyoma (his''ter-o-mi-o'mah) leiomyoma of the uterus.

hysteromyomectomy (-mi''o-mek'to-me) excision of a leiomyoma of the uterus.

hysteromyotomy (-mi-ot'o-me) incision of uterus for removal of a solid tumor.

hysteropathy (his''tě-rop'ah-the) metropathy.

hysteropexy (his'ter-o-pek''se) surgical fixation of a displaced uterus.

hysteropia (his''tě-ro'pe-ah) a hysterical disorder of vision.

hysteroptosis (his''ter-op-to'sis) metroptosis.

hysterorrhaphy (his''tě-ror'ah-fe) 1. suture of the uterus. 2. hysteropexy.

hysterorrhexis (his''ter-o-rek'sis) metrorrhexis.

hysterosalpingectomy (-sal''pin-jek'to-me) excision of the uterus and uterine tubes.

hysterosalpingography (-sal''ping-gog'rah-fe) radiography of the uterus and uterine tubes.

hysterosalpingo-oophorectomy (-sal''ping-go-o''of-o-rek'to-me) excision of the uterus, uterine tubes, and ovaries.

hysterosalpingostomy (-sal''ping-gos'to-me) anastomosis of a uterine tube to the uterus.

hysteroscope (his'ter-o-skōp'') an endoscope for direct visual examination of the cervical canal and uterine cavity.

hysterospasm (-spazm'') spasm of the uterus.

hysterotomy (his''tě-rot'o-me) incision of the uterus, performed either transabdominally (*abdominal h.*) or vaginally (*vaginal h.*).

hysterotrachelorrhaphy (his''ter-o-tra''kel-or'rah-fe) suture of the uterine cervix.

hysterotrachelotomy (-tra''kel-ot'o-me) incision of the uterine cervix.

hysterotraumatism (-traw'mah-tizm) hysteric symptoms following injury.

hysterotubography (-tu-bog'rah-fe) hysterosalpingography.

Hytakerol (hi-tak'er-ol) trademark for preparations of dihydrotachysterol.

Hz hertz.

I

I chemical symbol, *iodine*.

[131]I, I 131 symbol for radioactive isotope of iodine of atomic mass 131, half-life, 8.07 days; also written I^{131}.

-ia word element, *state; condition*.

IAEA International Atomic Energy Agency.

I.A.G.P. International Association of Geographic Pathology.

I.A.G.U.S. International Association of Genito-Urinary Surgeons.

I.A.M.M. International Association of Medical Museums.

I.A.P.B. International Association for Prevention of Blindness.

I.A.P.P. International Association for Preventive Pediatrics.

-iasis word element [Gr.], *condition; state*.

iatr(o)- word element [Gr.], *medicine; physician*.

iatric (i-at'rik) pertaining to medicine or to a physician.

iatrochemistry (i-at''ro-kem'is-tre) a school of medicine (17th century) which espoused the theory that all phenomena of life and disease are based on chemical action.

iatrogenic (-jen'ik) resulting from the activity of physicians; said of any adverse condition in a patient resulting from treatment by a physician or surgeon.

iatrophysics (-fiz'iks) 1. treatment of disease by physical or mechanical means. 2. medical physics. 3. the early theory that all vital phenomena are controlled by laws of physics.

iatrotechnics (-tek'niks) the techniques of medical and surgical practice.

ICD intrauterine contraceptive device.

ichor (i'kor) watery discharge from wounds or sores. **i'chorous,** adj.

ichoroid (i'ko-roid) resembling ichor.

ichorrhea (i''ko-re'ah) copious discharge of ichor.

ichthammol (ik-tham'ol) a reddish brown to brownish black viscous fluid obtained by destructive distillation of certain bituminous schists, sulfonated and neutralized with ammonia; used as a local skin anti-infective.

ichthy(o)- word element [Gr.], *fish*.

ichthyismus (ik''the-iz'mus) ichthyotoxism.

ichthyoid (ik'the-oid) fishlike.

Ichthyol (-ol) trademark for a preparation of ichthammol.

ichthyology (ik''the-ol'o-je) the study of fishes.

ichthyophagous (ik''the-of'ah-gus) eating or subsisting on fish.

ichthyosarcotoxin (ik''the-o-sar''ko-tok'sin) a toxin found in the flesh of poisonous fishes.

ichthyosarcotoxism (-sar''ko-tok'sizm) poisoning due to ingestion of poisonous fish, marked by various gastrointestinal and neurological disturbances.

ichthyosis (ik''the-o'sis) 1. any of several generalized skin disorders marked by dryness, roughness, and scaliness, due to hypertrophy of the horny layer resulting from excessive production or retention of keratin, or a molecular defect in the keratin. 2. i. vulgaris. **ichthyot'ic,** adj. **i. hys'trix,** a rare form of epidermolytic hyperkeratosis, marked by generalized, dark brown, linear verrucoid ridges somewhat like porcupine skin. **lamellar i.,** a hereditary disease present at or soon after birth, with large, quadrilateral, grayish brown scales; it may be associated with short stature, oligophrenia, spastic paralysis, genital hypoplasia, hypotrichia, and shortened life-span. **i. sauroder′ma,** lamellar exfoliation of the newborn persisting into childhood, in which the skin is covered with thick plates somewhat like crocodile skin. **i. sim′plex,** i. vulgaris. **i. u′teri,** transformation of the columnar epithelium of the endometrium into stratified squamous epithelium. **i. vulga′ris,** hereditary ichthyosis present at or shortly after birth, with large, thick, dry scales on the neck, ears, scalp, face, and flexural surfaces, or occurring after three months of age and rarely involving the flexural surfaces.

ichthyotoxin (ik″the-o-tok′sin) any toxic substance derived from fish.

ichthyotoxism (-tok′sizm) any intoxication due to an ichthyotoxin.

I.C.N. International Council of Nurses.

I.C.S. International College of Surgeons.

ICSH interstitial cell-stimulating hormone.

ictal (ik′tal) pertaining to, marked by, or due to a stroke or an acute epileptic seizure.

icterogenic (ik″ter-o-jen′ik) causing jaundice.

icterohepatitis (-hep″ah-ti′tis) inflammation of the liver with marked jaundice.

icteroid (ik′ter-oid) resembling jaundice.

icterus (ik′ter-us) [L.] jaundice. **icter′ic,** adj. **febrile i., i. febri′lis,** infectious hepatitis. **i. gra′vis,** acute yellow atrophy. **i. neonato′rum,** jaundice in newborn children.

ictus (ik′tus) a seizure, stroke, blow, or sudden attack. **ic′tal,** adj.

ICU intensive care unit.

I.D.₅₀ median infective dose.

id (id) 1. the self-preservative tendencies and instincts of an individual as a totality; the true unconscious. 2. a rash associated with but remote from the main lesion of the disease; considered to be an allergic reaction to the causative agent of the disease. Often used as a suffix of a root representing the causative factor, as *syphilid.*

-id [Gr.] 1. a suffix meaning having the shape of, or resembling. 2. see *id* (2).

-ide (īd) a suffix indicating a binary chemical compound.

idea (i-de′ah) a mental impression or conception. **autochthonous i.,** a strange idea which comes into the mind in some unaccountable way, but is not a hallucination. **compulsive i.,** one that persists despite reason and will, and impels toward some inappropriate act. **dominant i.,** a morbid or other impression that controls or colors every action and thought. **fixed i.,** a persistent morbid impression or belief that cannot be changed by reason. **i. of reference,** the incorrect idea that words and actions of others refer to one's self or the projection of the causes of one's own imaginary difficulties upon someone else.

ideal (i-de′al) a pattern or concept of perfection. **ego i.,** the standard of perfection unconsciously created by a person for himself.

ideation (i″de-a′shun) the formation of ideas or images. **idea′tional,** adj.

idée fixe (e-da′ fēks′) [Fr.] fixed idea.

identification (i-den″ti-fi-ka′shun) an unconscious defense mechanism by which one person patterns himself after another.

identity (i-den′ti-te) the aggregate of characteristics by which an individual is recognized by himself and others.

ideogenetic, ideogenous (i″de-o-jĕ-net′ik; i″-de-oj′ĕ-nus) induced by or related to vague sense impressions rather than organized images.

ideology (i″de-ol′o-je, id″e-) 1. the science of the development of ideas. 2. the body of ideas characteristic of an individual or of a social unit.

ideomotion (i″de-o-mo′shun) muscular action induced by a dominant idea.

ideomotor (-mo′tor) aroused by an idea or thought; said of involuntary motion so aroused.

idio- word element [Gr.], *self; peculiar to a substance or organism.*

idiocy (id′e-o-se) severe mental retardation. **amaurotic familial i.,** a group of hereditary disorders due to an inborn defect of lipid metabolism in which sphingolipids accumulate in the brain, and marked by cerebromacular degeneration, blindness, progressive dementia; paralysis, and death. They are classified according to age of onset; see *Tay-Sachs disease, Bielschowsky's disease, Spielmeyer-Vogt disease,* and *Kufs' disease.* **Aztec i.,** microcephalic i. **cretinoid i.,** cretinism. **epileptic i.,** that combined with epilepsy. **hydrocephalic i.,** that combined with chronic hydrocephalus. **microcephalic i.,** that associated with microcephaly. **mongolian i.,** Down's syndrome. **sensorial i.,** that associated with early loss of any special sense. **traumatic i.,** that due to injury received at birth or in infancy.

idioglossia (id″e-o-glos′e-ah) imperfect articulation, with the utterance of meaningless vocal sounds. **idioglot′tic,** adj.

idiogram (id′e-o-gram) a drawing or photograph of the chromosomes of a particular cell.

idiopathic (id″e-o-path′ik) self-originated; occurring without known cause.

idiopathy (id″e-op′ah-the) a morbid state arising without known cause.

idiosome (id′e-o-sōm) the centrosome of a spermatocyte, together with the surrounding Golgi apparatus and mitochondria.

idiosyncrasy (id″e-o-sin′krah-se) 1. a habit or quality of body or mind peculiar to an individual. 2. an abnormal susceptibility to an agent (e.g., a drug) peculiar to an individual. **idiosyncrat′ic,** adj.

idiot (id′e-ot) a person afflicted with severe mental retardation. **mongolian i.,** former name for a person affected with Down's syndrome. **i.-savant,** a person who is severely mentally retarded in some respects, yet has a particular mental faculty developed to an unusually high degree, as for mathematics, music, etc.

idiotrophic (id″e-o-trof′ik) capable of selecting its own nourishment.

idioventricular (-ven-trik′u-ler) pertaining to the cardiac ventricle alone.

idoxuridine (i″doks-ūr′ĭ-den) a pyrimidine analogue that prevents replication of DNA viruses; used topically in herpes simplex keratitis.

I.D.S. Investigative Dermatological Society.

IDU idoxuridine.

Ig immunoglobulin of any of the five classes: IgA, IgD, IgE, IgG, and IgM.

ignipuncture (ig″nĭ-pungk′tūr) therapeutic puncture with hot needles.

I.L.A. International Leprosy Association.

ile(o)- word element [L.], *ileum.*

ileac (il′e-ak) 1. of the nature of ileus. 2. pertaining to the ileum.

ileal (il′e-al) pertaining to the ileum.

ileectomy (il″e-ek′to-me) excision of the ileum.

ileitis (-i′tis) inflammation of the ileum. **regional i.,** a chronic granulomatous inflammatory disease, commonly involving the terminal ileum with scarring and thickening of the bowel wall, often leading to ileus and abscess formation.

ileocecal (il″e-o-se′kal) pertaining to the ileum and cecum.

ileocecostomy (-se-kos′to-me) surgical anastomosis of the ileum to the cecum.

ileocolic (-kol′ik) pertaining to ileum and colon.

ileocolitis (-ko-li′tis) inflammation of the ileum and colon. **i. ulcero′sa chron′ica,** chronic ileocolitis with fever, rapid pulse, anemia, diarrhea, and right iliac pain.

ileocolostomy (-ko-los′to-me) surgical anastomosis of the ileum to the colon.

ileocolotomy (-ko-lot′o-me) incision of the ileum and colon.

ileocystoplasty (-sis′to-plas″te) repair of the wall of the urinary bladder with an isolated segment of the wall of the ileum.

ileocystostomy (-sis-tos′to-me) use of an isolated segment of ileum to create a passage from the urinary bladder to an opening in the abdominal wall.

ileoileostomy (-il″e-os′to-me) surgical anastomosis between two parts of the ileum.

ileorectal (il″e-o-rek′tal) pertaining to or communicating with the ileum and rectum.

ileorrhaphy (il″e-or′ah-fe) suture of the ileum.

ileosigmoidostomy (il″e-o-sig″moi-dos′to-me) surgical anastomosis of the ileum to the sigmoid colon.

ileostomy (il″e-os′to-me) surgical creation of an opening into the ileum, with a stoma on the abdominal wall.

ileotomy (-ot′o-me) incision of the ileum.

Iletin (il′ĕ-tin) trademark for preparations of insulin for injection.

ileum (il′e-um) the distal portion of the small intestine, extending from the jejunum to the cecum. **duplex i.,** congenital duplication of the ileum.

ileus (il′e-us) intestinal obstruction. **adynamic i.,** that due to inhibition of bowel motility. **dynamic i., hyperdynamic i., spastic i. mechanical i.,** that due to mechanical causes, such as hernia, adhesions, volvulus, etc. **meconium i.,** ileus in the newborn due to blocking of the bowel with thick meconium. **occlusive i.,** mechanical i. **paralytic i., i. paralyt′icus,** adynamic i. **spastic i.,** mechanical ileus due to persistent contracture of a bowel segment. **i. subpar′ta,** that due to pressure of the gravid uterus on the pelvic colon.

ili(o)- word element [L.], *ilium.*

iliac (il′e-ak) pertaining to the ilium.

iliadelphus (il″e-ah-del′fus) iliopagus.

Ilidar (il′ĭ-dar) trademark for a preparation of azapetine.

iliococcygeal (il″e-o-kok-sij′e-al) pertaining to the ilium and coccyx.

iliofemoral (-fem′o-ral) pertaining to the ilium and femur.

ilioinguinal (-ing′gwĭ-nal) pertaining to the iliac and inguinal regions.

iliolumbar (-lum′bar) pertaining to the iliac and lumbar regions.

iliopagus (il″e-op′ah-gus) symmetrical conjoined twins united in the iliac region.

iliopectineal (il″e-o-pek-tin″e-al) pertaining to the ilium and pubes.

iliotrochanteric (-tro″kan-ter′ik) pertaining to the ilium and femoral trochanter.

ilium (il′e-um), pl. *il′ia* [L.] see *Table of Bones.*

ill (il) 1. not well; sick. 2. a disease or disorder. **colt i.,** navel ill in colts. **leaping i.,** gid. **louping i.,** a tickborne viral encephalomyelitis of sheep. **navel i.,** generalized septicemia affecting foals, calves, and lambs, usually with omphalophlebitis and abscesses in the joints causing polyarthritis; due to infection through the open navel by various organisms.

illness (il′nes) a condition marked by pronounced deviation from the normal healthy state; sickness. **mental i.,** see under *disorder.*

illumination (ĭ-lu″mĭ-na′shun) the lighting up of a part, organ, or object for inspection. **axial i.,** light transmitted or reflected along the axis of a microscope. **darkfield i., dark-ground i.,** the casting of peripheral light rays upon a microscopical object from the side, the center rays being blocked out; the object appears bright on a dark background. **direct i.,** light thrown from above or from the direction of observation. **focal i.,** light thrown upon the focus of a lens or mirror. **oblique i.,** light from a source at one side of the object. **through i.,** light from a source behind and shining through the object.

illuminator (ĭ-lu″mĭ-na′tor) the source of light for viewing an object.

illusion (ĭ-lu′zhun) a mental impression derived from misinterpretation of an actual experience. **illu′sional,** adj.

Ilotycin (i″lo-ti′sin) trademark for preparations of erythromycin.

im- 1. a prefix, replacing *in-* before words beginning *b, m,* and *p.* 2. a chemical prefix indicating the bivalent group >NH.

I.M. intramuscularly.

I.M.A. Industrial Medical Association.

image (im′ij) a picture or concept with more or less likeness to an objective reality. **body i.,** the three-dimensional concept of one's self, recorded in the cortex by perception of ever-changing body postures, and constantly changing with them. **direct i., erect i.,** virtual i. **false i.,** that formed by the deviating eye in strabismus. **inverted i.,** real i. **mirror i.,** 1. the image of light made visible by the reflecting surface of the cornea and lens when illuminated through the slit lamp. 2. one with right and left relations reversed, as in the reflection of an object in a mirror. **motor i.,** the organized cerebral model of the possible movements of the body. **Purkinje's i's, Purkinje-Sanson i's,** three reflected images of an object seen in observing the pupil of the eye: two on the posterior and anterior surfaces of the lens, one on the anterior surface of the cornea. **real i.,** one formed where the emanating rays are collected, in which the object is pictured as being inverted. **virtual i.,** a picture from projected light rays that are intercepted before focusing.

imago (ĭ-ma′go), pl. *ima′goes,* or *imag′ines* [L.] 1. the adult or definitive form of an insect. 2. a childhood memory or fantasy of a loved person which persists in adult life.

imbalance (im-bal′ans) lack of balance; especially lack of balance between muscles, as in insufficiency of ocular muscles. **autonomic i.,** defective coordination between the sympathetic and parasympathetic nervous systems, especially with respect to vasomotor activities. **sympathetic i.,** vagotonia. **vasomotor i.,** autonomic i.

imbecile (im′bĕ-sil) defective mentally; a person exhibiting imbecility.

imbecility (im″bĕ-sil′ĭ-te) mental retardation less severe than in idiocy but more severe than in moronity.

imbibition (im″bĭ-bish′un) absorption of a liquid.

imbricated (im′brĭ-kāt″ed) overlapping like shingles.

imidazole (im″id-az′ōl) a base found combined with alanine in histidine.

imide (im′īd) any compound containing the bivalent group, $>NH$, to which are attached only acid radicals.

iminazole (im″in-az′ōl) imidazole.

imipramine (ĭ-mip′rah-mēn) an antidepressant, $C_{19}H_{24}N_2$, used as the hydrochloride salt.

immature (im″ah-tūr) not fully developed; unripe.

immersion (ĭ-mer′shun) 1. the plunging of a body into a liquid. 2. the use of the microscope with the object and object glass both covered with a liquid.

immiscible (ĭ-mis′ĭ-b'l) not susceptible of being mixed.

immobilization (im-mo″bĭ-li-za′shun) the rendering of a part incapable of being moved.

immobilize (im-mo′bil-īz) to render incapable of being moved, as by a cast.

immune (ĭ-mūn′) 1. being highly resistant to a disease because of the formation of humoral antibodies or the development of cellular immunity, or both, or as a result of some other mechanism, as interferon activity in viral infections. 2. characterized by the development of humoral antibodies or cellular immunity, or both, following antigenic challenge. 3. produced in response to antigenic challenge as, immune serum globulin.

immunifacient (ĭ-mu″nĭ-fa′shent) producing immunity.

immunity (ĭ-mu′nĭ-te) 1. the condition of being immune; security against a particular disease; nonsusceptibility to the invasive or pathogenic effects of foreign microorganisms or to the toxic effect of antigenic substances. See also *active i., nonspecific i.,* and *passive i.* 2. heightened responsiveness to antigenic challenge that leads to more rapid binding or elimination of antigen than in the nonimmune state; it includes both humoral and cell-mediated immunity. 3. the capcity to distinguish foreign material from self, and to neutralize, eliminate, or metabolize that which is foreign by the physiologic mechanisms of the immune response. **acquired i.,** that occurring as a result of prior exposure to an infectious agent or its antigens (*active i.*), or of passive transfer of antibody or immune lymphoid cells (*passive i.*). **active i.,** see *acquired i.* **artificial i.,** active or passive immunity produced artificially, in contrast to natural immunity. **cell-mediated i., cellular i.,** acquired immunity in which the role of small lymphocytes of thymic origin is predominant. **genetic i.,** innate i. **herd i.,** the resistance of a group to attack by a disease to which a large proportion of the members are immune. **humoral i.,** acquired immunity in which the role of circulating antibodies (immunoglobulins) is predominant. **inherent i., innate i.,** that determined by the genetic constitution of the individual. **local i.,** that manifested predominantly in a restricted anatomical area or type of tissue. **natural i.,** the resistance of the normal animal to infection. **nonspecific i.,** that which does not involve humoral or cell-mediated immunity, but includes lysozyme and interferon activity, phagocytosis, inflammatory response, etc. **passive i.,** see *acquired i.* **specific i.,** immunity against a particular disease or antigen.

immunization (im″u-ni-za′shun) the process of rendering a subject immune, or of becoming immune. **active i.,** inoculation with specific antigen to induce an immune response. **passive i.,** the conferral of specific immune reactivity on previously nonimmune individuals by administration of sensitized lymphoid cells or serum from immune individuals.

immunize (im′u-nīz) to render immune.

immunoassay (im″u-no-as′sa) the measurement of antigen-antibody interaction, as by immunofluorescent techniques, radioimmunoassay, etc.

immunobiology (-bi-ol′o-je) that branch of biology dealing with immunologic effects on such phenomena as infectious disease, growth and development, recognition phenomena, hypersensitivity, heredity, aging, cancer, and transplantation.

immunochemistry (-kem′is-tre) the study of the

HUMAN IMMUNOGLOBULIN CLASSES: SOME PHYSICAL AND BIOLOGIC PROPERTIES

CLASS	MEAN SERUM CONCEN- TRATION (mg/100 ml)	MOLECULAR WEIGHT	$S_{20,w}$	MEAN SURVIVAL T/2 (days)	BIOLOGIC FUNCTION	HEAVY CHAIN DESIG- NATION	NO. OF SUB- CLASSES
γG or IgG	1240	150,000	7	23	1. Fix complement 2. Cross placenta 3. Heterocytotropic antibody	γ	4
γA or IgA	280	170,000	7, 10, 14	6	1. Secretory antibody	α	2
γM or IgM	120	890,000	19	5	1. Fix complement 2. Efficient agglutination	μ	2
γD or IgD	3	150,000	7	2.8	?	δ	—
γE or IgE	.03	196,000	8	1.5	1. Reaginic antibody 2. Homocytotropic antibody	ϵ	—

From Bellanti: Immunology.

physical chemical basis of immune phenomena and their interactions.

immunocompetence (-kom′pĕ-tens) the capacity to develop an immune response following antigenic challenge. **immunocom′petent,** adj.

immunocyte (im′u-no-sīt″) any cell of the lymphoid series which can react with antigen to produce antibody or to participate in cell-mediated reactions.

immunodeficiency (im″mu-no-dĕ-fish′en-se) a deficiency of the immune response due to hypoactivity or decreased numbers of lymphoid cells. **immunodefi′cient,** adj.

immunodiffusion (-dĭ-fu′zhun) the diffusion of antigen and antibody from separate reservoirs to form decreasing concentration gradients in hydrophilic gels.

immunoelectrophoresis (-e-lek″tro-fo-re′sis) a method of distinguishing proteins and other materials on the basis of their electrophoretic mobility and antigenic specificities.

immunoferritin (-fer′ĭ-tin) an antibody labeled with ferritin.

immunofiltration (-fil-tra′shun) the extraction of antibodies in pure form by subjection of serum to insoluble specific antigen, the antigen then being removed from the antibody by treatment with soluble carriers.

immunofluorescence (-floo″o-res′ens) a method of determining the location of antigen (or antibody) in a tissue section or smear by the pattern of fluorescence resulting when the specimen is exposed to the specific antibody (or antigen) labeled with a fluorochrome.

immunogen (im′u-no-jen) any substance capable of eliciting an immune response.

immunogenetics (im″u-no-jĕ-net′iks) the study of the genetic factors controlling the individual's immune response and the transmission of those factors from generation to generation. **immunogenet′ic,** adj.

immunogenicity (-jĕ-nis′ĭ-te) the ability of a substance to provoke an immune response. **immunogen′ic,** adj.

immunoglobulin (-glob′u-lin) a protein of animal origin with known antibody activity, synthesized by lymphocytes and plasma cells and found in serum and in other body fluids and tissues; abbreviated Ig. There are five distinct classes based on structural and antigenic properties: IgA, IgD, IgE, IgG, and IgM.

immunohematology (-hem″ah-tol′o-je) the study of antigen-antibody reactions and analogous phenomena as they relate to blood disorders.

immunologist (im″u-nol′o-jist) a specialist in immunology.

immunology (im″u-nol′o-je) the science dealing with all aspects of immunity, including allergy, hypersensitivity, etc. **immunolog′ic,** adj.

immunopathology (im″u-no-pah-thol′o-je) that branch of biomedical science concerned with immune reactions associated with disease, whether the reactions be beneficial, without effect, or harmful. **immunopatholog′ic,** adj.

immunoprecipitation (-pre-sip″ĭ-ta′shun) precipitation resulting from interaction of specific antibody and antigen.

immunoproliferative (-pro-lif′er-ah-tiv) characterized by the proliferation of the lymphoid cells producing immunoglobulins, as in the gammopathies.

immunosorbent (-sor′bent) an insoluble support for antigen, used to adsorb homologous antibodies from a mixture.

immunosuppressant (-su-pres′ant) immunosuppressive.

immunosuppression (-su-presh′un) the artificial prevention or dimunution of the immune response, as by use of radiation, antimetabolites, etc.

immunosuppressive (-su-pres′iv) 1. pertaining to or inducing immunosuppression. 2. an agent that induces immunosuppression.

immunosurveillance (-ser-va′lens) the monitoring function of the immune system whereby it recognizes and reacts against aberrant cells arising within the body.

immunotherapy (-ther′ah-pe) the production of passive immunity.

immunotoxin (-tok′sin) any antitoxin.

immunotransfusion (-trans-fu′zhun) transfusion of blood from a donor previously rendered immune to the disease affecting the patient.

impacted (im-pak′ted) being wedged in firmly. In obstetrics, denoting twins so situated during delivery that pressure of one against the other prevents complete engagement of either.

impaction (im-pak′shun) the condition of being impacted. **dental i.,** prevention of eruption, normal occlusion, or routine removal of a tooth because of its being locked in position by bone, dental restoration, or surfaces of adjacent teeth. **fecal i.,** a collection of hardened feces in the rectum or sigmoid.

impalpable (im-pal′pah-b'l) not detectable by touch.

impar (im′par) unpaired; azygous.

impatent (im-pa′tent) not open; closed.

impeaance (im-pe′dans) obstruction or opposition to passage or flow, as of an electric current or other form of energy. **acoustic i.,** an expression of the opposition to passage of sound waves, being the product of the density of a substance and the velocity of sound in it.

imperforate (im-per′fo-rāt) not open; abnormally closed.

impermeable (im-per′me-ah-b'l) not permitting passage, as of fluid.

impetigo (im″pĕ-ti′go) impetigo contagiosa; a streptococcal or staphylococcal skin infection marked by vesicles or bullae that become pustular, rupture and form yellow crusts. **impetig′inous,** adj. **i. bullo′sa, bullous i.,** impetigo in which the developing vesicles progress to form bullae, which collapse and become covered with crusts. **i. contagio′sa,** impetigo. **i. herpetifor′mis,** a very rare, acute dermatitis with symmetrically ringed, pustular lesions, occurring chiefly in pregnant women and associated with severe constitutional symptoms. **neonatal i., i. neonato′rum,** bulbous impetigo of newborn infants. **i. vulga′ris,** impetigo.

implant 1. (im-plant′) to insert or to graft (tissue, or inert or radioactive material) into intact tissues or a body cavity. 2. (im′plant) any material so inserted or grafted into the body.

implantation (im″plan-ta′shun) 1. the insertion of an organ or tissue in a new site in the body. 2. the attachment and embedding of the fertilized ovum in the endometrium. 3. the insertion or grafting into the body of biological, living, inert, or radioactive material.

impotence (im′po-tens) lack of power, chiefly of copulative power in the male. **im′potent,** adj.

impregnation (im″preg-na′shun) 1. the act of fertilizing or of rendering pregnant. 2. saturation.

impressio (im-pres′e-o), pl. *impressio′nes* [L.] impression (1).

impression (im-presh′un) 1. a slight indentation or depression, as one produced in the surface of one organ by pressure exerted by another. 2. a

negative imprint of an object made in some plastic material that later solidifies. 3. an effect produced upon the mind, body, or senses by some external stimulus or agent. **basilar i.,** a developmental deformity of the occipital bone and upper cervical spine, in which the latter seems to have pushed the floor of the occipital bone upward. **cardiac i.,** an impression made by the heart on another organ. **complete denture i.,** one made of the entire maxilla or mandible for the purpose of construction of a complete denture. **dental i.,** one made of the jaw and/or teeth in some plastic material, which is later filled in with plaster of Paris to produce a facsimile of the oral structures present.

imprinting (im′print-ing) a species-specific, rapid kind of learning during a critical period of early life in which social attachment and identification are established.

impulse (im′puls) 1. a sudden pushing force. 2. a sudden uncontrollable determination to act. 3. nerve i. **cardiac i.,** movement of the chest wall caused by the heart beat. **nerve i.,** the electrochemical process propagated along nerve fibers.

impulsion (im-pul′shun) an abnormal impulse to perform certain acts, usually of a disagreeable nature.

In chemical symbol, *indium.*

in- 1. a prefix, *in, within,* or *into.* 2. an intensive prefix. 3. a negative or privative prefix.

I.N.A. International Neurological Association.

inactivation (in-ak″tĭ-va′shun) the destruction of biological activity, as of a virus, by the action of heat or other agent.

inanimate (-an′ĭ-mat) 1. without life. 2. lacking in animation.

inanition (in″ah-nish′un) the exhausted state due to prolonged undernutrition; starvation.

inappetence (in-ap′ĕ-tens) lack of appetite or desire.

inarticulate (in″ar-tik′u-lāt) 1. not having joints; disjointed. 2. uttered so as to be unintelligible; incapable of articulate speech.

inassimilable (-ah-sim′ĭ-lah-b'l) not susceptible of being utilized as nutriment.

inborn (in′born) inherited; formed or implanted during intrauterine life.

inbreeding (-brēd-ing) the mating of closely related individuals or of individuals having closely similar genetic constitutions.

incarceration (in-kar″sĕ-ra′shun) unnatural retention or confinement of a part.

incest (in′sest) sexual activity between persons so closely related that marriage between them is legally or culturally prohibited.

incidence (-si-dens) the rate at which a certain event occurs, as the number of new cases of a specific disease occurring during a certain period.

incident (-sĭ-dent) impinging upon, as incident radiation.

incipient (in-sip′e-ent) beginning to exist; coming into existence.

incision (-sizh′un) 1. a cut or a wound made by cutting with a sharp instrument. 2. the act of cutting.

incisive (-si′siv) 1. having the power of cutting; sharp. 2. pertaining to the incisor teeth.

incisor (-si′zor) 1. adapted for cutting. 2. any of the four front teeth in either jaw.

incisura (in″si-su′rah), pl. *incisu′rae* [L.] incisure.

incisure (in-si′zher) a cut, incision, or notch. **i's of Lanterman, i's of Lanterman-Schmidt,** oblique slashes or lines on the sheath of the medullated nerve fibers. **Rivinus' i.,** tympanic notch; a defect in the upper tympanic part of the temporal bone, filled by the upper portion of the tympanic membrane.

inclinatio (in″kli-na′she-o), pl. *inclinatio′nes* [L.] inclination.

inclination (-kli-na′shun) a sloping or leaning; the angle of deviation from a particular line or plane of reference; in dentistry, the deviation of a tooth from the vertical. **pelvic i.,** the angle between the plane of the pelvic inlet and the horizontal plane.

inclusion (in-kloo′zhun) 1. the act of enclosing or the condition of being enclosed. 2. anything that is enclosed; a cell inclusion. **cell i.,** a usually lifeless, often temporary, constituent in the cytoplasm of a cell. **dental i.,** 1. a tooth so surrounded with bony tissue that it is unable to erupt. 2. a cyst of oral soft tissue or bone. **intranuclear i's,** inclusion bodies.

incoagulability (in″ko-ag″u-lah-bil′i-te) the state of being incapable of coagulation. **incoag′ulable,** adj.

incompatibility (-kom-pat″i-bil′i-te) the quality of being incompatible.

incompatible (-kom-pat′i-b′l) not suitable for combination, simultaneous administration, or transplantation; mutually repellent.

incompetence (in-kom′pĕ-tens) 1. inability to function properly. 2. the legal status of an incompetent.

incompetent (-kom′pĕ-tent) 1. unable to function properly. 2. a person determined by the courts to be unable to manage his own affairs.

incontinence (-kon′ti-nens) 1. inability to control excretory functions. 2. immoderation or excess. **incon′tinent,** adj. **fecal i.,** involuntary passage of feces and flatus. **stress i.,** involuntary escape of urine due to strain on the orifice of the bladder, as in coughing or sneezing. **urinary i.,** inability to control the voiding of urine.

incontinentia (-kon″ti-nen′she-ah) [L.] incontinence. **i. al′vi,** fecal incontinence. **i. pigmen′ti,** a hereditary disorder in which early vesicular and later verrucous and bizarrely pigmented skin lesions are associated with eye, bone, and central nervous system defects. **i. uri′nae,** urinary incontinence.

incoordination (in″ko-or″di-na′shun) lack of normal adjustment of muscular motions; failure to work harmoniously.

incorporation (in-kor″po-ra′shun) 1. the union of a substance with another, or with others, in a composite mass. 2. an unconscious mental mechanism in which a person figuratively ingests the psychic representation of another person, or parts of him.

increment (in′kre-ment) increase or addition; the amount by which a value or quantity is increased. **incremen′tal,** adj.

incrustation (in″krus-ta′shun) 1. the formation of a crust. 2. a crust, scab, or scale.

incubate (in′ku-bāt) 1. to subject to or to undergo incubation. 2. material that has undergone incubation.

incubation (in″ku-ba′shun) 1. the provision of proper conditions for growth and development, as for bacterial or tissue cultures. 2. the development of an infectious disease from time of the entrance of the pathogen to the appearance of clinical symptoms. 3. the development of the embryo in the eggs of oviparous animals. 4. the maintenance of an artificial environment for an infant, especially a premature infant.

incubator (-ku-ba′ter) an apparatus for maintaining optimal conditions (temperature, humidity, etc.) for growth and development, as one used in the early care of premature infants, or one used for cultures.

incubus (in′ku-bus) 1. nightmare. 2. a heavy mental burden.

incudal (-ku-dal) pertaining to the incus.

incudectomy (in″ku-dek′to-me) excision of the incus.

incudiform (in-ku′di-form) anvil-shaped.

incudomalleal (in″ku-do-mal′e-al) pertaining to the incus and malleus.

incudostapedial (-stah-pe′de-al) pertaining to the incus and stapes.

incurable (in-kūr′ah-b′l) 1. not susceptible of being cured. 2. a person with a disease which cannot be cured.

incus (ing′kus) [L.] see *Table of Bones.*

incyclophoria (in″si-klo-fo′re-ah) cyclophoria in which the upper pole of the visual axis deviates toward the nose.

incyclotropia (-tro′pe-ah) cyclotropia in which the upper pole of the visual axis deviates toward the nose.

Indecidua (in″de-sid′u-ah) a division of the class Mammalia, comprising the mammals without a decidua, including whales and ungulates.

index (in′deks), pl. *indexes* or *in′dices* [L.] 1. the second digit of the hand, the forefinger. 2. the numerical ratio of measurement of any part in comparison with a fixed standard. **alveolar i.,** gnathic i. **cephalic i.,** 100 times the maximum breadth of the skull divided by its maximum length. **cerebral i.,** ratio of greatest transverse to greatest anteroposterior diameter of the cranial cavity. **color i.,** the relative amount of hemoglobulin in an erythrocyte compared with that of a normal individual of the same age and sex. **dental i.,** 100 times the dental length, divided by the length of the basinasal line. **gnathic i.,** the degree of prominence of the jaws; the distance from the basion to the front of the jaw expressed as a percentage of the distance from the basion to the midpoint of the nasal suture. **hemolytic i.,** a formula for calculating increased erythrocyte destruction. **icteric i.,** the ratio of bilirubin in the blood. **length-breadth i.,** cephalic i. **length-height i.,** vertical i. **leukopenic i.,** a fall of 1000 or more in the total leukocyte count within 1½ hours after ingestion of food indicates allergic hypersensitivity to that food. **nasal i.,** 100 times the width of the nose, divided by its length. **opsonic i.,** a measure of opsonic activity determined by the ratio of the number of microorganisms phagocytized by normal leukocytes in the presence of serum from an individual infected by the microorganism, to the number phagocytized in serum from a normal individual. **orbital i. (of Broca),** 100 times the height of the opening of the orbit divided by its width. **phagocytic i.,** the average number of bacteria ingested per leukocyte of the patient's blood. **refractive i.,** the refractive power of a medium compared with that of air (assumed to be 1). **refractive i., absolute,** an expression of the ratio of the velocity of light in air to its velocity in a specific substance. **refractive i., relative,** an expression of the ratio of the absolute refractive indexes of two different optically dense substances. **sacral i.,** 100 times the breadth of the sacrum divided by the length. **thoracic i.,** the ratio of the anteroposterior diameter of the thorax to the transverse diameter. **uricolytic i.,** the percentage of uric acid oxidized to allantoin before being secreted. **vertical i.,** 100 times the height of the skull divided by its length. **vital i.,** the ratio of births to deaths within a given time in a population. **volume i.,** the index indicating the size of the erythrocytes as compared to the normal.

indican (in'dĭ-kan) 1. a yellow glycoside, $C_{14}H_{17}NO_6$, from indigo plants, which yields glucose and indoxyl on hydrolysis. 2. potassium indoxyl sulfate, $C_8H_6NSO_4K$, formed by decomposition of tryptophan in the intestines and excreted in the urine.

indicanuria (in''dĭ-kan-u're-ah) an excess of indican in the urine.

indication (in''dĭ-ka'shun) a sign or circumstance that points to or shows the cause, treatment, etc., of a disease.

indicator (in'dĭ-ka''ter) 1. the index finger, or the extensor muscle of the index finger. 2. any substance that indicates the appearance or disappearance of a chemical by a color change or attainment of a certain pH.

indigestion (in''dĭ-jes'chun) lack or failure of digestion; commonly used to denote vague abdominal discomfort after meals. **acid i.,** hyperchlorhydria. **fat i.,** steatorrhea. **gastric i.,** that taking place in, or due to a disorder of, the stomach. **intestinal i.,** disorder of the digestive function of the intestine. **sugar i.,** defective ability to digest sugar, resulting in fermental diarrhea.

indigitation (in-dij''ĭ-ta'shun) intussusception (1).

indigo (in'dĭ-go) a blue dyeing material from various leguminous and other plants, being the aglycone of indican and also made synthetically; sometimes found in the sweat and urine.

indigotin (in''dĭ-go'tin) a neutral tasteless, insoluble, dark blue powder, $C_{16}H_{10}N_2O_2$, the principal ingredient of commercial indigo.

indium (in'de-um) chemical element (*see table*), at. no. 49, symbol In.

individuation (in''dĭ-vid''u-a'shun) 1. the process of developing individual characteristics. 2. differential regional activity in the embryo occurring in response to organizer influence.

indole (in'dōl) a compound obtained from coal tar and indigo and produced by decomposition of tryptophan in the intestine, where it contributes to the peculiar odor of feces. It is excreted in the urine in the form of indican.

indolent (in'do-lent) causing little pain; slow growing.

indomethacin (in''do-meth'ah-sin) an anti-inflammatory, antipyretic, and analgesic agent, $C_{19}H_{16}ClNO_4$, used in arthritic disorders and degenerative joint disease.

indoxyl (in-dok'sil) an oxidation product of indole, C_8H_7NO, formed in tryptophan decomposition, and excreted in the urine as indican.

indoxyluria (in-dok''sil-u're-ah) an excess of indoxyl in the urine.

inducer (in-dūs'er) in biosynthesis, a compound that induces synthesis of a specific enzyme or sequence of enzymes, by antagonizing the corresponding repressor, or by some other mechanism.

induction (-duk'shun) 1. the process or act of inducing, or causing to occur, especially the production of a specific morphogenetic effect in the embryo through evocators or organizers, or the production of anesthesia or unconsciousness by use of appropriate agents. 2. the generation of an electric current or magnetic properties in a body because of its proximity to an electrified or magnetized object.

inductor (-duk'tor) a tissue elaborating a chemical substance that acts to determine growth and differentiation of embryonic parts.

indulin (in'du-lin) a coal tar dye used as a histologic stain.

indurated (in'du-rāt''ed) hardened; abnormally hard.

induration (in''du-ra'shun) quality of being hard; process of hardening; an abnormally hard spot or place. **indura'tive,** adj. **black i.,** hardening and pigmentation of lung tissue, as in pneumonia. **brown i.,** 1. a deposit of altered blood pigment in the lung in pneumonia. 2. increase of pulmonary connective tissue and excessive pigmentation, due to chronic congestion from valvular heart disease or to anthracosis. **cyanotic i.,** hardening of an organ from chronic venous congestion. **granular i.,** cirrhosis. **gray i.,** induration of lung tissue in or after pneumonia, without pigmentation. **red i.,** interstitial pneumonia in which the lung is red and congested.

indusium griseum (in-du'ze-um gris'e-um) [L.] a thin layer of gray matter on the dorsal surface of the corpus callosum.

inebriant (in-e'bre-ant) 1. causing drunkenness. 2. an agent that causes drunkenness.

inebriation (-e''bre-a'shun) the condition of being drunk.

inelastic (in''e-las'tik) lacking elasticity.

inert (in-ert') inactive.

inertia (-er'she-ah) [L.] inactivity; inability to move spontaneously. **colonic i.,** weak muscular activity of the colon, leading to distention of the organ and constipation. **uterine i.,** sluggishness of uterine contractions in labor.

in extremis (in ek-stre′mis) [L.] at the point of death.

infancy (in′fan-se) the first two years of life.

infant (-fant) the human young from the time of birth to two years of age. **floppy i.,** see under *syndrome.* **immature i.,** one weighing between 17 ounces and 2.2 lbs. (500–999 gm.) at birth, with little chance of survival. **mature i.,** one weighing 5½ lbs. (2500 gm.) or more at birth, with optimal chance of survival. **newborn i.,** the human young during the first two to four weeks after birth. **postmature i.,** one carried for more than 294 days from the beginning of the last menstrual period or 280 days from the date of conception. **premature i.,** one weighing between 2½ and 5½ lbs. (1000–2499 gm.) at birth, with poor to good chance of survival.

infantile (-fan-tīl) relating to infancy; having features or traits characteristic of early childhood.

infantilism (in′fan-tĭ-lizm″, in-fan′tĭ-lizm) persistence of childhood characters into adult life, marked by mental retardation, underdevelopment of sex organs and, often dwarfism. **cachectic i.,** that due to chronic infection or poisoning. **celiac i.,** that due to the infantile form of nontropical sprue. **dysthyroidal i.,** that due to defective thyroid activity. **hepatic i.,** that associated with hepatic cirrhosis. **hypophyseal i.,** that due to deficiency of growth hormone and gonadotropic hormones of the anterior pituitary gland. **myxedematous i.,** cretinism. **pancreatic i.,** that associated with defective pancreatic action. **pituitary i.,** hypophyseal i. **renal i.,** see under *osteodystrophy.* **sexual i.,** continuance of prepuberal sex characters and behavior after the usual age of puberty. **universal i.,** general dwarfishness in stature, with absence of secondary sex characteristics.

infarct (in′farkt) a localized area of ischemic necrosis produced by occlusion of the arterial supply or the venous drainage of the part. **anemic i.,** one due to the sudden arrest of circulation in a vessel, or to decoloration of hemorrhagic blood. **bland i.,** an uninfected infarct. **hemorrhagic i.,** one that is red owing to oozing of erythrocytes into the injured area. **pale i.,** anemic i. **red i.,** hemorrhagic i. **septic i.,** one in which the tissues have been invaded by pathogenic organisms. **white i.,** anemic i.

infarction (in-fark′shun) 1. the formation of an infarct. 2. an infarct. **cardiac i.,** myocardial i. **cerebral i.,** an ischemic condition of the brain, causing a persistent focal neurologic deficit in the area affected. **myocardial i.,** gross necrosis of the myocardium, due to interruption of the blood supply to the area. **pulmonary i.,** localized necrosis of lung tissue, due to obstruction of the arterial blood supply.

infection (-fek′shun) 1. invasion and multiplication of microorganisms in body tissues, especially that causing local cellular injury due to competitive metabolism, toxins, intracellular replication, or antigen-antibody response. 2. an infectious disease. **airborne i.,** infection by inhalation of organisms suspended in air on water droplets or dust particles. **cross i.,** infection transmitted between persons infected with different pathogenic microorganisms. **cryptogenic i.,** infection whose pathogenesis is unclear or undefinable. **droplet i.,** infection due to inhalation of respiratory pathogens suspended on liquid particles exhaled by someone already infected. **dustborne i.,** infection by inhalation of pathogens that have become affixed to particles of dust. **endogenous i.,** that due to reactivation of organisms present in a dormant focus, as occurs in tuberculosis, etc. **exogenous i.,** that caused by organisms not normally present in the body but which have gained entrance from the environment. **mixed i.,** infection with more than one kind of organisms at the same time. **pyogenic i.,** infection by pus-producing organisms. **secondary i.,** infection by a pathogen following an infection by a pathogen of another kind. **terminal i.,** an acute infection occurring near the end of a disease and often causing death. **waterborne i.,** infection by microorganisms transmitted in water.

infectious (in-fek′shus) caused by or capable of being communicated by infection.

infective (-fek′tiv) infectious; capable of producing infection; pertaining to or characterized by the presence of pathogens.

inferior (in-fe′rĭ-or) situated below, or directed downward; in anatomy, used in reference to the lower surface of a structure, or to the lower of two (or more) similar structures.

infertility (in″fer-til′ĭ-te) diminution or absence of ability to produce offspring. **infer′tile,** adj.

infestation (-fes-ta′shun) parasitic attack or subsistance on the skin and/or its appendages, as by insects, mites, or ticks; sometimes used to denote parasitic invasion of the organs and tissues, as by helminths.

infiltrate (in-fil′trāt) 1. to penetrate the interstices of a tissue or substance. 2. material deposited by infiltration.

infiltration (in″fil-tra′shun) the diffusion or accumulation in a tissue or cells of substances not normal to it or in amounts in excess of the normal; also, the material so accumulated. **adipose i.,** fatty i. **calcareous i.,** deposit of lime and magnesium salts in the tissues. **cellular i.,** the migration and accumulation of cells within the tissues. **fatty i.,** 1. a deposit of fat in tissues, especially between cells. 2. the presence of fat vacuoles in the cell cytoplasm. **serous i.,** abnormal presence of serum in a tissue. **urinous i.,** the extravasation of urine into a tissue.

infirm (in-ferm′) weak; feeble, as from disease or old age.

infirmary (-fer′mah-re) a hospital or place where the sick or infirm are maintained or treated.

inflammation (in″flah-ma′shun) a protective tissue response to injury or destruction of tissues, which serves to destroy, dilute, or wall off both the injurious agent and the injured tissues. The classical signs of acute inflammation are pain (dolor), heat (calor), redness (rubor), swelling (tumor), and loss of function (functio laesa). **inflam′matory,** adj. **acute i.,** inflammation, usually of sudden onset, marked by the classical signs (see *inflammation*), in which vascular and exudative processes predominate. **catarrhal i.,** a form affecting mainly a mucous surface, marked by a copious discharge of mucus and epithelial debris. **chronic i.,** prolonged and persistent inflammation marked chiefly by new connective tissue formation; it may be a continuation of an acute form or a prolonged low-grade form. **exudative i.,** one in which the prominent feature is an exudate. **fibrinous i.,** one marked by an exudate of coagulated fibrin. **granulomatous i.,** a form, usually chronic, marked by granuloma formation. **hyperplastic i.,** proliferative i. **interstitial i.,** one affecting chiefly the stroma of an organ. **parenchymatous i.,** one affecting chiefly the essential tissue elements of an organ. **productive i., proliferative i.,** one leading to the production of new connective tissue fibers. **pseudomembranous i.,** an acute inflammatory response to a powerful necrotizing toxin, e.g., diphtheria toxin, with formation, on a mucosal surface, of a false membrane composed of precipitated fibrin, necrotic epithelium, and inflammatory white cells. **purulent i.,** suppurative i. **serous i.,** one producing a serous exudate. **specific i.,** one due to a particular microorganism. **subacute i.,** a condition intermediate between chronic and acute inflammation, exhibiting some of the characteristics of each. **suppurative i.,** one marked by pus formation. **toxic i.,** one due to a poison, e.g., a bacterial product. **traumatic i.,** one due to an injury. **ulcerative i.,** that in which necrosis on or near the surface leads to loss of tissue and creation of a local defect (ulcer).

inflation (in-fla′shun) distention, or the act of distending, with air, gas, or fluid.

inflection, inflexion (-flek′shun) the act of bending inward, or the state of being bent inward.

influenza (in″floo-en′zah) an acute viral infection of the respiratory tract, occurring in isolated cases, epidemics, and pandemics, with inflammation of the nasal mucosa, pharynx, and conjunctiva, headache, and severe, often generalized, myalgia. **influen′zal,** adj. **summer i. of Italy,** phlebotomus fever.

infra- word element [L.], *beneath.*

infra-axillary (in″frah-ak′sĭ-ler″e) below the axilla.

infrabulge (in′frah-bulj) the surfaces of a tooth gingival to the height of contour, or sloping cervically.

infraclavicular (in″frah-klah-vik′u-lar) below the clavicle.

infraclusion (-kloo′zhun) a condition in which the occluding surface of a tooth does not reach the normal occlusal plane and is out of contact with the opposing tooth.

infracostal (-kos′tal) below a rib.

infraction (in-frak′shun) incomplete bone fracture without displacement.

infradentale (in″frah-den-ta′le) a cephalometric landmark, being the highest anterior point

on the gingiva between the mandibular medial (central) incisors.

infrahyoid (-hi′oid) below the hyoid bone.

inframaxillary (-mak′sĭ-ler″e) beneath the maxilla.

infranuclear (-nu′kle-ar) below a nucleus.

infraocclusion (-ŏ-kloo′zhun) infraclusion.

infraorbital (-or′bĭ-tal) lying under or on the floor of the orbit.

infrapatellar (-pah-tel′ar) beneath the patella.

infraplacement (-plās′ment) infraclusion.

infrared (-red′) denoting electromagnetic radiation of wavelength greater than that of the red end of the spectrum, having wavelengths of 0.75–1000 μ; sometimes subdivided into *long-wave* or *far i.* (about 3.0–1000 μ) and *short-wave* or *near i.* (about 0.75–3.0 μ).

infrascapular (-skap′u-lar) below the scapula.

infrasonic (-son′ik) below the frequency range of sound waves.

infraspinous (-spi′nus) beneath the spine of the scapula.

infrasternal (-ster′nal) beneath the sternum.

infratrochlear (-trok′le-ar) beneath the trochlea.

infraversion (-ver′zhun) 1. downward deviation of the eye. 2. infraclusion.

infundibuliform (in″fun-dib′u-lĭ-form″) shaped like a funnel.

infundibuloma (in″fun-dib″u-lo′mah) a tumor of the stalk (infundibulum) of the hypophysis.

infundibulum (in″fun-dib′u-lum), pl. *infundib′-ula* [L.] 1. any funnel-shaped passage. 2. conus arteriosus. **infundib′ular,** adj. **ethmoidal i.,** 1. a passage connecting the nasal cavity with anterior ethmoidal cells and frontal sinus. 2. a sinuous passage connecting the middle nasal meatus with the anterior ethmoidal cells and often with the frontal sinus. **i. of hypothalamus,** a hollow, funnel-shaped mass in front of the tuber cinereum, extending to the posterior lobe of the pituitary gland. **i. of uterine tube,** the distal, funnel-shaped portion of the uterine tube.

infusion (in-fu′zhun) 1. the steeping of a substance in water to obtain its soluble principles. 2. the product obtained by this process. 3. the slow therapeutic introduction of fluid other than blood into a vein.

ingesta (-jes′tah) material taken into the body by mouth.

ingestant (-jes′tant) a substance that is or may be taken into the body by mouth or through the digestive system.

ingestion (-jes′chun) the taking of food, drugs, etc., into the body by mouth.

ingravescent (in″grah-ves′ent) gradually becoming more severe.

inguen (in′gwen), pl. *in′guina* [L.] the groin.

inguinal (in′gwĭ-nal) pertaining to the groin.

inguinocrural (ing″gwĭ-no-kroo′ral) pertaining to the groin and thigh.

inguinolabial (-la′be-al) pertaining to the groin and labium.

inguinoscrotal (-skro′tal) pertaining to the groin and scrotum.

INH trademark for preparations of isoniazid.

inhalant (in-ha′lant) a substance that is or may be taken into the body by way of the nose and trachea (through the respiratory system). **antifoaming i.,** an agent that is inhaled as a vapor to prevent the formation of foam in the respiratory passages of a patient with pulmonary edema.

inhalation (in″hah-la′shun) 1. the act of breathing in. 2. an agent to be inhaled as a vapor.

inhaler (in-ha′ler) an apparatus for administering vaporized or volatilized agents by inhalation, or for protecting the lungs from harmful substances in the air.

inheritance (-her′ĭ-tans) 1. the acquisition of characters or qualities by transmission from parent to offspring. 2. that which is transmitted from parent to offspring. **cytoplasmic i.,** transmission of characters dependent on self-perpetuating elements not nuclear in origin. **dominant i.,** see under *gene.* **maternal i.,** the transmission of characters that are dependent on peculiarities of the egg cytoplasm produced, in turn, by nuclear genes. **recessive i.,** see under *gene.* **sex-linked i., X-linked i.,** see under *gene.*

inhibition (in″ĭ-bish′un, -hĭ-bish′un) arrest or restraint of a process; in psychiatry, the unconscious restraining of an instinctual drive. **inhib′itory,** adj. **competitive i.,** inhibition of enzyme activity in which the inhibitor (a substrate analogue) competes with the substrate for binding sites on the enzymes. **contact i.,** inhibition of cell division in normal animal cells when in close contact with each other. **endproduct i.,** inhibition of an activity resulting from the effect of the end product of a biosynthetic process on an earlier step in the process. **false feed-back i.,** inhibition of the initial steps of a process by an analogue of the end product of the specific process. **feedback i.,** endproduct i. **noncompetitive i.,** inhibition of enzyme activity by substances that combine with the enzyme at a site other than that utilized by the substrate.

inhibitor (in-hib′ĭ-tor) 1. any substance that interferes with a chemical reaction, growth, or other biologic activity. 2. a chemical substance that inhibits or checks the action of a tissue organizer or the growth of microorganisms.

inion (in′e-on) the external occipital protuberance. **in′ial,** adj.

iniopagus (in″e-op′ah-gus) a twin monster joined at the occiput.

iniops (in′e-ops) a double-faced monster with a posterior face incomplete.

initis (ĭ-ni′tus) inflammation of the substance of a muscle.

injected (in-jek′ted) 1. introduced by injection. 2. congested.

injection (-jek′shun) 1. the forcing of a liquid into a part, as into the subcutaneous tissues, the vacular tree, or an organ. 2. a substance so forced or administered; in pharmacy, a solution of a medicament suitable for injection. 3. congestion. **Brown-Séquard i.,** injection of testic-ular extract. **circumcorneal i.,** dilatation of the ciliary and conjunctival blood vessels close to the limbus, and diminishing toward the periphery. **dextrose i.,** a sterile solution of dextrose in water; used as a fluid and nutrient replenisher. **fructose i.,** a sterile solution of fructose in water; used as a fluid and nutrient replenisher. **hypodermic i.,** injection into the subcutaneous tissues. **insulin i.,** a sterile solution of the active principle of the pancreas which affects the metabolism of glucose; a prompt-acting hypoglycemic used in treatment of diabetes mellitus. **intracutaneous i., intradermal i.,** one made into the corium or substance of the skin. **intramuscular i.,** one made into the substance of a muscle. **intravenous i.,** one made into a vein. **opacifying i.,** injection of a radiopaque substance into the vessels or a body cavity for diagnostic radiologic study. **oxytocin i.,** a sterile solution of an oxytocic principle prepared by synthesis or obtained from the posterior pituitary of domestic animals; used to stimulate contraction of smooth muscle, particularly the pregnant uterus. **parathyroid i.,** a sterile solution of water-soluble principles of parathyroid glands, administered intramuscularly to maintain blood calcium levels. **posterior pituitary i.,** a sterile solution in water of the principles from the posterior lobe of the pituitary gland of domestic animals used for food by man; used as an oxytocic, in the treatment of diabetes insipidus, and to stimulate intestinal peristalsis. **protamine sulfate i.,** a sterile isotonic solution from sperm or mature testes of certain fish; used to counteract the action of heparin. **protein hydrolysate i.,** a sterile solution of amino acids and short-chain peptides; used as a fluid and nutrient replenisher. **Ringer's i.,** a sterile solution of sodium chloride, potassium chloride, and calcium chloride in water for injection; used as a fluid and electrolyte replenisher. **sodium chloride i.,** a sterile isotonic solution of sodium chloride in water for injection; used as a fluid and electrolyte replenisher, as an irrigating solution, and as a vehicle for drugs. **sodium chromate Cr 51 i.,** a sterile solution of radioactive chromium of mass number 51, processed in the form of sodium chromate, in water for injection; used as a diagnostic aid to determine erythrocyte volume and survival time, total blood volume, and plasma volume, and to detect gastrointestinal bleeding and to determine the site of placental implantation. **sodium radiochromate i.,** sodium chromate Cr 51 i. **subcutaneous i.,** hypodermic i. **vasopressin i.,** a sterile solution of the water-soluble, pressor principle of the posterior lobe of the pituitary gland of healthy domestic animals; used as an antidiuretic.

injury (in′ju-re) harm or hurt; a wound or maim; usually applied to damage inflicted on the body by an external force. **birth i.,** impairment of body function or structure due to adverse influences to which the infant has been subjected at birth. **Goyrand's i.,** pulled elbow. **whiplash i.,** a nonspecific term applied to injury to the spine and spinal cord due to sudden extension of the neck.

inlay (in′la) material laid into a defect in tissue; in dentistry, a filling made outside the tooth to correspond with the cavity form and then cemented into the tooth.

inlet (-let) a means or route of entrance. **pelvic i.,** the upper limit of the pelvic cavity.

I.N.N. International Nonproprietary Names, the designations recommended by the World Health Organization for pharmaceuticals.

innate (in′āt) inborn; hereditary; congenital.

innervation (in″er-va′shun) 1. the distribution or supply of nerves to a part. 2. the supply of nervous energy or of nerve stimulation sent to a part.

innidiation (ĭ-nid″e-a′shun) development of cells in a part to which they have been carried by metastasis.

innocent (in′o-sent) not malignant; benign.

innocuous (ĭ-nok′u-us) harmless.

innominate (ĭ-nom′ĭ-nāt) nameless.

inochondritis (in″o-kon-dri′tis) inflammation of a fibrocartilage.

inoculability (ĭ-nok″u-lah-bil′ĭ-te) the quality of being inoculable.

inoculable (ĭ-nok′u-lah-b'l) 1. susceptible of being inoculated; transmissible by inoculation. 2. not immune against a disease transmissible by inoculation.

inoculation (ĭ-nok″u-la′shun) introduction of microorganisms, infective material, serum, or other substances into tissues of living organisms, or culture media; introduction of a disease agent into a healthy individual to produce a mild form of the disease followed by immunity.

inoculum (ĭ-nok′u-lum), pl. *inoc′ula* [L.] material used in inoculation.

inocyte (in′o-sīt) a cell of fibrous tissue.

inogenesis (in″o-jen′ĕ-sis) the formation of fibrous tissue.

inogenous (in-oj′ĕ-nus) produced from or forming fibrous tissue.

inoperable (-op′er-ah-b'l) not susceptible to treatment by surgery.

inorganic (in″or-gan′ik) 1. having no organs. 2. not of organic origin.

inoscopy (in-os′ko-pe) the diagnosis of disease by artificial digestion and examination of the fibers or fibrinous matter of the sputum, blood, effusions, etc.

inose (in′ōs) inositol.

inosemia (in″o-se′me-ah) 1. the presence of inositol in the blood. 2. an excess of fibrin in the blood.

inosine (in′o-sin) a nucleoside resulting from cleavage of inosinic acid, composed of hypoxanthine and ribose.

inosite (-sīt) inositol.

inositol (in-o′sĭ-tol) a sugar-like vitamin of the B complex found in many animal and plant tissues; it is concerned in the growth of yeast and certain bacteria, and has been shown to have lipotropic action on fatty liver in rats and to be curative of mouse alopecia.

inosituria (in″o-si-tu′re-ah) the presence of inositol in the urine.

inotropic (in′o-trop″ik) affecting the force of muscular contractions.

inquest (in′kwest) a legal inquiry before a coroner or medical examiner, and usually a jury, into the manner of death.

insalubrious (in″sah-lu′bre-us) injurious to health.

insanity (in-san′ĭ-te) a legal term for mental illness, roughly equivalent to psychosis and implying inability to be responsible for one's acts. **insane′,** adj.

inscriptio (in-skrip′she-o) [L.] inscription. **i. tendin′ea,** see under *intersectio.*

inscription (-skrip′shun) 1. a mark, or line. 2. that part of a prescription containing the names and amounts of the ingredients.

insect (in′sekt) any member of the Insecta.

Insecta (in-sek′tah) a class of arthropods whose members are characterized by division into three parts: head, thorax, and abdomen.

insecticide (-sek′tĭ-sīd) an agent which kills insects. **insec′ticidal,** adj.

Insectivora (in″sek-tiv′o-rah) an order of small, terrestrial mammals, including moles, shrews, etc., which feed primarily on insects.

insectivore (in-sek′tĭ-vōr) an individual of the order Insectivora. **insec′tivorous,** adj.

insemination (-sem″ĭ-na′shun) the deposit of seminal fluid within the vagina or cervix. **artificial i.,** that done by artificial means.

insensible (-sen′sĭ-b'l) 1. devoid of sensibility or consciousness. 2. not perceptible to the senses.

insertion (-ser′shun) 1. the act of implanting, or condition of being implanted. 2. the site of attachment, as of a muscle to the bone that it moves. **velamentous i.,** attachment of the umbilical cord to the membranes.

insidious (-sid′ĭ-ous) coming on stealthily; of gradual and subtle development.

insight (in′sīt) self-understanding; in psychiatry, referring to the extent to which the patient is aware of his illness and understands its nature.

in situ (in si′tu) [L.] in its normal place; confined to the site of origin.

insoluble (in-sol′u-b'l) not susceptible of being dissolved.

insomnia (-som′ne-ah) inability to sleep; abnormal wakefulness.

insorption (-sorp′shun) movement of a substance into the blood, especially from the gastrointestinal tract into the circulating blood.

inspersion (-sper′shun) sprinkling, as with powder.

inspiration (in″spĭ-ra′shun) the drawing of air into the lungs. **inspi′ratory,** adj.

inspissated (in-spis′āt-ed) being thickened, dried, or made less fluid by evaporation.

instar (in′stahr) any stage of an arthropod between molts.

instep (-step) the dorsal part of the arch of the foot.

instillation (in″stĭ-la′shun) administration of a liquid drop by drop.

instinct (in'stinkt) a complex of unlearned responses characteristic of a species. **death i.,** in psychoanalysis, the latent instinctive impulse toward death. **herd i.,** the instinct or urge to be one of a group and to conform to its standards of conduct and opinion.

instrumentation (in"stroo-men-ta'shun) the use of instruments; work performed with instruments.

insufficiency (-su-fish'en-se) inability to perform properly an allotted function. **adrenal i.,** hypoadrenalism. **aortic i.,** see under *regurgitation*. **cardiac i.,** heart failure. **coronary i.,** decrease in flow of blood through the coronary blood vessels. **i. of the externi,** deficient power in the externi muscles of the eye, resulting in esophoria. **ileocecal i.,** inability of the ileocecal valve to prevent backflow of contents from the cecum into the ileum. **i. of the interni,** deficient power in the interni muscles of the eye, resulting in exophoria. **mitral i.,** see under *regurgitation*. **pulmonary i.,** see under *regurgitation*. **thyroid i.,** hypothyroidism. **tricuspid i.,** see under *regurgitation*. **valvular i.,** see under *regurgitation*. **velopharyngeal i.,** failure of velopharyngeal closure due to cleft palate, muscular dysfunction, etc., resulting in defective speech. **venous i.,** inadequacy of the venous valves with impairment of venous drainage, resulting in edema.

insufflation (-su-fla'shun) the blowing of a powder, vapor, or gas into a body cavity. **perirenal i.,** injection of air around the kidney for roentgen examination of the adrenal glands. **tubal i.,** see *Rubin's test*.

insufflator (-su-fla'tor) an instrument used in insufflation.

insula (in'su-lah), pl. *in'sulae* [L.] a triangular area of the cerebral cortex forming the floor of the lateral cerebral fossa.

insular (in'su-lar) pertaining to the insula or to an island, as the islands of Langerhans.

insulation (in"su-la'shun) 1. the surrounding of a space or body with material designed to prevent the entrance or escape of radiant or electrical energy. 2. the material so used.

insulin (in'su-lin) a protein hormone secreted by the beta cells of the islands of Langerhans of the pancreas into the blood, where it regulates carbohydrate, lipid, and amino acid metabolism; also, a preparation of the active principle of the pancreas, used therapeutically in diabetes and sometimes in other conditions. **i. lente,** a sterile suspension of insulin modified by the addition of zinc chloride. **isophane i., NPH i.,** a neutral, crystalline protamine zinc insulin. **protamine zinc i.,** insulin modified by addition of zinc chloride and protamine. **regular i.,** the active principle of the pancreas of slaughter-house animals (cattle or swine), used in sterile acidified solution.

insulinemia (in"su-lin-e'me-ah) the presence of insulin in the blood.

insulinogenesis (in"su-lin"o-jen'ĕ-sis) the formation and release of insulin by the islands of Langerhans.

insulinogenic (-jen'ik) relating to insulinogenesis.

insulinoma (in"su-lin-o'mah) a tumor of the beta cells of the islands of Langerhans; although usually benign, it is one of the chief causes of hypoglycemia.

insulitis (in"su-li'tis) cellular infiltration of the islands of Langerhans, possibly in response to invasion by an infectious agent.

insuloma (in"su-lo'mah) insulinoma.

insusceptibility (in"su-sep"tǐ-bil'ǐ-te) the state of being unaffected; immunity.

intake (in'tāk) the substances, or the quantities thereof, taken in and utilized by the body.

integration (in"tĕ-gra'shun) harmonious assimilation into a common body or activity; anabolic activity.

integument (in-teg'u-ment) a covering or investment; the skin.

integumentary (in-teg"u-men'tar-e) 1. pertaining to or composed of skin. 2. serving as a covering.

integumentum (in-teg"u-men'tum) [L.] integument.

intellect (in'tĕ-lekt) the mind, thinking faculty, or understanding.

intellectualization (in"tĕ-lek"chu-al-ǐ-za'shun) the mental process in which reasoning is used as a defense against confronting unconscious conflict and its stressful emotions.

intelligence (in-tel'ǐ-jens) the ability to comprehend or understand.

intensimeter (in"ten-sim'ĕ-ter) a device for measuring intensity of roentgen rays.

intention (in-ten'shun) a manner of healing; see under *healing*.

inter- word element [L.], *between*.

interarticular (in"ter-ar-tik'u-ler) between articulating surfaces.

interatrial (-a'tre-al) between the atria of the heart.

interbrain (in'ter-brān) 1. thalamencephalon. 2. diencephalon.

intercalary (in-ter'kah-ler"e) inserted between; interposed.

intercalated (-kah-la"ted) inserted between.

intercartilaginous (in"ter-kar"tǐ-laj'ǐ-nus) between, or connecting, cartilages.

intercellular (-sel'u-lar) between the cells.

interchondral (-kon'dral) intercartilaginous.

intercilium (-sil'e-um) the space between the eyebrows.

interclavicular (-klah-vik'u-ler) between the clavicles.

intercondylar (-kon'dǐ-lar) between two condyles.

intercostal (-kos'tal) between two ribs.

intercourse (in'ter-kōrs) mutual exchange. **sexual i.,** coitus.

intercricothyrotomy (in"ter-kri"ko-thi-rot'o-me) incision of the larynx through the cricothyroid membrane; inferior laryngotomy.

intercurrent (-kur'ent) occurring during and modifying the course of another disease.

intercusping (-kusp'ing) the occlusion of the

cusps of the teeth of one jaw with the depressions in the teeth of the other jaw.

interdental (-den′tal) between the proximal surfaces of adjacent teeth in the same arch.

interdentium (-den′she-um) the interproximal space.

interdigital (-dij′ĭ-tal) between two digits (fingers or toes).

interdigitation (-dij″ĭ-ta′shun) 1. an interlocking of parts by finger-like processes. 2. one of a set of finger-like processes.

interface (in′ter-fās) the boundary between two systems or phases.

interfascicular (in″ter-fah-sik′u-lar) between adjacent fascicles.

interfemoral (-fem′o-ral) between the thighs.

interferon (-fēr′on) a class of small soluble proteins released by cells invaded by virus, which induces in noninfected cells the formation of an antiviral protein that inhibits viral multiplication.

interfibrillar (-fi′bril-ar) between fibrils.

interfilar (-fi′lar) between or among the fibrils of a reticulum.

interictal (-ik′tal) occurring between attacks or paroxysms.

interkinesis (-ki-ne′sis) the period between the first and second divisions in meiosis.

interlobar (-lo′bar) between lobes.

interlobitis (-lo-bi′tis) interlobular pleurisy.

interlobular (-lob′u-lar) between lobules.

intermaxillary (-mak′sĭ-ler″e) between the maxillae.

intermediate (-me′de-at) 1. between; intervening; resembling, in part, each of two extremes. 2. a substance formed in a chemical process that is essential to formation of the end product of the process.

intermedin (-me′din) melanocyte-stimulating hormone.

intermedius (-me′de-us) [L.] intermediate; in anatomy, denoting a structure lying between a lateral and a medial structure.

intermeningeal (-mĕ-nin′je-al) between the meninges.

intermittent (-mit′ent) marked by alternating periods of activity and inactivity.

intermural (-mu′ral) situated between the walls of an organ or organs.

intermuscular (-mus′ku-lar) between muscles.

intern (in′tern) a medical graduate serving and residing in a hospital preparatory to being licensed to practice medicine.

internal (in-ter′nal) situated or occurring on the inside; in anatomy, many structures formerly called internal are now termed medial.

internalization (in-ter″nal-i-za′shun) a mental mechanism whereby certain external attributes, attitudes, or standards of others are unconsciously taken as one's own.

internatal (in″ter-na′tal) between the nates, or buttocks.

interneuron (-nu′ron) a neuron between the primary afferent neuron and the final motoneuron.

internist (in-ter′nist) a specialist in internal medicine.

internode (in′ter-nōd) a space between two nodes.

internship (in′tern-ship) the position or term of service of an intern in a hospital.

internuclear (in″ter-nu′kle-ar) situated between nuclei or between nuclear layers of the retina.

internuncial (-nun′shal) transmitting impulses between two different parts.

internus (in-ter′nus) [L.] internal; in anatomy, denoting a structure nearer to the center of an organ or part.

interocclusal (in″ter-ŏ-kloo′zal) situated between the occlusal surfaces of opposing teeth in the two dental arches.

interoceptor (-sep′tor) a sensory nerve ending that is located in and transmits impulses from the viscera. **interocep′tive,** adj.

interofective (-fek′tiv) affecting the interior of the organism—a term applied to the autonomic nervous system.

interolivary (in″ter-ol′ĭ-var″e) between the olivary bodies.

interorbital (-or′bĭ-tal) between the orbits.

interosseous (-os′e-us) between two bones.

interpalpebral (-pal′pĕ-bral) between the eyelids.

interparietal (-pah-ri′ĕ-tal) 1. intermural. 2. between the parietal bones.

interparoxysmal (-par″ok-siz′mal) between paroxysms.

interphalangeal (-fah-lan′je-al) between two contiguous phalanges.

interphase (in′ter-fāz) the interval between two successive cell divisions, during which the chromosomes are not individually distinguishable.

interplant (-plant) an embryonic part isolated by transference to an indifferent environment provided by another embryo.

interpolation (in-ter″po-la′shun) 1. surgical implantation of tissue. 2. the determination of intermediate values in a series on the basis of observed values.

interproximal (in″ter-prok′sĭ-mal) between two adjoining surfaces.

interpubic (-pu′bik) between the pubic bones.

interpupillary (-pu′pĭ-ler″e) between the pupils.

interscapular (-skap′u-lar) between the scapulae.

intersectio (-sek′she-o), pl. *intersectio′nes*[L.] intersection. **i. tendin′ea,** a fibrous band traversing the belly of a muscle, dividing it into two parts.

intersection (-sek′shun) a site at which one structure crosses another.

intersex (in′ter-seks) 1. intersexuality. 2. an individual who exhibits intersexuality. **female i.,** a female pseudohermaprodite. **male i.,** a male pseudohermaphrodite. **true i.,** a true hermaphrodite.

intersexuality (in″ter-seks″u-al′ĭ-te) an intermingling, in varying degrees, of the characters of each sex, including physical form, reproductive tissue, and sexual behavior, in one individual, as a result of some flaw in embryonic development; see *hermaphroditism* and *pseudohermaphroditism.* **intersex′ual,** adj.

interspace (in′ter-spās) a space between similar structures.

interspinal (in″ter-spi′nal) between two spinous processes.

interstice (in-ter′stis) a small interval, space, or gap in a tissue or structure.

interstitial (in″ter-stish′al) pertaining to or situated between parts or in the interspaces of a tissue.

interstitium (-stish′ĭ-um) 1. interstice. 2. interstitial tissue.

intertransverse (-trans-vers′) between transverse processes of the vertebrae.

intertrigo (-tri′go) an erythematous skin eruption occurring on apposed skin surfaces.

intertubular (-tu′bu-lar) between tubules.

interureteral (-u-re′ter-al) interureteric.

interureteric (-u-rĕ-ter′ik) between ureters.

intervaginal (-vaj′ĭ-nal) between sheaths.

interval (in′ter-val) the space between two objects or parts; the lapse of time between two events. **atrioventricular i., A–V i.,** P–R i. **c.-a. i., cardioarterial i.,** the time between the apex beat and arterial pulsation. **lucid i.,** a brief period of remission of symptoms in a psychosis. **postsphygmic i.,** see under *period.* **P–R i.,** the time between the onset of the P wave (atrial activity) and the QRS complex (ventricular activity). **presphygmic i.,** see under *period.* **QRST i., Q–T i.,** the duration of ventricular electrical activity.

intervalvular (in″ter-val′vu-lar) between valves.

intervascular (-vas′ku-lar) between blood vessels.

interventricular (-ven-trik′u-lar) between the ventricles of the heart.

intervertebral (-ver′tĕ-bral) between two contiguous vertebrae.

intervillous (-vil′us) between or among villi.

intestine (in-tes′tin) the part of the alimentary canal extending from the pyloric opening of the stomach to the anus. See Plates *IV, V,* and *XV.* **intes′tinal,** adj. **large i.,** the distal portion of the intestine, about 5 feet long, extending from its junction with the small intestine to the anus and comprising the cecum, colon, rectum, and anal canal. **small i.,** the proximal portion of the intestine about 20 feet long, smaller in caliber than the large intestine, extending from the pylorus to the cecum and comprising the duodenum, jejunum, and ileum.

intestinum (in″tes-ti′num), pl. *intesti′na* [L.] intestine.

intima (in′tĭ-mah) an innermost structure; see *tunica intima.* **in′timal,** adj.

intimitis (in″tĭ-mi′tis) endarteritis.

Intocostrin (in″to-kos′trin) trademark for a preparation of tubocurarine.

intolerance (in-tol′er-ans) inability to withstand or consume; inability to absorb or metabolize nutrients.

intorsion (-tor′shun) tilting of the upper part of the vertical meridian of the eye toward the midline of the face.

intoxication (-tok″sĭ-ka′shun) 1. poisoning; the state of being poisoned. 2. the condition produced by excessive use of alcohol.

intra- word element [L.], *inside of; within.*

intra-abdominal (in″trah-ab-dom′ĭ-nal) within the abdomen.

intra-arterial (-ar-te′re-al) within an artery.

intra-articular (-ar-tik′u-lar) within a joint.

intra-atrial (-a′tre-al) within an atrium.

intracanalicular (-kan″ah-lik′u-lar) within canaliculi.

intracapsular (-kap′su-lar) within a capsule.

intracardiac (-kar′de-ak) within the heart.

intracartilaginous (-kar″tĭ-laj′ĭ-nus) within a cartilage.

intracellular (-sel′u-lar) within a cell or cells.

intracerebral (-ser′ĕ-bral) within the cerebrum.

intracervical (-ser′vĭ-kal) within the canal of the cervix uteri.

intracisternal (-sis-ter′nal) within a subarachnoid cistern.

intracranial (-kra′ne-al) within the cranium.

intractable (in-trak′tah-b′l) resistant to cure, relief, or control.

intracutaneous (in″trah-ku-ta′ne-us) within the substance of the skin.

intracystic (-sis′tik) within the bladder or a cyst.

intradermal (-der′mal) within the dermis.

intraductal (-duk′tal) within a duct.

intradural (-du′ral) within or beneath the dura mater.

intrafusal (-fu′zal) pertaining to the striated fibers within a muscle spindle.

intrahepatic (-hĕ-pat′ik) within the liver.

intralobar (-lo′bar) within a lobe.

intralobular (-lob′u-lar) within a lobule.

intraluminal (-lu′mĭ-nal) within the lumen of a tubular structure.

intramedullary (-med′u-lār″e) within (1) the spinal cord, (2) the medulla oblongata, or (3) the marrow cavity of a bone.

intramural (-mu′ral) within the wall of an organ.

intramuscular (-mus′ku-lar) within the muscular substance.

intraocular (-ok′u-lar) within the eye.

intraoperative (-op′er-a″tiv) occurring during a surgical operation.

intraoral (-o′ral) within the mouth.

intraorbital (-or′bĭ-tal) within the orbit.

intraparietal (-pah-ri′ĕ-tal) 1. intramural. 2. within the parietal region of the brain.

intrapartum (-par′tum) occurring during childbirth or during delivery.

intraperitoneal (-per″ĭ-to-ne′al) within the peritoneal cavity.

intrapleural (-ploo′ral) within the pleura.

intrapsychic (-si′kik) taking place within the mind.

intrapulmonary (-pul′mo-ner″e) within the substance of the lung.

intraspinal (-spi′nal) within the spinal column.

intrasternal (-ster′nal) within the sternum.

intrathecal (-the′kal) within a sheath; through the theca of the spinal cord into the subarachnoid space.

intrathoracic (-tho-ras′ik) within the thorax.

intratracheal (-tra′ke-al) endotracheal.

intratubal (-tu′bal) within a tube.

intratympanic (-tim-pan′ik) within the tympanic cavity.

intrauterine (-u′ter-in) within the uterus.

intravasation (in-trav″ah-sa′shun) the entrance of foreign material into vessels.

intravascular (in″trah-vas′ku-lar) within a vessel or vessels.

intravenous (-ve′nus) within a vein.

intraventricular (-ven-trik′u-lar) within a ventricle.

intravital (-vi′tal) occurring during life.

intra vitam (in′trah vi′tam) [L.] during life.

intrinsic (in-trin′sik) situated entirely within or pertaining exclusively to a part.

introitus (-tro′ĭ-tus), pl. *intro′itus* [L.] the entrance to a cavity or space.

introjection (in″tro-jek′shun) a mental mechanism in which loved or hated external objects are unconsciously and symbolically taken within oneself.

intromission (-mish′un) the entrance of one part or object into another.

introspection (-spek′shun) contemplation or observation of one's own thoughts and feelings; self-analysis. **introspec′tive,** adj.

introsusception (-sŭ-sep′shun) intussusception.

introversion (-ver′zhun) 1. the turning outside in, more or less completely, of an organ. 2. preoccupation with oneself, with reduction of interest in the outside world.

introvert (in′tro-vert) a person whose interests are turned inward upon himself.

intubate (in′tu-bāt) to perform intubation.

intubation (in″tu-ba′shun) the insertion of a tube, as into the larynx. **endotracheal i.,** insertion of a tube through the trachea to assure a clear airway and prevent entrance of foreign material into the tracheobronchial tree. **nasal i.,** insertion of a tube into the respiratory or gastrointestinal tract through the nose. **oral i.,** insertion of a tube into the respiratory or gastrointestinal tract through the mouth.

intumescence (in″tu-mes′ens) 1. a swelling, normal or abnormal. 2. the process of swelling. **intumes′cent,** adj.

intumescentia (in-tu″mĕ-sen′she-ah) intumescence.

intussusception (in″tŭ-sŭ-sep′shun) 1. prolapse of one part of the intestine into the lumen of an immediately adjacent part. 2. the reception into an organism of matter, such as food, and its transformation into new protoplasm.

intussusceptum (-sep′tum) the portion of intestine that has prolapsed in intussusception.

intussuscipiens (-sip′e-ens) the portion of intestine containing the intussusceptum.

inulase (in′u-lās) an enzyme that converts inulin to fructose.

inulin (in′u-lin) a starch occurring in the rhizome of certain plants, yielding fructose on hydrolysis, and used in tests of renal function.

inunction (in-unk′shun) 1. the act of anointing or applying an ointment by friction. 2. an ointment made with lanolin as a menstruum.

in utero (in u′ter-o) [L.] within the uterus.

invaginate (in-vaj′ĭ-nāt) to infold one portion of a structure within another portion.

invagination (-vaj″ĭ-na′shun) 1. the infolding of one part within another part of a structure, as of the blastula during gastrulation. 2. intussusception.

invasiveness (-va′siv-nes) 1. the ability of microorganisms to enter the body and spread in the tissues. 2. the ability to infiltrate and actively destroy surrounding tissue, a property of malignant tumors. **inva′sive,** adj.

Inversine (-ver′sēn) trademark for a preparation of mecamylamine.

inversion (-ver′zhun) 1. a turning inward, inside out, or other reversal of the normal relation of a part. 2. homosexuality. 3. a chromosomal aberration due to the inverted reunion of the middle segment after breakage of a chromosome at two points, resulting in a change in sequence of genes or nucleotides. **carbohydrate i.,** hydrolysis of disaccharides or polysaccharides to monosaccharides. **sexual i.,** homosexuality. **i. of uterus,** a turning of the uterus whereby the fundus is forced through the cervix, protruding into or completely outside of the vagina. **visceral i.,** the more or less complete right and left transposition of the viscera.

invert (in′vert) a homosexual.

invertase (in-ver′tās) β-fructofuranosidase.

invertebrate (-ver′tĕ-brāt) 1. having no spinal column. 2. any animal having no spinal column.

invertin (-ver′tin) β-fructofuranosidase.

investment (-vest′ment) material in which a denture, tooth, crown, or model for a dental restoration is enclosed for curing, soldering, or casting, or the process of such enclosure.

inveterate (-vet′er-āt) confirmed and chronic; long-established and difficult to cure.

in vitro (in ve′tro) [L.] within a glass; observable in a test tube; in an artificial environment.

in vivo (in ve′vo) [L.] within the living body.

involucrum (in″vo-lu′krum), pl. *involu′cra* [L.] a covering or sheath, as of a sequestrum.

involution (-lu′shun) 1. a rolling or turning inward. 2. one of the movements involved in the gastrulation of many animals. 3. a retrograde change of the entire body or in a particular organ, as the retrograde changes in the female genital organs that result in normal size after delivery. 4. the progressive degeneration occurring naturally with advancing age, resulting in shriveling of organs or tissues. **involu′tional,** adj.

Io chemical symbol, *ionium.*

Iodamoeba (i-o″dah-me′bah) a genus of amebas, including *I. buetschlii,* parasitic in man, and *I. suis,* found in pigs.

iodate (i′o-dāt) a salt of iodic acid.

iodide (-dīd) a binary compound of iodine.

iodination (i″o-din-a′shun) the incorporation or addition of iodine in a compound.

iodine (i′o-dīn) chemical elements (*see table*), at. no. 53, symbol I; it is essential in nutrition, being especially prevalent in the colloid of the thyroid gland. **protein-bound i.,** iodine firmly bound to protein in the serum, determination of which constitutes one test of thyroid function. **radioactive i.,** radioiodine.

iodinophilous (i″o-din-of′ĭ-lus) easily stainable with iodine.

iodipamide (i″o-dip′ah-mīd) a radiopaque medium, $C_{20}H_{14}I_6N_2O_6$, used in the form of its meglumine and sodium salts in cholecystography.

iodism (i′o-dizm) chronic poisoning by iodine or iodides, with coryza, ptyalism, frontal headache, emaciation, weakness, and skin eruptions.

iodochlorhydroxyquin (i-o″do-klōr″hi-drok′-se-kwin) an anti-infective, C_9H_5ClINO, used topically in the treatment of amebiasis, *Trichomonas vaginalis* infection, and eczema.

iododerma (-der′mah) any skin lesion resulting from iodism.

iodoform (i-o′do-form) a local anti-infective, CHI_3.

iodoglobulin (i-o″do-glob′u-lin) an iodine-containing globulin (protein).

iodomethamate (-meth′ah-māt) an acid compound, $C_8H_3I_2NO_5$, used as the sodium salt as a radiopaque medium in urography.

iodophilia (-fil′e-ah) a reaction shown by leuko-cytes in certain pathologic conditions, as in toxemia and severe anemia, in which the polymorphonuclears show diffuse brownish coloration when treated with iodine or iodides.

iodophthalein (-thal′e-in) a radiopaque medium, $C_{20}H_{10}I_4O_4$, used as the disodium salt in cholecystography.

iodopsin (i″o-dop′sin) a photosensitive violet pigment found in the retinal cones of some animals and important for color vision.

iodopyracet (i-o″do-pi′rah-set) a radiopaque medium, $C_{11}H_{16}I_2N_2O_5$, used in urography.

iodotherapy (-ther′ah-pe) treatment with iodine or iodides.

iodum (i-o′dum) [L.] iodine.

ion (i′on) an atom or group of atoms having a charge of positive (cation) or negative (anion) electricity by virtue of having gained or lost an electron. **ion′ic,** adj. **dipolar i.,** zwitterion.

ionium (i-o′ne-um) the radioactive isotope of thorium, which emits both alpha and gamma rays; symbol Io.

ionization (i″on-i-za′shun) 1. the dissociation of a substance in solution into ions. 2. iontophoresis.

ionometer (i″o-nom′ĕ-ter) an instrument for measuring the intensity or quantity of radiation from an ionizing radiation source.

ionophose (i′o-no-fōz″) a violet phose.

ionotherapy (i″o-no-ther′ah-pe) 1. iontophoresis. 2. treatment with ultraviolet rays.

iontophoresis (i-on″to-fo-re′sis) the introduc-tion of ions of soluble salts into the body by means of electric current.

iophendylate (i″o-fen′dĭ-lāt) a radiopaque medium, $C_{19}H_{29}IO_2$, used in myelography.

iothalamate (-thal′ah-māt) a radiopaque medium for angiography and urography.

iothiouracil (-thi″o-u′rah-sil) a drug that inhibits thyroid activity.

I.P. intraperitoneally; isoelectric point.

I.P.A.A. International Psychoanalytical Association.

ipecac (ip′ĕ-kak) the dried rhizome and roots of *Cephaelis ipecacuanha* or *Cephaelis acuminata;* used as an emetic or expectorant.

ipomea (i″po-me′ah) the dried root of *Ipomaea orizabensis;* used as a cathartic.

IPPB intermittent positive pressure breathing.

Ipral (ip′ral) trademark for preparations of probarbital.

iproniazid (i″pro-ni′ah-zid) a psychic stimulant, $C_9H_{13}N_3O$.

ipsi- word element [L.], *same; self.*

ipsilateral (ip″sĭ-lat′er-al) situated on or affecting the same side.

I.Q. intelligence quotient.

Ir chemical symbol, *iridium.*

Ircon (ir′kon) trademark for a preparation of ferrous fumarate.

irid(o)- word element [Gr.], *iris of the eye; a colored circle.*

iridal (i′rĭ-dal) pertaining to the iris.

iridalgia (i″rĭ-dal′je-ah) pain in the iris.

iridauxesis (ir″id-awk-se′sis) thickening of the iris.

iridectomesodialysis (ir″ĭ-dek″to-me″so-di-al′-ĭ-sis) excision and separation of adhesions around the inner edge of the iris.

iridectomize (ir″ĭ-dek′to-mīz) to subject to iridectomy.

iridectomy (ir″ĭ-dek′to-me) excision of part of the iris.

iridectropium (ir″ĭ-dek-tro′pe-um) eversion of the iris.

iridemia (ir″ĭ-de′me-ah) hemorrhage from the iris.

iridencleisis (ir″ĭ-den-kli′sis) surgical incarcer-ation of a slip of the iris within a corneal or limbal incision to act as a wick for aqueous drainage in glaucoma.

iridentropium (ir″ĭ-den-tro′pe-um) inversion of the iris.

irideremia (ir″ĭ-der-e′me-ah) congenital absence of the iris.

irides (ir′ĭ-dēz) [Gr.] plural of *iris.*

iridescence (ir″ĭ-des′ens) the condition of gleaming with bright and changing colors. **irides′cent,** adj.

iridesis (i-rid′ĕ-sis) repositioning of the pupil by fixation of a sector of iris in a corneal or limbal incision.

iridic (i-rid′ik) pertaining to the iris.

iridium (ĭ-rid′e-um, i-rid′e-um) chemical element (*see table*), at. no. 77, symbol Ir.

iridoavulsion (ir″ĭ-do-ah-vul′shun) complete tearing away of the iris from its periphery.

iridocapsulitis (-kap″su-li′tis) inflammation of the iris and lens capsule.

iridocele (i-rid′o-sēl) hernial protrusion of part of the iris through the cornea.

iridochoroiditis (ir″i-do-ko″roi-di′tis) inflammation of the iris and choroid.

iridocoloboma (-kol″o-bo′mah) congenital fissure or coloboma of the iris.

iridoconstrictor (-kon-strik′tor) a muscle element or an agent which acts to constrict the pupil of the eye.

iridocyclectomy (-si-klek′to-me) excision of part of the iris and of the ciliary body.

iridocyclitis (-si-kli′tis) inflammation of the iris and ciliary body. **heterochromic i.,** a unilateral low-grade form leading to depigmentation of the iris of the affected eye.

iridocyclochoroiditis (-si″klo-ko″roi-di′tis) inflammation of the iris, ciliary body, and choroid.

iridocystectomy (-sis-tek′to-me) excision of part of the iris to form an artificial pupil.

iridodesis (ir″i-dod′e-sis) iridesis.

iridodialysis (ir″i-do-di-al′i-sis) the separation or loosening of the iris from its attachments.

iridodilator (-di-la′tor) a muscle element or an agent which acts to dilate the pupil of the eye.

iridodonesis (-do-ne′sis) tremulousness of the iris on movement of the eye, occurring in subluxation of the lens.

iridokeratitis (-ker″ah-ti′tis) inflammation of the iris and cornea.

iridokinesia, iridokinesis (-ki-ne′ze-ah; -ki-ne′sis) contraction and expansion of the iris. **iridokinet′ic,** adj.

iridoleptynsis (-lep-tin′sis) thinning or atrophy of the iris.

iridology (ir″i-dol′o-je) the study of the iris as associated with disease.

iridomalacia (ir″i-do-mah-la′she-ah) softening of the iris.

iridomesodialysis (-me″so-di-al′i-sis) surgical loosening of adhesions around the inner edge of the iris.

iridomotor (-mo′tor) pertaining to movements of the iris.

iridoncus (ir″i-dong′kus) tumor or swelling of the eye.

iridoparalysis (ir″i-do-pah-ral′i-sis) iridoplegia.

iridoperiphakitis (-per″i-fah-ki′tis) inflammation of the lens capsule.

iridoplegia (-ple′je-ah) paralysis of the sphincter of the iris.

iridoptosis (ir″i-dop-to′sis) prolapse of the iris.

iridopupillary (ir″i-do-pu′pĭ-ler′e) pertaining to the iris and pupil.

iridorhexis (-rek′sis) 1. rupture of the iris. 2. the tearing away of the iris.

iridoschisis (ir″i-dos′kĭ-sis) splitting of the mesodermal stroma of the iris into two layers, with fibrils of the anterior layer floating in the aqueous.

iridosclerotomy (ir″i-do-skle-rot′o-me) incision of the sclera and edge of the iris in glaucoma.

iridosteresis (-stĕ-re′sis) removal of all or part of the iris.

iridotasis (ir″i-dot′ah-sis) surgical stretching of the iris for glaucoma.

iridotomy (ir″i-dot′o-me) incision of the iris.

iris (i′ris) the circular pigmented membrane behind the cornea, perforated by the pupil. See Plate XIII.

iritis (i-ri′tis) inflammation of the iris. **irit′ic,** adj. **serous i.,** iritis with a serous exudate.

iritoectomy (ir″ĭ-to-ek′to-me) iridectomy.

iritomy (i-rit′o-me) iridotomy.

irium (ir′e-um) sodium lauryl sulfate.

iron (i′ern) chemical element (*see table*), at. no. 26, symbol Fe; it is an essential constituent of hemoglobin, cytochrome, and other components of respiratory enzyme systems. **i. choline citrate,** ferrocholinate. **i. gluconate,** ferrous gluconate. **i. protosulfate,** ferrous sulfate. **radioactive i.,** radioiron. **reduced i.,** finely powdered metallic iron obtained by precipitation with hydrogen from a solution of any soluble salt of iron.

Ironate (i′ron-āt) trademark for a preparation of ferrous sulfate.

Irosul (i′ro-sul) trademark for preparations of ferrous sulfate.

irotomy (i-rot′o-me) iridotomy.

irradiate (ĭ-ra′de-āt) to treat with radiant energy.

irradiation (ĭ-ra″de-a′shun) exposure to radiant energy (heat, light, roentgen rays, etc.) for therapeutic or diagnostic purposes.

irreducible (ir″re-doo′sĭ-b'l) not susceptible to reduction, as a fracture, hernia, or chemical substance.

irrigation (ir″i-ga′shun) washing by a stream of water or other fluid.

irritability (ir″i-tah-bil′i-te) the quality of being irritable. **myotatic i.,** the ability of a muscle to contract in response to stretching.

irritable (ir′i-tah-b'l) 1. capable of reacting to a stimulus. 2. abnormally sensitive to stimuli.

irritant (ir′i-tant) 1. causing irritation. 2. an agent causing irritation.

irritation (ir″i-ta′shun) 1. the act of stimulating. 2. a state of overexcitation and undue sensitivity. **ir′ritative,** adj.

IRV inspiratory reserve volume.

ischemia (is-ke′me-ah) deficiency of blood in a part, due to functional constriction or actual obstruction of a blood vessel. **ische′mic,** adj.

ischi(o)- word element [Gr.], *ischium.*

ischiadic (is″ke-ad′ik) ischiatic.

ischial (is′ke-al) ischiatic.

ischialgia (is″ke-al′je-ah) pain in the ischium.

ischiatic (is″ke-at′ik) pertaining to the ischium.

ischidrosis (is″kĭ-dro′sis) anhidrosis.

ischiobulbar (is″ke-o-bul′bar) pertaining to the ischium and the bulb of the urethra.

ischiocapsular (-kap′su-lar) pertaining to the ischium and the capsular ligament of the hip joint.

ischiocele (is′ke-o-sēl″) hernia through the sacrosciatic notch.

ischiococcygeal (is″ke-o-kok-sij′e-al) pertaining to the ischium and coccyx.

ischiodidymus (-did′ĭ-mus) conjoined twins united at the pelvis.

ischiodynia (-din′e-ah) pain in the ischium.

ischiofemoral (-fem′o-ral) pertaining to the ischium and femur.

ischiohebotomy (-he-bot′o-me) surgical division of the ischiopubic ramus and ascending ramus of the pubes.

ischiopagus (is″ke-op′ah-gus) conjoined twins fused at the ischial region.

ischiopubic (is″ke-o-pu′bik) pertaining to the ischium and pubes.

ischiorectal (-rek′tal) pertaining to ischium and rectum.

ischium (is′ke-um), pl. *is′chia* [L.] see *Table of Bones* and Plate II.

ischuria (is-ku′re-ah) retention or suppression of the urine. **ischuret′ic,** adj.

iseikonia (is″i-ko′ne-ah) iso-iconia. **iseikon′ic,** adj.

island (i′land) a cluster of cells or isolated piece of tissue. **blood i's,** aggregations of mesenchymal cells in the angioblast of the embryo, developing into vascular endothelium and blood cells. **i's of Langerhans,** irregular microscopic structures scattered throughout the pancreas, composed of alpha cells, which secrete glucagon; beta cells, which secrete insulin; and delta cells, which secrete gastrin. **i. of Reil,** insula.

islet (i′let) an island. **i's of Langerhans,** see under *island*. **Walthard's i's,** microscopic inclusions of the ovarian germinal epithelium, which have been implicated in the development of Brenner tumors.

Ismelin (is′me-lin) trademark for a preparation of guanethidine.

iso- word element [Gr.], *equal; alike; same.*

isoagglutinin (i″so-ah-gloo′tĭ-nin) an isoantigen that acts as an agglutinin.

isoalloxazine (-ah-lok′sah-zēn) an isomer of alloxazine from which riboflavin and other flavins are derived.

isoamyl nitrite (-am′il ni-trīt) amyl nitrite.

isoanaphylaxis (-an″ah-fi-lak′sis) anaphylaxis produced by serum from an individual of the same species.

isoantibody (-an″tĭ-bod′e) an antibody produced by one individual that reacts with isoantigens of another individual of the same species.

isoantigen (-an′tĭ-jen) an antigen existing in alternative (allelic) forms in a species, thus inducing an immune response when one form is transferred to members of the species who lack it; typical isoantigens are the blood group antigens.

isobar (i′so-bahr) 1. one of two or more chemical species with the same atomic weight but different atomic numbers. 2. a line on a map or chart depicting the boundries of an area of constant atmospheric pressure.

isobornyl thiocyanoacetate (i″so-bor′nil thi″-o-si″ah-no-as′ĕ-tāt) a pediculicide, $C_{13}H_{19}NO_2S$.

isobucaine (-bu′kān) a local anesthetic, $C_{15}H_{23}$-NO_2, used as the hydrochloride salt.

isocaloric (-kah-lo′rik) providing the same number of calories.

isocarboxazid (-kar-bok′sah-zid) an antidepressant, $C_{12}H_{13}N_3O_2$.

isocellular (-sel′u-lar) made up of identical cells.

isochromatic (-kro-mat′ik) of the same color throughout.

isochromatophil (-kro-mat′o-fil) staining equally with the same stain.

isochromosome (-kro′mo-sōm) an abnormal chromosome having a median centromere and two identical arms, formed by transverse, rather than normal longitudinal, splitting of a replicating chromosome.

isochronic, isochronous (-kron′ik; i-sok′ro-nus) performed in equal times; said of motions and vibrations occurring at the same time and being equal in duration.

isocoria (i″so-ko′re-ah) equality of size of the pupils of the two eyes.

isocortex (-kor′teks) neopallium.

isocytolysin (-si-tol′ĭ-sin) an isoantigen that acts as a cytolysin.

isocytosis (-si-to′sis) equality of size of cells, especially of erythrocytes.

isodactylism (-dak′tĭ-lizm) relatively even length of the fingers.

isodiametric (-di″ah-met′rik) measuring the same in all diameters.

isodontic (-don′tik) having all the teeth alike.

isodose (i′so-dōs) a radiation dose of equal intensity to more than one body area.

isoelectric (i″so-e-lek′trik) showing no variation in electric potential.

isoenergetic (-en″er-jet′ik) exhibiting equal energy.

isoenzyme (-en′zīm) one of the many forms in which a protein catalyst may exist in a single species, the various forms differing chemically, physically, and/or immunologically, but catalyzing the same reaction.

isoflurophate (-floo′ro-fāt) diisopropyl flurophosphate or diisopropyl phosphorofluoridate: an anticholinesterase, $C_6H_{14}FO_3P$, used topically as a miotic in glaucoma.

isogamety (-gam′ĕ-te) production by an individual of one sex of gametes identical with respect to the sex chromosome. **isogamet′ic,** adj.

isogamy (i-sog′ah-me) reproduction resulting from union of two gametes identical in size and structure, as in protozoa. **isog′amous,** adj.

isogeneic (i″so-jĕ-ne′ik) syngeneic.

isogeneric (-jĕ-ner′ik) of the same kind; belonging to the same species.

isogenesis (-jen′ĕ-sis) similarity in the processes of development.

isograft (i′so-graft) a graft between genetically identical individuals.

isohemagglutination (i″so-hem″ah-gloo″tĭ-na′-shun) agglutination of erythrocytes caused by an isohemagglutinin.

isohemagglutinin (-hem″ah-gloo′tĭ-nin) an isoantigen that agglutinates erythrocytes.

isohemolysin (-he-mol′ĭ-sin) an isoantigen that causes hemolysis.

isohemolysis (-he-mol′ĭ-sis) hemolysis produced by isohemolysin. **isohemolyt′ic,** adj.

isohypercytosis (-hi″per-si-to′sis) increase in the number of leukocytes with normal proportions of neutrophil cells.

isohypocytosis (-hi″po-si-to′sis) decrease in the number of leukocytes, with normal relation between the number of various forms.

iso-iconia (-i-ko′ne-ah) a condition in which the image of an object is the same in both eyes. **iso-icon′ic,** adj.

isoimmunization (-im″u-ni-za′shun) development of antibodies in response to isoantigens.

isolate (i′so-lāt) 1. to separate from others; to set apart. 2. a group of individuals prevented by geographic, genetic, ecologic, social, or artificial barriers from interbreeding with others of their kind.

isolation (i″so-la′shun) the act of isolating or state of being isolated, such as (a) the physiologic separation of a part, as by tissue culture or by interposition of inert material; (b) the segregation of patients with a communicable disease; (c) the successive propagation of a growth of microorganisms until a pure culture is obtained; (d) the chemical extraction of an unknown substance in pure form from a tissue; (e) the defensive failure to connect behavior with motives, or contradictory attitudes and behavior with each other.

isolecithal (-les′ĭ-thal) having a small amount of yolk evenly distributed throughout the cytoplasm of the ovum.

isoleucine (-lu′sēn) an amino acid produced by hydrolysis of fibrin and other proteins; essential for optimal infant growth and for nitrogen equilibrium in adults.

isologous (i-sol′o-gus) characterized by an identical genotype.

isolysin (i-sol′ĭ-sin) a lysin acting on cells of animals of the same species as that from which it is derived.

isolysis (i-sol′ĭ-sis) lysis of cells by isolysins. **isolyt′ic,** adj.

isomer (i′so-mer) any compound exhibiting, or capable of exhibiting isomerism. **isomer′ic,** adj.

isomerase (i-som′er-ās) a major class of enzymes comprising those that catalyze the process of isomerization.

isomerism (i-som′ĕ-rizm) the possession by two or more distinct compounds of the same molecular formula, each molecule having the same number of atoms of each element, but in different arrangement. **chain i.,** that in which the compounds differ in the linkages in the basic chain of carbon atoms. **geometric i.,** stereoisomerism said to be dependent upon some form of resticted rotation, enabling the molecular components to occupy different spatial positions. **optical i.,** stereoisomerism in which an appreciable number of molecules exhibit different effects on polarized light. **stereochemical i.,** stereoisomerism. **structural i.,** isomerism in which the compounds have the same molecular but different structural formula, the linkages of the atoms being different.

isomerization (i-som″er-i-za′shun) the process whereby any isomer is converted into another isomer, usually requiring special conditions of temperature, pressure, or catalysts.

isometheptene (i″so-meth′ep-tēn) a sympathomimetic, $C_9H_{19}N$, used as an antispasmodic and vasoconstrictor.

isometric (-met′rik) maintaining, or pertaining to, the same measure of length; of equal dimensions.

isometropia (-mĕ-tro′pe-ah) equality in refraction of the two eyes.

isomorphism (-mor′fizm) identity in form; in genetics, referring to genotypes of polyploid organisms which produce similar gametes even though containing genes in different combinations on homologous chromosomes. **isomor′phous,** adj.

isoniazid (-ni′ah-zid) a tuberculostatic, C_6H_7-N_3O.

isonicotinoylhydrazine (-nik″o-tin″o-il-hi′-drah-zēn) isoniazid.

isopathy (i-sop′ah-the) the treatment of disease by means of products of the disease or with material from the affected organ. **isopath′ic,** adj.

isophoria (i″so-fo′re-ah) equality in the tension of the vertical muscles of each eye.

Isophrine (i′so-frin) trademark for a preparation of phenylephrine.

isoprecipitin (i″so-pre-sip′ĭ-tin) an isoantingen that acts as a precipitin.

isoprenaline (-pren′ah-lēn) isoproterenol.

isopropamide iodide (-pro′pah-mīd) an anticholinergic, $C_{23}H_{33}IN_2O$, used as an antisecretory and antispasmodic in gastrointestinal disorders.

isopropanol (-pro′pah-nol) isopropyl alcohol.

isoproterenol (-pro″tĕ-re′nol) a sympathomimetic, $C_{11}H_{17}NO_3$, used chiefly, in the form of the hydrochloride and sulfate salts, as a bronchodilator.

isopter (i-sop′ter) a curve representing areas of equal visual acuity in the field of vision.

isopyknosis (i″so-pik-no′sis) the quality of showing uniform density throughout, especially the uniformity of condensation observed in comparison of different chromosomes or in different areas of the same chromosome. **isopyknot′ic,** adj.

Isordil (i′sor-dil) trademark for preparations of isosorbide dinitrate.

isorrhea (i″so-re′ah) an equilibrium between the intake and output, by the body, of water and solutes. **isorrhe′ic,** adj.

isosexual (-sek′su-al) pertaining to or characteristic of the same sex.

isosmotic (i″sos-mot′ik) having the same osmotic pressure.

isosorbide (i″so-sor′bīd) an osmotic diuretic, $C_6H_{10}O_4$; the dinitrate of isosorbide is used as a coronary vasodilator in coronary insufficiency and angina pectoris.

Isospora (i-sos′po-rah) a genus of sporozoan parasites (order Coccidia), found in birds, amphibians, reptiles, and various mammals, including man; *I. bel′li* and *I. hom′inis* cause coccidiosis in man.

isospore (i'so-spōr) 1. an isogamete of organisms that reproduce by spores. 2. an asexual spore produced by a homosporous organism.

isosthenuria (i″sos-thĕ-nu're-ah) maintenance of a constant osmolality of the urine, regardless of changes in osmotic pressure of the blood.

isotherapy (i″so-ther'ah-pe) isopathy.

isotherm (i'so-therm) a line on a map or chart depicting the boundaries of an area in which the temperature is the same.

isothermal, isothermic (i″so-ther'mal; -ther'-mik) having the same temperature.

isotone (i'so-tōn) one of several nuclides having the same number of neutrons, but differing in number of protons in their nuclei.

isotonia (i″so-to'ne-ah) 1. a condition of equal tone, tension, or acitivity. 2. equality of osmotic pressure between two elements of a solution or between two different solutions.

isotonic (-ton'ik) 1. of equal tension. 2. denoting a solution in which body cells can be bathed without net flow of water across the semipermeable cell membrane; also, denoting a solution having the same tonicity as another solution with which it is compared.

isotope (i'so-tōp) a chemical element having the same atomic number as another (i.e., the same number of nuclear protons), but having a different atomic mass (i.e., a different number of nuclear neutrons). **radioactive i.,** radioisotope. **stable i.,** one that does not transmute into another element with emission of corpuscular or electromagnetic radiations.

isotropic (i″so-trop'ik) 1. having like properties in all directions, as in a cubic crystal or a piece of glass. 2. being singly refractive.

isotropy (i-sot'ro-pe) the quality or condition of being isotropic.

isotypical (i″so-tip'e-kal) of the same type.

isoxsuprine (i-sok'su-prēn) a vasodilator, C_{18}-$H_{23}NO_3$, used as the hydrochloride salt.

isozyme (i'so-zīm) isoenzyme.

issue (ish'ū) a discharge of pus, blood, or other matter; a suppurating lesion emitting such a discharge.

isthmectomy (is-mek'to-me) excision of an isthmus, especially the isthmus of the thyroid.

isthmoparalysis (is″mo-pah-ral'ĭ-sis) isthmoplegia.

isthmoplegia (-ple'je-ah) paralysis of the isthmus of the fauces.

isthmus (is'mus) a narrow connection between two larger bodies or parts. **is'thmian,** adj. **i. of auditory tube, i. of eustachian tube,** the narrowest part of the auditory tube at the junction of its bony and cartilaginous parts. **i. of fauces,** the constricted aperture between the cavity of the mouth and the pharynx. **i. of rhombencephalon,** the narrow segment of the fetal brain, forming the plane of separation between the rhombencephalon and cerebrum. **i. of thyroid,** the band of tissue joining the lobes of the thyroid. **i. of uterine tube,** the narrower, thicker-walled portion of the uterine tube closest to the uterus. **i. of uterus,** the constricted part of the uterus between the cervix and the body of the uterus.

Isuprel (i'su-prel) trademark for a preparation of isoproterenol.

isuria (i-su're-ah) excretion of urine at a uniform rate.

itch (ich) a skin disorder attended with itching. **Aujesky's i.,** pseudorabies. **bakers' i.,** any of several inflammatory dermatoses of the hands, especially chronic monilial paronychia, seen with special frequency in bakers. **barbers' i.,** sycosis barbae. **copra i.,** a dermatitis affecting coconut workers, caused by a mite. **dew i.,** ground i. **dhobie i.,** allergic contact dermatitis due to the catechols in the marking fluid used on laundry by native washermen (dhobie) of India. **foot i.,** ground i. **grain i.,** itching dermatitis due to a mite, *Pyemotes ventricosus,* which preys on certain insect larvae which live on straw, grain, and other plants. **grocers' i.,** a vesicular dermatitis caused by certain mites found in stored hides, dried fruits, grain, copra, and cheese. **ground i.,** the itching eruption caused by the entrance into the skin of the larvae of *Ancylostoma duodenale* or *Necator americanus;* see *hookworm disease.* **jock i.,** tinea cruris. **mad i.,** pseudorabies. **millers' i.,** grain i. **miners' i.,** ground i. **seven-year i.,** scabies. **straw i.,** grain i. **swimmers' i.,** an itching dermatitis due to penetration into the skin of larval forms (cercaria) of schistosomes, occurring in bathers in waters infested with these organisms. **winter i.,** itching of the skin in cold weather, unassociated with structural lesions.

itching (ich'ing) pruritus; an unpleasant cutaneous sensation, provoking the desire to scratch or rub the skin.

iter (i'ter) a tubular passage. **i'teral,** adj. **i. ad infundib'ulum,** the passage from the third ventricle of the brain to the infundibulum (1). **i. den'tium,** the passage through which a permanent tooth erupts through the gums. **i. e ter'tio ad quar'tum ventric'ulum,** cerebral aqueduct.

iteroparity (it″er-o-par'ĭ-te) the state, in an individual organism, of reproducing repeatedly, or more than once in a lifetime. **iterop'arous,** adj.

-itis, pl. **it'ides.** Word element [Gr.], *inflammation.*

ITP idiopathic thrombocytopenic purpura.

Itrumil (it'roo-mil) trademark for a preparation of iothiouracil.

I.U. immunizing unit; international unit.

IUCD intrauterine contraceptive device.

IUD intrauterine contraceptive device.

I.V. intravenously.

I.V.T. intravenous transfusion.

Ixodes (iks-o'dēz) a genus of parasitic ticks (family Ixodidae); some species are disease vectors.

ixodiasis (ik″so-di'ah-sis) any disease or lesion due to tick bites; infestation with ticks.

ixodic (ik-sod'ik) pertaining to or caused by ticks.

Ixodidae (iks-od'ĭ-de) a family of ticks (superfamily Ixodoidea), comprising the hard-bodied ticks.

Ixodides (iks-od′ĭ-dēz) the ticks, a suborder of Acarina, including the superfamily Ixodoidea.
Ixodoidea (iks″o-doi′de-ah) a superfamily of arthropods (suborder Ixodides), comprising both the hard- and soft-bodied ticks.

J

J symbol, *Joule's equivalent.*

jacket (jak′et) an enveloping structure or garment for the trunk or upper part of the body. **plaster-of-Paris j.,** a casing of plaster of Paris enveloping the body, for the purpose of giving support or correcting deformities. **Sayre's j.,** a plaster-of-Paris jacket used as a support for the vertebral column. **strait j.,** see *straitjacket.*

jackscrew (jak′skroo) a device operated by means of a screw to expand the dental arch and move individual teeth.

jactitation (jak″tĭ-ta′shun) restless tossing to and fro in acute illness.

janiceps (jan′ĭ-seps) a double monster with one head and two opposite faces.

jaundice (jawn′dis) icterus; yellowness of the skin, sclerae, and excretions due to hyperbilirubinemia and deposition of bile pigments. **acholuric j.,** jaundice without bilirubinemia, associated with elevated unconjugated bilirubin that is not excreted by the kidney. **acholuric familial j.,** hereditary spherocytosis. **acute febrile j., acute infectious j.,** infectious hepatitis. **cholestatic j.,** that resulting from abnormality of bile flow in the liver. **hematogenous j., hemolytic j.,** jaundice associated with hemolytic anemia. **hemorrhagic j.,** leptospiral j. **hepatocellular j.,** that due to injury to or disease of liver cells. **hepatogenic j., hepatogenous j.,** that due to disease or disorder of the liver. **homologous serum j.,** serum hepatitis. **infectious j., infective j.,** 1. infectious hepatitis. 2. leptospiral j. **leptospiral j.,** severe leptospirosis with fever, jaundice, myalgia, and occasionally meningitis and nephritis. **malignant j.,** acute yellow atrophy. **mechanical j.,** obstructive j. **j. of the newborn,** icterus neonatorum. **nonhemolytic j.,** that due to an abnormality in bilirubin metabolism. **nuclear j.,** kernicterus. **obstructive j.,** that due to blocking of bile flow. **physiologic j.,** mild icterus neonatorum lasting the first few days of life. **retention j.,** that due to inability of the liver to dispose of the bilirubin provided by the circulating blood. **spirochetal j.,** leptospiral j.

jaw (jaw) either of the two bony structures (mandible and maxilla) in the head of dentate vertebrates, bearing the teeth and enabling carnivores to seize their prey and others to bite and chew. **Hapsburg j.,** a mandibular prognathous jaw, often accompanied by Hapsburg lip. **lumpy j.,** actinomycosis of cattle. **phossy j.,** phosphonecrosis. **rubber j.,** a softened condition of the jaw in animals, due to resorption and replacement of the bone by fibrous tissue, occurring in association with renal osteodystrophy.

jejunectomy (jĕ″joo-nek′to-me) excision of the jejunum.

jejunitis (-ni′tis) inflammation of the jejunum.

jejunocecostomy (jĕ-joo″no-se-kos′to-me) anastomosis of the jejunum to the cecum.

jejunocolostomy (-ko-los′to-me) anastomosis of the jejunum to the colon.

jejunoileitis (-il″e-i′tis) inflammation of the jejunum and ileum.

jejunoileostomy (-il″e-os′to-me) surgical anastomosis of the jejunum to the ileum.

jejunojejunostomy (-jĕ″joo-nos′to-me) surgical anastomosis between two portions of the jejunum.

jejunorrhaphy (jĕ″joo-nor′ah-fe) operative repair of the jejunum.

jejunostomy (-nos′to-me) the creation of a permanent opening between the jejunum and the surface of the abdominal wall.

jejunotomy (-not′o-me) incision of the jejunum.

jejunum (jĕ-joo′num) that part of the small intestine extending from the duodenum to the ileum. **jeju′nal,** adj.

jelly (jel′e) a soft, coherent, resilient substance; generally, a colloidal semisolid mass. **cardiac j.,** a jelly present between the endothelium and myocardium of the embryonic heart that transforms into the connective tissue of the endocardium. **contraceptive j.,** a nongreasy jelly used in the vagina for prevention of conception. **enamel j.,** stellate reticulum. **petroleum j.,** petrolatum. **Wharton's j.,** the soft, jelly-like intracellular substance of the umbilical cord.

jerk (jerk) a sudden reflex or involuntary movement. **Achilles j., ankle j.,** triceps surae j. **biceps j.,** see under *reflex.* **elbow j.,** involuntary flexion of the elbow on striking the tendon of the biceps or triceps muscle. **jaw j.,** see under *reflex.* **knee j.,** a kick reflex produced by sharply tapping the patellar ligament. **tendon j.,** see under *reflex.* **triceps surae j.,** plantar flexion of the foot elicited by a tap on the Achilles tendon, preferably while the patient kneels on a bed or chair, the feet hanging free over the edge.

joint (joint) the site of junction or union between two or more bones, especially one that admits of motion of one or more bones. **amphidiarthrodial j.,** amphidiarthrosis. **arthrodial j.,** plane j. **ball-and-socket j.,** spheroidal j. **biaxial j.,** one with two chief axes of movement, at right angles to each other. **bilocular j.,** one with two synovial compartments separated by an interarticular cartilage. **Brodie's j.,** hysteric j. **cartilaginous j.,** one in which the bones are united by cartilage. **Charcot's j.,** see under *arthropathy.* **Chopart's j.,** one between the calcaneus and the cuboid bone and the talus and navicular bone. **cochlear j.,** a form of hinge joint which permits of some rotation or lateral motion. **composite j., compound j.,** one in which several bones articulate. **condyloid j.,** one in which an ovoid head of one bone moves in an elliptical cavity of another, permitting all movements except axial rotation. **diarthrodial j.,** synovial j. **elbow j.,** the articulation between the humerus, ulna, and radius. **ellipsoidal j.,** one resembling a spheroidal joint, but having an ellipsoidal articular surface. **enarthrodial j.,** spheroidal j. **false j.,** pseudarthrosis. **fibrocartilaginous j.,** symphysis. **fibrous j.,** one in which the bones are united by fibrous tissue. **flail j.,** an unusually mobile joint. **ginglymoid j.,** ginglymus. **gliding j.,** plane j. **hinge j.,** ginglymus. **hip j.,** the spheroidal joint between the head of the femur and the acetabulum of the hip bone. **hysteric j.,** a condition resembling arthritis, but of psychic origin. **immovable j.,** fibrous j. **intercarpal j's,** the articulations between the carpal bones. **irritable j.,** one subject to attacks of inflammation without known cause. **knee j.,** the compound joint between the femur, patella, and tibia. **Lisfranc's j.,** the articulation between the tarsal and metatarsal bones. **mixed j.,** one combining features of different types of joints. **multiaxial j.,** spheroidal j. **pivot j.,** a uniaxial joint in which one bone pivots within a bony or an osseoligamentous ring. **plane j.,** a synovial joint in which the opposed surfaces are flat or only slightly curved. **polyaxial j.,** spheroidal j. **rotary j.,** pivot j. **saddle j.,** one having two saddle-shaped surfaces at right angles to each other. **simple j.,** one in which only two bones articulate. **spheroidal j.,** a synovial joint in which a spheroidal surface on one bone ("ball") moves within a concavity ("socket") on the other bone. **spiral j.,** cochlear j. **stifle j.,** the articulation in quadrupeds corresponding with the knee joint of man, consisting of two joints, one between the femur and tibia and one between the femur and patella. **synarthrodial j.,** fibrous j. **synovial j.,** a special form of articulation permitting more or less free motion, the union of the bony elements being surrounded by an articular capsule enclosing a cavity lined by synovial membrane. **trochoid j.,** pivot j. **uniaxial j.,** one which permits movement in one axis only. **unilocular j.,** a synovial joint having only one cavity.

joule (jōōl) the SI unit of energy, being the work done by a force of one newton acting over a distance of one meter.

jugal (joo′gal) pertaining to the cheek.

jugale (joo-ga′le) jugal point.

jugular (jug′u-lar) 1. pertaining to the neck. 2. the jugular vein.

jugum (joo′gum), pl. *ju′ga* [L.] a depression or ridge connecting two structures. **j. pe′nis,** a forceps for compressing the penis.

juice (jōōs) any fluid from animal or plant tissue. **gastric j.,** the liquid secretion of the gastric glands. **intestinal j.,** the liquid secretion of glands in the intestinal lining. **pancreatic j.,** the enzyme-containing secretion of the pancreas, conducted through its ducts to the duodenum. **prostatic j.,** the liquid secretion of the prostate, which contributes to semen formation.

jumping (jump′ing) Gilles de la Tourette's syndrome.

junction (junk′shun) the place of meeting or coming together. **junc′tional,** adj. **amelodentinal j.,** dentinoenamel j. **dentinocemental j.,** the line of meeting of the dentin and cementum on the root of a tooth. **dentinoenamel j.,** the plane of meeting between dentin and enamel on the crown of a tooth. **mucogingival j.,** the histologically distinct line marking the separation of the gingival tissue from the oral mucosa. **myoneural j.,** the site of junction of a nerve fiber with the muscle it innervates. **sclerocorneal j.,** the line of union of the sclera and cornea.

junctura (junk-tu′rah), pl. *junctu′rae* [L.] a junction or joint.

jurisprudence (jōōr″is-proo′dens) the science of the law. **medical j.,** the science of the law as applied to the practice of medicine.

jury-mast (jōōr′e mast) upright bar used in supporting the head in cases of tuberculosis of the spine (Pott's disease).

juvenile (ju′vĕ-nīl) 1. pertaining to youth or childhood; young or immature. 2. a youth or child; a young animal.

juxta-articular (juks″tah-ar-tik′u-lar) near or in the region of a joint.

juxtaglomerular (-glo-mer′u-lar) near to or adjoining a glomerulus of the kidney.

juxtaposition (-po-zish′un) apposition.

juxtapyloric (-pi-lor′ik) near the pylorus.

juxtaspinal (-spi′nal) near the spinal column.

K

K chemical symbol, *potassium* (L. *kalium*).

K. cathode; Kelvin (scale).

Ka (*Kathode*) cathode.

kak- for words beginning thus, see those beginning *cac-*.

kakosmia (kak-oz'me-ah) cacosmia.

kala-azar (kah"lah-ah-zar') a highly fatal infectious disease endemic in the tropics and subtropics, caused by *Leishmania donovani*, and marked by fever, anemia, wasting, splenomegaly, and hepatomegaly.

kalemia (kah-le'me-ah) the presence of potassium in the blood.

kaliemia (ka"le-e'me-ah) kalemia.

kaligenous (kah-lij'ĕ-nus) producing potash.

kalimeter (kah-lim'ĕ-ter) alkalimeter.

kaliopenia (ka"le-o-pe'ne-ah) hypokalemia. kaliope'nic, adj.

kalium (ka'le-um) [L.] potassium (symbol K).

kaliuresis (ka"le-u-re'sis) excretion of potassium in the urine.

kaliuretic (-ret'ik) 1. pertaining to or promoting kaliuresis. 2. a kaliuretic agent.

kallak (kal'ak) a pustular dermatitis occurring among Eskimos.

kallidin (kal'lĭ-din) a kinin liberated by the action of kallikrein on a plasma globulin. Kallidin I is the same as bradykinin.

kallikrein (kal"lĭ-kre'in) one of a group of enzymes present in plasma, various glands, urine, and lymph, the major action of which is liberation of kinins from α-2-globulins.

kallikreinogen (-kri'no-jen) the inactive precursor of kallikrein which is normally present in blood.

kanamycin (kan"ah-mi'sin) a broad-spectrum antibiotic derived from *Streptomyces kanamyceticus*.

Kantrex (kan'treks) trademark for preparations of kanamycin.

kaolin (ka'o-lin) native hydrated aluminum silicate, powdered and freed from gritty particles by elutriation; used as an absorbent and in kaolin mixture with pectin.

kaolinosis (ka"o-lin-o'sis) pneumoconiosis from inhaling particles of kaolin.

Kappadione (kap"pah-di'ōn) trademark for preparation of menadiol sodium diphosphate.

karyo- word element [Gr.], *nucleus*.

karyochrome (kar'e-o-krōm") a nerve cell the nucleus of which is deeply stainable, while the body is not.

karyocyte (kar'e-o-sīt") a nucleated cell.

karyogamy (kar"e-og'ah-me) cell conjugation with union of nuclei.

karyogenesis (kar"e-o-jen'ĕ-sis) the formation of a cell nucleus. karyogen'ic, adj.

karyokinesis (-ki-ne'sis) division of the nucleus, usually an early stage in the process of cell division, or mitosis. karyokinet'ic, adj.

karyoklasis (kar"e-ok'lah-sis) the breaking

down of the cell nucleus or nuclear membrane. karyoklas'tic, adj.

karyolymph (kar'e-o-limf") the liquid portion of the nucleus of a cell, in which the other elements are dispersed.

karyolysis (kar"e-ol'ĭ-sis) the dissolution of the nucleus of a cell. karyolyt'ic, adj.

karyomegaly (kar"e-o-meg'ah-le) abnormal enlargement of a cell nucleus.

karyomere (kar'e-o-mēr") 1. chromomere (1). 2. a vesicle containing only a small portion of the typical nucleus, usually after abnormal mitosis.

karyomitome (kar"e-om'ĭ-tōm) nuclear chromatin network.

karyomitosis (kar"e-o-mi-to'sis) division of the cell nucleus preceding mitosis.

karyomorphism (-mor'fizm) the shape of a cell nucleus.

karyon (kar'e-on) the nucleus of a cell.

karyophage (kar'e-o-fāj") a protozoon that phagocytizes the nucleus of the cell it infects.

karyoplasm (-plazm") nucleoplasm.

karyopyknosis (kar"e-o-pik-no'sis) shrinkage of a cell nucleus, with condensation of the chromatin. karyopyknot'ic, adj.

karyorrhexis (-rek'sis) rupture of the cell nucleus in which the chromatin disintegrates into formless granules that are extruded from the cell. karyorrhec'tic, adj.

karyosome (kar'e-o-sōm") any of the condensed irregular clumps of chromatin dispersed in the chromatin network of a cell.

karyostasis (kar"e-os'tah-sis) the so-called resting stage of the nucleus between mitotic divisions.

karyotype (kar'e-o-tīp") the chromosomal constitution of the cell nucleus; by extension, the photomicrograph of chromosomes arranged according to the Denver classification.

kat(a)- word element [Gr.], *down; against*. See also words beginning *cat(a)-*.

katathermometer (kat"ah-ther-mom'ĕ-ter) a thermometer with a wet bulb and a dry bulb, for detecting cooling rates.

kc. kilocycle.

kc.p.s. kilocycles per second.

keloid (ke'loid) a sharply elevated, irregularly shaped, progressively enlarging scar due to excessive collagen formation in the corium during connective tissue repair. keloid'al, adj. Addison's k., morphea.

kelosomus (ke"lo-so'mus) celosomus.

Kemadrin (kem'ah-drin) trademark for a preparation of procyclidine.

Kenacort (ken'ah-kort) trademark for preparations of triamcinolone.

Kenalog (-ah-log) trademark for preparations of triamcinolone acetonide.

keno- word element [Gr.], *empty*.

kenotoxin (ke"no-tok'sin) the toxin of fatigue,

thought to be produced by muscular contractions.

kerasin (ker′ah-sin) a cerebroside from brain tissue, yielding galactose, sphingosine, and lignoceric acid on hydrolysis.

kerat(o)- word element [Gr.], *horny tissue; cornea.*

keratalgia (ker″ah-tal′je-ah) pain in the cornea.

keratectasia (ker″ah-tek-ta′ze-ah) protrusion of a thinned, scarred cornea.

keratectomy (ker″ah-tek′to-me) excision of a portion of the cornea.

keratic (kĕ-rat′ik) 1. pertaining to keratin. 2. pertaining to the cornea.

keratin (ker′ah-tin) a scleroprotein that is the main constituent of epidermis, hair, nails, horny tissues, and the organic matrix of tooth enamel.

keratinase (-ās″) a proteolytic enzyme that hydrolyzes keratin.

keratinization (ker″ah-tin″i-za′shun) the development of or conversion into keratin.

keratinocyte (kĕ-rat′ĭ-no-sīt) the epidermal cell that synthesizes keratin, known in its successive stages in the layers of the skin as basal cell, prickle cell, and granular cell.

keratinous (kĕ-rat′ĭ-nus) containing or of the nature of keratin.

keratitis (ker″ah-ti′tis) inflammation of the cornea. **k. bullo′sa,** presence of large or small blebs upon the cornea. **dendritic k.,** herpetic keratitis which results in a branching ulceration of the cornea. **herpetic k.,** 1. keratitis, commonly with dendritic ulceration, due to infection with herpes simplex virus. 2. keratitis occurring in herpes zoster ophthalmicus. **interstitial k.,** chronic keratitis with deep deposits in the cornea, which becomes hazy. **lattice k.,** bilateral hereditary corneal dystrophy with formation of interwoven filamentous lesions. **neuroparalytic k.,** that due to injury to the trifacial nerve which prevents proper closing of the eyelids, marked by dryness and fissuring of the corneal epithelium. **phlyctenular k.,** see under *keratoconjunctivitis.* **punctate k.,** that marked by discrete punctate opacities. **sclerosing k.,** keratitis with scleritis. **trachomatous k.,** pannus trachomatosus.

keratoacanthoma (ker″ah-to-ak″an-tho′mah) a rapidly growing benign papular lesion, with a crater filled with a keratin plug; it resolves spontaneously.

keratocele (ker′ah-to-sēl″) hernial protrusion of Descemet's membrane.

keratocentesis (ker″ah-to-sen-te′sis) puncture of the cornea.

keratoconjunctivitis (-kon-junk″tĭ-vi′tis) inflammation of the cornea and conjunctiva. **epidemic k.,** a highly infectious form, commonly with regional lymph node involvement, occurring in epidemics; an adenovirus has been repeatedly isolated from affected patients. **phlyctenular k.,** a form marked by formation of a small, gray, circumscribed lesion at the corneal limbus. **k. sic′ca,** a condition marked by hyperemia of the conjunctiva, thickening and drying of the corneal epithelium, itching and

burning of the eye and, often, reduced visual acuity. **viral k.,** epidemic k.

keratoconus (-ko′nus) conical protrusion of the central part of the cornea.

keratoderma (-der′mah) hypertrophy of the horny layer of the skin. **k. blennorrha′gicum,** pustular psoriasis associated with gonorrhea. **k. climacter′icum, endocrine k.,** circumscribed hyperkeratosis of palms and soles, occurring in menopausal women.

keratodermia (-der′me-ah) keratoderma.

keratogenous (ker″ah-toj′ĕ-nus) giving rise to a growth of horny material.

keratoglobus (ker″ah-to-glo′bus) a bilateral anomaly in which the cornea is enlarged and globular in shape.

keratohelcosis (-hel-ko′sis) ulceration of the cornea.

keratohemia (-he′me-ah) deposition of blood in the cornea.

keratohyalin (-hi′ah-lin) granules in the stratum granulosum of the epidermis. **keratohy′aline,** adj.

keratoid (ker′ah-toid) resembling horn or corneal tissue.

keratoiridoscope (ker″ah-to-i-rid′o-skōp) a compound microscope for examining the eye.

keratoiritis (-i-ri′tis) inflammation of the cornea and iris.

keratoleptynsis (-lep-tin′sis) removal of the anterior portion of the cornea and replacement with bulbar conjunctiva.

keratoleukoma (-lu-ko′mah) a white opacity of the cornea.

keratolysis (ker″ah-tol′ĭ-sis) loosening or separation of the horny layer of the epidermis. **pitted k., k. planta′re sulca′tum,** a tropical disease marked by thickening and deep fissuring of the skin of the soles, occurring during the rainy season.

keratolytic (ker″ah-to-lit′ik) 1. pertaining to or promoting keratolysis. 2. an agent that promotes keratolysis.

keratoma (ker″ah-to′mah) keratosis.

keratomalacia (ker″ah-to-mah-la′she-ah) softening and necrosis of the cornea associated with vitamin A deficiency.

keratome (ker′ah-tōm) a knife for incising the cornea.

keratometer (ker″ah-tom′ĕ-ter) an instrument for measuring the curves of the cornea.

keratometry (ker″ah-tom′ĕ-tre) measurement of corneal curves. **keratomet′ric,** adj.

keratomycosis (ker″ah-to-mi-ko′sis) fungal infection of the cornea. **k. lin′guae,** black tongue.

keratonyxis (-nik′sis) keratocentesis.

keratopathy (ker″ah-top′ah-the) noninflammatory disease of the cornea. **band k.,** a condition characterized by an abnormal gray circumcorneal band.

keratoplasty (ker′ah-to-plas″te) plastic surgery of the cornea; corneal grafting. **optic k.,** transplantation of corneal material to replace scar tissue which interferes with vision. **tectonic k.,** transplantation of corneal material to replace tissue which has been lost.

keratorhexis (ker″ah-to-rek′sis) rupture of the cornea.

keratoscleritis (-skle-ri′tis) inflammation of the cornea and sclera.

keratoscope (ker′ah-to-skōp″) an instrument for examining the cornea.

keratoscopy (ker″ah-tos′ko-pe) inspection of the cornea.

keratosis (ker″ah-to′sis) any horny growth, such as a wart or callosity. **keratot′ic,** adj. **actinic k.,** a sharply outlined verrucous or keratotic growth, which may develop into a cutaneous horn, and may become malignant; it usually occurs in the middle aged or elderly and is due to excessive exposure to the sun. **k. blennor-rha′gica,** keratoderma blennorrhagicum. **k. follicula′ris,** a hereditary form marked by areas of crusting, itching, verrucous papular growths. **gonorrheal k.,** keratoderma blennorrhagicum. **k. lin′guae,** leukoplakia of the tongue. **k. palma′ris et planta′ris,** congenital, hereditary thickening of the skin of the palms and soles, sometimes with painful lesions resulting from fissuring; often associated with other anomalies. **k. pila′ris,** hyperkeratosis limited to the hair follicles. **k. pharyn′gea,** horny projections from the tonsils and pharyngeal walls. **k. puncta′ta,** a hereditary hyperkeratosis in which the lesions are localized in multiple points on the palms and soles. **sebor-rheic k., k. seborrhe′ica,** a benign, noninvasive tumor of epidermal origin, marked by numerous yellow or brown, sharply marginated, oval, raised lesions. **senile k., solar k.,** actinic k.

keratotomy (ker″ah-tot′o-me) incision of the cornea.

keratotorus (ker″ah-to-to′rus) a vaultlike protrusion of the cornea.

kerectomy (kĕ-rek′to-me) keratectomy.

kerion (ke′re-on) a boggy, exudative tumefaction covered with pustules.

kernicterus (ker-nik′ter-us) a condition with severe neural symptoms, associated with high levels of bilirubin in the blood.

ketamine (kēt′ah-mēn) a rapid-acting general anesthetic, $C_{13}H_{16}ClNO.$

keto- word element, *ketone group.*

ketoacidosis (ke″to-ah″sĭ-do′sis) acidosis due to accumulation of ketone bodies.

ketoaciduria (-as″ĭ-du′re-ah) excretion of an excess of ketonic acid in the urine.

ketogenesis (-jen′ĕ-sis) the production of ketone bodies. **ketogenet′ic,** adj.

ketogenic (-jen′ik) forming or capable of being converted into ketone bodies.

ketolysis (ke-tol′ĭ-sis) the splitting up of ketone bodies. **ketolyt′ic,** adj.

ketone (ke′tōn) any compound containing the carbonyl group, CO, and having hydrocarbon groups attached to the carbonyl carbon. See also under *body.*

ketonemia (ke″to-ne′me-ah) an excess of ketone bodies in the blood.

ketonuria (-nu′re-ah) an excess of ketone bodies in the urine.

ketose (ke′tōs) any sugar that contains a ketone group.

ketosis (ke-to′sis) accumulation of excessive amounts of ketone bodies in body tissues and fluids. **ketot′ic,** adj.

ketosteroid (ke″to-stēr′oid) a steroid having ketone groups on functional carbon atoms. The *17-ketosteroids* found in normal urine and in excess in certain tumors, have a ketone group on the 17th carbon atom, and include certain androgenic and adrenocortical hormones.

ketosuria (-su′re-ah) ketose in the urine.

kev kilo (1000) electron volts (3.82×10^{-17} gram-calories, or 1.6×10^{-9} ergs).

kg. kilogram.

kg.-m. kilogram-meter.

khellin (kel′in) an active principle of the fruit of the plant *Ammi visnaga,* used as a coronary vasodilator and bronchodilator.

kHz kilohertz.

kidney (kid′ne) either of the two organs in the lumbar region that filter the blood, excreting the end-products of body metabolism in the form of urine, and regulating the concentrations of hydrogen, sodium, potassium, phosphate, and other ions in the extracellular fluid. **amyloid k.,** one marked by deposition of amyloid. **artificial k.,** an extracorporeal device through which blood may be circulated for removal of elements that normally are excreted in the urine; a hemodialyzer. **cake k.,** a solid, irregularly lobed organ of bizarre shape, formed by fusion of the two renal anlagen. **cicatricial k.,** a shriveled, irregular, and scarred kidney due to suppurative pyelonephritis. **contracted k.,** an atrophic kidney which may be scarred and granular. **fatty k.,** one affected with fatty degeneration. **flea-bitten k.,** one with small, randomly scattered petechiae on its surface. **floating k.,** hypermobile k. **fused k.,** a single anomalous organ developed as a result of fusion of the renal anlagen. **Goldblatt k.,** one with obstruction of its blood flow, resulting in renal hypertension. **head k.,** pronephros. **horseshoe k.,** an anomalous organ resulting from fusion of the corresponding poles of the renal anlagen. **hypermobile k.,** one that is freely movable. **lump k.,** cake k. **middle k.,** mesonephros. **pelvic k.,** one displaced into the pelvis. **polycystic k.,** a hereditary congenital condition marked by bilateral multiple renal cysts. **primordial k.,** pronephros. **sigmoid k.,** a deformed and fused kidney, the upper pole of one kidney being fused with the lower pole of the other. **sponge k.,** a congenital condition in which multiple small cystic dilatations of the collecting tubules of the medullary portion of the renal pyramids give the organ a spongy, porous feeling and appearance. **wandering k.,** hypermobile k. **waxy k.,** amyloid k.

kilo- word element [Gr.], *one thousand* (10^3), used in naming units of measurement.

kilocalorie (kil′o-kal″o-re) large calorie.

kilocycle (-si′k′l) a unit of 1000 (10^3) cycles; e.g., 1000 cycles per second; applied to the frequency of electromagnetic waves.

kilogram (-gram) a unit of mass (weight) of the

metric system, 1000 grams; equivalent to 15,432 grains, or 2.205 pounds (avoirdupois) or 2.679 pounds (apothecaries' weight).

kilogram-meter (-gram-me'ter) a unit of work, representing the energy required to raise 1 kg. of weight 1 meter vertically against gravitational force, equivalent to about 7.2 foot pounds and to 1000 gram-meters.

kilohertz (-hertz) one thousand (10³) hertz; abbreviated kHz.

kiloliter (-le''ter) 1000 liters, 264.18 gallons.

kilometer (-me''ter) 1000 meters; 3280.83 feet; five-eighths of a mile.

kilounit (kil''o-u'nit) a quantity equivalent to 1000 (10³) units.

kilovolt (kil'o-volt) 1000 volts.

kinanesthesia (kin''an-es-the'ze-ah) loss of power of perceiving sensations of movement.

kinase (ki'nās) 1. a subclass of the transferases, comprising the enzymes that catalyze the transfer of a high-energy group from a donor (usually ATP) to an acceptor, and named, according to the acceptor, as *creatine kinase, fructokinase*, etc. 2. an enzyme that activates a zymogen, and named, according to its source, as *enterokinase, streptokinase*, etc.

kine- word element [Gr.], *movement.* See also words beginning *cine-.*

kinematics (kin''ĕ-mat'iks) that phase of mechanics which deals with the possible motions of a material body.

kinematograph (-mat'o-graf) an instrument for showing pictures of objects in motion.

kineplasty (kin'ĕ-plas''te) utilization of the stump of an amputated extremity for producing motion of the prosthesis.

kinesalgia (kin''ĕ-sal'je-ah) pain on muscular exertion.

kinescope (kin'ĕ-skōp) an instrument for ascertaining ocular refraction.

kinesi(o)- word element [Gr.], *movement.*

kinesia (ki-ne'se-ah) motion sickness.

kinesialgia (ki-ne''se-al'je-ah) kinesalgia.

kinesiatrics (-at'riks) kinesitherapy.

kinesimeter (kin''ĕ-sim'ĕ-ter) 1. an instrument for quantitative measurement of motions. 2. an instrument for exploring the body surface to test cutaneous sensibility.

kinesiology (ki-ne''se-ol'o-je) scientific study of movement of body parts.

kinesioneurosis (ki-ne''se-o-nu-ro'sis) a functional nervous disorder marked by motor disturbances.

kinesitherapy (ki-ne''sĭ-ther'ah-pe) treatment of disease by movements or exercise.

kinesthesia (kin''es-the'ze-ah) the sense by which position, weight, and movement are perceived. **kinesthet'ic**, adj.

kinesthesiometer (kin''es-the''ze-om'ĕ-ter) an apparatus for testing kinesthesia.

kinesthesis (kin''es-the'sis) kinesthesia.

kinetic (kĭ-net'ik) pertaining to or producing motion.

kineticist (ki-net'ĭ-sist) a specialist in kinetics.

kinetics (kĭ-net'iks, ki-net'iks) the scientific study of the turnover, or rate of change, or a specific factor in the body, commonly expressed as units of amount per unit time. **chemical k.,** the study of the rates and mechanisms of chemical reactions.

kinetin (ki-ne'tin) a plant growth factor.

kinetocardiogram (ki-ne''to-kar'de-o-gram) the record produced by kinetocardiography.

kinetocardiography (-kar''de-og'rah-fe) the graphic recording of slow vibrations of the anterior chest wall in the region of the heart, the vibrations representing the absolute motion at a given point on the chest.

kinetochore (ki-ne'to-kōr) centromere.

kinetogenic (ki-ne''to-jen'ik) causing or producing movement.

kinetoplasm (ki-ne'to-plazm) the most highly contractile portion of the cytoplasm; applied to the chromatophilic elements in the nervous system.

kinetoplast (-plast) an accessory body found in many protozoa, primarily the Mastigophora, consisting of the blepharoplast and parabasal body, united by a delicate membrane; loosely called *micronucleus.*

kinetosis (ki''nĕ-to'sis) any disorder due to unaccustomed motions; see *motion sickness.*

kinetosome (ki-ne'to-sōm) basal corpuscle.

kinetotherapy (ki-ne''to-ther'ah-pe) kinesitherapy.

kingdom (king'dum) one of the three major categories into which natural objects are usually classified: the animal (including all animals), plant (including all plants), and mineral (including all substance and objects without life). A fourth, the Protista, includes all single-celled organisms.

kinin (ki'nin) any of a group of endogenous peptides that act on blood vessels, smooth muscles, and nociceptive nerve endings. **venom k.,** a peptide found in the venom of insects.

kinocilium (ki''no-sil'e-um), pl. *kinocil'ia.* A motile, protoplasmic filament on the free surface of a cell.

kinosphere (kin'o-sfēr) aster.

kinotoxin (ki''no-tok'sin) a fatigue toxin; kenotoxin.

kinship (kin'ship) a group of individuals of varying degrees of descent from a common ancestor.

kiotomy (ki-ot'o-me) excision of the vulva.

kl. kiloliter.

Klebsiella (kleb''se-el'ah) a genus of gram-negative bacteria (tribe Escherichieae), including *K. pneumo'niae* (*K. friedlän'deri*), the etiologic agent of Friedländer's pneumonia and other respiratory infections.

kleptomania (klep''to-ma'ne-ah) compulsive stealing, the objects taken usually having a symbolic value of which the subject is unconscious, rather than an intrinsic value.

kleptomaniac (-ma'ne-ak) a person exhibiting kleptomania.

km. kilometer.

kMc.p.s. kilomegacycles per second.

knee (ne) genu; the point of articulation of the femur with the tibia. Also, any kneelike structure. **housemaid's k.,** inflammation of the bursa of the patella, with fluid accumulating within it. **knock k.,** knock-knee.

knock-knee (nok′ne) genu valgum; a deformity of the thigh or leg, or both, in which the knees are abnormally close together and the space between the ankles is increased.

knot (not) 1. an intertwining of the ends or parts of one or more threads, sutures, or strip of cloth. 2. in anatomy, a knoblike swelling or protuberance. **net k.,** karyosome. **primitive k.,** a mass of cells at the cranial end of the primitive streak in the early embryo. **surgeon's k., surgical k.,** a knot in which the thread is passed twice through the first loop.

knuckle (nuk″l) the dorsal aspect of any phalangeal joint, or any similarly bent structure.

knuckling (nuk′ling) upward and forward displacement of the fetlock joint of a horse.

koilo- word element [Gr.], *hollowed; concave.*

koilonychia (koi″lo-nik′e-ah) dystrophy of the fingernails in which they are thinned and concave, with raised edges.

koilorrhachic (-rak′ik) having a vertebral column in which the lumbar curvature is anteriorly concave.

koilosternia (-ster′ne-ah) funnel chest.

kolp- for words beginning thus, see those beginning *colp-.*

kolypeptic (ko″le-pep′tik) hindering or checking digestion.

Konakion (kon″ah-ki′on) trademark for a preparation of phytonadione (vitamin K₁).

konometer (ko-nom′ĕ-ter) an apparatus for counting the dust particles in the air.

koumiss (koo′mis) a fermented drink prepared from milk.

Kr chemical symbol, *krypton.*

kraurosis (kraw-ro′sis) a dried, shriveled condition. **k. vul′vae,** atrophy of the female external genitalia, resulting in drying and shriveling, with leukoplakic patches on the mucosa and intense itching.

kreo- for words beginning thus, see also those beginning *creo-.*

kreotoxism (kre″o-tok′sizm) meat poisoning.

krypton (krip′ton) chemical element (*see table*), at. no. 36, symbol Kr.

kuru (koo′roo) a chronic, progressive, uniformly fatal central nervous system disorder due to a virus and transmissible to subhuman primates; seen only in the Fore and neighboring peoples of New Guinea.

kv. kilovolt.

kvp. kilovolt peak.

kwashiorkor (kwash″e-or′kor) a syndrome due to severe protein deficiency; symptoms include retarded growth, changes in skin and hair pigment, edema, and pathologic changes in the liver. **marasmic k.,** a condition in which there is a deficiency of both calories and protein, with severe tissue wasting, loss of subcutaneous fat, and usually dehydration.

Kwell (kwel) trademark for preparations of gamma benzene hexachloride.

kyestein (ki-es′te-in) a film sometimes seen on stale urine.

kymatism (ki′mah-tizm) myokymia.

kymogram (ki′mo-gram) the graphic record made by a kymograph.

kymograph (-graf) an instrument for recording variations and undulations, arterial or other.

kymography (ki-mog′rah-fe) the use of the kymograph.

Kynex (ki′neks) trademark for preparations of sulfamethoxypyridazine.

kynocephalus (ki″no-sef′ah-lus) a monster with a head like that of a dog.

kynurenine (kin″u-re′nin) a metabolite of tryptophan found in microorganisms and in the urine of normal animals; it is a precursor of kynurenic acid and an intermediate in the conversion of tryptophan to niacin.

kyphos (ki′fos) the hump in the spine in kyphosis.

kyphoscoliosis (ki″fo-sko″le-o′sis) backward and lateral curvature of the spinal column.

kyphosis (ki-fo′sis) abnormally increased convexity in the curvature of the thoracic spine as viewed from the side. **kyphot′ic,** adj. **k. dorsa′lis juveni′lis,** juvenile k., Scheuermann's k., osteochondrosis of the vertebrae.

kyrtorrhachic (kir″to-rak′ik) having a vertebral column in which the lumbar curvature is convex anteriorly.

kyto- for words beginning thus, see those beginning *cyto-.*

L

L. Latin; left; length; libra (*pound, balance*), licentiate; light sense; limes (*boundary*), liter; lumbar; coefficient of induction.

L₀ Ehrlich's symbol for a toxin-antitoxin mixture which is completely neutralized and will not kill an animal.

L₁ Ehrlich's symbol for a toxin-antitoxin mixture which contains one fatal dose in excess and which will kill the experimental animal.

L- chemical prefix (small capital) specifying that the substance corresponds in chemical composition to the standard substance L-glyceraldehyde. Opposed to D-.

l. liter.

l- chemical abbreviation, *levo-* (i.e., left or counterclockwise).

λ lambda, the eleventh letter of the Greek alphabet; symbol for *decay constant*.

La chemical symbol, *lanthanum*.

L. & A. light and accommodation (reaction of pupils).

labia (la′be-ah) plural of *labium*.

labial (la′be-al) pertaining to a lip, or labium.

labialism (la′be-ah-lizm″) defective speech with use of labial sounds.

labile (la′bīl) 1. gliding; moving from point to point over the surface; unstable. 2. chemically unstable.

lability (la-bil′ĭ-te) the quality of being labile; in psychiatry, emotional instability.

labio- word element [L.], *lip*.

labioalveolar (la″be-o-al-ve′o-lar) 1. pertaining to the lip and dental alveoli. 2. pertaining to the labial side of a dental alveolus.

labiocervical (-ser′vĭ-kal) 1. pertaining to the labial surface of the neck of an anterior tooth. 2. labiogingival.

labiochorea (-ko-re′ah) a choreic affection of the lips in speech, with stammering.

labioclination (-kli-na′shun) deviation of an anterior tooth from the vertical, in the direction of the lips.

labiodental (-den′tal) pertaining to the lips and teeth.

labiogingival (-jin-ji′val) pertaining to or formed by the labial and gingival walls of a tooth cavity.

labioglossolaryngeal (-glos″o-lah-rin′je-al) pertaining to the lips, tongue, and larynx.

labioglossopharyngeal (-fah-rin′je-al) pertaining to the lips, tongue, and pharynx.

labiograph (la′be-o-graf″) an instrument for recording lip motions in speaking.

labiomental (la″be-o-men′tal) pertaining to the lip and chin.

labionasal (-na′zal) pertaining to the lip and nose.

labiopalatine (-pal′ah-tīn) pertaining to the lip and palate.

labioplacement (-plās′ment) displacement of a tooth toward the lip.

labioplasty (la′be-o-plas″te) cheiloplasty.

labioversion (la″be-o-ver′zhun) labial displacement of a tooth from the line of occlusion.

labium (la′be-um), pl. *la′bia* [L.] a fleshy border or edge; a lip. **la′bial**, adj. **l. ma′jus** (pl. *la′bia majo′ra*), an elongated fold in the female, one on either side of the rima pudendi. **l. mi′nus** (pl. *la′bia mino′ra*), a small skin fold on either side, between the labium majus and the vaginal opening. **la′bia o′ris**, the lips of the mouth.

labor (la′bor) the function of the female organism by which the product of conception is expelled through the vagina to the outside world: the *first stage* begins with onset of regular uterine contractions and ends when the os is completely dilated and flush with the vagina; the *second* extends from the end of the first stage until the expulsion of the infant is completed; the *third* extends from expulsion of the infant until the placenta and membranes are expelled and contraction of the uterus is completed. **artificial l.**, induced l. **dry l.**, that in which the amniotic fluid escapes before the onset of uterine contractions. **false l.**, see under *pain*. **induced l.**, that brought on by extraneous means. **instrumental l.**, delivery facilitated by use of instruments. **missed l.**, that in which contractions begin and then cease, the fetus being retained for weeks or months. **postmature l.**, **postponed l.**, that occurring two weeks or more after the expected date of confinement. **precipitate l.**, that occurring with undue rapidity. **premature l.**, expulsion of a viable infant before the normal end of gestation; usually applied to interruption of pregnancy between the twenty-eighth and thirty-seventh week. **spontaneous l.**, delivery without artificial aid.

laboratory (lab′o-rah-tor″e) a place equipped for making tests or doing experimental work.

labrum (la′brum), pl. *la′bra* [L.] an edge, rim, or lip.

labyrinth (lab′ĭ-rinth) the internal ear, made up of the vestibule, cochlea, and canals. See Plate XII. **labyrin′thine**, adj. **bony l.**, the bony part of the internal ear. **ethmoid e.**, either of the paired lateral masses of the ethmoid bone, consisting of many thin-walled cellular cavities, the ethmoidal cells. **membranous l.**, a system of communicating epithelial sacs and ducts within the bony labyrinth, containing the endolymph. **osseous l.**, bony l.

labyrinthectomy (lab″ĭ-rin-thek′to-me) excision of the labyrinth.

labyrinthitis (lab″ĭ-rin-thi′tis) inflammation of the labyrinth; otitis interna.

labyrinthotomy (lab″ĭ-rin-thot′o-me) incision of the labyrinth.

labyrinthus (lab″ĭ-rin′thus), pl. *labyrin′thi* [L.] labyrinth.

lac (lak), pl. *lac′ta* [L.] milk.

laccase (lak′ās) a copper-containing enzyme that catalyzes the oxidation of phenols to quinones.

laceration (las"ĕ-ra'shun) 1. the act of tearing. 2. a torn, ragged, mangled wound.

lacertus (lah-ser'tus), pl. *lacer'ti* [L.] a name given certain fibrous attachments of muscles.

lacrimal (lak'rĭ-mal) pertaining to tears.

lacrimation (lak"rĭ-ma'shun) secretion and discharge of tears.

lacrimator (lak'rĭ-ma"tor) an agent, as a gas, that induces the flow of tears.

lacrimatory (lak'rĭ-mah-to"re) causing a flow of tears.

lacrimonasal (lak"rĭ-mo-na'zal) pertaining to the lacrimal sac and nose.

lacrimotomy (lak"rĭ-mot'o-me) incision of the lacrimal gland, duct, or sac.

lact(o)- word element [L.], *milk.*

lactacidemia (lak-tas"ĭ-de'me-ah) an excess of lactic acid in the blood.

lactaciduria (-du're-ah) lactic acid in the urine.

lactagogue (lak'tah-gog) galactagogue.

lactalbumin (lak"tal-bu'min) an albumin from milk.

lactam (lak'tam) a cyclic amide formed from aminocarboxylic acids by elimination of water; lactams are isomeric with lactims, which are enol forms of lactams.

lactase (lak'tās) β-galactosidase.

lactate (lak'tāt) 1. any salt or ester of lactic acid. 2. to secrete milk.

lactation (lak-ta'shun) 1. the secretion of milk. 2. the period of milk secretion.

lacteal (lak'te-al) 1. pertaining to milk. 2. any of the intestinal lymphatics that transport chyle.

lactescence (lak-tes'ens) resemblance to milk.

lactic (lak'tik) pertaining to milk.

lacticemia (lak"tĭ-se'me-ah) lactic acid in the blood.

lactiferous (lak-tif'er-us) conveying milk.

lactifuge (lak'tĭ-fūj) checking or stopping milk secretion; also an agent that so acts.

lactigenous (lak-tij'ĕ-nus) producing milk.

lactigerous (lak-tij'er-us) lactiferous.

lactim (lak'tim) see *lactam.*

lactivorous (lak-tiv'o-rus) feeding or subsisting upon milk.

Lactobacillaceae (lak"to-bas"il-la'se-e) a family of schizomycetes (order Eubacteriales).

Lactobacilleae (-bah-sil'le-e) a tribe of schizomycetes (family Lactobacillaceae).

Lactobacillus (-bah-sil'lus) a genus of the tribe Lactobacilleae, some of which are considered to be etiologically related to dental caries, but are otherwise nonpathogenic; they produce lactic acid by fermentation.

lactobacillus (-bah-sil'us), pl. *lactobacil'li* [L.] an organism of the genus *Lactobacillus.*

lactocele (lak'to-sēl) galactocele.

lactogen (lak'to-jen) any substance that enhances lactation. **human placental l.,** a hormone secreted by the placenta; it has lactogenic, luteotropic, and growth-promoting activity, and inhibits maternal insulin activity.

lactogenic (lak"to-jen'ik) stimulating milk production.

lactoglobulin (lak"to-glob'u-lin) a globulin oc-

curring in milk. **immune l's,** antibodies (immunoglobulins) occurring in the colostrum of animals.

lactometer (lak-tom'ĕ-ter) galactometer.

lactone (lak'tōn) 1. an aromatic liquid from lactic acid. 2. a cyclic organic compound in which the chain is closer by ester formation between a carboxyl and a hydroxyl group in the same molecule.

lactophosphate (lak"to-fos'fāt) any salt of lactic and phosphoric acids.

lactoprotein (-pro'te-in) a protein derived from milk.

lactorrhea (-re'ah) galactorrhea.

lactose (lak'tōs) a sugar derived from milk, $C_{12}H_{22}O_{11}$, which on hydrolysis yields glucose and galactose.

lactosuria (lak"to-su're-ah) lactose in the urine.

lactotherapy (-ther'ah-pe) treatment by milk diet.

lactovegetarian (-vej"ĕ-ta're-an) 1. a person who subsists on a diet of milk (or milk products) and vegetables. 2. pertaining to such a diet.

lactulose (lak'tu-lōs) a synthetic disaccharide used as a cathartic.

lacuna (lah-ku'nah), pl. *lacu'nae* [L.] 1. a small pit or hollow cavity. 2. a defect or gap, as in the field of vision (scotoma). **lacu'nar,** adj. **absorption l.,** a pit or groove in developing bone that is undergoing resorption; frequently found to contain osteoclasts. **Howship's l.,** absorption l. **intervillous l.,** one of the blood spaces of the placenta in which the fetal villi are found. **l. mag'na,** navicular fossa (2). **l. pharyn'gis,** a depression at the pharyngeal end of the eustachian tube. **trophoblastic l.,** intervillous l.

lacunule (lah-ku'nūl) a minute lacuna.

lacus (la'kus), pl. *la'cus* [L.] lake. **l. lacrima'lis,** lacrimal lake.

lae- for words beginning thus, see those beginning *le-*.

laeve (le've) [L.] nonvillous.

lag (lag) 1. the time elapsing between application of a stimulus and the resulting reaction. 2. the early period after inoculation of bacteria into a culture medium, in which growth or cell division is slow.

lagena (lah-je'nah) 1. a part of the upper extremity of the cochlear duct. 2. the organ of hearing in nonmammalian vertebrates.

lageniform (lah-jen'ĭ-form) flask-shaped.

lagophthalmos (lag"of-thal'mos) inability to shut the eyes completely.

lake (lāk) 1. to undergo separation of hemoglobin from erythrocytes. 2. a circumscribed collection of fluid in a hollow or depressed cavity. See also *lacuna.* **lacrimal l.,** the triangular space at the medial angle of the eye, where the tears collect.

lal(o)- word element [Gr.], *speech; babbling.*

laliatry (lah-li'ah-tre) the study and treatment of disorders of speech.

lallation (lah-la'shun) a babbling, infantile form of speech.

lalognosis (lal"og-no'sis) the understanding of speech.

lalopathology (-o-pah-thol′o-je) the branch of medicine dealing with disorders of speech.

lalopathy (lah-lop′ah-the) any speech disorder.

laloplegia (lal″o-ple′je-ah) paralysis of the organs of speech.

lalorrhea (-re′ah) excessive flow of words.

lambda (lam′dah) point of union of the lambdoid and sagittal sutures.

lambdacism (-sizm) 1. the substitution of *l* for *r* sounds. 2. inability to utter correctly the sound of *l*.

lambdoid (lam′doid) shaped like the Greek letter lambda, Λ or λ.

Lamblia (lam′ble-ah) *Giardia*.

lambliasis (lam-bli′ah-sis) giardiasis.

lame (lām) incapable of normal locomotion; deviation from normal gait.

lamella (lah-mel′ah), pl. *lamel′lae* [L.] 1. a thin leaf or plate, as of bone. 2. a medicated disk or wafer to be inserted under the eyelid. **lamel′lar**, adj. **circumferential l.**, one of the layers of bone that underlie the periosteum and endosteum. **concentric l.**, haversian l. **endosteal l.**, one of the bony plates lying beneath the endosteum. **ground l.**, interstitial l. **haversian l.**, one of the concentric bony plates surrounding a haversian canal. **intermediate l., interstitial l.**, one of the bony plates that fill in between the haversian systems. **vitreous l.**, lamina basalis.

lamina (lam′ĭ-nah), pl. *lam′inae* [L.] a thin, flat plate or layer, used in anatomic nomenclature to designate such a structure, or a layer of a composite structure. **l. basa′lis**, one of the pair of longitudinal zones of the embryonic neural tube, from which develop the ventral gray columns of the spinal cord and the motor centers of the brain. **l. basila′ris**, the posterior wall of the cochlear duct, separating it from the scala tympani. **Bowman's l.**, see under *membrane*. **l. choroidocapilla′ris**, the inner layer of the choroid, composed of a single-layered network of small capillaries. **l. cribro′sa**, 1. fascia cribrosa. 2. (of *ethmoid bone*) the horizontal plate of ethmoid bone forming the roof of the nasal cavity, and perforated by many foramina for passage of olfactory nerves. 3. (*of sclera*) the perforated part of the sclera through which pass the axons of the retinal ganglion cells. **dental l.**, a thickened epithelial band along the margin of the gum in the embryo, from which the enamel organs are developed. **elastic l.**, 1. Bowman's membrane. 2. Descemet's membrane. **epithelial l.**, the layer of ependymal cells covering the choroid plexus. **l. fus′ca**, the pigmentary layer of the sclera. **l. pro′pria**, 1. the connective tissue layer of mucous membrane. 2. the middle fibrous layer of the tympanic membrane. **l. reticula′ris**, the perforated hyaline membrane covering the organ of Corti. **l. spira′lis**, 1. a double plate of bone winding spirally around the modiolus, dividing the spiral canal of the cochlea into the scala tympani and scali vestibuli. 2. a bony projection on the outer wall of the cochlea in the lower part of the first turn. **terminal l. of hypothalamus**, the thin plate derived from the telencephalon, forming the anterior wall of the third ventricle of the cerebrum. **l. of vertebral arch**, one of the paired dorsal parts of the vertebral arch connected to the pedicles of the vertebra. **vitreal l., vitreous l.**, Bruch's membrane.

laminagraphy (lam″ĭ-nag′rah-fe) see *body-section roentgenography*.

laminar (lam′ĭ-nar) made up of laminae or layers; pertaining to a lamina.

Laminaria (lam″ĭ-na′re-ah) a genus of seaweeds, the kelps, various species of which are used as sources of alginates.

laminated (lam′ĭ-nāt″ed) made up of laminae or thin layers.

lamination (lam″ĭ-na′shun) a laminated structure or arrangement.

laminectomy (lam″ĭ-nek′to-me) excision of the posterior arch of a vertebra.

laminography (lam″ĭ-nog′rah-fe) see *body-section roentgenography*.

laminotomy (lam″ĭ-not′o-me) transection of a lamina of a vertebra.

lamp (lamp) an apparatus for furnishing heat or light. **annealing l.**, an alcohol lamp for heating gold leaf for tooth fillings. **carbon arc l.**, one that produces an intense white light from an electric arc between carbon rods; used in artificial light therapy. **Finsen's l.**, a carbon arc lamp operating at 50 volts and 50 amperes so constructed that radiation is concentrated on an area 1 inch square; a water-cooled quartz system is used to remove caloric radiation and a compression quartz piece to dehematize the skin. **Gullstrand's slit l.**, an apparatus for projecting a narrow, flat beam of intense light into the eye. **Kromayer's l.**, a small water-cooled mercury vapor lamp with a quartz window that produces ultraviolet radiation. **mercury vapor l.**, one in which the arc is in mercury vapor, enclosed in a quartz burner; used in light therapy; it may be air or water-cooled. **quartz l.**, a mercury vacuum lamp made of melted quartz glass embedded in a running water bath; used for applying ultraviolet light treatment. **slit l.**, Gullstrand's slit l. **tungsten arc l.**, an electric arc lamp with tungsten electrodes; has been used in the treatment of acne, alopecia, etc. **ultraviolet l.**, one producing ultraviolet rays.

lamziekte (lam′zēk-te) a disease of cattle in South Africa, characterized by motor paralysis and due to ingestion by phosphorus-deficient animals of bones, contaminated by toxin produced by *Clostridium botulinum*.

lanatoside C (lah-nat′o-sīd) a cardiotonic glycoside, $C_{49}H_{76}O_{20}$, from the leaves of *Digitalis lanata;* used where digitalis is recommended.

lance (lans) 1. lancet. 2. to cut or incise with a lancet.

lancet (lan′set) a small, pointed, two-edged surgical knife.

lancinating (lan′sĭ-nāt″ing) tearing, darting, or sharply cutting; said of pain.

lanolin (lan′o-lin) a purified, fatlike substance from the wool of sheep, *Ovis aries*, mixed with 25 to 30% water; used as a water-in-oil ointment base. **anhydrous l.**, lanolin containing not more than 0.25% water; used as an absorbent ointment base.

Lanoxin (lah-nok′sin) trademark for preparations of digoxin.

lanthanum (lan′thah-num) chemical element (*see table*), at. no. 57, symbol La.

lanugo (lah-nu′go) the fine hair on the body of the fetus.

laparo- word element [Gr.], *loin* or *flank; abdomen* (loosely).

laparorrhaphy (lap″ah-ror′ah-fe) suture of the abdominal wall.

laparoscope (lap′ah-ro-skōp″) an endoscope for examining the peritoneal cavity.

laparoscopy (lap″ah-ros′ko-pe) examination by means of the laparoscope. **laparoscop′ic,** adj.

laparotomy (lap″ah-rot′o-me) incision through the flank or, more generally, through any part of the abdominal wall.

laparotrachelotomy (lap″ah-ro-tra″kĕ-lot′o-me) low cervical cesarean section, with incision into the lower uterine segment.

lapinization (lap″in-i-za′shun) serial passage of a virus or vaccine through rabbits to modify its characteristics.

lapinize (lap′in-īz) to attenuate (as a virus or vaccine) by serial passage through rabbits.

lapis (la′pis, lap′is) [L.] stone.

lard (lard) purified internal fat of the abdomen of the hog. **benzoinated l.,** a preparation of lard containing 1% benzoin; used as a vehicle for drugs and in ointments.

lardacein (lar-da′se-in) a protein found in tissues affected with amyloid degeneration.

lardaceous (lar-da′shus) 1. resembling lard. 2. containing lardacein.

larva (lar′vah), pl. *lar′vae* [L.] an independent, immature stage in the life cycle of an animal in which it is unlike the parent and must undergo changes in form and size to reach the adult stage. **l. cur′rens,** a variant of larva migrans caused by *Strongyloides stercoralis,* in which the progression of the linear lesion is much more rapid. **l. mi′grans,** creeping eruption; a convoluted threadlike skin eruption that appears to migrate, caused by the burrowing beneath the skin of roundworm larvae, particularly *Ancylostoma* larvae. Similar lesions are caused by the larvae of botflies. **l. mi′grans, visceral,** a condition due to prolonged migration of nematode larvae in human tissue other than skin.

larval (lar′val) 1. pertaining to larvae. 2. larvate.

larvate (lar′vāt) masked; concealed; said of a disease or symptom of disease.

larvicide (lar′vĭ-sīd) an agent that kills insect larvae.

laryng(o)- word element [Gr.], *larynx.*

laryngalgia (lar″in-gal′je-ah) pain in the larynx.

laryngeal (lah-rin′je-al) pertaining to the larynx.

laryngectomee (lar″in-jek′to-me) a person whose larynx has been removed.

laryngectomy (-jek′to-me) excision of the larynx.

laryngemphraxis (lar″in-jem-frak′sis) obstruction or closure of the larynx.

laryngismus (-jiz′mus) spasm of the larynx. **laryngis′mal,** adj. **l. paralyt′icus,** roaring. **l. strid′ulus,** sudden laryngeal spasm with crowing inspiration.

laryngitis (-ji′tis) inflammation of the larynx. **laryngit′ic,** adj. **atrophic l.,** an extreme form of chronic catarrhal laryngitis. **chronic catarrhal l.,** a form marked by atrophy of the glands of the mucous membrane. **subglottic l.,** inflammation of the under surface of the vocal cords.

laryngocele (lah-ring′go-sēl) a congenital anomalous air sac communicating with the cavity of the larynx, which may bulge outward on the neck.

laryngocentesis (lah-ring″go-sen-te′sis) surgical puncture of the larynx.

laryngofissure (-fish′er) median laryngotomy.

laryngogram (lah-ring′go-gram) a roentgenogram of the larynx.

laryngography (lar″ing-gog′rah-fe) radiography of the larynx.

laryngology (-gol′o-je) that branch of medicine having to do with the throat, pharynx, larynx, nasopharynx, and tracheobronchial tree.

laryngopathy (-gop′ah-the) any disorder of the larynx.

laryngophantom (lah-ring″go-fan′tom) an artificial model of the larynx.

laryngopharnygeal (-fah-rin′je-al) pertaining to the larynx and pharynx.

laryngopharyngectomy (-far″in-jek′to-me) excision of the larynx and pharynx.

laryngopharyngitis (-far″in-ji′tis) inflammation of the larynx and pharynx.

laryngopharynx (-far′inks) the portion of the pharynx below the upper edge of the epiglottis, opening into the larynx and esophagus.

laryngophony (lar″ing-gof′o-ne) the vocal sound heard in auscultating the larynx.

laryngoplasty (lah-ring′go-plas″te) plastic repair of the larynx.

laryngoplegia (lah-ring″go-ple′je-ah) paralysis of the larynx.

laryngoptosis (-to′sis) lowering and mobilization of the larynx.

laryngorhinology (-ri-nol′o-je) the branch of medicine that deals with the larynx and nose.

laryngoscleroma (-skle-ro′mah) scleroma of the larynx.

laryngoscope (lah-ring′go-skōp) an endoscope for examining the larynx.

laryngoscopy (lar″ing-gos′ko-pe) visual examination of the interior larynx. **laryngoscop′ic,** adj. **direct l.,** that performed with a speculum or laryngoscope. **indirect l., mirror l.,** examination of the larynx by observing its reflection in a mirror.

laryngospasm (lah-ring′go-spazm) spasmodic closure of the larynx.

laryngostenosis (lah-ring″go-stĕ-no′sis) narrowing or stricture of the larynx.

laryngostomy (lar″ing-gos′to-me) surgical fistulization of the larynx.

laryngotomy (-got′o-me) incision of the larynx. **inferior l.,** laryngotomy through the cricothyroid membrane. **median l.,** laryngotomy through the thyroid cartilage. **superior l., sub-hyoid l.,** laryngotomy through the thyrohyoid membrane.

laryngotracheal (lah-ring″go-tra′ke-al) pertaining to the larynx and trachea.

laryngotracheitis (-tra″ke-i′tis) inflammation of the larynx and trachea.

laryngotracheotomy (-tra″ke-ot′o-me) incision of the larynx and trachea.

laryngoxerosis (-ze-ro′sis) dryness of the larynx.

larynx (lar′inks) the organ of voice; the air passage between the lower pharynx and the trachea, containing the vocal cords and formed by nine cartilages: the thyroid, cricoid, and epiglottis and the paired arytenoid, corniculate, and cuneiform cartilages. See Plates VI and VII.

laser (la′zer) a device that transfers light of various frequencies into an extremely intense, small, and nearly nondivergent beam of monochromatic radiation in the visible region, with all the waves in phase; capable of mobilizing immense heat and power when focused at close range, it is used as a tool in surgery, in diagnosis, and in physiologic studies.

lassitude (las′ĭ-tūd) weakness; exhaustion.

latency (la′ten-se) the state of being latent.

latent (la′tent) dormant or concealed; not manifest; potential.

laterad (lat′er-ad) toward the lateral aspect.

lateral (lat′er-al) 1. denoting a position farther from the median plane or midline of the body or a structure. 2. pertaining to a side.

lateralis (lat″er-a′lis) [L.] lateral.

laterality (lat″er-al′ĭ-te) a tendency to use preferentially the organs (hand, foot, ear, eye) of the same side in voluntary motor acts. **crossed l.,** the preferential use of contralateral members of the different pairs of organs in voluntary motor acts, e.g., right eye and left hand.

lateroduction (lat″er-o-duk′shun) movement of an eye to either side.

lateroflexion (-flek′shun) flexion to one side.

laterotorsion (-tor′shun) twisting of the vertical meridian of the eye to either side.

lateroversion (-ver′zhun) abnormal turning to one side.

latex (la′teks) a viscid, milky juice secreted by some seed plants.

lathyrism (lath′ĭ-rizm) a morbid condition marked by spastic paraplegia, pain, hyperesthesia, and paresthesia, due to ingestion of the seeds of leguminous plants of the genus *Lathyrus*, which includes many kinds of peas. **lathyrit′ic,** adj.

lathyrogenic (lath″ĭ-ro-jen′ik) causing symptoms similar to those of lathyrism.

latissimus (lah-tis′ĭ-mus) [L.] widest; in anatomy, denoting a broad structure.

latrodectism (lat″ro-dek′tizm) intoxication due to venom of spiders of the genus *Latrodectus*.

Latrodectus (-dek′tus) a genus of poisonous spiders, including *L. mac′tans*, the black widow spider, whose bite may cause severe symptoms or even death.

LATS long-acting thyroid stimulator.

latus (la′tus) [L.] 1. broad, wide. 2. the side or flank.

Lauron (law′ron) trademark for a preparation of aurothioglycanide.

lavage (lah-vahzh′) 1. the irrigation or washing out of an organ, as of the stomach or bowel. 2. to wash out, or irrigate.

Lavema (lah-ve′mah) trademark for preparations of oxyphenisatin.

law (law) a uniform or constant fact or principle. **all-or-none l.,** see *all-or-none*. **Allen's paradoxic l.,** the more sugar a normal person is given the more is utilized; the reverse is true in diabetics. **l's of articulation,** a set of rules to be followed in arranging teeth to produce a balanced articulation. **Avogadro's l.,** equal volumes of perfect gases at the same temperature and pressure contain the same number of molecules. **Behring's l.,** blood and serum of an immunized person when transferred to another subject will render the latter immune. **Bell's l.,** the anterior roots of spinal nerves are motor roots, the posterior are sensory. **biogenetic l.,** recapitulation theory. **Boyle's l.,** at a constant temperature the volume of a perfect gas varies inversely as the pressure, and the pressure varies inversely as the volume. **Charles' l.,** at a constant pressure the volume of a given mass of a perfect gas varies directly with the absolute temperature. **Colles' l.,** a child affected with congenital syphilis, the mother showing no signs of the disease, will not infect the mother. **Dalton's l.,** the pressure exerted by a mixture of nonreacting gases is equal to the sum of the partial pressures of the separate components. **Donders' l.,** the rotation of the eye around the line of sight is not voluntary. **Fechner's l.,** the sensation produced by a stimulus varies as the logarithm of the stimulus. **Gay-Lussac's l.,** Charles' l. **Graham's l.,** the rate of diffusion of a gas through porous membranes varies inversely with the square root of its density. **Hellin's l.,** one in about 89 pregnancies ends in the birth of twins; one in 89 / 89 (7921), of triplets; one in 89 / 89 / 89 (704,969), of quadruplets. **Henry's l.,** the solubility of a gas in a liquid solution is proportionate to the partial pressure of the gas. **Hilton's l.,** a nerve trunk which supplies any given joint also supplies the muscles which move the joint and the skin over the insertion of such muscles. **l. of independent assortment,** the members of gene pairs segregate independently during meiosis. **Koch's l.,** Koch's postulate. **Listings l.,** when the eyeball is moved from a resting position, the rotational angle in the second position is the same as if the eye were turned about a fixed axis perpendicular to the first and second positions of the visual line. **malthusian l.,** the hypothesis that the human population tends to outrun the means available to sustain it. **Mariotte's l.,** Boyle's l. **Mendel's l., mendelian l.,** in the inheritance of certain traits or characters, offspring are not intermediate in type between the parents, but inherit from one or the other parent in this respect. Thus, if a plant with the factor tallness (TT) is mated with one with the factor shortness (SS), then the offspring will inherit these factors in the ratio TT, 2TS, SS. This law is usually expressed as the *law of independent assortment* and the *law of segregation*. **Müller-Haeckel l.,** recapitulation theory. **Nysten's l.,** rigor mortis affects first the muscles of mastication, next those of the face and neck, then those of the trunk and arms, and last those of the legs and feet. **Ohm's l.,** the strength of an electric current varies directly as the electromotive force and inversely as the resistance. **Profeta's l.,** the apparently nonsyphilitic child born of syphilitic parents is immune. **psychophysical l.,** Weber-Fechner l. **Raoult's l.,** 1. (*for freezing points*) the depression of the freezing point for the same type of electrolyte dissolved in a given solvent is proportional to the molecular concentration of the solute. 2. (*for vapor pressures*) *a,* the vapor pressure of a volatile substance from a liquid solution is equal to the mole fraction of that substance times its vapor pressure in the pure state. *b,* when a nonvolatile nonelectrolyte is dissolved in a solvent, the decrease in vapor pressure of that solvent is equal to the mole fraction of the solute times the vapor pressure of the pure solvent. **Ritter-Valli l.,** the primary increase and secondary loss of irritability in a nerve produced by a section which separates it from the nerve center, travel in a peripheral direction. **l. of segregation,** in each generation the ratio of (*a*) pure dominants, (*b*) dominants giving descendants in the proportion of three dominants to one recessive, and (*c*) pure recessives is 1 : 2 : 1. This ratio follows from the fact that the two alleles of a gene cannot be a part of a single gamete, but must segregate to different gametes. **l. of sines,** the sine of the angle of incidence is equal to the sine of the angle of reflection multiplied by a constant quantity. **Talbot's l.,** when complete fusion occurs and the sensation is uniform, the intensity is the same as it would be were the same amount of light spread uniformly over the disk. **van't Hoff's l.,** see under *rule.* **Weber's l.,** the variation of stimulus which causes the smallest appreciable change in sensation maintains an approximately fixed ratio to the whole stimulus. **Weber-Fechner l.,** for a sensation to increase by arithmetical progression, the stimulus must increase by geometrical progression. **Wolff's l.,** a bone, normal or abnormal, develops the structure most suited to resist the forces acting upon it.

lawrencium (law-ren'se-um) chemical element (*see table*), at. no. 103, symbol Lw.

laxative (lak'sah-tiv) 1. aperient; mildly cathartic. 2. a cathartic or purgative. **bulk l.,** one promoting bowel evacuation by increasing fecal volume.

laxator (lak-sa'tor) that which slackens or relaxes.

layer (la'er) stratum; a sheetlike mass of tissue of nearly uniform thickness, several of which may be superimposed, one above the other, as in the epidermis. **ameloblastic l.,** the inner layer of cells of the enamel organ, which forms the enamel prisms. **bacillary l.,** l. of rods and cones. **basal l.,** 1. the deepest layer of the epidermis.

2. the deepest layer of the uterine mucosa. **Bernard's glandular l.,** the stratum of cells lining the acini of the pancreas. **blastodermic l.,** germ l. **clear l.,** the clear translucent layer of the epidermis, just beneath the horny layer. **columnar l.,** 1. l. of rods and cones. 2. mantle l. **cortical l.,** the cortex of an organ, as of the brain or ovary. **cuticular l.,** a striate border of modified cytoplasm at the free end of some columnar cells. **enamel l.,** the outermost layer of cells of the enamel organ. **ganglionic l. of cerebellum,** the thin middle gray layer of the cerebral cortex, consisting of a single layer of Purkinje cells. **germ l.,** any of the three primary layers of cells of the embryo (ectoderm, entoderm, and mesoderm), from which the tissues and organs develop. **germinative l.,** 1. malpighian l. 2. the lower layer of the nail, from which the nail grows. **granular l.,** 1. the layer of epidermis between the clear and prickle-cell layers. 2. the deep layer of the cortex of the cerebellum. 3. the layer of follicle cells lining the theca of the vesicular ovarian follicle. **half-value l.,** the thickness of a given substance which, when introduced in the path of a given beam of rays, will reduce its intensity by one half. **Haller's l.,** the portion of the vascular layer of the choroid made up of large vessels. **Henle's l.,** the outermost layer of the inner root sheath of the hair follicle. **horny l.,** 1. stratum corneum; the outermost layer of the epidermis, consisting of dead and desquamating cells. 2. the outer, compact layer of the nail. **Langhans' l.,** cytotrophoblast. **malpighian l.,** the basal layer and prickle-cell layer of the epidermis considered together. **mantle l.,** the middle layer of the wall of the primitive neural tube, containing primitive nerve cells and later forming the gray substance of the central nervous system. **nervous l.,** all of the retina except the pigment layer; the inner layer of the optic cup. **neuroepidermal l.,** ectoderm. **odontoblastic l.,** the epithelioid layer of odontoblasts in contact with the dentin of teeth. **Ollier's l., osteogenetic l.,** the innermost layer of the periosteum. **prickle-cell l.,** stratum spinosum; the layer of the epidermis between the granular and basal layers, marked by the presence of prickle cells. **Rauber's l.,** the most external of the three layers forming the blastodisc in the early embryo. **l. of rods and cones,** a layer of the retina immediately beneath the pigment epithelium, between it and external limiting membrane, containing the rods and cones. **spinous l.,** prickle-cell l. **subendocardial l.,** the layer of loose fibrous tissue uniting the endocardium and myocardium. **zonal l. of thalamus,** a layer of myelinated fibers covering the dorsal surface of the thalamus.

lb. [L.] *li'bra* (pound).

L.D. lethal dose; light difference (difference in light perception between the two eyes).

L.D.₅₀ median lethal dose.

LDH lactic dehydrogenase.

LDL low-density lipoproteins.

L-dopa see *dopa.*

L.E. lupus erythematosus.

lead¹ (led) chemical element (*see table*), at. no. 82,

symbol Pb. Poisoning is caused by absorption or ingestion of lead, and affects the brain, nervous and digestive systems, and blood. **l. acetate,** a reagent and astringent, $Pb(C_2H_3O_2)_2 \cdot 3H_2O$. **l. monoxide,** a binary compound, PbO, used as a reagent. **sugar of l.,** l. acetate.

lead² (lēd) any of the conductors connected to the electrocardiograph; also any of the records made by the electrocardiograph, varying with the part of the body from which the current is led off. Usually, three peripheral leads are used: lead I, right arm and left arm; lead II, right arm and left leg; lead III, left arm and left leg. **bipolar l.,** an array involving two electrodes placed at different body sites. **esophageal l.,** one attached to an electrode inserted within the esophagus. **limb l's,** any of the three leads customarily used in electrocardiography. **precordial l's,** leads in which the exploring electrode is placed on the chest and the other is connected to one or more extremities, indicated as follows: CR = chest + right arm; CL = chest + left arm; CF = chest + left leg; V = chest + junction of leads from right and left arms and left leg. Subscript numbers 1 to 6 indicate at which points on the chest the lead is taken. **unipolar l.,** an array of two electrodes, only one of which transmits potential variation.

lecithal (les′ĭ-thal) having a yolk; used especially as a word termination (*isolecithal*, etc.).

lecithin (les′ĭ-thin) any of a group of phospholipids found in animal tissues, especially nerve tissue, the liver, semen, and egg yolk, consisting of esters of glycerol with two molecules of long-chain aliphatic acids and one of phosphoric acid, the latter being esterified with the alcohol group of choline.

lecithinase (-ās) phospholipase.

lecitho- word element [Gr.], *the yolk of an egg* or *ovum.*

lecithoblast (les′ĭ-tho-blast″) the primitive entoderm of a two-layered blastodisc.

lecithoprotein (les′ĭ-tho-pro′te-in) a conjugated protein having lecithin as the prosthetic group.

lectin (lek′tin) a term applied to hemagglutinating substances present in saline extracts of certain plant seeds, which specifically agglutinate erythrocytes of certain blood groups.

Ledercillin (led″er-sil′lin) trademark for preparations of procaine penicillin G.

leech (lēch) any of the annelids of the class Hirudinea, especially *Hirudo medicinalis;* some species are bloodsuckers, and were formerly used for drawing blood.

leg (leg) the lower limb, especially the part from knee to foot. **bandy l.,** bowleg. **Barbados l.,** elephantiasis of the leg. **bayonet l.,** ankylosis of the knee after backward displacement of the tibia and fibula. **black l.,** symptomatic anthrax. **bow l.,** see *bowleg.* **deck l's,** edema of lower legs occurring in ship passengers in the tropics. **elephant l.,** elephantiasis of the leg. **milk l.,** phlegmasia alba dolens. **restless l's,** a disagreeable, creeping, irritating sensation in the legs, usually the lower legs, relieved only by walking or keeping the legs moving. **scissor l.,** deformity with crossing of the legs in walking.

legume (leg′ūm) the pod or fruit of a leguminous plant, such as peas or beans.

legumin (lĕ-gu′min) a globulin characteristically found in the seeds of leguminous plants.

leiodermia (li″o-der′me-ah) abnormal smoothness and glossiness of the skin.

leiomyofibroma (-mi″o-fi-bro′mah) epithelioid leiomyoma.

leiomyoma (-mi-o′mah) a benign tumor derived from smooth muscle, most often of the uterus. **epithelioid l.,** leiomyoma, usually of the stomach, in which the cells are polygonal rather than spindle shaped.

leiomyosarcoma (-mi″o-sar-ko′mah) a sarcoma containing cells of smooth muscle.

Leishmania (lēsh-ma′ne-ah) a genus of parasitic protozoa, including *L. brazilien′sis,* the cause of mucocutaneous leishmaniasis; *L. brazilien′sis pifa′noi,* the cause of leishmaniasis tegmentaria diffusa; *L. donova′ni,* the cause of kala-azar; and *L. trop′ica,* the cause of cutaneous leishmaniasis.

leishmaniasis (lēsh″mah-ni′ah-sis) infection with *Leishmania.* **American l.,** mucocutaneous l. **cutaneous l.,** a chronic ulcerative granuloma endemic in the tropics and subtropics, caused by *Leishmania tropica.* **mucocutaneous l.,** a disease endemic in South and Central America caused by *Leishmania braziliensis,* marked by ulceration of the mucous membranes of the nose and throat; widespread destruction of soft tissues in nasal and oral regions may occur. **l. tegmenta′ria diffu′sa,** a generalized cutaneous disease endemic in South America and Mexico, caused by *Leishmania braziliensis pifanoi,* in which the lesions resemble those of nodular leprosy or of keloid. **visceral l.,** kala-azar.

lemmoblastic (lem″o-blas′tik) forming or developing into neurilemma tissue.

lemmocyte (lem′o-sīt) a cell which develops into a neurilemma cell.

lemniscus (lem-nis′kus), pl. *lemnis′ci* [L.] a ribbon or band; in anatomy, a band or bundle of fibers in the central nervous system.

length (length) an expression of the longest dimension of an object, or of the measurement between the two ends. **basialveolar l.,** the distance from the basion to the lower end of the intermaxillary suture. **basinasal l.,** the distance from the basion to the center of the suture between the frontal and nasal bones. **crown-heel l.,** the distance from the crown of the head to the heel in embryos, fetuses, and infants; the equivalent of standing height in older persons. **crown-rump l.,** the distance from the crown of the head to the breech in embryos, fetuses, and infants; the equivalent of sitting height in older persons. **focal l.,** the distance between a lens and an object from which all rays of light are brought to a focus. **wave l.,** see *wavelength.*

lens (lenz) 1. a piece of glass or other transparent material so shaped as to converge or scatter light rays; see also *glasses.* 2. crystalline lens; the transparent, biconvex body separating the posterior chamber and vitreous body, and constituting part of the refracting mechanism of the eye; see Plate XIII. **achromatic l.,** one corrected for chromatic aberration. **acrylic l.,** a plastic lens used to replace the crystalline lens after cataract surgery. **aplanatic l.,** one that serves to correct shperical aberrations. **apochromatic l.,** one corrected for chromatic and spheric aberration. **biconcave l.,** one concave on both faces. **biconvex l.,** one convex on both faces. **bifocal l.,** see under *glasses.* **concave l.,** one with one or both (biconvex) faces curved like a section of the interior of a hollow sphere; it disperses light rays. **concavoconcave l.,** biconcave l. **concavoconvex l.,** one with one concave and one convex face. **contact l.,** a curved shell of glass or plastic applied directly over the globe or cornea to correct refractive errors. **converging l., convex l.,** one curved like the exterior of a hollow sphere; it brings light to a focus. **convexoconcave l.,** one having one convex and one concave face. **crystalline l.,** lens (2). **cylindrical l.,** one that is a section of a cylinder cut parallel to its axis, with one surface plane and the other concave or convex. **decentered l.,** one in which the visual line does not pass through the center. **dispersing l.,** concave l. **omnifocal l.,** one whose power increases continuously and regularly in a downward direction, avoiding the discontinuity in field and power inherent in bifocal and trifocal lenses. **orthoscopic l.,** one that gives a flat and undistorted field of vision. **periscopic l.,** a concavoconvex or biconcave lens. **planoconcave l.,** a lens with one plane and one concave side. **planoconvex l.,** a lens with one plane and one convex side. **spherical l.,** one that is a segment of a sphere. **trial l's,** lenses used in determining visual acuity. **trifocal l.,** see under *glasses.*

lentectomize (len-tek′to-mīz) to remove the crystalline lens by surgical excision.

lentectomy (-tek′to-me) excision of the lens of the eye.

lenticonus (len″tĭ-ko′nus) a congenital conical bulging, anteriorly or posteriorly, of the lens of the eye.

lenticular (len-tik′u-ler) 1. pertaining to or shaped like a lens. 2. pertaining to the lens of the eye. 3. pertaining to the lenticular nucleus.

lenticulostriate (len-tik″u-lo-stri′āt) pertaining to lenticular nucleus and corpus striatum.

lenticulothalamic (-thah-lam′ik) relating to the lenticular nucleus and the thalamus.

lentiform (len′tĭ-fōrm) lens-shaped.

lentigines (len-tij′ĭ-nēz) plural of *lentigo.*

lentiginosis (len-tĭj″ĭ-no′sis) a condition marked by multiple lentigines.

lentiglobus (len″tĭ-glo′bus) exaggerated curvature of the lens of the eye, producing an anterior spherical bulging.

lentigo (len-ti′go), pl. *lentig′ines* [L.] a flat brownish pigmented spot on the skin due to increased deposition of melanin and an increased number of melanocytes. **l. malig′na, malignant l.,** melanotic freckle of Hutchinson.

leontiasis (le″on-ti′ah-sis) the leonine facies of lepromatous leprosy, due to nodular invasion of the subcutaneous tissue. **l. os′sea,** hypertrophy of the bones of the cranium and face, giving it a vaguely leonine appearance.

leper (lep′er) a person with leprosy; a term now in disfavor.

lepidic (lĕ-pid′ik) pertaining to scales.

lepothrix (lep′o-thriks) trichomycosis axillaris.

lepra (lep′rah) leprosy; prior to about 1850, psoriasis.

leprechaunism (lep′rĕ-kon″izm) a lethal familial congenital condition in which the infant is small and has elfin facies and severe endocrine disorders, as indicated by enlarged clitoris and breasts.

leprid (lep′rid) cutaneous lesion or lesions of tuberculoid leprosy: hypopigmented or erythematous nodules or plaques, lacking bacilli.

leprology (lep-rol′o-je) the study of leprosy.

leproma (lep-ro′mah) a superficial granulomatous nodule rich in leprosy bacilli, the characteristic lesion of lepromatous leprosy.

lepromatous (-tus) pertaining to lepromas; see under *leprosy.*

lepromin (lep′ro-min) a repeatedly boiled, autoclaved, gauze-filtered suspension of finely triturated lepromatous tissue and leprosy bacilli, used in the skin test for tissue resistance to leprosy.

leprosarium (lep″ro-sa′re-um) a hospital or colony for treatment and isolation of patients with leprosy.

leprostatic (-stat′ik) inhibiting the growth of *Mycobacterium leprae;* an agent that so acts.

leprosy (lep′ro-se) a chronic communicable disease caused by *Mycobacterium leprae* and characterized by the production of granulomatous lesions of the skin, mucous membranes, and peripheral nervous system. Two principal, or polar, types are recognized: lepromatous and tuberculoid. **borderline l.,** a form transitional between lepromatous and tuberculoid leprosy. **cutaneous l.,** lepromatous l. **dimorphous l.,** borderline l. **indeterminate l.,** leprosy in which hypopigmented macules of uncharacteristic histology occur; it may develop into lepromatous, tuberculoid, or borderline type. **lazarine l.,** a pure diffuse variant of lepromatous leprosy in which lepromas are absent but the entire skin may become infiltrated, and localized gangrenous macules may occur. Loosely used to refer to bullous or ulcerating manifestations of leprosy. **lepromatous l.,** that form marked by the development of lepromas and by an abundance of leprosy bacilli from the onset; nerve damage occurs only slowly, and the skin reaction to lepromin is negative. It is the only form which may regularly serve as a source of infection. **macular l., maculoanesthetic l.,** tuberculoid leprosy with hypopigmented, anesthetic macular skin lesions. **neural l.,** tuberculoid l. **nodular l.,** lepromatous l. **reactional l.,** leprosy during one of the recurring phases of acute exacerbation of lesions, accompanied in the lepromatous form by fever and often erythema multiforme. **trophoneurotic l.,** tuberculoid leprosy in which the visible lesions result entirely from the effects of denervation of tissue. **tuberculoid l.,** the form in which leprosy bacilli are few or lacking and nerve damage occurs early, so that all skin lesions are denervated from the onset, often with dissociation of sensation; the skin reaction to lepromin is positive, and the patient is rarely a source of infection to others.

leptazol (lep′tah-zol) pentylenetetrazol.

lepto- word element [Gr.], *slender; delicate.*

leptocephalus (lep″to-sef′ah-lus) a person with an abnormally tall, narrow skull.

leptochromatic (-kro-mat′ik) having a fine chromatin network.

leptocyte (lep′to-sīt) an erythrocyte characterized by a hemoglobinated border surrounding a clear area containing a center of pigment.

leptocytosis (lep″to-si-to′sis) leptocytes in the blood.

leptodactyly (-dak′tĭ-le) abnormal slenderness of the digits. **leptodac′tylous,** adj.

leptomeninges (-mĕ-nin′jēz) the pia mater and arachnoid taken together. **leptomenin′geal,** adj.

leptomeningitis (-men″in-ji′tis) inflammation of the leptomeninges.

leptomeningopathy (-men″ing-gop′ah-the) any disease of the leptomeninges.

leptomonad (-mo′nad) 1. of or pertaining to *Leptomonas.* 2. denoting the leptomonad form; see *promastigote.* 3. a protozoon exhibiting the leptomonad (promastigote) form.

Leptomonas (-mo′nas) a genus of protozoa of the family Trypanosomatidae, parasitic in the digestive track of insects.

leptopellic (-pel′ik) having a narrow pelvis.

leptophonia (-fo′ne-ah) weakness or feebleness of the voice. **leptophon′ic,** adj.

leptorrhine (lep′to-rīn) having a nasal index below 48.

leptoscope (-skōp) an optical apparatus for measuring the thickness of cell membranes.

Leptospira (lep″to-spi′rah) a genus of bacteria (family Treponemataceae), certain serotypes of which cause leptospirosis.

leptospire (lep′to-spīr) an individual organism of the genus *Leptospira.*

leptospirosis (lep″to-spi-ro′sis) any infectious disease due to certain serotypes of *Leptospira,* manifested by lymphocytic meningitis, hepatitis, and nephritis, separately or in combination.

leptotene (lep′to-tēn) the stage of meiosis in which the chromosomes are threadlike in shape.

leptothricosis (lep″to-thrĭ-ko′sis) leptotrichosis. **l. conjuncti′vae,** Parinaud's oculoglandular syndrome caused by *Leptothrix.*

Leptothrix (lep′to-thriks) a genus of schizomycetes (family Chlamydobacteriaceae), widely distributed and usually found in fresh water.

leptotrichosis (lep″to-trĭ-ko′sis) any infection with *Leptothrix.*

Leritine (ler′ĭ-tīn) trademark for preparations of anileridine.

lesbian (lez′be-an) 1. pertaining to lesbianism. 2. a female homosexual.

lesbianism (lez′be-ah-nizm″) homosexuality between women.

lesion (le′zhun) any pathological or traumatic discontinuity of tissue or loss of function of a part. **Armanni-Ebstein l.,** vacuolization of the renal tubular epithelium in diabetes. **Blumenthal l.,** a proliferative vascular lesion in the smaller arteries in diabetes. **central l.,** any lesion of the central nervous system. **Ghon's primary l.,** see under *tubercle.* **Janeway l.,** a small erythematous or hemorrhagic lesion, usually on the palms or soles, in bacterial endocarditis. **primary l.,** the original lesion manifesting a disease, as a chancre.

lethal (le′thal) deadly; fatal.

lethargy (leth′ar-je) a condition of drowsiness or indifference. **African l.,** see under *trypanosomiasis.*

leucine (lu′sēn) an amino acid, $C_6H_{13}NO_2$, essential for optimal growth in infants and for nitrogen equilibrium in adults.

leucinuria (lu″sin-u′re-ah) leucine in the urine.

leuco- for words beginning thus, see also those beginning *leuko-.*

Leuconostoc (lu″ko-nos′tok) a genus of slime-forming saprophytic bacteria (tribe Streptococceae) found in milk and fruit juices, including *L. citro′vorum, L. dextran′icum,* and *L. mesenteroi′des.*

leucovorin (-vo′rin) folinic acid.

leuk(o)- word element [Gr.], *white; leukocyte.*

leukapheresis (lu″kah-fĕ-re′sis) the selective removal of leukocytes from withdrawn blood, which is then retransfused into the patient.

leukemia (lu-ke′me-ah) a progressive, malignant disease of the blood-forming organs, marked by distorted proliferation and development of leukocytes and their precursors in the blood and bone marrow. **leuke′mic,** adj. **acute promyelocytic l.,** promyelocytic l. **aleukemic l.,** that in which the leukocyte count is normal or below normal. **basophilic l.,** leukemia in which the basophilic leukocytes predominate. **l. cu′tis,** leukemia with leukocytic invasion of the skin marked by pink, reddish brown, or purple macules, papules, and tumors. **embryonal l.,** stem cell l. **eosinophilic l.,** a form in which eosinophils are the predominating cells. **granulocytic l.,** myelocytic l. **histiocytic l.,** monocytic l. **leukopenic l.,** aleukemic l. **lymphatic l., lymphoblastic l., lymphocytic l., lymphogenous l., lymphoid l.,** a form associated with hyperplasia and overactivity of the lymphoid tissue, in which the leukocytes are lymphocytes or lymphoblasts. **lymphosarcoma cell l.,** a form marked by large numbers of lymphosarcoma cells in the peripheral blood; depending on degree of bone marrow involvement, it may be a variant of lymphosarcoma. **mast cell l.,** a form marked by overwhelming numbers of tissue mast cells in the peripheral blood. **megakaryocytic l.,** hemorrhagic thrombocythemia. **micromyeloblastic l.,** a form marked by the presence of large numbers of micromyeloblasts. **monocytic l.,** that in which the predominating leukocytes are monocytes. **myeloblastic l.,** leukemia in which myeloblasts predominate. **myelocytic l., myelogenous l., myeloid granulocytic l.,** a form arising from myeloid tissue in which the granular polymorphonuclear leukocytes and their precursors predominate. **plasma cell l., plasmacytic l.,** a form in which the predominating cell in the peripheral blood is the plasma cell. **promyelocytic l.,** a form in which the predominant cells are promyeloblasts, rather than myeloblasts, often associated with abnormal bleeding secondary to thrombocytopenia, hypofibrinogenemia, and decreased levels of coagulation Factor V. **Rieder cell l.,** myeloblastic leukemia in which the blood contains asynchronously developed cells with immature cytoplasm and a lobulated, relatively more mature nucleus. **stem cell l.,** a form in which the predominating cell is so immature and primitive that its classification is difficult. **subleukemic l.,** aleukemic l.

leukemid (lu-ke'mid) any of the polymorphic skin eruptions associated with leukemia; clinically, they may be nonspecific, i.e., papular, macular, purpuric, etc., but histopathologically they may represent true leukemic infiltrations.

leukemogen (lu-ke'mo-jen) any substance which produces leukemia. **leukemogen'ic,** adj.

leukemogenesis (lu-ke''mo-jen'ĕ-sis) the induction or development of leukemia.

leukemoid (lu-ke'moid) exhibiting blood and sometimes clinical findings resembling those of true leukemia, but due to some other cause.

leukin (lu'kin) a bactericidal substance from leukocyte extract.

leukoagglutinin (lu''ko-ah-gloo'tĭ-nin) an agglutinin which acts upon leukocytes.

leukoblast (lu'ko-blast) an immature granular leukocyte. **granular l.,** promyelocyte.

leukoblastosis (lu''ko-blas-to'sis) a general term for proliferation of leukocytes.

leukocidin (-si'din) a substance produced by some pathogenic bacteria that is toxic to polymorphonuclear leukocytes (neutrophils).

leukocyte (lu'ko-sīt) white cell; a colorless blood corpuscle capable of ameboid movement, whose chief function is to protect the body against microorganisms causing disease and which may be classified in two main groups: *granular* and *nongranular.* **leukocyt'ic,** adj. **agranular l's,** nongranular l's. **basophilic l.,** basophil (2). **endothelial l.,** Mallory's name for the large wandering cells of the circulating blood and the tissues which have notable phagocytic properties; see *endotheliocyte.* **eosinophilic l.,** eosinophil (2). **granular l's,** granulocytes; leukocytes containing abundant granules in their cytoplasm, including neutrophils, eosinophils, and basophils. **hyaline l.,** monocyte. **lymphoid l's,** nongranular l's. **neutrophilic l.,** neutrophil (2). **nongranular l's,** leukocytes without specific granules in their cytoplasm, including lymphocytes and monocytes. **polymorphonuclear l.,** neutrophil (2).

leukocythemia (lu''ko-si-the'me-ah) leukemia.

leukocytoblast (-si'to-blast) leukoblast.

leukocytogenesis (-si''to-jen'ĕ-sis) the formation of leukocytes.

leukocytolysin (-si-tol'ĭ-sin) a lysin that leads to disruption of leukocytes.

leukocytolysis (-si-tol'ĭ-sis) disintegration of leukocytes. **leukocytolyt'ic,** adj.

leukocytoma (-si-to'mah) a tumor-like mass of leukocytes.

leukocytometer (-si-tom'ĕ-ter) an instrument for counting leukocytes.

leukocytopenia (-si''to-pe'ne-ah) leukopenia.

leukocytoplania (-si''to-pla'ne-ah) wandering of leukocytes; passage of leukocytes through a membrane.

leukocytopoiesis (-si''to-poi-e'sis) leukopoiesis.

leukocytosis (-si-to'sis) a transient increase in the number of leukocytes in the blood, due to various causes. **basophilic l.,** increase in number of basophilic leukocytes in the blood. **mononuclear l.,** mononucleosis. **pathologic l.,** that due to some morbid reaction, e.g., infection or trauma.

leukocytotaxis (-si''to-tak'sis) leukotaxis.

leukocytotoxin (si-to-tok'sin) a toxin which destroys leukocytes.

leukocyturia (-si-tu're-ah) leukocytes in the urine.

leukoderma (-der'mah) an acquired condition with localized loss of pigmentation of the skin. **l. acquisi'tum centrif'ugum,** halo nevus. **syphilitic l.,** indistinct coarsely mottled hypopigmentation, usually on the sides of the neck, in late secondary syphilis.

leukodystrophy (-dis'tro-fe) disturbance of the white substance of the brain; see *leukoencephalopathy.* **metachromatic l.,** a hereditary leukoencephalopathy, marked by accumulation of a sphingolipid (sulfatide) in tissues, with diffuse loss of myelin in the central nervous system and progressive dementia and paralysis; classified according to age of onset as infantile, juvenile, and adult.

leukoedema (-ĕ-de'mah) an abnormality of the buccal mucosa, consisting of an increase in thickness of the epithelium and intracellular edema of the spinous or malpighian layer.

leukoencephalitis (-en-sef''ah-li'tis) 1. inflammation of the white substance of the brain. 2. forage poisoning, a contagious disease of horses.

leukoencephalopathy (-en-sef''ah-lop'ah-the) any of a group of diseases affecting the white substance of the brain. The term *leukodystrophy* is used to denote such disorders due to defective formation and maintenance of myelin in infants and children.

leukoerythroblastosis (-ĕ-rith''ro-blas-to'sis) an anemic condition associated with space-occupying lesions of the bone marrow, marked by a variable number of immature erythroid and myeloid cells in the circulation.

leukokeratosis (-ker''ah-to'sis) leukoplakia.

leukokoria (-ko're-ah) any condition marked by the appearance of a whitish reflex or mass in the pupillary area behind the lens.

leukokraurosis (-kraw-ro'sis) kraurosis vulvae.

leukolymphosarcoma (-lim''fo-sar-ko'mah) lymphosarcoma cell leukemia.

leukolysin (lu-kol'ĭ-sin) leukocytolysin.

leukolysis (lu-kol'ĭ-sis) leukocytolysis.

leukoma (lu-ko'mah) 1. a dense, white corneal

opacity. 2. leukoplakia of the buccal mucosa. **leukom′atous,** adj. **l. adhae′rens,** a white tumor of the cornea enclosing a prolapsed adherent iris.

leukomyelitis (lu″ko-mi″ĕ-li′tis) inflammation of the white substance of the spinal cord.

leukomyelopathy (-mi″ĕ-lop′ah-the) any disease of the white matter of the spinal cord.

leukomyoma (-mi-o′mah) lipomyoma.

leukonecrosis (-nĕ-kro′sis) gangrene with formation of a white slough.

leukonychia (-nik′e-ah) abnormal whiteness of the nails, either total or in spots or streaks.

leukopathia (-path′e-ah) 1. leukoderma. 2. disease of the leukocytes. **l. un′guium,** leukonychia.

leukopedesis (-pĕ-de′sis) diapedesis of leukocytes through blood vessel walls.

leukopenia (-pe′ne-ah) reduction of the number of leukocytes in the blood, the count being 5000 or less. **leukope′nic,** adj. **basophilic l.,** abnormal reduction of number of basophilic leukocytes in the blood. **malignant l., pernicious l.,** agranulocytosis.

leukoplakia (-pla′ke-ah) a disease marked by the development on the mucous membranes of the cheeks (*l. buccalis*), gums, or tongue (*l. lingualis*) of white thickened patches which sometimes show a tendency to fissure and to become malignant. **l. vul′vae,** the presence of hypertrophic grayish-white infiltrated patches on the vulvar mucosa.

leukopoiesis (-poi-e′sis) the production of leukocytes. **leukopoiet′ic,** adj.

leukopsin (lu-kop′sin) visual white; the colorless matter into which rhodopsin is changed by exposure to white light.

leukorrhagia (lu″ko-ra′je-ah) profuse leukorrhea.

leukorrhea (-re′ah) a whitish, viscid discharge from the vagina and uterine cavity.

leukosarcoma (-sar-ko′mah) the development of leukemia in patients originally having a well-differentiated, lymphocytic type of malignant lymphoma.

leukosarcomatosis (-sar-ko″mah-to′sis) the development of multiple sarcomas composed of leukemic cells.

leukosis (lu-ko′sis) proliferation of leukocyte-forming tissue. **avian l., fowl l.,** a group of transmissible, viral diseases of chickens, marked by proliferation of immature erythroid, myeloid, and lymphoid cells.

leukotaxine (lu″ko-tak′sin) a polypeptide that appears in injured tissue and inflammatory exudates; it promotes leukocytosis and leukotaxis and increases capillary permeability.

leukotaxis (-tak′sis) cytotaxis of leukocytes; the tendency of leukocytes to collect in regions of injury and inflammation. **leukotac′tic,** adj.

leukotomy (lu-kot′o-me) incision of the white matter of the frontal lobe of the brain.

leukotoxic (lu″ko-tok′sik) destructive to leukocytes.

leukotoxin (-tok′sin) a cytoxin destructive to leukocytes.

leukotrichia (-trik′e-ah) whiteness of the hair.

leukourobilin (-u″ro-bi′lin) a colorless decomposition product of urobilin.

leukovirus (-vi′rus) any of a group of RNA viruses causing leukemia and tumors in animals, including avian leukosis virus, Rous sarcoma virus, and murine leukemia virus.

levallorphan (lev″al-lor′fan) an antidote to narcotic overdosage, $C_{19}H_{25}NO$, used as the tartrate salt.

levamfetamine (le″vam-fet′ah-mēn) the levorotatory form of amphetamine; used as an anorexic drug in the form of the succinate salt.

levarterenol (lev″ar-tĕ-re′nol) norepinephrine. **l. bitartrate,** a vasopressor, $C_8H_{11}NO_3 \cdot C_4H_6O_6 \cdot H_2O$.

levator (lĕ-va′tor), pl. *levato′res* [L.] 1. a muscle that elevates an organ or structure. 2. an instrument for raising depressed osseous fragments in fractures.

levigation (lev″ĭ-ga′shun) the grinding to a powder of a moist or hard substance.

levo- word element [L.], *left.*

levocardia (le″vo-kar′de-ah) a term denoting normal position of the heart associated with transposition of other viscera (situs inversus).

levoclination (-kli-na′shun) rotation of the upper poles of the vertical meridians of the two eyes to the left.

levodopa (-do′pah) a synthetic compound of L-dopa, $C_9H_{11}NO_4$, used as an antiparkinsonian drug.

Levo-Dromoran (-dro′mo-ran) trademark for preparations of levorphanol.

levoduction (-duk′shun) movement of an eye to the left.

levogyration (-ji-ra′shun) levorotation.

levonordefrin (-nor′dĕ-frin) a vasoconstrictor, $C_9H_{13}NO_3$.

Levophed (lev′o-fed) trademark for a preparation of levarterenol bitartrate.

levopropoxyphene (le″vo-pro-pok′sĭ-fēn) an antitussive, $C_{32}H_{37}NO_5$; used as the napsylate salt.

levorotation (-ro-ta′shun) a turning to the left.

levorotatory (-ro′tah-to″re) turning the plane of polarization of polarized light to the left.

levorphanol (lēv-or′fah-nol) a narcotic analgesic, $C_{17}H_{23}NO$; used as the bitartrate salt.

levothyroxine (le″vo-thi-rok′sin) the levorotatory isomer of thyroxine, $C_{15}H_{10}I_4NO_4$; used as the sodium salt in thyroid replacement therapy.

levotorsion (-tor′shun) levoclination.

levoversion (-ver′zhun) a turning toward the left.

levulose (lev′u-lōs) fructose.

levurid (lev′u-rid) an allergic dermatitis ("id") thought to be caused by infection at a remote site by *Candida* or *Cryptococcus.*

L.F.A. left frontoanterior (position of the fetus).

L.F.P. left frontoposterior (position of the fetus).

L.F.T. left frontotransverse (position of the fetus).

L.H. luteinizing hormone.

Li chemical symbol, *lithium.*

libidinous (lĭ-bid′ĭ-nus) lustful; salacious.

libido (lĭ-be′do, lĭ-bi′do), pl. *libid′ines* [L.] 1. sexual desire. 2. the energy derived from the primitive impulses. In psychoanalysis the term is applied to the motive power of the sex life; in freudian psychology to psychic energy in general. **libid′inal,** adj.

libra (li′brah) [L.] 1. pound. 2. balance.

Librium (lib′re-um) trademark for preparations of chlordiazepoxide.

lice (līs) plural of *louse.*

licentiate (li-sen′she-āt) one holding a license from an authorized agency entitling him to practice a particular profession.

lichen (li′ken) 1. any of certain plants formed by the mutualistic combination of an alga and a fungus. 2. any of various papular skin diseases in which the lesions are typically small, firm papules set very close together, the specific kind being indicated by a modifying term. **l. amyloido′sus,** a condition characterized by localized cutaneous amyloidosis. **l. chron′icus sim′plex,** l. simplex chronicus. **l. fibromucinoido′sus, l. myxedemato′sus,** a condition resembling myxedema but unassociated with hypothyroidism, marked by mucinosis and a widespread eruption of asymptomatic, soft, pale red or yellowish, discrete papules. **l. nit′idus,** a skin eruption consisting of many, pinhead-sized pale, flat, sharply marginated, glistening, discrete papules, scarcely raised above the skin level. **l. pila′ris,** l. spinulosus. **l. planopila′ris,** a variant of lichen planus characterized by formation of acuminate horny papules around the hair follicles, in addition to the typical lesions of ordinary lichen planus. **l. pla′nus,** an inflammatory skin disease with wide, flat, violaceous, shiny papules in circumscribed patches; it may involve the hair follicles, nails, and buccal mucosa. **l. ru′ber monilifor′mis,** a variant of lichen simplex chronicus with papules arranged in linear beaded bands. **l. ru′ber pla′nus,** l. planus. **l. sclero′sus et atroph′icus,** a chronic atrophic skin disease marked by white papules with an erythematous halo and keratotic plugging. It sometimes affects the vulva (*kraurosis vulvae*) or penis (*balanitis xerotica obliterans*). **l. scrofuloso′rum, l. scrofulo′sus,** any eruption of minute reddish lichenoid follicular papules in children and young adults with tuberculosis. **l. sim′plex chron′icus,** a dermatosis of psychogenic origin, marked by a pruritic discrete or, more often, confluent papular eruption, usually confined to a localized area. **l. spinulo′sus,** a condition in which there is a horn or spine in the center of each hair follicle. **l. stria′tus,** a self-limited condition characterized by a linear lichenoid eruption, usually in children. **l. trop′icus,** miliaria rubra. **l. urtica′tus,** papular urticaria.

lichenification (li-ken″ĭ-fi-ka′shun) thickening and hardening of the skin, with exaggeration of its normal markings.

licheniformin (-ĭ-for′min) a group of antibiotic substances (licheniformin A, B, and C) from *Bacillus subtilis.*

lichenoid (li′kĕ-noid) resembling lichen.

licorice (lik′or-is) glycyrrhiza.

lidocaine (li′do-kān) a topical anesthetic, C_{14}-$H_{22}N_2O$, used as the hydrochloride salt.

lie (li) the situation of the long axis of the fetus with respect to that of the mother; see *presentation.* **transverse l.,** the situation during labor when the long axis of the fetus crosses the long axis of the mother; see table under *position.*

lien (li′en) [L.] spleen. **lie′nal,** adj. **l. acces-so′rius,** an accessory spleen. **l. mo′bilis,** an abnormally movable spleen.

lien(o)- word element [L.], *spleen;* see also words beginning *splen(o)-.*

lienocele (li-e′no-sēl) hernia of the spleen.

lienography (li″ĕ-nog′rah-fe) splenograhy.

lienomalacia (li-e″no-mah-la′she-ah) splenomalacia.

lienomedullary (-med′u-ler″e) splenomedullary.

lienomyelogenous (-mi″ĕ-loj′ĕ-nus) splenomyelogenous.

lienomyelomalacia (-mi″ĕ-lo-mah-la′she-ah) splenomyelomalacia.

lienotoxin (-tok′sin) splenotoxin.

lientery (li′en-ter″e) diarrhea with passage of undigested food. **lienter′ic,** adj.

lienunculus (li″en-ung′ku-lus) accessory spleen.

life (līf) the aggregate of vital phenomena; the quality or principle by which living things are distinguished from inorganic matter, as manifested by such phenomena as metabolism, growth, reproduction, adaptation, etc.

ligament (lig′ah-ment) 1. a band of fibrous tissue connecting bones or cartilages, serving to support and strengthen joints. 2. a double layer of peritoneum extending from one visceral organ to another. 3. cordlike remnants of fetal tubular structures that are nonfunctional after birth. **ligamen′tous,** adj. **accessory l.,** one that strengthens or supports another. **alar l's,** 1. two bands passing from the apex of the dens to the medial side of each occipital condyle. 2. a pair of folds of the synovial membrane of the knee joint. **alveolodental l.,** periodontal l. **arcuate l's,** the arched ligaments which connect the diaphragm with the lowest ribs and the first lumbar vertebra. **Barkow's l.,** anterior and posterior ligaments of the elbow joint. **Bérard's l.,** the suspensory ligament of the pericardium. **Bertin's l., Bigelow's l.,** iliofemoral l. **Botallo's l.,** a strong thick fibromuscular cord extending from the pulmonary artery to the aortic arch; it is the remains of the ductus arteriosus. **Bourgery's l.,** oblique popliteal ligament; a broad band of fibers extending from the medial condyle of the tibia across the back of the knee joint to the lateral epicondyle of the femur. **broad l.,** a broad fold of peritoneum supporting the uterus, extending from the uterus to the wall of the pelvis on either side. **Brodie's l.,** transverse humeral l. **Burns' l.,** falciform process (1). **Campbell's l.,** suspensory l. (2). **Camper's l.,** urogenital diaphragm. **capsular l.,** the fibrous layer of a joint capsule. **cardinal l.,** part of a thickening of the visceral pelvic fascia beside the cervix and vagina, passing laterally to merge with the upper fascia of the pelvic diaphragm. **Colles' l.,** a triangular band of fibers arising from the lacunar ligament and pubic bone and passing to the linea alba. **conoid l.,** the posteromedial portion of the coracoclavicular ligament, extending from the coracoid process to the inferior surface of the clavicle. **Cooper's l.,** pectineal l. **coracoclavicular l.,** a band joining the coracoid process of the scapula and the acromial extremity of the clavicle, consisting of two ligaments, the conoid and trapezoid. **costotransverse l's,** three ligaments (lateral, middle, and superior) that connect the neck of a rib to the transverse process of the vertebrae. **cotyloid l.,** a ring of fibrocartilage connected with the rim of the acetabulum. **cruciate l's of knee,** more or less cross-shaped ligaments, one anterior and one posterior which arise from the femur and pass through the intercondylar space to attach to the tibia. **crural l.,** inguinal l. **cysticoduodenal l.,** an anomalous fold of peritoneum extending between the gallbladder and the duodenum. **deltoid l.,** medial l. **diaphragmatic l.,** the involuting urogenital ridge that becomes the suspensory ligament of the ovary. **falciform l.,** a sickle-shaped sagittal fold of peritoneum that helps attach the liver to the diaphragm. **Flood's l.,** superior glenohumeral l. **Gerdy's l.,** suspensory l. of axilla. **Gimbernat's l.,** lacunar l. **glenohumeral l's,** bands, usually three, on the inner surface of the articular capsule of the humerus, extending from the glenoid lip to the anatomical neck of the humerus. **glenoid l.,** 1. a ring of fibrocartilage connected with the rim of the mandibular fossa. 2. (pl.) dense bands on the plantar surfaces of the metacarpophalangeal joints. 3. see under *lip.* **Henle's l.,** a lateral expansion of the lateral edge of the rectus abdominis which attaches to the pubic bone. **Hey's l's,** falciform process (1). **iliofemoral l.,** a very strong triangular or inverted Y-shaped band covering the anterior and superior portions of the hip joint. **iliotrochanteric l.,** a portion of the articular capsule of the hip joint. **inguinal l.,** a fibrous band running from the anterior superior spine of the ilium to the spine of the pubis. **lacunar l.,** a membrane with its base just medial to the femoral ring, one side attached to the inguinal ligament and the other to the pectineal line of the pubis. **lienorenal l.,** a fold of peritoneum connecting the spleen and the left kidney. **Lisfranc's l.,** a fibrous band extending from the medial cuneiform bone to the second metatarsal. **Lockwood's l.,** a suspensory sheath supporting the eyeball. **medial l.,** a large fan-shaped ligament on the medial side of the ankle. **meniscofemoral l's,** two small fibrous bands of the knee joint attached to the lateral meniscus, one (the anterior) extending to the anterior cruciate ligament and the other (the posterior) to the medial femoral condyle. **nephrocolic l.,** fasciculi from the fatty capsule of the kidney passing down on the right side to the posterior wall of the ascending colon and on the left side to the posterior wall of the descending colon. **nuchal l.,** a broad, fibrous, roughly triangular sagittal septum in the back of the neck, separating the right and left sides.

patellar l., the continuation of the central portion of the tendon of the quadriceps femoris muscle distal to the patella, extending from the patella to the tuberosity of the tibia. **pectineal l.,** a strong aponeurotic lateral continuation of the lacunar ligament along the pectineal line of the pubis. **periodontal l.,** the connective tissue structure that surrounds the roots of the teeth and holds them in place in the dental alveoli. **Petit's l.,** uterosacral l. **phrenicocolic l.,** a peritoneal fold passing from the left colic flexure to the adjacent part of the diaphragm. **Poupart's l.,** inguinal l. **pulmonary l.,** a vertical fold extending from the hilus to the base of the lung. **rhomboid l.,** a ligament connecting cartilage of the first rib to undersurface of clavicle. **Robert's l.,** anterior meniscofemoral l. **round l.,** 1. (*of femur*) a broad ligament arising from the fatty cushion of the acetabulum and inserted on the head of the femur. 2. (*of liver*) a fibrous cord from the navel to anterior border of the liver. 3. (*of uterus*) a fibromuscular band attached to the uterus near the uterine tube, passing through the inguinal ring to the labium majus. **Schlemm's l's,** two ligamentous bands of the capsule of the shoulder joint. **spring l.,** the ligament joining the calcaneus and navicular bone. **subflaval l.,** any of a series of bands of yellow elastic tissue between the ventral portions of the laminae of two adjacent vertebrae. **suspensory l.,** 1. (*of lens*) ciliary zonule. 2. (*of axilla*) a layer ascending from the axillary fascia and ensheathing the pectoralis minor muscle. 3. (*of ovary*) the portion of the broad ligament lateral to and above the ovary. **sutural l.,** a band of fibrous tissue between the opposed bones of a suture or immovable joint. **synovial l.,** a large synovial fold. **tendinotrochanteric l.,** a portion of the capsule of the hip joint. **transverse humeral l.,** a band of fibers bridging the intertubercular groove of the humerus and holding the tendon in the groove. **trapezoid l.,** the anterolateral portion of the coracoclavicular ligament, extending from the upper surface of the coracoid process to the trapezoid line of the clavicle. **umbilical l., medial,** a fibrous cord, the remains of the obliterated umbilical artery, running cranialward beside the bladder to the umbilicus. **uteropelvic l's,** expansions of muscular tissue in the broad ligament, radiating from the fascia over the obturator internus to the side of the uterus and the vagina. **uterosacral l.,** a part of the thickening of the visceral pelvic fascia beside the cervix and vagina. **ventricular l.,** vestibular l. **vesicoumbilical l.,** medial umbilical l. **vesicouterine l.,** a ligament that extends from the anterior aspect of the uterus to the bladder. **vestibular l.,** the membrane extending from the thyroid cartilage in front to the anterolateral surface of the arytenoid cartilage behind. **vocal l.,** the elastic tissue membrane extending from the thyroid cartilage in front to the vocal process of the arytenoid cartilage behind. **Weitbrecht's l.,** a small ligamentous band extending from the ulnar tuberosity to the radius. **Wrisberg's l.,** posterior meniscofemoral l. **Y l.,** iliofemoral l.

ligamentopexy (lig″ah-men′to-pek″se) fixation

of the uterus by shortening the round ligament.

ligamentum (lig″ah-men′tum), pl. *ligamen′ta* [L.] ligament.

ligand (li′gand, lig′and) an organic molecule that donates the necessary electrons to form coordinate covalent bonds with metallic ions. Also, an ion or molecule that reacts to form a complex with another molecule.

ligase (li′gās, lig′ās) any of a class of enzymes that catalyze the joining together of two molecules coupled with the breakdown of a pyrophosphate bond in ATP or a similar triphosphate.

ligate (li′gāt) to apply a ligature.

ligation (li-ga′shun) application of a ligature.

ligature (lig′ah-tūr) any material, such as thread or wire, used for tying a vessel or to constrict a part.

light (līt) electromagnetic radiation with a range of wavelength between 3900 (violet) and 7700 (red) angstroms, capable of stimulating the subjective sensation of sight; sometimes considered to include ultraviolet and infrared radiation as well. **axial l., central l.,** light whose rays are parallel to each other and to the optic axis. **cold l.,** a light transmitted through a quartz or plastic structure to dissipate the heat; this lamp may be applied directly to the skin, and used for transillumination of tissues for cancer diagnosis. **diffused l.,** light whose rays have been scattered by reflection and refraction. **Finsen l.,** light consisting mainly of violet and ultraviolet rays given off by Finsen's lamp; used in treatment of lupus and similar diseases. **idioretinal l., intrinsic l.,** the sensation of light in the complete absence of external stimuli. **Minin l.,** a lamp for therapeutic administration of violet and ultraviolet rays. **oblique l.,** light falling obliquely on a surface. **polarized l.,** light of which the vibrations are made over one plane or in circles or ellipses. **reflected l.,** light whose rays have been turned back from an illuminated surface. **refracted l.,** light whose rays have been bent out of their original course by passing from one transparent medium to another of different density. **transmitted l.,** light which passes or has passed through an object. **white l.,** that produced by a mixture of all wavelengths of electromagnetic energy perceptible as light. **Wood's l.,** ultraviolet radiation from a mercury vapor source, transmitted through a nickel-oxide filter (Wood's filter, or glass), which holds back all but a few violet rays and passes ultraviolet wavelengths of about 365 nm; used in diagnosis of fungal infections of the scalp and erythrasma, and to reveal the presence of porphyrins and fluorescent minerals.

lightening (līt′en-ing) the sensation of decreased abdominal distention produced by the descent of the uterus into the pelvic cavity, two to three weeks before labor begins.

lignin (lig′nin) a polysaccharide which along with cellulose forms the cell wall of plants and thus of wood.

lignocaine (lig′no-kān) lidocaine.

limb (lim) 1. one of the paired appendages of the body used in locomotion or grasping; in man, an arm or leg with all its component parts. 2. a structure or part resembling an arm or leg. **anacrotic l.,** the ascending portion of an arterial pulse tracing. **catacrotic l.,** the descending portion of an arterial pulse tracing. **pectoral l.,** the arm, or a homologous part. **pelvic l.,** the leg, or a homologous part. **phantom l.,** sensation, such as paresthesia or pain, subjectively perceived as originating in an absent limb after amputation. **thoracic l.,** pectoral l.

limbic (lim′bik) pertaining to a limbus, or margin; see also under *system.*

limbus (lim′bus), pl. *lim′bi*[L.] an edge, fringe, or border. **l. cor′neae,** the edge of the cornea where it joins the sclera. **l. lam′inae spira′lis,** the thickened periosteum of the osseous spiral lamina of the cochlea.

lime (līm) 1. a corrosively alkaline earth, CaO, used for absorbing carbon dioxide from air. 2. the acid fruit of the tropical tree, *Citrus aurantifolia;* its juice contains ascorbic acid. **l. arsenate,** a solution of white arsenic and soda in water, used as an insecticide. **chlorinated l.,** a compound produced by passing chlorine gas over calcium hydroxide; used as a bleaching agent and disinfectant. **slaked l.,** calcium hydroxide. **soda l.,** a mixture of calcium oxide with sodium hydroxide. **sulfurated l.,** a mixture of calcium sulfide, calcium sulfate, and carbon, used in skin diseases and as a depilatory.

limen (li′men), pl. *lim′ina* [L.] a threshold or boundary. **l. of insula, l. in′sulae,** the point at which the cortex of the insula is continuous with the cortex of the frontal lobe. **l. na′si,** the boundary line between the bony and cartilaginous portions of the nasal cavity walls.

liminal (lim′ĭ-nal) barely perceptible; pertaining to a threshold.

liminometer (lim″ĭ-nom′ĕ-ter) an instrument for measuring the strength of a stimulus that just induces a tendon reflex.

limitans (lim′ĭ-tanz) [L.] limiting.

lincomycin (lin′ko-mi″sin) an antibiotic produced by *Streptomyces lincolnensis;* used as the hydrochloride salt in infections with gram-positive cocci and gram-negative bacilli.

lindane (lin′dān) gamma benzene hexachloride.

line (līn) a stripe, streak, mark, or narrow ridge; often an imaginary line connecting different anatomic landmarks. **lin′ear,** adj. **absorption l's,** dark lines in the spectrum due to absorption of light by the substance through which the light has passed. **alveolonasal l.,** one from nasion to prosthion. **anocutaneous l.,** pectinate l. **base l.,** 1. one from the infraorbital ridge to the external auditory meatus and to the middle line of occiput. 2. a known quantity or a set of known quantities used as a reference point in evaluating similar data. **basinasal l.,** one from basion to nasion. **Beau's l's,** transverse furrows on the fingernails, usually a sign of a systemic disease but also due to other causes. **blood l.,** a line of direct descent through several generations. **cement l.,** a line visible in microscopic examination of bone in cross section, marking the boundary of an osteon (haversian system).

cervical l., an anatomic landmark determined by the junction of the enamel- and cementum-covered portions of a tooth (cementoenamel junction). **cleavage l's,** linear clefts in the skin indicative of direction of the fibers. **costoclavicular l.,** parasternal l. **l. of Douglas,** a crescentic line marking the termination of the posterior layer of the sheath of the rectus abdominis muscle. **epiphyseal l.,** one on the surface of an adult long bone, marking the junction of the epiphysis and diaphysis. **Fraunhofer's l's,** dark lines on the solar spectrum. **gingival l.,** 1. a line determined by the level to which the gingiva extends on a tooth. 2. any linear mark visible on the surface of the gingiva. **gluteal l.,** any of the three rough curved lines (anterior, inferior, and posterior) on the gluteal surface of the ala of the ilium. **gum l.,** gingival l. (1). **Hensen's l.,** M band. **Hilton's white l.,** pectinate l. **iliopectineal l.,** a ridge on the ilium and pubes showing the brim of the true pelvis. **incremental l's,** lines supposedly showing the successive layers deposited in a tissue, as in the tooth enamel. **intertrochanteric l.,** a line running obliquely from the greater to the lesser trochanter on the anterior surface of the femur. **Krause's l.,** Z band. **Langer's l's,** cleavage l's. **lead l.,** a bluish line at the edge of the gums in lead poisoning. **lip l.,** a line at the level to which the margin of either lip extends on the teeth. **mamillary l.,** an imaginary vertical line passing through the center of the nipple. **mammary l.,** 1. a line from one nipple to the other. 2. milk l. **median l.,** an imaginary line dividing the body surface equally into right and left sides. **milk l.,** the line of thickened epithelium in the embryo along which the mammary glands are developed. **mylohyoid l.,** a ridge on inner surface of lower jaw from the base of the symphysis to the ascending rami behind the last molar tooth. **nasobasilar l.,** one through the basion and nasion. **Nélaton's l.,** one from the anterior superior spine of the ilium to the most prominent part of tuberosity of the ischium. **nipple l.,** mamillary l. **nuchal l's,** three lines (inferior, superior, highest) on the outer surface of the occipital bone; see also *external occipital crest.* **parasternal l.,** an imaginary line midway between the mamillary line and the border of the sternum. **pectinate l.,** one marking the junction of the zone of the anal canal lined with stratified squamous epithelium and the zone lined with columnar epithelium. **pectineal l.,** 1. a line running down the posterior surface of the shaft of the femur, giving attachment to the pectineus muscle. 2. the anterior border of the superior ramus of the pubis. **Poupart's l.,** an imaginary line on the abdominal surface, passing perpendicularly through the midpoint of the inguinal ligament. **Retzius' l's,** incremental l's. **semilunar l.,** a curved line along the lateral border of each rectus abdominis muscle, marking the meeting of the aponeuroses of the internal oblique and transverse abdominal muscles. **Shenton's l.,** a curved line seen in radiographs of the normal hip, formed by the top of the obturator foramen. **Spieghel's l.,** semilunar l. **sternal l.,** an imaginary vertical line on the anterior body surface, corresponding to the lateral border of the sternum. **subcostal l.,** a transverse line on the surface of the abdomen at the level of the lower edge of the tenth costal cartilage. **temporal l's,** curved ridges, inferior and superior, on the outside of the parietal bone, continuous with the temporal line of the frontal bone, a ridge extending upward and backward from the zygomatic process of the frontal bone. **terminal l.,** one on the inner surface of each pelvic bone, from the sacroiliac joint to the iliopubic eminence anteriorly, separating the false from the true pelvis. **trapezoid l.,** a ridge on the inferior surface of the clavicle for attachment of the trapezoid ligament. **visual l.,** see under *axis.* **white l.,** linea alba. **Z l.,** see under *band.*

linea (lin′e-ah), pl. *lin′eae* [L.] line; in anatomy, a narrow ridge or streak on the surface of a structure. **l. al′ba,** white line; the tendinous median line on the anterior abdominal wall between the two rectus muscles. **lin′eae albi-can′tes,** see *atrophic striae.* **l. as′pera,** a rough longitudinal line on the back of the femur for muscle attachments. **lin′eae atroph′icae,** atrophic striae. **l. epiphysia′lis,** epiphyseal line. **l. glu′tea,** gluteal line. **l. ni′gra,** the linea alba when it has become pigmented in pregnancy. **l. splen′dens,** the sheath for the anterior spinal artery formed by the pia mater in the anterior median fissure of the spinal cord.

liner (līn′er) material applied to the inside of the walls of a cavity or container for protection or insulation of the surface.

lingua (ling′gwah), pl. *lin′guae* [L.] tongue. **lin′gual,** adj. **l. geograph′ica,** geographic tongue. **l. ni′gra,** black tongue. **l. plica′ta,** fissured tongue.

lingual (ling′gwal) pertaining to or near the tongue.

Linguatula (lin-gwat′u-lah) a genus of wormlike arthropods, the adults of which inhabit the respiratory tract of vertebrates; the larvae are found in the lungs and other internal organs. It includes *L. serra′ta* (*L. rhina′ria*), which parasitizes dogs and cats and sometimes man.

lingula (ling′gu-lah), pl. *lin′gulae* [L.] a small, tonguelike structure, such as the projection from the lower portion of the upper lobe of the left lung (*l. pulmo′nis sin′istra*), or the bony ridge between the body and great wing of the sphenoid (*l. sphenoida′lis*). **ling′ular,** adj.

lingulectomy (ling″gu-lek′to-me) excision of the lingula of the left lung.

linguo- word element [L.], *tongue.*

linguoclusion (ling″gwo-kloo′zhun) lingual occlusion.

linguodistal (-dis′tal) pertaining to the lingual and distal surfaces of a tooth, or the lingual and distal walls of a tooth cavity.

linguogingival (-jin′ji-val) pertaining to the tongue and gingiva or to the lingual and gingival walls of a tooth cavity.

linguopapillitis (-pap″ĭ-li′tis) inflammation or ulceration of the papillae of the edges of the tongue.

linguoversion (-ver′zhun) displacement of a tooth lingually from the line of occlusion.

liniment (lin′ĭ-ment) a medicinal preparation in an oily, soapy, or alcoholic vehicle, intended to be rubbed on the skin as a counterirritant or anodyne. **camphor l.,** a preparation of camphor and cottonseed oil used as a local irritant. **camphor and soap l.,** a mixture of green soap, camphor, rosemary oil, alcohol, and purified water, used as a local irritant. **chloroform l.,** a mixture of chloroform with camphor and soap liniment, used as a local irritant. **medicinal soft soap l.,** green soap tincture.

linin (li′nin) a substance of the achromatic nuclear reticulum of a cell.

linitis (lĭ-ni′tis) inflammation of gastric cellular tissue. **l. plas′tica,** diffuse fibrous proliferation of the submucous connective tissue of the stomach, resulting in thickening and fibrosis so that the organ is constricted, inelastic, and rigid (like a leather bottle).

linkage (lingk′ij) 1. the connection between different atoms in a chemical compound, or the symbol representing it in structural formulas; see also *bond.* 2. in genetics, the association of genes having loci on the same chromosome, which results in the tendency of a group of such nonallelic genes to be associated in inheritance. 3. in psychology, the connection between a stimulus and its response.

linseed (lin′sēd) dried ripe seed of *Linum usitatissimum;* used as a protective.

lint (lint) an absorbent surgical dressing material.

liothyronine (li′′o-thi′ro-nēn) the levorotatory isomer of triiodothyronine; used as the sodium salt in treatment of hypothyroidism.

lip (lip) 1. the upper or lower fleshy margin of the mouth. 2. any liplike part; labium. **cleft l.,** harelip. **double l.,** redundancy on the submucous tissue and mucous membrane on the lip on either side of the median line. **glenoid l.,** a ring of fibrocartilage joined to the rim of the glenoid cavity. **Hapsburg l.,** a thick, overdeveloped lower lip that often accompanies Hapsburg jaw.

lip(o)- word element [Gr.], *fat; lipid.*

lipacidemia (lip′′as-ĭ-de′me-ah) an excess of fatty acids in the blood.

lipaciduria (-du′re-ah) fatty acids in the urine.

lipase (li′pās, lip′ās) fat-splitting enzyme; any enzyme that catalyzes the splitting of fats into glycerol and fatty acids. **pancreatic l.,** steapsin.

lipectomy (li-pek′to-me) excision of a mass of subcutaneous adipose tissue.

lipedema (lip′′ĕ-de′mah) an accumulation of excess fat and fluid in subcutaneous tissues.

lipemia (li-pe′me-ah) an excess of lipids in the blood. **alimentary l.,** that occurring after ingestion of food. **l. retina′lis,** that manifested by a milky appearance of the veins and arteries of the retina.

lipid (lip′id) any of a group of organic substances, including fatty acids, neutral fats, waxes, steroids, and phosphatides, which are insoluble in water, but soluble in alcohol, ether, chloroform, and other fat solvents; lipids are a source of body fuel and an important constituent of cells.

lipidemia (lip′′ĭ-de′me-ah) lipemia.

lipidosis (lip′′ĭ-do′sis) any disorder of lipid metabolism involving abnormal accumulation of lipids, including Hand-Schüller-Christian disease, Niemann-Pick disease, Tay-Sachs disease, Gaucher's disease, etc.

lipiduria (lip′′ĭ-du′re-ah) lipids in the urine.

lipoarthritis (lip′′o-ar-thri′tis) inflammation of fatty tissue of a joint.

lipoatrophy (-at′ro-fe) atrophy of subcutaneous fatty tissues of the body.

lipoblast (lip′o-blast) a connective tissue cell which develops into a fat cell.

lipocaic (lip′′o-ka′ik) a substance extracted from the pancreas which prevents deposit of fat in the liver of animals after pancreatectomy.

lipocardiac (-kar′de-ak) relating to a fatty heart.

lipocatabolic (-kat′′ah-bol′ik) pertaining to or effecting catabolism of fat.

lipochondrodystrophy (-kon′′dro-dis′tro-fe) Hurler's syndrome.

lipochondroma (-kon-dro′mah) a tumor composed of mature lipomatous and cartilaginous elements.

lipochrome (lip′o-krōm) any of a group of fat-soluble hydrocarbon pigments, such as carotene, xanthophyll, lutein, chromophane, and the natural coloring material of butter, egg yolk, and yellow corn.

lipocyte (-sīt) a fat cell.

lipodystrophia (lip′′o-dis-tro′fe-ah) lipodystrophy. **l. progressi′va,** progressive lipodystrophy.

lipodystrophy (-dis′tro-fe) 1. any disturbance of fat metabolism. 2. progressive l. **intestinal l.,** Whipple's disease. **progressive l.,** progressive and symmetrical loss of subcutaneous fat from the parts above the pelvis, facial emaciation, and abnormal accumulation of fat about the thighs and buttocks.

lipofibroma (-fi-bro′mah) a lipoma containing areas of fibrosis.

lipofuscin (-fus′in) any of a class of fatty pigments formed by the solution of a pigment in fat.

lipogenesis (-jen′ĕ-sis) the formation of fat; the transformation of nonfat food materials into body fat. **lipogenet′ic,** adj.

lipogenic (-jen′ik) forming, producing, or caused by fat.

lipogenous (lĭ-poj′ĕ-nus) producing fatness.

lipogranuloma (lip′′o-gran′′u-lo′mah) a nodule of lipoid material associated with granulomatous inflammation.

lipogranulomatosis (-gran′′u-lo′′mah-to′sis) a condition of faulty lipid metabolism in which yellow nodules of lipoid material are deposited in the skin and mucosae, giving rise to granulomatous reactions.

lipoid (lip′oid) 1. fatlike. 2. lipid.

lipoidemia (lip′′oi-de′me-ah) lipemia.

lipoidosis (-do′sis) a disturbance of lipid metabolism with abnormal deposit of lipids in the cells.

lipoiduria (-du′re-ah) lipiduria.

Lipo-Lutin (li′′po-lu′tin) trademark for preparations of progesterone.

lipolysis (lǐ-pol′ǐ-sis) the splitting up or decomposition of fat. **lipolyt′ic,** adj.

lipoma (lǐ-po′mah) a benign fatty tumor usually composed of mature fat cells.

lipomatosis (lip″o-mah-to′sis) a condition marked by abnormal localized, or tumor-like, accumulations of fat in the tissues.

lipomatous (lǐ-po′mah-tus) affected with, or of the nature of, lipoma.

lipomeria (lip″o-me′re-ah) congenital absence of a limb.

lipometabolism (-mě-tab′o-lizm) metabolism of fat. **lipometabol′ic,** adj.

lipomyoma (-mi-o′mah) a benign mesenchymoma composed of leiomyomatous and lipomatous tissues.

lipomyxoma (-mik-so′mah) a myxoma containing fatty elements.

lipopenia (-pe′ne-ah) deficiency of lipids in the body.

lipopeptid (-pep′tid) any substance composed of amino acids and fatty acids.

lipophage (lip′o-fāj) a cell which absorbs or ingests fat.

lipophagia (lip″o-fa′je-ah) lipophagy. **l. granulomato′sis,** intestinal lipodystrophy.

lipophagy (lǐ-pof′ah-je) the absorption of fat; lipolysis. **lipopha′gic,** adj.

lipophil (lip′o-fil) an element which has an affinity for fat.

lipophilia (lip″o-fil′e-ah) affinity for fat. **lipophil′ic,** adj.

lipopolysaccharide (-pol″e-sak′ah-rīd) a molecule in which lipids and polysaccharides are linked.

lipoprotein (-pro′te-in) a combination of a lipid and a protein, having the general properties (e.g., solubility) of proteins.

liposarcoma (-sar-ko′mah) a malignant tumor characterized by large anaplastic lipoblasts, sometimes with foci of normal fat cells.

liposis (lǐ-po′sis) lipomatosis.

liposoluble (lip″o-sol′u-b'l) soluble in fats.

lipothymia (-thi′me-ah) syncope.

lipotrophy (li-pot′ro-fe) increase of bodily fat. **lipotroph′ic,** adj.

lipotropic (lip″o-trop′ik) acting on fat metabolism by hastening removal or decreasing the deposit of fat in the liver; also, an agent having such effects.

lipotropism (li-pot′ro-pizm) the condition of being lipotropic.

lipotropy (lǐ-pot′ro-pe) lipotropism.

lipovaccine (lip″o-vak′sēn) a vaccine in a vegetable oil vehicle.

lipoxidase (lǐ-pok′sǐ-dās) lipoxygenase.

lipoxygenase (lǐ-poks′ǐ-jě-nās) an enzyme that catalyzes the oxidation of polyunsaturated fatty acids to form a peroxide of the acid.

lipping (lip′ing) 1. a wedge-shaped shadow in the roentgenogram of chondrosarcoma between the cortex and the elevated periosteum. 2. the development of a bony overgrowth in osteoarthritis.

lipuria (lǐ-pu′re-ah) lipids in the urine.

Liquaemin (lik′wah-min) trademark for preparations of heparin.

Liquamar (-mar) trademark for a preparation of phenprocoumon.

liquefacient (lik″wě-fa′shent) 1. producing or pertaining to liquefaction. 2. an agent that produces liquefaction.

liquefaction (-fak′shun) conversion into a liquid form.

liquescent (lǐ-kwes′ent) tending to become liquid or fluid.

liquid (lik′wid) 1. a substance that flows readily in its natural state. 2. flowing readily; neither solid nor gaseous.

liquor (lik′er, li′kwor) 1. a liquid, especially an aqueous solution, or a solution not obtained by distillation. 2. a term applied to certain body fluids. **l. am′nii,** amniotic fluid. **l. cerebrospina′lis,** cerebrospinal fluid. **l. cotun′nii,** perilymph. **l. follic′uli,** the fluid in a developing ovarian follicle. **mother l.,** the liquid remaining after removal of crystals from a solution. **l. pu′ris,** the fluid portion of pus. **l. san′guinis,** blood plasma. **l. scar′pae,** endolymph.

Lissencephala (lis″en-sef′ah-lah) a group of placental mammals characterized by having a brain that is smooth or marked by only a few shallow gyri, as bats, rodents, etc.

lissencephaly (-sef′ah-le) agyria. **lissencephal′ic,** adj.

Listerella (lis-ter-el′ah) *Listeria.*

Listeria (lis-te′re-ah) a genus of gram-negative bacteria (family Corynebacterium); the single species, *L. monocytog′enes,* is found chiefly in lower animals. In man, it produces upper respiratory disease, septicemia, and encephalitic disease.

listeriosis (lis-tēr″e-o′sis) infection with organisms of the genus *Listeria.*

listerism (lis′ter-izm) the principles and practice of antiseptic and aseptic surgery.

liter (le′ter) the unit of volume in the metric system, equal to 1000 cubic centimeters or 1 cubic decimeter, or to 1.0567 quarts liquid measure.

lith(o)- word element [Gr.], *stone; calculus.*

lithagogue (lith′ah-gog) 1. expelling calculi. 2. an agent that promotes expulsion of calculi.

lithectasy (lǐ-thek′tah-se) extraction of calculi through the mechanically dilated urethra.

lithectomy (lǐ-thek′to-me) lithotomy.

lithemia (lǐ-the′me-ah) an excess of uric acid in the blood.

lithiasis (lǐ-thi′ah-sis) 1. a condition marked by formation of calculi and concretions. 2. gouty diathesis.

lithium (lith′e-um) chemical element (*see table*), at. no. 3, symbol Li. Its salts, especially *l. carbonate,* are used in the treatment of manic and other psychiatric disorders.

lithoclast (lith′o-klast) a lithotrite.

lithocystotomy (lith″o-sis-tot′o-me) incision of the bladder for removal of stone.

lithodialysis (-di-al′ĭ-sis) 1. the solution of calculi in the bladder by injected solvents. 2. litholapaxy.

lithogenesis (-jen′ĕ-sis) formation of calculi. **lithog′enous,** adj.

litholapaxy (lĭ-thol″ah-pak′se) the crushing of a stone in the bladder and washing out of the fragments.

litholysis (lĭ-thol′ĭ-sis) dissolution of calculi.

lithonephritis (lith″o-nĕ-fri′tis) inflammation of the kidney due to irritation by calculi.

lithonephrotomy (-nĕ-frot′o-me) excision of a renal calculus.

lithopedion (-pe′de-on) a calcified fetus.

lithophone (lith′o-fōn) a device for detecting calculi in the bladder by sound.

lithoscope (-skōp) an instrument for detecting calculi in the bladder.

lithotomy (lĭ-thot′o-me) incision of a duct or organ for removal of calculi.

lithotripsy (lith′o-trip″se) litholapaxy.

lithotriptic (-trip″tik) dissolving vesical calculi; also, an agent that so acts.

lithotrite (-trīt) an instrument for crushing calculi in the bladder.

lithotrity (lĭ-thot′rĭ-te) lithotripsy.

lithous (lith′us) pertaining to or of the nature of a calculus.

lithuresis (lith″u-re′sis) the passage of gravel in the urine.

litmus (lit′mus) a pigment prepared from *Rocella tinctoria* and other lichens; used as an acid-base (pH) indicator.

litter (lit′er) 1. a stretcher for carrying sick or wounded. 2. the offspring produced at one birth by a multiparous animal.

livedo (lĭ-ve′do) a discolored patch on the skin. **l. annula′ris, l. racemo′sa, l. reticula′ris,** a reddish blue, netlike mottling of the skin.

livedoid (liv′ĕ-doid) resembling livedo.

liver (liv′er) the large, dark-red gland in the upper part of the abdomen on the right side, just beneath the diaphragm. See Plate IV. Its manifold functions include storage and filtration of blood, secretion of bile, conversion of sugars into glycogen, and many other metabolic activities. **albuminoid l., amyloid l.,** one with albuminoid or amyloid degeneration. **biliary cirrhotic l.,** one in which the bile ducts are clogged and distended, the substance of the organ being inflamed; due to biliary cirrhosis. **fatty l.,** one affected with fatty infiltration. **floating l.,** wandering l. **foamy l.,** a liver seen post mortem, marked by the presence of numerous gas bubbles. **hobnail l.,** a liver whose surface is marked with nail-like points from cirrhosis. **lardaceous l.,** amyloid l. **nutmeg l.,** one presenting a mottled appearance when cut. **sago l.,** one affected with amyloid degeneration, the acini resembling boiled sago grains, i.e., translucent granules 2 or 3 mm. in diameter. **wandering l.,** a displaced and movable liver. **waxy l.,** albuminoid l.

livid (liv′id) discolored, as from a contusion or bruise; black and blue.

lividity (lĭ-vid′ĭ-te) the quality of being livid; discoloration, as of dependent parts, by gravitation of blood. **postmortem l.,** livor mortis.

livor (li′vor) discoloration. **l. mor′tis,** discoloration of dependent parts of the body after death.

lixiviation (liks″iv-e-a′shun) separation of soluble from insoluble material by use of an appropriate solvent, and drawing off the solution.

L.M. Licentiate in Midwifery.

L.M.A. left mentoanterior (position of fetus).

L.M.P. left mentoposterior (position of fetus).

L.M.T. left mentotransverse (position of fetus).

L.O.A. left occipitoanterior (position of fetus).

Loa (lo′ah) a genus of filarial nematodes, including *L. lo′a,* a West African species that migrates freely throughout the subcutaneous connective tissue, seen especially about the orbit and even under the conjunctiva, and occasionally causing edematous swellings.

loading (lōd′ing) administering sufficient quantities of a substance to test a subject's ability to metabolize or absorb it.

loaiasis (lo″ah-i′ah-sis) loiasis.

lobate (lo′bāt) divided into lobes.

lobe (lōb) 1. a more or less well-defined portion of an organ or gland. 2. one of the main divisions of a tooth crown. **lo′bar,** adj. **azygos l.,** a small accessory or anomalous lobe at the apex of the right lung. **caudate l.,** a small lobe of the liver between the inferior vena cava on the right and the left lobe. **cuneate l.,** cuneus. **ear l.,** the lower fleshy part of the external ear. **frontal l.,** the rostral (anterior) portion of the cerebral hemisphere. **hepatic l.,** one of the lobes of the liver, designated the right and left and the caudate and quadrate. **linguiform l.,** Riedel's l. **occipital l.,** the most posterior portion of the cerebral hemisphere, forming a small part of its dorsolateral surface. **parietal l.,** the upper central portion of the cerebral hemisphere, between the frontal and occipital lobes, and above the temporal lobe. **prefrontal l.,** the part of the frontal lobe of the brain anterior to the ascending convolution. **quadrate l.,** 1. precuneus. 2. a small lobe of the liver, between the gallbladder on the right, and the left lobe. **Riedel's l.,** an anomalous tongue-shaped mass of tissue projecting from the right lobe of the liver. **spigelian l.,** caudate l. **temporal l.,** the lower lateral lobe of the cerebral hemisphere.

lobectomy (lo-bek′to-me) excision of a lobe, as of the lung, brain, or liver.

lobelia (lo-be′le-ah) the dried leaves and tops of *Lobelia inflata,* a herb with properties resembling those of nicotine.

lobeline (lob′ĕ-lin) the principal alkaloid of *Lobelia inflata,* $C_{22}H_{27}NO_2$; used in certain anti-smoking preparations.

lobitis (lo-bi′tis) inflammation of a lobe, as of the lung.

lobocyte (lo′bo-sīt) a granulocyte with a segmented nucleus.

lobopodium (lo″bo-po′de-um), pl. *lobopo′dia* [Gr.] a blunt pseudopodium composed of ectoplasm or of ectoplasm and endoplasm.

lobotomy (lo-bot′o-me) incision of a lobe; in psychosurgery, section of the central core of white matter in the frontal lobe of the brain.

lobulated (lob′u-lāt″ed) made up of lobules.

lobule (lob′ūl) a small segment or lobe, especially one of the smaller divisions making up a lobe. **lob′ular,** adj. **l's of epididymis,** the wedge-shaped parts of the head of the epididymis, each comprising an efferent ductule of the testis. **hepatic l's,** the small vascular units comprising the substance of the liver. **l's of lung,** bronchopulmonary segments. **paracentral l.,** a lobe on the medial surface of the cerebral hemisphere, continuous with the pre- and postcentral gyri, limited below by the cingulate sulcus. **parietal l.,** one of the two divisions, inferior and superior, of the parietal lobe of the lung. **primary l. of lung, respiratory l.,** the functional unit of the lung, including a respiratory bronchiole, alveolar ducts and sacs, and alveoli. See Plate VII.

lobulus (lob′u-lus), pl. *lob′uli* [L.] lobule.

lobus (lo′bus), pl. *lo′bi* [L.] lobe.

local (lo′k'l) restricted to or pertaining to one spot or part; not general.

localization (lo″kah-li-za′shun) 1. the determination of the site or place of any process or lesion. 2. restriction to a circumscribed or limited area. **cerebral l.,** determination of areas of the cortex involved in performance of certain functions. **germinal l.,** the location on a blastoderm of prospective organs.

locator (lo′ka-tor) a device for determining the site of foreign objects within the body. **electroacoustic l.,** a device which amplifies into an audible click the contact of the probe with a solid object in tissue.

lochia (lo′ke-ah) a vaginal discharge occurring during the first week or two after childbirth. **lo′chial,** adj. **l. al′ba,** the final vaginal discharge after childbirth, when the amount of blood is decreased and the leukocytes are increased. **l. cruen′ta,** l. rubra. **l. purulen′ta,** l. alba. **l. ru′bra,** that occurring immediately after childbirth, consisting almost entirely of blood. **l. sanguinolen′ta,** l. serosa. **l. sero′sa,** the serous vaginal discharge occurring four or five days after childbirth.

lochiocolpos (lo″ke-o-kol′pos) distention of the vagina by retained lochia.

lochiometra (-me′trah) distention of the uterus by retained lochia.

lochiometritis (-me-tri′tis) puerperal metritis.

lochiorrhagia (-ra′je-ah) lochiorrhea.

lochiorrhea (-re′ah) an abnormally profuse lochia.

lochioschesis (lo″ke-os′kĕ-sis) retention of the lochia.

lockjaw (lok′jaw) 1. tetanus. 2. trismus.

loco (lo′ko) [Sp.] 1. any of various leguminous plants of the genera *Astragalus, Hosackia, Sophora,* and *Oxytropis,* poisonous to livestock in arid regions because of the selenium they contain. 2. locoism.

locoism (-izm) poisoning of livestock by loco, marked by locomotor disturbances, trembling, depression, and, in pregnant animals, abortion.

locomotion (lo″ko-mo′shun) movement, or the ability to move, from one place to another. **locomo′tive,** adj. **brachial l.,** brachiation.

locomotor (-mo′tor) of or pertaining to locomo-

tion; pertaining to or affecting the locomotive apparatus of the body.

loculus (lok′u-lus), pl. *loc′uli* [L.] 1. a small space or cavity. 2. a local enlargement of the uterus in some mammals, containing an embryo. **loc′ular,** adj.

locum (lo′kum) [L.] place. **l. ten′ens, l. ten′ent,** a practitioner who temporarily takes the place of another.

locus (lo′kus), pl. *lo′ci* [L.] place; site; in genetics, the specific site of a gene on a chromosome. **l. ceru′leus,** a pigmented eminence in the superior angle of the floor of the fourth ventricle of the brain.

löffleria (lef-le′re-ah) presence of the diphtheria bacillus without the ordinary symptoms of diphtheria.

log(o)- word element [Gr.], *words; speech.*

logadectomy (log″ah-dek′to-me) excision of a portion of the conjunctiva.

logagnosia (-ag-no′ze-ah) central word defect, as asphasia or alogia.

logagraphia (-ah-graf′e-ah) inability to express ideas in writing.

logamnesia (-am-ne′ze-ah) receptive aphasia.

logaphasia (-ah-fa′ze-ah) expressive aphasia.

logasthenia (-as-the′ne-ah) disturbance of the mental processes necessary to speech.

logoclonia (log′o-klon″e-ah) spasmodic repetition of the end-syllables of words.

logokophosis (log″o-ko-fo′sis) word deafness.

logomania (-ma′ne-ah) overtalkativeness.

logopathy (log-op′ah-the) any disorder of speech due to derangement of the central nervous system.

logopedia (log″o-pe′de-ah) logopedics.

logopedics (-pe′diks) the study and treatment of speech defects.

logoplegia (-ple′je-ah) paralysis of speech organs.

logorrhea (-re′ah) excessive or abnormal volubility.

logospasm (log′o-spazm) the spasmodic utterance of words.

-logy word element [Gr.], *science; treatise; sum of knowledge in a particular subject.*

loiasis (lo-i′ah-sis) infection with nematodes of the genus *Loa.*

loin (loin) the part of the back between the thorax and pelvis.

Lomotil (lo′mo-til) trademark for preparations of diphenoxylate.

longissimus (lon-jis′ĭ-mus) [L.] longest.

longitudinalis (lon″jĭ-tu″dĭ-na′lis) [L.] lengthwise.

longus (long′gus) [L.] long.

loop (lōōp) a turn or sharp curve in a cordlike structure. **capillary l's,** minute endothelial tubes that carry blood in the papillae of the skin. **closed l.,** a system in which the input to one or more of the subsystems is affected by its own output. **Henle's l.,** the U-shaped loop of the uriniferous tubule of the kidney.

L.O.P. left occipitoposterior (position of fetus).

lophotrichous (lo-fot′rĭ-kus) having two or more flagella at one end (of a bacterial cell).

lordoscoliosis (lor″do-sko″le-o′sis) lordosis complicated with scoliosis.

lordosis (lor-do′sis) forward curvature of the lumbar spine. **lordot′ic,** adj.

Lorfan (lor′fan) trademark for preparations of levallorphan.

L.O.T. left occipitotransverse (position of fetus).

lotio (lo′she-o) [L.] lotion. **l. al′ba, l. sulfura′ta,** white lotion.

lotion (lo′shun) a liquid suspension or dispersion for external application to the body. **benzyl benzoate l.,** a preparation of benzyl benzoate, triethanolamine, and oleic acid; scabicide. **calamine l.,** a mixture of calamine, zinc oxide, glycerin, bentonite magma, and calcium hydroxide solution; used as a topical protectant. **calamine l., phenolated,** calamine lotion with liquefied phenol added. **white l.,** a preparation of zinc sulfate and sulfurated potash in purified water; astringent and protectant.

Lotusate (lo′tu-sāt) trademark for a preparation of talbutal.

loupe (lōōp) [Fr.] a magnifying lens.

louse (lows), pl. *lice* [L.] any of various parasitic insects; species parasitic upon man are *Pediculus humanus* var. *capitis* (head l.), *P. humanus* var. *corporis* (body, or clothes, l.), and *Phthirus pubis* (crab, or pubic, l.). Lice are major vectors of typhus, relapsing fever, and trench fever.

loxoscelism (lok-sos′sĕ-lizm) a morbid condition due to the bite of the spiders *Loxosceles laeta* and *L. reclusa,* beginning with a painful erythematous vesicle and progressing to a gangrenous slough of the affected area.

loxotomy (lok-sot′o-me) oval amputation.

lozenge (loz′enj) troche.

L.P.N. Licensed Practical Nurse.

L.R.C.P. Licentiate of Royal College of Physicians.

L.R.C.S. Licentiate of Royal College of Surgeons.

LRF leuteinizing hormone releasing factor.

L.S.A. left sacroanterior (position of fetus).

L.Sc.A. left scapuloanterior (position of fetus).

L.Sc.P. left scapuloposterior (position of fetus).

LSD lysergic acid diethylamide; see *lysergide.*

L.S.P. left sacroposterior (position of fetus).

L.S.T. left sacrotransverse (position of fetus).

LTH luteotropic hormone.

Lu chemical symbol, *lutetium.*

lucanthone (loo-kan′thōn) an antischistosomal, $C_{20}H_{24}N_2OS$, used as the hydrochloride salt.

lucidity (lu-sid′ĭ-te) clearness of mind. **lu′cid,** adj.

luciferase (lu-sif′er-ās) an enzyme that catalyzes the bioluminescent reaction of luciferin in animals capable of luminescence.

luciferin (lu-sif′er-in) the organic substrate of luciferase which, when acted upon by luciferase in the presence of ATP and molecular oxygen, produces light.

lucifugal (lu-sif′u-gal) avoiding, or repelled by, bright light.

lucipetal (lu-sip′ĕ-tal) seeking, or attracted to, bright light.

lues (lu′ēz) syphilis. **luet′ic,** adj.

lumb(o)- word element [L.], *loin.*

lumbago (lum-ba′go) pain in the lumbar region.

lumbar (lum′bar) pertaining to the loins.

lumbarization (lum″bar-i-za′shun) nonfusion of the first and second segments of the sacrum so that there is one additional articulated vertebra, the sacrum consisting of only four segments.

lumbocolostomy (lum″bo-ko-los′to-me) colostomy through the lumbar region.

lumbocostal (-kos′tal) pertaining to the loin and ribs.

lumbodynia (-din′e-ah) lumbago.

lumboinguinal (-ing′gwĭ-nal) pertaining to the loin and groin.

lumbosacral (-sa′kral) pertaining to the lumbar and sacral region, or to the lumbar vertebrae and sacrum.

lumbricide (lum′brĭ-sīd) an agent that kills lumbrici (ascarides).

lumbricoid (lum′brĭ-koid) resembling the earthworm; designating the ascaris.

lumbricosis (lum″brĭ-ko′sis) infection with lumbrici (ascarides).

lumbricus (lum-bri′kus), pl. *lumbri′ci* [L.] 1. the earthworm. 2. ascaris.

lumbus (lum′bus) [L.] loin.

lumen (lu′men), pl. *lu′mina* [L.] the cavity or channel within a tube or tubular organ. **lu′minal,** adj. **residual l.,** the remains of Rathke's pouch, between the pars distalis and pars intermedia of the hypophysis.

luminescence (lu″mĭ-nes′ens) the property of giving off light without a corresponding degree of heat.

luminophore (lu″mĭ-no-fōr″) a chemical group which gives the property of luminescence to organic compounds.

lumirhodopsin (loo″mĭ-ro-dop′sin) an intermediate product of exposure of rhodopsin to light.

lunate (lu′nāt) 1. moon-shaped or crescentic. 2. lunate bone; see *Table of Bones.*

lung (lung) the organ of respiration; either of the pair of organs that effect aeration of blood, lying on either side of the heart within the chest cavity. See Plates VI and VII. **black l., coalminer's l.,** pneumoconiosis of coal workers. **farmer's l.,** a morbid condition due to inhalation of moldy hay dust. **iron l.,** popular name for the Drinker respirator. **white l.,** pneumonia alba.

lungmotor (lung′mo-tor) an apparatus for forcing air, or air and oxygen, into the lungs.

lungworm (-werm) any parasitic worm that invades the lungs, e.g., *Paragonimus westermani* in man.

lunula (lu′nu-lah), pl. *lu′nulae* [L.] a small, crescentic or moon-shaped area or structure, e.g., the white area at the base of the nail of a finger or toe, or one of the segments of the semilunar valves of the heart.

lupiform (lu′pĭ-form) resembling lupus.

lupoid (lu′poid) 1. pertaining to lupus vulgaris.

2. a variant of sarcoidosis marked by small papular lesions.

lupus (lu′pus) any of a group of skin diseases in which the lesions are characteristically eroded. **discoid l. erythemato′sus (D.L.E.)**, lupus erythematosus limited to cutaneous manifestations, with red macules covered with scanty adherent scales which fall off, leaving scars; the lesions typically form a butterfly pattern over the bridge of the nose and cheeks, but other areas may be involved. **l. erythemato′sus**, a chronic connective tissue disease manifested in two main types; see *discoid l. erythematosus* and *systemic l. erythematosus*. **disseminated l. erythemato′sus**, systemic l. erythematosus. **l. erythemato′sus profun′dus**, a form with deep brawny indurations or nodules under normal skin or under typical patches of lupus erythematosus; ulceration may occur. **l. milia′ris dissemina′tus fa′ciei**, a form marked by multiple, discrete, superficial nodules on the face, particularly on the eyelids, upper lip, chin, and nares. **l. per′nio**, a distinctive soft violaceous skin lesion occurring in sarcoidosis. **systemic l. erythemato′sus (S.L.E.)**, a chronic generalized connective tissue disorder, ranging from mild to fulminating, marked by skin eruptions, arthralgia, fever, leukopenia, visceral lesions, other constitutional symptoms, and many autoimmune phenomena, including hypergammaglobulinemia, with the presence of antinuclear antibodies and LE cells. **l. vulga′ris**, tuberculosis of the skin marked by formation of brownish nodules in the corium, chronic ulceration, and severe scarring.

lusus (lu′sus) [L.] a game, sport. **l. natu′rae**, a sport; a minor congenital anomaly.

luteal (lu′te-al) pertaining to or having the properties of the corpus luteum or its active principle.

lutein (lu′te-in) 1. a lipochrome from the corpus luteum, fat cells, and egg yolk. 2. any lipochrome.

luteinic (lu″te-in′ik) pertaining to the corpus luteum, to lutein, or to luteinization.

luteinization (lu″te-in″i-za′shun) the process by which a postovulatory ovarian follicle transforms into a corpus luteum through vascularization, follicular cell hypertrophy, and lipid accumulation, the latter in some species giving the yellow color indicated by the term.

luteohormone (lu″te-o-hor′mōn) progesterone.

luteoma (lu″te-o′mah) 1. a luteinized granulosa-theca cell tumor. 2. nodular hyperplasia of ovarian lutein cells sometimes occurring in the last trimester of pregnancy.

luteotrophic (lu″te-o-trof′ik) luteotropic.

luteotropic (-trop′ik) stimulating formation of the corpus luteum.

luteotropin (-trop′in) a hormone of the anterior pituitary which stimulates formation of the corpus luteum; identical with prolactin.

lutetium (lu-te′she-um) chemical element (*see table*), at. no. 71, symbol Lu.

Lutocylol (lu″to-si′lol) trademark for preparations of ethisterone.

Lutrexin (lu-trek′sin) trademark for a preparation of lututrin.

Lutromone (lu′tro-mōn) trademark for a preparation of progesterone.

lututrin (loo′tu-trin) a protein or polypeptide substance from the corpus luteum of sow ovaries; used as a uterine relaxant in treatment of functional dysmenorrhea.

luxation (luk-sa′shun) dislocation. **Malgaigne's l.**, pulled elbow.

luxus (luk′sus) [L.] excess.

L.V.N. licensed vocational nurse.

Lw chemical symbol, *lawrencium*.

lyase (lī′as) any of a class of enzymes that remove groups from their substrates (other than by hydrolysis), leaving double bonds, or that conversely add groups to double bonds.

lycanthropy (li-kan′thro-pe) delusion in which the patient believes himself a wolf.

lycomania (li″ko-ma′ne-ah) lycanthropy.

lycopene (li′ko-pēn) the red carotenoid pigment of tomatoes and various berries and fruits.

lycoperdonosis (li″ko-per″do-no′sis) a respiratory disease due to inhalation of spores of the puffball fungus, *Lycoperdon*.

lying-in (li′ing-in) 1. puerperal. 2. puerperium.

lymph (limf) 1. a transparent, usually slightly yellow, often opalescent liquid found within the lymphatic vessels, and collected from tissues in all parts of the body and returned to the blood via the lymphatic system. Its cellular component consists chiefly of lymphocytes. **aplastic l., corpuscular l.**, lymph that contains an excess of leukocytes and does not tend to become organized. **euplastic l.**, that which tends to coagulate and become organized. **inflammatory l.**, lymph produced by inflammation, as in wounds. **Koch's l.**, see *New* and *Old tuberculin*. **plastic l.**, inflammatory lymph having a tendency to become organized. **tissue l.**, lymph derived from body tissues and not from the blood. **vaccine l.**, material containing vaccinia virus collected from vaccinial vesicles of calves; used for active immunization against smallpox.

lympha (lim′fah) [L.] lymph.

lymphadenectasis (lim-fad″ĕ-nek′tah-sis) enlargement of a lymph node.

lymphadenectomy (-nek′to-me) excision of one or more lymph nodes.

lymphadenia (lim″fah-de′ne-ah) hypertrophy of lymph nodes.

lymphadenitis (lim-fad″ĕ-ni′tis) inflammation of the lymph nodes.

lymphadenocele (lim-fad′ĕ-no-sel) a cyst of a lymph node.

lymphadenogram (-no-gram″) the film produced by lymphadenography.

lymphadenography (lim″fad-ĕ-nog′rah-fe) radiography of lymph nodes after injection of a contrast medium in a lymphatic vessel.

lymphadenoid (lim-fad′ĭ-noid) resembling the tissue of lymph nodes; see under *tissue*.

lymphadenoma (lim-fad″ĕ-no′mah) lymphoma.

lymphadenopathy (-nop′ah-the) disease of the lymph nodes. **dermatopathic l.**, regional lymph node enlargement associated with melanoderma and other dermatoses marked by chronic erythroderma. **giant follicular l.,** see under *lymphoma.*

lymphadenosis (-no′sis) hypertrophy or proliferation of lymphoid tissue. **l. benig′na cu′tis,** a benign inflammatory hyperplasia of lymphocytes in the skin, principally on the face or ears, in the form of solitary or disseminated yellowish brown to bluish red nodules that usually involute spontaneously.

lymphadenotomy (-not′o-me) incision of a lymph node.

lymphagogue (lim′fah-gog) an agent promoting the production of lymph.

lymphangial (lim-fan′je-al) pertaining to a lymphatic vessel.

lymphangiectasia, lymphangiectasis (lim-fan″je-ek-ta′ze-ah; -ek′tah-sis) dilatation of the lymphatic vessels. **lymphangiectat′ic,** adj.

lymphangiectomy (-ek′to-me) excision of one or more lymphatic vessels.

lymphangiitis (-i′tis) lymphangitis.

lymphangioendothelioma (lim-fan″je-o-en″-do-the″le-o′mah) lymphangioma in which endothelial cells are the main component.

lymphangiofibroma (-fi-bro′mah) a fibrosing lymphangioma.

lymphangiogram (lim-fan′je-o-gram″) the film produced by lymphangiography.

lymphangiography (lim-fan″je-og′rah-fe) radiography of lymphatic channels after introduction of a contrast medium. **pedal l.,** radiography of the lymphatic channels of the lower extremity after injection of contrast medium into the first and second interdigital spaces of the foot.

lymphangiology (lim-fan″je-ol′o-je) the scientific study of the lymphatic system.

lymphangioma (lim-fan″je-o′mah) a tumor composed of new-formed lymph spaces and channels. **cavernous l.,** dilatation of the lymphatic vessels resulting in cavities filled with lymph. **cystic l., l. cys′ticum,** a cystic growth usually found in the neck or groin, thought to originate from a developmental anomaly of the primitive lymphatic spaces; symptoms are largely due to compression of adjoining structures by the mass.

lymphangiophlebitis (lim-fan″je-o-fle-bi′tis) inflammation of the lymphatic vessels and the veins.

lymphangioplasty (lim-fan′je-o-plas″te) surgical restoration of lymphatic channels.

lymphangiosarcoma (lim-fan″je-o-sar-ko′mah) a malignant tumor of lymphatic vessels, usually arising in a limb that is the site of chronic lymphedema.

lymphangiotomy (lim-fan″je-ot′o-me) incision of a lymphatic vessel.

lymphangitis (lim″fan-ji′tis) inflammation of a lymphatic vessel.

lymphatic (lim-fat′ik) 1. pertaining to lymph or to a lymphatic vessel. 2. a lymphatic vessel.

lymphaticostomy (lim-fat″ĭ-kos′to-me) surgical creation of an opening into a lymphatic duct, usually the thoracic duct.

lymphatism (lim′fah-tizm) a morbid condition due to excessive production or growth of lymphoid tissues, resulting in impaired development and lowered vitality.

lymphatitis (lim″fah-ti′tis) inflammation of some part of the lymphatic system.

lymphatolysis (-tol′ĭ-sis) destruction of lymphatic tissue. **lymphatolyt′ic,** adj.

lymphectasia (lim″fek-ta′ze-ah) distention with lymph.

lymphedema (lim″fĕ-de′mah) chronic swelling of a part due to accumulation of interstitial fluid (edema) secondary to obstruction of lymphatic vessels or lymph nodes. **congenital l.,** Milroy's disease.

lymphemia (lim-fe′me-ah) the presence of an undue number of lymphocytes or their precursors in the blood.

lymphenteritis (lim″fen-ter-i′tis) enteritis with serous infiltration.

lymphnoditis (limf″no-di′tis) inflammation of a lymph node.

lymphoblast (lim′fo-blast) the immature, nucleolated precursor of the mature lymphocyte. **lymphoblas′tic,** adj.

lymphoblastoma (lim″fo-blas-to′mah) poorly differentiated lymphocytic malignant lymphoma.

lymphoblastomatosis (-blas″to-mah-to′sis) the condition produced by the presence of lymphoblastomas.

lymphoblastosis (-blas-to′sis) an excess of lymphoblasts in the blood.

lymphocyte (lim′fo-sīt) a mononuclear, nongranular leukocyte having a deeply staining nucleus containing dense chromatin and a pale-blue–staining cytoplasm. Chiefly a product of lymphoid tissue, it participates in immunity. **lymphocyt′ic,** adj. **B-l's,** bursa-equivalent lymphocytes; those that migrate to tissues without passing through or being influenced by the thymus; they mature into plasma cells that synthesize humoral antibody. **T-l's,** thymus-dependent lymphocytes; those that pass through or are influenced by the thymus before migrating to tissues; they are responsible for cell-mediated immunity and delayed hypersensitivity.

lymphocythemia (lim″fo-si-the′me-ah) excess of lymphocytes in the blood.

lymphocytoblast (-si′to-blast) a lymphoblast.

lymphocytoma (-si-to′mah) well-differentiated lymphocytic malignant lymphoma. **lymphocyto′matous,** adj.

lymphocytopenia (-si″to-pe′ne-ah) reduction of the number of lymphocytes in the blood.

lymphocytopoiesis (-poi-e′sis) the formation of lymphocytes. **lymphocytopoiet′ic,** adj.

lymphocytosis (-si-to′sis) an excess of normal lymphocytes in the blood or an effusion.

lymphoduct (lim′fo-dukt) a lymphatic vessel.

lymphoepithelioma (lim″fo-ep″ĭ-the″le-o′mah) a pleomorphic, poorly differentiated carcinoma arising from modified epithelium overlying lymphoid tissue of the nasopharynx.

lymphogenous (lim-foj′ĕ-nus) 1. producing

lymph. 2. produced from lymph or in the lymphatics.

lymphoglandula (lim″fo-glan′du-lah), pl. *lymphoglan′dulae* [L.] a lymph node.

lymphogonia (-go′ne-ah) large lymphocytes having a large nucleus, little chromatin, and nongranular cytoplasm.

lymphogram (lim′fo-gram) a roentgenogram of the lymphatic channels and lymph nodes.

lymphogranuloma (lim″fo-gran″u-lo′mah) Hodgkin's disease. **l. inguina′le, venereal l., l. vene′reum,** a venereal infection due to a strain of *Chlamydia trachomatis,* marked by a primary transient ulcerative lesion of the genitals, followed by swelling of the regional lymph nodes; later, lymphatic obstruction may result in elephantiasis of the external genitals, while scarring accounts for rectal stricture.

lymphogranulomatosis (-gran″u-lo″mah-to′-sis) 1. infectious granuloma of the lymphatic system. 2. Hodgkin's disease.

lymphography (lim-fog′rah-fe) roentgenography of the lymphatic channels and lymph nodes after injection of radiopaque material.

lymphoid (lim′foid) resembling or pertaining to lymph or to tissue of the lymphatic system.

lymphoidectomy (lim″foi-dek′to-me) excision of lymphoid tissue.

lymphoidocyte (lim-foi′do-sīt) an embryonic cell considered by some to be the stem cell of all blood cells; hemocytoblast.

lymphokine (lim′fo-kīn) a general term for soluble protein mediators postulated to be released by sensitized lymphocytes on contact with antigen, and believed to play a role in macrophage activation, lymphocyte transformation, and cell-mediated immunity.

lymphokinesis (lim″fo-ki-ne′sis) 1. movement of endolymph in the semicircular canals. 2. the circulation of lymph in the body.

lymphology (lim-fol′o-je) the study of the lymphatic system.

lymphoma (lim-fo′mah) any neoplastic disorder of lymphoid tissue. Often used to denote *malignant l.,* classifications of which are based on predominant cell type and degree of differentiation; various categories may be subdivided into nodular and diffuse types depending on the predominant pattern of cell arrangement. **Burkitt's l.,** a form of undifferentiated malignant lymphoma, usually occurring in Africa, manifested usually as a large osteolytic lesion in the jaw or as an abdominal mass. **clasmocytic l.,** histiocytic malignant l. **giant follicular l.,** nodular well-differentiated lymphocytic malignant lymphoma, microscopically characterized by multiple, proliferative, follicle-like nodules which disturb the normal architecture of the lymph nodes. **granulomatous l.,** Hodgkin's disease. **lymphoblastic l.,** poorly differentiated lymphocytic malignant lymphoma. **lymphocytic l.,** well-differentiated lymphocytic malignant l. **malignant l., histiocytic,** a form in which the predominant cell is the primitive mesenchymal cell or one that has differentiated into the identifiable reticulum cell. **malignant l., mixed cell,** a form containing proliferations of both histiocytes and lymphocytes. **malignant l., poorly differentiated lymphocytic,** a form in which the predominant cell is morphologically similar to the lymphoblast, containing a fine nuclear chromatin structure and one or more nucleoli. **malignant l., undifferentiated,** a form in which relatively large stems cells with large nuclei, pale, scanty cytoplasm, and indistinct borders predominate. **malignant l., well-differentiated lymphocytic,** a form in which the predominant cell is the mature lymphocyte.

lymphomatosis (lim″fo-mah-to′sis) the formation of multiple lymphomas in the body. **avian l., l. of fowl,** avian leukosis involving chiefly the lymphocytes.

lymphomatous (lim-fo′mah-tus) pertaining to, or of the nature of, lymphoma.

lymphonodus (lim″fo-no′dus) lymph node.

lymphopathia (-path′e-ah) lymphopathy. **l. vene′reum,** see under *lymphogranuloma.*

lymphopathy (lim-fop′ah-the) any disease of the lymphatic system.

lymphopenia (lim″fo-pe′ne-ah) decrease in the number of lymphocytes of the blood.

lymphoplasmia (-plaz′me-ah) absence of hemoglobin from red blood cells.

lymphopoiesis (-poi-e′sis) the development of lymphocytes or of lymphatic tissue. **lymphopoiet′ic,** adj.

lymphoproliferative (-pro-lif′er-ah″tiv) pertaining to or characterized by proliferation of lymphoid tissue.

lymphoreticular (-rĕ-tik′u-lar) pertaining to reticuloendothelial cells of lymph nodes.

lymphoreticulosis (-re-tik″u-lo′sis) proliferation of the reticuloendothelial cells of the lymph nodes. **benign l.,** cat-scratch fever.

lymphorrhagia (-ra′je-ah) lymphorrhea.

lymphorrhea (-re′ah) flow of lymph from cut or ruptured lymph vessels.

lymphorrhoid (lim′fo-roid) a localized dilatation of a perianal lymph channel, resembling a hemorrhoid.

lymphosarcoma (lim″fo-sar-ko′mah) a general term applied to malignant neoplastic disorders of lymphoid tissue, but not including Hodgkin's disease; see *lymphoma.*

lymphosarcomatosis (-sar″ko-mah-to′sis) a condition characterized by the presence of multiple lesions of lymphosarcoma.

lymphostasis (lim-fos′tah-sis) stoppage of lymph flow.

lymphotaxis (lim″fo-tak′sis) the property of attracting or repulsing lymphocytes.

lymph-vascular (limf-vas′ku-ler) pertaining to lymphatic vessels.

lynestrenol (lin-es′trĕ-nōl) a progestin, $C_{20}H_{28}O$.

Lynoral (lin′or-al) trademark for a preparation of ethinyl estradiol.

lyophil (li′o-fil) a lyophilic substance.

lyophile (-fil) 1. lyophil. 2. lyophilic.

lyophilic (li″o-fil′ik) having an affinity for, or stable in, solution.

lyophilization (li-of″ĭ-li-za′shun) the creation of

a stable preparation of a biological substance by rapid freezing and dehydration of the frozen product under high vacuum.

lyophobe (li′o-fōb) a lyophobic substance.

lyophobic (li″o-fo′bik) not having an affinity for, or unstable in, solution.

lyotropic (-trop′ik) readily soluble.

lypressin (li-pres′in) a synthetic preparation of lysine vasopressin used as an antidiuretic.

lyse (līz) 1. to cause or produce disintegration of a compound, substance, or cell. 2. to undergo lysis.

lysemia (li-se′me-ah) disintegration of the blood.

lysergide (li′ser-jīd) LSD; a hallucinogenic compound, $C_{20}H_{25}N_3O$, derived from lysergic acid, which has been used experimentally in the study and treatment of mental disorders, and has been found to be antagonistic to serotonin in its action on smooth muscle. The side effects include bizarre behavior and, reportedly, psychosis and chromosomal damage.

lysin (li′sin) an antibody capable of causing dissolution of cells, including hemolysin, bacteriolysin, etc.

lysine (li′sēn) a naturally occurring amino acid, essential for optimal growth in human infants and for maintenance of nitrogen equilibrium in adults.

lysinogen (li-sin′o-jen) lysogen.

lysis (li′sis) 1. destruction or decomposition, as of a cell or other substance, under influence of a specific agent. 2. mobilization of an organ by division of restraining adhesions. 3. gradual abatement of the symptoms of a disease.

-lysis (li′sis) word element [Gr.], *dissolution.* **-lyt′ic,** adj.

lysocephalin (li″so-sef′ah-lin) a cephalin from which a fatty acid radical has been removed.

lysogen (li′so-jen) an antigen inducing the formation of lysin.

lysogenesis (li″so-jen′ĕ-sis) 1. the production of lysis or lysins. 2. lysogenicity.

lysogenic (-jen′ik) 1. producing lysins or causing lysis. 2. pertaining to lysogenicity.

lysogenicity (-jĕ-nis′ĭ-te) 1. the ability to produce lysins or cause lysis. 2. the potentiality of a bacterium to produce phage. 3. the specific association of the phage genome (prophage) with the bacterial genome in such a way that only a few, if any, phage genes are transcribed.

lysogeny (li-soj′ĭ-ne) lysogenicity.

lysokinase (li″so-ki′nās) general term for substances of the fibrinolytic system that activates plasma proactivators.

lysolecithin (-les′ĭ-thin) a lecithin from which the terminal fatty acid radical has been removed.

lysosome (li′so-sōm) one of the minute bodies occurring in many types of cells, containing various hydrolytic enzymes and normally involved in the process of localized intracellular digestion. **lysoso′mal,** adj.

lysotype (-tīp) phage type.

lysozyme (-zīm) a crystalline basic enzyme present in saliva, tears, egg white, and many animal fluids, which functions as an antibacterial agent.

lyssa (lis′ah) rabies. **lys′sic,** adj.

lyssoid (lis′oid) resembling rabies.

lyssophobia (lis″o-fo′be-ah) morbid fear of rabies.

lytic (lit′ik) 1. pertaining to lysis or to a lysin. 2. producing lysis.

lyze (līz) lyse.

M

M symbol, *molar* (solution), as M/10, M/100, etc., denote tenth molar, hundredth molar, etc.

M. macerate, maximal, member, meter, minim, muscle, myopia; [L.] mil or mille (*thousand*), misce (*mix*), mistura (*mixture*).

m. meter.

m- meta-.

μ symbol, *micron.*

M.A. Master of Arts; meter angle; mental age.

ma. milliampere.

Macaca (mah-kak′ah) a genus of Old World monkeys.

macerate (mas′er-āt) to soften by wetting or soaking.

maceration (mas″ĕ-ra′shun) the softening of a solid or tissue by soaking.

machine (mah-shēn′) a mechanical contrivance for doing work or generating energy. **heart-lung m.,** a combination blood pump (artificial heart) and blood oxygenator (artificial lung) used in open-heart surgery.

macies (ma′she-ēz) [L.] wasting.

macr(o)- word element [Gr.], *large; abnormal size.*

Macracanthorhynchus (mak″rah-kan″tho-ring′kus) a genus of parasitic worms (phylum Acanthocephala), including *M. hirudina′ceus,* found in swine.

macrencephaly (mak″ren-sef′ah-le) hypertrophy of the brain.

macroamylase (mak″ro-am′ĭ-lās) a complex in which normal serum amylase is bound to a variety of specific binding proteins, forming a complex too large for renal excretion.

macroamylasemia (-am″ĭ-la-se′me-ah) the presence of macroamylase in the blood. **macroamylase′mic,** adj.

macrobiota (-bi-o′tah) the macroscopic living organisms of a region. **macrobiot′ic,** adj.

macroblast (mak′ro-blast) an abnormally large, nucleated red blood cell; a large young normoblast with megaloblastic features.

macroblepharia (mak″ro-blĕ-fa′re-ah) abnormal largeness of the eyelid.

macrocardius (-kar′de-us) a fetus with an extremely large heart.

macrocephalous (-sef″ah-lus) having an abnormally large head.

macrocephalus (-sef′ah-lus) macrocephaly.

macrocephaly (-sef′ah-le) excessive size of the head.

macrocheilia (-ki′le-ah) excessive size of lip.

macrocheiria (-ki′re-ah) megalocheiria.

macrochemistry (-kem′is-tre) chemistry in which the reactions may be seen with the naked eye.

macrocolon (-ko′lon) megacolon.

macrocrania (-kra′ne-ah) excessive size of the skull in relation to the face.

macrocyte (mak′ro-sīt) an abnormally large erythrocyte. **macrocyt′ic,** adj.

macrocythemia (mak″ro-si-the′me-ah) the presence of macrocytes in the blood.

macrocytosis (-si-to′sis) macrocythemia.

macrodactyly (-dak′tĭ-le) megalodactyly.

macrodontia (-don′she-ah) abnormal increase in size of one or more teeth. **mac′rodont, macrodon′tic,** adj.

macrofauna (-faw′nah) the macroscopic animal organisms of a region.

macroflora (-flo′rah) the macroscopic vegetable organisms of a region.

macrogamete (-gam′ēt) see *gamete* (2).

macrogametocyte (-gah-me′to-sīt) see *gametocyte.*

macrogenitosomia (-jen″ĭ-to-so′me-ah) excessive bodily development, with unusual enlargement of the genital organs. **m. pre′cox,** macrogenitosomia occurring at an early age.

macroglia (mak-rog′le-ah) astroglia.

macroglobulin (mak″ro-glob′u-lin) a globulin of unusually high molecular weight, in the range of 1,000,000.

macroglobulinemia (-glob″u-lĭ-ne′me-ah) increased levels of macroglobulins in the blood. **Waldenström's m.,** a progressive syndrome of the endothelial system seen chiefly in males past age 50, associated with macroglobulinemia, adenopathy, hepatosplenomegaly, hemorrhagic phenomena, anemia, and lymphocytosis and plasmacytosis of bone marrow.

macroglossia (-glos′e-ah) excessive size of the tongue.

macrognathia (-nath′e-ah) enlargment of the jaw. **macrognath′ic,** adj.

macrogyria (-ji′re-ah) moderate reduction in the number of sulci of the cerebrum, sometimes with increase in the brain substance, resulting in excessive size of the gyri.

macrolide (mak′ro-līd) any antibiotic with molecules having many-membered lactone rings.

macromastia (mak″ro-mas′te-ah) excessive size of the breasts.

macromelia (-me′le-ah) enlargement of one or more limbs.

macromelus (mak-rom′ĕ-lus) a fetus with abormally large or long limbs.

macromere (mak′ro-mēr) one of the large blastomeres formed by unequal cleavage of the fertilized ovum (at the vegetal pole).

macromethod (-meth″od) a chemical method using customary (not minute) quantities of the substance being analyzed.

macromolecule (mak″ro-mol′ĕ-kūl) a very large molecule having a polymeric chain structure, as in proteins, polysaccharides, etc. **macromolec′ular,** adj.

macromonocyte (-mon′o-sīt) a giant monocyte.

macromyeloblast (-mi′ĕ-lo-blast″) a large myeloblast.

macronormoblast (-nor′mo-blast) macroblast.

macronucleus (-nu′kle-us) in ciliate protozoa, the larger of two types of nucleus in each cell, which governs nonreproductive functions.

macronychia (-nik′e-ah) abnormal length of the fingernails.

macrophage (mak′ro-fāj) any of the highly phagocytic cells in the wall of blood vessels and in loose connective tissue; they are usually immobile (histiocytes, or fixed macrophages), but when stimulated by inflammation become actively mobile (free macrophages).

macrophthalmia (mak″rof-thal′me-ah) abnormal enlargement of the eyeball.

macropolycyte (mak″ro-pol′ĭ-sīt) a hypersegmented polymorphonuclear leukocyte of greater than normal size.

macroprosopia (-pro-so′pe-ah) excessive size of the face.

macropsia (mah-krop′se-ah) a disorder of visual perception in which objects appear larger than their actual size.

macrorrhinia (mak″ro-rin′e-ah) excessive size of the nose.

macroscopic (-skop′ik) of large size; visible to the unaided eye.

macroscopy (mah-kros′ko-pe) examination with the unaided eye.

macrosigmoid (mak″ro-sig′moid) excessive size of the sigmoid.

macrosomatia (-so-ma′she-ah) great bodily size.

macrostomia (-sto′me-ah) greatly exaggerated width of the mouth.

macrotia (mak-ro′she-ah) abnormal enlargement of the pinna of the ear.

macula (mak′u-lah), pl. *mac′ulae* [L.] 1. a stain, spot, or thickening; in anatomy, an area distinguishable by color or otherwise from its surroundings. 2. a macule: a discolored spot on the skin that is not raised above the surface. 3. a corneal scar, appreciated as a gray spot. 4. macula lutea. **mac′ular, mac′ulate,** adj. **mac′ulae acus′ticae,** the macula sacculi and macula utriculi considered together. **m. adher′ens,** desmosome. **mac′ulae atroph′icae,** white scarlike patches formed on the skin by atrophy. **mac′ulae caeru′leae,** faint grayish blue spots, sometimes found peripheral to the axilla or groin in pediculosis corporis or pubis. **cerebral**

m., tache cérébrale. **m. cor′neae,** a circumscribed opacity of the cornea. **m. cribro′sa,** one of three perforated areas (inferior, medial, and superior) on the vestibular wall through which branches of the vestibulocochlear nerve pass to the saccule, utricle, and semicircular canals. **m. den′sa,** a zone of heavily nucleated cells in the distal renal tubule. **m. fla′va,** a yellow nodule at one end of a vocal cord. **m. follic′uli,** the point on the surface of a vesicular ovarian follicle where rupture occurs. **m. germinati′va,** germinal area. **m. lu′tea, m. ret′inae,** an irregular yellowish depression on the retina, lateral to and slightly below the optic disk. **m. sac′culi,** a thickening on the wall of the saccule where the epithelium contains hair cells that receive and transmit vestibular impulses. **m. utric′uli,** a thickening in the wall of the utricle where the epithelium contains hair cells that receive and transmit vestibular impulses.

macule (mak′ūl) a macula.

maculocerebral (mak″u-lo-ser′ĕ-bral) pertaining to the macula lutea and the brain.

maculopapular (-pap′u-lar) both macular and papular.

madarosis (mad″ah-ro′sis) loss of eyelashes or eyebrows.

Madurella (mad″u-rel′ah) a genus of imperfect fungi. *M. gris′ea* and *M. myceto′mi* are etiologic agents of maduromycosis.

maduromycosis (mah-du″ro-mi-ko′sis) a chronic disease due to various fungi or actinomycetes, affecting the foot, hands, legs, or other parts, including the internal organs; the most common form is that of the foot (*Madura foot*), marked by sinus formation, necrosis, and swelling.

mafenide (maf′en-īd) an antibacterial, $C_7H_{10}N_2$-O_2S, used topically in superficial infections.

magaldrate (mag′al-drāt) a combination of aluminum hydroxide and magnesium hydroxide used as an antacid.

magenta (mah-jen′tah) fuchsin or other salt of rosaniline.

maggot (mag′ot) the soft-bodied larva of an insect, especially a form living in decaying flesh.

magma (mag′mah) 1. a suspension of finely divided material in a small amount of water. 2. a thin, pastelike substance composed of organic material. **bentonite m.,** a preparation of bentonite and purified water, used as a suspending agent. **bismuth m.,** milk of bismuth. **magnesia m.,** magnesium hydroxide; used as a laxative and antacid.

Magnacort (mag′nah-kort) trademark for a preparation of hydrocortamate.

magnesia (mag-ne′zhe-ah) magnesium oxide.

magnesium (mag-ne′ze-um) chemical element (*see table*), at. no. 12, symbol Mg; its salts are essential in nutrition, being required for the activity of many enzymes, especially those concerned with oxidative phosphorylation. **m. carbonate,** a basic hydrated magnesium carbonate containing the equivalent of 40–43.5% magnesium oxide; an antacid. **m. citrate,** a mild cathartic. **m. hydroxide,** $Mg(OH)_2$; a laxative and antacid. **m. oxide,** MgO; an antacid. **m.**

phosphate, tribasic m. phosphate: Mg_3-$(PO_4)_2 \cdot 5H_2O$; an antacid. **m. phosphate, dibasic,** $MgHPO_4 \cdot 3H_2O$; a mild saline laxative. **m. stearate,** a combination of magnesium with stearic and palmitic acids; a dusting powder and tablet lubricant. **m. sulfate,** Epsom salt: $MgSO_4 \cdot 7H_2O$; a cathartic. **m. trisilicate,** a combination of magnesium oxide and silicon dioxide with varying proportions of water; an antacid.

magnet (mag′net) an object having polarity and capable of attracting iron.

magnetism (mag′nĕ-tizm) magnetic attraction or repulsion.

magnetotherapy (mag-ne″to-ther′ah-pe) treatment of disease by magnetic currents.

magnetropism (mag-net′ro-pizm) a growth response in a nonmotile organism under the influence of a magnet.

magnification (mag″nĭ-fĭ-ka′shun) 1. apparent increase in size, as under the microscope. 2. the process of making something appear larger, as by use of lenses. 3. the ratio of apparent (image) size to real size.

main (mān) [Fr.] hand. **m. en griffe** (ma-non-grif′), clawhand.

mal (mal) [Fr.] illness; disease. **m. de caderas,** a trypanosomiasis of horses, mules, and dogs in South America, with weakness, especially of the hind quarters, and a staggering, swinging gait. **grand m.,** see under *epilepsy.* **m. de Meleda,** symmetrical keratosis of the palms and soles associated with an ichthyotic thickening of the wrists and ankles. **m. de mer,** seasickness. **petit m.,** see under *epilepsy.* **m. del pinto,** pinta.

mala (ma′lah) 1. the cheek. 2. the zygomatic bone. **ma′lar,** adj.

malabsorption (mal″ab-sorp′shun) impaired intestinal absorption of nutrients.

malacia (mah-la′she-ah) 1. morbid softening or softness of a part or tissue; also used as word termination, as in osteomalacia. 2. morbid craving for highly spiced foods.

malacoma (mal″ah-ko′mah) a morbidly soft part or spot.

malacoplakia (mal″ah-ko-pla′ke-ah) the formation of soft patches of the mucous membrane of a hollow organ. **m. vesi′cae,** a soft, yellowish, fungus-like growth on the mucosa of the bladder and ureters.

malacosis (mal″ah-ko′sis) malacia.

malacosteon (mal″ah-kos′te-on) osteomalacia.

malacotic (mal″ah-kot′ik) inclined to malacia; soft; said of teeth.

maladjustment (mal″ad-just′ment) in psychiatry, defective adaptation to the environment, marked by anxiety.

malady (mal′ah-de) a disease or illness.

malaise (mal-āz′) [Fr.] a vague feeling of bodily discomfort.

malalignment (mal″ah-līn′ment) displacement out of line, especially displacement of teeth from their normal relation to the line of the dental arch.

malaria (mah-lār′e-ah) an infectious febrile disease caused by protozoa of the genus *Plasmodium,* which are parasitic in red blood cells; it is transmitted by *Anopheles* mosquitoes and marked by attacks of chills, fever, and sweating occurring at intervals that depend on the time required for development of a new generation of parasites in the body. **malar'ial,** adj. **cerebral m.,** falciparum malaria with delirium or coma. **falciparum m.,** the most serious form, due to *Plasmodium falciparum,* with severe constitutional symptoms and sometimes causing death. **hemolytic m.,** blackwater fever. **hemorrhagic m.,** falciparum malaria with hemorrhages. **ovale m.,** a mild form due to *Plasmodium ovale,* with recurring tertian febrile paroxysms and a tendency to end in spontaneous recovery. **pernicious m.,** falciparum m. **quartan m.,** that in which the febrile paroxysms occur every 72 hours, or every fourth day counting the day of occurrence as the first day of each cycle; due to *Plasmodium malariae.* **quotidian m.,** vivax malaria in which the febrile paroxysms occur daily. **tertian m.,** vivax malaria in which the febrile paroxysms occur every 42 to 47 hours, or every third day counting the day of occurrence as the first day of the cycle. **vivax m.,** that due to *Plasmodium vivax,* in which the febrile paroxysms commonly occur every other day (*tertian m.*), but may occur daily (*quotidian m.*), if there are two broods of parasites segmenting on alternate days.

malariologist (mah-lār"e-ol'o-jist) a specialist in malariology.

malariology (-ol'o-je) the study of malaria.

malariotherapy (mah-lār"e-o-ther'ah-pe) treatment of paralytic dementia by infecting the patient with malarial parasites, usually *Plasmodium vivax* or *P. malariae.*

Malassezia (mal"ah-se'ze-ah) *Pityrosporon.* **M. fur'fur, M. trop'ica,** *Pityrosporon orbiculare.*

malassimilation (mal"ah-sim"ĭ-la'shun) defective or faulty assimilation.

malate (ma'lāt) any salt of malic acid.

malaxation (mal"ak-sa'shun) an act of kneading.

male (māl) an individual of the sex that produces spermatozoa.

maleate (mal'e-āt) any salt or ester of maleic acid.

maleruption (mal"e-rup'shun) eruption of a tooth out of its normal position.

malformation (-for-ma'shun) defective or abnormal formation; deformity.

malignancy (mah-lig'nan-se) tendency to progress in virulence; the quality of being malignant.

malignant (mah-lig'nant) tending to become progressively worse and to result in death. Having the properties of anaplasia, invasiveness, and metastasis; said of tumors.

malingerer (mah-ling'ger-er) one who is guilty of malingering.

malingering (-ing) willful, deliberate, and fraudulent feigning or exaggeration of the symptoms of illness or injury to attain a consciously desired end.

malleable (mal'e-ah-b'l) susceptible of being beaten out into a thin plate.

malleoincudal (mal"e-o-ing'ku-dal) pertaining to the malleus and incus.

malleolus (mah-le'o-lus), pl. *malle'oli* [L.] a rounded process, such as the protuberance on either side of the ankle joint, at the lower end of the fibula, or of the tibia. **malle'olar,** adj.

malleotomy (mal"e-ot'o-me) 1. operative division of the malleus. 2. operative separation of the malleoli.

malleus (mal'e-us) [L.] 1. see *Table of Bones.* 2. glanders.

malnutrition (mal"nu-trish'un) any disorder of nutrition.

malocclusion (-o-kloo'zhun) absence of proper relations of apposing teeth when the jaws are in contact.

malposition (-po-zish'un) abnormal or anomalous placement.

malpractice (mal-prak'tis) improper or injurious practice; unskillful and faulty medical or surgical treatment.

malpresentation (mal"prez-en-ta'shun) faulty fetal presentation.

malrotation (-ro-ta'shun) abnormal or pathologic rotation, as of the spine.

malt (mawlt) grain, for the most part barley, which has been soaked, made to germinate, and then dried; it contains dextrin, maltose, and diastase and is used as a nutritive and digestant agent.

maltase (mawl'tās) see *glucosidase.*

maltose (mawl'tōs) a dissaccharide formed when starch is hydrolyzed by amylase.

malum (ma'lum) [L.] disease. **m. articulo'rum seni'lis,** a painful degenerative state of a joint as a result of aging. **m. cox'ae seni'lis,** osteoarthritis of the hip joint. **m. per'forans pe'dis,** perforating ulcer of the foot.

malunion (mal-ūn'yon) faulty union of the fragments of a fractured bone.

mamilla (mah-mil'ah), pl. *mamil'lae* [L.] 1. the nipple of the breast. 2. any nipple-like prominence. **mam'illary,** adj.

mamillated (mam"ĭ-lāt'ed) having nipple-like projections or prominences.

mamillation (mam"ĭ-la'shun) 1. the condition of being mamillated. 2. a nipple-like elevation or projection.

mamilliform (mah-mil'ĭ-form) nipple-like.

mamilliplasty (-plas"te) theleplasty.

mamillitis (mam"ĭ-li'tis) thelitis.

mamm(o)- word element [L.], *breast; mammary gland.*

mamma (mam'ah), pl. *mam'mae* [L.] the breast.

mammal (mam'al) an individual of Mammalia.

mammalgia (mah-mal'je-ah) mastalgia.

Mammalia (mah-ma'le-ah) a class of warm-blooded vertebrate animals, including all that have hair and suckle their young.

mammaplasty (mam'ah-plas"te) mammoplasty.

mammary (mam'ar-e) pertaining to the mammary gland, or breast.

mammectomy (mah-mek′to-me) mastectomy.

mammilla (mah-mil′ah) mamilla.

mammillated (mam″ĭ-lāt′ed) mamillated.

mammilliplasty (mah-mil′i-plas″te) theleplasty.

mammillitis (mam″ĭ-li′tis) thelitis.

mammiplasia (mam″ĭ-pla′ze-ah) mammoplasia.

mammitis (mah-mi′tis) mastitis.

mammogram (mam′o-gram) a radiograph of the mammary gland.

mammography (mah-mog′rah-fe) radiography of the mammary gland.

mammoplasia (mam″o-pla′ze-ah) development of breast tissue.

mammoplasty (mam′o-plas″te) plastic reconstruction of the breast, either to augment or reduce its size.

mammose (mam′ōs) 1. having large breasts. 2. mamillated.

mammotomy (mah-mot′o-me) mastotomy.

mammotrophic (mam″o-trof′ik) mammotropic.

mammotropic (-trop′ik) having a stimulating effect on the mammary gland.

mammotropin (-trōp′in) prolactin.

Mandelamine (man-del′ah-mēn) trademark for a preparation of methenamine mandelate.

mandible (man′dĭ-b′l) the lower jaw; see *Table of Bones.* **mandib′ular,** adj.

mandibula (man-dib′u-lah), pl. *mandib′ulae*[L.] mandible.

mandrel (man′drel) the shaft on which a dental tool is held in the dental handpiece, for rotation by the dental engine.

mandrin (man′drin) a metal guide for a flexible catheter.

maneuver (mah-noo′ver) a skillful or dextrous procedure. **Bracht's m.,** a method of extraction of the aftercoming head in breech presentation. **Brandt-Andrews m.,** a method of expressing the placenta from the uterus. **Heimlich m.,** to force food or other material from the throat of a choking victim: wrap one's arms around the victim from behind, making a fist with one hand and grasping it with the other; place both hands against the victim's abdomen just above the navel and below the ribs, and forcefully press into the abdomen with a quick upward thrust. **Løvset's m.,** extraction of the arms in breech birth by clockwise and counterclockwise rotation of the fetus. **Müller's m.,** an inspiratory effort with a closed glottis after expiration, used during fluoroscopic examination to cause a negative intrathoracic pressure with engorgement of intrathoracic vascular structures. **Müller-Hillis m.,** a method of ascertaining the relation between the size of the fetal head and the maternal pelvis. **Pajot's m.,** a method of forceps extraction of the fetal head. **Pinard's m.,** a method of bringing down the foot in breech extraction. **Prague m.,** a method of extracting the aftercoming head in breech presentation. **Scanzoni's m.,** double application of forceps blades for delivery of a fetus in the occiput posterior position. **Schatz m.,** a method of changing a face presentation to a brow presentation. **Valsalva's m.,** increase in intrathoracic pressure by forcible exhalation effort against the closed glottis. **Van Hoorn's m.,** a modified Prague maneuver.

manganese (man′gah-nēs) chemical element (*see table*), at. no. 25, symbol Mn; its salts occur in the body tissue in very small amounts and serve as an activator of liver arginase and other enzymes. Poisoning, usually due to inhalation of manganese dust, is manifested by symptoms including mental disorders accompanying a syndrome resembling paralysis agitans, and inflammation of the respiratory system.

mange (mānj) a skin disease of domestic animals, due to mites.

mania (ma′ne-ah) disordered mental state of extreme excitement; specifically, the manic type of manic-depressive psychosis. Also used as a word termination to denote obsessive preoccupation with something, as in tomomania. **mani′acal, ma′nic,** adj.

maniac (ma′ne-ak) one affected with mania.

manic-depressive (man″ik-de-pres′iv) alternating between attacks of mania and depression; see under *psychosis.*

manikin (man′ĭ-kin) a model to illustrate anatomy or on which to practice surgical or other manipulations.

manipulation (mah-nip″u-la-shun) skillful or dextrous treatment by the hands.

mannitol (man′ĭ-tol) a sugar alcohol widely distributed in plants and fungi; used in diagnostic tests of kidney function and as a diuretic. **m. hexanitrate,** a compound formed by nitration of mannitol; used as a vasodilator.

mannose (man′ōs) a monosaccharide produced by oxidation of mannitol.

manometer (mah-nom′ĕ-ter) an instrument for measuring the pressure of liquids or gases. **manomet′ric,** adj.

Mansonella (man″so-nel′ah) a genus of filarial nematodes. *M. ozzar'di* is found in the mesentery and visceral fat of man in Panama, Yucatan, Guyana, Surinam, and Argentina.

Mansonia (man-so′ne-ah) a genus of mosquitoes, several species of which transmit *Brugia malayi;* some may also transmit viruses, such as those of equine encephalomyelitis.

mantle (man′t′l) an enveloping cover or layer, such as the brain mantle, or cerebral cortex.

manubrium (mah-nu′bre-um), pl. *manu'bria* [L.] the handle-like part of the sternum or malleus. **m. of malleus,** the longest process of the malleus; it is attached to the inner surface of the tympanic membrane and has the tensor tympani muscle attached to it. **m. of sternum,** the cranial part of the sternum, articulating with the clavicles and first two pairs of ribs.

manudynamometer (man″u-di″nah-mom′ĕ-ter) an apparatus for measuring the force of the thrust of an instrument.

manus (ma′nus), pl. *ma'nus* [L.] hand.

map (map) a two-dimensional graphic representation of arrangement in space. **fate m.,** a graphic representation of a blastula or other early stage of an embryo, showing prospective significance of certain areas in normal development. **genetic m.,** a graphic representation of the linear arrangement of genes on a chromosome. **linkage m.,** a graphic representation of the relative positions of, and distances between, genes on the same chromosome.

marasmus (mah-raz′mus) a form of protein-calorie malnutrition occurring chiefly in the first year of life, with growth retardation and wasting of subcutaneous fat and muscle. **maran′tic, maras′mic,** adj.

margin (mar′jin) an edge or border. **mar′ginal,** adj. **dentate m.,** pectinate line. **gingival m., gum m.,** the border of the gingivia surrounding, but unattached to, the substance of the teeth.

margination (mar″ji-na′shun) adhesion of leukocytes to blood vessel walls in the early stages of inflammation.

marginoplasty (mar′jin-o-plas″te) surgical restoration of a border, as of the eyelid.

margo (mar′go), pl. *mar′gines* [L.] margin.

marihuana, marijuana (mar″ĭ-wahn′ah) a preparation of the leaves and flowering tops of hemp plants (*Cannabis sativa*), usually smoked in cigarettes for its euphoric properties.

mark (mark) a spot, blemish, or other circumscribed area visible on a surface. **birth m.,** see *birthmark*. **port-wine m.,** nevus flammeus. **strawbery m.,** cavernous hemangioma.

Marplan (mar′plan) trademark for a preparation of isocarboxazid.

marrow (mar′o) the soft organic material filling the cavities of bones (*bone marrow*). **spinal m.,** the spinal cord.

marsupial (mar-su′pe-al) a member of the Marsupialia.

Marsupialia (mar-su″pe-a′le-ah) an order of mammals characterized by the possession of a marsupium, including opossums, kangaroos, wallabies, koala bears, and wombats.

marsupialization (mar-su″pe-ah-lĭ-za′shun) conversion of a closed cavity into an open pouch, by incising it and suturing the edges of its wall to the edges of the wound.

marsupium (mar-su′pe-um), pl. *marsu′pia* [L.] 1. the scrotum. 2. an external abdominal pouch or skin fold for carrying the young and containing the mammary gland; it occurs in marsupials and spiny anteaters; also, a similar structure for carrying eggs and/or young, as in the male sea horse.

masculine (mas′ku-lin) pertaining to the male sex, or having qualities normally characteristic of the male.

masculinity (mas″ku-lin′ĭ-te) the possession of masculine qualities.

masculinization (mas″ku-lin-i-za′shun) the normal induction or development of male sex characters in the male; also, the induction or development of male secondary sex characters in the female.

masculinize (mas′ku-lĭ-nīz″) to produce masculine qualities in women.

masculinovoblastoma (mas″ku-lin-o″vo-blasto′mah) lipoid cell tumor of the ovary.

maser (ma′zer) a device which produces an extremely intense, small and nearly nondivergent beam of monochromatic radiation in the microwave region, with all the waves in phase.

mask (mask) 1. to cover or conceal, as the masking of the nature of a disorder by the presence of unrelated signs, organisms, etc.; in audiometry, to obscure or diminish a sound by the presence of another sound of different frequency. 2. an appliance for shading, protecting, or medicating the face. 3. in dentistry, to camouflage metal parts of a prosthesis by covering with opaque material. **ecchymotic m.,** cyanosis of the head and neck due to traumatic asphyxia. **Hutchinson's m.,** a sensation as if the skin of the face were compressed by a mask, often a symptom of tabes dorsalis. **m. of pregnancy,** see *melasma*.

masochism (mas′o-kizm) a perversion in which infliction of physical or psychological pain gives sexual gratification to the recipient. **masochis′tic,** adj.

masochist (mas-o-kist) a person exhibiting or characterized by masochism.

mass (mas) 1. a lump or collection of cohering particles. 2. a cohesive mixture suitable for being made up into pills. 3. that characteristic of matter which gives it inertia. **atomic m.,** the mass of a neutral atom of a nuclide, usually expressed as atomic mass units (amu). **body cell m.,** the total weight of the cells of the body, constituting the total mass of oxygen-utilizing, carbohydrate-burning, and energy-exchanging cells of the body; regarded as proportional to total exchangeable potassium in the body. **inner cell m.,** the cell cluster at the animal pole of a blastocyst from which the embryo proper develops. **intermediate cell m.,** nephrotome. **lean body m.,** that part of the body including all its components except neutral storage lipid; in essence, the fat-free mass of the body. **tigroid m's,** Nissl bodies.

massa (mas′ah), pl. *mas′sae* [L.] mass (1).

massage (mah-sahzh′) systematic therapeutic friction, stroking, or kneading of the body. **auditory m.,** massage of the tympanic membrane. **cardiac m.,** intermittent compression of the heart by pressure applied over the sternum (*closed cardiac m.*) or directly to the heart through an opening in the chest wall (*open cardiac m.*); done to reinstate and maintain circulation. **electrovibratory m.,** massage by means of an electric vibrator. **vibratory m.,** massage by rapidly repeated light percussion with a vibrating hammer or sound.

masseter (mas-se′ter) see *Table of Muscles*. **masseter′ic,** adj.

masseur (mah-ser′) [Fr.] 1. a man who performs massage. 2. an instrument for performing massage.

masseuse (mah-suhz′) [Fr.] a woman who performs massage.

massotherapy (mas″o-ther′ah-pe) treatment of disease by massage.

mastadenitis (mas″tad-ĕ-ni′tis) mastitis.

mastadenoma (mas″tad-ĕ-no′mah) a tumor of the breast.

mastalgia (mas-tal′je-ah) pain in the breast.

mastatrophy (mas-tat′ro-fe) atrophy of the breast.

mastectomy (mas-tek′to-me) excision of the breast. **radical m.,** amputation of the breast with wide excision of the pectoral muscles and axillary lymph nodes.

mastication (mas″tĭ-ka′shun) the process of chewing food.

masticatory (mas′tĭ-kah-tor″e) 1. pertaining to mastication. 2. a substance to be chewed, but not swallowed.

Mastigophora (mas″tĭ-gof′o-rah) a subphylum of Protozoa comprising those having one or more flagella throughout most of their life cycle, and a simple, centrally located nucleus; many are parasitic in both invertebrates and vertebrates, including man.

mastigote (mas′tĭ-gōt) any member of the Mastigophora.

mastitis (mas-ti′tis) inflammation of the breast. **m. neonato′rum,** any abnormal condition of the breast in the newborn. **periductal m.,** inflammation of the tissues about the ducts of the mammary gland. **plasma cell m.,** infiltration of the breast stroma with plasma cells and proliferation of the cells lining the ducts.

masto- word element [Gr.], *breast; mastoid process.*

mastocyte (mas′to-sīt) a mast cell.

mastocytoma (mas′to-si-to′mah) mast cell tumor.

mastocytosis (-si-to′sis) an accumulation, local or systemic, of mast cells in the tissues; known as *urticaria pigmentosa* when widespread in the skin.

mastodynia (-din′e-ah) mastalgia.

mastoid (mas′toid) 1. breast-shaped. 2. mastoid process. 3. pertaining to the mastoid process.

mastoidalgia (mas″toi-dal′je-ah) pain in the mastoid region.

mastoidectomy (mas″toi-dek′to-me) excision of the mastoid cells or the mastoid process.

mastoideocentesis (mas-toi″de-o-sen-te′sis) paracentesis of the mastoid cells.

mastoiditis (mas″toi-di′tis) inflammation of the mastoid antrum and cells.

mastoidotomy (mas″toi-dot′o-me) incision of the mastoid antrum.

mastoncus (mas-tong′kus) a tumor or swelling of the breast.

masto-occipital (mas″to-ok-sip′ĭ-tal) pertaining to mastoid process and occipital bone.

mastopathy (mas-top′ah-the) any disease of the mammary gland.

mastoparietal (mas″to-pah-ri′ĕ-tal) pertaining to the mastoid process and parietal bone.

mastopexy (mas′to-pek″se) surgical fixation of a pendulous breast.

mastoplasia (mas″to-pla′ze-ah) mammoplasia.

mastoplasty (mas′to-plas″te) mammoplasty.

mastoptosis (mas″to-to′sis) pendulous breasts.

mastorrhagia (-ra′je-ah) hemorrhage from the mammary gland.

mastoscirrhus (-skir′us) hardening of the mammary gland.

mastosquamous (-skwa′mus) pertaining to the mastoid and squama of the temporal bone.

mastotomy (mas-tot′o-me) incision of a mammary gland.

masturbation (mas″ter-ba′shun) induction of orgasm by self-stimulation of the genitals.

matching (mach′ing) comparison for the purpose of selecting objects having similar or identical characteristics; in transplantation immunology, a method of measuring degree of tissue compatibility between individuals. **cross m.,** determination of the compatibility of the blood of a donor and that of a recipient before transfusion by placing the donor's red cells in the recipient's serum and the recipient's red cells in the donor's serum; absence of agglutination indicates compatibility.

materia (mah-tēr′e-ah) [L.] material; substance. **m. al′ba,** whitish deposits on the teeth, composed of mucus and epithelial cells containing bacteria and filamentous organisms. **m. med′ica,** pharmacology.

maternal (mah-ter′nal) pertaining to the mother.

maternity (mah-ter′nĭ-te) 1. motherhood. 2. a lying-in hospital.

mating (māt′ing) pairing of individuals of opposite sexes, especially for reproduction. **assortative m., assorted m., assortive m.,** the mating of individuals having similar qualities or constitutions. **random m.,** the mating of individuals without regard to any similarity between them.

matrix (ma′triks), pl. *mat′rices* [L.] 1. the groundwork on which anything is cast, or the basic material from which a thing develops. 2. a metal band used to provide form to a dental restoration. **bone m.,** the intercellular substance of bone consisting of collagenous fibers, ground substance, and inorganic salts. **interterritorial m.,** a paler staining region among the darker territorial matrices. **nail m.,** m. unguis. **territorial m.,** basophilic matrix about groups of cartilage cells. **m. un′guis,** nail bed; also, the proximal part of the nail bed where growth chiefly occurs.

matter (mat′er) 1. substance; anything that occupies space. 2. pus. **gray m.,** see under *substance*. **white m.,** see under *substance*.

maturation (mat″u-ra′shun) 1. the stage or process of becoming mature; attainment of emotional and intellectual maturity. In biology, a process of cell division during which the number of chromosomes in the germ cells is reduced to one half the number characteristic of the species. 2. suppuration.

mature (mah-tūr′) 1. to develop to maturity; to ripen. 2. fully developed; ripe.

maturity (mah-tu′rĭ-te) the period of attainment of maximal development.

matutinal (mah-tu′tĭ-nal) occurring in the morning.

maxilla (mak-sil′ah), pl. *maxil′lae* [L.] the bone of the upper jaw; see *Table of Bones.* **max′illary,** adj. **inferior m.,** the mandible.

maxillofacial (mak-sil″o-fa′shal) pertaining to the maxilla and the face.

maxillomandibular (-man-dib′u-lar) pertaining to the upper and lower jaws.

maxillotomy (mak″sĭ-lot′o-me) surgical sectioning of the maxilla which allows movement of all or part of the maxilla into the desired position.

maximum (mak′sĭ-mum) 1. the greatest possible or actual effect or quantity. 2. largest; utmost. **maximal**, adj. **tubular m.**, the highest rate in milligrams per minute at which the renal tubules can transfer a substance either from the tubular luminal fluid to the interstitial fluid or from the latter to the former.

Maxitate (mak′sĭ-tāt) trademark for preparations of mannitol hexanitrate.

maze (māz) a complicated system of intersecting paths used in intelligence tests and in demonstrating learning in experimental animals.

mazopexy (ma′zo-pek″se) mastopexy.

mazoplasia (ma″zo-pla′ze-ah) degenerative epithelial hyperplasia of the mammary acini.

M.B. [L.] Medici′nae Baccalau′reus (*Bachelor of Medicine*).

M.C. [L.] Ma′gister Chirur′giae (*Master of Surgery*); Medical Corps.

Mc. megacycle.

mc. millicurie.

μc. microcurie.

mcg. microgram.

MCH mean corpuscular hemoglobin, an expression of the average hemoglobin content of a single cell in micromicrograms, obtained by multiplying the hemoglobin in grams by ten and dividing by the number of red cells (in millions).

μc.h. microcurie-hour.

MCHC mean corpuscular hemoglobin concentration, an expression of the average hemoglobin concentration in per cent, obtained by multiplying the hemoglobin in grams by 100 and dividing by the hematocrit determination.

mcoul. millicoulomb.

Mc.p.s. megacycles per second.

M.C.S.P. Member of the Chartered Society of Physiotherapists (Brit.).

MCV 1. mean corpuscular volume, an expression of the average volume of individual red cells in cubic microns, obtained by multiplying the hematocrit determination by ten and dividing by the number of red cells (in millions). 2. mean clinical value, obtained by assigning a numerical value to the response noted in a number of patients receiving a specific treatment, adding these numbers, and dividing by the number of patients treated.

M.D. [L.] Medici′nae Doc′tor (*Doctor of Medicine*).

Md chemical symbol, *mendelevium.*

meal (mēl) a portion of food or foods taken at some particular and usually stated or fixed time. **Boyden m.**, a test meal for the study of gallbladder evacuation, containing three or four egg yolks combined with milk and seasoned with sugar, port wine, etc. **test m.**, a meal containing material given to aid in diagnostic examination of the stomach.

mean (mēn) an average; a numerical value intermediate between two extremes. **arithmetical m.**, the arithmetical average. **geometrical m.**, the antilogarithm of the arithmetical mean of the logarithm of a series of values.

measles (me′zelz) rubeola; a highly contagious viral infection, usually of childhood, involving primarily the respiratory tract and reticuloendothelial tissues, marked by an eruption of discrete, red papules, which become confluent, flatten, turn brown, and desquamate. **black m.**, a severe form in which the eruption is very dark and petechial. **German m.**, rubella. **hemorrhagic m.**, black m.

measure (mezh′er) see *Tables of Weights and Measures,* accompanying *weight.*

meatorrhaphy (me″ah-tor′ah-fe) suture of the wound made in meatotomy.

meatoscopy (me″ah-tos′ko-pe) inspection of any meatus, especially the urethral meatus.

meatotomy (me″ah-tot′o-me) incision of the urinary meatus in order to enlarge it.

meatus (me-a′tus), pl. *mea′tus* [L.] an opening or passage. **mea′tal**, adj. **acoustic m., m. acus′ticus**, either of two passages in the ear, one leading to the tympanic membrane (*external acoustic m.*), and one through which the facial, intermediate, and vestibulocochlear nerves and the labyrinthine artery pass (*internal acoustic m.*). **auditory m.**, acoustic m. **m. na′si, m. of nose**, one of the four portions (common, inferior, middle, and superior) of the nasal cavity on either side of the septum. **m. urina′rius, urinary m.**, the opening of the urethra on the body surface through which urine is discharged.

Mebaral (meb′ah-ral) trademark for a preparation of mephobarbital.

mebeverine (mĕ-bev′er-ēn) a smooth muscle relaxant, $C_{25}H_{35}NO_5$, used as the hydrochloride salt.

mebutamate (mĕ-bu′tah-māt) an antihypertensive, $C_{10}H_{20}N_2O_4$.

mecamine (mek′ah-min) mecamylamine.

mecamylamine (mek″ah-mil′ah-min) a ganglionic blocking agent, $C_{11}H_{21}N$, used in the form of the hydrochloride salt as an antihypertensive.

mechanics (mĕ-kan′iks) the science dealing with the motions of material bodies. **body m.**, the application of kinesiology to use the body in daily life activities and to the prevention and correction of problems related to posture.

mechanism (mek′ah-nizm) 1. a machine or machine-like structure. 2. the manner of combination of parts, processes, etc., which subserve a common function. **defense m.**, a mental mechanism by which psychic tension is diminished, e.g., repression, rationalization, etc. **mental m.**, 1. the organization of mental operations. 2. an unconscious and indirect manner of gratifying a repressed desire.

mechanoreceptor (mek″ah-no-re-sep′tor) a receptor that is excited by mechanical pressures or distortions, as those responding to touch and muscular contractions.

mechanotherapy (-ther′ah-pe) use of mechanical apparatus for therapeutic exercises.

mechlorethamine (mĕ″klōr-eth′ah-mēn) one of the nitrogen mustards, $C_5H_{11}Cl_2N$; used in the form of the hydrochloride salt as an antineoplastic.

Mecholyl (me′ko-lil) trademark for preparations of methacholine.

meclizine (mek′lĭ-zēn) an antinauseant, $C_{25}H_{27}$-ClN_2, used as the hydrochloride salt.

mecloqualon (mek′lo-kwal′ōn) a sedative and hypnotic, $C_{15}H_{11}ClN_2O$.

meconate (mek′o-nāt) any salt of meconic acid.

meconium (mĕ-ko′ne-um) dark green mucilaginous material in the intestine of the full-term fetus.

medazepam (mĕ-daz′ĕ-pam) a minor tranquilizer, $C_{16}H_{15}ClN_2$.

media (me′de-ah) 1. plural of *medium*. 2. middle.

medial (me′de-al) situated toward the midline of the body or a structure.

medialis (me″de-a′lis) [L.] medial.

median (me′de-an) pertaining to or situated in the midline.

medianus (me″de-a′nus) [L.] median.

mediastinitis (me″de-as″tĭ-ni′tis) inflammation of the mediastinum.

mediastinogram (me″de-as-ti′no-gram) a roentgenogram of the mediastinum.

mediastinography (me″de-as″tĭ-nog′rah-fe) radiography of the mediastinum.

mediastinopericarditis (me″de-as″tĭ-no-per″ĭ-kar-di′tis) pericarditis with adhesions extending from the pericardium to the mediastinum.

mediastinoscopy (me″de-as″ti-nos′ko-pe) endoscopic examination of the mediastinum.

mediastinotomy (me″de-as″ti-not′o-me) incision of the mediastinum.

mediastinum (me″de-ah-sti′num), pl. *mediasti′na* [L.] 1. a median septum or partition. 2. the mass of tissues and organs separating the sternum in front and the vertebral column behind, containing the heart and its large vessels, trachea, esophagus, thymus, lymph nodes, and other structures and tissues; it is divided into anterior, middle, posterior, and superior regions. **mediasti′nal**, adj. **m. tes′tis**, a partial septum of the testis formed near its posterior border by a continuation of the tunica albuginea.

mediate (me′de-āt) 1. to serve as an intermediate agent. 2. indirect; accomplished by means of an intervening medium.

mediator (me′de-a″tor) an agent by which a process or reaction is mediated.

medicable (med′ĭ-kah-b'l) subject to treatment with reasonable expectation of cure.

medical (med′ĭ-kal) pertaining to medicine.

medicament (mĕ-dik′ah-ment, med′ĭ-kah-ment) a medicinal agent.

Medicare (med′ĭ-kār) a program of the Social Security Administration which provides medical care to the aged.

medicated (med′ĭ-kāt″ed) imbued with a medicinal substance.

medication (med″ĭ-ka′shun) 1. impregnation with a medicine. 2. the administration of remedies. 3. a medicament. **ionic m.,** iontophoresis.

medicinal (mĕ-dis′ĭ-nal) having healing qualities; pertaining to a medicine.

medicine (med′ĭ-sin) 1. any drug or remedy. 2. the art and science of the diagnosis and treatment of disease and the maintenance of health. 3. the nonsurgical treatment of disease. **aviation m.,** that dealing with the physiologic, medical, psychologic, and epidemiologic problems involved in aviation. **clinical m.,** 1. the study of disease by direct examination of the living patient. 2. the last two years of the usual curriculum in a medical college. **environmental m.,** that dealing with the effects of the environment on man, including rapid population growth, water and air pollution, travel, etc. **experimental m.,** the study of diseases based on experimentation in animals. **family m.,** the medical specialty concerned with planning and provision of comprehensive primary health care for all family members, regardless of age or sex, on a continuing basis. **forensic m.,** medical jurisprudence. **group m.,** the practice of medicine by a group of physicians, usually representing various specialties, who are associated together for the cooperative diagnosis, treatment, and prevention of disease. **internal m.,** that dealing especially with diagnosis and medical treatment of diseases and disorders of internal structures of the body. **ionic m.,** treatment by electrochemical means, such as cataphoresis, iontophoresis. **legal m.,** medical jurisprudence. **nuclear m.,** that branch of medicine concerned with the use of radionuclides in the diagnosis and treatment of disease. **patent m.,** a drug or remedy protected by a trademark, available without a prescription. **physical m.,** physiatrics. **preclinical m.,** 1. preventive m. 2. the first two years of the usual curriculum in a medical college. **preventive m.,** science aimed at preventing disease. **proprietary m.,** a remedy whose formula is owned exclusively by the manufacturer and which is marketed usually under a name registered as a trademark. **psychosomatic m.,** the study of the interrelations between bodily processes and emotional life. **socialized m.,** a system of medical care regulated and controlled by the government. **space m.,** that branch of aviation medicine concerned with conditions to be encountered in space. **state m.,** socialized m. **tropical m.,** medical science as applied to diseases occurring primarily in the tropics and subtropics. **veterinary m.,** the diagnosis and treatment of diseases of animals.

medicolegal (med″ĭ-ko-le′gal) pertaining to medical jurisprudence.

medicus (med′ĭ-kus) [L.] physician.

mediolateral (me″de-o-lat′er-al) pertaining to the midline and one side.

medionecrosis (-nĕ-kro′sis) necrosis of the tunica media of a blood vessel.

mediotarsal (-tar′sal) pertaining to the center of the tarsus.

medium (me′de-um), pl. *mediums, me′dia* [L.] 1. a means. 2. a substance that transmits impulses. 3. culture medium; see under *C.* 4. a preparation used in treating histological specimens. **clearing m.,** a substance for rendering histologic specimens transparent. **contrast m.,** radiopaque substance used in roentgenography to permit visualization of internal body structures. **culture m.,** see under *C*. **dioptric media,** refracting media. **disperse m., dispersion m.,** the continuous phase of a colloid system; the medium in which a colloid is dispersed, corresponding to the solvent in a true solution. **nutrient m.,** a culture medium to which nutrient materials have been added. **refracting media,** the transparent tissues and fluid in the eye through which light rays pass and by which they are refracted and brought to a focus on the retina.

medius (me′de-us) [L.] situated in the middle.

Medomin (med′o-min) trademark for a preparation of heptabarbital.

medrogestone (med″ro-jes′tōn) a progestational agent, $C_{23}H_{32}O_2$.

Medrol (med′rol) trademark for a preparation of methylprednisolone.

medroxyprogesterone (med-rok″sĭ-pro-jes′ter-ōn) a progestational agent, $C_{24}H_{34}O_4$, used as the acetate salt.

medulla (mĕ-dul′ah), pl. *medul′lae* [L.] the innermost part; marrow; applied to the marrow of bones (*m. os′sium*), the spinal cord (*m. spina′lis*), and the central portion of such organs as the adrenal gland and the kidney (*m. re′nis*). **med′-ullary,** adj. **adrenal m.,** the inner, reddish brown, soft part of the adrenal gland; it synthesizes, stores, and releases catecholamines. **m. of bone,** bone marrow. **m. neph′rica,** m. renis. **m. oblonga′ta,** that part of the brain stem continuous with the pons above and the spinal cord below. **m. os′sium,** bone marrow. **m. re′nis,** the inner part of the kidney substance, composed chiefly of collecting elements and loops of Henle, organized grossly into pyramids. **m. spina′lis,** spinal cord.

medullated (med′u-lāt″ed) myelinated.

medullization (med″u-li-za′shun) enlargement of marrow spaces, as in rarefying osteitis.

medulloadrenal (mĕ-dul″o-ah-dre′nal) pertaining to the adrenal medulla.

medulloblast (mĕ-dul′o-blast) an undifferentiated cell of the neural tube which may develop into either a neuroblast or spongioblast.

medulloblastoma (mĕ-dul″o-blas-to′mah) a cerebellar tumor composed of medulloblasts.

medulloepithelioma (-ep″ĭ-the″le-o′mah) a brain tumor composed of primitive neuroepithelial cells lining the tubular spaces.

mega- word element [Gr.], *large;* used in naming units of measurement to designate an amount 10^6 (one million) times the size of the unit to which it is joined, as megacuries (10^6 curies); symbol M.

megabladder (meg″ah-blad′er) permanent overdistention of the bladder.

megacaryocyte (-kar′e-o-sīt) megakaryocyte.

megacephaly (-sef′ah-le) megalocephaly.

megacolon (-ko′lon) dilatation and hypertrophy of the colon. **acquired m.,** colonic enlargement associated with chronic constipation, but with normal ganglion cell innervation. **aganglionic m., congenital m.,** that due to congenital ab-

sence of myenteric ganglion cells in a distal segment of the large bowel, with resultant loss of motor function in the aganglionic segment and massive hypertrophic dilatation of the normal proximal colon. **idiopathic m.,** acquired m. **toxic m.,** that associated with amebic or ulcerative colitis.

megacycle (-si″k'l) one million (10^6) cycles; megahertz.

megadont (-dont) having very large teeth.

megadyne (-dīn) one million dynes.

megaesophagus (meg″ah-ĕ-sof′ah-gus) see *achalasia.*

megahertz (meg′ah-hertz) one million (10^6) hertz; abbreviated MHz.

megakaryoblast (meg″ah-kar′e-o-blast″) the cell from which the mature megakaryocyte is derived.

megakaryocyte (-kar′e-o-sīt″) the giant cell of bone marrow containing a greatly lobulated nucleus, from which mature blood platelets originate.

megakaryocytosis (-kar″e-o-si-to′sis) the presence of megakaryocytes in the blood or of excessive numbers in the bone marrow.

megakaryophthisis (-thi′sis) deficiency of megakaryocytes in bone marrow or blood.

megal(o)- word element [Gr.], *large; abnormal enlargement.*

megalgia (meg-al′je-ah) a severe pain.

megaloblast (meg′ah-lo-blast″) a large, nucleated, immature progenitor of an abnormal erythrocytic series. **megaloblas′tic,** adj.

megalocardia (meg″ah-lo-kar′de-ah) cardiomegaly.

megalocephaly (-sef′ah-le) 1. macrocephaly. 2. leontiasis ossea. **megalocephal′ic,** adj.

megalocheiria (-ki′re-ah) abnormal largeness of the hands.

megalocornea (-kor′ne-ah) congenital abnormal enlargement of the cornea.

megalocystis (-sis′tis) an abnormally enlarged bladder.

megalocyte (meg′ah-lo-sīt″) an extremely large erythrocyte.

megalodactyly (meg″ah-lo-dak′tĭ-le) excessive size of the fingers or toes. **megalodac′tylous,** adj.

megalodontia (-don′she-ah) macrodontia.

megaloenteron (-en′ter-on) enlargement of the intestine.

megaloesophagus (-ĕ-sof′ah-gus) see *achalasia.*

megalogastria (-gas′tre-ah) enlargement or abnormally large size of the stomach.

megaloglossia (-glos′e-ah) macroglossia.

megalohepatia (-hĕ-pat′e-ah) hepatomegaly.

megalokaryoblast (-kar′e-o-blast″) megakaryoblast.

megalokaryocyte (-kar′e-o-sīt″) megakaryocyte.

megalomania (-ma′ne-ah) unreasonable conviction of one's own extreme greatness, goodness, or power.

megalomaniac (-ma′ne-ak) a person exhibiting megalomania.

megalomelia (-me′le-ah) macromelia.

megalopenis (-pe′nis) abnormal largeness of the penis.

megalophthalmos (meg″ah-lof-thal′mos) buphthalmos.

megalopia (meg″al-o′pe-ah) macropsia.

megalopodia (meg″ah-lo-po′de-ah) abnormal largeness of the feet.

megalopsia (meg″ah-lop′se-ah) macropsia.

megalosplenia (meg″ah-lo-sple′ne-ah) splenomegaly.

megalosyndactyly (-sin-dak′tĭ-le) a condition in which the digits are very large and more or less webbed together.

megaloureter (-u-re′ter) enlargement of the ureter.

-megaly word element [Gr.], *enlargement.*

megarectum (meg″ah-rek′tum) a greatly dilated rectum.

megavitamin (-vi′tah-min) a term denoting massive doses of vitamins.

megavolt (meg′ah-volt) one million volts.

megestrol (mĕ-jes′trŏl) a synthetic progestational agent, $C_{24}H_{32}O_4$.

Megimide (meg′i-mīd) trademark for a preparation of bemegride.

meglumine (meg′lu-mēn) methylglucamine; a crystalline base, $C_7H_{17}NO_5$, used in preparing salts of certain acids for use as diagnostic radiopaque media (*m. diatrizoate, m. iodipamide, m. iothalamate*).

megohm (meg′ōm) one million ohms.

megophthalmos (meg″of-thal′mos) buphthalmos; hydrophthalmos.

megrim (me′grim) migraine.

meibomianitis (mi-bo″me-ah-ni′tis) inflammation of the meibomian glands.

meiosis (mi-o′sis) a special method of cell division occurring in maturation of sex cells, wherein, over two successive cell divisions, each daughter nucleus receives half the number of chromosomes typical of the somatic cells of the species, so that the gametes are haploid. **meiot′ic,** adj.

mel (mel) [L.] honey.

melagra (mel-ag′rah) muscular pain in the limbs.

melalgia (mel-al′je-ah) pain in the limbs.

melan(o)- word element [Gr.], *black; melanin.*

melancholia (mel″an-ko′le-ah) a depressed and unhappy emotional state with abnormal inhibition of mental and bodily activity. **acute m.,** an acute form marked, in addition to the usual symptoms, by loss of appetite, emaciation, insomnia, and subnormal temperature. **m. agita′ta, agitated m.,** a form with constant motion and signs of great emotional excitement. **m. hypochondri′aca,** extreme hypochondria. **involutional m.,** an affective disorder occurring in late middle life, with agitation, worry, anxiety, somatic preoccupations, insomnia, and sometimes paranoid reactions. **recurrent m.,** that occurring at more or less regular intervals. **m. sim′plex,** a mild form without delusions or great excitement. **stuporous m.,** a form in which the patient lies motionless and silent, with fixed eyes and indifference to surroundings, sometimes with hallucinations.

mélangeur (ma-lan-zher′) [Fr.] an instrument for drawing and diluting specimens of blood for examination.

melaniferous (mel″ah-nif′er-us) containing melanin or other black pigment.

melanin (mel′ah-nin) the dark pigment of the skin, hair, choroid coat of the eye, substantia nigra, and various tumors; it is produced by polymerization of oxidation products of tyrosine and dihydroxyphenol compounds.

melanism (mel′ah-nizm) excessive pigmentation or blackening of the integuments or other tissues, usually of genetic origin.

melanoameloblastoma (mel″ah-no-ah-mel″o-blas-to′mah) melanotic neuroectodermal tumor.

melanoblast (mel′ah-no-blast″) a cell originating from the neural crest, which develops into a melanocyte.

melanoblastoma (mel″ah-no-blas-to′mah) melanotic neuroectodermal tumor.

melanocarcinoma (-kar″sĭ-no′mah) malignant melanoma.

melanocyte (mel′ah-no-sīt, mĕ-lan′o-sīt) the cell which produces the melanin-synthesizing organelle melanosome. **melanocyt′ic,** adj.

melanocytoma (mel″ah-no-si-to′mah) a neoplasm or hamartoma composed of melanocytes.

melanoderma (-der′mah) an abnormally increased amount of melanin in the skin.

melanodermatitis (-der″mah-ti′tis) dermatitis with deposit of melanin in the skin.

melanogen (mĕ-lan′o-jen) a colorless chromogen, convertible into melanin, which may occur in the urine in certain diseases.

melanogenesis (mel″ah-no-jen′ĕ-sis) the production of melanin.

melanoglossia (-glos′e-ah) black tongue.

melanoid (mel′ah-noid) 1. resembling melanin. 2. a substance resembling melanin.

melanoleukoderma (mel″ah-no-lu″ko-der′-mah) a mottled appearance of the skin. **m. col′li,** syphilitic leukoderma about the neck.

melanoma (mel″ah-no′mah) 1. any tumor composed of melanin-pigmented cells. 2. malignant melanoma. **juvenile m.,** a benign, pink to purplish red papule, usually on the face, especially the cheeks, most commonly originating before puberty; histologically, it suggests and has been mistaken for malignant melanoma. **malignant m.,** a malignant tumor usually developing from a nevus and consisting of black masses of cells with a marked tendency to metastasis.

melanomatosis (mel″ah-no-mah-to′sis) the formation of widespread melanomas.

melanonychia (-nik′e-ah) blackening of the nails by melanin pigmentation.

melanophage (mel′ah-no-fāj″) a histiocyte laden with phagocytosed melanin.

melanophore (-fōr″) a pigment cell containing melanin, especially such a cell in fishes, amphibians, and reptiles.

melanoplakia (mel″ah-no-pla′ke-ah) the formation of melanotic patches on the oral mucosa.

melanosarcoma (-sar-ko′mah) malignant melanoma.

melanosis (mel″ah-no′sis), pl. *melano′ses.* 1. a condition characterized by dark pigmentary deposits. 2. disorder of pigment metabolism. **m. co′li,** black or dark brown discoloration of the mucosa of the colon, due to the presence of pigment-laden (not true melanin) macrophages within the lamina propria.

melanosome (mel′ah-no-sōm″) any of the granules within melanocytes that contain melanin.

melanotic (mel″ah-not′ik) characterized by the presence of melanin; pertaining to melanosis.

melanotrichia (mel″ah-no-trik′e-ah) abnormal hyperpigmentation of the hair.

melanuria (mel″ah-nu′re-ah) the excretion of darkly stained urine. **melanu′ric,** adj.

melasma (mě-laz′mah) dark pigmentation of the skin. **m. gravida′rum,** that occurring on the face during pregnancy (*mask of pregnancy*).

melatonin (mel″ah-to′min) a hormone formed by the mammalian pineal body which produces marked lightening of skin pigmentation; it seems to be inactive in humans.

melena (mě-le′nah) the passage of dark stools stained with altered blood.

melengestrol (mel″en-jes′trōl) a progestin and antineoplastic, $C_{25}H_{32}O_4$.

melibiase (mel″ĭ-bi′ās) see *galactosidase.*

melibiose (mel″ĭ-bi′ōs) a disaccharide from melitose, which yields galactose and dextrose on hydrolysis.

melioidosis (mel″e-oi-do′sis) a glanders-like disease of rodents, transmissible to man, and caused by *Pseudomonas pseudomallei.*

melitoptyalism (mel″ĭ-to-ti′al-izm) secretion of saliva containing glucose.

melitose (mel′ĭ-tōs) a crystalline sugar, $C_{18}H_{32}$-$O_{16}5H_2O$, from cottonseed meal, Australian manna, and various species of *Eucalyptus,* which on hydrolysis yields dextrose, fructose, and galactose.

melituria (mel″ĭ-tu′re-ah) the presence of any sugar in the urine.

Mellaril (mel′ah-ril) trademark for a preparation of thioridazine.

melodidymus (mel″o-did″ĭ-mus) an individual with a supernumary limb.

melomelus (mě-lom′ě-lus) a fetus with normal limbs and rudimentary supernumary limbs.

meloplasty (mel′o-plas″te) plastic surgery of the cheek.

melorheostosis (mel″o-re″os-to′sis) a form of osteosclerosis, with linear tracks extending through a long bone; see *rheostosis.*

melotia (mě-lo′she-ah) congenital displacement of the ear onto the cheek.

melphalan (mel′fah-lan) an alkylating antineoplastic agent, $C_{13}H_{18}Cl_2N_2O_2$.

member (mem′ber) a distinct part of the body, especially a limb.

membra (mem′bra) [L.] plural of *membrum.*

membrana (mem-bra′nah), pl. *membra′nae* [L.] membrane.

membrane (mem′brān) a thin layer of tissue that covers a surface, lines a cavity, or divides a space or organ. **mem′branous,** adj. **accidental m.,** false m. **alveolodental m.,** periodontium. **arachnoid m.,** arachnoid (2). **atlanto-occipital m.,** either of two midline ligamentous structures, one (the *anterior*) passing from the anterior arch of the atlas to the anterior margin of the foramen magnum, the other (the *posterior*) connecting the posterior aspects of the same structures. **basement m.,** the delicate layer underlying the epithelium of mucous membranes and secreting glands. **basilar m.,** lamina basilaris. **Bichat's m.,** fenestrated m. **Bowman's m.,** a thin layer of cornea between the outer layer of stratified epithelium and the substantia propria. **Bruch's m.,** the inner layer of the choroid, separating it from the pigmentary layer of the retina. **Brunn's m.,** the epithelium of the olfactory region of the nose. **cell m.,** the condensed protoplasm which forms the enveloping capsule of a cell. **cloacal m.,** the thin temporary barrier between the embryonic hindgut and the exterior. **Corti's m.,** a gelatinous mass resting on the organ of Corti, connected with the hairs of the hair cells. **croupous m.,** the false membrane of true croup. **decidual m., deciduous m.,** decidua. **Descemet's m.,** a thin hyaline membrane between the substantia propria and epithelial layer of the cornea. **diphtheritic m.,** a false membrane characteristic of diphtheria, formed by coagulation necrosis. **drum m.,** tympanic m. **elastic m.,** one made up largely of elastic fibers. **enamel m.,** 1. dental cuticle. 2. the inner layer of cells within the enamel organ of the fetal dental germ. **extraembryonic m's,** fetal m's. **false m.,** a morbid pellicle or skinlike layer resembling an organized and living membrane, but made up of coagulated fibrin with bacteria and leukocytes, such as may be formed on mucous membranes in diphtheria. **fenestrated m.,** one of the perforated elastic sheets of the tunica intima and tunica media of arteries. **fetal m's,** those that protect the embryo or fetus and provide for its nutrition, respiration, and excretion; the yolk sac (umbilical vesicle), allantois, amnion, chorion, decidua, and placenta. **fibroelastic m.,** the fibroelastic layer beneath the mucous coat of the larynx. **germinal m.,** blastoderm. **Henle's m.,** fenestrated m. **hyaline m.,** 1. a membrane between the outer root sheath and inner fibrous layer of a hair follicle. 2. a layer of eosinophilic hyaline material lining alveoli, alveolar ducts, and bronchioles, found at autopsy in infants who have died of respiratory distress syndrome of the newborn. **hyaloid m.,** vitreous m. (1). **hyoglossal m.,** a fibrous lamina connecting the undersurface of the tongue with the hyoid bone. **Jackson's m.,** a web of adhesions sometimes covering the cecum and causing obstruction of the bowel. **keratogenous m.,** matrix unguis. **Krause's m.,** Z band. **limiting m.,** one which constitutes the border of some tissue or structure. **medullary m.,** endosteum. **mucous m.,** the membrane lining various canals and cavities of the body. **Nasmyth's m.,** dental cuticle. **nictitating m.,** a transparent fold of skin lying deep to the eyelids, which may be drawn over the front of the eyeball; found in reptiles, birds, and many mammals. **nuclear**

m., the condensed double layer enclosing the nucleoplasm, separating it from the cytoplasm. **olfactory m.,** the olfactory portion of the mucous membrane lining the nasal fossa. **ovular m.,** vitelline m. **peridental m.,** periodontium. **periodontal m.,** see under *ligament.* **placental m.,** the semipermeable membrane separating the fetal from the maternal blood in the placenta. **plasma m.,** cell m. **pupillary m.,** a mesodermal layer attached to the rim or front of the iris of the embryo, sometimes persisting in the adult. **Reissner's m.,** the thin anterior wall of the cochlear duct, separating it from the scala vestibuli. **reticular m.,** a netlike membrane over the spiral organ of the ear, through which pass the free ends of the outer hair cells. **Ruysch's m., ruyschian m.,** lamina choroidocapillaris. **Scarpa's m.,** secondary tympanic m. **schneiderian m.,** the mucous membrane lining the nose. **semipermeable m.,** one permitting passage through it of some but not all substances. **serous m.,** tunica serosa. **Shrapnell's m.,** the thin upper part of the tympanic membrane. **striated m.,** zona pellucida. **synaptic m.,** the layer separating the neuroplasm of an axon from that of the body of the nerve cell with which it makes synapsis. **synovial m.,** the inner of the two layers of the articular capsule of a synovial joint, composed of loose connective tissue, having a free smooth surface that lines the joint cavity. **tectorial m.,** Corti's m. **tympanic m.,** the thin partition between the external acoustic meatus and the middle ear. **tympanic m., secondary,** the membrane enclosing the fenestra cochlearis. **undulating m.,** a protoplasmic membrane running like a fin along the bodies of certain protozoa. **unit m.,** a trilaminar structure common to all cell membranes, probably consisting of two layers of protein with a layer of lipid between them. **vestibular m.,** the thin anterior wall of the cochlear duct, separating it from the scala vestibuli. **virginal m.,** hymen. **vitelline m.,** the external envelope of the ovum. **vitreous m.,** 1. a delicate boundary layer investing the vitreous body. 2. Bruch's m. 3. Descemet's m. 4. hyaline m. (1). **yolk m.,** vitelline m. **Zinn's m.,** ciliary zonule.

membraniform (mem-bran′ĭ-form) resembling a membrane.

membranocartilaginous (mem″brah-no-kar″tĭ-laj′ĭ-nus) 1. developed in both membrane and cartilage. 2. partly cartilaginous and partly membranous.

membranoid (mem′brah-noid) resembling a membrane.

membrum (mem′brum), pl. *mem′bra* [L.] a limb or member of the body; an entire arm or leg. **m. mulie′bre,** clitoris. **m. viri′le,** penis.

memory (mem′o-re) that mental faculty by which sensations, impressions, and ideas are stored and recalled.

menacme (mĕ-nak′me) the period of a woman's life which is marked by menstrual activity.

menadiol (men″ah-di′ol) a vitamin K analogue; its sodium diphosphate salt is used as a prothrombinogenic vitamin.

menadione (men″ah-di′ōn) a prothrombino-

genic compound, $C_{11}C_8O_2$, used as a vitamin K supplement.

menaphthene (men-af′thēn) menadione.

menaphthone (men-af′thōn) menadione.

menarche (mĕ-nar′ke) establishment or beginning of the menstrual function. **menar′chial,** adj.

mendelevium (men″dĕ-le′ve-um) chemical element (*see table*), at. no. 101, symbol Md.

Menformon (men′for-mon) trademark for a preparation of estrone.

mening(o)- word element [Gr.], *meninges; membrane.*

meningeal (mĕ-nin′je-al) pertaining to the meninges.

meningeorrhaphy (mĕ-nin″je-or′ah-fe) suture of the meninges.

meninges (mĕn-in′jēz) (plural of *meninx*) the three membranes covering the brain and spinal cord: dura mater, arachnoid, and pia mater. **menin′geal,** adj.

meningioma (mĕ-nin″je-o′mah) a hard, usually vascular tumor, occurring mainly along the meningeal vessels and superior longitudinal sinus, invading the dura and skull and leading to erosion and thinning of the skull. **angioblastic m.,** angioblastoma.

meningism (men′in-jizm) 1. the symptoms and signs of meningitis associated with acute febrile illness or dehydration with infection of the meninges. 2. hysterical simulation of meningitis.

meningismus (men″in-jiz′mus) meningism.

meningitis (men″in-ji′tis), pl. *meningit′ides* [Gr.] inflammation of the meninges. **meningit′ic,** adj. **m. of the base, basilar m.,** that affecting the meninges at the base of the brain. **cerebral m.,** inflammation of the membranes of the brain. **cerebrospinal m.,** inflammation of the meninges of the brain and spinal cord. **epidemic cerebrospinal m.,** an acute infectious, usually epidemic, disease attended by a seropurulent meningitis, due to *Neisseria meningitides,* usually with an erythematous, herpetic, or hemorrhagic skin eruption. **meningococcic m.,** epidemic cerebrospinal m. **occlusive m.,** leptomeningitis of children, with closure of the lateral and median apertures of the fourth ventricle. **m. ossif′icans,** ossification of the cerebral meninges. **otitic m.,** that secondary to otitis media. **septicemic m.,** that due to septic blood poisoning. **serous m.,** that with serous exudation into the ventricles and subarachnoid spaces and slight to moderate spinal fluid changes. **spinal m.,** inflammation of the membranes of the spinal cord. **tubercular m., tuberculous m.,** severe meningitis due to *Mycobacterium tuberculosis.* **viral m.,** that due to various viruses, e.g., coxsackieviruses and the virus of lymphocytic choriomeningitis, marked by malaise, fever, headache, nausea, cerebrospinal fluid pleocytosis (mainly lymphocytic), abdominal pain, stiff neck and back, and a short uncomplicated course.

meningoarteritis (mĕ-ning″go-ar″ter-i′tis) inflammation of the meningeal arteries.

meningocele (mĕ-ning′go-sēl) hernial protrusion of the meninges through a defect in the cranium or vertebral column.

meningocerebritis (mĕ-ning″go-ser″ĕ-bri′tis) meningoencephalitis.

meningococcemia (-kok-se′me-ah) invasion of the blood by meningococci. **acute fulminating m.,** Waterhouse-Friderichsen syndrome.

meningococcus (-kok′us), pl. *meningococ′ci.* An individual organism of *Neisseria meningitidis.* **meningococ′cal, meningococ′cic,** adj.

meningocortical (-kor′tĭ-kal) pertaining to the meninges and cortex of the brain.

meningocyte (mĕ-ning′go-sīt) a histiocyte of the meninges.

meningoencephalitis (mĕ-ning″go-en-sef″ah-li′tis) inflammation of the brain and meninges.

meningoencephalocele (-en-sef′ah-lo-sēl″) hernial protrusion of the meninges and brain substance through a skull defect.

meningoencephalomyelitis (-en-sef″ah-lo-mi″ĕ-li′tis) inflammation of the meninges, brain and spinal cord.

meningoencephalopathy (-en-sef″ah-lop′ah-the) noninflammatory disease of the cerebral meninges and brain.

meningomalacia (-mah-la′she-ah) softening of a membrane.

meningomyelitis (-mi″ĕ-li′tis) inflammation of the spinal cord and meninges.

meningomyelocele (-mi′ĕ-lo-sēl) myelomeningocele.

meningo-osteophlebitis (-os″te-o-fle-bi′tis) periostitis with inflammation of the veins of a bone.

meningopathy (men″in-gop′ah-the) any disease of the meninges.

meningoradicular (mĕ-ning″go-rah-dik′u-lar) pertaining to the meninges and the cranial or spinal nerve roots.

meningoradiculitis (-rah-dik″u-li′tis) inflammation of the meninges and spinal nerve roots.

meningorhachidian (-rah-kid′e-an) pertaining to spinal cord and meninges.

meningorrhagia (-ra′je-ah) hemorrhage from cerebral or spinal membranes.

meningorrhea (-re′ah) effusion of blood between or upon the meninges.

meningosis (men″in-go′sis) attachment of bones by membrane.

meningovascular (mĕ-ning″go-vas′ku-lar) pertaining to the meningeal blood vessels.

meninx (me′ninks), pl. *menin′ges* [Gr.] a membrane, especially one of the membranes of the brain or spinal cord—the dura mater, arachnoid, and pia mater.

meniscectomy (men″ĭ-sek′to-me) excision of a meniscus, as of the knee joint.

meniscitis (men″ĭ-si′tis) inflammation of a meniscus of the knee joint.

meniscocyte (mĕ-nis′ko-sīt) a sickle cell.

meniscocytosis (mĕ-nis″ko-si-to′sis) sickle cell anemia.

meniscus (mĕ-nis′kus), pl. *menis′ci* [L.] something of crescent shape, as the concave or convex surface of a column of liquid in a pipet or buret, or a crescent-shaped fibrocartilage in the knee joint.

meno- word element [Gr.], *menstruation.*

menoctone (mĕ-nok′tōn) an antimalarial, $C_{24}H_{32}O_3$.

menolipsis (men″o-lip′sis) temporary cessation of menstruation.

menometrorrhagia (-met″ro-ra′je-ah) excessive uterine bleeding at and between menstrual periods.

menopause (men′o-pawz) cessation of menstruation. **men′opausal,** adj.

menorrhagia (men″o-ra′je-ah) excessive menstruation.

menorrhalgia (-ral′je-ah) dysmenorrhea.

menoschesis (mĕ-nos′kĕ-sis, men″o-ske′sis) retention of the menses.

menostasis (mĕ-nos′tah-sis) amenorrhea.

menostaxis (men″o-stak′sis) a prolonged menstrual period.

menotropins (-tro′pins) a purified extract of postmenopausal urine containing chiefly follicle-stimulating hormone with a trace of luteinizing hormone; used as a fertility drug.

menses (men′sēz) the monthly flow of blood from the female genital tract. **men′strual,** adj.

menstruate (men′stroo-āt) to undergo menstruation.

menstruation (men″stroo-a′shun) the cyclic, physiologic discharge of blood from the nonpregnant uterus, occurring usually at approximately four-week intervals during the reproductive period of the female of humans and a few other primates. **anovular m., anovulatory m.,** periodic uterine bleeding without preceding ovulation. **vicarious m.,** discharge of blood from an extragenital source at the time menstruation is normally expected.

menstruum (men′stroo-um) a solvent medium.

mensuration (men″su-ra′shun) the act or process of measuring.

mental (men′tal) 1. pertaining to the mind. 2. pertaining to the chin.

menthol (men′thol) an alcohol from various mint oils or produced synthetically; used locally to relieve itching.

mentum (men′tum) [L.] chin.

mepacrine (mep′ah-krin) quinacrine.

mepazine (mep′ah-zēn) a neuroleptic and antinauseant, $C_{19}H_{22}N_2S$.

mepenzolate (me-pen′zo-lāt) an anticholinergic, $C_{21}H_{26}NO_3$, used to relieve abdominal pain, gaseous distention, and diarrhea associated with colonic disease.

meperidine (mĕ-per′ĭ-dēn) a narcotic analgesic, $C_{15}H_{21}NO_2$, used as the hydrochloride salt.

mephenoxalone (mef″en-ok′sah-lōn) an antianxiety agent, $C_{11}H_{13}NO_4$.

mephentermine (mĕ-fen′ter-mēn) a sympathomimetic and pressor substance, $C_{11}H_{17}N$, used as the sulfate salt.

mephenytoin (mĕ-fen′ĭ-to″in) an anticonvulsant, $C_{12}H_{14}N_2O_2$.

mephitic (mĕ-fit′ik) emitting a foul odor.

mephobarbital (mef″o-bar′bĭ-tal) an anticonvulsant and sedative, $C_{13}H_{14}N_2O_3$.

Mephyton (mef′ĭ-ton) trademark for preparations of phytonadione (vitamin K_1).

mepivacaine (mĕ-piv′ah-kān) a lidocaine analogue, $C_{14}H_{21}NO_2$; its hydrochloride salt is used as a local anesthetic.

Meprane (me′prān) trademark for preparations of promethestrol.

meprednisone (mĕ-pred′nĭ-sōn) an oral glucocorticoid, $C_{22}H_{28}O_5$, used as an anti-inflammatory, antiallergic, and antineoplastic steroid.

meprobamate (mĕ-pro′bah-māt, mep″ro-bam′āt) a minor tranquilizer, $C_9H_{18}N_2O_4$.

meprylcaine (mep′ril-kān) a local anesthetic, $C_{14}H_{21}NO_2$; used in dentistry in the form of the hydrochloride salt.

mepyramine (me-pir′ah-mēn) pyrilamine.

mEq. milliequivalent.

meralgia (mĕ-ral′je-ah) pain in the thigh. **m. paresthet′ica,** paresthesia, pain, and numbness in the outer surface of the thigh due to entrapment of the lateral femoral cutaneous nerve at the inguinal ligament.

meralluride (mer-al′lu-rīd) a mercurial diuretic, $C_9H_{16}HgN_2O_6$.

Meratran (mer′ah-tran) trademark for a preparation of pipradrol.

merbromin (mer-bro′min) a topical antibacterial, $C_{20}H_8Br_2HgNa_2O_6$.

mercaptan (mer-kap′tan) any compound containing the —SH group bound to carbon.

mercaptol (mer-kap′tol) a compound formed from ketone by introducing two thio-alkyl groups in place of bivalent oxygen.

mercaptomerin (mer-kap″to-mer′in) an organic mercurial diuretic; used as the disodium salt, $C_{16}H_{25}HgNNa_2O_6S$.

mercaptopurine (-pu′rēn) an antineoplastic, $C_5H_4N_4S$.

mercocresol (mer″ko-kre′sol) a combination of cresol derivatives and an organic mercury, having germicidal, fungicidal, and bacteriostatic properties.

Mercodinone (-di′nōn) trademark for a preparation of hydrocodone.

Mercuhydrin (mer″ku-hi′drin) trademark for preparations of meralluride.

mercurial (mer-ku′re-al) 1. pertaining to mercury. 2. a preparation containing mercury.

mercurialism (mer-ku′re-al-izm″) mercury poisoning; see *mercury.*

mercuric (mer-ku′rik) pertaining to mercury as a bivalent element. **m. chloride,** mercury bichloride. **m. oxide, yellow,** an anti-infective, HgO, used in ophthalmology.

Mercurochrome (mer-ku′ro-krōm) trademark for preparations of merbromin.

mercurophylline (mer″ku-ro-fil′lin) a mercurial diuretic.

mercurous (mer′ku-rus) pertaining to mercury as a monovalent element. **m. chloride,** calomel.

mercury (mer′ku-re) chemical element (*see table*), at. no. 80, symbol Hg. Acute mercury poisoning, due to ingestion, is marked by severe abdominal pain, vomiting, bloody diarrhea with watery stools, oliguria or anuria, and corrosion and ulceration of the digestive tract; in the chronic form, due to absorption through skin and mucous membranes, inhalation, or ingestion, there is stomatitis, blue line along the gum border, sore hypertrophied gums that bleed easily, loosening of teeth, erethrism, ptyalism, tremors, and incoordination. **ammoniated m.,** a topical anti-infective, $HgNH_2Cl$. **m. bichloride,** an extremely poisonous compound, $HgCl_2$, used as a disinfectant. **m. chloride, mild,** calomel. **m. oleate,** a mixture of yellow mercuric oxide and oleic acid, used topically in various skin diseases. **m. perchloride,** m. bichloride.

merergastic (mer″er-gas′tik) pertaining to the simplest type of disorder of psychic function, marked by emotional instability and anxiety.

merethoxylline (mer″ĕ-thok′sĭ-lēn) a mercurial diuretic.

meridian (mĕ-rid′e-an) an imaginary line on the surface of a globe or sphere, connecting the opposite ends of its axis. **merid′ional,** adj.

meridianus (mĕ-rid″e-a′nus), pl. *meridia′ni* [L.] meridian.

mero- word element [Gr.], *part.*

meroblastic (mer-o-blas′tik) partially dividing; undergoing cleavage in which only part of the ovum participates.

merocrine (mer′o-krin) discharging only the secretory product and maintaining the secretory cell intact (e.g., salivary glands, pancreas).

merogenesis (mer″o-jen′ĕ-sis) cleavage of an ovum. **merogenet′ic,** adj.

merogony (mĕ-rog′o-ne) the development of only a portion of an ovum. **merogon′ic,** adj.

meromelia (mer″o-me′le-ah) congenital absence of any part, but not all, of a limb.

meromicrosomia (-mi″kro-so′me-ah) unusual smallness of some part of the body.

meromyosin (-mi′o-sin) a fragment of the myosin molecule isolated by treatment with proteolytic enzyme; there are two types, heavy (H-meromyosin) and light (L-meromyosin).

meropia (mĕ-ro′pe-ah) partial blindness.

merorhachischisis (me″ro-rah-kis′kĭ-sis) fissure of part of the spinal cord.

merosmia (mĕ-roz′me-ah) inability to perceive certain odors.

merotomy (mĕ-rot′o-me) dissection into segments, especially dissection of a cell.

merozoite (mer″o-zo′īt) one of the organisms formed by multiple fission (schizogony) of a sporozoite within the body of the host.

mersalyl (mer′sah-lil) a mercurial diuretic.

Merthiolate (mer-thi′o-lāt) trademark for preparations of thimerosal.

merycism (mer′ĭ-sizm) rumination.

mes(o)- word element [Gr.], *middle.*

mesangium (mes-an′je-um) the thin membrane supporting the capillary loops in renal glomeruli. **mesan′gial,** adj.

Mesantoin (mĕ-san′to-in) trademark for preparations of mephenytoin.

mesarteritis (mes″ar-ter-i′tis) inflammation of the middle coat of an artery.

mesaticephalic (mes-at″ĭ-sĕ-fal′ik) mesocephalic (2).

mesatipellic (-pel′ik) having a transverse diameter of the pelvic inlet almost the same as that of the true conjugated diameter.

mesaxon (mes-ak′son) a pair of parallel membranes marking the line of edge-to-edge contact of Schwann cells encircling an axon.

mescaline (mes′kah-lēn) a poisonous alkaloid from the flowering heads (mescal buttons) of a Mexican cactus, *Lophophora williamsii;* it produces an intoxication with delusions of color and sound.

mescalism (mes′kah-lizm) intoxication due to mescal buttons or mescaline.

mesectoderm (mĕ-sek′to-derm) embryonic migratory cells derived from the neural crest of the head that contribute to the formation of the meninges and become pigment cells.

mesencephalitis (mes″en-sef″ah-li′tis) inflammation of the mesencephalon.

mesencephalon (-en-sef′ah-lon) the midbrain. **mesencephal′ic,** adj.

mesencephalotomy (-en-sef″ah-lot′o-me) surgical production of lesions in the midbrain, especially for relief of intractable pain.

mesenchyma (mĕ-seng′kĭ-mah) the meshwork of embryonic connective tissue in the mesoderm from which are formed the connective tissues of the body and the blood and lymphatic vessels. **mesen′chymal,** adj.

mesenchyme (mes′eng-kīm) mesenchyma.

mesenchymoma (mes″en-ki-mo′mah) a mixed mesenchymal tumor composed of two or more cellular elements not commonly associated, exclusive of fibrous tissue.

mesenterectomy (mes″en-tĕ-rek′to-me) resection of the mesentery.

mesenteriopexy (-en-ter′e-o-pek″se) fixation or suspension of a torn mesentery.

mesenteriorrhaphy (-en-ter″e-or′ah-fe) suture or repair of the mesentery.

mesenteriplication (-en-ter″ĭ-pli-ka′shun) shortening of the mesentery by plication.

mesenteritis (-en-tĕ-ri′tis) inflammation of the midgut.

mesenterium (-en-te′re-um) [L.] mesentery.

mesenteron (mes-en′ter-on) the midgut.

mesentery (mes′en-ter″e) a membranous fold attaching various organs to the body wall; especially the peritoneal fold attaching the small intestine to the dorsal body wall. **mesenter′ic,** adj.

mesiad (me′ze-ad) toward the middle or center.

mesial (me′ze-al) nearer the center of the dental arch.

mesially (me′ze-al″e) toward the median line.

mesiobuccal (me″ze-o-buk′kal) pertaining to or formed by the mesial and buccal surfaces of a tooth, or the mesial and buccal walls of a tooth cavity.

mesiocervical (-ser′vĭ-kal) pertaining to the mesial surface of the neck of a tooth.

mesioclusion (-kloo′zhun) anteroclusion; malrelation of the dental arches with the mandibular arch anterior to the maxillary arch (prognathism).

mesiodens (me′ze-o-dens), pl. *mesioden′tes.* A small supernumerary tooth, occurring singly or paired, generally palatally between the maxillary central incisors.

mesiodistal (me″ze-o-dis′tal) pertaining to the mesial and distal surfaces of a tooth.

mesiolabial (-la′be-al) pertaining to the mesial and labial surfaces of a tooth or a tooth cavity.

mesion (me′ze-on) the plane dividing the body into right and left symmetrical halves.

mesio-occlusal (me″ze-o-ŏ-kloo′zal) pertaining to the mesial and occlusal surfaces of a tooth or a tooth cavity.

mesioversion (-ver′zhun) displacement of a tooth along the dental arch toward the midline of the face.

mesmerism (mes′mer-izm) hypnotism.

mesoappendix (mes″o-ah-pen′diks) the peritoneal fold connecting the appendix to the ileum.

mesobilirubin (-bil″ĭ-roo′bin) a compound formed by reduction of bilirubin.

mesobilirubinogen (-bil″ĭ-roo-bin′o-jen) a reduced form of bilirubin, formed in the intestine, which on oxidation forms stercobilin.

mesobiliviolin (-bil″ĭ-vi′o-lin) an oxidation product of mesobilirubinogen and of stercobilin.

mesoblast (mes′o-blast) the mesoderm, especially in the early stages.

mesoblastema (mes″o-blas-te′mah) the cells composing the mesoblast.

mesobronchitis (-brong-ki′tis) inflammation of middle coat of bronchi.

mesocardia (-kar′de-ah) atypical location of the heart, with the apex in the midline of the thorax.

mesocardium (-kar′de-um) 1. that part of the embryonic mesentery connecting the heart with the body wall in front and the foregut behind. 2. myocardium.

mesocecum (-se′kum) the occasionally occurring mesentery of the cecum.

mesocephalic (-sĕ-fal′ik) 1. mesencephalic. 2. having a cephalic index of 76.0–80.9.

mesocephalon (-sef′ah-lon) the midbrain.

mesocolon (-ko′lon) the peritoneal process attaching the colon to the posterior abdominal wall, and called, ascending, descending, etc., according to the portion of colon to which it attaches. **mesocol′ic,** adj.

mesocolopexy (-ko′lo-pek″se) suspension or fixation of the mesocolon.

mesocoloplication (-ko″lo-pli-ka′shun) plication of the mesocolon to limit its mobility.

mesocord (mes′o-kord) an umbilical cord adherent to the placenta.

mesoderm (-derm) the middle of the three primary germ layers of the embryo, lying between the ectoderm and entoderm; from it are derived the connective tissue, bone, cartilage, muscle, blood and blood vessels, lymphatics, lymphoid organs, notochord, pleura, pericardium, peritoneum, kidneys, and gonads. **mesoder′mal, mesoder′mic,** adj.

mesodiastolic (mes″o-di″ah-stol′ik) pertaining to the middle of the diastole.

mesoduodenum (-du″o-de′num) the mesenteric fold enclosing the duodenum of the early fetus.

mesoepididymis (-ep″ĭ-did′ĭ-mis) a fold of tunica vaginalis sometimes connecting the epididymis and testis.

mesogaster (-gas′ter) mesogastrium.

mesogastrium (-gas′tre-um) the portion of the primitive mesentery which encloses the stomach and from which the greater omentum develops. **mesogas′tric,** adj.

mesoglia (me-sog′le-ah) 1. microglia. 2. oligodendroglia.

mesogluteus (mes″o-gloo′te-us) gluteus medius muscle; see Table of Muscles. **mesoglu′teal,** adj.

mesognathous (mĕ-sog′nah-thus) having a gnathic index of 98–103.

mesoileum (mes″o-il′e-um) the mesentery of the ileum.

mesojejunum (-jĕ-ju′num) the mesentery of the jejunum.

mesolymphocyte (-lim′fo-sīt) a medium-sized lymphocyte.

mesomere (mes′o-mēr) 1. a blastomere of size intermediate between a macromere and a micromere. 2. a midzone of the mesoderm between the epimere and hypomere.

mesomerism (mĕ-som′er-izm) the existence of organic chemical structures differing only in the position of electrons rather than atoms. **mesomer′ic,** adj.

mesometrium (mes″o-me′tre-um) the portion of the broad ligament below the mesovarium.

mesomorph (mez′o-morf, mes′o-morf) 1. an individual having the type of body build in which mesodermal tissues predominate: there is relative preponderance of muscle, bone, and connective tissue, usually with heavy, hard physique of rectangular outline. 2. a well-proportioned individual.

mesomorphy (mes″o-mor′fe) the condition of being a mesomorph. **mesomor′phic,** adj.

meson (me′zon, mes′on) 1. mesion. 2. a subatomic particle having a rest mass intermediate between the mass of the electron and that of the proton, carrying either a positive or a negative electric charge.

mesonephroma (mez″o-nĕ-fro′mah) a malignant tumor of the female genital tract, usually the ovary, formerly thought to arise from mesonephric rests. Two types are recognized: one of müllerian duct derivation, the other an embryonal tumor occurring chiefly in children; the latter may also arise in the testis.

mesonephros (-nef′ros), pl. mesoneph′roi [Gr.] the excretory organ of the embryo, arising caudad to the pronephric rudiments or the pronephros and using its ducts. **mesoneph′ric,** adj.

mesopexy (mes′o-pek″se) mesenteriopexy.

mesophile (-fīl) an organism which grows best at 20°–55° C. **mesophil′ic,** adj.

mesophlebitis (mes″o-fle-bi′tis) inflammation of the middle coat of a vein.

mesophryon (mes-of′re-on) the glabella, or its central point.

Mesopin (mes′o-pin) trademark for a preparation of homatropine.

mesoporphyrin (mes″o-por′fĭ-rin) a crystalline iron-free porphyrin, $C_{34}H_{38}O_4N_4$, from heme, obtained by a process of reduction.

mesopulmonum (-pul-mo′num) the embryonic mesentery enclosing the laterally expanding lung.

mesorchium (mes-or′ke-um) the portion of the primitive mesentery enclosing the fetal testis, represented in the adult by a fold between the testis and epididymis. **mesor′chial,** adj.

mesorectum (mes″o-rek′tum) the fold of peritoneum connecting the upper portion of the rectum with the sacrum.

mesoridazine (-rid′ah-zēn) a member of the phenothiazine group, $C_{21}H_{26}N_2OS_2$, used as a major tranquilizer.

mesoropter (-rop′ter) the normal position of the eyes with their muscles at rest.

mesorrhaphy (mes-or′ah-fe) mesenteriorrhaphy.

mesorrhine (mes′o-rīn) having a nasal index of 48–53.

mesosalpinx (mes″o-sal′pinks) the portion of the broad ligament above the mesovarium.

mesosigmoid (-sig′moid) the peritoneal fold attaching the sigmoid flexure to the posterior abdominal wall.

mesosigmoidopexy (-sig-moi′do-pek″se) fixation of the mesosigmoid for prolapse of the rectum.

mesosome (mes′o-sōm) an invagination of the bacterial cell membrane, forming organelles thought to be the site of cytochrome enzymes and the enzymes of oxidative phosphorylation and the citric acid cycle.

mesosternum (mes″o-ster′num) corpus sterni.

mesotendineum (-ten-din′e-um) the connective tissue sheath attaching a tendon to its fibrous sheath.

mesotendon (-ten′don) mesotendineum.

mesothelioma (-the″le-o′mah) a tumor arising from mesothelial tissue.

mesothelium (-the′le-um) the layer of cells, derived from mesoderm, lining the body cavity of the embryo; in the adult, forming the simple squamous-cell layer of epithelium covering the surface of all true serous membranes (peritoneum, pericardium, pleura). **mesothe′lial,** adj.

mesovarium (-va′re-um) the portion of the broad ligament between the mesometrium and mesosalpinx, which encloses and holds the ovary in place.

Mesozoa (-zo′ah) a small group of tiny parasites whose relationship to the Protozoa and Metazoa is uncertain.

mestranol (mes′trah-nōl) an estrogenic agent, $C_{21}H_{26}O_2$, used in combination with various progestogens as an oral contraceptive.

mesuprine (mes′u-prēn) a vasodilator and smooth muscle relaxant, $C_{19}H_{26}N_2O_5S$, used as the hydrochloride salt.

meta- word element [Gr.], (1) change; transfor-

mation; exchange; (2) *after; next;* (3) the 1,3-position in derivatives of benzene.

metabasis (mě-tab′ah-sis) a change in the manifestations or course of a disease.

metabiosis (met″ah-bi-o′sis) dependence of one organism upon another for its existence; commensalism.

metabolimeter (met″ah-bo-lim′ĕ-ter) an apparatus for measuring basal metabolism.

metabolism (mě-tab′o-lizm) the sum of all the physical and chemical processes by which living organized substance is produced and maintained (anabolism), and also the transformation by which energy is made available for the uses of the organism (catabolism). **metabol′ic,** adj. **basal m.,** the minimal energy expended for the maintenance of respiration, circulation, peristalsis, muscle tonus, body temperature, glandular activity, and the other vegetative functions of the body. The rate of basal metabolism (basal metabolic rate) is measured by means of a calorimeter, in a subject at absolute rest, 14 to 18 hours after eating, and is expressed in calories per hour per square meter of body surface. **inborn error of m.,** a genetically determined biochemical disorder in which a specific enzyme defect causes a metabolic block that may have pathologic consequences at birth or in later life.

metabolite (mě-tab′o-līt) any substance produced by metabolism or by a metabolic process.

metabolize (mě-tab′o-līz) to subject to or be transformed by metabolism.

metabutethamine (met″ah-bu-teth′ah-min) a local anesthetic, $C_{13}H_{20}N_2O_2$; used in dentistry as the hydrochloride salt.

metabutoxycaine (-bu-tok′sĭ-kān) a local anesthetic, $C_{17}H_{28}N_2O_3$.

metacarpal (-kar′pal) 1. pertaining to the metacarpus. 2. a bone of the metacarpus.

metacarpectomy (-kar-pek′to-me) excision or resection of a metacarpal bone.

metacarpophalangeal (-kar″po-fah-lan′je-al) pertaining to the metacarpus and the phalanges of the fingers.

metacarpus (-kar′pus) the part of the hand between the wrist and fingers, its skeleton being five bones (metacarpals) extending from the carpus to the phalanges.

metacentric (-sen′trik) having the centromere near the middle, so that the arms of the replicating chromosome are approximately equal in length.

metacercaria (-ser-ka′re-ah), pl. *metacerca′riae.* The encysted resting or maturing stage of a trematode parasite in the tissues of an intermediate host or on vegetation.

metachromasia (-kro-ma′ze-ah) 1. failure to stain true with a given stain. 2. the different coloration of different tissues produced by the same stain. 3. change of color produced by staining. **metachromat′ic,** adj.

metachromatism (-kro′mah-tizm) metachromasia.

metachromophil (-kro′mo-fil) not staining in the usual manner with a given stain.

metachrosis (-kro′sis) change of color in animals.

metacone (met′ah-kōn) the distobuccal cusp of an upper molar tooth.

metaconid (met″ah-ko′nid) the mesiolingual cusp of a lower molar tooth.

metaconule (-ko′nūl) the distal intermediate cusp of an upper molar tooth in animals.

metacresol (-kre′sol) one of the three isomeric forms of cresol, the most strongly antiseptic of the group.

metagenesis (-jen′ĕ-sis) alternation of generations; alternation in regular sequence of asexual with sexual reproductive methods, as in certain fungi.

Metagonimus (-gon′ĭ-mus) a genus of trematodes, including *M. yokoga′wai,* which is parasitic in the small intestine of man and mammals in Japan, China, Indonesia, the Balkans, and Israel.

metal (met′al) any element marked by luster, malleability, ductility, and conductivity of electricity and heat and which will ionize positively in solution. **metal′lic,** adj. **alkali m.,** any of a group of monovalent metals, including lithium, sodium, potassium, rubidium, and cesium. **Babbitt m.,** an alloy of tin, copper, and antimony, sometimes used in dentistry.

metalbumin (met″al-bu′min) pseudomucin.

metalloenzyme (mě-tal″o-en′zīm) any enzyme containing tightly bound metal atoms, e.g., the cytochromes.

metalloid (met′ah-loid) 1. any element with both metallic and nonmetallic properties. 2. any metallic element having not all the characters of a typical metal.

metalloporphyrin (mě-tal″o-por′fĭ-rin) a combination of a metal with porphyrin, as in heme.

metalloprotein (-pro′te-in) a protein molecule bound to a metal ion, e.g., hemoglobin.

metallurgy (met″al-er′je) the science and art of using metals.

metalol (met′ah-lōl) an antiadrenergic (β-receptor antagonist), $C_{11}H_{18}N_2O_3S$; used as the hydrochloride salt.

metamer (met′ah-mer) a compound exhibiting, or capable of exhibiting, metamerism.

metamere (-mēr) one of a series of homologous segments of the body of an animal. In genetic theory, one of a varying number of common repeating units that make up the repressor segment of a chromosome segment.

metamerism (mě-tam′er-izm) 1. a type of structural isomerism in which different radicals of the same chemical type are attached to the same polyvalent element and yet give rise to compounds having identical molecular formulas. 2. arrangement into metameres by the serial repetition of a structural pattern. **metamer′ic,** adj.

Metamine (met′ah-mēn) trademark for preparations of trolnitrate.

metamorphopsia (met″ah-mor-fop′se-ah) defective vision, with distortion of shape.

metamorphosis (-mor′fŏ-sis) change of structure or shape, particularly, transition from one developmental stage to another, as from larva to adult form. **metamor′phic,** adj. **fatty m.,** any normal or pathologic transformation of fat. **platelet m.,** structural m. **retrograde m.,** degeneration; a retrograde metabolic change. **structural m., viscous m.,** the progressive, irreversible aggregation and fusion of blood platelets during coagulation.

metamyelocyte (-mi′ĕ-lo-sīt″) an immature polymorphonuclear leukocyte with a horseshoe- or sausage-shaped nucleus, developmentally preceded by the myelocyte and followed by the mature leukocyte.

Metandren (mĕ-tan′dren) trademark for preparations of methyltestosterone.

metanephrine (met″ah-nef′rin) a metabolite of epinephrine excreted in urine and found in certain tissues.

metanephrogenic (-nef″ro-jen′ik) capable of giving rise to the metanephros.

metanephros (-nef′ros), pl. *metaneph′roi* [Gr.] the permanent embryonic kidney, developing later than and caudad to the mesonephros. **metaneph′ric,** adj.

metaneutrophil (-nu′tro-fil) staining abnormally with neutral stains.

metaphase (met′ah-fāz) the second stage of cell division (mitosis or meiosis), in which the chromosomes, each consisting of two chromatids, are arranged in the equatorial plane of the spindle prior to separation.

Metaphedrin (met″ah-fed′rin) trademark for a preparation of nitromersol and ephedrine.

Metaphen (met′ah-fen) trademark for preparations of nitromersol.

metaphysis (mĕ-taf′ĭ-sis), pl. *metaph′yses* [Gr.] the wider part at the end of the shaft of a long bone, adjacent to the epiphyseal disk. **metaphys′eal,** adj.

metaplasia (met″ah-pla′ze-ah) the change in the type of adult cells in a tissue to a form abnormal for that tissue. **metaplas′tic,** adj. **myeloid m., agnogenic,** a condition characterized by foci of extramedullary hematopoiesis and by splenomegaly, immature blood cells in the peripheral blood, and mild to moderate anemia.

metaplasm (met′ah-plazm) deutoplasm.

metapneumonic (met″ah-nu-mon′ik) succeeding or following pneumonia.

metaproterenol (-pro-ter′ĕ-nōl) a bronchodilator, $(C_{11}H_{17}NO_3)_2$, used as the sulfate salt.

metapsychology (-si-kol′o-je) the branch of speculative psychology that deals with the significance of mental processes that are beyond empirical verification.

metaraminol (-ram′ĭ-nol) a sympathomimetic and pressor agent, $C_9H_{13}NO_2$.

metarhodopsin (-ro-dop′sin) an intermediate formed as rhodopsin absorbs light and eventually dissociates to opsin and *trans*-retinal.

metarubricyte (-roo″brĭ-sīt) orthochromatic normoblast.

metastasis (mĕ-tas′tah-sis) 1. transfer of disease from one organ or part of the body to another not directly connected with it, due either to transfer of pathogenic microorganisms or to transfer of cells; all malignant tumors are capable of metastasizing. 2. (pl. *metas′tases*) a growth of pathogenic microorganisms or of abnormal cells distant from the site primarily involved by the morbid process. **metastat′ic,** adj.

metastasize (mĕ-tas′tah-sīz) to form new foci of disease in a distant part by metastasis.

metatarsal (met″ah-tar′sal) 1. pertaining to the metatarsus. 2. a bone of the metatarsus.

metatarsalgia (-tar-sal′je-ah) pain in the metatarsus.

metatarsectomy (-tar-sek′to-me) excision or resection of the metatarsus.

metatarsophalangeal (-tar″so-fah-lan′je-al) pertaining to a metatarsal bone and a phalanx.

metatarsus (-tar′sus) the part of the foot between the ankle and the toes, its skeleton being the five bones (metatarsals) extending from the tarsus to the phalanges. **m. pri′mus va′rus,** angulation of the first metatarsal bone toward the midline of the body, producing an angle sometimes of 20 degrees or more between its base and that of the second metatarsal bone.

metathalamus (-thal′ah-mus) the part of the thalamencephalon composed of the medial and lateral geniculate bodies.

metathesis (mĕ-tath′ĕ-sis) 1. artificial transfer of a morbid process. 2. a chemical reaction in which an element or radical in one compound exchanges places with another element or radical in another compound.

metatrophic (met″ah-trof′ik) utilizing organic matter for food.

metaxalone (mĕ-taks′ah-lōn) a smooth muscle relaxant, $C_{12}H_{15}NO_3$.

Metazoa (met″ah-zo′ah) that division of the animal kingdom embracing the multicellular animals whose cells differentiate to form tissues, i.e., all animals except the Protozoa. **metazo′al, metazo′an,** adj.

metazoon (-zo′on), pl. *metazo′a* [Gr.] an individual organism of the Metazoa.

metencephalon (met″en-sef′ah-lon) [Gr.] 1. the anterior part of the hindbrain, comprising the cerebellum and pons. 2. the anterior of two brain vesicles formed by specialization of the hindbrain in embryonic development.

meteorism (me′te-o-rizm″) tympanites.

meteorotropism (me″te-o-rot′ro-pizm) response to influence by meteorologic factors noted in certain biological events. **meteorotrop′ic,** adj.

meter (me′ter) 1. the basic unit of linear measure of the metric system, being the equivalent of 39.371 inches. 2. an apparatus devised to measure the quantity of anything passing through it.

-meter word element [Gr.], *relationship to measurement; instrument for measuring.*

metestrus (met-es′trus) the period of subsiding follicular function following estrus in female mammals.

metformin (-for′min) an oral hypoglycemic, $C_4H_{11}N_5$.

methacholine (meth″ah-ko′lēn) a parasympathomimetic, $C_8H_{18}NO_2$, used as the chloride and bromide salts in management of cardiovascular disorders.

methacrylate (meth-ak′rĭ-lāt) an acrylic resin widely used in denture bases and as an adhesive for joint prostheses.

methacycline (meth″ah-si′klēn) a semisynthetic tetracycline derivative; its hydrochloride is used as an oral broad-spectrum antibiotic.

methadone (meth′ah-dōn) a synthetic compound, $C_{21}H_{27}NO$, with pharmacologic action similar to that of morphine and heroin and almost equal in addiction liability; the hydrochloride is used as an antitussive and analgesic and as a substitute narcotic in the management of heroin addiction.

methallenestril (meth″al-lĕ-nes′tril) a nonsteroid estrogenic agent, $C_{18}H_{22}O_3$.

methalthiazide (-al-thi′ah-zīd) a diuretic and antihypertensive, $C_{12}H_{16}ClN_3O_4S_3$.

methamphetamine (-am-fet′ah-mēn) a central nervous system stimulant and pressor substance, $C_{10}H_{15}N$, used as the hydrochloride salt. Abuse may lead to dependence.

methandriol (meth-an′dre-ol) an anabolic stimulant, $C_{20}H_{32}O_2$.

methandrostenolone (-an″dro-sten′o-lōn) an anabolic steroid with androgenic effects, $C_{20}H_{28}O_2$.

methane (meth′ān) an inflammable, explosive gas, CH_4, from decomposition of organic matter.

methanol (meth′ah-nol) a clear, colorless, flammable liquid, CH_3OH, used as a solvent.

methantheline (mě-than′thě-lin) an anticholinergic, $C_{21}H_{26}NO$, used to depress gastric activity.

methapyrilene (meth″ah-pir′ĭ-lēn) an antihistaminic, $C_{14}H_{19}N_3S$, with sedative action; the hydrochloride salt is used in the treatment of allergic disorders and insomnia, and as a local anesthetic.

methaqualone (kwa′lōn) a hypnotic, $C_{16}H_{14}N_2O$.

metharbital (meth-ar′bĭ-tal) an anticonvulsant, $C_9H_{14}N_2O_3$, used in controlling myoclonic seizures and in conditions due to organic brain damage.

methazolamide (meth″ah-zo′lah-mīd) a carbonic anhydrase inhibitor, $C_5H_8N_4O_3S_2$, given orally to reduce intraocular pressure.

methdilazine (meth-di′lah-zēn) an antihistaminic, $C_{18}H_{20}N_2S$.

methemalbumin (met″hem-al-bu′min) a brownish pigment formed in the blood by the binding of albumin with heme; indicative of intravascular hemolysis.

methemoglobin (met-he″mo-glo′bin) a compound formed from hemoglobin by oxidation of the ferrous to the ferric state with essentially ionic bonds; it does not combine reversibly with oxygen.

methemoglobinemia (-glo″bĭ-ne′me-ah) the presence of methemoglobin in the blood.

methemoglobinuria (-glo″bĭ″nu′re-ah) the presence of methemoglobin in the urine.

methenamine (meth″en-am′in) an antibacterial, $C_6H_{12}N_6$, used in urinary tract infections.

m. mandelate, a salt of methenamine and mandelic acid, used in infections of the urinary tract.

Methergine (meth′er-jin) trademark for preparations of methylergonovine.

methicillin (meth″ĭ-sil′in) a semisynthetic penicillin which is highly resistant to inactivation by penicillinase; its sodium salt is used parenterally.

methimazole (meth-im′ah-zōl) a thyroid inhibitor, $C_4H_6N_2S$.

methiodal (-i′o-dal) an iodine-containing compound, CH_2IO_3S, whose sodium salt is used as a radiopaque medium in excretory urography.

methionine (mě-thi′o-nin) a sulfur-bearing amino acid, $C_5H_{11}NO_2S$, essential for optimal growth in infants and for nitrogen equilibrium in adults; used therapeutically as a dietary supplement with lipotropic action.

methisazone (mě-this′ah-zōn) an antiviral agent, $C_{10}H_{10}N_4OS$, used to treat vaccinia.

Methium (meth′e-um) trademark for preparations of hexamethonium.

methixene (mě-thiks′ēn) a smooth muscle relaxant, $C_{20}H_{23}NS$, used as the hydrochloride salt.

methocarbamol (meth″o-kar′bah-mol) a skeletal muscle relaxant, $C_{11}H_{15}NO_5$.

method (meth′od) the manner of performing any act or operation; a procedure or technique.

methodology (meth″o-dol′o-je) the science of method; the science dealing with principles of procedure in research and study.

methohexital (-hek′sĭ-tal) an ultrashort-acting barbiturate; its sodium salt, $C_{14}H_{17}N_2NaO_3$, is used intravenously as a general anesthetic.

methopholine (-fo′lēn) an analgesic, $C_{20}H_{24}ClNO_2$.

methopromazine (-pro′mah-zēn) methoxypromazine.

methotrexate (-trek′sāt) an antineoplastic agent, $C_{20}H_{22}N_8O_5$.

methotrimeprazine (-tri-mep′rah-zēn) an analgesic, $C_{19}H_{24}N_2OS$, given intramuscularly.

methoxamine (mě-thok′sah-mēn) an adrenergic vasopressor, $C_{11}H_{17}NO_3$, used as the hydrochloride salt.

methoxsalen (mě-thok′sah-len) an acrylic acid compound, $C_{12}H_8O_4$, which induces melanin production on exposure of the skin to ultraviolet light; used in the treatment of idiopathic vitiligo and as a suntan accelerator and protectant.

methoxyflurane (mě-thok″se-floo′rān) a general inhalation anesthetic, $C_3H_4Cl_2F_2O$.

methoxyphenamine (-fen′ah-mēn) a sympathomimetic, $C_{11}H_{17}NO$, used as a bronchodilator and nasal decongestant in the form of the hydrochloride salt.

methscopolamine bromide (meth″sko-pol′ah-min) an anticholinergic, $C_{18}H_{24}BrNO_4$.

methsuximide (meth-suk′sĭ-mīd) an anticonvulsant, $C_{12}H_{13}NO_2$, used to treat petit mal and psychomotor epilepsy.

methyclothiazide (meth″ĭ-klo-thi′ah-zīd) a diuretic and antihypertensive, $C_9H_{11}Cl_2N_3O_4S_2$.

methyl (meth′il) the chemical group or radical

CH₃—. **m. salicylate,** an oily liquid obtained from leaves of *Gaultheria procumbens* or bark of *Betula lenta,* or produced synthetically; used as a flavoring agent and as a topical analgesic in rheumatic disorders, lumbago, and sciatica.

methylamine (meth″il-am′in) a gaseous ptomaine from decaying fish and from cultures of *Vibrio cholerae.*

methylate (meth′ĭ-lāt) 1. a compound of methyl alcohol and a base. 2. to add a methyl group to a substance.

methylation (meth″ĭ-la′shun) treatment with reagent to add a methyl group to a compound.

methylatropine (meth″il-at′ro-pēn) an atropine derivative; *m. nitrate,* the quaternary ammonium derivative, has strong antimuscarinic effects and strong ganglionic blocking activity.

methylbenzethonium (-ben″zĕ-tho′ne-um) a local anti-infective, $C_{28}H_{44}NO_2$; used as the chloride salt.

methylcellulose (-sel′u-lōs) a methyl ester of cellulose; used as a bulk laxative and as a suspending agent for drugs.

methylcholanthrene (-ko-lan′thrēn) a carcinogenic hydrocarbon, $C_{21}H_{16}$, from deoxycholic acid, cholic acid, and cholesterol.

methyldopa (-do′pah) an antihypertensive, $C_{10}H_{13}NO_4$.

methyldopate (-do′pāt) the ethyl ester of methyldopa; its hydrochloride salt is given intravenously as an antihypertensive.

methylene (meth″ĭ-lēn) the divalent hydrocarbon radical CH₂.

methylergonovine (meth″il-er″go-no′vin) an oxytocic, $C_{20}H_{25}N_3O_2$, used as the maleate salt.

methylglucamine (-gloo′kah-min) 1. a compound prepared from D-glucose and methylamine, used in the synthesis of pharmaceuticals. 2. meglumine.

methylhexaneamine (-hek-sān′ah-min) a sympathomimetic, $C_7H_{17}N$, used as a nasal decongestant.

methylmercaptan (-mer-kap-tan) a gas, CH₃··SH, formed in the intestine by decomposition of proteins and having a disagreeable odor.

methylparaben (-par′ah-ben) an antifungal preservative, $C_8H_8O_3$.

methylparafynol (-par″ah-fi′nol) a sedative, $C_6H_{10}O$.

methylphenidate (-fen′i-dāt) a central stimulant, $C_{14}H_{19}NO_2$; used as the hydrochloride salt.

methylprednisolone (-pred-nis′o-lōn) a glucocorticoid, $C_{22}H_{30}O_5$, with anti-inflammatory activity slightly greater than prednisolone; also used as the 21-acetate ester and sodium succinate salt.

methylrosaniline (-ro-zan′ĭ-lēn) gentian violet.

methyltestosterone (-tes-tos′ter-ōn) a synthetic androgenic hormone with actions and uses similar to those of testosterone.

methylthiouracil (-thi″o-u′rah-sil) a thyroid suppressant, $C_5H_6N_2OS$.

methyltransferase (-trans′fer-ās) any enzyme that catalyzes transmethylation.

methyprylon (meth″ĭ-pri′lon) a sedative, $C_{10}H_{17}NO_2$.

methysergide (-ser′jĭd) a potent serotonin antagonist used in prophylaxis of migraine; also available as the maleate salt.

Meticortelone (met″ĭ-kor′tĕ-lōn) trademark for preparations of prednisolone.

Meticorten (-kor′ten) trademark for a preparation of prednisone.

metmyoglobin (met-mi″o-glo′bin) a compound formed from myoglobin by oxidation of the ferrous to the ferric state.

metopic (mĕ-top′ik) pertaining to the forehead.

metopion (mĕ-to′pe-on) glabella.

metopon (met-o′pon) a morphine derivative, used as an analgesic.

metopopagus (met″o-pop′ah-gus) conjoined twins united at the forehead.

metoxenous (mĕ-tok′sĕ-nus) requiring two hosts for the life cycle; said of parasites.

metoxeny (mĕ-tok′sĕ-ne) the condition of being metoxenous.

metra (me′trah) the uterus.

metra-, metro- word element [Gr.], *uterus.*

metralgia (me-tral′je-ah) pain in the uterus.

metratonia (me″trah-to′ne-ah) uterine atony.

metratrophia (-tro′fe-ah) atrophy of the uterus.

Metrazol (met′rah-zol) trademark for preparations of pentylenetetrazol.

metrectasia (me″trek-ta′ze-ah) dilatation of the nonpregnant uterus.

metrectopia (me″trek-to′pe-ah) uterine displacement.

metreurynter (me″troo-rin′ter) an inflatable bag for dilating the cervical canal.

metreurysis (me-troo′rĭ-sis) dilation of the cervix uteri by means of the metreurynter.

metric (met′rik) 1. pertaining to measures or measurement. 2. having the meter as a basis.

metriocephalic (me″tre-o-sĕ-fal′ik) having a vertical index of 72–77.

metritis (me-tri′tis) inflammation of the uterus. **m. dis′secans,** metritis with necrosis of portions of the uterine wall. **puerperal m.,** infection of the uterus of the puerperal woman.

metrocele (me′tro-sēl) hernia of the uterus.

metrocolpocele (me″tro-kol′po-sēl) hernia of uterus with prolapse into the vagina.

metrocystosis (-sis-to′sis) formation of cysts in the uterus.

metrocyte (me′tro-sīt) a mother cell.

metrodynia (me″tro-din′e-ah) metralgia.

metroleukorrhea (-lu″ko-re′ah) leukorrhea of uterine origin.

metrology (me-trol′o-je) the science dealing with measurements.

metrolymphangitis (me″tro-limf″an-ji′tis) inflammation of the uterine lymphatic vessels.

metromalacia (-mah-la′she-ah) abnormal softening of the uterus.

metronidazole (-ni′dah-zōl) a trichomonacide, $C_6H_9N_3O_3$.

metroparalysis (-pah-ral′ĭ-sis) paralysis of the uterus.

metropathia (-path′e-ah) metropathy. **m. hemorrha′gica,** essential uterine hemorrhage.

MULTIPLES AND SUBMULTIPLES OF THE METRIC SYSTEM

MULTIPLES AND SUBMULTIPLES	PREFIX	PRONUNCIATION	SYMBOL
$1,000,000,000,000 = 10^{12}$	tera	ter'a	T
$1,000,000,000 = 10^9$	giga	ji'ga	G
$1,000,000 = 10^6$	mega	meg'a	M
$1,000 = 10^3$	kilo	kil'o	k
$100 = 10^2$	hecto	hek'to	h
$10 = 10$	deka	dek'a	dk
[The unit = one]			
$0.1 = 10^{-1}$	deci	des'i	d
$0.01 = 10^{-2}$	centi	sen'ti	c
$0.001 = 10^{-3}$	milli	mil'i	m
$0.000\ 001 = 10^{-6}$	micro	mi'kro	μ
$0.000\ 000\ 001 = 10^{-9}$	nano	nan'o	n
$0.000\ 000\ 000\ 001 = 10^{-12}$	pico	pe'co	p
$0.000\ 000\ 000\ 000\ 001 = 10^{-15}$	femto	fem'to	f
$0.000\ 000\ 000\ 000\ 000\ 001 = 10^{-18}$	atto	at'to	a

International Committee on Weights and Measures, 1962. From Style Manual for Biological Journals.

metropathy (me-trop'ah-the) any uterine disease or disorder. **metropath'ic,** adj.

metroperitonitis (me"tro-per"ĭ-to-ni'tis) inflammation of the peritoneum about the uterus.

metrophlebitis (-fle-bi'tis) inflammation of the uterine veins.

Metropine (met'ro-pin) trademark for preparations of methylatropine.

metroplasty (me'tro-plas"te) reconstructive surgery on the uterus.

metroptosis (me"tro-to'sis) downward displacement, or prolapse of the uterus.

metrorrhagia (-ra'je-ah) uterine bleeding, usually of normal amount, occurring at completely irregular intervals, the period of flow sometimes being prolonged.

metrorrhea (-re'ah) a free or abnormal uterine discharge.

metrorrhexis (-rek'sis) rupture of the uterus.

metrosalpingitis (-sal"pin-ji'tis) inflammation of the uterus and oviducts.

metrosalpingography (-sal"ping-gog'rah-fe) hysterosalpingography.

metroscope (me'tro-skōp) hysteroscope.

metrostaxis (me"tro-stak'sis) slight but persistent uterine bleeding.

metrostenosis (-stĕ-no'sis) contraction or stenosis of the uterine cavity.

-metry word element [Gr.], *measurement.*

Metubine (mĕ-tu'bin) trademark for a preparation of tubocurarine.

Metycaine (met'ĭ-kān) trademark for preparations of piperocaine.

metyrapone (mĕ-ter'ah-pōn) a compound, $C_{14}H_{14}N_2O$, used as a diagnostic aid in determining anterior pituitary function (corticotropin secretion).

Mev. million electron volts.

μf. microfarad.

M.F.D. minimum fatal dose.

Mg chemical symbol, *magnesium.*

mg. milligram.

μg. microgram.

μγ micromicrogram.

MHz megahertz.

mianserin (me-an'ser-in) a sertonin inhibitor and antihistaminic, $C_{18}H_{20}N_2$, used as the hydrochloride salt.

mication (mi-ka'shun) a quick motion, such as winking.

micr(o)- word element [Gr.], *small;* used in naming units of measurement to designate an amount 10^{-6} (one millionth) the size of the unit to which it is joined, e.g., microgram.

micracoustic (mi"krah-koos'tik) 1. rendering very faint sounds audible. 2. an instrument for rendering faint sounds audible.

micrencephaly (mi"kren-sef'ah-le) abnormal smallness and underdevelopment of the brain.

microabscess (mi"kro-ab'ses) a very small, localized collection of pus.

microaerophilic (-a"er-o-fil'ik) growing best in the presence of very little free oxygen.

microaerotonometer (-a"er-o-to-nom'ĕ-ter) an instrument for measuring the volume of gases in the blood.

microanalysis (-ah-nal'ĭ-sis) the chemical analysis of minute quantities of material.

microanatomy (-ah-nat'o-me) histology.

microaneurysm (-an'u-rizm) a microscopic aneurysm, a characteristic of thrombotic purpura.

microangiopathy (-an"je-op'ah-the) disease of the small blood vessels. **microangiopath'ic,** adj. **thrombotic m.,** formation of thrombi in the arterioles and capillaries.

Microbacterium (-bak-te're-um) a genus of bacteria (family Corynebacteriaceae) found in dairy products, characterized by relatively high heat resistance.

microbe (mi′krōb) a microorganism, especially a pathogenic bacterium. **micro′bial, micro′bic,** adj.

microbicidal (mi-kro″bĭ-si′dal) destroying microbes.

microbicide (mi-kro′bĭ-sīd) an agent that destroys microbes.

microbiologist (mi″kro-bi-ol′o-jist) a specialist in microbiology.

microbiology (-bi-ol′o-je) the science dealing with the study of microorganisms. **microbiolog′ical,** adj.

microbiota (-bi-o′tah) the microscopic living organisms of a region. **microbiot′ic,** adj.

microblast (mi′kro-blast) an erythroblast of 5 microns or less in diameter.

microblepharia (mi″kro-blĕ-fār′e-ah) abnormal shortness of the vertical dimensions of the eyelids.

microbody (mi′kro-bod″e) any of the cytoplasmic particles found in kidney and liver cells and in certain other cells, surrounded by a limiting membrane, and containing dense crystalline-like inclusions and oxidases.

microbrachius (mi″kro-bra′ke-us) a fetus with abnormally small arms.

microburet (-bu-ret′) a buret with a capacity of the order of 0.1 to 10 ml., with graduated intervals of 0.001 to 0.02 ml.

microcalorie (-kal′o-re) the heat required to raise 1 ml. of distilled water from 0° to 1° C.

microcardia (-kar′de-ah) abnormal smallness of the heart.

microcentrum (-sen′trum) centrosome.

microcephalus (-sef′ah-lus) an individual with an abnormally small head.

microcephaly (-sef′ah-le) abnormal smallness of the head. **microcephal′ic,** adj.

microcheilia (-ki′le-ah) abnormal smallness of the lip.

microcheiria (-ki′re-ah) abnormal smallness of the hands.

microchemistry (-kem′is-tre) chemistry concerned with exceedingly small quantities of chemical substances.

microcinematography (-sin″ĕ-mah-tog′rah-fe) moving picture photography of microscopic objects.

microcirculation (-ser″ku-la′shun) the flow of blood through the fine vessels (arterioles, capillaries, and venules). **microcirculato′ry,** adj.

Micrococcaceae (-kok-a′se-e) a family of bacteria (order Eubacteriales).

Micrococcus (-kok′us) a genus of gram-positive bacteria (family Micrococcaceae) found in soil, water, etc.

micrococcus (-kok′us), pl. *micrococ′ci.* 1. an organism of the genus *Micrococcus.* 2. a very small, spherical microorganism.

microcolon (-ko′lon) abnormal smallness of the colon.

microcoria (-ko′re-ah) smallness of the pupil.

microcornea (-kor′ne-ah) unusual smallness of the cornea, usually bilateral.

microcoulomb (-koo′lomb) one millionth of a coulomb.

microcrystalline (-kris′tah-lin) made up of minute crystals.

microcurie (-ku′re) one millionth (10^{-6}) curie; abbreviated μC., μ.c.h.

microcurie-hour (mi′kro-ku″re-owr″) a unit of exposure equivalent to that obtained by exposure for one hour to radioactive material disintegrating at the rate of 3.7×10^4 atoms per second; abbreviated μC hr., μc.

microcyst (mi′kro-sist) a very small cyst.

microcyte (-sīt) an erythrocyte 5 microns or less in diameter.

microcythemia (mi″kro-si-the′me-ah) a condition in which the erythrocytes are smaller than normal.

microcytosis (-si-to′sis) microcythemia.

microdactyly (-dak′tĭ-le) abnormal smallness of fingers or toes.

microdetermination (-de-ter″mĭ-na′shun) chemical examination of minute quantities of substance.

microdissection (-dĭ-sek′shun) dissection of tissue or cells under the microscope.

microdont (mi′kro-dont) having a dental index below 42.

microdontia (mi″kro-don′she-ah) abnormal smallness of the teeth.

microdrepanocytic (-drep″ah-no-sit′ik) containing microcytic and drepanocytic elements.

microerythrocyte (-ĕ-rith′ro-sīt) microcyte.

microfarad (-far′ad) one millionth (10^{-6}) farad; abbreviated μf.

microfauna (-faw′nah) the microscopic animal organisms of a special region.

microfibril (-fi′bril) an extremely small fibril.

microfilament (-fil′ah-ment) any of the filaments about 60 Å in diameter, in the cytoplasmic ground substance.

microfilaremia (-fil″ah-re′me-ah) the presence of microfilariae in the circulating blood.

microfilaria (-fi-la′re-ah), pl. *microfila′riae* [L.] the prelarval stage of Filarioidea in the blood of man and in the tissues of the vector; sometimes incorrectly used as a genus name.

microflora (-flo′rah) the microscopic vegetable organisms of a special region.

microgamete (-gam′ēt) see *gamete* (2).

microgametocyte (-gah-me′to-sīt) see *gametocyte.*

microgastria (-gas′tre-ah) congenital smallness of the stomach.

microgenia (-je′ne-ah) abnormal smallness of the chin.

microgenitalism (-jen′ĭ-tal-izm) smallness of the external genitals.

microglia (mi-krog′le-ah) non-neural cells forming part of the adventitial structure of the central nervous system. They are migratory and act as phagocytes to waste products. **microg′lial,** adj.

microgliocyte (mi-krog′le-o-sīt) a precursor of a microglial cell.

microglioma (mi″kro-gli-o′mah) a tumor composed of microglial cells.

microglossia (-glos′e-ah) abnormal smallness of the tongue.

micrognathia (-nath′e-ah) unusual smallness of the jaws, especially the lower jaw. **micrognath′ic**, adj.

microgonioscope (-go′ne-o-skōp) a gonioscope with a magnifying lens.

microgram (mi′kro-gram) one millionth (10^{-6}) gram; abbreviated μg. or mcg.

micrograph (-graf) 1. an instrument for recording very minute movements by making a greatly magnified photograph of the minute motions of a diaphragm. 2. a photograph of a minute object or specimen as seen through a microscope.

micrography (mi-krog′rah-fe) an account of microscopic objects.

microgyria (mi″kro-ji′re-ah) polymicrogyria.

microgyrus (-ji′rus), pl. *microgy′ri.* An abnormally small, malformed convolution of the brain.

microhm (mi′krōm) one millionth (10^{-6}) ohm.

microincineration (mi″kro-in-sin″er-a′shun) the oxidation of a small quantity of material, for identification from the ash of the elements composing it.

microinjector (-in-jek′tor) an instrument for infusion of very small amounts of fluids or drugs.

microlesion (mi′kro-le″zhun) a minute lesion.

microliter (-le″ter) one millionth (10^{-6}) liter; abbreviated μl.

microlith (-lith) a minute concretion or calculus.

microlithiasis (mi″kro-lĭ-thi′ah-sis) the formation of minute concretions in an organ. **m. alveola′ris pulmo′num,** pulmonary alveolar **m.,** a condition due to deposition of minute calculi in the pulmonary alveoli, appearing radiographically as fine, sandlike mottling.

micromanipulation (-mah-nip″u-la′shun) the use of the micromanipulator.

micromanipulator (-mah-nip′u-la″tor) an instrument for the moving, dissecting, etc., of minute specimens under the microscope.

micromastia (-mas′te-ah) abnormal smallness of the mammary gland.

micromelia (-me′le-ah) abnormal smallness or shortness of the limbs.

micromelus (mi-krom′ĕ-lus) an individual exhibiting micromelia.

micromere (mi′kro-mēr) one of the small blastomeres formed by unequal cleavage of a fertilized ovum (at the animal pole).

micrometer[1] (mi-krom′ĕ-ter) an instrument for measuring objects seen through the microscope.

micrometer[2] (mi′kro-me″ter) micron; one thousandth (10^{-3}) of a millimeter or one millionth (10^{-6}) of a meter. Abbreviated μm.

micromethod (-meth″od) any technique dealing with exceedingly small quantities of material.

micrometry (mi-krom′ĕ-tre) measurement of microscopic objects.

micromicro- word element designating 10^{-12} (one trillionth); now supplanted by *pico-.*

micromicron (mi″kro-mi′kron) one millionth (10^{-6}) micron, or 1 picometer; symbol $\mu\mu$.

micromillimeter (-mil′ĭ-me″ter) one millionth (10^{-6}) millimeter, or 1 nanometer; abbreviated μmm.

micromolecular (-mo-lek′u-lar) composed of small molecules.

micromyelia (-mi-e′le-ah) abnormal smallness of the spinal cord.

micromyeloblast (-mi′ĕ-lo-blast) a small, immature myelocyte. **micromyeloblas′tic,** adj.

micron (mi′kron) micrometer; one thousandth (10^{-3}) of a millimeter or one millionth (10^{-6}) of a meter; abbreviated μ.

microneedle (mi″kro-ne′d'l) a fine glass needle used in micromanipulation.

micronodular (-nod′u-lar) marked by the presence of small nodules.

micronucleus (-nu′kle-us) 1. in ciliate protozoa, the smaller of two types of nucleus in each cell, which functions in sexual reproduction; cf. *macronucleus.* 2. a small nucleus. 3. nucleolus.

micronutrient (-nu′tre-ent) a dietary element essential only in small quantities.

micronychia (-nik′e-ah) abnormal smallness of the nails.

microorganism (-or′gah-nizm) a microscopic organism; those of medical interest include bacteria, rickettsiae, viruses, fungi, and protozoa.

micropathology (-pah-thol′o-je) 1. the sum of what is known about minute pathologic change. 2. pathology of diseases caused by microorganisms.

microphage (mi′kro-fāj) a small phagocyte; an actively motile neutrophilic leukocyte capable of phagocytosis.

microphakia (mi″kro-fa′ke-ah) abnormal smallness of the crystalline lens.

microphallus (-fal′us) abnormal smallness of the penis.

microphone (mi′kro-fōn) a device to pick up sound for purposes of amplification or transmission.

microphonia (mi″kro-fo′ne-ah) marked weakness of voice.

microphotograph (-fo′to-graf) a photograph of small size.

microphthalmia (mi″krof-thal′me-ah) abnormal smallness of the eyeball.

micropipet (mi″kro-pi-pet′) a pipet for handling small quantities of liquids (up to 1 ml.).

microplethysmography (-pleth″is-mog′rah-fe) the recording of minute changes in the size of a part as produced by circulation of blood.

micropodia (-po′de-ah) abnormal smallness of the feet.

microprobe (mi′kro-prōb″) a minute probe, as one used in microsurgery.

micropsia (mi-krop′se-ah) a visual disorder in which objects appear smaller than their actual size.

micropyle (mi′kro-pīl) an opening in the investing membrane of certain ova, through which a spermatozoon enters.

microradiography (mi″kro-ra″de-og′rah-fe) radiography under conditions which permit subsequent microscopic examination or enlargement of the radiograph up to several hundred linear magnifications.

microrefractometer (-re″frak-tom′ĕ-ter) a refractometer for the discernment of variations in minute structures.

microrespirometer (-res″pĭ-rom′ĕ-ter) an apparatus for investigating oxygen utilization in isolated tissues.

microscope (mi′kro-skōp) an instrument used to obtain an enlarged image of small objects and reveal details of structure not otherwise distinguishable. **binocular m.,** one with two eyepieces, permitting use of both eyes simultaneously. **compound m.,** one consisting of two lens systems. **corneal m.,** one with a lens of high magnifying power, for observing minute changes in the cornea and iris. **darkfield m.,** one designed to permit diversion of light rays and illumination from the side, so that details appear light against a dark background. **electron m.,** one in which an electron beam, instead of light, forms an image for viewing on a fluorescent screen, or for photography. **infrared m.,** one in which radiation of 800 nm. or longer wavelength is used as the image-forming energy. **light m.,** one in which the specimen is viewed under visible light. **phase m., phase-contrast m.,** one altering the phase relationships of the light passing through and that passing around the object, the contrast permitting visualization without the necessity of staining or other special preparation. **simple m.,** one consisting of a single lens. **slit lamp m.,** a corneal microscope with a special attachment that permits examination of the endothelium on the posterior surface of the cornea. **stereoscopic m.,** a binocular microscope modified to give a three-dimensional view of the specimen. **ultraviolet m.,** one that utilizes reflecting optics or quartz and other ultraviolet-transmitting lenses. **x-ray m.,** one in which x-rays are used instead of light, the image usually being reproduced on film.

microscopic (mi″kro-skop′ik) of extremely small size; visible only by aid of a microscope.

microscopical (-skop′ĭ-kal) 1. pertaining to microscopy. 2. microscopic.

microscopist (mi-kros′ko-pist) a person skilled in using the microscope.

microscopy (mi-kros′ko-pe) examination with a microscope. **television m.,** a special technique in which a magnified image produced by a microscope is projected on a television screen.

microsecond (mi′kro-sek″und) one millionth (10^{-6}) of a second; abbreviated μs. or μsec.

microseme (-sēm) having an orbital index of less than 83.

microsmatic (mi″kros-mat′ik) having a feebly developed sense of smell, as in man.

microsome (mi′kro-sōm) any of the vesicular fragments of endoplasmic reticulum produced during homogenization of cells.

microsomia (mi″kro-so′me-ah) abnormally small size of the body.

microspectroscope (-spek′tro-skōp) a spectroscope and microscope combined.

microspherocyte (-sfe′ro-sīt) spherocyte.

microspherocytosis (-sfe″ro-si-to′sis) spherocytosis.

microsphygmia (-sfig′me-ah) a pulse that is difficult to perceive by the finger.

microsplenia (-sple′ne-ah) smallness of the spleen.

microsporid (mi-kros′po-rid) a secondary skin eruption which is an expression of hypersensitivity to *Microsporum* infection.

Microsporon (mi″kro-spo′ron) *Microsporum.*

microsporosis (-spo-ro′sis) a ringworm infection due to *Microsporum.*

Microsporum (-spo′rum) a genus of fungi which cause various diseases of skin and hair, including *M. audoui′ni, M. ca′nis, M. ful′vum,* and *M. gyp′seum.*

microstomia (-sto′me-ah) unusual smallness of the mouth.

microsurgery (-ser′jer-e) dissection of minute structures under the microscope by means of hand-held instruments.

microsyringe (-sēr′inj) a syringe fitted with a screw-thread micrometer for accurate measurement of minute quantities.

microtia (mi-kro′she-ah) abnormal smallness of the pinna of the ear.

microtome (mi′kro-tōm) an instrument for cutting thin sections for microscopic study.

microtomy (mi-krot′o-me) the cutting of thin sections.

microtonometer (mi″kro-to-nom′ĕ-ter) an instrument for measuring the oxygen and carbon dioxide tension of arterial blood.

microtrauma (-traw′mah) a microscopic lesion or injury.

microtubule (-tu′bul) a cylindrical structure in the cytoplasmic substance of many motile cells; they increase in number during mitosis. Also, similar structures having a constant number and arrangement in cilia of cells.

microvasculature (-vas′ku-lah-tūr) the finer vessels of the body, as the arterioles, capillaries, and venules.

microvillus (-vil′us), pl. *microvil′li.* A minute process or protrusion from the free surface of a cell, especially cells of the proximal convolution in renal tubules and of the intestinal epithelium.

microvolt (mi′kro-volt) one millionth of a volt; symbol μv.

microwave (-wāv) a wave typical of electromagnetic radiation between far infrared and radio waves, generally regarded as extending from 300,000 to 100 megacycles (wavelength of 1 mm. to 30 cm.).

microzoon (mi″kro-zo′on) a microscopic animal organism.

micrurgy (mi′krur-je) manipulative technique in the field of a microscope. **micrur′gic,** adj.

micturate (mik′tu-rāt) urinate.

micturition (mik″tu-rish′un) urination.

midbrain (mid′brān) mesencephalon; the part of the brain developed from the middle of the three primary brain vesicles, comprising the tectum and the cerebral peduncles and traversed by the aqueduct.

midget (mij'et) a normal dwarf; a person who is undersized but perfectly formed.

midgut (mid'gut) the region in the developing embryo between the foregut and hindgut, opening into the yolk sac.

Midicel (-ĭ-sel) trademark for preparations of sulfamethoxypyridazine.

midriff (-rif) the diaphragm; the region between the breast and waistline.

midwife (-wīf) a women who assists at childbirth but who is not a physician.

midwifery (-wi-fer-e) the practice of a midwife.

migraine (mi'grān, me'grān) a symptom complex of periodic headaches, usually temporal and unilateral, often with irritability, nausea, vomiting, constipation or diarrhea, and photophobia, preceded by constriction of the cranial arteries, usually with resultant prodromal sensory (especially ocular) symptoms, and commencing with the vasodilation that follows. **mi'grainous,** adj. **abdominal m.,** that in which abdominal symptoms are predominant.

migration (mi-gra'shun) 1. an apparently spontaneous change of place, as of symptoms. 2. diapedesis.

Mikedimide (mi-ked'ĭ-mīd) trademark for a preparation of bemegride.

mikro- for words beginning thus, see those beginning *micro-*.

mildew (mil'dew) vernacular term for any superficial fungous growth on plants or any organic material.

miliaria (mil"e-a're-ah) a cutaneous condition with retention of sweat, which is extravasated at different levels in the skin; when used alone, it refers to *m. rubra*. **m. ru'bra,** heat rash; prickly heat; a condition due to obstruction of the ducts of the sweat glands; the sweat escapes into the epidermis, producing pruritic red papulovesicles.

miliary (mil'e-er"e) 1. like millet seeds. 2. characterized by lesions resembling millet seeds.

Milibis (mil"ĭ-bis) trademark for preparations of glycobiarsol.

milieu (me-lyuh') [Fr.] surroundings; environment. **m. exté'rieur,** external environment. **m. inté'rieur,** internal environment; the blood and lymph in which the cells are bathed.

milium (mil'e-um), pl. *mil'ia* [L.] a whitish nodule in the skin, especially of the face, usually 1 to 4 mm. in diameter.

milk (milk) 1. the fluid secretion of the mammary gland forming the natural food of young mammals. 2. a liquid (emulsion or suspension) resembling the secretion of the mammary gland. **acidophilus m.,** milk fermented with cultures of *Lactobacillus acidophilus;* used in gastrointestinal disorders to modify the bacterial flora of the intestinal tract. **m. of bismuth,** a suspension of bismuth hydroxide and bismuth subcarbonate in water; used as an astringent and antacid. **certified m.,** milk whose purity is certified by a committee of physicians or a medical milk commission. **condensed m.,** milk which has been partly evaporated and sweet-ened with sugar. **evaporated m.,** milk prepared by evaporation of half of its water content. **fortified m.,** milk made more nutritious by addition of cream, egg white, or vitamins. **homogenized m.,** milk treated so that the fats form a permanent emulsion. **m. of magnesia,** a suspension containing 7–8.5 per cent of magnesium hydroxide; used as an antacid and cathartic. **modified m.,** cow's milk made to correspond to the composition of human milk. **skim m., skimmed m.,** milk from which the cream has been removed. **m. of sulfur,** precipitated sulfur. **vitamin D m.,** cow's milk fortified by addition of vitamin D. **witch's m.,** milk secreted in the breast of the newborn infant.

milking (milk'ing) the pressing out of the contents of a tubular structure by running the finger along it.

milkpox (-poks) variola minor.

milli- word element [Fr.], *one thousandth;* used in naming units of measurement to designate an amount 10^{-3} the size of the unit to which it is joined, e.g., milligram.

milliampere (mil"e-am'pēr) one thousandth of an ampere.

millicurie (mil"ĭ-ku're) one thousandth (10^{-3}) curie; abbreviated mc.

milliequivalent (mil"e-e-kwiv'ah-lent) the number of grams of a solute in 1 ml. of a normal solution; abbreviated mEq.

milligram (mil'ĭ-gram) one thousandth (10^{-3}) gram; abbreviated mg.

milliliter (-le"ter) one thousandth (10^{-3}) liter; abbreviated ml.

millimeter (-me"ter) one thousandth (10^{-3}) meter; abbreviated mm.

millimicro- word element designating 10^{-9} (one billionth) part of the unit to which it is joined; nano-.

millimicron (mil"ĭ-mi'kron) nanometer; one thousandth (10^{-6}) micron, or one billionth (10^{-9}) meter; abbreviated mμ.

millimole (mil'ĭ-mōl) one thousandth part of a mole; symbol mmol.

millinormal (mil"ĭ-nor'mal) having a concentration one-thousandth of normal; abbreviated mN.

milliosmole (mil"e-os'mōl) one thousandth of an osmole.

millisecond (mil"ĭ-sek'ond) one thousandth (10^{-3}) of a second; abbreviated ms. or msec.

millivolt (mil'ĭ-volt) one thousandth of a volt; abbreviated mv.

Milontin (mi-lon'tin) trademark for preparations of phensuximide.

Milpath (mil'path) trademark for a preparation of meprobamate and tridihexethyl chloride.

milphae, milphosis (mil'fe; mil-fo'sis) the falling out of the eyelashes.

Miltown (mil'town) trademark for a preparation of meprobamate.

mimesis (mi-me'sis) stimulation of one disease or bodily process by another.

mimetic (mi-met'ik) pertaining to mimesis. Also used as a word termination indicating simulation of a function, process, etc.

min. minim; minimum; minute.

mind (mīnd) the psyche; the faculty, or brain function, by which one is aware of his surroundings, and by which one experiences feelings, emotions, and desires, and is able to attend, reason, and make decisions.

mineral (min'er-al) any nonorganic homogeneous solid substance of the earth's crust.

mineralocorticoid (min''er-al-o-kor'tĭ-koid) a corticoid effective in causing the retention of sodium and loss of potassium.

minim (min'im) a unit of capacity (liquid measure), being $\frac{1}{60}$ fluid dram, or the equivalent of 0.0616 ml.

miocardia (mi''o-kar'de-ah) systole.

miopus (mi'o-pus) a monster with two fused heads, one face being rudimentary.

miosis (mi-o'sis) contraction of the pupil.

miotic (mi-ot'ik) 1. pertaining to, characterized by, or producing miosis. 2. an agent that causes contraction of the pupil.

miracidium (mi''rah-sid'e-um), pl. *miracid'ia* [Gr.] the first stage larva of a trematode which undergoes further development in the body of a snail.

mire (mēr) [Fr.] one of the figures on the arm of an ophthalmometer whose images are reflected on the cornea; measurement of their variations measures the amount of corneal astigmatism.

mirror (mir'or) a polished surface that reflects sufficient light to yield images of objects in front of it. **concave m.,** one with a concave reflecting surface. **convex m.,** one with a convex reflecting surface. **dental m.,** mouth m. **frontal m., head m.,** a circular mirror strapped to the head; used to reflect light into a cavity, especially in nasal, pharyngeal, and laryngeal examinations. **Glatzel m.,** a plate of cold metal held below the nostrils; the patch of moisture deposited by breathing on its surface indicates the patency or nonpatency of the nasal passages. **mouth m.,** a small mirror attached at an angle to a handle, for use in dentistry. **nasographic m.,** Glatzel m. **plane m.,** one with a flat reflecting surface.

misanthropy (mis-an'thro-pe) hatred of mankind.

miscarriage (mis-kar'ij) loss of the products of conception from the uterus before the fetus is viable; spontaneous abortion.

miscegenation (mis''ĕ-jĕ-na'shun) intermarriage or interbreeding between persons of different races.

miscible (mis'ĭ-b'l) susceptible of being mixed.

misogamy (mĭ-sog'ah-me) morbid aversion to marriage.

misogyny (mĭ-soj'ĭ-ne) aversion to women.

mite (mīt) any arthropod of the order Acarina except the ticks; they are minute animals, usually transparent or semitransparent, and may be parasitic on man and domestic animals, causing various skin irritations. **harvest m.,** chigger. **itch m., mange m.,** see *Notoedres* and *Sarcoptes*.

mithramycin (mith''rah-mi'sin) an antineoplastic antibiotic produced by *Streptomyces argillaceus* and *S. tanashiensis*.

mithridatism (mith'rĭ-da''tizm) acquisition of immunity to a poison by ingestion of gradually increasing amounts of it.

miticide (mi'tĭ-sīd) an agent destructive to mites.

mitochondria (mi''to-kon'dre-ah), sing. *mitochon'drion* [Gr.] small, spherical to rod-shaped components (organelles) of the cytoplasm; they are the principal sites of the generation of energy resulting from oxidation of foodstuffs, and contain enzymes of the Krebs and fatty acid cycles and the respiratory pathway.

mitogen (mi'to-jen) an agent that induces mitosis. **mitogen'ic,** adj.

mitogenesis (mi''to-jen'ĕ-sis) the induction of mitosis in a cell. **mitogenet'ic,** adj.

mitome (mi'tōm) a thready network of the protoplasm; the more solid portion of the protoplasm.

mitomycin (mi''to-mi'sin) a group of antitumor antibiotics (mitomycin A, B, and C) produced by *Streptomyces caespitosus*.

mitosis (mi-to'sis) a method of indirect cell division in which the two daughter nuclei normally receive identical complements of the number of chromosomes characteristic of the somatic cells of the species. **mitot'ic,** adj.

mitral (mi'tral) shaped like a miter; pertaining to the mitral valve.

mitralization (mi''tral-i-za'shun) a straightening of the left border of the cardiac shadow, commonly seen radiographically in mitral stenosis.

mittelschmerz (mit'el-shmerts) pain midway between the menstrual periods.

mixture (miks'tūr) a combination of different drugs or ingredients, as a fluid with other fluids or solids, or of a solid with a liquid. **brown m.,** a preparation of glycyrrhiza fluidextract, antimony potassium tartrate, paregoric, alcohol, glycerin, and purified water; used as an expectorant. **chalk m.,** prepared chalk, with bentonite magma, cinnamon water, and saccharin sodium; used as an antacid. **kaolin m. with pectin,** a preparation containing kaolin, pectin, powdered tragacanth, benzoic acid, saccharin sodium, glycerin, and peppermint oil in purified water; used as an adsorbent and demulcent.

Miyagawanella (mi''yah-gah''wah-nel'ah) a genus of organisms, the species of which are now assigned to the genus *Chlamydia* as follows: *M. lymphogranulomato'sis* and *M. bronchopneumo'niae* are assigned to *C. trachomatis,* and *M. bo'vis, M. fe'lis, M. illi'nii, M. louisia'nae, M. opos'sumi, M. ornitho'sis, M. o'vis, M. pe'coris, M. pneumo'niae,* and *M. psit'taci* are assigned to *C. psittaci.*

M.L. Licentiate in Medicine.

ml. milliliter.

μl. microliter.

M.L.A. Medical Library Association.

M.L.D. minimum lethal dose.

mm. millimeter; muscles.

mμ millimicron.

Mn chemical symbol, *manganese*.

mnemonics (ne-mon′iks) improvement of memory by special methods or techniques. **mnemon′ic,** adj.

M.O. Medical Officer.

Mo chemical symbol, *molybdenum.*

mobilization (mo″bĭ-li-za′shun) the rendering of a fixed part movable. **stapes m.,** surgical correction of immobility of the stapes in treatment of deafness.

modality (mo-dal′ĭ-te) 1. in homeopathy, a condition that modifies drug action; a condition under which symptoms develop, becoming better or worse. 2. a method of application of, or the employment of, any therapeutic agent; limited usually to physical agents. 3. a specific sensory entity, such as taste.

mode (mōd) in statistics, the value or item in a variations curve showing the maximum frequency of occurrence.

Moderil (mod′er-il) trademark for a preparation of rescinnamine.

modiolus (mo-di′o-lus) the central pillar or columella of the cochlea.

Modumate (mod′u-māt) trademark for a preparation of arginine and glutamic acid.

M.O.H. Medical Officer of Health.

moiety (moi′ĕ-te) any equal part; a half; also any part or portion, as a portion of a molecule.

mol (mol) mole (3).

molal (mo′lal) containing one mole of solute per 1000 grams of solvent.

molality (mo-lal′ĭ-te) the number of moles of a solute per kilogram of pure solvent.

molar (mo′lar) 1. pertaining to a mass; not molecular. 2. adapted for grinding; see under *tooth* and see Plate XV. 3. containing one mole of solute per liter of solution.

molarity (mo-lar′ĭ-te) the number of moles of a solute per liter of solution.

mold (mōld) 1. any of a group of parasitic and saprophytic fungi causing a cottony growth on organic substances; also the deposit or growth produced by such fungi. 2. a form in which an object is shaped, or cast. 3. in dentistry, the shape of an artificial tooth.

molding (mold′ing) the adjusting of the shape and size of the fetal head to the birth canal during labor.

mole (mōl) 1. a fleshy mass formed in the uterus by degeneration or abortive development of an ovum. 2. a nevocytic nevus; also, any pigmented fleshy growth. 3. that amount of a chemical compound whose mass in grams is equivalent to its formula mass. **hairy m.,** see under *nevus.* **hydatid m., hydatidiform m.,** a condition resulting from deterioration of circulation of the chorionic villi in a pathologic ovum, marked by trophoblastic proliferation and by edematous dissolution and cystic cavitation of the avascular stroma of the villi, which come to resemble grapelike cysts. **pigmented m.,** see under *nevus.*

molecular (mo-lek′u-lar) of, pertaining to, or composed of molecules.

molecule (mol′ĕ-kūl) a very small mass of matter; the smallest amount of a substance which can exist alone; an aggregation of atoms, specifically a chemical combination of two or more atoms which form a specific chemical substance.

molimen (mo-li′men), pl. *molim′ina* [L.] a laborious effort made for the performance of any normal body function, especially that manifested by a variety of unpleasant symptoms preceding or accompanying menstruation.

mollities (mo-lish′e-ēz) [L.] softness; abnormal softening. **m. os′sium,** osteomalacia.

molluscum (mŏ-lus′kum) 1. any of various skin diseases marked by the formation of soft rounded cutaneous tumors. 2. m. contagiosum. **mollus′cous,** adj. **m. contagio′sum,** a viral skin disease, with firm, round, translucent, crateriform papules containing caseous matter and peculiar capsulated bodies.

molt (mōlt) to shed skin, cuticle, or feathers.

mol. wt. molecular weight.

molybdate (mo-lib′dāt) any salt of molybdic acid.

molybdenum (mo-lib′dĕ-num) chemical element (*see table*), at. no. 42, symbol Mo.

monad (mo′nad) 1. a single-celled protozoon or coccus. 2. a univalent radical or element. 3. in meiosis, one member of a tetrad.

monarthric (mon-ar′thrik) pertaining to a single joint.

monarthritis (mon″ar-thri′tis) inflammation of a single joint.

monarticular (-tik′u-ler) pertaining to a single joint.

monaster (mon-as′ter) the single star-shaped figure at the end of prophase in mitosis.

monathetosis (-ath″ĕ-to′sis) athetosis of one limb.

monatomic (mon″ah-tom′ik) 1. univalent. 2. monobasic. 3. containing one atom.

monecious (mon-e′shus) monoecious.

monesthetic (mon″es-thet′ik) pertaining to or affecting a single sense or sensation.

mongolism (mon′go-lizm) Down's syndrome.

monilethrix (mo-nil′ĕ-thriks) a hereditary condition in which the hairs exhibit marked multiple constrictions, giving a beading effect, and are very brittle.

Monilia (mo-nil′e-ah) *Candida.*

monilial (mo-nil′e-al) pertaining to or caused by *Monilia (Candida).*

moniliasis (mo″nĭ-li′ah-sis) candidiasis.

moniliform (mo-nil′ĭ-form) beaded.

Moniliformis (mo-nil″ĭ-for′mis) a genus of acanthocephalan worms. *M. monilifor′mis,* a parasite of rodents, is an occasional facultative parasite of man.

moniliid (mo-nil′e-id) candidid.

monitor (mon′ĭ-tor) 1. to check constantly on a given condition or phenomenon, e.g., blood pressure or heart or respiratory rate. 2. an apparatus by which such conditions can be constantly observed or recorded.

mono- word element [Gr.] *one; single; limited to one part; combined with one atom.*

monoamide (mon″o-am′īd) an amide compound with only one amide group.

monoamine (-am′ēn) an amine containing only one amino group.

monobasic (-ba′sik) having but one atom of replaceable hydrogen.

monobenzone (-ben′zōn) a depigmenting agent, $C_{13}H_{12}O_2$.

monoblast (mon′o-blast) the cell which is the precursor of the mature monocyte.

monoblepsia (mon″o-blep′se-ah) 1. a condition in which vision is better when only one eye is used. 2. blindness to all colors but one.

monobrachius (-bra′ke-us) an individual with but one arm.

monocephalus (-sef′ah-lus) a monster with one head but with some duplication of its other parts.

monochorea (-ko-re′ah) chorea affecting but a simple part of the body.

monochorionic (-ko″re-on′ik) having a common chorion; said of identical twins.

monochromatic (-kro-mat′ik) 1. existing in or having only one color. 2. pertaining to or characterized by perception of a single color band in the spectrum. 3. staining with only one dye at a time.

monochromatophil (-kro-mat′o-fil) 1. stainable with only one kind of stain. 2. any cell or other element taking only one stain.

monoclonal (-klōn′al) derived from a single cell; pertaining to a single clone.

monocular (mon-ok′u-lar) 1. pertaining to or having but one eye. 2. having but one eyepiece, as in a microscope.

monoculus (-ok′u-lus) 1. a bandage for one eye. 2. a cyclops.

monocyte (mon′o-sīt) a mononuclear, phagocytic leukocyte, 13μ to 25μ in diameter, having an ovoid or kidney-shaped nucleus, containing chromatin, and an abundant cytoplasm filled with fine reddish and azurophilic granules. **monocyt′ic**, adj.

monocytopenia (mon″o-si″to-pe′ne-ah) deficiency of monocytes in the blood.

monocytosis (-si-to′sis) excess of monocytes in the blood.

monodactyly (-dak′tĭ-le) the presence of only one finger or toe on a hand or foot.

monodermoma (-der-mo′mah) a tumor developed from one germinal layer.

monodiplopia (-dĭ-plo′pe-ah) double vision in one eye.

Monodral (mon′o-dral) trademark for a preparation of penthienate.

monoecious (mon-e′shus) having reproductive organs typical of both sexes in a single individual.

monoethanolamine (mon″o-eth″ah-nōl′ah-mēn) a moderately viscous liquid, C_2H_7NO, used as a surfactant.

monogerminal (-jer′mĭ-nal) developed from one ovum; said of identical twins.

monoiodotyrosine (-i-o″do-ti′ro-sēn) an iodinated amino acid intermediate in the synthesis of thyroxine and triiodothyronine.

monolayer (-la′er) pertaining to or consisting of a single layer of molecules.

monolocular (-lok′u-lar) having but one cavity or compartment, as a cyst.

monomania (-ma′ne-ah) psychosis on a single subject or class of subjects.

monomelic (-mel′ik) affecting one limb.

monomer (mon′o-mer) a simple molecule of relatively low molecular weight, capable of reacting to form by repetition a dimer, trimer, or polymer.

monomeric (mon″o-mer′ik) 1. pertaining to a single segment. 2. in genetics, determined by a gene or genes at a single locus. 3. consisting of monomers.

monomolecular (-mo-lek′u-lar) pertaining to a single molecule or to a layer one molecule thick.

monomorphic (-mor′fik) existing in only one form; maintaining the same form throughout all developmental stages.

monomphalus (mon-om′fah-lus) a double monster joined at the navel.

monomyoplegia (mon″o-mi″o-ple′je-ah) paralysis of a single muscle.

monomyositis (-mi″o-si′tis) inflammation of a single muscle.

mononeural (-nu′ral) supplied by a single nerve.

mononeuritis (-nu-ri′tis) inflammation of a single nerve. **m. mul′tiplex,** simultaneous inflammation of individual peripheral nerves at sites remote from one another.

mononeuropathy (-nu-rop′ah-the) disease affecting a single nerve.

mononuclear (-nu′kle-ar) having but one nucleus.

mononucleosis (-nu″kle-o′sis) excess of mononuclear leukocytes (monocytes) in the blood. **infectious m.,** an acute infectious disease associated with the Epstein-Barr virus; symptoms include fever, malaise, sore throat, lymphadenopathy, atypical lymphocytes (resembling monocytes) in the peripheral blood, and high titers of agglutinins against sheep cells.

mononucleotide (-nu′kle-o-tīd″) nucleotide. **flavin m. (FMN),** a derivative of riboflavin that serves as a coenzyme for a number of oxidative enzymes.

monoparesis (-pah-re′sis) paresis of a single part.

monoparesthesia (-par″es-the′ze-ah) paresthesia of a single part.

monopathy (mo-nop′ah-the) a disease affecting a single part.

monophasia (mon″o-fa′ze-ah) aphasia with ability to utter but one word or phrase. **monopha′sic,** adj.

monophthalmus (mon″of-thal′mus) cyclops.

monophyletic (mon″o-fi-let′ik) descended from a common ancestor or stem cell.

monoplegia (-ple′je-ah) paralysis of a single part. **monople′gic,** adj.

monops (mon′ops) a cyclops.

monopus (mon′o-pus) an individual with congenital absence of a foot or leg.

monorchid (mon-or′kid) a person with monorchidism.

monorchidism, monorchism (mon-or′kid-izm; mon′or-kizm) the condition of having only one testis or one descended testis.

monosaccharide (mon″o-sak′ah-rīd) a simple sugar; a carbohydrate that cannot be decomposed by hydrolysis.

monosomy (-so′me) existence in a cell of only one instead of the normal diploid pair of a particular chromosome. **monoso′mic,** adj.

monospasm (mon′o-spazm) spasm of a single limb or part.

Monosporium (mon″o-spo′re-um) a genus of fungi, including *M. apiosper′mum,* a cause of maduromycosis.

monostotic (mon″os-tot′ik) pertaining to or affecting a single bone.

monostratal (mon″o-stra′tal) pertaining to a single layer or stratum.

monosymptomatic (-simp″to-mat′ik) manifested by only one symptom.

monosynaptic (-sĭ-nap′tik) pertaining to or passing through a single synapse.

Monotheamin (-the′ah-min) trademark for preparations of theophylline ethanolamine.

monothermia (-ther′me-ah) maintenance of the same body temperature throughout the day.

monotocous (mo-not′o-kus) giving birth to but one offspring at a time.

monotrichous (mon-ot′rĭ-kus) having a single polar flagellum.

monovalent (mon″o-va′lent) 1. having a valency of one. 2. capable of combining with only one antigenic specificity or with only one antibody specificity.

monoxenic (-zen′ik) associated with a single known species of microorganisms; said of otherwise germ-free animals.

monoxenous (mo-nok′sĕ-nus) requiring only one host to complete the life cycle.

monoxide (mon-ok′sīd) an oxide with one oxygen atom in the molecule.

monozygotic (mon″o-zi-got′ik) derived from a single zygote (fertilized ovum); said of twins.

mons (mons), pl. *mon′tes* [L.] a prominence. **m. pu′bis, m. ven′eris,** the rounded fleshy prominence over the symphysis pubis in the female.

monster (mon′ster) a fetus or infant with such pronounced developmental anomalies as to be grotesque and usually nonviable. **autositic m.,** one capable of independent life, the circulation of which supplies nutrition to its parasitic partner. **compound m.,** one showing some duplication of parts. **double m.,** one arising from a single ovum but with duplication or doubling of head, trunk, or limbs. **parasitic m.,** an imperfect fetus unable to exist alone and attached to an autositic partner. **triplet m.,** one with triplication of body parts. **twin m.,** double m.

monstrosity (mon-stros′ĭ-te) 1. great congenital deformity. 2. a monster or teratism.

monticulus (mon-tik′u-lus), pl. *montic′uli* [L.] a small eminence. **m. cerebel′li,** the projecting or superior part of the vermis.

mood (mōōd) the emotional state of an individual.

morantel (mo-ran′tel) an anthelmintic, $C_{12}H_{16}N_2S$; used as the tartrate salt.

Moraxella (mo-rak-sel′ah) a genus of bacteria found as parasites and pathogens in warm-blooded animals. **M. lacuna′ta,** *Hemophilus duplex.*

morbid (mor′bid) 1. pertaining to, affected with, or inducing disease; diseased. 2. unhealthy or unwholesome.

morbidity (mor-bid′ĭ-te) 1. the condition of being diseased or morbid. 2. the sick rate; the ratio of sick to well persons in a community.

morbific (mor-bif′ik) causing or inducing disease.

morbilli (mor-bil′i) [L.] measles.

morbilliform (mor-bil′ĭ-form) measles-like; resembling the eruption of measles.

morbus (mor′bus) [L.] disease. **m. cadu′cus,** epilepsy. **m. caeru′leus,** severe cyanosis, resulting from congenital malformation of the heart. **m. coxa′rius,** hip-joint disease. **m. maculo′sus werlho′fii, m. werlho′fii,** idiopathic thrombocytopenic purpura.

morcellation (mor″sĕ-la′shun) division of a tumor or organ, with piecemeal removal.

mordant (mor′dant) 1. a substance capable of intensifying or deepening the reaction of a specimen to a stain. 2. to subject to the action of a mordant before staining.

morgue (morg) a place where dead bodies may be kept for identification or until claimed for burial.

moria (mo′re-ah) dementia or fatuity; in psychiatry, a morbid tendency to joke.

moribund (mor′ĭ-bund) in a dying state.

Mornidine (mor′nĭ-dēn) trademark for preparations of pipamazine.

moron (mo′ron) a person exhibiting moronity.

moronity (mo-ron′ĭ-te) former category of mental retardation comprising persons with an I.Q. of 50–69.

morphea (mor-fe′ah) a condition in which there is connective tissue replacement of the skin and sometimes the subcutaneous tissues, with formation of firm ivory white or pinkish patches, bands, or lines.

morphine (mor′fēn) the principal and most active alkaloid of opium, $C_{17}H_{19}NO_3$; its hydrochloride and sulfate salts are used as narcotic analgesics.

morphinism (mor′fĭ-nizm) morbid state due to habitual misuse of morphine.

morphogenesis (mor″fo-jen′ĕ-sis) the evolution and development of form, as the development of the shape of a particular organ or part of the body, or the development undergone by individuals who attain the type to which the majority of the individuals of the species approximate. **morphogenet′ic,** adj.

morphology (mor-fol′o-je) the science of organic forms and structure. **morpholog′ic,** adj.

morphometry (mor-fom′ĕ-tre) the measurement of the forms of organisms.

morphosis (mor-fo′sis) the process of formation of a part or organ. **morphot′ic,** adj.

-morphous word element [Gr.], *shape; form.*

mors (mōrs) [L.] death.

morsus (mor′sus) [L.] bite. **m. diab′oli,** the fimbriae at the ovarian end of an oviduct.

mortal (mor′tal) 1. destined to die. 2. causing or terminating in death; fatal.

mortality (mor-tal′ĭ-te) 1. the quality of being mortal. 2. see *death rate.* 3. the ratio of actual deaths to expected deaths.

mortar (mor′tar) a bell- or urn-shaped vessel in which drugs are beaten, crushed, or ground with a pestle.

mortification (mor″tĭ-fĭ-ka′shun) gangrene.

morula (mor′u-lah) the solid mass of cells formed by cleavage of a fertilized ovum.

morulation (mor″u-la′shun) formulation of a morula.

mosaic (mo-za′ik) a pattern made of numerous small pieces fitted together; in genetics, an individual exhibiting mosaicism.

mosaicism (mo-za′ĭ-sizm) in genetics, the presence in an individual of two or more cell lines that are karyotypically or genotypically distinct and are derived from a single zygote.

mosquito (mos-ke′to) a bloodsucking and venomous insect of the family Culicidae, including the genera *Aedes, Anopheles, Culex,* and *Mansonia.*

motility (mo-til′ĭ-te) the ability to move spontaneously. **mo′tile,** adj.

motoneuron (mo″to-nu′ron) motor neuron; a neuron having a motor function; an efferent neuron conveying motor impulses. **lower m′s,** peripheral neurons whose cell bodies lie in the ventral gray columns of the spinal cord and whose terminations are in skeletal muscles. **peripheral m′s,** neurons in a peripheral reflex arc that receive impulses from interneurons and transmit them to voluntary muscles. **upper m′s,** neurons in the cerebral cortex that conduct impulses from the motor cortex to the motor nuclei of the cerebral nerves or to the ventral gray columns of the spinal cord.

motor (mo′tor) 1. a muscle, nerve, or center that effects or produces motion. 2. producing or subserving motion.

mottling (mot′ling) discoloration in irregular areas.

moulage (moo-lahzh′) [Fr.] the making of molds or models in wax or plaster; also, a mold or model so produced.

mounding (mownd′ing) the rising in a lump of a wasting muscle when struck.

mount (mownt) to prepare specimens and slides for study.

mouse (mows) 1. a small rodent, various species of which are used in laboratory experiments. 2. a small weight or movable structure. **joint m.,** a movable fragment of cartilage or other body within a joint. **peritoneal m.,** a free body in the peritoneal cavity, probably a small detached mass of omentum, sometimes visible radiographically.

mouth (mowth) an opening, especially the anterior opening of the alimentary canal, the cavity containing the tongue and teeth. **trench m.,** necrotizing ulcerative gingivitis.

mouthwash (mowth′wawsh) a solution for rinsing the mouth, e.g., a preparation of potassium bicarbonate, sodium borate, thymol, eucalyptol, methyl salicylate, amaranth solution, alcohol, glycerin, and purified water.

movement (moov′ment) 1. an act of moving; motion. 2. an act of defecation. **ameboid m.,** movement like that of an ameba, accomplished by protrusion of cytoplasm of the cell. **angular m.,** movement which changes the angle between two bones. **associated m.,** movement of parts which act together, as the eyes. **brownian m.,** the dancing motion of minute particles suspended in a liquid, due to thermal agitation. **forced m.,** a movement caused by injury to a motor center or conducting path. **index m.,** a movement of the cephalic part of the body about the fixed caudal part. **molecular m.,** brownian m. **passive m.,** an body movement effected by a force entirely outside of the organism. **vermicular m′s,** the wormlike movements of the intestines in peristalsis.

moxa (mok′sah) a tuft of soft, combustible substance to be burned upon the skin as a cautery.

moxibustion (mok″sĭ-bus′chun) cauterization by the burning of a moxa.

M.P.D. maximum permissible dose.

M.P.H. Master of Public Health.

M.Phys.A Member of the Physiotherapists′ Association (Brit.).

mR milliroentgen.

M.R.C. Medical Reserve Corps.

M.R.C.P. Member of Royal College of Physicians.

M.R.C.S. Member of Royal College of Surgeons.

M.R.L. Medical Record Librarian.

mRNA messenger RNA.

MS multiple sclerosis.

M.S. Master of Science; Master of Surgery.

MSH melanocyte-stimulating hormone.

M.T. Medical Technologist.

m.u. mouse unit.

muciferous (mu-sif′er-us) secreting mucus.

muciform (mu′sĭ-form) resembling mucus.

mucigen (mu′sĭ-jen) the substance from which mucin is derived.

mucilage (mu′sĭ-lij) an aqueous solution of a gummy substance, used as a vehicle or demulcent. **mucilag′inous,** adj. **acacia m.,** a preparation of acacia and benzoic acid in purified water; used as a suspending agent for drugs. **tragacanth m.,** a preparation of tragacanth, benzoic acid, glycerin, and purified water; used as a protective.

mucilaginous (mu″sĭ-laj′ĭ-nus) of the nature of mucilage.

mucin (mu′sin) a mucopolysaccharide or glycoprotein, the chief constituent of mucus.

mucinase (mu′sĭ-nās) an enzyme which acts upon mucin.

mucinogen (mu-sin′o-jen) a precursor of mucin.

mucinoid (mu′sĭ-noid) 1. resembing mucin. 2. mucoid (2).

mucinosis (mu″si-no′sis) a state with abnormal deposits of mucins in the skin. **follicular m.,** a disease of unknown cause, characterized by plaques of folliculopapules and usually alopecia.

mucinous (mu′sĭ-nus) resembling, or marked by formation of, mucin.

muciparous (mu-sip′ah-rus) secreting mucin.

mucocele (mu′ko-sēl) 1. dilatation of a cavity with mucous secretion. 2. a mucous polyp.

mucocutaneous (mu″ko-ku-ta′ne-us) pertaining to mucous membrane and skin.

mucoenteritis (-en″tĕ-ri′tis) mucous colitis.

mucoglobulin (-glob′u-lin) one of the class of glycoproteins.

mucoid (mu′koid) 1. mucinoid. 2. any of a group of mucus-like conjugated proteins of animal origin, differing from mucin in solubility.

mucolytic (mu″ko-lit′ik) destroying or dissolving mucus.

mucomembranous (-mem′brah-nus) pertaining to mucous membrane.

mucoperiosteum (-per″ĭ-os′te-um) periosteum having a mucous surface. **mucoperios′teal,** adj.

mucopolysaccharide (-pol″ĭ-sak′ah-rīd) a group of polysaccharides which contain hexosamine, which may or may not be combined with protein, and which, dispersed in water, form many of the mucins.

mucopolysaccharidosis (-pol″ĭ-sak″ah-rĭ-do′sis) any of a group of genetically determined disorders due to a defect in mucopolysaccharide metabolism, marked by skeletal changes, mental retardation, visceral involvement, corneal clouding, with widespread tissue deposits and mucopolysacchariduria.

mucopolysacchariduria (-pol″ĭ-sak″ah-rĭ-du′re-ah) an excess of mucopolysaccharides in the urine.

mucoprotein (-pro′te-in) a compound present in all connective and supporting tissues, containing mucopolysaccharides as prosthetic groups; they are relatively resistant to denaturation.

mucopurulent (-pu′roo-lent) containing both mucus and pus.

mucopus (mu′ko-pus) mucus blended with pus.

Mucor (mu′kor) a genus of fungi, some species of which cause mucormycosis.

Mucorales (mu″kor-a′lēz) an order of fungi, including bread molds and related fungi, most of which are saprophytic.

mucormycosis (-mi-ko′sis) mycosis due to fungi of the order Mucorales, including species of *Absidia, Mucor,* and *Rhizopus,* usually occurring in debilitated patients, often beginning in the upper respiratory tract or lungs, from which mycelial growths metastasize to other organs.

mucosa (mu-ko′sah), pl. *muco′sae* [L.] mucous membrane. **muco′sal,** adj.

mucosanguineous (mu″ko-sang-gwin′e-us) composed of mucus and blood.

mucoserous (-se′rus) pertaining to or producing both mucus and serum.

mucosin (mu-ko′sin) a form of mucin found in tenacious mucus.

mucous (mu′kus) pertaining to or resembling mucus; secreting mucus.

mucoviscidosis (mu″ko-vis″ĭ-do′sis) cystic fibrosis of the pancreas.

mucus (mu′kus) the free slime of the mucous membranes, composed of secretion of the glands, various salts, desquamated cells, and leukocytes.

multangular (mul-tang′gu-lar) having many angles or corners.

multi- word element [L.], *many.*

multiarticular (mul″te-ar-tik′u-lar) pertaining to or affecting many joints.

multicapsular (mul″tĭ-kap′su-lar) having many capsules.

multicellular (-sel′u-lar) composed of many cells.

Multiceps (mul′tĭ-seps) a genus of tapeworms, including *M. mul′ticeps,* whose adult stage is parasitic in dogs and whose larval stage (*Coenurus cerebralis*) usually develops in the central nervous system of goats and sheep and occasionally in man.

multicuspidate (mul″tĭ-kus′pĭ-dāt) having numerous cusps.

multifid (mul′tĭ-fid) cleft into many parts.

multifocal (mul″tĭ-fo′kal) arising from or pertaining to many foci.

multiform (mul′tĭ-form) polymorphic.

multiglandular (mul″tĭ-glan′du-lar) affecting several glands; pluriglandular.

multigravida (-grav′ĭ-dah) a woman who is pregnant and has been pregnant at least twice before.

multi-infection (mul″te-in-fek′shun) infection with several kinds of pathogens.

multilobar (mul″tĭ-lo′bar) having numerous lobes.

multilobular (-lob′u-lar) having many lobules.

mutilocular (-lok′u-lar) having many loculi.

multinodular (-nod′u-lar) having many nodules.

multinucleate (-nu′kle-āt) having many nuclei.

multipara (mul-tip′ah-rah) a woman who has had two or more pregnancies resulting in viable fetuses whether or not the offspring were alive at birth. **multip′arous,** adj. **grand m.,** a woman who has had six or more pregnancies resulting in viable fetuses.

multiparity (mul″tĭ-par′ĭ-te) 1. the condition of being a multipara. 2. the production of several offspring in one gestation.

multipolar (-po′lar) having more than two poles or processes.

multisynaptic (-sĭ-nap′tik) polysynaptic.

multiterminal (-ter′mĭ-nal) having several sets of terminals so that several electrodes may be used.

multivalent (-va′lent) 1. having the power of combining with three or more univalent atoms. 2. active against several strains of an organism.

mummification (mum″ĭ-fĭ-ka′shun) the shriveling up of a tissue, as in dry gangrene, or of a dead, retained fetus.

mumps (mumps) an acute contagious myxovirus disease seen mainly in childhood, involving chiefly the salivary glands, most often the parotids, but other tissues, e.g., the meninges and testes (in postpubertal males) may be affected.

mural (mu′rel) pertaining to or occurring in the wall of a body cavity.

muramidase (mu-ram′ĭ-das) lysozyme.

Murel (mu′rel) trademark for preparations of valethamate bromide.

murexine (mu-rek′sin) a neurotoxin from the hypobranchial gland of the snail *Murex*.

murine (mu′rēn) pertaining to mice or rats.

murmur (mer′mer) an auscultatory sound, particularly a periodic sound of short duration of cardiac or vascular origin. **anemic m.,** a cardiac murmur heard in anemia. **aortic m.,** a sound generated by blood flowing through a diseased aorta or aortic valve. **apex m.,** one heard over the apex of the heart. **arterial m.,** a murmur over an artery, sometimes aneurysmal and sometimes constricted. **Austin Flint m.,** a presystolic murmur heard at the apex in aortic regurgitation. **blood m.,** one due to an abnormal, commonly anemic, condition of the blood. **cardiac m.,** a murmur of finite length generated by blood flow through the heart. **cardiopulmonary m.,** a sound generated within lung tissue and related to heart movement. **Carey-Coombs m.,** a rumbling mid-diastolic murmur occurring in the early stages of rheumatic fever. **continuous m.,** a humming murmur heard throughout systole and diastole. **crescendo m.,** one marked by progressively increasing loudness. **Cruveilhier-Baumgarten m.,** one heard at the abdominal wall over veins connecting the portal and caval systems. **diastolic m.,** one heard during diastole; due to mitral obstruction, or to aortic or pulmonary regurgitation. **Duroziez's m.,** a double murmur over the femoral or other large peripheral artery; due to aortic insufficiency. **ejection m.,** systolic murmurs heard predominantly in midsystole when ejection volume and velocity of blood flow are at their maximum. **Flint's m.,** Austin Flint m. **friction m.,** see *rub.* **functional m.,** a cardiac murmur generated within a structurally normal heart. **Gibson m.,** a long, rumbling sound occupying most of systole and diastole, usually localized in the second left interspace near the sternum, and usually indicative of patent ductus arteriosus. **Graham Steell's m.,** one due to pulmonary regurgitation in patients with pulmonary hypertension and mitral stenosis. **heart m.,** cardiac m. **hemic m.,** blood m. **innocent m.,** functional m. **machinery m.,** Gibson m. **mitral m.,** one due to diseased mitral valve. **musical m.,** a cardiac murmur having a periodic harmonic pattern. **organic m.,** one due to structural change in the heart, a vessel, or the lung. **pansystolic m.,** one heard throughout systole. **pericardial m.,** see under *rub.* **prediastolic m.,** one occurring just before and with diastole; due to mitral obstruction, or to aortic or pulmonary regurgitation. **presystolic m.,** one shortly before the onset of ventricular ejection, usually associated with a narrowed atrial ventricular valve. **pulmonic m.,** one due to disease of the valves of the pulmonary artery. **regurgitant m.,** one due to regurgitation of blood through a diseased valvu-

lar orifice. **seagull m.,** a raucous murmur with musical qualities heard occasionally in aortic insufficiency. **Still's m.,** a functional cardiac murmur of childhood, heard in midsystole. **systolic m.,** one heard during systole; usually due to mitral or tricuspid regurgitation, or to aortic or pulmonary obstruction. **tricuspid m.,** one caused by disease of the tricuspid valve. **vascular m.,** one heard over a blood vessel. **vesicular m.,** the normal breath sounds heard over the lungs.

murrina (moo-re′nah) trypanosomiasis of mules and horses in Panama.

Musca (mus′kah) a genus of flies, including the common housefly, *M. domes′tica*, which may serve as a mechanical vector of various pathogens; its larvae may cause myiasis.

musca (mus′kah), plural *mus′cae* [L.] a fly. **mus′cae volitan′tes,** specks seen as floating before the eyes.

muscarine (-rin) a deadly alkaloid from various mushrooms, e.g., *Amanita muscaria* (the fly agaric), and also from rotten fish.

muscle (mus′el) a organ which by contraction produces movement of an animal organism; see *Table of Muscles,* and see Plates I and XIV. **agonistic m.,** one opposed in action by another muscle (the antagonist). **antagonistic m.,** one that counteracts the action of another muscle (agonist). **antigravity m's,** those that by their tone resist the constant pull of gravity in the maintenance of normal posture. **appendicular m's,** the muscles of a limb. **articular m.,** one that has one end attached to a joint capsule. **Bell's m.,** the muscular strands between the ureteric orifices and the uvula vesicae, bounding the trigone of the urinary bladder. **Brücke's m.,** the longitudinal fibers of the ciliary muscle. **cardiac m.,** the muscle of the heart, composed of striated muscle fibers. **cutaneous m.,** striated muscle that inserts into the skin. **extraocular m's,** the six voluntary muscles that move the eyeball: superior, inferior, middle, and lateral recti, and superior and inferior oblique muscles. **extrinsic m.,** one not originating in the limb or part in which it is inserted. **fixation m's, fixator m's,** accessory muscles that serve to steady a part. **fusiform m.,** a spindle-shaped muscle. **Gavard's m.,** the oblique muscular elements of the stomach wall. **Guthrie's m.,** sphincter muscle of the urethra. **hamstring m's,** the muscles of the back of the thigh: biceps femoris, semitendinous, and semimembranous muscles. **Horner's m.,** the lacrimal part of the orbicularis oculi muscle. **Houston's m.,** fibers of the bulbocavernosus muscle compressing the dorsal vein of the penis. **inspiratory m's,** those that act in inspiration. **intraocular m's,** the intrinsic muscles of the eyeball. **intrinsic m.,** one whose origin and insertion are in the same part or organ. **involuntary m.,** one that is not under the control of the will. **Landström's m.,** minute muscle fibers in the fascia around and behind the eyeball, attached in front to the anterior orbital fascia and eyelids. **Langer's m.,** muscular fibers from the insertion of the pectoralis major muscle over the bicipital groove to the insertion of the latissimus dorsi. **Müller's m.,** the circular fibers of the ciliary muscle. **nonstriated m.,** a muscle without transverse striations on its constituent fibers; such muscles are almost always involuntary. **orbicular m.,** one that encircles a body opening, e.g., the eye or mouth. **postaxial m.,** one on the dorsal side of a limb. **preaxial m.,** one on the ventral side of a limb. **red m.,** the darker-colored muscle tissue of some mammals, composed of fibers rich in sarcoplasm, but with only faint cross-striping. **Reisseisen's m's,** the smooth muscle fibers of the smallest bronchi. **rider's m's,** the adductor muscles of the thigh. **Ruysch's m.,** the muscular tissue of the fundus uteri. **skeletal m's,** striated muscles attached to bones, which cross at least one joint. **smooth m.,** nonstriated, involuntary muscle. **striated m., striped m.,** any muscle whose fibers are divided by transverse bands into striations; such muscles are voluntary. **synergistic m's,** those that assist one another in action. **thenar m's,** the abductor and flexor muscles of the thumb. **m. of Treitz,** suspensory muscle of duodenum. **unstriated m.,** nonstriated m. **vestigial m.,** one that was once well developed but through evolution has become rudimentary. **visceral m.,** muscle fibers associated chiefly with the hollow viscera. **voluntary m.,** any muscle that is normally under the control of the will. **white m.,** the paler muscle tissue of some mammals, composed of fibers with little sarcoplasm and prominent cross-striping. **yoked m's,** those that normally act simultaneously and equally, as in moving the eyes.

muscular (mus′ku-lar) 1. pertaining to or composing muscle. 2. having a well-developed musculature.

muscularis (mus″ku-la′ris) [L.] relating to muscle, specifically a muscular layer (lamina muscularis) or coat (tunica muscularis).

musculature (mus′ku-lah-tūr) the muscular apparatus of the body or of a part.

musculocutaneous (mus″ku-lo-ku-ta′ne-us) pertaining to or supplying muscle and skin.

musculomembranous (-mem′brah-nus) both muscular and membranous.

musculophrenic (-fren′ik) pertaining to or supplying the diaphragm and adjoining muscles.

musculoskeletal (-skel′ĕ-tal) pertaining to or comprising the skeleton and muscles.

musculotendinous (-ten′dĭ-nus) pertaining to or composed of muscle and tendon.

musculotropic (-trop′ik) having a special affinity for or exerting its principal effect on muscular tissue.

musculus (mus′ku-lus), pl. *mus′culi* [L.] muscle; see NA terms in *Table of Muscles.*

musicogenic (mu″zĭ-ko-jen′ik) induced by musical sounds.

musicotherapy (-ther′ah-pe) treatment of disease by music.

mustard (mus′tard) 1. a plant of the genus *Brassica.* 2. the ripe seeds of *Bassica alba* and *B. nigra,* whose oils have irritant and stimulant properties. **nitrogen m's,** a class of chemical compounds, some of which have been used as antineoplastics.

Mustargen (mus′tar-jen) trademark for a preparation of mechlorethamine.

mutacism (mu′tah-sizm) mytacism.

mutagen (mu′tah-jen) an agent which induces genetic mutation.

mutagenesis (mu″tah-jen′ĕ-sis) the induction of genetic mutation.

mutagenic (-jen′ik) inducing genetic mutation.

mutagenicity (-jĕ-nis′ĭ-te) the property of being able to induce genetic mutation.

mutant (mu′tant) 1. an organism who has undergone genetic mutation. 2. produced by mutation.

mutarotase (mu″tah-ro′tās) an enzyme that catalyzes the conversion of α-D- to β-D-glucose.

mutarotation (-ro-ta′shun) the change in optical rotation of an optically active compound in solution.

mutase (mu′tās) an enzyme that catalyzes intramolecular transfer of a group.

mutation (mu-ta′shun) a permanent transmissible change in the genetic material. Also, an individual exhibiting such change; a sport. **induced m.,** one caused by application of external factors. **point m.,** a mutation not accompanied by a morphologically demonstrable change in the chromosome. **somatic m.,** a genetic mutation occurring in a somatic cell, providing the basis for a mosaic condition.

mute (mūt) 1. unable to speak. 2. a person who is unable to speak.

mutilation (mu″tĭ-la′shun) the act of depriving an individual of a limb, member, or other important part. Also, the condition resulting therefrom.

mutism (mu′tizm) inability or refusal to speak. **akinetic m.,** a state in which the person makes no spontaneous movement or vocal sound.

muton (mu′ton) the smallest element of DNA whose alteration can give rise to a mutant organism.

mutualism (mu′tu-al-izm″) the biologic association of two individuals or populations of different species, both of which are benefited by the relationship and sometimes unable to exist without it.

mutualist (-ist) an organism or species living in a state of mutualism.

M.V. [L.] *Medicus Veterinarius* (veterinary physician).

Mv chemical symbol, *mendelevium.*

mv. millivolt.

μv. microvolt.

Mx Medex.

my(o)- word element [Gr.], *muscle.*

myalgia (mi-al′je-ah) muscular pain. **epidemic m.,** see under *pleurodynia.*

myasthenia (mi″as-the′ne-ah) muscular debility or weakness. **myasthen′ic,** adj. **angiosclerotic m.,** intermittent claudication. **m. gas′trica,** weakness and loss of tone in the muscular coats of the stomach; atony of the stomach. **m. gra′vis,** fatigue and exhaustion of the muscular system with progressive muscular paralysis but without sensory disturbance of atrophy,

TABLE OF MUSCLES

COMMON NAME*	NA TERM†	ORIGIN*	INSERTION*	INNERVATION	ACTION
abductor m. of great toe	m. abductor hallucis	medial tubercle of calcaneus, plantar fascia	medial side of base of proximal phalanx of great toe	medial plantar	abducts, flexes great toe
abductor m. of little finger	m. abductor digiti minimi manus	pisiform bone, tendon of ulnar flexor m. of wrist	medial side of base of proximal phalanx of little finger	ulnar	abducts little finger
abductor m. of little toe	m. abductor digiti minimi pedis	medial and lateral tubercle of calcaneus, plantar fascia	lateral side of base of proximal phalanx of little toe	lateral plantar	abducts little toe
abductor m. of thumb, long	m. abductor pollicis longus	posterior surfaces of radius and ulna	lateral side of base of first metacarpal bone and trapezium	posterior interosseous	abducts, extends thumb
abductor m. of thumb, short	m. abductor pollicis brevis	tubercles of scaphoid and trapezium, flexor retinaculum of hand	lateral side of base of proximal phalanx of thumb	median	abducts thumb
adductor m., great	m. adductor magnus	*deep part*—inferior ramus of pubis, ramus of ischium; *superficial part*—ischial tuberosity	*deep part*—linea aspera of femur; *superficial part*—adductor tubercle of femur	*deep part*—obturator; *superficial part*—sciatic	*deep part* — adducts thigh; *superficial part* —extends thigh
adductor m. of great toe	m. adductor hallucis	*oblique head*—long plantar ligament; *transverse head*—plantar ligaments	lateral side of base of proximal phalanx of great toe	lateral plantar	flexes, adducts great toe
adductor m., long	m. adductor longus	body of pubis	linea aspera of femur	obturator	adducts, rotates, flexes thigh
adductor m., short	m. adductor brevis	body and inferior ramus of pubis	upper part of linea aspera of femur	obturator	adducts, rotates, flexes thigh
adductor m. of thumb	m. adductor pollicis	*oblique head*—second metacarpal, capitate, and trapezoid; *transverse head*—front of third metacarpal	medial side of base of proximal phalanx of thumb	ulnar	adducts, opposes thumb
anconeus m.	m. anconeus	back of lateral epicondyle of humerus	olecranon and posterior surface of ulna	radial	extends forearm
antitragus m.	m. antitragicus	outer part of antitragus	caudate process of helix and anthelix	temporal, posterior auricular branches of facial	

*m. = muscle; m's = (pl.) muscles   † = musculus; mm. = (L. pl.) musculi

427

COMMON NAME*	NA TERM†	ORIGIN*	INSERTION*	INNERVATION	ACTION
arrector m's of hair	mm. arrectores pilorum	dermis	hair follicles	sympathetic	elevate hairs of skin
articular m. of elbow	m. articularis cubiti	a name applied to a few fibers of the deep surface of the triceps m. of arm that insert into the posterior ligament and synovial membrane of the elbow joint			
articular m. of knee	m. articularis genus	front of lower part of femur	upper part of capsule of knee joint	femoral	raises capsule of knee joint
aryepiglottic m.	m. aryepiglotticus	a name applied to inconstant fibers of oblique arytenoid m., from apex of arytenoid cartilage to lateral margin of epiglottis			
arytenoid m., oblique	m. arytenoideus obliquus	muscular process of arytenoid cartilage	apex of opposite arytenoid cartilage	recurrent laryngeal	closes inlet of larynx
arytenoid m., transverse	m. arytenoideus transversus	medial surface of arytenoid cartilage	medial surface of opposite arytenoid cartilage	recurrent laryngeal	approximates arytenoid cartilage
auricular m., anterior	m. auricularis anterior	superficial temporal fascia	cartilage of ear	facial	draws auricle forward
auricular m., posterior	m. auricularis posterior	mastoid process	cartilage of ear	facial	draws auricle backward
auricular m., superior	m. auricularis superior	galea aponeurotica	cartilage of ear	facial	raises auricle
biceps m. of arm	m. biceps brachii	*long head*—supraglenoid tubercle of scapula; *short head*—apex of coracoid process	tuberosity of radius, antebrachial fascia, ulna	musculocutaneous	flexes, supinates forearm
biceps m. of thigh	m. biceps femoris	*long head*—ischial tuberosity; *short head*—linea aspera of femur	head of fibula, lateral condyle of tibia	*long head* — tibial; *short head*—peroneal, popliteal	flexes, rotates leg laterally, extends thigh
brachial m.	m. brachialis	anterior aspect of humerus	coronoid process of ulna	musculocutaneous, radial	flexes forearm
brachioradial m.	m. brachioradialis	lateral supracondylar ridge of humerus	lateral surface of lower end of radius	radial	flexes forearm
bronchoesophageal m.	m. bronchoesophageus	a name applied to muscle fibers arising from wall of left bronchus, reinforcing musculature of esophagus			
buccinator m.	m. buccinator	buccinator ridge of mandible, alveolar processes of maxilla, pterygomandibular ligament	orbicular m. of mouth at angle of mouth	buccal branch of facial	compresses cheek and retracts angle of mouth

Common name	NA term	Origin	Insertion	Nerve	Action
bulbocavernous m.	m. bulbocavernosus, m. bulbospongiosus	tendinous center of perineum, median raphe of bulb	fascia of penis or clitoris	pudendal	constricts urethra in male, vagina in female
canine m. *See* levator m. of angle of mouth					
ceratocricoid m.	m. ceratocricoideus	a name applied to muscle fibers from cricoid cartilage to inferior horn of thyroid cartilage			
chin m.	m. mentalis	incisive fossa of mandible	skin of chin	facial	wrinkles skin of chin
chondroglossus m.	m. chondroglossus	lesser horn and body of hyoid bone	substance of tongue	hypoglossal	depresses, retracts tongue
ciliary m.	m. ciliaris	*longitudinal division* (Brücke's m's)—junction of cornea and sclera; *circular division* (Müller's m.)—sphincter of ciliary body	outer layers of choroid and ciliary processes	short ciliary	makes lens more convex in visual accommodation
coccygeus m.	m. coccygeus	ischial spine	lateral border of lower part of sacrum, coccyx	third and fourth sacral	supports and raises coccyx
constrictor m. of pharynx, inferior	m. constrictor pharyngis inferior	undersurfaces of cricoid and thyroid cartilages	median raphe of posterior wall of pharynx	glossopharyngeal, pharyngeal plexus, external branch of superior laryngeal and recurrent laryngeal	constricts pharynx
constrictor m. of pharynx, middle	m. constrictor pharyngis medius	horns of hyoid bone, stylohyoid ligament	median raphe of posterior wall of pharynx	pharyngeal plexus of vagus, glossopharyngeal	constricts pharynx
constrictor m. of pharynx, superior	m. constrictor pharyngis superior	pterygoid plate, pterygomandibular raphe, mylohyoid ridge of mandible, mucous membrane of floor of mouth	median raphe of posterior wall of pharynx	pharyngeal plexus of vagus	constricts pharynx
coracobrachial m.	m. coracobrachialis	coracoid process of scapula	medial surface of shaft of humerus	musculocutaneous	flexes, adducts arm
corrugator m., superciliary	m. corrugator supercilii	medial end of superciliary arch	skin of eyebrow	facial	draws eyebrow downward and medially
cremaster m.	m. cremaster	inferior margin of internal oblique m. of abdomen	pubic tubercle	genital branch of genitofemoral	elevates testis

TABLE OF MUSCLES (*Continued*)

COMMON NAME*	NA TERM†	ORIGIN*	INSERTION*	INNERVATION	ACTION
cricoarytenoid lateral m.,	m. cricoarytenoideus lateralis	lateral surface of cricoid cartilage	muscular process of arytenoid cartilage	recurrent laryngeal	approximates vocal folds
cricoarytenoid posterior m.,	m. cricoarytenoideus posterior	back of lamina of cricoid cartilage	muscular process of arytenoid cartilage	recurrent laryngeal	separates vocal folds
cricothyroid m.	m. cricothyroideus	front and side of cricoid cartilage	lamina and inferior horn of thyroid cartilage	external branch of superior laryngeal	tenses vocal folds
deltoid m.	m. deltoideus	clavicle, acromion, spine of scapula	deltoid tuberosity of humerus	axillary	abducts, flexes, or extends arm
depressor m. of angle of mouth	m. depressor anguli oris	lateral border of mandible	angle of mouth	facial	pulls down angle of mouth
depressor m. of lower lip	m. depressor labii inferioris	anterior surface of lower border of mandible	orbicular m. of mouth and skin of lower lip	facial	depresses lower lip
depressor m. of septum of nose	m. depressor septi nasi	incisive fossa of maxilla	ala and septum of nose	facial	constricts nostril and depresses ala
depressor m., superciliary	m. depressor supercilii	a name applied to a few fibers of orbital part of orbicular m. of eye that are inserted into the eyebrow, which they depress			
detrusor urinae. *See* pubovesical m.					
diaphragm	diaphragma	back of xiphoid process, inner surfaces of lower 6 costal cartilages and lower 4 ribs, medial and lateral arcuate ligaments, bodies of upper lumbar vertebrae	central tendon of diaphragm	phrenic	increases volume of thorax in inspiration
digastric m.	m. digastricus	*anterior belly*—digastric fossa on lower border of mandible near symphysis; *posterior belly*—mastoid notch of temporal bone	intermediate tendon on hyoid bone	*anterior belly*—mylohyoid branch of inferior alveolar; *posterior belly*—digastric branch of facial	elevates hyoid bone, lowers jaw
dilator m. of pupil	m. dilator pupillae	a name applied to fibers extending radially from sphincter of pupil to ciliary margin		sympathetic	dilates iris
epicranial m.	m. epicranius	a name applied to muscular covering of scalp, including occipitofrontal and temporoparietal m's and galea aponeurotica			

erector m. of spine	m. erector spinae	a name applied to fibers of more superficial of deep muscles of back, originating from sacrum, spines of lumbar and eleventh and twelfth thoracic vertebrae, and iliac crest, which split and insert as iliocostal, longissimus, and spinal m's			
extensor m. of fingers	m. extensor digitorum	lateral epicondyle of humerus	extensor expansion of 4 medial fingers	deep branch of radial	extends wrist joint and phalanges
extensor m. of great toe, long	m. extensor hallucis longus	front of fibula, interosseous membrane	base of distal phalanx of great toe	deep peroneal	extends great toe, dorsiflexes ankle joint
extensor m. of great toe, short	m. extensor hallucis brevis	a name applied to portion of short extensor m. of toes that goes to great toe			
extensor m. of index finger	m. extensor indicis	posterior surface of ulna, interosseous membrane	extensor expansion of index finger	posterior interosseous	extends index finger
extensor m. of little finger	m. extensor digiti minimi	lateral epicondyle of humerus	extensor aponeurosis of little finger	deep branch of radial	extends little finger
extensor m. of thumb, long	m. extensor pollicis longus	posterior surface of ulna and interosseous membrane	back of distal phalanx of thumb	posterior interosseous	extends, adducts thumb
extensor m. of thumb, short	m. extensor pollicis brevis	posterior surface of radius	back of proximal phalanx of thumb	posterior interosseous	extends thumb
extensor m. of toes, long	m. extensor digitorum longus	anterior surface of fibula, lateral condyle of tibia, interosseous membrane	extensor expansion of 4 lateral toes	deep peroneal	extends toes
extensor m. of toes, short	m. extensor digitorum brevis	upper surface of calcaneus	extensor tendons of first, second, third, fourth toes	deep peroneal	extends toes
extensor m. of wrist, radial, long	m. extensor carpi radialis longus	lateral supracondylar ridge of humerus	back of base of second metacarpal bone	radial	extends, abducts wrist joint
extensor m. of wrist, radial, short	m. extensor carpi radialis brevis	lateral epicondyle of humerus	back of bases of second and third metacarpal bones	radial or its deep branch	extends, abducts wrist joint
extensor m. of wrist, ulnar	m. extensor carpi ulnaris	*humeral head*—lateral epicondyle of humerus; *ulnar head*—posterior border of ulna	base of fifth metacarpal bone	deep branch of radial	extends, abducts wrist joint
fibular m. *See* peroneal m.					
flexor m. of fingers, deep	m. flexor digitorum profundus	shaft of ulna, coronoid process, interosseous membrane	bases of distal phalanges of 4 medial fingers	anterior interosseous, ulnar	flexes distal phalanges
flexor m. of fingers, superficial	m. flexor digitorum superficialis	*humeroulnar head*—medial epicondyle of humerus, coronoid process of ulna; *radial head*—anterior border of radius	sides of middle phalanges of 4 medial fingers	median	flexes middle phalanges

431

COMMON NAME*	NA TERM†	ORIGIN*	INSERTION*	INNERVATION	ACTION
flexor m. of great toe, long	m. flexor hallucis longus	posterior surface of fibula	base of distal phalanx of great toe	tibial	flexes great toe
flexor m. of great toe, short	m. flexor hallucis brevis	undersurface of cuboid, lateral cuneiform	both sides of base of proximal phalanx of great toe	medial plantar	flexes great toe
flexor m. of little finger, short	m. flexor digiti minimi brevis manus	hook of hamate bone, transverse carpal ligament	medial side of proximal phalanx of little finger	ulnar	flexes little finger
flexor m. of little toe, short	m. flexor digiti minimi brevis pedis	sheath of long peroneal	lateral surface of base of proximal phalanx of little toe	lateral plantar	flexes little toe
flexor m. of thumb, long	m. flexor pollicis longus	anterior surface of radius, medial epicondyle of humerus, coronoid process of ulna	base of distal phalanx of thumb	anterior interosseous	flexes thumb
flexor m. of thumb, short	m. flexor pollicis brevis	tubercle of trapezium, flexor retinaculum	lateral side of base of proximal phalanx of thumb	median, ulnar	flexes, adducts thumb
flexor m. of toes, long	m. flexor digitorum longus	posterior surface of shaft of tibia	distal phalanges of 4 lateral toes	tibial	flexes toes, extends foot
flexor m. of toes, short	m. flexor digitorum brevis	medial tuberosity of calcaneus, plantar fascia	middle phalanges of 4 lateral toes	medial plantar	flexes toes
flexor m. of wrist, radial	m. flexor carpi radialis	medial epicondyle of humerus	bases of second and third metacarpal bones	median	flexes, abducts wrist joint
flexor m. of wrist, ulnar	m. flexor carpi ulnaris	*humeral head* — medial epicondyle of humerus; *ulnar head*—olecranon and posterior border of ulna	pisiform bone, hook of hamate bone, base of fifth metacarpal bone	ulnar	flexes, adducts wrist joint
gastrocnemius m.	m. gastrocnemius	*medial head*—popliteal surface of femur, upper part of medial condyle, capsule of knee; *lateral head*—lateral condyle, capsule of knee	aponeurosis unites with tendon of soleus to form Achilles tendon	tibial	plantar flexes foot, flexes knee joint
gemellus m., inferior	m. gemellus inferior	tuberosity of ischium	internal obturator tendon	nerve to quadrate m. of thigh	rotates thigh laterally
gemellus m., superior	m. gemellus superior	spine of ischium	internal obturator tendon	nerve to internal obturator	rotates thigh laterally

Common name	Latin name	Origin	Insertion	Nerve	Action
genioglossus m.	m. genioglossus	superior genial tubercle	hyoid bone, undersurface of tongue	hypoglossal	protrudes, depresses tongue
geniohyoid m.	m. geniohyoideus	inferior genial tubercle	body of hyoid bone	a branch of first cervical nerve through hypoglossal	draws hyoid bone forward
glossopalatine m. *See* palatoglossus m.					
gluteus maximus m., (gluteal m., greatest)	m. gluteus maximus	dorsal aspect of ilium, dorsal surfaces of sacrum, coccyx, sacrotuberous ligament	iliotibial tract of fascia lata, gluteal tuberosity of femur	inferior gluteal	extends, abducts, rotates thigh laterally
gluteus medius m., (gluteal m., middle)	m. gluteus medius	dorsal aspect of ilium between anterior and posterior gluteal lines	greater trochanter of femur	superior gluteal	abducts, rotates thigh medially
gluteus minimus m., (gluteal m., least)	m. gluteus minimus	dorsal aspect of ilium between anterior and posterior gluteal lines	greater trochanter of femur	superior gluteal	abducts, rotates thigh medially
gracilis m.	m. gracilis	body and inferior ramus of pubis	medial surface of shaft of tibia	obturator	adducts thigh, flexes knee joint
m. of helix, greater	m. helicis major	spine of helix	anterior border of helix	auriculotemporal, posterior auricular	tenses skin of acoustic meatus
m. of helix, smaller	m. helicis minor	anterior rim of helix	concha	temporal, posterior auricular	
hyoglossus m.	m. hyoglossus	body and greater horn of hyoid bone	side of tongue	hypoglossal	depresses, retracts tongue
iliac m.	m. iliacus	iliac fossa, ala of sacrum	greater psoas tendon, lesser trochanter of femur	femoral	flexes thigh, trunk on limb
iliococcygeus m.	m. iliococcygeus	a name applied to posterior portion of levator ani m., including fibers originating as far forward as obturator canal, and inserting on side of coccyx and in anococcygeal ligaments			
iliocostal m.	m. iliocostalis	a name applied to lateral division of erector m. of spine			
iliocostal m. of loins	m. iliocostalis lumborum	iliac crest	angles of lower 6 or 7 ribs	thoracic and lumbar	extends lumbar spine
iliocostal m. of neck	m. iliocostalis cervicis	angles of third, fourth, fifth, and sixth ribs	transverse processes of lower fourth, fifth, and sixth cervical vertebrae	cervical	extends cervical spine
iliocostal m. of thorax	m. iliocostalis thoracis	upper borders of angles of 6 lower ribs	angles of upper ribs and transverse process of seventh cervical vertebra	thoracic	keeps thoracic spine erect
iliopsoas m.	m. iliopsoas	a name applied collectively to iliac and greater psoas m's			

TABLE OF MUSCLES (*Continued*)

COMMON NAME*	NA TERM†	ORIGIN*	INSERTION*	INNERVATION	ACTION
incisive m's of inferior lip	mm. incisivi labii inferioris	incisive fossae of mandible	angle of mouth	facial	make vestibule of mouth shallow
incisive m's of superior lip	m. incisivi labii superioris	incisive fossae of maxilla	angle of mouth	facial	make vestibule of mouth shallow
m. of incisure of helix	m. incisurae helicis	a name applied to inconstant slips of fibers continuing forward from m. of tragus to bridge notch of cartilaginous part of meatus			
infraspinous m.	m. infraspinatus	infraspinous fossa of scapula	greater tubercle of humerus	suprascapular	rotates arm laterally
intercostal m's	mm. intercostales	a name applied to the layer of muscle fibers separated from the internal intercostal m's by the intercostal nerves and vessels			
intercostal m's, external	mm. intercostales externi	inferior border of rib	superior border of rib below	intercostal	elevate ribs in inspiration
intercostal m's, internal	mm. intercostales interni	inferior border of rib and costal cartilage	superior border of rib and costal cartilage below	intercostal	act on ribs in expiration
interosseous m's of foot, dorsal	mm. interossei dorsales pedis	sides of adjacent metatarsal bones	base of proximal phalanges of second, third, and fourth toes	lateral plantar	flex, abduct toes
interosseous m's of hand, dorsal	mm. interossei dorsales manus	each by two heads from adjacent sides of metacarpal bones	extensor tendons of second, third, and fourth fingers	ulnar	abduct, flex proximal, extend middle and distal phalanges
interosseous m's, palmar	mm. interossei palmares	sides at first, second, fourth, and fifth metacarpal bones	extensor tendons of first, second, fourth, and fifth fingers	ulnar	adduct, flex proximal, extend middle and distal phalanges
interosseous m's, plantar	mm. interossei plantares	medial side of third, fourth, and fifth metatarsal bones	medial side of base of proximal phalanges of third, fourth, and fifth toes	lateral plantar	flex, abduct toes
interspinal m's	mm. interspinales	a name applied to short bands of muscle fibers extending on each side between spinous processes of contiguous vertebrae		spinal	extend vertebral column
intertransverse m's	mm. intertransversarii	a name applied to small muscles passing between transverse processes of adjacent vertebrae		spinal	bend vertebral column laterally
ischiocavernous m.	m. ischiocavernosus	ramus of ischium	crus of penis or clitoris	perineal	maintains erection of penis or clitoris

latissimus dorsi m.	m. latissimus dorsi	spines of lower thoracic vertebrae, spines of lumbar and sacral vertebrae through attachment to thoracolumbar fascia, iliac crest, lower ribs, inferior angle of scapula	floor of intertubercular groove of humerus	thoracodorsal	adducts, extends, rotates humerus medially
levator m. of angle of mouth	m., levator anguli oris	canine fossa of maxilla	orbicular m. of mouth, skin at angle of mouth	facial	raises angle of mouth
levator ani m.	m. levator ani	a name applied collectively to important muscular components of pelvic diaphragm, arising mainly from back of body of pubis and running backward toward coccyx; includes pubococcygeus (levator m. of prostate in male and pubovaginal in female), puborectal, and iliococcygeus m's		third and fourth sacral	helps support pelvic viscera and resist increases in intra-abdominal pressure
levator m. of palatine velum	m. levator veli palatini	apex of pars petrosa of temporal bone and cartilage of auditory tube	aponeurosis of soft palate	pharyngeal plexus	raises and draws back soft palate
levator m. of prostate	m. levator prostatae	a name applied to part of anterior portion of pubococcygeus m., which in male is inserted into prostate and tendinous center of perineum		sacral, pudendal	supports, compresses prostate, helps control micturition
levator m's of ribs	mm. levatores costarum	transverse processes of seventh cervical and first 11 thoracic vertebrae	medial to angle of rib below	intercostal	aid elevation of ribs in respiration
levator m. of scapula	m. levator scapulae	transverse processes of 4 upper cervical vertebrae	vertebral border of scapula	third and fourth cervical	raises scapula
levator m. of thyroid gland	m. levator glandulae thyroideae	isthmus or pyramidal lobule of thyroid gland	body of hyoid bone	external branch of superior laryngeal	
levator m. of upper eyelid	m. levator palpebrae superioris	sphenoid bone above optic foramen	skin and tarsal plate of upper eyelid	oculomotor	raises upper eyelid
levator m. of upper lip	m. levator labii superioris	lower margin of orbit	musculature of upper lip	facial	raises upper lip
levator m. of upper lip and ala of nose	m. levator labii superioris alaeque nasi	frontal process of maxilla	skin and cartilage of ala of nose, upper lip	infraorbital branch of facial	raises upper lip, dilates nostril
long m. of head	m. longus capitis	transverse processes of third to sixth cervical vertebrae	basilar portion of occipital bone	cervical	flexes head

COMMON NAME*	NA TERM†	ORIGIN*	INSERTION*	INNERVATION	ACTION
long m. of neck	m. longus colli	*superior oblique portion*—transverse processes of third to fifth cervical vertebrae; *inferior oblique portion*—bodies of first to third thoracic vertebrae; *vertical portion*—bodies of 3 upper thoracic and 3 lower cervical vertebrae	*superior oblique portion*—tubercle of anterior arch of atlas; *inferior oblique portion*—transverse processes of fifth and sixth cervical vertebrae; *vertical portion*—bodies of second to fourth cervical vertebrae	anterior cervical	flexes, supports cervical vertebrae
longissimus m. of head	m. longissimus capitis	transverse processes of 4 or 5 upper thoracic vertebrae, articular processes of 3 or 4 lower cervical vertebrae	mastoid process of temporal bone	cervical	draws head backward, rotates head
longissimus m. of neck	m. longissimus cervicis	transverse processes of 4 or 5 upper thoracic vertebrae	transverse processes of second or third to sixth cervical vertebrae	lower cervical and upper thoracic	extends cervical vertebrae
longissimus m. of thorax	m. longissimus thoracis	transverse and articular processes of lumbar vertebrae and thoracolumbar fascia	transverse processes of all thoracic vertebrae, 9 or 10 lower ribs	lumbar and thoracic	extends thoracic vertebrae
longitudinal m. of tongue, inferior	m. longitudinalis inferior linguae	undersurface of tongue at base	tip of tongue	hypoglossal	changes shape of tongue in mastication and deglutition
longitudinal m. of tongue, superior	m. longitudinalis superior linguae	submucosa and septum of tongue	margins of tongue	hypoglossal	changes shape of tongue in mastication and deglutition
lumbrical m's of foot	mm. lumbricales pedis	tendons of long flexor m. of toes	medial side of base of proximal phalanges of 4 lateral toes	medial and lateral plantar	flex metatarsophalangeal joints, extend distal phalanges
lumbrical m's of hand	mm. lumbricales manus	tendons of deep flexor m. of fingers	extensor tendons of 4 lateral fingers	median, ulnar	flex metacarpophalangeal joints, extend middle and distal phalanges

masseter m.	m. masseter	*superficial part*—zygomatic process of maxilla, lower border of zygomatic arch; *deep part*—lower border and medial surface of zygomatic arch	*superficial part*—angle and ramus of mandible; *deep part*—upper half of ramus and lateral surface of coronoid process of mandible	masseteric, from mandibular division of trigeminal	raises mandible, closes jaws
multifidus m's	mm. multifidi	sacrum, sacroiliac ligament, mamillary processes of lumbar, transverse processes of thoracic, and articular processes of cervical vertebrae	spines of contiguous vertebrae above	spinal	extend, rotate vertebral column
mylohyoid m.	m. mylohyoideus	mylohyoid line of mandible	body of hyoid bone, median raphe	mylohyoid branch of inferior alveolar	elevates hyoid bone, supports floor of mouth
nasal m.	m. nasalis	maxilla	*alar part*—ala of nose; *transverse part*—by aponeurotic expansion with fellow of opposite side	facial	*alar part*—aids in widening nostril; *transverse part*—depresses cartilage of nose
oblique m. of abdomen, external	m. obliquus externus abdominis	lower 8 ribs at costal cartilages	crest of ilium, linea alba through rectus sheath	lower thoracic	flexes, rotates vertebral column, compresses abdominal viscera
oblique m. of abdomen, internal	m. obliquus internus abdominis	thoracolumbar fascia, iliac crest, iliac fascia, inguinal fascia	lower 3 or 4 costal cartilages, linea alba, conjoined tendon to pubis	lower thoracic	flexes, rotates vertebral column, compresses abdominal viscera
oblique m. of auricle	m. obliquus auriculae	cranial surface of concha	cranial surface of auricle above concha	posterior auricular, temporal	
oblique m. of eyeball, inferior	m. obliquus inferior bulbi	orbital surface of maxilla	sclera	oculomotor	abducts, rotates eyeball upward and outward
oblique m. of eyeball, superior	m. obliquus superior bulbi	lesser wing of sphenoid above optic foramen	sclera	trochlear	abducts, rotates eyeball downward and outward
oblique m. of head, inferior	m. obliquus capitis inferior	spinous process of axis	transverse process of atlas	spinal	rotates atlas and head
oblique m. of head, superior	m. obliquus capitis superior	transverse process of atlas	occipital bone	spinal	extends and moves head laterally
obturator m., external	m. obturatorius externus	pubis, ischium, external surface of obturator membrane	trochanteric fossa of femur	obturator	rotates thigh laterally

TABLE OF MUSCLES *(Continued)*

COMMON NAME*	NA TERM†	ORIGIN*	INSERTION*	INNERVATION	ACTION
obturator m., internal	m. obturatorius internus	pelvic surface of hip bone and obturator membrane, margin of obturator foramen	greater trochanter of femur	fifth lumbar, first and second sacral	rotates thigh laterally
occipitofrontal m.	m. occipitofrontalis	*frontal belly*—galea aponeurotica; *occipital belly* —highest nuchal line of occipital bone	*frontal belly*—skin of eyebrow, root of nose; *occipital belly*—galea aponeurotica	*frontal belly*—temporal branch of facial; *occipital belly*—posterior auricular branch of facial	*frontal belly*—raises eyebrow; *occipital belly*—draws scalp backward
omohyoid m.	m. omohyoideus	superior border of scapula	body of hyoid bone	upper cervical through ansa cervicalis	depresses hyoid bone
opposing m. of little finger	m. opponens digiti minimi manus	hook of hamate bone	front of fifth metacarpal	eighth cervical through ulnar	abducts, flexes, rotates fifth metacarpal
opposing m. of thumb	m. opponens pollicis	tubercle of trapezium, flexor retinaculum	lateral side of first metacarpal	sixth and seventh metacarpal through median	flexes, opposes thumb
orbicular m. of eye	m. orbicularis oculi	*orbital part*—medial margin of orbit, including frontal process of maxilla; *palpebral part*—medial palpebral ligament; *lacrimal part*—posterior lacrimal crest	*orbital part*—near origin after encircling orbit; *palpebral part*—orbital tubercle of zygomatic bone; *lacrimal part*— lateral palpebral raphe	facial	closes eyelids, wrinkles forehead, compresses lacrimal sac
orbicular m. of mouth	m. orbicularis oris	a name applied to complicated sphincter muscle of mouth, comprising 2 parts: *labial part*—consisting of fibers restricted to lips; *marginal part*—consisting of fibers blending with those of adjacent muscles		facial	closes, protrudes lips
orbital m.	m. orbitalis	bridges inferior orbital fissure	fascia of inferior orbital fissure	sympathetic fibers	protrudes eye
palatoglossus m.	m. palatoglossus	undersurface of soft palate	side of tongue	pharyngeal plexus	elevates tongue, constricts fauces
palatopharyngeal m.	m. palatopharyngeus	posterior border of bony palate, palatine aponeurosis	posterior border of thyroid cartilage, side of pharynx and esophagus	pharyngeal plexus	constricts pharynx, aids swallowing
palmar m., long	m. palmaris longus	medial epicondyle of humerus	flexor retinaculum, palmar aponeurosis	median	tenses palmar aponeurosis
palmar m., short	m. palmaris brevis	palmar aponeurosis	skin of medial border of hand	ulnar	assists in deepening hollow of palm-

438

papillary m's	mm. papillares	a name applied to conical muscular projections from walls of cardiac ventricles, attached to cusps of atrioventricular valves by chordae tendineae		steady and strengthen atrioventricular valves and prevent eversion of their cusps
pectinate m's	mm. pectinati	a name applied to small ridges of muscular fibers projecting from inner walls of auricles of heart, and extending in right atrium from auricle to crista terminalis		
pectineal m.	m. pectineus	pectineal line of pubis	femoral, obturator	flexes, adducts thigh
pectoral m., greater	m. pectoralis major	clavicle, sternum, 6 upper costal cartilages, aponeurosis of external oblique m. of abdomen — crest of greater tubercle of humerus	lateral and medial pectoral	adducts, flexes, rotates arm medially
pectoral m., smaller	m. pectoralis minor	second, third, fourth, and fifth ribs — coracoid process of scapula	medial and lateral pectoral	draws shoulder forward and downward, raises third, fourth, and fifth ribs in forced inspiration
peroneal m., long	m. peroneus longus	lateral condyle of tibia, head of fibula, lateral surface of fibula — medial cuneiform, first metatarsal	superficial peroneal	plantar flexes, everts, abducts foot
peroneal m., short	m. peroneus brevis	lateral surface of fibula — tuberosity of fifth metatarsal bone	superficial peroneal	everts, abducts, plantar flexes foot
peroneal m., third	m. peroneus tertius	anterior surface of fibula, interosseous membrane — fascia or base of fifth (or fourth) metatarsal	deep peroneal	everts, dorsiflexes foot
piriform m.	m. piriformis	ilium, second to fourth sacral vertebrae — greater trochanter of femur	first and second sacral	rotates thigh laterally
plantar m.	m. plantaris	popliteal surface of femur — Achilles tendon or back of calcaneus	tibial	plantar flexes foot, flexes leg
platysma	platysma	a name applied to a platelike muscle originating from the fascia of cervical region and inserting on mandible, and skin around mouth	cervical branch of facial	wrinkles skin of neck, depresses jaw
pleuroesophageal m.	m. pleuroesophageus	a name applied to a bundle of smooth muscle fibers, usually connecting esophagus with left mediastinal pleura		
popliteal m.	m. popliteus	lateral condyle of femur, posterior surface of tibia, lateral meniscus	tibial	flexes leg, rotates leg medially
procerus m.	m. procerus	fascia over nasal bones — skin of forehead	facial	draws medial angle of eyebrows down

TABLE OF MUSCLES (*Continued*)

COMMON NAME*	NA TERM†	ORIGIN*	INSERTION*	INNERVATION	ACTION
pronator m., quadrate	m. pronator quadratus	anterior surface and border of distal third or fourth of shaft of ulna	anterior surface and border of distal fourth of shaft of radius	anterior interosseous	pronates forearm
pronator m., round	m. pronator teres	*humeral head*—medial epicondyle of humerus; *ulnar head*—coronoid process of ulna	lateral surface of radius	median	pronates and flexes forearm
psoas m., greater	m. psoas major	lumbar vertebrae	lesser trochanter of femur	second and third lumbar	flexes thigh or trunk
psoas m., smaller	m. psoas minor	last thoracic and first lumbar vertebrae	arcuate line of hip bone	first lumbar	assists greater psoas m.
pterygoid m., lateral (external)	m. pterygoideus lateralis	*upper head*—infratemporal surface of greater wing of sphenoid; *lower head*—lateral surface of lateral pterygoid plate	neck of mandible, capsule of temporomandibular joint	mandibular	protrudes mandible, opens jaws, moves mandible from side to side
pterygoid m., medial (internal)	m. pterygoideus medialis	medial surface of lateral pterygoid plate, tuber of maxilla	medial surface of ramus and angle of mandible	mandibular	closes jaw
pubococcygeus m.	m. pubococcygeus	a name applied to anterior portion of levator ani m., originating in front of obturator canal and inserting in anococcygeal ligament and side of coccyx		third and fourth sacral	helps support pelvic viscera and resist increases in intra-abdominal pressure
puboprostatic m.	m. puboprostaticus	a name applied to smooth muscle fibers contained within medial puboprostatic ligament, which pass from prostate anteriorly to pubis			
puborectal m.	m. puborectalis	a name applied to portion of levator ani m., with a more lateral origin from pubic bone, and continuous posteriorly with corresponding muscle of opposite side		third and fourth sacral	helps support pelvic viscera and resist increases in intra-abdominal pressure
pubovaginal m.	m. pubovaginalis	a name applied to part of anterior portion of pubococcygeus m., which is inserted into urethra and vagina		sacral and pudendal	helps control micturition
pubovesical m.	m. pubovesicalis	a name applied to smooth muscle fibers extending from neck of urinary bladder to pubis			
pyramidal m.	m. pyramidalis	body of pubis	linea alba	last thoracic	tenses abdominal wall
pyramidal m. of auricle	m. pyramidalis auriculae	a name applied to inconstant prolongation of fibers of m. of tragus to spine of helix			

Common name	Latin name	Origin	Insertion	Nerve	Action
quadrate m. of loins	m. quadratus lumborum	iliac crest, thoracolumbar fascia	twelfth rib, transverse processes of lumbar vertebrae	first and second lumbar, twelfth thoracic	flexes trunk laterally
quadrate m. of lower lip. See depressor m. of lower lip.					
quadrate m. of sole	m. quadratus plantae	calcaneus, plantar fascia	tendons of long flexor m. of toes	lateral plantar	aids in flexing toes
quadrate m. of thigh	m. quadratus femoris	tuberosity of ischium	intertrochanteric crest and quadrate tubercle of femur	fourth and fifth lumbar, first sacral	adducts, rotates thigh laterally
quadrate m. of upper lip. See levator m. of upper lip.					
quadriceps m. of thigh	m. quadriceps femoris	a name applied collectively to rectus m. of thigh and intermediate, lateral, and medial vastus m's, inserting by a common tendon that surrounds patella and ends on tuberosity of tibia		femoral	extends leg upon thigh
rectococcygeus m.	m. rectococcygeus	a name applied to smooth muscle fibers originating on anterior surface of second and third coccygeal vertebrae and inserting on posterior surface of rectum		autonomic	retracts, elevates rectum
rectourethral m.	m. rectourethralis	a name applied to band of smooth muscle fibers in male, extending from perineal flexure of rectum to membranous part of urethra			
rectouterine m.	m. rectouterinus	a name applied to band of fibers in female, running between cervix uteri and rectum, in rectouterine fold			
rectovesical m.	m. rectovesicalis	a name applied to band of fibers in male, connecting longitudinal musculature of rectum with external muscular coat of bladder			
rectus m. of abdomen	m. rectus abdominis	pubic crest and symphysis	xiphoid process, fifth, sixth, and seventh costal cartilages	lower thoracic	flexes lumbar vertebrae, supports abdomen
rectus m. of eyeball, inferior	m. rectus inferior bulbi	common tendinous ring	underside of sclera	oculomotor	adducts, rotates eyeball downward and medially
rectus m. of eyeball, lateral	m. rectus lateralis bulbi	common tendinous ring	lateral side of sclera	abducens	abducts eyeball
rectus m. of eyeball, medial	m. rectus medialis bulbi	common tendinous ring	medial side of sclera	oculomotor	adducts eyeball
rectus m. of eyeball, superior	m. rectus superior bulbi	common tendinous ring	upper side of sclera	oculomotor	adducts, rotates eyeball upward and medially

441

COMMON NAME*	NA TERM†	ORIGIN*	INSERTION*	INNERVATION	ACTION
rectus m. of head, anterior	m. rectus capitis anterior	lateral mass of atlas	basilar part of occipital bone	first and second cervical	flexes, supports head
rectus m. of head, lateral	m. rectus capitis lateralis	transverses process of atlas	jugular process of occipital bone	first and second cervical	flexes, supports head
rectus m. of head, posterior, greater	m. rectus capitis posterior major	spinous process of axis	occipital bone	suboccipital, greater occipital	extends head
rectus m. of head, posterior, smaller	m. rectus capitis posterior minor	posterior tubercle of atlas	occipital bone	suboccipital, greater occipital	extends head
rectus m. of thigh	m. rectus femoris	anterior inferior iliac spine, rim of acetabulum	base of patella, tuberosity of tibia	femoral	extends leg, flexes thigh
rhomboid m., greater	m. rhomboideus major	spinous processes of second, third, fourth, and fifth thoracic vertebrae	vertebral margin of scapula	dorsal scapular	retracts and fixes scapula
rhomboid m., smaller	m. rhomboideus minor	spinous processes of seventh cervical and first thoracic vertebrae, lower part of nuchal ligament	vertebral margin of scapula at root of spine	dorsal scapular	retracts and fixes scapula
risorius m.	m. risorius	fascia over masseter	skin at angle of mouth	buccal branch of facial	draws angle of mouth laterally
rotator m's	mm. rotatores	a name applied to a series of small muscles deep in groove between spinous and transverse processes of vertebrae		spinal	extend and rotate vertebral column toward opposite side
sacrococcygeal m., dorsal (posterior)	m. sacrococcygeus dorsalis	a name applied to muscular slip passing from dorsal surface of sacrum to coccyx			
sacrococcygeal m., ventral (anterior)	m. sacrococcygeus ventralis	a name applied to musculotendinous slip passing from lower sacral vertebrae to coccyx			
sacrospinal m. *See* erector m. of spine					
salpingopharyngeal m.	m. salpingopharyngeus	cartilage of auditory tube	posterior part of palatopharyngeus	pharyngeal plexus	raises pharynx
sartorius m.	m. sartorius	anterior superior iliac spine	upper part of medial surface of tibia	femoral	flexes thigh and leg
scalene m., anterior	m. scalenus anterior	transverse processes of third to sixth cervical vertebrae	scalene tubercle of first rib	second to seventh cervical	raises first rib, flexes cervical vertebrae laterally
scalene m., middle	m. scalenus medius	transverse processes of first to seventh cervical vertebrae	upper surface of first rib	second to seventh cervical	raises first rib, flexes cervical vertebrae laterally

scalene m. of pleura. *See* scalene m., smallest					
scalene m., posterior	m. scalenus posterior	transverse processes of fourth to sixth cervical vertebrae	second rib	second to seventh cervical	raises first and second ribs, flexes cervical vertebrae laterally
scalene m., smallest	m. scalenus minimus	a name applied to muscular band occasionally found between anterior and middle scalene m's			
semimembranous m.	m. semimembranosus	tuberosity of ischium	lateral condyle of femur, medial condyle and border of tibia	sciatic	flexes leg, extends thigh
semispinal m. of head	m. semispinalis capitis	transverse processes of upper thoracic and lower cervical vertebrae	occipital bone	suboccipital, greater occipital, branches of cervical	extends head
semispinal m. of neck	m. semispinalis cervicis	transverse processes of upper thoracic vertebrae	spinous processes of second to fifth (or fourth) cervical vertebrae	branches of cervical	extends, rotates vertebral column
semispinal m. of thorax	m. semispinalis thoracis	transverse processes of lower thoracic vertebrae	spinous processes of lower cervical and upper thoracic vertebrae	spinal	extends, rotates vertebral column
semitendinous m.	m. semitendinosus	tuberosity of ischium	upper part of medial surface of tibia	sciatic	flexes and rotates leg medially, extends thigh
serratus m., anterior	m. serratus anterior	8 upper ribs	vertebral border of scapula	long thoracic	draws scapula forward, rotates scapula to raise shoulder in abduction of arm
serratus m., posterior, inferior	m. serratus posterior inferior	spines of lower thoracic and upper lumbar vertebrae	4 lower ribs	ninth to twelfth (or eleventh) thoracic	lower ribs in expiration
serratus m., posterior, superior	m. serratus posterior superior	nuchal ligament, spinous processes of upper thoracic vertebrae	second, third, fourth, and fifth ribs	upper 4 thoracic	raises ribs in inspiration
soleus m.	m. soleus	fibula, tendinous arch, tibia	calcaneus by Achilles tendon	tibial	plantar flexes foot
sphincter m. of anus, external	m. sphincter ani externus	tip of coccyx, anococcygeal ligament	tendinous center of perineum	inferior rectal, perineal branch of fourth sacral	closes anus
sphincter m. of anus, internal	m. sphincter ani internus	a name applied to a thickening of circular layer of muscular tunic at caudal end of rectum			
sphincter m. of bile duct	m. sphincter ductus choledochi	a name applied to annular sheath of muscle fibers investing bile duct within wall of duodenum			

443

Table of Muscles (*Continued*)

COMMON NAME*	NA TERM†	ORIGIN*	INSERTION*	INNERVATION	ACTION
sphincter m. of hepatopancreatic ampulla	m. sphincter ampullae hepatopancreaticae	a name applied to annular band of muscle fibers investing hepatopancreatic ampulla			
sphincter m. of pupil	m. sphincter pupillae	a name applied to circular fibers of iris		parasympathetic through ciliary	constricts pupil
sphincter m. of pylorus	m. sphincter pylori	a name applied to a thickening of circular muscle of stomach around its opening into duodenum pylorus			
sphincter m. of urethra	m. sphincter urethrae	inferior ramus of pubis	median raphe behind and in front of urethra	perineal	compresses membranous urethra
sphincter m. of urinary bladder	m. sphincter vesicae urinariae	a name applied to circular layer of fibers surrounding internal urethral orifice		vesical	closes internal orifice of urethra
spinal m. of head	m. spinalis capitis	spinous processes of upper thoracic and lower cervical vertebrae	occipital bone	spinal	extends head
spinal m. of neck	m. spinalis cervicis	spinous process of seventh cervical vertebra, nuchal ligament	spinous processes of axis	branches of cervical	extends vertebral column
spinal m. of thorax	m. spinalis thoracis	spinous processes of upper lumbar and lower thoracic vertebrae	spinous processes of upper thoracic vertebrae	branches of spinal	extends vertebral column
splenius m. of head	m. splenius capitis	lower half of nuchal ligament, spinous processes of seventh cervical and upper thoracic vertebrae	mastoid part of temporal bone, occipital bone	cervical	extends, rotates head
splenius m. of neck	m. splenius cervicis	spinous process of upper thoracic vertebrae	transverse processes of upper cervical vertebrae	cervical	extends, rotates head and neck
stapedius m.	m. stapedius	interior of pyramidal eminence of tympanic cavity	neck of stapes	facial	dampens movement of stapes
sternal m.	m. sternalis	a name applied to muscular band occasionally found parallel to sternum on sternocostal head of greater pectoral m.			
sternocleidomastoid m.	m. sternocleidomastoideus	*sternal head*—manubrium; *clavicular head*—medial third of clavicle	mastoid process, superior nuchal line of occipital bone	accessory, cervical plexus	flexes vertebral column, rotates head to opposite side
sternocostal m. *See* transverse m. of thorax					

		Origin	Insertion	Nerve	Action
sternohyoid m.	m. sternohyoideus	manubrium sterni and/or clavicle	body of hyoid bone	ansa cervicalis	depresses hyoid bone and larynx
sternothyroid m.	m. sternothyroideus	manubrium sterni	lamina of thyroid cartilage	ansa cervicalis	depresses thyroid cartilage
styloglossus m.	m. styloglossus	styloid process	margin of tongue	hypoglossal	raises, retracts tongue
stylohyoid m.	m. stylohyoideus	styloid process	body of hyoid bone	facial	draws hyoid bone and tongue upward and backward
stylopharyngeus m.	m. stylopharyngeus	styloid process	thyroid cartilage, side of pharynx	glossopharyngeal, pharyngeal plexus	raises, dilates pharynx
subclavius m.	m. subclavius	first rib and its cartilage	lower surface of clavicle	nerve to subclavius	depresses lateral end of clavicle
subcostal m's	mm. subcostales	lower border of ribs	upper border of second or third rib below	intercostal	raise ribs in inspiration
subscapular m.	m. subscapularis	subscapular fossa of scapula	lesser tubercle of humerus	subscapular	rotates arm medially
supinator m.	m. supinator	lateral epicondyle of humerus, ligaments of elbow	radius	deep branch of radial	supinates forearm
supraspinous m.	m. supraspinatus	supraspinous fossa of scapula	greater tubercle of humerus	suprascapular	abducts arm
suspensory m.	m. suspensorius	a name applied to flat band of smooth muscle fibers originating from left crus of diaphragm and inserting continuous with muscular coat of duodenum at its junction with jejunum			
tarsal m., inferior	m. tarsalis inferior	inferior rectus m. of eyeball	tarsal plate of lower eyelid	sympathetic	widens palpebral fissure
tarsal m., superior	m. tarsalis superior	levator m. of upper eyelid	tarsal plate of upper eyelid	sympathetic	widens palpebral fissure
temporal m.	m. temporalis	temporal fossa and fascia	coronoid process of mandible	mandibular	closes jaws
temporoparietal m.	m. temporoparietalis	temporal fascia above ear	galea aponeurotica	temporal branches of facial	tightens scalp
tensor m. of fascia lata	m. tensor fasciae latae	iliac crest	iliotibial tract of fascia lata	superior gluteal	flexes, rotates thigh medially
tensor m. of palatine velum	m. tensor veli palatini	scaphoid fossa and spine of sphenoid	aponeurosis of soft palate, wall of auditory tube	mandibular	tenses soft palate, opens auditory tube
tensor m. of tympanum	m. tensor tympani	cartilaginous portion of auditory tube	handle of malleus	mandibular	tenses tympanic membrane
teres major m.	m. teres major	inferior angle of scapula	crest of lesser tubercle of humerus	lower subscapular	adducts, extends, and rotates arm medially

445

COMMON NAME*	NA TERM†	ORIGIN*	INSERTION*	INNERVATION	ACTION
teres minor m.	m. teres minor	lateral margin of scapula	greater tubercle of humerus	axillary	rotates arm laterally
thyroarytenoid m.	m. thyroarytenoideus	medial surface of lamina of thyroid cartilage	muscular process of arytenoid cartilage	recurrent laryngeal	relaxes, shortens vocal folds
thyroepiglottic m.	m. thyroepiglotticus	lamina of thyroid cartilage	epiglottis	recurrent laryngeal	closes inlet to larynx
thyrohyoid m.	m. thyrohyoideus	lamina of thyroid cartilage	greater horn of hyoid bone	ansa cervicalis	raises and changes form of larynx
tibial m., anterior	m. tibialis anterior	lateral condyle and surface of tibia, interosseous membrane	medial cuneiform, base of first metatarsal	deep peroneal	dorsiflexes, inverts foot
tibial m., posterior	m. tibialis posterior	tibia, fibula, interosseous membrane	bases of second to fourth metatarsal bones and tarsal bones, except talus	tibial	plantar flexes, inverts foot
tracheal m.	m. trachealis	a name applied to transverse smooth muscle fibers filling gap at back of each cartilage of trachea		autonomic	lessens caliber of trachea
m. of tragus	m. tragicus	a name applied to short, flattened vertical band on lateral surface of tragus, innervated by auriculotemporal and posterior auricular nerves			
transverse m. of abdomen	m. transversus abdominis	lower 6 costal cartilages, thoracolumbar fascia, iliac crest	linea alba through rectus sheath, conjoined tendon to pubis	lower thoracic	compresses abdominal viscera
transverse m. of auricle	m. transversus auriculae	cranial surface of auricle	circumference of auricle	posterior auricular branch of facial	retracts helix
transverse m. of chin	m. transversus menti	a name applied to superficial fibers of depressor m. of angle of mouth which turn medially and cross to opposite side			
transverse m. of nape	m. transversus nuchae	a name applied to small muscle often present, passing from occipital protuberance to posterior auricular m.; it may be either superficial or deep to trapezius			
transverse m. of perineum, deep	m. transversus perinei profundus	ramus of ischium	tendinous center of perineum	perineal	fixes tendinous center of perineum
transverse m. of perineum, superficial	m. transversus perinei superficialis	ramus of ischium	tendinous center of perineum	perineal	fixes tendinous center of perineum
transverse m. of thorax	m. transversus thoracis	posterior surface of body of sternum and of xiphoid process	second to sixth costal cartilages	intercostal	perhaps narrows chest
transverse m. of tongue	m. transversus linguae	median septum of tongue	dorsum and margins of tongue	hypoglossal	changes shape of tongue in mastication and swallowing

Common name	Latin name	Origin	Insertion	Nerve	Action
transversospinal m.	m. transversospinalis	a name applied collectively to semispinal, multifidus and rotator m's			
trapezius m.	m. trapezius	occipital bone, nuchal ligament, spinous processes of seventh cervical and all thoracic vertebrae	clavicle, acromion, spine of scapula	accessory, cervical plexus	elevates shoulder, rotates scapula to raise shoulder in abduction of arm, draws scapula backward
triangular m. *See* depressor m. of angle of mouth					
triceps m. of arm (triceps brachii m.)	m. triceps brachii	*long head*—infraglenoid tubercle of scapula; *lateral head*—posterior surface of humerus; *medial head*—posterior surface of humerus below groove for radial nerve	olecranon of ulna	radial	extends forearm; *long head* adducts, extends arm
triceps m. of calf (triceps surae m.)	m. triceps surae	a name applied collectively to gastrocnemius and soleus m's			
m. of uvula	m. uvulae	posterior nasal spine of palatine bone and aponeurosis of soft palate	uvula	pharyngeal plexus	raises uvula
vastus m., intermediate	m. vastus intermedius	anterior and lateral surfaces of femur	patella, common tendon of quadriceps m. of thigh	femoral	extends leg
vastus m., lateral	m. vastus lateralis	lateral aspect of femur	patella, common tendon of quadriceps m. of thigh	femoral	extends leg
vastus m., medial	m. vastus medialis	medial aspect of femur	patella, common tendon of quadriceps m. of thigh	femoral	extends leg
vertical m. of tongue	m. verticalis linguae	dorsal fascia of tongue	sides and base of tongue	hypoglossal	changes shape of tongue in mastication and deglutition
vocal m.	m. vocalis	angle between laminae of thyroid cartilage	vocal process of arytenoid cartilage	recurrent laryngeal	causes local variations in tension of vocal fold
zygomatic m., greater	m. zygomaticus major	zygomatic bone	angle of mouth	facial	draws angle of mouth upward and backward
zygomatic m., smaller	m. zygomaticus minor	zygomatic bone	orbicular m. of mouth, levator m. of upper lip	facial	draws upper lip upward and laterally

affecting any muscle, especially those of the face and throat.

myatonia (-ah-to'ne-ah) amyotonia. **m. congen'ita,** amyotonia congenita.

myatrophy (mi-at'ro-fe) atrophy of a muscle.

myc(o)- word element [Gr.], *fungus.*

mycelium (mi-se'le-um), pl. *myce'lia.* The mass of threadlike processes (hyphae) constituting the fungal thallus. **myce'lial,** adj.

mycete (mi'sēt) a fungus.

mycethemia (mi''sě-the'me-ah) presence of fungi in the blood.

mycetismus (mi''sě-tiz'mus) fungus poisoning, especially mushroom poisoning; see also *Amanita.*

mycetogenic (mi-se''to-jen'ik) caused by fungi.

mycetoma (mi''sě-to'mah) maduromycosis.

Mycobacteriaceae (mi''ko-bak-te''re-a'se-e) a family of bacteria (order Actinomycetales) found in soil and dairy products and as parasites in man and other animals.

Mycobacterium (-bak-te're-um) a genus of gram-positive, acid-fast bacteria (family Mycobacteriaceae), including *M. bal'nei* (*M. mari'-num*), the cause of swimming pool granuloma; *M. bo'vis,* the cause of cattle tuberculosis, transmitted to man through milk; *M. kansas'ii,* the cause of a tuberculosis-like disease in man; *M. lep'rae,* the cause of leprosy; *M. paratuberculo'-sis,* the cause of Johne's disease; and *M. tuberculo'sis* (the tubercle bacillus), the cause of tuberculosis, most commonly of the lungs, in man.

mycobacterium (-bak-te're-um), pl. *mycobac-te'ria* [L.] 1. an individual organism of the genus *Mycobacterium.* 2. a slender, acid-fast microorganism resembling *Mycobacterium tuberculo-sis.* **anonymous mycobacteria,** acid-fast bacteria resembling the tubercle bacilli, found in human pulmonary infections, for which species names have not been established; they are divided into the chromogens (including photochromogens [Group I] and scotochromogens [Group II]) and nonchromogens (subdivided into filamentous forms [Group III] and rapid growers [Group IV]). **Group I–IV m.,** see *anonymous m.*

mycocidin (-si'din) an antibiotic extracted from a mold, active against *Mycobacterium tuberculosis.*

mycodermatitis (-der''mah-ti'tis) candidiasis.

mycologist (mi-kol'o-jist) a specialist in mycology; a student of mycology.

mycology (mi-kol'o-je) the science and study of fungi.

mycomyringitis (mi''ko-mir''in-ji'tis) myringomycosis.

Mycoplasma (-plaz'mah) a genus of microorganisms (family Mycoplasmataceae) including the pleuropneumonia-like organisms (PPLO), separated into 15 species, including *M. hom'-inis,* found associated with nongonococcal urethritis and reported to cause mild pharyngitis in humans; *M. mycoi'des,* the type species, which causes pleuropneumonia (2); and *M. pneumo'niae,* a cause of primary atypical pneumonia.

mycoplasma (-plaz'mah) any member of *Mycoplasma.*

Mycoplasmataceae (-plaz''mah-ta'se-e) a family of schizomycetes, made up of a single genus, *Mycoplasma.*

mycosis (mi-ko'sis) any disease caused by fungi. **m. fungoi'des,** a chronic, malignant, lymphoreticular neoplasm of the skin and, in late stages, lymph nodes and viscera, with development of large, painful, ulcerating tumors.

mycotic (mi-kot'ik) pertaining to a mycosis; caused by fungi.

mycotoxicosis (mi''ko-tok-sǐ-ko'sis) 1. poisoning due to a fungal or bacterial toxin. 2. poisoning due to ingestion of fungi.

mycotoxin (-tok'sin) a fungal toxin.

mydriasis (mǐ-dri'ah-sis) dilatation of the pupil.

mydriatic (mid''re-at'ik) 1. dilating the pupil. 2. a drug that dilates the pupil.

myectomy (mi-ek'to-me) excision of a muscle.

myectopia (mi''ek-to'pe-ah) displacement of a muscle.

myel(o)- word element [Gr.], *marrow* (often with specific reference to the *spinal cord*).

myelalgia (mi''ě-lal'je-ah) pain in the spinal cord.

myelapoplexy (mi''el-ap'o-plek''se) hemorrhage within the spinal cord.

myelatelia (-ah-te'le-ah) imperfect development of the spinal cord.

myelatrophy (-at'ro-fe) atrophy of the spinal cord.

myelemia (-e'me-ah) myelocytosis.

myelencephalon (-en-sef'ah-lon) 1. the posterior part of the hindbrain, comprising the medulla oblongata and the lower part of the fourth ventricle. 2. the posterior of two brain vesicles formed by specialization of the hindbrain in embryonic development.

myelin (mi'ě-lin) 1. the lipid substance surrounding the axon of myelinated nerve fibers. 2. any of a certain group of lipid substances found in various normal and pathologic tissues, differing from fats in being doubly refractive. **myelin'ic,** adj.

myelinated (mi'ě-lǐ-nāt''ed) having a myelin sheath.

myelination (mi''ě-lǐ-na'shun) myelinization.

myelinization (mi''ě-lin''ǐ-za'shun) production of myelin around an axon.

myelinolysis (mi''ě-lin-ol'ǐ-sis) destruction of myelin; demyelination.

myelinosis (mi''ě-lǐ-no'sis) fatty degeneration, with formation of myelin.

myelitis (mi''ě-li'tis) inflammation of the spinal cord or bone marrow (osteomyelitis). **myelit'ic,** adj. **ascending m.,** see under *myelopathy.* **bulbar m.,** that involving the medulla oblongata. **cavitary m.,** syringomyelitis. **central m.,** that affecting chiefly the gray substance of the spinal cord. **disseminated m.,** that which has several distinct foci in the spinal cord. **focal m.,** see under *myelopathy.* **transverse m.,** see under *myelopathy.*

myeloblast (mi'ě-lo-blast'') an immature cell of bone marrow, not normally found in peripheral blood; it is the precursor of the promyelocyte, having evenly distributed chromatin, several nucleoli, and nongranular basophilic cytoplasm.

myeloblastemia (mi″ĕ-lo-blas-te′me-ah) the presence of myeloblasts in the blood.

myeloblastoma (-blas-to′mah) a focal malignant tumor composed of myeloblasts observed in acute myelocytic leukemia.

myeloblastosis (-blas-to′sis) excess of myeloblasts in the blood.

myelocele (mi′ĕ-lo-sēl″) hernial protrusion of the spinal cord through a defect in the vertebral column.

myelocyst (-sist″) a benign cyst developed from rudimentary medullary canals.

myelocystocele, myelocystomeningocele (mi″ĕ-lo-sis′to-sēl; -sis″to-mĭ-ning′go-sēl) myelomeningocele.

myelocyte (mi′ĕ-lo-sīt″) 1. an immature cell of the bone marrow, developed from the promyelocyte and developing into the metamyelocyte. In this stage, differentiation into specific cytoplasmic granules has begun. 2. any cell of the gray matter of the nervous system. **myelocyt′ic,** adj.

myelocythemia (mi″ĕ-lo-si-the′me-ah) an excess of myelocytes in the circulating blood.

myelocytoma (-si-to′mah) myeloma.

myelocytosis (-si-to′sis) increase of myelocytes in the blood.

myelodysplasia (-dis-pla′ze-ah) defective development of any part of the spinal cord.

myeloencephalitis (-en-sef″ah-li′tis) inflammation of the spinal cord and brain.

myelofibrosis (-fi-bro′sis) replacement of bone marrow by fibrous tissue.

myelogenesis (-jen′ĕ-sis) 1. development of the central nervous system. 2. the deposition of myelin around the axon.

myelogenic (-jen′ik) myelogenous.

myelogenous (mi″ĕ-loj′ĕ-nus) produced in bone marrow.

myelogone (mi′ĕ-lo-gōn″) a white blood cell of the myeloid series having a reticulate violaceous nucleus, well-stained nucleolus, and deep blue rim of cytoplasm. **myelogon′ic,** adj.

myelogram (-gram) 1. the film produced by myelography. 2. a graphic representation of the differential count of cells found in a stained representation of bone marrow.

myelography (mi″ĕ-log′rah-fe) radiography of the spinal cord after injection of a contrast medium into the subarachnoid space.

myeloid (mi′ĕ-loid) 1. pertaining to, derived from, or resembling bone marrow. 2. pertaining to the spinal cord. 3. having the appearance of myelocytes, but not derived from bone marrow.

myeloidosis (mi″ĕ-loi-do′sis) formation of myeloid tissue, especially hyperplastic development of such tissue.

myelolipoma (mi″ĕ-lo-lip′o-mah) a rare benign tumor of the adrenal gland composed of adipose tissue, lymphocytes, and primitive myeloid cells.

myeloma (mi″ĕ-lo′mah) a tumor composed of cells of the type normally found in the bone marrow. **giant cell m.,** see under *tumor* (1). **multiple m., plasma cell m.,** a malignant neoplasm of plasma cells, usually arising in bone marrow, manifested by skeletal destruction, pathologic fractures, bone pain, the presence of anomalous circulating immunoglobulins, Bence-Jones proteinuria, and anemia; see also *plasmacytoma.*

myelomalacia (mi″ĕ-lo-mah-la′she-ah) morbid softening of the spinal cord.

myelomatosis (-mah-to′sis) multiple myeloma.

myelomenia (-me′ne-ah) vicarious menstruation into the spinal cord.

myelomeningitis (-men″in-ji′tis) inflammation of the spinal cord and meninges.

myelomeningocele (-mĕ-ning′go-sēl) hernial protrusion of the spinal cord and its meninges through a defect in the vertebral column.

myelomere (-mēr″) any segment of the embryonic brain or spinal cord.

myeloneuritis (-nu-ri′tis) inflammation of the spinal cord and peripheral nerves.

myelopathy (mi″ĕ-lop′ah-the) 1. any functional disturbance and/or pathological change in the spinal cord; often used to denote nonspecific lesions, as opposed to *myelitis.* 2. pathological bone marrow changes. **myelopath′ic,** adj. **ascending m.,** that progressing cephalad along the spinal cord. **descending m.,** that progressing caudad along the spinal cord. **focal m.,** that affecting a small area only, or several small areas. **sclerosing m.,** that marked by hardening of the spinal cord and overgrowth of the glia. **transverse m.,** that extending across the spinal cord. **traumatic m.,** that following spinal cord injury.

myelopetal (mi″ĕ-lop′ĕ-tal) moving toward the spinal cord.

myelophthisis (mi″ĕ-lo-thi′sis) 1. wasting of the spinal cord. 2. reduction of the cell-forming functions of bone marrow.

myeloplast (mi′ĕ-lo-plast″) any leukocyte of the bone marrow.

myelopoiesis (mi″ĕ-lo-poi-e′sis) the formation of marrow or the cells arising from it. **myelopoiet′ic,** adj. **ectopic m., extramedullary m.,** the formation of myeloid tissue outside the bone marrow.

myeloproliferative (-pro-lif′er-ah″tiv) pertaining to or characterized by medullary and extramedullary proliferation of bone marrow constituents; see under *syndrome.*

myeloradiculitis (-rah-dik″u-li′tis) inflammation of the spinal cord and posterior nerve roots.

myeloradiculodysplasia (-rah-dik″u-lo-dis-pla′ze-ah) abnormal development of the spinal cord and spinal nerve roots.

myeloradiculopathy (-rah-dik″u-lop′ah-the) disease of the spinal cord and spinal nerve roots.

myelorrhagia (-ra′je-ah) spinal hemorrhage.

myelosarcoma (-sar-ko′mah) a sarcomatous growth made up of myeloid tissue or bone marrow cells.

myelosclerosis (-skle-ro′sis) 1. sclerosis of the

spinal cord. 2. obliteration of the marrow cavity by small spicules of bone. 3. myelofibrosis.

myelosis (mi''ĕ-lo'sis) 1. proliferation of bone marrow tissue, producing the blood changes of myelocytic leukemia. 2. formation of a tumor of the spinal cord. **erythremic m.,** a malignant blood dyscrasia, one of the myeloproliferative disorders, with progressive anemia, megaloblastic erythroid hyperplasia, myeloid dysplasia, hepatosplenomegaly, and hemorrhagic phenomena.

myelospongium (mi''ĕ-lo-spun'je-um) a network developing into the neuroglia.

myelotomy (mi''ĕ-lot'o-me) severance of nerve tracts in the spinal cord.

myelotoxin (mi''ĕ-lo-tok'sin) a cytotoxin destructive to bone marrow cells. **myelotox'ic,** adj.

myenteron (mi-en'ter-on) the muscular coat of the intestine. **myenter'ic,** adj.

myesthesia (mi''es-the'ze-ah) muscle sensibility; sensibility to impressions coming from the muscles.

myiasis (mi-i'ah-sis) invasion of the body by the larvae of flies, characterized as cutaneous (subdermal tissue), gastrointestinal, nasopharyngeal, ocular, or urinary, depending on the region invaded.

Myleran (mil'er-an) trademark for a preparation of busulfan.

mylohyoid (mi''lo-hi'oid) pertaining to the hyoid bone and molar teeth.

myo- word element [Gr.], *muscle.*

myoalbumin (mi''o-al-bu'min) an albumin in muscle tissue.

myoarchitectonic (-ar''kĭ-tek-ton'ik) pertaining to structural arrangement of muscle fibers.

myoatrophy (-at'ro-fe) muscular atrophy.

myoblast (mi'o-blast) an embryonic cell which becomes a cell of muscle fiber. **myoblas'tic,** adj.

myoblastoma (mi''o-blas-to'mah) a benign circumscribed tumor-like lesion of soft tissue; see *granular cell tumor.* **granular cell m.,** see under *tumor.*

myobradia (-bra'de-ah) slow reaction of muscle to stimulation.

myocardiograph (-kar'de-o-graf'') instrument for making tracings of heart movements.

myocardiopathy (-kar''de-op'ah-the) any noninflammatory disease of the myocardium.

myocarditis (-kar-di'tis) inflammation of the myocardium. **acute isolated m., Fiedler's m.,** a frequently fatal, idiopathic, acute myocarditis affecting chiefly the interstitial fibrous tissue.

myocardium (-kar'de-um) the middle and thickest layer of the heart wall, composed of cardiac muscle. **myocar'dial,** adj.

myocardosis (-kar-do'sis) any degenerative, noninflammatory disease of the myocardium.

myocele (mi'o-sēl) protrusion of a muscle through its ruptured sheath.

myocellulitis (mi''o-sel''u-li'tis) myositis with cellulitis.

myoceptor (mi'o-sep''tor) end-plate.

myocerosis (mi''o-se-ro'sis) waxy degeneration of muscle.

Myochrysine (-kri'sin) trademark for a preparation of gold sodium thiomalate.

myoclonia (-klo'ne-ah) any disorder characterized by myoclonus.

myoclonus (-klo'nus) shocklike contractions of a muscle or a group of muscles. **myoclon'ic,** adj. **palatal m.,** rapid rhythmic, up-and-down movement of one or both sides of the palate, often with ipsilateral synchronous clonic movements of the face, tongue, pharynx, and diaphragm muscles.

myocoele (mi'o-sēl) the cavity within a myotome (2).

myocyte (-sīt) a muscle cell. **Anichkov's m.,** a myocyte found in Aschoff's bodies, having a serrated bar of chromatin in its nucleus.

myocytoma (mi''o-si-to'mah) a tumor composed of myocytes.

myodemia (-de'me-ah) fatty degeneration of muscle.

myodystonia (-dis-to'ne-ah) disorder of muscular tone.

myodystrophy (-dis'tro-fe) 1. muscular dystrophy. 2. myotonic dystrophy.

myoedema (-ĕ-de'mah) 1. mounding. 2. edema of a muscle.

myoelectric (-e-lek'trik) pertaining to the electric or electromotive properties of muscle.

myoendocarditis (-en''do-kar-di'tis) combined myocarditis and endocarditis.

myoepithelioma (-ep''ĭ-the''le-o'mah) a tumor composed of outgrowths of myoepithelial cells from a sweat gland.

myoepithelium (-ep''ĭ-the'le-um) tissue made up of contractile epithelial cells. **myoepithe'lial,** adj.

myofascitis (-fah-si'tis) inflammation of a muscle and its fascia.

myofibril (-fi'bril) a muscle fibril, one of the slender threads of a muscle fiber, composed of numerous myofilaments. See Plate XIV.

myofibroma (-fi-bro'mah) a tumor containing muscular and fibrous elements.

myofibrosis (-fi-bro'sis) replacement of muscle tissue by fibrous tissue.

myofibrositis (-fi''bro-si'tis) perimysiitis.

myofilament (-fil'ah-ment) any of the ultramicroscopic threadlike structures composing the myofibrils of striated muscle fibers; thick ones contain myosin, thin ones actin. See Plate XIV.

myogen (mi'o-jen) a water-soluble mixture of proteins from muscle.

myogenesis (mi''o-jen'ĕ-sis) the development of muscle tissue, especially its embryonic development. **myogenet'ic,** adj.

myogenic (-jen'ik) giving rise to or forming muscle tissue.

myogenous (mi-oj'ĕ-nus) originating in muscular tissue.

myoglia (mi-og'le-ah) a fibrillar substance formed by embryonic muscle cells, present only during early embryogenesis of muscle fibers.

myoglobin (mi''o-glo'bin) a ferrous protoporphyrin globin complex resembling hemoglobin, present in sarcoplasm of muscle; it contributes to the color of muscle and acts as a store of oxygen.

myoglobinuria (-glo″bin-u′re-ah) the presence of myoglobin in the urine.

myoglobulin (-glob′u-lin) a globulin from muscle serum.

myogram (mi′o-gram) a record produced by myography.

myograph (-graf) apparatus for recording effects of muscular contraction.

myography (mi-og′rah-fe) 1. the use of a myograph. 2. description of muscles. 3. radiography of muscle tissue after injection of a radiopaque medium. **myograph′ic,** adj.

myohematin (mi″o-hem′ah-tin) the cytochrome of muscle tissue.

myohemoglobin (-he″mo-glo′bin) myoglobin.

myoid (mi′oid) resembling muscle.

myokinase (mi″o-ki′nās) adenylate kinase; an enzyme of muscle that catalyzes the phosphorylation of ADP to molecules of ATP and AMP.

myokinesimeter (-kin″ĕ-sim′ĕ-ter) an apparatus for measuring muscular contraction aroused by electrical stimulation.

myokinetic (-ki-net′ik) pertaining to the motion or kinetic function of muscle, as contrasted with the myotonic or tonic function.

myokymia (-ki′me-ah) persistent quivering of the muscles.

myolipoma (-lĭ-po′mah) myoma with fatty or lipomatous elements.

myologia (-lo′je-ah) myology.

myology (mi-ol′o-je) the scientific study or description of the muscles and accessory structures (bursae and synovial sheath).

myolysis (mi-ol′ĭ-sis) disintegration or degeneration of muscle tissue.

myoma (mi-o′mah) a tumor formed of muscular tissue. **myom′atous,** adj.

myomalacia (mi″o-mah-la′she-ah) morbid softening of a muscle.

myomatosis (-mah-to′sis) the formation of multiple myomas.

myomectomy (-mek′to-me) 1. excision of a myoma. 2. myectomy.

myomelanosis (-mel″ah-no′sis) melanosis of muscle tissue.

myomere (mi′o-mēr) myotome (2).

myometer (mi-om′ĕ-ter) an apparatus for measuring muscle contraction.

myometritis (mi″o-me-tri′tis) inflammation of the myometrium.

myometrium (-me′tre-um) the tunica muscularis of the uterus. **myome′trial,** adj.

myonecrosis (-nĕ-kro′sis) necrosis of individual muscle fibers.

myoneme (mi′o-nēm) a fine contractile fiber found in the cytoplasm of certain protozoa.

myoneural (mi″o-nu′ral) pertaining to nerve terminations in muscles.

myoneuralgia (-nu-ral′je-ah) neuralgic pain in a muscle.

myopalmus (-pal′mus) muscle twitching.

myoparalysis (-pah-ral′ĭ-sis) paralysis of a muscle.

myoparesis (-pah-re′sis) slight muscle paralysis.

myopathia (-path′e-ah) myopathy.

myopathy (mi-op′ah-the) any disease of muscle. **myopath′ic,** adj. **centronuclear m.,** myotubular m. **late distal m.,** hereditary muscular dystrophy starting in the hands and feet and spreading proximally. **myotubular m.,** that marked by myofibers resembling those of early fetal muscle, i.e., myotubules. **nemaline m.,** a congenital abnormality of myofibrils in which small threadlike fibers are scattered through the muscle fibers; marked by hypotonia and proximal muscle weakness. **ocular m.,** a slowly progressive form affecting the extraocular muscles, with ptosis and progressive immobility of the eyes.

myope (mi′ōp) a person affected with myopia.

myopericarditis (mi″o-per″ĭ-kar-di′tis) myocarditis combined with pericarditis.

myopia (mi-o′pe-ah) nearsightedness; ametropia in which parallel rays come to a focus in front of the retina, vision being better for near objects than for far. **myop′ic,** adj. **curvature m.,** myopia due to changes in curvature of the refracting surfaces of the eye. **index m.,** myopia due to abnormal refractivity of the media of the eye. **malignant m., pernicious m.,** progressive myopia with disease of the choroid, leading to retinal detachment and blindness. **progressive m.,** myopia that continues to increase in adult life.

myoplasm (mi′o-plazm) the contractile part of a muscle cell, or myofibril.

myoplasty (-plas″te) plastic surgery on muscle. **myoplas′tic,** adj.

myopsychopathy, myopsychosis (mi″o-si-kop′ah-the; -si-ko′sis) any neuromuscular affection associated with mental disorder.

myorrhaphy (mi-or′ah-fe) suture of a muscle.

myorrhexis (mi″o-rek′sis) rupture of a muscle.

myosarcoma (-sar-ko′mah) a malignant tumor derived from myogenic cells.

myosclerosis (-skle-ro′sis) hardening of muscle tissue.

myosin (mi′o-sin) a protein of the myofibril, occurring chiefly in the A band; with actin it forms actomyosin, which is responsible for the contractile properties of muscle.

myositis (mi″o-si′tis) inflammation of a voluntary muscle. **epidemic m.,** see under *pleurodynia.* **m. fibro′sa,** a type in which connective tissue forms within the muscle. **multiple m.,** polymyositis. **m. ossif′icans,** myositis marked by bony deposits or by ossification of muscle. **trichinous m.,** that due to the presence of *Trichinella spiralis.*

myospasm (mi′o-spazm) spasm of a muscle.

myotactic (mi″o-tak′tik) pertaining to the proprioceptive sense of muscles.

myotasis (mi-ot′ah-sis) stretching of muscle. **myotat′ic,** adj.

myotenositis (mi″o-te″no-si′tis) inflammation of a muscle and tendon.

myotenotomy

myotenotomy (-te-not′o-me) surgical division of the tendon of a muscle.

myotome (mi′o-tōm) 1. an instrument for performing myotomy. 2. the muscle plate or portion of a somite, from which voluntary muscles develop. 3. a group of muscles innervated from a single spinal segment.

myotomy (mi-ot′o-me) cutting or dissection of muscular tissue or of a muscle.

myotonia (mi″o-to′ne-ah) any disorder involving tonic spasm of muscle. **myoton′ic,** adj. **m. atroph′ica,** myotonic dystrophy. **m. congen′ita,** a hereditary disease marked by tonic spasm and rigidity of certain muscles when attempts are made to move them after rest. **m. dystroph′ica,** myotonic dystrophy.

myotonoid (mi-ot′o-noid) denoting muscle reactions marked by slow contraction or relaxation.

myotonus (mi-ot′o-nus) tonic spasm of a muscle or a group of muscles.

myotrophic (mi′o-tro″fik) 1. increasing the weight of muscle. 2. pertaining to myotrophy.

myotrophy (mi-ot′ro-fe) nutrition of muscle.

myotubule (mi″o-tu′būl) a developing muscle fiber with a centrally located nucleus. **myotu′bular,** adj.

Myriapoda (mir″e-ap′o-dah) a superclass of arthropods, including centipedes and millipedes.

myring(o)- word element [L.], *tympanic membrane.*

myringa (mĭ-ring′gah) the tympanic membrane.

myringectomy (mir″in-jek′to-me) myringodectomy.

myringitis (mir″in-ji′tis) inflammation of the tympanic membrane. **m. bullo′sa, bullous m.,** a form of viral otitis media in which serous or hemorrhagic blebs appear on the tympanic membrane and often on the adjacent wall of the auditory meatus.

myringodectomy (mĭ-ring″go-dek′to-me) excision of the tympanic membrane.

myringomycosis (-mi-ko′sis) fungal disease of the tympanic membrane.

myringoplasty (mĭ-ring′go-plas″te) surgical restoration of the tympanic membrane.

myringotomy (mir″ing-got′o-me) incision of the tympanic membrane.

myrmesia (mur-me′she-ah) a wart somewhat resembling an anthill.

myrosinase (mi-ro′sĭ-nās) thioglucosidase.

Mysoline (mi′so-lēn) trademark for preparations of primidone.

mysophilia (mi″so-fil′ĭ-ah) paraphilia marked by lustful attitude toward excretions.

mysophobia (-fo′be-ah) morbid dread of contamination and filth.

mytacism (mi′tah-sizm) too free use of the *m* sound in speaking.

Mytelase (mi′tĕ-lās) trademark for a preparation of ambenonium.

mythomania (mith″o-ma′ne-ah) morbid tendency to lie or exaggerate.

mytilotoxin (mit″ĭ-lo-tok′sin) a neurotoxin from mussels of the genus *Mytilus;* see *gonyaulax poison.*

myx(o)- word element [Gr.], *mucus; slime.*

myxadenitis (mik″sad-ĕ-ni′tis) inflammation of a mucous gland.

myxadenoma (-sad-ĕ-no′mah) an epithelial tumor with the structure of a mucous gland.

myxasthenia (-sas-the′ne-ah) deficient secretion of mucus.

myxedema (-sĕ-de′mah) a dry, waxy type of swelling (nonpitting edema) with abnormal deposits of mucin in the skin (mucinosis) and other tissues, associated with hypothyroidism; the facial changes are distinctive, with swollen lips and thickened nose. **myxedem′atous,** adj. **congenital m.,** cretinism. **papular m.,** lichen myxedematosus. **pituitary m.,** that due to deficient secretion of the pituitary hormone thyrotropin. **pretibial m.,** localized edema associated with preceding hyperthyroidism and exophthalmos, occurring typically on the anterior (pretibial) surface of the legs, the mucin deposits appearing as both plaques and papules.

myxedematoid (-sĕ-dem′ah-toid) resembling myxedema.

myxochondroma (mik″so-kon-dro′mah) chondroma with stroma resembling primitive mesenchymal tissue.

myxocyte (mik′so-sīt) one of the cells of mucous tissue.

myxofibroma (mik″so-fi-bro′mah) a fibroma containing myxomatous tissue.

myxofibrosarcoma (-fi″bro-sar-ko′mah) fibrosarcoma with myxomatous areas.

myxoid (mik′soid) resembling mucus.

myxolipoma (mik″so-lĭ-po′mah) lipoma with foci of myxomatous degeneration.

myxoma (mik-so′mah) a tumor composed of primitive connective tissue cells and stroma resembling mesencyhma. **myxo′matous,** adj. **odontogenic m.,** a uncommon tumor of the jaw, possibly produced by myxomatous degeneration of an odontogenic fibroma.

myxomatosis (mik″so-mah-to′sis) 1. the development of multiple myxomas. 2. myxomatous degeneration.

myxomyoma (-mi-o′mah) a myoma with myxomatous degeneration.

myxopoiesis (-poi-e′sis) the formation of mucus.

myxorrhea (-re′ah) excessive flow of mucus.

myxosarcoma (-sar-ko′mah) a sarcoma with myxomatous tissue.

Myxosporidia (-spo-rid′e-ah) an order of ameboid sporozoa endoparasitic in lower vertebrates.

myxovirus (-vi′rus) any of a group of RNA viruses, including the viruses of influenza, parainfluenza, mumps, and Newcastle disease, characteristically causing agglutination of erythrocytes.

N

N 1. symbol, *refractive index*. 2. chemical symbol, *nitrogen*. 3. symbol, *normal* (solution); the expressions 2N (double normal), N/2 or 0.5N (half-normal), N/10 or 0.1N (tenth-normal), etc., denote the strength of a solution in comparison with the normal.

n 1. symbol, *refractive index*. 2. chemical symbol, *normal*.

NA Nomina Anatomica.

Na chemical symbol, *sodium* (L. *natrium*).

nacreous (na'kre-us) having a pearl-like luster.

Nacton (nak'ton) trademark for a preparation of poldine.

NAD nicotinamide-adenine dinucleotide.

NADH the reduced form of NAD.

NADP nicotinamide-adenine dinucleotide phosphate.

NADPH the reduced form of NADP.

naepaine (ne'pān) a local anesthetic, $C_{14}H_{22}N_2$-O_2, used as the hydrochloride salt.

nafcillin (naf-sil'in) a semisynthetic, acid- and penicillinase-resistance penicillin that is effective against staphylococcal infections.

nagana (nah-gah'nah) a rapidly fatal trypanosomiasis of equines, pigs, goats, sheep, camels, and elephants in Africa.

nail (nāl) 1. the horny cutaneous plate on the dorsal surface of the distal end of a finger or toe. 2. a rod of metal, bone, or other material for fixation of fragments of fractured bones. **ingrown n.,** aberrant growth of a toenail, with one or both lateral margins pushing deeply into adjacent soft tissue. **racket n.,** a short broad thumbnail. **Smith-Petersen n.,** a flanged nail for fixing the head of the femur in fracture of the femoral neck. **spoon n.,** one with a concave surface.

Nalline (nal'lēn) trademark for a preparation of nalorphine.

nalorphine (nal'or-fēn) a semisynthetic congener of morphine, used as a narcotic antagonist.

naloxone (nal-oks'ōn) a synthetic congener of oxymorphone, $C_{19}H_{21}NO_4$, whose hydrochloride salt is used as a narcotic antagonist.

nandrolone (nan'dro-lōn) an androgenic, anabolic steroid, $C_{18}H_{26}O_2$; used as the decanoate and phenpropionate esters.

nanism (na'nizm) dwarfism.

nano- word element [Gr.], *dwarf; small size;* used in naming units of measurement to designate an amount 10^{-9} (one billionth) the size of the unit to which it is joined, e.g., nanocurie.

nanocephaly (na"no-sef'ah-le) microcephaly. **nanoceph'alous,** adj.

nanocormia (-kor'me-ah) abnormal smallness of the body or trunk.

nanogram (na'no-gram) one billionth (10^{-9}) gram.

nanoid (na'noid) dwarfish.

nanomelus (na-nom'ĕ-lus) micromelus.

nanometer (na"no-me'ter) one billionth (10^{-9}) meter.

nanosecond (-sek'und) one billionth (10^{-9}) second.

nanosomia (-so'me-ah) nanism.

nanous (na'nus) dwarfed; stunted.

nanukayami (nah"nu-kah-yah'me) a leptospirosis marked by fever and jaundice, first reported in Japan, due to *Leptospira hebdomidis*.

nanus (na'nus) a dwarf.

nape (nāp) the back of the neck.

napelline (na-pel'in) an analgesic alkaloid, C_{22}-$H_{33}O_3N$, from aconite.

naphazoline (naf-az'o-lēn) a vasoconstrictor, $C_{14}H_{14}N_2$, used as the hydrochloride salt to decongest nasal and ocular mucosae.

naphtha (naf'thah) petroleum benzin.

naphthalene (naf'thah-lēn) a hydrocarbon from coal tar oil; antiseptic.

naphthol (naf'thol) a crystalline antiseptic substance, $C_{10}H_7 \cdot OH$, from coal tar, occurring in two forms, alphanaphthol and betanaphthol. Excessive or continued use causes a toxic condition, marked by anemia, jaundice, convulsions, and coma.

N.A.P.N.E.S. National Association for Practical Nurse Education and Services.

Naqua (nak'wah) trademark for a preparation of trichlormethiazide.

narcissism (nar'si-sizm) dominant interest in one's self; self-love. **narcissis'tic,** adj.

narco- word element [Gr.], *stupor; stuporous state.*

narcoanalysis (nar"ko-ah-nal'ĭ-sis) psychotherapy utilizing barbiturates to release suppressed or repressed thoughts.

narcohypnia (-hip'ne-ah) numbness felt on waking from sleep.

narcohypnosis (-hip-no'sis) hypnotic suggestions made while the patient is narcotized.

narcolepsy (nar'ko-lep"se) recurrent uncontrollable desire for sleep. **narcolep'tic,** adj.

narcosis (nar-ko'sis) stuporous state induced by a drug. **basal n., basis n.,** narcosis with complete unconsciousness, amnesia, and analgesia.

narcosynthesis (nar"ko-sin'thĕ-sis) narcoanalysis.

narcotic (nar-kot'ic) 1. pertaining to or producing narcosis. 2. a drug that produces insensibility or stupor.

narcotine (nar'ko-tin) noscapine.

narcotize (-tīz) to put under the influence of a narcotic.

Nardil (nar'dil) trademark for a preparation of phenelzine.

nares (na'rēs), sing. *na'ris* [L.] the nostrils; the external openings of the nasal cavity.

Narone (nar'ōn) trademark for preparations of dipyrone.

nasal (na'zal) pertaining to the nose.

nasalis (na-za'lis) [L.] nasal.

nascent (nas'ent, na'sent) 1. being born; just coming into existence. 2. just liberated from a chemical combination, and hence more reactive because uncombined.

nasion (na'ze-on) the middle point of the fronto-nasal suture.

naso- word element [L.], *nose.*

nasoantral (na''zo-an'tral) pertaining to the nose and maxillary antrum.

nasociliary (-sil'e-a''re) pertaining to the eyes, brow, and root of the nose.

nasofrontal (-frun'tal) pertaining to the nasal and frontal bones.

nasolabial (-la'be-al) pertaining to the nose and lip.

nasolacrimal (-lak'rĭ-mal) pertaining to the nose and lacrimal apparatus.

naso-oral (-o'ral) pertaining to the nose and mouth.

nasopalatine (-pal'ah-tīn) pertaining to the nose and palate.

nasopharyngitis (-far''in-ji'tis) inflammation of the nasopharynx.

nasopharynx (-far'inks) the part of the pharynx above the soft palate. **nasopharyn'geal**, adj.

nasosinusitis (-si''nŭ-si'tis) inflammation of the accessory sinuses of the nose.

nasospinale (-spi-na'le) the point at which the midsagittal plane intersects a line tangent to the lower margin of the nasal apertures.

nasus (na'sus) nose.

natal (na'tal) 1. pertaining to birth. 2. pertaining to the nates (buttocks).

natality (na-tal'ĭ-te) the birth rate.

nates (na'tēz) (pl.) the buttocks.

natimortality (na''te-mor-tal'ĭ-te) the proportion of stillbirths to the general birth rate.

National Formulary a book of standards for certain pharmaceuticals and preparations not included in the USP; revised every 5 years, and recognized as a book of official standards by the Pure Food and Drug Act of 1906. Abbreviated NF.

natremia (na-tre'me-ah) hypernatremia.

natrium (na'tre-um) [L.] sodium (symbol Na).

natriuresis (na''tre-u-re'sis) excretion of abnormal amounts of sodium in the urine.

natriuretic (-u-ret'ik) 1. pertaiing to or promoting natriuresis. 2. an agent that promotes natriuresis.

natron (na'tron) native sodium carbonate.

Naturetin (nat''u-re'tin) trademark for preparations of bendroflumethiazide.

naturopath (na'tūr-o-path'') a practitioner of naturopathy.

naturopathy (na''tūr-op'ah-the) a drugless system of healing by the use of physical methods.

nausea (naw'ze-ah) an unpleasant sensation vaguely referred to the epigastrium and abdomen, with a tendency to vomit. **n. gravida'rum,** the morning sickness of pregnancy. **n. mari'na, n. nava'lis,** seasickness.

nauseant (naw'ze-ant) 1. inducing nausea. 2. an agent causing nausea.

nauseate (naw'ze-āt) to affect with nausea.

nauseous (naw'shus, naw'ze-us) pertaining to or producing nausea.

navel (na'vel) the umbilicus.

navicular (nah-vik'u-ler) boat-shaped, as the navicular bone.

NB chemical symbol, *niobium.*

N.C.I. National Cancer Institute.

N.C.N. National Council of Nurses.

Nd chemical symbol, *neodymium.*

N.D.A. National Dental Association.

Ne chemical symbol, *neon.*

nearsightedness (nēr-sīt'ed-nes) myopia.

nearthrosis (ne''ar-thro'sis) a false or artificial joint.

nebramycin (neb''rah-mi'sin) an aminoglycoside antibiotic complex consisting of eight components, produced by *Streptomyces tenebrarius.*

nebula (neb'u-lah) 1. a slight corneal opacity. 2. an oily preparation for use in an atomizer.

nebulization (neb''u-li-za'shun) 1. conversion into a spray. 2. treatment by a spray.

nebulizer (neb'u-līz''er) an atomizer; a device for throwing a spray.

Necator (ne-ka'tor) a genus of hookworms, including *N. america'nus* (American or New World hookworm), a cause of hookworm disease.

necatoriasis (ne-ka''to-ri'ah-sis) infection with *Necator;* see *hookworm disease.*

neck (nek) a constricted portion, such as the part connecting the head and trunk, or the constricted part of an organ or other structure. **anatomic n.,** a constriction of the humerus just below its proximal articular surface. **n. of femur,** the heavy column of bone connecting the head of the femur and the shaft. **Madelung's n.,** diffuse symmetrical lipomas of the neck. **surgical n.,** the constricted part of the humerus just below the tuberosities. **n. of tooth,** the narrowed part of a tooth between the crown and the root. **uterine n., n. of uterus,** cervix uteri. **webbed n.,** pterygium colli. **wry n.,** torticollis.

necklace (nek'las) a structure encircling the neck. **Casal's n.,** an eruption in pellagra, encircling the lower part of the neck.

necrectomy (nĕ-krek'to-me) excision of necrotic tissue.

necro- word element [Gr.], *death.*

necrobacillosis (nek''ro-bas''ĭ-lo'sis) infection of animals with *Bacteroides funduliformis* (q.v.).

necrobiosis (-bi-o'sis) swelling, basophilia, and distortion of collagen bundles in the dermis, sometimes with obliteration of normal structure, but short of actual necrosis. **necrobiot'ic,** adj. **n. lipoi'dica diabetico'rum,** necrobiosis of elastic and connective tissue of the skin, with degenerated collagen occurring in irregular patches, especially in the dermis, most often located on the mid or lower shins, and usually seen in diabetics.

necrocytosis (-si-to'sis) death and decay of cells.

necrogenic (-jen'ik) productive of necrosis or death.

necrogenous (nĕ-kroj'ĕ-nus) originating or arising from dead matter.

necrology (ně-krol′o-je, ne-krol′o-je) statistics or records of death.

necrolysis (ně-krol′ĭ-sis) separation or exfoliation of necrotic tissue.

necromania (nek″ro-ma′ne-ah) necrophilia.

necrophagous (ne-krof′ah-gus) feeding upon carrion.

necrophilia (nek″ro-fil′e-ah) morbid attraction to death or to dead bodies; sexual intercourse with a dead body.

necrophilic (-fil′ik) 1. pertaining to necrophilia. 2. necrophilous.

necrophilous (ně-krof′ĭ-lus) showing a preference for dead tissue; said of microorganisms.

necrophobia (nek″ro-fo′be-ah) morbid dread of death or of dead bodies.

necropneumonia (-nu-mo′ne-ah) gangrene of the lung.

necropsy (nek′rop-se) examination of a body after death; autopsy.

necrose (ne-krōs′) to become necrotic or to undergo necrosis.

necrosin (ne-kro′sin) a toxic substance occurring in inflammatory exudates.

necrosis (ně-kro′sis, ne-kro′sis) death of individual cells or groups of cells, or of localized areas of tissue. **necrot′ic,** adj. **aseptic n.,** necrosis without infection. **Balser's fatty n.,** gangrenous pancreatitis with omental bursitis and disseminated patches of necrosis of fatty tissues. **caseous n.,** that in which the tissue is soft, dry, and cheesy. **central n.,** that affecting the central portion of an affected bone, cell, or lobule of the liver. **cheesy n.,** that in which the tissue resembles cottage cheese; most often seen in tuberculosis and syphilis. **coagulation n.,** death of cells, the protoplasm of the cells becoming fixed and opaque by coagulation of the protein elements, the cellular outline persisting for a long time. **colliquative n.,** liquefactive n. **fat n.,** necrosis of fatty tissue in small white areas. **liquefactive n.,** that in which the necrotic material becomes softened and liquefied. **phosphorus n.,** phosphonecrosis. **postpartum pituitary n.,** necrosis of the pituitary during the postpartum period, often associated with shock and excessive uterine bleeding during delivery, and leading to variable patterns of hypopituitarism. **subcutaneous fat n. of newborn,** a benign condition seen in the first few weeks of life, in which there is induration of the subcutaneous fat. **n. ustilagin′ea,** that due to ergotism. **Zenker's n.,** see under *degeneration.*

necrospermia (nek″ro-sper′me-ah) a condition in which the spermatozoa of the semen are dead or motionless. **necrosper′mic,** adj.

necrotizing (nek′ro-tīz″ing) causing necrosis.

necrotomy (ně-krot′o-me) 1. dissection of a dead body. 2. excision of a sequestrum.

necrotoxin (nek″ro-tok′sin) a factor or substance produced by certain staphylococci which kills tissue cells.

needle (ne′d'l) 1. a sharp instrument for suturing or puncturing. 2. to puncture or separate with a needle. **aneurysm n.,** one with a handle, used in ligating blood vessels. **aspirating n.,** a long, hollow needle for removing fluid from a cavity. **cataract n.,** one used in removing a cataract. **discission n.,** a special form of cataract needle. **Hagedorn's n.,** a form of flat suture needle. **hypodermic n.,** a short, slender, hollow needle, used in injecting drugs beneath the skin. **knife n.,** a slender knife with a needle-like point, used in ophthalmic operations. **ligature n.,** a long-handled, slender steel needle with an eye in its curved end, used for passing a ligature underneath an artery. **Reverdin's n.,** a surgical needle with an eye that can be opened by means of a slide. **stop n.,** one with a shoulder that prevents too deep penetration.

negative (neg′ah-tiv) having a value of less than zero; indicating lack or absence, as chromatin-negative; characterized by denial or opposition.

negativism (neg′ah-tĭ-vizm″) opposition to suggestion or advice; behavior opposite to that appropriate to a specific situation.

negatron (neg′ah-tron) a negatively charged electron.

Neisseria (ni-se′re-ah) a genus of gram-negative bacteria (family Neisseriaceae), including *N. gonorrhoe′ae,* the etiologic agent of gonorrhea, *N. meningi′tidis,* a prominent cause of meningitis and the specific etiologic agent of meningococcal meningitis.

Neisseriaceae (ni-se″re-a′se-e) a family of parasitic bacteria (order Eubacteriales).

nem (nem) a unit of nutrition equivalent to the nutritive value of 1 gm. of breast milk.

Nema (ne′mah) trademark for a preparation of tetrachloroethylene.

Nemathelminthes (nem″ah-thel-min′thēz) in some classifications, a phylum including the Acanthocephala and Nematoda.

nematocide (nem′ah-to-sīd″) 1. destroying nematodes. 2. an agent which destroys nematodes.

Nematoda (nem″ah-to′dah) a class of helminths (phylum Aschelminthes), the roundworms many of which are parasites; in some classifications, considered to be a phylum, and sometimes known as Nemathelminthes, or a class of that phylum.

nematode (nem′ah-tōd) a roundworm; any individual of the class Nematoda.

Nembutal (nem′bu-tal) trademark for a preparation of pentobarbital.

neo- word element [Gr.], *new; recent.*

Neo-Antergan (ne″o-an′ter-gan) trademark for a preparation of pyrilamine.

neoantigen (-an′tĭ-jen) an intranuclear antigen, e.g., a T antigen, present in cells infected by oncogenic viruses.

neoarthrosis (-ar-thro′sis) nearthrosis.

neoblastic (-blas′tik) originating in or of the nature of new tissue.

neocerebellum (-ser″ě-bel′um) phylogenetically, the newer parts of the cerebellum, consisting of those parts predominately supplied by corticopontocerebellar fibers.

neocinetic (-si-net′ik) neokinetic.

neocortex (-kor′teks) neopallium.

neodymium (-dim′e-um) chemical element (*see table*), at. no. 60, symbol Nd.

neogenesis (-jen′ĕ-sis) tissue regeneration. **neogenet′ic,** adj.

Neohetramine (-he′trah-min) trademark for a preparation of thonzylamine.

Neo-Hombreol (-hom′bre-ol) trademark for preparations of testosterone.

Neohydrin (-hi′drin) trademark for a preparation of chlormerodrin.

neokinetic (-ki-net′ik) pertaining to the nervous motor mechanism regulating voluntary muscular control.

neologism (ne-ol′o-jizm) a newly coined word; in psychiatry, a new word whose meaning may be known only to the patient using it.

neomembrane (ne″o-mem′brān) a false membrane.

neomycin (-mi′sin) an antibacterial substance produced by growth of *Streptomyces fradiae;* used as an intestinal antiseptic and in treatment of systemic infections due to gram-negative microorganisms.

neon (ne′on) chemical element (*see table*), at. no. 10, symbole Ne.

neonatal (ne″o-na′tal) pertaining to the first four weeks after birth.

neonate (ne′o-nāt) a newborn infant.

neontologist (ne″o-na-tol′o-jist) a physician who specializes in neonatology.

neonatology (-na-tol′o-je) the diagnosis and treatment of disorders of the newborn.

neopallium (-pal′le-um) that part of the pallium (cerebral cortex) showing stratification and organization of the most highly evolved type; cf. *archipallium* and *paleopallium.*

neoplasia (-pla′ze-ah) the formation of a neoplasm.

neoplasm (ne′o-plazm) tumor; any new and abnormal growth, specifically one in which cell multiplication is uncontrolled and progressive. Neoplasms may be benign or malignant.

neoplastic (ne″o-plas′tik) pertaining to neoplasia or to a neoplasm.

Neorickettsia (-rĭ-ket′sĭ-ah) a genus of rickettsiae (tribe Ehrlichieae), including a single species, *N. helmin′thoeca.* It is found in the salmon fluke (*Troglotrema salmincola*), a parasite of various fish, especially salmon and trout, and causes hemorrhagic enteritis in those ingesting raw infected fish.

neostigmine (-stig′min) a cholinergic used orally as the bromide salt ($C_{12}H_{19}BrN_2O_2$) and parenterally as the methylsulfate salt ($C_{13}H_{22}N_2O_6S$) in prevention and treatment of postoperative abdominal distention and urinary retention, in treatment of myasthenia gravis, glaucoma, and delayed menstruation, as a screening test for early pregnancy, and as an antidote for excessive curarization.

neostriatum (-stri-a′tum) the caudate nucleus and the putamen combined.

Neo-Synephrine (-sĭ-nef′rin) trademark for a preparation of phenylephrine.

neoteny (ne-ot′ĕ-ne) prolongation of the larval form in a sexually mature organism. **neoten′ic,** adj.

neothalamus (ne″o-thal′ah-mus) the part of the thalamus connected to the neocortex.

Neothylline (-thil′lin) trademark for preparations of dyphylline.

nephelometer (nef″ĕ-lom′ĕ-ter) an instrument for measuring the concentration of substances in suspension.

nephelometry (nef″ĕ-lom′ĕ-tre) measurement of the concentration of a suspension by means of a nephelometer. **nephelomet′ric,** adj.

nephelopia (nef″ĕ-lo′pe-ah) a visual defect due to cloudiness of the cornea.

nephr(o)- word element [Gr.], *kidney.*

nephralgia (ne-fral′je-ah) pain in a kidney.

nephrectasia (nef″rek-ta′ze-ah) distention of the kidney.

nephrectomy (ne-frek′to-me) excision of a kidney.

nephrelcosis (nef″rel-ko′sis) ulceration of the kidney.

nephric (nef′rik) pertaining to the kidney.

nephridium (nĕ-frid′e-um), pl. *nephrid′ia* [L.] either of the paired excretory organs of certain invertebrates, having the inner end of the tubule opening into the coelomic cavity.

nephritic (nĕ-frit′ik) 1. pertaining to or affected with nephritis. 2. pertaining to the kidneys; renal. 3. an agent useful in kidney disease.

nephritis (nĕ-fri′tis), pl. *nephrit′ides* [Gr.] inflammation of the kidney; a focal or diffuse proliferative or destructive disease that may involve the glomerulus, tubule, or interstitial renal tissue. **glomerular n.,** glomerulonephritis. **interstitial n.,** primary or secondary disease of the renal interstitial tissue. **parenchymatous n.,** that affecting the parenchyma of kidney. **salt-losing n.,** intrinsic renal disease causing abnormal urinary sodium loss in persons ingesting normal amounts of sodium chloride, with vomiting, dehydration, and vascular collapse. **scarlatinal n.,** an acute nephritis due to scarlet fever. **suppurative n.,** a form accompanied by abscess of kidney. **transfusion n.,** nephropathy following transfusion from an incompatible donor.

nephritogenic (nĕ-frit″o-jen′ik) causing nephritis.

nephroblastoma (nef″ro-blas-to′mah) Wilms' tumor.

nephrocalcinosis (-kal″sĭ-no′sis) precipitation of calcium phosphate in the renal tubules, with resultant renal insufficiency.

nephrocapsectomy (-kap-sek′to-me) excision of the renal capsule.

nephrocardiac (-kar′de-ak) pertaining to the kidney and heart.

nephrocele (nef′ro-sēl) hernia of a kidney.

nephrocolic (nef″ro-kol′ik) 1. pertaining to the kidney and colon. 2. renal colic.

nephrocoloptosis (-ko″lop-to′sis) downward displacement of the kidney and colon.

nephrocystitis (-sis-ti′tis) inflammation of the kidney and bladder.

nephrogenic (-jen′ik) producing kidney tissue.

nephrogenous (nĕ-froj′ĕ-nus) arising in a kidney.

nephrogram (nef'ro-gram) a roentgenogram of the kidney.

nephrography (ně-frog'rah-fe) roentgenography of the kidney.

nephroid (nef'roid) resembling a kidney.

nephrolith (nef'ro-lith) a calculus in a kidney.

nephrolithiasis (nef″ro-lǐ-thi'ah-sis) a condition marked by the presence of renal calculi.

nephrolithotomy (-lǐ-thot'o-me) incision of the kidney for removal of calculi.

nephrology (ně-frol'o-je) the branch of medical science that deals with the kidneys.

nephrolysine (ně-frol'ǐ-sin) nephrotoxin.

nephrolysis (ně-frol'ǐ-sis) 1. freeing of a kidney from adhesions. 2. destruction of kidney substance. **nephrolyt'ic**, adj.

nephroma (ně-fro'mah) a tumor of kidney tissue.

nephromegaly (nef″ro-meg'ah-le) enlargement of the kidney.

nephron (nef'ron) the structural and functional unit of the kidney, numbering about a million in the renal parenchyma, each being capable of forming urine; see also *renal tubules*.

nephropathy (ně-frop'ah-the) disease of the kidneys. **nephropath'ic**, adj.

nephropexy (nef'ro-pek″se) fixation or suspension of a hypermobile kidney.

nephroptosis (nef″rop-to'sis) downward displacement of a kidney.

nephropyelitis (nef″ro-pi″ě-li'tis) pyelonephritis.

nephropyelography (-pi″ě-log'rah-fe) radiography of the kidney and its pelvis.

nephropyosis (-pi-o'sis) suppuration of a kidney.

nephrorrhagia (-ra'je-ah) hemorrhage from the kidney.

nephrorrhaphy (nef-ror'ah-fe) suture of the kidney.

nephrosclerosis (nef″ro-skle-ro'sis) hardening of the kidney; the condition of the kidney due to renovascular disease. **arteriolar n.,** that involving chiefly the arterioles, with degeneration of the renal tubules and fibrotic thickening of the glomeruli; the benign form is often associated with benign hypertension and hyaline arteriolosclerosis, the malignant with malignant hypertension and hyperplastic arteriolosclerosis.

nephrosis (ně-fro'sis), pl. *nephro'ses* [Gr.] any kidney disease, especially disease marked by purely degenerative lesions of the renal tubules. **nephrot'ic**, adj. **amyloid n.,** chronic nephrosis with amyloid degeneration of the median coat of the arteries and glomerular capillaries. **lipid n.,** nephrosis marked by edema, albuminuria, and changes in the protein and lipids of the blood and accumulation of globules of cholesterol esters in the tubular epithelium of the kidney. **lower nephron n.,** renal insufficiency leading to uremia, due to necrosis of the lower nephron cells, blocking the tubular lumens of this region; seen after severe injuries, especially crushing injury to muscles (*crush syndrome*).

nephrosonephritis (ně-fro″so-ně-fri'tis) renal disease with nephrotic and nephritic components.

nephrostoma (ně-fros'to-mah) one of the ciliated funnel-shaped openings of excretory tubules that open into the coelom; best seen in lower vertebrates.

nephrostomy (ně-fros'to-me) creation of a permanent fistula leading into the renal pelvis.

nephrotome (nef'ro-tōm) one of the segmented divisions of the mesoderm connecting the somite with the lateral plates of unsegmented mesoderm; the source of much of the urogenital system.

nephrotomography (nef″ro-to-mog'rah-fe) body-section roentgenography for visualization of the kidney. **nephrotomograph'ic**, adj.

nephrotomy (ně-frot'o-me) incision of a kidney.

nephrotoxic (nef″ro-tok'sik) destructive to kidney cells.

nephrotoxin (-tok'sin) a toxin having a specific destructive effect on kidney cells.

nephrotropic (-trop'ik) having a special affinity for kidney tissue.

nephrotuberculosis (-tu-ber″ku-lo'sis) renal disease due to *Mycobacterium tuberculosis*.

neptunium (nep-tu'ne-um) chemical element (*see table*), at. no. 93, symbol Np.

nerve (nerv) a macroscopic, cordlike structure comprising a collection of nerve fibers that convey impulses between a part of the central nervous system and some other body region. See *Table of Nerves* and Plates X and XI. **accelerator n's,** the cardiac sympathetic nerves, which, when stimulated, accelerate action of the heart. **afferent n.,** any nerve that transmits impulses from the periphery toward the central nervous system; see *sensory n*. **centrifugal n.,** efferent n. **centripetal n.,** afferent n. **depressor n.,** 1. one that lessens the activity of an organ. 2. an inhibitory nerve whose stimulation depresses a motor center. **efferent n.,** any that carries impulses from the central nervous system to the periphery, e.g., a motor nerve. **exciter n.,** one that transmits impulses resulting in an increase in functional activity. **excitoreflex n.,** a visceral nerve that produces reflex action. **furcal n.,** the fourth lumbar nerve. **gangliated n.,** any nerve of the sympathetic nervous system. **inhibitory n.,** one that transmits impulses resulting in a decrease in functional activity. **Jacobson's n.,** tympanic n. **mixed n.,** one composed of both sensory and motor fibers. **motor n.,** an efferent nerve that stimulates muscle contraction. **pilomotor n's,** those that supply the arrectores pilorum muscles. **pressor n.,** an afferent nerve irritation of which stimulates a vasomotor center and increases intravascular tension. **secretory n.,** any efferent nerve whose stimulation increases glandular activity. **sensory n.,** a peripheral nerve that conducts impulses from a sense organ to the spinal cord or brain. **somatic n's,** the motor and sensory nerves supplying skeletal muscle and somatic tissues. **splanchnic n's,** those of the blood vessels and viscera, especially the visceral branches of the thoracic, lumbar, and pelvic parts of the sympathetic trunks. **sudomotor n's,** those innervating the sweat glands. **sympathetic n.,** 1. see under *trunk.* 2. any nerve of the sympathetic nervous system. **trophic n.,** one concerned with regulation of nutrition. **vasoconstrictor n.,** one whose stimulation contracts blood vessels. **vasodilator n.,** one whose stimulation dilates blood vessels. **vasomotor n.,** one concerned in controlling the caliber of vessels, whether as a vasoconstrictor or vasodilator. **vasosensory n.,** any nerve supplying sensory fibers to the vessels.

nervimotor (ner″vĭ-mo′tor) pertaining to a motor nerve.

nervone (ner′vōn) a cerebroside, $C_{48}H_{91}O_8N$, isolated from nerve tissue.

nervous (ner′vus) 1. pertaining to a nerve or nerves. 2. unduly excitable.

nervousness (-nes) a state of excitability, with great mental and physical unrest.

nervous system see under *system.*

nervus (ner′vus), pl. *ner′vi* [L.] nerve.

Nesacaine (nes′ah-kān) trademark for preparations of chloroprocaine.

nesidiectomy (ne-sid″e-ek′to-me) excision of the islet cells of the pancreas.

nesidioblast (ne-sid′e-o-blast″) any of the cells giving rise to islet cells of the pancreas.

network (net′werk) a meshlike structure of interlocking fibers or strands.

neur(o)- word element [Gr.], *nerve.*

neurad (nu′rad) toward the neural axis or aspect.

neural (nu′ral) pertaining to a nerve or to the nerves.

neuralgia (nu-ral′je-ah) paroxysmal pain extending along the course of one or more nerves. **neural′gic,** adj. **n. facia′lis ve′ra,** geniculate n. **Fothergill's n.,** trigeminal n. **geniculate n.,** that involving the geniculate ganglion, the pain being limited to the middle ear and auditory canal. **Hunt's n.,** geniculate n. **idiopathic n.,** that of unknown etiology, unaccompanied by any structual change. **intercostal n.,** neuralgia of the intercostal nerves. **mammary n.,** neuralgic pain in the breast. **migrainous n.,** cluster headache. **Morton's n.,** traumatic neuroma of the interdigital nerve of the foot. **nasociliary n.,** pain in the eyes, brow, and root of the nose. **red n.,** erythromelalgia. **trifacial n., trigeminal n.,** excruciating episodic pain in the area of the trigeminal nerve, often precipitated by stimulation of well-defined trigger points.

neuraminidase (nūr″ah-min′ĭ-dās) an enzyme of the surface coat of myxoviruses that destroys the neuraminic acid of the cell surface during attachment, thereby preventing hemagglutination.

neuranagenesis (nu″ran-ah-jen′ĕ-sis) regeneration of nerve tissue.

neurapophysis (nu″rah-pof′ĭ-sis) a structure forming either side of the neural arch; also, the part supposedly homologous with this structure in a so-called cranial vertebra.

neurapraxia (-prak′se-ah) nerve injury in which paralysis occurs in the absence of structural changes.

neurarthropathy (nūr″ar-throp′ah-the) neuroarthropathy.

neurasthenia (nu″ras-the′ne-ah) a neurosis marked by chronic abnormal fatigability, lack of energy, feelings of inadequacy, moderate depression, inability to concentrate, loss of appetite, insomnia, etc. **neurasthen′ic,** adj. **gastric n.,** a form marked by functional stomach complications. **sexual n.,** a form associated with disorders of sexual function. **traumatic n.,** neurasthenia following shock or injury.

neuratrophia (nu″rah-tro′fe-ah) impaired nutrition of the nervous system.

neuratrophic (-trof′ik) characterized by atrophy of the nerves; also, a person so affected.

neuraxis (nu-rak′sis) 1. axon. 2. central nervous system. **neurax′ial,** adj.

neuraxon (nu-rak′son) axon.

neurectasia (nu″rek-ta′ze-ah) neurotony.

neurectomy (nu-rek′to-me) excision of a part of a nerve.

neurectopia (nu″rek-to′pe-ah) displacement of or abnormal situation of a nerve.

neurenteric (nu″ren-ter′ik) pertaining to the neural tube and archenteron of the embryo.

neurergic (nu-rer′jik) pertaining to or dependent on nerve action.

neurexeresis (nūr″ek-ser-e′sis) operation of tearing out (avulsion) of a nerve.

neurilemma (nu″rĭ-lem′ah) the thin membrane spirally enwrapping the myelin layers of myelinated nerve fibers and the axons of unmyelinated nerve fibers.

neurilemmitis (-lĕ-mi′tis) inflammation of the neurilemma.

neurilemoma (-lĕ-mo′mah) a tumor of a peripheral nerve sheath (neurilemma).

neurinoma (-no′mah) neurilemoma.

neuritis (nu-ri′tis), pl. *neurit′ides.* Inflammation of a nerve; also used to denote noninflammatory lesions of the peripheral nervous system (see *neuropathy*). **neurit′ic,** adj. **endemic n.,** beriberi. **interstitial n.,** inflammation of the connective tissue of a nerve trunk. **multiple n.,** polyneuritis. **optic n.,** inflammation of the optic nerve, affecting part of the nerve within the eyeball (*neuropapillitis*) or the part behind the eyeball (*retrobulbar n.*). **parenchymatous n.,** that affecting chiefly the axons and myelin of the peripheral nerves. **retrobulbar n.,** see *optic n.* **toxic n.,** that due to some poison. **traumatic n.,** that following and due to an injury.

neuroanastomosis (nu″ro-ah-nas″to-mo′sis) surgical anastomosis of one nerve to another.

neuroanatomy (-ah-nat′o-me) anatomy of the nervous system.

neuroarthropathy (-ar-throp′ah-the) any disease of joint structures associated with disease of the central or peripheral nervous system.

neuroastrocytoma (-as″tro-si-to′mah) a glioma composed mainly of astrocytes, found mostly in the floor of the third ventricle and the temporal lobes.

neurobiology (-bi-ol′o-je) biology of the nervous system.

neurobiotaxis (-bi″o-tak′sis) the theory that

TABLE OF NERVES

COMMON NAME* [MODALITY]	NA TERM†	ORIGIN*	BRANCHES*	DISTRIBUTION*
abducent n. (6th cranial) [motor]	n. abducens	a nucleus in the pons, beneath floor of fourth ventricle		lateral rectus muscle of eyeball
accessory n. (11th cranial) [parasympathetic, motor]	n. accessorius	by cranial roots from side of medulla oblongata, and by spinal roots of spinal cord		internal branch to vagus, thereby to palate, pharynx, larynx, and thoracic viscera; external to sternocleiodomastoid and trapezius muscles
acoustic n. See vestibulocochlear n.				
alveolar n., inferior [motor, general sensory]	n. alveolaris inferior	mandibular n.	inferior dental, mental, and inferior gingival nerves; mylohyoid n.	teeth and gums of lower jaw, skin of chin and lower lip, mylohyoid muscle and anterior belly of digastric muscle
alveolar n's, superior	nn. alveolares superiores	superior alveolar branches (anterior, middle, and posterior) that arise from infraorbital and maxillary n's, innervating teeth of upper jaw and maxillary sinus, and forming superior dental plexus		
ampullary n., anterior	n. ampullaris anterior	branch of vestibular part of eighth cranial (vestibulocochlear) n. that innervates ampulla of anterior semicircular duct, ending around hair cells of ampullary crest		
ampullary n., inferior. See ampullary n., posterior				
ampullary n., lateral	n. ampullaris lateralis	branch of vestibular part of eighth cranial (vestibulocochlear) n. that innervates ampulla of lateral semicircular duct, ending around hair cells of ampullary crest		
ampullary n., posterior	n. ampullaris posterior	branch of vestibular part of eighth cranial (vestibulocochlear) n. that innervates ampulla of posterior semicircular duct, ending around hair cells of ampullary crest		
ampullary n., superior. See ampullary n., anterior				
anococcygeal n's [general sensory]	nn. anococcygei	coccygeal plexus		sacrococcygeal joint, coccyx, skin over coccyx
auditory n. See vestibulocochlear n.				

*n. = nerve; n's = (pl.) nerves.
†n. = [L.] nervus; nn. = [L. (pl.)] nervi.

459

COMMON NAME* [MODALITY]	NA TERM†	ORIGIN*	BRANCHES*	DISTRIBUTION*
auricular n's, anterior [general sensory]	nn. auriculares anteriores	auriculotemporal n.		skin of anterosuperior part of external ear
auricular n., great [general sensory]	n. auricularis magnus	cervical plexus—C2–C3	anterior and posterior branches	skin over parotid gland and mastoid process, and both surfaces of auricle
auricular n., posterior [motor, general sensory]	n. auricularis posterior	facial n.	occipital branch	posterior auricular and occipitofrontal muscles, skin of external acoustic meatus
auriculotemporal n. [general sensory]	n. auriculotemporalis	by two roots from mandibular n.	anterior auricular n., n. of external acoustic meatus, parotid branches, branch to tympanic membrane, branch communicating with facial n.; terminal branches superficial temporal branches to scalp	parotid gland, scalp in temporal region, tympanic membrane. *See also* auricular n., anterior, *and* n. of external acoustic meatus
axillary n. [motor, general sensory]	n. axillaris	posterior cord of brachial plexus—C5–C6	lateral superior brachial cutaneous n., muscular branches	deltoid and teres minor muscles, skin over back of arm
buccal n. [general sensory]	n. buccalis	mandibular n.		skin and mucous membrane of cheeks, gums, and perhaps first two molars and the premolars
cardiac n., cervical, inferior [sympathetic (accelerator), visceral afferent (chiefly pain)]	n. cardiacus cervicalis inferior	cervicothoracic ganglion		heart via cardiac plexus
cardiac n., cervical, middle [sympathetic (accelerator), visceral afferent (chiefly pain)]	n. cardiacus cervicalis medius	middle cervical ganglion		heart
cardiac n., cervical, superior [sympathetic (accelerator)] cardiac n., inferior. *See* cardiac n., cervical, inferior cardiac n., middle. *See* cardiac n., cervical, middle cardiac n., superior. *See* cardiac n., cervical, superior	n. cardiacus cervicalis superior	superior cervical ganglion		heart

common name	NA term	origin	branches	distribution
cardiac n's, thoracic [sympathetic (accelerator), visceral afferent (chiefly pain)]	nn. cardiaci thoracici	ganglia T2–T4 or T5 of sympathetic trunk		heart
caroticotympanic n's [sympathetic]	nn. caroticotympanici	internal carotid plexus	together with tympanic n. forms tympanic plexus	tympanic region, parotid gland
carotid n's, external [sympathetic]	nn. carotici externi	superior cervical ganglion	help form tympanic plexus	cranial blood vessels and glands via external carotid plexus
carotid n., internal [sympathetic]	n. caroticus internus	superior cervical ganglion		cranial blood vessels and glands via internal carotid plexus
cavernous n's of clitoris [parasympathetic, sympathetic, visceral afferent]	nn. cavernosi clitoridis	uterovaginal plexus		erectile tissue of clitoris
cavernous n's of penis [sympathetic, parasympathetic, visceral afferent]	nn. cavernosi penis	prostatic plexus		erectile tissue of penis
cerebral n's. See cranial n's				
cervical n's	nn. cervicales	the 8 pairs of n's that arise from cervical segments of spinal cord and, except last pair, leave vertebral column above correspondingly numbered vertebra; the ventral branches of upper 4, on either side, unite to form cervical plexus; those of lower 4, together with ventral branch of first thoracic n., form most of brachial plexus		
cervical n., transverse [general sensory]	n. transversus colli	cervical plexus—C2–C3	superior and inferior branches	skin on side and front of neck
ciliary n's, long [sympathetic, general sensory]	nn. ciliares longi	nasociliary n., from ophthalmic n.		dilator muscle of pupil, uvea, cornea
ciliary n's, short [parasympathetic, sympathetic, general sensory]	nn. ciliares breves	ciliary ganglion		smooth muscle and tunics of eye
clunial n's, inferior [general sensory]	nn. clunium inferiores	posterior femoral cutaneous n.		skin of lower part of buttock
clunial n's, middle [general sensory]	nn. clunium medii	plexus formed by lateral branches of dorsal branches of first 4 sacral nerves behind sacrum and coccyx		ligaments of sacrum and skin over posterior part of buttock

Table of Nerves (*Continued*)

COMMON NAME* [MODALITY]	NA TERM†	ORIGIN*	BRANCHES*	DISTRIBUTION*
clunial n's, superior [general sensory]	nn. clunium superiores	lateral branches of dorsal branch of upper lumbar n's		skin of upper part of buttock
coccygeal n.	n. coccygeus	one of the pair of nerves arising from coccygeal segment of spinal cord		
cochlear n. *See* vestibulocochlear n.				
cranial n's	nn. craniales	the 12 pairs of n's connected with brain, including olfactory (I), optic (II), oculomotor (III), trochlear (IV), trigeminal (V), abducens (VI), facial (VII), vestibulocochlear (VIII), glossopharyngeal (IX), vagus (X), accessory (XI), and hypoglossal (XII) nerves		
cubital n. *See* ulnar n.				
cutaneous n. of arm, lateral, inferior [general sensory]	n. cutaneus brachii lateralis inferior	radial n.		skin of lateral surface of lower arm
cutaneous n. of arm, lateral, superior [general sensory]	n. cutaneus brachii lateralis superior	axillary n.		skin of back of arm
cutaneous n. of arm, medial [general sensory]	n. cutaneus brachii medialis	medial cord of brachial plexus (T1)		skin on medial and posterior aspects of arm
cutaneous n. of arm, posterior [general sensory]	n. cutaneus brachii posterior	radial n. in axilla		skin on back of arm
cutaneous n. of calf, lateral [general sensory]	n. cutaneus surae lateralis	common peroneal n.		skin of lateral side of back of leg, rarely may continue as sural n.
cutaneous n. of calf, medial [general sensory]	n. cutaneus surae medialis	tibial n.; usually joins peroneal communicating branch of common peroneal n. to form sural n.		may continue as sural n.
cutaneous n., dorsal, intermediate [general sensory]	n. cutaneus dorsalis intermedius	superficial peroneal n.	dorsal digital n's of foot	skin of front of lower third of leg and dorsum of foot; ankle; skin and joints of adjacent sides of third and fourth, and of fourth and fifth toes
cutaneous n., dorsal, lateral [general sensory]	n. cutaneus dorsalis lateralis	continuation of sural n.		skin and joints of lateral side of foot and fifth toe

cutaneous n's, dorsal, medial [general sensory]	n. cutaneus dorsalis medialis	superficial peroneal n.		skin and joints of medial side of foot and big toe; adjacent sides of second and third toes
cutaneous n. of forearm, lateral [general sensory]	n. cutaneus antebrachii lateralis	continuation of musculocutaneous n.		skin over radial side of forearm; sometimes an area of skin of back of hand
cutaneous n. of forearm, medial [general sensory]	n. cutaneus antebrachii medialis	medial cord of brachial plexus (C8, T1)	anterior and ulnar	skin of front, medial, and posteromedial aspects of forearm
cutaneous n. of forearm, posterior [general sensory]	n. cutaneus antebrachii posterior	radial n.		skin of dorsal aspect of forearm
cutaneous n. of thigh, lateral [general sensory]	n. cutaneus femoris lateralis	lumbar plexus—L2–L3		skin of lateral aspect and front of thigh
cutaneous n. of thigh, posterior [general sensory]	n. cutaneus femoris posterior	sacral plexus—S1–S3	inferior clunial n's; perineal branches	skin of buttock, external genitalia, back of thigh and calf
digital n's, dorsal, radial. See digital n's of radial n., dorsal				
digital n's, dorsal, ulnar. See digital n's of ulnar n., dorsal				
digital n's of foot, dorsal [general sensory]	nn. digitales dorsales pedis	intermediate dorsal cutaneous n.		skin and joints of adjacent sides of third and fourth, and of fourth and fifth toes
digital n's of lateral plantar n., common plantar, common [general sensory]	nn. digitales plantares communes nervi plantaris lateralis	superficial branch of lateral plantar n.	medial n. gives rise to 2 proper plantar digital n's	lateral one to short flexor muscle of little toe, skin and joints of little toe; lateral side of sole and little toe; medial one to adjacent sides of fourth and fifth toes
digital n's of lateral plantar n., plantar, proper [motor, general sensory]	nn. digitales plantares proprii nervi plantaris lateralis	common plantar digital n's		short flexor muscle of little toe, skin and joints of lateral side of sole and little toe, and adjacent surfaces of fourth and fifth toes
digital n's of lateral surface of great toe and medial surface of second toe, dorsal [general sensory]	nn. digitales dorsales hallucis lateralis et digiti secundi medialis	medial terminal division of deep peroneal n.		skin and joints of adjacent sides of great and second toes

TABLE OF NERVES (Continued)

COMMON NAME* [MODALITY]	NA TERM†	ORIGIN*	BRANCHES*	DISTRIBUTION*
digital n's of medial plantar n., plantar, common [motor, general sensory]	nn. digitales plantares communes nervi plantaris medialis	medial plantar n.	muscular and proper plantar digital n's	flexor hallucis brevis muscle and first lumbrical muscles, skin and joints of medial side of foot and big toe, and adjacent sides of first and second, second and third, and third and fourth toes
digital n's of medial plantar n., plantar, proper [motor, general sensory]	nn. digitales plantares proprii nervi plantaris medialis	common plantar digital n's		skin and joints of first toe, and adjacent sides of first and second, second and third, and third and fourth toes; the nerves extend to the dorsum to supply nail beds and tips of toes
digital n's of median n., palmar, common [motor, general sensory]	nn. digitales palmares communes nervi mediani	lateral and medial divisions of median n.	proper palmar digital n's	thumb, index, middle, and ring fingers, and first two lumbrical muscles
digital n's of median n., palmar, proper [motor, general sensory]	nn. digitales palmares proprii nervi mediani	common palmar digital n's		first two lumbrical muscles, skin and joints of both sides and palmar aspect of thumb, index, and middle fingers, radial side of ring finger, back of distal aspect of these digits
digital n's of radial n., dorsal [general sensory]	nn. digitales dorsales nervi radialis	superficial branch of radial n.		skin and joints of back of thumb, index finger, and part of middle finger, as far distally as digital phalanx
digital n's of ulnar n., dorsal [general sensory]4c4h	nn. digitales dorsales nervi ulnaris	dorsal branch of ulnar n.		skin and joints of medial side of little finger, dorsal aspects of adjacent sides of little and ring fingers and of ring and middle fingers
digital n's of ulnar n., palmar, common [general sensory]	nn. digitales palmares communes nervi ulnaris	superficial branch of ulnar n.	proper palmar digital n's	little and ring fingers

Common name [type]	NA term	Origin	Branches	Distribution
digital n's of ulnar n., palmar, proper [general sensory]	nn. digitales palmares proprii nervi ulnaris	the lateral of the two common palmar digital n's from superficial branch of ulnar n.		skin and joints of adjacent sides of fourth and fifth fingers
dorsal n. of clitoris [general sensory, motor]	n. dorsalis clitoridis	pudendal n.		deep transverse muscle of perineum, sphincter muscle of urethra, corpus cavernosum of clitoris, and skin, prepuce, and glans of clitoris
dorsal n. of penis [general sensory, motor]	n. dorsalis penis	pudendal n.		deep transverse muscle of perineum, sphincter muscle of urethra, corpus cavernosum of penis, and skin, prepuce, and glans of penis
dorsal scapular n. [motor]	n. dorsalis scapulae	brachial plexus—ventral branch of C5		rhomboid muscles and occasionally the levator muscle of scapula
ethmoidal n., anterior [general sensory]	n. ethmoidalis anterior	continuation of nasociliary n., from ophthalmic n.	internal, external, lateral, and medial nasal branches	mucosa of upper and anterior nasal septum, lateral wall of nasal cavity, skin of lower bridge and tip of nose
ethmoidal n., posterior [general sensory]	n. ethmoidalis posterior	nasociliary n., from ophthalmic n.		mucosa of posterior ethmoid cells and of sphenoidal sinus
n. of external acoustic meatus [general sensory]	n. meatus acustici externi	auriculotemporal n.		skin lining external acoustic meatus, and tympanic membrane
facial n. (7th cranial) [motor, parasympathetic, general sensory, special sensory]. See also intermediate n.	n. facialis	inferior border of pons, between olive and inferior cerebellar peduncle	stapedius n.; posterior auricular n.; parotid plexus; digastric, temporal, zygomatic, buccal, lingual, marginal mandibular, and cervical branches, and communicating branch with tympanic plexus	various structures of face, head, and neck (see also individual branches in this table)
femoral n. [general sensory, motor]	n. femoralis	lumbar plexus—L2-L4; descending behind inguinal ligament to femoral triangle	saphenous n., muscular and anterior cutaneous branches	skin of thigh and leg, muscles of front of thigh, and hip and knee joints (see also individual branches in this table)

TABLE OF NERVES (*Continued*)

COMMON NAME* [MODALITY]	NA TERM†	ORIGIN*	BRANCHES*	DISTRIBUTION*
fibular n. *See* entries under peroneus n.	n. fibularis (NA alternative for n. peroneus)			
frontal n. [general sensory]	n. frontalis	ophthalmic division of trigeminal n.; enters orbit through superior orbital fissure	supraorbital and supratrochlear n's	chiefly to forehead and scalp (see individual branches listed in this table)
genitofemoral n. [general sensory, motor]	n. genitofemoralis	lumbar plexus—L1–L2	genital and femoral branches	cremaster muscle, skin of scrotum or labium majus and of adjacent area of thigh and femoral triangle
glossopharyngeal n. (9th cranial) [motor, parasympathetic, general sensory, special sensory, visceral sensory]	n. glossopharyngeus	several rootlets from lateral side of upper medulla oblongata, between olive and inferior cerebellar peduncle	tympanic n., pharyngeal, stylopharyngeal, tonsillar, and lingual branches, branch to carotid sinus, communicating branch with auricular branch of vagus n.	has two enlargements (superior and inferior ganglia) and supplies tongue, pharynx, and parotid nerve (see also individual branches in this table)
gluteal n., inferior [motor]	n. gluteus inferior	sacral plexus—L5–S2		gluteus maximus muscle
gluteal n., superior [motor, general sensory]	n. gluteus superior	sacral plexus—L4–S1		gluteus medius and minimus muscles, tensor fasciae latae, and hip joint
hemorrhoidal n's, inferior. *See* rectal n's, inferior				
hypogastric n.	n. hypogastricus (dexter et sinister)	a nerve trunk situated on either side (right and left), interconnecting superior and inferior hypogastric plexuses		
hypoglossal n. (12th cranial) [motor]	n. hypoglossus	several rootlets in anterolateral sulcus between olive and pyramid of medulla oblongata; passes through hypoglossal canal to tongue	lingual branches	styloglossus, hyoglossus, and genioglossus muscles, intrinsic muscles of tongue
iliohypogastric n. [motor, general sensory]	n. iliohypogastricus	lumbar plexus—L1 (sometimes T12)	lateral and anterior cutaneous branches	skin above pubis and over lateral side of buttock, and occasionally pyramidal muscle

ilioinguinal n. [general sensory]	n. ilioinguinalis	lumbar plexus—L1 (sometimes T12); accompanies spermatic cord through inguinal canal	anterior scrotal or labial branches	skin of scrotum or labia majora, and adjacent part of thigh
infraoccipital n. See suboccipital n.				
infraorbital n. [general sensory]	n. infraorbitalis	continuation of maxillary n., entering orbit through inferior orbital fissure, occupying in succession infraorbital groove, canal, and foramen	middle and anterior superior alveolar, inferior palpebral, internal and external nasal, and superior labial branches	incisor, cuspid, and premolar teeth of upper jaw, skin and conjunctiva of lower eyelid, mobile septum and skin of side of nose, mucous membrane of mouth, skin of upper lip
infratrochlear n. [general sensory]	n. infratrochlearis	nasociliary n., from ophthalmic n.	palpebral branches	skin of root and upper bridge of nose and lower eyelid, conjunctiva, lacrimal duct
intercostobrachial n's [general sensory]	nn. intercostobrachiales	second and third intercostal n's		skin on back and medial aspect of arm
intermediate n. [parasympathetic, special sensory]	n. intermedius	smaller root of facial n., between main root and vestibulocochlear n.	greater petrosal n., chorda tympani	lacrimal, nasal, palatine, submandibular, and sublingual glands, and anterior two thirds of tongue
interosseous n. of forearm, anterior [motor, general sensory]	n. interosseous [antebrachii] anterior	median n.		flexor pollicis longus, flexor digitorum profundus, and pronator quadratus muscles, wrist and intercarpal joints
interosseous n. of forearm, posterior [motor, general sensory]	n. interosseus [antebrachii] posterior	continuation of deep branch of radial n.		long abductor muscle of thumb, extensor muscles of thumb and index finger, and wrist and intercarpal joints
interosseous n. of leg [general sensory]	interosseus cruris	tibial n.		interosseous membrane and tibiofemoral syndesmosis
ischiadic n. See sciatic n.				
jugular n.	n. jugularis	a branch of the superior cervical which communicates with glossopharyngeal and vagus n's		
labial n's, anterior [general sensory]	nn. labiales anteriores	ilioinguinal n.		skin of anterior labial region of labia majora and adjacent part of thigh
labial n's, posterior [general sensory]	nn. labiales posteriores	pudendal n.		labium majus
lacrimal n. [general sensory]	n. lacrimalis	ophthalmic division of trigeminal n. entering orbit through superior orbital fissure		lacrimal gland, conjunctiva, lateral commissure of eye, skin of upper eyelid

TABLE OF NERVES (Continued)

COMMON NAME* [MODALITY]	NA TERM†	ORIGIN*	BRANCHES*	DISTRIBUTION*
laryngeal n., inferior [motor]	n. laryngeus inferior	recurrent laryngeal n., especially the terminal portion		intrinsic muscles of larynx, except cricothyroid communicates with internal laryngeal n.
laryngeal n., recurrent [parasympathetic, visceral afferent, motor]	n. laryngeus recurrens	vagus n. (chiefly the cranial part of the accessory n.)	inferior laryngeal n., tracheal, esophageal, and inferior cardiac branches	tracheal mucosa, esophagus, cardiac plexus (see also individual branches in this table)
laryngeal n., superior [motor, general sensory, visceral afferent, parasympathetic]	n. laryngeus superior	inferior ganglion of vagus n.	external, internal, and communicating branches	cricothyroid muscle and inferior constrictor muscle of pharynx, mucous membrane of back of tongue and larynx
lingual n. [general sensory]	n. lingualis	mandibular n., descending to tongue, first medial to mandible and then under cover of mucosa of mouth	sublingual n., lingual branch, branch to isthmus of fauces, branch communicating with hypoglossal n. and chorda tympani	anterior two thirds of tongue, adjacent areas of mouth, gums, isthmus of fauces
lumbar n's	nn. lumbales	the 5 pairs of n's that arise from lumbar segments of spinal cord, each pair leaving vertebral column below correspondingly numbered vertebrae; ventral branches of these nerves participate in formation of lumbosacral plexus		
mandibular n. (third division of trigeminal n.) [general sensory, motor]	n. mandibularis	trigeminal ganglion	meningeal branch, masseteric, deep temporal, lateral and medial pterygoid, buccal, auriculotemporal, lingual and inferior alveolar n's	extensive distribution to muscles of mastication, skin of face, mucous membrane of mouth, and teeth (see also individual branches in this table)
masseteric n. [motor, general sensory]	n. massetericus	mandibular division of trigeminal n.		masseter muscle, temporomandibular joint
maxillary n. (second division of trigeminal n.) [general sensory]	n. maxillaris	trigeminal ganglion	meningeal branch, zygomatic n., posterior superior alveolar branches, infraorbital n., pterygopalatine n's, and indirectly branches of pterygopalatine ganglion	extensive distribution to skin of face and scalp, mucous membrane of maxillary sinus and nasal cavity, and teeth

Nerve [type]	Origin	Branches	Distribution
median n. [general sensory]	lateral and medial cords of brachial plexus—C6–T1	anterior interosseous n. of forearm, common palmar digital n's, and muscular and palmar branches, and a communicating branch with ulnar n.	ultimately, skin on front of lateral part of hand, most of flexor muscles of front of forearm, most of short muscles of thumb, elbow joint, and many joints of hand
mental n. [general sensory]	inferior alveolar n.	mental and inferior labial branches	skin of chin, lower lip
musculocutaneous n. [general sensory, motor]	lateral cord of brachial plexus—C5–C7	lateral cutaneous n. of forearm, muscular branches	coracobrachial, biceps, brachial muscles, elbow joint, skin of radial side of forearm
mylohyoid n. [motor]	inferior alveolar n.		mylohyoid muscle, anterior belly of digastric muscle
nasociliary n. [general sensory]	ophthalmic division of trigeminal nerve	long ciliary, posterior ethmoidal, anterior ethmoidal, and infratrochlear n's and a communicating branch to ciliary ganglion	(see individual branches in this table)
nasopalatine n. [parasympathetic, general sensory]	pterygopalatine ganglion		mucosa and glands of most of nasal septum and anterior part of hard palate
obturator n. [general sensory, motor]	lumbar plexus—L3–L4	anterior, posterior, and muscular branches	gracilis and adductor muscles, skin of medial part of thigh, and hip joints
occipital n., greater [general sensory, motor]	medial branch of dorsal branch of C2		semispinal muscle of head and skin of head as far forward as vertex
occipital n., lesser [general sensory]	superficial cervical plexus—C2–C3		ascends behind auricle and supplies some of the skin of side of head and on cranial surface of auricle
occipital n., third [general sensory]	medial branch of dorsal branch of C3		skin of upper part of back of neck and head
oculomotor n. (3rd cranial) [motor, parasympathetic]	brain stem, emerging medial to cerebral peduncles, running forward in the cavernous sinus	superior and inferior branches	entering orbit through superior orbital fissure, the branches supply levator muscle of upper lid, all extrinsic muscles except lateral rectus and superior oblique, and carry parasympathetic fibers from ciliary muscle to sphincter of pupil

TABLE OF NERVES (*Continued*)

COMMON NAME* [MODALITY]	NA TERM†	ORIGIN*	BRANCHES*	DISTRIBUTION*
olfactory n's (1st cranial) [special sensory]	nn. olfactorii	the n's of smell, consisting of about 20 bundles arising in the olfactory epithelium and passing through the cribriform plate of ethmoid bone to olfactory bulb		
ophthalmic n. (first division of trigeminal n.) [general sensory]	n. ophthalmicus	trigeminal ganglion	tentorial branches, frontal, lacrimal, nasociliary n's	eyeball and conjunctiva, lacrimal sac and gland, nasal mucosa and frontal sinus, external nose, eyelid, forehead, and scalp (see also individual branches in this table)
optic n. (2nd cranial) [special sensory]	n. opticus	the nerve of sight, consisting chiefly of axons and central processes of cells of the ganglionic layer of retina leaving the orbit through the optic canal, joining the optic chiasm (the medial ones crossing over to opposite side), and continuing as the optic tract		
palatine n., anterior. *See* palatine n., greater				
palatine n., greater [parasympathetic, sympathetic, general sensory]	n. palatinus major	pterygopalatine ganglion	posterior inferior [lateral] nasal branches	emerges through greater palatine foramen and supplies palate
palatine n's, lesser [parasympathetic, sympathetic, general sensory]	nn. palatini minores	pterygopalatine ganglion		emerge through lesser palatine foramen and supply soft palate and tonsil
perineal n's [general sensory, motor]	nn. perineales	pudendal n. in pudendal canal	muscular branches and posterior scrotal or labial nerves	muscular branches supply bulbospongiosus, ischiocavernosus, superficial transverse perinei muscles and bulb of penis and, in part, sphincter ani externi and levator ani; the scrotal (labial) n's supply the scrotum or labium majus
peroneal n., common [general sensory, motor]	n. peroneus communis	sciatic n. in lower thigh	supplies short head of biceps femoris muscle (while still incorporated in sciatic nerve); gives off lateral sural cutaneous n. and peroneal communicating branch descends in popliteal fossa, supplies knee and superior tibiofibular joints and anterior tibial muscle, and divides into superficial and deep peroneal n's	

Common name [modality]	Latin name	Origin	Branches	Distribution
peroneal n., deep [general sensory, motor]	n. peroneus profundus	a terminal branch of common peroneal n.		winds around neck of fibula and descends on interosseous membrane to front of ankle; gives off muscular branches to tibialis anterior, extensor digitorum longus, and peroneus tertius muscles, and a twig to ankle joint; lateral terminal division supplies extensor digitorum brevis muscle and tarsal joints; medial terminal division (digital branch) divides into dorsal digital nerves for skin and joints of adjacent sides of big and second toes
peroneal n., superficial [general sensory, motor]	n. peroneus superficialis	a terminal branch of common peroneal n.		descends in front of fibula and, in lower leg, divides into muscular branches and, medial and intermediate dorsal cutaneous n's (see also individual branches in this table)
petrosal n., deep [sympathetic]	n. petrosus profundus	internal carotid plexus		joins greater petrosal n. to form n. of pterygoid canal, and supplies lacrimal, nasal, and palatine glands via pterygopalatine ganglion and its branches
petrosal n., greater [parasympathetic, general sensory]	n. petrosus major	intermediate n. via geniculate ganglion		running forward from geniculate ganglion, joins deep petrosal n. of pterygoid canal, and reaches lacrimal, nasal, and palatine glands and nasopharynx via pterygopalatine ganglion and its branches
petrosal n. lesser [parasympathetic]	n. petrosus minor	tympanic plexus		parotid gland via otic ganglion and auriculotemporal n.
phrenic n. [general sensory, motor]	n. phrenicus	cervical plexus—C4–C5	pericardial and phrenico-abdominal branches	pleura, pericardium, diaphragm, peritoneum, sympathetic plexuses
phrenic n's, accessory	nn. phrenici accessorii	inconstant contribution of fifth cervical n. to phrenic n.; when present, they run a separate course to root of neck or into thorax before joining phrenic n.		
plantar n., lateral [general sensory, motor]	n. plantaris lateralis	smaller of terminal branches of tibial n.	muscular, superficial, and deep branches	lying between first and second layers of muscles of sole, supplies quadratus plantae, abductor digiti minimi, flexor digiti minimi brevis, adductor hallucis, interossei, and second, third, and fourth lumbrical muscles, and gives off cutaneous and articular twigs to lateral side of sole and fourth and fifth toes (see also individual branches in this table)

TABLE OF NERVES (Continued)

COMMON NAME* [MODALITY]	NA TERM†	ORIGIN*	BRANCHES*	DISTRIBUTION*
plantar n., medial [general sensory, motor]	n. plantaris medialis	larger of terminal branches of tibial n.	common plantar digital n's and muscular branches	abductor hallucis, flexor digitorum brevis, and first lumbrical muscles and cutaneous and articular twigs to medial side of sole and first to fourth toes (see also individual branches in this table)
pneumogastric n. See vagus n.				
pterygoid n., lateral [motor]	n. pterygoideus lateralis	mandibular n.		lateral pterygoid, tensor tympani, and tensor veli palatini muscles
pterygoid n., medial [motor]	n. pterygoideus medialis	mandibular n.		medial pterygoid muscle
n. of pterygoid canal [parasympathetic, sympathetic]	n. canalis pterygoidei	union of deep and greater petrosal n's		pterygopalatine ganglion and branches
pterygopalatine n's [general sensory]	nn. pterygopalatini	two nerves connecting maxillary n. to pterygopalatine ganglion; they are the sensory roots of the ganglion		
pudendal n. [general sensory, motor, parasympathetic]	n. pudendus	sacral plexus—S2–S4	enters pudendal canal, gives off inferior rectal n., then divides into perineal n. and dorsal n. of penis (clitoris)	muscles, skin, and erectile tissue of perineum (see also individual branches in this table)
radial n. [general sensory, motor]	n. radialis	posterior cord of brachial plexus—C6–C8, and sometimes C5 and T1	posterior cutaneous and inferior lateral cutaneous n's of arm, posterior cutaneous n. of forearm, muscular, deep, and superficial branches	descending in back of arm and forearm, ultimately distributed to skin on back of forearm, arm, and hand, extensor muscles on back of arm and forearm, and elbow joint and many joints of hand
rectal n's, inferior [general sensory, motor]	nn. rectales inferiores	pudendal n., or independently from sacral plexus		sphincter ani externus muscle, skin around anus, lining of anal canal up to pectinate line
recurrent n. See laryngeal n., recurrent				

n. saccularis	saccular n.	the branch of vestibular part of eighth cranial (vestibulocochlear) nerve that innervates macula of saccule		
nn. sacrales	sacral n's	the 5 pairs of n's that arise from sacral segments of spinal cord; the ventral branches of first 4 pairs participate in formation of sacral plexus		
n. saphenus	saphenous n. [general sensory]	termination of femoral n.	infrapatellar and medial crural cutaneous	knee joint, subsartorial and patellar plexuses, skin on medial side of leg and foot
n. ischiadicus	sciatic n. [general sensory, motor]	sacral plexus—L4–S3; leaves pelvis through greater sciatic foramen	divides into common peroneal and tibial n's, usually in lower third of thigh	(see individual branches in this table)
nn. scrotales anteriores	scrotal n's, anterior [general sensory]	ilioinguinal n.		skin of anterior scrotal region
nn. scrotales posteriores	scrotal n's, posterior [general sensory]	perineal n's		skin of scrotum
nn. spinales	spinal n's	the 31 pairs of n's that arise from spinal cord, and pass between the vertebrae, including 8 cervical, 12 thoracic, 5 lumbar, 5 sacral, and 1 coccygeal		
n. splanchnicus major	splanchnic n., greater [preganglionic sympathetic, visceral afferent]	thoracic sympathetic trunk and thoracic ganglia T5–T10 of sympathetic trunk		descending through diaphragm or its aortic opening, ends in celiac ganglia and plexuses, with a splanchnic ganglion commonly near the diaphragm
n. splanchnicus minor	splanchnic n., lesser [preganglionic sympathetic, visceral afferent]	thoracic ganglia T9, T10 or sympathetic trunk	renal branch	pierces diaphragm, joins aorticorenal ganglion and celiac plexus, and communicates with renal and superior mesenteric plexuses
n. splanchnicus imus	splanchnic n., lowest [sympathetic, visceral afferent]	last ganglion of sympathetic trunk, or lesser splanchnic n.		aorticorenal ganglion and adjacent plexus
nn. splanchnici lumbales	splanchnic n's, lumbar [preganglionic sympathetic, visceral afferent]	lumbar ganglia or sympathetic trunk		upper nerves join celiac and adjacent plexuses, middle ones go to mesenteric and adjacent plexuses, lower ones descend to superior hypogastric plexus
nn. splanchnici pelvini	splanchnic n's, pelvic [preganglionic parasympathetic, visceral afferent]	sacral plexus—S3–S4		leaving sacral plexus, they enter inferior hypogastric plexus and supply pelvic organs

COMMON NAME* [MODALITY]	NA TERM†	ORIGIN*	BRANCHES*	DISTRIBUTION*
splanchnic n's, sacral [preganglionic sympathetic, visceral afferent]	nn. splanchnici sacrales	sacral part of sympathetic trunk		pelvic organs and blood vessels via inferior hypogastric plexus
stapedius n. [motor]	n. stapedius	facial n.		stapedius muscle
subclavian n. [motor, general sensory]	n. subclavius	upper trunk of brachial plexus—C5		subclavius muscle, sternoclavicular joint
subcostal n. [generally sensory, motor]	n. subcostalis	ventral branch of T12		skin of lower abdomen and lateral side of gluteal region, parts of transverse, oblique, and rectus muscles, and usually pyramidal muscle, and adjacent peritoneum
sublingual n. [parasympathetic, general sensory]	n. sublingualis	lingual n.		sublingual gland and overlying mucous membrane
suboccipital n. [motor]	n. suboccipitalis	dorsal branch of C1		emerges above posterior arch of atlas, supplies muscles of suboccipital triangle and semispinal muscle of head
subscapular n. [motor]	n. subscapularis	posterior cord of brachial plexus—C5		usually two or more nerves, upper and lower, supplying subscapular and teres major muscles
supraclavicular n's, anterior. *See supraclavicular n's, medial*				
supraclavicular n's, intermediate [general sensory]	nn. supraclaviculares intermedii	cervical plexus—C3–C4		descends in posterior triangle, crosses clavicle, supplying skin over pectoral and deltoid regions
supraclavicular n's, lateral [general sensory]	nn. supraclaviculares laterales	cervical plexus—C3–C4		descends in posterior triangle, crosses clavicle, supplying skin of superior and posterior aspects of shoulder
supraclavicular n's, medial [general sensory]	nn. supraclaviculares mediales	cervical plexus—C3–C4		descends in posterior triangle, crosses clavicle, supplying skin of medial infraclavicular region

supraclavicular n's, middle. *See* supraclavicular n's, intermediate		
supraclavicular n's, posterior. *See* supraclavicular n's, lateral		
supraorbital n. [general sensory]	continuation of frontal n., from ophthalmic n.	lateral and medial branches	leaves orbit through supraorbital notch or foramen, supplying skin of upper eyelid, forehead, anterior part of scalp (to vertex), mucosa of frontal sinus
suprascapular n. [motor, general sensory]	brachial plexus—C5–C6		descends through suprascapular and spinoglenoid notches, supplying acromioclavicular and shoulder joints, and supraspinous and infraspinous muscles
supratrochlear n. [general sensory]	frontal n., from ophthalmic n.		leaves orbit at end of supraorbital margin, supplying forehead and upper eyelid
sural n. [general sensory]	medial sural n. and communicating branch of common peroneal n.	lateral dorsal cutaneous n. and lateral calcaneal branches	skin on back of leg, and skin and joints on lateral side of foot and heel
temporal n's, deep [motor]	nn. temporales profundi		temporal muscles
n. of tensor tympani [motor]	mandibular n. via n. to medial pterygoid muscle and otic ganglion		tensor muscle of tympanum
n. of tensor veli palatini [motor]	mandibular n. via n. to medial pterygoid muscle and otic ganglion		tensor muscle of palatine velum
thoracic n's	the 12 pairs of spinal n's that arise from thoracic segments of spinal cord, each pair leaving vertebral column below correspondingly numbered vertebra		body wall of thorax and upper part of abdomen
thoracic n., long [motor]	brachial plexus—ventral branches of C5–C7		descends behind brachial plexus to anterior serratus muscle
thoracodorsal n. [motor]	posterior cord of brachial plexus—C7–C8		latissimus dorsi muscle

TABLE OF NERVES (Concluded)

COMMON NAME* [MODALITY]	NA TERM†	ORIGIN*	BRANCHES*	DISTRIBUTION*
tibial n. [general sensory, motor]	n. tibialis	sciatic n. in lower thigh	interosseous n. of leg, medial cutaneous n. of calf, sural and medial and lateral plantar n's, and muscular and medial calcaneal branches	while still incorporated in sciatic n., supplies semimembranous and semitendinous muscles, long head of biceps, and adductor magnus muscle; supplies knee joint as it descends in popliteal fossa continuing into leg, supplies muscles and skin of calf, sole, and toes (see also individual branches in this table)
trigeminal n. (5th cranial) [general sensory, motor]	n. trigeminus	emerges from lateral surface of pons as a motor and a sensory root, the latter expanding into trigeminal ganglion, from which the 3 divisions of nerve arise (see mandibular n., maxillary n., and ophthalmic n.)		face, teeth, mouth, nasal cavity, muscles of mastication
trochlear n. (4th cranial) [motor]	n. trochlearis	fibers of each nerve (one on either side) decussate across median plane, and emerge from back of brain stem below corresponding inferior colliculus		runs forward in lateral wall of cavernous sinus, traverses superior orbital fissure, supplying superior oblique muscle of eyeball
tympanic n. [general sensory, parasympathetic]	n. tympanicus	inferior ganglion of glossopharyngeal n.	helps form tympanic plexus	mucous membrane of tympanic cavity, mastoid air cells, auditory tube, and, via lesser petrosal n. and otic ganglion, parotid gland
ulnar n. [general sensory, motor]	n. ulnaris	medial and lateral cords of brachial plexus—C7–T1	muscular, dorsal, palmar, superficial, and deep branches	ultimately to skin on front and medial part of hand, some flexor muscles on front of forearm, many short muscles of hand, elbow joint, many joints of hand
utricular n.	n. utricularis	the branch of vestibular part of eighth cranial (vestibulocochlear) n. that innervates macula of utricle		
utriculoampullary n.	n. utriculoampullaris	a n. that arises by peripheral division of vestibular part of eighth cranial (vestibulocochlear) nerve, and supplies utricle and ampullae of semicircular ducts		

vaginal n's [sympathetic, parasympathetic]	nn. vaginales	uterovaginal plexus		vagina
vagus n. (10th cranial) [parasympathetic, visceral afferent, motor, general sensory]	n. vagus	by numerous rootlets from lateral side of medulla oblongata in groove between olive and inferior cerebellar peduncle	superior and recurrent laryngeal n's, meningeal, auricular, pharyngeal, cardiac, bronchial, gastric, hepatic, celiac, and renal branches, pharyngeal, pulmonary, and esophageal plexuses, and anterior and posterior trunks	descending through jugular foramen, presents as a superior and an inferior ganglion, continues through neck and thorax into abdomen, supplying sensory fibers to ear, tongue, pharynx, and larynx, motor fibers to pharynx, larynx, esophagus, and parasympathetic and visceral fibers to thoracic and abdominal viscera (see also individual branches in this table)
vertebral n. [sympathetic]	n. vertebralis	cervicothoracic and vertebral		ascends with vertebral artery and gives fibers to spinal meninges, cervical n's, and posterior cranial fossa
vestibulocochlear n. (8th cranial)	n. vestibulocochlearis	emerges from brain between pons and medulla oblongata, at cerebellopontine angle and behind facial n.; it consists of 2 sets of fibers, the vestibular part from utricle, saccule, and semicircular ducts, and the cochlear part, from the cochlea, and is connected with the brain by corresponding superior and inferior roots		
vidian n. *See* n. of pterygoid canal				
vidian n., deep. *See* petrosal n., deep				
zygomatic n. [general sensory]	n. zygomaticus	maxillary n., entering orbit through inferior orbital fissure	zygomaticofacial and zygomaticotemporal branches	communicates with lacrimal nerve, supplying skin of temple and adjacent part of face

nerve cell bodies have a tendency during development to migrate toward the source of their stimulation. **neurobiotac′tic,** adj.

neuroblast (nu′ro-blast) an embryonic cell from which nervous tissue is formed.

neuroblastoma (nu″ro-blas-to′mah) sarcoma of nervous system origin, composed chiefly of neuroblasts, affecting mostly infants and children up to 10 years of age, usually arising in the autonomic nervous system (sympathicoblastoma) or in the adrenal medulla.

neurocanal (-kah-nal′) vertebral canal.

neurocardiac (-kar′de-ak) pertaining to the nervous system and the heart.

neurocentrum (-sen′trum) one of the embryonic vertebral elements from which the spinous processes of the vertebrae develop. **neurocen′tral,** adj.

neurochemistry (kem′is-tre) that branch of neurology dealing with the chemistry of the nervous system.

neurochorioretinitis (-ko″re-o-ret″ĭ-ni′tis) inflammation of the optic nerve, choroid, and retina.

neurochoroiditis (-ko″roi-di′tis) inflammation of the optic nerve and choroid.

neurocirculatory (-sir′ku-lah-to″re) pertaining to the nervous and circulatory systems.

neurocladism (nu-rok′lah-dizm) the formation of new branches by the process of a neuron.

neuroclonic (nu″ro-klon′ik) marked by nervous spasm.

neurocoele (nu′ro-sēl) vertebral canal.

neurocranium (nu″ro-kra′ne-um) the part of the cranium enclosing the brain. **neurocra′nial,** adj.

neurocrine (nu′ro-krĭn) 1. denoting an endocrine influence on or by the nerves. 2. pertaining to neurosecretion.

neurocutaneous (nu″ro-ku-ta′ne-us) pertaining to the nerves and skin, or the cutaneous nerves.

neurocyte (nu′ro-sīt) a nerve cell of any kind.

neurocytolysin (nu″ro-si-tol′ĭ-sin) a constituent of certain snake venoms which lyses nerve cells.

neurocytoma (-si-to′mah) a brain tumor consisting of undifferentiated nerve cells of nervous origin, i.e., cells resembling medullary neural epithelium.

neurodendrite (-den′drīt) dendrite.

neurodendron (-den′dron) dendrite.

neurodermatitis (-der″mah-ti′tis), pl. *neurodermatit′ides* [Gr.] a general term for a dermatosis presumed to be caused by itching due to emotional causes; also used to refer to n. circumscripta (*lichen simplex chronicus*) and sometimes n. disseminata (*atopic dermatitis*).

neurodynamic (-di-nam′ik) pertaining to nervous energy.

neurodynia (-din′e-ah) pain in a nerve.

neuroencephalomyelopathy (-en-sef″ah-lo-mi″ĕ-lop′ah-the) disease involving the nerves, brain, and spinal cord.

neuroendocrine (-en′do-krin) pertaining to neural and endocrine influence, and particularly to the interaction between the nervous and endocrine systems.

neuroendocrinology (-en″do-kri-nol′o-je) the study of the interactions of the nervous and endocrine systems.

neuroepithelioma (-ep″ĭ-the″le-o′mah) neurocytoma.

neuroepithelium (-ep″ĭ-the′le-um) 1. epithelium made up of cells specialized to serve as sensory cells for reception of external stimuli. 2. the ectodermal epithelium, from which the cerebrospinal axis is derived.

neurofibril, neurofibrilla (-fi′bril; -fi-bril′ah) one of the delicate threads running in every direction through the cytoplasm of a nerve cell, extending into the axon and dendrites.

neurofibroma (-fi-bro′mah) a tumor of peripheral nerves due to abnormal proliferation of Schwann cells.

neurofibromatosis (-fi″bro-mah-to′sis) a familial condition characterized by developmental changes in the nervous system, muscles, bones, and skin, and marked by the formation of neurofibromas over the entire body associated with areas of pigmentation.

neurogenesis (-jen′ĕ-sis) the development of nervous tissue.

neurogenic (-jen′ik) 1. forming nervous tissue, or stimulating nervous energy. 2. originating in the nervous system.

neurogenous (nu-roj′ĕ-nus) arising in the nervous system, or from some lesion of the nervous system.

neuroglia (nu-rog′le-ah) the supporting structure of nervous tissue, consisting, in the central nervous system, of astrocytes, oligodendrocytes, and microglia. **neurog′lial,** adj.

neurogliocyte (nu-rog′le-o-sīt) one of the cells composing the neuroglia.

neuroglioma (nu″ro-gli-o′mah) a tumor composed of neuroglial tissue. **n. gangliona′re,** ganglioneuroma.

neurogliosis (nu-rog″le-o′sis) a condition marked by numerous neurogliomas.

neurogram (nu′ro-gram) the imprint left on the brain by past mental experiences.

neurohistology (nu″ro-his-tol′o-je) histology of the nervous system.

neurohormone (nu′ro-hor″mōn) a hormone stimulating the neural mechanism.

neurohumor (nu″ro-hu′mor) a chemical substance formed in a neuron and able to activate or modify the function of a neighboring neuron, muscle, or gland. **neurohu′moral,** adj.

neurohypophysis (-hi-pof′ĭ-sis) the posterior (or neural) lobe of the pituitary gland. **neurohypophys′eal,** adj.

neuroid (nu′roid) resembling a nerve.

neuroinduction (nu″ro-in-duk′shun) mental suggestion.

neurokeratin (-ker′ah-tin) a protein network seen in histological specimens of the myelin sheath.

neurolemma (-lem′ah) neurilemma.

neurolemmitis (-lĕ-mi′tis) neurilemmitis.

neurolemmoma (-lĕ-mo′mah) neurilemoma.

neuroleptanalgesia (-lep″tan-al-je′ze-ah) a state of quiescence, altered awareness, and analgesia produced by a combination of a narcotic analgesic and a neuroleptic.

neuroleptic (-lep′tik) 1. denoting a neuropharmacologic agent having antipsychotic action affecting mainly psychomotor activity. 2. an agent producing such action.

neurologist (nu-rol′o-jist) a specialist in neurology.

neurology (nu-rol′o-je) that branch of medical science which deals with the nervous system, both normal and in disease. **neurolog′ic**, adj. **clinical n.**, that especially concerned with the diagnosis and treatment of disorders of the nervous system.

neurolysin (nu-rol′ĭ-sin) a cytolysin with a specific destructive action on neurons.

neurolysis (nu-rol′ĭ-sis) 1. release of a nerve sheath by cutting it longitudinally. 2. operative breaking up of perineural adhesions. 3. relief of tension upon a nerve obtained by stretching. 4. exhaustion of nervous energy. 5. destruction or dissolution of nerve tissue. **neurolyt′ic**, adj.

neuroma (nu-ro′mah) a tumor or new growth largely made up of nerve cells and nerve fibers; a tumor growing from a nerve. **neurom′atous**, adj. **acoustic n.**, a benign tumor within the auditory canal arising from the eighth cranial (acoustic) nerve. **amputation n.**, traumatic neuroma occurring after amputation of an extremity or part. **n. cu′tis**, neuroma in the skin. **false n.**, one which does not contain nerve elements. **plexiform n.**, one made up of contorted nerve trunks. **n. telangiecto′des**, one containing an excess of blood vessels. **traumatic n.**, an unorganized bulbous or nodular mass of nerve fibers and Schwann cells produced by hyperplasia of nerve fibers and their supporting tissues after accidental or purposeful sectioning of the nerve.

neuromalacia (nu″ro-mah-la′she-ah) morbid softening of the nerves.

neuromatosis (-mah-to′sis) a condition marked by the presence of many neuromas.

neuromechanism (-mek′ah-nizm) the structure and arrangement of the nervous system in relation to function.

neuromere (nu′ro-mēr) 1. any of a series of transitory segmental elevations in the wall of the neural tube in the developing embryo; also, such elevations in the wall of the mature rhombencephalon. 2. a part of the spinal cord to which a pair of dorsal roots and a pair of ventral roots are attached.

neuromuscular (nu″ro-mus′ku-ler) pertaining to nerves and muscles.

neuromyelitis (-mi″ĕ-li′tis) inflammation of nervous and medullary substance; myelitis attended with neuritis. **n. op′tica**, combined demyelination of the optic nerve and spinal cord, with diminution of vision and possible blindness, flaccid paralysis of extremities, and sensory and genitourinary disturbances.

neuromyositis (-mi″o-si′tis) neuritis blended with myositis.

neuron (nu′ron) nerve cell; any of the conducting cells of the nervous system, consisting of a cell body, containing the nucleus and its surrounding cytoplasm and the axon and dendrites. See Plate XI. **neuro′nal**, adj. **afferent n.**, one that conducts a nervous impulse from a receptor to a center. **efferent n.**, one that conducts a nervous impulse from a center to an organ of response. **Golgi n's**, 1. (*type I*): pyramidal cells with long axons, which leave the gray matter of the central nervous system, traverse the white matter, and terminate in the periphery. 2. (*type II*): stellate neurons with short axons in the cerebral and cerebellar cortices and in the retina. **motor n.**, motoneuron. **postganglionic n's**, neurons whose cell bodies lie in the autonomic ganglia and whose purpose is to relay impulses beyond the ganglia. **preganglionic n's**, neurons whose cell bodies lie in the central nervous system and whose efferent fibers terminate in the autonomic ganglia. **sensory n.**, any neuron having a sensory function; an afferent neuron conveying sensory impulses.

neuronevus (nu″ro-ne′vus) a cellular or nevocytic nevus, especially a mature one with differentiation toward neural skin structures.

neuronophage (nu-ron′o-fāj) a phagocyte that destroys nerve cells.

neuronophagia (nu″ron-o-fa′je-ah) phagocytic destruction of nerve cells.

neuro-ophthalmology (nu″ro-of″thal-mol′o-je) the specialty dealing with the portions of the nervous system related to the eye.

neuropapillitis (-pap″ĭ-li′tis) optic neuritis.

neuroparalysis (-pah-ral′ĭ-sis) paralysis due to disease of a nerve or nerves.

neuropathogenicity (-path″o-jĕ-nis′ĭ-te) the quality of producing or the ability to produce pathologic changes in nerve tissue.

neuropathology (-pah-thol′o-je) pathology of diseases of the nervous system.

neuropathy (nu-rop′ah-the) any functional disturbances and/or pathological changes in the peripheral nervous system; also used to denote nonspecific lesions, in contrast to inflammatory lesions (see *neuritis*). **neuropath′ic**, adj. **ascending n.**, that progressing from the feet upwards to affect thigh, hip, trunk, etc. **descending n.**, that starting proximately (shoulder, hip) and spreading distally toward the limb extremities (hands, feet). **entrapment n.**, any of a group of neuropathies, e.g., carpal tunnel syndrome, due to mechanical pressure on a peripheral nerve. **progressive hypertrophic interstitial n.**, a slowly progressive familial disease beginning in early life, marked by hyperplasia of interstitial connective tissue, causing thickening of peripheral nerve trunks and posterior roots, and by sclerosis of the posterior columns of the spinal cord, with atrophy of distal parts of the legs and diminution of tendon reflexes and sensation.

neuropharmacology (nu″ro-far″mah-kol′o-je) the scientific study of the effects of drugs on the nervous system.

neurophthisis (nu-rof′thĭ-sis) wasting of nerve tissue.

neurophysiology (nu″ro-fiz″e-ol′o-je) physiology of the nervous system.

neuropil (nu′ro-pīl) a feltwork of interwoven

dendrites and axons and of neuroglial cells in the central nervous system and in some parts of the peripheral nervous system.

neuroplasm (-plazm) the protoplasm of a nerve cell. **neuroplas′mic,** adj.

neuroplasty (-plas″te) plastic repair of a nerve.

neuropodium (nu″ro-po′de-um) a bullous termination of an axon in one type of synapse.

neuropore (nu′ro-pōr) the open anterior or posterior end of the neural tube of the early embryo; they close as the embryo develops.

neuropotential (nu″ro-po-ten′shal) nerve energy; nerve potential.

neuropsychiatrist (-si-ki′ah-trist) a specialist in neuropsychiatry.

neuropsychiatry (-si-ki′ah-tre) the combined specialties of neurology and psychiatry.

neuropsychopathy (-si-kop′ah-the) a combined nervous and mental disease.

neuroradiology (-ra″de-ol′o-je) radiology of the nervous system.

neurorecidive (-res″ĭ-dēv′) neurorelapse.

neurorecurrence (-re-ker′ens) neurorelapse.

neurorelapse (nu′ro-re-laps″) acute nervous symptoms precipitated by insufficient treatment of syphilis with arsphenamine.

neuroretinitis (nu″ro-ret″ĭ-ni′tis) inflammation of the optic nerve and retina.

neuroretinopathy (ret″ĭ-nop′ah-the) pathologic involvement of the optic disk and retina.

neuroroentgenography (-rent″gen-og′rah-fe) neuroradiology.

neurorrhaphy (nu-ror′ah-fe) suture of a divided nerve.

neurosarcokleisis (nu″ro-sar″ko-kli′sis) an operation performed for neuralgia, done by relieving pressure on the affected nerve by partial resection of the bony canal through which it passes, and transplanting the nerve among soft tissues.

neurosarcoma (-sar-ko′mah) a sarcoma with neuromatous elements.

neurosclerosis (-skle-ro′sis) hardening of nerve tissue.

neurosecretion (-se-kre′shun) secretory activities of nerve cells. **neurosecre′tory,** adj.

neurosis (nu-ro′sis), pl. *neuro′ses.* An emotional disorder due to unresolved conflicts, anxiety being its chief characteristic; in contrast with psychoses, neuroses do not involve gross distortions of external reality or disorganization of personality. **neurot′ic,** adj. **accident n.,** a neurosis with hysterical symptoms caused by accident or injury. **anxiety n.,** anxiety reaction; neurosis characterized by morbid and unjustified dread, sometimes extending to panic and often associated somatic symptoms. **cardiac n.,** neurocirculatory asthenia. **character n.,** a neurosis in which certain personality traits have become exaggerated or overdeveloped. **combat n.,** a neurosis resulting from battle experiences and conditions of military life. **compensation n.,** a neurosis following injury and motivated in part by prospects of financial compensation. **compulsive n.,** an urge to perform unacceptable or senseless acts. **conversion n.,** see under *reac-*

tion. **obsessional n.,** that marked by obsessions that dominate the patient's conduct. **obsessive-compulsive n.,** that marked by the persistent intrusion of repetitive thoughts or urges, compelling the performance of ritual acts. **occupational n.,** neurosis in which the symptoms are related to the patient's occupation and interfere with its pursuit. **traumatic n.,** neurosis resulting from an injury. **vegetative n.,** acrodynia.

neuroskeletal (nu″ro-skel′ĕ-tal) pertaining to nervous tissue and skeletal muscular tissue.

neuroskeleton (-skel′ĕ-ton) endoskeleton.

neurosome (nu′ro-sōm) 1. the body of a nerve cell. 2. any of a set of small particles in the ground substance of neurons.

neurospasm (-spazm) nervous twitching of a muscle.

neurosplanchnic (nu″ro-splangk′nik) pertaining to the cerebrospinal and sympathetic nervous systems.

neurospongioma (-spun″je-o′mah) neuroglioma.

neurospongium (-spun″je-um) 1. the fibrillar component of neurons. 2. a meshwork of nerve fibers, especially the inner reticular layer of the retina.

Neurospora (nu-ros′po-rah) a genus of fungi, comprising the bread molds, capable of converting tryptophan to niacin; used in genetic and enzyme research.

neurosurgeon (nu″ro-ser′jun) a physician who specializes in neurosurgery.

neurosurgery (-ser′jer-e) surgery of the nervous system.

neurosuture (nu′ro-su″tūr) neurorrhaphy.

neurosyphilis (nu″ro-sif′ĭ-lus) syphilis of the central nervous system. **paretic n.,** dementia paralytica. **tabetic n.,** tabes dorsalis.

neurotendinous (-ten′dĭ-nus) pertaining to both nerve and tendon.

neurotherapy (-ther′ah-pe) the treatment of nervous disorders.

neurotic (nu-rot′ik) 1. pertaining to or affected with a neurosis. 2. pertaining to the nerves. 3. a nervous person in whom emotions predominate over reason.

neuroticism (nu-rot″ĭ-sizm) a neurotic condition or trait.

neurotization (nu-rot″ĭ-za′shun) 1. regeneration of a nerve after its division. 2. the implantation of a nerve into a paralyzed muscle.

neurotmesis (nu″rot-me′sis) damage to a nerve, producing complete division of all the essential structures.

neurotome (nu′ro-tōm) 1. a needle-like knife for dissecting nerves. 2. neuromere.

neurotomy (nu-rot′o-me) dissection or cutting of nerves.

neurotonic (nu″ro-ton′ik) having a tonic effect upon the nerves.

neurotony (nu-rot′o-ne) stretching of a nerve.

neurotoxicity (nu″ro-tok-sis′ĭ-te) the quality of exerting a destructive or poisonous effect upon nerve tissue. **neurotox′ic,** adj.

neurotoxin (-tok′sin) a substance that is poisonous or destructive to nerve tissue.

neurotransmitter (-trans′mit-er) a substance released at the synapse of a neuron that induces activity in susceptible cells.

neurotrauma (-traw′mah) mechanical injury to a nerve.

neurotrophy (nu-rot′ro-fe) nutrition and maintenance of tissues as regulated by nervous influence. **neurotroph′ic,** adj.

neurotropism (nu-rot′ro-pizm) 1. the quality of having a special affinity for nervous tissue. 2. the alleged tendency of regenerating nerve fibers to grow toward specific portions of the periphery. **neurotrop′ic,** adj.

neurotubule (nu″ro-tu′būl) any of the long, straight, parallel tubules or canaliculi, 20 to 30 μm. in diameter, found in the axon, dendrites, and perikaryon of a neuron.

neurovaccine (-vak′sēn) vaccine virus prepared by growing the virus in a rabbit's brain.

neurovascular (-vas′ku-ler) pertaining to both nervous and vascular elements, or to nerves controlling the caliber of blood vessels.

neurovisceral (-vis′er-al) neurosplanchnic.

neurula (nu′roo-lah) the early embryonic stage following the gastrula, marked by the first appearance of the nervous system.

neurulation (nu″roo-la′shun) formation in the early embryo of the neural plate, followed by its closure with development of the neural tube.

neutral (nu′tral) neither basic nor acid.

neutralize (-īz) to render neutral.

Neutrapen (nu′trah-pen) trademark for a lyophilized preparation of penicillinase.

neutrino (nu-tre′no) a subatomic particle with an extremely small mass and no electric charge.

neutrocyte (nu′tro-sīt) neutrophil (2).

neutron (nu′tron) an electrically neutral or uncharged particle of matter existing along with protons in the atoms of all elements except the mass 1 isotope of hydrogen.

neutropenia (nu″tro-pe′ne-ah) diminished number of neutrophils in the blood. **cyclic n.,** periodic n. **malignant n.,** agranulocytosis. **periodic n.,** a chronic form marked by regular, periodic episodic recurrences, associated with malaise, fever, stomatitis, and various infections.

neutrophil (nu′tro-fil) 1. a granular leukocyte having a nucleus with three to five lobes connected by threads of chromatin, and cytoplasm containing very fine granules; cf. *heterophil.* 2. any cell, structure, or histologic element readily stainable with neutral dyes. **stab n.,** one whose nucleus is not divided into segments.

neutrophilia (nu″tro-fil′e-ah) increase in the number of neutrophils in the blood.

neutrophilic (-fil′ik) 1. pertaining to neutrophils. 2. stainable by neutral dyes.

nevocarcinoma (ne″vo-kar″sin-o′mah) malignant melanoma.

nevoid (ne′void) resembling a nevus.

nevoxanthoendothelioma (ne″vo-zan″tho-en″do-the″le-o′mah) a condition in which

groups of yellow-brown papules or nodules occur on the extensor surfaces of the extremities of infants.

nevus (ne′vus), pl. *ne′vi* [L.] a circumscribed stable malformation of the skin and occasionally of the oral mucosa, which is not due to external causes; the excess (or deficiency) of tissue may involve epidermal, connective tissue, adnexal, nervous, or vascular elements. **n. arachnoi′deus, n. araneo′sus, n. ara′neus,** vascular spider. **blue n.,** a dark blue nodular lesion composed of closely grouped melanocytes and melanophages situated in the mid-dermis. **blue rubber bleb n.,** a hereditary condition marked by multiple bluish cutaneous hemangiomas with soft raised centers, frequently associated with hemangiomas of the gastrointestinal tract. **n. comedon′icus,** a rare epidermal nevus marked by one or more patches 2 to 5 cm. or more in diameter, in which there are collections of large comedones or comedo-like lesions. **connective tissue n.,** any nevus occurring in the dermal connective tissue and characterized by nodules, papules, or plaques, or by combinations of such lesions. Histologically, there is inconstant focal or diffuse thickening and abnormal staining of collagen fibers. **epidermal nevi,** congenital skin tumors that do not contain melanocytes, which vary widely in appearance, size, and distribution, and which are commonly hyperkeratotic. **n. flam′meus,** portwine stain; a poorly defined, pink to dark bluish red area involving otherwise normal skin. **hairy n.,** a more or less pigmented nevus with hairs growing from its surface. **halo n.,** a pigmented nevus surrounded by a ring of depigmentation. **intradermal n.,** a nevocytic nevus in which the nevus cells occur in nests in the upper part of the dermis, with no evidence of the proliferative process by which they originated. **n. of Ito,** a mongolian spot in the distribution of the posterior supraclavicular and lateral cutaneous brachial nerves, over the shoulder. **junction n.,** a brownish, smooth, flat or slightly raised nevocytic nevus; histologically, there are nests of melanin-containing nevus cells at the dermoepidermal junction. **n. lipomato′sus,** one containing much fibrofatty tissue. **melanocytic n.,** any nevus, usually pigmented, composed of melanocytes. **nevocytic n., nevus-cell n.,** the common mole; a usually more or less hyperpigmented nevus, initially flat but soon becoming elevated, composed of nests of nevus cells. **n. of Ota,** a mongolian spot, usually unilateral, involving the conjunctiva and lids, as well as adjacent facial skin, sclera, ocular muscles, and periosteum; rarely malignant melanoma may develop, usually in the iris. **pigmented n.,** one containing melanin; the term is usually restricted to nevocytic nevi (moles), but may be applied to other pigmented nevi. **sebaceous n., sebaceous n. of Jadassohn,** an epidermal nevus of the scalp or less often the face, frequently growing larger during puberty or early adult life, and rarely giving rise to a variety of new growths, including basal cell carcinoma. **spider n.,** vascular spider. **n. spi′lus,** a smooth, tan to brown, macular nevus composed of melanocytes, and speckled with smaller, darker macules. **n. spongio′sus al′bus,** white sponge n. **n. un′ius lat′eris,** a verrucous epidermal nevus occurring as a linear band, patch, or streak, usually along the margin between two neuromeres. **vascular n., n. vasculo′sus,** a reddish swelling or patch on the skin due to hypertrophy of the skin capillaries. **white sponge n.,** a white spongy nevus of a mucous membrane, occurring as a hereditary condition.

newborn (nu′born) 1. recently born. 2. a recently born infant.

newton (nu′ton) the SI unit of force: the force which, when acting continuously upon a mass of 1 kilogram, will impart to it an acceleration of 1 meter per second per second.

nexus (nek′sus) a bond, as between members of a series or group.

NF National Formulary.

N.F.L.P.N. National Federation for Licensed Practical Nurses.

ng. nanogram.

N.H.I. National Health Insurance; National Heart Institute.

N.H.L.I. National Heart and Lung Institute.

Ni chemical symbol, *nickel.*

niacin (ni′ah-sin) nicotinic acid; a water-soluble vitamin of the B complex found in various animal and plant tissues, and first prepared by oxidation of nicotine. Important because of its biochemical role in the body, its pellagra-curative property, and its vasodilating action.

niacinamide (ni″ah-sin-am′mīd) the amide of niacin, $C_6H_6N_2O$, differing from niacin in not having its vasodilating action, occurring naturally in the body and interconvertible with niacin; a preparation is used in treating pellagra.

NIAID National Institute of Allergy and Infectious Diseases.

nialamide (ni-al′ah-mīd) a monoamine oxidase inhibitor, $C_{16}H_{18}N_4O_2$, used as an antidepressant.

NIAMD National Institute of Arthritis and Metabolic Diseases.

Niamid (ni′ah-mid) trademark for a preparation of nialamide.

niche (nich) a defect in an otherwise even surface, especially a depression or recess in the wall of a hollow organ, as seen in a roentgenogram, or such a depression in an organ visible to the naked eye. **ecologic n.,** the place of an organism within its community or ecosystem. **enamel n.,** either of two depressions between the dental lamina and the developing tooth germ, one pointing distally (*distal enamel n.*) and the other mesially (*mesial enamel n.*). **Haudek's n.,** see under *sign.*

NICHHD National Institute of Child Health and Human Development.

nickel (nik′el) chemical element (*see table*), at. no. 28, symbol Ni.

nicking (nik′ing) localized constriction of the retinal blood vessels.

niclosamide (nĭ-klo′sah-mīd) an anthelminthic, $C_{13}H_8Cl_2N_2O_4$.

Niconyl (ni′ko-nil) trademark for a preparation of isoniazid.

nicotinamide (nik″o-tin′ah-mīd) niacinamide. **n.-adenine dinucleotide (NAD),** see under *dinucleotide.*

nicotine (nik′o-tēn, nik′o-tin) a very poisonous alkaloid, $C_{10}H_{14}N_2$, obtained from tobacco or produced synthetically; used as an agricultural insecticide. See also *nicotinism.*

nicotinism (nik′o-tin-izm″) nicotine poisoning, marked by stimulation and subsequent depression of the central and autonomic nervous systems, with death due to respiratory paralysis.

nicoumalone (ni-koo′mah-lōn) acenocoumarol.

nictitation (nik″tĭ-ta′shun) the act of winking.

nidal (ni′dal) pertaining to a nidus.

nidation (ni-da′shun) implantation of the conceptus in the endometrium.

NIDR National Institute of Dental Research.

nidus (ni′dus), pl. *ni′di* [L.] 1. the point of origin or focus of a morbid process. 2. nucleus (2). **n. a′vis, n. hirun′dinis** [L., swallow's nest], a depression in the cerebellum between the posterior velum and uvula.

nifuroxime (ni″fūr-ok′sim) an antibacterial and antitrichomonal agent, $C_5H_4N_2O_4$.

nightmare (nīt′mār) a terrifying dream.

nightshade (-shād) a plant of the genus *Solanum.* **deadly n.,** belladonna leaf.

NIGMS National Institute of General Medical Sciences.

nigra (ni′grah) [L., black] substantia nigra. **ni′gral,** adj.

nigrities (ni-grish′e-ēz) blackness. **n. lin′guae,** black tongue.

nigrosin (ni′gro-sin) an aniline dye, $C_{36}H_{27}N_3$, having a special affinity for ganglion cells.

N.I.H. National Institutes of Health.

nihilism (ni′ĕ-lizm) the delusion of nonexistence of the self, part of the self, or of some object in external reality.

nikethamide (nĭ-keth′ah-mīd) a central and respiratory stimulant, $C_{10}H_{14}N_2O$.

Nilevar (ni′le-var) trademark for preparations of norethandrolone.

NIMH National Institute of Mental Health.

NINDB National Institute of Neurological Diseases and Blindness.

niobium (ni-o′be-um) chemical element (*see table*), at. no. 41, symbol Nb.

Nionate (ni′o-nāt) trademark for a preparation of ferrous gluconate.

niphablepsia (nif″ah-blep′se-ah) snow blindness.

nipple (nip′l) the pigmented projection on the anterior surface of the mammary gland, surrounded by the areola; it gives outlet to milk from the breast. Also, any similarly shaped structure.

niridazole (nĭ-rid′ah-zōl) an antischistosomal, $C_6H_6N_4O_3S$.

Nisentil (ni′sen-til) trademark for a preparation of alphaprodine.

nisobamate (ni″so-bam′āt) a minor tranquilizer, sedative, and hypnotic, $C_{13}H_{26}N_2O_4$.

Nisulfazole (ni-sul'fah-zōl) trademark for a preparation of para-nitrosulfathiazole.

nisus (ni'sus) [L.] an effort, strong tendency, or molimen.

nit (nit) the egg of a louse.

niter (ni'ter) potassium nitrate.

niton (ni'ton) radon.

Nitranitol (ni'trah-ni''tol) trademark for preparations of mannitol.

nitrate (ni'trāt) any salt of nitric acid; organic nitrates are used in the treatment of angina pectoris.

nitre (ni'ter) potassium nitrate.

Nitretamin (ni-tre'tah-min) trademark for a preparation of trolnitrate.

nitric (ni'trik) pertaining to or containing nitrogen in one of its higher valences.

nitride (ni'trīd) a binary compound of nitrogen with a metal.

nitrification (ni''trĭ-fĭ-ka'shun) the bacterial oxidation of ammonia to nitrite and nitrate in the soil.

nitrifying (ni'trĭ-fi''ing) oxidizing nitrites into nitrates; said of certain nitrogen bacteria.

nitrile (ni'trīl) an organic compound containing trivalent nitrogen attached to one carbon atom, ·C∷N.

nitrite (ni'trīt) any salt of nitrous acid; organic nitrites are used in the treatment of angina pectoris.

Nitrobacter (ni''tro-bak'ter) a genus of bacteria (family Nitrobacteraceae) which oxidize nitrites to nitrates.

Nitrobacteraceae (-bak''te-ra'se-e) a family of bacteria (order Pseudomonadales), deriving energy solely from oxidation of ammonia to nitrite, or of nitrite to nitrate; known informally as *nitrifying bacteria*.

nitrobenzene (-ben'zēn) a poisonous benzol derivative, $C_6H_5NO_2$.

nitrocellulose (-sel'u-lōs) pyroxylin.

Nitrocystis (-sis'tis) a genus of nitrifying bacteria (family Nitrobacteraceae), which are embedded in slime to form zooglea.

nitrodan (ni'tro-dan) an anthelminthic, $C_{10}H_8N_4O_3S_2$.

nitrofuran (ni''tro-fu'ran) any of a group of antibacterials, including nitrofurantoin, nitrofurazone, etc., that are effective against a wide range of bacteria.

nitrofurantoin (-fu-ran'to-in) an antibacterial, $C_8H_4N_4O_5$, used in urinary tract infections.

nitrofurazone (-fu'rah-zōn) a local anti-infective, $C_6H_6N_4O_4$.

nitrogen (ni'tro-jen) chemical element (*see table*), at. no. 7, symbol N. It forms about 78% of the atmosphere and is a constituent of all proteins and nucleic acids. **n. dioxide,** a brownish irritant gas generated by decomposition of nitrogen peroxide or the reaction of metals with concentrated nitric acid. **n. monoxide,** nitrous oxide. **n. mustards,** see under *mustard*. **nonprotein n.,** the nitrogenous constituents of the blood exclusive of the protein bodies, consisting of the nitrogen of urea, uric acid, creatine, creatinine, amino acids, polypeptides, and an undetermined part known as *rest nitrogen*. **n. pentoxide,** a crystalline compound, nitric anhydride, which combines with water to form nitric acid. **n. peroxide,** a poisonous volatile liquid, decomposing at room temperature to nitrogen dioxide. **rest n.,** see *nonprotein n.* **n. tetroxide,** n. peroxide. **urea n.,** see under *urea*.

nitrogenous (ni-troj'ĕ-nus) containing nitrogen.

nitroglycerin (ni''tro-glis'er-in) a vasodilator, $C_3H_5N_3O_9$, used especially in the prophylaxis and treatment of angina pectoris.

Nitroglyn (ni'tro-glin) trademark for a preparation of nitroglycerin.

Nitrol (ni'trol) trademark for a preparation of nitroglycerin.

nitromannite (ni''tro-man'īt) mannitol hexanitrate.

nitromersol (-mer'sol) a local anti-infective, $C_7H_5HgNO_3$, used topically in solution or tincture.

nitrous (ni'trus) pertaining to nitrogen in its lowest valency. **n. oxide,** a gas, N_2O, used as a general anesthetic and analgesic.

Nitrovas (ni'tro-vas) trademark for a preparation of nitroglycerin.

nl. nanoliter.

N.L.N. National League for Nursing.

nm. nanometer.

N.M.S.S. National Multiple Sclerosis Society.

nn. nervi (L. pl.), *nerves*.

No chemical symbol, *nobelium*.

nobelium (no-be'le-um) chemical element (*see table*), at. no. 102, symbol No.

Nocardia (no-kar'de-ah) a genus of bacteria (family Actinomycetaceae), including *N. asteroi'des*, which produces a tuberculosis-like infection in man, and *N. farci'nica* (probably identical with *N. asteroides*), which produces a tuberculosis-like infection in cattle.

nocardial (no-kar'de-al) pertaining to or caused by *Nocardia*.

nocardiosis (no-kar''de-o'sis) infection with *Nocardia*.

noci- word element [L.], *harm; injury*.

nociassociation (no''se-ah-so''se-a'shun) unconscious discharge of nervous energy under the stimulus of trauma.

nociceptor (-sep'tor) a receptor that is stimulated by injury; a receptor for pain. **nocicep'tive,** adj.

noci-influence (-in'floo-ens) injurious or traumatic influence.

nociperception (-per-sep'shun) the perception of traumatic stimuli.

noctalbuminuria (nok''tal-bu''mĭ-nu're-ah) excess of albumin in urine secreted at night.

Noctec (nok'tek) trademark for preparations of chloral hydrate.

noctiphobia (nok''tĭ-fo'be-ah) morbid dread of night.

nocturia (nok-tu're-ah) excessive urination at night.

node (nōd) a small mass of tissue in the form of a swelling, knot, or protuberance, either normal or pathological. **no'dal,** adj. **n. of Aschoff**

and Tawara, atrioventricular n. **atrioventricular n.,** a collection of Purkinje fibers beneath the endocardium of the right atrium, continuous with the atrial muscle fibers and atrioventricular bundle. **Bouchard's n's,** cartilaginous and bony enlargements of the proximal interphalangeal joints of the fingers in degenerative joint disease. **Delphian n.,** a lymph node encased in the fascia in the midline just anterior to the thyroid isthmus, so called because it is exposed first at operation and, if diseased, is indicative of disease of the thyroid gland. **Dürck's n's,** granulomatous perivascular infiltrations in the cerebral cortex in trypanosomiasis. **Ewald n.,** sentinel n. **Flack's n.,** sinoatrial n. **Haygarth's n's,** joint swelling in arthritis deformans. **Heberden's n's,** small hard nodules, usually at the distal interphalangeal joints of the fingers, formed by calcific spurs of the articular cartilage and associated with osteoarthritis. **hemal n's,** nodes with a rich content of erythrocytes within sinuses, found near large blood vessels along the ventral side of the vertebrae in various mammals, especially ruminants, having functions probably like those of the spleen; their presence in man is doubtful. **Hensen's n.,** primitive knot. **Keith's n., Keith-Flack n.,** sinoatrial n. **lymph n.,** any of the accumulations of lymphoid tissue organized as definite lymphoid organs along the course of lymphatic vessels, consisting of an outer cortical and an inner medullary part; they are the main source of lymphocytes of the peripheral blood and, as part of the reticuloendothelial system, serve as a defense mechanism by removing noxious agents, e.g., bacteria and toxins, and probably play a role in antibody formation. **Meynet's n's,** nodules in the capsules of joints and in tendons in rheumatic conditions, especially in children. **Osler's n's,** small, raised, swollen, tender areas, bluish or sometimes pink or red, occurring commonly in the pads of the fingers or toes, in the thenar or hypothenar eminences or the soles of the feet; they are practically pathognomonic of subacute bacterial endocarditis. **Parrot's n.,** bony nodes on the outer table of the skull of infants with congenital syphilis. **n's of Ranvier,** constrictions of myelinated nerve fibers at regular intervals at which the myelin sheath is absent and the axon is enclosed only by Schwann cell processes; see Plate XI. **Schmorl's n.,** an irregular or hemispherical bone defect in the upper or lower margin of the body of a vertebra. **sentinel n., signal n.,** an enlarged supraclavicular lymph node; often the first sign of a malignant abdominal tumor. **singer's n.,** a small, white nodule on the vocal cord in those who use their voice excessively. **sinoatrial n., sinus n.,** a collection of atypical muscle fibers (Purkinje fibers) at the junction of the superior vena cava and right atrium, in which the cardiac rhythm normally originates and which is therefore called the pacemaker of the heart. **syphilitic n.,** a swelling upon a bone due to syphilitic periostitis. **n. of Tawara,** atrioventricular n. **teacher's n.,** singer's n. **Troisier's n., Virchow's n.,** sentinel n.

nodi (no′di) plural of *nodus*.

nodose (no′dōs) having nodes or projections.

nodosity (no-dos′ĭ-te) 1. a node. 2. the quality of being nodose.

nodular (nod′u-ler) marked with, or resembling, nodules.

nodulation (nod″u-la′shun) the formation of or presence of nodules.

nodule (nod′ūl) a small node or boss which is solid and can be detected by touch. **Albini's n's,** gray nodules of the size of small grains, sometimes seen on the free edges of the atrioventricular valves of infants; they are remains of fetal structures. **apple jelly n's,** minute, yellowish or reddish brown, translucent nodules, seen on diascopic examination of the lesions of lupus vulgaris. **n's of Arantius,** see under *body.* **Aschoff's n's,** see under *body.* **Bianchi's n's,** bodies of Arantius. **Gamna's n's, Gandy-Gamna n's,** brown or yellow pigmented nodules sometimes seen in the enlarged spleen, e.g., in Gamna's disease and siderotic splenomegaly. **Jeanselme's n's, juxta-articular n's,** gummata of tertiary syphilis and of nonvenereal treponemal diseases, located on joint capsules, bursae, or tendon sheaths. **lymphatic n.,** 1. lymph node. 2. lymph follicle. **milker's n's,** hard circumscribed nodules on the hands of those who milk cows affected with cowpox. **Morgagni's n's,** bodies of Arantius. **pulp n.,** denticle (2). **rheumatic n's,** small round or oval, mostly subcutaneous nodules composed chiefly of a mass of Aschoff bodies; seen in rheumatic fever. **Schmorl's n.,** an irregular or hemispherical bone defect in the upper or lower margin of the body of the vertebra. **surfer's n's,** hyperplastic, fibrosing granulomas occurring over bony prominences of the feet and legs as a result of repeated trauma from kneeling on surfboards. **triticeous n.,** see under *cartilage.* **typhus n's,** minute nodes in the skin, formed by perivascular infiltration of mononuclear cells in typhus. **n. of vermis,** the part of the vermis of the cerebellum, on the ventral surface, where the inferior medullary velum attaches.

nodulus (nod′u-lus), pl. *nod′uli* [L.] nodule.

nodus (no′dus), pl. *no′di* [L.] node.

nogalamycin (no-gal″ah-mi′sin) an antineoplastic antibiotic produced by *Streptomyces nogalater.*

Noguchia (no-goo′che-ah) a genus of gram-negative bacteria (family Brucellaceae) found in the conjunctiva of man and animals having a follicular type of disease.

Noludar (nol′u-dar) trademark for preparations of methyprylon.

noma (no′mah) gangrenous processes of the mouth or genitalia. In the mouth (*cancrum oris, gangrenous stomatitis*), it begins as a small gingival ulcer and results in gangrenous necrosis of surrounding facial tissues; on the genitalia (*cancrum pudendi, n. pudendi, n. vulvae*), it affects one labium majus and then the other.

nomenclature (no′men-kla″chur, no-men′kla″-chur) a classified system of names, as of anatomical structures, organisms, etc. **binomial**

n., the system of designating plants and animals by two latinized words signifying the genus and species.

Nomina Anatomica (no′mĭ-nah an-ah-tom′ĭ-kah) [L.] the internationally approved official body of anatomical nomenclature; abbreviated NA.

nomogram (nom′o-gram) the graphic representation produced in nomography.

nomography (no-mog′rah-fe) a graphic method of representing the relation between any number of variables.

nomotopic (no″mo-top′ik) occurring at a normal place.

nonan (no′nan) recurring every ninth day.

non compos mentis (non kom′pos men′tis) [L.] not of sound mind.

nonconductor (non″kon-duk′tor) a substance that does not readily transmit electricity, light, or heat.

nondisjunction (-dis-junk′shun) failure (*a*) of two homologous chromosomes to pass to separate cells during the first division of meiosis, or (*b*) of the two chromatids of a chromosome to pass to separate cells during mitosis or during the second meiotic division. As a result, one daughter cell has two chromosomes or two chromatids, and the other has none.

nonelectrolyte (-e-lek′tro-līt) a substance which in solution is a nonconductor of electricity.

nonigravida (no″ne-grav′ĭ-dah) a woman pregnant for the ninth time.

nonipara (no-nip′ah-rah) a woman who has had nine pregnancies which resulted in viable offspring.

nonoxynol (no-noks′ĭ-nōl) a group of compounds of the general composition, $C_{15}H_{24}O(C_2H_4O)_n$, which are assigned a number according to the value of *n*. Nonoxynol 4, 15, and 30 are nonionic surfactants; nonoxynol 9 is a spermaticide.

nonsecretor (non″se-kre′tor) a person with A or B type blood whose body secretions do not contain the particular (A or B) substance.

nonunion (-ūn′yun) failure of the ends of a fractured bone to unite.

nonviable (-vi′ah-b'l) not capable of living.

noopsyche (no′o-si″ke) the intellectual processes of the mind.

N.O.P.H.N. National Organization for Public Health Nursing.

noracymethadol (nor″ah-si-meth′ah-dōl) an analgesic, $C_{22}H_{29}NO_2$, used as the hydrochloride salt.

noradrenalin (-ah-dren′ah-lin) norepinephrine.

norbolethone (nor-bol′ĕ-thōn) an anabolic steroid, $C_{21}H_{32}O_2$.

nordefrin (nor′dĕ-frin) a sympathomimetic, $C_9H_{13}O_3$, used as a vasoconstrictor in the form of the hydrochloride salt.

norepinephrine (nor″ep-ĭ-nef′rin) a hormone secreted by neurons which acts as a transmitter substance of the peripheral sympathetic nerve endings and probably of certain synapses in the central nervous system; also secreted by the adrenal medulla in response to splanchnic stimulation and released predominantly in response

to hypotension. A synthetic compound is used as a sympathomimetic vasopressor.

norethandrolone (-eth-an′dro-lōn) a synthetic androgen, $C_{20}H_{30}O_2$, equal to testosterone in anabolic activity, but having less androgenic activity.

norethindrone (nor-eth′in-drōn) a progestational agent, $C_{22}H_{28}O_3$, similar in action to progesterone; also used in combination with mestranol as an oral contraceptive.

norethynodrel (nor″ĕ-thi′no-drel) a progestin, $C_{20}H_{26}O_2$, used alone as a gestational agent and, in combination with mestranol, as an oral contraceptive.

norflurane (nor-floor′ān) an inhalation anesthetic, $C_2H_2F_4$.

norgestrel (-jes′trel) a potent progestin, $C_{21}H_{28}O_2$, used as an antifertility agent.

Norisodrine (-i′so-drin) trademark for preparations of isoproterenol.

norleucine (-lu′sēn) a nonessential amino acid extracted from the leucine fraction of nervous tissue proteins; it has been synthesized.

Norlutin (-lu′tin) trademark for a preparation of norethindrone.

norm (norm) a fixed or ideal standard.

norm(o)- word element [L.], *normal; usual; conforming to the rule.*

normal (nor′mal) 1. agreeing with the regular and established type; when said of a solution, denoting one containing in each 1000 ml., 1 gram equivalent weight of the active substance; see also *N* (3). 2. in bacteriology, not immunized or otherwise bacteriologically treated.

normetanephrine (nor″met-ah-nef′rin) a metabolite of norepinephrine excreted in the urine and found in certain tissues.

normoblast (nor′mo-blast) a nucleated precursor cell in the erythrocytic series; four developmental stages are recognized: the *pronormoblast* (q.v.); the *basophilic n.*, in which the cytoplasm is basophilic, the nucleus is large with clumped chromatin, and the nucleoli have disappeared; the *polychromatic n.*, in which the nuclear chromatin shows increased clumping and the cytoplasm begins to acquire hemoglobin and takes on an acidophilic tint; and the *orthochromatic n.*, the final stage before nuclear loss, in which the nucleus is small and ultimately becomes a blue-black, homogenous structureless mass. **normoblas′tic,** adj.

normoblastosis (nor″mo-blas-to′sis) excessive production of normoblasts by the bone marrow.

normocalcemia (-kal-se′me-ah) a normal level of calcium in the blood. **normocalce′mic,** adj.

normochromia (-kro′me-ah) normal color of erythrocytes.

normocyte (nor′mo-sīt) an erythrocyte that is normal in size, shape, and color.

Normocytin (nor″mo-si′tin) trademark for preparations of concentrated crystalline cyanocobalamine (vitamin B_{12}).

normocytosis (-si-to′sis) a normal state of the blood in respect to erythrocytes.

normoglycemia (-gli-se′me-ah) normal glucose content of the blood. **normoglyce′mic,** adj.

normokalemia (-kah-le′me-ah) a normal level of potassium in the blood. **normokale′mic,** adj.

normospermic (-sper′mik) producing spermatozoa normal in number and motility.

normotensive (-ten′siv) 1. characterized by normal tone, tension, or pressure, as by normal blood pressure. 2. a person with normal blood pressure.

normothermia (-ther′me-ah) a normal state of temperature. **normother′mic,** adj.

normotonia (-to′ne-ah) normal tone or tension. **normoton′ic,** adj.

normovolemia (-vo-le′me-ah) normal blood volume.

Norodin (nor′o-din) trademark for a preparation of methamphetamine.

nortriptyline (nor-trip′tĭ-lēn) an antidepressant, $C_{19}H_{21}N$, used as the hydrochloride salt.

nos(o)- word element [Gr.], *disease.*

noscapine (nos′kah-pēn) an alkaloid present in opium; used as a nonaddictive antitussive.

nose (nōz) the specialized facial structure serving as an organ of the sense of smell and as part of the respiratory apparatus; see Plate XVI. **saddle n.,** a nose with a sunken bridge.

nosebleed (nōz′blēd) bleeding from the nose; epistaxis.

Nosema (no-se′mah) a genus of sporozoan parasites, including *N. a′pis,* causing disease in bees, and *N. bomby′cis,* causing disease in silkworms.

nosencephalus (no″sen-sef′ah-lus) a fetus with defective cranium and brain.

nosepiece (nōz′pēs) the portion of a microscope nearest to the stage, which bears the objective or objectives.

nosocomial (nos″o-ko′me-al) pertaining to or originating in a hospital.

nosogeny (no-soj′ĕ-ne) pathogenesis.

nosology (no-sol′o-je) the science of the classification of diseases. **nosolog′ic,** adj.

nosomania (nos″o-ma′ne-ah) the incorrect belief that one has some special disease; hypochondriasis.

nosomycosis (-mi-ko′sis) any fungal disease; mycosis.

nosonomy (no-son′o-me) the classification of diseases.

nosoparasite (nos″o-par′ah-sīt) an organism found in a disease which it is able to modify, but not to produce.

nosophilia (-fil′e-ah) morbid desire to be sick.

nosophobia (-fo′be-ah) morbid dread of sickness or of a specific disease.

nosopoietic (-poi-et′ik) causing disease.

Nosopsyllus (-sil′us) a genus of fleas, including *N. fascia′tus,* the common rat flea of North America and Europe, a vector of murine typhus and probably of plague.

nosotaxy (nos′o-tak″se) the classification of disease.

nostril (nos′tril) either of the nares.

nostrum (nos′trum) a quack, patent, or secret remedy.

Nostyn (nos′tin) trademark for a preparation of ectylurea.

not(o)- word element [Gr.], *the back.*

notalgia (no-tal′je-ah) pain in the back.

notancephalia (no″tan-sĕ-fa′le-ah) congenital absence of the back of the skull.

notch (noch) an indentation on the edge of a bone or other organ. **aortic n.,** dicrotic n. **dicrotic n.,** a small downward deflection in the arterial pulse or pressure contour immediately following the closure of the semilunar valves, sometimes used as a marker for the end of systole or the ejection period. **parotid n.,** the notch between the ramus of the mandible and the mastoid process of the temporal bone.

notencephalocele (no″ten-sef′ah-lo-sēl″) hernial protrusion of the brain at the back of the head.

notencephalus (no″ten-sef′ah-lus) a fetus affected with notencephalocele.

notifiable (ni″tĭ-fi′ah-b'l) required to be reported to the board of health.

notochord (no′to-kord) the rod-shaped cord of cells below the primitive groove of the embryo, defining the primitive axis of the body; the common factor of all chordates.

Notoedres (no″to-ed′rēz) a genus of mites, including *N. ca′ti,* an itch mite causing a persistent, often fatal, mange in cats; it also infests domestic animals, and may temporarily infest man.

notomelus (no-tom′ĕ-lus) a fetus with accessory limbs attached to the back.

not-self (not′self) a term denoting antigenic constituents foreign to the organism (self), which are eliminated through humoral or cell-mediated immunity.

Novaldin (no-val′din) trademark for preparations of dipyrone.

novobiocin (no″vo-bi′o-sin) an antibacterial, $C_{13}H_{36}N_2O_{11}$, produced by *Streptomyces niveus;* used in treatment of infections due to cocci and other gram-positive organisms.

Novocain (no′vo-kān) trademark for preparations of procaine.

Novrad (nov′rad) trademark for preparations of levopropoxyphene.

noxious (nok′shus) hurtful; injurious.

Np chemical symbol, *neptunium.*

NPN nonprotein nitrogen.

ns. nanosecond.

N.S.A. Neurosurgical Society of America.

N.S.C.C. National Society for Crippled Children.

N.S.N.A. National Student Nurse Association.

N.S.P.B. National Society for the Prevention of Blindness.

N.T.A. National Tuberculosis Association.

nucha (nu′kah) the nape, or back, of the neck. **nu′chal,** adj.

nuclear (nu′kle-ar) pertaining to a nucleus.

nuclease (nu′kle-ās) any of a group of enzymes that split nucleic acids into nucleotides and other products.

nucleated (nu′kle-āt″ed) having a nucleus or nuclei.

nuclei (nu′kle-i) plural of *nucleus.*

nuclein (nu′kle-in) a decomposition product of

nucleoprotein intermediate between native nucleoprotein and nucleic acid.

nucleocapsid (nu″kle-o-kap′sid) a unit of viral structure, consisting of a capsid with the enclosed nucleic acid.

nucleofugal (nu″kle-of′u-gal) moving away from a nucleus.

nucleohistone (nu″kle-o-his′tōn) a nucleoprotein found in the nuclei of the spermatozoa of various animals, the avian erythrocyte, and somatic cells in general.

nucleoid (nuk′kle-oid) 1. resembling a nucleus. 2. a nucleus-like body sometimes seen in the center of an erythrocyte. 3. the genetic material (nucleic acid) of a virus situated in the center of the virion.

nucleolonema (nu″kle-o″lo-ne′mah) a network of strands formed by organization of a finely granular substance, perhaps containing RNA, in the nucleolus of a cell.

nucleolus (nu-kle′o-lus), pl. *nucle′oli* [L.] a vacuole-like achromatic body, rich in RNA, within the nucleus of a cell; multiple nucleoli occur in some cells.

nucleon (nu′kle-on) a particle of an atomic nucleus; a proton or neutron, the total number of which constitutes the mass number of the isotope.

nucleonics (nu″kle-on′iks) the study of atomic nuclei and their reactions; nuclear physics.

nucleopetal (nu″kle-op′ĕ-tal) moving towad a nucleus.

nucleophilic (nu″kle-o-fil′ik) having an affinity for nuclei.

nucleoplasm (nu′kle-o-plazm″) the protoplasm of the nucleus of a cell.

nucleoprotein (nu″kle-o-pro′te-in) a substance composed of a simple basic protein (e.g., a histone) combined with a nucleic acid.

nucleosidase (-si′dās) an enzyme that catalyzes the splitting of nucleosides.

nucleoside (nu′kle-o-sīd″) one of the compounds into which a nucleotide is split by the action of nucleotidase or by chemical means; it consists of a sugar (a pentose) with a purine or pyrimidine base.

nucleotidase (nu″kle-ot′ĭ-dās) an enzyme that splits nucleotides into nucleosides and phosphoric acid.

nucleotide (nu′kle-o-tīd″) one of the compounds into which nucleic acid is split by action of nuclease; nucleotides are composed of a base (purine or pyrimidine), a sugar (ribose or deoxyribose), and a phosphate group. **diphosphopyridine n.,** nicotinamide-adenine dinucleotide. **triphosphopyridine n.,** nicotinamide-adenine dinucleotide phosphate.

nucleotidyl (nu″kle-o-tīd′il) a nucleotide residue.

nucleotoxin (nu″kle-o-tok′sin) 1. a toxin from cell nuclei. 2. any toxin affecting cell nuclei.

nucleus (nu′kle-us), pl. *nu′clei* [L.] 1. a spheroid body within a cell, consisting of a thin nuclear membrane, organelles, one or more nucleoli, chromatin, linin, and nucleoplasm. 2. a group of nerve cells, usually within the central nervous system, bearing a direct relationship to the fibers of a particular nerve. 3. in organic chemistry, the combination of atoms forming the central element or basic framework of the molecule of a specific compound or class of compounds. 4. see *atomic n.* **nu′clear,** adj. **ambiguous n.,** the nucleus of origin of motor fibers of the vagus, glossopharyngeal, and accessory nerves in the medulla oblongata. **arcuate nuclei, nu′clei arcua′ti,** small irregular areas of gray substance on the ventromedial aspect of the pyramid of the medulla oblongata. **atomic n.,** the central core of an atom, constituting most of its mass, but only a small part of its volume, and containing an excess of electricity. **caudate n., n. cauda′tus,** an elongated, arched gray mass closely related to the lateral ventricle throughout its entire extent, which, together with the putamen, forms the neostriatum. **central n. of thalamus, n. centra′lis thal′ami,** a collection of cells close to the wall of the third ventricle, between the medial and posterior ventral nuclei of the thalamus. **cleavage n.,** segmentation n. **cochlear nuclei, ventral and dorsal,** the nuclei of termination of sensory fibers of the cochlear part of the vestibulocochlear nerve, which partly encircle the inferior cerebellar peduncle at the junction of the medulla oblongata and pons. **conjugation n.,** fertilization n. **cuneate n., n. cunea′tus,** a nucleus in the medulla oblongata, in which the fibers of the fasciculcus cuneatus synapse. **Deiters′ n.,** lateral vestibular n. **dentate n., n. denta′tus,** the largest of the deep cerebellar nuclei lying in the white matter of the cerebellum. **diploid n.,** a cell nucleus containing the number of chromosomes typical of the somatic cells of the particular species. **n. dorsa′lis,** n. thoracicus. **fastigial n., n. fasti′gii,** the most medial of the deep cerebellar nuclei, near the midline in the roof of the fourth ventricle. **fertilization n.,** one produced by fusion of the male and female pronuclei in the fertilized ovum. **germ n., germinal n.,** pronucleus. **gonad n.,** micronucleus (1). **n. gra′cilis,** a nucleus in the medulla oblongata, in which the fibers of the fasciculus gracilis of the spinal cord synapse. **hypoglossal n.,** the nucleus of origin of the hypoglossal nerve in the medulla oblongata. **interpeduncular n., n. interpeduncula′re,** a nucleus between the cerebral peduncles immediately dorsal to the interpeduncular fossa. **lenticular n., lentiform n.,** the part of the corpus striatum just lateral to the internal capsule, comprising the putamen and globus pallidus. **motor n.,** any collection of cells in the central nervous system giving origin to a motor nerve. **nutrition n.,** macronucleus. **olivary n., n. oliva′ris,** 1. a folded band of gray substance enclosing a white core and producing the elevation (olive) of the medulla oblongata. 2. olive (2). **n. of origin,** any collection of nerve cells giving origin to the fibers, or a part of the fibers, of a peripheral nerve. **paraventricular n., n. paraventricula′ris,** a band of cells in the wall of the third ventricle in the supraoptic part of the hypothalamus; many of its cells are neurosecretory in function and project to the neurohypophysis. **pontine nuclei, nu′clei pon′tis,**

groups of nerve cell bodies in the part of the pyramidal tract within the ventral part of the pons upon which the fibers of the corticopontine tract synapse, and whose axons in turn cross to the opposite side and form the middle cerebellar peduncle. **n. pulpo'sus, pulpy n.,** a semifluid mass of fine white and elastic fibers forming the center of an intervertebral disk. **red n.,** a distinctive oval nucleus (pink in fresh specimens) centrally placed in the upper mesencephalic reticular formation. **reproductive n.,** micronucleus. **n. of roof of cerebellum,** fastigial n. **n. ru'ber,** red n. **segmentation n.,** the fertilization nucleus after cleavage has begun. **sensory n.,** the nucleus of termination of the afferent (sensory) fibers of a peripheral nerve. **somatic n.,** macronucleus. **sperm n.,** the male pronucleus. **subthalamic n., n. subthalam'icus,** a nucleus on the medial side of the junction of the internal capsule and crus cerebri. **supraoptic n., n. supraop'ticus,** one just above the lateral part of the optic chiasm; many of its cells are neurosecretory in function and project to the neurohypophysis. **tegmental nuclei,** several nuclear masses of the reticular formations of the pons and midbrain, especially of the latter, where they are in close approximation to the superior cerebellar penduncles. **terminal nuclei,** groups of nerve cells within the central nervous system on which the axons of primary afferent neurons of various cranial nerves synapse. **thoracic n., n. thorac'icus,** a column of cells in the posterior gray column of the spinal cord, extending from the 7th or 8th cervical segments to the 2nd or 3rd lumbar level. **triangular n.,** medial vestibular n. **trophic n.,** macronucleus. **vestibular nuclei, nu'clei vestibula'res,** the four (superior, lateral, medial, and inferior) cellular masses in the floor of the fourth ventricle in which the branches of the vestibulocochlear nerve terminate.

nuclide (nu'klīd) a species of atom characterized by the charge, mass, number, and quantum state of its nucleus, and capable of existing for a measurable lifetime (usually more than 10^{-10} sec.).

nullipara (nu-lip'ah-rah) para 0; a women who has never borne a viable child. See *para*. **nullip'arous,** adj.

nulliparity (nul"ĭ-par'ĭ-te) the state of being a nullipara.

number (num'ber) a symbol, as a figure or word, expressive of a certain value or a specified quantity determined by count. **atomic n.,** a number expressive of the number of protons in an atomic nucleus, or the positive charge of the nucleus expressed in terms of the electronic charge. **Avogadro's n.,** see under *constant*. **mass n.,** the number expressive of the mass of a nucleus, being the total number of nucleons—protons and neutrons—in the nucleus of an atom or nuclide.

numbness (num'nes) a lack or diminution of sensation in a part.

nummular (num'u-lar) 1. coin-sized and coin-shaped. 2. made up of round, flat disks. 3. arranged like a stack of coins.

Numorphan (nu-mor'fan) trademark for preparations of oxymorphone.

nunnation (nun-a'shun) the too frequent use of *n* sounds.

Nupercaine (nu'per-kān) trademark for preparations of dibucaine.

nurse 1. one who is especially prepared in the scientific basis of nursing and who meets certain prescribed standards of education and clinical competence. 2. to provide services essential to or helpful in the promotion, maintenance, and restoration of health and well-being. 3. to breast-feed an infant. **charge n.,** one who is in charge of a patient care unit of a hospital or similar health agency. **clinical n. specialist,** n. specialist. **community n.,** in Great Britain, a public health nurse. **community health n.,** public health n. **district n.,** community n. **general duty n.,** a registered nurse, usually one who has not undergone training beyond the basic nursing program, who sees to the general nursing care of patients in a hospital or other health agency. **graduate n.,** a graduate of a school of nursing; often used to designate one who has not been registered or licensed. **head n.,** charge n. **licensed practical n.,** a graduate of a school of practical nursing whose qualifications have been examined by a state board of nursing and who has been legally authorized to practice as a licensed practical or vocational nurse (L.P.N. or L.V.N.), under supervision of a physician or registered nurse. **licensed vocational n.,** see *licensed practical n.* **practical n.,** one who has had practical experience in nursing care but who is not a graduate of a nursing school; cf. *licensed practical n.* **private n., private duty n.,** one who attends an individual patient, usually on a fee-for-service basis, and who may specialize in a specific class of diseases. **probationer n.,** a person who has entered a school of nursing and is under observation to determine fitness for the nursing profession; applied principally to nursing students enrolled in hospital schools of nursing. **public health n.,** an especially prepared registered nurse employed in a community agency to safeguard the health of persons in the community, giving care to the sick in their homes, promoting health and well-being by teaching families how to keep well, and assisting in programs for the prevention of disease. **Queen's Nurse,** in Great Britain, a district nurse who has been trained at or in accordance with the regulations of the Queen Victoria Jubilee Institute for Nurses. **registered n.,** a graduate nurse who has been legally authorized (registered) to practice after examination by a state board of nurse examiners or similar regulatory authority, and who is legally entitled to use the designation R.N. **scrub n.,** one who directly assists the surgeon in the operating room. **n. specialist,** a registered nurse with training at the master's degree level in one of the clinical specialties. **trained n.,** graduate n. **visiting n.,** public health n. **wet n.,** a woman who breast-feeds the infant of another.

nursery (ner'sĕ-re) the department in a hospital where the newborn are cared for. **day n.,** an institution devoted to the care of young children during the day.

nursing (nurs′ing) the provision, at various levels of preparation, of services essential to or helpful in the promotion, maintenance, and restoration of health and well-being or in prevention of illness, as of infants, of sick and injured, or of others for any reason unable to provide such services for themselves.

nutation (nu-ta′shun) the act of nodding, especially involuntary nodding.

nutgall (nut′gawl) an excrescence growing on certain oak trees, produced by insect eggs and larvae embedded in the plant tissues; a source of gallic and tannic acids.

nutrient (nu′tre-ent) 1. nourishing; aiding nutrition. 2. a nourishing substance, or food.

nutriment (nu′trĭ-ment) nourishment; nutritious material; food.

nutrition (nu-trish′un) 1. the sum of the processes involved in taking in nutriments and assimilating and utilizing them. 2. nutriment. **nutri′tional,** adj.

nutritious (nu-trish′us) affording nourishment.

nutritive (nu′trĭ-tiv) pertaining to or promoting nutrition.

nutriture (nu′trĭ-tūr) the status of the body in relation to nutrition.

Nuttallia (nŭ-tal′e-ah) *Babesia.*

nux (nuks) [L.] nut. **n. vom′ica,** the dried ripe seed of *Strychnos nox-vomica,* containing several alkaloids, chiefly strychnine and brucine; see *strychnine.*

nyct(o)- word element [Gr.], *night; darkness.*

nyctalgia (nik-tal′je-ah) pain that occurs only in sleep.

nyctalope (nik′tah-lōp) a person affected with nyctalopia.

nyctalopia (nik″tah-lo′pe-ah) 1. night blindness. 2. in French (and incorrectly in English), day blindness.

nycterine (nik′ter-in) occurring at night.

nyctohemeral (nik″to-hem′er-al) pertaining to both day and night.

nyctophilia (-fil′e-ah) a preference for darkness or for night.

nyctophobia (-fo′be-ah) morbid dread of darkness.

nyctophonia (-fo′ne-ah) loss of voice during the day but not at night.

nyctotyphlosis (-tif-lo′sis) nyctalopia.

Nydrazid (ni′drah-zid) trademark for preparations of isoniazid.

nylidrin (nil′ĭ-drin) a peripheral vasodilator, $C_{19}H_{25}NO_2$, used as the hydrochloride salt.

nymph (nimf) a developmental stage in certain arthropods, e.g., ticks, between the larval form and the adult, and resembling the latter in appearance.

nymph(o)- word element [Gr.], *nymphae* (labia minora).

nympha (nim′fah), pl. *nym′phae* [L.] labium minus.

nymphectomy (nim-fek′to-me) excision of the nymphae (labia minora).

nymphitis (nim-fi′tis) inflammation of the nymphae (labium minora).

nymphomania (nim″fo-ma′ne-ah) exaggerated sexual desire in a female.

nymphoncus (nim-fong′kus) swelling of the nymphae (labia minora).

nymphotomy (nim-fot′o-me) surgical incision of the nymphae (labia minora) or clitoris.

nystagmiform (nis-tag′mĭ-form) nystagmoid.

nystagmograph (nis-tag′mo-graf) an instrument for recording the movements of the eyeball in nystagmus.

nystagmoid (nis-tag′moid) resembling nystagmus.

nystagmus (nis-tag′mus) involuntary rapid movement (horizontal, vertical, rotatory, or mixed, i.e., of two types) of the eyeball. **nystag′mic,** adj. **aural n.,** labyrinthine n. **caloric n.,** Bárány's symptom (2). **Cheyne's n.,** a peculiar rhythmical eye movement. **dissociated n.,** that in which the movements in the two eyes are dissimilar. **end-position n.,** that occurring only at extremes of gaze. **fixation n.,** that occurring only on gazing fixedly at an object. **labyrinthine n.,** vestibular nystagmus due to labyrinthine disturbance. **latent n.,** that occurring only when one eye is covered. **lateral n.,** involuntary horizontal movement of the eyes. **miners' n.,** that occurring in coal miners after years of exposure to cramped and dark conditions. **opticokinetic n.,** that induced by looking at a moving object. **pendular n.,** that which consists of to-and-fro movements of equal velocity. **retraction n., n. retracto′rius,** a spasmodic backward movement of the eyeball occurring on attempts to move the eye; a sign of midbrain disease. **rotatory n.,** involuntary rotation of eyes about the visual axis. **undulatory n.,** pendular n. **vertical n.,** involuntary up-and-down movement of the eyes. **vestibular n.,** that due to disturbance of the labyrinth or of the vestibular nuclei; the movements are usually jerky.

nystatin (nis′tah-tin) an antifungal agent, $C_{46}H_{77}NO_{19}$, produced by growth of *Streptomyces noursei;* used in treatment of infections with *Candida albicans.*

nyxis (nik′sis) puncture, or paracentesis.

O

O chemical symbol, *oxygen.*

O. [L.] oculus (*eye*); [L.] octarius (*pint*); opening.

o- symbol, *ortho-.*

O₂ 1. chemical symbol, *molecular* (diatomic) *oxygen.* 2. symbol, *both eyes.*

O₃ chemical symbol, *ozone* (triatomic oxygen).

O.B. obstetrics.

ob- word element [L.], *against; in front of; toward.*

obcecation (ob″se-ka′shun) incomplete blindness.

obelion (o-be′le-on) a point at the juncture of the sagittal suture and a line connecting the parietal foramina. **obe′liac**, adj.

obesity (o-bēs′ĭ-te) an increase in body weight beyond the limitation of skeletal and physical requirements, as the result of excessive accumulation of body fat. **obese′**, adj.

obex (o′beks) the ependyma-lined junction of the teniae of the fourth ventricle of the brain at the inferior angle.

objective (ob-jek′tiv) 1. perceptible by the external senses. 2. a result for whose achievement an effort is made. 3. the lens or system of lenses of a microscope (or telescope) nearest the object that is being examined. **achromatic o.**, one in which the chromatic aberration is corrected for two colors and the spherical aberration for one color. **apochromatic o.**, one in which chromatic aberration is corrected for three colors and the spherical aberration for two colors. **immersion o.**, one designed to have its tip and the coverglass over the specimen connected by a liquid instead of air.

obligate (ob′lĭ-gāt) [L.] not facultative; necessary; compulsory; pertaining to or characterized by the ability to survive only in a particular environment or to assume only a particular role, as an obligate anaerobe.

oblique (o-blēk′, o-blīk′) slanting; inclined.

obliquity (ob-lik′wĭ-te) the state of being oblique or slanting. **Litzmann's o.**, inclination of the fetal head so that the posterior parietal bone presents to the birth canal. **Nägele's o.**, presentation of the anterior parietal bone to the birth canal, the biparietal diameter being oblique to the brim of the pelvis.

obliteration (ob-lit″er-a′shun) complete removal by disease, degeneration, surgical procedure, irradiation, etc.

oblongata (ob-long-gah′tah) medulla oblongata. **oblonga′tal**, adj.

obsession (ob-sesh′un) an persistent unwanted idea or impulse that cannot be eliminated by reasoning. **obses′sive**, adj.

obsessive-compulsive (ob-ses′iv-kom-pul′siv) marked by compulsion to repetitively perform certain acts, or carry out certain rituals.

obstetrician (ob″stĕ-trish′an) one who practices obstetrics.

obstetrics (ob-stet′riks) the branch of medicine dealing with pregnancy, labor, and the puerperium. **obstet′ric, obstet′rical**, adj.

obstipation (ob″stĭ-pa′shun) intractable constipation.

obstruction (ob-struk′shun) the act of blocking or clogging; the state of being clogged.

obstruent (ob′stroo-ent) 1. causing obstruction. 2. an agent that causes obstruction.

obtund (ob-tund′) to render dull or blunt.

obtundent (ob-tun′dent) 1. having the power to dull sensibility or to soothe pain. 2. a soothing or partially anesthetic medicine.

obturator (ob″tu-ra′tor) a disk or plate, natural or artificial, that closes an opening.

obtusion (ob-tu′zhun) a deadening or blunting of sensitiveness.

occipitalization (ok-sip″ĭ-tal-i-za′shun) synostosis of the atlas with the occipital bone.

occipitocervical (ok-sip″ĭ-to-ser′vĭ-kal) pertaining to the occiput and neck.

occipitofrontal (-fron′tal) pertaining to the occiput and the face.

occipitomastoid (-mas′toid) pertaining to the occipital bone and mastoid process.

occipitomental (-men′tal) pertaining to the occiput and chin.

occipitoparietal (-pah-ri′ĕ-tal) pertaining to the occipital and parietal bones or lobes of the brain.

occipitotemporal (-tem′po-ral) pertaining to the occipital and temporal bones.

occipitothalamic (-thah-lam′ik) pertaining to the occipital lobe and thalamus.

occiput (ok′si-put) the back part of the head. **occip′ital**, adj.

occlude (o-klood′) to fit close together; to close tight; to obstruct or close off.

occlusal (ŏ-kloo′zal) pertaining to closure; applied to the masticating surfaces of the premolar and molar teeth, or to the contacting surfaces of opposing occlusion rims, or designating a position toward the hypothetical plane passing between the mandibular and maxillary teeth when the jaws are brought into approximation.

occlusion (ŏ-kloo′zhun) 1. the act of closure or state of being closed; an obstruction or a closing off. 2. the relation of the teeth of both jaws when in functional contact during activity of the mandible. **abnormal o.**, malocclusion. **afunctional o.**, malocclusion which prevents mastication. **balanced o.**, occlusion in which the teeth are in harmonious working relation. **central o., centric o.**, occlusion of the teeth when the mandible is in centric relation to the maxilla, with full occlusal surface contact of the upper and lower teeth in habitual occlusion. **coronary o.**, complete obstruction of an artery of the heart. **eccentric o.**, occlusion of the teeth when the lower jaw has moved from the centric position. **functional o.**, occlusion providing the highest efficiency during all the excursive

490

movements of the jaws essential to the function of mastication without producing trauma. **habitual o.,** the consistent relationship of the teeth in the maxilla to those of the mandible when the teeth in both jaws are brought into maximum contact. **hyperfunctional o.,** traumatic o. **lateral o.,** occlusion of the teeth when the lower jaw is moved to the right or left of centric occlusion. **lingual o.,** malocclusion in which the tooth is lingual to the line of the normal dental arch. **mesial o.,** the position of a lower tooth when it is mesial to its opposite number in the maxilla. **normal o.,** the contact of the upper and lower teeth in the centric relationship. **protrusive o.,** anteroclusion. **retrusive o.,** distoclusion. **traumatic o.,** occlusion in which the contact relation of the masticatory surfaces of the teeth is directly due to trauma.

occlusive (ŏ-kloo′siv) pertaining to or effecting occlusion.

occult (ŏ-kult′) obscure or hidden from view.

ocellus (o-sel′us) [L.] 1. a small simple eye in insects and other invertebrates. 2. one of the elements of a compound eye of insects. 3. a roundish, eyelike patch of color.

ochrometer (o-krom′ĕ-ter) an instrument for measuring capillary blood pressure.

ochronosis (o″kro-no′sis) a peculiar discoloration of certain body tissues caused by deposit of alkapton bodies as the result of a metabolic disorder. **ochronot′ic,** adj. **ocular o.,** brown or gray discoloration of the sclera, sometimes involving also the conjunctivae and eyelids.

octa- word element [Gr., L.], *eight.*

octabenzone (ok″tah-ben′zōn) a sun-screening agent, $C_{21}H_{26}O_3$.

octamethyl pyrophosphoramide (-meth′il pir″o-fos-for′ah-mīd) a potent cholinesterase inhibitor and a systemic insecticide, $C_8N_{24}N_4O_3$-P_2.

octan (ok′tan) recurring on the eighth day (every seven days).

octapeptide (ok″tah-pep′tīd) a peptide which on hydrolysis yields eight amino acids.

octaploid (ok′tah-ploid) 1. pertaining to or characterized by octaploidy. 2. an individual or cell having eight sets of chromosomes.

octaploidy (-ploi″de) the state of having eight sets of chromosomes (8n).

octavalent (ok″tah-va′lent) having a valency of eight.

octigravida (ok″tĭ-grav′ĭ-dah) a woman pregnant for the eighth time.

Octin (ok′tin) trademark for preparations of isometheptene.

octipara (ok-tip′ah-rah) a woman who has had eight pregnancies which resulted in viable offspring; para VIII.

octodrine (ok′to-drēn) a vasoconstrictor and local anesthetic, $C_8H_{19}N$.

octoxynol (ok-toks′ĭ-nol) a surfactant, $C_{34}H_{62}$-O_{11}.

ocul(o)- word element [L.], *eye.*

ocular (ok′u-lar) 1. pertaining to the eye. 2. eyepiece.

oculist (ok′u-list) ophthalmologist.

oculocutaneous (ok″u-lo-ku-ta′ne-us) pertaining to or affecting the eyes and the skin.

oculofacial (-fa′shal) pertaining to the eyes and the face.

oculogyration (-ji-ra′shun) movement of the eye about the anteroposterior axis.

oculogyric (-ji′rik) pertaining to or causing movement of the eyeballs.

oculomotor (-mo′tor) pertaining to or effecting eye movements.

oculomotorius (-mo-to′re-us) the oculomotor nerve.

oculomycosis (-mi-ko′sis) any fungal disease of the eye.

oculonasal (-na′zal) pertaining to the eye and the nose.

oculopupillary (-pu′pĭ-ler″e) pertaining to the pupil of the eye.

oculozygomatic (-zi″go-mat′ik) pertaining to the eye and the zygoma.

oculus (ok′u-lus), pl. *oc′uli* [L.] eye.

O.D. Doctor of Optometry; [L.] *oc′ulus dex′ter* (right eye).

odont(o)- word element [Gr.], *tooth.*

odontalgia (o″don-tal′je-ah) toothache.

odontectomy (o″don-tek′to-me) excision of a tooth.

odontic (o-don′tik) pertaining to the teeth.

odontoblast (o-don′to-blast) one of the connective tissue cells that deposit dentin and form the outer surface of the dental pulp adjacent to the dentin.

odontoblastoma (o-don″to-blas-to′mah) a tumor made up of odontoblasts.

odontoclast (o-don′to-klast) an osteoclast associated with absorption of the roots of deciduous teeth.

odontogenesis (o-don″to-jen′ĕ-sis) the origin and histogenesis of the teeth. **odontogenet′ic,** adj. **o. imperfec′ta,** dentinogenesis imperfecta.

odontogenic (-jen′ik) 1. forming teeth. 2. arising in tissues that give origin to the teeth.

odontogeny (o″don-toj′ĕ-ne) odontogenesis.

odontograph (o-don′to-graf) an instrument for recording the unevenness of the surface of tooth enamel.

odontography (o″don-tog′rah-fe) 1. a description of the teeth. 2. the use of the odontograph.

odontoid (o-don′toid) like a tooth.

odontology (o″don-tol′o-je) 1. scientific study of the teeth. 2. dentistry.

odontolysis (o″don-tol′ĭ-sis) the resorption of dental tissue.

odontoma (o″don-to′mah) any odontogenic tumor, especially a composite odontoma. **ameloblastic o.,** a rare neoplasm composed of enamel, dentin, and an odontogenic epithelium like that seen in ameloblastoma. **composite o.,** one consisting of both enamel and dentin in an abnormal pattern. **radicular o.,** one associated with a tooth root, or formed when the root was developing.

odontopathy (o″don-top′ah-the) any disease of the teeth.

odontosis (o″don-to′sis) formation or eruption of the teeth.

odontotomy (o″don-tot′o-me) incision of a tooth.

odor (o′dor) a volatile emanation perceived by the sense of smell.

odynacusis (o-din″ah-ku′sis) painful hearing.

-odynia word element [Gr.], *pain.*

odynometer (o″din-om′ĕ-ter) an instrument for measuring pain.

odynophagia (o-din″o-fa′je-ah) painful swallowing of food.

oe- for words beginning thus, see also those beginning *e-.*

oedipal (ed′ĭ-pal) pertaining to the Oedipus complex.

Oedipus complex (ed′ĭ-pus) see under *complex.*

oesophagostomiasis (e-sof″ah-go-sto-mi′ah-sis) infection with *Œsophagostomum.*

Œsophagostomum (e-sof″ah-gos′to-mum) a genus of nematode worms found in the intestines of various animals.

Oestrus (es′trus) a genus of botflies, including *O. o′vis,* a species whose larvae may infest nasal cavities and sinuses of sheep, and may cause ocular myiasis in man.

official (ŏ-fish′al) authorized by pharmacopeias and recognized formularies.

officinal (o-fis′ĭ-nal) regularly kept for sale in druggists' shops.

OH hydroxyl group; (with negative sign) hydroxyl ion; a hydroxide.

ohm (ōm) a unit of electric resistance, being that of a column of mercury 1 sq. mm. in cross section and 106.25 cm. long.

ohmmeter (ōm′me-ter) an instrument that measures electrical resistance in ohms.

-oid word element [Gr.], *resembling.*

oil (oil) 1. an unctuous, combustible substance that is liquid, or easily liquefiable, on warming, and is soluble in ether but not in water. Oils may be animal, vegetable, or mineral in origin, and volatile or nonvolatile (fixed). 2. a fat that is liquid at room temperature. **almond o.,** fixed oil from kernels of varieties of *Prunus amygdalus;* used as an emollient and perfume and as an ingredient of rose water ointment. **anise o.,** volatile oil from dried ripe fruit of *Pimpinella anisum* or *Ilicium verum;* used as a flavoring agent for drugs. **apricot kernel o.,** persic o. **arachis o.,** peanut o. **Benne o.,** sesame o. **betula o., birch o., sweet,** methyl salicylate. **cade o.,** juniper tar. **camphorated o.,** camphor liniment. **caraway o.,** volatile oil from dried ripe fruit of *Carum carvi;* used as a flavoring agent. **cassia o.,** cinnamon o. **castor o.,** a fixed oil obtained from the seed of *Ricinus communis;* used as a cathartic and, externally, as an emollient in seborrheic dermatitis and other dermatoses. **castor o., aromatic,** castor oil mixed with cinnamon and clove oils, saccharin, vanillin, and alcohol; used as a cathartic. **chaulmoogra o.,** a fixed oil from ripe seeds of *Taraktogenos kurzii* or species of *Hydnocarpus;* see also *ethyl chaulmoograte.* **cinnamon o.,** a volatile oil from leaves and twigs of *Cinnamonum cassia;* used as a flavoring agent and carminative.

citronella o., a fragrant oil used as an insect repellent. **clove o.,** a volatile oil from cloves (dried flowerbuds of *Eugenia caryophyllus*); used as a topical dental analgesic, flavoring agent, germicide, and counterirritant. **cod liver o.,** partially destearinated, fixed oil from fresh livers of *Gadus morrhua* and other fish of the family Gadidae; used as a source of vitamins A and D. **cod liver o., nondestearinated,** entire fixed oil from fresh livers of *Gadus morrhua* and other fish of the family Gadidae; used as a source of vitamins A and D. **coriander o.,** a volatile oil from dried ripe fruit of *Coriandrum sativum;* used as a flavoring agent. **corn o.,** refined, fixed oil from the embryo of *Zea mays;* used as a solvent and vehicle for various medicinal agents and as a vehicle for injections. **cottonseed o.,** refined, fixed oil from seeds of cultivated plants of various species of *Gossypium;* used as a solvent and vehicle for drugs. **croton o.,** an oil from seeds of the Asiatic plant *Croton tiglium;* a drastic purgative and counterirritant, unsafe for human use, it is used as a standard irritant in pharmacological research. **distilled o.,** volatile o. **essential o., ethereal o.,** volatile o. **ethiodized o.,** an iodine addition product of the ethyl ester of fatty acids of poppyseed oil; used as a radiopaque medium iin bronchography. **eucalyptus o.,** a volatile oil from fresh leaf of species of *Eucalyptus;* used as a flavoring agent, expectorant, local antiseptic, and vermifuge. **expressed o., fatty o.,** fixed o. **fennel o.,** a volatile oil from dried ripe fruit of the herb *Foeniculum vulgare;* used as a flavoring agent and carminative. **fixed o.,** a nonvolatile oil, i.e., one that does not evaporate on warming; such oils consist of a mixture of fatty acids and their esters, and are classified as solid, semisolid, and liquid. **flaxseed o.,** linseed o. **gaultheria o.,** methyl salicylate. **gingilli o.,** sesame o. **halibut liver o.,** a fixed oil from fresh or suitably preserved livers of halibut species; used as a source of vitamins A and D. **hydnocarpus o.,** chaulmoogra o. **iodized o.,** a sterile preparation of vegetable oil or oils containing 38–42% of organically combined iodine; used as a contrast medium in hysterosalpingography. **lavender o.,** a volatile oil from fresh flowering tops of *Lavandula officinalis;* used as a perfuming agent and flavoring agent. **lemon o.,** a volatile oil from fresh peel of fruit of *Citrus limon;* used as a flavoring agent. **linseed o.,** a fixed oil from dried ripe seed of *Linum usitatissimum;* used as an emollient in liniments, pastes, and medicinal soaps. **mineral o.,** a mixture of liquid hydrocarbons from petroleum; used as a levigating agent, lubricant laxative, and drug vehicle. **mineral o., light,** a mixture of hydrocarbons from petrolatum; used as a drug vehicle and laxative. **myristica o., nutmeg o.,** a volatile oil distilled with steam from dried kernels of ripe seeds of *Myristica fragrans;* used as a flavoring agent. **olive o.,** a fixed oil obtained from ripe fruit of *Olea europaea;* used as an emollient, laxative, and cholagogue. **orange o.,** a volatile oil from fresh peel of ripe fruit of *Citreus sinensis;* used as a flavoring agent. **orange flower o.,** a volatile oil from fresh flowers of *Citrus aurantium;* used as a flavoring and perfuming agent. **peach kernel o.,** persic o. **peanut o.,** a refined fixed oil from seed kernels of cultivated varieties of *Arachis hypogaea;* used as a solvent for drugs. **peppermint o.,** a volatile oil from fresh overground parts of flowering plant of *Mentha piperita;* used as a flavoring agent and carminative. **persic o.,** oil expressed from kernels of varieties of *Prunus armeniaca* (apricot) or *P. persica* (peach); used as a drug vehicle. **pine o.,** a volatile oil from *Pinus palustris* and other species of *Pinus;* used as a deodorant and disinfectant. **pine needle o.,** a volatile oil from fresh leaf of *Pinus mugo;* used as a perfuming and flavoring agent. **rose o.,** a volatile oil from fresh flowers of *Rosa gallica* and other species of *Rosa;* used as a perfuming agent. **safflower o.,** an oily liquid from the seeds of *Carthamus tinctorius;* used as a dietary supplement in the management of hypercholesterolemia. **sesame o.,** a refined, fixed oil from seeds of cultivated varieties of *Sesamum indicum;* used as a solvent for drugs. **spearmint o.,** a volatile oil from fresh parts of flowering plants of *Mentha spicata* or *M. cardiaca;* used as a flavoring agent. **sweet o.,** olive o. **tar o., rectified,** a volatile oil from pine tar rectified by steam distillation. **teel o.,** sesame o. **theobroma o.,** fat from roasted seed of the tropical American tree *Theobroma cacao;* used as a base in suppositories. **turpentine o.,** a volatile oil from an oleoresin obtained from *Pinus;* used as a counterirritant and rubefacient. **volatile o.,** a readily evaporating substance of plant origin, containing aromatic hydrocarbons, aldehydes, alcohols, ethers, acids, terpenes, or camphors. **wintergreen o.,** methyl salicylate.

ointment (oint′ment) a semisolid preparation for external application to the body, usually containing a medicinal substance. **ammoniated mercury o.,** a preparation of ammoniated mercury, mineral oil, and white ointment; used as a topical anti-infective. **blue o.,** a preparation of mercury and mercury oleate in solid bases; used as a topical parasiticide. **calamine o.,** a mixture of calamine, yellow wax, anhydrous lanolin, and petrolatum; used as an astringent protectant. **chrysarobin o.,** a preparation of chrysarobin, chloroform, and white ointment; used in topical treatment of psoriatic lesions. **coal tar o.,** a preparation of coal tar, polysorbate 80, and zinc oxide paste; used as an antieczematic. **hydrophilic o.,** a water-in-oil emulsion consisting of methylparaben, propylparaben, sodium lauryl sulfate, propylene glycol, stearyl alcohol, white petrolatum, and purified water; used as an ointment base. **pine tar o.,** a preparation of pine tar, yellow wax, and yellow ointment; used as a local irritant and antibacterial. **polyethylene glycol o.,** a mixture of polyethylene glycol 4000 and polyethylene glycol 400; used as a water-soluble ointment base. **rose water o.,** a preparation of spermaceti, white wax, almond oil, sodium borate, stronger rose water, purified water, and rose oil; used as an emollient and ointment base. **sulfur o.,** a mixture of precipitated sulfur, mineral oil, and white ointment; used as a scabicide.

undecylenic acid o., compound, 1. a preparation of undecylenic acid, zinc undecylenate, and polyethylene glycol ointment; used as a topical antifungal. 2. a preparation of clove and cinnamon oils, salicylic acid, undecylenic acid, benzoic acid, and white petrolatum; used in podiatry. **white o.,** an oleaginous ointment base prepared from white wax and white petrolatum. **yellow o.,** a mixture of yellow wax and petrolatum; used as an ointment base. **zinc o., zinc oxide o.,** a preparation of zinc oxide and mineral oil in white ointment; used topically as an astringent and protective.

O.L. [L.] *oc′ulus lae′vus* (left eye).

-ol word termination indicating an alcohol or a phenol.

oleaginous (o″le-aj′ĭ-nus) oily; greasy.

oleandomycin (o″le-an″do-mi′sin) an antibiotic produced by *Streptomyces antibioticus;* used chiefly in treatment of infections by gram-positive organisms.

oleate (o′le-āt) 1. a salt of oleic acid. 2. a solution of a substance in oleic acid.

olecranarthritis (o-lek″ran-ar-thri′tis) inflammation of the elbow joint.

olecranarthrocace (-ar-throk′ah-se) tuberculosis of the elbow joint.

olecranarthropathy (-ar-throp′ah-the) disease of the elbow joint.

olecranoid (o-lek′rah-noid) resembling the olecranon.

olecranon (o-lek′rah-non) bony projection of the ulna at the elbow. **olec′ranal,** adj.

oleo- word element [L.], *oil.*

oleoresin (o″le-o-rez′in) 1. a compound of a resin and a volatile oil, such as exudes from pines, etc. 2. a compound extracted from a drug by percolation with a volatile solvent, such as acetone, alcohol, or ether, and evaporation of the solvent.

oleotherapy (-ther′ah-pe) treatment by injections of oil.

oleothorax (-tho′raks) intrapleural injection of oil to compress the lung in pulmonary tuberculosis.

oleovitamin (-vi′tah-min) a preparation of fish liver oil or edible vegetable oil containing one or more fat-soluble vitamins or their derivatives.

oleum (o′le-um), pl. *o′lea* [L.] oil.

olfact (ol′fakt) a unit of odor, the *minimum perceptible odor,* being the minimum concentration of a substance in solution that can be perceived by a large number of normal individuals; expressed in grams per liter.

olfaction (ol-fak′shun) 1. the act of smelling. 2. the sense of smell.

olfactology (ol″fak-tol′o-je) the science of the sense of smell.

olfactometer (ol″fak-tom′ĕ-ter) an instrument for testing the sense of smell.

olfactory (ol-fak′to-re) pertaining to the sense of smell.

olig(o)- word element [Gr.], *few; little; scanty.*

oligemia (ol″ĭ-ge′me-ah) deficiency in volume of the blood. **olige′mic,** adj.

oligoblast (ol′ĭ-go-blast″) a primitive oligodendrocyte.

oligocardia (ol″ĭ-go-kar′de-ah) bradycardia.

oligochromemia (-kro-me′me-ah) deficiency of hemoglobin in the blood.

oligocystic (-sis′tik) containing few cysts.

oligocythemia (-si-the′me-ah) deficiency of the cellular elements of the blood. **oligocythe′mic,** adj.

oligodactyly (-dak′tĭ-le) congenital absence of one or more fingers or toes.

oligodendria (-den′dre-ah) oligodendroglia.

oligodendrocyte (-den′dro-sīt) a cell of oligodendroglia.

oligodendroglia (-den-drog′le-ah) 1. the nonneural cells of ectodermal origin forming part of the adventitial structure of the central nervous system. 2. the tissue composed of such cells.

oligodendroglioma (-den″dro-gli-o′mah) a neoplasm derived from and composed of oligodendrocytes.

oligodipsia (-dip′se-ah) abnormally diminished thirst.

oligodontia (-don′she-ah) presence of fewer than the normal number of teeth.

oligodynamic (-di-nam′ik) active in a small quantity.

oligogalactia (-gah-lak′she-ah) deficient secretion of milk.

oligogenic (-jen′ik) produced by a few genes at most; used in reference to certain hereditary characters.

oligohemia (-he′me-ah) oligemia.

oligohydramnios (-hi-dram′ne-os) deficiency in the amount of amniotic fluid.

oligohydruria (-hi-droo′re-ah) abnormally high concentration of urine.

oligolecithal (-les′ĭ-thal) having only a little yolk.

oligomenorrhea (-men″o-re′ah) abnormally infrequent menstruation.

oligomorphic (-mor′fik) passing through only a few forms of growth.

oligonucleotide (-nu′kle-o-tīd) a polymer made up of a few (2–10) nucleotides.

oligophosphaturia (-fos″fah-tu′re-ah) deficiency of phosphates in the urine.

oligophrenia (-fre′ne-ah) mental deficiency. **oligophren′ic,** adj. **phenylpyruvic o., o. phenylpyru′vica,** mental deficiency associated with phenylketonuria.

oligoplasmia (-plaz′me-ah) deficiency of blood plasma.

oligopnea (ol″ĭ-gop′ne-ah) hypoventilation.

oligoptyalism (ol″ĭ-go-ti′al-izm) diminished secretion of saliva.

oligosaccharide (-sak′ah-rīd) a carbohydrate that, on acid hydrolysis, yields two to ten monosaccharides.

oligospermia (-sper′me-ah) deficiency of spermatozoa in the semen.

oligotrophia, oligotrophy (-tro′fe-ah; ol″ĭ-got′ro-fe) a state of poor (insufficient) nutrition.

oligozoospermia (ol″ĭ-go-zo″o-sper′me-ah) oligospermia.

oliguria (ol″ĭ-gu′re-ah) diminished urine secretion in relation to fluid intake. **oligu′ric,** adj.

oliva (o-li′vah), pl. *oli′vae* [L.] olive.

olivary (ol′ĭ-ver″e) shaped like an olive.

olive (ol′iv) 1. the tree *Olea europaea* and its fruit. 2. olivary body; a rounded elevation lateral to the upper part of each pyramid of the medulla oblongata.

olivifugal (ol″ĭ-vif′u-gal) moving or conducting away from the olive.

olivipetal (ol″ĭ-vip′ĕ-tal) moving or conducting toward the olive.

olivopontocerebellar (ol″ĭ-vo-pon″to-ser″ĕ-bel′ar) pertaining to the olive, the middle peduncles, and the cerebellar cortex.

olophonia (ol″o-fo′ne-ah) defective speech due to malformed vocal organs.

-oma word element [Gr.], *tumor; neoplasm.*

omagra (o-mag′rah) gout in the shoulder.

omalgia (o-mal′je-ah) pain in the shoulder.

omarthritis (o″mar-thri′tis) inflammation of the shoulder joint.

omasitis (o″mah-si′tis) inflammation of the omasum.

omasum (o-ma′sum) the third division of the stomach of a ruminant animal.

omentectomy (o″men-tek′to-me) excision of all or part of the omentum.

omentitis (o″men-ti′tis) inflammation of the omentum.

omentofixation (o-men″to-fik-sa′shun) omentopexy.

omentopexy (o-men′to-pek″se) fixation of the omentum, especially to establish collateral circulation in portal obstruction.

omentorrhaphy (o″men-tor′ah-fe) suture or repair of the omentum.

omentum (o-men′tum), pl. *omen′ta* [L.] a fold of peritoneum extending from the stomach to adjacent abdominal organs. **omen′tal,** adj. **gastrocolic o.,** greater o. **gastrohepatic o.,** lesser o. **greater o.,** a peritoneal fold attached to the anterior surface of the transverse colon. **lesser o.,** a peritoneal fold joining the lesser curvature of the stomach and the first part of the duodenum to the porta hepatis. **o. ma′jus,** greater o. **o. mi′nor,** lesser o.

omitis (o-mi′tis) inflammation of the shoulder.

omnivorous (om-niv′o-rus) eating both plant and animal foods.

omoclavicular (o″mo-klah-vik′u-lar) pertaining to the shoulder and clavicle.

omodynia (-din′e-ah) pain in the shoulder.

omohyoid (-hi′oid) pertaining to the shoulder and the hyoid bone.

omphal(o)- word element [Gr.], *umbilicus.*

omphalectomy (om″fah-lek′to-me) excision of the umbilicus.

omphalelcosis (om″fal-el-ko′sis) ulceration of the umbilicus.

omphalic (om-fal′ik) pertaining to the umbilicus.

omphalitis (om″fah-li′tis) inflammation of the umbilicus.

omphaloangiopagus (om″fah-lo-an″je-op′ah-gus) twin fetuses, one of which derives its blood supply from the umbilicus or placenta of the other.

omphalocele (om′fal-o-sēl″) protrusion, at birth, of part of the intestine through a defect in the abdominal wall at the umbilicus.

omphalomesenteric (om″fah-lo-mes″en-ter′ik) pertaining to the umbilicus and mesentery.

omphalophlebitis (-fle-bi′tis) 1. inflammation of the umbilical veins. 2. an infectious condition characterized by markedly suppurative lesions of the umbilicus in young animals; see *navel ill*.

omphalorrhagia (-ra′je-ah) hemorrhage from the umbilicus.

omphalorrhea (-re′ah) effusion of lymph at the umbilicus.

omphalorrhexis (-rek′sis) rupture of the umbilicus.

omphalosite (om′fal-o-sīt″) the underdeveloped member of allantoidoangiopagous twins, joined t᠎ the more developed member (autosite) by the vessels of the umbilical cord.

omphalotomy (om″fah-lot′o-me) the cutting of the umbilical cord.

onanism (o′nah-nizm) coitus interruptus; sometimes used incorrectly to mean masturbation.

Onchocerca (ong″ko-ser′kah) a genus of nematode parasites of the superfamily Filarioidea, including *O. vol′vulus*, which causes human infection by invading the skin, subcutaneous tissues, and other tissues, producing fibrous nodules; blindness occurs after ocular invasion.

onchocerciasis (-ser-ki′ah-sis) infection by nematodes of the genus *Onchocerca*.

onchocercosis (-ser-ko′sis) onchocerciasis.

onco- word element [Gr.], *tumor; swelling; mass*.

oncogenesis (ong″ko-jen′ĕ-sis) the production or causation of tumors. **oncogenet′ic**, adj.

oncogenic (-jen′ik) giving rise to tumors or causing tumor formation; said especially of tumor-inducing viruses.

oncogenous (ong-koj′ĕ-nus) arising in or originating from a tumor.

oncology (ong-kol′o-je) the sum of knowledge regarding tumors; the study of tumors.

oncolysis (ong-kol′ĭ-sis) destruction or dissolution of a neoplasm. **oncolyt′ic**, adj.

oncoma (ong-ko′mah) a tumor.

oncosis (ong-ko′sis) a morbid condition marked by the development of tumors.

oncosphere (ong′ko-sfēr) the larva of the tapeworm contained within the external embryonic envelope and armed with six hooks.

oncotherapy (ong″ko-ther′ah-pe) the treatment of tumors.

oncotic (ong-kot′ik) pertaining to swelling.

oncotomy (ong-kot′o-me) the incision of a tumor or swelling.

oncotropic (ong″ko-trop′ik) having special affinity for tumor cells.

oneir(o)- word element [Gr.], *dream*.

oneiric (o-ni′rik) pertaining to dreams.

oneirism (o-ni′rizm) a waking dream state.

oneirodynia (o-ni″ro-din′e-ah) nightmare.

oneirology (o″ni-rol′o-je) the science of dreams.

oneiroscopy (o″ni-ros′ko-pe) analysis of dreams for diagnosis of the mental state.

onlay (on′la) a graft applied or laid on the surface of an organ or structure.

onomatology (on″o-mah-tol′o-je) the science of names and nomenclature.

onomatomania (on″o-mat″o-ma′ne-ah) mental derangement with regard to words or names.

onomatophobia (-fo′be-ah) morbid aversion to a certain word or name.

ontogenesis (on″to-jen′ĕ-sis) ontogeny.

ontogeny (on-toj′ĕ-ne) the complete developmental history of an individual organism. **ontogenet′ic, ontogen′ic**, adj.

onyalai, onyalia (o″ne-al′a-e; o″ne-a′le-ah) a form of thrombopenic purpura due to a nutritional disorder occurring in Africa, marked by blebs on the buccal and palatal mucosa which contain semicoagulated blood.

onych(o)- word element [Gr.], *the nails*.

onychatrophia (o-nik″ah-tro′fe-ah) atrophy of a nail or the nails.

onychauxis (on″ĭ-kawk′sis) hypertrophy of the nails.

onychectomy (on″ĭ-kek′to-me) excision of a nail or nail bed.

onychia (o-nik′e-ah) inflammation of the nail bed, resulting in loss of the nail.

onychitis (on″ĭ-ki′tis) onychia.

onychodystrophy (on″ĭ-ko-dis′tro-fe) malformation of a nail.

onychogenic (-jen′ik) producing nail substance.

onychograph (o-nik′o-graf) an instrument for observing and recording the nail pulse and capillary circulation.

onychogryphosis, onychogryposis (on″ĭ-ko-grĭ-fo′sis; -grĭ-po′sis) hypertrophy and curving of the nails, giving them a clawlike appearance.

onychoheterotopia (-het″er-o-to′pe-ah) abnormal location of the nails.

onychoid (on′ĭ-koid) resembling a fingernail.

onycholysis (on″ĭ-kol′ĭ-sis) loosening or separation of a nail from its bed.

onychomadesis (on″ĭ-ko-mah-de′sis) complete loss of the nails.

onychomalacia (-mah-la′she-ah) softening of the fingernail.

onychomycosis (-mi-ko′sis) fungal disease of the fingernails; the nails become opaque, white, thickened, and friable.

onychopathy (on″ĭ-kop′ah-the) any disease of the nails. **onychopath′ic**, adj.

onychophagia, onychophagy (on″ĭ-ko-fa′je-ah; on″ĭ-kof′ah-je) biting of the nails.

onychorrhexis (on″ĭ-ko-rek′sis) spontaneous splitting or breaking of the nails.

onychoschizia (-skiz′e-ah) onycholysis.

onychosis (on″ĭ-ko′sis) disease or deformity of a nail or the nails.

onychotillomania (on″ĭ-ko-til″o-ma′ne-ah) neurotic picking or tearing at the nails.

onychotomy (on″ĭ-kot′o-me) incision into a fingernail or toenail.

onyx (on′iks) 1. a variety of hypopyon. 2. a fingernail or toenail.

oo- word element [Gr.], *egg; ovum.*

ooblast (o′o-blast) a primitive cell from which an ovum ultimately develops.

oocyst (-sist) the encysted or encapsulated ookinete in the wall of a mosquito's stomach; also, the analogous stage in the development of any sporozoon.

oocyte (-sīt) an immature ovum; it is derived from an oogonium, and is called a *primary o.* prior to completion of the first maturation division, and a *secondary o.* in the period between the first and second maturation division.

oogenesis (o″o-jen′ĕ-sis) the process of formation of female gametes (ova). **oogenet′ic,** adj.

oogonium (-go′ne-um), pl. *oogo′nia* [Gr.] an ovarian egg during fetal development; near the time of birth it becomes a primary oocyte.

ookinesis (-ki-ne′sis) the mitotic movements of an ovum during maturation and fertilization.

ookinete (-kĭ-nēt′) the fertilized form of the malarial parasite in a mosquito's body, formed by fertilization of a macrogamete by a microgamete and developing into an oocyst.

oolemma (-lem′ah) zona pellucida.

oophor(o)- word element [Gr.], *ovary.*

oophorectomy (o″of-o-rek′to-me) excision of one or both ovaries.

oophoritis (-ri′tis) inflammation of an ovary.

oophorocystectomy (o-of″o-ro-sis-tek′to-me) excision of an ovarian cyst.

oophorocystosis (-sis-to′sis) the formation of ovarian cysts.

oophorohysterectomy (-his″ter-ek′to-me) excision of the ovaries and uterus.

oophoron (o-of′o-ron) an ovary.

oophoropexy (o-of′o-ro-pek″se) ovariopexy.

oophoroplasty (-plas″te) plastic repair of an ovary.

oophorostomy (o-of″o-ros′to-me) incision of an ovarian cyst for drainage purposes.

oophorotomy (o-of″o-rot′o-me) incision of an ovary.

ooplasm (o′o-plazm) cytoplasm of an ovum.

oosperm (-sperm) a fertilized ovum.

ootid (-tid) the cell produced by meiotic division of a secondary oocyte, which develops into the ovum. In mammals, this second maturation division is not completed unless fertilization occurs.

opacification (o-pah″sĭ-fĭ-ka′shun) the development of an opacity.

opacity (o-pas′ĭ-te) 1. the condition of being opaque. 2. an opaque area.

opalescent (o″pal-es′ent) showing a milky iridescence, like an opal.

opaque (o-pāk′) impervious to light rays or, by extension, to x-rays or other electromagnetic radiation.

opening (o′pen-ing) an aperture, orifice, or open space. **aortic o.,** 1. the aperture of the ventricle into the aorta. 2. the aperture in the diaphragm for passage of the descending aorta. **cardiac o.,** the opening from the esophagus into the stomach. **pyloric o.,** the opening between the stomach and duodenum. **saphenous o.,** see under *hiatus.*

operable (op′er-ah-b'l) subject to being operated upon with a reasonable degree of safety; appropriate for surgical removal.

operate (op′er-āt) 1. to perform an operation. 2. the subject of an experiment which has undergone a specific surgical procedure.

operation (op″er-a′shun) 1. any action performed with instruments or by the hands of a surgeon; a surgical procedure. 2. any effect produced by a therapeutic agent. **Abbé-Estlander o.,** the transfer of a full-thickness flap from one lip to fill a defect in the other. **Albee's o.,** an operation for ankylosis of the hip. **Babcock's o.,** a technique for eradication of varicose veins by extirpation of the saphenous vein. **Bassini's o.,** plastic repair of inguinal hernia. **Beck o.,** a one-stage (*Beck I o.*) or a two-stage (*Beck II o.*) operation for supplying collateral circulation to the heart. **Beer's o.,** a flap method for cataract. **Billroth's o.,** partial resection of the stomach with anastomosis to the duodenum (Billroth I) or to the jejunum (Billroth II). **Blalock-Taussig o.,** anastomosis of the subclavian artery to the pulmonary artery to shunt some of the systemic circulation into the pulmonary circulation; done in congenital pulmonary stenosis. **Bricker's o.,** surgical creation of an ileal conduit for the collection of urine. **Brunschwig's o.,** pancreatoduodenectomy performed in two stages. **Cotte's o.,** removal of the presacral nerve. **Daviel's o.,** extraction of a cataract through a corneal incision without cutting the iris. **Dührssen's o.,** vaginal fixation of the uterus. **Dupuy-Dutemps o.,** blepharoplasty of the lower lid with tissue from the upper lid. **Caldwell-Luc o.,** radical maxillary sinusotomy. **Elliot's o.,** sclerectomy by trephine. **equilibrating o.,** tenotomy of the direct antagonist of a paralyzed eye muscle. **exploratory o.,** incision into a body area to determine the cause of unexplained symptoms. **flap o.,** any operation involving the raising of a flap of tissue. **Fothergill o.,** an operation for uterine prolapse by fixation of the cardinal ligaments. **Frazier-Spiller o.,** division of the sensory root of the gasserian ganglion for relief of trigeminal neuralgia. **Fredet-Ramstedt o.,** pyloromyotomy. **Freyer's o.,** suprapubic enucleation of the hypertrophied prostate. **Frost-Lang o.,** insertion of a gold ball in place of an enucleated eyeball. **Gonin's o.,** thermocautery of the fissure in the retina, for retinal detachment. **Kelly's o., King's o.,** arytenoidopexy. **Kondoleon's o.,** excision of fascia in treatment of elephantiasis. **Kraske's o.,** removal of the coccyx and part of the sacrum for access to a rectal carcinoma. **Lagrange's o.,** sclerectoiridectomy. **Le Forte's o.,** partial colpectomy. **Lorenz's o.,** an operation for congenital dislocation of the hip. **McBurney's o.,** radical surgery for the cure of inguinal hernia. **Macewen's o.,** supracondylar section of the femur for genu valgum. **McGill's o.,** suprapubic transvesical prostatectomy. **Madlener o.,** sterilization by crushing and ligating the middle portion of the fallopian tube. **Manchester o.,** Fothergill o. **Motais o.,** transplantation of a portion of the tendon of the superior rectus muscle of the eyeball into the upper lid, for ptosis. **Partsch o.,** a technique for marsupialization of a dental cyst. **Pomeroy's o.,** sterilization by ligation of a loop of fallopian tube and resection of the tied loop. **radical o.,** one involving extensive resection of tissue for complete extirpation of disease. **Ramstedt o.,** pyloromyotomy. **Saemisch's o.,** transfixion of the cornea and of the base of the ulcer for cure of hypopyon. **Semb's o.,** extrafascial apicolysis. **Torkildsen's o.,** ventriculocisternostomy. **Verhoeff's o.,** posterior sclerotomy followed by electrolytic punctures, for detachment of the retina. **Wertheim's o.,** radical hysterectomy. **Ziegler's o.,** V-shaped iridectomy for forming an artificial pupil.

operative (op′er-ă-tiv) pertaining to an operation.

operculum (o-per′ku-lum), pl. *oper′cula*[L.] a lid or covering; the folds of pallium from the frontal, parietal, and temporal lobes of the cerebrum overlying the insula. **oper′cular,** adj. **dental o.,** the hood of gingival tissue overlying the crown of an erupting tooth. **trophoblastic o.,** the plug of trophoblast that helps close the gap in the endometrium made by the implanting blastocyst.

operon (op′er-on) a segment of a chromosome comprising an operator gene and closely linked structural genes having related functions.

ophiasis (o-fi′ah-sis) a form of alopecia areata involving the temporal and occipital margins of the scalp in a continuous band.

ophidism (o′fĭ-dizm) poisoning by snake venom.

ophryon (o′fre-on) the middle point of the transverse supraorbital line.

ophryosis (of″re-o′sis) spasm of the eyebrow.

Ophthaine (of′thān) trademark for preparations of proparacaine.

ophthalm(o)- word element [Gr.], *eye.*

ophthalmagra (of″thal-mag′rah) sudden pain in the eye.

ophthalmalgia (of″thal-mal′je-ah) pain in the eye.

ophthalmectomy (of″thal-mek′to-me) excision of an eye; enuceation of the eyeball.

ophthalmencephalon (of″thal-men-sef′ah-lon) the retina, optic nerve, and visual apparatus of the brain.

ophthalmia (of-thal′me-ah) severe inflammation of the eye. **Egyptian o.,** trachoma. **gonorrheal o.,** acute and severe purulent ophthalmia due to gonorrheal infection. **o. neonato′rum,** any hyperacute purulent conjunctivitis occurring during the first 10 days of life, usually contracted during birth from infected vaginal discharge of the mother. **periodic o.,** a form of uveitis affecting horses. **phlyctenular o.,** see under *keratoconjunctivitis.* **purulent o.,** a form with a purulent discharge, commonly due to gonorrheal infection. **sympathetic o.,** granulomatous inflammation of the uveal tract of the uninjured eye following a wound involving the uveal tract of the other eye, resulting in bilateral granulomatous inflammation of the entire uveal tract.

ophthalmic (of-thal′mik) pertaining to the eye.

ophthalmitis (of″thal-mi′tis) inflammation of the eyeball. **ophthalmit′ic,** adj.

ophthalmoblennorrhea (of-thal″mo-blen″ŏ-re′ah) gonorrheal ophthalmia.

ophthalmocele (of-thal′mo-sēl) exophthalmos.

ophthalmodonesis (of-thal″mo-do-ne′sis) trembling motion of the eyes.

ophthalmodynamometry (-di″nah-mom′ĕ-tre) determination of the blood pressure in the retinal artery.

ophthalmodynia (-din′e-ah) pain in the eye.

ophthalmoeikonometer (-i-ko-nom′ĕ-ter) an instrument for determining both the refraction of the eye and the relative size and shape of the ocular images.

ophthalmography (of″thal-mog′rah-fe) description of the eye and its diseases.

ophthalmogyric (of-thal″mo-ji′rik) oculogyric.

ophthalmolith (of-thal′mo-lith) a lacrimal calculus.

ophthalmologist (of″thal-mol′o-jist) a physician who specializes in ophthalmology.

ophthalmology (of″thal-mol′o-je) that branch of medicine dealing with the eye, its anatomy, physiology, pathology, etc. **ophthalmolog′ic,** adj.

ophthalmomalacia (of-thal″mo-mah-la′she-ah) abnormal softness of the eyeball.

ophthalmometer (of″thal-mom′ĕ-ter) an instrument used in ophthalmometry.

ophthalmometry (of″thal-mom′ĕ-tre) determination of the refractive powers and defects of the eye.

ophthalmomycosis (of-thal″mo-mi-ko′sis) any disease of the eye caused by a fungus.

ophthalmomyotomy (-mi-ot′o-me) surgical division of the muscles of the eyes.

ophthalmoneuritis (-nu-ri′tis) inflammation of the ophthalmic nerve.

ophthalmopathy (of″thal-mop′ah-the) any disease of the eye.

ophthalmoplasty (of-thal′mo-plas″te) plastic surgery of the eye or its appendages.

ophthalmoplegia (of-thal″mo-ple′je-ah) paralysis of the eye muscles. **ophthalmople′gic,** adj. **o. exter′na,** paralysis of extraocular muscles. **o. inter′na,** paralysis of the iris and ciliary apparatus. **nuclear o.,** that due to a lesion of nuclei of motor nerves of eye. **Parinaud's o.,** paralysis of conjugate upward movement of the eyes without paralysis of convergence, associated with midbrain lesions. **partial o.,** that affecting some of the eye muscles. **progressive o.,** gradual paralysis of all the eye muscles. **total o.,** paralysis of all the eye muscles, both intraocular and extraocular.

ophthalmoptosis (of-thal″mop-to′sis) exophthalmos.

ophthalmoreaction (of-thal″mo-re-ak′shun) ophthalmic reaction.

ophthalmorrhagia (-ra′je-ah) hemorrhage from the eye.

ophthalmorrhea (-re′ah) oozing of blood from the eye.

ophthalmorrhexis (-rek′sis) rupture of an eyeball.

ophthalmoscope (of-thal′mo-skōp) an instrument containing a perforated mirror and lenses used to examine the interior of the eye. **direct o.,** one that produces an upright, or unreversed, image of approximately 15 times magnification. **indirect o.,** one that produces an inverted, or reversed, direct image of two to five times magnification.

ophthalmoscopy (of″thal-mos′ko-pe) examination of the eye by means of the ophthalmoscope. **medical o.,** that performed for diagnostic purposes. **metric o.,** that performed for measurement of refraction.

ophthalmostasis (of″thal-mos′tah-sis) fixation of the eye with the ophthalmostat.

ophthalmostat (of-thal′mo-stat) an instrument for holding the eye steady during operation.

ophthalmosteresis (of-thal″mo-stĕ-re′sis) loss of an eye.

ophthalmosynchysis (-sin′kĭ-sis) effusion into the eye.

ophthalmotomy (of″thal-mot′o-me) incision of the eye.

ophthalmotrope (of-thal′mo-trōp) a mechanical eye that moves like a real eye.

ophthalmoxerosis (of-thal″mo-ze-ro′sis) xerophthalmia.

opianine (o-pi′ah-nin) noscapine.

opiate (o′pe-ăt) a remedy containing opium; also, any sleep-inducing drug.

opiomania (o″pe-o-ma′ne-ah) intense craving for opium.

opipramol (o-pip′rah-mōl) an antidepressant and tranquilizer, $C_{23}H_{29}N_3O$.

opisthion (o-pis′the-on) the midpoint of the lower border of the foramen magnum.

opisthorchiasis (o″pis-thor-ki′ah-sis) a diseased condition of the liver due to the presence of flukes of the genus *Opisthorchis.*

Opisthorchis (o″pis-thor′kis) a genus of flukes parasitic in the liver and biliary tract of various birds and mammals, including man; *O. sinen′sis* is found in China, Japan, Korea, Taiwan, and Indochina.

opisthotonos (o″pis-thot′o-nos) a form of spasm in which the head and heels are bent backward and the body bowed forward. **opisthoton′ic,** adj.

opium (o′pe-um) air-dried milky exudation from incised unripe capsules of *Papaver somniferum* or its variety *album,* yielding not less than 9.5% of anhydrous morphine, and containing some 25 alkaloids, the more important being morphine, narcotine, codeine, papaverine, thebaine, and narceine; the alkaloids are used for their narcotic and analgesic effect. *Powdered opium* (containing not less than 10% of anhydrous morphine) is the standarized form. Because it is highly addictive, opium production is restricted. **granulated o.,** opium reduced to a coarse powder.

opocephalus (o″po-sef′ah-lus) a monster with

the ears fused to the head, one orbit, no mouth, and no nose.

opodidymus (-did′ĭ-mus) a monster with two fused heads and sense organs partly fused.

opportunistic (op″or-tu-nis′tik) capable of adapting to a tissue or host other than the normal one; said of microorganisms.

opsin (op′sin) a protein of the retinal rods (scotopsin) and cones (photopsin) that combines with 11-*cis*-retinal to form visual pigments.

opsinogen (op-sin′o-jen) a substance (antigen) capable of inducing the formation of opsonins. **opsinog′enous,** adj.

opsiuria (op″se-u′re-ah) excretion of urine more rapidly during fasting than after a meal.

opsoclonia, opsoclonus (op″so-clo′ne-ah; -clo′nus) involuntary, nonrhythmic horizontal and vertical oscillations of the eyes.

opsogen (op′so-jen) opsinogen.

opsomania (op″so-ma′ne-ah) an abnormal craving for some special food.

opsonin (op′so-nin) an antibody which renders bacteria and other cells susceptible to phagocytosis. **opson′ic,** adj. **immune o.,** an antibody which sensitizes a particulate antigen to phagocytosis, after combination with the homologous antigen *in vivo* or *in vitro.*

opsonization (op″so-ni-za′shun) the rendering of bacteria and other cells subject to phagocytosis.

opsonize (op′so-nīz) to subject to opsonization.

opsonocytophagic (op″so-no-si″to-faj′ik) denoting the phagocytic activity of blood in the presence of serum opsonins and homologous leukocytes.

opsonometry (op″so-nom′ĕ-tre) measurement of the opsonic index.

opsonotherapy (op″so-no-ther′ah-pe) treatment by use of bacterial vaccines to increase the opsonic index.

optesthesia (op″tes-the′ze-ah) visual sensibility; ability to perceive visual stimuli.

optic (op′tik) of or pertaining to the eye.

optical (op′tĭ-kal) pertaining to vision.

optician (op-tish′an) a specialist in opticianry.

opticianry (op-tish′an-re) the translation, filling, and adapting of ophthalmic prescriptions, products, and accessories.

opticist (op′tĭ-sist) a specialist in the science of optics.

opticociliary (op″tĭ-ko-sil′e-er″e) pertaining to the optic and ciliary nerves.

opticokinetic (-ki-net′ik) pertaining to movement of the eyes.

opticopupillary (-pu′pĭ-ler″e) pertaining to the optic nerve and pupil.

optics (op′tiks) the science of light and vision.

opto- word element [Gr.], *visible; vision; sight.*

optogram (op′to-gram) the retinal image formed by the bleaching of visual purple under the influence of light.

optometer (op-tom′ĕ-ter) a device for measuring the power and range of vision.

optometrist (op-tom′ĕ-trist) a specialist in optometry.

optometry (op-tom′ĕ-tre) measurement of the powers of vision and the adaptation of lenses or prisms for the aid thereof, utilizing any means other than drugs.

optomyometer (op″to-mi-om′ĕ-ter) a device for measuring the power of ocular muscles.

O.R. operating room.

ora¹ (o′rah), pl. *o′rae* [L.] an edge or margin. **o. serra′ta ret′inae,** the zigzag margin of the retina of the eye.

ora² (o′rah) [L.] plural of *os,* mouth.

orad (o′rad) toward the mouth.

oral (o′ral) pertaining to the mouth.

orange (or′anj) 1. the tree, *Citrus aurantium,* and its edible yellow fruit; the peel of two varieties is used in making various pharmaceuticals. 2. a color between yellow and red. 3. a dye or stain that produces an orange color. **methyl o.,** an orange-yellow aniline dye, used as an indicator with a pH range of 3.2–4.4 and a color change from pink to yellow.

orbicular (or-bik′u-lar) circular; rounded.

orbiculare (or-bik″u-la′re) a small oval knob on the long limb of the incus, articulating with or ossified to the head of the stapes.

orbiculus (or-bik′u-lus), pl. *orbic′uli* [L.] a small disk.

orbit (or′bit) the bony cavity containing the eyeball and its associated muscles, vessels, and nerves. **or′bital,** adj.

orbita (or′bĭ-tah), pl. *or′bitae* [L.] orbit.

orbitale (or″bĭ-ta′le) the lowest point on the inferior edge of the orbit.

orbitalis (or″bĭ-ta′lis) [L.] pertaining to the orbit.

orbitonasal (or″bĭ-to-na′zal) pertaining to the orbit and nose.

orbitonometer (-nom′ĕ-ter) an instrument for measuring backward displacement of the eyeball produced by a given pressure on its anterior aspect.

orbitotomy (or″bĭ-tot′o-me) incision into the orbit.

orcein (or-se′in) a brownish-red coloring substance obtained from orcinol; used as a stain for elastic tissue.

orchi(o)- word element [Gr.], *testis.*

orchialgia (or″ke-al′je-ah) pain in a testis.

orchidectomy (or″kĭ-dek′to-me) orchiectomy.

orchidic (or-kid′ik) pertaining to a testis.

orchidorrhaphy (or″kĭ-dor′ah-fe) orchiopexy.

orchiectomy (or″ke-ek′to-me) excision of one or both testes.

orchiencephaloma (-en-sef″ah-lo′mah) embryonal carcinoma.

orchiepididymitis (-ep″ĭ-did″ĭ-mi′tis) inflammation of the testis and epididymis.

orchiocele (or′ke-o-sēl) 1. hernial protrusion of a testis. 2. scrotal hernia. 3. tumor of a testis.

orchiomyeloma (or″ke-o-mi″ĕ-lo′mah) plasmacytoma of the testis.

orchiopathy (or″ke-op′ah-the) any disease of the testis.

orchiopexy (or′ke-o-pek″se) fixation of an undescended testis in the scrotum.

orchioplasty (-plas″te) plastic surgery of a testis.

orchioscheocele (or″ke-os′ke-o-sēl″) scrotal tumor with scrotal hernia.

orchiotomy (or″kĭ-ot′o-me) incision and drainage of a testis.

orchitis (or-ki′tis) inflammation of a testis. **orchit′ic,** adj. **mumps o.,** that occurring before, or as the only manifestation of, mumps.

orcinol (or′sĭ-nol) an antiseptic principle, $C_7H_8O_2 \cdot H_2O$, derived mainly from lichens; used as a reagent.

order (or′der) 1. arrangement systematically or in proper sequence. 2. a taxonomic category subordinate to a class and superior to a family (or suborder).

orderly (or′der-le) a male hospital attendant who does general work, attending especially to needs of male patients.

ordinate (or′dĭ-nāt) the vertical line in a graph along which is plotted one of two sets of factors considered in the study.

Oretic (o-ret′ik) trademark for a preparation of hydrochlorothiazide.

Oreton (or′ĕ-ton) trademark for preparations of testosterone.

orexigenic (o-rek″sĭ-jen′ik) increasing or stimulating the appetite.

orf (orf) a contagious pustular viral dermatitis of sheep, communicable to man.

organ (or′gan) a somewhat independent body part that performs a special function. **o. of Corti,** the organ lying against the basilar membrane in the cochlear duct, containing special sensory receptors for hearing, and consisting of neuroepithelial hair cells and several types of supporting cells. **enamel o.,** a process of epithelium forming a cap over a dental papilla and developing into the enamel. **genital o's,** reproductive o's. **o. of Giraldés,** the paradidymis. **Golgi tendon o.,** any of the mechanoreceptors arranged in series with muscle in the tendons of mammalian muscles, being the receptor for stimuli responsible for the lengthening reaction. **Jacobson's o.,** vomeronasal o. **lateral line o's,** a system of sense organs arranged in longitudinal canals in the skin of fishes and amphibians which are sensitive to changes in pressure and current and to vibrations of low frequency and thus aid in localizing objects. **reproductive o's,** the various organs, internal and external, concerned with reproduction. **o. of Rosenmüller,** epoophoron. **sense o's, sensory o's,** organs that receive stimuli that give rise to sensations, i.e., organs that translate certain forms of energy into nerve impulses which are perceived as special sensations. **spiral o.,** o. of Corti. **target o.,** the organ affected by a particular hormone. **vestigial o.,** an undeveloped organ that, in the embryo or in some ancestor, was well developed and functional. **vomeronasal o.,** a small sac just above the vomeronasal cartilage; rudimentary in adult man but well developed in many lower animals. **Weber's o.,** prostatic utriculus. **o's of Zuckerkandl,** paraaortic bodies.

organelle (or″gah-nel′) 1. a specific particle of

membrane-bound organized living substance present in practically all cells, including mitochondria, the Golgi complex, etc. 2. one of the minute organs of protozoa concerned with such functions as locomotion, metabolism, or the like.

organic (or-gan′ik) 1. pertaining to an organ or organs. 2. having an organized structure. 3. arising from an organism. 4. pertaining to substances derived from living organisms. 5. denoting chemical substances containing carbon. 6. pertaining to or cultivated by use of animal or vegetable fertilizers, rather than synthetic chemicals.

organism (or′gah-nizm) an individual living thing, whether animal or plant.

organization (or″gah-ni-za′shun) 1. the process of organizing or of becoming organized. 2. the replacement of blood clots by fibrous tissue. 3. an organized body, group, or structure.

organize (or′gah-nīz) to provide with an organic structure; to form into organs.

organizer (or′gah-nīz″er) a special region of the embryo which is capable of determining the differentiation of other regions. **primary o.,** the dorsal lip region of the blastopore.

organo- word element [Gr.], *organ.*

organogel (or-gan′o-jel) a gel in which an organic liquid replaces water.

organogenesis, organogeny (or″gah-no-jen′-ĕ-sis; or″gah-noj′ĕ-ne) the development or growth of organs.

organoid (or′gah-noid) 1. resembling an organ. 2. a structure that resembles an organ.

organology (or″gah-nol′o-je) the sum of what is known regarding the body organs.

organometallic (or″gah-no-mĕ-tal′ik) consisting of a metal combined with an organic radical.

organon (or′gah-non), pl. *or′gana* [Gr.] organ.

organotherapy (or″gah-no-ther′ah-pe) therapeutic administration of animal endocrine organs or their extracts.

organotropism (or-gah-not′ro-pizm) the special affinity of chemical compounds or pathogenic agents for particular tissues or organs of the body. **organotrop′ic,** adj.

organ-specific (or′gan-spĕ-sif′ik) restricted to, or having an effect only on, a particular organ, as an organ-specific antigen.

organum (or′gah-num), pl. *or′gana* [L.] organ.

orgasm (or′gazm) the apex and culmination of sexual excitement.

orientation (o″re-en-ta′shun) the recognition of one's position in relation to time and space.

orifice (or′ĭ-fis) 1. the entrance or outlet of any body cavity. 2. any foramen, meatus, or opening. **orific′ial,** adj. **cardiac o.,** see under *opening.* **root canal o.,** an opening in the pulp chamber of a tooth, leading to the root canal.

orificium (or″i-fish′e-um), pl. *orific′ia* [L.] orifice.

origin (or′ĭ-jin) [L.] the source or beginning of anything, especially the more fixed end or attachment of a muscle (as distinguished from its

insertion), or the site of emergence of a peripheral nerve from the central nervous system.

Orinase (or′ĭ-nās) trademark for a preparation of tolbutamide.

ornithine (or′nĭ-thēn) an amino acid obtained from arginine by splitting of urea; it is an intermediate in urea biosynthesis.

Ornithodoros (or″nĭ-thod′o-ros) a genus of soft-bodied ticks, many species of which are reservoirs and vectors of the spirochetes (*Borrelia*) of relapsing fevers.

Ornithonyssus (or″nĭ-tho-nis′us) a genus of mites, including *O. baco′ti,* the rat mite; *O. bur′sa,* the tropical fowl mite; and *O. sylvia′rum,* the northern fowl mite.

ornithosis (or″nĭ-tho′sis) a disease of birds and domestic fowl, transmissible to man, caused by a strain of *Chlamydia psittaci;* the human disease is called *psittacosis.*

orolingual (o″ro-ling′gwal) pertaining to the mouth and tongue.

oronasal (-na′zal) pertaining to the mouth and nose.

oropharynx (-phar′inks) the part of the pharynx between the soft palate and the upper edge of the epiglottis.

orphenadrine (or-fen′ah-drēn) a drug, $C_{18}H_{23}$-NO, having antihistaminic, antitremor, and antispasmodic activities; its citrate and hydrochloride salts are used as skeletal muscle relaxants.

orth(o)- word element [Gr.], *straight; normal; correct.* In chemistry, *ortho-* indicates an isomer; also, a cyclic derivative having two substitutes in adjacent positions.

orthergasia (or″ther-ga′ze-ah) normal mental functioning.

orthesis (or-the′sis), pl. *orthe′ses* [Gr.] orthosis.

orthetics (or-thet′iks) orthotics.

orthetist (or′thĕ-tist) orthotist.

orthocephalic (or″tho-sĕ-fal′ik) having a vertical index of 70.1–75.

orthochorea (-ko-re′ah) choreic movements in the erect posture.

orthochromatic (-kro-mat′ik) staining normally.

orthodentin (-den′tin) straight-tubed dentin, as in mammalian teeth.

orthodontia (-don′she-ah) orthodontics.

orthodontics (-don′tiks) that branch of dentistry concerned with irregularities of teeth and malocclusion, and associated facial abnormalities. **orthodon′tic,** adj.

orthodontist (-don′tist) a dentist who specializes in orthodontics.

orthodromic (-drom′ik) conducting impulses in the normal direction; said of nerve fibers.

orthognathous (or-thog′nah-thus) having a gnathic index below 98.

orthograde (or′tho-grād) walking with the body upright.

orthometer (or-thom′ĕ-ter) instrument for determining relative protrusion of the eyeballs.

orthomyxovirus (or″tho-mik″so-vi′rus) a subgroup of myxoviruses that includes the viruses of human and animal influenza.

orthopedic (-pe′dik) pertaining to the correction of deformities of the musculoskeletal system; pertaining to orthopedics.

orthopedics (-pe′diks) that branch of surgery dealing with the preservation and restoration of the function of the skeletal system, its articulations, and associated structures.

orthopedist (-pe′dist) an orthopedic surgeon.

orthopercussion (-per-kush′un) percussion with the distal phalanx of the finger held perpendicularly to the body wall.

orthophenolase (-fe′no-lās) an enzyme in sweet potatoes that oxidizes catechol and orthocresol.

orthophoria (-fo′re-ah) normal equilibrium of the eye muscles, or muscular balance. **orthophor′ic,** adj.

orthopnea (or″thop-ne′ah) difficult breathing except in the upright position. **orthopne′ic,** adj.

orthopraxis, orthopraxy (or″tho-prak′sis; -prak′se) mechanical correction of deformities.

orthopsychiatry (-si-ki′ah-tre) that branch of psychiatry dealing with mental and emotional development, embracing child psychiatry and mental hygiene.

orthoptic (or-thop′tik) correcting obliquity of one or both visual axes.

orthoptics (or-thop′tiks) treatment of strabismus by exercise of the ocular muscles.

orthoscope (or′tho-skōp) an apparatus which neutralizes corneal refraction by means of a layer of water.

orthoscopic (or″tho-skop′ik) 1. affording a correct and undistorted view. 2. pertaining to orthoscopy.

orthoscopy (or-thos′ko-pe) examination by means of an orthoscope.

orthosis (or-tho′sis), pl. *ortho′ses.* An orthopedic appliance or apparatus used to support, align, prevent, or correct deformities or to improve function of movable parts of the body.

orthostatic (or″tho-stat′ik) pertaining to or caused by standing erect.

orthostatism (or′tho-stat″izm) an erect standing position of the body.

orthotast (-tast) an apparatus for straightening curvatures of bone.

orthotic (or-thot′ik) serving to protect or to restore or improve function; pertaining to the use or application of an orthosis.

orthotics (or-thot′iks) the field of knowledge relating to orthoses and their use.

orthotist (or′tho-tist) a person skilled in orthotics, and practicing its application in individual cases.

orthotonos, orthotonus (or-thot′o-nus) tetanic spasm which fixes the head, body, and limbs in a rigid straight line.

orthotopic (or″tho-top′ik) occurring at the normal place.

orthovoltage (-vol′tij) voltage in the range of 30 to 400 kv.

Orthoxine (or-thok′sēn) trademark for preparations of methoxyphenamine.

O.S. [L.] *oc′ulus sinis′ter* (left eye).

Os chemical symbol, *osmium.*

os[1] (os), pl. *o′ra* [L.] 1. any body orifice. 2. the mouth.

os[2] (os), pl. *os′sa* [L.] bone; see *Table of Bones.*

osazone (o′sah-zōn) any one of a series of compounds obtained by heating sugars with phenylhydrazine and acetic acid.

osche(o)- word element [Gr.], *scrotum.*

oscheitis (os″ke-i′tis) inflammation of the scrotum.

oscheocele (os′ke-o-sēl″) a swelling or tumor of the scrotum.

oscheoma (os″ke-o′mah) tumor of the scrotum.

oscheoplasty (os′ke-o-plas″te) plastic surgery of the scrotum.

oscillation (os″ĭ-la′shun) a backward and forward motion, like that of a pendulum; also vibration, fluctuation, or variation.

oscillo- word element [L.], *oscillation.*

oscillogram (ŏ-sil′o-gram) a graphic record made by an oscillograph.

oscillograph (-graf) an instrument for recording electric oscillations.

oscillometer (os″ĭ-lom′ĕ-ter) an instrument for measuring oscillations.

oscillometry (os″ĭ-lom′ĕ-tre) the measurement of oscillations.

oscillopsia (os″ĭ-lop′se-ah) a visual sensation that stationary objects are swaying back and forth.

oscilloscope (ŏ-sil′o-skōp) an instrument that displays a visual representation of electrical variations on the fluorescent screen of a cathode-ray tube.

oscitation (os″ĭ-ta′shun) the act of yawning.

osculum (os′ku-lum) [L.] a small aperture or minute opening.

-osis word element [Gr.], *disease; morbid state; abnormal increase.*

osm(o)- word element [Gr.], (1) *odor; smell* (2) *impulse; osmosis.*

osmate (oz′māt) a salt of osmic acid.

osmatic (oz-mat′ik) pertaining to the sense of smell.

osmics (oz′miks) the science dealing with the sense of smell.

osmidrosis (oz″mĭ-dro′sis) bromhidrosis.

osmium (oz′me-um) chemical element (*see table*), at. no. 76, symbol Os. **o. tetroxide,** a fixative used in preparing histologic specimens, OsO_4.

osmolality (os″mo-lal′ĭ-te) the concentration of the solute in a solution per unit of solvent.

osmolar (oz-mo′lar) pertaining to the concentration of osmotically active particles in solution.

osmolarity (os″mo-lar′ĭ-te) the concentration of osmotically active particles in solution.

osmole (os′mōl) the standard unit of osmotic pressure.

osmometer (oz-mom′ĕ-ter) 1. a device for testing the sense of smell. 2. an instrument for measuring osmotic pressure.

osmophilic (oz″mo-fil′ik) having an affinity for solutions of high osmotic pressure.

osmophore (oz′mo-fōr) the group of atoms responsible for the odor of a compound.

osmoreceptor (oz″mo-re-sep′tor) 1. a specialized sensory nerve ending which is stimulated by changes in osmotic pressure of the surrounding medium. 2. a specialized sensory nerve ending sensitive to stimulation giving rise to the sensation of odors.

osmoregulation (-reg″u-la′shun) adjustment of internal osmotic pressure of a simple organism or body cell in relation to that of the surrounding medium. **osmoreg′ulatory**, adj.

osmose (oz′mōs) to diffuse by osmosis.

osmosis (oz-mo′sis, os-mo′sis) [Gr.] the passage of pure solvent from a solution of lesser to one of greater solute concentration when the two solutions are separated by a membrane which selectively prevents the passage of solute molecules, but is permeable to the solvent. **osmot′ic**, adj.

osphresiology (os-fre″ze-ol′o-je) the science of odors and the sense of smell.

osphresiometer (os-fre″ze-om′ĕ-ter) an instrument for measuring acuteness of the sense of smell.

osphresis (os-fre′sis) the sense of smell. **osphret′ic**, adj.

ossein (os′e-in) the collagen of bone.

osseocartilaginous (os″e-o-kar″tĭ-laj′ĭ-nus) composed of bone and cartilage.

osseofibrous (-fi′brus) made up of fibrous tissue and bone.

osseomucin (-mu′sin) the ground substance that binds together the collagen and elastic fibrils of bone.

osseous (os′e-us) of the nature or quality of bone; bony.

ossicle (os′ĭ-k'l) a small bone, especially one of those in the middle ear. **ossic′ular**, adj. **Andernach's o's**, sutural bones. **auditory o's**, the small bones of the middle ear: incus, malleus, and stapes. See Plate XII.

ossiculectomy (os″ĭ-ku-lek′to-me) excision of one or more ossicles of the middle ear.

ossiculotomy (os″ĭ-ku-lot′o-me) incision of the auditory ossicles.

ossiculum (ŏ-sik′u-lum), pl. *ossic′ula* [L.] ossicle.

ossiferous (ŏ-sif′er-us) producing bone.

ossific (ŏ-sif′ik) forming or becoming bone.

ossification (os″ĭ-fĭ-ka′shun) formation of or conversion into bone or a bony substance. **endochondral o.**, ossification which occurs in and replaces cartilage. **intramembranous o.**, ossification that occurs in and replaces connective tissue.

ossify (os′ĭ-fi) to change or develop into bone.

oste(o)- word element [Gr.], *bone*.

ostealgia (os″te-al′je-ah) pain in the bones.

ostearthritis (-ar-thri′tis) osteoarthritis.

ostearthrotomy (-ar-throt′o-me) excision of an articular end of a bone.

ostectomy (os-tek′to-me) excision of a bone or part of a bone.

osteectopia (os″te-ek-to′pe-ah) displacement of a bone.

ostein (os′te-in) ossein.

osteitis (os″te-i′tis) inflammation of bone.

o. conden′sans generalisa′ta, osteopoikilosis. **condensing o.**, osteitis with hard deposits of earthy salts in affected bone. **o. defor′mans**, rarefying osteitis leading to bowing of the long bones and deformation of the flat bones. **o. fibro′sa cys′tica**, **o. fibro′sa cys′tica generalisa′ta**, **o. fibro′sa osteoplas′tica**, rarefying osteitis with fibrous degeneration and formation of cysts and with the presence of fibrous nodules on the affected bones, due to marked osteoclastic activity secondary to hyperparathyroidism. **o. fragil′itans**, osteogenesis imperfecta. **o. fungo′sa**, chronic osteitis in which the haversian canals are dilated and filled with granulation tissue. **parathyroid o.**, o. fibrosa cystica. **pedal o.**, inflammation of the pedal bone in horses. **rarefying o.**, a bone disease in which the inorganic matter is diminished and the hard bone becomes cancellated. **sclerosing o.**, 1. sclerosing nonsuppurative osteomyelitis. 2. condensing o.

ostempyesis (os″tem-pi-e′sis) suppuration within a bone.

osteoanagenesis (os″te-o-an′ah-jen″ĕ-sis) regeneration of bone.

osteoarthritis (-ar-thri′tis) degenerative joint disease marked by degeneration of the articular cartilage, hypertrophy of bone at the margins, and changes in the synovial membrane, accompanied by pain and stiffness.

osteoarthropathy (-ar-throp′ah-the) any disease of the joints and bones. **hypertrophic pulmonary o.**, **secondary hypertrophic o.**, symmetrical osteitis of the four limbs, chiefly localized to the phalanges and terminal epiphyses of the long bones of the forearm and leg; it is often secondary to chronic lung and heart conditions.

osteoarthrosis (-ar-thro′sis) chronic noninflammatory bone disease.

osteoarthrotomy (-ar-throt′o-me) ostearthrotomy.

osteoblast (os′te-o-blast″) a cell arising from a fibroblast, which, as it matures, is associated with bone production.

osteoblastoma (os″te-o-blas-to′mah) a benign, rather vascular tumor of bone marked by formation of osteoid tissue and primitive bone.

osteocampsia (-kamp′se-ah) curvature of a bone.

osteochondral (-kon′dral) pertaining to bone and cartilage.

osteochondritis (-kon-dri′tis) inflammation of bone and cartilage. **o. defor′mans juveni′lis**, osteochondrosis of the capitular epiphysis of the femur. **o. defor′mans juveni′lis dor′si**, osteochondrosis of vertebrae. **o. dis′secans**, that resulting in splitting of pieces of cartilage into the affected joint.

osteochondrodystrophia (-kon″dro-dis-tro′fe-ah) Morquio's syndrome.

osteochondrodystrophy (-kon″dro-dis′tro-fe) Morquio's syndrome. **familial o.**, Morquio's syndrome.

osteochondrolysis (-kon-drol′ĭ-sis) osteochondritis dissecans.

osteochondroma (-kon-dro′mah) a benign bone

tumor consisting of projecting adult bone capped by cartilage.

osteochondromatosis (-kon″dro-mah-to′sis) occurrence of multiple osteochondromas.

osteochondrosarcoma (-kon″dro-sar-ko′mah) sarcoma blended with osteoma and chondroma.

osteochondrosis (-kon-dro′sis) a disease of the growth ossification centers in children, beginning as a degeneration or necrosis followed by regeneration or recalcification; known by various names, depending on the bone involved. **o. defor′mans tib′iae,** aseptic necrosis of the medial tibial condyle, producing lateral bowing of the leg.

osteoclasis (os″te-ok′lah-sis) surgical fracture or refracture of bones.

osteoclast (os′te-o-klast″) 1. a large multinuclear cell associated with absorption and removal of bone. 2. an instrument used for osteoclasis. **osteoclas′tic,** adj.

osteoclastoma (os″te-o-klas-to′mah) giant cell tumor of bone.

osteocope (os′te-o-kōp″) severe pain in a bone. **osteocop′ic,** adj.

osteocranium (os″te-o-kra′ne-um) the fetal skull during the period of ossification.

osteocystoma (-sis-to′mah) a bone cyst.

osteocyte (os′te-o-sīt″) an osteoblast that has become embedded within the bone matrix, occupying a flat oval cavity and sending, through openings in its walls, cytoplasmic processes that connect with other osteocytes in developing bone.

osteodentin (os″te-o-den′tin) dentin that resembles bone.

osteodermia (-der′me-ah) osteoma cutis.

osteodiastasis (-di-as′tah-sis) the separation of two adjacent bones.

osteodynia (-din′e-ah) ostealgia.

osteodystrophia (-dis-tro′fe-ah) osteodystrophy.

osteodystrophy (-dis′tro-fe) abnormal development of bone. **renal o.,** a condition due to chronic kidney disease, marked by impaired kidney function, elevated serum phosphorus levels, and low or normal serum calcium levels, and by stimulation of parathyroid function, resulting in a variable admixture of bone disease, including osteitis fibrosa cystica, osteomalacia, osteoporosis, and sometimes osteosclerosis; if the onset is in childhood, renal dwarfism may result.

osteoepiphysis (-e-pif′ĭ-sis) any bony epiphysis.

osteofibroma (-fi-bro′mah) osteoma blended with fibroma.

osteogen (os′te-o-jen″) the substance composing the inner layer of the periosteum, from which bone is formed.

osteogenesis (os″te-o-jen′ĕ-sis) the formation of bone; the development of the bones. **o. imperfec′ta,** an inherited condition marked by abnormally brittle bones that are subject to fracture; *o. imperfec′ta congen′ita* occurs during intrauterine life and the child is born with deformities; in *o. imperfec′ta tar′da,* the fractures occur when the child begins to walk. It is usually

attended by blue coloration of the sclera (Lobstein's disease) and sometimes by otosclerotic deafness (van der Hoeve's syndrome).

osteogenic (-jen′ik) derived from or composed of any tissue concerned in bone growth or repair.

osteogeny (os″te-oj′ĕ-ne) osteogenesis.

osteography (os″te-og′rah-fe) description of the bones.

osteohalisteresis (os″te-o-hah-lis″ter-e′sis) deficiency in mineral elements of bone.

osteoid (os′te-oid) 1. resembling bone. 2. the organic matrix of bone; young bone that has not undergone calcification.

osteolathyrism (os″te-o-lath′ĭ-rizm) a skeletal disorder in animals caused by diets containing the sweet pea (*Lathyrus odoratus*) or its active principle, or other aminonitriles.

osteolipochondroma (-lip″o-kon-dro′mah) osteochondroma with fatty elements.

osteologia (-lo′je-ah) osteology.

osteologist (os″te-ol′o-jist) a specialist in osteology.

osteology (os″te-ol′o-je) scientific study of the bones.

osteolysis (os″te-ol′ĭ-sis) dissolution of bone; applied especially to the removal or loss of the calcium of bone. **osteolyt′ic,** adj.

osteoma (os″te-o′mah) a tumor composed of bony tissue; a hard tumor of bonelike structure developing on a bone (*homoplastic o.*) and sometimes on other structures (*heteroplastic o.*). **o. cu′tis,** a condition in which bone-containing nodules form in the skin. **o. du′rum, o. ebur′-neum,** one containing hard bony tissue. **o. medulla′re,** one containing marrow spaces. **osteoid o.,** a benign tumor of spongy bone occurring in the bones of the extremities and vertebrae in young persons. **o. spongio′sum,** one containing cancellated bone.

osteomalacia (os″te-o-mah-la′she-ah) softening of the bones (due to impaired mineralization, with excess accumulation of osteoid), resulting from vitamin D deficiency. **osteomala′cic,** adj. **infantile o., juvenile o.,** late rickets.

osteomatoid (os″te-o′mah-toid) resembling an osteoma.

osteomere (os′te-o-mēr″) one of a series of similar bony structures, such as the vertebrae.

osteometry (os″te-om′ĕ-tre) measurement of the bones.

osteomyelitis (os″te-o-mi″ĕ-li′tis) inflammation of bone, localized or generalized, due to pyogenic infection. **osteomyelit′ic,** adj. **Garré's o., sclerosing nonsuppurative o.,** a chronic form involving the long bones, especially the tibia and femur, marked by a diffuse inflammatory reaction, increased density and spindle-shaped sclerotic thickening of the cortex, and an absence of suppuration.

osteomyelodysplasia (-mi″ĕ-lo-dis-pla′ze-ah) a condition characterized by thinning of the osseous tissue of bones and increase in size of the marrow cavities, attended with leukopenia and fever.

osteon (os′te-on) the basic unit of structure of

compact bone, comprising a haversian canal and its concentrically arranged lamellae.

osteonecrosis (os″te-o-nĕ-kro′sis) necrosis of a bone.

osteoneuralgia (-nu-ral′je-ah) neuralgia of a bone.

osteopath (os′te-o-path″) a practitioner of osteopathy.

osteopathia (os″te-o-path′e-ah) osteopathy (1). **o. conden′sans dissemina′ta,** osteopoikilosis. **o. stria′ta,** an asymptomatic condition characterized radiographically by multiple condensations of cancellous bone tissue, giving a striated appearance.

osteopathology (-pah-thol′o-je) osteopathy (1).

osteopathy (os″te-op′ah-the) 1. any disease of a bone. 2. a system of therapy based on the theory that the body is capable of making its own remedies against disease and other toxic conditions when it is in normal structural relationship and has favorable environmental conditions and adequate nutrition; it utilizes generally accepted physical methods of diagnosis and therapy, while emphasizing the importance of normal body mechanics and manipulative methods of detecting and correcting faulty structure. **osteopath′ic,** adj. **disseminated condensing o.,** osteopoikilosis.

osteopenia (os″te-o-pe′ne-ah) any condition involving reduced bone mass.

osteoperiosteal (-per″e-os′te-al) pertaining to bone and its periosteum.

osteoperiostitis (-per″e-os-ti′tis) inflammation of a bone and its periosteum.

osteopetrosis (-pĕ-tro′sis) a hereditary disease marked by abnormally dense bone, and by the common occurrence of fractures of affected bone. It may lead to obliteration of the narrow spaces, causing leukemia.

osteophage (os′te-o-fāj″) osteoclast (1).

osteophlebitis (os″te-o-fle-bi′tis) inflammation of the veins of a bone.

osteophony (os″te-of′o-ne) bone conduction.

osteophore (os′te-o-fōr) a bone-crushing forceps.

osteophyma, osteophyte (os″te-o-fi′mah; os′-te-o-fīt″) a bony excrescence or outgrowth.

osteoplasty (os′te-o-plas″te) plastic surgery of the bones.

osteopoikilosis (os″te-o-poi″kĭ-lo′sis) a mottled condition of bones, apparent radiographically, due to the presence of multiple sclerotic foci and scattered stippling. **osteopoikilot′ic,** adj.

osteoporosis (-po-ro′sis) abnormal rarefaction of bone; it may be idiopathic or occur secondary to other diseases. **osteoporot′ic,** adj. **o. of disuse,** that occurring when the normal laying down of bone is slowed because of lack of the normal stimulus of functional stress on the bone. **post-traumatic o.,** loss of bone substance after an injury in which there is nerve damage, sometimes due to increased blood supply caused by the neurogenic insult, or to disuse secondary to pain.

osteoradionecrosis (-ra″de-o-nĕ-kro′sis) necrosis of bone as a result of excessive exposure to radiation.

osteorrhagia (-ra″je-ah) hemorrhage from bone.

osteorrhaphy (os″te-or′ah-fe) fixation of fragments of bone with sutures or wires.

osteosarcoma (os″te-o-sar-ko′mah) osteogenic sarcoma. **osteosarco′matous,** adj.

osteosclerosis (-skle-ro′sis) the hardening or abnormal density of bone. **osteosclerot′ic,** adj. **o. congen′ita,** achondroplasia. **o. frag′ilis,** osteopetrosis. **o. frag′ilis generalisa′ta,** osteopetrosis.

osteosis (os″te-o′sis) the formation of bony tissue. **o. cu′tis,** osteoma cutis.

osteostixis (os″te-o-stik′sis) surgical puncture of a bone.

osteosuture (-su′tūr) osteorrhaphy.

osteosynovitis (-sin″o-vi′tis) synovitis with osteitis of neighboring bones.

osteosynthesis (-sin′thĕ-sis) surgical fastening of the ends of a fractured bone.

osteotabes (-ta′bēz) a disease, chiefly of infants, in which bone marrow cells are destroyed and the marrow disappears.

osteothrombosis (-throm-bo′sis) thrombosis of the veins of a bone.

osteotome (os′te-o-tōm″) a chisel-like knife for cutting bone.

osteotomoclasis (os″te-o-to-mok′lah-sis) correction of bone curvature by partial division with the osteotome, followed by forcible fracture.

osteotomy (os″te-ot′o-me) incision or transection of a bone. **cuneiform o.,** removal of a wedge of bone. **linear o.,** the sawing or linear cutting of a bone. **Macewen's o.,** see under *operation.*

ostitis (os-ti′tis) osteitis.

ostium (os′te-um), pl. *os′tia* [L.] a mouth or orifice. **os′tial,** adj. **o. abdomina′le,** the fimbriated end of an oviduct. **o. inter′num,** o. uterinum tubae. **o. pharyn′geum,** the pharyngeal opening of the auditory tube. **o. pri′mum,** an opening in the lower portion of the membrane dividing the embryonic heart into right and left sides. **o. secun′dum,** an opening high in the septum of the embryonic heart, approximately where the foramen ovale will later appear. **tympanic o., o. tympan′icum,** the opening of the auditory tube on the carotid wall of the tympanic cavity. **o. u′teri,** the external opening of the uterine cervix into the vagina. **o. uteri′num tu′bae,** the point where the cavity of the uterine tube becomes continuous with that of the uterus. **o. vagi′nae,** external orifice of the vagina.

ostomate (os′to-māt) one who has undergone enterostomy or ureterostomy.

ostomy (os′to-me) general term for an operation in which an artificial opening is formed, as in colostomy, ureterostomy, etc.

O.T. occupational therapy; Old tuberculin.

ot(o)- word element [Gr.], ear.

otalgia (o-tal′je-ah) pain in the ear; earache.

OTC over the counter; said of drugs not required by law to be sold on prescription only.

otectomy (o-tek′to-me) excision of tissues of the internal and middle ear.

othelcosis (ōt″hel-ko′sis) 1. ulceration of the auricle or external meatus of the ear. 2. suppuration of the middle ear.

othemorrhea (ōt″hem-o-re′ah) otorrhagia.

otic (o′tik) pertaining to the ear; aural.

otitis (o-ti′tis) inflammation of the ear. **otit′ic,** adj. **aviation o.,** barotitis media. **o. exter′na,** inflammation of the external ear. **furuncular o.,** formation of furuncles in the external meatus. **o. inter′na, o. labyrin′thica,** labyrinthitis. **o. mastoi′dea,** inflammation of the mastoid spaces. **o me′dia,** inflammation of the middle ear. **o. me′dia, secretory,** a painless accumulation of mucoid or serous fluid in the middle ear, due to obstruction of the eustachian tube and causing conduction deafness. **o. mycot′ica,** that due to parasitic fungi. **o. parasit′ica,** otoacariasis. **o. sclerot′ica,** otitis marked by hardening of the ear structures.

otoacariasis (o″to-ak″ah-ri′ah-sis) infection of the ears of cats, dogs, and domestic rabbits with mites of the genus *Otodectes.*

otoantritis (-an-tri′tis) inflammation of the attic of the tympanum and the mastoid antrum.

Otobius (o-to′be-us) a genus of soft-bodied ticks parasitic in the ears of various animals and known also to infest man.

otoblennorrhea (o″to-blen″o-re′ah) mucous discharge from the ear.

otocephalus (-sef′ah-lus) a monster lacking a lower jaw and having ears united below the face.

otocleisis (-kli′sis) closure of the auditory passages.

otoconia (-ko′ne-ah) statoconia.

otocranium (-kra′ne-um) 1. the chamber in the petrous bone lodging the internal ear. 2. the auditory portion of the cranium. **otocra′nial,** adj.

otocyst (o′to-sist) 1. the auditory vesicle of the embryo. 2. the auditory sac of some lower animals.

Otodectes (o″to-dek′tēz) a genus of mites; see also *otoacariasis.*

otodynia (-din′e-ah) otalgia.

otoencephalitis (-en-sef″ah-li′tis) inflammation of the brain due to extension from an inflamed middle ear.

otoganglion (-gang′gle-on) the otic ganglion.

otogenic, otogenous (o″to-jen′ik; o-toj′ĕ-nus) originating within the ear.

otography (o-tog′rah-fe) description of the ear.

otolaryngology (o″to-lar″in-gol′o-je) that branch of medicine dealing with disease of the ear, nose, and throat.

otolith (o′to-lith) 1. see *statoconia.* 2. a calcareous mass in the inner ear of vertebrates or in the otocyst of invertebrates.

otologist (o-tol′o-jist) a specialist in otology.

otology (o-tol′o-je) the branch of medicine dealing with the ear, its anatomy, physiology, and pathology. **otolog′ic,** adj.

Oto-Microscope (o″to-mi′kro-skōp) trademark for an operating microscope devised to improve visualization of the surgical field in operations on the ear.

otomucormycosis (-mu″kor-mi-ko′sis) mucormycosis of the ear.

otomycosis (-mi-ko′sis) fungal infection of the external auditory meatus and ear canal.

otopathy (o-top′ah-the) any disease of the ear.

otopharyngeal (o″to-fah-rin′je-al) pertaining to the ear and pharynx.

otoplasty (o′to-plas″te) plastic surgery of the ear.

otopolypus (o″to-pol′ĭ-pus) polyp in the ear.

otopyorrhea (-pi″o-re′ah) a copious purulent discharge from the ear.

otopyosis (-pi-o′sis) suppurative disease of the ear.

otorhinolaryngology (-ri″no-lar″in-gol′o-je) the branch of medicine dealing with the ear, nose, and throat.

otorhinology (-ri-nol′o-je) the branch of medicine dealing with the ear and nose.

otorrhagia (-ra′je-ah) hemorrhage from the ear.

otorrhea (-re′ah) a discharge from the ear.

otosclerosis (-skle-ro′sis) the formation of spongy bone in the capsule of the labryrinth of the ear. **otosclerot′ic,** adj.

otoscope (o′to-skōp) an instrument for inspecting or auscultating the ear.

otoscopy (o-tos′ko-pe) examination of the ear by means of the otoscope.

otosteal (o-tos′te-al) pertaining to the ossicles of the ear.

ototomy (o-tot′o-me) dissection of the ear.

ototoxic (o″to-tok′sik) having a deleterious effect upon the eighth nerve or on the organs of hearing and balance.

ototoxicity (-tok-sis′ĭ-te) the property of being ototoxic.

Otrivin (o′trĭ-vin) trademark for preparations of xylometazoline.

O.U. [L.] *oculi uterque* (each eye).

ouabain (wah-ba′in) a glycoside, $C_{29}H_{44}$-$O_{12}\cdot 8H_2O$, chiefly from *Strophanthus gratus;* used as a cardiotonic.

ounce (owns) a measure of weight in both the avoirdupois ($\frac{1}{16}$ lb., 437.5 gr., 28.3495 gm.) and apothecaries ($\frac{1}{12}$ lb., 480 gr., 31.103 gm.) system; abbreviated oz. **fluid o.,** a unit of liquid measure of the apothecaries' system, being 8 fluiddrams, or the equivalent of 29.57 ml.

outlet (owt′let) a means or route of exit or egress. **pelvic o.,** the inferior opening of the pelvis.

outpatient (owt-pa′shent) a patient who comes to the hospital, clinic, or dispensary for diagnosis and/or treatment but does not occupy a bed.

outpocketing (-pok′et-ing) evagination.

outpouching (owt′powch″ing) obtrusion of a layer or part to form a pouch; evagination.

output (-put) the yield or total of anything produced by any functional system of the body. **cardiac o.,** the effective volume of blood expelled by either ventricle of the heart per unit of time (usually volume per minute); it is equal to the stroke output multiplied by the number of beats per the time unit used in the computation. **energy o.,** the energy a body is able to manifest in work or activity. **stroke o.,** the amount of blood ejected by each ventricle at each beat of the heart. **urinary o.,** the amount of urine excreted by the kidneys.

ova (o'vah) plural of *ovum.*

ovalbumin (ov″al-bu'min) egg albumin.

ovalocyte (o'vah-lo-sīt″) elliptocyte.

ovalocytosis (o-val″o-si-to'sis) elliptocytosis.

ovari(o)- word element [Gr.], *ovary.*

ovariectomy (o-va″re-ek'to-me) oophorectomy.

ovariocele (o-va're-o-sēl″) hernia of an ovary.

ovariocentesis (o-va″re-o-sen-te'sis) surgical puncture of an ovary.

ovariocyesis (-si-e'sis) ovarian pregnancy.

ovariopexy (-pek'se) the operation of elevating and fixing an ovary to the abdominal wall.

ovariorrhexis (-rek'sis) rupture of an ovary.

ovariosalpingectomy (-sal″pin-jek'to-me) excision of an ovary and oviduct.

ovariostomy (o-va″re-os'to-me) oophorostomy.

ovariotomy (-ot'o-me) surgical removal of an ovary, or removal of an ovarian tumor.

ovariotubal (o-va″re-o-tu'bal) pertaining to an ovary and oviduct.

ovaritis (o″vah-ri'tis) oophoritis.

ovarium (o-va're-um), pl. *ova'ria* [L.] ovary.

ovary (o'var-e) the female gonad: either of the paired female sexual glands in which ova are formed. **ova'rian,** adj. **polycystic o.,** one containing multiple, small follicular cysts filled with yellow or bloodstained, thin serous fluid.

overbite (o'ver-bīt) the extension of the upper incisor teeth over the lower ones vertically when the opposing posterior teeth are in contact.

overcompensation (o″ver-kom″pen-sa'shun) exaggerated correction of a real or imagined physical or psychologic defect.

overdetermination (-de-ter″min-a'shun) the unconscious mechanism through which every emotional reaction or symptom is the result of multiple factors.

overhydration (-hi-dra'shun) a state of excess fluids in the body.

overjet (o'ver-jet) extension of the incisal or buccal cusp ridges of the upper teeth labially or buccally to the incisal margins and ridges of the lower teeth when the jaws are closed normally.

overlay (-la) a later component superimposed on a preexisting state or condition. **psychogenic o.,** an emotionally determined increment to a preexisting symptom or disability of organic or physically traumatic origin.

overventilation (o″ver-ven″tĭ-la'shun) hyperventilation.

ovi-, ovo- word element [L.], *egg; ovum.*

ovicide (o'vĭ-sīd) an agent destructive to the ova of certain organisms.

oviduct (-dukt) a passage through which ova leave the maternal body or pass to an organ communicating with exterior of the body; see *uterine tube.* **ovidu'cal, oviduct'al,** adj.

oviferous (o-vif'er-us) producing ova.

oviform (o'vĭ-form) egg-shaped.

ovigenesis (o″vĭ-jen'ĕ-sis) oogenesis. **ovigenet'ic,** adj.

ovine (o'vīn) pertaining to, characteristic of, or derived from sheep.

oviparous (o-vip'ah-rus) producing eggs in which the embryo develops outside the maternal body, as in birds.

oviposition (o″vĭ-po-zish'un) the act of laying or depositing eggs.

ovipositor (-pos'ĭ-tor) a specialized organ by which many female insects deposit their eggs.

ovisac (o'vĭ-sak) a vesicular ovarian follicle.

Ovocylin (o″vo-sil'in) trademark for a preparation of estradiol.

ovoflavin (-fla'vin) riboflavin derived from eggs.

ovoglobulin (-glob'u-lin) the globulin of white of egg.

ovomucoid (-mu'koid) a mucoid principle from egg albumin.

ovoplasm (o'vo-plazm) the cytoplasm of an unfertilized ovum.

ovotestis (o″vo-tes'tis) a gonad containing both testicular and ovarian tissue.

ovoviviparous (-vi-vip'ah-rus) bearing living young that hatch from eggs inside the maternal body, the embryo being nourished by food stored in the egg; said of lizards, etc.

ovular (o'vu-lar) pertaining to an ovule or an ovum.

ovulation (o″vu-la'shun) the discharge of the ovum from the vesicular (graafian) follicle. **ov'ulatory,** adj.

ovule (o'vūl) 1. the ovum within a vesicular ovarian follicle. 2. any small, egglike structure.

ovum (o'vum), pl. *o'va* [L.] an egg; the female reproductive or germ cell which, after fertilization, is capable of developing into a new member of the same species. **centrolecithal o.,** one with the yolk massed centrally surrounded by a peripheral shell of cytoplasm, and with an island of cytoplasm surrounding the nucleus. **holoblastic o.,** one that undergoes total cleavage. **isolecithal o.,** one with a small amount of yolk evenly distributed throughout the cytoplasm. **meroblastic o.,** one that undergoes partial cleavage. **primitive o., primordial o.,** an egg cell very early in its development. **telolecithal o.,** one with a comparatively large amount of yolk massed at one pole.

oxacillin (ok″sah-sil'in) a semisynthetic penicillin used as the sodium salt in infections due to penicillin-resistant, gram-positive organisms.

Oxaine (ok'sān) trademark for a preparation of oxethazaine.

oxalate (ok'sah-lāt) any salt of oxalic acid. **potassium o.,** $K_2C_2O_4 \cdot H_2O$; used extensively as a reagent.

oxalemia (ok″sah-le'me-ah) excess of oxalates in the blood.

oxalism (ok'sah-lizm) poisoning by oxalic acid or by an oxalate.

oxalosis (ok″sah-lo'sis) primary hyperoxaluria.

oxaluria (ok″sah-lu're-ah) hyperoxaluria.

oxanamide (ok-san'ah-mīd) a tranquilizer, $C_8H_{15}NO_2$.

oxandrolone (ok-san'dro-lōn) an androgenic steroidal lactone, $C_{19}H_{30}O_3$, used to accelerate anabolism and/or to arrest excessive catabolism.

oxazepam (oks-az′ĕ-pam) a minor tranquilizer, $C_{15}H_{11}ClN_2O_2$.

oxethazaine (ok-seth′ah-zān) a gastric mucosal anesthetic, $C_{28}H_{39}N_3O_3$; used as the hydrochloride salt.

oxidant (ok′sĭ-dant) the electron acceptor in an oxidation-reduction (redox) reaction.

oxidase (ok′sĭ-dās) any of a class of enzymes that catalyze the reduction of molecular oxygen independently of hydrogen peroxide.

oxidation (ok″sĭ-da′shun) the act of oxidizing or state of being oxidized.

oxidation-reduction (-re-duk′shun) the chemical reaction whereby electrons are removed (oxidation) from atoms of the substance being oxidized and transferred to those being reduced (reduction).

oxide (ok′sīd) a compound of oxygen with an element or radical.

oxidize (ok′sĭ-dīz) to cause to combine with oxygen or to remove hydrogen.

oxidoreductase (ok″sĭ-do-re-duk′tās) a class of enzymes that catalyze the reversible transfer of electrons from one substance to another (oxidation-reduction, or redox reaction).

oxim, oxime (ok′sim) any of a series of compounds formed by action of hydroxylamine on an aldehyde or ketone.

oximeter (ok-sim′ĕ-ter) a photoelectric device for determining oxygen saturation of the blood.

oxogestone (ok″so-jes′tōn) a progestin, $C_{29}H_{38}O_3$.

oxophenarsine (-phen-ar′sin) an antitrypanosomal, $C_6H_6AsNO_2$.

oxprenolol (oks-pren′o-lōl) a coronary vasodilator, $C_{15}H_{23}NO_3$.

Oxsoralen (ok-sor′ah-len) trademark for preparations of methoxsalen.

oxtriphylline (oks-trif′ĭ-lēn) a bronchodilator, $C_{12}H_{21}N_5O_3$.

oxy- word element [Gr.], *sharp; quick; sour; presence of oxygen in a compound.*

oxyblepsia (ok″sĭ-blep′se-ah) unusual acuity of vision.

Oxycel (ok′sĭ-sel) trademark for preparations of oxidized cellulose.

oxycephalia (ok″sĭ-sĕ-fa′le-ah) oxycephaly.

oxycephaly (-sef′ah-le) a high, pointed condition of the skull, with a vertical index of 77 or more. **oxycephal′ic,** adj.

oxychloride (-klo′rīd) an element or radical combined with oxygen and chlorine.

oxychromatic (-kro-mat′ik) staining with acid dyes; acidophilic.

oxychromatin (-kro′mah-tin) that part of chromatin that stains with acid aniline dyes.

oxycinesia (-si-ne′ze-ah) pain on motion.

oxyesthesia (ok″se-es-the′ze-ah) abnormal acuteness of the senses.

oxygen (ok′sĭ-jen) chemical element (*see table*), at. no. 8, symbol O. It constitutes about 20% of atmospheric air, and is the essential agent in the respiration of plants and animals, and, although noninflammable, is necessary to support combustion. **o. debt,** deficiency of oxygen occurring in violent exercise. **heavy o.,** an isotope of oxygen of atomic weight 18. **hyperbaric o.,** oxygen under greater than atmospheric pressure. **molecular o.,** oxygen whose atoms are joined in pairs, as in the atmosphere; symbol O_2.

oxygenase (-jĕ-nās″) any oxidoreductase that catalyzes the incorporation of both atoms of molecular oxygen into the substrate.

oxygenate (-jĕ-nāt) to saturate with oxygen.

oxygenation (ok″sĭ-je-na′shun) saturation with oxygen.

oxygeusia (-gu′ze-ah) extreme acuteness of the sense of taste.

oxyhematoporphyrin (-hem″ah-to-por′fĭ-rin) a pigment sometimes found in the urine, closely allied to hematoporphyrin.

oxyhemoglobin (-he″mo-glo′bin) hemoglobin charged with oxygen.

oxyiodide (ok″se-i′o-dīd) an element or radical combined with oxygen and iodine.

oxylalia (ok″sĭ-la′le-ah) rapidity of speech.

Oxylone (ok′sĭ-lōn) trademark for a preparation of fluorometholone.

oxymetazoline (ok″sĭ-met-az′o-lēn) a vasoconstrictor, $C_{16}H_{24}N_2O$, used topically as the hydrochloride salt in nasal congestion.

oxymetholone (-meth′o-lōn) an anabolic-androgenic steroid, $C_{21}H_{32}O_3$, which promotes retention of nitrogen, phosphorus, and calcium.

oxymorphone (-mor′fōn) a narcotic analgesic, $C_{17}H_{19}NO_4$; used as the hydrochloride salt.

oxymyoglobin (-mi″o-glo′bin) myoglobin charged with oxygen.

oxyopia (ok″si-o′pe-ah) abnormal acuteness of sight.

oxypertine (ok″sĭ-per′tēn) an antidepressant, $C_{23}H_{29}N_3O_2$.

oxyphenbutazone (-fen-bu′tah-zōn) a nonsteroid anti-inflammatory agent, $C_{19}H_{20}N_2O_3H_2O$.

oxyphencyclimine (-si′klĭ-mēn) an anticholinergic, $C_{20}H_{28}N_2O_3$, with antisecretory, antimotility, and antispasmodic actions; the hydrochloride salt is used in the treatment of peptic ulcer and other gastrointestinal disorders.

oxyphenisatin (-fĕ-ni′sah-tin) a compound used as an enema for cleansing the colon.

oxyphenonium (-fĕ-no′ne-um) an anticholinergic, $C_{21}H_{34}NO_3$, used as the bromide ester in the treatment of peptic ulcer and gastrointestinal hypermotility or spasm.

oxyphil (ok′sĭ-fil) 1. Hürthle cell. 2. oxyphilic.

oxyphilic, oxyphilous (ok″sĭ-fil′ik; ok-sif′ĭ-lus) stainable with an acid dye.

oxyphonia (ok″sĭ-fo′ne-ah) an abnormally sharp quality or pitch of the voice.

oxypurine (-pu′rēn) a purine containing oxygen.

oxypurinol (-pūr′ĭ-nol) a xanthine oxidase inhibitor, $C_5H_4N_4O_2$.

oxytalan (oks-it′ah-lan) a connective tissue fiber found in the periodontal membrane.

oxytetracycline (ok″sĭ-tet-rah-si′klēn) a broad-spectrum antibiotic, $C_{22}H_{24}N_2O_9 \cdot 2H_2O$, produced by *Streptomyces rimosus.*

oxytocia (-to′se-ah) rapid labor.

oxytocic (-to′sik) 1. pertaining to, marked by, or promoting oxytocia. 2. an agent that promotes rapid labor by stimulating contractions of the myometrium.

oxytocin (-to′sin) a hypothalamic hormone stored in the posterior pituitary, which stimulates uterine contractions and milk ejection. It is also produced synthetically.

oxyuriasis (ok″se-u-ri′ah-sis) infection with *Enterobius vermicularis* (in humans) or with other oxyurids; enterobiasis.

oxyuricide (-u′ri-sīd) an agent that destroys oxyurids.

oxyurid (-u′rid) a pinworm, seatworm, or threadworm; any individual of the superfamily Oxyuroidea.

Oxyuris (-u′ris) a genus of intestinal nematode worms (superfamily Oxyuroidea). **O. e′qui,** a species found in horses. **O. vermicula′ris,** *Enterobius vermicularis.*

Oxyuroidea (-u″roi-de′ah) a superfamily of small nematodes—the pinworms, seatworms, or threadworms—usually parasitic in the cecum and colon of vertebrates, but may infect invertebrates.

oz. ounce.

ozena (o-ze′nah) a condition of the nose associated with a foul-smelling discharge.

ozone (o′zōn) a bluish explosive gas or blue liquid, being an allotropic form of oxygen, O_3; it is antiseptic and disinfectant, and irritating and toxic to the pulmonary system.

ozonometer (o″zo-nom′ĕ-ter) an apparatus for measuring ozone in the atmosphere.

ozostomia (-sto′me-ah) foulness of the breath.

P

P chemical symbol, *phosphorus.*

P. Pharmacopeia; position; presbyopia; [L.] proximum (*near*); pulse, [L.] punctum (*point*); pupil.

P₁ parental generation.

P₂ pulmonic second sound.

³²P the radioactive isotope of phosphorus of atomic mass 32; also written P³² and P 32.

p- symbol, *para-.*

Pa chemical symbol, *protactinium.*

PAB, PABA para-aminobenzoic acid.

pabulum (pab′u-lum) food or aliment.

Pacatal (pak′ah-tal) trademark for a preparation of mepazine.

pacemaker (pās′māk-er) that which sets the pace at which a phenomenon occurs; often used alone to indicate the cardiac pacemaker. **cardiac p.,** the group of cells rhythmically initiating the heart beat, characterized physiologically by a slow loss of membrane potential during diastole. Usually the pacemaker site is the sinoatrial node. **cardiac p., artificial,** a device designed to stimulate, by electrical impulses, contraction of the heart muscle at a certain rate; worn by or implanted in the body of the patient. **demand p.,** an implanted cardiac pacemaker in which the generator stimulus is inhibited by a signal derived from the heart's electrical activation (depolarization), thus minimizing the risk of pacemaker-induced fibrillation. **fixed-rate p.,** an implanted cardiac pacemaker in which the generator stimulates the heart at a predetermined rate, regardless of cardiac rhythm. **wandering p.,** a condition in which the site of origin of the impulses controlling the heart rate shifts from the head of the sinoatrial node to a lower part of the node or to another part of the atrium.

pachy- word element [Gr.], *thick.*

pachyacria (pak″e-a′kre-ah) enlargement of the soft parts of the extremities.

pachyblepharon (pak″ĭ-blef′ah-ron) thickening of the eyelids.

pachycephaly (-sef′ah-le) abnormal thickness of the bones of the skull. **pachycephal′ic,** adj.

pachycheilia (-ki′le-ah) thickening of the lips.

pachychromatic (-kro-mat′ik) having the chromatin in thick strands.

pachydactyly (-dak′tĭ-le) enlargement of the fingers and toes.

pachyderma (-der′mah) abnormal thickening of the skin. **pachyder′matous,** adj. **p. circumscrip′ta, p. laryn′gis,** localized warty epithelial thickenings on the vocal cords. **p. ves′icae,** thickening of the bladder mucosa.

pachydermatocele (-der-mat′o-sēl) plexiform neuroma attaining large size, producing an elephantiasis-like condition.

pachydermoperiostosis (-der″mo-per″e-os-to′sis) pachyderma affecting the face and scalp, thickening of the bones of the distal extremities, and acropachy.

pachyglossia (-glos′e-ah) abnormal thickness of the tongue.

pachygyria (-ji′re-ah) macrogyria.

pachyhematous (-hem′ah-tus) pertaining to or having thickened blood.

pachyleptomeningitis (-lep″to-men″in-ji′tis) inflammation of dura mater and pia mater.

pachymeningitis (-men″in-ji′tis) inflammation of the dura mater.

pachymeningopathy (-men″ing-gop′ah-the) noninflammatory disease of the dura mater.

pachymeninx (-me′ninks) the dura mater.

pachynsis (pah-kin′sis) an abnormal thickening. **pachyn′tic,** adj.

pachyonychia (pak″e-o-nik′e-ah) abnormal thickening of the nails. **p. congen′ita,** a hereditary congenital anomaly marked by great thickening of the nails, hyperkeratosis of palms and soles, and leukoplakia.

pachyperiostitis (pak″ĭ-per″e-os-ti′tis) periostitis of the long bones resulting in abnormal thickness of affected bones.

pachyperitonitis (-per″ĭ-to-ni′tis) inflammation and thickening of the peritoneum.

pachypleuritis (-ploo-ri′tis) fibrothorax.

pachysalpingitis (-sal″pin-ji′tis) chronic salpingitis with thickening.

pachysalpingo-ovaritis (-sal-ping″go-o″var-i′tis) chronic inflammation of the ovary and uterine tube, with thickening.

pachysomia (-so′me-ah) abnormal thickening of parts of the body.

pachytene (pak′ĭ-tēn) in meiosis, the stage following synapsis, in which the homologous chromosome threads shorten, thicken, and intertwine.

pachyvaginalitis (pak″ĭ-vaj″ĭ-nal-i′tis) inflammation and thickening of the tunica vaginalis.

pachyvaginitis (-vaj″ĭ-ni′tis) chronic vaginitis with thickening of the vaginal walls.

pack (pak) 1. treatment by wrapping a patient in blankets or sheets or a limb in towels, wet or dry and either hot or cold; also, the blankets or towels used for this purpose. 2. a tampon.

packer (pak′er) an instrument for introducing a dressing into a cavity or a wound.

packing (pak′ing) the filling of a wound or cavity with gauze, sponges, pads, or other material; also, the material used for this purpose.

pad (pad) a cushion-like mass of soft material. **abdominal p.,** a pad for the absorption of discharges from abdominal wounds, or for packing off abdominal viscera to improve exposure during surgery. **dinner p.,** a pad placed over the stomach before a plaster jacket is applied; the pad is then removed, leaving space under the jacket to take care of expansion of the stomach after eating. **fat p.,** a large pad of fat lying behind and below the patella. **knuckle p's,** nodular thickenings of the skin on the dorsal surface of the interphalangeal joints. **Mikulicz's p.,** a pad made of folded gauze, used in surgical procedures. **retromolar p.,** a cushion-like mass of tissue situated at the distal termination of the mandibular residual ridge. **sucking p., suctorial p.,** a lobulated mass of fat which occupies the space between the masseter and the external surface of the buccinator; it is well developed in infants.

pae- for words beginning thus, see those beginning with *pe-*.

pagetoid (paj′ĕ-toid) resembling Paget's disease.

Pagitane (paj′i-tān) trademark for a preparation of cycrimine.

-pagus word element [Gr.], *conjoined twins.*

PAH, PAHA para-aminohippuric acid.

pain (pān) a feeling of distress, suffering, or agony, caused by stimulation of specialized nerve endings. **bearing-down p.,** pain accompanying uterine contractions during the second stage of labor. **boring p.,** a sensation as of being pierced with a long, slender twisting object. **false p's,** ineffective pains resembling labor pains, not accompanied by cervical dilatation. **fulgurant p's,** lightning p's. **gas p's,** pains caused by distention of the stomach or intestines with accumulations of air or other gases. **growing p's,**

recurrent quasirheumatic limb pains peculiar to early youth. **hunger p.,** pain coming on at the time for feeling hunger for a meal; a symptom of gastric disorder. **intermenstrual p.,** pain accompanying ovulation, occurring during the period between the menses, usually about midway. **labor p's,** the rhythmic pains of increasing severity and frequency due to contraction of the uterus at childbirth. **lancinating p.,** sharp darting pain. **lightning p's,** the cutting and intense darting pains of tabes dorsalis. **phantom limb p.,** pain felt as though arising in an absent (amputated) limb. **referred p.,** pain felt in a part other than that in which the cause that produced it is situated. **root p.,** pain due to disease of the sensory nerve roots and felt in the cutaneous areas supplied by the affected roots. **shooting p's,** lightning p's. **terebrant p., terebrating p.,** boring p.

paint (pānt) 1. a liquid designed for application to a surface, as of the body or a tooth. 2. to apply a liquid to a specific area as a remedial or protective measure. **Castellani's p.,** carbolfuchsin solution.

palat(o)- word element [L.], *palate.*

palate (pal′at) roof of the mouth; the partition separating the nasal and oral cavities. **pal′atal, pal′atine,** adj. **cleft p.,** congenital fissure of median line of palate. **hard p.,** the anterior portion of the palate, separating the oral and nasal cavities, consisting of the bony framework and covering membranes. **soft p.,** the fleshy part of the palate, extending from the posterior edge of the hard palate; the uvula projects from its free inferior border.

palatitis (pal″ah-ti′tis) inflammation of the palate.

palatoglossal (pal″ah-to-glos′al) pertaining to the palate and tongue.

palatognathous (pal″ah-tog′nah-thus) having a congenitally cleft palate.

palatomaxillary (pal″ah-to-mak′sĭ-ler-e) pertaining to the palate and maxilla.

palatopharyngeal (-fah-rin′je-al) pertaining to the palate and pharynx.

platoplasty (pal′ah-to-plas″te) plastic reconstruction of the palate.

palatoplegia (pal″ah-to-ple′je-ah) paralysis of the palate.

palatorrhaphy (pal″ah-tor′ah-fe) surgical correction of a cleft palate.

palatoschisis (pal″ah-tos′kĭ-sis) cleft palate.

palatum (pal-ah′tum) [L.] palate.

pale(o)- word element [Gr.], *old.*

paleencephalon (pa″le-en-sef′ah-lon) the (phylogenetically) old brain; all of the brain except the cerebral cortex and its dependencies.

paleocerebellum (pa″le-o-ser″ĕ-bel′um) originally, the phylogenetically older parts of the cerebellum; the term is now applied specifically to those parts whose afferent inflow is predominantly supplied by spinocerebellar fibers. **paleocerebel′lar,** adj.

paleocortex (-kor′teks) paleopallium.

paleogenetic (-jĕ-net′ik) originated in the past; not newly acquired; said of traits, structures, etc., of species.

paleokinetic (-ki-net′ik) old kinetic; applied to the nervous motor mechanism concerned in automatic associated movements.

paleopallium (-pal′e-um) that part of the pallium (cerebral cortex) developing with the archipallium in association with the olfactory system; it is phylogenetically older and less stratified than the neopallium, and composed chiefly of the piriform cortex and parahippocampal gyrus.

paleopathology (-pah-thol′o-je) study of disease in bodies which have been preserved from ancient times.

paleostriatum (-stri-a′tum) the phylogenetically older portion of the corpus striatum, represented by the globus pallidus. **paleostria′tal,** adj.

paleothalamus (-thal′ah-mus) the phylogenetically older part of the thalamus, i.e., the medial portion which lacks reciprocal connections with the neopallium.

pali(n)- word element [Gr.], *again; pathologic repetition.*

palikinesia (pal″ĭ-ki-ne′ze-ah) pathologic repetition of movements.

palilalia (-la′le-ah) a condition in which a phrase or word is repeated with increasing rapidity.

palindromia (pal″in-dro′me-ah) a recurrence of relapse. **palindrom′ic,** adj.

palingraphia (-gra′fe-ah) pathologic repetition of letters or words in writing.

palinphrasia (-fra′ze-ah) pathologic repetition of words or phrases in speaking.

palladium (pah-la′de-um) chemical element (*see table*), at. no. 46, symbol Pd.

pallanesthesia (pal″an-es-the′ze-ah) loss or absence of pallesthesia.

pallesthesia (pal″es-the′ze-ah) sensibility to vibrations; the peculiar vibrating sensation felt when a vibrating tuning-fork is placed against a subcutaneous bony prominence of the body. **pallinesthet′ic,** adj.

palliate (pal′e-āt) to relieve symptoms.

palliative (pal′e-ah-tiv, -a″tiv) affording relief; also, a drug that so acts.

pallidectomy (pal″ĭ-dek′to-me) extirpation of the globus pallidus.

pallidotomy (-dot′o-me) production of lesions in the globus pallidus for treatment of extrapyramidal disorders.

pallidum (pal′ĭ-dum) the globus pallidus. **pal′-lidal,** adj.

pallium (pal′e-um) the cerebral cortex viewed in its entirety, i.e., the mantle of gray matter covering both cerebral hemispheres. Also, the cerebral cortex during its development.

pallor (pal′or) paleness, as of the skin.

palm (pahm) the hollow or flexor surface of the hand. **pal′mar,** adj.

palma (pahl′mah), pl. *pal′mae* [L.] palm.

palmaris (pahl-ma′ris) palmar.

palmus (pahl′mus) 1. palpitation. 2. clonic spasm of leg muscles, producing jumping motion.

palpable (pal′pah-b'l) perceptible by touch.

palpate (pal′pāt) to perform palpation.

palpation (pal-pa′shun) the act of feeling with the hand; the application of the fingers with light pressure to the surface of the body for the purpose of determining the condition of the parts beneath in physical diagnosis.

palpebra (pal′pĕ-brah), pl. *pal′pebrae* [L.] eyelid. **pal′pebral,** adj. **p. ter′tius,** nictitating membrane.

palpebralis (pal″pĕ-bra′lis) [L.] palpebral.

palpebritis (pal″pĕ-bri′tis) blepharitis.

palpitation (pal″pĭ-ta′shun) disagreeable subjective awareness of the heart beat.

palsy (pawl′ze) paralysis. **Bell's p.,** facial paralysis due to lesion of the facial nerve, resulting in characteristic facial distortion. **birth p.,** see under *paralysis.* **bulbar p.,** see under *paralysis.* **cerebral p.,** persisting qualitative motor disorder appearing before age three, due to nonprogressive damage to the brain. **Erb's p.,** Erb-Duchenne paralysis. **facial p.,** Bell's p. **shaking p.,** paralysis agitans. **wasting p.,** spinal muscular atrophy.

paludal (pal′u-dal) pertaining to, or arising from, marshes.

paludism (pal′u-dizm) malaria.

Paludrine (pal′u-drin) trademark for a preparation of proguanil.

Pamine (pam′ēn) trademark for preparations of methscopolamine bromide.

Pamisyl (pam′ĭ-sil) trademark for preparations of aminosalicylc acid.

pampiniform (pam-pin′ĭ-form) shaped like a tendril.

pan- word element [Gr.], *all.*

panacea (pan″ah-se′ah) a remedy for all diseases.

panagglutinin (pan″ah-gloo′tĭ-nin) an agglutinin which agglutinates the erythrocytes of all human blood groups.

panangiitis (-an-je-i′tis) inflammation involving all the coats of a vessel.

panarthritis (-ar-thri′tis) inflammation of all the joints.

panatrophy (pan-at′ro-fe) atrophy of several parts; diffuse atrophy.

pancarditis (pan″kar-di′tis) diffuse inflammation of the heart.

pancolectomy (-ko-lek′to-me) excision of the entire colon, with creation of an outlet from the ileum on the body surface.

pancreas (pan′kre-as), pl. *pan′creata* [Gr.] a large, elongated, racemose gland situated transversely behind the stomach, between the spleen and duodenum. Its external secretion contains digestive enzymes. An internal secretion, insulin, is produced by the beta cells, and glucagon is produced by the alpha cells. The alpha and beta cells form aggregates, called islands of Langerhans. See Plate IV. **pancreat′ic,** adj. **annular p.,** one which forms a ring surrounding the duodenum. **lesser p.,** small, partially detached portion of the pancreas lying dorsad to its head. **ventral p.,** an outgrowth on the ventral side of the embryonic intestine. **Willis' p., Winslow's p.,** lesser p.

pancreatalgia (pan″kre-ah-tal′je-ah) pain in the pancreas.

pancreatectomy (-tek′to-me) excision of the pancreas.

pancreatico- word element [Gr.], *pancreatic duct.*

pancreaticoduodenal (pan″kre-at″ĭ-ko-du″o-de′nal) pertaining to the pancreas and duodenum.

pancreaticoduodenostomy (-du″o-dĕ-nos′to-me) anastomosis of the pancreatic duct to a different site on the duodenum.

pancreaticoenterostomy (-en″ter-os′to-me) anastomosis of the pancreatic duct to the intestine.

pancreaticogastrostomy (-gas-tros′to-me) anastomosis of the pancreatic duct to the stomach.

pancreaticojejunostomy (-je″joo-nos′to-me) anastomosis of the pancreatic duct to the jejunum.

pancreatin (pan′kre-ah-tin) a substance from the pancreas of the hog or ox containing enzymes, principally amylase, protease, and lipase; used as a digestive aid.

pancreatitis (pan″kre-ah-ti′tis) inflammation of the pancreas. **acute hemorrhagic p.,** a condition due to autolysis of pancreatic tissue caused by escape of enzymes into the substance, resulting in hemorrhage into the parenchyma and surrounding tissues.

pancreato- word element [Gr.], *pancreas.*

pancreatoduodenectomy (pan″kre-ah-to-du″-o-dĕ-nek′to-me) excision of the head of the pancreas along with the encircling loop of the duodenum.

pancreatogenic (-jen′ik) pancreatogenous.

pancreatogenous (pan″kre-ah-toj′ĕ-nus) arising in the pancreas.

pancreatography (-tog′rah-fe) roentgenography of the pancreas.

pancreatolithectomy (pan″kre-ah-to-lĭ-thek′-to-me) excision of a calculus from the pancreas.

pancreatolithiasis (-lĭ-thi′ah-sis) presence of calculi in the ductal system or parenchyma of the pancreas.

pancreatolithotomy (-lĭ-thot′o-me) incision of the pancreas for the removal of calculi.

pancreatolysis (pan″kre-ah-tol′ĭ-sis) destruction of pancreatic tissue. **pancreatolyt′ic,** adj.

pancreatotomy (-tot′o-me) incision of the pancreas.

pancreatotropic (pan″kre-ah-to-trop′ik) having an affinity for the pancreas.

pancreolithotomy (pan″kre-o-lĭ-thot′o-me) pancreatolithotomy.

pancreolysis (pan″kre-ol′ĭ-sis) pancreatolysis. **pancreolyt′ic,** adj.

pancreoprivic (pan″kre-o-priv′ik) lacking a pancreas.

pancreozymin (-zi′min) a hormone of the duodenal mucosa that stimulates the external secretory activity of the pancreas, especially its production of amylase; identical with cholecystokinin.

pancuronium (pan″ku-ro′ne-um) a skeletal muscle relaxant used as the bromide salt, $C_{35}H_{60}Br_2N_2O_4$.

pancytopenia (pan″si-to-pe′ne-ah) abnormal depression of all the cellular elements of the blood.

pandemic (pan-dem′ik) a widespread epidemic disease; widely epidemic.

panencephalitis (pan″en-sef″ah-li′tis) encephalitis, probably of viral origin, which produces intranuclear or intracytoplasmic inclusion bodies that result in parenchymatous lesions of both the gray and white matter of the brain.

panendoscope (pan-en′do-skōp) a cystoscope which gives a wide view of the bladder.

panesthesia (pan″es-the′ze-ah) the sum of the sensations experienced. **panesthet′ic,** adj.

panhypopituitarism (pan-hi″po-pĭ-tu′ĭ-tar-izm) generalized hypopituitarism due to absence or damage of the pituitary gland, which, in its complete form, leads to absence of gonadal function and insufficiency of thyroid and adrenal function. When cachexia is a prominent feature, it is called *Simmonds' disease* or *pituitary cachexia.*

panhysterectomy (pan″his-tĕ-rek′to-me) total hysterectomy.

panhysterosalpingectomy (-his-ter-o-sal″pin-jek′to-me) excision of the body of the uterus, cervix, and uterine tubes.

panhysterosalpingo-oophorectomy (-sal-ping″go-o″of-o-rek′to-me) excision of the uterus, cervix, uterine tubes, and ovaries.

panic (pan′ik) extreme and unreasoning fear and anxiety.

panimmunity (pan″ĭ-mu′nĭ-te) immunity to several bacterial and viral infections.

panleukopenia (-lu-ko-pe′ne-ah) a viral disease of cats, marked by leukopenia and by inactivity, refusal of food, diarrhea, and vomiting.

Panmycin (pan-mi′sin) trademark for preparations of tetracycline.

panmyeloid (-mi′ĕ-loid) pertaining to all the elements of the bone marrow.

panmyelophthisis (-mi-ĕ-lof′thĭ-sis) aplastic anemia.

panmyelosis (-mi″ĕ-lo′sis) proliferation of all the elements of the bone marrow.

panniculitis (pah-nik″u-li′tis) inflammation of the panniculus adiposus, especially of the abdomen. **nodular nonsuppurative p., relapsing febrile nonsuppurative p.,** a disease marked by fever and the formation of crops of tender nodules in subcutaneous fatty tissues.

panniculus (pah-nik′u-lus), pl. *pannic′uli* [L.] a layer of membrane. **p. adipo′sus,** the subcutaneous fat: a layer of fat underlying the corium. **p. carno′sus,** a muscular layer in the superficial fascia of certain lower animals; represented in man mainly by the platysma.

pannus (pan′us) 1. superficial vascularization of the cornea with infiltration of granulation tissue. 2. an inflammatory exudate overlying the synovial cells on the inside of a joint. **p. trachomato′sus,** pannus of the cornea secondary to trachoma.

panophobia (pan″o-fo′be-ah) panphobia.

panophthalmitis (pan″of-thal-mi′tis) inflammation of all the eye structures or tissues.

panosteitis (-os-te-i′tis) inflammation of every part of a bone.

panotitis (-o-ti′tis) inflammation of all the parts or structures of the ear.

Panparnit (pan-par′nit) trademark for a preparation of caramiphen.

panphobia (-fo′be-ah) fear of everything; vague and persistent dread of an unknown evil.

pansinusitis (pan″si-nu-si′tus) inflammation involving all the paranasal sinuses.

Panstrongylus (pan-stron′ji-lus) a genus of hemipterous insects, species of which transmit trypanosomes.

pant(o)- word element [Gr.], *all; the whole.*

pantalgia (pan-tal′je-ah) pain over the whole body.

pantetheine (pan″tĕ-the′in) an amide of pantothenic acid, an intermediate in the biosynthesis of CoA, a growth factor for *Lactobacillus bulgaricus,* and a cofactor in certain enzyme complexes.

pantothenate (pan″to-then′āt) any salt of pantothenic acid.

pantotropic, pantropic (pan″to-trop′ik; pan-trop′ik) having affinity for tissues derived from all three germ layers.

panzootic (pan″zo-ot′ik) occurring pandemically among animals.

papain (pah-pa′in, pah-pi′in) a proteolytic enzyme from the latex of papaw, *Carica papaya.*

Papaver (pah-pav′er) a genus of herbs, the poppies. *P. somniferum* and its variety *al′bum* are the source of opium.

papaverine (-in) an alkaloid, $C_{20}H_{21}NO_4$, obtained from opium or prepared synthetically; the hydrochloride salt is used as a smooth muscle relaxant.

paper (pa′per) a material manufactured in thin sheets from fibrous substances which have first been reduced to a pulp. **litmus p.,** moisture-absorbing paper impregnated with a solution of litmus: if slightly acid, it is red, and alkalis turn it blue; if slightly alkaline, it is blue and acid turns it red. **test p.,** paper stained with a compound which changes visibly on occurrence of a chemical reaction.

papilla (pah-pil′ah), pl. *papil′lae*[L.] a small nipple-shaped projection or elevation. **pap′illary,** adj. **circumvallate p.,** vallate p. **conical p.,** one of the sparsely scattered elevations on the tongue, often considered to be modified filiform papillae. **papillae of corium,** conical extensions of the fibers, capillary blood vessels, and sometimes nerves of the corium into corresponding spaces among downward- or inward-projecting rete ridges on the undersurface of the epidermis. **dental p., dentinal p.,** the small mass of condensed mesenchyme capped by each of the enamel organs. **duodenal p.,** either of the small elevations (major and minor) on the mucosa of the duodenum, the *major* at the entrance of the conjoined pancreatic and common bile ducts, the *minor* at the entrance of the accessory pancreatic duct. **filiform p.,** one of the threadlike elevations covering most of the tongue surface. **foliate p.,** one of the parallel mucosal folds on the tongue margin at the junction of its body and root. **fungiform p.,** one of the knoblike projections of the tongue scattered among the filiform papillae. **gingival p.,** the triangular pad of the gingiva filling the space between the proximal surfaces of two adjacent teeth. **hair p.,** the fibrovascular mesodermal papilla enclosed within the hair bulb. **incisive p.,** an elevation at the anterior end of the raphe of the palate. **interdental p.,** gingival p. **lacrimal p.,** an elevation on the margin of either eyelid, near the medial angle of the eye. **lingual p.,** see *conical, filiform, foliate, fungiform,* and *vallate p.* **mammary p.,** the nipple of the breast. **optic p.,** optic disk. **palatine p.,** incisive p. **p. pi′li,** hair p. **renal p.,** the blunted apex of a renal pyramid. **p. of Santorini,** duodenal p. (major). **tactile papillae,** see under *corpuscle.* **urethral p.,** a slight elevation in the vestibule of the vagina at the external orifice of the urethra. **vallate p.,** one of the 8 to 12 large papillae arranged in a V near the base of the tongue. **p. of Vater,** duodenal p. (major).

papillectomy (pap″i-lek′to-me) excision of a papilla.

papilledema (pap″il-ĕ-de′mah) edema of the optic disk.

papillitis (pap″ĭ-li′tis) inflammation of the optic disk.

papilloadenocystoma (pap″ĭ-lo-ad″ĕ-no-sis-to′-mah) papillary cystadenoma.

papillocarcinoma (-kar″sĭ-no′mah) papillary carcinoma.

papilloma (pap″ĭ-lo′mah) a benign tumor derived from epithelium. **papillo′matous,** adj. **rabbit p., Shope p.,** a viral disease of rabbits marked by formation of warty growths.

papillomatosis (pap″ĭ-lo′mah-to′sis) development of multiple papillomas.

papilloretinitis (pap″ĭ-lo-ret″ĭ-ni′tis) inflammation of the optic disk and retina.

papovavirus (pap″o-vah-vi′rus) a group of relatively small, ether-resistant DNA viruses, many of which are oncogenic or potentially oncogenic.

papulation (pap″u-la′shun) the formation of papules.

papule (pap′ūl) a small circumscribed, solid, elevated lesion of the skin. **pap′ular,** adj.

papulopustular (pap″u-lo-pus′tu-lar) marked by papules and pustules.

papulosis (pap″u-lo′sis) the presence of multiple papules.

papulosquamous (pap″u-lo-skwa′mus) both papular and scaly.

papulovesicular (-vĕ-sik′u-lar) marked by papules and vesicles.

papyraceous (pap″ĭ-ra′shus) like paper.

par (par) [L.] pair.

para (par′ah) a woman who has produced one or more viable offspring. **p. I,** primipara. **p. II,** secundipara, etc.

para- word element [Gr.], *beside; beyond; accessory to; apart from; against, etc.* In chemistry, indicating the substitution in a derivative of the benzene ring of two atoms linked to opposite carbon atoms in the ring.

para-anesthesia (par″ah-an″es-the′ze-ah) anesthesia of the lower part of the body.

parabiosis (-bi-o′sis) 1. the union of two individuals, as conjoined twins, or of experimental animals by surgical operation. 2. temporary suppression of conductivity and excitability. **parabiot′ic,** adj.

parablepsia (-blep′se-ah) false or perverted vision.

parabulia (-bu′le-ah) perversion of will.

paracasein (-ka′se-in) the chemical product of the action of rennin on casein.

paracenesthesia (-se″nes-the′ze-ah) any disturbance of the general sense of well-being.

paracentesis (-sen-te′sis) surgical puncture of a cavity for the aspiration of fluid. **paracentet′ic,** adj.

paracephalus (-sef′ah-lus) a fetus with a defective head and imperfect sense organs.

parachlorophenol (-klo″ro-fe′nol) a local anti-infective, C_6H_5ClO, used in dentistry.

paracholera (-kol′er-ah) a disease resembling Asiatic cholera but not caused by *Vibrio cholerae.*

parachordal (-kor′dal) beside the notochord.

parachromatopsia (-kro″mah-top′se-ah) color blindness.

Paracoccidioides (-kok-sid″ĭ-oi′dēz) a genus of fungi that proliferate by multiple budding yeast cells in the tissues; it includes *P. brasilien′sis,* the etiologic agent of paracoccidioidomycosis.

paracoccidioidomycosis (-kok-sid″e-oi″do-mi-ko′sis) an often fatal, chronic granulomatous disease caused by *Paracoccidioides brasiliensis,* primarily involving the lungs, but spreading to the skin, mucous membranes, lymph nodes, and internal organs.

paracolitis (-ko-li′tis) inflammation of the outer coat of the colon.

Paracort (par′ah-kort) trademark for a preparation of prednisone.

Paracortol (par″ah-kor′tol) trademark for a preparation of prednisolone.

paracusia (-ku′se-ah) paracusis.

paracusis (-ku′sis) any perversion of hearing. **p. of Willis,** ability to hear best in a loud din.

paracystic (-sis′tik) situated near the bladder.

paracystitis (-sis-ti′tis) inflammation of tissues around the bladder.

paradental (-den′tal) 1. having some association with dentistry. 2. periodontal.

paradidymis (-did′ĭ-mis) a small, vestigial structure found occasionally in the adult in the anterior spermatic cord.

Paradione (-di′ōn) trademark for preparations of paramethadione.

paradipsia (-dip′se-ah) a perverted appetite for fluids.

paradox (par′ah-doks) a seemingly contradictory occurrence. **paradox′ic, paradox′ical,** adj. **Weber's p.,** elongation of a muscle which has been so stretched that it cannot contract.

paraffin (-fin) a purified mixture of solid hydro-

carbons obtained from petroleum. **light liquid p.,** light mineral oil. **liquid p.,** mineral oil.

paraffinoma (par″ah-fĭ-no′mah) a chronic granuloma produced by prolonged exposure to paraffin.

Paraflex (par′ah-fleks) trademark for a preparation of chlorzoxazone.

paragammacism (par″ah-gam′ah-sizm) faulty enunciation of *g, k,* and *ch* sounds.

paraganglioma (-gang″gle-o′mah) a tumor of the tissue composing the paraganglia. **nonchromaffin p.,** chemodectoma.

paraganglion (-gang′gle-on), pl. *paragan′glia.* A collection of chromaffin cells derived from neural ectoderm, occurring outside the adrenal medulla, usually near the sympathetic ganglia and in relation to the aorta and its branches.

parageusia (-gu′ze-ah) perversion of the sense of taste. **parageu′sic,** adj.

paraglobulin (-glob′u-lin) a globulin from blood serum, blood cells, lymph, and various connective tissues.

paraglossia (-glos′ĭ-ah) inflammation of the oral tissues under the tongue.

paragonimiasis (-gon′ĭ-mi′ah-sis) infection with flukes of the genus *Paragonimus.*

Paragonimus (-gon′ĭ-mus) a genus of trematode parasites, having two invertebrate hosts, the first a snail, the second a crab or crayfish; it includes *P. westerman′i,* the lung fluke, occurring especially in Asia, found in cysts in the lungs and sometimes the pleura, liver, abdominal cavity, and elsewhere in man and lower animals who ingest infected freshwater crayfish and crabs.

paragrammatism (-gram′ah-tizm) a disorder of speech, with confusion in the use and order of words and grammatical forms.

paragranuloma (-gran″u-lo′mah) the most benign form of Hodgkin's disease, largely confined to the lymph nodes.

paragraphia (-graf′e-ah) slight impairment of ability to express thoughts in writing.

parahemophilia (-he″mo-fil′e-ah) a hereditary hemorrhagic tendency due to deficiency of coagulation Factor V.

parahormone (-hor′mōn) a substance, not a true hormone, which has a hormone-like action in controlling the functioning of some distant organ.

parakeratosis (-ker″ah-to′sis) persistence of the nuclei of keratinocytes as they rise into the horny layer of the skin, marked by scaling.

parakinesia (-ki-ne′se-ah) perversion of motor function; in ophthalmology, irregular action of an individual ocular muscle.

paralalia (-la′le-ah) a disorder of speech, especially the production of a vocal sound different from the one desired, or the substitution in speech of one letter for another.

paralambdacism (-lam′dah-sizm) faulty enunciation of the *l* sound.

paralbumin (par″al-bu′min) an albumin or protein substance found in ovarian cysts.

paraldehyde (pah-ral′dĕ-hīd) a polymerization product of acetaldehyde, $C_6H_{12}O$, used as a hypnotic, especially in the treatment of alcoholism.

paralexia (par″ah-lek′se-ah) impairment of reading ability, with transposition of words and syllables into meaningless combinations.

paralgesia (par″al-je′ze-ah) an abnormal and painful sensation.

parallagma (par″ah-lag′mah) displacement of a bone or of the fragments of a broken bone.

parallax (par′ah-laks) an apparent displacement of an object due to change in the observer's position.

parallergy (par-al′er-je) a condition in which an allergic state, produced by specific sensitization, predisposes the body to react to other allergens with clinical manifestations that differ from the original reaction. **paraller′gic,** adj.

paralogia (par″ah-lo′je-ah) derangement of the reasoning faculty.

paralysis (pah-ral′ĭ-sis) loss or impairment of motor function in a part due to lesion of the neural or muscular mechanism; also, by analogy, impairment of sensory function (*sensory p.*). **p. of accommodation,** paralysis of the ciliary muscles of the eye so as to prevent accommodation. **p. ag′itans,** a slowly progressive form of parkinsonism, usually seen in late life, marked by masklike facies, tremor of resting muscles, slowing of voluntary movements, festinating gait, peculiar posture, muscular weakness, and sometimes excessive sweating and feelings of heat. **ascending p.,** spinal paralysis which progresses cephalad. **birth p.,** that due to injury received at birth. **brachial p.,** paralysis of an arm. **bulbar p.,** that due to changes in motor centers of the medulla oblongata; the chronic form is marked by progressive paralysis and atrophy of the lips, tongue, pharynx, and larynx, and is due to degeneration of the nerve nuclei of the floor of the fourth ventricle. **central p.,** that due to a lesion of the brain or spinal cord. **cerebral p.,** that caused by some intracranial lesion. **compression p.,** that caused by pressure on a nerve. **conjugate p.,** loss of ability to perform some parallel ocular movements. **crossed p.,** that affecting one side of face and the other side of body. **decubitus p.,** that due to pressure on a nerve from lying for a long time in one position. **divers' p.,** that resulting from too rapid reduction of pressure on deep-sea divers. **Duchenne's p.,** 1. Erb-Duchenne p. 2. progressive bulbar p. **Erb-Duchenne p.,** paralysis of the upper roots of the brachial plexus due to destruction of the fifth and sixth cervical roots, without involvement of the small muscles of the hand. **facial p.,** weakening or paralysis of the facial nerve, as in Bell's palsy. **familial periodic p.,** a hereditary disease with recurring attacks of rapidly progressive flaccid paralysis, associated with a fall in (hypokalemic type), a rise in (hyperkalemic type), or normal (normokalemic type) serum potassium levels. **flaccid p.,** paralysis with loss of muscle tone of the paralyzed part and absence of tendon reflexes. **hyperkalemic periodic p.,** see *familial periodic p.* **hypokalemic periodic p.,** see *familial periodic p.* **immunological p.,** the absence of immune response to a specific antigen. **infantile p.,** the major form of polio-

myelitis. **infantile cerebral ataxic p.,** a congenital condition due to defective development of the frontal regions of the brain, affecting all extremities. **ischemic p.,** local paralysis due to impairment of the circulation. **jake p., Jamaica ginger p.,** paralysis of the extremities, especially the legs, after ingestion of the beverage Jamaica ginger. **Klumpke's p., Klumpke-Dejerine p.,** atrophic paralysis of the lower arm and hand, due to lesion of the eighth cervical and first dorsal nerves. **Landry's p.,** acute febrile polyneuritis. **lead p.,** wristdrop due to lead poisoning. **mixed p.,** combined motor and sensory paralysis. **motor p.,** paralysis of voluntary muscles. **musculospiral p.,** paralysis of the extensor muscles of the wrist and fingers. **normokalemic periodic p.,** see *familial periodic p.* **obstetric p.,** birth p. **periodic p.,** a recurrent paralysis; see also *familial periodic p.* **progressive bulbar p.,** see *bulbar p.* **pseudobulbar p.,** spastic weakness of the muscles innervated by the cranial nerves, i.e., the facial muscles, the pharynx, and tongue, due to bilateral lesions of the corticospinal tract, often accompanied by uncontrolled weeping or laughing. **pseudohypertrophic muscular p.,** see under *dystrophy.* **sensory p.,** loss of sensation due to a morbid process. **spastic p.,** spasticity of the muscles of the paralyzed part and increased tendon reflexes, due to upper motor neuron lesions. **spastic spinal p.,** lateral sclerosis. **tick p.,** progressive ascending flaccid motor paralysis following the bite of certain ticks, usually *Dermacentor andersoni,* in children and domestic animals in Oregon, British Columbia, and other parts of the world. **Todd's p.,** transient hemiplegia or monoplegia occurring after an epileptic seizure. **vasomotor p.,** cessation of vasomotor control. **Volkmann's ischemic p.,** ischemic p. **Weber's p.,** see under *syndrome.*

paralytic (par″ah-lit′ik) 1. pertaining to paralysis. 2. a person affected with paralysis.

paralyzant (par′ah-līz″ant) 1. causing paralysis. 2. a drug that causes paralysis.

paramania (par″ah-ma′ne-ah) parathymia in which one manifests joy by complaining.

paramastigote (-mas′tĭ-gōt) having an accessory flagellum by the side of a larger one.

paramastitis (-mas-ti′tis) inflammation of tissues around the mammary gland.

Paramecium (-me′she-um) a genus of ciliate protozoa.

paramecium (-me′she-um), pl. *parame′cia.* An organism of the genus *Paramecium.*

paramedical (-med′ĭ-kal) related to the science or practice of medicine; especially, pertaining to personnel, such as physical therapists, laboratory technicians, etc., who perform adjunctive medical duties.

paramenia (-me′ne-ah) disordered or difficult menstruation.

parameter (pah-ram′ĕ-ter) a variable whose measure is indicative of a quantity or function that cannot itself be precisely determined by direct methods.

paramethadione (par″ah-meth″ah-di′ōn) an

anticonvulsant, $C_7H_{11}NO_3$, used in petit mal epilepsy.

paramethasone (-meth′ah-sōn) a glucocorticoid, $C_{22}H_{29}FO_5$, used as the 21-acetate ester for its anti-inflammatory and antiallergic effects.

parametric (-met′rik) near the uterus.

parametritis (-me-tri′tis) inflammation of parametrium.

parametrium (-me′tre-um) loose connective tissue between the two serous layers of the broad ligament. **parame′trial,** adj.

paramimia (-mim′e-ah) the use of improper or inappropriate gestures when speaking.

paramnesia (par″am-ne′ze-ah) an unconsciously false memory.

paramucin (par″ah-mu′sin) a colloid substance from ovarian cysts, differing from mucin and pseudomucin in that it reduces Fehling's solution before boiling with acid.

paramutation (-mu-ta′shun) a permanent transmissible change in an allele after passage through a heterozygote.

paramyloidosis (par-am″ĭ-loi-do′sis) accumulation of an atypical form of amyloid in tissues.

paramyoclonus (par″ah-mi-ok′lo-nus) a condition characterized by myoclonic contractions of various muscles. **p. mul′tiplex,** a condition characterized by sudden shocklike muscular contractions.

paramyotonia (-mi″o-to′ne-ah) a disease marked by tonic spasms due to disorder of muscular tonicity, especially a hereditary and congenital affection. **p. congen′ita,** see under *myotonia*.

paramyxovirus (-mik″so-vi′rus) any of a subgroup of myxoviruses, including the viruses of human and animal parainfluenza, mumps, and Newcaste disease.

paranephric (-nef′rik) 1. near the kidney. 2. pertaining to the adrenal gland.

paranephritis (-nĕ-fri′tis) 1. inflammation of the adrenal gland. 2. inflammation of the connective tissue around the kidney.

paranephros (-nef′ros) an adrenal gland.

paranesthesia (par″an-es-the′ze-ah) para-anesthesia.

paraneural (par″ah-nu′ral) beside or alongside a nerve.

para-nitrosulfathiazole (-ni″tro-sul″fah-thi′-ah-zōl) an antibacterial, $NO_2C_6H_4SO_2NH \cdot C_3$-$H_2NS$, used by rectal instillation as an adjunct in the treatment of ulcerative colitis and proctitis.

paranoia (-noi′ah) a mental disorder marked by well systematized delusions of grandeur and persecution. **parano′ic,** adj.

paranoiac (-noi′ak) a person affected with paranoia.

paranoid (par′ah-noid) 1. resembling paranoia. 2. paranoiac.

paranomia (par″ah-no′me-ah) aphasia marked by inability to name objects felt (*myotactic p.*) or seen (*visual p.*).

paranosis (-no′sis) the primary advantage that is to be gained by illness.

paranucleus (-nu′kle-us) a body sometimes seen in cell protoplasm near the nucleus. **paranu′-clear,** adj.

paraparesis (-pah-re′sis) partial paralysis of the lower extremities.

paraphasia (-fa′ze-ah) partial aphasia in which the patient employs wrong words, or uses words in wrong and senseless combinations (*choreic p.*).

paraphemia (-fe′me-ah) aphasia marked by the employment of the wrong words.

paraphia (par-a′fe-ah) perversion of the sense of touch.

paraphilia (par″ah-fil′e-ah) expression of the sexual instinct in practices socially prohibited or unacceptable, or biologically undesirable.

paraphiliac (-fil′e-ak) 1. pertaining to paraphilia. 2. a person exhibiting paraphilia; a sexual deviant.

paraphimosis (-fi-mo′sis) retraction of a phimotic foreskin, causing painful swelling of the glans.

paraphrasia (-fra′ze-ah) disorderly arrangement of spoken words.

paraplasm (par′ah-plazm) 1. any abnormal growth. 2. hyaloplasm (1).

paraplastic (-plas″tik) exhibiting a perverted formative power; of the nature of a paraplasm.

paraplectic (par″ah-plek′tik) paraplegic.

paraplegia (-ple′je-ah) paralysis of the lower part of the body including the legs.

paraplegic (-plej′ik) 1. pertaining to or of the nature of paraplegia. 2. a person affected with paraplegia.

paraplegiform (-plej′ĭ-form) resembling paraplegia.

parapoplexy (par-ap′o-plek″se) a condition resembling apoplexy.

parapraxia (par″ah-prak′se-ah) 1. irrational behavior. 2. inability to perform purposive movements properly.

paraprotein (-pro′te-in) immunoglobulin produced by a clone of neoplastic plasma cells proliferating abnormally, e.g., myeloma proteins and cryoglobulins.

paraproteinemia (-pro″te-in-e′me-ah) presence in the blood of paraproteins.

parapsis (par-ap′sis) paraphia.

parapsoriasis (par″ah-so-ri′ah-sis) a group of slowly developing, persistent, maculopapular scaly erythrodermas, devoid of subjective symptoms and resistant to treatment.

parapsychology (-si-kol′o-je) the branch of psychology dealing with psychical effects and experiences that appear to fall outside the scope of physical law, e.g., telepathy and clairvoyance.

parareflexia (-re-flek′se-ah) any disorder of the reflexes.

pararhotacism (-ro′tah-sizm) faulty enunciation of *r* sound.

pararosaniline (-ro-zan′ĭ-lin) a basic dye; a triphenylmethane derivative, $HOC(C_6H_4NH_2)_3$, one of the components of basic fuchsin.

pararrhythmia (-rith′me-ah) parasystole.

pararthria (par-ar′thre-ah) imperfect utterance of words.

parasacral (par″ah-sa′kral) situated near the sacrum.

Parasal (par′ah-sal) trademark for preparations of para-aminosalicylic acid.

parasigmatism (par″ah-sig′mah-tizm) faulty enunciation of *s* and *z* sounds.

parasinoidal (-si-noi′dal) situated along the course of a sinus.

parasite (par′ah-sīt) 1. a plant or animal that lives upon or within another living organism at whose expense it obtains some advantage; see *symbiosis*. 2. the smaller, less complete member of asymmetrical conjoined twins, attached to and dependent upon the autosite. **parasit′ic,** adj. **accidental p.,** one that parasitizes an organism other than the usual host. **facultative p.,** one that may be parasitic upon another organism but can exist independently. **incidental p.,** accidental p. **malarial p.,** *Plasmodium*. **obligate p., obligatory p.,** one that is entirely dependent upon a host for its survival. **periodic p.,** one that parasitizes a host for short periods. **temporary p.,** one that lives free of its host during part of its life cycle.

parasitemia (par″ah-si-te′me-ah) the presence of parasites, especially malarial forms, in the blood.

parasiticide (par″ah-sit′ĭ-sīd) destructive to parasites; also, an agent that destroys parasites.

parasitism (par′ah-sī″tizm) 1. symbiosis in which one population (or individual) adversely affects another, but cannot live without it. 2. infection or infestation with parasites.

parasitize (par′ah-sĭ-tīz″) to live on or within a host as a parasite.

parasitogenic (par″ah-si′to-jen′ik) due to parasites.

parasitologist (-si-tol′o-jist) a person skilled in parasitology.

parasitology (-si-tol′o-je) the scientific study of parasites and parasitism.

parasitotropic (-si″to-trop′ik) having an affinity for parasites.

paraspadias (-spa′de-as) a congenital condition in which the urethra opens on one side of the penis.

parasternal (-ster′nal) beside the sternum.

parasympathetic (-sim″pah-thet′ik) see under *system*.

parasympatholytic (-sim″pah-tho-lit′ik) anticholinergic: producing effects resembling those of interruption of the parasympathetic nerve supply of a part; having a destructive effect on the parasympathetic nerve fibers or blocking the transmission of impulses by them. Also, an agent that produces such effects.

parasympathomimetic (-mi-met′ik) producing effects resembling those of stimulation of the parasympathetic nerve supply of a part. Also, an agent that produces such effects.

parasynapsis (par″ah-sĭ-nap′sis) the union of chromosomes side by side during meiosis.

parasynovitis (-sin″o-vi′tis) inflammation of tissues about a synovial sac.

parasystole (-sis′to-le) a cardiac irregularity attributed to the interaction of two foci independently initiating cardiac impulses at different rates.

paratenon (-ten′on) the fatty areolar tissue filling the interstices of the fascial compartment in which a tendon is situated.

parathion (-thi′on) an agricultural insecticide, $C_{10}H_{14}NO_5PS$, highly toxic to humans and animals.

parathormone (-thor′mōn) parathyroid hormone.

parathymia (-thi′me-ah) a perverted, contrary, or inappropriate mood.

parathyroid (-thi′roid) see under *gland*.

parathyroidectomy (-thi″roi-dek′to-me) excision of a parathyroid gland.

parathyrotropic (-thi″ro-trop′ik) having an affinity for the parathyroid glands.

paratope (par′ah-tōp) the site on the antibody molecule that attaches to an antigen.

paratrophy (par-at′ro-fe) dystrophy.

paratuberculosis (par″ah-tu-ber″ku-lo′sis) 1. a tuberculosis-like disease not due to *Mycobacterium tuberculosis*. 2. Johne's disease.

paratyphoid (-ti′foid) infection due to *Salmonella* of all groups except *S. typhosa*.

paraurethral (-u-re′thral) near the urethra.

paravaginitis (-vaj″ĭ-ni′tis) inflammation of the tissues alongside the vagina.

paravertebral (-ver′tĕ-bral) near the vertebrae.

paravitaminosis (-vi″tah-mĭ-no′sis) vitamin deficiency without the usual symptoms.

paraxial (par-ak′se-al) alongside an axis.

parazone (par′ah-zōn) one of the white bands alternating with dark bands (diazones) seen in cross section of a tooth.

Paredrine (-drēn) trademark for preparations of hydroxyamphetamine.

paregoric (par″ĕ-gor′ik) a mixture of powdered opium, anise oil, benzoic acid, camphor, diluted alcohol, and glycerin; used as an antiperistaltic, especially in the treatment of diarrhea.

parenchyma (pah-reng′kĭ-mah) the essential or functional elements of an organ, as distinguished from its stroma or framework. **paren′chymal,** adj.

parenchymatitis (par″eng-kim″ah-ti′tis) inflammation of a parenchyma.

parenchymatous (-tus) pertaining to or of the nature of parenchyma.

Parenogen (pah-ren′o-jen) trademark for a preparation of fibrinogen.

parenteral (pah-ren′ter-al) not through the alimentary canal, but rather by injection through some other route, as subcutaneous, intramuscular, etc.

parepididymis (par″ep-ĭ-did′ĭ-mis) paradidymis.

paresis (pah-re′sis, par′ĕ-sis) 1. slight or incomplete paralysis. 2. dementia paralytica. **paret′ic,** adj. **general p.,** dementia paralytica.

paresthesia (par″es-the′ze-ah) morbid or perverted sensation; an abnormal sensation, as burning, prickling, formication, etc.

pargyline (par′gĭ-lēn) an antihypertensive, $C_{11}H_{13}N$, used as the hydrochloride salt.

paries (pa're-ez), pl. *pari'etes* [L.] a wall, as of an organ or cavity.

parietal (pah-ri'ĕ-tal) 1. of or pertaining to the walls of a cavity. 2. pertaining to or located near the parietal bone.

parietofrontal (pah-ri"ĕ-to-fron'tal) pertaining to the parietal and frontal bones, gyri, or fissures.

parietography (pah-ri"ĕ-tog'rah-fe) radiologic visualization of the walls of an organ.

parity (par'ĭ-te) 1. para; the condition of a women with respect to having borne viable offspring. 2. equality; close correspondence or similarity.

parkinsonism (par'kin-sun-izm") a group of neurological disorders marked by hypokinesia, tremor, and muscular rigidity; see *parkinsonian syndrome*, under *syndrome*, and see *paralysis agitans*. **parkinson'ian**, adj.

Parnate (par'nāt) trademark for a preparation of tranylcypromine.

paroccipital (par"ok-sip'ĭ-tal) beside the occipital bone.

paromomycin (par'o-mo-mi"sin) a broad-spectrum antibiotic derived from *Streptomyces rimosus* var. *paromomycinus;* the sulfate salt is used as an antiamebic.

paromphalocele (par"om-fal'o-sēl) hernia near the navel.

paronychia (-o-nik'e-ah) inflammation involving the folds of tissue around the fingernail.

paronychial (-o-nik'e-al) pertaining to paronychia or to the nail folds.

paroophoron (-o-of'o-ron) an inconstantly present, small group of coiled tubules between the layers of the mesosalpinx, being a remnant of the excretory part of the mesonephros.

parophthalmia (-of-thal'me-ah) inflammation of the connective tissue around the eye.

paropsis (par-op'sis) a disorder of vision.

parorchidium (par"or-kid'e-um) displacement of a testis or testes.

parorexia (-o-rek'se-ah) nervous perversion of the appetite, with craving for special articles of food or for articles not suitable for food.

parosmia (par-oz'me-ah) perversion of the sense of smell.

parostosis (par"os-to'sis) ossification of tissues outside the periosteum.

parotid (pah-rot'id) near the ear.

parotidectomy (pah-rot"ĭ-dek'to-me) excision of a parotid gland.

parotiditis (pah-rot"ĭ-di'tis) parotitis.

parotitis (par"o-ti'tis) inflammation of the parotid gland. **epidemic p.**, mumps.

parovarian (par"o-va're-an) 1. beside the ovary. 2. pertaining to the parovarium.

parovarium (-va're-um) epoophoron.

paroxysm (par'ok-sizm) 1. a sudden recurrence or intensification of symptoms. 2. a spasm or seizure. **paroxys'mal**, adj.

pars (pars), pl. *par'tes* [L.] a division or part. **p. mastoi'dea**, the mastoid portion of the temporal bone, being the irregular, posterior part. **p. petro'sa**, the petrous portion of the temporal bone, containing the inner ear and located at the base of the cranium. **p. pla'na**, the thin part of the ciliary body; the ciliary disk. **p. squamo'sa**, the flat scalelike, anterior and superior portion of the temporal bone. **p. tympan'ica**, the part of the temporal bone forming the anterior and inferior walls and part of the posterior wall of the external acoustic meatus.

pars planitis (pars pla-ni'tis) granulomatous uveitis of the pars plana of the ciliary body.

Parsidol (par'sĭ-dol) trademark for a preparation of ethopropazine.

parthenogenesis (par"thĕ-no-jen'ĕ-sis) asexual reproduction in which an egg develops without its being fertilized by a spermatozoon, as in certain lower animals, especially arthropods; it may occur as a natural phenomenon or be induced by chemical or mechanial stimulation (*artificial p.*).

particle (par'tĭ-k'l) a tiny mass of material. **Dane p.**, a particle 42 nm. in diameter, containing hepatitis B (HB) antigen on its surface (HB$_S$) and in its core (HB$_C$). **viral p.**, virion.

particulate (par-tik'u-lāt) composed of separate particles.

parturient (par-tu're-ent) giving birth or pertaining to birth; by extension, a woman in labor.

parturiometer (par-tu"re-om'ĕ-ter) device used in measuring expulsive power of the uterus.

parturition (par"tu-rish'un) the act or process of giving birth to a child; see *labor*.

parulis (pah-roo'lis) a subperiosteal abscess of the gum.

parumbilical (par"um-bil'ĭ-kal) alongside the navel.

parvicellular (par"vĭ-sel'u-lar) composed of small cells.

parvovirus (par"vo-vi'rus) a group of extremely small, morphologically similar, ether-resistant DNA viruses, including the adeno-associated viruses.

PAS, PASA para-aminosalicylic acid.

paste (pāst) a semisolid preparation, generally for external use, of a fatty base, a viscous or mucilaginous base, or a mixture of starch and petrolatum.

pastern (pas'tern) the part of a horse's foot occupied by the first and second phalanges.

Pasteurella (pas"tĕ-rel'ah) a genus of gram-negative bacteria (family Brucellaceae), including *P. multoci'da*, the etiologic agent of the hemorrhagic septicemias, and *P. pes'tis*, the etiologic agent of plague.

pasteurellosis (pas"ter-ĕ-lo'sis) infection with organisms of the genus *Pasteurella*.

pasteurization (pas"tūr-ĭ-za'shun) heating of milk or other liquids to moderate temperature for a definite time, often 60° C. for 30 min., which kills most pathogenic bacteria and considerably delays other bacterial development.

patch (pach) a small area differing from the rest of a surface. **Peyer's p's**, oval elevated patches of closely packed lymph follicles on the mucosa of the small intestines.

patella (pah-tel'ah), pl. *patel'lae* [L.] see *Table of Bones*. **patel'lar**, adj.

patellectomy (pat″ĕ-lek′to-me) excision of the patella.

patelliform (pah-tel′ĭ-form) shaped like the patella.

patency (pa′ten-se) the condition of being wide open.

patent (pa′tent) 1. open, unobstructed, or not closed. 2. apparent, evident.

path(o)- word element [Gr.], *disease.*

pathergasia (path″er-ga′ze-ah) mental malfunction, implying functional or structural damage, marked by abnormal behavior.

pathergy (path′er-je) 1. a condition in which the application of a stimulus leaves the organism unduly susceptible to subsequent stimuli of a different kind. 2. a condition of being allergic to numerous antigens. **pather′gic,** adj.

pathfinder (path′find-er) 1. an instrument for locating urethral strictures. 2. a dental instrument for tracing the course of root canals.

pathobiology (path″o-bi-ol′o-je) pathology.

pathoclisis (-klis′is) a specific sensitivity to specific toxins, or a specific affinity of certain toxins for certain systems or organs.

pathogen (path′o-jen) any disease-producing agent or microorganism. **pathogen′ic,** adj.

pathogenesis (path″o-jen′ĕ-sis) the development of morbid conditions or of disease; more specifically the cellular events and reactions and other pathologic mechanisms occurring in the development of disease. **pathogenet′ic,** adj.

pathogenicity (-jĕ-nis′ĭ-te) the quality of producing or the ability to produce pathologic changes or disease.

pathognomonic (path″og-no-mon′ik) specifically distinctive or characteristic of a disease or pathologic condition; denoting a sign or symptom on which a diagnosis can be made.

pathologic (path″o-loj′ik) indicative of or caused by some morbid condition.

pathological (-loj′ĭ-k'l) pertaining to pathology; pathologic.

pathologist (pah-thol′o-jist) a specialist in pathology.

pathology (pah-thol′o-je) that branch of medicine treating of the essential nature of disease, especially of the changes in body tissues and organs which cause or are caused by disease. **cellular p.,** that which regards the cells as starting points of the phenomena of disease and which recognizes that every cell descends from some preexisting cell. **clinical p.,** pathology applied to the solution of clinical problems, especially the use of laboratory methods in clinical diagnosis. **comparative p.,** that which considers human disease processes in comparison with those of the lower animals. **experimental p.,** the study of artifically induced pathologic processes. **general p.,** that taking cognizance of processes which may occur in various diseases and in different organs. **oral p.,** that treating of conditions causing or resulting from morbid anatomic or functional changes in the structures of the mouth. **special p.,** that dealing with changes produced by certain diseases or in a specific organ. **surgical p.,** the pathology of disease processes that are surgically accessible for diagnosis or treatment.

pathomimesis (path″o-mi-me′sis) malingering.

pathomorphism (-mor′fizm) perverted or abnormal morphology.

pathonomia (-no′me-ah) the sum of knowledge regarding the laws of disease.

pathophysiology (-fiz″e-ol′o-je) the physiology of disordered function.

pathopsychology (-si-kol′o-je) the psychology of mental disease.

pathosis (pah-tho′sis) a diseased condition.

pathway (path′wa) a course usually followed. In neurology, the nerve structures through which a sensory impression is conducted to the cerebral cortex (*afferent p.*) or through which an impulse passes from the brain to the skeletal musculature (*efferent p.*). Also used alone to indicate a sequence of reactions that convert one biological material to another (*metabolic p.*). **biosynthetic p.,** a sequence of enzymatic steps in the synthesis of a specific end-product in a living organism. **Embden-Meyerhof p.** (of glucose metabolism), the series of enzymatic reactions in the anaerobic conversion of glucose to lactic acid, resulting in energy in the form of adenosine triphosphate (ATP). **pentose phosphate p.,** a pathway of hexose oxidation in which glucose-6-phosphate undergoes two successive oxidations by NADP, the final forming a pentose phosphate.

-pathy word element [Gr.], *morbid condition* or *disease;* generally used to designate a noninflammatory condition.

patient (pa′shent) a person who is ill or is undergoing treatment for disease.

patrilineal (pat″rĭ-lin′e-al) descended through the male line.

patulin (pat′u-lin) a toxic antibiotic, $C_7H_6O_4$, from various fungi, especially *Aspergillus* and *Penicillium;* used as an antimicrobial.

patulous (pat′u-lus) spread widely apart; open; distended.

pause (pawz) an interruption, or rest. **compensatory p.,** the pause after a premature ventricular systole, related to blockage of one beat of the basic pacemaker.

Paveril (pav′er-il) trademark for preparations of dioxyline.

pavor (pa′vor) [L.] terror. **p. diur′nus,** attacks of fear in children during a daytime nap. **p. noctur′nus,** a nightmare of children causing them to cry out in fright and awake in panic.

P.B. *Pharmacopoeia Britannica* (British Pharmacopoeia).

Pb chemical symbol, *lead* (L. *plumbum*).

PBI protein-bound iodine.

p.c. [L.] *post ci′bum* (after meals).

PCG phonocardiogram.

PCO_2 carbon dioxide partial pressure or tension; also written P_{CO_2}, pCO_2, or pCO_2.

P.C.V. packed-cell volume.

Pd chemical symbol, *palladium.*

p.d. potential difference; prism diopter.

pearl (perl) 1. a small medicated granule, or a glass globule with a single dose of volatile medicine, as amyl nitrite. 2. a rounded mass of tough sputum as seen in the early stages of an attack of bronchial asthma. **epidermic p's, epithelial p's,** rounded concentric masses of epithelial cells found in certain papillomas and epitheliomas. **Laennec's p's,** soft casts of the smaller bronchial tubes expectorated in bronchial asthma.

pecazine (pe'kah-zēn) mepazine.

pectase (pek'tās) pectinesterase.

pecten (pek'ten), pl. *pec'tines* [L.] 1. a comb; in anatomy, applied to certain comblike structures. 2. a narrow zone in the anal canal, bounded above by the pectinate line. **p. os'sis pu'bis,** pectineal line.

pectenitis (pek"tĕ-ni'tis) inflammation of the pecten of the anus.

pectenosis (pek"tĕ-no'sis) stenosis of the anal canal due to an inelastic ring of tissue between the anal groove and anal crypts.

pectin (pek'tin) a homosaccharidic polymer of sugar acids of fruit that forms gels with sugar at the proper pH; a purified form obtained from the acid extract of the rind of citrus fruits or from apple pomace is used as a protectant and in cooking. **pec'tic,** adj.

pectinase (pek'tĭ-nās) polygalacturonase.

pectinate (pek'tĭ-nāt) comb-shaped.

pectineal (pek-tin'e-al) pertaining to the os pubis.

pectinesterase (pek"tin-es'ter-ās) an enzyme that catalyzes the hydrolysis of methyl ester groups of pectic substances, releasing the free acid.

pectiniform (pek-tin'ĭ-form) comb-shaped.

pectoral (pek'to-ral) 1. of or pertaining to the breast or chest. 2. relieving disorders of the respiratory tract, as an expectorant.

pectoralis (pek"to-ra'lis) [L.] pertaining to the chest or breast.

pectoriloquy (pek"to-ril'o-kwe) transmission of the sound of spoken words through the chest wall.

pectose (pek'tōs) a principle in unripe fruits and plants from which pectin is derived.

pectus (pek'tus) the breast, chest, or thorax. **p. carina'tum,** pigeon breast. **p. excava'tum,** funnel chest.

ped(o)- word element, (1) [Gr.], *child*; (2) [L.], *foot*.

pedal (ped'al) pertaining to the foot or feet.

pederast (ped'er-ast) one who practices pederasty.

pederasty (ped'er-as'te) homosexual anal intercourse between men and boys as the passive partners.

pedia- word element [Gr.], *child*.

pediatrician (pe"de-ah-trish'an) a specialist in pediatrics.

pediatrics (pe"de-at'riks) that branch of medicine dealing with the child and its development and care and with the diseases of children and their treatment. **pediat'ric,** adj.

pedicel (ped'ĭ-sel) a footlike part, especially any of the secondary processes of a podocyte.

pedicellation (ped"ĭ-sel-la'shun) the development of a pedicle.

pedicle (ped'ĭ-k'l) a footlike, stemlike, or narrow basal part or structure.

pedicular (pĕ-dik'u-lar) pertaining to or caused by lice.

pediculation (pĕ-dik"u-la'shun) 1. the process of forming a pedicle. 2. infestation with lice.

pediculicide (pĕ-dik'u-lĭ-sīd) 1. destroying lice. 2. an agent that destroys lice.

pediculosis (pĕ-dik"u-lo'sis) infestation with lice.

pediculous (pĕ-dik'u-lus) infested with lice.

Pediculus (pĕ-dik'u-lus) a genus of lice. *P. huma'nus,* a species feeding on human blood, is a major vector of typhus, trench fever, and relapsing fever; two subspecies are recognized: *P. huma'nus* var. *capitis* (head louse) found on the scalp hair, and *P. huma'nus* var. *corporis* (body, or clothes, louse) found on the body.

pediculus (pĕ-dik'u-lus), pl. *pedic'uli* [L.] pedicle.

peditis (pĕ-di'tis) pedal osteitis.

pedodontia (pe"do-don'she-ah) pedodontics.

pedodontics (-don'tiks) that branch of dentistry dealing with the teeth and mouth conditions of children.

pedodontist (-don'tist) a dentist who specializes in pedodontics.

pedodynamometer (-di"nah-mom'ĕ-ter) an instrument for measuring leg strength.

pedophilia (-fil'e-ah) abnormal fondness for children; sexual activity of adults with children as the objects. **pedophil'ic,** adj.

peduncle (pĕ-dung'k'l) a stemlike connecting part, especially, (*a*) a collection of nerve fibers coursing between different areas in the central nervous system, or (*b*) the stalk by which a nonsessile tumor is attached to normal tissue. **pedun'cular,** adj. **cerebellar p's,** three sets of paired bundles of the hindbrain (*superior, middle,* and *inferior*) connecting the cerebellum to the midbrain, pons, and medulla oblongata, respectively. **cerebral p.,** the ventral half of the midbrain, divisible into a dorsal part (*tegmentum*) and a ventral part (*crus cerebri*), which are separated by the substantia nigra. **pineal p.,** habenula (2).

pedunculated (pĕ-dung'ku-lāt"ed) having a peduncle.

pedunculotomy (pĕ-dung"ku-lot'o-me) incision of a cerebral peduncle.

pedunculus (pĕ-dung'ku-lus) [L.] peduncle.

peg (peg) a projecting structure. **rete p's,** inward projections of the epidermis into the dermis, as seen histologically in verticle sections.

Peganone (peg'ah-nōn) trademark for a preparation of ethotoin.

pelage (pel'ij, pĕ-lahzh') [Fr.] the hairy coat of mammals; hairs of the body, limbs, and head collectively.

peliosis (pe"le-o'sis) purpura. **p. hep'atis,** mottled blue liver, due to blood-filled lacunae in the parenchyma.

pellagra (pĕ-la'grah, pĕ-lag'rah) a syndrome due to niacin deficiency (or failure to convert tryptophan to niacin), marked by dermatitis on parts of the body exposed to light or trauma, inflammation of the mucous membranes, diarrhea, and psychic disturbances. **pellag′rous,** adj.

pellagroid (pĕ-lag′roid) resembling pellagra.

pellet (pel′et) a small pill or granule.

pellicle (pel′ĭ-k'l) a thin scum forming on the surface of liquids.

pellucid (pel-lu′sid) translucent.

pelotherapy (pe″lo-ther′ah-pe) therapeutic use of mud baths.

pelvicephalometry (pel″vĭ-sef″ah-lom′ĕ-tre) measurement of the fetal head in relation to the maternal pelvis.

pelvifixation (-fik-sa′shun) surgical fixation of a displaced pelvic organ.

pelvimeter (pel-vim′ĕ-ter) an instrument for measuring the pelvis.

pelvimetry (pel-vim′ĕ-tre) measurement of the capacity and diameter of the pelvis.

pelviotomy (pel″ve-ot′o-me) 1. incision or transection of a pelvic bone. 2. pyelotomy.

pelviperitonitis (pel″vĭ-per″ĕ-to-ni′tis) inflammation of the pelvic peritoneum.

pelvirectal (-rek′tal) pertaining to the pelvis and rectum.

pelvis (pel′vis), pl. *pel′ves.* The lower (caudal) portion of the trunk of the body, bounded anteriorly and laterally by the hip bones and posteriorly by the sacrum and coccyx. Also applied to any basin-like structure, e.g., the renal pelvis. **pel′vic,** adj. **android p.,** one with a wedge-shaped inlet and narrow anterior segment, typically found in the male. **anthropoid p.,** one in which the anteroposterior diameter of the inlet equals or exceeds the transverse diameter. **assimilation p.,** one in which the ilia articulate with the vertebral column higher (*high assimilation p.*) or lower (*low assimilation p.*) than normal, the number of lumbar vertebrae being correspondingly decreased or increased. **beaked p.,** one with the pelvic bones laterally compressed and their anterior junction pushed forward. **brachypellic p.,** one in which the transverse diameter exceeds the anteroposterior diameter by 1 to 3 cm. **contracted p.,** one showing a decrease of 1.5 to 2 cm. in any important diameter; when all dimensions are proportionately diminished it is a *generally contracted p.* **cordate p.,** a heart-shaped pelvis. **dolichopellic p.,** an elongated pelvis, the anteroposterior diameter being greater than the transverse diameter. **extrarenal p.,** see *renal p.* **false p.,** the part of the pelvis superior to a plane passing through the ileopectineal lines. **flat p.,** one in which the anteroposterior dimension is abnormally reduced. **frozen p.,** a condition, due to infection or carcinoma, in which the adnexa and uterus are fixed in the pelvis. **funnel p.,** one with a normal inlet but a greatly narrowed outlet. **gynecoid p.,** the normal female pelvis: a rounded oval pelvis with well rounded anterior and posterior segments. **infantile p.,** a generally contracted pelvis with an oval inlet, a high sacrum, and inclination of the walls. **p. jus′to ma′jor,** an unusually large gynecoid pelvis, with all dimensions increased. **p. jus′to mi′nor,** a small gynecoid pelvis, with all dimensions symmetrically reduced. **juvenile p.,** infantile p. **kyphotic p.,** a deformed pelvis marked by increase of conjugate diameter at the brim with decrease of transverse diameter at outlet. **p. ma′jor,** false p. **mesatipellic p.,** one in which the transverse diameter is equal to the anteroposterior diameter or exceeds it by no more than 1 cm. **p. mi′nor,** true p. **Nägele's p., oblique p.,** one contracted in an oblique diameter, with complete ankylosis of the sacroiliac synchondrosis of one side and imperfect development of the sacrum and coxa on the same side. **Otto p.,** one in which the acetabulum is depressed, with protrusion of the femoral head into the pelvis. **platypellic p., platypelloid p.,** one shortened in the anteroposterior aspect, with a flattened transverse, oval shape. **Prague p.,** spondylolisthetic p. **rachitic p.,** one distorted as a result of rickets. **renal p.,** the funnel-shaped expansion of the upper end of the ureter into which the renal calices open; it is usually within the renal sinus, but under certain conditions, a large part of it may be outside the kidney (*extrarenal p.*). **Robert's p.,** a transversely contracted pelvis caused by osteoarthritis affecting both sacroiliac joints, the inlet becoming a narrow wedge. **Rokitansky's p.,** spondylolisthetic p. **scoliotic p.,** one deformed as a result of scoliosis. **split p.,** one with a congenital separation at the symphysis pubis. **spondylolisthetic p.,** one deformed by sliding of the body of one of the lower lumbar vertebrae over the first sacral and into the pelvis. **true p.,** the part of the pelvis inferior to a plane passing through the ileopectineal lines.

pelvospondylitis (pel″vo-spon″dĭ-li′tis) inflammation of the pelvic portion of the spine. **p. ossif′icans,** rheumatoid spondylitis.

pemoline (pem′o-lēn) a central nervous system stimulant, $C_9H_8N_2O_2$.

pemphigoid (pem′fĭ-goid) 1. resembling pemphigus. 2. a group of dermatological syndromes similar to but clearly distinguishable from the pemphigus group. 3. bullous p. **bullous p.,** a chronic generalized bullous eruption, most often occurring in the elderly, and usually not fatal.

pemphigus (pem′fĭ-gus) 1. a distinctive group of diseases marked by successive crops of bullae. 2. p. vulgaris. **benign familial p.,** a hereditary, recurrent vesiculobullous dermatitis, usually involving the axillae, groin, and neck, with crops of lesions that regress over several weeks or months. **p. erythemato′sus,** a chronic form in which the lesions, limited to the face and chest, resemble those of disseminated lupus erythematosus. **p. folia′ceus,** a chronic, generalized, vesicular and scaling eruption somewhat resembling dermatitis herpetiformis or, later in its course, exfoliative dermatitis. **p. neonato′rum,** impetigo neonatorum. **p. veg′etans,** a variant of pemphigus vulgaris in which the bullae are replaced by verrucoid hypertrophic vegetative masses. **p. vulga′ris,** a rare relapsing disease with suprabasal, intraepidermal bullae of the skin and mucous membranes; invariably fatal if untreated.

pempidine (pem′pĭ-dēn) a ganglionic blocking agent, $C_{10}H_{21}N$, used in hypertension.

pendulous (pen′joo-lus, pen′dŭ-lus) hanging loosely; dependent.

penetrance (pen′ĕ-trans) the frequency with which a heritable trait is manifested by individuals carrying the principal gene or genes conditioning it.

penetrometer (pen″ĕ-trom′ĕ-ter) an instrument for measuring the penetrating power of x-rays.

-penia word element [Gr.], *deficiency.*

penicillamine (pen″ĭ-sil-am′in) a product of penicillin, $C_5H_{11}NO_2S$, which chelates copper and other metals; used mainly to remove excess copper from the body in hepatolenticular degeneration.

penicillin (pen″ĭ-sil′in) an antibiotic substance extracted from cultures of certain molds of the genera *Penicillium* and *Aspergillus* that have been grown on certain media; also prepared synthetically. **chloroprocaine p. O,** a combination of 2-chloroprocaine and penicillin O which has long-sustained activity, for intramuscular administration. **p. G,** the first antibiotic developed industrially for medical use, effective against gram-positive bacteria (except penicillinase-resistant staphylococci), gram-negative cocci, *Treponema pallidum, Actinomyces israelii,* and in treating various other infections; used mainly in the form of its sodium, potassium, benzathine, and procaine salts. **isoxazolyl p.,** a group of semisynthetic penicillins, e.g., cloxacillin, dicloxacillin, and oxacillin, which combine resistance to penicillinase with acid stability and activity to gram-positive bacteria. **p. O,** a penicillin produced biosynthetically by adding a precursor to the fermentation medium; also available in the form of its potassium and sodium salts. **phenoxymethyl p.,** a biosynthetically or semisynthetically produced antibiotic, similar to penicillin G, used orally for mild to moderately severe infections due to susceptible gram-positive bacteria; available in the form of its potassium and hydrabamine salts. **procaine p. G,** a compound of penicillin and procaine used as a long-acting antibacterial. **p. V,** phenoxymethyl p.

penicillinase (pen″ĭ-sil′ĭ-nās) an enzyme produced by certain bacteria which inactivates penicillin, thus increasing resistance to the antibiotic; a purified form from *Bacillus cereus* is used in the treatment reactions to penicillin.

Penicillium (-sil′e-um) a genus of fungi.

penicilloyl-polylysine (pen″ĭ-sil′oil-pol″ĕ-li′-sēn) an agent prepared from polylysine and a penicillenic acid; intradermal reaction elicits a wheal and erythema response in those sensitive to penicillin.

penicillus (pen″ĭ-sil′us), pl. *penicil′li* [L.] any of the brushlike groups of arterial branches in the lobules of the spleen.

penile (pe′nīl) of or pertaining to the penis.

penis (pe′nis) the male organ of urination and copulation.

penitis (pe-ni′tis) inflammation of the penis.

penniform (pen′ĭ-form) shaped like a feather.

pent(a)- word element [Gr.], *five.*

pentaerythritol (pen″tah-ĕ-rith′rĭ-tol) an alcohol, $(CH_2OH)_4C$, used in the form of the tetranitrate ester as a vasodilator in the treatment of angina pectoris.

pentagastrin (-gas′trin) a synthetic pentapeptide consisting of β-alanine and the C-terminal tetrapeptide of gastrin; used as a test of gastric secretory function.

pentamidine (pen-tam′ĭ-dēn) a trypanosomicide, $C_{19}H_{24}N_4O_2$, used as the isethionate salt in the prophylaxis and treatment of African trypanosomiasis and in the treatment of leishmaniasis.

pentapeptide (pen″tah-pep′tīd) a polypeptide containing five amino acids.

pentaploid (pen′tah-ploid) 1. pertaining to or characterized by pentaploidy. 2. an individual or cell having five sets of chromosomes.

pentaploidy (-ploi′de) the state of having five sets of chromosomes (5n).

pentavalent (pen″tah-va′lent, pen-tav′ah-lent) having a valence of five.

pentazocine (pen-taz′o-sēn) a synthetic narcotic, $C_{27}H_{27}NO$, used as an analgesic.

penthienate (pen-thi′ĕ-nāt) an anticholinergic, $C_{18}H_{30}NO_3S$; the bromide is used as an antispasmodic in peptic ulcer.

Penthrane (pen′thrān) trademark for a preparation of methoxyflurane.

Pentids (pen′tidz) trademark for preparations of potassium penicillin G.

pentobarbital (pen″to-bar′bĭ-tal) a short- to intermediate-acting barbiturate, $C_{11}H_{17}N_2O_3$; the sodium salt is used as a hypnotic and sedative.

pentolinium (-lin′e-um) a ganglionic blocking agent, $C_{23}H_{42}N_2O_{12}$, used as the tartrate salt in the management of hypertension.

pentose (pen′tōs) a monosaccharide containing five carbon atoms in a molecule.

pentosuria (pen″to-su′re-ah) a benign inborn error of metabolism due to a defect in the activity of the enzyme L-xylulose dehydrogenase, resulting in high levels of L-xylulose in the urine.

Pentothal (pen′to-thal) trademark for preparations of thiopental.

pentylenetetrazol (pen″tĭ-lēn-tet′rah-zol) a convulsant analeptic, $C_6H_{10}N_4$.

Pen-Vee (pen′ve) trademark for a preparation of phenoxymethyl penicillin.

peotillomania (pe″o-til″o-ma′ne-ah) constant but nonmasturbatory, pulling at the penis.

peplomer (pep′lo-mer) a subunit of a peplos.

peplos (pep′lohs) the lipoprotein envelope of some types of virions, assembled in some cases from subunits (peplomers).

peppermint (pep′er-mint) the dried leaves and flowering tops of *Mentha piperita,* used as a flavoring vehicle for drugs.

pepsin (pep′sin) the proteolytic enzyme of gastric juice which catalyzes the hydrolysis of native or denatured proteins to form a mixture of polypeptides; it is formed from pepsinogen in the presence of acid or, autocatalytically, in the presence of pepsin.

pepsinogen (pep-sin′o-jen) a zymogen secreted by the chief cells of the gastric glands and converted into pepsin in the presence of gastric acid or of pepsin itself.

peptic (pep′tik) pertaining to pepsin or to digestion or to the action of gastric juices.

peptidase (pep′tĭ-dās) any of a subclass of proteolytic enzymes that catalyze the hydrolysis of peptide linkages.

peptide (pep′tīd, pep′tid) any of a class of compounds of low molecular weight which yield two or more amino acids on hydrolysis; known as di-, tri-, tetra-, (etc.) peptides, depending on the number of amino acids in the molecule. Peptides form the constituent parts of proteins.

peptidolytic (pep″tĭ-do-lit′ik) capable of splitting peptide bonds.

peptogenic (pep″to-jen′ik) 1. producing pepsin or peptones. 2. promoting digestion.

peptolysis (pep-tol′ĭ-sis) the splitting up of peptones. **peptolyt′ic,** adj.

peptone (pep′tōn) a derived protein, or a mixture of cleavage products produced by partial hydrolysis of native protein. **pepton′ic,** adj.

peptonize (pep′to-nīz) to convert a native protein into peptone.

peptotoxin (pep″to-tok′sin) any toxin or poisonous base developed from a peptone; also, a poisonous alkaloid or ptomaine occurring in certain peptones and putrefying proteins.

per- word element [L.], (1) *throughout; completely; extremely;* (2) in chemistry, *a large amount; combination of an element in its highest valence.*

peracid (per-as′id) an acid containing more than the usual quantity of oxygen.

peracute (per″ah-kūt′) very acute.

Perandren (per-an′dren) trademark for a preparation of testosterone.

per anum (per a′num) [L.] through the anus.

Perazil (per′ah-zil) trademark for preparations of chlorcyclizine.

percept (per′sept) the object perceived; the mental image of an object in space perceived by the senses.

perception (per-sep′shun) the conscious mental registration of a sensory stimulus. **percep′tive,** adj. **depth p.,** the ability to recognize depth or the relative distances to different objects in space. **extrasensory p.,** knowledge of, or response to, an external thought or objective event not achieved as the result of stimulation of the sense organs.

perceptivity (per″sep-tiv′ĭ-te) ability to receive sense impressions.

percolate (per′ko-lāt) 1. to strain; to submit to percolation. 2. to trickle slowly through a substance. 3. a liquid that has been submitted to percolation.

percolation (per″ko-la′shun) the extraction of soluble parts of a drug by passing a solvent liquid through it.

percolator (per″ko-la′tor) vessel used in percolation.

Percorten (per-kor′ten) trademark for preparations of desoxycorticosterone.

percuss (per-kus′) to perform percussion.

percussible (per-kus′ĭ-b′l) detectable on percussion.

percussion (per-kush′un) the act of striking a part with short, sharp blows as an aid in diagnosing the condition of the underlying parts by the sound obtained. **auscultatory p.,** auscultation of the sound produced by percussion. **immediate p.,** that in which the blow is struck directly against the body surface. **mediate p.,** that in which a pleximeter is used. **palpatory p.,** a combination of palpation and percussion, affording tactile rather than auditory impressions.

percussor (per-kus′or) an instrument for performing percussion.

percutaneous (per″ku-ta′ne-us) performed through the skin.

perencephaly (per″en-sef′ah-le) porencephaly.

perfectionism (per-fek′shun-izm) the setting of impossible high standards for oneself.

perforans (per′fo-rans) [L.] penetrating; applied to various muscles and nerves.

perfusate (per-fu′zāt) a liquid that has been subjected to perfusion.

perfusion (per-fu′zhun) 1. the act of pouring over or through, especially the passage of a fluid through the vessels of a specific organ. 2. a liquid poured over or through an organ or tissue.

peri- word element [Gr.], *around; near.* See also words beginning *para-.*

periacinal, periacinous (per″e-as′ĭ-nal; -as′ĭ-nus) around an acinus.

Periactin (-ak′tin) trademark for a preparation of cyproheptadine.

periadenitis (-ad″ĕ-ni′tis) inflammation of tissues around a gland. **p. muco′sa necrot′ica recur′rens,** the more severe form of aphthous stomatitis, marked by recurrent attacks of aphtha-like lesions that begin as small, firm nodules, which enlarge, ulcerate, and heal by scar formation, leaving numerous atrophied scars on the oral mucosa.

perianal (-a′nal) around the anus.

periangiitis (-an″je-i′tis) inflammation of the tissue around a blood or lymph vessel.

periangiocholitis (-an″je-o-ko-li′tis) pericholangitis.

periaortitis (-a″or-ti′tis) inflammation of tissues around the aorta.

periapical (-a′pĭ-kal) surrounding the apex of the root of a tooth.

periappendicitis (-ah-pen″dĭ-si′tis) inflammation of the tissues around the vermiform appendix.

periarterial (-ar-te′re-al) around an artery.

periarteritis (-ar″tĕ-ri′tis) inflammation of the outer coat of an artery and of the tissues around it. **p. nodo′sa,** an inflammatory disease of the coats of small and medium-sized arteries, associated with a variety of systemic symptoms.

periarthritis (-ar-thri′tis) inflammation of tissues around a joint.

periarticular (-ar-tik′u-lar) around a joint.

periaxial (-ak′se-al) around an axis.

periaxillary (-ak′sĭ-ler″e) around the axilla.

periblast (per′ĭ-blast) the portion of the blastoderm of telolecithal eggs the cells of which lack complete cell membranes.

peribronchial (per″ĭ-brong′ke-al) around a bronchus or bronchi.

peribronchiolar (-brong″ke-o′lar) around the bronchioles.

peribronchiolitis (-brong″ke-o-li′tis) inflammation of tissues around the bronchioles.

peribronchitis (-brong-ki′tis) a form of bronchitis consisting of inflammation and thickening of the tissues around the bronchi.

pericardial (-kar′de-al) of or pertaining to the pericardium.

pericardiac (-kar′de-ak) pericardial.

pericardicentesis (-kar″dĭ-sen-te′sis) pericardiocentesis.

pericardiectomy (-kar″de-ek′to-me) excision of a portion of the pericardium.

pericardiocentesis (-kar″de-o-sen-te′sis) surgical puncture of the pericardial cavity for the aspiration of fluid.

pericardiolysis (-kar″de-ol′ĭ-sis) the operative freeing of adhesions between the visceral and parietal pericardium.

pericardiophrenic (-kar″de-o-fren′ik) pertaining to the pericardium and diaphragm.

pericardiopleural (-ploo′ral) pertaining to the pericardium and pleura.

pericardiorrhaphy (per″ĭ-kar″de-or′ah-fe) suture of the pericardium.

pericardiostomy (-kar″de-os′to-me) creation of an opening into the pericardium, usually for the drainage of effusions.

pericardiotomy (-kar″de-ot′o-me) incision of the pericardium.

pericarditis (-kar-di′tis) inflammation of the pericardium. **pericardit′ic**, adj. **adhesive p.,** a condition due to the presence of dense fibrous tissue between the parietal and visceral layers of the pericardium. **p. calculo′sa,** that with a calcareous deposit in the pericardium. **constrictive p.,** pericarditis leading to thickening and sometimes calcification, with impaired diastolic filling, inflow stasis, or constrictive effect. **fibrinous p., fibrous p.,** chronic pericarditis with formation of fibrous tissue and probably adhesions. **p. oblit′erans, obliterating p.,** adhesive pericarditis that leads to obliteration of the pericardial cavity.

pericardium (-kar′de-um) the fibroserous sac enclosing the heart and the roots of the great vessels. **pericar′dial,** adj. **adherent p.,** one abnormally connected with the heart by dense fibrous tissue. **fibrous p.,** the external layer of the pericardium, consisting of fibrous tissue. **parietal p.,** the parietal layer of the serous pericardium, which is in contact with the fibrous pericardium. **serous p.,** the inner, serous portion of pericardium, consisting of two layers, the parietal and visceral pericardium; the space between the layers is the pericardial cavity. **visceral p.,** the inner layer of the serous pericardium, which is in contact with the heart and roots of the great vessels.

pericecal (-se′kal) around the cecum.

pericecitis (-se-si′tis) inflammation of the tissues around the cecum.

pericellular (-sel′u-lar) surrounding a cell.

pericementitis (-se″men-ti′tis) periodontitis.

pericholangitis (-ko″lan-ji′tis) inflammation of the tissues around the bile ducts.

pericholecystitis (-ko″le-sis-ti′tis) inflammation of tissues around the gallbladder.

perichondritis (-kon-dri′tis) inflammation of perichondrium.

perichondrium (-kon′dre-um) the layer of fibrous connective tissue investing all cartilage except the articular cartilage of synovial joints. **perichon′dral,** adj.

perichordal (-kor′dal) surrounding the notochord.

perichoroidal (-ko-roi′dal) surrounding the choroid coat.

Periclor (pār′ĭ-klōr) trademark for a preparation of petrichloral.

pericolic (per″ĭ-ko′lik) around the colon.

pericolitis, pericolonitis (-ko-li′tis; -ko″lon-i′tis) inflammation around the colon, especially of its peritoneal coat.

pericolpitis (-kol-pi′tis) inflammation of tissues around the vagina.

periconchal (-kong′kal) around the concha.

pericorneal (-kor′ne-al) around the cornea.

pericoronal (-kŏ-ro′nal) around the crown of a tooth.

pericranitis (-kra-ni′tis) inflammation of the pericranium.

pericranium (-kra′ne-um) the periosteum of the skull. **pericra′nial,** adj.

pericystic (-sis′tik) about a bladder or cyst.

pericystitis (-sis-ti′tis) inflammation of tissues about the bladder.

pericyte (per′ĭ-sīt) one of the peculiar elongated, contractile cells found wrapped about precapillary arterioles outside the basement membrane.

pericytial (per″ĭ-si′shal) around a cell.

periderm (per′ĭ-derm) the outer layer of the bilaminar fetal epidermis, generally disappearing before birth.

peridesmitis (per″ĭ-dez-mi′tis) inflammation of the peridesmium.

peridesmium (-dez′me-um) the areolar membrane that covers the ligaments.

perididymis (-did′ĭ-mis) tunica vaginalis.

perididymitis (-did″ĭ-mi′tis) inflammation of the tunica vaginalis.

peridiverticulitis (-di″ver-tik″u-li′tis) inflammation around an intestinal diverticulum.

periductal (-duk′tal) around a duct.

periduodenitis (-du″o-dĕ-ni′tis) inflammation around the duodenum.

periencephalitis (per″e-en-sef″ah-li′tis) inflammation of the surface of the brain.

periencephalomeningitis (-en-sef″ah-lo-men″in-ji′tis) inflammation of the cerebral cortex and meninges.

perienteritis (-en″ter-i′tis) inflammation of the peritoneal coat of the intestines.

periesophagitis (-e-sof″ah-ji′tis) inflammation of tissues around the esophagus.

perifistular (per″ĭ-fis′tu-lar) around a fistula.

perifollicular (-fŏ-lik′u-lar) surrounding a follicle.

perifolliculitis (-fŏ-lik″u-li′tis) inflammation around the hair follicles.

perigangliitis (-gang″gle-i′tis) inflammation of tissues around a ganglion.

perigastric (-gas′trik) around the stomach; pertaining to the peritoneal coat of the stomach.

perigastritis (-gas-tri′tis) inflammation of the peritoneal coat of stomach.

perihepatic (-hĕ-pat′ik) around the liver.

perihepatitis (-hep″ah-ti′tis) inflammation of the peritoneal capsule of the liver and the surrounding tissue.

perijejunitis (-je″ju-ni′tis) inflammation around the jejunum.

perikaryon (-kar′e-on) the cell body of a neuron.

perilabyrinthitis (-lab″ĭ-rin-thi′tis) inflammation of tissues around the labyrinth.

perilaryngitis (-lar″in-ji′tis) inflammation of tissues around the larynx.

perilymph, perilympha (per′ĭ-limf; per″ĭ-lim′-fah) the fluid within the space separating the membranous and osseous labyrinth of the ear.

perilymphangitis (per″ĭ-lim″fan-ji′tis) inflammation around a lymphatic vessel.

perimeningitis (-men″in-ji′tis) pachymeningitis.

perimeter (pĕ-rim′ĕ-ter) 1. the boundary of a plane figure. 2. an apparatus for determining the extent of the peripheral visual field.

perimetrium (per″ĭ-me′tre-um) the serous membrane enveloping the uterus.

perimetry (pĕ-rim′ĕ-tre) determination of the extent of the peripheral visual field. **perimet′ric,** adj.

perimyelitis (per″ĭ-mi″ĕ-li′tis) inflammation of (*a*) the pia of the spinal cord, or (*b*) the endosteum.

perimyositis (-mi″o-si′tis) inflammation of connective tissue around a muscle.

perimysiitis (-mis″e-i′tis) inflammation of the perimysium.

perimysium (-mis′e-um) the connective tissue demarcating a fascicle of skeletal muscle fibers. See Plate XIV. **perimys′ial,** adj.

perinatal (-na′tal) relating to the period shortly before and after birth; from the twenty-ninth week of gestation to one to four weeks after birth.

perineal (-ne′al) pertaining to the perineum.

perineocele (-ne′o-sēl) a hernia between the rectum and the prostate or between the rectum and the vagina.

perineoplasty (-ne′o-plas″te) plastic repair of the perineum.

perineorrhaphy (-ne-or′ah-fe) suture of the perineum.

perineotomy (-ne-ot′o-me) incision of the perineum.

perineovaginal (-ne″o-vaj′ĭ-nal) pertaining to or communicating with the perineum and vagina.

perinephric (-nef′rik) around the kidney.

perinephritis (-nĕ-fri′tis) inflammation of the perinephrium.

perinephrium (-nef′re-um) the peritoneal envelope and other tissues around the kidney. **perineph′rial,** adj.

perineum (-ne′um) the pelvic floor and associated structures occupying the pelvic outlet, bounded anteriorly by the pubic symphysis, laterally by the ischial tuberosities, and posteriorly by the coccyx.

perineuritis (-nu-ri′tis) inflammation of the perineurium.

perineurium (-nu′re-um) the sheath surrounding each bundle of fibers in a peripheral nerve. See Plate XI. **perineu′rial,** adj.

perinuclear (-nu′kle-ar) around a nucleus.

periocular (per″e-ok′u-lar) around the eye.

period (pe′re-od) an interval or division of time. **child-bearing p.,** the duration of the reproductive ability in the human female, roughly from puberty to menopause. **gestational p.,** the duration of pregnancy; in the human female about 266 days. **incubation p.,** the interval required for development; especially, the time between invasion of the body by a pathogenic organism and appearance of the first symptoms of disease. **isoelectric p.,** the moment in muscular contraction when no deflection of the galvanometer is produced. **latency p.,** 1. latent p. 2. the period from the ages of five to seven years to adolescence when there is cessation of psychosexual development. **latent p.,** a seemingly inactive period, as that between exposure of tissue to an injurious agent and the manifestations of response, or that between the instant of stimulation and the beginning of response. **menstrual p., monthly p.,** menstruation. **postsphygmic p.,** the short period (0.08 second) of ventricular diastole, after the sphygmic period, and lasting until the atrioventricular valves open. **presphygmic p.,** the first phase of ventricular systole, being the period (0.04–0.06 sec.) immediately after closure of the atrioventricular valves and lasting until the semilunar valves open. **refractory p.,** the period of depolarization and repolarization of the cell membrane after excitation; during the first portion (*absolute refractory p.*), the nerve or muscle fiber cannot respond to a second stimulus, whereas during the *relative refractory period,* it can respond only to a strong stimulus. **safe p.,** the period during the menstrual cycle (about 10 days before menstruation begins until 10 days after it begins) when conception is considered least likely to occur. **sphygmic p.,** the second phase of ventricular systole (0.21–0.30 sec.), between the opening and closing of the semilunar valves, while the blood is discharged into the aorta and pulmonary artery. **Wenckebach p.,** a usually repetitive sequence seen in partial heart block, marked by progressive lengthening of the P-R interval until ventricular response occurs.

periodic (pe″re-od′ik) recurring at regular intervals of time.

periodicity (pe″re-o-dis′ĭ-te) recurrence at regular intervals of time.

periodontal (per″e-o-don′tal) around a tooth; pertaining to the periodontium.

peridontics (-don′tiks) the branch of dentistry dealing with the study and treatment of diseases of the periodontium.

periodontist (-don′tist) a dentist who specializes in periodontics.

periodontitis (-don-ti′tis) inflammation of periodontium. **compound p.,** that in which the combination of local irritants and occlusal trauma produces an exacerbation of simple periodontitis. **simple p.,** that due to various local irritants, e.g., calculus, impacted food, etc., with chronic gingivitis, periodontal pocket formation usually with pus formation, horizontal bone resorption, destruction of the periodontal ligament, and loss of teeth.

periodontium (-don′she-um) the tissues investing and supporting the teeth, including the cementum, periodontal ligament, alveolar bone, and gingiva. In NA, restricted to the periodontal ligament.

periodontoclasia (-don″to-kla′ze-ah) any degenerative or destructive disease of the periodontium.

periodontosis (-don-to′sis) a degenerative disorder of the periodontal structures, marked by tissue destruction.

periomphalic (per″e-om-fal′ik) around the umbilicus.

perionychium (-o-nik′e-um) the epidermis bordering a nail.

perioophoritis (-o″of-o-ri′tis) inflammation of tissues around the ovary.

perioophorosalpingitis (-o-of″o-ro-sal″pin-ji′tis) inflammation of tissues around an ovary and uterine tube.

periophthalmic (-of-thal′mik) around the eye.

periople (per′e-o″p'l) the smooth, shiny layer on the outer surface of the hoofs of ungulates.

perioptometry (per″e-op-tom′ĕ-tre) measurement of acuity of peripheral vision or of limits of the visual field.

perioral (-o′ral) around the mouth.

periorbit (-or′bit) periorbita.

periorbita (-or′bĭ-tah) periosteum of the bones of the orbit, or eye socket. **perior′bital,** adj.

periorbital (-or′bĭ-tal) around the eye socket.

periorbitis (-or-bi′tis) inflammation of the periorbita.

periorchitis (-or-ki′tis) vaginalitis.

periosteitis (-os″te-i′tis) periostitis.

periosteoma (-os-te-o′mah) a morbid bony growth surrounding a bone.

periosteomyelitis (-os″te-o-mi″ĕ-li′tis) inflammation of the entire bone, including periosteum and marrow.

periosteophyte (-os′te-o-fīt″) a bony growth on the periosteum.

periosteotomy (-os″te-ot′o-me) incision of the periosteum.

periosteum (-os′te-um) a specialized connective tissue covering all bones and having bone-forming potentialities. **perios′teal,** adj.

periostitis (-os-ti′tis) inflammation of the periosteum. **dental p.,** periodontitis. **diffuse p.,** widespread periostitis of the long bones.

periostosis (-os-to′sis) abnormal deposition of periosteal bone.

periotic (-o′tik) 1. situated about the ear, especially the internal ear. 2. the petrous and mastoid portions of the temporal bone, at one stage a distinct bone.

peripachymeningitis (per″ĭ-pak″ĭ-men″in-ji′tis) inflammation of tissue between the dura mater and its bony covering.

peripancreatitis (-pan″kre-ah-ti′tis) inflammation of tissues about the pancreas.

peripapillary (-pap′ĭ-ler″e) around the optic papilla.

periphacitis (-fah-si′tis) inflammation of the capsule of the eye lens.

peripherad (pĕ-rif′er-ad) toward the periphery.

periphery (pĕ-rif′er-e) an outward surface or structure; the portion of a system outside the central region. **periph′eral,** adj.

periphlebitis (per″ĭ-fle-bi′tis) inflammation of tissues around a vein, or of the external coat of a vein.

periplocin (-plo′sin) a cardiotonic glycoside from the woody vine *Periploca graeca.*

periplocymarin (-plo-si′mah-rin) a cardiac glycoside from the woody vine *Periploca graeca.*

periportal (-por′tal) around the portal vein.

periproctitis (-prok-ti′tis) inflammation of tissues around the rectum and anus.

periprostatic (-pros-tat′ik) around the prostate.

periprostatitis (-pros″tah-ti′tis) inflammation of tissues around the prostate.

peripylephlebitis (-pi″le-fle-bi′tis) inflammation of tissues around the portal vein.

peripyloric (-pi-lo′rik) around the pylorus.

perirectal (-rek′tal) around the rectum.

perirectitis (-rek-ti′tis) periproctitis.

perirenal (-re′nal) around the kidney.

perirhinal (-ri′nal) around the nose.

perisalpingitis (-sal″pin-ji′tis) inflammation of tissues around the uterine tube.

periscopic (-skop′ik) affording a wide range of vision.

perisigmoiditis (-sig″moi-di′tis) inflammation of the peritoneum of sigmoid flexure.

perisinusitis (-si″nu-si′tis) inflammation of tissues about a sinus.

perispermatitis (-sper″mah-ti′tis) inflammation of tissues about the spermatic cord.

perisplanchnic (-splangk′nik) around a viscus or viscera.

perisplanchnitis (-splangk-ni′tis) inflammation of tissues around the viscera.

perisplenic (-splen′ik) around the spleen.

perisplenitis (-sple-ni′tis) inflammation of the peritoneal surface of the spleen.

perispondylitis (-spon″dĭ-li′tis) inflammation of tissues around a vertebra.

peristalsis (per″ĭ-stal′sis) the wormlike movement by which the alimentary canal or other tubular organs having both longitudinal and circular muscle fibers propel their contents, consisting of a wave of contraction passing along the tube for variable distances. **peristal'tic,** adj. **reversed p.,** that which impels the contents of the intestine cephalad.

peristaphyline (-staf'ĭ-līn) around the uvula.

perisynovial (-sĭ-no've-al) around a synovial structure.

peritectomy (-tek'to-me) excision of a ring of conjunctiva around the cornea in treatment of pannus.

peritendineum (-ten-din'e-um) connective tissue investing larger tendons and extending between the fibers composing them.

peritendinitis, peritenonitis (-ten"dĭ-ni'tis; -ten"on-ni'tis) tenosynovitis.

perithelioma (-the"le-o'mah) hemangiopericytoma.

perithelium (-the'le-um) the connective tissue layer surrounding the capillaries and smaller vessels.

perithyroiditis (-thi"roi-di'tis) inflammation of the capsule of the thyroid gland.

peritomy (pĕ-rit'o-me) 1. incision of the conjunctiva and subconjunctival tissue about the entire circumference of the cornea. 2. circumcision.

peritoneal (per"ĭ-to-ne'al) pertaining to the peritoneum.

peritonealgia (per"ĭ-to"ne-al'je-ah) pain in the peritoneum.

peritoneocentesis (-to"ne-o-sen-te'sis) paracentesis of the abdominal cavity.

peritoneoclysis (-to"ne-ok'lĭ-sis) injection of fluid into the peritoneal cavity.

peritoneopathy (-to"ne-op'ah-the) any disease of the peritoneum.

peritoneopericardial (-to-ne"o-per"ĭ-kar'de-al) pertaining to the peritoneum and pericardium.

peritoneoscope (-to'ne-o-skōp") an endoscope for use in peritoneoscopy.

peritoneoscopy (-to"ne-os'ko-pe) visual examination of the organs of the abdominal (peritoneal) cavity with a peritoneoscope.

peritoneotomy (-to-ne-ot'o-me) incision into the peritoneum.

peritoneum (per"ĭ-to-ne'um) the serous membrane lining the walls of the abdominal and pelvic cavities (*parietal p.*) and investing the contained viscera (*visceral p.*), the two layers enclosing a potential space, the peritoneal cavity. **peritone'al,** adj.

peritonitis (-to-ni'tis) inflammation of the peritoneum, which may be due to chemical irritation or bacterial invasion. **adhesive p.,** that marked by adhesions between adjacent serous surfaces. **bile p., biliary p.,** choleperitoneum. **silent p.,** asymptomatic peritonitis.

peritonsillar (-ton'sĭ-lar) around a tonsil.

peritonsillitis (-ton"sĭ-li'tis) inflammation of peritonsillar tissues.

peritracheal (-tra'ke-al) around the trachea.

Peritrate (per'ĭ-trāt) trademark for a preparation of pentaerythritol.

peritrichous (pĕ-rit'rĭ-kus) 1. having flagella around the entire surface; said of bacteria. 2. having flagella around the cytostome only; said of Ciliophora.

periumbilical (per"e-um-bil'ĭ-kal) around the umbilicus.

periureteral (-u-re'ter-al) around the ureter.

periureteritis (-u-re"tĕ-ri'tis) inflammation of tissues around the ureter.

periurethral (-u-re'thral) around the urethra.

periuterine (-u'ter-īn) around the uterus.

perivaginal (per"ĭ-vaj'ĭ-nal) around the vagina.

perivaginitis (-vaj"ĭ-ni'tis) pericolpitis.

perivascular (-vas'ku-lar) around a vessel.

perivasculitis (-vas"ku-li'tis) inflammation of a perivascular sheath and surrounding tissue.

perivesical (-ves'ĭ-kal) around the bladder.

perivesiculitis (-vĕ-sik"u-li'tis) inflammation of tissues around the seminal vesicles.

perlèche (per-lesh') inflammation with exudation, maceration, and fissuring at the labial commissures.

permanganate (per-man'gah-nāt) a salt of permanganic acid.

permeability (per"me-ah-bil'ĭ-te) the property or state of being permeable.

permeable (per'me-ah-b'l) not impassable; pervious.

permease (per'me-ās) the genetically controlled mechanism responsible for active transport of nutrient substances across the bacterial membrane.

pernicious (per-nish'us) tending to a fatal issue.

pernio (per'ne-o) chilblain.

pero- word element [Gr.], *deformity; maimed.*

perobrachius (pe'ro-bra'ke-us) a fetus with deformed arms.

perocephalus (-sef'ah-lus) a fetus with a deformed head.

perochirus (-ki'rus) a fetus with deformed hands.

peromelia (-me'le-ah) congenital deformity of the limbs.

peromelus (pe-rom'ĕ-lus) a fetus with deformed limbs.

peroneal (per"o-ne'al) pertaining to the fibula or to the outer side of the leg; fibular.

peropus (pe'ro-pus) a fetus with malformed legs and feet.

peroral (per-o'ral) performed or administered through the mouth.

per os (per os) [L.] by mouth.

peroxidase (pĕ-rok'sĭ-dās) any of a group of iron-porphyrin enzymes that catalyze the oxidation of some organic substrates in the presence of hydrogen peroxide.

peroxide (pĕ-rok'sīd) that oxide of any element containing more oxygen than any other; more correctly applied to compounds having such linkage as —O—O—.

peroxisome (pĕ-roks'ĭ-sōm) a cellular microbody isolated from mitochondrial and lysosomal fractions that contains urate oxidase, amino acid oxidase, catalase, and other enzymes.

perphenazine (per-fen′ah-zēn) a major tranquilizer and antiemetic, $C_{21}H_{26}ClN_3OS$.

per primam (intentionem) (per pri′mam in-ten″she-o′nem) [L.] by first intention.

per rectum (per rek′tum) [L.] by way of the rectum.

Persantine (per-san′tēn) trademark for preparations of dipyridamole.

per secundam (intentionem) (per se-kun′dam in-ten″she-o′nem) [L.] by second intention.

perseveration (per-sev″er-a′shun) persistent repetition of the same verbal or motor response to varied stimuli; continuance of activity after cessation of the causative stimulus.

persona (per-so′nah) Jung's term for the personality "mask" or facade presented by a person to the outside world, as opposed to the anima.

personality (per″su-nal′ĭ-te) that which constitutes, distinguishes, and characterizes a person as an entity over a period of time; the total reaction of a person to his environment. **alternating p.,** see *multiple p.* **antisocial p.,** a personality disorder in which repetitive antisocial behavior is associated with ego eccentricity, lack of guilt or anxiety, and imperviousness to punishment. **cyclothymic p.,** a personality marked by alternate moods of elation and dejection. **double p., dual p.,** see *multiple p.* **multiple p.,** a dissociative reaction in which an individual adopts two or more personalities, alternatively, in none of which is he aware of the experiences of the other(s). **psychopathic p.,** antisocial p. **schizoid p.,** a personality disorder marked by timidness, self-consciousness, introversion, feelings of isolation and loneliness, and failure to form close interpersonal relationships; the individual is frequently ambitious, meticulous, and a perfectionist.

perspiration (per″spĭ-ra′shun) 1. sweating; the functional secretion of sweat. 2. sweat. **insensible p.,** that which evaporates before it becomes perceptible. **sensible p.,** the noticeable excretion of the sweat glands, which appears as moisture upon the skin.

persulfate (per-sul′fāt) a salt of persulfuric acid.

Pertofrane (per′to-frān) trademark for a preparation of desipramine.

per tubam (per tu′bam) [L.] through a tube.

pertussis (per-tus′is) whooping cough.

pertussoid (per-tus′oid) 1. resembling whooping cough. 2. an influenzal cough resembling that of whooping cough.

per vaginam (per vah-ji′nam) [L.] through the vagina.

perversion (per-ver′zhun) deviation from the normal course. **sexual p.,** paraphilia.

pervert (per′vert) a deviant person, especially a paraphiliac.

pes (pes), pl. *pe′des,* gen. *pe′dis* [L.] foot; the terminal organ of the leg, or lower limb; any footlike part. **p. abduc′tus,** a deformity in which the anterior part of the foot is displaced and lies laterally to the vertical axis of the leg. **p. adduc′tus,** a deformity in which the anterior part of the foot is displaced and lies medially to the vertical axis of the leg. **p. ca′vus,** a foot with an abnormally high longitudinal arch. **p. hip-**

pocam′pi, a formation of two or three elevations on the ventricular surface of the hippocampus. **p. pla′nus,** flatfoot. **p. val′gus,** flatfoot. **p. va′rus,** talipes varus.

pessary (pes′ah-re) 1. an instrument placed in the vagina to support the uterus or rectum or as a contraceptive device. 2. a medicated vaginal suppository.

pesticide (pes′tĭ-sīd) a poison used to destroy pests of any sort.

pestilence (pes′tĭ-lens) a virulent contagious epidemic or infectious epidemic disease. **pestilen′tial,** adj.

pestle (pes′'l) an implement for pounding drugs in a mortar.

-petal word element [L.], *directed* or *moving toward.*

petechia (pe-te′ke-ah), pl. *pete′chiae* [L.] a minute red spot due to escape of a small amount of blood. **pete′chial,** adj.

pethidine (peth′ĭ-dēn) meperidine.

petiole (pet′e-ōl) a stalk or pedicle. **epiglottic p.,** the pointed lower end of the epiglottic cartilage, attached to the thyroid cartilage.

petiolus (pĕ-ti′o-lus) petiole.

petit mal (pĕ-te′ mahl′) [Fr.] see under *epilepsy.*

petrichloral (pet″rĭ-klo′ral) a hypnotic and sedative, $C_{13}H_{16}Cl_{12}O_8$.

petrissage (pa-trĭ-sahzh′) [Fr.] foulage.

petrolatum (pet″ro-la′tum) a purified mixture of semisolid hydrocarbons obtained from petroleum; used as an ointment base, protective dressing, and soothing application to the skin. **hydrophilic p.,** a mixture of cholesterol, stearyl alcohol, white wax, and white petrolatum; used as an absorbent ointment base and topical protectant. **liquid p., liquid p., heavy,** mineral oil. **liquid p., light,** light mineral oil. **white p.,** a wholly or nearly decolorized, purified mixture of semisolid hydrocarbons from petroleum, used as an oleaginous ointment base and topical protectant.

petroleum (pĕ-tro′le-um) a thick natural oil obtained from beneath the earth, consisting of a mixture of various hydrocarbons of the paraffin and olefin series.

petromastoid (pet″ro-mas′toid) 1. pertaining to the petrous portion of the temporal bone and its mastoid process. 2. otocranium (2).

petro-occipital (-ok-sip′ĭ-tal) pertaining to the petrous portion of the temporal bone and to the occipital bone.

petrosal (pĕ-tro′sal) pertaining to the petrous portion of the temporal bone.

petrositis (pet″ro-si′tis) inflammation of the petrous portion of the temporal bone.

petrosphenoid (-sfe′noid) pertaining to the petrous portion of the temporal bone and to the sphenoid bone.

petrosquamous (-skwa′mus) pertaining to the petrous and squamous portions of the temporal bone.

petrous (pet′rus) resembling rock; stony.

pexis (pek′sis) 1. the fixation of matter by a tissue. 2. surgical fixation. **pex′ic,** adj.

-pexy word element [Gr.], *surgical fixation.* **-pec′tic,** adj.

peyote (pa-o′te) a stimulant drug from mescal buttons, whose active principle is mescaline; used by North American Indians in certain ceremonies to produce an intoxication marked by feelings of ecstasy.

pg. picogram.

PGA pteroylglutamic (folic) acid.

pH the symbol relating the hydrogen ion (H⁺) concentration or activity of a solution to that of a given standard solution. Numerically the pH is approximately equal to the negative logarithm of H⁺ concentration expressed in molarity. pH 7 is neutral; above it alkalinity increases and below it acidity increases.

phac(o)- word element [Gr.], *lens.* See also words beginning *phako-.*

phacitis (fah-si′tis) phakitis.

phacoanaphylaxis (fak″o-an″ah-fi-lak′sis) hypersensitivity to the protein of the crystalline lens of the eye, induced by escape of material from the lens capsule.

phacocele (fak′o-sēl) hernia of the eye lens.

phacocystectomy (fak″o-sis-tek′to-me) excision of part of lens capsule for cataract.

phacocystitis (-sis-ti′tis) inflammation of capsule of eye lens.

phacoemulsification (-e-mul″sĭ-fĭ-ka′shun) emulsification and aspiration of a cataract.

phacoerysis (-er′ĭ-sis) removal of the eye lens in cataract by suction.

phacoid (fak′oid) shaped like a lens.

phacoiditis (fak″oi-di′tis) phakitis.

phacoidoscope (fah-koi′do-skōp) phacoscope.

phacolysis (fah-kol′ĭ-sis) dissolution or discission of the eye lens. **phacolyt′ic,** adj.

phacoma (fah-ko′mah) phakoma.

phacomalacia (fak″o-mah-la′she-ah) softening of the lens; a soft cataract.

phacometachoresis (-met″ah-ko-re′sis) displacement of the eye lens.

phacosclerosis (-skle-ro′sis) hardening of the eye lens; a hard cataract.

phacoscope (fak′o-skōp) instrument for viewing accommodative changes of the eye lens.

phacotoxic (fak′o-tok′sik) exerting a deleterious effect upon the crystalline lens.

phag(o)- word element [Gr.], *eating; ingestion.*

phage (fāj) bacteriophage.

-phagia, -phagy word element [Gr.], *eating; swallowing.*

phagocyte (fag′o-sīt) any cell that ingests microorganisms or other cells and foreign particles. **phagocyt′ic,** adj.

phagocytin (fag″o-si′tin) a bactericidal substance from neutrophilic leukocytes.

phagocytize (fag′o-sĭ-tīz) phagocytose.

phagocytoblast (fag″o-si′to-blast) a cell giving rise to phagocytes.

phagocytolysis (-si-tol′ĭ-sis) destruction of phagocytes. **phagocytolyt′ic,** adj.

phagocytose (-si′tōs) to envelop and destroy bacteria and other foreign material.

phagocytosis (-si-to′sis) the engulfing of microorganisms or other cells and foreign particles by phagocytes.

phagodynamometer (-di″nah-mom′ĕ-ter) an apparatus for measuring the force exerted in chewing food.

phagokaryosis (-kar″e-o′sis) the alleged phagocytic action of the cell nucleus.

phagomania (-ma′ne-ah) an insatiable craving for food or an obsessive preoccupation with the subject of eating.

phagosome (fag′o-sōm) a membrane-bound vesicle in a phagocyte containing the phagocytized material.

phagotype (-tīp) phage type; see under *type.*

phak(o)- see *phac(o)-.*

phakitis (fa-ki′tis) inflammation of the crystalline lens.

phakoma (fah-ko′mah) 1. an occasional small, grayish white tumor seen microscopically in the retina in tuberous sclerosis. 2. a patch of myelinated nerve fibers seen very infrequently in the retina in neurofibromatosis.

phakomatosis (fak″o-mah-to′sis) any of four hereditary syndromes (neurofibromatosis, tuberous sclerosis, Sturge-Weber syndrome, and von Hippel-Lindau disease) marked by disseminated hamartomas of the eye, skin, and brain.

phalangeal (fah-lan′je-al) pertaining to a phalanx.

phalangectomy (fal″an-jek′to-me) excision of a phalanx.

phalangitis (fal″an-ji′tis) inflammation of one or more phalanges.

phalanx (fa′lanks), pl. *phalan′ges* [Gr.] any bone of a finger or toe; see *phalanges* in *Table of Bones.* **phalan′geal,** adj.

phallectomy (fal-ek′to-me) amputation of the penis.

phallitis (fal-li′tis) penitis.

phallocampsis (fal″o-kamp′sis) curvature of penis during erection.

phalloidin, phalloidine (fah-loid′in) a hexapeptide poison from the mushroom *Amanita phalloides,* which causes asthenia, vomiting, diarrhea, convulsions, and death.

phallus (fal′us) the penis. **phal′lic,** adj.

phanerosis (fan″er-o′sis) the process of becoming visible.

Phanodorn (fan′o-dorn) trademark for a preparation of cyclobarbital.

phantasm (fan′tazm) phantom (1).

phantom (fan′tom) 1. an image or impression not evoked by actual stimuli. 2. a model of the body or of a specific part thereof. 3. a device for simulating the *in vivo* effect of radiation on tissues.

phar., pharm. *pharmacy; pharmaceutical; pharmacopeia.*

pharmac(o)- word element [Gr.], *drug; medicine.*

pharmaceutical (fahr″mah-su′tĭ-kal) 1. pertaining to pharmacy or drugs. 2. a medicinal drug.

pharmaceutics (fahr″mah-su′tiks) 1. pharmacy (1). 2. pharmaceutical preparations.

pharmacist (fahr′mah-sist) one who is licensed

to prepare and sell or dispense drugs and compounds, and to make up prescriptions.

pharmacodiagnosis (fahr″mah-ko-di″ag-no′sis) use of drugs in diagnosis.

pharmacodynamics (-di-nam′iks) the study of the actions of drugs on living systems. **pharmacodynam′ic,** adj.

pharmacogenetics (-jĕ-net′iks) the study of the relationship between genetic factors and the nature of responses to drugs.

pharmacognosy (fahr″mah-kog′no-se) the branch of pharmacology dealing with natural drugs and their constituents.

pharmacologist (fahr″mah-kol′o-jist) a specialist in pharmacology.

pharmacology (-kol′o-je) the scientific study of the action of drugs on living systems. **pharmacolog′ic,** adj.

pharmacomania (fahr″mah-ko-ma′ne-ah) uncontrollable desire to take or to administer medicines.

pharmacopeia (-pe′ah) an authoritative treatise on drugs and their preparations. See also *U.S.P.* **pharmacopei′al,** adj.

pharmacophobia (-fo′be-ah) morbid dread of medicines or drugs.

pharmacophore (fahr′mah-ko-for″) the group of atoms in a drug molecule responsible for the drug's action.

pharmacopoeia (fahr″mah-ko-pe′ah) pharmacopeia.

pharmacopsychosis (-si-ko′sis) any of a group of mental diseases due to alcohol, drugs, or poisons.

pharmacotherapy (-ther′ah-pe) treatment of disease with medicines.

pharmacy (fahr′mah-se) 1. the art of preparing, compounding, and dispensing medicines. 2. a place for the preparation, compounding, and dispensing of drugs and medicinal supplies.

pharyng(o)- word element [Gr.], *pharynx.*

pharyngalgia (far″ing-gal′je-ah) pain in the pharynx.

pharyngeal (fah-rin′je-al) pertaining to the pharynx.

pharyngectomy (far″in-jek′to-me) excision of part of the pharynx.

pharyngemphraxis (far″in-jem-frak′sis) obstruction of the pharynx.

pharyngismus (far″in-jiz′mus) muscular spasm of the pharynx.

pharyngitis (far″in-ji′tis) inflammation of the pharynx. **pharyngit′ic,** adj.

pharyngocele (fah-ring′go-sēl) herniation or cystic deformity of the pharynx.

pharyngodynia (fah-ring″go-din′e-ah) pharyngalgia.

pharyngoesophageal (-ĕ-sof″ah-je′al) pertaining to the pharynx and esophagus.

pharyngoglossal (-glos′al) pertaining to the pharynx and tongue.

pharyngokeratosis (-ker″ah-to′sis) keratosis of the pharynx.

pharyngolaryngitis (-lar″in-ji′tis) inflammation of the pharynx and larynx.

pharyngomycosis (-mi-ko′sis) any fungal infection of the pharynx.

pharyngonasal (-na′zal) pertaining to the pharynx and nose.

pharyngoparalysis (-pah-ral′ĭ-sis) paralysis of the pharyngeal muscles.

pharyngoperistole (-pĕ-ris′to-le) pharyngostenosis.

pharyngoplasty (fah-ring′go-plas″te) plastic repair of the pharynx.

pharyngoplegia (fah-ring″go-ple′je-ah) pharyngoparalysis.

pharyngorhinitis (-ri-ni′tis) inflammation of the nasopharynx.

pharyngorrhea (-re′ah) mucous discharge from the pharynx.

pharyngoscleroma (-skle-ro′mah) scleroma of the pharynx.

pharyngoscope (fah-ring′go-skōp) an instrument for inspecting the pharynx.

pharyngoscopy (far″ing-gos′ko-pe) direct visual examination of the pharynx.

pharyngospasm (fah-ring′go-spazm) spasm of the pharyngeal muscles.

pharyngostenosis (fah-ring″go-ste-no′sis) narrowing of the pharynx.

pharyngotomy (far″ing-got′o-me) incision of the pharynx.

pharynx (far′ingks) the throat; the musculomembranous cavity behind the nasal cavities, mouth, and larynx, communicating with them and with the esophagus.

phase (fāz) 1. one of the aspects or stages through which a varying entity may pass. 2. in physical chemistry, any physically or chemically distinct, homogeneous, and mechanically separable part of a system, e.g., the ice and steam phases of water. **continuous p.,** one that is physically continuous; the continuous portion of a colloid system (see *dispersion medium*). **disperse p.,** the internal or discontinuous phase of a colloid system, analogous to the solute in a solution; cf. *dispersion medium*.

phasmid (faz′mid) 1. either of the two caudal chemoreceptors occurring in certain nematodes (Phasmidia). 2. any nematode containing phasmids.

Phe-Mer-Nite (fe′mer-nīt) trademark for preparations of phenylmercuric nitrate.

Phemerol (-ol) trademark for preparations of benzethonium.

phenacaine (fen′ah-kān) a topical anesthetic, $C_{18}H_{22}N_2O_2$; the hydrochloride salt is used in ophthalmology.

phenacemide (fĕ-nas′ĕ-mīd) an anticonvulsant, $C_9H_{10}N_2O_2$, used in psychomotor and grand mal epilepsy.

phenacetin (fĕ-nas′ĕ-tin) an analgesic, $C_{10}H_{13}NO_2$.

phenaglycodol (fen″ah-gli′ko-dol) a sedative, $C_{11}H_{15}ClO_2$.

phenanthrene (fe-nan′thrēn) a colorless, crystalline hydrocarbon, $(C_6H_4 \cdot CH)_2$.

phenazocine (fĕ-naz′o-sēn) a narcotic analgesic, $C_{22}N_{27}NO$, used as the hydrobromide salt.

phenazopyridine (fen″ah-zo-pēr′ĭ-dēn) a urinary analgesic, $C_{11}H_{11}N_5$, used as the hydrochloride salt.

phencarbamide (fen-kar'bah-mīd) an anticholinergic, $C_{19}H_{24}N_2OS$.

phencyclidine (-si'klǐ-dēn) an anesthetic, $C_{17}H_{25}N$.

phenelzine (fen'el-zēn) an antidepressant, $C_8H_{12}N_2$, used as the sulfate salt.

Phenergan (-er-gan) trademark for a preparation of promethazine.

phenethicillin (fĕ-neth"ĭ-sil'in) phenoxymethyl penicillin.

phenetidin (fĕ-net'ĭ-din) the ethyl ester of para-aminophenol; it appears in the urine after administration of acetophenetidin.

phenformin (fen-for'min) an oral hypoglycemic, $C_{10}H_{15}N_5$, used as the hydrochloride salt.

phenindamine (fĕ-nin'dah-min) an antihistaminic, $C_{19}H_{19}N$, used as the tartrate salt.

phenindione (fen-in'di-ōn) an anticoagulant, $C_{15}H_{10}O_2$.

pheniramine (fe-nir'ah-min) an antihistaminic, $C_{16}H_{20}N_2$, used as the maleate salt.

phenmetrazine (fen-met'rah-zēn) a central nervous stimulant, $C_{11}H_{15}NO$, used as an anorexic in the form of the hydrochloride salt.

phenobarbital (fe"no-bar'bǐ-tal) an anticonvulsant, sedative, and hypnotic, $C_{12}H_{12}N_2O_3$; also used as the sodium salt.

phenocopy (fe'no-kop"e) 1. an environmentally induced phenotype mimicking one usually produced by a specific genotype. 2. an individual exhibiting such a phenotype; the simulated trait in a phenocopy.

phenol (fe'nol) 1. an extremely poisonous compound, $C_6H_5 \cdot OH$, obtained by distillation of coal tar; used as an antimicrobial. Ingestion or absorption of phenol through the skin causes colic, weakness, collapse, and local irritation and corrosion. 2. any organic compound containing one or more hydroxyl groups attached to an aromatic or carbon ring. **liquefied p.,** an aqueous solution containing not less than 89% of phenol; used as a topical antipruritic. **p. red,** phenolsulfonphthalein.

phenolase (fe'no-lās) a copper-containing enzyme that catalyzes the oxidation of monophenols and dihydroxybenzenes to quinones.

phenolate (-lāt) 1. to treat with phenol for purposes of sterilization. 2. a salt formed by union of a base with phenol, in which a monovalent metal, such as sodium or potassium, replaces the hydrogen of the hydroxyl group.

phenolphthalein (fe"nol-tha'lēn) a cathartic, $C_{20}H_{14}O_4$.

phenolsulfonphthalein (-sul"fōn-tha'lēn) a red powder, $C_{19}H_{14}O_5S$, used as a test of renal function.

phenomenon (fe-nom'ĕ-non) any sign or objective symptom; any observable occurrence or fact. **Litten's diaphragm p.,** a movable horizontal depression of the lower part of the sides of the thorax, seen in respiration. **Raynaud's p.,** intermittent attacks of severe pallor of the fingers or toes and sometimes of the ears and nose, produced characteristically by cold and sometimes by emotion. **rebound p.,** on sudden withdrawal of resistance applied to a limb, it rebounds strongly in the direction of the resistance; a sign of cerebellar dysfunction. **second set p.,** occurrence in a recipient of a more severe immunologic reaction to a second graft of tissue from the same donor. **Shwartzman p.,** a severe local or general reaction observed in rabbits injected twice under specified conditions with bacterial cultures or endotoxic filtrates. **Trousseau's p.,** spasmodic contractions of muscles provoked by pressure upon the nerves which go to them; seen in tetany.

phenopropazine (fe"no-pro'pah-zēn) ethopropazine.

phenothiazine (-thi'ah-zēn) a veterinary anthelmintic; also used to denote a group of major tranquilizers resembling phenothiazine in molecular structure.

phenotype (fe'no-tīp) 1. the entire physical, biochemical, and physiological makeup of an individual as determined both genetically and environmentally. Also, any one or any group of such traits. 2. an individual or group of individuals exhibiting a certain phenotype. **phenotyp'ic,** adj.

Phenoxene (fen-ok'sēn) trademark for a preparation of chlorphenoxamine.

phenoxybenzamine (fĕ-nok"se-ben'zah-mēn) an adrenergic blocking agent, $C_{18}H_{22}ClNO$; the hydrochloride salt is used as a vasodilator and sometimes as an antihypertensive.

phenozygous (fe"no-zi'gus) having the calvaria narrower than the face, so that the zygomatic arches are visible when the head is viewed from above.

phenprocoumon (fen-pro'koo-mon) an anticoagulant of the coumarin type, $C_{18}H_{16}O_3$.

phensuximide (-suk'sǐ-mīd) an anticonvulsant, $C_{11}H_{11}NO_2$.

phentermine (fen'ter-mēn) an anorexic, $C_{10}H_{15}N$.

phentetiothalein (fen"tĕ-ti"o-thal'e-in) a compound whose sodium salt, $C_{20}H_8I_4O_4Na_2$, is used as a radiopaque medium and as a test of liver function.

phentolamine (fen-tol'ah-mēn) a potent alpha-adrenergic blocking agent; it blocks the hypertensive action of epinephrine and norepinephrine and most responses of smooth muscles that involve alpha-adrenergic cell receptors. Its hydrochloride and mesylate salts are used in the diagnosis of hypertension due to pheochromocytoma.

Phenurone (fen'u-rōn) trademark for a preparation of phenacemide.

phenyl (fen'il, fe'nil) the monovalent radical, C_6H_5. **phenyl'ic,** adj.

phenylalanine (fen"il-al'ah-nīn) a naturally occurring amino acid essential for optimal growth in infants and for nitrogen equilibrium in human adults.

phenylbutazone (-bu'tah-zōn) an antirheumatic, $C_{19}H_{20}N_2O_2$.

phenylephrine (-ef'rin) an adrenergic, $C_9H_{13}NO_2$, used as the hydrochloride salt for its potent vasoconstrictor properties.

phenylhydrazine (-hi′drah-zēn) a reagent for sugars, ketones, and aldehydes, $C_6H_5NH \cdot NH_2$; the hydrochloride salt is used in the treatment of polycythemia vera.

phenylketonuria (-ke″to-nu′re-ah) an inborn error of metabolism marked by an inability to convert phenylalanine into tyrosine, permitting accumulation of phenylalanine and its metabolic products in body fluids; it results in mental retardation, neurologic manifestations, light pigmentation, eczema, and mousy odor, unless treated by a diet low in phenylalanine. **phenylketonu′ric**, adj.

phenylmercuric (-mer-ku′rik) denoting a compound containing the radical C_6H_5Hg—, forming various antiseptic, antibacterial, and fungicidal salts; compounds of the acetate and nitrate salts are used as bacteriostatics, and the former is used as a herbicide.

phenylpropanolamine (-pro″pah-nol′am-in) an adrenergic, $C_9H_{13}NO$, used chiefly as a nasal and sinus decongestant in the form of the hydrochloride salt.

phenylpropylmethylamine (-pro″pil-meth″il-am′ēn) a vasoconstrictor, $C_{10}H_{15}N$; its hydrochloride salt is used as a nasal decongestant.

phenylthiocarbamide (-thi″o-kar-bam′īd) phenylthiourea.

phenylthiourea (-thi″o-u-re′ah) a compound used in genetics research; the ability to taste it is inherited as a dominant trait. It is intensely bitter to about 70% of the population, and nearly tasteless to the rest.

phenyltoloxamine (-tol-ok′sah-mēn) an antihistaminic, $C_{17}H_{21}NO$.

phenyramidol (fen″ĭ-ram′ĭ-dol) an analgesic and skeletal muscle relaxant, $C_{13}H_{14}N_2O$, used as the hydrochloride salt.

phenytoin (fen′ĭ-to-in) diphenylhydantoin.

pheochrome (fe′o-krōm) chromaffin.

pheochromoblast (fe″o-kro′mo-blast) any of the embryonic structures that develop into chromaffin (pheochrome) cells.

pheochromocyte (-kro′mo-sīt) a chromaffin cell.

pheochromocytoma (-kro″mo-si-to′mah) a tumor of chromaffin tissue of the adrenal medulla or sympathetic paraganglia; symptoms, notably hypertension, reflect the increased secretion of epinephrine and norepinephrine.

pheromone (fer′o-mōn) a substance secreted to the outside of the body and perceived (as by smell) by other individuals of the same species, releasing specific behavior in the percipient.

Ph.G. Graduate in Pharmacy.

Phialophora (fi″ah-lof′o-rah) a genus of imperfect fungi. *P. verrucosa* is a cause of chromomycosis; *P. jeanselmi* is a cause of maduromycosis.

-philia word element [Gr.], *affinity for; morbid fondness of.* **-phil′ic**, adj.

philtrum (fil′trum) the vertical groove in the median portion of the upper lip.

phimosis (fi-mo′sis) constriction of the orifice of the prepuce so that it cannot be drawn back over the glans. **phimot′ic**, adj.

pHisoHex (fi′so-heks) trademark for an emulsion containing hexachlorophene.

phleb(o)- word element [Gr.], *vein.*

phlebangioma (fleb″an-je-o′mah) a venous aneurysm.

phlebarteriectasia (-ar-te″re-ek-ta′ze-ah) general dilatation of veins and arteries.

phlebectasia (-ek-ta′ze-ah) dilatation of a vein; a varicosity.

phlebectomy (flĕ-bek′to-me) excision of a vein, or a segment of a vein.

phlebemphraxis (fleb″em-frak′sis) stoppage of a vein by a plug or clot.

phlebismus (flĕ-biz′mus) obstruction and consequent turgescence of veins.

phlebitis (flĕ-bi′tis) inflammation of a vein. **phlebit′ic**, adj. **sinus p.,** inflammation of a cerebral sinus.

phleboclysis (flĕ-bok′lĭ-sis) injection of fluid into a vein.

phlebogram (fleb′o-gram) 1. a radiogram of a vein filled with contrast medium. 2. a phlebographic or sphygmographic tracing of the venous pulse.

phlebograph (-graf) an instrument for recording the venous pulse.

phlebography (flĕ-bog′rah-fe) 1. radiography of a vein filled with contrast medium. 2. the graphic recording of the venous pulse. 3. a description of the veins.

phlebolith (fleb′o-lith) a venous calculus or concretion.

phlebolithiasis (fleb″o-lĭ-thi′ah-sis) the development of phleboliths.

phlebomanometer (-mah-nom′ĕ-ter) an instrument for the direct measurement of venous blood pressure.

phlebophlebostomy (-flĕ-bost′to-me) operative anastomosis of one vein to another.

phleboplasty (fleb′o-plas″te) plastic repair of a vein.

phleborrhaphy (flĕ-bor′ah-fe) suture of a vein.

phleborrhexis (fleb″o-rek′sis) rupture of a vein.

phlebosclerosis (-skle-ro′sis) fibrous thickening of the walls of veins.

phlebostasis (flĕ-bos′tah-sis) 1. retardation of blood flow in veins. 2. temporary sequestration of a portion of blood from the general circulation by compressing the veins of an extremity.

phlebothrombosis (fleb″o-throm-bo′sis) the development of venous thrombi in the absence of associated inflammation.

Phlebotomus (flĕ-bot′o-mus) a genus of biting sandflies, the females of which suck blood. They are vectors of various diseases, including kala-azar (*P. argen′tipes, P. chinen′sis, P. marti′ni, P. orienta′lis, P. pernicio′sus*), Carrión's disease (*P. nogu′chi, P. verruca′rum*), cutaneous leishmaniasis (*P. sergen′ti*), and phlebotomus fever (*P. papatas′ii*).

phlebotomy (flĕ-bot′o-me) incision of a vein.

phlegm (flem) viscid mucus excreted in abnormally large quantities from the respiratory tract.

phlegmasia (fleg-ma′ze-ah) [Gr.] inflammation. **p. al′ba do′lens,** phlebitis of the femoral vein, with swelling of the leg, usually without redness (milk leg), occasionally following parturition or an acute febrile illness. **p. ceru'lea do'lens,** an acute fulminating form of deep venous thrombosis, with pronounced edema and severe cyanosis of the extremity.

phlegmatic (fleg-mat'ik) of dull and sluggish temperament.

phlegmon (fleg'mon) cellulitis. **phleg'monous,** adj.

phlog(o)- word element [Gr.], *inflammation.*

phlogogenic (flo''go-jen'ik) producing inflammation.

phlorhizin (flo-ri'zin) a bitter glycoside from the root bark of apple, cherry, plum, and pear trees, which causes glycosuria by blocking tubular reabsorption of glucose.

phloroglucin (flo''ro-gloo'sin) the aglycone of many glycosides, obtained from the bark of apple and other trees; used as a reagent for hydrochloric acid in gastric juice and as a decalcifier of bone specimens.

phlyctena (flik-te'nah) 1. a small blister made by a burn. 2. a small vesicle containing lymph seen on the conjunctiva in certain conditions. **phlyc'tenar,** adj.

phlyctenoid (flik'tĕ-noid) resembling a phlyctena.

phlyctenular (flik-ten'u-lar) associated with the formation of phlyctenules, or of vesicle-like prominences.

phlyctenule (flik'ten-ūl) a minute vesicle; an ulcerated nodule of cornea or conjunctiva.

phlyctenulosis (flik-ten''u-lo'sis) a condition marked by formation of phlyctenules.

phobia (fo'be-ah) any persistent abnormal dread or fear; also, a word termination denoting abnormal fear or aversion. **pho'bic,** adj.

phobophobia (fo''bo-fo'be-ah) morbid fear of being afraid.

phocomelia (fo''ko-me'le-ah) congenital absence of the proximal portion of a limb or limbs, the hands or feet being attached to the trunk by a small, irregularly shaped bone. **phocome'lic,** adj.

phocomelus (fo-kom'ĕ-lus) an individual exhibiting phocomelia.

phon(o)- word element [Gr.], *sound; voice; speech.*

phonal (fo'nal) pertaining to the voice.

phonasthenia (fo''nas-the'ne-ah) weakness of the voice; difficult phonation from fatigue.

phonation (fo-na'shun) the utterance of vocal sounds.

phonatory (fo'nah-to''re) subserving or pertaining to phonation.

phoneme (fo'nēm) the smallest unit of sound in speech; the basic unit of spoken language.

phonendoscope (fo-nen'do-skōp) a stethoscopic device that intensifies auscultatory sounds.

phonetic (fo-net'ik) pertaining to the voice or to articulate sounds.

phonetics (fo-net'iks) science of vocal sounds.

phoniatrics (fo''ne-at'riks) the treatment of speech defects.

phonic (fon'ik, fo'nik) pertaining to the voice.

phonism (fo'nizm) a sensation of hearing produced by the effect of something seen, felt, tasted, smelled, or thought of.

phonocardiogram (fo''no-kar'de-o-gram) the record produced by phonocardiography.

phonocardiograph (-kar'de-o-graf'') the instrument used in phonocardiography.

phonocardiography (-kar''de-og'rah-fe) graphic recording of the sounds produced by the action of the heart. **phonocardiograph'ic,** adj.

phonocatheter (-kath'ĕ-ter) a device similar to a conventional catheter, with a microphone at the tip.

phonogram (fo'no-gram) a graphic record of a sound.

phonomassage (fo''no-mah-sahzh') the treatment of ear disease by an apparatus which carries a more or less musical vibration into the auditory canal.

phonometer (fo-nom'ĕ-ter) a device for measuring intensity of sounds.

phonomyoclonus (fo''no-mi-ok'lŏ-nus) myoclonus in which a sound is heard on auscultation of an affected muscle, indicating fibrillar contractions.

phonomyogram (-mi'o-gram) a record produced by phonomyography.

phonomyography (-mi-og'rah-fe) the recording of sounds produced by muscle contraction.

phonopathy (fo-nop'ah-the) any disease or disorder of the organs of speech.

phonophobia (fo''no-fo'be-ah) morbid dread of sounds or of speaking aloud.

phonophotography (-fo-tog'rah-fe) photographic recording of the movements of a diaphragm set up by sound waves.

phonopneumomassage (-nu''mo-mah-sahzh') air massage of the middle ear.

phonopsia (fo-nop'se-ah) a visual sensation caused by the hearing of sounds.

phonoreceptor (fo''no-re-sep'tor) a receptor for sound stimuli.

phonorenogram (-re'no-gram) a record of sounds produced by pulsation of the renal artery obtained by a phonocatheter passed through a ureter into the kidney pelvis.

phonostethograph (-steth'o-graf) an instrument by which chest sounds are amplified, filtered, and recorded.

-phore word element [Gr.], *a carrier.*

-phoresis word element [Gr.], *transmission.*

phoria (fo're-ah) tendency of the visual axis of one eye to deviate when the other eye is covered and fusion is prevented.

phorometer (fo-rom'ĕ-ter) an instrument for measuring heterophoria.

Phoroptor (fo-rop'ter) trademark for a phorometer fitted with a battery of cylindrical lenses.

phose (fōz) any subjective visual sensation.

phosgene (fos'jēn) a suffocating and highly poisonous war gas, carbonyl chloride, $COCl_2$.

phosphagen (fos'fah-jen) a group of compounds, including phosphocreatine and phosphoarginine, present in tissue which yield high-energy phosphate on cleavage.

Phosphaljel (fos′fal-jel) trademark for a preparation of aluminum phosphate gel.

phosphatase (fos′fah-tās) any of a group of enzymes capable of catalyzing the hydrolysis of esterified phosphoric acid, with liberation of inorganic phosphate. **acid p.**, a type showing optimal activity at a pH between 3 and 6. **alkaline p.**, a type showing optimal activity at a pH of about 9.3.

phosphate (fos′fāt) any salt or ester of phosphoric acid. **phosphat′ic**, adj. **acid p.**, any in which only one or two of the three replaceable hydrogen atoms are taken up or replaced. **arginine p.**, phosphoarginine. **calcium p.**, a compound containing calcium and the phosphate radical (PO_4). **creatine p.**, phosphocreatine. **earthy p.**, a phosphate of any of the alkaline earth metals. **high-energy p's**, those which, on hydrolysis, yield high levels of negative free energy, and thus are basic to the energy supply of living organisms; they include ATP, acetyl CoA, etc. **normal p.**, a phosphate in which all the hydrogen atoms of the acid have been replaced. **triple p.**, a calcium, ammonium, and magnesium phosphate, sometimes found in urine.

phosphatemia (fos″fah-te′me-ah) an excess of phosphates in the blood.

phosphaturia (fos″fah-tu′re-ah) an excess of phosphates in the urine.

phosphene (fos′fēn) a sensation of light due to a stimulus other than light rays, e.g., a mechanical stimulus.

phosphide (fos′fīd) a binary compound of phosphorus and another element or radical.

phosphite (fos′fīt) any salt of phosphorous acid.

phosphoamidase (fos″fo-am′ĭ-dās) an enzyme that catalyzes the conversion of phosphocreatine to creatine and orthophosphate.

phosphoarginine (-ar′jĭ-nin) an arginine–phosphoric acid compound homologous with phosphocreatine but found in invertebrate muscles.

phosphocreatine (-kre′ah-tin) a creatine–phosphoric acid compound occurring in muscle, being the most important storage form of high-energy phosphate, the energy source in muscle contraction.

phosphofructokinase (-fruk″to-ki′nās) an enzyme of spermatozoa, which enables them to utilize fructose as an energy source.

phospholipase (-lip′ās) any of four enzymes (phospholipase A to D), which catalyze the hydrolysis of a phospholipid.

phospholipid (-lip′id) a lipid containing phosphorus, which on hydrolysis yields fatty acids, glycerin, and a nitrogenous compound.

phospholipin (-lip′in) phospholipid.

phosphonecrosis (-ně-kro′sis) necrosis of the jaw bone due to exposure to phosphorus.

phosphoprotein (-pro′te-in) a conjugated protein in which phosphoric acid is esterified with a hydroxy amino acid.

phosphorated (fos′fo-rāt″ed) charged or combined with phosphorus.

phosphorescence (fos″fo-res′ens) the emission of light without appreciable heat; the property of continuing to be luminous in the dark after exposure to light or other radiation. **phosphores′cent**, adj.

phosphoribokinase (fos″fo-ri″bo-ki′nās) an enzyme that catalyzes the conversion of ATP and ribose 5-phosphate to ADP and ribose 1,5-diphosphate.

phosphoribulokinase (-ri″bu-lo-ki′nās) an enzyme that catalyzes the conversion of ATP and D-ribulose 5-phosphate to ADP and D-ribulose 1,5-diphosphate.

phosphorism (fos′fo-rizm) chronic phosphorus poisoning; see *phosphorus*.

phosphorolysis (fos″fo-rol′ĭ-sis) cleavage of a chemical bond with simultaneous addition of the elements of phosphoric acid to the residues.

phosphoruria (fos″for-u′re-ah) free phosphorus in the urine.

phosphorus (fos′fo-rus) chemical element (*see table*), at. no. 15, symbol P. Ingestion or inhalation produces toothache, phosphonecrosis (phossy jaw), anorexia, weakness, and anemia. **phos′phorous**, adj. **amorphous p.**, red p. **^{32}P**, **^{33}P**, **radioactive p.**, radiophosphorus. **red p.**, a nonpoisonous, dark red amorphous powder.

phosphoryl (fos′fōr-il) the trivalent chemical radical $\equiv P:O$.

phosphorylase (fos-fōr′ĭ-lās) an enzyme which, in the presence of inorganic phosphate, catalyzes reversibly the conversion of glycogen into glucose-1-phosphate.

phosphorylation (fos″fōr-ĭ-la′shun) the process of introducing the trivalent PO group into an organic molecule.

phosphotransacetylase (fos″fo-trans″ah-set′ĭ-lās) an enzyme which catalyzes the transfer of an acetyl group between acetylphosphate and acetyl coenzyme A.

phosphotransferase (-trans′fer-ās) any of a subclass of enzymes that catalyze the transfer of a phosphate group.

phot(o)- word element [Gr.], *light.*

photalgia (fo-tal′je-ah) pain, as in the eye, caused by light.

photic (fo′tik) pertaining to light.

photism (fo′tizm) a visual sensation produced by the effect of something heard, felt, tasted, smelled, or thought of.

photobiology (fo″to-bi-ol′o-je) the branch of biology dealing with the effect of light on organisms.

photobiotic (-bi-ot′ik) living only in the light.

photocatalysis (-kah-tal′ĭ-sis) promotion or stimulation of a chemical reaction by light. **photocatalyt′ic**, adj.

photocatalyst (-kat′ah-list) a substance, e.g., chlorophyll, that brings about a chemical reaction to light.

photochemistry (-kem′is-tre) the branch of chemistry dealing with the chemical properties or effects of light rays or other radiation. **photochem′ical**, adj.

photochromogen (-kro′mo-jen) a microorganism whose pigmentation develops as a result of exposure to light. **photochromogen′ic**, adj.

photocoagulation (-ko-ag″u-la′shun) condensation of protein material by controlled use of light rays, as in treatment of eye disorders.

photodermatitis (-der″mah-ti′tis) an abnormal state of the skin in which light is an important causative factor.

photodermatosis (-der″mah-to′sis) photodermatitis.

photodynamics (-di-nam′iks) the science of the activating effects of light. **photodynam′ic**, adj.

photodynesis (-di-ne′sis) initiation of cyclosis in plant cells by visible light.

photodynia (-din′e-ah) photalgia.

photofluorography (-floo″or-og′rah-fe) the photographic recording of fluoroscopic images on small films, using a fast lens.

photogenic (-jen′ik) 1. produced by light. 2. producing or emitting light.

photokinetic (-ki-net′ik) moving in response to the stimulus of light.

photolysis (fo-tol′ĭ-sis) chemical decomposition by light. **photolyt′ic**, adj.

photoluminescence (fo″to-lu″mĭ-nes′ens) the quality of being luminescent after exposure to light.

photolyte (fo′to-līt) a substance decomposed by light.

photometer (fo-tom′ĕ-ter) a device for measuring intensity of light.

photometry (fo-tom′ĕ-tre) measurement of the intensity of light.

photomicrograph (fo″to-mi′kro-graf) a photograph of an object as seen through an ordinary light microscope.

photon (fo′ton) a particle (quantum) of radiant energy.

photo-ophthalmia (fo″to-of-thal′me-ah) photophthalmia.

photoperceptive (-per-sep′tiv) able to perceive light.

photoperiod (-pēr′e-od) the period of time per day that an organism is exposed to daylight (or to artificial light). **photoperiod′ic**, adj.

photoperiodism (-pēr″e-o-dizm) the physiologic and behavioral reactions brought about in organisms by changes in the duration of daylight and darkness.

photophilic (-fil′ik) thriving in light.

photophobia (-fo′be-ah) abnormal visual intolerance to light. **photopho′bic**, adj.

photophthalmia (fo″tof-thal′me-ah) ophthalmia due to exposure to intense light, as in snow blindness.

photopia (fo-to′pe-ah) day vision. **photop′ic**, adj.

photopsia (fo-top′se-ah) appearance as of sparks or flashes, in retinal irritation.

photopsin (fo-top′sin) the protein moiety of the cones of the retina that combines with retinal to form photochemical pigments.

photopsy (fo′top-se) photopsia.

photoptarmosis (fo″to-tar-mo′sis) sneezing caused by the influence of light.

photoptometer (fo″top-tom′ĕ-ter) an instrument for measuring visual acuity by determining the smallest amount of light that will render an object just visible.

photoreactivation (fo″to-re-ak″tĭ-va′shun) reversal of the biological effects of ultraviolet radiation on cells by subsequent exposure to visible light.

photoreception (-re-sep′shun) the process of detecting radiant energy, usually of wavelengths between 3900 and 7700 angstroms, being the range of visible light.

photoreceptive (-re-sep′tiv) sensitive to stimulation by light.

photoreceptor (-re-sep′tor) a nerve end-organ or receptor sensitive to light.

photoretinitis (-ret″ĭ-ni′tis) retinitis due to exposure to intense light.

photoscan (fo′to-skan) a two-dimensional representation of gamma rays emitted by a radioactive isotope in body tissue, produced by a print-out mechanism utilizing a light source to expose a photographic film.

photosensitive (fo″to-sen′sĭ-tiv) exhibiting abnormally heightened sensitivity to sunlight.

photosensitization (-sen″sĭ-ti-za′shun) the development of abnormally heightened reactivity of the skin to sunlight.

photostable (fo′to-sta″b′l) unchanged by the influence of light.

photosynthesis (fo″to-sin′thĕ-sis) a chemical combination caused by the action of light; specifically, the formation of carbohydrates from carbon dioxide and water in the chlorophyll tissue of plants under the influence of light. **photosynthet′ic**, adj.

phototaxis (-tak′sis) the movement of cells and microorganisms under the influence of light. **phototac′tic**, adj.

phototherapy (-ther′ah-pe) treatment of disease by exposure to light.

phototoxic (-tok′sik) having a toxic effect triggered by exposure to light.

phototrophic (-trof′ik) utilizing light in metabolism.

phototropism (fo-tot′ro-pizm) 1. the tendency of an organism to turn or move toward or away from light. 2. color change produced in a substance by the action of light. **phototrop′ic**, adj.

photuria (fo-tu′re-ah) the excretion of urine having a luminous appearance.

phren(o)- word element [Gr.], (1) *diaphragm;* (2) *mind.*

phrenalgia (fre-nal′je-ah) 1. pain in the diaphragm. 2. melancholia.

phrenemphraxis (fren″em-frak′sis) phrenicotripsy.

phrenetic (frĕ-net′ik) maniacal.

phrenic (fren′ik) pertaining to the diaphragm or to the mind.

phrenicectomy (fren″ĭ-sek′to-me) resection of the phrenic nerve.

phrenicoexeresis (fren″ĭ-ko-ek-ser′ĕ-sis) avulsion of the phrenic nerve.

phrenicotomy (-kot′o-me) surgical division of the phrenic nerve.

phrenicotripsy (fren″ĭ-ko-trip′se) surgical crushing of the phrenic nerve.

phrenitis (frĕ-ni′tis) 1. delirium or frenzy. 2. diaphragmitis.

phrenocolic (fren″o-kol′ik) pertaining to the diaphragm and colon.

phrenogastric (-gas′trik) pertaining to the diaphragm and stomach.

phrenohepatic (-hĕ-pat′ik) pertaining to the diaphragm and liver.

phrenology (frĕ-nol′o-je) the study of the faculties and qualities of mind from the shape of the skull.

phrenoplegia (fren″o-ple′je-ah) 1. a sudden attack of mental disorder. 2. loss or paralysis of the mental faculties. 3. paralysis of the diaphragm.

phrenosin (fren′o-sin) a cerebroside containing cerebronic acid attached to the sphingosine.

phrenotropic (fren″o-trop′ik) exerting its principal effect upon the mind.

phrynoderma (frin″o-der′mah) a follicular hyperkeratosis probably due to deficiency of vitamin A or of essential fatty acids.

phthalein (thal′e-in) any one of a series of coloring matters formed by the condensation of phthalic anhydride with the phenols.

phthalylsulfacetamide (thal″il-sul″fah-set′ah-mīd) an intestinal antibacterial, $C_{16}H_{14}N_2O_6S$.

phthalylsulfathiazole (-thi′ah-zōl) an intestinal antibacterial, $C_{17}H_{13}N_3O_5S_2$.

phthalylsulfonazole (thal″il-sul-fon′ah-zōl) phthalylsulfacetamide.

phthiriasis (thi-ri′ah-sis) infestation with *Phthirus pubis*.

Phthirus (thir′us) a genus of lice, including *P. pu'bis* (the pubic, or crab, louse), which infests the hair of the pubic region, and sometimes the eyebrows and eyelashes.

phthisis (thi′sis) 1. a wasting of the body. 2. tuberculosis. **p. bul′bi**, shrinkage of eyeball. **grinder's p.**, a combination of tuberculosis and pneumoconiosis occurring among grinders in the cutlery trade. **miner's p.**, pneumoconiosis of coal workers.

phyco- word element [Gr.], *seaweed; algae.*

phycobilin (fi″ko-bil′in) a group of protein-linked pigments found in the red and the blue-green algae.

phycochrome (fi′ko-krōm) a blue-green pigment from algae.

phycocyanin (fi″ko-si′ah-nin) a blue chromoprotein found in blue-green algae.

phycoerythrin (-er′ĭ-thrin) a red chromoprotein found in red algae.

phycology (fi-kol′o-je) the scientific study of algae.

Phycomycetes (fi″ko-mi-se′tēz) a group of fungi comprising the common water, leaf, and bread molds.

phycomycosis (-mi-ko′sis) any of a group of acute fungal diseases caused by members of Phycomycetes.

phylloquinone (fil″o-kwin′ōn) phytonadione.

phylogeny (fi-loj′ĕ-ne) the complete developmental history of a race or group of organisms. **phylogen′ic,** adj.

phylum (fi′lum), pl. *phy'la.* A primary division of the plant or animal kingdom, grouping organisms which are assumed to have a common ancestry.

phyma (fi′mah) [Gr.] a skin tumor or tubercle.

physiatrics (fiz″e-at′riks) that branch of medicine using physical therapy, physical agents, such as light, heat, water, and electricity, and mechanical apparatus, in the diagnosis, prevention, and treatment of bodily disorders.

physiatrist (-at′rist) a physician who specializes in physiatrics.

physic (fiz′ik) 1. the art of medicine and of therapeutics. 2. a medicine, especially a cathartic.

physical (fiz′ĭ-kal) pertaining to the body, to material things, or to physics.

physician (fi-zish′un) an authorized practitioner of medicine, as one graduated from a college of medicine or osteopathy and licensed by the appropriate board; see also *doctor.* **attending p.,** one who attends a hospital at stated times to visit the patients and give directions as to their treatment. **family p.,** a medical specialist who plans and provides the comprehensive primary health care of all members of a family, regardless of age or sex, on a continuous basis. **resident p.,** a graduate and licensed physician resident in a hospital.

physicochemical (fiz″ĭ-ko-kem′ĭ-kal) pertaining to both physics and chemistry.

physics (fiz′iks) the study of the laws and phenomena of nature, especially of forces and general properties of matter and energy.

physio- word element [Gr.], *nature; physiology; physical.*

physiochemical (fiz″e-o-kem′ĭ-kal) pertaining to both physiology and chemistry.

physiognomy (fiz″e-og′no-me) 1. determination of mental or moral character and qualities by the face. 2. the countenance, or face. 3. the facial expression and appearance as a means of diagnosis.

physiologic, physiological (fiz″e-o-loj′ik; -loj′-ĭ-kal) pertaining to physiology; normal; not pathologic.

physiologist (fiz″e-ol′o-jist) a specialist in physiology.

physiology (fiz″e-ol′o-je) 1. the science which treats of the functions of the living organism and its parts, and of the physical and chemical factors and processes involved. 2. the basic processes underlying the functioning of a species or class of organism, or any of its parts or processes. **cell p.,** scientific study of phenomena involved in cell growth and maintenance, self-regulation and division of cells, interactions between nucleus and cytoplasm, and general behavior of protoplasm. **comparative p.,** a study of organ functions in various animals to find fundamental relations in the physiology of all animals. **general p.,** the science of the general laws of life and functional activity. **morbid p., pathologic p.,** the study of disordered function or of function in diseased tissues. **special p.,** the physiology of particular organs.

physiopathologic (fiz″e-o-path″o-loj′ik) pertaining to pathologic physiology.

physiotherapist (-ther′ah-pist) physical therapist.

physiotherapy (-ther′ah-pe) physical therapy.

physique (fĭ-zēk′) the body organization, development, and structure.

physo- word element [Gr.], *air; gas.*

physohematometra (fi″so-hem″ah-to-me′trah) gas and blood in the uterine cavity.

physohydrometra (-hi″dro-me′trah) gas and serum in the uterine cavity.

physometra (-me′trah) gas in the uterine cavity.

physopyosalpinx (-pi″o-sal′pinks) gas and pus in the uterine tube.

physostigmine (-stig′min) an alkaloid usually obtained from dried ripe seed of *Physostigma venenosum;* used as a topical miotic in the form of the base and of the salicylate and sulfate salts.

phyt(o)- word element [Gr.], *plant; an organism of the vegetable kingdom.*

phytase (fi′tās) an enzyme of plants that catalyzes the hydrolysis of phytic acid to inositol and phosphoric acid.

phytoagglutinin (fi″to-ah-gloo′tĭ-nin) an agglutinin of plant origin.

phytobezoar (-be′zōr) a bezoar composed of vegetable fibers.

phytochemistry (-kem′is-tre) the study of plant chemistry, including the chemical processes that take place in plants, the nature of plant chemicals, and the various applications of such chemicals to science and industry.

phytogenous (fi-toj′ĕ-nus) derived from plants, or caused by a vegetable growth.

phytohemagglutinin (fi″to-hem″ah-gloo′tĭ-nin) a hemagglutinin of plant origin.

phytohormone (-hōr′mōn) plant hormone; any of the hormones produced in plants which are active in controlling growth and other functions at a site remote from their place of production.

phytoid (fi′toid) resembling a plant.

phytol (fi′tol) an unsaturated aliphatic alcohol present in chlorophyll as an ester; used in the preparation of vitamins E and K.

phytomenadione (fi″to-men″ah-di′ōn) phytonadione.

phytonadione (-nah-di′ōn) vitamin K_1: a vitamin found in green plants or prepared synthetically, used as a prothrombinogenic agent.

phytoparasite (-par″ah-sīt) any parasitic vegetable organism or species.

phytopathogenic (-path″o-jen′ik) producing disease in plants.

phytopathology (-pah-thol′o-je) 1. the pathology of plants. 2. pathology of diseases caused by schizomycetes.

phytophotodermatitis (-fo″to-der″mah-ti′tis) phototoxic dermatitis induced by exposure to certain plants and then to sunlight.

phytoplankton (-plank′ton) the minute plant (vegetable) organisms which, with those of the animal kingdom, make up the plankton of natural waters.

phytoplasm (fi′to-plazm) protoplasm of plants.

phytoprecipitin (fi″to-pre-sip′ĭ-tin) a precipitin formed in response to vegetable antigen.

phytosis (fi-to′sis) any disease caused by a phytoparasite.

phytosterol (fi″to-ste′rol) a sterol of vegetable origin.

phytotoxic (-tok′sik) 1. pertaining to phytotoxin. 2. poisonous to plants.

phytotoxin (-tok′sin) an exotoxin produced by certain species of higher plants; any toxin of plant origin.

pia-arachnitis (pi″ah-ar″ak-ni′tis) leptomeningitis.

pia-arachnoid (-ah-rak′noid) the pia mater and arachnoid considered together.

pial (pi′al) pertaining to the pia mater.

pia mater (pi′ah ma′ter) [L.] the innermost of the three meninges covering the brain and spinal cord.

pian (pe-ahn′) yaws.

piarachnitis (pi″ar-ak-ni′tis) leptomeningitis.

piarachnoid (pi″ar-ak′noid) pia-arachnoid.

pica (pi′kah) craving for unnatural articles as food; a depraved appetite.

piceous (pi′se-us) of the nature of pitch.

pico- word element designating 10^{-12} (one trillionth) part of the unit to which it is joined.

picogram (pi′ko-gram) one trillionth (10^{-12}) gram. Abbreviated pg.

picometer (pi″ko-me′ter) a unit of length, 10^{-12} meter. Abbreviated pm.

picornavirus (pi-kor″nah-vi′rus) an extremely small, ether-resistant RNA virus, one of the group comprising the enteroviruses and the rhinoviruses.

picrate (pik′rāt) any salt of picric acid.

picrocarmine (pik″ro-kar′min) a histological stain consisting of a mixture of carmine, ammonia, distilled water, and aqueous solution of picric acid.

picrotoxin (-tok′sin) an active principle, $C_{30}H_{34}O_{13}$, from the seed of *Anamirta cocculus,* used as a central and respiratory stimulant in barbiturate poisoning.

piebaldism (pi-bawld′izm) a condition in which the skin is partly brown and partly white, as in partial albinism and vitiligo.

piedra (pe-a′drah) a fungal disease of the hair in which white or black nodules of fungi form on the shafts.

piesesthesia (pi-e″zes-the′ze-ah) the sense by which pressure stimuli are felt.

piesimeter (pi″ĕ-sim′ĕ-ter) instrument for testing the sensitiveness of the skin to pressure.

-piesis word element [Gr.], *pressure.* **-pies′ic,** adj.

pigment (pig′ment) 1. any coloring matter of the body. 2. a stain or dyestuff. 3. a paintlike medicinal preparation to be applied to the skin. **pig′-mentary,** adj. **bile p.,** any of the coloring matters of the bile, including bilirubin, biliverdin, etc. **blood p.,** any of the pigments derived from hemoglobin. **respiratory p's,** substances, e.g., hemoglobin, myoglobin, or cytochromes, which take part in the oxidative processes of the animal body.

pigmentation (pig″men-ta′shun) the deposition of coloring matter; the coloration or discoloration of a part by a pigment. **hematogenous p.,** pigmentation produced by accumulation of hemoglobin derivatives, such as hematoidin or hemosiderin.

pigmented (pig′ment-ed) colored by deposit of pigment.

pigmentolysin (pig″men-tol′ĭ-sin) a lysin which destroys pigment.

pigmentophage (pig-men′to-fāj) any pigment-destroying cell, especially such a cell of the hair.

piitis (pi-i′tis) inflammation of the pia mater.

pilar, pilary (pi′lar; pil′ah-re) pertaining to the hair.

pile (pīl) 1. hemorrhoid. 2. in nucleonics, a chain-reacting fission device for producing slow neutrons and radioactive isotopes. **sentinel p.,** a hemorrhoid-like thickening of the mucous membrane at the lower end of an anal fissure.

piles (pīlz) hemorrhoids.

pileus (pil′e-us) caul.

pili (pi′li) plural of *pilus.*

pill (pil) a small globular or oval medicated mass to be swallowed; a tablet. **enteric-coated p.,** one enclosed in a substance that dissolves only when it has reached the intestines. **hexylresorcinol p.,** one containing hexylresorcinol, with a rupture-resistant coating which disintegrates in the digestive tract.

pillar (pil′ar) a supporting column, usually occurring in pairs. **p's of the fauces,** folds of mucous membrane at sides of fauces.

pillion (pil′yon) a temporary artificial leg.

pilo- word element [L.], *hair; composed of hair.*

pilocarpine (pi″lo-kar′pin) a cholinergic alkaloid, $C_{11}H_{16}N_2O_2$, from leftlets of *Pilocarpus jaborandi* and *P. microphyllus;* used as an ophthalmic miotic in the form of the hydrochloride and nitrate salts.

pilocystic (-sis′tik) hollow or cystlike, and containing hair; said of dermoid tumors.

piloerection (-e-rek′shun) erection of the hair.

pilojection (-jek′shun) introduction of one or more hairs into an aneurysmal sac, to promote formation of a blood clot.

pilomatrixoma (-ma-trik′so-mah) a benign, circumscribed, calcifying epithelial neoplasm derived from hair matrix cells, manifested as a small firm intracutaneous spheroid mass, usually on the face, neck, or arms.

pilomotor (-mo′tor) pertaining to the arrector muscles, the contraction of which produces cutis anserina (goose flesh) and piloerection.

pilonidal (-ni′dal) having a nidus of hairs.

pilose (pi′lōs) hairy; covered with hair.

pilosebaceous (pi″lo-se-ba′shus) pertaining to the hair follicles and the sebaceous glands.

pilus (pi′lus), pl. *pi′li* [L.] 1. a hair. 2. fimbria (2). **p. cunicula′tus** (pl. *pi′li cunicula′ti*), burrowing hair. **p. incarna′tus** (pl. *pi′li incarna′ti*), ingrown hair. **p. tor′tus** (pl. *pi′li tor′ti*), twisted hair.

pimelitis (pim″ĕ-li′tis) inflammation of the adipose tissue.

pimelopterygium (pim″ĕ-lo-ter-ij′e-um) a fatty outgrowth on the conjunctiva.

pimelosis (pim″ĕ-lo′sis) 1. conversion into fat. 2. fatness, or obesity.

piminodine (pi-min′o-dēn) a narcotic analgesic, $C_{23}H_{30}N_2O_2$, used as the esylate salt.

pimple (pim′p'l) a papule or pustule.

pin (pin) a slender, elongated piece of metal used for securing fixation of parts. **Steinmann p.,** a metal rod for the internal fixation of fractures.

pincement (pans-maw′) [Fr.] pinching of the flesh in massage.

pindolol (pin′do-lōl) a vasodilator, $C_{14}H_{28}N_2O_2$.

pineal (pin′e-al) 1. pertaining to the pineal body. 2. shaped like a pine cone.

pinealectomy (pin″e-al-ek′to-me) excision of the pineal body.

pinealism (pin′e-al-izm) the condition due to deranged secretion of the pineal body.

pinealoblastoma (pin″e-ah-lo-blas-to′mah) pinealoma in which the pineal cells are not well differentiated.

pinealocyte (pin′e-ah-lo-sīt″) an epithelioid cell of the pineal body.

pinealoma (pin″e-ah-lo′mah) a tumor of the pineal body composed of neoplastic nests of large epithelial cells; it may cause hydrocephalus, precocious puberty, and gait disturbances.

pinguecula (pin-gwek′u-lah) a benign yellowish spot on the bulbar conjunctiva.

piniform (pin′ĭ-form) conical or cone shaped.

pinkeye (pink′i) acute contagious conjunctivitis.

pinna (pin′ah) auricle: the part of the ear outside the head. **pin′nal,** adj.

pinocyte (pin′o-sīt) a cell that exhibits pinocytosis. **pinocyt′ic,** adj.

pinocytosis (pi″no-si-to′sis) a mechanism by which cells ingest extracellular fluid and its contents; it involves the formation of invaginations by the cell membrane, which close and break off to form fluid-filled vacuoles in the cytoplasm. **pinocytot′ic,** adj.

pinosome (pi′no-sōm) the intracellular vacuole formed by pinocytosis.

pint (pīnt) a unit of liquid measure in the apothecaries' system, 16 fluid ounces or equivalent to 473.17 milliliters.

pinta (pin′tah) a treponemal infection characterized by bizarre pigmentary changes in the skin, occurring in tropical America.

pinworm (pin′werm) any oxyurid, especially *Enterobius vermicularis.*

pipamazine (pi-pam′ah-zēn) an antiemetic, $C_{21}H_{24}ClN_3OS$.

Pipanol (pip′ah-nol) trademark for a preparation of trihexyphenidyl.

pipazethate (pi-paz′ĕ-thāt) an antitussive, $C_{21}H_{25}N_3O_3S$.

pipenzolate (pi-pen′zo-lāt) an anticholinergic, $C_{22}H_{28}NO_3$, used as the bromide salt in peptic ulcer and gastritis.

piperacetazine (pi″per-ah-set′ah-zēn) a tranquilizer, $C_{24}H_{30}N_2O_2S$.

piperazine (pi-per′ah-zēn) a compound, C_4H_{10}-

N_2, various salts of which are used as anthelmintics.

piperidine (pi-per′ĭ-dēn) a colorless liquid, $C_5H_{22}N$, used as a pharmaceutical intermediate.

piperidolate (pi″per-id′o-lāt) an anticholinergic, $C_{21}H_{25}NO_2$; its hydrochloride salt is used as a gastrointestinal antispasmodic.

piperocaine (pi′per-o-kān″) a local anesthetic, $C_{16}H_{23}NO_2$, used as the hydrochloride salt.

piperoxan (pi″per-oks′an) an α-adrenergic blocking agent, $C_{14}H_{19}NO_2$, used in the diagnosis and surgical removal of pheochromocytoma.

pipet (pi-pet′) pipette.

pipette (pi-pet′) [Fr.] 1. a glass or transparent plastic tube used in measuring or transferring small quantities of liquid or gas. 2. to dispense by means of a pipette.

Pipizan (pi′pĭ-zan) trademark for a preparation of piperazine.

pipobroman (pi″po-bro′man) an antineoplastic, $C_{10}H_{16}Br_2N_2O_2$.

pipradrol (pi′prah-drol) a central stimulant, $C_{18}H_{21}NO$, used as the hydrochloride salt.

Piptal (pip′tal) trademark for preparations of pipenzolate.

piriform (pir′ĭ-form) pear-shaped.

Piroplasma (pi″ro-plaz′mah) *Babesia.*

piroplasmosis (-plaz-mo′sis) babesiasis. **canine p.,** infectious jaundice of dogs caused by *Babesia canis.*

pisiform (pi′sĭ-form) resembling a pea in shape and size.

pit (pit) 1. a hollow fovea or indentation. 2. a pockmark. 3. to indent, or to become and remain for a few minutes indented, by pressure. **anal p.,** proctodeum. **auditory p.,** a distinct depression in each auditory placode, marking the beginning of the embryonic development of the internal ear. **lens p.,** a pitlike depression in the fetal head where the lens develops. **nasal p., olfactory p.,** the primordium of a nasal cavity. **p. of stomach,** the epigastric fossa or epigastric region.

pitch (pich) 1. a dark, more or less viscous residue from distillation of tar and other substances. 2. natural asphalt of various kinds. 3. the quality of sound dependent on the frequency of vibration of the waves producing it. **Burgundy p.,** an aromatic, oily resin much used in plasters. **mineral p.,** bitumen.

pitchblend (pich′blend) a black mineral containing uranium oxide; from it are obtained radium, polonium, and uranium.

pithecoid (pith′ĕ-koid) apelike.

Pitocin (pĭ-to′sin) trademark for a solution of oxytocin for injection.

Pitressin (pĭ-tres′in) trademark for a solution of vasopressin for injection.

pitting (pit′ting) 1. the formation, usually by scarring, of a small depression. 2. the removal from erythrocytes, by the spleen, of such structures as iron granules, without destruction of the cells. 3. remaining indented for a few minutes after removal of firm finger-pressure, distinguishing fluid edema from myxedema.

pituicyte (pĭ-tu′ĭ-sīt) the distinctive fusiform cell composing most of the neurohypophysis.

pituitarism (pĭ-tu′ĭ-tar-izm″) disorder of pituitary function; see *hyper-* and *hypopituitarism.*

pituitary (pĭ-tu′ĭ-tār″e) 1. pituitary gland. 2. a preparation of the pituitary gland of animals, used therapeutically. **anterior p.,** the anterior lobe of the pituitary gland; also, a preparation of dried, partially defatted, powdered anterior pituitary of hogs, sheep, or cattle. **posterior p.,** the posterior lobe of the pituitary gland; also, a preparation of dried, partially defatted, powdered posterior pituitary of domesticated animals.

Pituitrin (pĭ-tu′ĭ-trin) trademark for a preparation of posterior pituitary injection.

pityriasis (pit″ĭ-ri′ah-sis) originally, a group of skin diseases marked by the formation of fine, branny scales, but now used only with a modifier. **p. al′ba,** a chronic condition with patchy scaling and hypopigmentation of the skin of the face. **p. ro′sea,** a dermatosis marked by scaling pink oval macules arranged with the long axes parallel to the cleavage lines of the skin. **p. ru′bra pila′ris,** a chronic inflammatory skin disease marked by pink scaling macules and fine acuminate, horny, follicular papules, beginning usually with severe seborrhea of the scalp and seborrheic dermatitis of the face, and associated with keratoderma of the palms and soles. **p. versic′olor,** tinea versicolor.

pityroid (pit′ĭ-roid) furfuraceous; branny.

Pityrosporon (pit″ĭ-ros′po-ron) a genus of yeastlike fungi, including *P. orbic′ulare,* a species customarily found on normal skin but capable of causing tinea versicolor in susceptible hosts.

Pityrosporum (pit″ĭ-ros′po-rum) *Pityrosporon.*

PKU phenylketonuria.

placebo (plah-se′bo) [L.] an inactive substance or preparation given to satisfy the patient's symbolic need for drug therapy, and used in controlled studies to determine the efficacy of medicinal substances. Also, a procedure with no intrinsic therapeutic value, performed for such purposes.

placenta (plah-sen′tah), pl. *placentas* or *placen′tae.* An organ characteristic of true mammals during pregnancy, joining mother and offspring, providing endocrine secretion and selective exchange of soluble bloodborne substances through apposition of uterine and trophoblastic vascularized parts. **placen′tal,** adj. **p. accre′ta,** one abnormally adherent to the uterine wall, with partial or complete absence of the decidua basalis. **battledore p.,** one with the umbilical cord inserted at the edge. **p. circumvalla′ta, circumvallate p.,** one encircled with a dense, raised, ring, the attached membranes being doubled back over the edge of the placenta. **p. fenestra′ta,** one which has spots where placental tissue is lacking. **fetal p.,** the part of the placenta derived from the chorionic sac that encloses the embryo, consisting of a chorionic plate and villi. **p. incre′ta,** placenta accreta with penetration of the uterine wall. **maternal p.,** the maternally contributed part of the placenta, derived from the decidua basalis. **p.**

membrana'cea, one that is abnormally thin and spread out over an unusually large area of the uterine wall. **p. percre'ta,** placenta accreta with invasion of the uterine wall to its serosal layer, sometimes causing rupture of the uterus. **p. pre'via,** one located in the lower uterine segment, so that it partially or entirely covers or adjoins the internal os. **p. reflex'a,** one in which the margin is thickened, appearing to turn back on itself. **p. spu'ria,** an accessory portion having no blood vessel attachment to the main placenta. **p. succenturia'ta,** an accessory portion attached to the main placenta by an artery and vein.

placentation (plas″en-ta'shun) the series of events following implantation of the embryo and leading to development of the placenta.

placentitis (-ti'tis) inflammation of the placenta.

placentography (-tog'rah-fe) radiological visualization of the placenta after injection of a contrast medium. **indirect p.,** that done to measure the space between the placenta and the presenting fetal head in placenta previa.

placentoid (plah-sen'toid) resembling the placenta.

placentolysin (plas″en-tol'ĭ-sin) an antibody (cytolysin) formed in reaction to injection of placenta cells.

Placidyl (plas'ĭ-dil) trademark for a preparation of ethchlorvynol.

placode (plak'ōd) a platelike structure, especially a thickened plate of ectoderm in the early embryo, from which a sense organ develops, e.g., *auditory p.* (ear), *lens p.* (eye), and *olfactory p.* (nose).

placoid (plak'oid) platelike or plaquelike.

plagiocephaly (pla″je-o-sef'ah-le) an unsymmetrical and twisted condition of the head, due to irregular closure of the cranial sutures. **plagiocephal'ic,** adj.

plague (plāg) an acute febrile, infectious, highly fatal disease due to *Pasteurella pestis,* beginning with chills and fever, quickly followed by prostration, and frequently attended by delirium, headache, vomiting, and diarrhea; primarily a disease of rats and other rodents, it is transmitted to man by flea bites, or communicated from patient to patient. **bubonic p.,** plague marked by swelling of the lymph nodes, forming buboes in the femoral, inguinal, axillary, and cervical regions; in the severe form (black death), septicemia occurs, producing petechial hemorrhages. **cattle p.,** a viral disease of cattle and sometimes of sheep and goats, marked by fever and croupous diphtheritic lesions of the intestinal tract. **hemorrhagic p.,** severe bubonic plague with petechial hemorrhages. **pneumonic p.,** that which extensively involves the lungs, the sputum being loaded with the causative organisms. **swine p.,** hemorrhagic septicemia of swine. **sylvatic p.,** plague in wild rodents, such as the ground squirrel, which serve as a reservoir from which man may be infected.

plane (plān) 1. a flat surface determined by the position of three points in space. 2. a specified level, as the plane of anesthesia. 3. to rub away or abrade; see *planing.* 4. a superficial incision in the wall of a cavity or between tissue layers, especially in plastic surgery, made so that the precise point of entry into the cavity or between the layers can be determined. **axial p.,** one parallel with the long axis of a structure. **axiobuccolingual p.,** one parallel with the long axis of a posterior tooth, passing through the buccal and lingual surfaces. **axiolabiolingual p.,** one parallel with the long axis of an anterior tooth, passing through its labial and lingual surfaces. **axiomesiodistal p.,** one parallel with the long axis of a tooth, passing through its mesial and distal surfaces. **base p.,** an imaginary plane upon which is estimated the retention of an artificial denture. **coronal p.,** frontal p. **datum p.,** a given horizontal plane from which craniometric measurements are made. **Frankfort horizontal p.,** a horizontal plane represented in profile by a line between the lowest point on the margin of the orbit and the highest point on the margin of the auditory meatus. **frontal p.,** one passing longitudinally through the body from side to side, at right angles to the median plane, dividing the body into front and back parts. **horizontal p.,** 1. one passing through the body, at right angles to both the frontal and median planes, dividing the body into upper and lower parts. 2. one passing through a tooth at right angles to its long axis. **median p.,** one passing longitudinally through the middle of the body from front to back, dividing it into right and left halves. **nuchal p.,** the outer surface of the occipital bone between the foramen magnum and the superior nuchal line. **occipital p.,** the outer surface of the occipital bone above the superior nuchal line. **orbital p.,** 1. the orbital surface of the maxilla. 2. visual p. **sagittal p.,** a vertical plane passing through the body parallel to the median plane (or to the sagittal suture), dividing the body into left and right portions. **sternal p.,** the anterior surface of the sternum. **temporal p.,** the depressed area on the side of the skull below the inferior temporal line. **transverse p.,** one passing horizontally through the body, at right angles to the sagittal and frontal planes, and dividing the body into upper and lower portions. **vertical p.,** one perpendicular to a horizontal plane, dividing the body into left and right, or front and back portions. **visual p.,** one passing through the visual axes of the two eyes.

planigraphy (plah-nig'rah-fe) see *body-section roentgenography.* **planigraph'ic,** adj.

planing (pla'ning) abrasion of disfigured skin to promote reepithelization with minimal scarring; done by mechanical means (dermabrasion) or by application of a caustic (chemabrasion).

plankton (plangk'ton) the minute, free-floating organisms, animal and vegetable, living in practically all natural waters.

planocellular (pla″no-sel'u-lar) composed of flat cells.

planoconcave (-kon'kāv) flat on one side and concave on the other.

planoconvex (-kon′veks) flat on one side and convex on the other.

planography (plah-nog′rah-fe) planigraphy.

planta pedis (plan′tah pe′dis) the sole of the foot.

Plantago (plan-ta′go) a genus of herbs, including *P. in′dica, P. psyl′lium* (Spanish psyllium), and *P. ova′ta* (blond psyllium); see *psyllium hydrophilic mucilloid* and *plantago seed.*

plantalgia (plan-tal′je-ah) pain in the sole of the foot.

plantar (plan′tar) pertaining to the sole of the foot.

plantaris (plan-ta′ris) [L.] plantar.

plantigrade (plan′tĭ-grād) walking on the full sole of the foot.

planula (plan′u-lah) a larval coelenterate.

planum (pla′num), pl. *pla′na* [L.] plane.

plaque (plak) any patch or flat area. **bacterial p., dental p.,** a deposit of material on a tooth surface, which may serve as a medium for bacterial growth or as a nucleus for formation of dental calculus. **Hollenhorst p′s,** atheromatous emboli containing cholesterol crystals in the retinal arterioles, a sign of impending serious cardiovascular disease.

Plaquenil (pla′kwĕ-nil) trademark for a preparation of hydroxychloroquine.

plasm (plazm) 1. plasma. 2. formative substance (cytoplasm, hyaloplasm, etc.). **germ p.,** the line of cells which by successive divisions give rise to the gametes.

plasma (plaz′mah) the fluid portion of the blood or lymph. **plasmat′ic,** adj. **antihemophilic human p.,** normal human plasma which has been processed promptly to preserve the antihemophilic properties of the original blood; used for temporary correction of bleeding tendency in hemophilia. **blood p.,** see under B. **normal human p.,** sterile plasma obtained by pooling approximately equal amounts of the liquid portion of citrated whole blood from eight or more adult humans; used as a blood volume replenisher.

plasmablast (plaz′mah-blast) the immature precursor of a plasma cell.

plasmacyte (-sīt) plasma cell.

plasmacytoma (plaz″mah-si-to′mah) any focal neoplasm of plasma cells, including those of multiple myeloma. Isolated plasmacytomas may occur outside the bone marrow (*extramedullary p′s*), affecting such tissues as the nasal, oral, and pharyngeal mucosa and the viscera.

plasmacytosis (-si-to′sis) an excess of plasma cells in the blood.

plasmagene (plaz′mah-jēn) a self-reproducing copy of a nuclear gene persisting in the cytoplasm of a cell.

plasmalemma (plaz″mah-lem′ah) cell membrane.

plasmalogen (plaz-mal′o-jen) a term applied to members of a group of phospholipids present in platelets which liberate higher fatty aldehydes on hydrolysis.

plasmapheresis (plaz″mah-fĕ-re′sis) removal of blood, separation of the blood cells by centrifu-

gation, and reinjection of the packed cells suspended in citrate-saline or other suitable medium.

plasmatorrhexis (-to-rek′sis) bursting of a cell from internal pressure.

plasmic (plaz′mik) plasmatic.

plasmin (plaz′min) a proteolytic enzyme with a high specificity for fibrin and the particular ability to dissolve formed fibrin clots.

plasminogen (plaz-min′o-jen) the inactive precursor of plasmin, occurring in plasma and converted to plasmin by the action of urokinase.

plasmocyte (plaz′mo-sīt) plasma cell.

plasmocytoma (plaz″mo-sĭ-to′mah) plasmacytoma.

plasmodesma (-dez′mah), pl. *plasmodes′mata.* A bridge of cytoplasm connecting adjacent cells.

plasmodicidal (plaz-mo″dĭ-si′dal) destructive to plasmodia; malariacidal.

Plasmodium (plaz-mo′de-um) a multispecies genus of sporozoa parasitic in the red blood cells of various animals; four species, *P. falcip′arum, P. mala′riae, P. ova′le,* and *P. vi′vax,* cause the four specific types of malaria in man.

plasmodium (plaz-mo′de-um), pl. *plasmo′dia* [Gr.] 1. a parasite of the genus *Plasmodium.* 2. a multinucleate continuous mass of protoplasm. **plasmo′dial,** adj.

plasmogen (plaz′mo-jen) bioplasm (2).

plasmolysis (plaz-mol′ĭ-sis) contraction of cell protoplasm due to loss of water by osmosis. **plasmolyt′ic,** adj.

plasmoma (plaz-mo′mah) plasmacytoma.

plasmon (plaz′mon) the hereditary factors of the egg cytoplasm.

plasmorrhexis (plaz″mo-rek′sis) erythrocytorrhexis.

plasmoschisis (plaz-mos′kĭ-sis) the splitting up of cell protoplasm.

plasmotropism (plaz-mot′ro-pizm) destruction of erythrocytes in the liver, spleen, or marrow, as contrasted with their destruction in the circulation. **plasmotrop′ic,** adj.

plaster (plas′ter) 1. plaster of Paris. 2. a paste-like mixture which can be spread over the skin and which is adhesive at body temperature; may be protectant, counterirritant, etc. **adhesive p.,** see under *tape.* **dental p.,** see *p. of Paris.* **p. of Paris,** calcined calcium sulfate; on addition of water it forms a porous mass that is used in making casts and bandages to support or immobilize body parts, and in dentistry for taking dental impressions. **salicylic acid p.,** a mixture of 10–40% salicylic acid in a suitable base, spread on paper, cloth, or other material; used as a keratolytic.

plastic (plas′tik) 1. tending to build up tissues to restore a lost part. 2. capable of being molded. 3. a substance produced by chemical condensation or by polymerization. 4. material that can be molded.

plasticity (plas-tis′ĭ-te) the quality of being plastic.

plastid (plas′tid) 1. any elementary constructive unit, as a cell. 2. any specialized organ of the cell other than the nucleus and centrosome, such as chloroplast or amyloplast.

-plasty word element [Gr.], *formation* or *plastic repair of.*

plate (plāt) 1. a flat structure or layer, as a thin layer of bone. 2. dental p. **axial p.,** primitive streak. **bite p.,** biteplate. **cribriform p.,** fascia cribrosa. **dental p.,** a plate of acrylic resin, metal, or other material which is fitted to the shape of the mouth, and serves to support artificial teeth. **dorsal p.,** roof p. **epiphyseal p.,** the thin plate of cartilage between the epiphysis and the metaphysis of a growing long bone. **equatorial p.,** the collection of chromosomes at the equator of the spindle in mitosis. **floor p.,** the unpaired ventral longitudinal zone of the neural tube. **foot p.,** the flat portion of the stapes. **medullary p.,** neural p. **motor p.,** end-plate. **muscle p.,** myotome (2). **neural p.,** the thickened plate of ectoderm in the embryo which develops into the neural tube. **polar p's,** platelike bodies at the end of the spindle in certain forms of mitosis. **roof p.,** the unpaired dorsal longitudinal zone of the neural tube. **sole p.,** a mass of protoplasm in which a motor nerve ending is embedded. **tarsal p.,** one of the plates of connective tissue forming the framework of either (upper or lower) eyelid. **tympanic p.,** the bony plate forming the floor and sides of the meatus auditorius. **ventral p.,** floor p.

platelet (plāt′let) blood platelet; any of the disk-shaped structures in the blood of all mammals, chiefly known for their role in blood coagulation. See also under *factor.*

platinum (plat′ĭ-num) chemical element (*see table*), at. no. 78, symbol Pt.

platy- word element [Gr.], *flat.*

platybasia (plat″ĭ-ba′ze-ah) basilar impression.

platycelous (-se′lus) having one surface flat and the other concave.

platycephalic, platycephalous (-sĕ-fal′ik; -sef′ah-lus) having a wide, flat head.

platycoria (-ko′re-ah) a dilated condition of the pupil of the eye.

platyhelminth (-hel′minth) one of the Platyhelminthes; a flatworm.

Platyhelminthes (-hel-min′thēz) a phylum of acoelomate, dorsoventrally flattened, bilaterally symmetrical animals, commonly known as flatworms; it includes the classes Cestoidea (tapeworms) and Trematoda (flukes).

platyhieric (-hi-er′ik) having a sacral index above 100.

platypellic, platypelloid (-pel′ik; -pel′oid) having a flat pelvis; see under *pelvis.*

platypodia (-po′de-ah) flatfoot.

platyrrhine (plat′ĭ-rīn) having a nasal index above 53.

platysma (plah-tiz′mah) see *Table of Muscles.*

pledge (plej) a solemn statement of intention. **Nightingale p.,** a statement of principles for the nursing profession, formulated by a committee in 1893 and subscribed to by student nurses at the time of the capping ceremonies.

pledget (plej′et) a small compress or tuft.

-plegia word element [Gr.], *paralysis; a stroke.*

pleiotropism, pleiotropy (pli-ot′ro-pizm; -rope) the production by a single gene of multiple phenotypic effects. **pleiotrop′ic,** adj.

pleo- word element [Gr.], *more.*

pleochromatism (ple″o-kro′mah-tizm) the property of some crystals of transmitting one color in one position and the complementary color in a position at right angles to the first. **pleochromat′ic,** adj.

pleocytosis (-si-to′sis) presence of a greater than normal number of cells in cerebrospinal fluid.

pleomastia (-mas′te-ah) polymastia.

pleomorphism (-mor′fizm) the occurrence of various distinct forms by a single organism or within a species. **pleomor′phic, pleomor′phous,** adj.

pleonasm (ple′o-nazm) an excess of parts.

pleonectic (ple″o-nek′tik) characterized by having a higher than normal O_2 content at a given PO_2; said of blood.

pleonexia (-nek′se-ah) morbid greediness.

pleonosteosis (ple″on-os″te-o′sis) abnormally increased ossification. **Léri's p.,** a hereditary syndrome of premature and excessive ossification, with short stature, limitation of movement, broadening and deformity of digits, and mongolian facies.

plessesthesia (ples″es-the′ze-ah) palpatory percussion.

plessimeter (plĕ-sim′ĕ-ter) pleximeter.

plessor (ples′or) plexor.

plethora (pleth′o-rah) an excess of blood. **plethor′ic,** adj.

plethysmograph (plĕ-thiz′mo-grah) an instrument for recording variations in volume of an organ, part, or limb.

plethysmography (pleth″iz-mog′rah-fe) the determination of changes in volume by means of a plethysmograph.

pleur(o)- word element [Gr.], *pleura; rib; side.*

pleura (ploor′ah), pl. *pleu′rae* [Gr.] serous membrane investing the lungs (*pulmonary p.*) and lining the walls of the thoracic cavity (*parietal p.*), the two layers enclosing a potential space, the pleural cavity. **pleu′ral,** adj.

pleuracotomy (ploor″ah-kot′o-me) incision into the pleural cavity.

pleuralgia (ploor-al′je-ah) pain in the pleura or in the side. **pleural′gic,** adj.

pleurapophysis (ploor″ah-pof′ĭ-sis) a rib, or a vertebral process corresponding to a rib.

pleurectomy (ploor-ek′to-me) excision of a portion of the pleura.

pleurisy (ploor′ĭ-se) inflammation of the pleura. **pleurit′ic,** adj. **adhesive p.,** that in which exudate forms dense adhesions which partially or totally obliterate the pleural space. **diaphragmatic p.,** that limited to parts near the diaphragm. **dry p.,** a variety with dry fibrinous exudate. **fibrinous p.,** that marked by deposition of large amounts of fibrin in the pleural cavity. **interlobular p.,** a form enclosed between the lobes of the lung. **plastic p.,** that characterized by deposition of a soft, semisolid exudate. **purulent p.,** thoracic empyema.

serous p., that marked by free exudation of fluid. **wet p., p. with effusion,** that marked by serous exudation.

pleuritis (ploo-ri′tis) pleurisy.

pleurocele (ploor′o-sēl) hernia of lung tissue or of pleura.

pleurocentesis (ploor″o-sen-te′sis) paracentesis of the thoracic (pleural) cavity.

pleurocentrum (-sen′trum) the lateral element of the vertebral column.

pleuroclysis (ploo-rok′lĭ-sis) injection of fluid into the pleural cavity.

pleurodont (ploor′o-dont) having teeth attached by one side on the inner surface of the jaw elements, as in certain lizards.

pleurodynia (ploor″o-din′e-ah) paroxysmal pain in the intercostal muscles. **epidemic p.,** an epidemic disease due to coxsackievirus B, marked by a sudden attack of violent pain in the chest, fever, and a tendency to recrudescence on the third day.

pleurogenic, pleurogenous (-jen′ik; ploor-oj′ĕ-nus) originating in the pleura.

pleurography (ploo-rog′rah-fe) radiography of the pleural cavity.

pleurohepatitis (ploor″o-hep″ah-ti′tis) hepatitis with inflammation of a portion of the pleura near the liver.

pleurolith (ploor′o-lith) a concretion in the pleura.

pleurolysis (ploo-rol′ĭ-sis) surgical separation of the pleura from its attachments.

pleuroparietopexy (ploor″o-pah-ri′ĕ-to-pek″se) fixation of the lung to the chest wall by adhesion of the visceral and parietal pleura.

pleuropericardial (-per″ĭ-kar′de-al) pertaining to the pleura and pericardium.

pleuropericarditis (-per″ĭ-kar-di′tis) inflammation involving the pleura and the pericardium.

pleuroperitoneal (-per″ĭ-to-ne′al) pertaining to the pleura and peritoneum.

pleuropneumonia (-nu-mo′ne-ah) 1. pleurisy complicated by pneumonia. 2. an infectious disease of cattle, combining pneumonia and pleurisy, due to *Mycoplasma mycoides.*

pleuropneumonia-like (-nu-mo′ne-ah-līk) a term applied to a group of filterable microorganisms similar to *Mycoplasma mycoides,* the cause of pleuropneumonia; such organisms have been isolated from sheep and goats, dogs, rats, mice, and man. See also *Mycoplasma.*

pleurosomus (-so′mus) a fetus with protrusion of the intestine and imperfect development of the arm of one side.

pleurothotonos (-thot′o-nus) tetanic bending of the body to one side.

pleurotomy (ploor-ot′o-me) incision of the pleura.

pleurovisceral (ploor″o-vis′er-al) pertaining to the pleura and viscera.

plexiform (plek′sĭ-form) resembling a plexus.

pleximeter (plek-sim′ĕ-ter) 1. a plate to be struck in mediate percussion. 2. diascope.

plexitis (plek-si′tis) inflammation of a nerve plexus.

plexor (plek′sor) a hammer used in diagnostic percussion.

plexus (plek′sus), pl. *plex′us, plex′uses* [L.] a network or tangle, chiefly of vessels or nerves. **plex′al,** adj. **brachial p.,** a nerve plexus originating from the ventral branches of the last four cervical and the first thoracic spinal nerves, giving off many of the principal nerves of the shoulder, chest, and arms. **cardiac p.,** the plexus around the base of the heart, chiefly in the epicardium, formed by cardiac branches from the vagus nerves and the sympathetic trunks and ganglia. **carotid p′s,** nerve plexuses surrounding the common, external, and internal carotid arteries. **celiac p.,** a network of ganglia and nerves lying in front of the aorta behind the stomach, supplying the abdominal viscera. **cervical p.,** a nerve plexus formed by the ventral branches of the first four cervical nerves, supplying structures in the neck region. **choroid p.,** the ependyma lining the ventricles of the brain with the vascular fringes of the pia mater invaginating them; concerned with formation of cerebrospinal fluid. **coccygeal p.,** a nerve plexus formed by the ventral branches of the coccygeal and fifth sacral nerve and by a communication from the fourth sacral nerve, giving off the anococcygeal nerves. **cystic p.,** a nerve plexus near the gallbladder. **dental p.,** either of two plexuses (inferior and superior) of nerve fibers, one from the inferior alveolar nerve, situated around the roots of the lower teeth, and the other from the superior alveolar nerve, situated around the roots of the upper teeth. **Exner's p.,** superficial tangential fibers in the molecular layer of the cerebral cortex. **Heller's p.,** an arterial network in the submucosa of the intestine. **lumbar p.,** one formed by the ventral branches of the second to fifth lumbar nerves in the psoas major muscle (the branches of the first lumbar nerve often are included). **lumbosacral p.,** the lumbar and sacral plexuses considered together, because of their continuous nature. **Meissner's p.,** a network of nerve fibers beneath the intestinal mucosa. **myenteric p.,** a nerve plexus within the muscular layers of the intestines. **nerve p.,** a plexus composed of intermingled nerve fibers. **pampiniform p.,** 1. a plexus of veins from the testicle and epididymis, constituting part of the spermatic cord. 2. a plexus of ovarian veins in the broad ligament. **phrenic p.,** a nerve plexus accompanying the inferior phrenic artery to the diaphragm and adrenal glands. **sacral p.,** one arising from the ventral branches of the last two lumbar and the first four sacral nerves. **solar p.,** celiac p. **tympanic p.,** a network of nerve fibers supplying the mucous lining of the tympanum, mastoid air cells, and pharyngotympanic tube.

plica (pli′kah), pl. *pli′cae* [L.] a fold.

plicate (pli′kāt) plaited or folded.

plication (pli-ka′shun) the operation of taking tucks in a structure to shorten it.

plicotomy (pli-kot′o-me) surgical division of the posterior fold of the tympanic membrane.

plombage (plom-bahzh′) [Fr.] the filling of a space or cavity in the body with inert material.

PLT *p*sittacosis-*l*ymphogranuloma venereum-trachoma (group); see *Chlamydia.*

plug (plug) an obstructing mass. **Dittrich's p's,** masses of fat globules, fatty acid crystals, and bacteria occurring in the bronchi in putrid bronchitis or bronchiectasis. **epithelial p.,** a mass of ectodermal cells that temporarily closes the external naris of the fetus. **mucous p.,** a plug formed by secretions of the mucous glands of the cervix uteri and closing the cervical canal during pregnancy. **vaginal p.,** one consisting of a mass of coagulated sperm and mucus which forms in the vagina of animals after coitus.

plugger (plug'er) an instrument for compacting filling material in a tooth cavity.

plumbic (plum'bik) pertaining to lead.

plumbism (plum'bizm) chronic lead poisoning; see *lead*[1].

plumbum (plum'bum) [L.] lead (symbol Pb).

pluri- word element [L.], *many.*

pluriglandular (ploor″ĭ-glan'du-lar) pertaining to several glands or their secretions.

plurigravida (-grav'ĭ-dah) multigravida.

plurilocular (-lok'u-lar) multilocular.

pluripara (ploo-rip'ah-rah) multipara.

pluriparity (ploor″ĭ-par'ĭ-te) multiparity.

pluripotentiality (-po-ten″she-al'ĭ-te) ability to develop in any one of several different ways, or to affect more than one organ or tissue. **pluripo'tent, pluripoten'tial,** adj.

plutonium (ploo-to'ne-um) chemical element (*see table*), at. no. 94, symbol Pu.

Pm chemical symbol, *promethium.*

P.M.I. point of maximal impulse (of the heart).

-pnea word element [Gr.], *respiration; breathing.* **-pneic,** adj.

pneo- word element [Gr.], *breath; breathing.*

pneogram (ne'o-gram) the tracing obtained by the pneograph.

pneograph (-graf) a device for registering chest movements in respiration.

pneometer (ne-om'ĕ-ter) a device for measuring the air inspired and expired.

pneoscope (ne'o-skōp) pneograph.

pneum(o)- word element [Gr.], *air or gas; lung.*

pneumarthrogram (nu-mar'thro-gram) a film obtained by pneumarthrography.

pneumarthrography (nu″mar-throg'rah-fe) radiography of a joint after injection of air or gas as a contrast medium.

pneumarthrosis (-thro'sis) gas or air in a joint.

pneumat(o)- word element [Gr.], *air or gas; lung.*

pneumatic (nu-mat'ik) pertaining to air or respiration.

pneumatization (nu″mah-ti-za'shun) the formation of pneumatic cells or cavities in tissue, especially such formation in the temporal bone.

pneumatocele (nu-mat'o-sēl) 1. hernia of lung tissue. 2. a usually benign, thin-walled air-containing cyst of the lung. 3. a tumor or sac containing gas, especially a gaseous swelling of the scrotum.

pneumatogram (-gram) pneogram.

pneumatograph (-graf) pneograph.

pneumatometer (nu″mah-tom'ĕ-ter) pneometer.

pneumatometry (-tom'ĕ-tre) measurement of the air inspired and expired.

pneumatorrhachis (-tor'ah-kis) presence of gas in the vertebral canal.

pneumatosis (-to'sis) air or gas in an abnormal location in the body. **p. cystoi'des intestina'-lis,** a condition characterized by the presence of thin-walled, gas-containing cysts in the wall of the intestine.

pneumatotherapy (nu″mah-to-ther'ah-pe) treatment by rarefied or compressed air.

pneumaturia (nu″mah-tu're-ah) gas or air in the urine.

pneumectomy (nu-mek'to-me) pneumonectomy.

pneumoangiogram (nu″mo-an'je-o-gram″) a composite of radiographs obtained by pneumoencephalography and cerebral angiography.

pneumoarthrography (-ar-throg'rah-fe) pneumarthrography.

pneumocephalus (-sef'ah-lus) air in the intracranial cavity.

pneumococcemia (-kok-se'me-ah) pneumococci in the blood.

pneumococcidal (-kok-si'dal) destroying pneumococci.

pneumococcosis (-kok-o'sis) infection with pneumococci.

pneumococcosuria (-kok″o-su're-ah) pneumococci in the urine.

pneumococcus (-kok'us), pl. *pneumococ'ci.* An individual organism of the species *Diplococcus pneumoniae.* **pneumococ'cal,** adj.

pneumoconiosis (-ko″ne-o'sis) any lung disease, e.g., anthracosis, silicosis, etc., due to permanent deposition of substantial amounts of particulate matter in the lungs.

pneumocranium (-kra'ne-um) pneumocephalus.

Pneumocystis (-sis'tis) a genus of organisms of uncertain status, but considered to be protozoa. *P. cari'nii* is the causative agent of interstitial plasma cell pneumonia.

pneumocystography (-sis-tog'rah-fe) radiography of the urinary bladder after injection of air or gas.

pneumoderma (-der'mah) subcutaneous emphysema.

pneumodynamics (-di-nam'iks) the dynamics of the respiratory process.

pneumoencephalogram (-en-sef'ah-lo-gram″) the radiograph obtained by pneumoencephalography.

pneumoencephalography (-en-sef″ah-log'-rah-fe) radiographic visualization of the fluid-containing structures of the brain after cerebrospinal fluid is intermittently withdrawn by lumbar puncture and replaced by air, oxygen, or helium.

pneumoenteritis (-en″ter-i'tis) inflammation of the lungs and intestine.

pneumography (nu-mog'rah-fe) 1. an anatomical description of the lungs. 2. graphic recording of the respiratory movements. 3. radiography of a part after injection of a gas.

pneumohemopericardium (nu″mo-he″mo-per″ĭ-kar′de-um) air or gas and blood in the pericardium.

pneumohemothorax (-tho′raks) gas or air and blood in the pleural cavity.

pneumohydrometra (nu″mo-hi″dro-me′trah) gas and fluid in the uterus.

pneumohydropericardium (-per″ĭ-kar′de-um) air or gas and fluid in the pericardium.

pneumohydrothorax (-tho′raks) air or gas with effused fluid in the thoracic cavity.

pneumolith (nu′mo-lith) a pulmonary concretion.

pneumolithiasis (nu″mo-lĭ-thi′ah-sis) the presence of concretions in the lungs.

pneumomediastinum (-me″de-as-ti′num) presence of air or gas in tissues of the mediastinum, occurring pathologically or introduced intentionally.

pneumometer (nu-mom′ĕ-ter) pneograph.

pneumomycosis (nu″mo-mi-ko′sis) any fungal disease of the lungs.

pneumomyelography (-mi″ĕ-log′rah-fe) radiography of the spinal canal after withdrawal of cerebrospinal fluid and injection of air or gas.

pneumonectomy (-nek′to-me) excision of lung tissue; it may be total, partial, or of a single lobe (*lobectomy*).

pneumonia (nu-mo′ne-ah) inflammation of the lungs with exudation and consolidation. **p. al′ba,** a fatal desquamative pneumonia of the newborn due to congenital syphilis, with fatty degeneration of the lungs, which appear pale and virtually airless. **aspiration p.,** that due to aspiration of foreign material into the lungs. **atypical p.,** primary atypical p. **bacterial p.,** that due to bacteria, chief among which are *Diplococcus pneumoniae, Streptococcus hemolytica, Staphylococcus aureus,* and *Klebsiella pneumoniae.* **bronchial p.,** bronchopneumonia. **desquamative p.,** chronic pneumonia with hardening of the fibrous exudate and proliferation of the interstitial tissue and epithelium. **desquamative interstitial p.,** chronic pneumonia with desquamation of large alveolar cells and thickening of the walls of distal air passages; marked by dyspnea and nonproductive cough. **double p.,** that affecting both lungs. **Friedländer's p., Friedländer's bacillus p.,** a form characterized by massive mucoid inflammatory exudates in a lobe of the lung, due to *Klebsiella pneumoniae.* **hypostatic p.,** that due to dorsal decubitus in weak or aged persons. **influenza virus p., influenzal p.,** an acute, severe, usually fatal disease due to influenza virus, with high fever, prostration, sore throat, aching pains, profound dyspnea and anxiety, and massive edema and consolidation. The term is also applied to influenza complicated by bacterial pneumonia. **inhalation p.,** 1. aspiration p. 2. bronchopneumonia due to inhalation of irritating vapors. **interstitial p.,** a chronic form with increase of the interstitial tissue and decrease of the proper lung tissue, with induration. **interstitial plasma cell p.,** a form affect-

ing infants and debilitated persons, including those receiving certain drugs, in which cellular detritus containing plasma cells appears in lung tissue; it is caused by *Pneumocystis carinii.* **lipid p., lipoid p.,** a pneumonia-like reaction of lung tissue to the aspiration of oil. **lobar p.,** an acute infectious disease due to the pneumococcus and marked by inflammation of one or more lobes of the lungs followed by consolidation. **lobular p.,** bronchopneumonia. **mycoplasmal p.,** primary atypical pneumonia caused by *Mycoplasma pneumoniae.* **parenchymatous p.,** desquamative p. **Pneumocystis p.,** interstitial plasma cell p. **primary atypical p.,** an acute infectious pulmonary disease caused by *Mycoplasma pneumoniae* and various viruses, with extensive but tenuous pulmonary infiltration, fever, malaise, myalgia, sore throat, and a cough that becomes productive and paroxysmal. **varicella p.,** that developing after the skin eruption in varicella (chickenpox) and apparently due to the same virus; symptoms may be severe, with violent cough, hemoptysis, and severe chest pain. **viral p.,** that due to a virus, e.g., adenovirus, or influenza, parinfluenza, or varicella virus; see *primary atypical p.* **white p.,** p. alba.

pneumonic (nu-mon′ik) pertaining to the lung or to pneumonia.

pneumonitis (nu″mo-ni′tis) inflammation of lung tissue.

pneumono- word element [Gr.], *lung.*

pneumonocentesis (nu-mo″no-sen-te′sis) surgical puncture of a lung for aspiration.

pneumonocyte (nu-mon′o-sīt) collective term for the alveolar epithelial cells (great alveolar cells and squamous alveolar cells) and alveolar phagocytes of the lungs.

pneumonolysis (nu″mo-nol′ĭ-sis) division of tissues attaching the lung to the wall of the chest cavity, to permit collapse of the lung.

pneumonopathy (nu″mo-nop′ah-the) any lung disease.

pneumonopexy (nu-mo′no-pek″se) surgical fixation of the lung to the thoracic wall.

pneumonorrhaphy (nu″mon-or′ah-fe) suture of the lung.

pneumonosis (nu″mo-no′sis) any lung disease.

pneumonotomy (nu″mo-not′o-me) incision of the lung.

pneumopericardium (-per″ĭ-kar′de-um) air or gas in the pericardial cavity.

pneumoperitoneum (-per″ĭ-to-ne′um) air or gas in the peritoneal cavity.

pneumoperitonitis (-per″ĭ-to-ni′tis) peritonitis with accumulation of air or gas in the peritoneal cavity.

pneumopleuritis (nu″mo-ploo-ri′tis) inflammation of the lungs and pleura.

pneumopyelography (-pi″ĕ-log′rah-fe) radiography after injection of oxygen or air into the renal pelvis.

pneumopyopericardium (-pi″o-per″ĭ-kar′de-um) air or gas and pus in the pericardium.

pneumopyothorax (-pi″o-tho′raks) air or gas and pus in the pleural cavity.

pneumoradiography (-ra″de-og′rah-fe) radiography after injection of air or oxygen.

pneumoretroperitoneum (-ret″ro-per″ĭ-tone′um) air in the retroperitoneal space.

pneumorrhagia (-ra′je-ah) hemorrhage from the lungs; severe hemoptysis.

pneumotachograph (-tak′o-graf) an instrument for recording the velocity of respired air.

pneumotachometer (-tah-kom′ĕ-ter) a transducer for measuring expired air flow.

pneumotaxic (-tak′sik) regulating the respiratory rate.

pneumotherapy (-ther′ah-pe) 1. treatment of disease of lungs. 2. pneumatotherapy.

pneumothorax (-tho′raks) air or gas in the pleural space, which may occur spontaneously (*spontaneous p.*), as a result of trauma or pathological process, or be introduced deliberately (*artifical p.*).

pneumotomy (nu-mot′o-me) pneumonotomy.

pneumoventriculography (nu″mo-ven-trik″u-log′rah-fe) radiography of the cerebral ventricles after injection of air or gas.

P.O. [L.] *per os* (by mouth; orally).

Po chemical symbol, *polonium.*

PO₂ oxygen partial pressure (tension); also written P_{O_2}, pO_2, and pO_2.

pock (pok) a pustule, especially of smallpox.

pockmark (pok′mark) a depressed scar left by a pustule.

pod(o)- word element [Gr.], *foot.*

podagra (po-dag′rah) gouty pain in the great toe.

podalgia (po-dal′je-ah) pain in the feet.

podalic (po-dal′ik) accomplished by means of the feet; see under *version.*

podarthritis (pod″ar-thri′tis) inflammation of the joints of the feet.

podencephalus (-en-sef′ah-lus) a monster whose brain, without a cranium, hangs by a pedicle.

podiatrist (po-di′ah-trist) chiropodist; a specialist in podiatry.

podiatry (po-di′ah-tre) chiropody; the specialized field dealing with the study and care of the foot, including its anatomy, pathology, medicial and surgical treatment, etc.

podium (po′de-um), pl. *po′dia* [L.] a footlike process; a sucker foot.

podocyte (pod′o-sīt) an epithelial cell of the visceral layer of a renal glomerulus, having a number of footlike radiating processes (pedicels).

pododynamometer (pod″o-di″nah-mom′ĕ-ter) a device for determining the strength of leg muscles.

pododynia (-din′e-ah) neuralgic pain of the heel and sole; burning pain without redness in the sole of the foot.

podology (po-dol′o-je) podiatry.

podophyllin (pod″o-fil′in) podophyllum resin.

podophyllum (-fil′um) the dried rhizome and roots of *Podophyllum peltatum;* see under *resin.*

poe- for words beginning thus, see those beginning *pe-*.

pogoniasis (po″go-ni′ah-sis) excessive growth of the beard, or growth of a beard on a woman.

pogonion (po-go′ne-on) the anterior midpoint of the chin.

-poiesis word element [Gr.], *formation.* **-poiet′ic,** adj.

poikilo- word element [Gr.], *varied; irregular.*

poikiloblast (poi′kĭ-lo-blast″) an abnormally shaped erythroblast.

poikilocyte (-sīt) an abnormally shaped erythrocyte.

poikilocytosis (poi″kĭ-lo-si-to′sis) poikilocytes in the blood.

poikiloderma (-der′mah) a condition characterized by pigmentary and atrophic changes in the skin, giving it a mottled appearance.

poikilotherm (poi′kĭ-lo-therm″) an animal that exhibits poikilothermy; a cold-blooded animal.

poikilothermy (poi′kĭ-lo-ther′me) the state of having a body temperature which varies with that of the environment. **poikilother′mal, poikilother′mic,** adj.

point (point) 1. a small area or spot; the sharp end of an object. 2. to approach the surface, like the pus of an abscess, at a definite spot or place. **p. A,** a roentgenograhic, cephalometric landmark, determined on the lateral head film; it is the most retruded part of the curved bony outline from the anterior nasal spine to the crest of the maxillary alveolar process. **auricular p.,** the center of the opening of the external auditory meatus. **p. B,** a roentgenograhic, cephalometric landmark, determined on the lateral head film; it is the most posterior midline point in the concavity between the infradentale and pogonium. **boiling p.,** the temperature at which a liquid will boil; at sea level, water boils at 100° C., or 212° F. **boiling p., normal,** the temperature at which a liquid boils at one atmosphere pressure. **cardinal p's,** 1. the points on the different refracting media of the eye which determine the direction of the entering or emerging light rays. 2. four points within the pelvic inlet—the two sacroiliac articulations and the two iliopectineal eminences. **corresponding p's,** points upon the two retinas whose impressions unite to produce a single perception; cf. *disparate p's.* **craniometric p's,** the established points of reference for measurement of the skull. **dew p.,** the atmospheric temperature at which moisture begins to be deposited as dew. **disparate p's,** points on the retina that are not paired exactly; cf. *corresponding p's.* **p's douloureux,** Valleix's p's. **far p.,** the remotest point at which an object is clearly seen when the eye is at rest. **fixation p.,** the point on which the vision is fixed. **freezing p.,** the temperature at which a liquid begins to freeze; for water, 0° C., or 32° F. **identical p's,** corresponding p's. **isoelectric p.,** the pH of a solution at which a dipolar ion does not migrate in an electric field. **isoionic p.,** the pH of a solution at which a specific ion contains as many negative charges as positive charges. **jugal p.,** the point at the angle formed by the masseteric and maxillary edges of the zygomatic bone. **lacrimal p.,** the opening on the lacrimal papilla of an eyelid, near the medial angle of the eye, into which tears from the lacrimal lake drain to enter the lacrimal canaliculi. **McBurney's p.,** a point of special tenderness in appendicitis, about $\frac{1}{2}$–2 inches from the right anterior iliac spine on a line between this spine and the navel. **p. of maximal impulse,** the point on the chest where the impulse of the left ventricle is felt most strongly, normally in the fifth costal interspace inside the mamillary line. **melting p.,** the minimum temperature at which a solid begins to liquefy. **near p.,** the nearest point of clear vision, the *absolute near p.* being that for either eye alone with accommodation relaxed, and the *relative near p.* that for both eyes with the employment of accommodation. **nodal p's,** two points on the axis of an optical system situated so that a ray falling on one will produce a parallel ray emerging through the other. **subnasal p.,** the central point at the base of the nasal spine. **trigger p.,** a spot on the body at which pressure or other stimulus gives rise to specific sensations or symptoms. **Valleix's p's,** tender points along the course of certain nerves in neuralgia.

pointer (point'er) contusion at a bony eminence. **hip p.,** a contusion of the bone of the iliac crest, or avulsion of muscle attachments at the iliac crest.

pointillage (pwahn-til-yahzh') [Fr.] massage with the points of the fingers.

poise (poiz) the unit of viscosity, being that of a fluid which would require a shearing force of one dyne to move a square centimeter area of a layer of fluid 1 cm. per second relative to a parallel layer of fluid 1 cm. distant.

poison (poi'zun) a substance which, on ingestion, inhalation, absorption, application, injection, or development within the body, in relatively small amounts, may cause structural damage or functional disturbance. **corrosive p.,** one that acts by directly destroying tissue. **whelk p.,** a toxic principle localized in the salivary gland of whelks; ingestion of whelks produces intoxication marked by headache, dizziness, nausea, and vomiting.

poisoning (poi'zuh-ning) the morbid condition produced by a poison. **blood p.,** septicemia. **callistin shellfish p.,** that due to ingestion of gastropods of the genus *Callista,* believed to be caused by a choline present in large amounts in the ovaries of the shellfish. **fish p.,** ichthyosarcotoxism. **food p.,** a group of acute illnesses due to ingestion of contaminated food. It may result from allergy; toxemia from foods, such as those inherently poisonous or those contaminated by poisons; foods containing poisons formed by bacteria; or foodborne infections. **forage p.,** a disease produced in animals, especially horses, as a result of eating moldy or fermented food. **gonyaulax p.,** a severe neurologic reaction that may end in paralysis and death, caused by ingestion of shellfish feeding on members of the genus *Gonyaulax* and related dinoflagellates, which produce a neurotoxic principle. **heavy metal p.,** poisoning with any of the heavy metals, particularly arsenic, antimony, lead, mercury, cadmium, or thallium. **mushroom p.,**

that due to ingestion of poisonous mushrooms; see *Amanita.* **salmon p.,** see *Neorickettsia.* **sausage p.,** allantiasis. **scombroid p.,** see *Scombroidea.* **shellfish p.,** see *callistin shellfish p.,* and *gonyaulax p.* **whelk p.,** see under *poison.*

Polaramine (po-lar'ah-mēn) trademark for preparations of dexchlorpheniramine.

polarimeter (po″lah-rim'ĕ-ter) a device for measuring the rotation of plane polarized light.

polarimetry (po″lah-rim'ĕ-tre) measurement of the rotation of plane polarized light.

polariscope (po-lar'ĭ-skōp) an instrument for measuring polarized light.

polarity (po-lar'ĭ-te) the condition of having poles or of exhibiting opposite effects at the two extremities.

polarization (po″lar-i-za'shun) the production of that condition in light in which its vibrations are parallel to each other in one plane, or in circles and ellipses.

polarizer (po'lah-rīz-er) an appliance for polarizing light.

poldine (pol'dēn) an anticholinergic, $C_{22}H_{29}NO_7S$, used as the methylsulfate salt to reduce gastric secretion of hydrochloric acid.

pole (pōl) 1. either extremity of any axis, as of the fetal ellipse or a body organ. 2. either one of two points which have opposite physical qualities. **po'lar,** adj. **animal p.,** that pole of an ovum to which the nucleus is approximated, and from which the polar bodies pinch off. **cephalic p.,** the end of the fetal ellipse at which the head of the fetus is situated. **frontal p.,** the most prominent part of the anterior end of each hemisphere of the brain. **germinal p.,** animal p. **negative p.,** cathode. **occipital p.,** the posterior end of the occipital lobe of the brain. **pelvic p.,** the end of the fetal ellipse at which the breech of the fetus is situated. **positive p.,** anode. **temporal p.,** the prominent anterior end of the temporal lobe of the brain. **vegetal p., vegetative p., vitelline p.,** that pole of an ovum at which the greater amount of food yolk is deposited.

poli(o)- word element [Gr.], *gray matter.*

policeman (po-lēs'man) a glass rod with a piece of rubber tubing on one end, used as a stirring rod and transfer tool in chemical analysis.

policlinic (pol″ĭ-klin'ik) a city hospital, infirmary, or clinic; cf. *polyclinic.*

polio (po'le-o) poliomyelitis.

polioclastic (po″le-o-klas'tik) destroying the gray matter of the nervous system.

poliodystrophia (-dis-tro'fe-ah) poliodystrophy. **p. cer'ebri,** a rare disease of young children, marked by neuron degeneration of the cerebral cortex and elsewhere, with progressive mental deterioration, motor disturbances, sometimes cortical deafness and blindness, and early death.

poliodystrophy (-dis'tro-fe) atrophy of the cerebral gray matter.

polioencephalitis (-en-sef″ah-li'tis) inflammatory disease of the gray matter of the brain. **inferior p.,** bulbar paralysis.

polioencephalomeningomyelitis (-en-sef″ah-lo-mĕ-ning″go-mi″ĕ-li′tis) inflammation of the gray matter of the brain and spinal cord and of the meninges.

polioencephalomyelitis (-mi″ĕ-li′tis) inflammation of the gray matter of the brain and spinal cord.

polioencephalopathy (-en-sef″ah-lop′ah-the) disease of the gray matter of the brain.

poliomyelitis (-mi″ĕ-li′tis) an acute viral disease marked clinically by fever, sore throat, headache, vomiting, and often stiffness of the neck and back; these may be the only symptoms of the minor illness. In the major illness (*acute anterior p.*), which may or may not be preceded by the minor illness, there is central nervous system involvement, stiff neck, pleocytosis in spinal fluid, and perhaps paralysis; there may be subsequent atrophy of muscle groups, ending in contraction and permanent deformity. **acute anterior p.,** see *poliomyelitis*. **ascending p.,** poliomyelitis with a cephalad progression. **bulbar p.,** a severe form affecting the medulla oblongata, which may result in dysfunction of the swallowing mechanism, respiratory embarrassment, and circulatory distress. **spinal paralytic p.,** the classic form of acute anterior poliomyelitis, in which the appearance of flaccid paralysis, usually of one or more limbs, makes the diagnosis definite.

poliomyelopathy (-mi″ĕ-lop′ah-the) any disease of the gray matter of the spinal cord.

poliosis (po″le-o′sis) premature grayness of the hair.

poliovirus (po″le-o-vi′rus) the causative agent of poliomyelitis, separable, on the basis of specificity of neutralizing antibody, into three serotypes designated types 1, 2, and 3.

politzerization (pol″it-zer-i-za′shun) inflation of the middle ear by means of a Politzer bag.

pollen (pol′en) the male fertilizing element of flowering plants.

pollenosis (pol″e-no′sis) pollinosis.

pollex (pol′eks) [L.] the thumb. **p. val′gus,** deviation of the thumb toward the ulnar side. **p. va′rus,** deviation of the thumb toward the radial side.

pollicization (pol″ĭ-si-za′shun) surgical construction of a thumb from a finger.

pollinosis (pol″ĭ-no′sis) an allergic reaction to pollen; hay fever.

pollution (pŏ-lu′shun) defiling or making impure.

polocyte (po′lo-sīt) see *polar bodies*.

polonium (po-lo′ne-um) chemical element (*see table*), at. no. 84, symbol Po.

poloxalkol (pol-ok′sal-kol) a pharmacologically inert oxyalkylene polymer used as a fecal softener.

polus (po′lus), pl. *po′li* [L.] pole.

poly- word element [Gr.], *many; much.*

polyadenitis (pol″e-ad″ĕ-ni′tis) inflammation of several glands.

polyadenosis (-ad″ĕ-no′sus) disorder of several glands, particularly endocrine glands.

polyangiitis (-an″je-i′tis) inflammation involving multiple blood or lymph vessels.

polyarteritis (-ar″tĕ-ri′tis) a condition marked by multiple sites of inflammatory and destructive lesions in the arterial system; see *periarteritis nodosa*.

polyarthric (-ar′thrik) polyarticular.

polyarthritis (-ar-thri′tis) inflammation of several joints. **chronic villous p.,** chronic inflammation of the synovial membrane of several joints. **p. rheumat′ica,** rheumatic fever.

polyarticular (-ar-tik′u-lar) affecting many joints.

polyatomic (-ah-tom′ik) made up of several atoms.

polybasic (-ba′sik) having several replaceable hydrogen atoms.

polyblast (pol′e-blast) free macrophage.

Polybrene (-brēn) trademark for a preparation of hexadimethrine bromide.

polycarbophil (pol″e-kar′bo-fil) polyacrylic acid cross-linked with divinyl glycol; used as a gastrointestinal absorbent.

polycholia (-ko′le-ah) excessive flow or secretion of bile.

polychondritis (-kon-dri′tis) inflammation of many cartilages of the body. **chronic atrophic p., p. chron′ica atro′phicans, relapsing p.,** an acquired, idiopathic chronic disease with a tendency to recurrence, marked by inflammatory and degenerative lesions of various cartilaginous structures.

polychromasia (-kro-ma′ze-ah) 1. variation in the hemoglobin content of erythrocytes. 2. polychromatophilia.

polychromatic (-kro-mat′ik) many-colored.

polychromatocyte (-kro-mat′o-sīt) a cell stainable with various kinds of stain.

polychromatophil (-kro-mat′o-fil) a structure stainable with many kinds of stain.

polychromatophilia (-kro-mat″o-fil′e-ah) 1. the property of being stainable with various stains; affinity for all sorts of stains. 2. a condition in which the erythrocytes, on staining, show various shades of blue combined with tinges of pink. **polychromatophil′ic,** adj.

polychromemia (-kro-me′me-ah) increase in the coloring matter of the blood.

polyclinic (-klin′ik) a hospital and school where diseases and injuries of all kinds are studied and treated.

polyclonal (-klōn′al) derived from different cells; pertaining to several clones.

polyclonia (-klo′ne-ah) a disease marked by many clonic spasms.

polycoria (-ko′re-ah) more than one pupil in an eye.

polycrotism (po-lik′ro-tizm) the quality of having several secondary waves to each beat of the pulse. **polycrot′ic,** adj.

Polycycline (pol″e-si′klēn) trademark for preparations of tetracycline.

polycyesis (-si-e′sis) multiple pregnancy.

polycystic (-sis′tik) containing many cysts.

polycythemia (-si-the′me-ah) an increase in the total cell mass of the blood. **p. hyperton′ica,** a syndrome of increased red cell mass (without splenomegaly, leukocytosis, or thrombocytosis), hypertrophy of the heart, and labile hypertension. **relative p.,** relative excess in the number of red cells due to decrease in the fluid portion of the blood. **p. ru′bra,** p. vera. **secondary p.,** any absolute increase in the total red cell mass other than polycythemia vera. **p. ve′ra,** a disease of unknown cause, marked by an absolute increase in red cell mass and total blood volume, associated often with splenomegaly, leukocytosis, and thrombocytopenia.

polydactylism, polydactyly (-dak′til-izm; -dak′tĭ-le) the presence of supernumerary digits on the hands or feet.

polydipsia (-dip′se-ah) excessive thirst.

polydysplasia (-dis-pla′ze-ah) faulty development of several tissues, organs, or systems.

polyemia (-e′me-ah) excessive blood in the body.

polyendocrine (-en′do-krīn) pertaining to several endocrine glands.

polyesthesia (-es-the′ze-ah) a sensation as if several points were touched on application of a stimulus to a single point.

polyethylene (-eth′ĭ-lēn) polymerized ethylene, $(CH_2—CH_2)_n$, a synthetic plastic material, forms of which have been used in reparative surgery. **p. glycol,** a polymer of ethylene oxide and water, available in liquid form (polyethylene glycol 300 or 400) or as waxy solids (polyethylene glycol 1540 or 4000), used in various pharmaceutical preparations.

polygalactia (-gah-lak′she-ah) excessive secretion of milk.

polygalacturonase (-gah-lak-tu′ro-nās) an enzyme that catylyzes the hyrolysis of pectin to sugars and galacturonic acid.

polygene (pol′ĕ-jēn) a group of nonallelic genes that interact to influence the same character with additive effect.

polygenic (pol′ĕ-jēn′ik) pertaining to or determined by several different genes.

polyglandular (-glan′du-lar) pertaining to or affecting several glands.

polygnathus (po-lig′nah-thus) a double monster in which a parasitic twin is attached to the autosite's jaw.

polygraph (pol′e-graf) an apparatus for simultaneously recording blood pressure, pulse, and respiration, and variations in electrical resistance of the skin; popularly known as a lie-detector.

polygyria (pol″e-ji′re-ah) excess of convolutions in the brain.

polyhedral (-he′dral) having many sides or surfaces.

polyhidrosis (-hi-dro′sis) hyperhidrosis.

polyhydramnios (-hi-dram′ne-os) hydramnios.

polyhydric (-hi′drik) containing more than two hydroxyl groups.

polyinfection (-in-fek′shun) infection with more than one organism.

Polykol (pol′e-kol) trademark for preparations of poloxalkol.

polyleptic (pol″e-lep′tik) having many remissions and exacerbations.

polylysine (-li′sin) a polypeptide composed of lysine molecules in peptide linkage; see *penicilloyl-polylysine.*

polymastia (-mas′te-ah) the presence of supernumerary mammary glands.

polymastigote (-mas′tĭ-gōt) 1. having several flagella. 2. a mastigote having several flagella.

polymelus (po-lim′ĕ-lus) an individual with supernumerary limbs.

polymenorrhea (pol″e-men″o-re′ah) abnormally frequent menstruation.

polymer (pol′ĭ-mer) a compound, usually of high molecular weight, formed by the linear combination of simpler molecules (monomeres); it may be formed without formation of any other product (*addition p.*) or with simultaneous elimination of water or other simple compound (*condensation p.*).

polymerase (pol-im′er-ās) an enzyme that catalyzes polymerization.

polymeric (pol″ĭ-mer′ik) exhibiting the characteristics of a polymer.

polymerization (po-lim″er-i-za′shun, -mer″i-za′shun) the combining of several simpler compounds to form a polymer.

polymicrobial, polymicrobic (pol″e-mi-kro′be-al; -mi-kro′bik) marked by the presence of several species of microorganisms.

polymicrogyria (-mi″kro-ji′re-ah) a brain malformation marked by development of numerous microgyri.

polymorph (pol′e-morf) colloquial term for polymorphonuclear leukocyte.

polymorphic (pol″e-mor′fik) occurring in several or many forms; appearing in different forms in different developmental stages.

polymorphism (-mor′fizm) the quality of existing in several different forms.

polymorphocellular (-mor″fo-sel′u-lar) having cells of many forms.

polymorphonuclear (-nu′kle-ar) 1. having a nucleus so deeply lobed or so divided as to appear to be multiple. 2. a polymorphonuclear leukocyte; see *neutrophil* (1).

polymorphous (-mor′fus) polymorphic.

polymyalgia (pol″e-mi-al′je-ah) pain involving many muscles.

polymyoclonus (-mi-ok′lo-nus) 1. a fine or minute muscular tremor. 2. polyclonia.

polymyopathy (-mi-op′ah-the) disease affecting several muscles simultaneously.

polymyositis (-mi″o-si′tis) inflammation of several or many muscles at once, attended by weakness, pain, tension, edema, deformity, insomnia, and sweats.

polymyxin (-mik′sin) generic term for antibiotics derived from *Bacillus polymyxa;* they are differentiated by affixing different letters of the alphabet. **p. B,** the least toxic of the polymyxins; its sulfate is used in the treatment of various gram-negative infections.

polynesic (-ne′sik) occurring in many foci.

polyneural (-nu′ral) pertaining to or supplied by many nerves.

polyneuralgia (-nu-ral′je-ah) neuralgia of several nerves.

polyneuritis (-nu-ri′tis) inflammation of many nerves simultaneously. **acute febrile p., acute infectious p.,** an acute, rapidly progressive, ascending paralysis, beginning in the feet and ascending to the other muscles, often occurring after an enteric or respiratory infection.

polyneuromyositis (-nu″ro-mi-o-si′tis) inflammation of the muscles and peripheral nerves, with loss of reflexes, sensory loss, and paresthesias.

polyneuropathy (-nu-rop′ah-the) a disease involving several nerves. **erythredema p.,** acrodynia.

polyneuroradiculitis (-nu″ro-rah-dik″u-li′tis) inflammation of spinal ganglia, nerve roots, and peripheral nerves.

polynuclear (-nu″kle-ar) 1. polynucleate. 2. polymorphonuclear.

polynucleate (-nu′kle-āt) polynuclear.

polynucleotidase (-nu″kle-o-ti′dās) an enzyme that catalyzes the depolymerization of nucleic acids.

polynucleotide (-nu′kle-o-tīd) any polymer of mononucleotides.

polyodontia (-o-don′she-ah) the presence of supernumerary teeth.

polyonychia (-o-nik′e-ah) the presence of supernumerary nails.

polyopia (-o′pe-ah) visual perception of several images of a single object.

polyorchidism (-or′kǐ-dizm) the presence of more than two testes.

polyorchis (-or′kis) a person exhibiting polyorchidism.

polyorchism (-or′kizm) polyorchidism.

polyostotic (-os-tot′ik) affecting several bones.

polyotia (-o′she-ah) the presence of more than two ears.

polyovulatory (-ov′u-lah-tor″e) discharging several ova in one ovarian cycle.

polyoxyl stearate (-oks′il) a group of surfactants consisting of a mixture of mono- and diesters of stearate and polyoxyethylene diols; they are numbered according to the average polymer length of oxyethylene units, e.g., polyoxyl 40 stearate.

polyp (pol′ip) any growth or mass protruding from a mucous membrane. **adenomatous p.,** a benign polypoid adenoma. **fibrinous p.,** intrauterine polyp made up of fibrin from retained blood. **juvenile p's,** small, benign hemispheric hamartomas of the large intestine occurring sporadically in children. **retention p's,** juvenile p's.

polyparesis (pol″e-pah-re′sis) dementia paralytica.

polypathia (-path′e-ah) the presence of several diseases at one time.

polypectomy (-pek′to-me) excision of a polyp.

polypeptidase (-pep′tǐ-dās) an enzyme which catalyzes the hydrolysis of polypeptides.

polypeptide (-pep′tīd) a peptide containing more than two amino acids linked by peptide bonds.

polypeptidemia (-pep″tǐ-de′me-ah) the presence of polypeptides in the blood.

polyphagia (-fa′je-ah) excessive ingestion of food.

polyphalangia, polyphalangism (-fah-lan′je-ah; -fah-lan′jizm) excess of phalanges in a finger or toe.

polypharmacy (-far′mah-se) 1. administration of many drugs together. 2. administration of excessive medication.

polyphenoloxidase (-fe″nol-ok′sǐ-dās) a copper-containing enzyme that oxidizes phenols and their amino compounds to quinones.

polyphobia (-fo′be-ah) abnormal fear of many things.

polyphrasia (-fra′ze-ah) morbid volubility.

polyplastic (-plas′tik) 1. containing many structural or constituent elements. 2. undergoing many changes of form.

polyplegia (-ple′je-ah) paralysis of several muscles.

polyploid (pol′e-ploid) 1. characterized by polyploidy. 2. an individual or cell characterized by polyploidy.

polyploidy (-ploi′de) possession of more than two sets of homologous chromosomes.

polypnea (pol″ip-ne′ah) hyperpnea.

polypodia (pol″e-po′de-ah) the presence of supernumerary feet.

polypoid (pol′ǐ-poid) resembling a polyp.

polyporous (pol-ip′o-rus) having many pores.

polyposia (pol′ǐ-po′ze-ah) ingestion of abnormally increased amounts of fluids for long periods of time.

polyposis (-po′sis) the formation of numerous polyps. **familial p.,** a hereditary condition marked by multiple adenomatous polyps with high malignant potential, lining the intestinal muscosa, especially that of the colon, beginning at about puberty. Multiple intestinal polyps occur in *Gardner's, Peutz-Jeghers, Canada-Cronkhite,* and *Turcot's syndromes.*

polypous (pol′ĕ-pus) polyp-like.

polyptychial (pol″e-ti′ke-al) arranged in several layers.

polypus (pol′ǐ-pus), pl. *pol′ypi* [L.] polyp.

polyradiculitis (pol″e-rah-dik″u-li′tis) inflammation of the nerve roots.

polyradiculoneuritis (-rah-dik″u-lo-nu-ri′tis) acute febrile polyneuritis which involves the peripheral nerves, the spinal nerve roots, and the spinal cord.

polyribosome (-ri′bo-sōm) a cluster of ribosomes connected with messenger RNA; they play a role in peptide synthesis.

polysaccharide (-sak′ah-rīd) a carbohydrate which, on acid hydrolysis, yields 10 or more monosaccharides. **immune p's,** ones that can function as specific antigens.

polyscelia (-se′le-ah) the presence of more than two legs.

polyserositis (-se″ro-si′tis) general inflammation of serous membranes, with effusion.

polysinusitis (-si″nu-si′tis) inflammation of several sinuses.

polysomaty (-so′mah-te) having reduplicated chromatin in the nucleus.

polysome (pol′e-sōm) polyribosome.

polysomia (pol″e-so′me-ah) doubling or tripling of the fetal body.

polysomus (-so′mus) a monster exhibiting polysomia. **polyso′mic,** adj.

polysomy (-so′me) an excess of a particular chromosome.

polysorbate 80 (-sor′bāt) an oleate ester of sorbitol and its anhydride (sorbitan) condensed with polymers of ethylene oxide, consisting of approximately 20 oxyethylene units; it is a surfactant used as an emulsifying, dispersing, and solubilizing agent.

polyspermia (-sper′me-ah) 1. excessive secretion of semen. 2. polyspermy.

polyspermy (-sper′me) fertilization of an ovum by more than one spermatozoon; occurring normally in certain species (*physiologic p.*) and sometimes abnormally in others (*pathologic p.*).

polystichia (-stik′e-ah) two or more rows of eyelashes on a lid.

polystyrene (-sti′rēn) the resin produced by polymerization of styrol, a clear resin of the thermoplastic type, used in the construction of denture bases.

polysynaptic (-sĭ-nap′tik) pertaining to or relayed through two or more synapses.

polysyndactyly (-sin-dak′tĭ-le) hereditary association of polydactyly and syndactyly.

polytene (pol′e-tēn) composed of or containing many strands of chromatin (chromonemata).

polythelia (pol″e-the′le-ah) the presence of supernumerary nipples.

polythiazide (-thi′ah-zīd) a diuretic and antihypertensive, $C_{11}H_{13}ClF_3N_3O_4S_3$.

polytocous (po-lit′ŏ-kus) giving birth to several offspring at one time.

polytrichia (pol″e-trik′e-ah) hypertrichiasis.

polyuria (-u′re-ah) excessive secretion of urine.

polyvalent (-va′lent) multivalent.

polyvinylpyrrolidine (-vi″nil-pi-rol′ĭ-dēn) povidone.

pompholyx (pom′fo-liks) an intensely pruritic skin eruption on the sides of the digits or on the palms and soles, consisting of small, discrete, round vesicles, typically occurring in repeated self-limited attacks.

pomum (po′mum), pl. *po′ma* [L.] apple. **p. ada′mi,** the prominence on the throat caused by thyroid cartilage.

pons (ponz) 1. any slip of tissue connecting two parts of an organ. 2. that part of the metencephalon lying between the medulla oblongata and the midbrain, ventral to the cerebellum; see *brain stem.* **p. hep′atis,** an occasional projection partially bridging the longitudinal fissure of the liver. **p. varo′lii,** pons (2).

pontic (pon′tik) the portion of a dental bridge which substitutes for an absent tooth.

ponticulus (pon-tik′u-lus), pl. *pontic′uli*[L.] delicate plates of white matter passing across the anterior end of the pyramid and just below the pons. **pontic′ular,** adj.

pontine (pon′tīn) pertaining to the pons.

pontobulbar (pon″to-bul′bar) pertaining to the pons and the region of the medulla oblongata dorsad to it.

Pontocaine (pon′to-kān) trademark for preparations of tetracaine.

pontocerebellar (pon″to-ser″ĕ-bel′ar) pertaining to the pons and cerebellum.

popliteal (pop″lĭ-te′al) pertaining to the area behind the knee.

poradenitis (pōr″ad-ĕ-ni′tis) inflammation of lymph nodes with formation of small abscesses.

porcine (por′sīn) pertaining to swine.

pore (pōr) a small opening or empty space.

porencephalia (po″ren-se-fa′le-ah) porencephaly.

porencephalitis (po″ren-sef″ah-li′tis) porencephaly associated with an inflammatory process.

porencephalous (po″ren-sef′ah-lus) characterized by porencephaly.

porencephaly (po″ren-sef′ah-le) development or presence of abnormal cysts or cavities in the brain tissue, usually communicating with a lateral ventricle. **porencephal′ic, porenceph′alous,** adj.

porocele (po′ro-sēl) scrotal hernia with thickening of the coverings of the testes.

porokeratosis (po″ro-ker″ah-to′sis) a hereditary dermatosis marked by a certrifugally spreading hypertrophy of the stratum corneum around the sweat pores followed by atrophy. Also known as *p. of Mibelli.* **porokeratot′ic,** adj.

poroma (po-ro′mah) a tumor arising in a pore. **eccrine p.,** a benign tumor arising from the intradermal portion of an eccrine sweat duct, usually on the sole.

porosis (po-ro′sis) 1. the formation of the callus in repair of a fractured bone. 2. cavity formation.

porosity (po-ros′ĭ-te) the condition of being porous; a pore.

porotomy (po-rot′o-me) meatotomy.

porous (po′rus) penetrated by pores and open spaces.

porphin (por′fin) the fundamental ring structure of four linked pyrrole nuclei around which porphyrins, hemin, cytochromes, and chlorophyll are built.

porphobilinogen (por″fo-bi-lin′o-jen) an intermediary product in the biosynethesis of heme.

porphyria (por-fēr′e-ah, por-fi′re-ah) a disturbance of porphyrin metabolism characterized by increase in formation and excretion of porphyrins or their precursors. **acute intermittent p.,** hereditary hepatic porphyria due to a defect of pyrrole metabolism, with recurrent attacks of abdominal pain, gastrointestinal and neurologic disturbances, and excessive amounts of aminolevulinic acid and porphobilinogen in the urine. **congenital erythropoietic p.,** hereditary erythropoietic porphyria, with cutaneous photosensitivity leading to mutilating lesions, hemolytic anemia, splenomegaly, excessive urinary excretion of uroporphyrin, and, invariably, erythrodontia and hypertrichosis. **p. cuta′nea tar′da heredita′ria,** hepatic porphyria resembling the variegate form except that abdominal and neurologic symptoms are absent or mild. **p. cuta′nea tar′da symptomat′ica,** a sporadic form, usually associated with chronic alcoholism, marked by chronic skin lesions ranging from slight fragility to severe scarring, and by hepatomegaly and excessive excretion of uro- and coproporphyrin. **erythropoietic p.,** that in which excessive formation of porphyrin or its precursors occurs in bone marrow normoblasts; it includes congenital erythropoietic porphyria and erythropoietic protoporphyria. **hepatic p.,** that in which the excess formation of porphyrin or its precursors occurs in the liver. **variegate p.,** hereditary hepatic porphyria, with chronic skin manifestations, chiefly extreme mechanical fragility of the skin, mainly of areas exposed to sunlight, episodes of abdominal pain, neuropathy, and, typically, an excess of coproporhyrin and protoporphyrin in bile and feces.

porphyrin (por′fĭ-rin) any of a group of iron- or magnesium-free cyclic tetrapyrrole derivatives, occurring universally in protoplasm, and forming the basis of the respiratory pigments of animals and plants.

porphyrinuria (por″fĭ-rĭ-nu′re-ah) an excess of porphyrin in the urine.

porta (por′tah), pl. *por′tae* [L.] an entrance or portal; especially the site of entrance to an organ of the blood vessels and other structures supplying or draining it. **p. hep′atis,** the transverse fissure on the visceral surface of the liver where the portal vein and hepatic artery enter and the hepatic ducts leave.

portacaval (por″tah-ka′val) pertaining to the portal vein and inferior vena cava.

portal (por′tal) 1. an avenue of entrance; porta. 2. pertaining to a porta, especially the porta hepatis. **p. of entry,** the pathway by which bacteria or other pathogenic agents gain entry to the body.

portio (por′she-o), pl. *portio′nes* [L.] a part or division. **p. du′ra,** the facial nerve. **p. interme′dia,** intermediate nerve. **p. mol′lis,** vestibulocochlear nerve. **p. supravagina′lis,** the part of the cervix uteri that does not protrude into the vagina. **p. vagina′lis,** the portion of the uterus projecting into the vagina.

portogram (por′to-gram) the film obtained by portography.

portography (por-tog′rah-fe) radiography of the portal vein after injection of opaque material into the superior mesenteric vein or one of its branches during operation (*portal p.*), or percutaneously into the spleen (*splenic p.*).

porus (po′rus), pl. *po′ri* [L.] an opening or pore. **p. acus′ticus exter′nus,** the outer end of the external acoustic meatus. **p. acus′ticus inter′nus,** the opening of the internal acoustic meatus. **p. op′ticus,** the opening in the sclera for passage of the optic nerve.

-posia word element [Gr.], *intake of fluids.*

position (po-zish′un) 1. a bodily posture or attitude. 2. the relationship of a given point on the presenting part of the fetus to a designated point of the maternal pelvis; see accompanying table. Cf. *presentation.* **anatomic p.,** that of the human body, standing erect, with palms turned forward, used as the position of reference in designating the site or direction of structures of the body. **Bonner's p.,** flexion, abduction, and outward rotation of the thigh in coxitis. **Bozeman's p.,** the knee-elbow position with straps used for support. **Brickner's p.,** the wrist is tied to the head of the bed to obtain abduction and external rotation for shoulder disability. **decubitus p.,** that of the body lying on a horizontal surface, designated according to the aspect of the body touching the surface, *dorsal decubitus* (on the back), *left lateral decubitus* (on the left side), *right lateral decubitus* (on the right side), or *ventral decubitus* (on the abdomen). **Fowler's p.,** that in which the head of the patient's bed is raised 18–20 inches above the level, with the knees also elevated. **genucubital p.,**

POSITIONS OF THE FETUS IN VARIOUS PRESENTATIONS

CEPHALIC PRESENTATION

Vertex—occiput the point of direction
  Left occipitoanterior (L.O.A.)
  Left occipitotransverse (L.O.T.)
  Right occipitoposterior (R.O.P.)
  Right occipitotransverse (R.O.T.)
  Right occipitoanterior (R.O.A.)
  Left occipitoposterior (L.O.P.)
Face—chin the point of direction
  Right mentoposterior (R.M.P.)
  Left mentoanterior (L.M.A.)
  Right mentotransverse (R.M.T.)
  Right mentoanterior (R.M.A.)
  Left mentotransverse (L.M.T.)
  Left mentoposterior (L.M.P.)
Brow—the point of direction
  Right frontoposterior (R.F.P.)
  Left frontoanterior (L.F.A.)
  Right frontotransverse (R.F.T.)
  Right frontoanterior (R.F.A.)
  Left frontotransverse (L.F.T.)
  Left frontoposterior (L.F.P.)

BREECH OR PELVIC PRESENTATION

Complete breech—sacrum, the point of direction (feet crossed and thighs flexed on abdomen)
  Left sacroanterior (L.S.A.)
  Left sacrotransverse (L.S.T.)
  Right sacroposterior (R.S.P.)
  Right sacroanterior (R.S.A.)
  Right sacrotransverse (R.S.T.)
  Left sacroposterior (L.S.P.)
Incomplete breech—sacrum, the point of direction. Same designations as above, adding the qualifications footling, knee, etc.

TRANSVERSE LIE OR SHOULDER PRESENTATION

Shoulder—scapula the point of direction

Left scapuloanterior (L.Sc.A.)	⎱	Back
Right scapuloanterior (R.Sc.A.)	⎰	anterior positions
Right scapuloposterior (R.Sc.P.)	⎱	Back
Left scapuloposterior (L.Sc.P.)	⎰	posterior positions

knee-elbow p. **genupectoral p.,** knee-chest p.
knee-chest p., the patient resting on his knees and upper chest. **knee-elbow p.,** the patient resting on his knees and elbows with the chest elevated. **lithotomy p.,** the patient on his back with hips and knees flexed and thighs abducted and externally rotated. **Rose's p.,** a supine position with the head over the table edge in full extension. **Sims' p.,** the patient on his left side and chest, the right knee and thigh drawn up, the left arm along the back. **Trendelenburg's p.,** the patient is supine on a surface inclined 45 degrees, his head at the lower end and his legs flexed over the upper end.

positive (poz′ĭ-tiv) having a value greater than zero; indicating existence or presence, as chromatin-positive; characterized by affirmation or cooperation.

positron (poz′ĭ-tron) a positively charged electron.

posology (po-sol′o-je) the science or system of dosage. **posolog′ic,** adj.

post- word element [L.], *after; behind.*

postaxial (pōst-ak′se-al) behind an axis; in anatomy, referring to the medial (ulnar) aspect of the upper arm, and the lateral (fibular) aspect of the lower leg.

postbrachial (-bra′ke-al) on the posterior part of the upper arm.

postcardiotomy (-kar″de-ot′o-me) occurring after open-heart surgery.

postcava (-ka′vah) the inferior vena cava. **postca′val,** adj.

postcibal (-si′bal) after eating.

postclavicular (pōst″klah-vik′u-lar) behind the clavicle.

postcoital (pōst-ko′ĭ-tal) after coitus.

postcordial (-kor′de-al) behind the heart.

postcornu (-kor′nu) the posterior horn of the lateral ventricle.

postdiastolic (-di″as-tol′ik) after diastole.

postdicrotic (pōst″di-krot′ik) after the dicrotic elevation of the sphygmogram.

postencephalitic (-en-sef″ah-lit′ik) occurring after or as a consequence of encephalitis.

postepileptic (-ep-ĭ-lep′tik) following an epileptic attack.

posterior (pos-tēr′e-or) directed toward or situated at the back; opposite of anterior.

postero- word element [L.], *the back; posterior to.*

posteroanterior (pos″ter-o-an-te′re-or) directed from the back toward the front.

posteroclusion (-kloo′zhun) distoclusion.

posteroexternal (-ek-ster′nal) situated on the outside of a posterior aspect.

posteroinferior (-in-fe′re-or) behind and below.

posterolateral (-lat′er-al) situated on the side and toward the posterior aspect.

posteromedian (-me′de-an) situated on the middle of a posterior aspect.

posterosuperior (-su-pēr′e-or) situated behind and above.

postesophageal (pōst″ĕ-sof″ah-ge′al) retroesophageal.

postfebrile (pōst-feb′ril) occurring after a fever.

postganglionic (pōst″gang-gle-on′ik) distal to a ganglion.

posthepatitic (-hep-ah-tit′ik) occurring after or as a consequence of hepatitis.

posthioplasty (pos′the-o-plas″te) plastic repair of the prepuce.

posthitis (pos-thi′tis) inflammation of the prepuce.

posthypnotic (pōst″hip-not′ik) following the hypnotic state.

postictal (pōst-ik′tal) following a seizure.

postmaturity (pōst″mah-tū′rĭ-te) the condition of an infant after a prolonged gestation period. **postmature′,** adj.

postmenopausal (-men-o-paw′zal) after the menopause.

postmitotic (-mi-tot′ik) occurring after or pertaining to the time following mitosis.

post mortem (pōst mor′tem) [L.] after death.

postmortem (pōst-mor′tem) performed or occurring after death.

postnatal (-na′tal) occurring after birth, with reference to the newborn.

postoperative (pōst-op′er-a″tiv) after a surgical operation.

postoral (-o′ral) in the back part of the mouth.

postparalytic (pōst″par-ah-lit′ik) following an attack of paralysis.

post partum (pōst par′tum) [L.] after parturition.

postpartum (pōst-par′tum) occurring after childbirth, with reference to the mother.

postprandial (-pran′de-al) after a meal.

postpuberal, postpubertal (-pu′ber-al; -tal) after puberty.

postpubescent (pōst″pu-bes′ent) after puberty.

postradiation (-ra-de-a′shun) following exposure to radiation.

postsphygmic (pōst-sfig′mik) after the pulse wave.

poststenotic (pōst″stĕ-not′ik) located or occurring distal to or beyond a stenosed segment.

postsynaptic (-sĭ-nap′tik) distal to or occurring beyond a synapse.

posttraumatic (-traw-mat′ik) following injury.

postulate (pos′tu-lāt) anything assumed or taken for granted. **Koch's p's,** a statement of the kind of experimental evidence required to establish the causative relation of a given microorganism to a given disease; the conditions include (1) the microorganism must be observed in every case of the disease; (2) it must be isolated and grown in pure culture; (3) inoculation of such culture must produce the disease in susceptible animals; (4) the microorganism must be observed in, and recovered from, the experimentally diseased animal.

posture (pos′tūr) an attitude of the body. **pos′tural,** adj.

postuterine (pōst-u′ter-īn) behind the uterus.

postvaccinal (-vak′sĭ-nal) occurring after vaccination for smallpox.

potable (po′tah-b'l) fit to drink.

potash (pot′ash) impure potassium carbonate. **caustic p.,** potassium hydroxide. **sulfurated p.,** a mixture of potassium polysulfides and potassium thiosulfate; a source of sulfide in pharmaceuticals.

potassemia (pot″ah-se′me-ah) hyperkalemia.

potassium (po-tas′e-um) chemical element (see *table*), at. no. 19, symbol K. For potassium salts not listed here, see under the acid or the active ingredient. **p. acetate,** a systemic and urinary alkalizer, $CH_3 \cdot COOK$. **p. aminosalicylate,** an antibacterial against tubercle bacilli, $C_7H_6\text{-}KNO_3$. **p. bicarbonate,** a transparent, crystalline salt used as an electrolyte replenisher. **p. chloride,** an electrolyte replenisher, KCL, for oral or intravenous administration. **p. citrate,** $C_6H_5K_3O_7 \cdot H_2O$, used in potassium deficiency and as a systemic alkalizer, diuretic, and expectorant. **p. gluconate,** $C_6H_{11}KO_7$, used as an electrolyte replenisher in the prophylaxis and treatment of hypokalemia. **p. guaiacolsulfonate,** an expectorant, $C_7H_7KO_5S$. **p. hydroxide,** a powerful alkaline and caustic compound, KOH, used as an alkalinizing agent and occasionally as an escharotic in bites of rabid animals. **p. iodide,** KI, used as an expectorant and as an antithyroid agent. **p. permanganate,** $KMnO_4$, used as a topical anti-infective, oxidizing agent, and antidote for many poisons. **p. phenethicillin,** $C_{17}H_{19}KN_2O_5S$, an oral penicillin. **p. phosphate,** a cathartic, K_2HPO_4. **p. sodium tartrate,** a mild cathartic, $C_4H_4\text{-}KNaO_6 \cdot 4H_2O$. **p. warfarin,** an anticoagulant, $C_{19}H_{15}KO_4$.

potency (po′ten-se) power, especially (1) the ability of the male to perform coitus; (2) the power of a drug to produce the desired effects; (3) the ability of an embryonic part to develop and complete its destiny. **po′tent,** adj.

potential (po-ten′shal) 1. existing and ready for action, but not active. 2. electric tension or pressure. **action p.,** the electrical activity developed in a muscle or nerve cell during activity. **after-p.,** the period following termination of the spike potential. **membrane p.,** the electric potential existing on the two sides of a membrane or across the cell wall. **resting p.,** the potential difference across the membrane of a normal cell at rest. **spike p.,** the initial, very large change in potential of an excitable cell membrane during excitation.

potentiation (po-ten″she-a′shun) enhancement of one agent by another so that the combined effect is greater than the sum of the effects of each one alone.

potion (po′shun) a large dose of liquid medicine.

pouch (powch) a pocket-like space or sac, as of the peritoneum. **abdominovesical p.,** one formed by reflection of the peritoneum from the abdominal wall to the anterior surface of the bladder. **p. of Douglas,** rectouterine p. **Prussak's p.,** a recess in the tympanic membrane between the flaccid part of the membrane and the neck of the malleus. **Rathke's p.,** a diverticulum from the embryonic buccal cavity from which the anterior pituitary is developed. **rectouterine p.,** the space between the bladder and uterus in the peritoneal cavity. **Seessel's p.,** an outpouching of the embryonic pharynx rostrad of the pharyngeal membrane and caudal to Rathe's pouch.

poudrage (poo-drahzh′) [Fr.] application of powder to a surface, as between the visceral and parietal pleura, to promote their fusion.

poultice (pōl′tis) a soft, moist, mass about the consistency of cooked cereal, spread between layers of muslin, linen, gauze, or towels and applied hot to a given area in order to create moist local heat or counterirritation.

pound (pownd) a unit of weight in the avoirdupois (453.6 grams, or 16 ounces) or apothecaries' (373.2 grams, or 12 ounces) system.

povidone (po′vĭ-don) polyvinylpyrrolidine, a synthetic polymer used as a dispersing and suspending agent; it has also been used as a plasma volume expander.

povidone-iodine (-i′o-dīn) a complex produced by reacting iodine with povidone; used as a topical anti-infective.

powder (pow′der) aggregation of particles obtained by grinding or triturating a solid. **aromatic p.,** powder of cinnamon, ginger, cardamon seed, and myristica. **dusting p.,** a fine powder used as a talc substitute. **effervescent p's, compound,** Seidlitz p's. **Goa p.,** a brownish yellow to umber brown powder deposited in the wood of the Brazilian tree *Andira araroba;* the source of chrysarobin. **Seidlitz p's,** a mixture of sodium bicarbonate, potassium sodium tartrate, and tartaric acid; used as a cathartic. **senna p., compound,** a powder prepared from fennel oil, sucrose, senna, glycyrrhiza, and washed sulfur; used as a laxative.

power (pow′er) 1. capability; potency; the ability to act. 2. a measure of magnification, as of a microscope. **defining p.,** the ability of a lens to make an object clearly visible. **resolving p.,** the ability of the eye or of a lens to make small objects that are close together, separately visible, thus revealing the structure of an object.

pox (poks) any eruptive or pustular disease, especially one caused by a virus, e.g., chickenpox, cowpox, etc.

poxvirus (poks-vi′rus) any of a group of morphologically similar and immunologically related DNA viruses, including the virus of vaccinia (cowpox), smallpox, and those producing pox diseases in lower animals.

P.P.D. purified protein derivative; see under *tuberculin.*

PPLO pleuropneumonia-like organisms; see *pleuropneumonia-like.*

p.p.m. parts per million.

Pr chemical symbol, *praseodymium.*

practice (prak′tis) the utilization of one's knowledge in a particular profession, the practice of medicine being the exercise of one's knowledge in the practical recognition and treatment of disease. **family p.,** see under *medicine.* **general p.,** the provision of comprehensive medical care as a continuing responsibility regardless of age of the patient or of the condition that may temporarily require the services of a specialist.

practitioner (prak-tish′un-er) one who has complied with the requirements and who is engaged in the practice of medicine. **nurse p.,** any person prepared and authorized by law to practice nursing, and therefore deemed competent to render safe nursing care.

prae- for words beginning thus, see those beginning *pre-*.

pragmatagnosia (prag″mat-ag-no′ze-ah) inability to recognize formerly known objects.

pragmatamnesia (-am-ne′ze-ah) loss of the power of remembering the appearance of objects.

pralidoxime (pral″ĭ-doks′ēm) a cholinesterase reactivator, $C_7H_9N_2O$, whose salts are used in treatment of organophosphate poisoning; it also has limited value in counteracting carbamate-type cholinesterase inhibitors.

pramoxine (pram-ok′sēn) a topical anesthetic, $C_{17}H_{27}NO_3$.

prandial (pran′de-al) pertaining to a meal.

Pranone (pra′nōn) trademark for a preparation of ethisterone.

Prantal (pran′tal) trademark for preparations of diphemanil methylsulfate.

praseodymium (pra″ze-o-dim′e-um) chemical element (*see table*), at. no. 59, symbol Pr.

praxiology (prak″se-ol′o-je) the science or study of conduct.

prazepam (praz′ĕ-pam) a muscle relaxant, $C_{15}H_{17}ClN_2O$.

pre- word element [L.], *before* (in time or space).

preagonal (pre-ag′o-nal) immediately before the death agony.

preanesthesia (pre″an-es-the′ze-ah) preliminary anesthesia; light anesthesia or narcosis induced by medication as a preliminary to administration of a general anesthetic.

preanesthetic (-an-es-thet′ik) 1. pertaining to preanesthesia. 2. an agent that induces preanesthesia.

preantiseptic (-an-tĭ-sep′tik) pertaining to the time before the discovery of antisepsis.

preauricular (-aw-rik′u-lar) in front of the auricle of the ear.

preaxial (pre-ak′se-al) situated before an axis; in anatomy, referring to the lateral (radial) aspect of the upper arm, and the medial (tibial) aspect of the lower leg.

precancerous (-kan′ser-us) pertaining to a pathologic process that tends to become malignant.

precapillary (-kap′ĭ-ler-e) a vessel lacking complete coats, intermediate between an arteriole and a capillary.

precava (-ka′vah) the superior vena cava. **preca′val,** adj.

prechordal (-kor′dal) in front of the notochord.

precipitant (-sip′ĭ-tant) a substance that causes precipitation.

precipitate (-sip′ĭ-tāt) 1. to cause settling in solid particles of substance in solution. 2. a deposit of solid particles settled out of a solution. 3. occurring with undue rapidity. **white p.,** ammoniated mercury.

precipitation (-sip″ĭ-ta′shun) the act or process of precipitating.

precipitin (-sip′ĭ-tin) an antibody to soluble antigen that specifically aggregates the macromolecular antigen *in vivo* or *in vitro* to give a visible precipitate.

precipitinogen (-sip″ĭ-tin′o-jen) a soluble antigen which stimulates the formation of and reacts with a precipitin.

preclinical (-klin′ĭ-kal) before a disease becomes clinically recognizable.

preclival (-kli′val) in front of the clivus.

precocity (-kos′ĭ-te) unusually early development of mental or physical traits. **preco′cious,** adj.

precognition (pre″kog-nish′un) extrasensory perception of a future event.

precoma (pre-ko′mah) the neuropsychiatric state preceding coma, as in hepatic encephalopathy. **precom′atose,** adj.

preconscious (-kon′shus) not present in consciousness, but readily recalled into it.

preconvulsive (pre″kon-vul′siv) preceding convulsions.

precordia (pre-kor′de-ah) precordium.

precordium (-kor′de-um) the region over the heart and lower thorax. **precor′dial,** adj.

precornu (-kor′nu) the anterior cornu of the lateral ventricle.

precostal (-kos′tal) in front of the ribs.

precuneus (-ku′ne-us), pl. *precu′nei* [L.] a small convolution on the medial surface of the parietal lobe of the cerebrum.

precursor (pre′kur-sor) something that precedes. In biological processes, a substance from which another, usually more active or mature substance is formed. In clinical medicine, a sign or symptom that heralds another.

predentin (pre-den′tin) the soft, primitive dentin.

prediabetes (-di″ah-be′tēz) a state of latent impairment of carbohydrate metabolism in which the criteria for diabetes mellitus are not all satisfied.

prediastole (pre″di-as′to-le) the interval immediately preceding diastole. **prediastol′ic,** adj.

predicrotic (-di-krot′ik) occurring before the dicrotic wave of the sphygmogram.

predigestion (-di-jes′chun) partial artificial digestion of food before its ingestion.

predisposition (pre-dis″po-zish′un) a latent susceptibility to disease which may be activated under certain conditions.

prednisolone (pred-nis′o-lōn) a glucocorticoid, $C_{21}H_{28}O_5$, used as an anti-inflammatory and antiallergic agent.

prednisone (pred′nĭ-sōn) a glucocorticoid, $C_{21}H_{26}O_5$, used like prednisolone.

preeclampsia (pre″e-klamp′se-ah) a toxemia of late pregnancy, characterized by hypertension, proteinuria, and edema.

preexcitation (pre-ek″si-ta′shun) premature excitation of a portion of the ventricle, occurring in Wolff-Parkinson-White syndrome and characterized by a short P-R interval and a wide QRS interval.

prefrontal (pre-fron′tal) 1. situated in the anterior part of the frontal lobe or region. 2. the central part of the ethmoid bone.

preganglionic (pre″gang-gle-on′ik) proximal to a ganglion.

pregenital (pre-jen′ĭ-tal) antedating the emergence of genital interests.

pregnancy (preg′nan-se) the condition of having a developing embryo or fetus in the body, after union of an ovum and spermatozoon. **abdominal p.,** ectopic pregnancy within the peritoneal cavity. **ampullar p.,** ectopic pregnancy in the ampulla of the uterine tube. **cervical p.,** ectopic pregnancy within the cervical canal. **combined p.,** simultaneous intrauterine and extrauterine pregnancies. **cornual p.,** pregnancy in a horn of the uterus. **ectopic p., extrauterine p.,** development of the fertilized ovum outside the cavity of the uterus. **false p.,** development of all the signs of pregnancy without the presence of an embryo. **interstitial p.,** pregnancy in the portion of the oviduct within the uterine wall. **intraligamentary p.,** ectopic pregnancy within the broad ligament. **multiple p.,** presence of more than one fetus in the uterus at the same time. **mural p.,** interstitial p. **ovarian p.,** pregnancy occurring in an ovary. **phantom p.,** false pregnancy due to psychogenic factors. **tubal p.,** ectopic pregnancy within a uterine tube. **tuboabdominal p.,** ectopic pregnancy occurring partly in the fimbriated end of the oviduct and partly in the abdominal cavity. **tubo-ovarian p.,** pregnancy at the fimbria of the uterine tube.

pregnane (preg′nān) a crystalline saturated steroid hydrocarbon, $C_{21}H_{36}$; *β-pregnane* is the form from which several hormones, including progesterone, are derived; *α-pregnane* is the form excreted in the urine.

pregnanediol (preg″nān′di-ol) a crystalline, biologically inactive dihydroxy derivative of pregnane, formed by reduction of progesterone and found especially in urine of pregnant women.

pregnanetriol (preg″nān-tri′ol) a metabolite of 17-hydroxyprogesterone; its excretion in the urine is greatly increased in certain disorders of the adrenal cortex.

pregnant (preg′nant) with child; gravid.

pregnene (preg′nēn) a compound which forms the chemical nucleus of progesterone.

pregneninolone (preg″nēn-in′o-lōn) ethisterone.

prehallux (pre-hal′uks) a supernumerary bone of the foot growing from the medial border of the scaphoid.

prehemiplegic (pre″hem-ĭ-ple′jik) preceding hemiplegia.

prehensile (pre-hen′sil) adapted for grasping or seizing.

prehension (-hen′shun) the act of grasping.

prehyoid (-hi′oid) in front of the hyoid bone.

prehypophysis (pre″hi-pof′ĭ-sis) the anterior lobe of the pituitary gland.

preictal (pre-ik′tal) occurring before a stroke, seizure, or attack.

preicteric (pre″ik-ter′ik) preceding the appearance of jaundice (icterus).

preinvasive (-in-va′siv) not yet invading tissues outside the site of origin.

preleukemia (-lu-ke′me-ah) a stage of bone marrow dysfunction preceding the development of acute myelogenous leukemia. **preleuke′mic,** adj.

prelimbic (pre-lim′bik) in front of a limbus.

premalignant (pre″mah-lig′nant) precancerous.

premature (-mah-tūr′) 1. occurring before the proper time. 2. a premature infant.

prematurity (-tūr′ĭ-te) underdevelopment; the condition of a premature infant.

premaxilla (pre″mak-sil′ah) incisive bone.

premaxillary (pre-mak′sĭ-ler″e) 1. in front of the maxilla. 2. pertaining to the premaxilla (incisive bone).

premedication (pre″med-ĭ-ka′shun) preliminary medication, particularly internal medication to produce narcosis prior to general anesthesia.

premenarchal (-mĕ-nar′kal) occurring before establishment of menstruation.

premenstrual (pre-men′stroo-al) preceding menstruation.

premenstruum (-men′stroo-um) the period immediately before menstruation.

premolar (-mo′lar) in front of the molar teeth; see under *tooth.*

premonocyte (-mon′o-sīt) promonocyte.

premorbid (-mor′bid) occurring before development of disease.

premunition (pre″mu-nish′un) resistance to infection by the same or closely related pathogen established after an acute infection has become chronic, and lasting as long as the infecting organisms are in the body. **premu′nitive,** adj.

premyeloblast (pre-mi′ĕ-lo-blast″) precursor of a myeloblast.

premyelocyte (-sīt″) promyelocyte.

prenatal (pre-na′tal) preceding birth.

preneoplastic (pre″ne-o-plas′tik) before the formation of a tumor.

prenylamine (prĕ-nil′ah-men) a coronary vasodilator, $C_{24}H_{27}N$.

preoperative (pre-op′er-a″tiv) preceding an operation.

preoptic (-op′tik) in front of the optic chiasm.

preoral (-o′ral) in front of the mouth.

preparalytic (pre″par-ah-lit′ik) preceding paralysis.

prepatellar (-pah-tel′ar) in front of the patella.

prepuberal, prepubertal (pre-pu′ber-al; -pu′ber-tal) before puberty; pertaining to the period of accelerated growth preceding gonadal maturity.

prepubescent (pre″pu-bes′ent) prepubertal.

prepuce (pre′pūs) the foreskin: a cutaneous fold over the glans penis. **prepu′tial,** adj. **p. of clitoris,** a fold capping the clitoris formed by union of the labia minora and the clitoris.

preputiotomy (pre-pu″she-ot′o-me) incision of the prepuce to relieve phimosis.

preputium (-pu′she-um) prepuce.

prepyloric (pre″pi-lor′ik) just proximal to the pylorus.

presacral (pre-sa′kral) anterior to the sacrum.

presby- word element [Gr.], *old age.*

presbyatrics (pres″be-at′riks) geriatrics.

presbycardia (pres″bĭ-kar′de-ah) impaired cardiac function attributed to aging, with senescent changes in the body and no evidence of other cause of heart disease.

presbycusis (-ku′sis) progressive, bilaterally symmetrical perceptive hearing loss occurring with age.

presbyope (pres′be-ōp) one who is presbyopic.

presbyophrenia (pres″be-o-fre′ne-ah) loss of memory, disorientation, and confabulation, occurring in old age.

presbyopia (-o′pe-ah) diminution of accommodation of the lens of the eye occurring normally with aging. **presbyop′ic,** adj.

prescription (pre-skrip′shun) a written directive for the preparation and administration of a remedy; see also *inscription, signature, subscription,* and *superscription.*

presenile (-se′nīl) pertaining to a condition resembling senility, but occurring in early or middle life.

presentation (prez″en-ta′shun) lie; the relationship of the long axis of the fetus to that of the mother. Cf. *position.* **breech p.,** presentation of the fetal buttocks or feet in labor; the feet may be alongside the buttocks (*complete breech p.*); the legs may be extended against the trunk and the feet lying against the face (*frank breech p.*); or one or both feet or knees may be prolapsed into the maternal vagina (*incomplete breech p.*). **brow p.,** presentation of the fetal brow in labor. **cephalic p.,** presentation of any part of the fetal head in labor, whether the vertex, face, or brow. **compound p.,** prolapse of an extremity of the fetus alongside the head in cephalic presentation or of one or both arms alongside a presenting breech at the beginning of labor. **footling p.,** presentation of the fetus with one (single footling) or both (double footling) feet prolapsed into the maternal vagina. **funic p.,** presentation of the umbilical cord in labor. **longitudinal p.,** that in which the long axis of the fetus lies parallel to that of the mother, with either the head or breech the presenting part. **oblique p.,** that in which the long axis of the fetal body lies obliquely to that of the mother; the shoulder presents first. **placental p.,** placenta previa. **shoulder p.,** see *oblique p.* and *transverse lie.* **transverse p.,** see under *lie.* **vertex p.,** that in which the vertex of the fetal head is the presenting part.

preservative (pre-zer′vah-tiv) a substance or preparation added to a product to destroy or inhibit multiplication of microorganisms.

presomite (-so′mīt) referring to embryos before the appearance of somites.

presphenoid (-sfe′noid) the anterior portion of the body of the sphenoid bone.

presphygmic (-sfig′mik) preceding the pulse wave.

prespinal (-spi′nal) in front of the spine.

pressor (pres′or) tending to increase blood pressure.

pressoreceptive (pres″o-re-sep′tiv) sensitive to stimuli due to vasomotor activity.

pressoreceptor (-re-sep′tor) a receptor or nerve ending sensitive to stimuli of vasomotor activity.

pressosensitive (-sen′sĭ-tiv) pressoreceptive.

pressure (presh′ur) stress or strain, by compression, expansion, pull, thrust, or shear. **arterial p.,** blood pressure in the arteries. **atmospheric p.,** the pressure exerted by the atmosphere, about 15 pounds to the square inch at sea level. **blood p.,** the pressure of the blood on the walls of the arteries, dependent on the energy of the heart action, elasticity of the arterial walls, and volume and viscosity of the blood; the *maximum* or *systolic* pressure occurs near the end of the stroke output of the left ventricle, and the *minimum* or *diastolic* late in ventricular diastole. **capillary p.,** blood pressure in the capillaries. **cerebrospinal p.,** the pressure or tension of the cerebrospinal fluid, normally 100–150 mm. as measured by the manometer. **intracranial p.,** pressure of the subarachnoidal fluid. **intraocular p.,** the pressure exerted against the outer coats by the contents of the eyeball. **negative p.,** pressure less than that of the atmosphere. **oncotic p.,** the osmotic pressure due to the presence of colloids in solution. **osmotic p.,** the potential pressure of a solution directly related to its solute osmolar concentration; it is the maximum pressure developed by osmosis in a solution separated from another by a semipermeable membrane, i.e., the pressure that will just prevent osmosis between two such solutions. **partial p.,** pressure exerted by each of the constituents of a mixture of gases. **positive p.,** pressure greater than that of the atmosphere. **pulse p.,** the difference between systolic and diastolic pressures. **venous p.,** blood pressure in the veins.

presternum (pre-ster′num) the manubrium of the sternum.

presubiculum (pre″su-bik′u-lum) a modified six-layered cortex between the subiculum and the main part of the parahippocampal gyrus.

presuppurative (pre-sup′u-ra″tiv) preceding suppuration.

presymptomatic (pre″simp-to-mat′ik) existing before the appearance of symptoms.

presynaptic (-sĭ-nap′tik) situated or occurring proximal to a synapse.

presystole (pre-sis′to-le) the interval just before systole.

presystolic (pre″sis-tol′ik) just before systole.

pretarsal (pre-tar′sal) in front of the tarsus.

pretibial (-tib′e-al) in front of the tibia.

prevalence (prev′ah-lens) the total number of cases of a specific disease in existence in a given population at a certain time.

preventive (pre-ven′tiv) prophylactic.

prevertebral (-ver′tĕ-bral) in front of a vertebra.

prevesical (-ves′ĭ-kal) anterior to the bladder.

prezygotic (pre″zi-got′ik) occurring before completion of fertilization.

priapism (pri′ah-pizm) persistent abnormal erection of penis, accompanied by pain and tenderness.

prilocaine (pril′o-kān) a local anesthetic, $C_{13}H_{20}N_2O$, used as the hydrochloride salt.

primaquine (pri′mah-kwin) a compound used as an antimalarial, $C_{15}H_{21}N_3O$, being gametocidal to all forms of malaria; used as the phosphate salt.

primate (pri′māt) an individual of the Primates.

Primates (pri-ma′tēz) the highest order of mammals, including man, apes, monkeys, and lemurs.

primidone (pri′mĭ-dōn) an anticonvulsant, $C_{12}H_{14}N_2O_2$.

primigravida (pri″mĭ-grav′ĭ-dah) a woman pregnant for the first time; gravida I.

primipara (pri-mip′ah-rah) para 1; a woman who has had one pregnancy that resulted in a viable young. See *para*. **primip′arous,** adj.

primiparity (pri″mĭ-par′ĭ-te) the state of being a primipara.

primitive (prim′ĭ-tiv) first in point of time; existing in a simple or early form; showing little evolution.

primordial (pri-mor′de-al) original or primitive; of the simplest and most undeveloped character.

primordium (pri-mor′de-um) the earliest indication during embryonic development of an organ or part.

Prinadol (prin′ah-dol) trademark for a preparation of phenazocine.

princeps (prin′seps) [L.] principal; chief.

principle (prin′sĭ-p'l) 1. a chemical component. 2. a substance on which certain of the properties of a drug depend. 3. a law of conduct. **active p.,** any constituent of a drug which helps to confer upon it a medicinal property. **antianemia p.,** the constituent in liver and certain other tissues (vitamin B_{12}) that produces the hematopoietic effect in pernicious anemia. **immediate p.,** any of the more or less complex substances of definite chemical constitution into which a heterogenous substance can be readily resolved. **pleasure p.,** the automatic instinct or tendency to avoid pain and secure pleasure. **proximate p.,** immediate p. **reality p.,** in freudian terminology, the mental activity which develops to control the pleasure principle under the pressure of necessity or the demands of reality.

Priodax (pri′o-daks) trademark for a preparation of iodoalphionic acid.

Priscoline (pris′ko-lēn) trademark for preparations of tolazoline.

prism (prizm) a solid with a triangular or polygonal cross section. **adamantine p's, enamel p's,** the microscopic prisms or columns, arranged perpendicular to the surface, which make up the tooth enamel. **Nicol p.,** one composed of two slabs of Iceland spar, for polarizing light. **Risley's p.,** a prism that rotates in a metal frame marked with a scale; for testing ocular muscles.

prismosphere (priz′mo-sfēr) a prism combined with a spherical lens.

Privine (pri′vēn) trademark for preparations of naphazoline.

p.r.n. [L.] *pro re na′ta* (according to circumstances).

Pro proline.

pro- word element [L., Gr.], *before; in front of; favoring.*

proaccelerin (pro″ak-sel′er-in) coagulation Factor V.

proactinomycin (pro-ak″tin-o-mi′sin) a group of antibiotics, designated A, B, and C, from cultures of *Nocardia gardneri,* active against gram-positive bacteria.

proactivator (-ak″tĭ-va′tor) a precursor of an activator; a factor which reacts with an enzyme to form an activator.

proatlas (-at′las) a rudimentary vertebra which in some animals lies in front of the atlas; sometimes seen in man as an anomaly.

proband (pro′band) propositus.

probang (-bang) a flexible rod with a ball, tuft, or sponge at one end; used to apply medications to or remove matter from the esophagus or larynx.

Pro-Banthine (pro-ban-thīn′) trademark for preparations of propantheline.

probarbital (-bar′bĭ-tal) a barbiturate $C_9H_{14}N_2O$, used as a sedative in the form of the calcium and sodium salts.

probe (prōb) a long, slender instrument for exploring wounds or body cavities or passages.

probenecid (pro-ben′ĕ-sid) a drug, $C_{13}H_{19}NO_4S$, used as a uricosuric agent in the treatment of gout; also used to increase serum concentration of certain antibiotics and other drugs.

procainamide (-kān′ah-mīd) a cardiac depressant, $C_{13}H_{21}N_3O$, used as the hydrochloride salt in the treatment of arrhythmias.

procaine (pro′kān) a local anesthetic, $C_{12}H_{20}N_2O_2$; the hydrochloride salt is used in solution for infiltration, nerve block, and spinal anesthesia.

procarboxypeptidase (pro″kar-bok″se-pep′tĭ-dās) the inactive precursor of carboxypeptidase, which is converted to the active enzyme by the action of trypsin.

procelous (pro-se′lus) having the anterior surface concave; said of vertebrae.

procentriole (-sen′tre-ōl) the immediate precursor of centrioles and ciliary basal bodies.

procephalic (pro″sĕ-fal′ik) pertaining to the anterior part of the head.

procercoid (pro-ser′koid) a larval stage of fish tapeworms.

process (pros′es) 1. a prominence or projection, as from a bone. 2. a series of operations, events, or steps leading to achievement of a specific result; also, to subject to such a series to produce desired changes. **acromial p.,** acromion. **alveolar p.,** the part of the bone in either the maxilla or mandible surrounding and supporting the teeth. **basilar p.,** a quadrilateral plate of the occipital bone projecting superiorly and anteriorly from the foramen magnum. **caudate p.,** the right of the two processes on the caudate lobe of the liver. **ciliary p's,** meridionally arranged ridges or folds projecting from the crown of the ciliary body. **clinoid p.,** any of the three (anterior, medial, and posterior) processes of the sphenoid bone. **coracoid p.,** a curved process arising from the upper neck of the scapula and overhanging the shoulder joint. **coronoid p.,** 1. the anterior part of the upper end of the ramus of the mandible. 2. a projection at the proximal end of the ulna. **ensiform p.,** xiphoid p. **ethmoid p.,** a bony projection above and behind the maxillary process of the inferior nasal concha. **falciform p.,** 1. the lateral margin of the saphenous hiatus. 2. falx cerebri. **frontonasal p.,** an expansive facial process in the embryo which develops into the forehead and bridge of the nose. **funicular p.,** the portion of the tunica vaginalis surrounding the spermatic cord. **lacrimal p.,** a process of the inferior nasal concha that articulates with the lacrimal bone. **malar p.,** zygomatic p. of maxilla. **mamillary p.,** a tubercle on each superior articular process of a lumbar vertebra. **mandibular p.,** one of the processes formed by bifurcation of the first branchial arch in the embryo, which unites ventrally with its fellow to form the lower jaw. **mastoid p.,** the conical projection at the base of the mastoid portion of the temporal bone. **maxillary p.,** 1. one of the processes formed by bifurcation of the first branchial arch in the embryo, which joins with the ipsilateral median nasal process in the formation of the upper jaw. 2. a bony process descending from the ethmoid process of the inferior nasal concha. **odontoid p.,** a toothlike projection of the axis which articulates with the atlas. **pterygoid p.,** one of the wing-shaped processes of the sphenoid. **spinous p. of vertebrae,** a part of the vertebrae projecting backward from the arch, giving attachment to the back muscles. **styloid p.,** a long pointed projection, especially a long spine projecting downward from the inferior surface of the temporal bone. **uncinate p.,** any hooklike process, as of vertebrae, the lacrimal bone, or the pancreas. **xiphoid p.,** the pointed process of cartilage, supported by a core of bone, connected with the lower end of the sternum. **zygomatic p.,** a projection from the frontal or temporal bone, or from the maxilla, by which they articulate with the zygomatic bone.

processus (pro-ses'us), pl. *proces'sus* [L.] process; used in official names of various anatomic structures.

prochlorperazine (pro-per'ah-zēn) a phenothiazine derivative, $C_{20}H_{24}ClN_3S$, used as a tranquilizer and antiemetic.

prochondral (-kon'dral) occurring before the formation of cartilage.

procidentia (pro"sĭ-den'she-ah) a state of prolapse, especially of the uterus.

proclonol (pro'klo-nōl) an anthelminthic and antifungal, $C_{16}H_{14}Cl_2O$.

procoagulant (pro"ko-ag'u-lant) 1. tending to promote coagulation. 2. a precursor of a natural substance necessary to coagulation of the blood.

proconvertin (-ver'tin) coagulation Factor VII.

procreation (-kre-a'shun) the act of begetting or generating.

proct(o)- word element [Gr.], *rectum;* see also words beginning *rect(o)-.*

proctalgia (prok-tal'je-ah) pain in the rectum.

proctatresia (prok"tah-tre'ze-ah) imperforate anus.

proctectasia (prok"tek-ta'ze-ah) dilatation of the rectum or anus.

proctectomy (prok-tek'to-me) excision of the rectum.

procteurynter (prok"tu-rin'ter) a baglike device used to dilate the rectum.

proctitis (prok-ti'tis) inflammation of the rectum.

proctocele (prok'to-sēl) rectocele.

proctoclysis (prok-tok'lĭ-sis) slow introduction of large quantities of liquid into the rectum.

proctocolonoscopy (prok"to-ko"lon-os'ko-pe) inspection of the interior of the rectum and lower colon.

proctocolpoplasty (-kol'po-plas"te) repair of a rectovaginal fistula.

proctocystoplasty (-sis'to-plas"te) repair of a rectovesical fistula.

proctocystotomy (-sis-tot'o-me) removal of a vesical stone through the rectum.

proctodeum (-de'um) the ectodermal depression of the caudal end of the embryo, where later the anus is formed.

proctodynia (-din'e-ah) proctalgia.

proctology (prok-tol'o-je) the branch of medicine concerned with disorders of the rectum and anus. **proctolog'ic,** adj.

proctoparalysis (prok"to-pah-ral'ĭ-sis) paralysis of the anal and rectal muscles.

proctopexy (prok'to-pek"se) surgical fixation of the rectum.

proctoplasty (-plas"te) plastic repair of the rectum.

proctoplegia (prok"to-ple'je-ah) proctoparalysis.

proctoptosis (prok"top-to'sis) prolapse of the rectum.

proctorrhaphy (prok-tor'ah-fe) surgical repair of the rectum.

proctorrhea (prok"to-re'ah) a mucous discharge from the anus.

proctoscope (prok'to-skōp) a speculum or tubular instrument with illumination for inspecting the rectum.

proctoscopy (prok-tos'ko-pe) inspection of the lower part of the intestine with a proctoscope.

proctosigmoidectomy (prok"to-sig"moi-dek'to-me) rectosigmoidectomy.

proctosigmoiditis (-sig"moi-di'tis) inflammation of the rectum and sigmoid colon.

proctosigmoidoscopy (-sig"moi-dos'ko-pe) examination of the rectum and sigmoid colon with the sigmoidoscope.

proctospasm (prok'to-spazm) spasm of the rectum.

proctostenosis (prok"to-stĕ-no'sis) stricture of the rectum.

proctostomy (prok-tos'to-me) creation of a permanent artificial opening from the body surface into the rectum.

proctotomy (prok-tot'o-me) incision of the rectum.

proctovalvotomy (prok"to-val-vot'o-me) incision of the rectal valves.

procumbent (pro-kum'bent) prone; lying on the face.

procursive (-ker'siv) tending to run forward.

procyclidine (-si′klĭ-dēn) a synthetic drug, C_{19}-$H_{29}NO$, used as the hydrochloride salt in treatment of parkinsonism.

prodrome (pro′drōm) a premonitory symptom; a symptom indicating the onset of a disease. **prodro′mal, prodro′mic,** adj.

product (prod′ukt) something produced. **cleavage p.,** a substance formed by splitting of a compound molecule into a simpler one. **fission p.,** an isotope, usually radioactive, of an element in the middle of the periodic table, produced by fission of a heavy element under bombardment with high-energy particles. **spallation p's,** the isotopes of many different chemical elements produced in small amounts in nuclear fission. **substitution p.,** a substance formed by substitution of one atom or radical in a molecule by another atom or radical.

productive (pro-duk′tiv) producing or forming; said especially of an inflammation that produces new tissue or of a cough that brings forth sputum or mucus.

proencephalus (pro″en-sef′ah-lus) a fetus with protrusion of the brain through a frontal fissure.

proenzyme (pro-en′zīm) zymogen; an inactive precursor of an enzyme.

proerythroblast (pro″ĕ-rith′ro-blast) pronormoblast.

proestrus (pro-es′trus) the period of heightened follicular activity preceding estrus.

profadol (pro′fah-dōl) a non-narcotic analgesic, $D_{14}H_{21}NO$.

profenamine (pro-fen′ah-mēn) ethopropazine.

profibrinolysin (-fi″brĭ-no-li′sin) plasminogen.

profile (pro′fīl) a simple outline as of the side view of the head or face; by extension, a graph representing quantitatively a set of characteristics determined by tests.

proflavine (pro-fla′vin) a constituent of acriflavine, $C_{13}H_{11}N_3$, used as a topical and urinary antiseptic in the form of the hemisulfate salt.

profundus (-fun′dus) [L.] deep.

progastrin (-gas′trin) an inactive precursor of gastrin.

progeria (pro-je′re-ah) premature old age, a condition occurring in childhood marked by small stature, absence of facial and pubic hair, wrinkled skin, gray hair, and eventual development of atherosclerosis.

progestational (pro″jes-ta′shun-al) 1. referring to that phase of the menstrual cycle just before menstruation, when the corpus luteum is active and the endometrium is secreting. 2. denoting a class of pharmaceutical preparations having effects similar to those of progesterone.

progesterone (pro-jes′tĕ-rōn) the steroid hormone produced by the corpus luteum, adrenal cortex, and placenta which serves to prepare the uterus for reception and development of the fertilized ovum by inducing secretion in the proliferated glands. A synthetic preparation is used in the treatment of functional uterine bleeding, menstrual cycle abnormalities, and threatened abortion.

progestin (-jes′tin) originally, the crude hormone of the corpus luteum; it has since been isolated in pure form and is now known as *progesterone*. Certain synthetic and natural progestational agents are called progestins.

progestogen (-jes′to-jen) any substance having progestational activity.

proglossis (-glos′is) the tip of the tongue.

proglottid (-glot′id) one of the segments making up the body of a tapeworm; see *strobila*.

proglottis (-glot′is) proglottid.

prognathism (prog′nah-thizm) abnormal protrusion of one or both jaws, especially the lower jaw, the gnathic index being above 103. **prognath′ic, prog′nathous,** adj.

prognose (prog-nōs′) to give a prognosis.

prognosis (prog-no′sis) a forecast of the probable course and outcome of a disorder. **prognos′tic,** adj.

progranulocyte (pro-gran′u-lo-sīt″) promyelocyte.

progravid (-grav′id) denoting the phase of the endometrium in which it is prepared for pregnancy.

progressive (-gres′iv) advancing; increasing in scope or severity.

proguanil (-gwan′il) an antimalarial, $C_{11}H_{16}Cl$-N_5, effective against *Plasmodium falciparum;* used as the hydrochloride salt.

Progynon (-jin′on) trademark for preparations of estradiol.

proinsulin (-in′su-lin) a precursor of insulin, having low biologic activity.

projection (pro-jek′shun) 1. a throwing forward, especially the reference of impressions made on the sense organs to their proper source, so as to locate correctly the objects producing them. 2. a connection between the cerebral cortex and other parts of the nervous system or organs of special sense. 3. the act of extending or jutting out, or a part that juts out. 4. a mental mechanism by which a repressed complex is regarded as belonging to the external world or to someone else.

prokaryon (-kar′e-on) 1. nuclear material scattered in the cytoplasm of the cell, rather than bounded by a nuclear membrane; found in some unicellular organisms, such as bacteria. 2. prokaryote.

prokaryote (-kar′e-ōt) an organism without a true nucleus, the nuclear material being scattered in the cytoplasm of the cell, and which reproduces by cell division. **prokaryot′ic,** adj.

prolabium (-la′be-um) the prominent central part of the upper lip.

prolactin (-lak′tin) a hormone of the anterior pituitary which stimulates and sustains lactation in postpartum mammals, and shows luteotropic activity in certain mammals.

prolamine (-lam′in) any of a class of simple proteins insoluble in water and absolute alcohol, but soluble in 70–80% alcohol; obtained principally from cereals.

prolapse (pro′laps) 1. the falling down, or downward displacement, of a part or viscus. 2. to undergo such displacement. **p. of cord,** protrusion of the umbilical cord ahead of the presenting part of the fetus in labor. **p. of the iris,**

protrusion of the iris through a wound in the cornea. **Morgagni's p.,** chronic inflammatory hyperplasia of the mucosa and submucosa of the sacculus laryngis. **rectal p., p. of rectum,** protrusion of the rectal mucous membrane through the anus. **p. of uterus,** downward displacement of the uterus so that the cervix is within the vaginal orifice (*first-degree p.*), the cervix is outside the orifice (*second-degree p.*), or the entire uterus is outside the orifice (*third-degree p.*).

prolapsus (pro-lap′sus) [L.] prolapse.

prolepsis (-lep′sis) recurrence of a paroxysm before the expected time. **prolep′tic,** adj.

prolidase (pro′lĭ-dās) an enzyme which catalyzes the hydrolysis of the imide bond between an α-carboxyl group and proline or hydroxyproline.

proliferation (-lif″ĕ-ra′shun) the reproduction or multiplication of similar forms, especially of cells. **prolif′erative, prolif′erous,** adj.

proligerous (pro-lij′er-us) producing offspring.

prolinase (pro′lĭ-nās) an enzyme that catalyzes the hydrolysis of dipeptides containing proline or hydroxyproline as N-terminal groups.

proline (-lēn) a naturally occurring amino acid discovered in 1901.

Prolixin (pro-lik′sin) trademark for preparations of fluphenazine.

Proluton (-lu′ton) trademark for preparations of progesterone.

prolymphocyte (-lim′fo-sīt) a cell of the lymphocytic series intermediate between the lymphoblast and lymphocyte.

promastigote (-mas′tĭ-gōt) the morphologic stage in the development of certain protozoa, characterized by a free anterior flagellum and resembling the typical adult form of *Leptomonas.*

promazine (pro′mah-zēn) a phenothiazine derivative, $C_{17}H_{20}N_2S$, used as a major tranquilizer in the form of the hydrochloride salt.

promegakaryocyte (pro″meg-ah-kar′e-o-sīt″) a developmental form of the platelet-producing megakaryocyte series, intermediate between the megakaryoblast and the megakaryocyte.

promegaloblast (pro-meg′ah-lo-blast″) the earliest form in the abnormal erythrocyte maturation sequence occurring in vitamin B_{12} and folic acid deficiencies; it corresponds to the pronormoblast, and develops into a megaloblast.

promethazine (-meth′ah-zēn) a phenothiazine derivative, $C_{17}H_{20}N_2S$; the hydrochloride salt is used as an antihistaminic, antiemetic, and tranquilizer.

promethestrol (-meth′es-trol) a synthetic estrogenic agent, $C_{20}H_{26}O_2$, used as the dipropionate ester.

promethium (-me′the-um) chemical element (*see table*), at. no. 61, symbol Pm.

Promin (pro′min) trademark for a preparation of glucosulfone.

promine (-mēn) a substance widely distributed in animal cells, characterized by its ability to promote cell division and growth.

prominence (prom′ĭ-nens) a protrusion or projection.

promonocyte (pro-mon′o-sīt) a cell of the monocytic series intermediate between the monoblast and monocyte, with coarse chromatin structure and one or two nucleoli.

promontory (prom′on-tor″e) a projecting process or eminence.

promoxolane (pro-mok′so-lān) a skeletal muscle relaxant and tranquilizer, $C_{10}H_{20}O_3$.

promyelocyte (-mi′ĕ-lo-sīt″) a precursor of the granular leukocytes, intermediate between myeloblast and myelocyte, containing a few, as yet undifferentiated, cytoplasmic granules.

pronate (pro′nāt) to subject to pronation.

pronation (pro-na′shun) the act of assuming the prone position, or the state of being prone. Applied to the hand, the act of turning the palm backward (posteriorly) or downward, performed by medial rotation of the forearm. Applied to the foot, a combination of eversion and abduction movements taking place in the tarsal and metatarsal joints and resulting in lowering of the medial margin of the foot, hence of the longitudinal arch.

pronator (-na′tor) a muscle that pronates.

prone (prōn) lying face downward.

pronephros (pro-nef′ros), pl. *proneph′roi* [Gr.] the primordial kidney; an excretory structure or its rudiments developing in the embryo before the mesonephros; its duct is later used by the mesonephros, which arises caudal to it.

Pronestyl (-nes′til) trademark for preparations of procainamide.

pronethalol (-neth′ah-lōl) a β-adrenergic blocking agent.

pronograde (pro′no-grād) walking with the body approximately horizontal; applied to quadrupeds.

pronormoblast (pro-nor′mo-blast) the earliest erythrocyte precursor, having a relatively large nucleus containing several nucleoli, surrounded by a small amount of cytoplasm; see also *normoblast.*

pronucleus (-nu′kle-us) the haploid nucleus of a sex cell. **female p.,** the haploid nucleus of the fully mature ovum which loses its nuclear envelope and liberates its chromosomes to meet in synapsis with those from the male pronucleus. **male p.,** the nuclear material of the head of a spermatozoon, after it has penetrated the ovum and acquired a pronuclear membrane.

prootic (-o′tik) in front of the ear.

Propadrine (pro′pah-drēn) trademark for a preparation of phenylpropanolamine.

propagation (prop″ah-ga′shun) reproduction. **prop′agative,** adj.

propane (pro′pān) a gaseous hydrocarbon from petroleum and natural gas.

propanolide (pro-pan′o-līd) propiolactone.

propantheline (-pan′thĕ-lēn) an anticholinergic, $C_{23}H_{30}NO_3$, used as the bromide salt, especially in the treatment of peptic ulcer.

proparacaine (-par′ah-kān) a topical anesthetic, $C_{16}H_{26}N_2O_3$, used as the hydrochloride salt.

propepsin (-pep′sin) pepsinogen.

propeptone (-pep′tōn) hemialbumose.

properdin (pro′per-din) a relatively heat-labile, normal serum protein (a euglobulin) that, in the presence of complement component C3 and magnesium ions, acts nonspecifically against gram-negative bacteria and viruses and plays a role in lysis of erythrocytes. It migrates as a β-globulin, and although not an antibody, may act in conjunction with complement-fixing antibody.

prophage (-fāj) the latent stage of a phage in a lysogenic bacterium, in which the viral genome becomes inserted into a specific portion of the host chromosome and is duplicated in each cell generation.

prophase (-fāz) the first stage in cell reduplication in either meiosis or mitosis.

prophenpyridamine (pro″fen-pi-rid′ah-mēn) pheniramine.

prophylactic (-fĭ-lak′tik) 1. tending to ward off disease; pertaining to prophylaxis. 2. an agent that tends to ward off disease.

prophylaxis (-fĭ-lak′sis) prevention of disease; preventive treatment.

propiolactone (pro″pe-o-lak′tōn) a disinfectant, $C_3H_4O_2$.

propiomazine (-ma′zēn) a phenothiazine derivative, $C_{20}H_{24}N_2OS$, used as a tranquilizer in the form of the hydrochloride salt.

Propionibacterium (-bak-te′re-um) a genus of gram-positive bacteria found as saprophytes in dairy products.

proplasmacyte (pro-plaz′mah-sīt) a cell intermediate between the plasmablast and the plasmacyte (plasma cell).

proplastid (-plas′tid) an organelle that develops into a plastid as the cell matures.

propositus (-poz′ĭ-tus), pl. *propos′iti* [L.] the original person presenting a mental or physical disorder who serves as the basis for a hereditary or genetic study.

propoxycaine (-pok′se-kān) a local anesthetic, $C_{16}H_{26}N_2O_3$, used as the hydrochloride salt.

propoxyphene (-pok′se-fēn) an analgesic, $C_{22}H_{29}NO_2$, used as the hydrochloride and napsylate salts.

propranolol (-pran′o-lōl) a β-adrenergic blocking agent, $C_{16}H_{21}NO_2$, used in the treatment of cardiac arrhythmias and hypertrophic subaortic stenosis.

proprietary (-pri′ĕ-ter″e) 1. denoting a medicine protected against free competition as to name, composition, or manufacturing process by patent, trademark, copyright, or secrecy. 2. a medicine so protected.

proprioceptor (pro″pre-o-sep′tor) any of the sensory nerve endings that give information concerning movements and position of the body; they occur chiefly in muscles, tendons, and the labyrinth. **propriocep′tive**, adj.

proptometer (pro-tom′ĕ-ter) an instrument for measuring the degree of exophthalmos.

proptosis (prop-to′sis) forward displacement or bulging, especially of the eye.

propulsion (pro-pul′shun) 1. a tendency to fall forward in walking. 2. festination.

propyl (pro′pil) the univalent radical CH_3CH_2-CH_2— from propane.

propylene (-pĭ-lēn) a gaseous hydrocarbon, $CH_3 \cdot CH{:}CH_2$, having anesthetic properties. **p. glycol,** a colorless, viscous liquid used as a humectant and solvent.

propylhexedrine (pro″pil-hek′sĕ-drēn) an adrenergic, $C_{10}H_{21}N$, given by inhalation to decongest the nasal mucosa.

propyliodone (-i′o-dōn) a radiopaque medium, $C_{10}H_{11}I_2NO_3$, used in bronchography.

propylparaben (-par′ah-ben) an antifungal preservative, $C_{10}H_{12}O_3$.

propylthiouracil (-thi″o-u′rah-sil) a thyroid inhibitor, $C_7H_{10}N_2OS$.

pro re nata (pro ra nah′tah) [L.] according to circumstances. Abbreviated p.r.n.

prorennin (pro-ren′in) the zymogen (proenzyme) in the gastric glands that is converted to rennin.

prorubricyte (-roo′brĭ-sīt) basophilic normoblast.

pros(o)- word element [Gr.], *forward; anterior.*

proscillaridin A (pro″sil-ar′ĭ-din) a cardiac glycoside, $C_{30}H_{42}O_8$, used as a cardiotonic.

prosecretin (-se-kre′tin) the precursor of secretin.

prosection (pro-sek′shun) carefully programmed dissection for demonstration of anatomic structure.

prosector (-sek′tor) one who performs prosection.

prosencephalon (pros″en-sef′ah-lon) forebrain.

prosodemic (pros″o-dem′ik) passing directly from one person to another; said of disease.

prosop(o)- word element [Gr.], *face.*

prosopagnosia (-pag-no′se-ah) inability to recognize faces.

prosopalgia (-pal′je-ah) trigeminal neuralgia. **prosopal′gic,** adj.

prosopectasia (-pek-ta′ze-ah) oversize of the face.

prosoplasia (-pla′se-ah) 1. abnormal differentiation of tissue. 2. development into a higher level of organization or function.

prosopodiplegia (pros″o-po-di-ple′je-ah) paralysis of the face and one lower extremity.

prosoponeuralgia (-nu-ral′je-ah) facial neuralgia.

prosopoplegia (-ple′je-ah) facial paralysis. **prosopople′gic,** adj.

prosoposchisis (pros″o-pos′kĭ-sis) congenital fissure of the face.

prosopospasm (pros′o-po-spazm″) spasm of the facial muscles.

prosoposternodymia (pros″o-po-ster″no-dim′-e-ah) a double monster joined face to face and sternum to sternum.

prosopothoracopagus (-tho″rah-kop′ah-gus) twin fetuses fused from the face to the thorax.

prostaglandin (pros″tah-glan′din) a group of naturally occurring fatty acids found in semen, menstrual fluid, and various tissues of many species, which stimulate contractility of the uterine and other smooth muscle and have the ability to lower blood pressure and to affect the action of certain hormones. Four types, F, E, A, and B, are subdivided according to side-chain saturation as F_1, F_2, etc.

prostata (pros′tah-tah) prostate.

prostatalgia (pros″tah-tal′je-ah) pain in the prostate.

prostate (pros′tāt) a gland surrounding the neck of the bladder and urethra in the male; it contributes a secretion to the semen. **prostat′ic,** adj.

prostatectomy (pros″tah-tek′to-me) excision of all or part of the prostate.

prostatism (pros′tah-tizm) the signs and symptoms associated with prostatic lesions that produce malfunction of the urinary tract.

prostatitis (pros″tah-ti′tis) inflammation of the prostate. **prostatit′ic,** adj.

prostatocystitis (pros″tah-to-sis-ti′tis) inflammation of the neck of the bladder (prostatic urethra) and the bladder cavity.

prostatocystotomy (-sis-tot′o-me) incision of the bladder and prostate.

prostatodynia (-din′e-ah) pain in the prostate.

prostatolith (pros-tat′o-lith) a calculus in the prostate.

prostatolithotomy (pros″tah-to-lĭ-thot′o-me) incision of the prostate for removal of a calculus.

prostatomegaly (-meg′ah-le) hypertrophy of the prostate.

prostatorrhea (-re′ah) catarrhal discharge from the prostate.

prostatotomy (pros″tah-tot′o-me) surgical incision of the prostate.

prostatovesiculectomy (pros″tah-to-vĕ-sik″u-lek′to-me) excision of the prostate and seminal vesicles.

prostatovesiculitis (-vĕ-sik″u-li′tis) inflammation of the prostate and seminal vesicles.

prosthesis (pros-the′sis), pl. *prosthe′ses* [Gr.] an artificial substitute for a missing body part, such as an arm or leg, eye, or tooth, used for functional or cosmetic reasons, or both. **Cape-Town p.,** an aortic valve replacement inserted in conjunction with a cardiopulmonary bypass. **Cutter SCDK p.,** a double-cage modification of the Starr-Edwards prosthesis. **Magovern-Cromie p.,** a Starr-Edwards prosthesis fitted with multiple recessed pins for ejection into adjacent tissue to eliminate suturing. **Sauerbruch's p.,** an artificial limb given motion by the stump. **Starr-Edwards p.,** a caged-ball cardiac valve replacement, which prevents reflux of blood.

prosthetic (pros-thet′ik) serving as a substitute; pertaining to prostheses or to prosthetics.

prosthetics (pros-thet′iks) the field of knowledge relating to prostheses, their design, use, etc.

prosthetist (pros′thĕ-tist) a person skilled in prosthetics and practicing its application.

prosthion (pros′the-on) the point on the maxil-lary alveolar process that projects most anteriorly in the midline.

prosthodontics (pros″tho-don′tiks) that branch of dentistry concerned with the construction of artificial appliances designed to restore and maintain oral function by replacing missing teeth and sometimes other oral structures or parts of the face.

prosthodontist (-don′tist) a specialist in prosthodontics.

prostholith (pros′tho-lith) a preputial concretion or calculus.

Prostigmin (pro-stig′min) trademark for preparations of neostigmine.

prostration (pros-tra′shun) extreme exhaustion or lack of energy or power. **heat p.,** see under *exhaustion.* **nervous p.,** neurasthenia.

protactinium (pro″tak-tin′e-um) chemical element (*see table*), at. no. 91, symbol Pa.

protamine (pro′tah-min) one of a class of basic proteins occurring in the sperm of certain fish, having the property of neutralizing heparin; the sulfate salt is used as an antidote to heparin overdosage.

protanope (-tah-nōp″) a person exhibiting protanopia.

protanopia (pro″tah-no′pe-ah) red blindness; imperfect perception of red, with confusion of reds and greens. **protanop′ic,** adj.

protean (pro′te-an) changing form or assuming different shapes.

protease (te-ās) any proteolytic enzyme; see *peptidase.*

protectant, protective (pro-tek′tant; pro-tek′tiv) 1. affording defense or immunity. 2. an agent affording defense against harmful influence.

proteid (pro′te-id) protein.

protein (pro′te-in) any of a group of organic nitrogenous compounds, widely distributed in plants and animals, which are the principal constituents of the cell protoplasm. They are essentially combinations of α-amino acids in peptide linkages. **protein′ic,** adj. **Bence Jones p.,** a low-molecular weight, heat-sensitive urinary protein found in multiple myeloma, which coagulates when heated to 45°–55° C. and redissolves partially or wholly on boiling. **carrier p.,** one which, when coupled to a hapten, renders it capable of eliciting an immune response. **conjugated p's,** those in which the protein molecule is united with nonprotein molecule(s) (the prosthetic group) otherwise than as a salt. **C-reactive p.,** a globulin that forms a precipitate with the C-polysaccharide of the pneumococcus; its demonstration in the serum is an indicator of inflammation of infectious or noninfectious origin. **denatured p.,** one whose structure has been so changed, as by heat, that it has lost its unique properties. **derived p's,** derivatives of proteins formed by hydrolytic changes. **immune p's,** immunoglobulins. **native p.,** an unchanged, naturally occurring animal or vegetable protein. **plasma p's,** all the proteins present in the blood plasma, including the immunoglobulins. **serum p's,** proteins in the blood serum, including immunoglobulins, albumin, complement, coagulation factors, and enzymes. **simple p's,** those that yield only α-amino acids on complete hydrolysis.

proteinaceous (pro″te-in-a′shus) pertaining to or of the nature of protein.

proteinase (pro′te-in-ās″) any enzyme that catalyzes the splitting of interior peptide bonds in a protein; an endopeptidase.

proteinemia (pro″te-ĭ-ne′me-ah) excess of protein in the blood.

proteinosis (pro″te-in-o′sis) the accumulation of excess protein in the tissues. **lipid p.,** a hereditary defect of lipid metabolism marked by yellowish deposits of hyaline lipid-carbohydrate mixture on the inner surface of the lips, under the tongue, on the oropharynx and larynx, and by skin lesions. **pulmonary alveolar p.,** a chronic lung disease in which the distal alveoli become filled with a bland, eosinophilic, probably endogenous proteinaceous material that prevents ventilation of affected areas.

proteinuria (-u′re-ah) an excess of serum proteins in the urine. **proteinu′ric,** adj. **adventitious p.,** that not due to kidney disease. **cardiac p.,** that caused by cardiac disease. **dietetic p., digestive p.,** that produced by ingestion of certain foods. **false p.,** adventitious p. **functional p.,** proteinuria that is not truly pathologic, e.g., transient proteinurias of pregnancy and adolescence. **orthostatic p.,** proteinuria that appears on standing erect and disappears on lying down. **prerenal p.,** that due primarily to a disease other than kidney disease. **true p.,** that in which some of the protein elements of the blood are discharged in the urine.

proteolipid (pro″te-o-lip′id) a combination of a peptide or protein with a lipid, having the solubility characteristic of lipids.

proteolysis (pro″te-ol′ĭ-sis) the splitting of proteins by hydrolysis of the peptide bonds with formation of smaller polypeptides.

proteolytic (pro″te-o-lit′ik) 1. pertaining to, characterized by, or promoting proteolysis. 2. a proteolytic enzyme.

proteometabolism (-mĕ-tab′o-lizm) the metabolism of protein.

proteopeptic (-pep′tik) digesting protein.

proteose (pro′te-ōs) any of a group of derived proteins intermediate between native proteins and peptones.

proteosuria (pro″te-o-su′re-ah) presence of proteose in the urine.

Proteus (pro′te-us) a genus of gram-negative, motile bacteria usually found in fecal and other putrefying matter, including *P. morga′ni,* found in the intestines and associated with summer diarrhea of infants, and *P. vulga′ris,* often found as a secondary invader in various localized suppurative pathologic processes; it is a cause of cystitis.

prothipendyl (pro-thi′pen-dil) a sedative and tranquilizer, $C_{16}H_{19}N_3S$.

prothrombin (-throm′bin) coagulation Factor II.

prothrombinase (-throm′bin-ās) thromboplastin.

prothrombinogenic (pro-throm″bĭ-no-jen′ik) promoting the production of prothrombin.

protist (pro′tist) any member of the Protista.

Protista (pro-tis′tah) a kingdom comprising bacteria, algae, slime molds, fungi, and protozoa; it includes all single-celled organisms.

protistologist (pro″tis-tol′o-jist) a microbiologist.

protistology (pro″tis-tol′o-je) microbiology.

protium (pro′te-um) see *hydrogen.*

proto- word element [Gr.], *first.*

protoalbumose (pro″to-al′bu-mōs) a primary proteose.

protoblast (pro′to-blast) 1. a cell with no cell wall; an embryonic cell. 2. the nucleus of an ovum. 3. a blastomere from which a particular organ or part develops. **protoblas′tic,** adj.

protocol (-kol) the original notes made on a necropsy, an experiment, or on a case of disease.

protodiastolic (pro″to-di″ah-stol′ik) pertaining to early diastole, i.e., immediately following the second heart sound.

protoduodenum (-du″o-de′num) the first or proximal portion of the duodenum, extending from the pylorus to the duodenal papilla.

protoelastose (-e-las′tōs) hemielastose.

protofibril (-fi′bril) the first elongated unit appearing in formation of any type of fiber.

protogaster (-gas′ter) archenteron.

protoglobulose (-glob′u-lōs) a primary product formed in the digestion of globulin.

protokylol (-ki′lol) a sympathomimetic, $C_{18}H_{21}$-NO_5, used as a bronchodilator in the form of the hydrochloride salt.

protomerite (-mer′īt) the anterior portion of certain gregarine protozoa.

proton (pro′ton) an elementary particle that is the core or nucleus of an ordinary hydrogen atom of mass 1; the unit of positive electricity, being equivalent to the electron in charge and approximately to the hydrogen ion in mass.

protoneuron (pro″to-nu′ron) the first neuron in a peripheral reflex arc.

protoplasm (pro′to-plazm) the viscid, translucent colloid material, the essential constituent of the living cell, including cytoplasm and nucleoplasm. **protoplas′mic,** adj.

protoplast (-plast) a bacterial or plant cell deprived of its rigid wall but with its plasma membrane intact; the cell is dependent for its integrity on an isotonic or hypertonic medium.

protoporphyria (pro″to-por-fēr′e-ah) erythropoietic p.: porphyria marked by excessive protoporphyrin in erythrocytes, plasma, and feces, and by intense itching, erythema, and edema on short exposure to sunlight; skin lesions usually fade without scarring or pigmentation but a chronic weatherbeaten appearance is characteristic.

protoporphyrin (-por′fĭ-rin) the porphyrin, C_{34}-$H_{34}N_4O_4$, whose iron complex united with protein occurs in hemoglobin and other respiratory pigments.

protoporphyrinuria (-por″fĭ-rĭ-nu′re-ah) protoporphyrin in the urine.

protospasm (pro′to-spazm) a spasm which begins in a limited area and extends to other parts.

prototroph (-trŏf) an organism with the same growth factor requirements as the ancestral strain; said of microbial mutants. **prototroph'ic,** adj.

prototype (-tīp) the original type or form that is typical of later individuals or species.

protoveratrine (pro″to-ver′ah-trēn) an antihypertensive alkaloid from *Veratrum album* and *V. viride,* occurring in two forms, designated A and B.

protovertebra (-ver′tĕ-brah) 1. somite. 2. the caudal half of a somite forming most of the vertebra.

Protozoa (-zo′ah) a phylum comprising the simplest organisms of the animal kingdom, consisting of unicellular organisms ranging in size from submicroscopic to macroscopic. It includes the Sarcodina, Mastigophora, Ciliophora, and Sporozoa.

protozoacide (-zo′ah-sīd) destructive to protozoa; an agent destructive to protozoa.

protozoal (-zo′al) pertaining to or caused by protozoa.

protozoan (-zo′an) 1. of or pertaining to protozoa. 2. an organism belonging to the Protozoa.

protozoiasis (-zo-i′ah-sis) any disease caused by protozoa.

protozoology (-zo-ol′o-je) the study of protozoa.

protozoon (-zo′on), pl. *protozo′a* [Gr.] any member of the Protozoa.

protozoophage (-zo′o-fāj) a cell having a phagocytic action on protozoa.

protraction (pro-trak′shun) a forward projection of a facial structure; in *mandibular p.,* the gnathion is anterior to the orbital plane; in *maxillary p.,* the subnasion is anterior to the orbital plane.

protractor (-trak′tor) an instrument for extracting foreign bodies from wounds.

protrusion (-troo′zhun) extension beyond the usual limits, or above a plane surface.

protuberance (-tu′ber-ans) a projecting part, or prominence.

protuberantia (-tu″ber-an′she-ah), pl. *protuberan′tiae* [L.] protuberance.

proud (prowd) characterized by exuberant granulation tissue.

Provera (pro-ver′ah) trademark for preparations of medroxyprogesterone acetate.

provertebra (-ver′tĕ-brah) somite.

provirus (-vi′rus) the genome of an animal virus integrated (by crossing over) into the chromosome of the host cell, and thus replicated in all of its daughter cells.

provitamin (-vi′tah-min) a substance, e.g., ergosterol, from which the animal organism can form vitamin.

proximad (prok′sĭ-mad) in a proximal direction.

proximal (prok′sĭ-mal) nearest to a point of reference, as to a center or median line or to the point of attachment or origin.

proximalis (prok″sĭ-ma′lis) [L.] proximal.

proximate (prok′sĭ-māt) immediate; nearest.

proximoataxia (prok″sĭ-mo-ah-tak′se-ah) ataxia of the proximal part of an extremity.

proximobuccal (-buk′al) pertaining to the proximal and buccal surfaces of a posterior tooth.

prozone (pro′zōn) the phenomenon exhibited by some sera, in which agglutination or precipitation occurs at higher dilution ranges, but is not visible at lower dilutions or when undiluted.

pruriginous (proo-rij′ĭ-nus) of the nature of or tending to cause prurigo.

prurigo (proo-ri′go) [L.] any of several itchy skin eruptions in which the characteristic lesion is dome-shaped with a small transient vesicle on top, followed by crusting or lichenification. **p. mi′tis,** prurigo of a mild type. **p. nodula′ris,** a form of neurodermatitis, usually occurring on the extremities in middle-aged women, marked by discrete, firm, rough-surfaced, dark brownish-gray, intensely itchy nodules. **p. sim′plex,** papular urticaria.

pruritogenic (proo″rĭ-to-jen′ik) causing pruritus, or itching.

pruritus (proo-ri′tus) itching. **prurit′ic,** adj. **p. a′ni,** intense chronic itching in the anal region. **essential p.,** that occurring without known cause. **p. hiema′lis,** winter itch. **p. seni′lis,** itching in the aged, due to degeneration of the skin. **symptomatic p.,** that occurring secondarily to another condition. **p. vul′vae,** intense itching of the female external genitals.

psalterium (sal-te′re-um) 1. omasum. 2. commissure of the fornix.

psammoma (sah-mo′mah) a tumor, especially a meningioma, containing psammoma bodies.

psammosarcoma (sam″o-sar-ko′mah) a sarcoma containing granular material.

psammous (sam′us) sandy.

pseud(o)- word element [Gr.], *false.*

pseudarthritis (su″dar-thri′tis) a hysterical joint affection.

pseudarthrosis (su″dar-thro′sis) a pathologic condition in which failure of callus formation following pathologic fracture through an area of deossification in a weight-bearing long bone results in formation of a false joint.

pseudencephalus (su″den-sef′ah-lus) a fetus with a tumor in place of a brain.

pseudesthesia (su″des-the′ze-ah) a subjective sensation occurring in the absence of the appropriate stimuli.

pseudoagraphia (su″do-ah-graf′e-ah) a condition in which the patient can copy writing, but cannot write independently except in a meaningless and illegible manner.

pseudoallele (-ah-lēl′) one of two or more genes which are seemingly allelic, but which can be shown to have distinctive but closely linked loci. **pseudoallel′ic,** adj.

pseudoanemia (-ah-ne′me-ah) marked pallor with no evidence of anemia.

pseudoaneurysm (-an′u-rizm) dilatation and tortuosity of a vessel, giving the appearance of an aneurysm.

pseudoangina (-an-ji′nah) a nervous disorder resembling angina.

pseudoankylosis (-ang"kĭ-lo'sis) a false ankylosis.

pseudoapoplexy (-ap'o-plek"se) a condition resembling apoplexy, but without hemorrhage.

pseudobulbar (-bul'bar) apparently, but not really, due to a bulbar lesion.

pseudocartilaginous (-kar"tĭ-laj'ĭ-nus) resembling cartilage.

pseudocast (su'do-kast) an accidental formation of urinary sediment resembling a true cast.

pseudocele (-sēl) the fifth ventricle.

pseudochancre (su"do-shang'ker) an indurated lesion resembling chancre.

pseudocholesteatoma (-ko"les-te"ah-to'mah) a horny mass of epithelial cells resembling cholesteatoma in the tympanic cavity in chronic middle ear inflammation.

pseudochorea (-ko-re'ah) a state of general incoordination resembling chorea.

pseudochromesthesia (-kro"mes-the'ze-ah) a false sensation of color.

pseudochromhidrosis (-krōm"hĭ-dro'sis) discoloration of sweat by surface contaminants, such as pigment-producing bacteria or chemical substances on the skin.

pseudocirrhosis (-sĭ-ro'sis) a condition suggestive of, but not due to, cirrhosis; often due to pericarditis (*pericardial p.*); see *Pick's disease* (2).

pseudocoarctation (-ko"ark-ta'shun) a condition radiographically resembling coarctation but without compromise of the lumen, as occurs in a congenital anomaly of the aortic arch.

pseudocoele (su'do-sēl) the fifth ventricle.

pseudocolloid (su"do-kol'oid) a mucoid substance sometimes found in ovarian cysts. **p. of lips,** Fordyce's disease.

pseudocoloboma (-kol"o-bo'mah) a line or scar on the iris resembling a coloboma.

pseudocoxalgia (-kok-sal'je-ah) osteochondrosis of the capitular epiphysis of the femur.

pseudocrisis (-kri'sis) sudden but temporary abatement of febrile symptoms.

pseudocroup (su'do-krōōp) 1. laryngismus stridulus. 2. thymic asthma.

pseudocyesis (su"do-si-e'sis) false pregnancy.

pseudocylindroid (-sĭ-lin'droid) a shred of mucin in the urine resembling a cylindroid.

pseudocyst (su'do-sist) an abnormal or dilated space resembling a cyst but not lined with epithelium.

pseudodementia (su"do-de-men'she-ah) a state of general apathy resembling dementia, but without defect of intelligence.

pseudodiphtheria (-dif-the're-ah) the presence of a false membrane not due to *Corynebacterium diphtheriae.*

pseudoedema (-ĕ-de'mah) a puffy state resembling edema.

pseudoemphysema (-em"fĭ-ze'mah) a condition resembling emphysema, but due to temporary obstruction of the bronchi.

pseudoephedrine (-ĕ-fed'rin) one of the optical isomers of ephedrine; the hydrochloride salt is used as a nasal decongestant.

pseudofracture (-frak'chur) a condition seen in the roentgenogram of a bone as a thickening of the periosteum and formation of new bone over what looks like an incomplete fracture.

pseudoganglion (-gang'gle-on) an enlargement on a nerve resembling a ganglion.

pseudogeusesthesia (-gūs"es-the'ze-ah) a false sensation of taste associated with a sensation of another modality.

pseudogeusia (-gu'ze-ah) a sensation of taste occurring in the absence of a stimulus, or inappropriate to the exciting stimulus.

pseudoglioma (-gli-o'mah) any condition mimicking retinoblastoma, e.g., retrolental fibroplasia or exudative retinopathy.

pseudoglobulin (-glob'u-lin) any of a class of globulins characterized by being soluble in water in the absence of neutral salts and thus not a euglobulin.

pseudogout (su'do-gowt) a condition resembling gout, but with calcium pyrophosphate rather than urate crystals in the synovial fluid.

pseudohemophilia (su"do-he"mo-fil'e-ah) angiohemophilia.

pseudohermaphrodite (-her-maf'ro-dīt) an individual exhibiting pseudohermaphroditism.

pseudohermaphroditism (-her-maf'ro-dīt-izm") a state in which the gonads are of one sex, but one or more contradictions exist in the morphologic criteria of sex. In *female p.* the individual is a genetic and gonadal female with partial masculinization; in *male p.* the individual is a genetic and gonadal male with incomplete masculinization.

pseudohernia (-her'ne-ah) an inflamed sac or gland simulating strangulated hernia.

pseudohypertrophy (-hi-per'tro-fe) increase in size without true hypertrophy. **pseudohypertroph'ic,** adj.

pseudohypoparathyroidism (-hi"po-par"ah-thi'roi-dizm) a hereditary condition clinically resembling hypoparathyroidism, but caused by failure of response to, rather than deficiency of, parathyroid hormone, marked by hypocalcemia and hyperphosphatemia and commonly by short stature, obesity, short metacarpals, and ectopic calcification.

pseudoisochromatic (-i"so-kro-mat'ik) seemingly of the same color throughout; applied to solution for testing color blindness, containing two pigments that can be distinguished by the normal eye.

pseudojaundice (-jawn'dis) skin discoloration due to blood changes and not to liver disease.

pseudologia (-lo'je-ah) the writing of anonymous letters to people of prominence, to one's self, etc. **p. fantas'tica,** a tendency to tell extravagant and fantastic falsehoods centered about one's self.

pseudomania (-ma'ne-ah) 1. false or pretended mental disorder. 2. pathologic lying.

pseudomelanosis (-mel"ah-no'sis) discoloration of tissue after death by blood pigments.

pseudomembrane (-mem'brān) false membrane. **pseudomem'branous,** adj.

Pseudomonas (-mo'nas) a genus of bacteria,

some species of which are pathogenic for plants and vertebrates. *P. aerugino'sa,* the only species pathogenic for man, produces the blue-green pigment, pyocyanin, which gives the color to "blue pus," and causes various human diseases; *P. mal'lei* causes glanders; *P. pseudomal'lei* causes melioidosis.

pseudomucin (-mu'sin) a mucin-like substance found in ovarian cysts.

pseudomyxoma (-mik-so'mah) a mass of epithelial mucus resembling a myxoma. **p. perito- ne'i,** the presence in the peritoneal cavity of mucoid matter from a ruptured ovarian cyst or a ruptured mucocele of the appendix.

pseudoneuritis (-nu-ri'tis) a congenital hyperemic condition of the optic papilla.

pseudopapilledema (-pap"ĭ-lĕ-de'mah) anomalous elevation of the optic disk.

pseudoparalysis (-pah-ral'ĭ-sis) apparent loss of muscular power without real paralysis. **arthritic general p.,** a condition resembling dementia paralytica, dependent on intracranial atheroma in arthritic patients. **Parrot's p., syphilitic p.,** pseudoparalysis of one or more extremities in infants, due to syphilitic osteochondritis of an epiphysis.

pseudoparaplegia (-par"ah-ple'je-ah) spurious paralysis of the lower limbs, as in hysteria or malingering.

pseudoparesis (-pah-re'sis) a hysterical or nonorganic condition simulating paresis.

pseudopelade (-pe'lād) patchy alopecia roughly simulating alopecia areata; it may be due to various disease of the hair follicles, some of which are associated with scarring.

pseudoplegia (-ple'je-ah) hysterical paralysis.

pseudopodium (-po'de-um) a temporary protrusion of the cytoplasm of an ameba, serving for purposes of locomotion or to engulf food.

pseudopolyp (-pol'ip) a hypertrophied tab of mucous membrane resembling a polyp.

pseudopolyposis (-pol"ĭ-po'sis) numerous pseudopolyps in the colon and rectum, due to long-standing inflammation.

pseudopregnancy (-preg'nan-se) false pregnancy.

pseudo-pseudohypoparathyroidism (-su"do-hi"po-par"ah-thi'roi-dizm) an incomplete form of pseudohypoparathyroidism marked by the same constitutional features but by normal levels of calcium and phosphorus in the blood serum.

pseudopsia (su-dop'se-ah) false or perverted vision.

pseudopterygium (su"do-ter-ij'e-um) an adhesion of the conjunctiva to the cornea following a burn or other injury.

pseudoptosis (-to'sis) decrease in the size of the palpebral aperture.

pseudorabies (-ra'bēz) a highly contagious disease of the central nervous system of dogs, cats, rats, cattle, and swine, due to a herpesvirus and marked by sudden onset, late paralysis, convulsions, and death within three days; in swine, it usually runs a milder course.

pseudoreaction (-re-ak'shun) a false or deceptive reaction; a skin reaction in intradermal tests which is not due to the specific test substance but to protein in the medium employed in producing the toxin.

pseudorickets (-rik'ets) renal osteodystrophy.

pseudoscarlatina (-skar"lah-te'nah) a septic condition with fever and eruption resembling scarlet fever.

pseudosclerosis (-skle-ro'sis) a condition with the symptoms but without the lesions of multiple sclerosis. **Strümpell-Westphal p., Westphal-Strümpell p.,** hepatolenticular degeneration.

pseudosmia (su-doz'me-ah) a sensation of odor without the appropriate stimulus.

pseudostoma (su-dos'to-mah) an apparent communication between silver-stained endothelial cells.

pseudotetanus (su"do-tet'ah-nus) persistent muscular contractions resembling tetanus but unassociated with *Clostridium tetani.*

pseudotruncus arteriosus (-trunk'us ar-te"re-o'sus) the most severe form of tetralogy of Fallot.

pseudotuberculosis (-tu-ber"ku-lo'sis) a fatal disease of rodents due to *Yersinia pseudotuberculosis,* with caseous swellings and nodules in various organs. Rarely, *Corynebacterium pseudotuberculosis* causes the disease in domestic animals.

pseudotumor (-tu'mor) phantom tumor. **p. cer'ebri,** cerebral edema and raised intracranial pressure without neurological signs except occasional sixth-nerve palsy.

pseudoxanthoma elasticum (-zan-tho'mah e-las'tĭ-kum) a dermatosis marked clinically by small yellowish macules and papules, individual or confluent, or massed into plaques, and histologically by masses of swollen, calcified elastic fibers with degeneration of the collagen fibers in the lower and middle dermis and in the gastrointestinal tract and heart.

p.s.i. pounds per square inch.

psilocin (si'lo-sin) a hallucinogenic substance closely related to psilocybin.

psilocybin (si"lo-si'bin) a hallucinogen, $C_{13}H_{18(20)}O_3N_2P_2$, having indole characteristics, isolated from the mushroom *Psilocybe mexicana.*

psittacosis (sit"ah-ko'sis) a disease due to a strain of *Chlamydia psittaci,* first seen in parrots and later in other birds and domestic fowl; it is transmissible to man, usually taking the form of a pneumonia accompanied by fever, cough, and often splenomegaly. See also *ornithosis.*

psoitis (so-i'tis) inflammation of a psoas muscle or its sheath.

psoralen (sor'ah-len) any of the constituents of certain plants (e.g., *Psoralea corylifolia*) that have the ability to produce phototoxic dermatitis when an individual is first exposed to a psoralen and then to sunlight; certain perfumes and drugs (e.g., methoxsalen) contain psoralens.

psoriasis (so-ri'ah-sis) a chronic, hereditary, recurrent dermatosis marked by discrete vivid red macules, papules, or plaques covered with silvery lamellated scales. **psoriat'ic,** adj.

P.S.P. phenolsulfonphthalein.

PSRO Professional Standards Review Organization.

psych(o)- word element [Gr.], *mind.*

psychalgia (si-kal'je-ah) pain of mental or hysterical origin; pain attending or due to mental effort. **psychal'gic,** adj.

psychanopsia (si″kah-nop'se-ah) psychic blindness.

psychataxia (si″kah-tak'se-ah) disordered mental state with confusion, agitation, and inability to fix the attention.

psyche (si'ke) the mind; the human faculty for thought, judgment, and emotion; the mental life, including both conscious and unconscious processes. **psy'chic,** adj.

psychedelic (si″kĕ-del'ik) pertaining to or causing hallucinations, distortions of perception, and, sometimes, psychotic-like behavior; also, a drug producing such effects.

psychiatrist (si-ki'ah-trist) a physician who specializes in psychiatry.

psychiatry (si-ki'ah-tre) that branch of medicine dealing with the study, treatment, and prevention of mental illness. **psychiat'ric,** adj. **descriptive p.,** that based on observation and study of external factors that can be seen, heard, or felt. **dynamic p.,** the study of emotional processes, their origins and the mental mechanisms underlying them. **forensic p.,** that dealing with the legal aspects of mental disorders. **orthomolecular p.,** the study of mental disease on the basis of the molecular environment of the brain.

psychic (si'kik) pertaining to the mind.

psychoanaleptic (si″ko-an″ah-lep'tik) exerting a stimulating effect upon the mind.

psychoanalysis (-ah-nal'ĭ-sis) a method of diagnosing and treating mental and emotional disorders through ascertaining and analyzing the facts of the patient's mental life. **psychoanalyt'ic,** adj.

psychoanalyst (-an'ah-list) a practitioner of psychoanalysis.

psychobiology (-bi-ol'o-je) study of the interrelations of body and mind in the formation and functioning of personality. **psychobiolog'ical,** adj.

psychocortical (-kor'tĭ-kal) pertaining to the mind and the cerebral cortex.

psychodiagnosis (-di″ag-no'sis) the diagnostic use of psychologic testing.

psychodrama (-drah'mah) group psychotherapy in which patients dramatize their individual conflicting situations of daily life.

psychodynamics (-di-nam'iks) the science of human behavior and motivation.

psychogalvanometer (-gal″vah-nom'ĕ-ter) a galvanometer for recording the electrical agitation produced by emotional stresses.

psychogenesis (-jen'ĕ-sis) 1. mental development. 2. production of a symptom or illness by psychic, as opposed to organic, factors.

psychogenic (-jen'ik) having an emotional or psychologic origin.

psychogram (si'ko-gram) psychograph.

psychograph (-graf) 1. a chart for recording graphically a person's personality traits. 2. a written description of a person's mental functioning.

psychokinesis (si″ko-ki-ne'sis) the production or alteration of motion by directed thought processes.

psycholepsy (-lep'se) a condition marked by sudden mood changes.

psycholeptic (-lep'tik) a drug that affects the mental state; cf. *neuroleptic.*

psychology (si-kol'o-je) the science dealing with the mind and mental processes, especially in relation to human and animal behavior. **psycholog'ic, psycholog'ical,** adj. **analytic p.,** psychology by introspective methods. **child p.,** the study of the development of the mind of the child. **clinical p.,** the use of psychologic knowledge and techniques in the treatment of persons with emotional difficulties. **criminal p.,** the study of the mentality, motivation, and social behavior of criminals. **depth p.,** psychoanalysis. **dynamic p.,** that stressing the element of energy in mental processes. **experimental p.,** the study of the mind and mental operations by the use of experimental methods. **genetic p.,** that dealing with the development of the mind in the individual and with its evolution in the race. **gestalt p.,** gestaltism. **physiologic p.,** that applying the facts taught in neurology to show the relation between the mental and the neural. **social p.,** that treating of the social aspects of mental life.

psychometrician (si″ko-mĕ-trish'an) a person skilled in psychometry.

psychometrics (-met'riks) psychometry.

psychometry (si-kom'ĕ-tre) the testing and measuring of mental and psychologic ability, efficiency, potentials, and functioning. **psychomet'ric,** adj.

psychomotor (si″ko-mo'tor) pertaining to motor effects of cerebral or psychic activity.

psychoneurosis (-nu-ro'sis) neurosis. **psychoneurot'ic,** adj.

psychonomy (si-kon'o-me) the science of the laws of mental activity.

psychopath (si'ko-path) a person who has an antisocial personality.

psychopathic (si″ko-path'ik) antisocial; pertaining to a psycopath.

psychopathology (-pah-thol'o-je) the branch of medicine dealing with the causes and processes of mental disorders.

psychopathy (si-kop'ah-the) any disease of the mind.

psychopharmacology (si″ko-fahr″mah-kol'o-je) the study of the action of drugs on the mind. **psychopharmacolog'ic,** adj.

psychophysical (-fiz'ĕ-kal) pertaining to the mind and its relation to physical manifestations.

psychophysics (-fiz'iks) scientific study of quantitative relations between characteristics or patterns of physical stimuli and the sensations induced by them.

psychophysiology (-fiz″e-ol′o-je) scientific study of the interaction an interrelations of psychic and physiologic factors. **psychophysiolog′ic,** adj.

psychoplegic (-ple′jik) an agent lessening cerebral activity or excitability.

psychosensory (-sen′sor-e) perceiving and interpreting sensory stimuli.

psychosexual (-seks′u-al) pertaining to the psychic or emotional aspects of sex.

psychosis (si-ko′sis), pl. *psycho′ses.* Any major mental disorder of organic or emotional origin marked by derangement of personality and loss of contact with reality, often with delusions, hallucinations, or illusions. Cf. *neurosis.* **affective p.,** one marked by severe disorder of mood, either elation or depression, with secondary effect upon behavior and thought. **alcoholic p.,** mental disorder caused by excessive use of alcohol. **circular p.,** manic-depressive psychosis in which there is no free interval between the manic and depressive reactions. **depressive p.,** one characterized by mental depression, melancholy, despondency, inadequacy, and feelings of guilt. **exhaustion p.,** one due to some exhausting or depressing occurrence, as an operation. **gestational p.,** one developing during pregnancy. **involutional p.,** see under *melancholia.* **Korsakoff's p.,** an alcoholic psychosis, believed to be a chronic form of Wernicke's encephalopathy, with amnesia, confabulation, disorientation, susceptibility to external stimulation and suggestion, hallucinations, and, usually, the signs of polyneuritis (wristdrop, etc.). **manic p.,** the stage of manic-depressive psychosis marked by flight of ideas, ideas of grandiosity, psychomotor activity, and euphoria. **manic-depressive p.,** an essentially benign affective psychosis, chiefly marked by emotional instability, striking mood swings and a tendency to recurrence; seen in depressive, manic, and circular types. **organic p.,** organic brain syndrome. **polyneuritic p.,** Korsakoff's p. **senile p.,** mental deterioration in old age, with organic brain changes, the symptoms including impaired memory for recent events, confabulation, irritability, etc. **situational p.,** one caused by an unbearable situation over which the patient has no control. **toxic p.,** one due to ingestion of toxic agents into the body, or to the presence of toxins within the body.

psychosomatic (si″ko-so-mat′ik) pertaining to the mind-body relationship; having bodily symptoms of psychic, emotional, or mental origin.

psychosurgery (-ser′jer-e) brain surgery done to relieve mental and psychic symptoms.

psychotherapy (-ther′ah-pe) treatment designed to produce a response by mental rather than by physical effects.

psychotic (si-kot′ik) 1. pertaining to, characterized by, or caused by psychosis. 2. a person exhibiting psychosis.

psychotogenic (si-kot″o-jen′ik) producing a psychosis.

psychotomimetic (-mi-met′ik) pertaining to, characterized by, or producing symptoms similar to those of a psychosis.

psychotropic (si″ko-trop′ik) exerting an effect on the mind; said especially of drugs.

psychr(o)- word element [Gr.], *cold.*

psychralgia (si-kral′je-ah) a painful sensation of cold.

psychrometer (si-krom′ĕ-ter) an instrument for measuring atmospheric moisture.

psychrophile (si′kro-fīl) an organism growing best at low temperatures.

psychrophilic (si″kro-fil′ik) fond of cold; said of bacteria growing best in the cold (15°–20° C.).

psychrophore (si′kro-fōr) a double catheter for applying cold.

psychrotherapy (si″kro-ther′ah-pe) treatment of disease by applying cold.

psyllium (sil′ĭ-um) a plant of the genus *Plantago.*

Pt chemical symbol, *platinum.*

pt. pint.

PTA plasma thromboplastin antecedent (coagulation Factor XI).

ptarmic (tar′mik) causing sneezing.

ptarmus (tar′mus) spasmodic sneezing.

PTC plasma thromboplastin component; phenylthiocarbamide.

pterin (ter′in) any of a class of nitrogenous compounds, including aminopterin and xanthopterin, first observed in butterfly wings.

pterion (te′re-on) a point of junction of frontal, parietal, temporal, and sphenoid bones.

pterygium (tĕ-rij′e-um) a winglike structure, especially an abnormal triangular fold of membrane in the interpalpebral fissure, extending from the conjunctiva to the cornea. **p. col′li,** webbed neck; a thick skin fold on the side of the neck, from the mastoid region to the acromion.

pterygoid (ter′ĭ-goid) shaped like a wing.

pterygomandibular (ter″ĭ-go-man-dib′u-lar) pertaining to the pterygoid process and the mandible.

pterygomaxillary (-mak′sĭ-ler″e) pertaining to the pterygoid process and the maxilla.

pterygopalatine (pal′ah-tīn) pertaining to the pterygoid process and the palate bone.

ptilosis (ti-lo′sis) falling out of the eyelashes.

ptomaine (to′mān, to-mān′) any of an indefinite class of toxic bases, usually considered to be formed by the action of bacterial metabolism or proteins.

ptosed (tōst) affected with ptosis.

ptosis (to′sis) 1. prolapse of an organ or part. 2. paralytic drooping of the upper eyelid. **ptot′ic,** adj.

-ptosis word element [Gr.], *downward displacement.* **-ptot′ic,** adj.

PTT partial thromboplastin time.

ptyal(o)- word element [Gr.], *saliva.*

ptyalagogue (ti-al′ah-gog) sialagogue.

ptyalectasis (ti″ah-lek′tah-sis) 1. a state of dilatation of a salivary duct. 2. surgical dilation of a salivary duct.

ptyalin (ti′ah-lin) α-amylase occurring in saliva.

ptyalism (ti′al-izm) excessive secretion of saliva.

ptyalocele (ti-al′o-sēl) a cystic tumor containing saliva.

ptyalogenic (ti″ah-lo-jen′ik) formed from or by the action of saliva.

ptyaloreaction (-re-ak′shun) a reaction occurring in or performed on the saliva.

ptyalorrhea (-re′ah) ptyalism.

Pu chemical symbol, *plutonium.*

pubarche (pu-bar′ke) the first appearance of pubic hair.

pubertas (pu-ber′tas) puberty. **p. prae′cox,** precocious puberty.

puberty (pu′ber-te) the period during which the secondary sex characteristics begin to develop and the capability of sexual reproduction is attained. **pu′beral, pu′bertal,** adj. **precocious p.,** unusually early sexual maturation, either idiopathic or pathologic.

pubes (pu′bez), sing. *pu′bis*[L.] 1. the hairs growing over the pubic region. 2. the pubic region.

pubescence (pu-bes′ens) 1. puberty. 2. lanugo.

pubescent (pu-bes′ent) 1. arriving at the age of puberty. 2. covered with down or lanugo.

pubic (pu′bik) pertaining to or lying near the pubes.

pubiotomy (pu″be-ot′o-me) surgical separation of the pubic bone lateral to the symphysis.

pubis (pu′bis) pubic bone; see *Table of Bones.*

pubofemoral (pu″bo-fem′o-ral) pertaining to the pubis and femur.

puboprostatic (-pros-tat′ik) pertaining to the pubis and prostate.

pubovesical (-ves′ĭ-kal) pertaining to the pubis and bladder.

pudendum (pu-den′dum), pl. *puden′da* [L.] vulva; the external genitalia of humans, especially of the female, including the mons pubis, labia majora and minora, vestibule, and clitoris. **puden′dal, pu′dic,** adj. **p. femini′num, p. mulie′bre,** the female pudendum; see *pudendum.*

puerile (pu′er-il) pertaining to childhood or to children; childish.

puerpera (pu-er′per-ah) a woman who has just given birth to a child.

puerperal (-per-al) pertaining to a puerpera or to the puerperium.

puerperalism (-per-al-izm″) morbid condition incident to childbirth.

puerperium (pu″er-pe′re-um) the period or state of confinement after childbirth.

Pulex (pu′leks) a genus of fleas, including *P. ir′ritans,* the common, or human flea, which attacks man and domestic animals, and may act as an intermediate host of certain helminths.

pulicicide (pu-lis′ĭ-sīd) an agent destructive to fleas.

pullulation (pul″u-la′shun) development by sprouting or budding.

pulmo (pul′mo), pl. *pulmo′nes* [L.] lung.

pulmoaortic (pul″mo-a-or′tik) pertaining to the lungs and aorta.

pulmonary (pul′mo-ner″e) pertaining to the lungs or the pulmonary artery.

pulmonic (pul-mon′ik) pulmonary.

pulmonitis (pul″mo-ni′tis) pneumonitis.

pulmotor (pul′mo-tor) an apparatus for forcing oxygen into the lungs and inducing artificial respiration.

pulp (pulp) any soft, juicy animal or vegetable tissue. **pul′pal,** adj. **coronal p.,** the part of the dental pulp contained in the crown portion of the pulp cavity. **dental p.,** richly vascularized and innervated connective tissue inside the pulp cavity of a tooth. **digital p.,** a cushion of soft tissue on the palmar or plantar surface of the distal phalanx of a finger or toe. **red p., splenic p.,** the dark reddish brown substance filling the interspaces of the splenic sinuses. **tooth p.,** dental p. **white p.,** sheaths of lymphatic tissue surrounding the arteries of the spleen.

pulpa (pul′pah), pl. *pul′pae* [L.] pulp.

pulpectomy (pul-pek′to-me) removal of dental pulp.

pulpefaction (pul″pě-fak′shun) conversion into pulp.

pulpitis (pul-pi′tis), pl. *pulpit′ides*[L.] inflammation of dental pulp.

pulpotomy (pul-pot′o-me) excision of the coronal pulp.

pulpy (pul′pe) soft; of the consistency of pulp.

pulsatile (pul′sah-tīl) characterized by a rhythmic pulsation.

pulsation (pul-sa′shun) a throb, or rhythmic beat, as of the heart.

pulse (puls) the rhythmic expansion of an artery which may be felt with the finger. **abdominal p.,** that over the abdominal aorta. **alternating p.,** one with regular alternation of weak and strong beats without changes in cycle length. **anacrotic p.,** one in which the ascending limb of the tracing shows a transient drop in amplitude. **bigeminal p.,** one in which two beats occur in rapid succession, the groups of two being separated by a longer interval. **cannon ball p.,** Corrigan's p. **capillary p.,** Quincke's p. **catadicrotic p.,** one in which the descending limb of the tracing shows two small notches. **Corrigan's p.,** jerky pulse with full expansion and sudden collapse. **dicrotic p.,** one in which the tracing shows two marked expansions in one beat of the artery. **entoptic p.,** a phose occurring with each pulse beat. **hard p.,** one characterized by high tension. **jerky p.,** one in which the artery is suddenly and markedly distended. **paradoxical p.,** one that markedly decreases in size during inspiration, as often occurs in constrictive pericarditis. **pistol-shot p.,** one in which the arteries are subject to sudden distention and collapse. **plateau p.,** one that is slowly rising and sustained. **quadrigeminal p.,** one with a pause after every fourth beat. **Quincke's p.,** alternate blanching and flushing of the nail bed due to pulsation of subpapillary arteriolar and venous plexuses, as seen in aortic insufficiency. **radial p.,** that felt over the radial artery. **Riegel's p.,** one which is smaller during respiration. **thready p.,** one that is very fine and scarcely perceptible. **tricrotic p.,** one in which the tracing shows three marked expansions in one beat of the artery. **trigeminal p.,** one with a pause after every third beat. **undulating p.,** one giving the sensation of successive waves. **vagus p.,** a slow pulse. **venous p.,** the pulsation over a vein, especially over the right jugular vein. **water-hammer p.,** Corrigan's p. **wiry p.,** a small, tense pulse.

pulsion (pul'shun) a pushing outward.

pulsus (pul'sus) [L.] pulse. **p. alter'nans,** alternating pulse. **p. bigem'inus,** bigeminal pulse. **p. ce'ler,** a swift, abrupt pulse. **p. dif'ferens,** inequality of the pulse observable at corresponding sites on either side of the body. **p. paradox'us,** paradoxical pulse. **p. par'vus et tar'dus,** a small hard pulse that rises and falls slowly. **p. tar'dus,** an abnormally slow pulse.

pultaceous (pul-ta'shus) like a poultice; pulpy.

pulverulent (pul-ver'u-lent) powdery; dustlike.

pulvinar (pul-vi'nar) the prominent medial part of the posterior end of the thalamus.

pumice (pum'is) a substance consisting of silicates of aluminum, potassium, and sodium; used in dentistry as an abrasive.

pump (pump) 1. an apparatus for drawing or forcing liquids or gases. 2. to draw or force liquids or gases. **air p.,** one for exhausting or forcing in air. **blood p.,** a machine used to propel blood through the tubing of extracorporeal circulation devices. **breast p.,** a manual or electric pump for abstracting breast milk. **sodium p.,** the mechanism of active transport by which sodium is extruded from a cell to maintain electrolyte balance across the cell membrane. **stomach p.,** pump for removing the stomach contents.

pump-oxygenator (pump'ok"sĭ-jĕ-na'tor) an apparatus consisting of a blood pump and oxygenator, plus filters and traps, for saturating the blood with oxygen during heart surgery.

punchdrunk (punch'drunk) a traumatic encephalopathy of prizefighters resulting from cumulative cerebral concussions, with general slowing of mental functions, bouts of confusion, and scattered memory loss.

punctate (punk'tāt) spotted; marked with points or punctures.

punctiform (-tĭ-form) like a point.

punctograph (-to-graf) an instrument for radiographic localization of foreign bodies.

punctum (-tum), pl. *punc'ta* [L.] a point or small spot. **p. cae'cum,** blind spot. **punc'ta do-loro'sa,** Valleix's points. **p. lacrima'le** lacrimal point. **p. prox'imum,** near point. **p. remo'-tum,** far point. **punc'ta vasculo'sa,** minute red spots which mark the cut surface of white substance of the brain.

puncture (-chur) the act of piercing or penetrating with a pointed object or instrument; a wound so made. **cisternal p.,** puncture of the cisterna cerebellomedullaris through the posterior atlanto-occipital membrane to obtain cerebrospinal fluid. **lumbar p., spinal p.,** the tapping of the subarachnoid space in the lumbar region, usually between the third and fourth lumbar vertebrae. **sternal p.,** removal of bone

marrow from the manubrium of the sternum through an appropriate needle.

P.U.O. pyrexia of unknown origin.

pupa (pu'pah), pl. *pu'pae* [L.] the second stage in the devlopment of an insect, between the larva and the imago. **pu'pal,** adj.

pupil (pu'pil) the opening in the center of the iris. See Plate XIII. **pu'pillary,** adj. **Adie's p.,** tonic p. **Argyll Robertson p.,** one which is miotic and responds to accommodative effort, but not to light. **fixed p.,** one that does not react either to light or on convergence, or in accommodation. **Hutchinson's p.,** one which is dilated while the other is not. **tonic p.,** one that responds to accommodation and convergence in a slow, delayed fashion, as in Adie's syndrome.

pupilla (pu-pil'ah) [L.] pupil.

pupillometer (pu"pĭ-lom'ĕ-ter) an instrument for measuring the width or diameter of the pupil.

pupillometry (-lom'ĕ-tre) measurement of the diameter or width of the pupil of the eye.

pupilloplegia (pu"pĭ-lo-ple'je-ah) tonic pupil.

pupilloscopy (pu"pĭ-los'ko-pe) retinoscopy.

pupillostatometer (pu"pĭ-lo-stah-tom'ĕ-ter) an instrument for measuring the distance between the pupils.

purgation (per-ga'shun) catharsis; purging effected by a cathartic medicine.

purgative (per'gah-tiv) 1. cathartic (1); causing bowel evacuation. 2. a cathartic, particularly one stimulating peristaltic action.

purge (perj) 1. a purgative medicine or dose. 2. to cause free evacuation of feces.

purinase (pu'rĭ-nās) an enzyme that catalyzes purine conversions.

purine (pu'rēn) a compound, $C_5H_4N_4$, not found in nature, but variously substituted to produce a group of compounds, *purines* or *purine bases*, of which uric acid is a metabolic end product.

Purinethol (-thol) trademark for a preparation of mercaptopurine.

Purodigin (pu"ro-di'jin) trademark for a preparation of digitoxin.

puromycin (-mi'sin) an antineoplastic and antitrypanosomal antibiotic, $C_{22}H_{29}N_7O_5$, produced by *Streptomyces alboniger.*

purple (pur'p'l) 1. a color between blue and red. 2. a substance of this color used as a dye or indicator. **visual p.,** rhodopsin.

purpura (per'pu-rah) a group of disorders characterized by purplish or brownish red discoloration, easily visible through the epidermis, caused by hemorrhage into the tissues. **pur-pu'ric,** adj. **allergic p., anaphylactoid p.,** Schönlein-Henoch p. **p. annula'ris telangiec-to'des,** a rare form in which punctate erythematous lesions coalesce to form an annular or serpiginous pattern. **fibrinolytic p.,** purpura associated with increased fibrinolytic activity of the blood. **p. ful'minans,** nonthrombocytopenic purpura seen mainly in children, usually after an infectious disease, marked by fever, shock, anemia, and sudden, rapidly spreading symmetrical skin hemorrhages of the lower limbs, often associated with extensive intravascular thromboses and gangrene. **p. hemorrha'gica,** idiopathic thrombocytopenic p. **Henoch's p.,** Schönlein-Henoch purpura in which abdominal symptoms predominate. **malignant p.,** epidemic cerebrospinal meningitis. **nonthrombocytopenic p.,** purpura without any decrease in the platelet count of the blood. **Schönlein's p.,** Schönlein-Henoch purpura in which articular symptoms predominate. **Schönlein-Henoch p.,** nonthrombocytopenic purpura of unknown cause, most often seen in children, associated with various clinical symptoms, such as urticaria and erythema, arthropathy and arthritis, gastrointestinal symptoms, and renal involvement. **p. seni'lis,** dark purplish red ecchymoses occurring on the forearms and backs of the hands in the elderly. **thrombocytopenic p.,** any form in which the platelet count is decreased, occurring as a primary disease (*idiopathic thrombocytopenic p.*) or as a consequence of a primary hematologic disorder (*secondary thrombocytopenic p.*). **thrombotic thrombocytopenic p.,** a disease marked by thrombocytopenia, hemolytic anemia, neurological manifestations, azotemia, fever, and thromboses in terminal arterioles and capillaries.

purpureaglycoside (per-pu″re-ah-gli′ko-sīd) a cardiac glycoside, $C_{47}H_{74}O_{18}$, from the leaves of *Digitalis purpurea.* **p. C,** deslanoside.

purpurin (per′pu-rin) 1. a dye, $C_{14}H_8O_5$, from madder root. 2. uroerythrin.

purpurinuria (pur″pu-rin-u′re-ah) purpurin (uroerythrin) in the urine.

purulence (pu′roo-lens) the formation or presence of pus.

purulent (pur′roo-lent) containing or forming pus.

puruloid (pu′roo-loid) resembling pus.

pus (pus) a protein-rich liquid inflammation product made up of cells (leukocytes), a thin fluid (liquor puris), and cellular debris. **blue p.,** pus with a bluish tint, produced by *Pseudomonas aeruginosa.*

pustula (pus′tu-lah), pl. *pus′tulae* [L.] pustule.

pustular (pus′tu-lar) pertaining to or of the nature of a pustule; consisting of pustules.

pustulation (pus″tu-la′shun) the formation of pustules.

pustule (pus′tūl) a small, elevated, circumscribed, pus-containing lesion of the skin.

pustulosis (pus″tu-lo′sis) a condition marked by an eruption of pustules.

putamen (pu-ta′men) the larger and more lateral part of the lentiform nucleus.

putrefaction (pu″trĕ-fak′shun) enzymatic decomposition, especially of proteins, with the production of foul-smelling compounds, such as hydrogen sulfide, ammonia, and mercaptans. **putrefac′tive,** adj.

putrefy (pu′trĕ-fi) to undergo putrefaction.

putrescence (pu-tres′ens) the condition of undergoing putrefaction. **putres′cent,** adj.

putrescine (pu-tres′in) a poisonous bacterial decomposition product found in decaying meat, formed by decarboxylation of ornithine.

putrid (pu′trid) rotten; putrefied.

PVP polyvinylpyrrolodine (see *povidone*).

PVP-I povidone-iodine.

pyarthrosis (pi″ar-thro′sis) suppuration within a joint cavity; acute suppurative arthritis.

pycno- see words beginning *pykn(o)-*.

pyel(o)- word element [Gr.], *renal pelvis.*

pyelectasis (pi″ĕ-lek′tah-sis) dilatation of the renal pelvis.

pyelitis (pi″ĕ-li′tis) inflammation of the renal pelvis. **pyelit′ic,** adj. **p. cys′tica,** pyelitis with formation of multiple submucosal cysts.

pyelocaliectasis (pi″ĕ-lo-kal″e-ek′tah-sis) dilatation of the renal pelvis and calices.

pyelocystitis (-sis-ti′tis) inflammation of the renal pelvis and bladder.

pyelogram (pi′ĕ-lo-gram″) the film produced by pyelography.

pyelography (pi″e-log′rah-fe) radiography of the renal pelvis and ureter after injection of contrast material. **retrograde p.,** pyelography after introduction of contrast material through the ureter.

pyelolithotomy (pi″ĕ-lo-lĭ-thot′o-me) incision of the renal pelvis for removal of calculi.

pyelonephritis (-nĕ-fri′tis) inflammation of the kidney and its pelvis due to bacterial infection.

pyelonephrosis (-nĕ-fro′sis) any disease of the kidney and its pelvis.

pyelopathy (pi″ĕ-lop′ah-the) any disease of the renal pelvis.

pyeloplasty (pi′ĕ-lo-plas″te) plastic repair of the renal pelvis.

pyeloplication (pi″ĕ-lo-pli-ka′shun) reduction in size of a dilated renal pelvis by surgical infolding of its walls.

pyelostomy (pi″ĕ-los′to-me) surgical formation of an opening into the renal pelvis.

pyelotomy (pi″ĕ-lot′o-me) incision of the renal pelvis.

pyelovenous (pi″ĕ-lo-ve′nus) pertaining to the renal pelvis and renal veins.

pyemesis (pi-em′ĕ-sis) the vomiting of pus.

pyemia (pi-e′me-ah) septicemia in which secondary foci of suppuration occur and multiple abscesses are formed. **pye′mic,** adj. **arterial p.,** that due to dissemination of septic emboli from the heart. **cryptogenic p.,** that in which the source of infection is in an unidentified tissue.

Pyemotes (pi″ĕ-mo′tēz) a genus of parasitic mites. *P. ventrico′sus* attacks certain insect larvae found on straw, grain, and other plants, and causes grain itch in man.

pyencephalus (pi″en-sef′ah-lus) abscess of the brain.

pyesis (pi-e′sis) suppuration.

pygal (pi′gal) pertaining to the buttocks.

pygalgia (pi-gal′je-ah) pain in the buttocks.

pygoamorphus (pi″go-ah-mor′fus) asymmetrical conjoined twins, in which the parasite is an amorphous mass attached to the sacral region of the autosite.

pygodidymus (-did′ĭ-mus) a fetus with double hips and pelvis.

pygomelus (pi-gom′ĕ-lus) a fetus with a supernumerary limb or limbs attached to or near the buttocks.

pygopagus (pi-gop′ah-gus) conjoined twins fused in the sacral region.

pykn(o)- word element [Gr.], *thick; compact; frequent.*

pyknic (pik′nik) having a short, thick, stocky build.

pyknocyte (pik′no-sīt) a distorted and contracted, occasionally spiculed erythrocyte.

pyknocytosis (pik″no-si-to′sis) conspicuous increase in the numbers of pyknocytes.

pyknodysostosis (-dis″os-to′sis) a hereditary syndrome of dwarfism, osteopetrosis, and skeletal anomalies of the cranium, digits, and mandible.

pyknometer (pik-nom′ĕ-ter) an instrument for determining the specific gravity of fluids.

pyknomorphous (pik″no-mor′fus) having the stained portions of the cell body compactly arranged.

pyknophrasia (-fra′ze-ah) thickness of speech.

pyknosis (pik-no′sis) a thickening, especially degeneration of a cell in which the nucleus shrinks in size and the chromatin condenses to a solid, structureless mass or masses. **pyknot′ic,** adj.

pyle- word element [Gr.], *portal vein.*

pylephlebectasis (pi″le-flĕ-bek′tah-sis) dilatation of the portal vein.

pylephlebitis (-flĕ-bi′tis) inflammation of the portal vein.

pylethrombophlebitis (-throm″bo-flĕ-bi′tis) thrombosis and inflammation of the portal vein.

pylethrombosis (-throm-bo′sis) thrombosis of the portal vein.

pylor(o)- word element [Gr.], *pylorus.*

pyloralgia (pi″lo-ral′je-ah) pain in the region of the pylorus.

pylorectomy (pi″lo-rek′to-me) excision of the pylorus.

pyloric (pi-lor′ik) pertaining to the pylorus or to the pyloric part of the stomach.

pyloristenosis (pi-lor″e-stĕ-no′sis) pyloric stenosis.

pylorodiosis (pi-lor″o-di-o′sis) dilation of a pyloric stricture with the finger during operation.

pyloroduodenitis (-du″o-de-ni′tis) inflammation of the pyloric and duodenal mucosa.

pylorogastrectomy (-gas-trek′to-me) excision of the pylorus and adjacent portion of the stomach.

pyloromyotomy (-mi-ot′o-me) incision of the longitudinal and circular muscles of the pylorus.

pyloroplasty (pi-lor′o-plas″te) plastic surgery of the pylorus. **Finney p.,** enlargement of the pyloric canal by establishment of an inverted U-shaped anastomosis between the stomach and duodenum after longitudinal incision. **Heineke-Mikulicz p.,** enlargement of a pyloric stricture by incising the pylorus longitudinally and suturing the incision transversely.

pyloroscopy (pi″lor-os′ko-pe) endoscopic inspection of the pylorus.

pylorospasm (pi-lor′o-spazm) spasm of the pylorus or the pyloric part of the stomach.

pylorostenosis (pi-lor″o-stĕ-no′sis) stenosis of the pylorus.

pylorostomy (pi″lor-os′to-me) surgical formation of an opening through the abdominal wall into the stomach near the pylorus.

pylorotomy (-ot′o-me) incision of the pylorus.

pylorus (pi-lo′rus) the distal aperture of the stomach, opening into the duodenum; variously used to mean pyloric part of the stomach, and pyloric antrum, canal, opening, or sphincter.

pyo- word element [Gr.], *pus.*

pyocele (pi′o-sēl) a collection of pus, as in the scrotum.

pyocephalus (pi″o-sef′ah-lus) purulent fluid in the cerebral ventricles.

pyochezia (-ke′ze-ah) pus in the feces.

pyococcus (-kok′us) any pus-forming coccus.

pyocolpocele (-kol′po-sēl) a vaginal tumor containing pus.

pyocolpos (-kol′pos) pus in the vagina.

pyocyanase (-si′ah-nās) an antibacterial material from cultures of *Pseudomonas aeruginosa* (*pyocyanea*)*;* bactericidal for many bacteria and lytic for some (*Vibrio cholerae*).

pyocyanic (-si-an′ik) pertaining to blue pus, or to *Pseudomonas aeruginosa.*

pyocyanin (-si′ah-nin) a blue-green antibiotic pigment produced by *Pseudomonas aeruginosa;* it gives the color to "blue pus."

pyocyst (pi′o-sist) a cyst containing pus.

pyoderma (pi″o-der′mah) any purulent skin disease. **p. gangreno′sum,** a rapidly evolving cutaneous ulcer or ulcers, with marked undermining of the border.

pyodermia (-der′me-ah) pyoderma.

pyogenesis (-jen′ĕ-sis) the formation of pus.

pyogenic (-jen′ik) producing pus.

pyohemia (-he′me-ah) pyemia.

pyohemothorax (-he″mo-tho′raks) pus and blood in the pleural space.

pyoid (pi′oid) resembling or like pus.

pyolabyrinthitis (pi″o-lab″ĭ-rin-thi′tis) inflammation of the labyrinth of the ear, with suppuration.

pyometra (-me′trah) accumulation of pus within the uterus.

pyometritis (-me-tri′tis) purulent inflammation of the uterus.

pyomyositis (-mi″o-si′tis) purulent myositis.

pyonephritis (-nĕ-fri′tis) purulent inflammation of the kidney.

pyonephrolithiasis (-nef″ro-lĭ-thi′ah-sis) pus and stones in the kidney.

pyonephrosis (-nĕ-fro′sis) suppurative destruction of the renal parenchyma, with total or almost complete loss of kidney function.

pyo-ovarium (-o-va′re-um) an abscess of the ovary.

pyopericarditis (-per″ĭ-kar-di′tis) purulent pericarditis.

pyopericardium (-per″ĭ-kar′de-um) pus in the pericardium.

pyoperitoneum (-per″ĭ-to-ne′um) pus in the peritoneal cavity.

pyoperitonitis (-per″ĭ-to-ni′tis) purulent inflammation of the peritoneum.

pyophthalmitis (pi″of-thal-mi′tis) purulent inflammation of the eye.

pyophysometra (pi″o-fi″so-me′trah) pus and gas in the uterus.

pyopneumocholecystitis (pi″o-nu″mo-ko″le-sis-ti′tis) distention of the gallbladder, with presence of pus and gas.

pyopneumohepatitis (-hep″ah-ti′tis) abscess of the liver with pus and gas in the abscess cavity.

pyopneumopericardium (-per″ĭ-kar′de-um) pus and gas in the pericardium.

pyopneumoperitonitis (-per″ĭ-to-ni′tis) peritonitis with presence of pus and gas.

pyopneumothorax (-tho′raks) pus and air or gas in the pleural cavity.

pyopoiesis (pi″o-poi-e′sis) pyogenesis.

pyoptysis (pi-op′tĭ-sis) expectoration of purulent matter.

pyopyelectasis (pi″o-pi″ĕ-lek′tah-sis) dilatation of the renal pelvis with pus.

pyorrhea (-re′ah) a copious discharge of pus. **pyorrhe′al,** adj. **p. alveola′ris,** compound periodontitis.

pyosalpingitis (-sal″pin-ji′tis) purulent salpingitis.

pyosalpingo-oophoritis (-sal-ping″go-o″of-o-ri′tis) purulent inflammation of the uterine tube and ovary.

pyosalpinx (-sal′pinks) accumulation of pus in a uterine tube.

pyostatic (-stat′ik) arresting suppuration; an agent that arrests suppuration.

pyothorax (-tho′raks) an accumulation of pus in the thorax; empyema.

pyourachus (-u′rah-kus) pus in the urachus.

pyoureter (-u-re′ter) pus in the ureter.

pyoxanthine (-zan′thēn) a brownish pigment from oxidation of pyocyanine.

pyoxanthose (-zan′thōs) a yellow pigment produced by the oxidation of pyocyanin.

pyramid (pir′ah-mid) a pointed or cone-shaped structure or part. **pyram′idal,** adj. **p. of cerebellum,** p. of vermis. **p. of Ferrein,** any of the intracortical prolongations of the renal pyramids. **Lalouette's p.,** p. of thyroid. **p. of light,** a triangular reflection seen upon the tympanic membrane. **malpighian p's,** renal p's. **p. of medulla oblongata,** either of two rounded masses, one on either side of the median fissure of the medulla oblongata. **petrous p.,** pars petrosa. **renal p's,** the conical masses composing the medullary substance of the kidney. **p. of thyroid,** an occasional third lobe of the thyroid gland, extending upward from the isthmus. **p. of tympanum,** the hollow elevation in the inner wall of the middle ear containing the stapedius muscle. **p. of vermis,** the part of the vermis cerebelli between the tuber vermis and the uvula.

pyramidal (pĭ-ram′ĭ-dal) shaped like a pyramid; see also under *tract.*

pyramis (pir′ah-mis), pl. *pyram′ides* [Gr.] pyramid.

pyran (pi′ran) a cyclic compound, C_5H_6O, in which the ring consists of 5 carbon atoms and 1 oxygen atom.

pyranisamine (pi″rah-nis′ah-mēn) pyrilamine.

pyranose (pi′rah-nōs) a hexose having a ring structure analogous to pyran.

pyrantel (pĭ-ran′tel) an anthelminthic, $C_{11}H_{14}$-N_2S, used as the pamoate and tartrate salts.

pyrathiazine (pi″rah-thi′ah-zēn) a phenothiazine derivative, $C_{18}H_{20}N_2S_4$; the hydrochloride salt is used as an antihistaminic.

pyrazinamide (-zin′ah-mīd) a tuberculostatic antibacterial, $C_5H_5N_3O$.

pyrectic (pi-rek′tik) 1. pertaining to fever; feverish. 2. a fever-inducing agent.

pyretic (pi-ret′ik) pertaining to fever.

pyretogenesis (pi-re″to-jen′ĕ-sis) the origin and causation of fever.

pyretogenous (pi″rĕ-toj′ĕ-nus) 1. caused by high body temperature. 2. pyrogenic.

pyretotherapy (pi-re″to-ther′ah-pe) 1. treatment by artifically increasing body temperature. 2. the treatment of fever.

pyrexia (pi-rek′se-ah) a fever, or febrile condition. **pyrex′ial,** adj.

Pyribenzamine (pir″ĭ-ben′zah-mēn) trademark for preparations of tripelennamine.

pyridine (pir″ĭ-din) 1. a coal tar derivative, C_5-H_5N, derived also from tobacco and various organic matter. 2. any of a group of substances homologous with normal pyridine.

pyridostigmine (pir″ĭ-do-stig′mēn) a cholinesterase inhibitor, $C_9H_{13}N_2O_2$; the bromide salt is used in treatment of myasthenia gravis.

pyridoxal (pir″ĭ-dok′sal) a form of vitamin B_6.

pyridoxamine (pir″ĭ-doks′ah-mēn) one of the three active forms of vitamin B_6.

pyridoxine (pir″ĭ-dok′sēn) one of the forms of vitamin B_6, $C_8H_{11}NO_3$, chiefly used, as the hydrochloride salt, in the prophylaxis and treatment of vitamin B_6 deficiency. It is also used in counteracting the neurotoxic effects of isoniazid, and sometimes in the treatment of myasthenia gravis.

pyrilamine (pi-ril′ah-mēn) an antihistaminic, $C_{17}H_{23}N_3O$, used as the maleate salt.

pyrimethamine (pi″rĭ-meth′ah-mēn) an antimalarial, $C_{12}H_{13}ClN_4$, used especially for suppressive prophylaxis.

pyrimidine (pi-rim′ĭ-dēn) an organic compound, $C_4H_4N_2$, the fundamental form of the pyrimidine bases, including uracil, cytosine, and thymine.

pyrithiamine (pir″ĭ-thi′ah-min) an analogue of thiamine which by metabolic competition can cause symptoms of thiamine deficiency.

pyro- word element [Gr.], *fire; heat;* (in chemistry) *produced by heating.*

pyrogallol (pi″ro-gal′ol) pyrogallic acid, derived from gallic acid and used externally as an antimicrobial and irritant.

pyrogen (pi′ro-jen) a fever-producing substance. **pyrogen′ic,** adj.

pyroglobulinemia (pi″ro-glob″u-lin-e′me-ah)

presence in the blood of an abnormal globulin constituent which is precipitated by heat.

pyromania (-ma'ne-ah) obsessive preoccupation with fires; compulsion to set fires.

pyrometer (pi-rom'ĕ-ter) a device for measuring high degrees of heat.

Pyronil (pi'ro-nil) trademark for a preparation of pyrrobutamine.

pyronine (-nin) a red aniline histologic stain.

pyrophobia (pi″ro-fo'be-ah) morbid dread of fire.

pyrophosphatase (-fos'fah-tās) any enzyme that catalyzes the hydrolysis of central pyrophosphate linkages.

pyrophosphate (-fos'fāt) a salt of pyrophosphoric acid.

pyrosis (pi-ro'sis) heartburn; a burning sensation in the esophagus and stomach, with sour eructation.

pyrotic (pi-rot'ik) caustic; burning.

pyroxylin (pi-rok'sĭ-lin) a product of the action of a mixture of nitric and sulfuric acids on cotton, consisting chiefly of cellulose tetranitrate; a necessary ingredient of collodion.

pyrrobutamine (pir″ro-bu'tah-min) an antihistaminic, $C_{20}H_{22}ClN$.

pyrrocaine (pir'o-kān) a local anesthetic, $C_{14}H_{20}N_2O$, used in dentistry as the hydrochloride salt.

pyrrole (pir'ōl) a basic, cyclic substance, $(CH)_4$-NH, obtained by destructive distillation of various animal substances.

pyrrolidine (pĭ-rol'ĭ-din) a simple base, $(CH_2)_4$-NH, obtained from tobacco or prepared from pyrrole.

pyruvate (pi'roo-vāt) a salt or ester of pyruvic acid; in biochemistry, the term is used interchangeably with pyruvic acid.

pyrvinium (pir-vin'e-um) an anthelmintic used for intestinal pinworms in the form of the pamoate salt, $C_{75}H_{70}N_6O_6$.

pyuria (pi-u're-ah) pus in the urine.

PZI protamine zinc insulin.

Q

q.d. [L.] *qua'que di'e* (every day).

q.h. *qua'que ho'ra* (every hour).

q.i.d. [L.] *qua'ter in di'e* (four times a day).

q.s. [L.] *quan'tum sa'tis* (a sufficient amount).

qt. quart.

quack (kwak) one who misrepresents his ability and experience in diagnosis and treatment of disease or effects to be achieved by his treatment.

quackery (kwak'er-e) the practice or methods of a quack.

quadr(i)- word element [L.], *four*.

quadrangular (kwod-rang'gu-lar) having four angles.

quadrant (kwod'rant) 1. one fourth of the circumference of a circle. 2. one of four corresponding parts, or quarters, as of the surface of the abdomen or of the field of vision.

quadrantanopia (kwod″ran-tah-no'pe-ah) defective vision or blindness in one fourth of the visual field.

quadrantanopsia (-nop'se-ah) quandrantanopia.

quadrate (kwod'rāt) square or squared.

quadriceps (kwod'rĭ-seps) having four heads.

quadrigemina (kwod″rĭ-jem'ĭ-nah) the corpora quadrigemina.

quadrigeminal (-jem'ĭ-nal) fourfold; in four parts; forming a group of four.

quadripara (kwod-rip'ah-rah) a woman who has had four pregnancies which resulted in viable offspring; para IV.

quadriplegia (kwod″rĭ-ple'je-ah) paralysis of all four limbs.

quadritubercular (-tu-ber'ku-lar) having four tubercles or cusps.

quadruped (kwod'roo-ped) 1. four-footed. 2. an animal having four feet.

quadruplet (-plet) one of four offspring produced at one birth.

qualimeter (kwah-lim'ĕ-ter) penetrometer (1).

quantimeter (kwon-tim'ĕ-ter) an instrument for measuring the quantity of roentgen rays generated by a tube.

quantum (kwon'tum), pl. *quan'ta* [L.] a unit of measure under the quantum theory (q.v.).

quarantine (kwor'an-tēn) 1. a place or period of detention of ships or persons coming from infected or suspected areas. 2. to detain or isolate on account of suspected contagion. 3. restrictions placed on entering or leaving premises where a case of communicable disease exists.

quartan (kwor'tan) recurring in four-day cycles; see *malaria*.

quart (kwort) one fourth of a gallon (946 ml.); abbreviated qt.

quarter (kwor'ter) the part of a horse's hoof between the heel and the toe. **false q.,** a cleft in a horse's hoof from the top to the bottom.

quartz (kworts) a crystalline form of silica (silicon dioxide).

quater in die (kwah'ter in de'a) [L.] four times a day.

quaternary (kwah'ter-ner″e, kwah-ter'nar-e) 1. fourth in order. 2. containing four elements or groups.

Quelicin (kwel'ĭ-sin) trademark for a preparation of succinylcholine.

quickening (kwik'en-ing) the first perceptible movement of the fetus in the uterus.

quinacrine (kwin'ah-krin) an anthelmintic for

tapeworms, $C_{23}H_{30}ClN_3O$, used as the hydrochloride salt.

quinalbarbitone (kwin″al-bar′bĭ-tōn) secobarbital.

quinestrol (kwin-es′trōl) a long-acting estrogen, $C_{25}H_{32}O_2$.

quinethazone (-eth′ah-zōn) a diuretic, $C_{10}H_{12}ClN_3O_3S$.

quingestanol (-jes′tah-nōl) a long-acting progestin, $C_{26}H_{38}O_2$.

quinidine (kwin′ĭ-din) the dextrorotatory isomer of quinine, $C_{20}H_{24}N_2O_2$, used in treatment of cardiac arrhythmias.

quinine (kwi′nin) an alkaloid, $C_{20}H_{24}N_2O_2 + 3H_2O$, from cinchona used as an antimalarial, especially against *Plasmodium falciparum;* also used for its analgesic, oxytocic, antipyretic, and sclerosing properties, and for alleviating muscle contractures and cramps.

quininism (kwin′ĭ-nizm) cinchonism.

quinone (kwi-non′, kwin′ōn) any benzene derivative in which two hydrogen atoms are replaced by two oxygen atoms.

quinsy (kwin′ze) peritonsillar abscess.

quint- word element [L.], *five.*

quintan (kwin′tan) recurring every fifth day, as a fever.

quintipara (kwin-tip′ah-rah) a woman who has had five pregnancies which resulted in viable offspring; para V.

quintuplet (kwin′tu-plet) one of five offspring produced at one birth.

quittor (kwit′or) a fistulous sore on the quarters or the coronet of a horse's foot.

Quotane (kwo′tān) trademark for a preparation of dimethisoquin.

quotidian (kwo-tid′e-an) recurring every day; see *malaria.*

quotient (kwo′shent) a number obtained by division. **achievement q.,** the achievement age divided by the mental age, indicating progress in learning. **caloric q.,** the heat evolved (in calories) divided by the oxygen consumed (in milligrams) in a metabolic process. **intelligence q.,** a measure of intelligence obtained by dividing the mental age by the chronological age and multiplying the result by 100. **respiratory q.,** the ratio of the volume of expired carbon dioxide to the volume of oxygen absorbed by the lungs per unit of time.

R

R symbol for *roentgen;* chemical symbol for an organic radical.

R. Rankine (scale), Réaumur (scale); L. *remo′tum* (far); respiration; *Rickettsia;* right.

℞ symbol, L. *rec′ipe* (take); prescription; treatment.

Ra chemical symbol, *radium.*

rabid (rab′id) affected with rabies; pertaining to rabies.

rabies (ra′bēz, ra′be-ēz) an acute infectious viral disease of the central nervous system of mammals, human infection resulting from the bite of a rabid animal (bats, dogs, etc.). In the later stages, it is marked by paralysis of the muscles of deglutition and glottal spasm provoked by the drinking or the sight of liquids, and by manical behavior, convulsions, tetany, and respiratory paralysis. **rab′ic,** adj.

racemase (ra′se-mās) an enzyme that catalyzes the racemization of an optically active substance.

racemate (ra′se-māt) a racemic compound.

racemic (ra-se′mik) optically inactive, being composed of equal amounts of dextrorotatory and levorotatory isomers.

racemization (ras″e-mĭ-za′shun) the transformation of one half of the molecules of an optically active compound into molecules having exactly the opposite configuration, with complete loss of rotatory power because of the statistical balance between equal numbers of dextro- and levorotatory molecules.

racemose (ras′e-mōs) shaped like a bunch of grapes.

racephedrine (ra-sef′e-drin) the racemic form of ephedrine, $C_{10}H_{15}NO$; the hydrochloride salt is used as a sympathomimetic.

rachi(o)- word element [Gr.], *spine.*

rachialgia (ra″ke-al′je-ah) pain in the spine.

rachicentesis (ra″kĭ-sen-te′sis) lumbar puncture.

rachidial, rachidian (rah-kid′e-al; rah-kid′e-an) pertaining to the spine.

rachigraph (ra′kĭ-graf) an instrument for recording the outlines of the spine and back.

rachilysis (rah-kil′ĭ-sis) correction of lateral curvature of the spine by combined traction and pressure.

rachiometer (ra″ke-om′e-ter) an apparatus for measuring spinal curvature.

rachiotomy (-ot′o-me) incision of a vertebra or the vertebral column.

rachis (ra′kis) the vertebral column.

rachischisis (rah-kis′kĭ-sis) congenital fissure of the vertebral column. **r. poste′rior,** spina bifida.

rachitic (rah-kit′ik) pertaining to rickets.

rachitis (rah-ki′tis) rickets.

rachitogenic (rah-kit″o-jen′ik) causing rickets.

rad (rad) *r*adiation *a*bsorbed *d*ose: a unit of measurement of the absorbed dose of ionizing radiation, corresponding to an energy transfer of 100 ergs per gram of any absorbing material.

rad. [L.] *ra′dix* (root).

radectomy (rah-dek′to-me) excision of the root of a tooth.

radiability (ra″de-ah-bil′ĭ-te) the property of being readily penetrated by roentgen or other rays.

radiad (ra′de-ad) toward the radius or radial side.

radial (ra′de-al) pertaining to the radius.

radialis (ra″de-a′lis) [L.] radial.

radiant (ra′de-ant) diverging from a center; emitting rays.

radiate (ra′de-āt) 1. to diverge or spread from a common point. 2. arranged in a radiating manner.

radiatio (ra″de-a′she-o), pl. *radiatio′nes* [L.] a radiation or radiating structure.

radiation (ra″de-a′shun) 1. divergence from a common center. 2. a structure made up of divergent elements, as one of the fiber tracts in the brain. 3. electromagnetic waves, such as those of light, or particulate rays, such as alpha, beta, and gamma rays, given off from some source. **acoustic r.,** a fiber tract arising in the medial geniculate nucleus and passing laterally to terminate in the transverse temporal gyri of the temporal lobe. **adaptive r.,** evolution from a generalized, primitive species to diverse, specialized species, each adapted to a distinct mode of life. **r. of corpus callosum,** the fibers of the corpus callosum radiating to all parts of the neopallium. **corpuscular r.,** particles emitted in nuclear disintegration, including alpha and beta particles, protons, neutrons, positrons, and deuterons. **electromagnetic r.,** see under *wave*. **interstitial r.,** energy emitted by radium or radon inserted directly into the tissue. **ionizing r.,** high-energy radiation (x-rays and gamma rays) which interacts to produce ion pairs in matter. **optic r.,** a fiber tract starting at the lateral geniculate body, passing through the pars retrolentiformis of the internal capsule, and terminating in the striate area on the medial surface of the occipital lobe, on either side of the calcarine sulcus. **pyramidal r.,** fibers extending from the pyramidal tract to the cortex. **tegmental r.,** fibers radiating laterally from the red nucleus. **thalamic r.,** fibers which reciprocally connect the thalamus and cerebral cortex by way of the internal capsule, usually grouped into four subradiations (peduncles): anterior or frontal, superior or centroparietal, posterior or occipital, and inferior or temporal.

radical (rad′ĭ-k'l) 1. directed to the root or cause; designed to eliminate all possible extensions of a morbid process. 2. a group of atoms which enters and goes out of chemical combination without change.

radicle (rad′ĭ-k'l) one of the smallest branches of a vessel or nerve.

radicotomy (rad″ĭ-kot′o-me) rhizotomy.

radiculalgia (rah-dik″u-lal′je-ah) pain due to disorder of the spinal nerve roots.

radicular (rah-dik′u-lar) pertaining to a root or radicle.

radiculitis (rah-dik″u-li′tis) inflammation of the spinal nerve roots.

radiculoganglionitis (rah-dik″u-lo-gang″gle-o-

ni′tis) inflammation of the posterior spinal nerve roots and their ganglia.

radiculomeningomyelitis (-mĕ-ning″go-mi″ĕ-li′tis) inflammation of the nerve roots, meninges, and spinal cord.

radiculomyelopathy (-mi″ĕ-lop′ah-the) disease of the nerve roots and spinal cord.

radiculoneuritis (-nu-ri′tis) acute febrile polyneuritis.

radiculoneuropathy (-nu-rop′ah-the) disease of the nerve roots and spinal nerves.

radiculopathy (rah-dik″u-lop′ah-the) disease of the nerve roots.

radio- word element [L.], *ray; radiation; emission of radiant energy; radium; radius* (bone of the forearm); affixed to the name of a chemical element to designate a radioactive isotope of that element.

radioactinium (ra″de-o-ak-tin′e-um) a disintegration product of actinium.

radioactive (-ak′tiv) characterized by radioactivity.

radioactivity (-ak-tiv′ĭ-te) emission of corpuscular or electromagnetic radiations consequent to nuclear disintegration, a natural property of all chemical elements of atomic number above 83 and possible of induction in all other known elements. **artificial r., induced r.,** that produced by bombarding an element with high-velocity particles.

radioautograph (-aw′to-graf) autoradiograph.

radioautography (-aw-tog′rah-fe) autoradiography.

radiobicipital (-bi-sip′ĭ-tal) pertaining to the radius and the biceps muscle.

radiobiologist (-bi-ol′o-jist) an expert in radiobiology.

radiobiology (-bi-ol′o-je) the branch of science concerned with effects of light and of ultraviolet and ionizing radiations on living tissue or organisms.

radiocalcium (-kal′se-um) a radioactive isotope of calcium, ^{45}Ca, with a half-life of 180 days; used as a tracer in the study of calcium metabolism.

radiocarbon (-kar′bon) a radioactive isotope of carbon, e.g., ^{14}C, with a half-life of over 5000 years.

radiocardiogram (-kar′de-o-gram) the graphic record produced by radiocardiography.

radiocardiography (-kar″de-og′rah-fe) graphic recording of variation with time of the concentration, in a selected chamber of the heart, of a radioactive isotope, usually injected intravenously.

radiocarpal (-kar′pal) pertaining to the radius and carpus.

radiochemistry (-kem′is-tre) the branch of chemistry dealing with radioactive materials.

radiocinematograph (-sin″ĕ-mat′o-graf) a moving picture camera combined with an x-ray machine, making possible moving pictures of internal organs.

radiocurable (-kūr′ah-b'l) curable by irradiation.

radiocystitis (-sis-ti′tis) inflammatory tissue

changes in the urinary bladder caused by irradiation.

radiode (ra'de-ōd) an apparatus for therapeutic application of radioactive substance.

radiodermatitis (ra"de-o-der"mah-ti'tis) a cutaneous inflammatory reaction to exposure to biologically effective levels of ionizing radiation.

radiodiagnosis (-di"ag-no'sis) diagnosis by means of x-rays or gamma rays.

radiodontics (-don'tiks) dental radiology.

radiodontist (-don'tist) a dentist who specializes in dental radiology.

radioelement (-el'ě-ment) any chemical element having radioactive properties.

radiogold (ra'de-o-gold") a radioactive isotope of gold, especially ^{198}Au, which has a half-life of 2.7 days and emits gamma and beta radiation.

radiogram (-gram") radiograph.

radiograph (-graf") the film produced by radiography.

radiography (ra"de-og'rah-fe) the making of film records (radiographs) of internal structures of the body by exposure of film specially sensitized to x-rays or gamma rays. **radiograph'ic,** adj.

radiohumeral (ra"de-o-hu'mer-al) pertaining to the radius and humerus.

radioimmunity (-ĭ-mu'nĭ-te) diminished sensitivity to radiation.

radioimmunoassay (-im"u-no-as'a) immunoassay using a radioactive-labeled substance that reacts with the substance under test.

radioimmunodiffusion (-im"u-no-dif-fu'zhun) immunodiffusion conducted with radioisotope-labeled antibodies or antigens.

radioiodine (-i'o-dīn) a radioactive isotope of iodine; ^{131}I and ^{125}I are used in diagnosis and treatment of disease of the thyroid gland and in scintiscanning of the lungs, liver, etc.

radioiron (-i'ern) a radioactive isotope of iron; a mixture of ^{55}Fe and ^{59}Fe has been used in blood studies.

radioisotope (-i'so-tōp) a radioactive isotope, i.e., one having an unstable nucleus and which emits characteristic radiation during its decay to a stable form.

radiologist (ra"de-ol'o-jist) a physician specializing in radiology.

radiology (ra"de-ol'o-je) the branch of medical science dealing with use of radiant energy in diagnosis and treatment of disease. **radiolog'ic, radiolog'ical,** adj.

radiolucent (ra"de-o-lu'sent) permitting the passage of radiant energy, such as x-rays, yet offering some resistance to it, the representative areas appearing dark on the exposed film.

radiometer (ra"de-om'ě-ter) 1. an instrument for estimating roentgen-ray quantity. 2. an instrument in which radiant heat and light may be directly converted into mechanical energy. 3. an instrument for measuring the penetrating power of radiant energy.

radiomimetic (ra"de-o-mi-met'ik) producing effects similar to those of ionizing radiations.

radion (ra'de-on) a particle given off by radioactive matter.

radionecrosis (ra"de-o-ně-kro'sis) tissue destruction due to radiant energy.

radioneuritis (-nu-ri'tis) neuritis from exposure to radiant energy.

radionuclide (-nu'klīd) a radioactive nuclide.

radiopacity (-pas'ĭ-te) the quality or property of obstructing the passage of radiant energy, such as x-rays, the representative areas appearing light or white on the exposed film. **radiopaque',** adj.

radiopathology (-pah-thol'o-je) the pathology of radiation effects on tissues.

radiopelvimetry (-pel-vim'ě-tre) measurement of the pelvis by radiography.

radiophosphorus (-fos'fo-rus) either of two radioactive isotopes of phosphorus, ^{32}P and ^{33}P; the former, a pure beta emitter, has a half-life of 14.3 days and is used in solution or colloidal form as a diagnostic and therapeutic agent.

radiopotentiation (-po-ten"she-a'shun) the action of a drug in enhancing the effects of irradiation.

radioreceptor (-re-sep'tor) a receptor which is stimulated by radiant energy, e.g., light.

radioresistance (-re-zis'tans) resistance, as of tissue or cells to irradiation. **radioresist'ant,** adj.

radioresponsive (-re-spon'siv) reacting favorably to irradiation.

radioscopy (ra"de-os'ko-pe) fluoroscopy.

radiosensitivity (ra"de-o-sen"sĭ-tiv'ĭ-te) sensitivity, as of the skin, tumor tissue, etc., to radiant energy, such as x-ray or other radiations. **radiosen'sitive,** adj.

radiosodium (-so'de-um) a radioactive isotope of sodium; ^{24}Na and ^{22}Na are used in the study of blood flow, water balance, and peripheral vascular diseases.

radiosurgery (-ser'jer-e) surgical treatment in which radium is used.

radiotelemetry (-tel-em'ě-tre) measurement based on data transmitted by radio waves from the subject to the recording apparatus.

radiotherapist (-ther'ah-pist) a specialist in radiotherapy.

radiotherapy (-ther'ah-pe) treatment of disease by means of ionizing radiation; tissue may be exposed to a beam of radiation, or a radioactive element may be contained in devices (e.g., needles or wire) and inserted directly into the tissues (*interstitial r.*), or it may be introduced into a natural body cavity (*intracavitary r.*).

radiothermy (-ther'me) short-wave diathermy.

radiotoxemia (-tok-se'me-ah) toxemia produced by radiant energy.

radiotransparent (-trans-pār'ent) permitting the passage of x-rays or other forms of radiation.

radiotropic (-trop'ik) influenced by radiation.

radioulnar (-ul'nar) pertaining to the radius and ulna.

radium (ra'de-um) a radioactive element (*see table*), at. no. 88, symbol Ra; it has a half-life of 1622 years, emitting alpha, beta, and gamma radiation. It decays to radon.

radius (ra'de-us), pl. *ra'dii* [L.] 1. a line from the

center of a circle to a point on its circumference. 2. see *Table of Bones*. **r. fix′us,** straight line from the hormion to inion.

radix (ra′diks), pl. *rad′ices* [L.] root.

radon (ra′don) a radioactive element (*see table*), at. no. 86, symbol Rn, resulting from decay of radium.

raffinase (raf′ĭ-nās) an enzyme that catalyzes the hydrolytic cleavage of raffinose (melitose).

raffinose (raf′ĭ-nōs) melitose.

rage (rāj) a state of violent anger. **sham r.,** a state resembling rage occurring in decorticated animals or in certain pathologic conditions in man.

rale (rahl) an abnormal respiratory sound heard on auscultation, indicating some pathologic condition. **amphoric r.,** a coarse, musical, and tinkling rale due to the splashing of fluid in a cavity connected with a bronchus. **clicking r.,** a small sticky sound heard on inspiration, due to the passage of air through secretions in the smaller bronchi. **crackling r.,** subcrepitant r. **crepitant r.,** a fine dry, crackling sound like that made by rubbing hairs between the fingers; heard at the end of inspiration. **dry r.,** a whistling, musical, or squeaky sound, heard in asthma and bronchitis. **moist r.,** a sound produced by fluid in the bronchial tubes. **sibilant r.,** a high-pitched hissing sound due to viscid secretions in the bronchial tubes or by thickening of the tube walls; heard in asthma and bronchitis. **subcrepitant r.,** a fine moist rale heard in conditions associated with liquid in the smaller tubes.

ramal (ra′mal) pertaining to a ramus.

ramification (ram″ĭ-fĭ-ka′shun) 1. distribution in branches. 2. a branching.

ramify (ram′ĭ-fi) 1. to branch; to diverge in different directions. 2. to traverse in branches.

ramisection (ram″ĭ-sek′shun) section of the appropriate rami communicantes of the sympathetic nervous system.

ramose (ra′mos) branching; having many branches.

ramulus (ram′u-lus), pl. *ram′uli* [L.] a small branch or terminal division.

ramus (ra′mus), pl. *ra′mi* [L.] a branch, as of a nerve, vein, or artery. **r. commu′nicans** (pl. *ra′mi communican′tes*), a branch connecting two nerves or two arteries.

rancid (ran′sid) having a musty, rank taste or smell, as of fats that have undergone decomposition.

ranine (ra′nīn) pertaining to (*a*) a frog; (*b*) a ranula, or to the lower surface of the tongue; (*c*) the sublingual vein.

ranula (ran′u-lah) a cystic tumor beneath the tongue. **ran′ular,** adj. **pancreatic r.,** a retention cyst of the pancreatic duct.

raphe (ra′fe) a seam; the line of union of the halves of various symmetrical parts.

rapport (rah-por′) a relation of harmony and accord, as between patient and physician.

rarefaction (rar″ĕ-fak′shun) condition of being or becoming less dense.

rash (rash) a temporary eruption on the skin.

butterfly r., a skin eruption across the nose and adjacent areas of the cheeks in the pattern of a butterfly, as in lupus erythematosus and seborrheic dermatitis. **diaper r.,** dermatitis occurring in infants on the areas covered by the diaper. **drug r.,** see under *eruption*. **heat r.,** miliaria rubra.

raspatory (ras′pah-to-re) a file or rasp for surgical use.

rate (rāt) the speed or frequency with which an event or circumstance occurs per unit of time, population, or other standard of comparison. **basal metabolic r.,** an expression of the rate at which oxygen is utilized in a fasting subject at complete rest as a percentage of a value established as normal for such a subject. **birth r.,** the number of births during one year for the total population (*crude birth r.*), for the female population (*refined birth r.*), or for the female population of childbearing age (*true birth r.*). **case fatality r.,** the number of deaths due to a specific disease compared to the total number of cases. **death r.,** the ratio of the total number of deaths to the population of a specified area in a given time period, generally figured in terms of number of deaths per 1,000, 10,000, or 100,000 of population. **dose r.,** the amount of any therapeutic agent administered per unit of time. **erythrocyte sedimentation r.,** an expression of the extent of settling of erythrocytes in a vertical column of blood per unit of time. **fatality r.,** the number of deaths caused by a specific circumstance or disease, expressed as the absolute or relative number among individuals encountering the circumstance or having the disease. **glomerular filtration r.,** a expression of the quantity of glomerular filtrate formed each minute in the nephrons of both kidneys, calculated by measuring the clearance of specific substances, e.g., inulin or creatinine. **growth r.,** an expression of the increase in size of an organic object per unit of time. **heart r.,** the number of contractions of the cardiac ventricles per unit of time. **morbidity r.,** the number of cases of a given disease occurring in a specified period per unit of population. **mortality r.,** death r. **pulse r.,** the number of pulsations noted in a peripheral artery per unit of time. **respiration r.,** the number of movements of the chest wall per unit of time, indicative of inspiration and expiration. **sedimentation r.,** the rate at which a sediment is deposited in a given volume of solution, especialy when subjected to the action of a centrifuge.

ratio (ra′she-o) [L.] an expression of the quantity of one substance or entity in relation to that of another; the relationship between two quantities expressed as the quotient of one divided by the other. **A-G r., albumin-globulin r.,** the ratio of albumin to globulin in blood serum, plasma, or the urine in various renal diseases. **cardiothoracic r.,** the ratio of the transverse diameter of the heart to the internal diameter of the chest at its widest point just above the dome of the diaphragm. **sex r.,** the number of males in a population per number of females, usually stated as the number of males per 100 females.

rational (rash'un-al) based upon reason; characterized by possession of one's reason.

rationalization (rash''un-al-i-za'shun) an unconscious defense mechanism by which one justifies attitudes and behavior that would otherwise be intolerable.

Rau-Sed (row'sed) trademark for a preparation of reserpine.

Rauwiloid (row'wĭ-loid) trademark for preparations of alseroxylon.

Rauwolfia (raw-wul'fe-ah) a genus of tropical trees and shrubs, including over 100 species, that provide numerous alkaloids, notably reserpine, of medical interest.

rauwolfia (raw-wul'fe-ah) any member of the genus *Rauwolfia;* the dried root, or extract of the dried root, of *Rauwolfia.* **r. serpenti'na,** the dried root of *Rauwolfia serpentina,* sometimes with fragments of rhizome and other parts, used as an antihypertensive and sedative.

ray (ra) a line emanating from a center, as a more or less distinct portion of radiant energy (light or heat), proceeding in a specific direction. **actinic r.,** a light ray which produces chemical changes. **alpha r's, α-r's,** high-speed helium nuclei ejected from radioactive substances; they have less penetrating power than beta rays. **beta r's, β-r's,** electrons ejected from radioactive substances with velocities as high as 0.98 of the velocity of light; they have more penetrating power than alpha rays, but less than gamma rays. **border r's,** grenz r's. **caloric r.,** radiant energy that is converted into heat when applied to the body. **cathode r's,** negative particles of electricity streaming out in a vacuum tube at right angles to the surface of the cathode and away from it irrespective of the anode's position, moving in a straight line unless deflected by a magnet; by striking on solids they generate roentgen rays. **cosmic r's,** very penetrating radiations apparently moving through interplanetary space in every direction. **gamma r's, γ-r's,** electromagnetic radiation of short wavelengths emitted by an atomic nucleus during a nuclear reaction, consisting of high energy photons, having no mass and no electric charge, and traveling with the speed of light and with great penetrating power. **grenz r's,** roentgen rays having wavelengths about 2 A.U., lying between roentgen rays and ultraviolet rays. **hertzian r's,** see under *wave.* **medullary r.,** any cortical extension of a bundle of tubules from a renal pyramid. **Millikan r's,** cosmic r's. **roentgen r's,** x-rays; electromagnetic radiations of wavelengths below 5 A.U., commonly generated by passing high voltage current (about 10,000 volts) through a Coolidge tube; they are able to penetrate most substances to some extent. **x-r's,** roentgen r's.

Rb chemical symbol, *rubidium.*

RBC red blood cells; red blood (cell) count.

R.B.E. relative biological effectiveness.

R.C.P. Royal College of Physicians.

R.C.S. Royal College of Surgeons.

Re chemical symbol, *rhenium.*

re- word element [L.], *back; again; contrary,* etc.

reabsorb (re''ab-sorb') to absorb again; to undergo or to subject to reabsorption; to resorb.

reabsorption (-sorp'shun) 1. the act or process of absorbing again, as the absorption by the kidneys of substances (glucose, proteins, sodium, etc.) already secreted into the renal tubules. 2. resorption.

react (re-akt') 1. to respond to a stimulus. 2. to enter into chemical action.

reactant (re-ak'tant) a substance entering into a chemical reaction.

reaction (re-ak'shun) 1. opposite action, or counterreaction; the response to stimuli. 2. a phenomenon caused by the action of chemical agents; a chemical process in which one substance is transformed into another substance or other substances. 3. the mental and/or emotional state that develops in any particular situation. **acute situational r.,** gross stress r. **alarm r.,** all of the nonspecific phenomena elicited by exposure to stimuli affecting large portions of the body and to which the organism is not adapted; rapid involution of lymphoid tissues due to hormonal action is a striking manifestation. **allergic r.,** a local or general reaction characterized by altered reactivity of the animal body to an antigenic substance. **antigen-antibody r.,** the specific combination of antigen with homologous antibody resulting in the reversible formation of antigen-antibody complexes that differ in solubility according to the antigen-antibody ratio. **anxiety r.,** see under *neurosis.* **Arias-Stella r.,** nuclear and cellular hypertrophy of the endometrial epithelium, associated with ectopic pregnancy. **Cannizzaro's r.,** the reaction that aldehydes may undergo in alkali or on contact with animal tissue, one molecule being reduced to the corresponding alcohol and another being oxidized to the corresponding acid. **Casoni's r.,** see under *test.* **chain r.,** one which is self-propagating, each step initiating the succeeding step. **conversion r.,** a loss or alteration of a sensory or motor function as an expression of anxiety. **cross r.,** interaction between an antibody and an antigen that is closely related to the one which specifically stimulated synthesis of the antibody. **defense r.,** a mental reaction which shuts out from consciousness ideas not acceptable to the ego. **r. of degeneration** the reaction to electrical stimulation of muscles whose nerves have degenerated, consisting of loss of response to a faradic stimulation in a muscle, and to galvanic and faradic stimulation in the nerve. **delayed r.,** a reaction, such as an allergic reaction, occurring hours to days after exposure to an inducer. **dissociative r.,** a neurotic reaction in which such dissociated behavior as fugues, somnambolism, amnesia, and dream states occur. **Ehrlich's diazo r.,** deep red color in urine produced by the diazo reagent in certain diseases. **false positive r.,** an erroneously positive reaction to a test. **gross stress r.,** an acute emotional reaction incident to severe environmental stress. **hemianopic pupillary r.,** in certain cases of hemianopia, light thrown upon one side of the retina causes the iris to contract, while light thrown upon the other side arouses no response. **Herxheimer's r.,** Jarisch-Herxheimer r. **immune r.,** 1. see under *response.* 2. formation of a papule and areola without development of a vesicle following smallpox vaccination. **Jarish-Herxheimer r.,** transiently increased discomfort in skin lesions and temperature rise within two hours after start of antibiotic therapy of secondary syphilis and relapsing fever. **lengthening r.,** reflex elongation of the extensor muscles which permits flexion of a limb. **leukemic r., leukemoid r.,** a peripheral blood picture resembling that of leukemia or indistinguishable from it on the basis of morphologic appearance alone. **Much-Holzmann r.,** inhibition of the hemolytic action of cobra venom on erythrocytes, reported to occur in schizophrenia and manic-depressive psychosis. **Neufeld's r.,** swelling of the capsules of pneumococci, seen under the microscope, on mixture with specific immune serum. **ophthalmic r.,** local reaction of the conjunctiva after instillation into the eye of toxins of organisms causing typhoid fever and tuberculosis, being more severe in those affected with these diseases. **Pirquet's r.,** appearance of a papule with a red areola 24–48 hours after introduction of two small drops of Old tuberculin by slight scarification of the skin; a positive test indicates previous infection. **Prausnitz-Küstner r.,** a local hypersensitivity reaction induced by intradermal injection into a normal person of serum from a hypersensitive individual; injection 24 hrs. later of the antigen to which the donor is allergic results in a wheal-and-flare response. **precipitin r.,** one involving the serologic precipitation of an antigen in solution with its antiserum in the presence of electrolytes. **psychotic depressive r.,** severe, nonrecurrent depression of psychotic intensity. **Schultz-Charlton r.,** disappearance of scarlet fever rash around the site of an injection of scarlet fever antitoxin. **serum r.,** seroreaction. **stress r.,** 1. alarm r. 2. gross stress r. **Wassermann r.,** a test for syphilis based upon fixation of complement. **Weil-Felix r.,** agglutination by blood serum of typhus patients of a bacillus of the proteus group from the urine and feces. **Wernicke's r.,** hemianopic pupillary r. **wheal-flare r.,** a cutaneous sensitivity reaction to skin injury or administration of antigen, due to histamine production and marked by edematous elevation and erythematous flare.

reaction-formation (re-ak′shun-for-ma′shun) a psychic mechanism by which a person consciously assumes an attitude which is the reverse of, and a substitute for, a repressed antisocial impulse.

reactivity (re″ak-tiv′ĭ-te) the process or property of reacting.

Reactrol (re-ak′trol) trademark for a preparation of clemizole.

reading (rēd′ing) understanding of written or printed symbols representing words. **lip r., speech r.,** understanding of speech through observation of the speaker's lip movements.

reagent (re-a′jent) a substance used to produce a chemical reaction so as to detect, measure, produce, etc., other substances. **diazo r., Ehr-** lich's diazo r., a mixture of aqueous solutions of sodium nitrite and of sulfanilic and hydrochloric acids. **Million's r.,** aqueous solution of mercury dissolved in fuming nitric acid. **Nessler's r.,** mercuric chloride, potassium iodide, and potash, dissolved in water; used in estimating small amounts of ammonia.

reagin (re′ah-jin) 1. antibody of a specialized immunoglobulin class (IgE) which attaches to tissue cells of the same species from which it is derived, and which interacts with its antigen to induce the release of histamine and other vasoactive amines. A form of cytotropic antibody, it is present in the serum of naturally hypersensitive individuals and can confer specific immediate hypersensitivity in nonreactive individuals. 2. a complement-fixing antibody interacting with cardiolipin in the Wassermann reaction. **re′aginic,** adj. **atopic r.,** the reagin of humans.

reamer (re′mer) an instrument used in dentistry for enlarging root canals.

recapitulation (re″kah-pit″u-la′shun) see under *theory.*

receptaculum (re″sep-tak′u-lum), pl. *receptac′ula* [L.] a vessel or receptacle. **r. chy′li,** cisterna chyli.

receptor (re-sep′tor) 1. a chemical grouping on the surface of an immunologically competent cell with the capability of combining specifically with antigen. 2. a sensory nerve ending that responds to various stimuli. **adrenergic r's,** postulated sites on effector organs innervated by postganglionic adrenergic fibers of the sympathetic nervous system, classified as α-adrenergic and β-adrenergic receptors according to their reaction to norepinephrine and epinephrine respectively, and to certain blocking and stimulating agents. **cholinergic r.,** receptor sites on effector organs innervated by cholinergic nerve fibers and which respond to the acetylcholine secreted by these fibers.

recess (re′ses) a small, empty space or cavity.

recessive (re-ses′iv) 1. tending to recede; in genetics, incapable of expression unless (the responsible allele is) carried by both members of a pair of homologous chromosomes. 2. a recessive allele or trait.

recessus (re-ses′us), pl. *reces′sus* [L.] a recess.

recidivation, recidivism (re-sid″ĭ-va′shun; -sid′ĭ-vizm) 1. the repetition of an offense or crime. 2. the relapse or recurrence of a disease.

recidivist (re-sid′ĭ-vist) a person who tends to relapse, especially one who tends to return to criminal habits after treatment or punishment.

recipe (res′ĭ-pe) [L.] take; used at the head of a prescription, indicated by the symbol ℞. 2. a formula for the preparation of a specific combination of ingredients.

recipient (re-sip′e-ent) one who receives, as a blood transfusion, or a tissue or organ graft. **universal r.,** a person thought to be able to receive blood of any "type" without agglutination of the donor cells.

recombination (re″kom-bĭ-na′shun) the reunion, in the same or different arrangement, of formerly united elements that have been separated; in genetics, the formation of new gene combinations due to crossing over by homologous chromosomes.

recompression (re″kom-presh′un) return to normal environmental pressure after exposure to greatly diminished pressure.

recon (re′kon) the smallest unit of genetic material capable of recombination.

recrement (rek′rĕ-ment) saliva, or other secretion, which is reabsorbed into the blood. **recrementi′tous,** adj.

recrudescence (re″kroo-des′ens) recurrence of symptoms after temporary abatement. **recrudes′cent,** adj.

recruitment (re-kroot′ment) the gradual increase to a maximum in a reflex when a stimulus of unaltered intensity is prolonged.

rect(o)- word element [L.], *rectum.* See also words beginning *proct(o)-.*

rectalgia (rek-tal′je-ah) proctalgia.

rectectomy (rek-tek′to-me) proctectomy.

rectification (rek″tĭ-fĭ-ka′shun) 1. the act of making straight, pure, or correct. 2. redistillation of a liquid to purify it.

rectified (rek′tĭ-fīd) refined; made straight.

rectitis (rek-ti′tis) proctitis.

rectoabdominal (rek″to-ab-dom′ĭ-nal) pertaining to the rectum and abdomen.

rectocele (rek′to-sēl) hernial protrusion of part of the rectum into the vagina.

rectocolitis (rek″to-co-li′tis) coloproctitis.

rectolabial (-la′be-al) relating to the rectum and a labium majus.

rectopexy (rek′to-pek″se) proctopexy.

rectoplasty (-plas″te) proctoplasty.

rectoscope (-skōp) proctoscope.

rectosigmoid (rek″to-sig′moid) the terminal portion of the sigmoid colon and the proximal portion of the rectum.

rectosigmoidectomy (-sig″moi-dek′to-me) excision of the rectosigmoid.

rectostomy (rek-tos′to-me) proctostomy.

rectourethral (rek″to-u-re′thral) pertaining to or communicating with the rectum and urethra.

rectouterine (-u′ter-in) pertaining to the rectum and uterus.

rectovaginal (-vaj′ĭ-nal) pertaining to or communicating with the rectum and vagina.

rectovesical (-ves′ĭ-kal) pertaining to or communicating with the rectum and bladder.

rectum (rek′tum) the distal portion of the large intestine. **rec′tal,** adj.

rectus (rek′tus) [L.] straight.

recumbent (re-kum′bent) lying down.

recuperation (re-ku″per-a′shun) recovery of health and strength.

recurrence (re-ker′ens) the return of symptoms after a remission.

recurrent (re-ker′ent) returning after a remission; reappearing.

recurvation (re″kur-va′shun) a backward bending or curvature.

red (red) 1. one of the primary colors, produced by the longest waves of the visible spectrum. 2. a red dye or stain. **Congo r.,** a dark red or

brownish powder used as a diagnostic aid in amyloidosis. **cresol r.,** an indicator, being yellow at pH 7.2 and red at pH 8.8. **methyl r.,** an indicator, being red at pH 4.4 and yellow at pH 6.0. **neutral r.,** an indicator, being red at pH 6.8 and yellow at pH 8.0. **phenol r.,** phenolsulfonphthalein. **scarlet r.,** an azo dye having some power to stimulate cell proliferation; it has been used to enhance wound healing. **vital r.,** a dye injected into the circulation to estimate blood volume by determining the concentration of the dye in the plasma.

redia (re′de-ah), pl. *re′diae* [L.] a larval stage of certain trematode parasites, which develops in the body of a snail host and gives rise to daughter rediae, or to the cercariae.

redintegration (red″in-tĕ-gra′shun) 1. the restoration or repair of a lost or damaged part. 2. a psychic process in which part of a complex stimulus provokes the complete reaction that was previously made only to the complex stimulus as a whole.

Redisol (red′ĭ-sol) trademark for a preparation of crystalline cyanocobalamin (vitamin B_{12}).

redox (red′oks) oxidation-reduction.

reduce (re-dūs′) 1. to restore to the normal place or relation of parts, as to reduce a fracture. 2. to undergo reduction. 3. to decrease in weight or size.

reducible (re-du′sĭ-b′l) permitting of reduction.

reductant (re-duk′tant) the electron donor in an oxidation-reduction (redox) reaction.

reductase (re-duk′tās) any enzyme that has a reducing action on chemicals.

reduction (re-duk′shun) 1. the correction of a fracture, luxation, or hernia. 2. the addition of hydrogen to a substance, or more generally, the gain of electrons. **closed r.,** the manipulative reduction of a fracture without incision. **r. of chromosomes,** the passing of the members of a chromosome pair to the daughter cells during meiosis, each daughter cell receiving half the diploid number. **open r.,** reduction of a fracture after incision into the fracture site.

reduplication (re″du-plĭ-ka′shun) 1. a doubling back. 2. the recurrence of paroxysms of a double type. 3. a doubling of parts, connected at some point, the extra part being usually a mirror image of the other.

reentry (re-en′tre) in cardiology, a postulated mechanism by which a premature beat can be coupled to the normal beat.

refection (re-fek′shun) recovery; repair: applied specifically to the ability of the flora of the cecum of rats to synthesize vitamins of the B group from deficient diets and supply them to the host animal.

refine (re-fīn′) to purify or free from foreign matter.

reflection (re-flek′shun) 1. a turning or bending back, as the turning back of a ray of light, sound, or heat when it strikes against a surface that it does not penetrate. 2. an image made by reflection.

reflector (re-flek′tor) a device for reflecting light or sound waves.

reflex (re′fleks) a reflected action or movement;

the sum total of any particular automatic response mediated by the nervous system. **abdominal r's,** contractions of the abdominal muscles on stimulating the abdominal skin. **accommodation r.,** adjustment of direction of the visual axis, size of pupil, and convexity of lens when an individual fixes his eyes on a point at a different distance. **Achilles tendon r.,** triceps surae jerk. **anal r.,** contraction of the anal sphincter on irritation of the anal skin. **ankle r.,** triceps surae jerk. **auditory r.,** any reflex caused by stimulation of the auditory nerve, especially momentary closure of both eyes produced by a sudden sound. **Babinski's r.,** dorsiflexion of the big toe on stimulation of the sole, occurring in lesions of the pyramidal tract. **biceps r.,** contraction of the biceps muscle when its tendon is tapped. **Brain's r.,** quadrupedal extensor r. **carotid sinus r.,** slowing of the heart beat on pressure on the carotid artery at the level of the cricoid cartilage. **Chaddock's r.,** in lesions of the pyramidal tract, stimulation below the external malleolus causes extension of the great toe. **chain r.,** a series of reflexes, each serving as a stimulus to the next one, representing a complete activity. **ciliary r.,** the movement of the pupil in accommodation. **ciliospinal r.,** dilation of the ipsilateral pupil on painful stimulation of the skin at the side of the neck. **conditioned r.,** an acquired reflex developed by regular association of some physiological function with an unrelated outside event. **conjunctival r.,** closure of the eyelid when the conjunctiva is touched. **corneal r.,** closure of the lids on irritation of the cornea. **cough r.,** the sequence of events initiated by the sensitivity of the lining of the passageways of the lung and mediated by the medulla as a consequence of impulses transmitted by the vagus nerve, resulting in coughing, i.e., the clearing of the passageways of foreign matter. **cremasteric r.,** stimulation of the skin on the front and inner thigh retracts the testis on the same side. **deep r.,** one elicited by a sharp tap on the appropriate tendon or muscle to induce brief stretch of the muscle. **digital r.,** Hoffmann's sign (2). **embrace r.,** Moro r. **gag r.,** pharyngeal r. **gastrocolic r.,** increase in intestinal peristalsis after food enters the empty stomach. **gastroileal r.,** increase in ileal motility and opening of the ileocecal valve when food enters the empty stomach. **grasp r.,** flexion or clenching of the fingers or toes on stimulation of the palm or sole. **Hoffmann's r.,** see under *sign* (2). **jaw r., jaw-jerk r.,** closure of the mouth caused by a downward blow on the passively hanging chin; rarely seen in health but very noticeable in corticospinal tract lesions. **knee r.,** see under *jerk.* **light r.,** 1. a luminous image reflected from the membrana tympani. 2. contraction of the pupil when light falls on the eye. **Magnus and de Kleijn neck r's,** extension of both ipsilateral limbs, or one, or part of a limb, and increase of tonus on the side to which the chin is turned when the head is rotated to the side, and flexion with loss of tonus on the side to which occiput points. Essentially a sign of *decerebrate rigidity.* **Mayer's r.,** opposition and adduction of the thumb combined with flexion at the metacarpo-

phalangeal joint and extension at the interphalangeal joint, on downward pressure of the index finger. **Mendel-Bechterew r.,** dorsal flexion of the second to fifth toes on percussion of the dorsum of the foot; in certain organic nervous disorders, plantar flexion occurs. **Moro r.,** flexion of an infant's thighs and knees, fanning and then clenching of fingers, with arms first thrown outward and then brought together as though embracing something; produced by a sudden stimulus and seen normally in the newborn. **myotactic r.,** stretch r. **nociceptive r.,** any reflex initiated by painful stimuli. **Oppenheim's r.,** see under *sign.* **palatal r.,** stimulation of the palate causes swallowing. **patellar r.,** knee jerk. **pharyngeal r.,** contraction of the pharyngeal constrictor muscle elicited by touching the back of the pharynx. **pilomotor r.,** the production of goose flesh on stroking the skin. **plantar r.,** irritation of the sole contracts the toes. **proprioceptive r.,** one initiated by stimuli arising from some function of the reflex mechanism itself. **psychogalvanic r.,** decreased electrical resistance of the body due to emotional or mental agitation. **pupillary r.,** a change in size of the pupil in response to various stimuli (change in illumination or point of fixation, or emotional stimulation). **quadriceps r.,** knee jerk. **quadrupedal extensor r.,** extension of a hemiplegic flexed arm on assumption of the quadrupedal position. **red r.,** a luminous red appearance seen upon the retina in retinoscopy. **righting r.,** the ability to assume an optimal position when there has been a departure from it. **Rossolimo's s.,** in pyramidal tract lesions, plantar flexion of the toes on tapping their plantar surface. **spinal r.,** any reflex action mediated through a center of the spinal cord. **startle r.,** Moro r. **stretch r.,** reflex contraction of a muscle in response to passive longitudinal stretching. **sucking r.,** sucking movements of the lips of an infant elicited by touching the lips or the skin near the mouth. **superficial r.,** one elicited by stimulation of superficial nerve endings, as in the skin. **swallowing r.,** palatal r. **tendon r.,** contraction of a muscle caused by percussion of its tendon. **tonic neck r.,** extensions of the arm and sometimes of the leg on the side to which the head is forcibly turned, with flexion of the contralateral limbs; seen normally in the newborn. **triceps r.,** contraction of the belly of the triceps muscle and slight extension of the arm when the tendon of the muscle is tapped directly, with the arm flexed and fully supported and relaxed. **triceps surae r.,** see under *jerk.*

reflexogenic (re-flek″so-jen′ik) producing or increasing reflex action.

reflexograph (re-flek′so-graf) an instrument for recording a reflex.

reflexometer (re″flek-som′ĕ-ter) an instrument for measuring the force required to produce myotatic contraction.

reflux (re′fluks) a backward or return flow. **hepatojugular r.,** distention of the jugular vein induced by applying manual pressure over the liver; it suggests insufficiency of the right heart. **vesicoureteral r.,** backward flow of urine from the bladder into a ureter.

refract (re-frakt′) 1. to cause to deviate. 2. to ascertain errors of ocular refraction.

refraction (re-frak′shun) 1. the act or process of refracting; specifically, the determination of the refractive errors of the eye and their correction with glasses. 2. the deviation of light in passing obliquely from one medium to another of different density. **double r.,** refraction in which incident rays are divided into two refracted rays. **dynamic r.,** the normal accommodation of the eye which is continually exerted without conscious effort. **ocular r.,** the refraction of light produced by the mediums of the normal eye and resulting in the focusing of images upon the retina. **static r.,** refraction of the eye when its accommodation is paralyzed.

refractionist (-ist) one skilled in determining the refracting power of the eyes and correcting refracting defects.

refractive (re-frak′tiv) pertaining to or subserving a process of refraction; having the power to refract.

refractometer (re″frak-tom′ĕ-ter) 1. an instrument for measuring the refractive power of the eye. 2. an instrument for determining the indexes of refraction of various substances, particularly for determining the strength of lenses for spectacles.

refractory (re-frak′to-re) not readily yielding to treatment.

refrangible (re-fran′jĭ-b'l) susceptible of being refracted.

refresh (re-fresh′) to denude an epithelial wound to enhance tissue repair.

refrigerant (re-frig′er-ant) 1. relieving fever and thirst. 2. a cooling remedy.

refrigeration (re-frij″er-a′shun) therapeutic application of low temperature.

refusion (re-fu′zhun) the temporary removal and subsequent return of blood to the circulation.

regeneration (re-jen″ĕ-ra′shun) the natural renewal of a structure, as of a lost tissue or part.

regimen (rej′ĭ-men) a strictly regulated scheme of diet, exercise, or other activity designed to achieve certain ends.

regio (re′je-o), pl. *regio′nes* [L.] region.

region (re′jun) a plane area with more or less definite boundaries. **re′gional,** adj. **abdominal r's,** the areas into which the anterior surface of the abdomen is divided, including the *epigastric, hypochondriac* (right and left), *inguinal* (right and left), *lateral* (right and left), *pubic,* and *umbilical.* **facial r's,** the areas into which the face is divided, including the *buccal* (side of oral cavity), *infraorbital* (below the eye), *mental* (chin), *nasal* (nose), *oral* (lips), *orbital* (eye), *parotideomasseter* (angle of the jaw), and *zygomatic* (cheek bone). **pectoral r's,** the areas into which the anterior surface of the chest is divided, including the *axillary, infraclavicular,* and *mammary.* **perineal r.,** the region overlying the pelvic outlet, including the *anal* and *urogenital.* **precordial r.,** the part of the ante-

rior surface of the body covering the heart and the pit of the stomach.

registrant (rej′is-trant) a nurse listed on the books of a registry as available for duty.

registrar (rej′is-trar) 1. an official keeper of records. 2. in British hospitals, a resident specialist who acts as assistant to the chief or attending specialist.

registration (rej″is-tra′shun) the act of recording; in dentistry, the making of a record of the jaw relations present or desired, in order to transfer them to an articulator to facilitate proper construction of a dental prosthesis.

registry (rej′is-tre) 1. an office where a nurse's name may be listed as being available for duty. 2. a central agency for the collection of pathologic material and related data in a specified field of pathology. **nurse's r.,** an office with lists of nurses available for duty.

Regitine (rej′ĭ-tēn) trademark for a preparation of phentolamine.

regression (re-gresh′un) 1. return to a former or earlier state. 2. subsidence of symptoms or of a disease process. 3. in biology, the tendency in successive generations toward the mean. 4. defensive retreat to an earlier pattern of behavior or stage of development. **regres′sive,** adj.

regurgitant (re-ger′jĭ-tant) flowing backward.

regurgitation (re-ger″jĭ-ta′shun) a backward flowing, as the casting up of undigested food, or the backflow of blood through a defective heart valve. **valvular r.,** backflow of blood through the orifices of the heart valves owing to imperfect closing of the valves; named, according to the valve affected, *aortic, mitral, pulmonic,* or *tricuspid r.*

rehabilitation (re″hah-bil″ĭ-ta′shun) restoration to useful activity of persons with physical or other disability.

rehalation (re″hah-la′shun) rebreathing.

rehydration (re″hi-dra′shun) the restoration of water or fluid content to a body or to a substance which has become dehydrated.

reimplantation (re″im-plan-ta′shun) replacement of tissue or a structure in the site from which it was previously lost or removed.

reinfection (re″in-fek′shun) a second infection by the same agent.

reinforcement (re″in-fors′ment) the increasing of force or strength; in behavioral science, the presentation of a stimulus so as to modify a response; the stimulus may be a reward or a punishment. **r. of reflex,** strengthening of a reflex response by the patient's performance of some action during elicitation of the reflex.

reinnervation (re″in-er-va′shun) restoration of nerve supply of an organ by anastomosis with a living nerve.

reintegration (re″in-te-gra′shun) 1. biological integration. 2. the resumption of normal mental and physical activity after disappearance of the catatonic state or other psychic disturbance.

rejection (re-jek′shun) an immune reaction against grafted tissue.

relapse (re-laps′) the return of a disease after its apparent cessation.

relaxant (re-lak′sant) 1. causing relaxation. 2. an agent which causes relaxation. **muscle r.,** an agent that specifically aids in reducing muscle tension.

relaxation (re″lak-sa′shun) a lessening of tension.

relaxin (re-lak′sin) a protein-like principle secreted by the corpus luteum during pregnancy, producing relaxation of the pubic symphysis and dilation of the uterine cervix in certain animal species.

Releasin (re-le′sin) trademark for a preparation of relaxin.

reline (re-lin′) to resurface the tissue side of a denture with new base material in order to achieve a more accurate fit.

REM rapid eye movements (see under *sleep*).

rem (rem) roentgen-equivalent–*man:* the amount of any ionizing radiation which has the same biological effectiveness of 1 rad of x-rays; 1 rem = 1 rad × RBE (relative biological effectiveness).

remedy (rem′ĕ-de) anything that cures or palliates disease. **reme′dial,** adj.

remineralization (re-min″er-al-i-za′shun) restoration of mineral elements, as of calcium salts to bone.

remission (re-mish′un) diminution or abatement of the symptoms of a disease; the period during which such diminution occurs.

remittent (re-mit′ent) having periods of abatement and of exacerbation.

ren (ren), pl. *re′nes* [L.] kidney. **r. mo′bilis,** hypermobile kidney.

renal (re′nal) pertaining to the kidney.

reniform (ren′ĭ-form) kidney-shaped.

renin (re′nin) a proteolytic enzyme liberated by renal ischemia or by disminished pulse pressure, which converts angiotensinogen into angiotensin.

renipelvic (ren″ĭ-pel′vik) pertaining to the pelvis of the kidney.

reniportal (-por′tal) pertaining to the portal system of the kidney.

renipuncture (-pungk′tūr) surgical incision of the capsule of the kidney.

rennet (ren′et) an extract of calf's stomach containing rennin; used to curdle milk in cheese making.

rennin (ren′in) the milk-curdling enzyme found in the gastric juice of human infants (before pepsin formation) and abundantly in that of the calf and other ruminants; a preparation from the stomach of the calf is used to coagulate milk protein to facilitate its digestion.

renninogen (rĕ-nin′o-jen) prorennin.

renogastric (re″no-gas′trik) pertaining to the kidney and stomach.

renography (re-nog′rah-fe) radiography of the kidney.

renointestinal (re″no-in-tes′tĭ-nal) pertaining to the kidney and intestine.

renopathy (re-nop′ah-the) nephropathy.

renoprival (re″no-pri′val) pertaining to or caused by lack of kidney function.

reovirus (re″o-vi′rus) any of a group of ether-resistant RNA viruses isolated from healthy children, children with febrile and afebrile upper respiratory disease, children with diarrhea, and many animals.

rep (rep) roentgen-equivalent-*physical,* a unit of radiation equivalent to the absorption of 93 ergs per gram of water or soft tissue.

repair (re-pār′) the physical or mechanical restoration of damaged or diseased tissues by the growth of healthy new cells or by surgical apposition.

repellent (re-pel′ent) able to repel or drive off; also, an agent that repels.

repercussion (re″per-kush′un) 1. the driving in of an eruption, or scattering of a swelling. 2. ballottement.

replantation (re″plan-ta′shun) reimplantation.

replication (rĕ″plĭ-ka′shun) 1. a turning back of a part so as to form a duplication. 2. repetition of an experiment to ensure accuracy. 3. the process of duplicating or reproducing, as replication of an exact copy of a polynucleotide strand of DNA or RNA.

repolarization (re-po″lar-ĭ-za′shun) the reestablishment of polarity, especially the return of cell membrane potential to resting potential after depolarization.

repositor (-poz′ĭ-tor) an instrument used in returning displaced organs to the normal position.

repression (re-presh′un) the act of restraining, inhibiting, or suppressing; in psychiatry, the thrusting back from consciousness into the unconscious of disagreeable ideas or perceptions. **coordinate r.,** parallel diminution of the concentrations of the several enzymes of a metabolic pathway, resulting from increases in the level of repressor. **enzyme r.,** interference, usually by the endproduct of a pathway, with synthesis of the enzymes of that pathway.

repressor (re-pres′sor) that which restrains or inhibits; a substance produced by a regulator gene that acts to prevent initiation by the operator gene of protein synthesis by the operon.

reproduction (re″pro-duk′shun) 1. the production of offspring by organized bodies. 2. the creation of a similar object or situation; duplication; replication. **asexual r.,** reproduction without the fusion of sexual cells. **cytogenic r.,** production of a new individual from a single germ cell or zygote. **sexual r.,** reproduction by the fusion of a female sexual cell with a male sexual cell or by the development of an unfertilized egg. **somatic r.,** production of a new individual from a multicellular fragment by fission or budding.

reproductive (-duk′tiv) subserving or pertaining to reproduction.

repulsion (re-pul′shun) 1. the act of driving apart or away; a force that tends to drive two bodies apart. 2. in genetics, the occurrence on opposite chromosomes in a double heterozygote of the two mutant alleles of interest.

RES reticuloendothelial system.

rescinnamine (re-sin′ah-min) an alkaloid, $C_{35}H_{42}N_2O_9$, from various species of *Rauwolfia;* used as an antihypertensive and tranquilizer.

resect (re-sekt′) to excise part of an organ or other structure.

resection (re-sek′shun) excision of a portion of an organ or other structure. **root r.,** apicoectomy. **transurethral r.,** resection of the prostate by means of an instrument passed through the urethra. **wedge r.,** removal of a triangular mass of tissue, as from the ovary.

resectoscope (re-sek′to-skōp) an instrument for transurethral prostatic resection.

reserpine (res′er-pēn) an alkaloid, $C_{33}H_{40}N_2O_9$, from various species of *Rauwolfia;* used as an antihypertensive and tranquilizer.

reserve (re-zerv′) 1. to hold back for future use. 2. a supply, beyond that ordinarily used, which may be utilized in emergency. **alkali r., alkaline r.,** the amount of conjugate base components of the blood buffers, the most important being bicarbonate. **cardiac r.,** potential ability of the heart to perform work beyond that necessary under basal conditions.

reservoir (rez′er-vwar) 1. a storage place or cavity. 2. an alternate host or passive carrier of a pathogenic organism. **r. of Pecquet,** cisterna chyli.

resident (rez′ĭ-dent) a graduate and licensed physician receiving training in a specialty in a hospital.

residual (re-zid′u-al) remaining or left behind.

residue (rez′ĭ-du) a remainder; that remaining after removal of other substances.

residuum (re-zid′u-um), pl. *resid′ua* [L.] a residue or remainder.

resin (rez′in) 1. a solid or semisolid, amorphous organic substance, of vegetable origin or produced synthetically. True resins are insoluble in water, but are readily dissolved in alcohol, ether, and volatile oils. 2. rosin. **res′inous,** adj. **acrylic r's,** products of the polymerization of acrylic or methacrylic acid or their derivatives, used in fabrication of medical prostheses and dental restorations and appliances. **activated r., autopolymer r.,** self-curing r. **anion-exchange r.,** see *ion-exchange r.* **cation-exchange r.,** see *ion-exchange r.* **cholestyramine r.,** a synthetic, strongly basic anion-exchange resin in the chloride form which chelates bile salts in the intestine, thus preventing their reabsorption; used in the symptomatic relief of pruritus associated with bile stasis. **ion-exchange r.,** a high molecular weight insoluble polymer of simple organic compounds capable of exchanging its attached ions for other ions in the surrounding medium; classified as (*a*) *cation-* or *anion-exchange r's,* depending on which ions the resin exchanges (the former are used to restrict intestinal sodium absorption in edematous states, and the latter as antacids in ulcer treatment); and (*b*) carboxylic, sulfonic, etc., depending on the nature of the active groups. **podophyllum r.,** a mixture of resins from podophyllum, used as a topical caustic in the treatment of certain papillomas. **quick-cure r., self-curing r.,** any resin which can be polymerized by addition of an activator and a catalyst without the use of external heat. **synthetic r.,** an amorphous, organic solid or semisolid material produced by polymerization or condensation of simpler compounds.

resistance (re-zis′tans) 1. opposition, or counteracting force, as opposition of a conductor to passage of electricity or other energy or substance. 2. the natural ability of a normal organism to remain unaffected by noxious agents in its environment; see also *immunity.* 3. in studies of respiration, an expression of the opposition to flow of air produced by the tissues of the air passages, in terms of pressure per amount of air per unit of time. 4. in psychoanalysis, opposition to the coming into consciousness of repressed material. **peripheral r.,** the resistance to the passage of the blood through the small blood vessels, especially the arterioles.

resolution (rez″o-lu′shun) 1. subsidence of a pathologic state. 2. perception as separate of two adjacent points; in microscopy, the smallest distance at which two adjacent objects can be distinguished as separate.

resolvent (re-zol′vent) 1. promoting resolution or the dissipation of a pathologic growth. 2. an agent that promotes resolution.

resonance (rez′o-nans) 1. the prolongation and intensification of sound produced by transmission of its vibrations to a cavity, especially such a sound elicited by percussion. Decrease of resonance is called *dullness;* its increase, *flatness.* 2. a vocal sound heard on auscultation. 3. mesomerism. **amphoric r.,** a sound resembling that produced by blowing over the mouth of an empty bottle. **skodaic r.,** increased percussion resonance at the upper part of the chest, with flatness below it. **tympanitic r.,** peculiar sound elicited by percussing a tympanitic abdomen. **vesicular r.,** normal pulmonary resonance. **vocal r.,** the sound of ordinary speech as heard through the chest wall.

resonant (rez′o-nant) giving an intense, rich sound on percussion.

resonator (rez′o-na″tor) 1. an instrument used to intensify sounds. 2. an electric circuit in which oscillations of a certain frequency are set up by oscillations of the same frequency in another circuit.

resorb (re-sorb′) to dissolve and assimilate; to reabsorb.

resorcin (rĕ-zor′sin) resorcinol.

resorcinism (rĕ-zor′sĭ-nizm) chronic poisoning by resorcinol, resulting in methemoglobinemia, paralysis, and damage to the capillaries, kidneys, heart, and nervous system.

resorcinol (rĕ-zor′sĭ-nol) a keratolytic, $C_6H_6O_2$, applied topically to the skin; the monoacetate salt is used as a keratolytic and antiseborrheic applied topically to the scalp.

resorcinolphthalein (-thal′e-in) fluorescein.

resorption (re-sorp′shun) 1. the lysis and assimilation of a substance, as of bone. 2. reabsorption.

respirable (rĕ-spīr′ah-b'l) suitable for respiration.

respiration (res″pĭ-ra′shun) the exchange of oxygen and carbon dioxide between the atmosphere and the body cells, including inspiration and expiration, diffusion of oxygen from alveoli to the blood and of carbon dioxide from the blood to the alveoli, and the transport of oxygen to and carbon dioxide from the body cells. **abdominal r.,** the inspiration and expiration accomplished mainly by the abdominal muscles and diaphragm. **aerobic r.,** the oxidative transformation of certain substrates into secretory products, the released energy being used in the process of assimilation. **anaerobic r.,** respiration in which energy is released from chemical reactions in which free oxygen takes no part. **artificial r.,** that which is maintained by force applied to the body, such as *Eve's method* (patient face down on a stretcher placed on a trestle, the ends being alternately lowered and raised); *Schafer's method* (pressure alternately applied and relaxed over the lower ribs, the patient lying face downward); or *Silvester's method* (patient supine, arms pulled firmly over head, raising ribs, until air no longer enters chest); stimulation of the phrenic nerve by application of electric current; or *mouth-to-mouth method* (resuscitation of an apneic victim by direct application of the mouth to his, regularly taking a deep breath and blowing into the victim's lungs). **Biot's r.,** rapid, short breathing, with pauses of several seconds. **cell r.,** the processes in the living cell by which organic substances are oxidized and chemical energy is released. **Cheyne-Stokes r.,** breathing characterized by rhythmic waxing and waning of respiration depth, with regularly recurring apneic periods. **cogwheel r.,** breathing with jerky inspiration. **diaphragmatic r.,** that performed mainly by the diaphragm. **electrophrenic r.,** induction of respiration by electric stimulation of the phrenic nerve. **external r.,** the exchange of gases between the lungs and the blood. **internal r.,** the exchange of gases between the body cells and the blood. **Kussmaul's r.,** air hunger. **paradoxical r.,** that in which a lung, or a portion of a lung, is deflated during inspiration and inflated during expiration. **tissue r.,** internal r.

respirator (res'pĭ-ra″tor) an apparatus to qualify the air breathed through it, or a device for giving artificial respiration or to assist in pulmonary ventilation. **cuirass r.,** a respirator applied only to the chest, either completely surrounding the trunk or applied only to the front of the chest and abdomen. **Drinker r.,** popularly, "iron lung": an apparatus for producing artificial respiration over long periods of time, consisting of a metal tank, enclosing the patient's body, with his head outside, and within which artificial respiration is maintained by alternating negative and positive pressure.

respiratory (rĕ-spi'rah-to-re) pertaining to respiration.

respirometer (res″pĭ-rom'ĕ-ter) an instrument for determining the nature of respiration.

response (re-spons') any action or change of condition evoked by a stimulus. **anamnestic r.,** the rapid reappearance of antibody in the blood following administration of an antigen to which the subject had previously developed a primary immune response. **autoimmune r.,** the immune response in which antibodies or immune lymphoid cells are produced against the body's own tissues. **galvanic skin r.,** the alteration in the electrical resistance of the skin associated with sympathetic nerve discharge. **immune r.,** specifically altered reactivity of the animal body after exposure to antigen, manifested as antibody-produced, cell-mediated immunity, or as immunologic tolerance. **triple r. (of Lewis),** a physiologic reaction of the skin to stroking with a blunt instrument: first a red line develops at the site of stroking, owing to the release of histamine or a histamine-like substance, then a flare develops around the red line, and lastly a wheal is formed as a result of local edema.

rest (rest) 1. repose after exertion. 2. a fragment of embryonic tissue retained within the adult organism. 3. an extension which helps support a removable partial denture. **adrenal r.,** accessory adrenal tissue. **incisal r., lingual r., occlusal r.,** a metallic extension from a removable partial denture to aid in supporting the appliance. **suprarenal r.,** adrenal r. **Walthard cell r's,** see under *islet.*

restenosis (re″stĕ-no'sis) recurrent stenosis, especially of a cardiac valve after surgical correction of the primary condition.

restibrachium (res″tĭ-bra'ke-um) the inferior peduncle of the cerebellum.

restiform (res'tĭ-form) shaped like a rope.

restis (res'tis) inferior peduncle of cerebellum.

restitution (res″tĭ-too'shun) the spontaneous realignment of the fetal head with the fetal body, after delivery of the head.

restoration (res″to-ra'shun) 1. induction of a return to a previous state, as a return to health or replacement of a part to normal position. 2. partial or complete reconstruction of a body part, or the device used in its place.

restorative (re-stor'ah-tiv) 1. promoting a return to health or to consciousness. 2. a remedy that aids in restoring health, vigor, or consciousness.

restraint (re-strānt') forcible control, as by means of a straitjacket.

resuscitation (re-sus″ĭ-ta'shun) restoration to life of one apparently dead.

resuscitator (re-sus'ĭ-ta″tor) an apparatus for initiating respiration in persons whose breathing has stopped.

retainer (re-tān'er) an appliance or device that keeps a tooth or partial denture in proper position.

retardate (re-tar'dāt) a mentally retarded person.

retardation (re″tar-da'shun) delay; hindrance; delayed development. **mental r.,** subnormal general intellectual development, associated with impairment either of learning and social adjustment or of maturation, or of both; classified according to I.Q. as *borderline* (68–83), *mild* (52–67), *moderate* (36–51), *severe* (20–35), or *profound* (less than 20).

retching (rech'ing) strong involuntary effort to vomit.

rete (re'te), pl. *re'tia* [L.] a network or meshwork, especially of blood vessels. **arterial r., r. arteri-o'sum,** an anastomotic network of minute arteries, just before they become capillaries. **articular r.,** a network of anastomosing blood vessels in or around a joint. **r. malpig'hii,** malpighian layer. **r. mirab'ile,** a vascular network formed by division of an artery or vein into many smaller vessels that reunite into a single vessel. **r. test'is,** a network formed in the mediastinum testis by the seminiferous tubules. **r. veno'sum,** an anastomotic network of small veins.

retention (re-ten'shun) the process of holding back or keeping in position, as persistence in the body of material normally excreted, or maintenance of a dental prosthesis in proper position in the mouth.

reticula (rĕ-tik'u-lah) [L.] plural of *reticulum.*

reticular, reticulated (rĕ-tik'u-lar; rĕ-tik'u-lāt″ed) resembling a net.

reticulation (rĕ-tik″u-la'shun) the formation or presence of a network.

reticulin (rĕ-tik'u-lin) a scleroprotein from the connective fibers of reticular tissue.

reticulitis (rĕ-tik″u-li'tis) inflammation of the reticulum of a ruminant animal.

reticulocyte (rĕ-tik'u-lo-sīt) a young erythrocyte showing a basophilic reticulum under vital staining.

reticulocytopenia (rĕ-tik″u-lo-si″to-pe'ne-ah) deficiency of reticulocytes in the blood.

reticulocytosis (-si-to'sis) an excess of reticulocytes in the peripheral blood.

reticuloendothelial (-en″do-the'le-al) pertaining to the reticuloendothelium or to the reticuloendothelial system.

reticuloendothelioma (-en″do-the″le-o'mah) malignant lymphoma.

reticuloendotheliosis (-en″do-the″le-o'sis) hyperplasia of reticuloendothelial tissue.

reticuloendothelium (-en″do-the'le-um) the tissue of the reticuloendothelial system.

reticulohistiocytoma (-his″te-o-si-to'mah) a granulomatous aggregation of lipid-laden histiocytes and multinucleated giant cells.

reticulopenia (-pe'ne-ah) reticulocytopenia.

reticulopodium (-po'de-um) a threadlike, branching pseudopod.

reticulosarcoma (-sar-ko'mah) malignant lymphoma, histiocytic or undifferentiated.

reticulosis (rĕ-tik″u-lo'sis) an abnormal increase in cells derived from or related to the reticuloendothelial cells. **familial histiocytic r., histiocytic medullary r.,** a fatal hereditary disorder marked by anemia, granulocytopenia, thrombocytopenia, phagocytosis of blood cells, diffuse proliferation of histiocytes, and enlargement of the liver, spleen, and lymph nodes.

reticulum (rĕ-tik'u-lum), pl. *retic'ula* [L.] 1. a small network, especially a protoplasmic network in cells. 2. reticular tissue. 3. the second stomach of a ruminant animal. **endoplasmic r.,** an ultramicroscopic organelle of nearly all higher plant and animal cells, consisting of a system of membrane-bound cavities in the cytoplasm; occurring in two types, rough-surfaced (*granular r.*), bearing large numbers of ribosomes on its outer surface, and smooth-surfaced

(*agranular r.*). **sarcoplasmic r.,** a form of agranular reticulum in the sarcoplasm of striated muscle, comprising a system of smooth-surfaced tubules surrounding each myofibril. **stellate r.,** the soft, middle part of the enamel organ of a developing tooth.

retiform (re'tĭ-form, ret'ĭ-form) reticular.

retina (ret'ĭ-nah) the innermost tunic of the eyeball, containing the neural elements for reception and transmission of visual stimuli.

retinaculum (ret″ĭ-nak'u-lum), pl. *retinac'ula* [L.] 1. a structure that retains an organ or tissue in place. 2. an instrument for retracting tissues during surgery. **r. flexo'rum ma'nus,** a fibrous band forming the carpal canal through which pass the tendons of the flexor muscles of the hand and fingers. **r. musculo'rum peroneo'-rum infe'rius,** a fibrous band across the peroneal tendons that holds them in place on the lateral calcaneus. **r. musculo'rum peroneo'-rum supe'rius,** a fibrous band across the peroneal tendons that helps hold them in place below and behind the lateral malleolus. **r. ten'dinum,** a tendinous restraining structure, such as an annular ligament.

retinal (ret'ĭ-nal) 1. pertaining to the retina. 2. the aldehyde of retinol, having vitamin A activity. One isomer (11-*cis* r.), combines with opsin in the retinal rods (scotopsin) to form rhodopsin (visual purple); another, all-*trans* r., or visual yellow, results from the bleaching of rhodopsin by light, in which the 11-*cis* form is converted to the all-*trans* form. Retinal also combines with opsins in the retinal cones to form the three pigments responsible for color vision.

retine (ret'ēn) a substance stated to be widely distributed in animal cells, capable of inhibiting cell division and growth.

retinene (ret'ĭ-nēn) the aldehyde of vitamin A, occurring in two forms: r_1 is retinal (2), and r_2 is dehydroretinal.

retinitis (ret″ĭ-ni'tis) inflammation of the retina. **r. circina'ta, circinate r.,** circinate retinopathy. **r. discifor'mis,** a bilateral, degenerative retinal disease, with an elevated grayish white mass in the macular area. **exudative r.,** Coats' disease. **r. haemorrha'gica,** that marked by profuse retinal hemorrhage. **r. pigmento'sa,** a group of diseases, often hereditary, marked by progressive loss of retinal response, retinal atrophy, attenuation of retinal vessels, clumping of pigment, and contraction of the visual field. **r. prolif'erans,** a condition sometimes due to intraocular hemorrhage, with formation of fibrous tissue extending into the vitreous from the retinal surface; retinal detachment may be a sequel. **suppurative r.,** that due to pyemic infection.

retinoblastoma (ret″ĭ-no-blas-to'mah) a tumor arising from retinal cells.

retinochoroiditis (-ko″roi-di'tis) inflammation of the retina and choroid. **r. juxtapapilla'ris,** a small area of inflammation on the fundus near the papilla; seen in young healthy individuals.

retinoid (ret'ĭ-noid) resembling the retina.

retinol (ret'ĭ-nol) vitamin A₁; the form $C_{20}H_{30}O$, of vitamin A found in mammals, which is reversibly dehydrogenated by enzymatic action into its aldehyde, retinal (2).

retinomalacia (ret″ĭ-no-mah-la′she-ah) softening of the retina.

retinopapillitis (-pap″ĭ-li′tis) inflammation of the retina and optic papilla.

retinopathy (ret″ĭ-nop′ah-the) any noninflammatory disease of the retina. **circinate r.,** a condition in which a circle of white spots encloses the macula, leading to complete foveal blindness. **exudative r.,** Coats' disease. **r. of prematurity,** retrolental fibroplasia.

retinoschisis (ret″ĭ-nos′kĭ-sis) splitting of the retina, occurring in the nerve fiber layer (in *juvenile form*), or in the external plexiform layer (in *adult form*).

retinoscope (ret′ĭ-no-skōp″) an instrument for performing retinoscopy.

retinoscopy (ret″ĭ-nos′ko-pe) observation of the pupil under a beam of light projected into the eye, as a means of determining refractive errors.

retinosis (ret″ĭ-no′sis) any degenerative, noninflammatory condition of the retina.

retothelium (re″to-the′le-um) reticuloendothelium.

retractile (re-trak′til) susceptible of being drawn back.

retraction (re-trak′shun) the act of drawing back, or condition of being drawn back. **clot r.,** the drawing away of a blood clot from a vessel wall, a function of blood platelets.

retractor (re-trak′tor) 1. an instrument for holding open the lips of a wound. 2. a muscle that retracts.

retro- word element [L.], *behind; backward.*

retroaction (ret″ro-ak′shun) action in a reversed direction; reaction.

retroauricular (-aw-rik′u-lar) behind the auricle of the ear.

retrobulbar (-bul′bar) behind the eyeball.

retrocecal (-se′kal) behind the cecum.

retrocervical (-ser′vĭ-kal) behind the cervix uteri.

retrocession (-sesh′un) a going backward; backward displacement.

retrocolic (-ko′lik) behind the colon.

retrocollic (-kol′ik) pertaining to the back of the neck; nuchal.

retrocollis (-kol′is) spasmodic wryneck in which the head is drawn back.

retrocursive (-ker′siv) marked by stepping backward.

retrodeviation (-de″ve-a′shun) a general term including retroversion, retroflexion, retroposition, etc.

retrodisplacement (-dis-plās′ment) backward or posterior displacement.

retroesophageal (-ĕ-sof″ah-je′al) behind the esophagus.

retroflexion (-flek′shun) the bending of an organ so that its top is thrust backward.

retrogasserian (-gas-se′re-an) pertaining to the sensory (posterior) root of the trigeminal (gasserian) ganglion.

retrognathia (-nath′e-ah) underdevelopment of the maxilla and/or mandible. **retrognath′ic,** adj.

retrograde (ret′ro-grād) going backward; retracing a former course; catabolic.

retrogression (ret″ro-gresh′un) degeneration; deterioration; regression; return to an earlier, less complex condition.

retroinsular (-in′su-lar) behind the insula.

retrolental (-len′tal) behind the lens of the eye.

retrolingual (-ling′gwal) behind the tongue.

retromammary (-mam′ar-e) behind the mammary gland.

retromandibular (-man-dib′u-lar) behind the lower jaw.

retromastoid (-mas′toid) behind the mastoid process.

retromorphosis (-mor-fo′sis) retrograde metamorphosis.

retronasal (-na′zal) pertaining to the back part of the nose.

retro-ocular (-ok′u-lar) behind the eye.

retroparotid (-pah-rot′id) behind the parotid gland.

retroperitoneal (-per″ĭ-to-ne′al) behind the peritoneum.

retroperitoneum (-per″ĭ-to-ne′um) the retroperitoneal space.

retroperitonitis (-per″ĭ-to-ni′tis) inflammation of the retroperitoneal space.

retropharyngeal (-fah-rin′je-al) behind the pharynx.

retropharyngitis (-far″in-ji′tis) inflammation of the posterior part of the pharynx.

retroplasia (-pla′ze-ah) retrograde metaplasia; degeneration of a tissue or cell into a more primitive type.

retroposed (-pōsd′) displaced backward.

retroposition (-po-zish′un) backward displacement.

retropulsion (-pul′shun) 1. a driving back, as of the fetal head in labor. 2. tendency to walk backward, as in some cases of tabes dorsalis. 3. an abnormal gait in which the body is bent backward.

retrotarsal (-tar′sal) behind the tarsus of the eye.

retrouterine (-u′ter-in) behind the uterus.

retroversion (-ver′zhun) the tipping backward of an entire organ.

reversion (re-ver′zhun) 1. a returning to a previous condition; regression. 2. in genetics, inheritance from some remote ancestor of a character which has not been manifest for several generations.

revulsant (re-vul′sant) revulsive.

revulsion (re-vul′shun) the act of drawing blood from one part to another, as in counterirritation; the diminution of morbid action in any part of the body by irritation in another.

revulsive (re-vul′siv) 1. causing revulsion. 2. an agent causing revulsion.

Rezipas (rez′ĭ-pas) trademark for a preparation of para-aminosalicylic acid.

Rf chemical symbol, *rutherfordium.*

R.F.A. right fronto-anterior (position of the fetus).

R.F.P. right frontoposterior (position of the fetus).

R.F.T. right frontotransverse (position of the fetus).

Rh 1. chemical symbol, *rhodium*. 2. symbol for *Rhesus factor*.

rhabd(o)- word element [Gr.], *rod; rod-shaped*.

Rhabditis (rab-di′tis) a genus of minute nematodes found mostly in damp earth, and as an accidental parasite in man.

rhabdocyte (rab′do-sīt) metamyelocyte.

rhabdoid (rab′doid) resembling a rod; rod-shaped.

rhabdomyoblastoma (rab″do-mi″o-blas-to′-mah) rhabdomyosarcoma.

rhabdomyolysis (-mi-ol′ĭ-sis) disintegration of striated muscle fibers with excretion of myoglobin in the urine.

rhabdomyoma (-mi-o′mah) a tumor containing striated muscle fibers.

rhabdomyosarcoma (-mi″o-sar-ko′mah) a highly malignant tumor of striated muscle derived from primitive mesenchymal cells and characterized by anaplastic striated cells.

Rhabdonema (-ne′mah) *Rhabditis*.

rhabdosarcoma (-sar-ko′mah) rhabdomyosarcoma.

rhabdovirus (-vi′rus) any of a group of morphologically similar bullet-shaped or bacilliform RNA viruses.

rhachi- for words beginning thus, see those beginning *rachi-*.

rhagades (rag′ah-dēz) fissures, cracks, or fine linear scars in the skin, especially such lesions around the mouth or other regions subjected to frequent movement.

rhaphe (ra′fe) raphe.

rhenium (re′ne-um) chemical element (*see table*), at. no. 75, symbol Re.

rheo- word element [Gr.], *electric current; flow* (as of fluids).

rheobase (re′o-bās) the minimum potential of electric current necessary to produce stimulation. **rheoba′sic,** adj.

rheology (re-ol′o-je) the science of the deformation and flow of matter, such as the flow of blood through the heart and blood vessels.

rheonome (re′o-nōm) apparatus for determining the effect of irritation on a nerve.

rheostosis (re″os-to′sis) a condition of hyperostosis marked by the presence of streaks in the bones; see also *melorheostosis*.

rheotaxis (re″o-tak′sis) the orientation of an organism in a stream of liquid, with its long axis parallel with the direction of flow, designated *negative* (moving in the same direction) or *positive* (moving in the opposite direction).

rhestocythemia (res″to-si-the′me-ah) the occurrence of broken-down erythrocytes in the blood.

rheum (rōōm) any watery or catarrhal discharge.

rheumarthritis (roo″mar-thri′tis) rheumatoid arthritis.

rheumatalgia (roo″mah-tal′je-ah) chronic rheumatic pain.

rheumatid (roo′mah-tid) any skin lesion etiologically associated with rheumatism.

rheumatism (roo′mah-tizm) any of a variety of disorders marked by inflammation, degeneration, or metabolic derangement of the connective tissue structures, especially the joints and related structures, and attended by pain, stiffness, or limitation of motion. **rheumat′ic,** adj. **acute articular r., inflammatory r.,** rheumatic fever. **muscular r.,** fibrositis. **palindromic r.,** repeated attacks of arthritis and periarthritis without fever and without causing irreversible joint changes.

rheumatoid (roo′mah-toid) resembling rheumatism.

rheumatologist (roo″mah-tol′o-jist) a specialist in rheumatology.

rheumatology (-tol′o-je) the study of rheumatism.

rhexis (rek′sis) the rupture of a blood vessel or of an organ.

rhigosis (ri-go′sis) the perception of cold.

rhin(o)- word element [Gr.], *nose; nose-like structure*.

rhinal (ri′nal) pertaining to the nose.

rhinalgia (ri-nal′je-ah) pain in the nose.

rhinencephalon (ri″nen-sef′ah-lon) 1. the part of the brain once thought to be concerned entirely with olfactory mechanisms, including olfactory nerves, bulbs, tracts, and subsequent connections (all olfactory in function) and the limbic system (not primarily olfactory in function); homologous with olfactory portions of the brain in lower animals. 2. one of the parts of the embryonic telencephalon.

rhinesthesia (ri″nes-the′ze-ah) the sense of smell.

rhineurynter (ri″nu-rin′ter) a dilatable rubber bag for distending a nostril.

rhinion (rin′e-on) the lower end of the suture between the nasal bones.

rhinitis (ri-ni′tis) inflammation of the nasal mucous membrane. **allergic r., anaphylactic r.,** any allergic reaction of the nasal mucosa, occurring perennially (*nonseasonal allergic r.*) or seasonally (*hay fever*). **atrophic r.,** chronic rhinitis with wasting of the mucous membrane and glands. **r. caseo′sa,** that with a caseous, gelatinous, and fetid discharge. **fibrinous r.,** rhinitis with development of a false membrane. **hypertrophic r.,** that with thickening and swelling of the mucous membrane. **membranous r.,** chronic rhinitis with a membranous exudate. **nonseasonal allergic r.,** allergic rhinitis occurring continuously or intermittently all year round, due to exposure to a more or less ever-present allergen, marked by sudden attacks of sneezing, swelling of the nasal mucosa with profuse watery discharge, itching of the eyes, and lacrimation. **purulent r.,** chronic rhinitis with formation of pus. **vasomotor r.,** 1. nonallergic rhinitis in which transient changes in vascular tone and permeability (with the same symptoms of allergic rhinitis) are brought on by such stimuli as mild chilling, fatigue, anger, and anxiety. 2. any condition of allergic or nonallergic rhinitis, as opposed to infectious rhinitis.

rhinoantritis (ri″no-an-tri′tis) inflammation of the nasal cavity and maxillary sinus.

rhinocanthectomy (-kan-thek′to-me) rhinommectomy.

rhinocele (ri′no-sēl) rhinocoele.

rhinocephalus (ri″no-sef′ah-lus) a fetus exhibiting rhinocephaly.

rhinocephaly (-sef′ah-le) a developmental anomaly characterized by the presence of a proboscis-like nose above eyes partially or completely fused into one.

rhinocheiloplasty (-ki′lo-plas″te) plastic surgery of the lip and nose.

rhinocleisis (-kli′sis) obstruction of the nasal passage.

rhinocoele (ri′no-sēl) the ventricle of the olfactory lobe of the brain.

rhinodacryolith (-ri″no-dak′re-o-lith″) lacrimal concretion in the nasal duct.

rhinodynia (-din′e-ah) pain in the nose.

rhinogenous (ri-noj′ĕ-nus) arising in the nose.

rhinokyphosis (ri″no-ki-fo′sis) an abnormal hump on the ridge of the nose.

rhinolalia (-la′le-ah) a nasal quality of the voice from some disease or defect of the nasal passages, such as undue patency (r. aper′ta) or undue closure (r. clau′sa) of the posterior nares.

rhinolaryngitis (-lar″in-ji′tis) inflammation of the mucosa of the nose and larynx.

rhinolith (ri′no-lith) a nasal calculus.

rhinolithiasis (ri″no-lĭ-thi′ah-sis) a condition associated with formation of rhinoliths.

rhinologist (ri-nol′o-jist) a specialist in rhinology.

rhinology (ri-nol′o-je) the sum of knowledge about the nose and its diseases.

rhinometer (ri-nom′ĕ-ter) an instrument for measuring the nose or its cavities.

rhinommectomy (ri″nom-mek′to-me) excision of the inner canthus of the eye.

rhinomycosis (ri″no-mi-ko′sis) fungal infection of the nasal mucosa.

rhinonecrosis (-nĕ-kro′sis) necrosis of the nasal bones.

rhinopathy (ri-nop′ah-the) any disease of the nose.

rhinopharyngitis (ri″no-far″in-ji′tis) inflammation of the nasopharynx.

rhinophonia (-fo′ne-ah) a nasal twang or quality of voice.

rhinophore (ri′no-fōr) a nasal cannula to facilitate breathing.

rhinophycomycosis (ri″no-fi″ko-mi-ko′sis) a fungal disease caused by Entomophora coronata, marked by formation of large polyps in the subcutaneous tissues of the nose and paranasal sinuses; orbital involvement and unilateral blindness may follow. Cerebral involvement is common.

rhinophyma (-fi′mah) a form of rosacea marked by redness, sebaceous hyperplasia, and nodular swelling and congestion of the skin of the nose.

rhinoplasty (ri′no-plas″te) plastic surgery of the nose.

rhinopolypus (ri″no-pol′ĭ-pus) a nasal polyp.

rhinorrhagia (-ra′je-ah) nosebleed; epistaxis.

rhinorrhea (-re′ah) the free discharge of a thin nasal mucus. **cerebrospinal r.,** discharge of cerebrospinal fluid through the nose.

rhinosalpingitis (-sal″pin-ji′tis) inflammation of the mucosa of the nose and eustachian tube.

rhinoscleroma (-skle-ro′mah) a granulomatous disease involving the nose and nasopharynx; the growth forms hard patches or nodules, which tend to enlarge and are painful to the touch. It is ascribed to the presence of Klebsiella rhinoscleromatis.

rhinoscope (ri′no-skōp) a speculum for use in nasal examination.

rhinoscopy (ri-nos′ko-pe) examination of the nose with a speculum, either through the anterior nares (anterior r.) or the nasopharynx (posterior r.).

rhinosporidiosis (ri″no-spo-rid″e-o′sis) a fungal disease caused by Rhinosporidium seeberi, marked by large polyps on the mucosa of the nose, eyes, ears, and sometimes the penis and vagina.

rhinotomy (ri-not′o-me) incision into the nose.

rhinovirus (ri″no-vi′rus) a subgroup of the picornaviruses, considered to be etiologically associated with the common cold and certain other upper respiratory ailments.

Rhipicephalus (ri″pĭ-sef′ah-lus) a genus of cattle ticks, many species of which transmit disease-producing organisms, such as Babesia ovis, B. canis, Theileria parva, Borrelia theileri, Rickettsia rickettsii, and R. conorii.

rhizo- word element [Gr.], root.

Rhizobium (ri-zo′be-um) a genus of symbiotic nitrogen-fixing schizomycetes (family Rhizobiaceae), producing nodules on the roots of leguminous plants.

rhizoid (ri′zoid) resembling a root.

rhizome (ri′zōm) the subterranean root stem of a plant.

rhizomelic (ri″zo-mel′ik) pertaining to the hips and shoulders (the roots of the limbs).

rhizomeningomyelitis (-mĕ-ning″go-mi″ĕ-li′tis) radiculomeningomyelitis.

rhizoneure (ri′zo-nūr) a nerve cell forming a nerve root.

Rhizopoda (ri-zop′o-dah) a class of protozoa of the subphylum Sarcodina, having pseudopodia and including the amebae.

Rhizopus (ri-zo′pus) a genus of fungi (order Mucorales), some species of which cause mucormycosis.

rhizotomy (ri-zot′o-me) division or transection of a nerve root.

rhod(o)- word element [Gr.], red.

rhodamine (ro-dah′min) a red fluorescent dye.

rhodium (ro′de-um) chemical element (see table), at. no. 45, symbol Rh.

Rhodnius prolixus (rod′ne-us pro-lik′sus) a winged hemipterous insect of South America capable of transmitting Trypanosoma cruzi, the cause of Chagas' disease.

rhodogenesis (ro″do-jen′ĕ-sis) regeneration of rhodopsin after its bleaching by light.

rhodophylaxis (-fi-lak′sis) the property of the retinal epithelium of facilitating rhodogenesis. **rhodophylac′tic**, adj.

rhodopsin (ro-dop′sin) visual purple; a photosensitive purple-red chromoprotein in the retinal rods that is bleached to visual yellow (all-*trans* retinal) by light, thereby stimulating retinal sensory endings.

RhoGAM (ro′gam) trademark for a preparation of Rh_o (D antigen) immune globulin.

rhombencephalon (romb″en-sef′ah-lon) hindbrain.

rhombocoele (rom′bo-sēl) the terminal expansion of the canal of the spinal cord.

rhomboid (rom′boid) shaped like a rectangle that has been skewed to one side so that the angles are oblique.

rhonchus (rong′kus) a rattling in the throat; also a dry, coarse rale in the bronchial tubes, due to a partial obstruction. See *rale*. **rhon′chal, rhon′chial**, adj.

rhubarb (roo′barb) the dried rhizome and root of *Rheum officinale;* used in fluidextract or aromatic tincture as a cathartic.

Rhus (rus) a genus of trees and shrubs; contact with certain species causes severe dermatitis. The most important species are: *R. diversilo′ba* and *R. toxicoden′dron*, or poison oak; *R. ra′dicans*, or poison ivy; and *R. ver′nix*, or poison sumac.

rhythm (rithm) a measured movement; the recurrence of an action or function at regular intervals. **rhyth′mic, rhyth′mical**, adj. **alpha r.**, electroencephalographic waves having a frequency of 8 to 13 per second, typical of a normal person awake in a quiet resting state. **beta r.**, electroencephalographic waves having a frequency of 18 to 30 per second, typical during periods of intense activity of the nervous system. **cantering r.**, gallop r. **circadian r.**, the regular recurrence in cycles of approximately 24 hours from one stated point to another, e.g., certain biological activities that occur at that interval regardless of constant darkness or other conditions of illumination. **coupled r.**, heart beats occurring in pairs, the second beat usually being a ventricular premature beat; see also *bigeminal pulse*. **delta r.**, 1. electroencephalographic waves having a frequency below $3\frac{1}{2}$ per second, typical in deep sleep, in infancy, and in serious brain disorders. 2. delta waves (1). **escape r.**, a heart rhythm initiated by lower centers when the sinoatrial node fails to initiate impulses, when its rhythmicity is depressed, or when its impulses are completely blocked. **gallop r.**, an auscultatory finding of three (*triple r.*) or four heart sounds, the extra sound(s) by convention being in diastole and related either to atrial contraction (*fourth sound, presystolic gallop*), to early rapid filling of a ventricle with an altered ventricular compliance (*protodiastolic gallop*), or to concurrence of atrial contraction and ventricular early rapid filling (*summation gallop*). **nodal r.**, heart rhythm initiated in the specialized junctional tissue, i.e., the atrioventricular node and the main (His) bundle. **sinus r.**, the normal heart rhythm originating in the sinoatrial node. **theta r.**, electroencephalographic waves having a frequency of 4 to 7 per second, occurring mainly in children but also in adults under emotional stress. **triple r.**, the cadence produced when three heart sounds recur in successive cardiac cycles; see also *gallop r.* **ventricular r.**, the ventricular contractions occurring in complete heart block.

rhythmicity (rith-mis′ĭ-te) in cardiology, the ability to beat, or the state of beating, rhythmically without external stimuli.

rhytidectomy (rit″ĭ-dek′to-me) excision of skin for elimination of wrinkles.

rhytidoplasty (rit′ĭ-do-plas″te) plastic sugery for the elimination of skin wrinkles.

rhytidosis (rit″ĭ-do′sis) a wrinkling, as of the cornea.

rib (rib) any one of the paired bones, 12 on either side, extending from the thoracic vertebrae toward the median line on the ventral aspect of the trunk, forming the major part of the thoracic skeleton; see also *Table of Bones*. **abdominal r's, asternal r's**, false r's. **cervical r.**, a supernumerary rib arising from a cervical vertebra. **false r's**, the five lower ribs on either side, not attached directly to the sternum. **floating r's**, the two lower false ribs on either side, usually without ventral attachment. **slipping r.**, one whose attaching cartilage is repeatedly dislocated. **true r's**, the seven upper ribs on either side, connected to the sternum by their costal cartilages.

riboflavin (ri″bo-fla′vin) vitamin B_2; the heat-stable factor of the vitamin B complex, found in milk, muscle, liver, kidney, eggs, grass, malt, and various algae; it functions as a coenzyme concerned with oxidative processes. Dietary deficiency results in angular stomatitis, cheilitis, corneal and other ocular changes, and seborrheic dermatitis.

ribonuclease (-nu′kle-ās) an enzyme which catalyzes the depolymerization of ribonucleic acid.

ribonucleoprotein (-nu″kle-o-pro′te-in) a substance composed of both protein and ribonucleic acid.

ribonucleoside (-nu′kle-o-sīd) a nucleoside in which the purine or pyrimidine base is combined with ribose.

ribonucleotide (-nu′kle-o-tīd) a nucleotide in which the purine or pyrimidine base is combined with ribose.

ribose (ri′bōs) an aldopentose present in ribonucleic acid (RNA).

ribosome (ri′bo-sōm) any of the intracellular ribonucleoprotein particles concerned with protein synthesis; they consist of reversibly dissociable units and are found either bound to cell membranes or free in the cytoplasm. They may occur singly or occur in clusters (polyribosomes).

ribosyl (-sil) a glycosyl radical formed from ribose.

ribulose (ri′bu-lōs) the 2-ketose isomer of ribose.

rice (rīs) the cereal plant, *Oryza sativa;* also its seed or grain.

ricin (ri′sin) a phytotoxin in the seeds of the castor oil plant (*Ricinus communis*), inhalation or ingestion of which causes intoxication producing superficial inflammation of the respiratory mucosa with hemorrhages into the lungs, or edema of the gastrointestinal tract with hemorrhages.

Ricinus (ris′ĭ-nus) a genus of euphorbiaceous plants, including *R. commu′nis,* or castor oil plant, the seeds of which afford castor oil. See also *ricin.*

rickets (rik′ets) a condition due to vitamin D deficiency, especially in infancy and childhood, with disturbance of normal ossification, marked by bending and distortion of the bones, nodular enlargements on the ends and sides of the bones, delayed closure of the fontanels, muscle pain, and sweating of the head. **adult r.,** a rickets-like disease affecting adults. **fetal r.,** achondroplasia. **late r.,** that occurring in older children. **renal r.,** renal osteodystrophy. **tardy r.,** late r. **vitamin D–resistant r.,** a condition almost indistinguishable from ordinary rickets clinically but resistant to unusually large doses of vitamin D; it is often familial but may occur sporadically. In *hypophosphatemic vitamin D–resistant r.,* hypophosphatemia is the main characteristic, while in *hypocalcemic vitamin D–resistant r.,* the serum concentration of phosphate is within normal limits or nearly so, and the concentration of calcium is abnormally low.

Rickettsia (rĭ-ket′se-ah) a genus of the tribe Rickettsieae, transmitted by lice, fleas, ticks, and mites to man and other animals, causing various diseases. **R. ak′ari,** the etiologic agent of rickettsialpox, transmitted by the mite *Allodermanyssus sanguineus* from the reservoir of infection in house mice. **R. austra′lis,** the etiologic agent of North Queensland tick typhus, possibly transmitted by *Ixodes* ticks. **R. cono′-rii,** the etiologic agent of boutonneuse fever (Marseilles fever, Mediterranean fever) and possibly of Indian tick typhus, Kenya typhus, and South American tick-bite fever; transmitted by *Rhipicephalus* and *Haemaphysalis* ticks. **R. prowaze′kii,** the etiologic agent of epidemic typhus and the latent infection Brill's disease, which are transmitted from man to man via *Pediculus humanus* var. *corporis.* **R. rickett′sii,** the etiologic agent of Rocky Mountain spotted fever, transmitted by *Dermacentor, Rhipicephalus, Haemaphysalis, Amblyomma,* and *Ixodes* ticks. **R. tsutsugamu′shi,** the etiologic agent of scrub typhus, transmitted by larval mites of the genus *Trombicula,* including *T. akamushi* and *T. deliensis,* from rodent reservoirs of infection.

rickettsia (rĭ-ket′se-ah), pl. *rickett′siae.* An individual organism of the Rickettsiaceae.

Rickettsiaceae (rĭ-ket″se-a′se-e) a family of the order Rickettsiales.

rickettsial (rĭ-ket′se-al) pertaining to or caused by rickettsiae.

Rickettsiales (rĭ-ket″se-a′lēz) an order of microorganisms occurring as elementary bodies, usually found intercellularly. Parasitic for verte-

brates and invertebrates, which serve as vectors, they may be pathogenic for man and other animals.

rickettsialpox (rik-et′se-al-poks″) a febrile disease with a vesiculopapular eruption, resembling chickenpox clinically, caused by *Rickettsia akari.*

rickettsicidal (rik-et″sĭ-si′dal) destructive to rickettsiae.

Rickettsieae (rik″et-si′e-e) a tribe of the family Rickettsiaceae.

Rickettsiella (rĭ-ket″se-el′lah) a genus of rickettsiae of the tribe Wolbachieae, parasitic on the Japanese beetle; nonpathogenic for mammals.

rickettsiosis (rik-et″se-o′sis) infection with rickettsiae.

Ricolesia (rik″o-le′ze-ah) a genus of uncertain taxonomic classification, the species of which cause a keratoconjunctivitis in cattle, goats, fowl, and swine.

ridge (rij) a linear projection or projecting structure; a crest. **dental r.,** any linear elevation on the crown of a tooth. **dermal r's,** cristae cutis. **genital r.,** the more medial part of the urogenital ridge, giving rise to the gonad. **interureteric r.,** a fold on mucous membrane extending across the bladder between the ureteric orifices. **mammary r.,** an ectodermal thickening in early embryos, along which the mammary glands subsequently develop. **mesonephric r.,** the more lateral portion of the urogenital ridge, giving rise to the mesonephros. **oblique r.,** a variable linear elevation obliquely crossing the occlusive surface of a maxillary molar. **urogenital r.,** a longitudinal ridge in the embryo, lateral to the mesentery.

ridgling (rij′ling) an animal, especially a horse, with one or both testes undescended.

rifamide (rif′ah-mīd) a semisynthetic antibacterial derived from rifamycin B, used in treatment of pulmonary tuberculosis.

rifampicin (rif′am-pĭ-sin) rifampin.

rifampin (rif′am-pin) a semisynthetic antibacterial derived from rifamycin SV, used in treatment of pulmonary tuberculosis and carriers of *Neisseria meningitidis.*

rifamycin (rif″ah-mi′sin) any of a family of antibiotics isolated from broths of *Streptomyces mediterranei,* effective against tubercle bacilli and certain other bacteria; the various forms are designated rifamycin B, C, D, E, O, S, SV, and X.

right-handed (rīt-hand′ed) using the right hand preferentially, or more skillfully than the left, in voluntary motor acts.

rigidity (rĭ-jid′ĭ-te) inflexibility or stiffness. **clasp-knife r.,** increased tension in the extensors of a joint when it is passively flexed, giving way suddenly on exertion of further pressure. **cogwheel r.,** tension in a muscle which gives way in little jerks when the muscle is passively stretched. **decerebrate r.,** rigid extension of an animal's legs as a result of decerebration; occurring in man as a result of lesions in the upper brain stem.

rigor (rig′or, ri′gor) [L.] a chill; rigidity. **r. mor′-**

tis, the stiffening of a dead body accompanying depletion of adenosine triphosphate in the muscle fibers.

rim (rim) a border or edge. **bite r., occlusion r., record r.,** a border constructed on temporary or permanent denture bases in order to record the maxillomandibular relation and for positioning of the teeth.

rima (ri′mah), pl. *ri′mae* [L.] a cleft or crack. **r. glot′tidis,** the elongated opening between the true vocal cords and between the arytenoid cartilages. **r. o′ris,** the opening of the mouth. **r. palpebra′rum,** palpebral fissure. **r. puden′di,** the cleft between the labia majora.

Rimifon (rim′ĭ-fon) trademark for a preparation of isoniazid.

rimula (rim′u-lah), pl. *rim′ulae* [L.] a minute fissure, as of the spinal cord or brain.

rinderpest (rin′der-pest) cattle plague.

ring (ring) 1. any annular or circular organ or area. 2. in chemistry, a collection of atoms united in a continuous or closed chain. **abdominal r., external,** superficial inguinal r. **abdominal r., internal,** deep inguinal r. **Albl's r.,** a ring-shaped shadow in radiographs of the skull, caused by aneurysm of a cerebral artery. **Bandl's r.,** pathologic retraction r.; see *retraction r.* **benzene r.,** the closed hexagon of carbon atoms in benzene, from which different benzene compounds are derived by replacement of hydrogen atoms. **Cannon's r.,** a focal contraction seen radiographically at the mid-third of the transverse colon, marking an area of overlap between the superior and inferior nerve plexuses. **conjunctival r.,** a ring at the junction of the conjunctiva and cornea. **constriction r.,** a contracted area of the uterus, where the resistance of the uterine contents is slight, as over a depression in the contour of the fetus, or below the presenting part. **deep inguinal r.,** an aperture in the transverse fascia for the spermatic cord or the round ligament. **Kayser-Fleischer r.,** a gray-green to red-gold pigmented ring at the outer margin of the cornea, seen in progressive lenticular degeneration and pseudosclerosis. **retraction r.,** a ringlike thickening and indentation occurring in normal labor at the junction of the isthmus and corpus uteri, delineating the upper contracting portion and the lower dilating portion (*physiologic retraction r.*), or a persistent retraction ring in abnormal or prolonged labor that obstructs expulsion of the fetus (*pathologic retraction r.*). **Schwalbe's r.,** a circular ridge composed of collagenous fibers surrounding the outer margin of Descemet's membrane. **superficial inguinal r.,** an opening in the aponeurosis of the external oblique muscle for the spermatic cord or the round ligament. **tympanic r.,** the bony ring forming part of the temporal bone at birth and developing into the tympanic plate. **umbilical r.,** the aperture in the fetal abdominal wall through which the umbilical cord communicates with the fetus. **vascular r.,** a developmental anomaly of the aortic arch wherein the trachea and esophagus are encircled by vascular structures, many variations being possible.

ring-bone (ring′bōn) exostosis involving the first or second phalanx of the horse.

ringworm (-werm) tinea. **Tokelau r.,** tinea imbricata.

Risa-131 (ri′sah) trademark for a preparation of iodinated I 131 serum albumin.

ristocetin (ris″to-se′tin) an antibiotic derived from culture of *Nocardia lurida;* effective against gram-positive cocci.

risus (ri′sus) [L.] laughter. **r. sardon′icus,** a grinning expression produced by spasm of facial muscles.

Ritalin (rit′ah-lin) trademark for preparations of methylphenidate.

riziform (riz′ĭ-form) resembling grains of rice.

R.L.L. right lower lobe (of lungs).

R.M.A. right mentoanterior (position of the fetus).

R.M.P. right mentoposterior (position of the fetus).

R.M.T. right mentotransverse (position of the fetus).

R.N. Registered Nurse.

Rn chemical symbol, *radon.*

RNA ribonucleic acid; see under *acid.*

RNase ribonuclease.

R.O.A. right occipitoanterior (position of the fetus).

roaring (rōr′ing) a condition in the horse marked by a rough sound on inspiration and sometimes on expiration.

Robalate (ro′bah-lāt) trademark for preparations of dihydroxyaluminum aminoacetate.

Robaxin (ro-bak′sin) trademark for preparations of methocarbamol.

Roccal (ro′kal) trademark for a preparation of benzalkonium chloride.

rod (rod) a straight, slim mass of substance, specifically one of the rodlike bodies of the retina. See *retinal r's.* **Corti's r's,** rodlike bodies in a double row in the inner ear, having their heads joined and their bases on the basilar membrane widely separated so as to form a spiral tunnel. **enamel r's,** the approximately parallel rods or prisms forming the enamel of the teeth. **retinal r's,** highly specialized cylindrical segments of the visual cells containing rhodopsin; together with the retinal cones, they form the light-sensitive elements of the retina.

rodenticide (ro-den′tĭ-sīd) 1. destructive to rodents. 2. an agent destructive to rodents.

roentgen (rent′gen) the international unit of x- or γ-radiation; it is the quantity of x- or γ-radiation such that the associated corpuscular emission per 0.001293 gm. of air produces, in air, ions carrying 1 electrostatic unit of electrical charge of either sign. Abbreviated R.

roentgenkymogram (rent″gen-ki′mo-gram) the film obtained by roentgenkymography.

roentgenkymograph (-ki′mo-graf) the apparatus used in roentgenkymography.

roentgenkymography (-ki-mog′rah-fe) a technique of graphically recording the movements of an organ on a single x-ray film.

roentgenogram (rent′gen-o-gram″) a film produced by roentgenography.

roentgenography (rent″gĕ-nog′rah-fe) the taking of pictures (roentgenograms) of internal structures of the body by passage of x-rays through the body to act on specially sensitized film. **roentgenograph′ic**, adj. **body-section r.**, a special technique to show in detail images and structures lying in a predetermined plane of tissue, while blurring or eliminating detail in images in other planes; various mechanisms and methods for such roentgenography have been given various names, e.g., laminagraphy, tomography, etc. **mucosal relief r.**, roentgenography after injection and evacuation of a barium enema and inflation of the intestine with air under light pressure, to reveal fine detail of the intestinal mucosa. **serial r.**, the making of several exposures of a particular area at arbitrary intervals. **spot-film r.**, the making of localized instantaneous roentgenographic exposures during fluoroscopy.

roentgenologist (rent″gĕ-nol′o-jist) a specialist in roentgenology; radiologist.

roentgenology (rent″gĕ-nol′o-je) that branch of radiology dealing with the diagnostic and therapeutic use of roentgen rays (x-rays).

roentgenometry (rent″gĕ-nom′ĕ-tre) 1. measurement of the intensity of x-rays. 2. the direct measurement of structures shown in the roentgenogram with or without the necessity of correcting for magnification.

roentgenoscope (rent′gen-o-skōp″) fluoroscope.

roentgenoscopy (rent″gĕ-nos′ko-pe) examination by means of roentgen rays (x-rays); fluoroscopy.

roentgenotherapy (rent″gen-o-ther′ah-pe) treatment by roentgen rays (x-rays).

roflurane (ro-floor′ān) an inhalation anesthetic, $C_3H_4BrF_3O$.

roletamide (ro-let′ah-mīd) a hypnotic, $C_{16}H_{19}NO_4$.

Rolicton (ro-lik′ton) trademark for a preparation of amisometradine.

rolitetracycline (ro″le-tet″rah-si′klēn) a highly soluble tetracycline compound used for intravenous or intramuscular injection.

rombergism (rom′berg-izm) Romberg's sign.

Romilar (ro′mil-ar) trademark for preparations of dextromethorphan.

rongeur (ron-zher′) [Fr.] an instrument for cutting tissue, particularly bone.

room (rŏŏm) a place in a building, enclosed and set apart for occupancy or for performance of certain procedures. **delivery r.**, one in which infants are delivered. **labor r.**, predelivery r. **operating r.**, one especially equipped for the performance of surgical operations. **postdelivery r.**, a recovery room for the care of obstetrical patients immediately after delivery. **predelivery r.**, a hospital room where an obstetrical patient remains during the first stage of labor, i.e., from the time the pains begin until she is ready for delivery. **recovery r.**, a hospital unit adjoining operating or delivery rooms, with special equipment and personnel for the care of patients immediately after operation or childbirth.

root (rŏŏt) 1. the descending and subterranean part of a plant. 2. that portion of an organ, such as a tooth, hair, or nail, that is buried in the tissues, or by which it arises from another structure. **anterior r.**, ventral r. **dorsal r.**, the posterior, or sensory, division of each spinal nerve, attached centrally to the spinal cord and joining peripherally with the ventral root to form the nerve before it emerges from the intervertebral foramen. **motor r.**, ventral r. **posterior r.**, dorsal r. **sensory r.**, dorsal r. **ventral r.**, the anterior, or motor, division of each spinal nerve, attached centrally to the spinal cord and joining peripherally with the dorsal root to form the nerve before it emerges from the intervertebral foramen.

R.O.P. right occipitoposterior (position of the fetus).

rosacea (ro-za′she-ah) a chronic disease of the skin of the nose, forehead, and cheeks, marked by flushing, followed by red coloration due to dilatation of the capillaries, with the appearance of papules and acne-like pustules.

rosaniline (ro-zan′ĭ-lin) a triphenylmethane derivative, $C_{20}H_{21}N_3O$, the basis of various dyes and a component of basic fuchsin.

rosary (ro′zah-re) a structure resembling a string of beads. **rachitic r.**, a succession of bead-like prominences along the costal cartilages, in rickets.

roseola (ro-ze′o-lah, ro″ze-o′lah) [L.] 1. any rose-colored rash. 2. exanthema subitum. **r. infan′tum**, exanthema subitum. **syphilitic r.**, eruption of rose-colored spots in early secondary syphilis. **r. typho′sa**, rose spots.

rosette (ro-zet′) [Fr.] any structure or formation resembling a rose, such as (a) the clusters of polymorphonuclear leukocytes around a globule of lipid nuclear material, as observed in the test for disseminated lupus erythematosus, or (b) a figure formed by the chromosomes in an early stage of mitosis.

rosin (roz′in) solid resin obtained from species of *Pinus;* used in preparation of ointments and plasters.

rostellum (ros-tel′um) a small protruberance or beak, especially the fleshy protuberance of the scolex of a tapeworm, which may or may not bear hooks.

rostrad (ros′trad) 1. toward a rostrum; nearer the rostrum in relation to a specific point of reference. 2. cephalad.

rostral (ros′tral) 1. pertaining to or resembling a rostrum; having a rostrum or beak. 2. rostrad.

rostrate (ros′trāt) beaked.

rostrum (ros′trum), pl. *ros′tra* [L.] a beak-shaped process.

rot (rot) 1. decay. 2. a disease of sheep, and sometimes of man, due to *Fasciola hepatica.*

rotation (ro-ta′shun) the process of turning around an axis. In obstetrics, the turning of the fetal head (or presenting part) for proper orientation to the pelvic axis. **optical r.**, the quality of certain optically active substances whereby the plane of polarized light is changed, so that it is rotated in an arc the length of which is characteristic of the substance.

rotavirus (ro′tah-vi″rus) any of a group of double-stranded RNA viruses having a wheel-like appearance and responsible for acute infantile gastroenteritis and for diarrhea in mice, calves, and pigs.

rotenone (ro'tĕ-nōn) a poisonous compound from derris root and other roots; used as an insecticide and as a scabicide.

rotoxamine (ro-toks'ah-mēn) an antihistaminic, $C_{16}H_{19}ClN_2O$.

rotular (rot'u-lar) patellar.

roughage (ruf'ij) indigestible material such as fibers, cellulose, etc., in the diet.

rouleau (roo-lo'), pl. *rouleaux'* [Fr.] a roll of red blood cells resembling a pile of coins.

roundworm (rownd'werm) any worm of the class Nematoda; a nematode.

Roux-en-Y (roo-ahn-wi) denoting any Y-shaped anastomosis in which the small intestine is included.

R.P.F. renal plasma flow.

rpm revolutions per minute.

R.Q. respiratory quotient.

-rrhage, -rrhagia word element [Gr.], *excessive flow*. **-rrhagic,** adj.

-rrhea word element [Gr.], *profuse flow*. **-rrheic,** adj.

rRNA ribosomal RNA (ribonucleic acid).

R.S.A. right sacroanterior (position of the fetus).

R.Sc.A. right scapuloanterior (position of the fetus).

R.Sc.P. right scapuloposterior (position of the fetus).

R.S.P. right sacroposterior (position of the fetus).

R.S.T. right sacrotransverse (position of the fetus).

Ru chemical symbol, *ruthenium*.

rub (rub) friction rub; an auscultatory sound caused by the rubbing together of two serous surfaces. **friction r.,** see *rub.* **pericardial r.,** a scraping or grating noise heard with the heart beat, usually a two-and-fro sound, associated with an inflamed pericardium.

rubber-dam (rub'er-dam) a sheet of thin latex rubber used by dentists to isolate teeth from the fluids of the mouth during dental treatment.

rubefacient (roo''bĕ-fa'shent) 1. reddening the skin. 2. an agent that reddens the skin.

rubella (roo-bel'ah) German measles: a mild viral infection marked by a pink macular rash, fever, and lymph node enlargement; transplacental infection of the fetus in the first trimester may produce developmental anomalies of the heart, eyes, brain, bone, and ears.

rubeola (roo-be'o-lah, ru''be-o'lah) a synonym of measles in English and of German measles in French and Spanish.

rubeosis (roo''be-o'sis) redness. **r. i'ridis,** a condition characterized by a new formation of vessels and connective tissue on the surface of the iris, frequently seen in diabetics.

ruber (roo'ber) [L.] red.

rubescent (roo-bes'ent) growing red; reddish.

rubidium (roo-bid'e-um) chemical element (*see table*), at. no. 37, symbol Rb.

rubor (roo'bor) [L.] redness, one of the cardinal signs of inflammation.

Rubramin (roo'brah-min) trademark for preparations of cyanocobalamin (vitamin B_{12}) activity concentrate.

rubriblast (roo'brĭ-blast) pronormoblast.

rubric (roo'brik) red; specifically, pertaining to the red nucleus.

rubricyte (roo'brĭ-sīt) polychromatic normoblast.

rubrospinal (roo''bro-spi'nal) pertaining to the red nucleus and the spinal cord.

rubrothalamic (-thah-lam'ik) pertaining to the red nucleus and the thalamus.

rubrum (roo'brum) [L.] red. **r. scarlati'num,** scarlet red.

rudiment (roo'dĭ-ment) 1. a vestigial organ. 2. primordium.

rudimentary (roo'dĭ-men'ter-e) 1. imperfectly developed. 2. vestigial.

rudimentum (roo''dĭ-men'tum) rudiment; in NA, the first indication of a structure in the course of its embryonic development.

ruga (roo'gah), pl. *ru'gae* [L.] a ridge or fold.

rugose (roo'gōs) marked by ridges; wrinkled.

rugosity (roo-gos'ĭ-te) 1. a condition of being rugose. 2. a fold, wrinkle, or ruga.

R.U.L. right upper lobe (of lung).

rule (roōl) a statement of conditions commonly observed in a given situation, or of a prescribed procedure to obtain a given result. **Clark's r.,** the dose of a drug for a child is obtained by multiplying the adult dose by the child's weight in pounds and dividing the result by 150. **Fried's r.,** the dose of a drug for an infant less than two years old is obtained by multiplying the child's age in months by the adult dose and dividing the result by 150. **M'Naghten r.,** "to establish a defense on the ground of insanity, it must be clearly proved that at the time of committing the act the party accused was laboring under such a defect of reason from disease of the mind as not to know the nature and quality of the act he was doing, or, if he did know it, that he did not know that what he was doing was wrong." **Nägele's r.,** (for predicting day of labor) subtract three months from the first day of the last menstruation and add seven days. **van't Hoff's r.,** the velocity of chemical reactions is increased twofold or more for each rise of 10° C. in temperature. **Young's r.,** the dose of a drug for a child is obtained by multiplying the adult dose by the child's age in years and dividing the result by the sum of the child's age plus 12.

rumbatron (rum'bah-tron) a high-efficiency radio oscillator in which atoms are shattered and which employs electrons as the bombarding particles.

rumen (roo'men) the first stomach of a ruminant.

rumenitis (roo''mĕ-ni'tis) inflammation of the rumen.

ruminant (roo'mĭ-nant) 1. chewing the cud. 2. one of the order of animals, including cattle, sheep, goats, deer, and antelopes, which have a stomach with four complete cavities (rumen, reticulum, omasum, abomasum), through which the food passes in digestion.

rumination (roo″mĭ-na′shun) 1. the casting up of the food to be chewed thoroughly a second time, as in cattle. 2. meditation.

rump (rump) the buttock or gluteal region.

rupia (roo′pe-ah) thick, dark, raised, lamellated, adherent crusts on the skin, somewhat resembling oyster shells, as in late recurrent secondary syphilis. **ru′pial,** adj.

rupture (rup′chur) 1. tearing or disruption of tissue. 2. hernia.

rush (rush) peristaltic rush; a powerful wave of contractile activity that travels very long distances down the small intestine, caused by intense irritation or unusual distention.

rut (rut) the period or season of heightened sexual activity in some male mammals, coinciding with estrus in females.

ruthenium (roo-the′ne-um) chemical element (*see table*), at. no. 44, symbol Ru.

rutherford (ruth′er-ford) a unit of radioactive disintegration, representing one million disintegrations per second.

rutherfordium (ruth″er-for′de-um) chemical element (*see table*), at. no. 104, symbol Rf.

RV residual volume.

℞, Rx symbol, [L.] *rec′ipe* (take); prescription; treatment.

rye (ri) the cereal plant *Secale cereale,* and its nutritious seed. **spurred r.,** see *ergot.*

S

S chemical symbol, *sulfur.*

S. [L.] *se′mis* (*half*); sight; [L.] *sig′na* (*sign*); [L.] *sin′ister* (*left*).

sabulous (sab′u-lus) gritty or sandy.

saburra (sah-bur′ah) foulness of the mouth or stomach.

saburral (sah-bur′al) 1. pertaining to saburra. 2. gritty; gravelly.

sac (sak) a pouch; a baglike organ or structure. **air s′s,** alveolar s′s. **allantoic s.,** the dilated portion of the allantois, becoming a part of the placenta in many mammals. **alveolar s′s,** the spaces into which the alveolar ducts open distally, and with which the alveoli communicate. **amniotic s.,** amnion. **conjunctival s.,** the potential space, lined by conjunctiva, between the eyelids and eyeball. **dental s.,** the dense fibrous layer of mesenchyme surrounding the enamel organ and dental papilla. **endolymphatic s.,** the blind, flattened cerebral end of the endolymphatic duct. **heart s.,** the pericardium. **hernial s.,** the peritoneal pouch enclosing a hernia. **Hilton's s.,** laryngeal saccule. **lacrimal s.,** the dilated upper end of the nasolacrimal duct. **yolk s.,** the extraembryonic membrane that connects with the midgut; in vertebrates below true mammals, it contains a yolk mass.

saccade (sah-kād′) the series of involuntary, abrupt, rapid, small movements or jerks of both eyes simultaneously in changing the point of fixation. **saccad′ic,** adj.

saccate (sak′āt) 1. shaped like a sac. 2. contained in a sac.

racchar(o)- word element [L.], *sugar.*

saccharase (sak′ah-rās) β-fructofuranosidase.

saccharate (sak′ah-rāt) a salt of saccharic acid.

saccharated (sak′ah-rāt″ed) charged with or containing sugar.

saccharide (sak′ah-rīd) one of a series of carbohydrates, including the sugars.

sacchariferous (sak″ah-rif′er-us) containing or yielding sugar.

saccharimeter (sak″ah-rim′ĕ-ter) a device for estimating the proportion of sugar in a solution.

saccharin (sak′ah-rin) a white, crystalline compound several hundred times sweeter than sucrose; used as a flavor and non-nutritive sweetener.

saccharogalactorrhea (sak″ah-ro-gah-lak″to-re′ah) secretion of milk containing an excess of sugar.

saccharolytic (-lit′ik) capable of splitting up sugar.

saccharometabolism (-mĕ-tab′o-lizm) metabolism of sugar. **saccharometabol′ic,** adj.

saccharometer (sak″ah-rom′ĕ-ter) saccharimeter.

Saccharomyces (sak″ah-ro-mi′sēz) a genus of yeasts, including *S. cerevis′iae,* or brewers' yeast.

saccharomycetic (-mi-set′ik) pertaining to or caused by yeast fungi.

saccharose (sak′ah-rōs) sucrose.

saccharum (sak′ah-rum) [L.] sugar. **s. lac′tis,** lactose.

sacciform (sak′sĭ-form) shaped like a bag or sac.

saccular (sak′u-lar) pertaining to or resembling a sac.

sacculated (sak′u-lāt″ed) containing saccules.

sacculation (sak″u-la′shun) 1. a saccule, or pouch. 2. the quality of being sacculated. 3. the formation of pouches.

saccule (sak′ūl) a little bag or sac; applied specifically to the smaller of the two divisions of the membranous labyrinth of the ear. **laryngeal s.,** a diverticulum extending upward from the front of the laryngeal ventricle.

sacculocochlear (sak″u-lo-kok′le-ar) pertaining to the saccule and cochlea.

sacculus (sak′u-lus), pl. *sac′culi* [L.] a saccule.

saccus (sak′us), pl. *sac′ci* [L.] a sac.

sacr(o)- word element [L.], *sacrum.*

sacrad (sa′krad) toward the sacrum.

sacral (sa′kral) pertaining to the sacrum.

sacralgia (sa-kral′je-ah) pain in the sacrum.

sacralization (sa″kral-i-za′shun) anomalous fusion of the fifth lumbar vertebra with the first segment of the sacrum.

sacrectomy (sa-krek′to-me) excision or resection of the sacrum.

sacrococcygeal (sa″kro-kok-sij′e-al) pertaining to the sacrum and coccyx.

sacrodynia (-din′e-ah) sacralgia.

sacroiliac (-il′e-ak) pertaining to the sacrum and ilium, or to their articulation.

sacrolumbar (-lum′bar) pertaining to the sacrum and loins.

sacrosciatic (-si-at′ik) pertaining to the sacrum and ischium.

sacrospinal (-spi′nal) pertaining to the sacrum and the spinal column.

sacrouterine (-u′ter-in) pertaining to the sacrum and uterus.

sacrovertebral (-ver′tĕ-bral) pertaining to the sacrum and vertebrae.

sacrum (sa′krum) [L.] see *Table of Bones*.

sadism (sad′izm) the derivation of sexual gratification through the infliction of pain or humiliation on others. **sadis′tic,** adj.

sadist (sad′ist) one who practices sadism.

sadomasochism (sad″o-mas′o-kizm) a state characterized by both sadistic and masochistic tendencies. **sadomasochis′tic,** adj.

sadomasochist (-kist) a person exhibiting sadomasochism.

Saff (saf) trademark for a preparation of safflower oil.

Safflor (saf′flor) trademark for a preparation of safflower oil.

sagittal (saj′ĭ-tal) 1. shaped like an arrow. 2. situated in the direction of the sagittal suture; said of an anteroposterior plane or section parallel to the median plane of the body.

sagittalis (saj″ĭ-ta′lis) [L.] sagittal.

sago (sa′go) starch from pith of various palm trees, chiefly of the genus *Sagus*.

sal (sal) [L.] salt. **s. ammo′niac,** ammonium chloride. **s. so′da,** sodium carbonate. **s. volat′ile,** ammonium carbonate.

salicylamide (sal″ĭ-sil-am′īd) an analgesic, C_7-H_7NO_2.

salicylanilide (-an′ĭ-līd) a local antifungal, C_{13}-$H_{11}NO_2$.

salicylate (sal′ĭ-sil″āt, sah-lis′ĭ-lāt) a salt of salicylic acid.

salicylated (sal′ĭ-sil-āt″ed) impregnated or charged with salicylic acid.

salicylazosulfapyridine (sal″ĭ-sil″ah-zo-sul″-fah-pir′ĭ-dēn) a salicylic acid compound, C_{18}-$H_{14}N_4O_5S$, used in treatment of chronic ulcerative colitis.

salicylic (sal″ĭ-sil′ik) containing the radical salicyl; see also under *acid*.

salicylism (sal′ĭ-sil″izm) toxic effects of overdosage with salicylic acid or its salts, usually marked by tinnitus, nausea, and vomiting.

salifiable (sal″ĭ-fi′ah-b'l) capable of combining with an acid to form a salt.

salimeter (sah-lim′ĕ-ter) a hydrometer for ascertaining the concentration of saline solutions.

saline (sa′līn) salty; of the nature of a salt. **physiological s.,** an isotonic aqueous solution of NaCl for temporarily maintaining living cells.

saliva (sah-li′vah) the enzyme-containing secretion of the salivary glands. **sal′ivary,** adj.

salivant (sal′ĭ-vant) provoking a flow of saliva.

salivation (sal″ĭ-va′shun) 1. the secretion of saliva. 2. ptyalism.

Salmonella (sal″mo-nel′ah) a genus of gram-negative bacteria (tribe Salmonellae), including *S. choleraesu′is,* an important secondary invader in hog cholera, which occasionally infects man; *S. enterit′idis,* a common cause of gastroenteritis in man; *S. paraty′phi,* the causative agent of paratyphoid; *S. typhimu′rium,* responsible for a food poisoning in man; and *S. typho′sa,* the causative agent of typhoid.

salmonella (-nel′ah), pl. *salmonel′lae.* Any organism of the genus *Salmonella.* **salmonel′lal,** adj.

Salmonelleae (-nel′e-e) a tribe of bacteria (family Enterobacteriaceae).

salmonellosis (-nel-lo′sis) infection with *Salmonella.*

salping(o)- word element [Gr.], *tube* (*eustachian tube* or *uterine tube*).

salpingectomy (sal″pin-jek′to-me) excision of a uterine tube.

salpingemphraxis (-jem-frak′sis) obstruction of a eustachian tube.

salpingian (sal-pin′je-an) pertaining to the auditory or the uterine tube.

salpingitis (sal″pin-ji′tis) inflammation of the auditory or the uterine tube. **salpingit′ic,** adj.

salpingocele (sal-ping′go-sēl) hernial protrusion of a uterine tube.

salpingography (sal″ping-gog′rah-fe) radiography of the uterine tubes after injection of a radiopaque medium.

salpingolithiasis (sal-ping″go-lĭ-thi′ah-sis) the presence of calcareous deposits in the wall of the uterine tubes.

salpingolysis (sal″ping-gol′ĭ-sis) surgical separation of adhesions involving the uterine tubes.

salpingo-oophorectomy (sal-ping″go-o″of-o-rek′to-me) excision of a uterine tube and ovary.

salpingo-oophoritis (-o″of-o-ri′tis) inflammation of a uterine tube and ovary.

salpingo-oophorocele (-o-of′o-ro-sēl″) hernia of a uterine tube and ovary.

salpingopexy (-pek′se) fixation of a uterine tube.

salpingopharyngeal (-fah-rin′je-al) pertaining to the auditory tube and the pharynx.

salpingoplasty (sal-ping′go-plas″te) plastic repair of a uterine tube.

salpingostomy (sal″ping-gos′to-me) 1. formation of an opening or fistula into a uterine tube for the purpose of drainage. 2. surgical restoration of the patency of a uterine tube.

salpingotomy (sal″ping-got′o-me) surgical incision of a uterine tube.

salpinx (sal′pinks) [Gr.] a tube; specifically, the auditory tube or the uterine tube.

salt (sawlt) 1. sodium chloride, or common salt.

2. any compound of a base and an acid; any compound of an acid some of whose replaceable atoms have been substituted. 3. [pl.] a saline purgative. **acid s.,** any salt in which the combining power of the acid is not entirely exhausted. **basic s.,** any salt with more than the normal proportion of the basic elements. **bile s's,** salts of bile acids occurring normally in the liver. **common s.,** sodium chloride. **double s.,** any salt in which two hydrogen atoms of a dibasic acid have been replaced by two separate metals or basic radicals. **Epsom s.,** magnesium sulfate. **Glauber's s.,** sodium sulfate. **neutral s., normal s.,** any salt that is neither acidic nor basic in reaction. **Rochelle s.,** potassium sodium tartrate. **smelling s's,** aromatized ammonium carbonate; stimulant and restorative.

saltation (sal-ta′shun) the action of leaping, especially (1) chorea, or the dancing which sometimes accompanies it; (2) conduction along myelinated nerves; (3) in genetics, an abrupt variation in species; a mutation. **sal′tatory,** adj.

salting out (sawl′ting-owt) the separation of protein fractions in the serum or plasma by precipitation in increasing concentrations of neutral salts.

saltpeter (sawlt-pe′ter) potassium nitrate.

salubrious (sah-lu′bre-us) conducive to health; wholesome.

saluresis (sal″u-re′sis) urinary excretion of sodium and chloride ions.

saluretic (-u-ret′ik) 1. pertaining to, characterized by, or promoting saluresis. 2. an agent that promotes saluresis.

salutary (sal′u-tār″e) healthful.

salvarsan (sal′var-san) arsphenamine.

salve (sav) a thick ointment or cerate.

Salyrgan (sal′er-gan) trademark for a preparation of mersalyl.

samarium (sah-ma′re-um) chemical element (*see table*), at. no. 62, symbol Sm.

sanative (san′ah-tiv) curative; healing.

sanatorium (san″ah-to′re-um) an institution for treatment of sick persons, especially a private hospital for convalescents or patients with chronic diseases or mental disorders.

sanatory (san′ah-tor″e) conducive to health.

sand (sand) material occurring in small, gritty particles. **brain s.,** acervulus cerebri.

sandfly (sand′fli) any of various two-winged flies, especially of the genus *Phlebotomus.*

Sandril (san′dril) trademark for preparations of reserpine.

sane (sān) sound in mind.

sangui- word element [L.], *blood.*

sanguifacient (sang″gwĭ-fa′shent) forming blood.

sanguine (sang′gwin) 1. abounding in blood. 2. ardent; hopeful.

sanguineous (sang-gwin′e-us) abounding in blood; pertaining to the blood.

sanguinolent (sang-gwin′o-lent) of a bloody tinge.

sanguis (sang′gwis) [L.] blood.

sanguivorous (sang-gwiv′o-rus) subsisting on blood.

sanies (sa′ne-ēz) a fetid ichorous discharge containing serum, pus, and blood. **sa′nious,** adj.

saniopurulent (sa″ne-o-pu′roo-lent) partly sanious and partly purulent.

sanioserous (-se′rus) partly sanious and partly serous.

sanitarian (san″ĭ-ta′re-an) one skilled in sanitation and public health science.

sanitarium (san″ĭ-ta′re-um) an institution for the promotion of health.

sanitary (san′ĭ-tār″e) promoting or pertaining to health.

sanitation (san″ĭ-ta′shun) the establishment of conditions favorable to health.

sanitization (san″ĭ-ti-za′shun) the process of making or the quality of being made sanitary.

sanitize (san′ĭ-tīz) to clean and sterilize.

sanity (san′ĭ-te) soundness of mind.

santonin (san′to-nin) a lactone from the unexpanded flower heads of *Artemisia cina;* has been used as an anthelmintic.

sap (sap) the natural juice of a living organism or tissue. **cell s.,** hyaloplasm (1). **nuclear s.,** karyolymph.

saphena (sah-fe′nah) [L.] the small sphenous or the great sphenous vein; see *Table of Veins.*

saphenous (sah-fe′nus) pertaining to or associated with a saphena; applied to certain arteries, nerves, veins, etc.

sapo (sa′po) [L.] soap.

sapogenin (sah-poj′ĕ-nin) the aglycone of saponin.

saponaceous (sa″po-na′shus) soapy; of soaplike feel or quality.

saponification (sah-pon″ĭ-fi-ka′shun) conversion of an oil or fat into a soap by combination with an alkali.

saponin (sap′o-nin) a group of glycosides widely distributed in plants, which form a durable foam when their watery solutions are shaken, and which dissolve erythrocytes even in high dilutions.

sapphism (saf′izm) lesbianism.

sapr(o)- word element [Gr.], decay; decayed matter.

saprophyte (sap′ro-fīt) any organism living upon dead or decaying organic matter. **saprophyt′ic,** adj.

saprozoic (sap″ro-zo′ik) living on decayed organic matter; said of animals, especially protozoa.

sarc(o)- word element [Gr.], *flesh.*

Sarcina (sar-si′nah) a genus of bacteria (family Micrococcaceae) found in soil and water as saprophytes.

sarcoblast (sar′ko-blast) a primitive cell which develops into a muscle cell.

sarcocele (-sēl) any fleshy swelling or tumor of the testis.

sarcocyst (-sist) any member of, or any cyst formed by, *Sarcocystis.*

Sarcocystis (sar″ko-sis′tis) a genus of parasitic sporozoa found in cysts in the muscle tissue of mammals, birds, and reptiles.

Sarcodina (-di′nah) a subphylum of Protozoa,

including all the amebae, both free-living and parasitic, characterized by the ability to produce pseudopodia during most of the life cycle; flagella, when present, develop only during the early stages.

sarcoid (sar′koid) 1. tuberculoid; characterized by noncaseating epithelioid cell tubercles. 2. pertaining to or resembling sarcoidosis. 3. sarcoidosis. **Boeck's s.**, sarcoidosis. **Spiegler-Fendt s.**, a sarcoid in the subcutaneous tissue in the form of a circumscribed cellular mass containing reticulated cells and lymphocytes; probably a solitary lymphocytoma.

sarcoidosis (sar″koi-do′sis) a chronic, progressive, generalized granulomatous reticulosis involving almost any organ or tissue, characterized histologically by the presence in all affected tissues of noncaseating epithelioid cell tubercles. **s. cor′dis**, that involving the heart, the lesions ranging from a few asymptomatic, microscopic granulomas to widespread infiltration of the myocardium by large masses of sarcoid tissue. **muscular s.**, that involving the skeletal muscles, with sarcoid tubercles, interstitial inflammation with fibrosis, and disruption and atrophy of the muscle fibers.

sarcolemma (sar″ko-lem′ah) the membrane covering a striated muscle fiber. **sarcolem′mic, sarcolem′mous**, adj.

sarcoma (sar-ko′mah) a malignant tumor of mesenchymal derivation. **Abernethy's s.**, a malignant fatty tumor occurring mainly on the trunk. **alveolar soft part s.**, one with a reticulated fibrous stroma enclosing groups of sarcoma cells enclosed in alveoli walled with connective tissue. **ameloblastic s.**, the malignant counterpart of ameloblastic fibroma. **botryoid s., s. botryoi′des**, an embryonal rhabdomyosarcoma arising in submucosal tissue, usually in the upper vagina, cervix uteri, or neck of urinary bladder in young children and infants, presenting grossly as a polypoid grapelike structure. **endometrial stromal s.**, a pale, polypoid, fleshy, malignant tumor of the endometrial stroma. **giant cell s.**, malignant giant cell tumor of bone. **Kaposi's s.**, a multifocal, metastasizing, malignant reticulosis with angiosarcoma-like features, chiefly involving the skin. **osteogenic s.**, a malignant primary tumor of bone composed of a malignant connective tissue stroma with evidence of osteoid, bone and/or cartilage formation; depending upon the dominant component, classified as osteoblastic, fibroblastic, and chondroblastic. **reticulocytic s., reticuloendothelial s., reticulum cell s.**, malignant lymphoma, histiocytic or undifferentiated. **Rous s.**, a virus-induced sarcoma of chickens.

sarcomatoid (-toid) resembling a sarcoma.

sarcomatosis (sar-ko″mah-to′sis) condition characterized by development of many sarcomas at various sites.

sarcomatous (sar-ko′mah-tus) pertaining to or of the nature of a sarcoma.

sarcomere (sar′ko-mēr) the unit of length of a myofibril, between two Z bands.

sarcomphalocele (sar″kom-fal′o-sēl) fleshy tumor of the umbilicus.

sarcoplasm (sar′ko-plazm) the interfibrillary matter of striated muscle. **sarcoplas′mic,** adj.

sarcoplast (-plast) an interstitial cell of muscle, itself capable of being transformed into muscle.

sarcopoietic (sar″ko-poi-et′ik) producing flesh or muscle.

Sarcoptes (sar-kop′tēz) a genus of mites, including *S. scabie′i,* the cause of scabies in man; other varieties cause mange in domestic animals.

sarcosine (sar′ko-sēn) an amino acid, *N*-methylglycine.

sarcosis (sar-ko′sis) abnormal increase of flesh.

Sarcosporidia (sar″ko-spo-rid′e-ah) an order of sporozoa parasitic in cardiac and striated muscles of vertebrates.

sarcosporidiosis (-spo-rid″e-o′sis) infection with sporozoa of the genus *Sarcocystis.*

sarcostosis (sar″kos-to′sis) ossification of fleshy tissue.

sarcotubules (sar″ko-tu′bŭlz) the membrane-limited structures of the sarcoplasm, forming a canalicular network around each myofibril.

sarcous (sar′kus) pertaining to flesh or muscle tissue.

satellite (sat′ĕ-līt) 1. a vein that closely accompanies an artery, such as the brachial. 2. a minor, or attendant, lesion situated near a larger one. 3. a globoid mass of chromatin attached at the secondary constriction to the ends of the short arms of acrocentric autosomes.

satellitosis (sat″ĕ-li-to′sis) accumulation of neuroglial cells about neurons; seen whenever neurons are damaged.

saturated (sat′u-rāt″ed) 1. having all the chemical affinities satisfied. 2. unable to hold in solution any more of a given substance.

saturation (sat″u-ra′shun) the state of being saturated, or the act of saturating.

saturnine (sat′ur-nīn) pertaining to lead or to lead poisoning.

saturnism (sat′urn-izm) lead poisoning.

satyriasis (sat″ĭ-ri′ah-sis) pathologic or exaggerated sexual desire in the male.

saucerization (saw″ser-i-za′shun) 1. the excavation of tissue to form a shallow shelving depression, usually performed to facilitate drainage from infected areas of bone. 2. the shallow saucer-like depression on the upper surface of a vertebra which has suffered a compression fracture.

saw (saw) a cutting instrument with a serrated edge. **Gigli's s.**, a flexible wire with saw teeth.

saxitoxin (sak″sĭ-tok′sin) a neurotoxin from poisonous mussels, clams, and plankton; see *gonyaulax poison.*

Sb chemical symbol, *antimony* (L. *stibium*).

Sc chemical symbol, *scandium.*

scab (skab) 1. the crust of a superficial sore. 2. to become covered with a crust or scab.

scabicide (ska′bĭ-sīd) 1. lethal to *Sarcoptes scabiei.* 2. an agent lethal to *Sarcoptes scabiei.*

scabies (ska′bēz) a contagious skin disease due to the itch mite, *Sarcoptes scabiei;* the female bores into the stratum corneum, forming burrows (cuniculi), attended by intense itching and eczema caused by scratching. **Norwegian s.,** a form associated with an immense number of mites with marked scales and crusts.

scabietic (ska″be-et′ik) pertaining to scabies.

scala (ska′lah), pl. *sca′lae* [L.] a ladder-like structure. **s. me′dia,** cochlear duct. **s. tym′pani,** the part of the cochlea below the lamina spiralis. **s. vestib′uli,** the part of the cochlea above the lamina spiralis.

scald (skawld) to burn with hot liquid or steam; a burn so produced.

scale (skāl) 1. a thin flake or compacted platelike structure, as of cornified epithelial cells on the body surface. 2. a scheme or device by which some property may be measured (as hardness, weight, linear dimension). 3. to remove material from a body surface, as incrustations from a tooth surface. **absolute s.,** a temperature scale with zero at the absolute zero of temperature. **Baumé's s.,** one for expressing specific gravity of fluids. **Celsius s.,** a temperature scale with the ice point at zero and the normal boiling point of water at 100 degrees (100° C.); see table accompanying *thermometer.* **centigrade s.,** one with 100 gradations or steps between two fixed points, as the Celsius scale; see table accompanying *thermometer.* **Fahrenheit s.,** a temperature scale with the ice point at 32 and the normal boiling point of water at 212 degrees (212° F.); see table accompanying *thermometer.* **French s.,** a scale used for denoting the size of catheters, sounds, etc., each unit being roughly equivalent to 0.33 mm. in diameter. **Kelvin s.,** an absolute centigrade scale on which the unit of measurement corresponds with that of the Celsius scale, but the ice point is at 273.15 degrees (273.15° K.). **Rankin s.,** an absolute scale on which the unit of measurement corresponds with that of the Fahrenheit scale, but the ice point is at 459.67 degrees (459.67° R.). **Réaumur s.,** a temperature scale with the ice point at zero and the normal boiling point of water at 80 degrees (80° R.). **temperature s.,** one for expressing degree of heat, based on absolute zero as a reference point, or with a certain value arbitrarily assigned to such temperatures as the ice point and boiling point of water. See table accompanying *thermometer.*

scalenectomy (ska″lĕ-nek′to-me) resection of the scalenus muscle.

scalenotomy (-not′o-me) division of the scalenus muscle.

scaler (skāl′er) a dental instrument for removal of calculus from teeth.

scalp (skalp) the skin covering the cranium.

scalpel (skal′pel) a small surgical knife usually having a convex edge.

scaly (skāl′e) characterized by scales; scalelike.

scan (skan) scintiscan.

scandium (skan′de-um) chemical element (*see table*), at. no. 21, symbol Sc.

scanning (skan′ning) 1. production of a scintiscan. 2. a manner of utterance characterized by somewhat regularly recurring pauses.

scanography (skan-og′rah-fe) a method of making radiographs by the use of a narrow slit beneath the tube so that, as the tube is moved over the target, all the rays of the central beam pass through the part being radiographed at the same angle.

scapha (ska′fah), pl. *sca′phae* [L.] the curved depression separating the helix and anthelix.

scaphocephaly (skaf″o-sef′ah-le) abnormal length and narrowness of the skull as a result of premature closure of the sagittal suture. **scaphocephal′ic, scaphoceph′alous,** adj.

scaphoid (skaf′oid) boat-shaped; see *Table of Bones.*

scaphoiditis (skaf″oi-di′tis) inflammation of the scaphoid bone.

scapula (skap′u-lah), pl. *scap′ulae* [L.] see *Table of Bones.* **scap′ular,** adj. **alar s.,** winged s. **scaphoid s.,** one with a more or less concave vertebral border. **winged s.,** one having a prominent vertebral border.

scapulalgia (skap″u-lal′je-ah) pain in the scapular region.

scapulectomy (skap″u-lek′to-me) excision or resection of the scapula.

scapuloclavicular (skap″u-lo-klah-vik′u-ler) pertaining to the scapula and clavicle.

scapulohumeral (-hu′mer-al) pertaining to the scapula and humerus.

scapulopexy (skap′u-lo-pek″se) surgical fixation of the scapula.

scapus (ska′pus), pl. *sca′pi* [L.] shaft.

scar (skahr) cicatrix; a mark remaining after the healing of a wound or other morbid process. By extension applied to other visible manifestations of an earlier event.

scarification (skar″ĭ-fĭ-ka′shun) production in the skin of many small superficial scratches or punctures, as for introduction of vaccine.

scarificator (-fĭ-ka′tor) scarifier.

scarifier (-fi′er) an instrument with many sharp points, used in scarification.

scarlatina (skahr″lah-te′nah) scarlet fever. **scarlat′inal,** adj. **s. angino′sa,** a form with severe throat symptoms. **s. haemorrha′gica,** a form in which there is extravasation of blood into the skin and mucous membranes.

scarlatinella (skahr-lat″ĭ-nel′ah) Duke's disease.

scarlatiniform (skahr″lah-tin′ĭ-form) resembling scarlet fever.

scat(o)- word element [Gr.], *dung; fecal matter.*

scatemia (skah-te′me-ah) alimentary toxemia in which chemical poisons are absorbed through the intestine.

scatology (skah-tol′o-je) study and analysis of feces, as for diagnostic purposes. **scatolog′ical,** adj.

scatophagy (skah-tof′ah-je) the eating of dung.

scatoscopy (skah-tos′ko-pe) examination of the feces.

scatter (skat′er) the diffusion or deviation of x-rays produced by a medium through which the rays pass; backward diffusion is called *backscatter.*

Sc.D. Doctor of Science.

schema (ske′mah) a plan, outline, or arrangement.

schindylesis (skin″dĭ-le′sis) an articulation in

which one bone is received into a cleft in another.

schist(o)- word element [Gr.], *cleft; split.*

schistocephalus (shis″to-sef′ah-lus) a fetus with a cleft head.

schistocoelia (-se′le-ah) congenital fissure of the abdomen.

schistocormus (-kor′mus) a fetus with a cleft trunk.

schistocyte (shis′to-sīt) a fragment of a red blood corpuscle, commonly observed in the blood in hemolytic anemia.

schistocytosis (shis″to-si-to′sis) an accumulation of schistocytes in the blood.

schistoglossia (-glos′e-ah) cleft tongue.

schistomelus (shis-tom′ĕ-lus) a fetus with a cleft limb.

schistoprosopus (shis″to-pros′o-pus) a fetus with a cleft face.

Schistosoma (-so′mah) a genus of blood flukes, including *S. haemato′bium* of Africa, *S. japon′i-cum* of the Far East, *S. manso′ni* of Africa, South America, and the West Indies, and *S. intercala′tum* of West Central Africa, which cause infection in man by penetrating the skin of persons coming in contact with infected waters; the invertebrate hosts are certain snails. See specific diseases under *schistosomiasis.*

schistosomal (-so′mal) pertaining to or caused by *Schistosoma.*

schistosome (shis′to-sōm) an individual of the genus *Schistosoma.*

schistosomiasis (shis″to-so-mi′ah-sis) infection with *Schistosoma.* **s. haemato′bia,** infection with *Schistosoma haematobium* in the vesical and pelvic venous plexuses, involving the urinary tract and causing cystitis and hematuria. **s. intercala′tum,** an endemic intestinal disease of West Central Africa due to infection with *Schistosoma intercalatum,* with abdominal pain, diarrhea, and other intestinal symptoms. **s. japon′ica,** infection with *Schistosoma japonica.* The acute form is marked by fever, allergic symptoms, and diarrhea; chronic effects, which may be severe, are due to fibrosis around eggs deposited in the liver, lungs, and central nervous system. **s. manso′ni,** infection with *Schistosoma mansoni,* living chiefly in the mesenteric veins but migrating to deposit eggs in venules, primarily of the large intestine; eggs lodging in the liver may lead to peripheral fibrosis, hepatosplenomegaly, and ascites.

schistosomicide (-so′mĭ-sīd) an agent lethal to schistosomes.

schistosomus (-so′mus) a fetus with a fissure of the abdomen and with rudimentary or absent lower limbs.

schistothorax (-tho′raks) congenital fissure of the chest or sternum.

schiz(o)- word element [Gr.], *divided; division.*

schizamnion (skiz-am′ne-on) an amnion formed by cavitation over or in the inner cell mass, as in human development.

schizaxon (-ak′son) an axon which divides into two nearly equal branches.

schizogenesis (skiz″o-jen′ĕ-sis) reproduction by fission. **schizog′enous,** adj.

schizogony (skĭ-zog′o-ne) the asexual reproduction of a sporozoan parasite (sporozoite) by multiple fission within the body of the host, giving rise to merozoites. **schizogon′ic,** adj.

schizogyria (skiz″o-ji′re-ah) a condition in which there are wedge-shaped cracks in the cerebral convolutions.

schizoid (skiz′oid, skit′soid) 1. resembling schizophrenia; see under *personality.* 2. a person with a schizoid personality.

schizomycete (skiz″o-mi-sēt′) an organism of the class Schizomycetes.

Schizomycetes (-mi-se′tēz) a taxonomic class comprising the bacteria; they are prokaryotic microorganisms, commonly multiplying by cell division; they may be free living, saprophytic, parasitic, or pathogenic.

schizont (skiz′ont) the stage in the development of the malarial parasite following the trophozoite whose nucleus divides into many smaller nuclei.

schizonychia (skiz″o-nik′e-ah) splitting of the nails.

schizophasia (-fa′ze-ah) incomprehensible, disordered speech.

schizophrenia (skit″so-, skiz″o-fre′ne-ah) any of a group of severe emotional disorders, usually of psychotic proportions, characterized by withdrawal from reality, delusions, hallucinations, ambivalence, inappropriate affect, and withdrawn, bizarre, or regressive behavior. **schizophren′ic,** adj. **catatonic s.,** a form marked by excessive and sometimes violent motor activity and excitement, or by generalized inhibition. **hebephrenic s.,** a form marked by shallow and inappropriate affect, giggling, silly behavior and mannerisms, regression, and hypochondriasis. **paranoid s.,** a psychotic state characterized by delusions of grandeur or persecution, often with hallucinations. **process s.,** severe progressive schizophrenia with a poor prognosis, attributed by many to organic brain changes; cf. *reactive s.* **reactive s.,** a form attributed chiefly to environmental conditions, with an acute onset and a favorable prognosis. **simple s.,** a slow, insidiously progressive form, marked by apathy, lack of initiative, and withdrawal.

schizotrichia (skiz″o-trik′e-ah) splitting of the hairs at the ends.

schwannoma (shwan-o′mah) neurilemoma. **granular cell s.,** see under *tumor.*

sciage (se-ahzh′) [Fr.] a sawing movement in massage.

sciatic (si-at′ik) pertaining to the ischium; see also *Table of Nerves.*

sciatica (si-at′ĭ-kah) neuralgia along the course of the sciatic nerve, most often with pain radiating into the buttock and lower limb, most commonly due to herniation of a lumbar disk.

science (si′ens) 1. the systematic observation of natural phenomena for the purpose of discovering laws governing those phenomena. 2. the body of knowledge accumulated by such means. **scientif′ic,** adj.

scientist (si′en-tist) one learned in science, especially one active in some particular field of investigation.

scieropia (si″er-o′pe-ah) defect of vision in which objects appear in a shadow.

scintigram (sin′tĭ-gram) scintiscan.

scintillation (sin″tĭ-la′shun) 1. an emission of sparks. 2. a subjective visual sensation, as of seeing sparks. 3. a particle emitted in disintegration of a radioactive element; see also under *counter.*

scintiscan (sin′tĭ-skan) a two-dimensional representation of the gamma rays emitted by a radioactive isotope, revealing its concentration in a specific organ or tissue.

scintiscanner (sin″tĭ-skan′er) the system of equipment used to make a scintiscan.

scirrhoid (skir′oid) resembling scirrhous carcinoma.

scirrhous (skir′us) hard or indurated; see under *carcinoma.*

scissura (sĭ-su′rah), pl. *scissu′rae* [L.] an incisure; a splitting.

scler(o)- word element [Gr.], *hard; sclera.*

sclera (skle′rah) the tough white outer coat of the eyeball, covering approximately the posterior five-sixths of its surface, continuous anteriorly with the cornea and posteriorly with the external sheath of the optic nerve. **scle′ral,** adj. **blue s.,** unusual blueness of the sclera, a prominent feature of osteogenesis imperfecta; also seen in certain other conditions.

scleradenitis (sklēr″ad-ĕ-ni′tis) inflammation and hardening of a gland.

sclerectasia (-ek-ta′ze-ah) a bulging state of the sclera.

sclerectoiridectomy (skle-rek″to-ir″ĭ-dek′to-me) excision of part of the sclera and of the iris.

sclerectoiridodialysis (-ir″ĭ-do-di-al′ĭ-sis) sclerectomy and iridodialysis.

sclerectomy (skle-rek′to-me) 1. excision of part of the sclera. 2. removal of sclerosed parts of the middle ear after otitis media.

scleredema (skler″ĕ-de′mah) chronic progressive thickening and induration of the skin occurring in children and in adults (*s. adulto′rum, Buschke′s s.*); typically it begins on the nape and upper back and slowly extends downward and anteriorly. **s. neonato′rum,** sclerema.

sclerema (skle-re′mah) induration of the skin. **s. adipo′sum, s. neonato′rum,** an often fatal condition marked by patchy or generalized progressive hardening of the subcutaneous fat, manifested as cold, yellowish, boardlike lesions; it affects premature and debilitated newborn infants.

scleriritomy (skle″rĭ-rit′o-me) incision of the sclera and iris in anterior staphyloma.

scleritis (skle-ri′tis) inflammation of the sclera; it may involve the part adjoining the limbus of the cornea (*anterior s.*) or the underlying retina and choroid (*posterior s.*).

scleroblastema (skle″ro-blas-te′mah) the embryonic tissue from which bone is formed. **scleroblastem′ic,** adj.

sclerochoroiditis (-ko″roi-di′tis) inflammation of the sclera and choroid.

sclerocornea (-kor′ne-ah) the sclera and choroid regarded as one.

sclerodactyly (-dak′tĭ-le) localized scleroderma of the digits.

scleroderma (-der′mah) chronic hardening and shrinkage of the connective tissues of any part of the body, including the skin, heart, esophagus, kidney, and lung; it may be circumscribed or generalized (*systemic s.*). **circumscribed s.,** morphea. **systemic s.,** systemic sclerosis; a progressive form involving large areas of the body surface and internal structures.

sclerogenous (skle-roj′ĕ-nus) producing sclerosis or sclerous tissue.

scleroiritis (skle″ro-i-ri′tis) inflammation of the sclera and iris.

sclerokeratitis (-ker″ah-ti′tis) inflammation of the sclera and cornea.

sclerokeratoiritis (-ker″ah-to-i-ri′tis) inflammation of the sclera, cornea, and iris.

scleroma (skle-ro′mah) a hardened patch or induration, especially of the nasal or laryngeal tissues. **respiratory s.,** rhinoscleroma.

scleromalacia (skle″ro-mah-la′she-ah) degeneration and thinning (softening) of the sclera, occurring in rheumatoid arthritis.

scleromere (skle′ro-mēr) 1. any segment or metamere of the skeletal system. 2. the caudal half of a sclerotome (2).

scleromyxedema (skle″ro-mik″sĕ-de′mah) a variant of lichen myxedematosus characterized by a generalized eruption of the nodules and diffuse thickening of the skin.

scleronyxis (-nik′sis) surgical puncture of the sclera.

sclero-oophoritis (-o″of-o-ri′tis) sclerosing inflammation of the ovary.

sclerophthalmia (skle″rof-thal′me-ah) encroachment of the sclera upon the cornea so that only the central part remains clear.

scleroprotein (skle″ro-pro′te-in) a simple protein characterized by its insolubility and its fibrous structure; it usually serves a supportive or protective function in the body.

sclerosant (skle-ro′sant) a chemical irritant producing inflammation and eventual fibrosis.

sclerose (skle′rōs) to become, or cause to become, hardened or sclerotic.

sclerosis (sklĕ-ro′sis) an induration or hardening, especially from inflammation and in diseases of the interstitial substance; applied chiefly to such hardening of the nervous system or to hardening of the blood vessels. **amyotrophic lateral s.,** progressive degeneration of the neurons that give rise to the corticospinal tract and of the motor cells of the brain stem and spinal cord, resulting in a deficit of upper and lower motor neurons; it usually has a fatal outcome. **arterial s.,** arteriosclerosis. **arteriolar s.,** arteriolosclerosis. **disseminated s.,** multiple s. **familial centrolobar s.,** a progressive familial form of leukoencephalopathy, marked by nystagmus, ataxia, tremor, parkinsonian facies, dysarthria, and mental deterioration. **lateral s.,** degeneration of the lateral columns of the spinal cord; it may be primary, with spastic paraplegia, limb rigidity, increase of the tendon reflexes, and no sensory disturbances, or secondary to myelitis, with spastic paraplegia and sensory and other disturbances. **Mönckeberg's s.**, see under *arteriosclerosis*. **multiple s.**, demyelination occurring in patches throughout the white matter of the central nervous system, sometimes extending into the gray matter; symptoms of lesions of the white matter are weakness, incoordination, paresthesias, speech disturbances, and visual complaints. **progressive systemic s.**, systemic scleroderma. **tuberous s.**, a congenital hereditary disease with tumors on the surfaces of the lateral ventricles of the brain and sclerotic patches on its surface, and marked by mental deterioration and epileptic attacks.

sclerostenosis (skle″ro-ste-no′sis) induration or hardening combined with contraction.

sclerostomy (skle-ros′to-me) incision of the sclera with drainage.

sclerotherapy (skle″ro-ther′ah-pe) injection of sclerosing solutions in the treatment of hemorrhoids or other varicose veins.

sclerotic (skle-rot′ik) 1. hard or hardening; affected with sclerosis. 2. sclera.

sclerotica (skle-rot′ĭ-kah) [L.] sclera.

sclerotitis (skle″ro-ti′tis) scleritis.

sclerotium (skle-ro′she-um) the hard, thickwalled blackish mass formed by certain fungi, such as the ergot of rye or the sclerotic cells seen in chromomycosis.

sclerotome (skle′ro-tōm) 1. an instrument used in the incision of the sclera. 2. the area of a bone innervated from a single spinal segment. 3. one of the paired masses of mesenchymal tissue, separated from the ventromedial part of a somite, which develop into vertebrae and ribs.

sclerotomy (skle-rot′o-me) incision of the sclera.

sclerous (skle′rus) hard; indurated.

scolex (sko′leks), pl. *sco′lices* [Gr.] the attachment organ of a tapeworm, generally considered the anterior, or cephalic, end.

scoli(o)- word element [Gr.], *crooked; twisted.*

scoliokyphosis (sko″le-o-ki-fo′sis) combined lateral (scoliosis) and posterior (kyphosis) curvature of the spine.

scoliosiometry (-se-om′ĕ-tre) measurement of spinal curvature.

scoliosis (sko″le-o′sis) lateral curvature of vertebral column. **scoliot′ic,** adj.

scombroid (skom′broid) of or pertaining to Scombroidea.

Scombroidea (skom-broid′de-ah) a suborder of marine fishes, including tunas, bonitos, mackerels, albacores, and skipjacks, the flesh of which contain a toxic histamine-like substance and, if ingested without being adequately preserved, can cause a condition marked by pain in the epigastric region, nausea, vomiting, headache, dysphagia, thirst, pruritus, and urticaria, usually subsiding within 12 hours.

scopograph (skop′o-graf) a combined fluoroscope and radiographic unit.

scopolamine (sko-pol′ah-mēn) an anticholiner-

gic alkaloid, $C_{17}H_{21}NO_4$, obtained from various solanaceous plants; the hydrobromide salt is used as a cerebral sedative, mydriatic, and cycloplegic.

scopometer (sko-pom′ĕ-ter) an instrument for measuring the turbidity of solutions, i.e., the density of a precipitate.

scopophilia (sko-po-fil′e-ah) 1. voyeurism (*active s.*). 2. exhibitionism (*passive s.*).

scopophobia (sko″po-fo′be-ah) morbid dread of being seen.

-scopy word element [Gr.], *examination of.*

scorbutic (skor-bu′tik) pertaining to or affected with scurvy.

scorbutigenic (skor-bu″tĭ-jen′ik) causing scurvy.

scorbutus (skor-bu′tus) [L.] scurvy.

scordinema (skor″dĭ-ne′mah) yawning and stretching with a feeling of lassitude, occurring as a preliminary symptom of some infectious disease.

score (skōr) a rating, usually expressed numerically, based on specific achievement or the degree to which certain qualities are manifest. **Apgar s.**, a numerical expression of an infant's condition, usually determined at 60 seconds after birth, based on heart rate, respiratory effort, muscle tone, reflex irritability, and color.

scoto- word element [Gr.], *darkness.*

scotochromogen (sko″to-kro′mo-jen) a microorganism whose pigmentation develops in the dark as well as in the light. **scotochromogen′ic,** adj.

scotodinia (-din′e-ah) dizziness with blurring of vision and headache.

scotogram, scotograph (sko′to-gram; -graf) 1. roentgenogram. 2. the effect produced upon a photographic plate in the dark by certain substances.

scotoma (sko-to′mah) an area of depressed vision in the visual field, surrounded by an area of less depressed or of normal vision. **scoto′matous,** adj. **absolute s.**, an area within the visual field in which perception of light is entirely lost. **annular s.**, a circular area of depressed vision surrounding the point of fixation. **arcuate s.**, an arc-shaped defect of vision arising in an area near the blind spot and extending toward it. **central s.**, an area of depressed vision corresponding with the point of fixation and interfering with central vision. **centrocecal s.**, a horizontal oval defect in the field of vision situated between and embracing both the point of fixation and the blind spot. **color s.**, an isolated area of depressed or defective vision for color. **negative s.**, one which appears as a blank spot or hiatus in the visual field. **peripheral s.**, an area of depressed vision toward the periphery of the visual field. **physiologic s.**, that area of the visual field corresponding with the optic disk, in which the photosensitive receptors are absent. **positive s.**, one which appears as a dark spot in the visual field. **relative s.**, an area of the visual field in which perception of light is only diminished, or loss is restricted to light of certain wavelengths. **ring s.**, annular s. **scintillating s.**, blurring of vision with sensation of a luminous appearance before the eyes, with zig-zag, wall-like outlines.

scotomagraph (sko-to′mah-graf) an instrument for recording a scotoma.

scotometer (sko-tom′ĕ-ter) an instrument for diagnosing and measuring scotomas.

scotometry (sko-tom′ĕ-tre) the measurement of scotomas.

scotophilia (sko″to-fil′e-ah) love of darkness.

scotophobia (-fo′be-ah) morbid fear of darkness.

scotopia (sko-to′pe-ah) 1. night vision. 2. dark adaptation. **scotop′ic,** adj.

scotopsin (sko-top′sin) the protein moiety in the retinal rods that combines with 11-*cis* retinal to form rhodopsin; see *retinal* (2).

scours (skowrz) diarrhea in newborn animals. **black s.,** acute dysentery in cattle, with intestinal hemorrhage producing dark feces. **white s.,** an acute infectious disease of newborn calves, lambs, and foals, due to enteropathogenic strains of *Escherichia coli*, marked by fever, dehydration, depression, and diarrhea with light-colored feces.

scrapie (skra′pe) a fatal disease of the nervous system of sheep and goats marked by pruritus, debility, and muscular incoordination.

scratches (skrach′ez) eczematous inflammation of the feet of a horse.

screen (skrēn) 1. a structure resembling a curtain or partition, used as a protection or shield; such a structure used in fluoroscopy, or on which light rays are projected. 2. to examine by fluoroscopy (Great Britain). 3. protectant (2). **Bjerrum s.,** tangent s. **fluorescent s.,** a plate in the fluoroscope coated with crystals of calcium tungstate. **tangent s.,** a large square of black cloth with a central mark for fixation; used with a campimeter in mapping the field of vision.

screening (skrēn′ing) 1. mass examination of a population to detect a particular disease. 2. fluoroscopy (Great Britain).

screwworm (skru′werm) the larva of *Cochliomyia hominivorax*.

scrobiculate (skro-bik′u-lāt) marked with pits.

scrobiculus (skro-bik′u-lus) [L.] pit. **s. cor′dis,** epigastric fossa.

scrofula (skrof′u-lah) primary tuberculosis of the cervical lymph nodes; the inflamed structures being subject to a cheesy degeneration.

scrofuloderma (skrof″u-lo-der′mah) suppurating abscesses and fistulous passages opening on the skin, secondary to tuberculosis of the lymph nodes, especially those of the neck (scrofula).

scrofulous (skrof′u-lus) pertaining to or characterized by scrofuloderma or scrofula.

scrotectomy (skro-tek′to-me) excision of part of the scrotum.

scrotitis (skro-ti′tis) inflammation of the scrotum.

scrotocele (skro′to-sēl) scrotal hernia.

scrotoplasty (-plas″te) plastic reconstruction of the scrotum.

scrotum (skro′tum) the pouch containing the testes and their accessory organs. **scro′tal,** adj. **lymph s.,** elephantiasis scroti.

scruple (skroo′p′l) 20 grains of the apothecaries′ system, or 1.296 gm.

scurvy (sker′ve) a disease due to deficiency of ascorbic acid (vitamin C), marked by anemia, spongy gums, a tendency to mucocutaneous hemorrhages, and brawny induration of calf and leg muscles.

scute (skūt) any squama or scalelike structure, especially the bony plate separating the upper tympanic cavity and mastoid cells (*tympanic s.*).

scutiform (sku′tĭ-form) shaped like a shield.

scutulum (sku′tu-lum), pl. *scu′tula* [L.] one of the disk- or saucer-like crusts characteristic of favus.

scutum (sku′tum) 1. scute. 2. a hard chitinous plate on the anterior dorsal surface of hard-bodied ticks.

scybalous (sib′ah-lus) of the nature of or composed of scybala.

scybalum (sib′ah-lum), pl. *scyb′ala* [Gr.] a hard mass of fecal matter in the intestines.

scyphoid (si′foid) shaped like a cup.

S.D. skin dose; standard deviation.

S.E. standard error.

Se chemical symbol, *selenium.*

searcher (serch′er) sound used in examining the bladder for calculi.

seasickness (se′sik-nes) motion sickness occasioned by ship travel.

seatworm (sēt′werm) any oxyurid, especially *Enterobius vermicularis.*

sebaceous (sĕ-ba′shus) pertaining to or secreting sebum.

sebiferous (sĕ-bif′er-us) sebiparous.

sebiparous (sĕ-bip′ah-rus) producing fatty secretion.

sebolith (seb′o-lith) calculus in a sebaceous gland.

seborrhea (seb″o-re′ah) 1. excessive secretion of sebum. 2. seborrheic dermatitis. **seborrhe′al, seborrhe′ic,** adj. **s. sic′ca,** dry, scaly seborrheic dermatitis.

seborrheid (seb″o-re′id) a seborrheic eruption.

sebum (se′bum) the oily secretion of the sebaceous glands, composed of fat and epithelial debris.

secobarbital (sek″o-bar′bĭ-tal) a short- to intermediate-acting barbiturate, $C_{12}H_{18}N_2O_3$, used as a hypnotic; also used as the sodium salt.

secodont (se′ko-dont) having molars whose tubercles have cutting edges.

Seconal (sek′ŏ-nal) trademark for preparations of secobarbital.

secreta (se-kre′tah) [L., pl.] secretion products.

secretagogue (se-krēt′ah-gog) stimulating secretion; an agent that so acts.

secrete (se-krēt′) to elaborate and release a secretion.

secretin (se-kre′tin) a hormone secreted by the duodenal and jejunal mucosa when acid chyme enters the intestine; it stimulates secretion of pancreatic juice and, to a lesser extent, bile and intestinal secretion.

secretinase (-ās) an enzyme of the serum that inactivates secretin.

secretion (se-kre′shun) 1. the cellular process of elaborating and releasing a specific product; this activity may range from separating a specific substance of the blood to the elaboration of a new chemical substance. 2. any substance produced by secretion. **external s.,** one that is discharged upon an external or internal body surface; see also *exocrine gland.* **internal s.,** hormone.

secretoinhibitory (se-kre″to-in-hib′ĭ-tor″e) inhibiting secretion.

secretomotor, secretomotory (-mo′tor; -mo′tor-e) stimulating secretion; said of nerves.

secretor (se-kre′tor) in genetics, one who secretes the ABH antigens of the ABO blood group in the saliva and other body fluids; also, the gene determining this trait.

secretory (se-kre′to-re) pertaining to secretion.

sectio (sek′she-o), pl. *sectio′nes* [L.] section.

section (sek′shun) 1. an act of cutting. 2. a cut surface. 3. a segment or subdivision of an organ. **abdominal s.,** laparotomy. **cesarean s.,** delivery of a fetus by incision through the abdominal wall and uterus. **frontal s.,** a section parallel with the long axis, dividing the body into dorsal and ventral parts. **frozen s.,** a specimen cut by microtome from tissue that has been frozen. **perineal s.,** external urethrotomy. **Pitres' s's,** a series of six frontal sections made at certain specified locations through the brain. **Saemisch's s.,** see under *operation.* **sagittal s.,** a section that follows the sagittal suture, dividing the head or the body into right and left halves. **serial s's,** histologic sections made in consecutive order and so arranged for the purpose of microscopic examination.

sectorial (sek-to′re-al) cutting.

secundigravida (se-kun″dĭ-grav′ĭ-dah) a woman pregnant the second time; gravida II.

secundines (se-kun′dīnz, -dēnz) afterbirth.

secundipara (se″kun-dip′ah-rah) a woman who has had two pregnancies which resulted in viable offspring; para II.

S.E.D. skin erythema dose.

Sedamyl (sed′ah-mil) trademark for a preparation of acetylcarbromal.

sedation (se-da′shun) 1. the allaying of irritability or excitement, especially by administration of a sedative. 2. the state so induced.

sedative (sed′ah-tiv) 1. allaying irritability and excitement. 2. a drug that so acts. Sedatives are classified, according to the organ most affected, as cardiac, gastric, etc.

sedentary (sed′en-ter″e) 1. sitting habitually; of inactive habits. 2. pertaining to a sitting posture.

sediment (sed′ĭ-ment) a precipitate, especially that formed spontaneously.

sedimentation (sed″ĭ-men-ta′shun) the settling out of sediment.

seed (sēd) 1. the mature ovule of a flowering plant. 2. semen. 3. a small cylindrical shell of gold or other suitable material, used in application of radiation therapy. 4. to inoculate a culture medium with microorganisms. **cardamom s.,** the dried ripe seed of *Elettaria cardamomum,* a plant of tropical Asia; used as a

flavoring agent. **plantago s., psyllium s.,** cleaned, dried ripe seed of species of *Plantago;* used as a cathartic.

segment (seg′ment) a demarcated portion of a whole. **segmen′tal,** adj. **bronchopulmonary s's,** the smaller subdivisions of the lobes of the lungs, separated by connective tissue septa and supplied by branches of the respective lobar bronchi. **hepatic s's,** subdivisions of the hepatic lobes based on arterial and biliary supply and venous drainage. **uterine s.,** either of the portions into which the uterus differentiates in early labor; the upper contractile portion (corpus uteri) becomes thicker as labor advances, and the lower noncontractile portion (the isthmus) is expanded and thin-walled.

segmentation (seg″men-ta′shun) 1. division into similar parts. 2. cleavage.

segmentum (seg-men′tum), pl. *segmen′ta* [L.] segment.

segregation (seg″re-ga′shun) 1. the separation of allelic genes during meiosis as homologous chromosomes begin to migrate toward opposite poles of the cell, so that eventually the members of each pair of allelic genes go to separate gametes. 2. the progressive restriction of potencies in the zygote to the various regions of the forming embryo.

segregator (seg′rĕ-ga″tor) an instrument for obtaining the urine from each kidney separately.

seismotherapy (sīz″mo-ther′ah-pe) treatment of disease by mechanical vibration.

seizure (se′zhur) a sudden attack, as of disease or epilepsy.

selection (sĕ-lek′shun) the play of forces that determines the relative reproductive performance of the various genotypes in a population. **natural s.,** the survival in nature of those individuals and their progeny best equipped to adapt to environmental conditions. **sexual s.,** natural selection in which certain characteristics attract male or female members of a species, thus ensuring survival of those characteristics.

selenium (sĕ-le′ne-um) chemical element (*see table*), at. no. 34, symbol Se; it causes alkali disease in animals that feed on vegetation grown on soils which contain it. **s. sulfide,** SeS_2, an antiseborrheic, applied topically to the scalp.

self-antigen (self-an′tĭ-jen) any constituent of the body's own tissues capable of stimulating autoimmunity.

self-limited (-lim′it-ed) limited by its own peculiarities, and not by outside influence; said of a disease that runs a definite limited course.

self-tolerance (-tol′er-ans) immunological tolerance to self-antigens.

sella (sel′ah), pl. *sel′lae* [L.] a saddle-shaped depression. **sel′lar,** adj. **s. tur′cica,** a depression on the upper surface of the sphenoid bone, lodging the pituitary gland.

semantics (sĕ-man′tiks) study of the meanings of words and the rules of their use; study of the relation between language and significance.

semeiography (se″mi-og′rah-fe) a description of the signs and symptoms of disease.

semeiotic (se″mi-ot′ik) 1. pertaining to signs or symptoms. 2. pathognomonic.

semeiotics (se″mi-ot′iks) symptomatology.

semelincident (sem″el-in′sĭ-dent) attacking only once, as an infectious disease which induces immunity thereafter.

semen (se′men) fluid discharged at ejaculation in the male, consisting of secretion of glands associated with the urogenital tract and containing spermatozoa. **sem′inal,** adj.

semi- word element [L.], *half.*

semicanal (sem″ĭ-kah-nal′) a channel open at one end.

semicoma (-ko′mah) a stupor from which the patient may be aroused. **semico′matose,** adj.

semiflexion (-flek′shun) position of a limb midway between flexion and extension; the act of bringing to such a position.

Semikon (sem′ĭ-kon) trademark for preparations of methapyrilene.

semilunar (sem″ĭ-lu′nar) resembling a crescent or half-moon.

semination (-na′shun) insemination.

seminiferous (-nif′er-us) producing or carrying semen.

seminoma (-no′mah) a malignant tumor of the testis thought to arise from primitive gonadal cells.

seminormal (-nor′mal) half of normal solution.

seminuria (se″mĭ-nu′re-ah) discharge of semen in the urine.

semipermeable (sem″ĭ-per′me-ah-b'l) permitting passage only of certain molecules.

semis (se′mis) [L.] half; abbreviated ss.

semisulcus (sem′ĭ-sul′kus) a depression which, with an adjoining one, forms a sulcus.

semisupination (-su″pĭ-na′shun) a position halfway toward supination.

semisynthetic (-sin-thet′ik) produced by chemical manipulation of naturally occurring substances.

Semoxydrine (sem-ok′sĭ-drin) trademark for a preparation of methamphetamine.

senescence (sĕ-nes′ens) the process of growing old. **senes′cent,** adj.

senile (se′nīl) pertaining to old age.

senilism (se′nil-izm) premature old age.

senility (sĕ-nil′ĭ-te) the physical and mental deterioration associated with old age.

senna (sen′ah) the dried leaflets of *Cassia senna* or of *C. angustifolia;* used chiefly as a cathartic.

sennoside (sen′o-sīd) either of two anthraquinone glucosides, sennoside A and B, from senna; used as a cathartic.

senopia (se-no′pe-ah) second sight; improvement of vision, especially near vision, in the aged, a sign of incipient cataract.

sensation (sen-sa′shun) an impression produced by impulses conveyed by an afferent nerve to the sensorium. **girdle s.,** zonesthesia. **gnostic s's,** sensations perceived by the more recently developed senses, such as those of light touch and the epicritic sensibility to muscle, joint, and tendon vibrations. **internal s.,** subjective s. **primary s.,** that resulting immediately and di-

rectly from application of a stimulus. **reflex s., referred s.,** one felt elsewhere than at the site of application of a stimulus. **subjective s.,** one perceptible only to the person himself, and not connected with any object external to his body.

sense (sens) a faculty by which the conditions or properties of things are perceived. **color s.,** the faculty by which colors are perceived and distinguished. **kinesthetic s.,** muscle s. **light s.,** the sense by which degrees of brilliancy are distinguished. **muscle s., muscular s.,** the sense by which muscular movements are perceived. **posture s.,** the muscular sense by which the position or attitude of the body or its parts is perceived. **pressure s.,** the sense by which pressure upon the surface of the body is perceived. **sixth s.,** cenesthesia. **space s.,** the sense by which relative positions and relations of objects in space are perceived. **special s.,** one of the five senses of seeing, feeling, hearing, taste, and smell. **stereognostic s.,** the sense by which form and solidity are perceived. **temperature s.,** the sense by which differences of temperature are appreciated.

sensibility (sen″sĭ-bil′ĭ-te) susceptibility of feeling; ability to feel or perceive. **deep s.,** the sensibility of deep tissue (muscle, tendon, etc.) to pressure, pain, and movement. **epicritic s.,** the sensibility to gentle stimulations permitting fine discriminations of touch and temperature, localized in the skin. **proprioceptive s.,** the sensibility afforded by receptors in muscles, joints, and other parts, by which one is made aware of their position and state. **protopathic s.,** sensibility to pain and temperature which is low in degree and poorly localized. **somesthetic s.,** proprioceptive s. **splanchnesthetic s.,** the sensibility to stimuli received by the splanchnic receptors.

sensible (sen′sĭ-b'l) capable of sensation; perceptible to the senses.

sensitive (sen′sĭ-tiv) 1. able to receive or respond to stimuli. 2. unusually responsive to stimulation, or responding quickly and acutely.

sensitivity (sen″sĭ-tiv′ĭ-te) the state or quality of being sensitive.

sensitization (sen″sĭ-ti-za′shun) 1. the initial exposure of an individual to a specific antigen, resulting in an immune response, subsequent exposure then inducing a much stronger immune response; said especially of such exposure resulting in a hypersensitivity reaction. 2. the coating of cells with antibody as a preparatory step in eliciting an immune reaction. 3. the preparation of a tissue or organ by one hormone so that it will respond functionally to the action of another. **active s.,** that resulting from the injection of antigen into an animal. **autoerythrocyte s.,** see under *syndrome.* **passive s.,** that which results when blood serum containing specific antibodies or immune lymphoid cells from a sensitized animal is injected into a normal animal. **protein s.,** that bodily state in which the individual is sensitive or hypersusceptible to some foreign protein.

sensitized (sen′sĭ-tīzd) rendered sensitive.

sensomobile (sen″so-mo′bil) moving in response to a stimulus.

sensomotor (-mo′tor) sensorimotor.

sensorial (sen-so′re-al) pertaining to the sensorium.

sensorimotor (sen″so-re-mo′tor) both sensory and motor.

sensorineural (-nu′ral) of or pertaining to a sensory nerve or mechanism; see also under *deafness.*

sensorium (sen-so′re-um) 1. the part of the cerebral cortex that receives and coordinates all the impulses sent to individual nerve centers. 2. the state of an individual as regards consciousness or mental awareness.

sensory (sen′so-re) pertaining to sensation.

sentient (sen′she-ent) able to feel; sensitive.

sepsis (sep′sis) the presence in the blood or other tissues of pathogenic microorganisms or their toxins; the condition associated with such presence. **puerperal s.,** that occurring after childbirth, due to matter absorbed from the birth canal; see also *puerperal fever.*

septa (sep′tah) plural of *septum.*

septal (sep′tal) pertaining to a septum.

septan (sep′tan) recurring every seventh day, as a fever.

septate (sep′tāt) divided by a septum.

septectomy (sep-tek′to-me) excision of part of the nasal septum.

septic (sep′tik) pertaining to sepsis.

septicemia (sep″tĭ-se′me-ah) blood poisoning; systemic disease associated with the presence and persistence of pathogenic microorganisms or their toxins in the blood. **septice′mic,** adj. **cryptogenic s.,** septicemia in which the focus of infection is not evident during life. **fowl s.,** a disease of fowl resembling fowl cholera, due to *Vibrio metchnikovii,* with diarrhea, hyperemia of the alimentary canal, and the presence of a blood-tinged, yellowish liquid in the small intestine. **hemorrhagic s.,** any of a group of animal diseases due to *Pasteurella multocida,* marked by hemorrhagic areas in various body organs and tissues. **puerperal s.,** see under *fever.*

septicophlebitis (sep″tĭ-ko-flĕ-bi′tis) septicemic inflammation of veins.

septicopyemia (-pi-e′me-ah) septicemia and pyemia combined. **septicopye′mic,** adj.

septipara (sep-tip′ah-rah) a woman who has had seven pregnancies which resulted in living offspring; para VII.

septivalent (sep″tĭ-va′lent) having a valence of seven.

septomarginal (sep″to-mar′jin-al) pertaining to the margin of a septum.

septonasal (-na′zal) pertaining to the nasal septum.

septotomy (sep-tot′o-me) incision of the nasal septum.

septulum (sep′tu-lum), pl. *sep′tula* [L.] a small separating wall or partition.

septum (sep′tum), pl. *sep′ta* [L.] a dividing wall or partition. **atrioventricular s.,** the part of the membranous portion of the interventricular septum between the left ventricle and the right atrium. **Bigelow's s.,** a layer of hard, bony tissue in the neck of the femur. **s. of Cloquet, crural s., femoral s.,** the thin fibrous membrane that helps close the femoral ring. **gingival s.,** the part of the gingiva interposed between adjoining teeth. **interalveolar s.,** one of the thin plates of bone separating the alveoli of the different teeth in the mandible and maxilla. **interatrial s.,** the partition separating the right and left atria of the heart. **interdental s.,** interalveolar s. **interventricular s.,** the partition separating the right and left ventricles of the heart. **s. lu′cidum,** pellucid s. **nasal s.,** the partition between the two nasal cavities. **s. pectinifor′me,** s. of penis. **pellucid s.,** the triangular double membrane separating the anterior horns of the lateral ventricles of the brain. **s. of penis,** the fibrous sheet between the corpora cavernosa of the penis. **rectovaginal s.,** the membranous partition between the rectum and vagina. **rectovesical s.,** a membranous partition separating the rectum from the prostate and urinary bladder. **s. of scrotum, s. scro′ti,** the partition between the two chambers of the scrotum.

septuplet (sep′tu-plet) one of seven offspring produced at one birth.

sequel (se′kwel) sequela.

sequela (se-kew′lah), pl. *seque′lae* [L.] a morbid condition following or occurring as a consequence of another condition or event.

sequester (se-kwes′ter) to detach or separate abnormally a small portion from the whole. See *sequestration* and *sequestrum.*

sequestration (se″kwes-tra′shun) 1. the formation of a sequestrum. 2. the isolation of a patient. 3. a net increase in the quantity of blood within a limited vascular area, occurring physiologically, with forward flow persisting or not, or produced artifically by the application of tourniquets. **pulmonary s.,** loss of connection of lung tissue with the bronchial tree and the pulmonary veins.

sequestrectomy (-trek′to-me) excision of a sequestrum.

sequestrum (se-kwes′trum), pl. *seques′tra* [L.] a piece of dead bone separated from the sound bone in necrosis.

sera (se′rah) plural of *serum.*

seralbumin (sēr″al-bu′min) serum albumin.

Serenium (sĕ-re′ne-um) trademark for a preparation of ethoxazene.

Serfin (ser′fin) trademark for a preparation of reserpine.

series (se′rēz) a group or succession of events, objects, or substances arranged in regular order or forming a kind of chain; in electricity, parts of a circuit connected successively end to end to form a single path for the current. **se′rial,** adj. **aliphatic s.,** the open chain or fatty series of chemical compounds. **aromatic s.,** the compounds derived from benzene. **erythrocytic s.,** the succession of developing cells which ultimately culminate in mature erythrocytes. **fatty s.,** methane and its derivatives and the homologous hydrocarbons. **granulocytic s.,** the succession of developing cells that ultimately culminate in mature granulocytes.

homologous s., a series of compounds each member of which differs from the one preceding it by the radical CH₂. **lymphocytic s.,** the succession of developing cells that ultimately culminate in mature lymphocytes. **monocytic s.,** the succession of developing cells that ultimately culminate in mature monocytes. **thrombocytic s.,** the succession of developing cells that ultimately culminate in mature blood platelets (thrombocytes).

serine (ser′ēn) a naturally occurring amino acid, C₃H₇NO₃, present in many proteins.

serocolitis (se″ro-ko-li′tis) inflammation of the serous coat of the colon.

seroconversion (-con-ver′zhun) the development of antibodies in response to administration of a vaccine.

seroculture (-kul′tūr) a bacterial culture on blood serum.

serodiagnosis (-di″ag-no′sis) diagnosis of disease based on serum reactions.

seroenteritis (-en″tĕ-ri′tis) inflammation of the serous coat of the intestine.

serofibrinous (-fi′bri-nus) composed of serum and fibrin, as a serofibrinous exudate.

seroflocculation (-flok″u-la′shun) flocculation produced in blood serum by an antigen.

seroimmunity (-ĭ-mu′nĭ-te) immunity produced by an antiserum; passive immunity.

serolipase (-li′pās) a lipase from blood serum.

serologist (se-rol′o-jist) a specialist in serology.

serology (se-rol′o-je) the study of antigen-antibody reactions *in vitro.* **serolog′ic,** adj.

serolysin (se-rol′ĭ-sin) a lysin of the blood serum.

seroma (se-ro′mah) a tumor-like collection of serosanguineous fluid in the tissues.

seromembranous (se″ro-mem′brah-nus) pertaining to or composed of serous membrane.

seromucous (-mu′kus) both serous and mucous.

seromuscular (-mus′ku-lar) pertaining to the serous and muscular coats of the intestine.

Seromycin (ser′o-mi″sin) trademark for preparations of cycloserine.

seronegative (se″ro-neg′ah-tiv) showing a negative serum reaction.

seropositive (-poz′ĭ-tiv) showing positive results on serologic examination.

seroprognosis (-prog-no′sis) prognosis of disease based on seroreactions.

seropurulent (-pu′roo-lent) both serous and purulent.

seropus (-pus′) serum mingled with pus.

seroreaction (-re-ak′shun) a reaction occurring in serum or as a result of the action of a serum.

seroresistant (-re-zis′tant) showing a seropositive reaction to a pathogen after treatment.

serosa (se-ro′sah, se-ro′zah) 1. any serous membrane (tunica serosa). 2. the chorion. **sero′sal,** adj.

serosamucin (se-ro″sah-mu′sin) a protein from inflammatory serous exudates.

serosanguineous (se″ro-sang-gwin′e-us) composed of serum and blood.

seroserous (-se′rus) pertaining to two or more serous membranes.

serositis (-si′tis) inflammation of a serous membrane.

serosity (se-ros′ĭ-te) the quality of serous fluids.

serosynovitis (se″ro-sin″o-vi′tis) synovitis with effusion of serum.

serotherapy (-ther′ah-pe) treatment of infectious disease by injection of antiserum.

serotonergic (-tōn-er′jik) containing or activated by serotonin.

serotonin (-to′nin) a vasoconstrictor present in blood, central nervous system, and other tissues. Produced enzymatically from tryptophan, it also stimulates smooth muscle and serves as a central neurotransmitter.

serotype (se′ro-tīp) the type of a microorganism determined by its constituent antigens; a taxonomic subdivision based thereon.

serous (se′rus) 1. pertaining to or resembling serum. 2. producing or containing serum.

serovaccination (se″ro-vak″sĭ-na′shun) injection of serum combined with bacterial vaccination to produce passive immunity by the former and active immunity by the latter.

Serpasil (ser″pah-sil) trademark for preparations of reserpine.

serpiginous (ser-pij′ĭ-nus) creeping; having a wavy or much indented border.

serrated (ser′āt-ed) having a sawlike edge.

Serratia (sĕ-ra′she-ah) a genus of bacteria (tribe Serratieae) made up of gram-negative rods which produce a red pigment. For the most part, they are free-living saprophytes, but have been found in association with pathological processes.

Serratieae (ser″ah-ti′e-e) a tribe of bacteria (order Eubacteriales, family Enterobacteriaceae) saprophytic on decaying plant or animal materials.

serration (sĕ-ra′shun) 1. the state of being serrated. 2. a serrated structure or formation.

serum (se′rum), pl. *se′ra, serums* [L.] 1. the clear portion of any liquid separated from its more solid elements; see *blood serum,* under B. 2. blood serum from animals inoculated with bacteria or their toxin which, when introduced into the body, produces passive immunization by virtue of its antibody content. **antilymphocyte s.,** serum from animals immunized with lymphocytes from a different species; a powerful immunosuppressive agent. **blood s.,** see under B. **foreign s.,** serum from an animal to be injected into one of another species. **immune s.,** serum from an immunized individual, containing specific antibody or antibodies. **muscle s.,** muscle plasma deprived of myosin. **polyvalent s.,** antiserum containing antibody to more than one kind of antigen. **pooled s.,** the mixed serum from a number of individuals.

serumal (se-roo′mal) pertaining to or formed from serum.

serum-fast (se′rum-fast) resistant to the effects of serum.

sesamoid (ses′ah-moid) 1. denoting a small nodular bone embedded in a tendon or joint capsule. 2. a sesamoid bone.

sesamoiditis (ses″ah-moi-di′tis) inflammation of the sesamoid bones of a horse's foot.

sesqui- word element [L.], *one and one-half.*

sesquioxide (ses″kwe-ok′sīd) a compound of three parts of oxygen with two of another element.

sessile (ses′il) attached by a broad base, as opposed to being pedunculated or stalked.

setaceous (se-ta′shus) bristle-like.

Setaria (se-ta′re-ah) a genus of filarial nematodes.

sex (seks) 1. a distinctive character of most animals and plants, based on the type of gametes produced by the gonads, ova (macrogametes) being typical of the female, and sperm (microgametes) of the male, or the category in which the individual is placed on such basis. 2. to determine the sex of an organism. **chromosomal s.,** sex as determined by the presence of the XX (female) or the XY (male) genotype in somatic cells, without regard to phenotypic manifestations. **gonadal s.,** the sex as determined on the basis of gonadal tissue present (ovarian or testicular). **morphologic s.,** that determined on the basis of the external genital organs. **nuclear s.,** that determined on the basis of the presence or absence of sex chromatin in somatic cells, its presence normally indicating the XX (female) genotype. **psychological s.,** the self-image of the gender role of an individual.

sexduction (seks-duk′shun) the process whereby part of the bacterial chromosome is attached to the autonomous F (sex) factor and thus is transferred from donor (male) bacterium to recipient (female).

sex-limited (-lim′ĭ-ted) affecting individuals of one sex only.

sex-linked (-linkt′) transmitted by a gene located on the X chromosome.

sexology (sek-sol′o-je) the scientific study of sex and sexual relations.

sextan (seks′tan) recurring in six-day cycles (every five days); said of fevers.

sextigravida (seks″tĭ-grav′ĭ-dah) a woman pregnant for the sixth time; gravida VI.

sextipara (seks-tip′ah-rah) a woman who has had six pregnancies that resulted in viable offspring; para VI.

sextuplet (seks′tu-plet) any one of six offspring produced at the same birth.

sexual (seks′u-al) pertaining to sex.

sexuality (seks″u-al′ĭ-te) 1. the characteristic of the male and female reproductive elements. 2. the constitution of an individual in relation to sexual attitudes and behavior.

S.G.O. Surgeon-General's Office.

SGOT serum glutamic oxaloacetic transaminase.

SGPT serum glutamic pyruvic transaminase.

shadow-casting (shad″o-kast′ing) application of a coating of gold, chromium, or other metal to ultramicroscopic structures to increase their visibility under the microscope.

shaft (shaft) a long slender part, such as the portion of a long bone between the wider ends or extremities.

shank (shangk) a leg, or leglike part.

sheath (shēth) a tubular case or envelope. **arachnoid s.,** the delicate membrane between the pial and dural sheath of the optic nerve. **carotid s.,** a portion of the cervical fascia enclosing the carotid artery, the internal jugular vein, and the vagus nerve. **connective tissue s. of Key and Retzius,** the endoneurium, especially the delicate continuation about terminal branches of nerve fibers. **crural s.,** see under *fascia.* **dentinal s.,** the layer of tissue forming the wall of a dentinal tubule. **dural s.,** the external investment of the optic nerve. **femoral s.,** the investing fascia of the proximal portion of the femoral vessels. **Henle's s.,** connective tissue s. of Key and Retzius. **Hertwig's s.,** root s. (1). **lamellar s.,** the perineurium. **Mauthner's s.,** axolemma. **medullary s., myelin s.,** the sheath surrounding the axon of some (myelinated) nerve fibers, consisting of myelin alternating with the spirally wrapped neurolemma. **pial s.,** the innermost of the three sheaths of the optic nerve. **root s.,** 1. an investment of epithelial cells around the unerupted tooth and inside the dental follicle. 2. the epithelial portion of a hair follicle. **s. of Schwann,** neurilemma. **synovial s.,** synovial membrane lining the cavity of a bone through which a tendon moves.

sheep-pox (shēp-poks) a highly infectious, sometimes fatal, eruptive viral disease of sheep.

sheet (shēt) an oblong piece of cotton, linen, etc., for a bed covering. **draw s.,** one folded and placed under a patient's body so it may be removed with minimal disturbance to the patient.

shield (shēld) any protecting structure. **Buller's s.,** a watch glass fitted over the eye to guard it from infection. **embryonic s.,** the double-layered disk of the blastoderm from which the primary organ rudiments are formed. **nipple s.,** a device to protect the nipple of the mammary gland.

shift (shift) a change or deviation. **chloride s.,** the exchange of chloride (Cl) and bicarbonate (HCO_3^-) between plasma and the erythrocytes occurring whenever HCO_3^- is generated or decomposed within the erythrocytes. **Doppler s.,** the magnitude of frequency change due to the Doppler effect. **s. to the left,** a change in the blood picture, with a preponderance of young neutrophils. **s. to the right,** a change in the blood picture, with a preponderance of older neutrophils.

Shigella (shĭ-gel′ah) a genus of gram-negative bacteria (tribe Salmonelleae) which cause dysentery. They are separated into four groups, each group making up a species: (A) *S. dysente′riae,* (B) *S. flexne′ri,* (C) *S. boy′dii,* and (D) *S. son′nei.*

shigella (shĭ-gel′ah), pl. *shigel′lae.* An individual organism of the genus *Shigella.*

shigellosis (shĭ″gel-lo′sis) infection with *Shigella;* bacillary dysentery.

shin (shin) the prominent anterior edge of the tibia or the leg. **saber s.,** marked anterior convexity of the tibia, seen in congenital syphilis and in yaws.

shingles (shing'gelz) herpes zoster.

shiver (shiv'er) 1. a slight tremor. 2. to tremble slightly, as from cold.

shivering (-ing) 1. involuntary shaking of the body, as with cold. 2. a disease of horses, with trembling or quivering of various muscles.

shock (shok) 1. a sudden disturbance of mental equilibrium. 2. acute peripheral circulatory failure due to derangement of circulatory control or loss of circulating fluid, marked by hypotension, coldness of skin, usually tachycardia, and often anxiety; see also under *therapy*. **allergic s., anaphylactic s.,** a violent attack of symptoms produced by a second injection of serum or protein and due to anaphylaxis. **electric s.,** shock produced by the passage of an electric current through the body. **insulin s.,** circulatory insufficiency resulting from overdosage with insulin, which causes too sudden reduction of blood sugar; marked by tremor, sweating, vertigo, diplopia, convulsions, and collapse. **irreversible s.,** a condition in which the changes produced cannot be corrected by treatment, and death is inevitable. **serum s.,** see *allergic s.* and see under *sickness*. **spinal s.,** the loss of spinal reflexes after injury of the spinal cord, which affects the muscles innervated by the cord segments situated below the site of the lesion.

shoulder (shōl'der) the junction of clavicle and scapula, where the arm joins the trunk. **frozen s.,** limited abduction and rotation of the arm, due to fibrositis.

shoulder-blade (-blād) scapula.

shoulder slip (-slip) inflammation and atrophy of the shoulder muscles and tendons in the horse.

show (sho) appearance of blood forerunning labor or menstruation.

shunt (shunt) 1. to turn to one side; to bypass. 2. a passage or anastomosis between two natural channels, especially between blood vessels, formed physiologically or anomalously. 3. a surgically created anastomosis; also, the operation of forming a shunt. **arteriovenous (A-V) s.,** the diversion of blood from an artery directly to a vein, bypassing the capillary network. **cardiovascular s.,** diversion of the blood flow through an anomalous opening from the left side of the heart to the right side or from the systemic to the pulmonary circulation (*left-to-right s.*), or from the right side to the left side or from the pulmonary to the systemic circulation (*right-to-left s.*). **left-to-right s.,** see *cardiovascular s.* **portacaval s.,** surgical anastomosis of the portal vein and the vena cava. **right-to-left s.,** see *cardiovascular s.*

SI Système International d'Unitès, or International System of Units. See *SI unit,* under *unit.*

Si chemical symbol, *silicon.*

sial(o)- word element [Gr.], *saliva; salivary glands.*

sialadenitis (si''al-ad''ĕ-ni'tis) inflammation of a salivary gland.

sialagogue (si-al'ah-gog) an agent which stimulates the flow of saliva. **sialagog'ic,** adj.

sialectasia (si''al-ek-ta'ze-ah) dilatation of a salivary duct.

sialine (si'ah-līn) pertaining to the saliva.

sialismus (si''ah-liz'mus) ptyalism.

sialitis (si''ah-li'tis) inflammation of a salivary gland or duct.

sialoadenectomy (si''ah-lo-ad''ĕ-nek'to-me) excision of a salivary gland.

sialoadenitis (-ad''ĕ-ni'tis) sialadenitis.

sialoadenotomy (-ad'ĕ-not'o-me) incision of a salivary gland.

sialoaerophagia (-a''er-o-fa'je-ah) the swallowing of saliva and air.

sialoangiectasis (-an''je-ek'tah-sis) sialectasia.

sialoangiitis (-an''je-i'tis) inflammation of a salivary duct.

sialoangiography (-an''je-og'rah-fe) radiography of the ducts of the salivary glands after injection of radiopaque material.

sialocele (si'ah-lo-sēl'') a salivary cyst.

sialodochitis (si''ah-lo-do-ki'tis) sialoangiitis.

sialodochoplasty (-do'ko-plas''te) plastic repair of a salivary duct.

sialoductitis (-duk-ti'tis) sialoangiitis.

sialogenous (si''ah-loj'ĕ-nus) producing saliva.

sialogogue (si-al'o-gog) sialagogue.

sialogram (-gram) a film produced by sialography.

sialography (si''ah-log'rah-fe) sialoangiography.

sialolith (si-al'o-lith) a salivary calculus.

sialolithiasis (si''ah-lo-lĭ-thi'ah-sis) the formation of salivary calculi.

sialolithotomy (-lĭ-thot'o-me) excision of a salivary calculus.

sialorrhea (-re'ah) ptyalism.

sialoschesis (si''ah-los'kĕ-sis) suppression of secretion of saliva.

sialosis (si''ah-lo'sis) 1. the flow of saliva. 2. ptyalism. **sialot'ic,** adj.

sialostenosis (si''ah-lo-ste-no'sis) stenosis of a salivary duct.

sialosyrinx (-si'rinks) 1. salivary fistula. 2. a syringe for washing out the salivary ducts, or a drainage tube for the salivary ducts.

sib (sib) 1. a blood relative; one of a group of persons all descended from a common ancestor. 2. sibling.

sibilant (sib'ĭ-lant) whistling or hissing.

sibling (sib'ling) any of two or more offspring of the same parents; a brother or sister.

sibship (-ship) relationship, especially between individuals born of the same parents.

siccative (sik'ah-tiv) 1. drying; removing moisture. 2. an agent which produces drying.

siccus (sik'us) [L.] dry.

sick (sik) 1. not in good health; afflicted by disease; ill. 2. nauseous.

sicklemia (sik-le'me-ah) sickle cell anemia.

sickling (sik'ling) the development of sickle cells in the blood.

sickness (sik'nes) any condition or episode marked by pronounced deviation from the normal healthy state. **African sleeping s.,** African trypanosomiasis. **air s.,** 1. motion sickness due to travel by airplane. 2. altitude s. **altitude s.,** a morbid condition due to diminished oxygen pressure at high altitudes. **car s.,** motion sickness due to automobile or other vehicular travel. **decompression s.,** joint pain, respiratory manifestations, skin lesions, and neurologic signs, due to rapid reduction of air pressure in a person's environment. **falling s.,** epilepsy. **milk s.,** 1. an acute, often fatal disease due to ingestion of milk, milk products, or flesh of cattle or sheep affected with trembles (q.v.), marked by weakness, anoxeria, vomiting, and sometimes muscular tremors. 2. trembles. **morning s.,** nausea of early pregnancy. **motion s.,** nausea and malaise due to unaccustomed motion, such as may be experienced in various modes of travel, as by airplane, automobile, ship, or train. **mountain s.,** oliguria, dyspnea, blood pressure and pulse rate changes, headache, and neurological disorders due to difficulty in adjusting to reduced oxygen pressure at high altitudes. **radiation s.,** malaise, nausea, vomiting, diarrhea, leukopenia, etc., sometimes produced by exposure to ionizing radiation. **serum s.,** a hypersensitivity reaction following a single, relatively large injection of foreign serum, with urticarial rashes, edema, adenitis, joint pains, high fever, and prostration. **sleeping s.,** increasing lethargy and drowsiness due to a protozoal infection, e.g., African trypanosomiasis, or by a viral infection, e.g., lethargic encephalitis.

side bone (sīd′bōn) a condition of horses marked by ossification of the lateral cartilages of the third phalanx of the foot.

side effect (-ef-fek″) a consequence other than that for which an agent is used, especially an adverse effect on another organ system.

sidero- word element [Gr.], *iron.*

sideroblast (sid′er-o-blast″) a nucleated erythrocyte containing iron granules in its cytoplasm.

siderocyte (-sīt″) an erythrocyte containing nonhemoglobin iron.

sideroderma (sid″er-o-der′mah) bronzed coloration of the skin due to disordered iron metabolism.

siderofibrosis (-fi-bro′sis) fibrosis associated with deposits of iron, as in the spleen. **siderofibrot′ic,** adj.

sideropenia (-pe′ne-ah) deficiency of iron in the body or blood. **siderope′nic,** adj.

siderophil (sid′er-o-fil) 1. siderophilous. 2. a siderophilous cell or tissue.

siderophilin (sid″er-of′ĭ-lin) transferrin.

siderophilous (sid″er-of′ĭ-lus) tending to absorb iron.

siderophore (sid′er-o-fōr″) a macrophage containing hemosiderin.

siderosis (sid″er-o′sis) 1. pneumoconiosis due to inhalation of iron particles. 2. excess of iron in the blood. 3. the deposit of iron in the tissues. **hepatic s.,** the deposit of an abnormal quantity of iron in the liver. **urinary s.,** the presence of hemosiderin granules in the urine.

sig. [L.] *sig′na* (mark).

sight (sīt) 1. the act or faculty of vision. 2. a thing seen. **far s.,** hyperopia. **near s.,** myopia. **night s.,** hemeralopia; day blindness. **second s.,** senopia.

sigmatism (sig′mah-tizm) faulty enunciation or too frequent use of the s sound.

sigmoid (sig′moid) 1. shaped like the letter C or S. 2. the sigmoid colon.

sigmoidectomy (sig″moi-dek′to-me) excision of part or all of the sigmoid colon.

sigmoiditis (sig″moi-di′tis) inflammation of the sigmoid colon.

sigmoidopexy (sig-moi′do-pek″se) fixation of the sigmoid colon, as for rectal prolapse.

sigmoidoproctostomy (sig-moi″do-prok-tos′to-me) surgical anastomosis of the sigmoid colon to the rectum.

sigmoidorectostomy (-rek-tos′to-me) sigmoidoproctostomy.

sigmoidoscope (sig-moi′do-skōp) an endoscope for use in sigmoidoscopy.

sigmoidoscopy (sig″moi-dos′ko-pe) direct examination of the interior of the sigmoid colon.

sigmoidosigmoidostomy (sig-moi″do-sig″moi-dos′to-me) surgical anastomosis of two portions of the sigmoid colon.

sigmoidostomy (sig″moi-dos′to-me) creation of an artificial opening from the sigmoid colon to the body surface.

sigmoidotomy (sig″moi-dot′o-me) incision of the sigmoid colon.

sigmoidovesical (sig-moi″do-ves″ĭ-kal) pertaining to or communicating with the sigmoid colon and the urinary bladder.

sign (sīn) an indication of the existence of something; any objective evidence of a disease, i.e., such evidence as is perceptible to the examining physician, as opposed to the subjective sensations (symptoms) of the patient. **Abadie's s.,** 1. spasm of the levator muscle of the upper lid in Graves' disease. 2. insensibility of the Achilles tendon to pressure in tabes dorsalis. **Babinski's s's,** 1. loss or lessening of the triceps surae jerk in organic sciatica. 2. in organic hemiplegia, failure of the platysma muscle to contract on the affected side in opening the mouth, whistling, etc. 3. see under *reflex.* 4. in organic hemiplegia, flexion of the thigh and lifting of the heel from the ground when the patient tries to sit up from a supine position with arms crossed upon his chest; this is repeated when the patient resumes the lying posture. 5. in organic paralysis, when the affected forearm is placed in supination, it turns over to pronation. **Babinski's toe s.,** Babinski's reflex. **Beevor's s.,** 1. in functional paralysis, inability to inhibit the antagonistic muscles. 2. in paralysis of the lower parts of the recti abdominis muscles, there is upward excursion of the umbilicus. **Biernacki's s.,** analgesia of the ulnar nerve in paralytic dementia and tabes dorsalis. **Blumberg's s.,** pain on abrupt release of steady pressure (rebound tenderness) over the site of a suspected abdominal lesion, indicative of peritonitis. **Branham's s.,** bradycardia produced by digital closure of an artery proximal to an arteriovenous fistula. **Braxton Hicks s.,** painless intermittent contractions of the uterus without cervical dilatation, after about the third month of pregnancy. **Broadbent's s.,** retraction on the left side of the back, near the eleventh and twelfth ribs, related to pericardial adhesion. **Brudzinski's s.,** 1. in meningitis, flexion of the neck usually causes flexion of the hip and knee. 2. in meningitis, on passive flexion of one lower limb, the contralateral limb shows a similar movement. **Cardarelli's s.,** transverse pulsation in the laryngotracheal tube in aneurysms and dilatation of the aortic arch. **Chaddock's s.,** see under *reflex*. **Chvostek's s., Chvostek-Weiss s.,** spasm of the facial muscles resulting from tapping the muscles or branches of the facial nerve; seen in tetany. **Cullen's s.,** bluish discoloration around the umbilicus sometimes associated with intraperitoneal hemorrhage, especially after rupture of the uterine tube in ectopic pregnancy; similar discoloration occurs in acute hemorrhagic pancreatitis. **Dalrymple's s.,** abnormal wideness of the palpebral opening in Graves' disease. **Delbet's s.,** in aneurysm of a limb's main artery, if nutrition of the part distal to the aneurysm is maintained, despite absence of the pulse, collateral circulation is sufficient. **de Musset's s.,** Musset's s. **Erb's s.,** 1. increased electric irritability of motor nerves in tetany. 2. dullness in percussion over the manubrium sterni in acromegaly. **Ewart's s.,** 1. undue prominence of the sternal end of the first rib in certain cases of pericardial effusion. 2. bronchial breathing and dullness on percussion at the lower angle of the left scapula in pericardial effusion. **fabere s.,** see *Patrick's test*. **Friedreich's s.,** 1. diastolic collapse of the cervical veins due to adhesion of the pericardium. 2. lowering of the pitch of the percussion note over an area of cavitation during forced inspiration. **Goodell's s.,** softening of the cervix and vagina; a sign of pregnancy. **Graefe's s.,** tardy or jerky downward movement of the upper eyelids when the gaze is directed downward; noted in thyrotoxicosis. **halo s.,** a halo effect produced in the roentgenogram of the fetal head between the subcutaneous fat and the cranium; said to be indicative of intrauterine death of the fetus. **harlequin s.,** reddening of the lower half of the laterally recumbent body and blanching of the upper half, due to temporary vasomotor disturbance in newborn infants. **Haudek's s.,** a projecting shadow in radiographs of penetrating gastric ulcer, due to settlement of bismuth in pathological niches of the stomach wall. **Hegar's s.,** softening of the lower uterine segment; indicative of pregnancy. **Hoffmann's s.,** 1. increased mechanical irritability of the sensory nerves in tetany; the ulnar nerve is usually tested. 2. a sudden nipping of the nail of the index, middle, or ring finger produces flexion of the terminal phalanx of the thumb and of the second and third phalanx of some other finger. **Homans' s.,** discomfort behind the knee on forced dorsiflexion of the foot, due to thrombosis in the calf veins. **Hoover's s.,** 1. in the normal state or in true paralysis, when the supine patient presses the leg against the surface on which he is lying, the other leg will lift. 2. movement of the costal

margins toward the midline in inspiration, occurring bilaterally in pulmonary emphysema and unilaterally in conditions causing flattening of the diaphragm. **Joffroy's s.,** in Graves' disease, absence of forehead wrinkling when the gaze is suddenly directed upward. **Kernig's s.,** in meningitis, inability to completely extend the leg when sitting or lying with the thigh flexed upon the abdomen; when supine, the leg can be easily and completely extended. **Klippel-Feil s.,** in pyramidal tract disease, flexion and adduction of the thumb when the flexed fingers are quickly extended by the examiner. **Ladin's s.,** softening of the medial anterior surface of the body of the uterus just above the junction of the body and cervix; indicative of pregnancy. **Lasègue's s.,** in sciatica, flexion of the hip is painful when the knee is extended, but painless when the knee is flexed. **Leri's s.,** absence of normal flexion of the elbow on passive flexion of the hand at the wrist of the affected side in hemiplegia. **Lhermitte's s.,** electric-like shocks spreading down the body on flexing the head forward; seen mainly in multiple sclerosis but also in compression and other cervical cord disorders. **Litten's s.,** see under *phenomenon*. **McBurney's s.,** tenderness at McBurney's point; indicative of appendicitis. **Macewen's s.,** a more than normal resonant note on percussion of the skull behind the junction of the frontal, temporal, and parietal bones in internal hydrocephalus and cerebral abscess. **McMurray's s.,** occurrence of a cartilage click on manipulation of the knee; indicative of menisceal injury. **Möbius' s.,** in Graves' disease, inability to keep the eyes converged due to insufficiency of the internal recti muscles. **Murphy's s.,** inability to take a deep breath when the physician's fingers are pressed deeply beneath the right costal arch, below the hepatic margin; a sign of gallbladder disease. **Musset's s.,** rhythmical jerking of the head in aortic aneurysm and aortic insufficiency. **Myerson's s.,** in Parkinson's disease, blepharospasm is readily induced on tapping the frontalis muscle. **Nikolsky's s.,** in pemphigus vulgaris and some other bullous diseases, the outer epidermis separates easily from the basal layer on exertion of firm sliding manual pressure. **obturator s.,** pain on outward pressure on the obturator foramen as a sign of inflammation in the sheath of the obturator nerve; probably due to appendicitis. **Oliver's s.,** tracheal tugging; see *tugging*. **Oppenheim's s.,** in pryamidal tract disease, dorsiflexion of the big toe on stroking downward the medial side of the tibia. **Piskacek's s.,** asymmetrical enlargement of the uterus; indicative of pregnancy. **Queckenstedt's s.,** when the veins in the neck are compressed on one or both sides, there is a rapid rise in the pressure of the cerebrospinal fluid of healthy persons, and this rise quickly disappears when compression ceases. In obstruction of the vertebral canal, the pressure of the cerebrospinal fluid is little or not at all affected. **Romberg's s.,** swaying of the body or falling when the eyes are closed while standing with the feet close together; observed in tabes dorsalis. **Rossolimo's s.,** see under *reflex*. **setting-sun s.,** downward deviation of the eyes so that each iris appears to "set" beneath the lower lid, with white sclera exposed between it and the upper lid; indicative of intracranial pressure or irritation of the brain stem. **Stellwag's s.,** infrequent or incomplete blinking, a sign of Graves' disease. **Tinel's s.,** a tingling sensation in the distal end of a limb when percussion is made over the site of a divided nerve. It indicates a partial lesion or the beginning regeneration of the nerve. **Troisier's s.,** in intra-abdominal malignancy or retrosternal tumor, enlargement of the lymph nodes about the clavicle. **Trousseau's s.,** 1. see under *phenomenon.* 2. tache cérébrale. **vital s's,** the pulse, respiration, and temperature. **Wartenberg's s.,** 1. in ulnar palsy, the little finger assumes a position of abduction. 2. in cerebellar disease, reduction or absence of pendulum movements of the arm while walking.

signa (sig′nah) [L.] mark, or write; abbreviated S. or sig. in prescriptions.

signature (-chur) that part of a prescription which gives directions as to the taking of the medicine.

Silastic (sĭ-las′tik) trademark for polymeric silicone substances having the properties of rubber; it is biologically inert and used in surgical prostheses.

silica (sil′ĭ-kah) silicon dioxide, SiO_2, occurring in various allotropic forms, some of which are used in dental materials.

silicate (sil′ĭ-kāt) a salt of any of the silicic acids.

silicatosis (sil″ĭ-kah-to′sis) pneumoconiosis due to inhalation of silicate dust.

silicoanthracosis (sil″ĭ-ko-an″thrah-ko′sis) silicosis combined with pneumoconiosis of coal workers.

silicon (sil′ĭ-kon) chemical element (*see table*), at. no. 14, symbol Si. **s. carbide,** a compound of silicon and carbon used in dentistry as an abrasive agent. **s. dioxide,** silica.

silicone (sil′ĭ-kōn) any organic compound in which all or part of the carbon has been replaced by silicon.

silicosiderosis (sil″ĭ-ko-sid″er-o′sis) pneumoconiosis in which the inhaled dust is that of silica and iron.

silicosis (sil″ĭ-ko′sis) pneumoconiosis due to inhalation of the dust of stone, sand, or flint containing silica, with formation of generalized nodular fibrotic changes in both lungs. **silicot′ic,** adj.

Silicote (sil′ĭ-kōt) trademark for preparations of dimethicone.

silicotuberculosis (sil″ĭ-ko-tu-ber″ku-lo′sis) tuberculous infection of the silicotic lung.

siliquose (sil′ĭ-kwōs) pertaining to or resembling a pod or husk.

silver (sil′ver) chemical element (*see table*), at. no. 47, symbol Ag. **colloidal s.,** a silver preparation in which the silver exists as free ions to only a small extent. **s. iodide,** AgI, used in treatment of syphilis, nervous diseases, and conjunctivitis. **s. nitrate,** $AgNO_3$, used as a local anti-infective, as in the prophylaxis of ophthalmia neonatorum. **s. nitrate, toughened,** a compound of silver nitrate, hydrochloric acid,

sodium chloride, or potassium nitrate; used as a caustic, applied topically after being dipped in water. **s. protein,** silver made colloidal by the presence of, or combination with, protein; an active germicide with a local irritant and astringent effect.

simethicone (sĭ-meth′ĭ-kōn) an antiflatulent substance consisting of a mixture of dimethyl polysiloxanes and silica gel.

simul (sim′ul) [L.] at the same time as.

simulation (sim″u-la′shun) 1. the act of counterfeiting a disease; malingering. 2. the mimicking of one disease by another.

Simulium (sĭ-mu′le-um) a genus of biting gnats; some species are intermediate hosts of *Onchocerca volvulus.*

Sinaxar (sin′ak-sar) trademark for a preparation of styramate.

sinciput (sin′sĭ-put) the upper and front part of the head. **sincip′ital,** adj.

sinew (sin′u) a tendon of a muscle. **weeping s.,** an encysted ganglion, chiefly on the back of the hand, containing synovial fluid.

Singoserp (sing′go-serp) trademark for preparations of syrosingopine.

singultus (sing-gul′tus) [L.] hiccup.

sinister (sin′is-ter) [L.] left; on the left side.

sinistr(o)- word element [L.], *left; left side.*

sinistrad (sin′is-trad) to or toward the left.

sinistral (sin′is-tral) 1. pertaining to the left side 2. a left-handed person.

sinistrality (sin″is-tral′ĭ-te) the preferential use, in voluntary motor acts, of the left member of the major paired organs of the body, as ear, eye, hand, and leg.

sinistraural (sin″is-traw′ral) hearing better with the left ear.

sinistrocardia (sin″is-tro-kar′de-ah) levocardia.

sinistrocerebral (-ser′ĕ-bral) pertaining to or situated in the left cerebral hemisphere.

sinistrocular (sin″is-trok′u-lar) having the left eye dominant.

sinistrogyration (sin″is-tro-ji-ra′shun) a turning to the left.

sinistromanual (-man′u-al) left-handed.

sinistropedal (sin″is-trop′ĕ-dal) using the left foot in preference to the right.

sinistrotorsion (sin″is-tro-tor′shun) a twisting toward the left, as of the eye.

sinoatrial (si″no-a′tre-al) pertaining to the sinus venosus and the atrium of the heart.

sinobronchitis (-brong-ki′tis) chronic paranasal sinusitis with recurrent episodes of bronchitis.

Sintrom (sin′trom) trademark for a preparation of acenocoumarol.

sinuitis (sin″u-i′tis) sinusitis.

sinuous (sin′u-us) bending in and out; winding.

sinus (si′nus) 1. a recess, cavity, or channel, as (*a*) one in bone or (*b*) a dilated channel for venous blood. 2. an abnormal channel or fistula, permitting escape of pus. **si′nusal,** adj. **air s.,** an air-containing space within a bone. **anal s's,** furrows with pouchlike openings at the distal end, separating the rectal columns. **aortic s's,** a dilatation between the aortic wall and each of the semilunar cusps of the aortic valve. **carotid s.,** a dilatation of the proximal portion of the internal carotid or distal portion of the common carotid artery, containing in its wall pressore-ceptors which are stimulated by changes in blood pressure. **cavernous s.,** an irregularly shaped venous channel between the layers of dura mater of the brain, one on either side of the body of the sphenoid bone and communicating across the midline; it contains the internal carotid artery and abducent nerve. **cerebral s.,** one of the ventricles of the brain. **cervical s.,** a temporary depression caudal to the embryonic hyoid arch, containing the succeeding branchial arches; it is overgrown by the hyoid arch and closes off as the cervical vesicle. **circular s.,** the venous channel encircling the hypophysis, formed by the two cavernous sinuses and the anterior and posterior intercavernous sinuses. **coccygeal s.,** a sinus or fistula just over or close to the tip of the coccyx. **coronary s.,** the terminal portion of the great cardiac vein, lying in the coronary sulcus between the left atrium and ventricle, and emptying into the right atrium. **dermal s.,** a congenital sinus tract extending from the surface of the body, between the bodies of two adjacent lumbar vertebrae, to the spinal canal. **ethmoidal s.,** that paranasal sinus consisting of the ethmoidal cells collectively, and communicating with the nasal meatuses. See Plate XVI. **frontal s.,** one of the paired paranasal sinuses in the frontal bone, each communicating with the middle meatus of the ipsilateral nasal cavity. See Plate XVI. **intercavernous s's,** channels connecting the two cavernous sinuses, one passing anterior and the other posterior to the infundibulum of the hypophysis. **lacteal s's, lactiferous s's,** enlargements of the lactiferous ducts just before they open on the mammary papilla. **lymphatic s's,** irregular, tortuous spaces within lymphoid tissue (nodes) through which lymph passes, to enter efferent lymphatic vessels. **marginal s.,** a venous channel near the edge of the placenta. **maxillary s.,** one of the paired paranasal sinuses in the body of the maxilla on either side, and opening into the middle meatus of the ipsilateral nasal cavity. See Plate XVI. **occipital s.,** a venous sinus between the layers of dura mater, passing upward along the midline of the cerebellum. **oral s.,** stomodeum. **paranasal s's,** mucosa-lined air cavities in bones of the skull, communicating with the nasal cavity and including ethmoidal, frontal, maxillary, and sphenoidal sinuses. See Plate XVI. **petrosal s., inferior,** a venous channel arising from the cavernous sinus and draining into the internal jugular vein. **petrosal s., superior,** one arising from the cavernous sinus and draining into the transverse sinus. **pilonidal s.,** a suppurating sinus containing hair, occurring chiefly in the coccygeal region. **s. pocula'ris,** prostatic utricle. **prostatic s.,** the posterolateral recess between the seminal colliculus and the wall of the urethra. **s's of pulmonary trunk,** slight dilatations in the wall of the pulmonary trunk just above the pulmonary valve. **renal s.,** a recess in the substance of the kidney, occupied by the renal pelvis, calices, vessels, nerves, and fat.

sagittal s., inferior, a small venous sinus of the dura mater, opening into the straight sinus. **sagittal s., superior,** a venous sinus of the dura mater which ends in the confluence of sinuses. **sigmoid s.,** a venous sinus of the dura mater on either side, continuous with the straight sinus and draining into the internal jugular vein of the same side. **sphenoidal s.,** one of the paired paranasal sinuses in the body of the sphenoid bone and opening into the highest meatus of the ipsilateral nasal cavity. See Plate XVI. **sphenoparietal s.,** a venous sinus of the dura mater, draining into the anterior part of the cavernous sinus. **s's of spleen,** dilated venous channels in the substance of the spleen. **straight s.,** a venous sinus of the dura mater formed by junction of the great cerebral vein and inferior sagittal sinus, commonly ending in the confluence of sinuses. **tarsal s.,** a space between the calcaneus and talus. **tentorial s.,** straight s. **terminal s.,** a vein which encircles the vascular area in the blastoderm. **transverse s.,** 1. either of two large venous sinuses of the dura mater. 2. a passage behind the aorta and pulmonary trunk and in front of the atria. **tympanic s.,** a deep recess on the medial wall of the tympanic cavity. **urogenital s.,** an elongated sac formed by division of the cloaca in the early embryo, forming the female vestibule and most of the male urethra. **uterine s's,** venous channels in the wall of the uterus in pregnancy. **uteroplacental s's,** blood spaces between the placenta and uterine sinuses. **s. of venae cavae,** the portion of the right atrium into which the inferior and the superior vena cava open. **venous s., s. veno'sus,** 1. the common venous receptacle in the embryonic midheart, attached to the posterior wall of the primitive atrium. 2. s. of venae cavae. **venous s's of dura mater,** large channels for venous blood forming an anastomosing system between the layers of the dura mater of the brain, receiving blood from the brain and draining into the veins of the scalp or deep veins at the base of the skull. **venous s. of sclera,** a branching, circumferential vessel in the internal scleral sulcus, a major component of the drainage pathway for aqueous humor.

sinusitis (si″nu-si′tis) inflammation of a sinus.

sinusoid (si′nu-soid) 1. resembling a sinus. 2. a form of terminal blood channel consisting of a large, irregular anastomosing vessel having a lining of reticuloendothelium and found in the liver, heart, spleen, pancreas, and the adrenal, parathyroid, carotid, and hemolymph glands.

sinusotomy (si″nu-sot′o-me) incision of a sinus.

siphon (si′fon) a bent tube with two arms of unequal length, used to transfer liquids from a higher to a lower level by the force of atmospheric pressure.

siphonage (si′fon-ij) the use of the siphon, as in gastric lavage or in draining the bladder.

sirenomelus (si″ren-om′ĕ-lus) a fetus with fused legs and no feet.

-sis word element [Gr.], *state; condition.*

sister (sis′ter) the nurse in charge of a hospital ward (Great Britain).

site (sīt) a place, position, or locus. **allosteric s.,** that subunit of an enzyme molecule which binds with a nonsubstrate molecule, inducing a conformational change that results in inactivation of the enzyme for its substrate.

sitology (sit″e-ol′o-je, si-tol′o-je) dietetics.

sito- word element [Gr.], *food.*

sitomania (si″to-ma′ne-ah) 1. excessive hunger, or morbid craving for food. 2. periodic bulimia.

sitosterol (si-tos′ter-ol) any of a group of closely related plant sterols, designated by Greek letters and sometimes by subscript numerals, e.g., α_1, β, γ, on the basis of differing characteristics; a preparation of β-sitosterol and related sterols of plant origin (called *sitosterols*) is used as an anticholesterolemic agent.

sitotherapy (si″to-ther′ah-pe) dietetic treatment.

sitotropism (si-tot′ro-pizm) response of living cells to the presence of nutritive elements.

situs (si′tus), pl. *si′tus* [L.] site or position. **s. inver′sus vis′cerum,** lateral transposition of the viscera of the thorax and abdomen. **s. transver′sus,** s. inversus viscerum.

SK streptokinase.

skatole (skat′ōl) a strong-smelling crystalline amine from human feces, produced by protein decomposition in the intestine and directly from tryptophan by decarboxylation.

skatoxyl (skah-tok′sil) oxidation product of skatole found in urine in certain diseases of the large intestine.

skein (skān) spireme.

skelalgia (ske-lal′je-ah) pain in the leg.

skeletization (skel″ĕ-te-za′shun) 1. extreme emaciation. 2. removal of soft parts from the skeleton.

skeletogenous (skel″ĕ-toj′ĕ-nus) producing skeletal structures or tissues.

skeleton (skel′ĕ-ton) the hard framework of the animal body, especially that of higher vertebrates; the bones of the body collectively. See Plate II. **skel′etal,** adj. **appendicular s.,** the bones of the limbs and supporting thoracic (pectoral) and pelvic girdles. **axial s.,** the bones of the body axis, including the skull, vertebral column, ribs, and sternum.

skenitis (ske-ni′tis) inflammation of the paraurethral ducts (Skene's glands).

skeocytosis (ske″o-si-to′sis) shift to the left.

skeptophylaxis (skep″to-fi-lak′sis) 1. a condition in which a minute dose of a substance poisonous to animals will produce immediate temporary immunity to the action of the poison, although the blood of the animal may be highly toxic during that period of immunity. 2. the method of allergic desensitization by the preliminary injection of a small amount of the allergen, as is commonly done before the injection of an antiserum.

skia- word element [Gr.], *shadow* (especially as produced by roentgen rays).

skiameter (ski-am′ĕ-ter) an instrument for measuring intensity of roentgen rays.

skiametry (ski-am′ĕ-tre) retinoscopy.

skiascope (ski′ah-skōp) retinoscopy.

skiascopy (ski-as′ko-pe) 1. retinoscopy. 2. fluoroscopy.

skin (skin) the outer protective covering of the body, consisting of the corium (or dermis) and the epidermis. **alligator s.,** ichthyosis sauroderma. **elastic s.,** Ehlers-Danlos syndrome. **false s.,** epidermis. **farmer's s.,** sailor's s. **lax s.,** cutis laxa. **marble s.,** cutis marmorata. **sailor's s.,** elastosis, atrophy, telangiectasis, and actinic keratosis of the skin, seen especially in fair-skinned persons, due to excessive exposure to the sun. **true s.,** corium.

Skiodan (ski′o-dan) trademark for a preparation of methiodal.

skler(o)- for words beginning thus; see those beginning *scler(o)-.*

skot(o)- for words beginning thus, see those beginning *scot(o)-.*

skull (skul) the cranium; the bony framework of the head, composed of the cranial and facial bones. See *Table of Bones.* **steeple s., tower s.,** oxycephaly.

S.L.E. systemic lupus erythematosus.

sleep (slēp) a period of rest for the body and mind, during which volition and consciousness are in partial or complete abeyance and bodily functions are partially suspended; also described as a behavioral state, with characteristic immobile posture and diminished but readily reversible sensitivity to external stimuli. **REM s.,** the stage of sleep in which dreaming is associated with mild involuntary muscle jerks and rapid eye movements (REM). **twilight s.,** analgesia and amnesia produced by injection of morphine and scopolamine; the patient responds to pain but does not retain it in memory.

sleepwalking (slēp′wok″ing) somnambulism (1).

slide (slīd) a piece of glass or other transparent substance on which material is placed for examination under the microscope.

sling (sling) a bandage or suspensory for supporting a part.

slough (sluf) 1. necrotic tissue in the process of separating from viable portions of the body. 2. to shed or cast off.

sludge (sluj) a suspension of solid or semisolid particles in a fluid which itself may or may not be a truly viscous fluid.

sludging (sluj′ing) settling out of solid particles from solution. **s. of blood,** intravascular agglutination.

Sm chemical symbol, *samarium.*

smallpox (smawl′poks) variola; an acute infectious disease due to a poxvirus, marked by sustained high fever and the appearance first of macules and later of papules on the skin, leaving small depressed, depigmented scars. **black s., hemorrhagic s.,** a form in which hemorrhage occurs into the lesions or from the mucous surfaces. **modified s.,** varioloid.

smear (smēr) a specimen for microscopic study prepared by spreading the material across the slide. **Pap s., Papanicolaou s.,** see under *tests.*

smegma (smeg′mah) the secretion of sebaceous glands, especially the cheesy secretion, consisting principally of desquamated epithelial cells, found chiefly beneath the prepuce. **smegmat′ic,** adj.

smog (smog) a mixture of smoke and fog.

Sn chemical symbol, *tin* (L. *stannum*).

snap (snap) a short, sharp sound. **opening s.,** a short, sharp sound in early diastole caused by movement of the mitral leaflet into the ventricle at the start of ventricular filling.

snare (snār) a wire loop for removing polyps and tumors by encircling them at the base and closing the loop.

sneeze (snēz) 1. to expel air forcibly and spasmodically through the nose and mouth. 2. an involuntary, sudden, violent, and audible expulsion of air through the mouth and nose.

snore (snōr) 1. rough, noisy breathing during sleep, due to vibration of the uvula and soft palate. 2. to produce such sounds during sleep.

snow (sno) a freezing or frozen mixture consisting of discrete particles or crystals. **carbon dioxide s.,** solid carbon dioxide formed by rapid evaporation of liquid carbon dioxide; it gives a temperature of about –110° F. (–79° C.), and is used as an escharotic in various skin diseases.

snowblindness (sno'blīnd-nes) see under *blindness*.

snuffles (snuf'elz) catarrhal discharge from the nasal mucous membrane in infants, generally in congenital syphilis.

soap (sōp) any compound of one or more fatty acids, or their equivalents, with an alkali. Soap is detergent and is much employed in liniments, enemas, and in making pills. It is also a mild aperient, antacid, and antiseptic. **green s.,** a potassium soap made by saponification of vegetable oils, excluding coconut oil and palm kernel oil, without the removal of glycerin; it is the chief ingredient of green soap tincture. **hard s.,** soda s. **soda s.,** soap made from soda and olive oil. **soft s.,** 1. a liquid soap made from potash and some oil. 2. green s. **soft s., medicinal,** green s.

sociologist (so"se-ol'o-jist) a specialist in sociology.

sociology (so"se-ol'o-je) the scientific study of social relationships and phenomena.

sociometry (so"se-om'ĕ-tre) the branch of sociology concerned with the measurement of human social behavior.

sociopath (so'se-o-path") a person with an antisocial personality; a psychopath. **sociopath'ic,** adj.

socket (sok'et) a hollow into which a corresponding part fits. **dry s.,** a condition sometimes occurring after tooth extraction, with exposure of bone, inflammation of an alveolar crypt, and severe pain. **tooth s's,** the dental alveoli.

soda (so'dah) a term loosely applied to sodium bicarbonate, sodium hydroxide, or sodium carbonate. **baking s.,** sodium bicarbonate. **caustic s.,** sodium hydroxide. **s. lime,** calcium hydroxide with sodium or potassium hydroxide, or both; used as adsorbent of carbon dioxide in equipment for metabolism tests, inhalant anesthesia, or oxygen therapy. **washing s.,** sodium carbonate.

sodium (so'de-um) chemical element (*see table*), at. no. 11, symbol Na; the chief cation of extracellular body fluids. For sodium salts not listed here, see under the acid or the active ingredient. **s. acetate,** a systemic and urinary alkalizer. **s. acid phosphate,** s. biphosphate. **s. alginate,** a product derived from brown seaweeds, used in formulating various pharmaceutical preparations. **s. aminosalicylate,** an antibacterial compound used in tuberculosis. **s. antimonyl-thioglycollate,** an organic compound of antimony, used in leishmaniasis and schistosomiasis. **s. ascorbate,** an antiscorbutic vitamin for parenteral administration. **s. benzoate,** a white, odorless granular or crystalline powder, used as an antifungal agent and as a test of liver function. **s. bicarbonate,** $NaHCO_3$, used as a gastric and systemic antacid and to alkalinize urine; also used, in solution, for washing the nose, mouth, and vagina, as a cleansing enema, and as a dressing for minor burns. **s. biphosphate,** the monohydrate salt of phosphoric acid, used as a urinary acidifier. **s. bisulfite,** a salt, $NaHSO_3$, used as an antioxidant in pharmaceuticals. **s. borate,** $Na_2B_4O_7$, used as an alkalizing agent in pharmaceuticals. **s. carbonate,** $Na_2CO_3 \cdot H_2O$, used as an alkalizing agent in pharmaceuticals, and has been used as a lotion or bath in the treatment of scaly skin and as a detergent. **s. carboxymethyl cellulose,** sodium salt of a carboxymethyl ether of cellulose, used as a suspending agent, bulk laxative, and gastric antacid. **s. chloride,** common salt, a white crystalline compound, a necessary constituent of the body and therefore of the diet; sometimes used parenterally in solution to replenish electrolytes in the body. **s. citrate,** a crystalline compound, largely used as an anticoagulant in blood for transfusion. **s. fluoride,** NaF, used in the fluoridation of water or applied locally to the teeth, in 2% solution, to reduce the incidence of dental caries. **s. folate,** a compound used in various anemias and in control of diarrhea in sprue. **s. glutamate,** the monosodium salt of L-glutamic acid; used in treatment of encephalopathies associated with liver diseases. Also used to enhance the flavor of foods. **s. hydrate, s. hydroxide,** a strongly alkaline and caustic compound, NaOH, used as an alkalinizing agent in pharmaceuticals. **s. iodide,** NaI, used as a source of iodine, and also as an expectorant. **s. iodipamide,** a water-soluble organic iodine compound used in roentgenography of the biliary tract. **s. iodohippurate,** a compound used as a contrast medium in roentgenography of the urinary tract. **s. lauryl sulfate,** a surface active agent, $CH_3(CH_2)_{10}CH_2OSONa$, used as a wetting agent, emulsifying aid, and detergent in various dermatologic and cosmetic preparations, and as a tooth paste ingredient. **s. nitrite,** a compound used as an antidote in cyanide poisoning. **s. perborate,** $NaBO_3 \cdot 4H_2O$, used as an oxidant and local anti-infective. **s. peroxide,** a white water-soluble powder, Na_2O_2, which liberates oxygen. **s. phosphate,** a cathartic, $Na_2HPO_4 \cdot 7H_2O$. **s. polystyrene sulfonate,** an ion-exchange resin used for treatment of hyperpotassemia. **s. propionate,** a compound used in fungal infections. **s. salicylate,** an analgesic compound. **s. sulfate,** a hydrogogue cathartic, $Na_2SO_4 \cdot 10H_2O$; also used as a diuretic and sometimes applied topically to wounds in solution to relieve edema and pain of infected wounds. **s. tetradecyl sulfate,** a sclerosing agent, C_{14}-$H_{29}NaSO_4$, used in solution for varicose veins that are not prolapsed or thrombosed. **s. thiosulfate,** a compound, $NaS_2O_3 \cdot 5H_2O$, used as an antidote (with s. nitrite) to cyanide poisoning, in the prophylaxis of ringworm (added to foot baths), and as a topical application in solution in tinea versicolor.

sodoku (so′do-koo) a relapsing form of rat-bite fever due to *Spirillum minus,* transmitted by the bite of an infected rat, with fever of sudden onset, delayed local inflammatory reaction at the site of the bite, lymphangitis, lymphadenitis, and rigors.

sodomist (sod′o-mist) one who practices sodomy.

sodomy (sod′o-me) anal intercourse; also used to denote bestiality and fellatio.

softening (sof′en-ing) the process of becoming soft; any morbid process of becoming soft, as of the brain or spinal cord. **red s.,** softening of a patch(es) of brain substance, with local redness due to congestion. **white s.,** the stage following yellow softening, in which the spot has become white from the presence of fatty deposit. **yellow s.,** the stage followng red softening, in which the patch has become yellow due to degenerative changes in the brain substance.

sol (sol) a liquid colloidal solution.

sol. solution.

Solanum (so-la′num) [L.] a genus of solanaceous plants, including the potato, tomato, egg plant, several of the nightshades, and many poisonous and medicinal species.

solar (so′lar) 1. pertaining to the sun. 2. denoting the great sympathetic plexus and its principal ganglia (especially the celiac); so called because of their radiating nerves.

solation (so-la′shun) the liquefaction of a gel.

sole (sōl) the bottom of the foot.

Solganal (sol′gah-nal) trademark for a preparation of aurothioglucose.

solid (sol′id) 1. not fluid or gaseous; not hollow. 2. a substance or tissue not fluid or gaseous.

solipsism (sōl′ip-sizm) the belief that the world exists only in the mind of the individual, or that it consists solely of the individual himself and his own experiences. **solipsis′tic,** adj.

soluble (sol′u-b′l) susceptible of being dissolved.

solubility (sol″u-bil′ĭ-te) quality of being soluble; susceptibility of being dissolved.

Solu-Cortef (sol″u-kor′tef) trademark for hydrocortisone sodium succinate.

solum (so′lum), pl. *so′la* [L.] the bottom or lowest part.

solute (sol′ūt) the substance dissolved in solvent to form a solution.

solution (so-loo′shun) 1. a homogeneous mixture of one or more substances (solutes) dispersed in a sufficient quantity of dissolving medium (solvent). 2. the process of dissolving. 3. a loosening or separation. **aluminum acetate s.,** a preparation of aluminum subacetate solution, glacial acetic acid, and water; applied topically to the skin as an astringent, and also used as a topical

antiseptic and antipruritic in various skin diseases. **aluminum subacetate s.,** a solution of aluminum sulfate, acetic acid, precipitated calcium carbonate, and water; applied topically to the skin as an astringent, and also as an antiseptic and a wet dressing. **ammonia s.,** a colorless, transparent liquid of alkaline reaction containing either 9–10 gm. of ammonia in each 100 ml. (*diluted ammonia s.*), or 20–30% of ammonia (*strong ammonia s.*); the former is a pharmaceutic necessity, the latter a solvent and source of ammonia. **ammoniacal silver nitrate s.,** a mixture of silver nitrate, purified water, and strong ammonia solution; used as a dental protective. **ammonium hydroxide s.,** ammonia s. **anisotonic s.,** one having an osmotic pressure differing from that of the standard of reference. **antiseptic s.,** a preparation of boric acid, thymol, chlorothymol, menthol, eucalyptol, methyl salicylate, thyme oil, and alcohol in purified water; used as an antibacterial. **aqueous s.,** one in which water is the solvent. **Benedict's s.,** a sodium citrate, sodium carbonate, and copper sulfate water solution; used to determine presence of glucose in urine. **buffer s.,** one which resists appreciable change in its hydrogen ion concentration when acid or alkali is added to it. **Burow's s.,** aluminum acetate s. **calcium hydroxide s.,** an aqueous solution of calcium hydroxide; used in preparation of various astringent solutions and lotions and as an antacid for infants. **carbol-fuchsin s.,** a mixture of basic fuchsin, phenol, resorcinol, acetone, and alcohol in purified water; used as an antifungal agent. **colloid s., colloidal s.,** a preparation consisting of minute particles of matter suspended in a solvent. **contrast s.,** a solution of a substance opaque to the roentgen ray, used to facilitate x-ray visualization of some organ or structure in the body. **cresol s., saponated,** a mixture of cresol, vegetable oil (excluding coconut and palm kernel oil), alcohol, potassium hydroxide, and purified water; used as a disinfectant. **Dakin's s.,** dilute sodium hypochlorite s. **Fehling's s.,** (1) 34.66 gm. cupric sulfate in water to make 500 ml.; (2) 173 gm. crystallized potassium and sodium tartrate and 50 gm. sodium hydroxide in water to make 500 ml.; mix equal volumes of (1) and (2) at time of use. **ferric subsulfate s.,** an aqueous solution of basic ferric sulfate, used as an astringent. **formaldehyde s.,** an aqueous solution containing not less than 37% formaldehyde; used as a disinfectant. **Fowler's s.,** potassium arsenite s. **gold** [198]**Au s.,** a sterile, pyrogen-free colloidal solution of radioactive gold ([198]Au); used by intracavitary or interstitial injection in the treatment of certain cancers. **hyperbaric s.,** one having a greater specific gravity than a standard of reference. **hypertonic s.,** one having an osmotic pressure greater than that of a standard of reference. **hypobaric s.,** one having a specific gravity less than that of a standard of reference. **hypotonic s.,** one having an osmotic pressure less than that of a standard of reference. **iodine s.,** a solution prepared with purified water, each 100 ml. containing 1.8–2.2 gm. of iodine and 2.1–2.6 gm. of sodium iodide; a local anti-infective. **iodine s., strong,** a solution containing, in each 100 ml., 4.5–5.5 gm. of iodine and 9.5–10.5 gm. of potassium iodide; a source of iodine. **isobaric s.,** a solution having the same specific gravity as a standard of reference. **isotonic s.,** one having an osmotic pressure the same as that of a standard of reference. **lead subacetate s.,** a solution of lead acetate and lead monoxide in distilled water; astringent and locally sedative. **Locke's s.,** a solution of sodium chloride, calcium chloride, potassium chloride, sodium bicarbonate, and dextrose; used in physiologic experiments to keep the mammalian heart beating. **Lugol's s.,** iodine solution, strong. **magnesium citrate s.,** a preparation of magnesium carbonate, anhydrous citric acid, with syrup, talc, lemon oil, and potassium bicarbonate in purified water; used as a cathartic. **molar s.,** a solution each liter of which contains 1 gram-molecule of the dissolved substance; designated M/1 or 1 M. The concentration of other solutions may be expressed in relation to that of molar solutions as tenth-molar (M/10 or 0.1 M), etc. **normal s.,** a solution each liter of which contains 1 gram equivalent weight of the dissolved substance; designated N/1 or 1 N. **ophthalmic s.,** a sterile solution, free from foreign particles, for instillation into the eye. **physiological salt s., physiological sodium chloride s.,** an aqueous solution of sodium chloride having an osmolality similar to that of blood serum. **potassium arsenite s.,** a solution of arsenic trioxide, potassium bicarbonate, and alcohol in water; has been used as an antileukemic agent. **Ringer's s.,** a solution of sodium chloride, potassium chloride, and calcium chloride in purified water; a physiological salt solution for topical use. **saline s., salt s.,** a solution of sodium chloride, or common salt, in purified water. **saturated s.,** one containing all of the solute which can be held in solution by the solvent. **sclerosing s.,** one containing an irritant substance which will cause obliteration of a space, as the lumen of a varicose vein or the cavity of a hernial sac. **sodium hypochlorite s.,** a solution containing 4–6% by weight of sodium hypochlorite; used to disinfect various utensils. For wound disinfection, *dilute sodium hypochlorite s.* (Dakin's s., or fluid), containing 0.45–0.50% sodium hypochloride, is used. **sodium phosphate P-32 s.,** a solution containing radioactive phosphorus (^{32}P); used as an antineoplastic, as a diagnostic aid in the location of tumors, and in the treatment of polycythemia vera and certain chronic leukemias. **standard s.,** one which contains in each liter a definitely stated amount of reagent; usually expressed in terms of normality (equivalent weights of solute per liter of solution) or molarity (g.mol.wts. of solute per liter of solution). **supersaturated s.,** an unstable solution containing more of the solute than it can permanently hold. **test s's,** standard solutions (in purity and concentration) of specified chemical substances used in performng certain test procedures. **volumetric s.,** one which contains a specific quantity of solvent per stated unit of volume.

solvent (sol′vent) 1. dissolving; effecting a solu-

tion. 2. a liquid that dissolves or is capable of dissolving; the component of a solution present in greater amount.

soma (so′mah) 1. the body as distinguished from the mind. 2. the body tissue as distinguished from the germ cells. 3. the cell body.

somal (so′mal) somatic.

somasthenia (so″mas-the′ne-ah) bodily weakness with poor appetite and poor sleep.

somat(o)- word element [Gr.], *body.*

somatalgia (so″mah-tal′je-ah) bodily pain.

somatesthesia (so″mat-es-the′ze-ah) body consciousness or awareness.

somatic (so-mat′ik) 1. pertaining to or characteristic of the soma or body. 2. pertaining to the body wall in contrast to the viscera.

somatization (so″mah-ti-za′shun) the conversion of mental experiences or states into bodily symptoms.

somatochrome (so-mat′o-krōm) any neuron which has a well marked cell body completely surrounding the nucleus, its colorable protoplasm having a distinct contour; used also adjectively.

somatogenic (so″mah-to-jen′ik) originating in the body.

somatology (so″mah-tol′o-je) the sum of what is known about the body; the study of anatomy and physiology.

somatome (so′mah-tōm) 1. an appliance for cutting the body of a fetus. 2. a somite.

somatomedin (so″mah-to-me′din) a peptide elaborated by the liver in response to stimulation by growth hormone; it stimulates skeletal growth by acting directly on cartilage cells.

somatometry (so″mah-tom′ĕ-tre) measurement of the body.

somatopagus (so″mah-top′ah-gus) a double fetus with trunks more or less fused.

somatopathy (so″mah-top′ah-the) a bodily disorder as distinguished from a mental one. **somatopath′ic,** adj.

somatoplasm (so-mat′o-plazm) the protoplasm of the body cells exclusive of the germ cells.

somatopleure (-plŏŏr) the embryonic body wall, formed by ectoderm and somatic mesoderm. **somatopleur′al,** adj.

somatopsychic (so″mah-to-si′kik) pertaining to both mind and body.

somatopsychosis (-si-ko′sis) any mental disease symptomatic of bodily disease.

somatoscopy (so″mah-tos′ko-pe) examination of the body.

somatosexual (so″mah-to-seks′u-al) pertaining to both physical and sex characteristics, or to physical manifestations of sexual development.

somatostatin (-stat′in) a polypeptide secreted by the hypothalamus that inhibits release of growth hormone from the pituitary, of insulin and glucagon from the pancreas, and of thyrotropin and gastrin; also produced synthetically.

somatotherapy (-ther′ah-pe) treatment aimed at relieving or curing ills of the body.

somatotonia (-to′ne-ah) a group of traits characterized by dominance of muscular activity and vigorous body assertiveness; considered typical of a mesomorph.

somatotopic (-top′ik) related to particular areas of the body; describing organization of motor area of the brain, control of the movement of different parts of the body being centered in specific regions of the cortex.

somatotrophin (-tro′fin) growth hormone. **somatotro′phic**, adj.

somatotropin (-tro′pin) growth hormone. **somatotro′pic**, adj.

somatotype (so-mat′o-tīp) a particular type of body build.

Sombulex (som′bu-leks) trademark for a preparation of hexobarbital.

somesthesia (so″mes-the′ze-ah) sensibility to bodily sensations. **somesthet′ic**, adj.

somite (so′mīt) one of the paired, blocklike masses of mesoderm, arranged segmentally alongside the neural tube of the embryo, forming the vertebral column and segmental musculature.

somnambulism (som-nam′bu-lizm) 1. sleepwalking; habitual walking in the sleep. 2. a hypnotic state in which the subject has full possession of his senses but no subsequent recollection.

somnifacient (som″nĭ-fa′shent) hypnotic (1).

somniferous (som-nif′er-us) producing sleep.

somniloquism (som-nil′o-kwizm) habitual talking in one's sleep.

somnipathy (som-nip′ah-the) any disorder of sleep; a condition of hypnotic trance.

somnolence (som′no-lens) sleepiness; also, unnatural drowsiness.

somnolentia (som″no-len′she-ah) 1. drowsiness, or somnolence. 2. sleep drunkenness; a condition of incomplete sleep with disorientation and excited or violent behavior.

Somnos (som′nos) trademark for preparations of chloral hydrate.

sonitus (son′ĭ-tus) tinnitus aurium.

sonometer (so-nom′ĕ-ter) 1. an apparatus for testing acuteness of hearing. 2. an instrument for measuring the ratios of sound vibrations in various bodies.

sonorous (so-nōr′us) resonant; sounding.

sopor (so′por) deep or profound sleep.

soporific (sop″ŏ-rif′ik, so″pŏ-rif′ik) producing deep sleep; an agent that so acts.

soporous (so′por-us) associated with coma or profound sleep.

sorbefacient (sōr″bĕ-fa′shent) 1. promoting absorption. 2. a sorbefacient agent.

sorbitan (sor′bĭ-tan) any of the anhydrides of sorbitol, the fatty acids of which are surfactants; see also *polysorbate 80*.

sorbitol (sor′bĭ-tol) a crystalline, hexahydric alcohol, $C_6H_8(OH)_6$, found in various berries and fruits; a pharmaceutical preparation is used as a flavoring agent and as an osmotic diuretic.

sordes (sōr′dēz) materia alba. **s. gas′tricae,** undigested food, mucus, etc., in the stomach.

sore (sōr) 1. popularly, almost any lesion of the skin or mucous membranes. 2. painful. **bed s.,** decubitus ulcer. **cold s.,** see *herpes simplex.*

Delhi s., cutaneous leishmaniasis. **desert s.,** a form of tropical ulcer occurring in desert areas of Africa, Australia, and the Near East. **natal s., oriental s.,** cutaneous leishmaniasis. **pressure s.,** decubitus ulcer.

sore throat (sōr thrōt) see *laryngitis, pharyngitis,* and *tonsillitis.* **septic s., t., streptococcal s. t.,** severe sore throat occurring in epidemics, usually due to *Streptococcus pyogenes,* with intense local hyperemia with or without a grayish exudate and enlargement of the cervical lymph glands.

sorption (sorp′shun) 1. incorporation of water in a colloid. 2. processes involved in net movement of components of adjoining substances across a boundary separating them, as various membranes of the body. 3. the adsorption or chemisorption of gases on the surface of a metal or other solid.

S.O.S. [L.] *si o′pus sit* (if necessary).

sotalol (so′tah-lōl) an antiadrenergic (β-receptor), $C_{12}H_{20}N_2O_3S$; used as the hydrochloride salt.

soterenol (so-ter′ĕ-nōl) an adrenergic with bronchodilator properties, $C_{12}H_{20}O_4S$; used as the hydrochloride salt.

souffle (soo′fel) a soft, blowing auscultatory sound. **cardiac s.,** any cardiac or vascular murmur of a blowing quality. **fetal s.,** murmur sometimes heard over the pregnant uterus, supposed to be due to compression of the umbilical cord. **funic s., funicular s.,** hissing souffle synchronous with fetal heart sounds, probably from the umbilical cord. **placental s.,** the sound supposed to be produced by the blood current in the placenta. **uterine s.,** a sound made by the blood within the arteries of the gravid uterus.

sound (sownd) 1. the effect produced on the organ of hearing by vibrations of the air or other medium. 2. mechanical radiant energy, the motion of particles of the material medium through which it travels being along the line of transmission (longitudinal); such energy, having frequency of 20–20,000 c.p.s., provides the stimulus for the subjective sensation of hearing. 3. an instrument to be introduced into a cavity to detect a foreign body or to dilate a stricture. 4. a noise, normal or abnormal, heard within the body. **ejection s's,** high-pitched clicking sounds heard very shortly after the first heart sound, attributed to sudden distention of a dilated pulmonary artery or aorta or to forceful opening of the pulmonic or aortic cusps. **friction s.,** one produced by rubbing of two surfaces. **heart s's,** the sounds produced by the functioning of the heart, the *first,* a dull, prolonged sound, occurring with ventricular systole; the *second,* a sharp, short sound, occurring with closure of the semilunar valves; the *third,* a very faint sound caused by rapid passive filling of the ventricle; and the *fourth,* a rarely audible, low-pitched sound caused by atrial contraction and ventricular filling. **hippocratic s.,** the succussion sound heard in pyopneumothorax or seropneumothorax. **Korotkoff s's,** sounds heard during auscultatory determination of blood pressure. **percussion s.,** any sound obtained by percussion. **respiratory s.,** any sound heard on auscultation over the respiratory tract. **succussion s's,** splashing sounds heard on succussion over a distended stomach or in hydropneumothorax. **to-and-fro s.,** a friction sound or murmur heard with both systole and diastole. **urethral s.,** a long, slender instrument for exploring and dilating the urethra. **white s.,** that produced by a mixture of all frequencies of mechanical vibration perceptible as sound.

space (spās) 1. a delimited area. 2. an actual or potential cavity of the body. 3. the areas of the universe beyond the earth and its atmosphere. **spa′tial,** adj. **apical s.,** the region between the wall of the alveolus and the apex of the root of a tooth. **axillary s.,** the axilla. **arachnoid s.,** see *subarachnoid s.* and *subdural s.* **bregmatic s.,** the anterior fontanel. **cartilage s's,** the spaces in hyaline cartilage containing the cartilage cells. **corneal s's,** the spaces between the lamellae of the substantia propria of the cornea containing corneal cells and interstitial fluid. **cupular s.,** the part of the attic above the malleus. **dead s.,** 1. the space remaining after incomplete closure of surgical or other wounds, permitting accumulation of blood or serum and resultant delay in healing. 2. in the respiratory tract: (1) *anatomical dead s.,* those portions, from the nose and mouth to the terminal bronchioles, not participating in oxygen–carbon dioxide exchange, and (2) *physiologic dead s.,* which reflects nonuniformity of ventilation and perfusion in the lung, is the anatomical dead space plus the space in the alveoli occupied by air that does not participate in oxygen–carbon dioxide exchange. **epidural s.,** the space between the dura mater and the lining of the vertebral canal. **episcleral s.,** the space between the bulbar fascia and the eyeball. **haversian s.,** see under *canal.* **intercostal s.,** the space between two adjacent ribs. **interglobular s's,** small irregular spaces on the outer surface of the dentin in the tooth root. **interpeduncular s.,** see under *fossa.* **interpleural s.,** mediastinum. **interproximal s.,** the space between the proximal surfaces of adjoining teeth. **intervillous s.,** the cavernous space of the placenta into which the chorionic villi project and through which the maternal blood circulates. **Kiernan's s's,** the triangular spaces bounded by invaginated Glisson's capsule between the liver lobules, containing the larger interlobular branches of the portal vein, hepatic artery, and hepatic duct. **lymph s.,** any space in tissue occupied by lymph. **Meckel's s.,** a recess in the dura mater which lodges the gasserian ganglion. **mediastinal s.,** mediastinum. **medullary s.,** the central cavity and the intervals between the trabeculae of bone which contain the marrow. **palmar s.,** a large fascial space in the hand, divided by a fibrous septum into a midpalmar and a thenar space. **parasinoidal s's,** lateral lacunae in the dura mater, along the superior sagittal sinus, which receive meningeal and diploic veins. **perforated s.,** see under *substance.* **perineal s's,** spaces on either side of the inferior fascia of the urogenital diaphragm, the *deep* between it and the superior fascia, the

superficial between it and the superficial perineal fascia. **perivascular s.,** a lymph space within the walls of an artery. **Petit's s's,** zonular s's. **pneumatic s.,** a portion of bone occupied by air-containing cells, especially the spaces constituting the paranasal sinuses. **Poiseuille's s.,** that part of the lumen of a tube, at its periphery, where no flow of liquid occurs. **retroperitoneal s.,** the space between the peritoneum and the posterior abdominal wall. **retropharyngeal s.,** the space behind the pharynx, containing areolar tissue. **retropubic s., Retzius s.,** the areolar space bounded by the reflection of peritoneum, symphysis pubis, and bladder. **subarachnoid s.,** the space between the arachnoid and the pia mater. **subdural s.,** the space between the dura mater and the arachnoid. **subgingival s.,** gingival crevice. **subphrenic s.,** the space between the diaphragm and subjacent organs. **subumbilical s.,** a somewhat triangular space in the body cavity beneath the umbilicus. **Tenon's s.,** episcleral s. **thenar s.,** the palmar space lying between the middle metacarpal bone and the tendon of the flexor pollicis longus. **zonular s's,** the lymph-filled spaces between the fibers of the ciliary zonule.

sparganosis (spar″gah-no′sis) infection with the larvae (spargana) of any of several species of tapeworms, which invade the subcutaneous tissues, causing inflammation and fibrosis.

sparganum (spar-ga′num), pl. *sparga′na* [Gr.] the larval stage of certain tapeworms, especially of the genera *Diphyllobothrium* and *Spirometra;* see also *sparganosis.* Also, a genus name applied to such larvae, usually when the adult stage is unknown.

Sparine (spar′ēn) trademark for preparations of promazine.

sparteine (spar′te-in) an alkaloid from the legumes *Cytisus scoparius* and *Lupinus luteus;* its sulfate salt has been used as a digitalis substitute and as an oxytocic.

spasm (spazm) 1. a sudden, violent, involuntary muscular contraction. 2. a sudden transitory constriction of a passage, canal, or orifice. **bronchial s.,** spasmodic contraction of the muscular coat of the bronchial tubes, as occurs in asthma. **carpopedal s.,** spasm of the hand or foot, or of the thumbs and great toes, seen in tetany. **clonic s.,** spasm with rigidity followed immediately by relaxation. **cynic s.,** risus sardonicus. **facial s.,** tonic spasm of the muscles supplied by the facial nerve, involving the entire side of the face or confined to a limited area about the eye. **habit s.,** tic. **intention s.,** muscular spasm on attempting voluntary movement. **myopathic s.,** spasm accompanying disease of the muscles. **nodding s.,** chronic spasm of the sternocleidomastoid muscles, causing a nodding motion of the head. **saltatory s.,** clonic spasm of the muscles of the legs, producing a peculiar jumping or springing motion when standing. **tetanic s.,** 1. muscular spasm occurring in tetanus. 2. tonic s. **tonic s.,** spasm with rigidity persisting for a long period. **toxic s.,** spasm caused by a toxin.

spasmodic (spaz-mod′ik) of the nature of a spasm; occurring in spasms.

spasmolysis (spaz-mol′ĭ-sis) the arrest of spasm. **spasmolyt′ic,** adj.

spasmophilia (spaz″mo-fil′e-ah) abnormal tendency to spasm or convulsions.

spasmus (spaz′mus) [L.] spasm. **s. nu′tans,** nodding spasm.

spastic (spas′tik) 1. of the nature of or characterized by spasms. 2. hypertonic, so that the muscles are stiff and movements awkward.

spasticity (spas-tis′ĭ-te) a state of increased muscle tone, with heightened deep tendon reflexes.

spatium (spa′she-um), pl. *spa′tia* [L.] space.

spatula (spach′ŭ-lah) a wide, flat, blunt, usually flexible instrument of little thickness, used for spreading material on a smooth surface.

spatulate (spach′ŭ-lāt) 1. having a flat blunt end. 2. to mix or manipulate with a spatula.

spatulation (spach″ŭ-la′shun) the combining of materials into a homogeneous mixture by continuously heaping together and smoothing out on a smooth surface with a spatula.

spavin (spav′in) in general, an exostosis, usually medial, of the tarsus of equines, distal to the tibiotarsal articulation and often involving the metatarsals. **bog s.,** a distention of the synovial capsule of the tibiotarsal joint in equines.

spavined (spav′ind) affected with spavin.

spay (spa) to remove the ovaries.

SPCA serum prothrombin conversion accelerator (blood coagulation Factor VII).

specialist (spesh′ah-list) a physician whose practice is limited to a particular branch of medicine or surgery, especially one who, by virture of advanced training, is certified by a specialty board as being qualified to so limit his practice.

specialty (spesh′al-te) the field of practice of a specialist.

speciation (spe″se-a′shun) the evolutionary formation of new species.

species (spe′shēz) a taxonomic category subordinate to a genus (or subgenus) and superior to a subspecies or variety. **type s.,** the original species from which the description of the genus is formulated.

species-specific (-spĕ-sif′ik) characteristic of a particular species; having a characteristic effect on, or interaction with, cells or tissues of members of a particular species; said of an antigen, drug, or infective agent.

specific (spĕ-sif′ik) 1. pertaining to a species. 2. produced by a single kind of microorganism. 3. restricted in application, effect, etc., to a particular structure, function, etc. 4. a remedy specially indicated for any particular disease. 5. in immunology, pertaining to the special affinity of antigen for the corresponding antibody.

specificity (spes″ĭ-fis′ĭ-te) the quality or state of being specific.

specimen (spes′ĭ-men) a small sample or part taken to show the nature of the whole, as a small quantity of urine for analysis, or a small fragment of tissue for microscopic study. **corrosion s.,** a preparation of an organ, such as the liver, by injection of certain of its structures (e.g., the arteries and veins) and chemical digestion of surrounding substance.

spectacles (spek′tĕ-kals) a pair of lenses in a frame to assist vision.

spectinomycin (spek″tĭ-no-mi′sin) an antibiotic derived from *Streptomyces spectabilis,* used in treatment of gonorrhea.

spectra (spek′trah) plural of *spectrum.*

spectral (spek′tral) pertaining to a spectrum; performed by means of a spectrum.

spectrocolorimeter (spek″tro-kul″ĕ-rim′ĕ-ter) an instrument for detecting color blindness.

spectrometry (spek-trom′ĕ-tre) determination of the place of lines in a spectrum.

spectrophotometer (spek″tro-fo-tom′ĕ-ter) 1. an apparatus for measuring light sense by means of a spectrum. 2. an apparatus for determining quantity of coloring matter in solution by measurement of transmitted light.

spectrophotometry (-fo-tom′ĕ-tre) the use of the spectrophotometer.

spectroscope (spek′tro-skōp) an instrument for developing and analyzing spectra.

spectroscopy (spek-tros′ko-pe) examination by means of a spectroscope; the propagation and analysis of spectra.

spectrum (spek′trum) a charted band of wavelengths of electromagnetic radiation obtained by refraction or diffraction; by extension, a measurable range of activity, as the range of bacteria affected by an antibiotic (*antibacterial s.*) or the complete range of manifestations of a disease. **absorption s.,** one obtained by passing radiation with a continuous spectrum through a selectively absorbing medium, showing spaces or dark lines for wavelengths for which the spectrum of the medium itself would be bright. **broad-s.,** effective against a wide range of microorganisms. **chromatic s.,** that portion of the electromagnetic spectrum including wavelengths of 7700–3900 A.U., giving rise to the perception of color by the normal eye. **electromagnetic s.,** the range of electromagnetic energy from cosmic rays to electric waves, including gamma, x- and ultraviolet rays, visible light, and infrared waves, and radio waves. **fortification s.,** scintillating scotoma. **invisible s.,** that made up of vibrations of wavelengths less than 3900 A.U. (ultraviolet, grenz rays, x-rays, and gamma rays) and between 7700 and 120,000 A.U. (infrared). **solar s.,** that portion of the electromagnetic spectrum including vibrations emanating from the sun. **visible s.,** that portion of the range of wavelengths of electromagnetic vibrations (from 7700 to 3900 A.U.) which is capable of stimulating specialized sense organs and is perceptible as light.

speculum (spek′u-lum) an intrument for opening or distending a body orifice or cavity to permit visual inspection.

speech (spēch) the expression of thoughts and ideas by vocal sounds. **esophageal s.,** that produced by vibration of the column of air in the esophagus against the contracting cricopharyngeal sphincter, after laryngectomy. **explosive s.,** loud, sudden enunciation, seen in certain brain diseases. **mirror s.,** a speech abnormality, the order of syllables in a sentence being reversed. **scanning s., staccato s.,** speech in which syllables of words are separated by noticeable pauses.

sperm (sperm) 1. semen. 2. spermatozoon.

spermaceti (sper″mah-set′e) a waxy substance obtained from the head of the sperm whale; an emollient used in cold cream.

spermatic (sper-mat′ik) pertaining to the semen; seminal.

spermatid (sper′mah-tid) a cell derived from a secondary spermatocyte by fission, and developing into a spermatozoon.

spermatitis (sper″mah-ti′tis) deferentitis.

spermato-, spermo- word element [Gr.], *seed;* specifically, the male germinative element.

spermatoblast (sper-mat′o-blast) spermatid.

spermatocele (-sēl) cystic distention of the epididymis or rete testis, containing spermatozoa.

spermatocelectomy (sper″mah-to-se-lek′to-me) excision of a spermatocele.

spermatocidal (-si′dal) spermicidal.

spermatocyst (sper-mat′o-sist) 1. a seminal vesicle. 2. spermatocele.

spermatocystectomy (sper″mah-to-sis-tek′to-me) excision of a seminal vesicle.

spermatocystitis (-sis-ti′tis) seminal vesiculitis.

spermatocystotomy (-sis-tot′o-me) incision of a seminal vesicle.

spermatocyte (sper-mat′o-sīt) a cell developed from a spermatogonium in spermatogenesis. **primary s.,** the original large cell into which a spermatogonium develops. **secondary s.,** a cell produced by meiotic division of the primary spermatocyte and which gives rise to the spermatid.

spermatocytogenesis (sper″mah-to-si″to-jen′-ĕ-sis) the first stage of formation of spermatozoa in which the spermatogonia develop into spermatocytes and then into spermatids.

spermatogenesis (-jen′ĕ-sis) the process of the formation of spermatozoa, including spermatocytogenesis and spermiogenesis.

spermatogenic (-jen′ik) giving rise to sperm.

spermatogonium (-go′ne-um), pl. *spermatogo′nia* [Gr.] an undifferentiated male germ cell, originating in a seminal tubule and dividing into two spermatocytes.

spermatoid (sper′mah-toid) resembling semen.

spermatolysin (sper″mah-tol′ĭ-sin) a substance causing spermatolysis.

spermatolysis (sper″mah-tol′ĭ-sis) destruction or dissolution of spermatozoa. **spermatolyt′ic,** adj.

spermatopathia (sper″mah-to-path′e-ah) abnormality of the semen.

spermatorrhea (-re′ah) involuntary escape of semen, without orgasm.

spermatoschesis (sper″mah-tos′kĕ-sis) suppression of the semen.

spermatoxin (sper″mah-tok′sin) spermotoxin.

spermatozoicide (sper″mah-to-zo′ĭ-sīd) spermicide.

spermatozoon (-zo′on), pl. *spermatozo′a* [Gr.] a mature male germ cell, the specific output of the testes, which impregnates the ovum in sexual reproduction. **spermatozo′al,** adj.

spermaturia (sper″mah-tu′re-ah) seminuria.

spermectomy (sper-mek′to-me) excision of a portion of the spermatic cord.

spermicide (sper′mĭ-sīd) an agent destructive to spermatozoa. **spermici′dal,** adj.

spermiduct (-dukt) the ejaculatory duct and vas deferens together.

spermine (sper′min) a leukomaine from semen and other animal substances.

spermiogenesis (sper″me-o-jen′ĕ-sis) the second stage in the formation of spermatozoa, in which the spermatids transform into spermatozoa.

spermiogram (sper′me-o-gram″) a diagram or chart of various cells formed in development of the spermatozoon, or of the cells present in a specimen of semen.

spermist (sper′mist) a believer in the theory of preformation, which held that the spermatozoon held a complete miniature individual.

spermolith (sper′mo-lith) a stone in the spermatic duct.

spermoneuralgia (sper″mo-nu-ral′je-ah) neuralgic pain in the spermatic cord.

spermophlebectasia (-fle″bek-ta′ze-ah) varicose state of the spermatic veins.

spermotoxin (-tok′sin) a toxin lethal to spermatozoa; especially in antibody produced by injection of an animal with spermatozoa.

sp.gr. specific gravity.

sphacelate (sfas′ĕ-lāt) to become gangrenous.

sphacelation (sfas″ĕ-la′shun) the formation of a sphacelus; mortification.

sphacelism (sfas′ĕ-lizm) sphacelation or necrosis; sloughing.

sphaceloderma (sfas″ĕ-lo-der′mah) gangrene of the skin.

sphacelous (sfas′ĕ-lus) gangrenous; sloughing.

sphacelus (sfas′ĕ-lus) a slough; a mass of gangrenous tissue.

Sphaerophorus (sfe-rof′o-rus) *Bacteroides.*

sphenion (sfe′ne-on) the point at the sphenoid angle of the parietal bone.

spheno- word element [Gr.], *wedge-shaped; sphenoid bone.*

sphenocephalus (sfe″no-sef′ah-lus) a fetus with a wedgelike head.

sphenoid (sfe′noid) 1. wedge-shaped. 2. see *Table of Bones.*

sphenoidal (sfe-noi′dal) relating to the sphenoid bone.

sphenoiditis (sfe″noi-di′tis) inflammation of the sphenoid sinus.

sphenoidotomy (sfe″noi-dot′o-me) incision of a sphenoid sinus.

sphenomaxillary (sfe″no-mak′sĭ-lār″e) pertaining to the sphenoid bone and maxilla.

sphenopalatine (-pal′ah-tīn) pertaining to the sphenoid and palatine bones.

sphenotresia (-tre′ze-ah) boring of the base of the skull in craniotomy.

sphenotribe (sfe′no-trīb) an instrument for crushing the base of the fetal skull.

sphere (sfēr) a ball or globe. **attraction s.,** centrosome. **segmentation s.,** 1. morula. 2. a blastomere.

sphero- word element [Gr.], *round; a sphere.*

spherocyte (sfe'ro-sīt) a small, globular, completely hemoglobinated erythrocyte without the usual central pallor characteristically found in hereditary spherocytosis but also in acquired hemolytic anemia. **spherocyt'ic,** adj.

spherocytosis (sfe"ro-si-to'sis) the presence of spherocytes in the blood. **hereditary s.,** a congenital hereditary form of hemolytic anemia characterized by spherocytosis, abnormal fragility of erythrocytes, jaundice, and splenomegaly.

spheroid (sfe'roid) a spherelike body.

spheroidal (sfe-roi'dal) resembling a sphere.

spheroma (sfe-ro'mah) a globular tumor.

spherometer (sfe-rom'ĕ-ter) an apparatus for measuring the curvature of a surface.

sphincter (sfingk'ter) a ringlike muscle which closes a natural orifice or passage. **anal s., s. a'ni,** see *sphincter muscle of anus* (*external* and *internal*) in *Table of Muscles*. **cardiac s.,** muscle fibers about the opening of the esophagus into the stomach. **O'Beirne's s.,** a band of muscle at the junction of the sigmoid colon and rectum. **Oddi's s.,** the sheath of muscle fibers investing the associated bile and pancreatic passages as they traverse the wall of the duodenum. **pyloric s.,** a thickening of the muscular wall of the stomach around the opening into the duodenum.

sphincteral, sphincteric (sfingk'ter-al; sfingkter'ik) pertaining to a sphincter.

sphincteralgia (sfingk"ter-al'je-ah) pain in a sphincter muscle.

sphincterectomy (-ek'to-me) excision of a sphincter.

sphincterismus (-iz'mus) spasm of a sphincter.

sphincteritis (-i'tis) inflammation of a sphincter.

sphincterolysis (-ol'ĭ-sis) surgical separation of the iris from the cornea in anterior synechia.

sphincteroplasty (sfingk'ter-o-plas"te) plastic reconstruction of a sphincter.

sphincterotomy (sfingk"ter-ot'o-me) incision of a sphincter.

sphingolipid (sfing"go-lip'id) a lipid containing sphingosine (e.g., ceramides, sphingomyelins, gangliosides, and cerebrosides), occurring in high concentrations in the brain and other nerve tissue.

sphingolipidosis (-lip"ĭ-do'sis), pl. *sphingolipido'ses* [Gr.] a group of diseases characterized by abnormal storage of sphingolipids, e.g., Gaucher's disease, Niemann-Pick disease, Hurler's syndrome, and Tay-Sachs disease.

sphingolipodystrophy (-lip"o-dis'tro-fe) any of a group of disorders of sphingolipid metabolism.

sphingomyelin (-mi'ĕ-lin) a group of phospholipids which on hydrolysis yield phosphoric acid, choline, sphingosine, and a fatty acid.

sphingosine (sfing'go-sin) a long-chain, monounsaturated aliphatic amino alcohol found in sphingolipids.

sphygmic (sfig'mik) pertaining to the pulse.

sphygmo- word element [Gr.], *the pulse.*

sphygmochronograph (-kro'no-graf) a self-registering sphygmograph.

sphygmodynamometer (-di"nah-mom'ĕ-ter) an instrument for measuring the force of the pulse.

sphygmogram (sfig'mo-gram) a record or tracing made by a sphygmograph.

sphygmograph (-graf) apparatus for registering the movements, form, and force of the arterial pulse. **sphygmograph'ic,** adj.

sphygmoid (sfig'moid) resembling the pulse.

sphygmomanometer (sfig"mo-mah-nom'ĕ-ter) an instrument for measuring arterial blood pressure.

sphygmometer (sfig-mom'ĕ-ter) an instrument for measuring the pulse.

sphygmoscope (sfig'mo-skōp) a device for rendering the pulse beat visible.

sphygmotonometer (sfig"mo-to-nom'ĕ-ter) an instrument for measuring elasticity of arterial walls.

sphyrectomy (sfi-rek'to-me) excision of the malleus.

sphyrotomy (sfi-rot'o-me) division of the malleus.

spica (spi'kah) a figure-of-8 bandage, with turns crossing each other.

spicule (spik'ūl) a sharp, needle-like body.

spiculum (spik'u-lum), pl. *spic'ula* [L.] spicule.

spider (spi'der) 1. an arthropod of the class Arachnida. 2. a spider-like nevus. **arterial s.,** vascular s. **black widow s.,** a spider, *Latrodectus mactans,* whose bite causes severe poisoning. **vascular s.,** a telangiectasis composed of small vessels radiating from a central arteriole, the whole resembling spider legs, occurring most often on the upper arms and chest, usually in children and pregnant women, but also in persons with liver disease.

spike (spīk) a sharp upward deflection in a curve or tracing, as on the encephalogram.

spina (spi'nah), pl. *spi'nae* [L.] a spine; in anatomy, a thornlike process or projection. **s. bif'ida,** a developmental anomaly marked by defective closure of the bony encasement of the spinal cord, through which the meninges may (*s. bif'ida cys'tica*) or may not (*s. bif'ida occul'ta*) protrude. **s. vento'sa,** dactylitis affecting mostly infants and young children, with enlargement of digits, caseation, sequestration, and sinus formation.

spinal (spi'nal) pertaining to a spine or to the vertebral column.

spinalgia (spi-nal'je-ah) pain in the spinal region.

spinate (spi'nāt) having thorns; thorn-shaped.

spindle (spin'd'l) 1. the fusiform figure occurring during metaphase of cell division, composed of microtubules radiating from the centrioles and connecting the chromosomes at their centromeres. 2. muscle s. **Krukenberg's s.,** a spindle-shaped, brownish-red opacity of the cornea. **muscle s.,** one of the mechanoreceptors arranged in parallel between the fibers of skeletal muscle, being the receptor of impulses responsible for the stretch reflex. **nuclear s.,** spindle (1). **tendon s.,** Golgi tendon organ.

spine (spīn) 1. a slender, thornlike process of bone. 2. the vertebral column. **alar s., angular s.,** s. of sphenoid. **bamboo s.,** the ankylosed spine produced by rheumatoid spondylitis. **bifid s., cleft s.,** spina bifida. **ischial s.,** a bony process projecting backward and medialward from the posterior border of the ischium. **mental s.,** any of the small projections (usually four) on the inner surface of the mandible, near the lower end of the midline, serving for attachment of the genioglossal and geniohyoid muscles. **nasal s., anterior,** the sharp anteriosuperior projection at the anterior extremity of the nasal crest of the maxilla. **nasal s., posterior,** a sharp, backward-projecting bony spine forming the medial posterior angle of the horizontal part of the palatine bone. **neural s.,** the spinous process of a vertebra. **palatine s's,** laterally placed ridges on the lower surface of the maxillary part of the hard palate, separating the palatine sulci. **poker s.,** the ankylosed spine produced by rheumatoid spondylitis. **rigid s.,** poker s. **s. of scapula,** a triangular bony plate attached by one end to the back of the scapula. **sciatic s.,** ischial s. **s. of sphenoid,** the posterior and downward projection from the lower aspect of the great wing of the sphenoid bone. **s. of tibia,** a longitudinally elongated, raised and roughened area on the anterior crest of the tibia. **trochlear s.,** a bony spicule on the anteromedial part of the orbital surface of the frontal bone for attachment of the trochlea of the superior oblique muscle.

spinipetal (spi-nip′ĕ-tal) conducting or moving toward the spinal cord.

spinnbarkeit (spin′bahr-kīt) mucous of low viscosity from the cervix uteri, indicative of ovulation.

spinobulbar (spi″no-bul′bar) pertaining to the spinal cord and medulla oblongata.

spinocellular (-sel′u-lar) pertaining to or composed of prickle cells.

spinocerebellar (-ser″ĕ-bel′ar) pertaining to the spinal cord and cerebellum.

spinous (spi′nus) pertaining to or like a spine.

spiradenoma (spi″rad-ĕ-no′mah) syringocystadenoma.

spiral (spi′ral) 1. winding like the thread of a screw. 2. a structure curving around a central point or axis. **Curschmann's s's,** coiled mucinous fibrils sometimes found in the sputum in bronchial asthma.

spireme (spi′rēm) the threadlike continuous or segmented figure formed by the chromosome material during prophase.

spirilla (spi-ril′ah) plural of *spirillum.*

spirillicidal (spi-ril″ĭ-si′dal) destroying spirilla.

spirillosis (spi″rĭ-lo′sis) a disease caused by presence of spirilla.

Spirillum (spi-ril′um) a genus of gram-negative bacteria, including one species, S. *mi′nus,* which is pathogenic for guinea pigs, rats, mice, and monkeys and is the cause of rat-bite fever (sodoku) in man.

spirillum (spi-ril′um), pl. *spiril′la* [L.] 1. a relatively rigid, spiral-shaped bacterium. 2. an organism of the genus *Spirillum.*

spirit (spir′it) 1. a volatile or distilled liquid. 2. a solution of a volatile material in alcohol. **proof s.,** a product containing 50 per cent by volume of C_2H_5OH. **rectified s.,** alcohol.

Spirochaeta (spi″ro-ke′tah) a genus of bacteria (family Spirochaetaceae) found in fresh- or sea-water slime, especially when hydrogen sulfide is present.

Spirochaetaceae (-ke-ta′se-e) a family of bacteria (order Spirochaetales) found in the intestinal tracts of bivalve mollusks and in stagnant fresh or salt water.

Spirochaetales (-ke-ta′lēz) an order of bacteria.

spirochete (spi′ro-kēt) 1. a spiral bacterium; any microorganism of the order Spirochaetales. 2. an organism of the genus *Spirochaeta.* **spiroche′tal,** adj.

spirocheticide (spi″ro-ke′tĭ-sīd) an agent which destroys spirochetes. **spirochetici′dal,** adj.

spirochetolysis (-ke-tol′ĭ-sis) the destruction of spirochetes by lysis.

spirochetosis (-ke-to′sis) infection with spirochetes. **avian s., fowl s.,** a septicemic disease of fowl caused by *Borrelia anserina* and transmitted by the tick *Argas persicus.*

spirogram (spi′ro-gram) pneogram.

spirograph (-graf) pneograph.

spiroid (spi′roid) resembling a spiral.

spirolactone (spi″ro-lak′tōn) a group of compounds capable of opposing the action of sodium-retaining steroids on renal transport of sodium and potassium.

spirometer (spi-rom′ĕ-ter) pneometer.

Spirometra (spi″ro-met′rah) a genus of tapeworms parasitic in fish-eating cats, dogs, and birds; larval infection (sparganosis) in man is caused by ingestion of inadequately cooked fish.

spirometry (spi-rom′ĕ-tre) pneumatometry. **spiromet′ric,** adj.

spironolactone (spi-ro″no-lak′tōn) one of the spirolactones, $C_{24}H_{32}O_4S$, an aldosterone inhibitor highly effective when given orally; used as a diuretic.

spissated (spis′āt-ed) inspissated.

splanchn(o)- word element [Gr.], *viscus (viscera); splanchnic nerve.*

splanchnapophysis (splangk″nah-pof′ĭ-sis) a skeletal element, such as the lower jaw, connected with the alimentary canal.

splanchnectopia (splangk″nek-to′pe-ah) displacement of one or more viscera.

splanchnesthesia (splangk″nes-the′ze-ah) visceral sensation. **splanchnesthet′ic,** adj.

splanchnic (splangk′nik) pertaining to the viscera.

splanchnicectomy (splangk″nĭ-sek′to-me) excision of part of the splanchnic nerve.

splanchnicotomy (-kot′o-me) transection of the splanchnic nerve.

splanchnocele (splangk′no-sēl) hernial protrusion of a viscus.

splanchnocoele (splangk′no-sēl) that portion of

the coelom from which the visceral cavities are formed.

splanchnodiastasis (splangk″no-di-as′tah-sis) displacement of a viscus or viscera.

splanchnography (splangk-nog′rah-fe) descriptive anatomy of the viscera.

splanchnolith (splangk′no-lith) intestinal calculus.

splanchnologia (splangk″no-lo′je-ah) splanchnology.

splanchnology (splangk-nol′o-je) the scientific study of the viscera of the body; applied also to the body of knowledge relating thereto.

splanchnomegaly (splangk″no-meg′ah-le) enlargement of the viscus; visceromegaly.

splanchnopathy (splangk-nop′ah-the) any disease of the viscera.

splanchnopleure (splangk′no-ploōr) the layer formed by union of the splanchnic mesoderm with entoderm; from it are developed the muscles and the connective tissue of the digestive tube.

splanchnoptosis (splangk″nop-to′sis) prolapse or downward displacement of the viscera.

splanchnosclerosis (splangk″no-skle-ro′sis) hardening of the viscera.

splanchnoskeleton (-skel′ĕ-ton) skeletal structures connected with the viscera.

splanchnotomy (splangk-not′o-me) anatomy or dissection of the viscera.

splanchnotribe (splangk′no-trīb) an instrument for crushing the intestine to obliterate its lumen.

splayfoot (spla′foot) flatfoot; talipes valgus.

spleen (splēn) a large, glandlike organ situated in the upper left part of the abdominal cavity, lateral to the cardiac end of the stomach. Among its functions are the disintegration of erythrocytes and the setting free of hemoglobin, which the liver converts into bilirubin; the genesis of new erythrocytes during fetal life and in the newborn; and serving as a blood reservoir. **splen′ic,** adj. **accessory s.,** a connected or detached outlying portion, or exclave, of the spleen. **diffuse waxy s.,** amyloid degeneration of the spleen involving especially the coats of the venous sinuses and the reticulum of the organ. **floating s., movable s.,** one displaced and preternaturally movable. **sago s.,** one with amyloid degeneration, the malpighian corpuscles looking like grains of sand. **wandering s.,** floating s. **waxy s.,** a spleen affected with amyloid degeneration.

splen(o)- word element [Gr.], *spleen.*

splenadenoma (splēn″ad-ĕ-no′mah) hyperplasia of the spleen pulp.

splenalgia (sple-nal′je-ah) pain in the spleen.

splenectasis (sple-nek′tah-sis) splenomegaly.

splenectomy (sple-nek′to-me) excision of the spleen.

splenectopia, splenectopy (sple″nek-to′pe-ah; sple-nek′to-pe) displacement of the spleen; floating spleen.

splenic (splen′ik) pertaining to the spleen.

splenitis (sple-ni′tis) inflammation of the spleen.

splenium (sple′ne-um) a compress or bandage; a bandlike structure. **s. cor′poris callo′si,** the posterior, rounded end of the callosum.

splenization (splen″i-za′shun) the conversion of a tissue, as of the lung, into tissue resembling that of the spleen, due to engorgement and condensation.

splenocele (sple′no-sēl) hernia of the spleen.

splenocolic (sple″no-kol′ik) pertaining to the spleen and colon.

splenocyte (splen′o-sīt) the monocyte characteristic of splenic tissue.

splenodynia (sple″no-din′e-ah) splenalgia.

splenography (sple-nog′rah-fe) 1. roentgenography of the spleen. 2. a description of the spleen.

splenohepatomegaly (sple″no-hep″ah-to-meg′-ah-le) enlargement of spleen and liver.

splenoid (sple′noid) resembling the spleen.

splenolysin (sple-nol′ĭ-sin) a lysin which destroys spleen tissue.

splenolysis (sple-nol′ĭ-sis) destruction of splenic tissue by a lysin.

splenoma (sple-no′mah) a splenic tumor.

splenomalacia (sple″no-mah-la′she-ah) abnormal softness of the spleen.

splenomedullary (-med′u-ler″e) of or pertaining to the spleen and bone marrow.

splenomegaly (-meg′ah-le) enlargement of the spleen. **congestive s.,** splenomegaly secondary to portal hypertension, with ascites, anemia, thrombocytopenia, leukopenia, and episodic hemorrhage from the intestinal tract. **hemolytic s.,** that associated with hemolytic anemia.

splenomyelogenous (-mi″ĕ-loj′ĕ-nus) formed in the spleen and bone marrow.

splenomyelomalacia (-mi″ĕ-lo-mah-la′she-ah) softening of the spleen and bone marrow.

splenoncus (sple-nong′kus) splenoma.

splenopancreatic (sple″no-pan″kre-at′ik) pertaining to the spleen and pancreas.

splenopathy (sple-nop′ah-the) any disease of the spleen.

splenopexy (sple′no-pek″se) surgical fixation of the spleen.

splenopneumonia (splen″o-nu-mo′ne-ah) pneumonia attended with splenization of the lung.

splenoptosis (sple″nop-to′sis) downward displacement of the spleen.

splenorrhagia (sple″no-ra′je-ah) hemorrhage from the spleen.

splenorrhaphy (sple-nor′ah-fe) suture of the spleen.

splenotomy (sple-not′o-me) incision of the spleen.

splenotoxin (sple″no-tok′sin) a toxin produced by or acting on the spleen.

splint (splint) 1. a rigid or flexible appliance for fixation of displaced or movable parts. 2. [pl.] exostosis of the rudimentary second or fourth metacarpal or metatarsal in the horse. **airplane s.,** one which holds the splinted limb suspended in the air. **anchor s.,** one for fracture of the jaw, with metal loops fitting over the teeth and held together by a rod. **Angle's s.,** one for fracture of the mandible. **Balkan s.,** an apparatus for continuous extension of fractures of the femur, consisting of an overhead bar, supported from the floor with pulleys attached, which supports the leg in a metal sling. **coaptation s's,** small splints adjusted about a fractured limb for the purpose of producing coaptation of fragments. **Denis Browne s.,** one for correction of clubfoot. **dynamic s.,** a supportive or protective apparatus which aids in initiation and performance of motion by the supported or adjacent parts. **functional s.,** dynamic s. **shin s's,** strain of the flexor digitorum longus muscle occurring in athletes, marked by pain along the shin bone. **Thomas' knee s.,** two round iron rods joined at the upper end by an oval iron ring, or half ring, and bent at the lower end to form the letter W; used to give support to the lower extremity.

splinting (splint'ing) 1. application of a splint, or treatment by use of a splint. 2. in dentistry, the application of a fixed restoration to join two or more teeth into a single rigid unit. 3. rigidity of muscles occurring as a means of avoiding pain caused by movement of the part.

spodogenous (spo-doj'ĕ-nus) caused by accumulation of waste material in an organ.

spondyl(o)- word element [Gr.], *vertebra; vertebral column.*

spondylalgia (spon"dĭ-lal'je-ah) pain in the vertebrae.

spondylarthritis (spon"dil-ar-thri'tis) arthritis of the spine.

spondylitic (spon"dĭ-lit'ik) pertaining to or marked by spondylitis.

spondylitis (spon"dĭ-li'tis) inflammation of vertebrae. **s. ankylopoiet'ica, ankylosing s., s. defor'mans,** rheumatoid s. **Kümmell's s.,** see under *disease.* **Marie-Strümpell s.,** rheumatoid s. **rheumatoid s.,** rheumatoid arthritis of the spine, affecting young males predominantly and producing pain and stiffness as a result of inflammation of the sacroiliac, intervertebral, and costovertebral joints; it may progress to cause complete spinal and thoracic rigidity. **s. tuberculo'sa,** tuberculosis of the spine. **s. typho'sa,** that following typhoid fever.

spondylizema (spon"dĭ-li-ze'mah) downward displacement of a vertebra because of destruction or softening of the one below it.

spondylocace (spon"dĭ-lok'ah-se) tuberculosis of the vertebrae.

spondylodymus (spon"dĭ-lod'ĭ-mus) twin fetuses united by the vertebrae.

spondylodynia (spon"dĭ-lo-din'e-ah) spondylalgia.

spondylolisthesis (-lis-the'sis) forward displacement of a vertebra over a lower segment, usually of the fourth or fifth lumbar. **spondylolisthet'ic,** adj.

spondylolysis (spon"dĭ-lol'ĭ-sis) the breaking down of a vertebra.

spondylopathy (spon"dĭ-lop'ah-the) any disease of the vertebrae.

spondylopyosis (spon"dĭ-lo-pi-o'sis) suppuration of a vertebra.

spondyloschisis (spon"dĭ-los'kĭ-sis) congenital fissure of a vertebral arch; spina bifida.

spondylosis (spon"dĭ-lo'sis) vertebral ankylosis; also, any degenerative changes in the spine. **rhizomelic s.,** rheumatoid spondylitis.

spondylosyndesis (spon"dĭ-lo-sin'dĕ-sis) surgical creation of ankylosis between contiguous vertebrae; spinal fusion.

sponge (spunj) a porous, absorbent mass, as a pad of gauze or cotton surrounded by gauze, or the elastic fibrous skeleton of certain species of marine animals. **gelatin s., absorbable,** a sterile, absorbable, water-insoluble, gelatin-base material, used as a local hemostatic.

spongi(o)- word element [L., Gr.], *sponge; sponge-like.*

spongiform (spun'ji-form) resembling a sponge.

spongioblast (spun'je-o-blast") 1. any of the embryonic epithelial cells developed about the neural tube, which become transformed, some into neuroglial and some into ependymal cells. 2. amacrine (2).

spongioblastoma (spun"je-o-blas-to'mah) a tumor containing spongioblasts; glioblastoma or gliosarcoma.

spongiocyte (spun'je-o-sīt") 1. a neuroglia cell. 2. one of the cells with spongy vacuolated protoplasm in the adrenal cortex.

spongioid (spun'je-oid) resembling a sponge.

spongioplasm (spun'je-o-plazm") 1. a substance forming the network of fibrils pervading the cell substance and forming the reticulum of the fixed cell. 2. the granular material of an axon.

spongiosis (spun"je-o'sis) intercellular edema within the epidermis.

spongiositis (spun"je-o-si'tis) inflammation of the corpus spongiosum of the penis.

spongy (spun'je) of spongelike appearance or texture.

sporadic (spo-rad'ic) occurring singly; widely scattered; not epidemic or endemic.

sporangium (spo-ran'je-um), pl. *sporan'gia* [Gr.] any encystment containing spores or sporelike bodies, as in certain fungi.

spore (spōr) the reproductive element of certain lower organisms, such as the protozoa, fungi, algae, etc.

sporicide (spo'rĭ-sīd) an agent which kills spores. **sporici'dal,** adj.

sporoagglutination (spo"ro-ah-gloo"tĭ-na'-shun) agglutination of spores in the diagnosis of sporotrichosis.

sporoblast (spo'ro-blast) one of the bodies formed in the oocyst of the malarial parasite in the mosquito and from which the sporozoite later develops; also, similar stages in certain other sporozoa.

sporocyst (-sist) 1. any cyst or sac containing spores or reproductive cells. 2. a saclike organism developing from a miracidium in the snail host, containing germ cells giving rise to other sporocyts or to rediae in the life cycle of certain helminths. 3. the stage formed within the oocyst, from a sporoblast, and which produces sporozoites.

sporogenic (spo"ro-jen'ik) producing spores.

sporogony (spo-rog'o-ne) the sexual cycle of sporozoa, especially the life-cycle of the malarial parasite in the stomach and body of the mosquito. **sporogon′ic**, adj.

sporont (spo′ront) a mature protozoon in its sexual cycle.

sporoplasm (spo′ro-plazm) protoplasm of reproductive cells.

Sporothrix (-thriks) a genus of fungi, including *S. schenck′ii* (see *sporotrichosis*), and *S. car′nis*, which causes formation of white mold on meat in cold storage.

sporotrichosis (spo″ro-trĭ-ko′sis) a chronic fungal disease caused by *Sporothrix schenckii*, occurring in three forms: a cutaneous lymphatic form, a disseminated form, and a pulmonary form.

Sporozoa (-zo′ah) a subphylum of endoparasitic protozoa, marked by the lack of locomotor organs in adult stages and a complex life cycle usually involving an alternation of a sexual with an asexual cycle.

sporozoan (-zo′an) 1. pertaining to sporozoa. 2. a sporozoon.

sporozoite (-zo′īt) the infective form of a sporozoon, which undergoes asexual reproduction (schizogony) in the body of the host.

sporozoon (-zo′on), pl. *sporozo′a* [Gr.] an individual organism of the Sporozoa.

sport (sport) a mutation.

sporulation (spor″u-la′shun) formation of spores.

sporule (spor′ūl) a small spore.

spot (spot) a circumscribed area; a small blemish; a macula. **Bitot's s′s**, foamy gray, triangular spots of keratinized epithelium on the conjunctiva, associated with vitamin A deficiency. **blind s.**, the area marking the site of entrance of the optic nerve on the retina; it is not sensitive to light. **café au lait s′s** (kah-fa′o-la′) [Fr.], macules, of a distinctive light brown color, occurring in neurofibromatosis and Albright's syndrome. **cherry-red s.**, the choroid appearing as a red circular area surrounded by gray-white retina, as viewed through the fovea centralis in Tay-Sachs disease. **cold s.**, see *temperature s′s*. **cotton-wool s′s**, white or gray soft-edged opacities in the retina composed of cytoid bodies; seen in hypertensive retinopathy, lupus erythematosus, and numerous other conditions. **focal s.**, the part of the target of an x-ray tube bombarded by the focused electron stream. **germinal s.**, the nucleolus of the fertilized ovum. **hot s.**, 1. see *temperature s′s*. 2. the sensitive area of a neuroma. 3. an area of increased density on an x-ray or thermographic film. **hypnogenetic s′s**, superficial areas, stimulation of which brings on sleep. **Koplik's s′s**, irregular, bright red spots on the buccal and lingual mucosa, with tiny bluish-white specks in the center of each; seen in the prodromal stage of measles. **liver s′s**, a lay term for brownish spots on the face, neck, or backs of the hands in many older people. **Mariotte's s.**, blind s. **mongolian s.**, a smooth, brown to grayish blue nevus, consisting of an excess of melanocytes, typically found at birth in the sacral region in Orientals, Negroes, American Indians, and many southern Europeans; it usually disap-

pears during childhood. **pain s′s**, spots on the skin where alone the sense of pain can be produced by a stimulus. **rose s′s**, an eruption of rose-colored spots on the abdomen and loins during the first seven days of typhoid fever. **Roth's s′s**, round or oval white spots sometimes seen in the retina early in the course of subacute bacterial endocarditis. **Soemmerring's s.**, macula lutea. **Tardieu's s′s**, spots of ecchymosis under the pleura after death by suffocation. **temperature s′s**, spots on the skin normally anesthetic to pain and pressure but sensitive respectively to heat and cold. **yellow s.**, macula retinae.

sprain (sprān) wrenching of a joint, with partial rupture of its ligaments.

spray (spra) a liquid minutely divided or nebulized, as by a jet of air or steam.

sprue (sproo) 1. a chronic form of malabsorption syndrome, occurring in both tropical and nontropical forms. 2. in dentistry, the hole through which metal or other material is poured or forced into a mold. **nontropical s.**, celiac disease: a malabsorption syndrome affecting both children and adults, precipitated by ingestion of gluten-containing foods and marked by diarrhea with bulky, frothy, fatty fetid stools, abdominal distention, weight loss, asthenia, deficiency of vitamins B, D, and K, and electrolyte depletion. **tropical s.**, a malabsorption syndrome occurring in the tropics and subtropics marked by stomatitis, diarrhea, and anemia; protein malnutrition is usually precipitated by the malabsorption, and the anemia by folic acid deficiency.

spur (sper) a projecting body, as from a bone; in dentistry, a piece of metal projecting from a plate, band, or other dental appliance. **calcaneal s.**, a bone excrescence on the lower surface of the calcaneus which frequently causes pain on walking.

spurious (spu′re-us) simulated; not genuine; false.

sputum (spu′tum) matter ejected from the trachea, bronchi, and lungs, through the mouth. **s. cruen′tum**, bloody sputum. **nummular s.**, sputum in rounded disks, shaped somewhat like coins. **rusty s.**, sputum stained with blood or blood pigments.

squalene (skwa′lēn) an unsaturated terpin hydrocarbon from the liver oil of sharks and other elasmobranch fishes; it is an intermediate in cholesterol biosynthesis in all animals examined, and is found in small amounts in blood plasma and in increased amounts in viral influenza.

squama (squa′mah), pl. *squa′mae* [L.] a scale, or thin, platelike structure.

squame (skwām) a scale or scalelike mass.

squamo-occipital (skwa″mo-ok-sip′ĭ-tal) pertaining to the squamous portion of the occipital bone.

squamoparietal (-pah-ri′ĕ-tal) pertaining to the squamous portion of the temporal bone and the parietal bone.

squamous (skwa′mus) scaly or platelike.

squatting (skwot′ing) a position with hips and

knees flexed, the buttocks resting on the heels; sometimes adopted by the parturient at delivery or by children with certain types of cardiac defects.

squill (skwil) the fleshy inner scales of the bulb of the white variety of *Urginea maritima;* it contains several cardioactive glycosides. The red variety is used as a rat poison.

squint (skwint) strabismus.

S.R. sedimentation rate.

Sr chemical symbol, *strontium.*

sRNA transfer RNA (soluble RNA).

SRS-A slow-reacting substance of anaphylaxis; see under *substance.*

ss. [L.] *se'mis* (one half).

S. T. 37 trademark for a solution of hexylresorcinol.

stabile (sta'bil, -bīl) stable; stationary; resistant to change; opposed to *labile.*

stability (stah-bil'ĭ-te) the quality of being stable or resistant to change.

stabilization (sta"bĭ-li-za'shun) the creation of a stable state.

stable (sta'b'l) not readily subject to change.

stadium (sta'de-um), pl. *sta'dia* [L.] stage. **s. decremen'ti,** the period of decrease of severity in a disease; the defervescence of fever. **s. incremen'ti,** the period of increase in the intensity of a disease; the stage of development of fever.

staff (staf) 1. a wooden rod or rodlike structure. 2. a grooved director used as a guide for the knife in lithotomy. 3. the professional personnel of a hospital. 4. see under *cell.* **s. of Æsculapius,** the rod or staff with entwining snake, symbolic of the god of healing, official insignia of the American Medical Association. See also *caduceus.* **attending s.,** the corps of attending physicians and surgeons of a hospital. **consulting s.,** specialists associated with a hospital and acting in an advisory capacity to the attending staff. **house s.,** the resident physicians and surgeons of a hospital.

stage (stāj) 1. a definite period or distinct phase, as of development of a disease or of an organism. 2. the platform of a microscope on which the slide containing the object to be studied is placed. **algid s.,** a period marked by flickering pulse, subnormal temperature, and varied nervous symptoms. **amphibolic s.,** the period between the acme and decline of an attack. **anal s.,** in psychoanalysis, the stage of psychosexual development from 12 months to as late as 36 months of age, characterized by libidinous experience of anal function; it follows the oral stage and precedes the genital stage. **cold s.,** the period of chill or rigor in a malarial paraoxysm. **first s.** (of labor), see *labor.* **fourth s.** (of labor), a name sometimes applied to the immediate postpartum period. **genital s.,** in psychoanalysis, the psychosexual stage in which libidinous pleasure is associated with the genitals; the adult sexual stage, which follows the anal stage. **hot s.,** period of pyrexia in a malarial paroxysm. **oral s.,** in psychoanalysis, the first stage of the infantile period in psychosexual development, lasting from birth to 12 months,

or even to 24 months of age, in which sensual or libidinous pleasure is associated with oral activities; it is followed by the anal stage. **second s.** (of labor), see *labor.* **third s.** (of labor), see *labor.*

staggers (stag'erz) 1. gid. 2. a form of vertigo occurring in decompression sickness.

stain (stān) 1. a substance used to impart color to tissues or cells, to facilitate microscopic study and identification. 2. an area of discoloration of the skin. **acid s.,** one that is acid in reaction and more readily colors the cell protoplasm. **basic s.,** one that is basic in reaction and shows an affinity for the cell nuclei. **contrast s.,** a stain used to color an unstained portion of a tissue after another portion has been stained with another dye. **differential s.,** one which facilitates differentiation of various elements in a specimen. **Giemsa s.,** a solution containing azure II-eosin, azure II, glycerin, and methanol; used for staining protozoan parasites, such as trypanosomes, *Leishmania,* etc., and *Leptospira, Borrelia,* viral inclusion bodies, and *Rickettsia.* **Gram's s.,** a staining procedure in which microorganisms are stained with crystal violet, treated with strong iodine solution, decolorized with ethanol or ethanol-acetone, and counterstained with a contrasting dye; those retaining the stain are *gram-positive,* and those losing the stain but staining with the counterstain are *gram-negative.* **hematoxylin-eosin s.,** a mixture of hematoxylin in distilled water and aqueous eosin solution, employed universally for routine tissue examination. **intravital s.,** vital s. **metachromatic s.,** one which produces in certain elements colors different from that of the stain itself. **neutral s.,** a combination of an acid and a basic stain for staining neutrophil tissues. **nuclear s.,** one which selectively stains cell nuclei, generally a basic stain. **port-wine s.,** nevus flammeus. **postvital s.,** a stain that appears after death of a tissue which has been previously stained by vital methods. **supravital s.,** a stain introduced in living tissue or cells that have been removed from the body. **tumor s.,** an area of increased density in a radiograph, due to collection of contrast material in distorted and abnormal vessels, prominent in the capillary and venous phase of arteriography, and presumed to indicate neoplasm. **vital s.,** a stain introduced into the living organism, and taken up selectively by various tissue or cellular elements. **Wright's s.,** a mixture of eosin and methylene blue, used for demonstrating blood cells and malarial parasites.

staining (stān'ing) artificial coloration of a substance to facilitate examination of tissues, microorganisms, or other cells under the microscope. For various techniques, see under *stain.* In dentistry, the modification of the color of a tooth or denture base.

stalagmometer (stal"ag-mom'ĕ-ter) an instrument for measuring surface tension by determining the exact number of drops in a given quantity of a liquid.

stalk (stawk) an elongated anatomical structure resembling a plant stalk. **allantoic s.,** the more slender tube interposed in most mammals between the urogenital sinus and allantoic sac.

yolk s., a narrow tube connecting the yolk sac (umbilical vesicle) with the midgut of the early embryo.

stammering (stam'er-ing) a speech problem characterized by involuntary pauses in speaking, often with repetition of sounds.

standard (stan'dard) something established as a measure or model to which other similar things should conform.

standstill (stand'stil) cessation of activity, as of the heart (*cardiac s.*) or chest (*respiratory s.*).

stannum (stan'um) [L.] tin (symbol Sn).

stanolone (stan'o-lōn) an androgen, $C_{19}H_{30}O_2$, having the same actions and uses as testosterone.

stanozolol (stan'o-zo-lol'') an androgen, $C_{21}H_{32}N_2O$, used to accelerate anabolism and/or to arrest excessive catabolism.

stapedectomy (sta''pĕ-dek'to-me) excision of the stapes.

stapedial (stah-pe'de-al) pertaining to the stapes.

stapediotenotomy (stah-pe''de-o-tĕ-not'o-me) cutting of the tendon of the stapedius muscle.

stapediovestibular (-ves-tib'u-lar) pertaining to the stapes and vestibule.

stapes (sta'pēz) [L.] see *Table of Bones* and Plate XII.

Staphcillin (staf-sil'in) trademark for a preparation of methicillin.

staphyl(o)- word element [Gr.], *uvula; resembling a bunch of grapes; staphylococci.*

staphylectomy (staf''ĭ-lek'to-me) uvulectomy.

staphyledema (staf''il-ĕ-de'mah) edema of the uvula.

staphyline (staf'ĭ-līn) 1. pertaining to the uvula. 2. shaped like a bunch of grapes.

staphylion (stah-fil'e-on) 1. the point at the midline of the posterior edge of the hard palate. 2. uvula.

staphylitis (staf''ĭ-li'tis) uvulitis.

staphylococcemia (staf''ĭ-lo-kok-se'me-ah) staphylococci in the blood.

Staphylococcus (-kok'us) a genus of gram-positive bacteria (family Micrococcaceae) constantly present on the skin and in the upper respiratory tract and the most common cause of localized suppurative infections; it includes *S. al'bus,* the white form, an occasional agent of pneumonia, but not very pathogenic; *S. au'reus,* the pigmented, coagulase-positive pathogenic form, and *S. pyog'enes* var. *al'bus,* the white form found occasionally in infectious processes.

staphylococcus (-kok'us,), pl. *staphylococ'ci* [Gr.] any organism of the genus *Staphylococcus.* **staphyloc'cal, staphylococ'cic,** adj.

staphyloderma (-der'mah) pyogenic skin infection by staphylococci.

staphylodialysis (-di-al'ĭ-sis) relaxation of the uvula.

staphylokinase (-ki'nās) a bacterial kinase produced by certain strains of staphylococci; it induces fibrinolysis by converting plasminogen to plasmin.

staphylolysin (staf''ĭ-lol'ĭ-sin) a hemolysin produced by staphylococci.

staphyloma (staf''ĭ-lo'mah) protrusion of the sclera or cornea, usually lined with uveal tissue, due to inflammation. **staphylom'atous,** adj. **anterior s.,** staphyloma in the anterior part of the eye. **corneal s.,** 1. bulging of the cornea with adherent uveal tissue. 2. one formed by protrusion of the iris through a corneal wound. **posterior s.,** backward bulging of the sclera at the posterior pole of the eye. **scleral s.,** protrusion of the contents of the eyeball where the sclera has become thinned.

staphyloncus (staf''ĭ-long'kus) a tumor or swelling of the uvula.

staphyloplasty (staf'ĭ-lo-plas''te) plastic repair of the soft palate and uvula.

staphyloptosia (staf''ĭ-lop-to-se-ah) elongation of the uvula.

staphylorrhaphy (staf''ĭ-lor'ah-fe) surgical correction of a midline cleft in the uvula and soft palate.

staphyloschisis (staf''ĭ-los'kĭ-sis) fissure of the uvula and soft palate.

staphylotomy (staf''ĭ-lot'o-me) 1. incision of the uvula. 2. excision of a staphyloma.

star (star) any star-like structure. **daughter s.,** amphiaster. **mother s.,** monaster. **s's of Verheyen,** stellate veins of kidney.

starch (starch) 1. any of a group of polysaccharides of the general formula, $(C_6H_{10}O_5)_n$; it is the chief storage form of carbohydrates in plants. 2. granular material separated from mature grain of *Zea mays,* Indian corn, or maize; used as a dusting powder and tablet disintegrant in pharmaceuticals. **animal s.,** glycogen. **s. glycerite,** a preparation of starch, benzoic acid, purified water, and glycerin, used topically as an emollient. **hydroxyethyl s.,** a starch product which has been suggested as a plasma substitute in man.

starvation (star-va'shun) prolonged deprival of food, and its morbid effects.

stasis (sta'sis) 1. a stoppage or diminution of flow, as of blood or other body fluid. 2. a state of equilibrium among opposing forces. **intestinal s.,** impairment of the normal passage of intestinal content, due to mechanical obstruction or to impaired intestinal motility. **urinary s.,** stoppage of the flow or discharge of urine, at any level of the urinary tract. **venous s.,** impairment or cessation of venous flow.

-stasis word element [Gr.], *maintenance of (or maintaining) a constant level; preventing increase or multiplication.* **-stat'ic,** adj.

stat. [L.] *sta'tim* (at once).

state (stāt) condition or situation. **dream s.,** a state of defective consciousness in which the environment is imperfectly perceived. **metastable s.,** the condition of a system (nucleus, atom, or molecule) capable of undergoing quantum transition to a state of lower energy. **refractory s.,** a condition of subnormal excitability of muscle and nerve following excitation. **resting s.,** the physiologic condition achieved by complete bed rest for at least one hour. **steady s.,** dynamic equilibrium.

statim (sta'tim) [L.] at once.

statistics (stah-tis'tiks) 1. numerical facts pertaining to a particular subject or body of objects. 2. the science dealing with the collection and tabulation of numerical facts. **vital s.,** numerical facts pertaining to human natality, morbidity, and mortality.

statoconia (stat″o-ko′ne-ah), sing. *statoco′nium* [Gr.] minute calciferous granules within the gelatinous membrane surrounding the acoustic maculae.

statolith (stat′o-lith) 1. a granule of the statoconia. 2. a solid or semisolid body occurring in the labyrinth of animals.

statolon (-lon) an antiviral agent derived from *Penicillium stoloniferum.*

statometer (stah-tom′ĕ-ter) an apparatus for measuring the degree of exophthalmos.

stature (stach′ur) the height or tallness of a person standing. **stat′ural,** adj.

status (sta′tus) [L.] condition or state. **s. asthmat′icus,** asthmatic crisis; a sudden intense and continuous asthmatic attack, with dyspnea to the point of exhaustion and no response to the usual therapy. **s. degenerati′vus,** a condition in which an unusual number of degenerative stigmata (developmental anomalies) occur in a single person. **s. epilep′ticus,** rapid succession of epileptic spasms without intervening periods of consciousness. **s. lymphat′icus,** lymphatism. **s. thymicolymphat′icus,** a condition resembling lymphatism, with enlargement of lymphadenoid tissue generally and of the thymus as the special influencing factor. **s. verruco′sus,** a wartlike appearance of the cerebral cortex, produced by disorderly arrangement of the neuroblasts so that the formation of fissures and sulci is irregular and unpredictable.

staurion (staw′re-on) intersection of the median and transverse palatine sutures.

stauroplegia (staw″ro-ple′je-ah) alternate hemiplegia.

staxis (stak′sis) hemorrhage.

steapsin (ste-ap′sin) the fat-splitting enzyme (lipase) of the pancreatic juice.

stear(o)- word element [Gr.], *fat.*

stearate (ste′ah-rāt) the ionic form of stearic acid; also, any compound of stearic acid.

stearin (ste′ah-rin) tristearin.

stearopten (ste″ah-rop′ten) a camphor, the more solid constituent of a volatile oil.

steat(o)- word element [Gr.], *fat; oil.*

steatitis (ste″ah-ti′tis) inflammation of adipose tissue.

steatocystoma (ste″ah-to-sis-to′mah) a keratin cyst. **s. mul′tiplex,** steatomatosis, a rare hereditary condition in which multiple sebaceous cysts occur on the trunk and limbs.

steatogenous (ste″ah-toj′ĕ-nus) lipogenic.

steatolysis (ste″ah-tol′ĭ-sis) the emulsification of fats preparatory to absorption. **steatolyt′ic,** adj.

steatoma (ste″ah-to′mah) 1. sebaceous cyst. 2. a sebaceous gland neoplasm.

steatomatosis (ste″ah-to″mah-to′sis) the presence of numerous sebaceous cysts; see *steatocystoma multiplex.*

steatonecrosis (-nĕ-kro′sis) fat necrosis.

steatopygia (ste″ah-to-pij′e-ah) excessive fatness of the buttocks. **steatop′ygous,** adj.

steatorrhea (-re′ah) excess fat in feces.

steatosis (ste″ah-to′sis) fatty degeneration.

Steclin (stek′lin) trademark for preparations of tetracycline.

stegnosis (steg-no′sis) constriction; stenosis. **stegnot′ic,** adj.

Stelazine (stel′ah-zēn) trademark for preparations of trifluoperazine.

stella (stel′ah), pl. *stel′lae* [L.] star.

stellate (stel′āt) star-shaped; arranged in rosettes.

stellectomy (stel-lek′to-me) excision of a portion of the stellate ganglion.

stellula (stel′u-lah), pl. *stel′lulae*[L.] a little star-like mass or figure. **stel′lulae of Verheyen,** stellate veins of the kidney.

stem (stem) a supporting structure comparable to the stalk of a plant. **brain s.,** see under *B.*

Stenediol (sten′di-ol) trademark for preparations of methandriol.

stenion (sten′e-on) the point at each end of the smallest transverse diameter of the head in the temporal region.

steno- word element [Gr.], *narrow; contracted; constriction.*

stenocardia (sten″o-kar′de-ah) angina pectoris.

stenocephaly (-sef′ah-le) narrowness of the head or cranium. **stenoceph′alous,** adj.

stenochoria (-ko′re-ah) stenosis.

stenocoriasis (-ko-ri′ah-sis) contraction of the pupil.

stenopeic (-pe′ik) having a narrow opening or slit.

stenosed (stĕ-nōst′, stĕ-nōzd′) narrowed; constricted.

stenosis (stĕ-no′sis) narrowing or contraction of a body passage or opening. **aortic s.,** a narrowing of the aortic orifice of the heart or of the aorta itself. **mitral s.,** a narrowing of the left atrioventricular orifice. **pulmonary s.,** narrowing of the opening between the pulmonary artery and the right ventricle. **pyloric s.,** obstruction of the pyloric orifice of the stomach; it may be congenital or acquired. **tricuspid s.,** narrowing or stricture of the tricuspid orifice of the heart.

stenostomia (sten″o-sto′me-ah) narrowing of the mouth.

stenothermal, stenothermic (-ther′mal; -ther′-mik) developing only within a narrow range of temperature; said of bacteria.

stenothorax (-tho′raks) abnormal narrowness of the chest.

stenotic (stĕ-not′ik) marked by stenosis; abnormally narrowed.

stent (stent) a device or mold of a suitable material, used to hold a skin graft in place or to support tubular structures that are being anastomosed.

stephanion (ste-fa′ne-on), pl. *stepha′nia*[Gr.] intersection of the superior temporal line and the coronal suture. **stepha′nial,** adj.

Sterane (ster′ān) trademark for preparations of prednisolone.

sterco- word element [L.], *feces.*

stercobilin (ster′ko-bi′lin) a bile pigment derivative formed by air oxidation of stercobilinogen; it is a brown-orange-red pigmentation contributing to the color of feces and urine.

stercobilinogen (-bi-lin′o-jen) a bilirubin metabolite and precursor of stercobilin, formed by reduction of urobilinogen.

stercolith (ster′ko-lith) fecalith.

stercoraceous (ster′ko-ra′shus) consisting of feces.

stercoroma (-ro′mah) a tumor-like mass of fecal matter in the rectum.

stercus (ster′kus) [L.] dung or feces. **ster′coral, ster′corous,** adj.

stere (stēr) a cubic meter.

stereo- word element [Gr.], *solid; three dimensional; firmly established.*

stereoarthrolysis (ste′′re-o-ar-throl′ĭ-sis) operative formation of a movable new joint in cases of bony ankylosis.

stereoauscultation (-aus′′kul-ta′shun) auscultation with two stethoscopes, on different parts of the chest.

stereocampimeter (-kam-pim′ĕ-ter) an instrument for studying unilateral central scotomas and central retinal defects.

stereochemistry (-kem′is-tre) the branch of chemistry treating of the space relations of atoms in molecules. **stereochem′ical,** adj.

stereocinefluorography (-sin′′e-floo′′or-og′-rah-fe) recording by motion picture camera of images observed by stereoscopic fluoroscopy.

stereoencephalotome (-en-sef′ah-lo-tōm′′) a guiding instrument used in stereoencephalotomy.

stereoencephalotomy (-en-sef′′ah-lot′o-me) the production of sharply circumscribed lesions in subcortical ganglia or pathways by means of accurately placed electrodes.

stereognosis (ste′′re-og-no′sis) 1. the faculty of perceiving and understanding the form and nature of objects by the sense of touch. 2. perception by the senses of the solidity of objects. **stereognos′tic,** adj.

stereoisomer (ste′′re-o-i′so-mer) a compound showing stereoisomerism.

stereoisomerism (-i-som′er-izm) isomerism in which the compounds have the same structural formula, but the atoms are distributed differently in space. **stereoisomer′ic,** adj.

Stereo-orthopter (-or-thop′ter) trademark for a mirror-reflecting instrument for correcting strabismus.

stereoroentgenography (-rent′′gen-og′′rah-fe) the making of a stereoscopic roentgenogram.

stereoscope (ste′re-o-skōp′′) an instrument for producing the appearance of solidity and relief by combining the images of two similar pictures of an object.

stereoscopic (ste′′re-o-skop′ik) having the effect of a stereoscope; giving objects a solid or three-dimensional appearance.

stereospecific (-spĕ-sif′ik) exhibiting structural specificity in interacting with a substrate or a limited class of substrates.

stereotactic (-tak′tik) 1. pertaining to or characterized by precise positioning in space; said especially of discrete areas of the brain that control specific functions. 2. pertaining to or exhibiting stereotaxis.

stereotaxis (-tak′sis) taxis in response to contact with a solid or rigid surface.

stereotropism (ste′′re-ot′ro-pizm) tropism in response to contact with a solid or rigid surface. **stereotrop′ic,** adj.

stereotypy (ste′re-o-ti′′pe) persistent repetition of senseless acts or words.

steric (ste′rik) pertaining to the arrangement of atoms in space; pertaining to stereochemistry.

sterile (ster′il) 1. not fertile; barren; not producing young. 2. aseptic; not producing microorganisms; free from living microorganisms.

sterility (stĕ-ril′ĭ-te) the state of being sterile.

sterilization (ster′′il-i-za′shun) 1. the complete elimination of microbial viability. 2. any procedure by which an individual is made incapable of reproduction.

sterilize (ster′ĭ-līz) to render sterile.

sterilizer (ster′ĭ-līz′er) an apparatus for the destruction of microorganisms.

Sterisil (ster′ĭ-sil) trademark for a preparation of hexetidine.

stern(o)- word element [Gr.], *sternum.*

sternal (ster′nal) of or relating to the sternum.

sternalgia (ster-nal′je-ah) pain in the sternum.

sternebra (ster′nĕ-brah), pl. *ster′nebrae* [L.] any of the segments of the sternum in early life, which later fuse to form the body of the sternum.

Sterneedle (ster′ne-d′l) trademark for a controlled-depth, multiple-puncture apparatus used in diagnosing tuberculosis; see *tuberculin test, Sterneedle.*

sternoclavicular (ster′′no-klah-vik′u-lar) pertaining to the sternum and clavicle.

sternoclavicularis (-klah-vik′′u-la′ris) [L.] sternoclavicular.

sternocleidomastoid (-kli′′do-mas′toid) pertaining to the sternum, clavicle, and mastoid process.

sternocostal (-kos′tal) pertaining to the sternum and ribs.

sternodymia (-dim′e-ah) union of two fetuses by the anterior chest wall.

sternodymus (ster-nod′ĭ-mus) conjoined twins united at the anterior chest wall.

sternohyoid (ster′′no-hi′oid) pertaining to the sternum and hyoid bone.

sternoid (ster′noid) resembling the sternum.

sternomastoid (ster′′no-mas′toid) pertaining to the sternum and mastoid process.

sternopagus (ster-nop′ah-gus) sternodymus.

sternopericardial (ster′′no-per′′ĭ-kar′de-al) pertaining to the sternum and pericardium.

sternoschisis (ster-nos′kĭ-sis) congenital fissure of the sternum.

sternothyroid (ster′′no-thy′roid) pertaining to the sternum and thyroid cartilage or gland.

sternotomy (ster-not′o-me) incision of the sternum.

sternum (ster′num) [L.] see *Table of Bones*.

sternutatory (ster-nu′tah-tor″e) 1. causing sneezing. 2. an agent that causes sneezing.

steroid (ster′oid, ste′roid) any of a group of compounds containing four carbon rings interlocked to form a hydrogenated cyclopentophenanthrene-ring system; it includes many hormones, cardiac aglycones, bile acids, sterols, etc.

steroidogenesis (ste-roi″do-jen′ĕ-sis) production of steroids, as by the adrenal glands.

sterol (ster′ol, ste′rol) a steroid, e.g., cholesterol and ergosterol, with long (8–10 carbons) aliphatic side-chains at position 17 an at least one alcohol hydroxyl group, usually at position 3; they have lipid-like solubility.

Sterosan (ster′o-san) trademark for preparations of chlorquinaldol.

stertor (ster′tor) the act of snoring; sonorous respiration. **ster′torous**, adj.

steth(o)- word element [Gr.], *chest*.

stethalgia (steth-al′je-ah) pain in the chest.

stethogoniometer (steth″o-go″ne-om′ĕ-ter) apparatus for measuring curvature of the chest.

stethometer (steth-om′ĕ-ter) an instrument for measuring the circular dimension or expansion of the chest.

stethoscope (steth′o-skōp) an instrument for performing mediate auscultation. **stethoscop′ic**, adj.

stethoscopy (steth-os′ko-pe) examination with the stethoscope.

stethospasm (steth′o-spazm) spasm of the chest muscles.

STH somatotropic hormone.

sthenia (sthe′ne-ah) a condition of strength and activity.

sthenic (sthen′ik) active; strong.

stibialism (stib′e-al-izm″) antimonial poisoning.

stibium (stib′e-um) [L.] antimony (symbol Sb).

stibophen (stib′o-fen) an antimony compound used as an antischistosomal and in the treatment of granuloma inguinale.

stichochrome (stik′o-krōm) any neuron having the stainable substance arranged in more or less regular layers.

stigma (stig′mah), pl. *stig′mas, stig′mata* [Gr.] 1. any mental or physical mark or peculiarity that aids in identification or diagnosis of a condition. 2. [pl.] purpuric or hemorrhagic lesions of the hands and/or feet, resembling crucifixion wounds. **stigmat′ic**, adj. **s. of degeneracy**, any of the developmental anomalies found in considerable number in status degenerativus. **hysterical s.**, a bodily mark or sign characteristic of hysteria. **malpighian stigmata**, the points where the smaller veins enter into the larger veins of the spleen.

stigmasterol (stig-mas′tĕ-rol) an unsaturated plant sterol from calabar and soya beans, cacao butter, and elsewhere; an important starting material for industrial synthesis of steroid hormones.

stigmatization (stig″mah-tĭ-za′shun) the formation of stigmas.

stilbestrol (stil-bes′trol) diethylstilbestrol.

Stilbetin (stil-be′tin) trademark for a preparation of diethylstilbestrol.

stilet (sti′let) stylet.

stillbirth (stil′berth) delivery of a dead child.

stillborn (-born) born dead.

stimulant (stim′u-lant) 1. producing stimulation. 2. an agent which stimulates. **central s.**, a stimulant affecting the central nervous system. **diffusible s.**, one which acts promptly, but transiently. **general s.**, one which acts upon the whole body. **local s.**, one that affects only, or mainly, the part to which it is applied.

stimulate (stim′u-lāt) to excite functional activity in a part.

stimulation (stim″u-la′shun) the act or process of stimulating; the condition of being stimulated.

stimulator (stim′u-la″tor) any agent that excites functional activity. **long-acting thyroid s. (LATS)**, a substance occurring in the blood in hyperthyroidism, which exerts a stimulating effect on the thyroid of longer duration than does thyrotropin; it is associated with IgG immunoglobulin and may function as an autoantibody.

stimulus (stim′u-lus) any agent, act, or influence which produces functional or trophic reaction in a receptor or an irritable tissue. **adequate s.**, a stimulus of the specific form of energy to which a given receptor is sensitive. **aversive s.**, one which, when applied following the occurrence of a response, decreases the strength of that response on later occurrences. **conditioned s.**, a neutral object or event which is psychologically related to a naturally stimulating object or event and which causes a conditioned response; abbreviated CS. **heterologous s.**, one that acts upon all the nerve elements of the sensory apparatus. **homologous s.**, adequate s. **thermal s.**, a stimulant application of heat. **threshold s.**, one just strong enough to elicit a response.

sting (sting) 1. injury due to a biotoxin introduced into an individual or with which he comes in contact, together with mechanical trauma incident to its introduction. 2. the organ used to inflict such injury.

stippling (stip′pling) a spotted condition or appearance, as an appearance of the retina as if dotted with light and dark points, or the appearance of red blood cells in basophilia.

stirrup (stir′up) stapes.

stitch (stich) 1. a sudden, transient cutting pain. 2. a suture.

stoichiology (stoi″ke-ol′o-je) the science of elements, especially the physiology of the cellular elements of tissues. **stoichiolog′ic**, adj.

stoichiometry (-om′ĕ-tre) the science of the numerical relations of chemical elements and compounds and the mathematical laws of chemical changes. **stoichiomet′ric**, adj.

stoma (sto′mah), pl. *sto′mas, sto′mata* [Gr.] a mouthlike opening, particularly an incised opening which is kept open for drainage or other purposes. **sto′mal,** adj.

stomach (stum′ak) the musculomembranous expansion of the alimentary canal between the esophagus and duodenum, consisting of a cardiac part, a fundus, a body, and a pyloric part. Its (gastric) glands secrete the gastric juice which, when mixed with food, forms chyme, a semifluid substance suitable for further digestion by the intestine. See Plates IV and V. **cascade s.,** an atypical form of hourglass stomach, characterized roentgenologically by a drawing up of the posterior wall; an opaque medium first fills the upper sac and then cascades into the lower sac. **hourglass s.,** one more or less completely divided into two parts, resembling an hourglass in shape; due to scarring which complicates chronic gastric ulcer. **leather bottle s.,** linitis plastica. **water-trap s.,** a stomach with an extremely high pylorus, so that it does not readily empty itself.

stomachal (stum′ah-kal) pertaining to the stomach; stomachic.

stomachalgia (stum″ah-kal′je-ah) pain in the stomach.

stomachic (sto-mak′ik) 1. stomachal. 2. a medicine that promotes functional activity of the stomach.

stomat(o)- word element [Gr.], *mouth.*

stomatalgia (sto″mah-tal′je-ah) pain in the mouth.

stomatitis (sto″mah-ti′tis) generalized inflammation of the oral mucosa. **angular s.,** superficial erosions and fissuring at the angles of the mouth; it may occur in riboflavin deficiency and in pellagra or result from overclosure of the jaws in denture wearers. **aphthous s.,** stomatitis with small whitish lesions surrounded by a red border (aphthae), chiefly associated with mild local trauma, allergy, endocrine-associated conditions, and emotional stress; the exact cause is unknown. **gangrenous s.,** see *noma.* **herpetic s.,** an acute infection of the oral mucosa with vesicle formation, due to the herpes simplex virus. **lead s.,** the oral manifestations of lead poisoning, including a bluish line along the free gingival margin, pigmentation of the mucosa in contact with the teeth, metallic taste, excessive salivation, and swelling of the salivary glands. **mercurial s.,** stomatitis arising from mercury poisoning. **mycotic s.,** thrush. **necrotizing ulcerative s.,** see under *gingivostomatitis.* **ulcerative s.,** stomatitis with shallow ulcers on the cheeks, tongue, and lips. **Vincent's s.,** necrotizing ulcerative gingivostomatitis.

stomatodynia (sto″mah-to-din′e-ah) pain in the mouth.

stomatogastric (-gas′trik) pertaining to the stomach and mouth.

stomatology (sto″mah-tol′o-je) that branch of medicine which treats of the mouth and its diseases. **stomatolog′ic,** adj.

stomatomalacia (sto″mah-to-mah-la′she-ah) softening of the structures of the mouth.

stomatomenia (-me′ne-ah) vicarious menstruation involving bleeding from the mouth.

stomatomycosis (-mi-ko′sis) any fungal disease of the mouth.

stomatonecrosis (-ně-kro′sis) see *noma.*

stomatopathy (sto″mah-top′ah-the) any disorder of the mouth.

stomatoplasty (sto′mah-to-plas″te) plastic reconstruction of the mouth. **stomatoplas′tic,** adj.

stomatorrhagia (sto″mah-to-ra′je-ah) hemorrhage from the mouth.

stomocephalus (sto″mo-sef′ah-lus) a fetus with rudimentary jaws and mouth.

stomodeum (-de′um) the ectodermal depression at the head end of the embryo, which becomes the front part of the mouth. **stomode′al,** adj.

-stomy word element [Gr.], *creation of an opening into* or *a communication between.*

stone (stōn) 1. a calculus. 2. a unit of weight, equivalent in the English system to 14 pounds avoirdupois.

stool (stōol) the fecal discharge from the bowels. **rice water s.,** the watery evacuations of cholera.

storax (sto′raks) a balsam from the trunk of *Liquidambar orientalis,* a tree of western Asia, or of *L. styraciflua* of North America; an ingredient of compound benzoin tincture.

storm (storm) a sudden and temporary increase in symptoms. **thyroid s., thyrotoxic s.,** a sudden and dangerous increase in the symptoms of thyrotoxicosis, especially after thyroidectomy.

strabismometer (strah-biz-mom′ě-ter) an apparatus for measuring strabismus.

strabismus (strah-biz′mus) squint; deviation of the eye which the patient cannot overcome; the visual axes assume a position relative to each other different from that required by the physiological conditions. **strabis′mic,** adj. **comitant s., concomitant s.,** that due to faulty insertion of the eye muscles, resulting in the same amount of deviation in whatever direction the eyes are looking. **convergent s.,** esotropia. **divergent s.,** exotropia. **noncomitant s., nonconcomitant s.,** that in which the amount of deviation of the squinting eye varies according to the direction of gaze. **vertical s.,** that in which the visual axis of the squinting eye deviates in the vertical plane (hypertropia or hypotropia).

strabotomy (strah-bot′o-me) section of an ocular tendon in treatment of strabismus.

strain (strān) 1. to overexercise; to use to an extreme and harmful degree. 2. to filter or subject to colation. 3. an overstretching or overexertion of some part of the musculature. 4. excessive effort. 5. a group of organisms within a species or variety, characterized by some particular quality, as rough or smooth strains of bacteria. **Vi s.,** a strain of *Salmonella typhosa* containing the Vi (virulence) antigen of Felix.

strait (strāt) a narrow passage. **s's of pelvis,** the pelvic inlet (*superior pelvic s.*) and pelvic outlet (*inferior pelvic s.*).

straitjacket (strāt′jak″et) a contrivance for restraining the limbs, especially the arms, of a violently disturbed person.

stramonium (strah-mo′ne-um) dried leaves and flowering or fruiting tops of *Datura stramonium,* which contain the anticholinergic alkaloids atropine, hyoscamine, and scopolamine; used in treatment of asthma.

strangles (strang′gelz) 1. an infectious disease of horses due to *Streptococcus equi,* with mucopurulent inflammation of the respiratory mucous membrane. 2. infection of the lymph nodes in swine, producing heavily encapsulated abscesses in the pharyngeal region.

strangulated (strang′gu-lāt″ed) congested by reason of constriction or hernial stricture.

strangulation (strang″gu-la′shun) 1. choking or throttling arrest of respiration by occlusion of the air passages. 2. arrest of circulation in a part due to compression.

strangury (strang′gu-re) slow and painful discharge of urine.

strap (strap) 1. a band or slip, as of adhesive plaster, used in attaching parts to each other. 2. to bind down tightly. **Montgomery's s's,** straps of adhesive tape used to secure dressings that must be changed frequently.

stratification (strat″ĭ-fi-ka′shun) arrangement in layers.

stratiform (strat′ĭ-form) occurring in layers.

stratigraphy (strah-tig′rah-fe) see *body-section roentgenograhy.* **stratigraph′ic,** adj.

stratum (stra′tum), pl. *stra′ta* [L.] a layer. **s. cor′neum,** horny layer. **s. germinati′vum,** 1. malpighian layer. 2. germinative layer. **s. granulo′sum,** granular layer. **s. lu′cidum,** clear layer. **s. malpig′hii, s. muco′sum, s. spino′sum,** prickle-cell layer.

streak (strēk) a line or stripe. **angioid s's,** red to black irregular bands in the ocular fundus running outward from the optic disk. **meningeal s.,** tache cérébrale. **primitive s.,** a faint white trace at the caudal end of the embryonic disk, formed by movement of cells at the onset of mesoderm formation, providing the first evidence of the embryonic axis.

strephosymbolia (stref″o-sim-bo′le-ah) 1. a perceptual disorder in which objects seem reversed as in a mirror. 2. a reading difficulty with confusion between similar but oppositely oriented letters (b-d, q-p) and a tendency to read backward.

strepogenin (strep″o-jen′in) a factor in casein and certain other proteins which is essential to optimal growth of animals.

strepto- word element [Gr.], *twisted.*

Streptobacillus (strep″to-bah-sil′lus) a genus of gram-negative bacteria (family Bacteroidaceae) said to be made up of pleomorphic bacteria; *S. monilifor′mis* is a cause of Haverhill fever.

streptobacillus (-bah-sil′lus), pl. *streptobacil′li.* 1. a rod-shaped bacterium remaining loosely attached end-to-end in long chains as a result of failure of daughter cells to separate after cell division. 2. an organism of the genus *Streptobacillus.*

streptococcemia (-kok-se′me-ah) occurrence of streptococci in the blood.

Streptococcus (-kok′us) a genus of gram-positive bacteria (tribe Streptococceae), separable into four groups: pyogenic, viridans, enterococcus, and lactic; the first includes the β-hemolytic human and animal pathogens, the second and third include α-hemolytic parasites occurring as normal flora in the upper respiratory and intestinal tracts, respectively, and the fourth consisting of saprophytes associated with souring of milk. **S. pyog′enes,** β-hemolytic, toxigenic streptococci causing septic sore throat, scarlet fever, rheumatic fever, puerperal fever, acute glomerulonephritis, and other conditions in man.

streptococcus (-kok′us), pl. *streptococ′ci* [Gr.] an organism of the genus *Streptococcus.* **streptococ′cal, streptococ′cic,** adj. **hemolytic s.,** any streptococcus capable of hemolyzing erythrocytes, classified as *α-hemolytic* or *viridans type,* producing a zone of greenish discoloration much smaller than the clear zone produced by the β type about the colony on blood agar; and the *β-hemolytic type,* producing a clear zone of hemolysis immediately around the colony on blood agar. The most virulent streptococci belong to the latter group.

streptodornase (-dor′nās) an enzyme produced by hemolytic streptococci which catalyzes the depolymerization of DNA.

streptokinase (-ki′nās) an enzyme produced by streptococci which catalyzes the conversion of plasminogen to plasmin. **s.-streptodornase,** a mixture of enzymes elaborated by hemolytic streptococci; used as a proteolytic and fibrinolytic agent.

streptolysin (strep-tol′ĭ-sin) the hemolysin of hemolytic streptococci.

Streptomyces (strep″to-mi′sēz) a genus of bacteria (order Actinomycetales), usually soil forms, but occasionally parasitic on plants and animals, and notable as the source of various antibiotics, e.g., the tetracyclines.

streptomycin (-mi′sin) an antibiotic produced by *Streptomyces griseus;* used chiefly in the treatment of tuberculosis.

streptonigrin (-ni′grin) an antineoplastic antibiotic produced by *Streptomyces flocculus.*

streptosepticemia (-sep″tĭ-se′me-ah) septicemia due to streptococci.

stress (stres) 1. forcibly exerted influence; pressure; in dentistry, the pressure of the upper teeth against the lower in mastication. 2. the sum of all nonspecific biological phenomena elicited by adverse external influences, including damage and defense.

stretcher (strech′er) a contrivance for carrying the sick or wounded.

stria (stri′ah), pl. *stri′ae* [L.] 1. a streak or line. 2. a narrow bandlike structure; in anatomy, a general term for longitudinal collections of nerve fibers in the brain. **acoustic striae,** striae medullares ventriculi quarti. **atrophic striae, stri′ae atroph′icae,** atrophic, pinkish or purplish, scarlike lesions, later becoming white (*lineae albicantes*), on the breasts, thighs, abdomen, and buttocks, due to weakening of elastic tissues, associated with pregnancy (*striae gravidarum*), overweight, rapid growth during puberty and adolescence, Cushing's syndrome, and topical or prolonged treatment with corticosteroids. **stri'ae gravida'rum,** see *atrophic striae.* **s. longitudina'lis latera'lis,** either of two slender bands of myelinated fibers across the upper aspect of each half of the corpus callosum. **stri'ae medulla'res,** bundles of white fibers across the floor of the fourth ventricle.

striate, striated (stri'āt; stri'āt-ed) having stripes or striae.

striation (stri-a'shun) 1. the quality of being marked by stripes or striae. 2. a streak or scratch, or a series of streaks.

Striatran (stri'ah-tran) trademark for a preparation of emylcamate.

striatum (stri-a'tum) corpus striatum. **stria'tal,** adj.

stricture (strik'chur) an abnormal narrowing of a duct or passage.

stridor (stri'dor) a harsh, high-pitched respiratory sound. **strid'ulous,** adj. **laryngeal s.,** that due to laryngeal obstruction. A *congenital* form, marked by stridor and dyspnea, is due to an infolding of a congenitally flabby epiglottis and aryepiglottic folds during inspiration; it is usually outgrown by two years of age.

striocerebellar (stri″o-ser″ĕ-bel'ar) pertaining to the corpus striatum and cerebellum.

strip (strip) 1. to press the contents from a canal, such as the urethra or a blood vessel, by running the finger along it. 2. to excise lengths of large veins and incompetent tributaries by subcutaneous dissection and the use of a stripper.

strobila (stro-bi'lah), pl. *strobi'lae* [L., Gr.] the chain of proglottids constituting the bulk of the body of adult tapeworms; considered by some to comprise the entire body, including the head, neck, and proglottids.

stroboscope (stro'bo-skōp) an apparatus for exhibiting the successive phases of animal movements. **stroboscop'ic,** adj.

stroke (strōk) a sudden and severe attack; see *stroke syndrome.* **apoplectic s.,** apoplexy (1). **heat s.,** a condition due to excessive exposure to heat, with dry skin, vertigo, headache, thirst, nausea, and muscular cramps; the body temperature may be dangerously elevated.

stroma (stro'mah), pl. *stro'mata* [Gr.] the supporting tissue or matrix of an organ. **stro'mal, stromat'ic,** adj.

stromuhr (strōm'oor) an instrument for measuring the velocity of blood flow.

Strongyloides (stron″jĭ-loi'dēz) a genus of widely distributed nematodes parasitic in the intestine of man and other mammals, including *S. stercora'lis,* found in the tropics and subtropics, where they cause diarrhea and intestinal ulceration.

strongyloidiasis (stron″jĭ-loi-di'ah-sis) infection with *Strongyloides stercoralis.*

strongyloidosis (-do'sis) strongyloidiasis.

strongylosis (stron″jĭ-lo'sis) infection with *Strongylus.*

Strongylus (stron'jĭ-lus) a genus of nematode parasites.

strontium (stron'she-um) chemical element (*see table*), at. no. 38, symbol Sr.

strophanthin (stro-fan'thin) a glycoside or a mixture of steroidal glycosides from the shrub *Strophanthus kombé;* used as a cardiotonic of rapid onset and short duration.

strophulus (strof'u-lus) papular urticaria.

struma (stroo'mah) goiter. **Hashimoto's s., s. lymphomato'sa,** a progressive disease of the thyroid gland with degeneration of its epithelial elements and replacement by lymphoid and fibrous tissue. **s. malig'na,** carcinoma of the thyroid gland. **s. ova'rii,** a teratoid ovarian tumor composed of thyroid tissue. **Riedel's s.,** a chronic, proliferating, fibrosing, inflammatory process involving usually one but sometimes both lobes of the thyroid gland, as well as the trachea and other adjacent structures.

strumectomy (stroo-mek'to-me) excision of a goiter.

strumitis (stroo-mi'tis) thyroiditis.

strychnine (strik'nīn) a very poisonous alkaloid, $C_{21}H_{22}N_2O_2$, obtained chiefly from *Strychnos nux-vomica* and other species of *Strychnos.*

S.T.S. serologic test for syphilis.

stump (stump) the distal end of a limb left after amputation.

stupe (stoōp) a hot, wet cloth or sponge, charged with a medication for external application.

stupefacient (stu″pĕ-fa'shent) 1. inducing stupor. 2. an agent that induces stupor.

stupefactive (-fak'tiv) producing narcosis or stupor.

stupor (stu'por) partial or nearly complete unconsciousness; in psychiatry, a disorder marked by reduced responsiveness.

stuttering (stut'er-ing) a speech problem characterized chiefly by spasmodic repetition of sounds, especially of initial consonants, and by prolongation of sounds and hesitation.

sty, stye (sti) pl. *sties, styes.* Hordeolum.

styl(o)- word element [L., Gr.], *stake; pole; styloid process of the temporal bone.*

stylet (sti'let) 1. a wire run through a catheter or cannula to render it stiff or to remove debris from its lumen. 2. a slender probe.

stylohyoid (sti″lo-hi'oid) pertaining to the styloid process and hyloid bone.

styloid (sti'loid) resembling a pillar; long and pointed; relating to the styloid process.

styloiditis (sti″loi-di'tis) inflammation of tissues around the styloid process.

stylomastoid (sti″lo-mas'toid) pertaining to the styloid and mastoid processes of the temporal bone.

stylomaxillary (-mak'sĭ-ler″e) pertaining to the styloid process of the temporal bone and the maxilla.

stylus (sti'lus) 1. stylet. 2. a pencil-shaped medicinal preparation, as of caustic.

stype (stīp) a tampon or pledget of cotton.

stypsis (stip'sis) 1. astringency; astringent action. 2. use of styptics.

styptic (stip'tik) 1. astringent; arresting hemorrhage by means of an astringent quality. 2. an astringent and hemostatic agent.

Stypven (stip'ven) trademark for a preparation of Russell's viper venom.

styramate (stir'ah-māt) a skeletal muscle relaxant, $C_9H_{11}NO_3$.

styrol (sti'rol) a liquid hydrocarbon from storax, or synthesized from benzene and ethylene.

Suavitil (swav'ĭ-til) trademark for a preparation of benactyzine.

sub- word element [L.], *under; near; almost; moderately.*

subabdominal (sub"ab-dom'ĭ-nal) below the abdomen.

subacetate (sub-as'ĕ-tāt) a basic acetate.

subacid (-as'id) somewhat acid.

subacromial (sub"ah-kro'me-al) below the acromion.

subacute (-ah-kūt) somewhat acute; between acute and chronic.

subalimentation (sub-al"ĭ-men-ta'shun) insufficient nourishment.

subaponeurotic (-ap"o-nu-rot'ik) below an aponeurosis.

subarachnoid (sub"ah-rak'noid) between the arachnoid and the pia mater.

subareolar (-ah-re'o-lar) beneath the areola of the nipple.

subastragalar (-as-trag'ah-lar) below the astragalus.

subastringent (-ah-strin'jent) moderately astringent.

subatomic (-ah-tom'ik) of or pertaining to the constituent parts of an atom.

subaural (sub-aw'ral) below the ear.

subaurale (sub"aw-ra'le) the lowest point on the inferior border of the ear lobule when the subject is looking straight ahead.

subcapsular (sub-kap'su-lar) below a capsule, especially the capsule of the cerebrum.

subcarbonate (-kar'bon-āt) a basic carbonate.

subcartilaginous (-kar"tĭ-laj'ĭ-nus) 1. below a cartilage. 2. partly cartilaginous.

subchronic (-kron'ik) between chronic and subacute.

subclavian (-kla've-an) below the clavicle.

subclavicular (sub"klah-vik'u-lar) subclavian.

subclinical (sub-klin'ĭ-kal) without clinical manifestations.

subconjunctival (sub"kon-jungk-ti'val) beneath the conjunctiva.

subconscious (sub-kon'shus) 1. imperfectly or partially conscious. 2. preconscious.

subconsciousness (-kon'shus-nes) 1. partial unconsciousness. 2. the area of mental activity below the level of conscious perception.

subcoracoid (-kor'ah-koid) situated under the coracoid process.

subcortex (-kor'teks) the brain substance underlying the cortex. **subcor'tical,** adj.

subcostal (-kos'tal) below a rib or ribs.

subcranial (-kra'ne-al) below the cranium.

subcrepitant (-krep'ĭ-tant) somewhat crepitant in nature; said of a rale.

subculture (-kul'chur) a culture of bacteria derived from another culture.

subcutaneous (sub"ku-ta'ne-us) beneath the skin.

subcuticular (-ku-tik'u-lar) subepidermal.

subdelirium (-dĕ-lir'e-um) mild delirium.

subdiaphragmatic (sub-di"ah-frag-mat'ik) below the diaphragm.

subduct (-dukt') to draw down.

subdural (-du'ral) between the dura mater and the arachnoid.

subendocardial (sub"en-do-kar'de-al) beneath the endocardium.

subendothelial (-en-do-the'le-al) beneath the endothelium.

subepidermal (ep-ĭ-der'mal) beneath the epidermis.

subepithelial (-ep-ĭ-the'le-al) beneath the epithelium.

subfamily (sub-fam'ĭ-le) a taxonomic division between a family and a tribe.

subfascial (-fash'al) beneath a fascia.

subgenus (-je'nus) a taxonomic category between a genus and a species.

subglenoid (-gle'noid) beneath the glenoid fossa.

subglossal (-glos'al) below the tongue.

subgrondation (sub"gron-da'shun) depression of one fragment of bone beneath another.

subhepatic (-hĕ-pat'ik) below the liver.

subhyoid (sub-hi'oid) below the hyoid bone.

subiculum (su-bik'u-lum) an underlying or supporting structure.

subiliac (sub-il'e-ak) below the ilium.

subilium (-il'e-um) the lowest portion of the ilium.

subinvolution (sub"in-vol-lu'shun) incomplete involution.

subiodide (sub-i'o-dīd) that iodide of any series containing the least iodine.

subjacent (-ja'sent) located beneath.

subject (sub'jekt) 1. a person or animal subjected to treatment, observation, or experiment. 2. a body for dissection.

subjective (sub-jek'tiv) perceived only by the affected individual and not by the examiner.

subjugal (-ju'gal) below the zygomatic bone.

sublatio retinae (-la'she-o ret'ĭ-ne) detachment of the retina.

sublethal (-le'thal) insufficient to cause death.

sublimate (sub'lĭ-māt) 1. a substance obtained by sublimation. 2. to accomplish sublimation.

sublimation (sub"lĭ-ma'shun) 1. the conversion of a solid directly into the gaseous state. 2. a mental mechanism operating outside of conscious awareness by which consciously unacceptable instinctual drives are expressed in personally and socially acceptable channels.

sublime (sub-līm') to volatilize a solid body by heat and then to collect it in a purified form as a solid or powder.

subliminal (-lim'ĭ-nal) below the threshold of sensation or conscious awareness.

sublingual (-ling'gwal) beneath the tongue.

sublinguitis (sub"ling-gwi'tis) inflammation of the sublingual gland.

subluxation (-luk-sa'shun) incomplete or partial dislocation.

submammary (sub-mam′ar-e) below the mammary gland.

submandibular (sub″man-dib′u-lar) below the mandible.

submaxilla (-mak-sil′ah) the mandible.

submaxillaritis (-mak-sĭ-lar-i′tis) inflammation of the submaxillary gland.

submaxillary (sub-mak′sĭ-ler″e) below the maxilla.

submental (-men′tal) beneath the chin.

submetacentric (-met″ah-sen′trik) having the centromere almost, but not quite, at the metacentric position.

submicron (-mi′kron) a colloidal particle visible with only the ultramicroscope.

submicroscopic (-mi″kro-skop′ik) too small to be visible with the miscroscope.

submorphous (-mor′fus) neither amorphous nor perfectly crystalline.

submucosa (sub″mu-ko′sah) areolar tissue situated beneath a mucous membrane.

submucous (sub-mu′kus) beneath a mucous membrane.

subnarcotic (sub″nar-kot′ik) moderately narcotic.

subnasale (-na-sa′le) the point at which the nasal septum merges, in the midsagittal plane, with the upper lip.

subneural (sub-nu′ral) beneath a nerve.

subnormal (-nor′mal) below normal.

subnormality (sub″nor-mal′ĭ-te) the state of being below normal.

subnucleus (sub-nu′kle-us) a partial or secondary nucleus.

suboccipital (sub″ok-sip′ĭ-tal) below the occiput.

suborbital (sub-or′bĭ-tal) beneath the orbit.

suborder (-or′der) a taxonomic category between an order and a family.

suboxide (-ok′sīd) that oxide in any series which contains the least oxygen.

subpapular (-pap′u-lar) indistinctly papular.

subpatellar (sub″pah-tel′ar) below the patella.

subpericardial (-per-ĭ-kar′de-al) beneath the pericardium.

subperiosteal (-per-e-os′te-al) beneath the periosteum.

subperitoneal (-per-ĭ-to-ne′al) beneath or deep to the peritoneum.

subpharyngeal (-fah-rin′je-al) beneath the pharynx.

subphrenic (sub-fren′ik) beneath the diaphragm.

subphylum (-fi′lum) a taxonomic category between a phylum and a class.

subplacenta (sub″plah-sen′tah) the decidua basalis.

subpleural (sub-ploor′al) beneath the pleura.

subpreputial (sub″pre-pu′shal) beneath the prepuce.

subpubic (sub-pu′bik) beneath the pubic bone.

subpulmonary (-pul′mo-nar″e) beneath the lung.

subretinal (-ret′ĭ-nal) beneath the retina.

subscapular (-skap′u-lar) below the scapula.

subscription (-skrip′shun) that part of a prescription giving the directions for compounding the ingredients.

subserous (-se′rus) beneath a serous membrane.

subspecies (sub′spe-sēz) a taxonomic category subordinate to a species, differing morphologically from others of the species but capable of interbreeding with them; a variety or race.

subspinale (sub″spi-na′le) point A.

substage (sub′stāj) the part of the microscope underneath the stage.

substance (sub′stans) material constituting an organ or body. α-**s.**, **alpha s.**, reticular s. β-**s.**, **beta s.**, Heinz bodies. **black s.**, substantia nigra. **cement s.**, material that holds different components of tissue together, as the intercellular substance in endothelium. **chromophil s.**, Nissl bodies. **depressor s.**, a substance that tends to decrease activity or blood pressure. **gray s.**, the gray nerve tissue composed of nerve cell bodies, unmyelinated nerve fibers, and supporting tissue. **ground s.**, the gel-like material in which connective tissue cells and fibers are embedded. **interstitial s.**, ground s. **medullary s.**, 1. the white matter of the central nervous system, consisting of axons and their myelin sheaths. 2. the soft, marrow-like substance of the interior of an organ. **Nissl s.**, see under *body*. **perforated s.**, 1. *anterior perforated s.*, an area anterolateral to each optic tract, pierced by branches of the anterior and middle cerebral arteries. 2. *posterior perforated s.*, an area between the cerebral peduncles, pierced by branches of the posterior cerebral arteries. **prelipid s.**, degenerated nerve tissue which has not yet been converted into fat. **pressor s.**, any substance that raises blood pressure. **reticular s.**, the netlike mass of threads seen in red blood cells after vital staining. **Rolando's gelatinous s.**, substantia gelatinosa. **sensibilizing s.**, **sensitizing s.**, antibody. **slow-reacting s. (SRS-A)**, a substance released in the anaphylactic reaction that induces slow, prolonged contraction of certain smooth muscles. **threshold s's**, those substances (e.g., glucose) excreted into the urine only when their concentration in plasma exceeds a certain value. **thromboplastic s.**, any substance with procoagulant activity. **tigroid s.**, Nissl bodies. **transmitter s.**, a chemical substance (mediator) which induces activity in an excitable tissue. **white s.**, the white nervous tissue, constituting the conducting portion of the brain and spinal cord, composed mostly of myelinated nerve fibers. **white s. of Schwann,** myelin (1). **zymoplastic s.**, thromboplastic s.

substantia (sub-stan′she-ah), pl. *substan′tiae* [L.] substance. **s. al′ba**, white substance. **s. ferrugin′ea**, locus ceruleus. **s. gelatino′sa**, the gelatinous-appearing cap forming the dorsal part of the posterior horn of the spinal cord. **s. gris′ea**, gray substance. **s. ni′gra**, the layer of gray substance separating the tegmentum of the midbrain from the crus cerebri. **s. pro′pria**, 1. the tough, fibrous, transparent main part of the cornea, between Bowman's membrane and Descemet's membrane. 2. the main part of the sclera, between the episcleral lamina and the lamina fusca.

substernal (sub-ster′nal) below the sternum.

substitution (sub″stĭ-tu′shun) 1. the act of putting one thing in place of another, especially the chemical replacement of one substance by another. 2. a defense mechanism, operating unconsciously, in which an unattainable or unacceptable goal, emotion, or object is replaced by one that is attainable or acceptable.

substrate (sub′strāt) a substance upon which an enzyme acts.

substructure (-struk-chur) the underlying or supporting portion of an organ or appliance; that portion of an implant denture embedded in the tissues of the jaw.

subsylvian (sub-sil′ve-an) situated deep in the lateral sulcus (sylvian fissure).

subtarsal (-tar′sal) below the tarsus.

subtentorial (sub″ten-to′re-al) beneath the tentorium of the cerebellum.

subthalamic (-thah-lam′ik) pertaining to the subthalamus.

subthalamus (sub-thal′ah-mus) the portion of the diencephalon between the thalamus and the tegmentum of the mesencephalon.

subtilin (sub′til-in) an antibiotic isolated from *Bacillus subtilis*, chiefly effective against gram-positive bacteria and certain acid-fast bacilli.

subtribe (-trīb) a taxonomic category between a tribe and a genus.

subtrochanteric (sub″tro-kan-ter′ik) below the trochanter.

subungual (sub-ung′gwal) beneath a nail.

suburethral (sub″u-re′thral) beneath the urethra.

subvaginal (sub-vaj′ĭ-nal) under a sheath, or below the vagina.

subvertebral (-ver′tĕ-bral) on the ventral side of the vertebrae.

subvirile (-vir′il) having deficient virility.

subvolution (sub″vo-lu′shun) the operation of turning over a flap to prevent adhesions.

Sucaryl (soo′kah-ril) trademark for preparations of calcium cyclamate and sodium cyclamate.

succenturiate (suk″sen-tu′re-at) accessory; serving as a substitute.

succinate (suk′sĭ-nāt) any salt of succinic acid.

succinylcholine (suk″sĭ-nil-ko′lēn) a skeletal muscle relaxant, $C_{14}H_{30}N_2O_4$, used as the chloride salt.

succinylsulfathiazole (-sul″fah-thi′ah-zōl) an intestinal antibacterial, $C_{13}H_{13}N_3O_5S_2$.

succorrhea (suk″o-re′ah) excessive flow of a natural secretion.

succus (suk′us), pl. *suc′ci* [L.] any fluid derived from a living tissue; juice. **s. enter′icus,** intestinal juice. **s. gas′tricus,** gastric juice. **s. pancreat′icus,** pancreatic juice. **s. prostat′icus,** prostatic juice.

succussion (sŭ-kush′un) a procedure in which the body is shaken, a splashing sound being indicative of the presence of fluid and air in a body cavity.

Sucostrin (su-kos′trin) trademark for a preparation of succinylcholine.

sucrase (soo′krās) β-fructofuranosidase.

sucrose (soo′krōs) a disaccharide, $C_{12}H_{22}O_{11}$, from sugar cane, sugar beet, or other sources; used as a food and sweetening agent.

sucrosuria (soo″kro-su′re-ah) sucrose in the urine.

suction (suk′shun) aspiration of gas or fluid by mechanical means. **post-tussive s.,** a sucking sound heard over a lung cavity just after a cough.

Suctoria (suk-to′re-ah) a class of protozoa (subphylum Ciliophora) whose members possess cilia only during the larval stage, the mature organism having suctorial tentacles that serve as locomotor and food-acquiring mechanisms; most are free-living, but some are parasites of other ciliates, of other protozoa, and of mammals.

suctorial (suk-to′re-al) adapted for sucking.

suctorian (suk-to′re-an) 1. any individual of the Suctoria. 2. of or pertaining to the Suctoria.

Sudafed (soo′dah-fed) trademark for preparations of pseudoephedrine.

sudamen (su-da′men), pl. *sudam′ina* [L.] a whitish vesicle caused by retention of sweat in the horny layer of the skin.

Sudan (su-dan′) a group of azo compounds used as biological stains for fats.

sudanophilia (su-dan″o-fil′e-ah) affinity for Sudan stain. **sudanophil′ic,** adj.

sudation (su-da′shun) the process of sweating.

sudatorium (su″dah-to′re-um), pl. *sudato′ria* [L.] 1. a hot air bath. 2. a room for the administration of hot air baths.

sudomotor (su″do-mo′tor) stimulating the sweat glands.

sudor (su′dor) sweat; perspiration.

sudoresis (su″do-re′sis) diaphoresis.

sudoriferous (-rif′er-us) 1. conveying sweat. 2. sudoriparous.

sudorific (-rif′ik) 1. promoting sweating; diaphoretic. 2. an agent that causes sweating.

sudoriparous (-rip′ah-rus) secreting or producing sweat.

suet (su′et) the fat from the abdominal cavity of ruminants, especially the sheep or ox, used in preparing cerates and ointments and as an emollient; the pharmaceutical preparation (*prepared s.*) is obtained from sheep.

suffocation (suf″ŏ-ka′shun) asphyxiation; the stoppage of respiration, or the asphyxia that results from it.

suffusion (sŭ-fu′zhun) 1. the process of overspreading, or diffusion. 2. the condition of being moistened or of being permeated through, as by blood.

sugar (shoog′ar) a sweet carbohydrate of both animal and vegatable origin, the two principal groups of which are the disaccharides and the monosaccharides. **beet s.,** sucrose obtained from the sugar beet. **cane s.,** sucrose from sugar cane. **fruit s.,** fructose. **grape s.,** dextrose. **invert s.,** mixture of dextrose and fructose. **liver s.,** dextrose from the liver. **malt s.,** maltose. **milk s.,** lactose. **muscle s.,** inositol. **starch s.,** dextrin. **wood s.,** xylose.

suggestibility (sug-jes″tĭ-bil′ĭ-te) susceptibility to suggestion. **sugges′tible,** adj.

suggestion (sug-jes′chun) 1. impartation of an idea to a individual from without. 2. an idea introduced from without. **posthypnotic s.,** implantation in the mind of a subject during hypnosis of a suggestion to be acted upon after recovery from the hypnotic state.

suggillation (sug″jĭ-la′shun) an ecchymosis.

suicide (soo′ĭ-sīd) the taking of one's own life.

Sulamyd (sul′am-id) trademark for a preparation of sulfacetamide.

sulcate (sul′kāt) furrowed; marked with sulci.

sulcus (sul′kus), pl. *sul′ci*[L.] a groove, trench, or furrow; in anatomy, a general term for such a depression, especially one on the brain surface, separating the gyri. **calcarine s.,** a sulcus of the medial surface of the occipital lobe, separating the cuneus from the lingual gyrus. **central s.,** one between the frontal and parietal lobes of the cerebral hemisphere. **cingulate s.,** one on the median surface of the hemisphere midway between the corpus callosum and the margin of the surface. **collateral s.,** one on the inferior surface of the cerebral hemisphere between the fusiform and parahippocampal gyri. **sul′ci cu′tis,** fine depressions of the skin between the ridges of the skin. **gingival s.,** the groove between the surface of the tooth and the epithelium lining the free gingiva. **hippocampal s.,** one extending from the splenium of the corpus callosum almost to the tip of the temporal lobe. **intraparietal s.,** one separating the parietal gyri. **lateral cerebral s.,** fissure of Sylvius. **s. of matrix of nail,** the skin fold in which the proximal part of the nail is embedded. **parieto-occipital s.,** 1. one marking the boundary between the cuneus and precuneus, and also between the parietal and occipital lobes of the cerebral hemisphere. 2. intraparietal s. **posterior median s.,** 1. a shallow vertical groove in the closed part of the medulla oblongata, continuous with the posterior median sulcus of the spinal cord. 2. a shallow vertical groove dividing the spinal cord throughout its whole length in the midline posteriorly. **precentral s.,** one separating the precentral gyrus from the remainder of the frontal lobe. **scleral s.,** a slight groove on the outer surface of the eyeball, at the junction of the sclera and cornea.

sulfacetamide (sul″fah-set′ah-mīd) an antibacterial sulfonamide, $C_8H_{10}N_2O_3S$, used in urinary tract infections; the sodium salt is used topically in ophthalmic infections.

sulfacytine (-si′tēn) a rapidly excreted, oral sulfonamide used in treatment of acute urinary tract infections.

sulfadiazine (-di′ah-zēn) an antibacterial sulfonamide, $C_{10}H_{10}N_4O_2S$, often used in combination with other sulfonamides; the sodium salt is used in solution for intravenous administration.

sulfadimethoxine (-di″mĕ-thoks′ēn) a long-acting sulfonamide, $C_{12}H_{14}N_4O_4S$.

sulfaethidole (-eth′ĭ-dōl) an antibacterial sulfonamide, $C_{10}H_{12}N_4O_2S_2$.

sulfaguanidine (-gwahn′ĭ-dēn) an antibacterial sulfonamide, $C_7H_{10}N_4O_2S$; used in infections of the gastrointestinal tract.

sulfamerazine (-mer′ah-zēn) an antibacterial sulfonamide, $C_{11}H_{12}N_4O_2S$, usually used in combination with other sulfonamides.

sulfameter (sul′fah-me″ter) a long-acting sulfonamide, $C_{11}H_{12}N_4O_3S$, used in urinary tract infections.

sulfamethazine (sul″fah-meth′ah-zēn) a readily acetylated antibacterial sulfonamide, $C_{12}H_{14}$-N_4O_2S; usually used in combination with other sulfonamides.

sulfamethizole (-meth′ĭ-zōl) an antibacterial sulfonamide, $C_9H_{10}N_4O_2S_2$, used mainly in urinary tract infections.

sulfamethoxazole (-meth-ok′sah-zōl) an antibacterial sulfonamide, $C_{10}H_{11}N_3O_3S$, especially useful in acute urinary tract infections and pyodermata and in infections of wounds and soft tissues.

sulfamethoxypyridazine (-meth-ok″se-pi-rid′-ah-zēn) an antibacterial sulfonamide, $C_{11}H_{12}$-N_4O_3S, used in urinary tract and other infections.

sulfamethyldiazine (-meth″il-di′ah-zēn) sulfamerazine.

sulfamethylthiadiazole (-thi″ah-di′ah-zōl) sulfamethizole.

Sulfamezathine (sul″fah-mez′ah-thēn) trademark for a preparation of sulfamethazine.

Sulfamylon (-mi′lon) trademark for preparations of mafenide.

sulfanilamide (-nil′ah-mīd) a potent antibacterial compound, the first of the sulfonamides discovered.

sulfanilate (sul-fan′ĭ-lāt) a salt of sulfanilic acid.

sulfapyridine (sul″fah-pir′ĭ-dēn) a sulfonamide, $C_{11}H_{11}N_3O_2S$, used as a suppressant in dermatitis herpetiformis.

sulfasalazine (-sal′ah-zēn) a combination of sulfapyridine and salicylic acid used in the treatment and prophylaxis of ulcerative colitis.

Sulfasuxidine (-suk′sĭ-dēn) trademark for preparations of succinylsulfathiazole.

sulfatase (sul′fah-tās) an enzyme which catalyzes the hydrolysis of sulfate esters.

sulfate (sul′fāt) a salt of sulfuric acid. **acid s.,** a bisulfate; one in which only half of the hydrogen of sulfuric acid is replaced. **cupric s.,** a crystalline salt of copper used as an emetic, astringent, and fungicide. **ferrous s.,** an iron-containing compound used in treatment of iron deficiency anemia.

Sulfathalidine (sul″fah-thal′ĭ-dēn) trademark for phthalylsulfathiazole.

sulfatide (sul′fah-tīd) any of a class of cerebroside sulfuric esters.

sulfhemoglobin (sulf″he-mo-glo′bin) sulfmethemoglobin.

sulfhemoglobinemia (-glo″bin-e′me-ah) sulfmethemoglobin in the blood.

sulfhydryl (sulf-hi′dril) the univalent radical, —SH.

sulfide (sul′fīd) any binary compound of sulfur; a compound of sulfur with another element or radical or base.

sulfinpyrazone (sul″fin-pi′rah-zōn) a uricosuric agent, $C_{23}H_{20}N_2O_3S$, used in the treatment of gout.

sulfisomidine (sul″fi-som′ĭ-dēn) a structural isomer of sulfamethazine, $C_{12}H_{14}N_4O_2S$, used in systemic and urinary tract infections.

sulfisoxazole (-sok′sah-zōl) an antibacterial sulfonamide, $C_{11}H_{13}N_3O_3S$, used in infections of the urinary and respiratory tracts and of soft tissues.

sulfite (sul′fīt) any salt of sulfurous acid.

sulfmethemoglobin (sulf″met-he″mo-glo′bin) a greenish substance formed by treating the blood with hydrogen sulfide or by absorption of this gas from the intestinal tract.

sulfobromophthalein (sul″fo-bro″mo-thal′e-in) a sulfur- and bromine-containing compound used as the disodium salt in liver function tests.

sulfonamide (sul-fon′ah-mīd) the chemical group SO_2NH_2; the sulfonamides are a group of compounds with one or more benzene rings, amino groups, and a sulfonamide group, including antibacterial drugs closely related to sulfanilamide.

sulfone (sul′fōn) 1. the radical SO_2. 2. any compound containing two hydrocarbon radicals attached to the radical SO_2.

sulfonethylmethane (sul″fōn-eth″il-meth′ān) a hypnotic, $(C_2H_5)(CH_3)C(SO_2C_2H_5)_2$.

sulfoxide (sul-fok′sīd) 1. the divalent radical $=SO$. 2. any of a group of compounds intermediate between the sulfides and the sulfones.

sulfoxone (sul-fok′sōn) a dapsone derivative; its sodium salt is used as a leprostatic and dermatitis herpetiformis suppressant.

sulfur (sul′fer) chemical element (*see table*), at. no. 16, symbol S. **s. dioxide**, a colorless, noninflammable gas, SO_2, used as an antioxidant in pharmaceutical preparations; a dry form is used as an insecticide and rodenticide. **s. lo′tum**, washed s. **precipitated s.**, a fine, pale yellow powder used in an ointment as a scabicide. **sublimed s.**, a fine yellow crystalline powder; used as a scabicide and parasiticide. **washed s.**, sublimed sulfur purified by washing with water.

sulfurated (sul′fu-rāt″ed) combined or charged with sulfur.

sulph- for words beginning thus, see those beginning *sulf-*.

Sul-Spansion (sul-span′shun) trademark for a suspension of sulfaethidole.

sumac (su′mak) name of various trees and shrubs of the genus *Rhus.* **poison s.**, a species, *Rhus vernix*, which causes an itching rash on contact with the skin.

summation (sum-ma′shun) the cumulative effect of a number of stimuli applied to a muscle, nerve, or reflex arc.

sunburn (sun′bern) injury to the skin, with erythema, tenderness, and sometimes blistering, after excessive exposure to sunlight, produced by unfiltered ultraviolet rays.

sunstroke (-strōk) a condition caused by excessive exposure to the sun, marked by high skin temperature, convulsions, and coma.

super- word element [L.], *above; excessive.*

superalimentation (su″per-al″ĭ-men-ta′shun) treatment of wasting diseases by feeding beyond appetite requirements.

superalkalinity (-al″kah-lin′ĭ-te) excessive alkalinity.

supercilia (-sil′e-ah) [pl., L.] the hairs on the arching protrusion over either eye.

supercilium (-sil′e-um) [sing., L.] eyebrow; the transverse elevation at the junction of the forehead and upper eyelid. **supercil′iary,** adj.

superclass (su′per-klas) a taxonomic category between a phylum and a class.

superego (su″per-e′go) a part of the psyche derived from both the id and the ego, which acts, largely unconsciously, as a monitor over the ego; the conscience.

superexcitation (-ek″si-ta′shun) extreme or excessive excitement.

superfamily (-fam′ĭ-le) a taxonomic category between an order and a family.

superfecundation (-fe″kun-da′shun) fertilization of two ova, liberated at the same time, by sperm of different fathers.

superfetation (-fe-ta′shun) fertilization and subsequent development of a ovum when a fetus is already present in the uterus.

superficial (-fish′al) situated on or near the surface.

superficialis (-fish″e-a′lis) [L.] superficial.

superficies (-fish′e-ēz) an outer surface.

superinduce (-indūs′) to bring on in addition to an already existing condition.

superinfection (-in-fek′shun) a new infection complicating the course of antimicrobial therapy of an existing infection, due to invasion by bacteria or fungi resistant to the drug(s) in use.

superinvolution (-in″vo-lu′shun) prolonged involution of the uterus, after delivery, to a size much smaller than the normal, occurring in nursing mothers.

superior (su-pe′rĭ-or) situated above, or directed upward.

superjacent (su″per-ja′sent) located just above.

superlactation (-lak-ta′shun) hyperlactation.

supermotility (-mo-til′ĭ-te) excess of motility.

supernatant (-na′tant) the liquid lying above a layer of precipitated insoluble material.

supernumerary (-nu′mer-ar″e) in excess of the regular or normal number.

supernutrition (-nu-trish′un) excessive nutrition.

superolateral (-o-lat′er-al) above and to the side.

superphosphate (-fos′fāt) an acid phosphate.

supersaturate (-sat′u-rāt) to add more of an ingredient than can be held in solution permanently.

superscription (-skrip′shun) the heading of a prescription, i.e., the symbol ℞ or the word Recipe, meaning "take."

supersonic (-son′ik) 1. traveling faster than the speed of sound. 2. ultrasonic.

superstructure (-struk′chur) the overlying or visible portion of an appliance.

supertension (-ten′shun) extreme tension.

supervoltage (su′per-vol″tij) very high voltage; in x-ray therapy, generally considered to be in the range of 1 to 2 million volts.

supinate (su′pĭ-nāt) the act of turning the palm forward or upward, or of raising the medial margin of the foot.

supination (su″pĭ-na′shun) the act of supinating.

supine (su′pīn) lying with the face upward, or on the dorsal surface.

suppository (sŭ-poz′ĭ-to″re) an easily fusible medicated mass to be introduced into a body orifice, as the rectum, urethra, or vagina. **glycerin s.,** one made up of a mixture of glycerin and sodium stearate; used as a rectal evacuant.

suppressant (sŭ-pres′sant) 1. inducing suppression. 2. an agent that stops secretion, excretion, or normal discharge.

suppression (sŭ-presh′un) 1. sudden stoppage of a secretion, excretion, or normal discharge. 2. conscious inhibition as contrasted with repression, which is unconscious. 3. in genetics, restoration of a lost function by a second mutation either in a gene other than that involved in the primary mutation, or within the same gene.

suppurant (sup′u-rant) 1. promoting suppuration. 2. an agent that causes suppuration.

suppuration (sup″u-ra′shun) formation or discharge of pus. **sup′purative,** adj.

supra- word element [L.], *above; over.*

supra-acromial (su″prah-ah-kro′me-al) above the acromion.

supra-auricular (-aw-rik′u-lar) above the auricle of the ear.

suprabulge (su′prah-bulj) the surfaces of a tooth occlusal to the height of contour, or sloping occlusally.

suprachoroid (su″prah-ko′roid) above or upon the choroid.

suprachoroidea (-ko-roi′de-ah) the outermost layer of the choroid.

supraclavicular (-klah-vik′u-lar) above the clavicle.

supraclusion (-kloo′zhun) projection of a tooth beyond the normal occlusal plane.

supracondylar (-kon′dĭ-lar) above a condyle.

supracostal (-kos′tal) above or outside the ribs.

supracotyloid (-kot′ĭ-loid) above the acetabulum.

supradiaphragmatic (-di″ah-frag-mat′ik) above the diaphragm.

supraduction (-duk′shun) sursumduction.

supraepicondylar (-ep″ĭ-kon′dĭ-lar) above an epicondyle.

suprahyoid (-hi′oid) above the hyoid bone.

supraliminal (-lim′ĭ-nal) above the threshold of sensation.

supralumbar (-lum′bar) above the loin.

supramalleolar (-mah-le′o-lar) above a malleolus.

supramaxilla (-mak-sil′ah) maxilla.

supramaxillary (-mak′sĭ-ler″e) 1. pertaining to the upper jaw. 2. above the maxilla.

supramentale (-men-ta′le) point B.

supraocclusion (-o-kloo′zhun) supraclusion.

supraorbital (-or′bĭ-tal) above the orbit.

suprapelvic (-pel′vik) above the pelvis.

suprapontine (-pon′tīn) above or in upper part of the pons.

suprapubic (-pu′bik) above the pubes.

suprarenal (-re′nal) 1. above a kidney. 2. pertaining to the suprarenal gland.

suprarenalectomy (-re″nal-ek′to-me) adrenalectomy; excision of one or both adrenal glands.

suprarenalism (-re′nal-izm) adrenalism.

Suprarenin (-ren′in) trademark for a preparation of epinephrine.

suprascapular (-skap′u-lar) above the scapula.

suprascleral (-skle′ral) on the outer surface of the sclera.

suprasellar (-sel′ar) above the sella turcica.

supraspinal (-spi′nal) above the spine.

suprasternal (-ster′nal) above the sternum.

supratrochlear (-trok′le-ar) above the trochlea.

supravaginal (-vaj′ĭ-nal) outside or above a sheath; specifically, above the vagina.

supraversion (-ver′zhun) abnormal elongation of a tooth from its socket.

sura (su′rah) [L.] calf of the leg. **su′ral,** adj.

suramin (soor′ah-min) an antitrypanosomal and antifilarial agent, $C_{51}H_{34}N_6O_{23}S_6$, used as the sodium salt.

surditas (ser′dĭ-tas) deafness.

Surfacaine (ser′fah-kān) trademark for preparations of cyclomethycaine.

surface (ser′fas) the outer part or external aspect of an object.

surfactant (ser-fak′tant) a surface-active agent, such as soap or a synthetic detergent. In pulmonary physiology, a mixture of lipoproteins (chiefly lecithin and sphingomyelin) secreted by the great alveolar (type II) cells into the alveoli and respiratory air passages, which reduces the surface tension of pulmonary fluids and thus contributes to the elastic properties of pulmonary tissue.

surgeon (ser′jun) 1. a physician who specializes in surgery. 2. the senior medical officer of a military unit.

surgery (ser′jer-e) 1. that branch of medicine which treats diseases, injuries, and deformities by manual or operative methods. 2. the place in a hospital, or doctor's or dentist's office where surgery is performed. 3. in Great Britain, a room or office where a doctor sees and treats patients. 4. the work performed by a surgeon. **sur′gical,** adj. **antiseptic s., aseptic s.,** surgery according to antiseptic or aseptic methods. **conservative s.,** surgery designed to preserve, or to remove with minimal risk, diseased or injured organs, tissues, or extremities. **dental s.,** operative dentistry. **major s.,** surgery involving the more important, difficult, and hazardous operations. **minor s.,** surgery restricted to management of minor problems and injuries. **operative s.,** the operative or mechanical aspect of surgery; that dealing with manual and manipulative methods or procedures. **oral s.,** that branch of medicine which deals with diagnosis and surgical and adjunctive treatment of diseases, injuries, and defects of the mouth, jaws, and associated structures. **orthopedic s.,** orthopedics. **physiologic s.,** the indirect treatment of certain disorders by surgically altering normal physiologic functions. **plastic s.,** surgery concerned with the restoration, reconstruction, correction, or improvement in the shape and appearance of body structures that are defective, damaged, or misshapened by injury, disease, or growth and development. **radical s.,** surgery designed to extirpate all areas of locally extensive disease and adjacent zones of lymphatic drainage. **veterinary s.,** the surgery of domestic animals.

Surital (sur′ĭ-tal) trademark for preparations of thiamylal.

surrogate (sur′o-gāt) a substitute; a thing or person that takes the place of something or someone else, as a drug used in place of another, or a person who takes the place of another in someone's affective existence.

sursumduction (sur″sum-duk′shun) the turning upward of a part, as of the eyes.

sursumvergence (-ver′jens) an upward movement, especially of an eye, the other eye not moving.

sursumversion (-ver′zhun) an act of turning or directing upward, especially the simultaneous and equal upward turning of the eyes.

susceptibility (sŭ-sep″tĭ-bil′ĭ-te) the state of being susceptible.

susceptible (sŭ-sep′tĭ-b′l) readily affected or acted upon; lacking immunity or resistance.

suscitate (sus′ĭ-tāt) to arouse to greater activity.

suscitation (sus″ĭ-ta′shun) arousal to greater activity.

suspension (sus-pen′shun) 1. a condition of temporary cessation, as of animation, of pain, or of any vital process. 2. treatment, chiefly of spinal disorders, by suspending the patient by the chin and the shoulders. 3. a preparation of a finely divided drug intended to be incorporated (suspended) in some suitable liquid vehicle before it is used, or already incorporated in such a vehicle.

suspensoid (sus-pen′soid) a colloid system in which the disperse phase consists of particles of any insoluble substance, as a metal, and the dispersion medium may be gaseous, liquid, or solid.

suspensory (sus-pen′sor-e) 1. serving to hold up a part. 2. a ligament, bone, muscle, sling, or bandage that serves to hold up a part.

sustentaculum (sus″ten-tak′u-lum), pl. *sustentac′uli* [L.] a support. **sustentac′ular,** adj.

susurrus (sŭ-sur′us) [L.] murmur.

sutura (su-tu′rah), pl. *sutu′rae* [L.] suture; in anatomy, a type of joint in which the apposed bony surfaces are united by fibrous tissue, permitting no movement; found only between

bones of the skull. **s. denta′ta,** s. serrata. **s. harmo′nia,** s. plana. **s. no′tha,** a type formed by apposition of the roughened surfaces of the two participating bones. **s. pla′na,** a type in which there is simple apposition of the contiguous surfaces, with no interlocking of the edges of the participating bones. **s. serra′ta,** a type in which the participating bones are united by interlocking processes resembling the teeth of a saw. **s. squamo′sa,** a type formed by overlapping of the broad beveled edges of the participating bones. **s. ve′ra,** a true suture; see *sutura*.

suturation (su″chŭ-ra′shun) process or act of suturing.

suture (su′cher) 1. sutura. 2. a stitch or series of stitches made to secure apposition of the edges of a surgical or accidental wound; used also as a verb to indicate application of such stitches. 3. material used in closing a wound with stitches. **su′tural,** adj. **absorbable s.,** a strand of material used for closing wounds which is subsequently dissolved by the tissue fluids. **apposition s.,** a superficial suture used for exact approximation of the cutaneous edges of a wound. **approximation s.,** a deep suture for securing apposition of the deep tissue of a wound. **basilar s.,** spheno-occipital fissure. **buried s.,** one placed deep in the tissues and concealed by the skin. **catgut s.,** see *catgut*. **coaptation s.,** apposition s. **cobblers′ s.,** one made with suture material threaded through a needle at each end. **continuous s.,** one in which a continuous, uninterrupted length of material is used. **coronal s.,** the line of junction of the frontal bone and the two parietal bones. **cranial s′s,** the lines of junction between the bones of the skull. **Czerny′s s.,** 1. an intestinal suture in which the thread is passed through the mucous membrane only. 2. union of a ruptured tendon by splitting one of the ends and suturing the other end into the slit. **Czerny-Lembert s.,** a combination of the Czerny and Lembert sutures. **false s.,** a line of junction between apposed surfaces without fibrous union of the bones. **figure-of-8 s.,** one in which the threads follow the contours of the figure 8. **Gély′s s.,** a continuous stitch for wounds of the intestine, made with a thread having a needle at each end. **glovers′ s.,** lock-stitch s. **Halsted s.,** a modification of the Lembert suture. **interrupted s.,** one in which each stitch is made with a separate piece of material. **lambdoid s.,** the line of junction between the occipital and parietal bones. **Lembert s.,** an inverting suture used in gastrointestinal surgery. **lock-stitch s.,** a continuous hemostatic suture used in intestinal surgery, in which the needle is, after each stitch, passed through the loop of the preceding stitch. **loop s.,** interrupted s. **mattress s.,** a method in which the stitches are parallel with (*horizontal mattress s.*) or at right angles to (*vertical mattress s.*) the wound edges. **nonabsorbable s.,** suture material which is not absorbed in the body. **pursestring s.,** a continuous, circular inverting suture used to bury the stump of the appendix. **relaxation s.,** any suture so formed that it may be loosened to relieve tension as necessary. **sagittal s.,** the line of junction between the two parietal bones. **subcuticular s.,** a method of skin closure involving placement of stitches in the subcuticular tissues parallel with the line of the wound. **uninterrupted s.,** continuous s.

Suvren (suv′ren) trademark for a preparation of captodiamine.

suxamethonium (suk″sah-mĕ-tho′ne-um) succinylcholine.

swab (swahb) a wad of cotton or other absorbable material attached to the end of a wire or stick, used for applying medication, removing material, collecting bacteriological material, etc.

swage (swāj) 1. to shape metal by hammering or by adapting it to a die. 2. to fuse, as suture material to the end of a suture needle.

sweat (swet) perspiration; the liquid secreted by the sweat glands.

sweeny (swe′ne) shoulder slip.

swelling (swel′ing) 1. transient abnormal enlargement of a body part or area not due to cell proliferation. 2. an eminence, or elevation. **cloudy s.,** an early stage of toxic degenerative changes, especially in protein constituents of organs in infectious diseases, in which the tissues appear swollen, parboiled, and opaque but revert to normal when the cause is removed.

sycosiform (si-ko′sĭ-form) resembling sycosis.

sycosis (si-ko′sis) papulopustular inflammation of hair follicles, especially of the beard. **s. bar′bae,** sycosis of the beard. **lupoid s.,** a chronic, scarring form of deep sycosis barbae. **s. vulga′ris,** sycosis of the beard due to staphylococci.

symballophone (sim-bal′o-fōn) a stethoscope with two chest pieces, making possible the comparison and localization of sounds.

symbiont (sim′bi-ont, sim′be-ont) an organism living in a state of symbiosis.

symbiosis (sim″bi-o′sis, -be-o′sis) 1. in parasitology, the close association of two dissimilar organisms, classified as mutualism, commensalism, parasitism, amensalism, or synnecrosis, depending on the advantage or disadvantage derived from the relationship. 2. in psychiatry, a mutually reinforcing relationship between persons who are dependent on each other. **symbiot′ic,** adj.

symbiote (sim′bi-ōt) symbiont.

symblepharon (sim-blef′ah-ron) adhesion of the eyelid(s) to the eyeball.

symblepharopterygium (-blef″ah-ro-tĕr-ij′e-um) symblepharon in which the adhesion is a cicatricial band resembling a pterygium.

symbolia (sim-bo′le-ah) ability to recognize the nature of objects by the sense of touch.

symbolism (sim′bo-lizm) 1. an unconscious mental state in which every occurrence is conceived of as a symbol of the patient's own thoughts. 2. an unconscious mechanism whereby the real meaning of an object or idea becomes transformed so as not to be recognized by the superego.

symbolization (sim″bol-i-za′shun) a mental mechanism of the subconscious which consists in the representation of one object, idea, or quality by another.

symmelus (sim′ĕ-lus) a fetus with fused legs and one, two, or three feet, or no feet.

symmetrical (sĭ-met′rĭ-kal) pertaining to or exhibiting symmetry.

symmetry (sim′ĕ-tre) correspondence in size, form, and arrangement of parts on opposite sides of a plane or around an axis. **bilateral s.,** the configuration of an irregularly shaped body (as the human body or that of higher animals) which can be divided by a longitudinal plane into halves that are mirror images of each other. **inverse s.,** correspondence as between a part and its mirror image, wherein the right (or left) side of one part corresponds with the left (or right) side of the other. **radial s.,** that in which the body parts are arranged regularly around a central axis.

sympathectomy (-thek′to-me) transection, resection, or other interruption of some portion of the sympathetic nervous pathway. **chemical s.,** that accomplished by means of a chemical agent. **periarterial s.,** surgical removal of the sheath of an artery containing the sympathetic nerve fibers; it produces temporary vasodilation.

sympathetic (sim″pah-thet′ik) 1. pertaining to or caused by sympathy. 2. pertaining to the sympathetic nervous system.

sympathicoblast (sim-path′ĭ-ko-blast″) the primitive pluripotential undifferentiated cell that develops into a sympathetic nerve cell.

sympathicoblastoma (sim-path″ĭ-ko-blas-to′mah) a malignant tumor containing sympathicoblasts: see *neuroblastoma*.

sympathicolytic (-lit′ik) sympatholytic.

sympathicomimetic (-mi-met′ik) sympathomimetic.

sympathicotonia (-to′ne-ah) a stimulated condition of the sympathetic nervous system, marked by vascular spasm, heightened blood pressure, and gooseflesh. **sympathicoton′ic,** adj.

sympathicotripsy (-trip′se) the surgical crushing of a nerve, ganglion, or plexus of the sympathetic nervous system.

sympathicotropic (-trop′ik) 1. having an affinity for the sympathetic nervous system. 2. an agent having such affinity.

sympathicus (sim-path′ĭ-kus) the sympathetic nervous system.

sympathin (sim′pah-thin) a neurohormonal mediator of nerve impulses at sympathetic nerve synapses; the term is used only when the nature of the mediator is unknown.

sympathism (sim′pah-thizm) suggestibility.

sympathoblast (sim-path′o-blast) sympathicoblast.

sympathoblastoma (sim″pah-tho-blast-to′mah) sympathicoblastoma.

sympathogonia (-go′ne-ah) sing. *sympathogo′nium* [Gr.] undifferentiated embryonic cells which develop into sympathetic cells.

sympathogonioma (-go″ne-o′mah) sympatheticoblastoma.

sympatholytic (-lit′ik) antiadrenergic: blocking transmission of impulses from the postganglionic fibers to effector organs or tissues, inhibiting smooth muscle contraction and glandular secretion. Also, an agent that produces such an effect.

sympathomimetic (-mi-met′ik) adrenergic: producing effects resembling those of impulses transmitted by the postganglionic fibers of the sympathetic nervous system. Also, an agent that produces such an effect.

sympathy (sim′pah-the) 1. an influence produced in any organ by disease or disorder in another part. 2. compassion for another's grief or loss. 3. the influence exerted by one individual upon another, or received by one from another, and the effects thus produced, as seen in hypnotism or in yawning.

symphalangia (sim″fah-lan′je-ah) congenital ankylosis of the proximal phalangeal joints.

symphyseal, symphysial (sim-fiz′e-al) pertaining to a symphysis.

symphysion (-fiz′e-on) the most anterior point of the alveolar process of the mandible.

symphysiorrhaphy (-fiz″e-or′ah-fe) suture of a divided symphysis.

symphysiotomy (-fiz″e-ot′o-me) division of the symphysis pubis to facilitate delivery.

symphysis (sim′fĭ-sis), pl. *sym′physes* [Gr.] 1. a site or line of union. 2. fibrocartilaginous joint; a type of joint in which the apposed bony surfaces are firmly united by a plate of fibrocartilage. **pubic s., s. pu′bica, s. pu′bis,** the line of union of the bodies of the pubic bones in the median plane.

sympodia (sim-po′de-ah) fusion of the lower extremities.

symptom (simp′tom) any subjective evidence of disease or of a patient's condition, i.e., such evidence as perceived by the patient; a change in a patient's condition indicative of some bodily or mental state. **abstinence s's,** withdrawal s's. **Bárány's s.,** 1. in disturbances of equilibrium of the vestibular apparatus, the direction of the fall is influenced by changing the position of the patient's head. 2. if the normal ear is irrigated with hot water, rotatory nystagmus is developed toward the side of the irrigated ear, but if cold water is used, rotatory nystagmus is developed away from the affected side; in labyrinthine disease, there is no nystagmus. **objective s.,** one that is evident to the observer; see *sign.* **presenting s.,** the symptom or group of symptoms about which the patient complains or from which he seeks relief. **signal s.,** a sensation, aura, or other subjective experience, indicative of an impending epileptic or other seizure. **subjective s.,** one perceptible only to the patient. **withdrawal s's,** symptoms caused by sudden withholding of a drug to which a person is habituated or addicted.

symptomatic (simp″to-mat′ik) 1. pertaining to or of the nature of a symptom. 2. indicative (of a particular disease or disorder). 3. exhibiting the symptoms of a particular disease but having a different cause. 4. directed at the allaying of symptoms, as symptomatic treatment.

symptomatology (simp″to-mah-tol′o-je) 1. the

branch of medicine dealing with symptoms. 2. the combined symptoms of a disease.

symptomatolytic (simp″to-mah-to-lit′ik) causing the disappearance of symptoms.

symptosis (simp-to′sis) gradual wasting of the body or of an organ.

sympus (sim′pus) a fetus with fused legs.

syn- word element [Gr.], *union; association; together with.*

Synalar (sin′ah-lar) trademark for a preparation of fluocinolone acetonide.

synapse (-aps) the region of junction between processes of two neurons, forming the place where a nervous impulse is transmitted from one neuron to another. **axodendritic s.,** one between the axon of one neuron and dendrites of another. **axodendrosomatic s.,** one between the axon of one neuron and dendrites and body of another. **axosomatic s.,** one between the axon of one neuron and the body of another.

synapsis (sĭ-nap′sis) the point-for-point pairing off of homologous chromosomes from male and female pronuclei during prophase of meiosis.

synaptic (sĭ-nap′tik) pertaining to a synapse or to synapsis.

synarthrodia (sin″ar-thro′de-ah) synarthrosis. **synarthro′dial,** adj.

synarthrophysis (-ar-thro-fi′sis) any ankylosing process.

synarthrosis (-ar-thro′sis), pl. *synarthro′ses* [Gr.] fibrous joint.

syncanthus (sin-kan′thus) adhesion of the eyeball to the orbital structures.

syncephalus (-sef′ah-lus) a twin monster with heads fused into one, there being a single face, with four ears.

synchilia (-ki′le-ah) congenital adhesion of the lips.

synchiria (-ki′re-ah) reference of sensation to the opposite side on application of a stimulus.

synchondrosis (sin″kon-dro′sis), pl. *synchondro′ses* [Gr.] a type of cartilaginous joint in which the cartilage is usually converted into bone before adult life.

synchondrotomy (-kon-drot′o-me) division of a synchondrosis.

synchronism (sin′kro-nizm) occurrence at the same time.

synchronous (-kro-nus) occurring at the same time.

synchysis (-kĭ-sis) a softening or fluid condition of the vitreous body of the eye. **s. scintil′lans,** floating cholesterol crystals in the vitreous, developing as a secondary degenerative change.

synclitism (-klĭ-tizm) parallelism between the planes of the fetal head and those of the maternal pelvis. **synclit′ic,** adj.

synclonus (-klo-nus) muscular tremor or successive clonic contraction of various muscles together.

syncope (-ko-pe) a faint; temporary loss of consciousness due to generalized cerebral ischemia. **syn′copal, syncop′ic,** adj. **carotid sinus s.,** see under *syndrome.* **laryngeal s., tussive s.,** brief loss of consciousness associated with paroxysms of coughing. **vasovagal s.,** see under *attack.*

Syncurine (-ku-rēn) trademark for a preparation of decamethonium.

syncytial (sin-sish′al) of or pertaining to a syncytium.

syncytiolysin (-sit″e-ol′ĭ-sin) a cytolysin formed in response to injection of emulsions of placental tissue.

syncytioma (-sit″e-o′mah) syncytial endometritis. **s. malig′num,** choriocarcinoma.

syncytiotrophoblast (-sit″e-o-trof′o-blast) the outer syncytial layer of the trophoblast.

syncytium (-sish′e-um) a multinucleate mass of protoplasm produced by the merging of cells.

syndactyly (-dak′tĭ-le) persistence of webbing between adjacent digits of the hand or foot, so that they are more or less completely fused together. **syndac′tylous,** adj.

syndectomy (-dek′to-me) peridectomy.

syndesis (sin′dĕ-sis) 1. arthrodesis. 2. synapsis.

syndesm(o)- word element [Gr.], *connective tissue; ligament.*

syndesmectomy (sin″des-mek′to-me) excision of a portion of ligament.

syndesmectopia (-mek-to′pe-ah) unusual situation of a ligament.

syndesmitis (-mi′tis) 1. inflammation of a ligament. 2. conjunctivitis.

syndesmography (-mog′rah-fe) a description of the ligaments.

syndesmology (-mol′o-je) the scientific study of ligaments; by extension including also study of the articulations and joints; applied to the body of knowledge relating thereto.

syndesmoma (-mo′mah) a tumor of connective tissue.

syndesmoplasty (sin-des′mo-plas″te) plastic repair of a ligament.

syndesmosis (sin″des-mo′sis), pl. *syndesmo′ses* [Gr.] a joint in which the bones are united by fibrous connective tissue forming an interosseous membrane or ligament.

syndesmotomy (-mot′o-me) incision of a ligament.

syndrome (sin′drōm) a set of symptoms occurring together; the sum of signs of any morbid state; a symptom complex. **abstinence s.,** withdrawal symptoms. **Adams-Stokes s.,** see under *disease.* **Adie's s.,** tonic pupil associated with absence or diminution of certain tendon reflexes. **adiposogenital s.,** see under *dystrophy.* **adrenogenital s.,** hyperfunction of the adrenal cortex, causing pseudohermaphroditism and virilism in the female, usually evident at birth, and precocious sexual development in the male, usually not evident until age three to four. **afferent loop s.,** chronic partial obstruction of the proximal loop (duodenum and jejunum) after gastrojejunostomy, resulting in duodenal distention, pain, and nausea following ingestion of food. **Albright's s.,** fibrous dysplasia of bone, melanotic pigmentation of the skin, and sexual precocity in the female. **Aldrich's s.,** Wiskott-Aldrich s. **Alport's s.,** a hereditary disorder marked by progressive nerve deafness, pro-

gressive pyelonephritis or glomerulonephritis, and occasionally ocular defects. **amyostatic s.,** hepatolenticular degeneration. **autoerythrocyte sensitization s.,** a purpuric reaction occurring chiefly in young women, in which spontaneous, painful, recurrent single or multiple ecchymoses occur on any part of the body without trauma or after insufficient trauma. Sensitivity to a component of the erythrocytes' structural framework is responsible in many cases, but in some cases the leukocytes seem to be responsible. Emotional upsets are believed to be a precipitating factor. **Avellis' s.,** ipsilateral paralysis of the vocal cord and soft palate, loss of pain and temperature sensibility in the contralateral leg, trunk, arm, neck, and in the skin over the scalp. **Banti's s.,** congestive splenomegaly. **Bartter's s.,** a hereditary disorder marked by juxtaglomerular cell hyperplasia, hyperaldosteronism, hypokalemic alkalosis, increased concentrations of plasma renin in the absence of hypertension, and by mental retardation and short stature. **Bassen-Kornzweig s.,** abetalipoproteinemia. **Behçet's s.,** severe uveitis and retinal vasculitis, optic atrophy, and aphtha-like lesions of the mouth and genitalia, often with other signs and symptoms suggesting a diffuse vasculitis; it most often affects young males. **Benedikt's s.,** ipsilateral oculomotor paralysis, contralateral hyperkinesia, contralateral tremor and paralysis of the arm and leg, and ipsilateral ataxia; due to damage to the third cranial nerve with involvement of the nucleus ruber and corticospinal tract. **Bloch-Sulzberger s.,** incontinentia pigmenti. **Bonnevie-Ullrich s.,** pterygium colli, lymphangiectatic edema of the hands and feet, ocular hypertelorism, short stature, and other developmental anomalies. **Bouillaud's s.,** the coincidence of pericarditis and endocarditis in acute articular rheumatism. **Bouveret's s.,** paroxysmal tachycardia. **brain s.,** see *organic brain s.* **Brock's s.,** middle lobe s. **Brown-Séquard s.,** ipsilateral paralysis and loss of discriminatory and joint sensation, and contralateral loss of pain and temperature sensation; due to damage to one half of the spinal cord. **Burnett's s.,** milk-alkali s. **Caffey's s.,** infantile cortical hyperostosis. **Canada-Cronkhite s.,** familial polyposis of the gastrointestinal tract associated with alopecia, nail dystrophy, and hyperpigmentation of the skin. **carcinoid s.,** a symptom complex associated with carcinoid tumors (argentaffinomas), marked by attacks of severe cyanotic flushing of the skin lasting from minutes to days and by diarrheal watery stools, bronchoconstrictive attacks, sudden drops in blood pressure, edema, and ascites; it is caused by a variety of catecholamines secreted by the agentaffinoma cells. **carotid sinus s.,** syncope sometimes associated with convulsions due to overactivity of the carotid sinus reflex when pressure is applied to one or both carotid sinuses. **carpal tunnel s.,** pain and burning or tingling paresthesias in the fingers and hand, sometimes extending to the elbow, due to compression of the median nerve in the carpal tunnel. **cervical rib s.,** scalenus s. **Cestan's s., Cestan-Chenais s.,** an association of contralateral hemiplegia, contralateral hemianesthesia, ipsilateral lateropulsion and hemiasynergia, Horner's syndrome, and ipsilateral laryngoplegia, due to scattered lesions of the pyramid, sensory tract, inferior cerebellar peduncle, nucleus ambiguus, and oculopupillary center. **Charcot's s.,** 1. amyotrophic lateral sclerosis. 2. intermittent claudication. **Chédiak-Higashi s.,** a hereditary disorder marked by massive leukocytic inclusions, decreased pigmentation of the skin, hair, and eyes, photophobia, nystagmus, susceptibility to infections, and early death; it may be associated with a predisposition to leukemia and malignant lymphoma. **Chinese restaurant s.,** transient arterial dilatation due to ingestion of monosodium glutamate, which is used liberally in seasoning Chinese food, marked by throbbing head, light-headedness, tightness of the jaw, neck, and shoulders, and backache. **Clarke-Hadfield s.,** congenital pancreatic infantilism, with hepatomegaly, bulky fatty stools, and extensive atrophy of the pancreas in an undersized and underweight child. **Claude's s.,** paralysis of the third (oculomotor) nerve on one side and asynergia on the other side, together with dysarthria. **Conn's s.,** primary hyperaldosteronism. **Costen's s.,** temporomandibular joint s. **cri du chat s.,** a hereditary congenital syndrome characterized by hypertelorism, microcephaly, severe mental deficiency, and a plaintive catlike cry, due to deletion of the short arm of a chromosome of the B group. **Crigler-Najjar s.,** a congenital hereditary nonhemolytic jaundice due to absence of the hepatic enzyme glucuronide transferase, marked by excessive amounts of unconjugated bilirubin in the blood, kernicterus, and severe central nervous system disorders. **crush s.,** the edema, oliguria, and other symptoms of renal failure that follow crushing of a part, especially a large muscle mass; see *lower nephron nephrosis.* **Cruveilhier-Baumgarten s.,** cirrhosis of the liver with portal hypertension associated with congenital patency of the umbilical and paraumbilical veins. **Cushing's s.,** a condition usually seen in women, due to hyperadrenocorticism caused by neoplasms of the adrenal cortex or the anterior pituitary; symptoms include adiposity of face, neck, and trunk, kyphosis, amenorrhea, hypertrichosis (in females), impotence (in males), hypertension, polycythemia, muscular weakness, etc. **Dandy-Walker s.,** congenital hydrocephalus due to obstruction of the foramina of Magendie and Luschka. **Down's s.,** mongoloid features, short phalanges, widened space between the first and second toes and fingers, and moderate to severe mental retardation; associated with a chromosomal abnormality, usually trisomy of chromosome 21. **Dubin-Johnson s.,** hereditary chronic nonhemolytic jaundice thought to be due to defective excretion of conjugated bilirubin and certain other organic anions by the liver; a brown, coarsely granular pigment in hepatic cells is pathognomonic. **dumping s.,** nausea, weakness, sweating, palpitation, syncope, often a sensation of warmth, and sometimes diarrhea, occurring after ingestion of food in patients who have undergone partial gastrectomy. **effort s.,**

neurocirculatory asthenia. **Ehlers-Danlos s.,** a congenital hereditary syndrome of joint hyperextensibility, hyperelasticity and fragility of the skin, poor wound healing leaving parchment-like scars, capillary fragility, and subcutaneous nodules after trauma. **Eisenmenger's s.,** ventricular septal defect with pulmonary hypertension and cyanosis due to right-to-left (reversed) shunt of blood. Sometimes defined as pulmonary hypertension (pulmonary vascular disease) and cyanosis with the shunt being at the atrial, ventricular, or great vessel area. **Ellis-van Creveld s.,** chondroectodermal dysplasia. **empty-sella s.,** a clinical syndrome in which the diaphragma sellae is vestigial, the sella turcica forms an extension of the subarachnoid space and is filled with cerebrospinal fluid, and the pituitary fossa appears to be empty, although the pituitary gland is present in a flattened form. **extrapyramidal s.,** any of a group of clinical disorders marked by abnormal involuntary movements, including parkinsonism, athetosis, and chorea. **Faber's s.,** hypochromic anemia. **Fanconi's s.,** 1. a hereditary disorder marked by pancytopenia, hypoplasia of bone marrow, patchy brown skin discoloration due to melanin deposition, and multiple musculoskeletal and genitourinary anomalies. 2. a hereditary disorder marked by aminoaciduria, glycosuria, hyperphosphaturia, deposition of cystine throughout the body, and by rickets, osteomalacia, and short stature. **Felty's s.,** chronic (rheumatoid) arthritis, splenomegaly, leukopenia, pigmented spots on the skin of the legs, and other inconsistent evidence of hypersplenism, namely, anemia and thrombocytopenia. **floppy infant s.,** a congenital myopathy of infants, marked clinically by myotonia and muscle weakness. **Franceschetti's s.,** see *mandibulofacial dysostosis.* **Frölich's s.,** adiposogenital dystrophy. **Ganser's s.,** amnesia, disturbance of consciousness, and hallucinations, associated with senseless answers to questions, and absurd acts. **Gardner's s.,** familial polyposis of the colon associated with osseous and soft tissue tumors. **general adaptation s.,** the total of all nonspecific reactions of the body to prolonged systemic stress. **Gilles de la Tourette's s.,** facial and vocal tics with onset in childhood, progressing to generalized jerking movements in any body part, with echolalia and coprolalia. **Goodpasture's s.,** glomerulonephritis associated with hemoptysis, an uncommon, rapidly progressive, usually fatal condition affecting chiefly young men. **Gradenigo's s.,** sixth nerve palsy and unilateral headache in suppurative disease of the middle ear, due to involvement of the abducens and trigeminal nerves by direct spread of the infection. **Guillain-Barré s.,** acute febrile polyneuritis. **Hallervorden-Spatz s.,** a hereditary disorder involving marked reduction in the number of myelin sheaths of the globus pallidus and substantia nigra, with accumulations of iron pigment, progressive rigidity beginning in the legs, choreoathetoid movements, dysarthria, and progressive mental deterioration. **Hamman-Rich s.,** the acute, rapidly fatal form of diffuse interstitial pulmonary fibrosis. **Hand-Schüller-**

Christian s., see under *disease*. **Harada's s.**, a syndrome, possibly caused by a virus, consisting of uveomeningitis associated with retinochoroidal detachment, temporary or permanent deafness and blindness, and sometimes, though often transiently, alopecia, vitiligo, and poliosis. **Horner's s.**, sinking in of the eyeball, ptosis of the upper lid, slight elevation of the lower lid, miosis, narrowing of palpebral fissure, and anhidrosis and flushing of the affected side of the face; due to paralysis of the cervical sympathetic nerves. **Hurler's s.**, the prototypical form of mucopolysaccharidosis, with gargoyle-like facies, dwarfism, severe somatic and skeletal changes, severe mental retardation, cloudy corneas, deafness, cardiovascular defects, hepatosplenomegaly, and joint contractures. **hyperkinetic s.**, a disorder of childhood, usually abating during adolescense, marked by overactivity, distractibility, restlessness, and low tolerance for frustration. **jugular foramen s.**, Vernet's s. **Kanner's s.**, infantile autism. **Kartagener's s.**, a hereditary syndrome consisting of dextrocardia, bronchiectasis, and sinusitis. **Kimmelstiel-Wilson s.**, intercapillary glomerulosclerosis. **Klinefelter's s.**, small testes with fibrosis and hyalinization of the seminiferous tubules, impairment of function and clumping of Leydig cells, and an increase in urinary gonadotropins; associated with an abnormality of the sex chromosomes. **Klippel-Feil s.**, shortness of the neck due to reduction in the number of cervical vertebrae or the fusion of multiple hemivertebrae into one osseous mass, with limitaion of neck motion and low hairline. **Korsakoff's s.**, see under *psychosis*. **Launois' s.**, gigantism due to excessive pituitary secretion, occurring before puberty and before the epiphyses close. **Laurence-Biedl s., Laurence-Moon-Biedl s.**, obesity, hypogenitalism, retinitis pigmentosa, mental retardation, skull defects, and sometimes syndactyly. **Leriche's s.**, fatigue in the hips, thighs, or calves on exercising, absence of pulsation in femoral arteries, impotence, and often pallor and coldness of the legs, usually affecting males and due to obstruction of the terminal aorta. **Lesch-Nyhan s.**, a hereditary disorder of purine metabolism with physical and mental retardation, compulsive self-mutilation of fingers and lips by biting, choreoathetosis, spastic cerebral palsy, and impaired renal function. **Libman-Sacks s.**, see under *disease*. **Lichtheim's s.**, subacute combined degeneration of the spinal cord. **Lowe's s.**, oculocerebrorenal s. **Lutembacher's s.**, atrial septal defect with mitral stenosis (usually rheumatic). **lymphoproliferative s.**, any of a group of diseases marked by proliferation of lymphoid tissue, as lymphocytic leukemia or malignant lymphoma. **McArdle's s.**, see under *disease*. **Maffucci's s.**, enchondromatosis with multiple cutaneous or visceral hemangiomas. **malabsorption s.**, a group of disorders marked by subnormal absorption of dietary constituents, and thus excessive loss of nutrients in the stool, which may be due to a digestive defect, a mucosal abnormality, or lymphatic obstruction. **Marchiafava-Micheli s.**, paroxysmal nocturnal hemoglobinuria; see *intermittent hemoglo-*

binuria. **Marfan's s.**, a hereditary syndrome of abnormal length of the extremities, especially of fingers and toes, with subluxation of the lens, cardiovascular abnormalities, and other disorders. **Marie's s.**, 1. a complex of symptoms due to excessive secretion of the anterior pituitary, with acromegaly a prominent feature. 2. hypertrophic pulmonary osteoarthropathy. **middle lobe s.**, atelectasis of the middle lobe of the right lung, with chronic pneumonitis. **Mikulicz's s.**, bilateral enlargement of the salivary and lacrimal glands due to various diseases, e.g., leukemia, tuberculosis, and sarcoidosis. **milk-alkali s.**, hypercalcemia without hypercalciuria or hypophosphatemia and with only mild alkalosis and other symptoms attributed to ingestion of milk and absorbable alkali for long periods. **Milkman's s.**, a generalized bone disease marked by multiple transparent stripes of absorption in the long and flat bones. **Möbius' s.**, agenesis or aplasia of the motor nuclei of the cranial nerves marked by congenital bilateral facial palsy, with unilateral or bilateral paralysis of the abductors of the eye, sometimes associated with cranial nerve involvement, and anomalies of the extremities. **Morel's s., Morgagni's s.**, frontal internal hyperostosis. **Morquio's s.**, a form of mucopolysaccharidosis becoming evident when the affected infant starts to walk, marked by severe dwarfism, prominent sternum, short neck, kyphosis, genu valgum, and waddling gait; mental retardation is absent or slight. **Munchausen s.**, habitual seeking of hospital treatment for apparent acute illness, the patient giving a plausible and dramatic history, all of which is false. **myeloproliferative s.**, a group of diseases related histogenetically and marked, at varying times in varying degrees, by medullary and extramedullary proliferation of one or more lines of bone marrow constitutents, including myelocytic, erythroblastic, and megakaryocytic forms, in addition to various cells derived from the reticulum and mesenchymal elements. **nephrotic s.**, a condition marked by massive edema, heavy proteinuria, hypoalbuminemia, and peculiar susceptibiliity to intercurrent infections. **Noonan's s.**, the male phenotype of Turner's syndrome, with short stature, webbed neck, low nuchal hairline, low-set ears, and cubitus valgus; valvular pulmonary stenosis, rather than coarctation of the aorta, is often present. **oculocerebrorenal s.**, a hereditary syndrome of males, with vitamin D–refractory rickets, hydrophthalmia, congenital glaucoma and cataracts, mental retardation, and renal tubule dysfunction as evidenced by hypophosphatemia, acidosis, and aminoaciduria. **organic brain s.**, any mental disorder, psychotic or nonpsychotic, caused by or associated with impairment of brain tissue function; it may be *acute* and reversible, arising in one previously psychologically normal and due to injury, infection, exogenous or endogenous intoxications, nutritional deficiency, etc., or *chronic,* resulting from or associated with relatively permanent and more or less irreversible diffuse organic impairment of brain tissue function. **orofaciodigital s.**, a syndrome occurring only in females, with mental retardation and anomalies of the mouth and tongue, the fingers, and frequently the face. **painful bruising s.,** autoerythrocyte sensitization s. **Pancoast's s.,** 1. roentgenographic shadow at the apex of the lung, neuritic pain in the arm, atrophy of the muscles of the arm and hand, and Horner's syndrome, observed in tumor near the apex of the lung; due to involvement of the brachial plexus. 2. osteolysis in the posterior part of one or more ribs and sometimes involving also the corresponding vertebra. **Parinaud's s.,** 1. see under *ophthalmoplegia.* 2. Parinaud's oculoglandular s. **Parinaud's oculoglandular s.,** a general term applied to conjunctivitis, usually unilateral and of the follicular type, followed by tenderness and enlargement of the preauricular lymph nodes; often due to leptotrichosis but may be associated with other infections. **parkinsonian s.,** a form of parkinsonism due to idiopathic degeneration of the corpus striatum or substantia nigra; frequently a sequel of lethargic encephalitis, but other factors have also been implicated. **Peutz-Jeghers s.,** familial gastrointestinal polyposis, especially in the small bowel, associated with mucocutaneous pigmentation. **pickwickian s.,** obesity, somnolence, hypoventilation, and erythrocytosis. **Pierre Robin s.,** micrognathia occurring in association with cleft palate, glossoptosis, and absent gag reflex. **Plummer-Vinson s.,** dysphagia with glossitis, hypochromic anemia, splenomegaly, and atrophy in the mouth, pharynx, and upper end of the esophagus. **postcommissurotomy s.,** fever, chest pain, pleuritis, pericarditis, and pneumonia, occurring after mitral commissurotomy, and sometimes related to cytomegalic inclusion disease. **postgastrectomy s.,** dumping s. **postpericardiectomy s.,** delayed pericardial or pleural reaction with fever, chest pains, and signs of pleural and/or pericardial inflammation, following opening of the pericardium. **preexcitation s.,** Wolff-Parkinson-White s. **Putnam-Dana s.,** subacute combined degeneration of the spinal cord. **Reiter's s.,** the triad of nongonococcal urethritis, conjunctivitis, and arthritis, frequently with mucocutaneous lesions. **respiratory distress s. of newborn,** a condition most often seen in premature infants, infants of diabetic mothers, and infants delivered by cesarean section, marked by dyspnea and cyanosis, and including two patterns: in *hyaline membrane disease,* affected infants often die of respiratory distress in the first few days of life and at autopsy have a hyaline-like membrane lining the terminal respiratory passages; in *idiopathic respiratory distress of newborn,* affected infants may live, but in those who die, only resorption atelectasis is seen. **Reye's s.,** an acute and often fatal childhood syndrome of encephalopathy and fatty degeneration of the liver, marked by rapid development of brain swelling and hepatomegaly and by disturbed consciousness and seizures. **Riley-Day s.,** dysautonomia. **rubella s.,** a congenital syndrome due to intrauterine rubella infection (German measles), commonly marked by cataracts, cardiac anomalies, deafness, microcephaly, and mental retardation. **salt-depletion s., salt-losing s.,** vomiting, de-

hydration, hypotension, and sudden death due to very large sodium losses from the body. It may be seen in abnormal losses of sodium into the urine (as in congenital adrenal hyperplasia, adrenocortical insufficiency, or one of the forms of salt-losing nephritis) or in large extrarenal sodium losses, usually from the gastrointestinal tract. **scalenus s., scalenus anticus s.,** pain over the shoulder, often extending down the arm or radiating up the back, due to compression of the nerves and vessels between a cervical rib and the scalenus anticus muscle. **Schaumann's s.,** sarcoidosis. **Scheie's s.,** a type of mucopolysaccharidosis considered to be an atypical form of Hurler's syndrome (q.v.), in which the principal sign is marked progressive corneal clouding; hirsutism, joint stiffness, mild deformities of the bones that may only affect the hands, disease of the aorta, and widemouthed facies occur, but there is no mental retardation. **Sertoli-cell–only s.,** congenital absence of the germinal epithelium of the testes, the seminiferous tubules containing only Sertoli cells, marked by testes slightly smaller than normal, azoospermia, and elevated titers of follicle-stimulating hormone or of general gonadotropins. **Sézary s., Sézary reticulosis s.,** an exfoliative erythroderma due to cutaneous infiltration of reticular lymphocytes, with alopecia, edema, hyperkeratosis, and pigment and nail changes. **Sheehan's s.,** postpartum pituitary necrosis. **shoulder-hand s.,** a disorder of the upper extremity characterized by pain and stiffness in the shoulder, with puffy swelling and pain in the ipsilateral hand, sometimes occurring after myocardial infarction, but also produced by other causes. **sick-sinus s.,** a complex cardiac arrhythmia manifested as severe sinus bradycardia alone, sinus bradycardia alternating with tachycardia, or sinus bradycardia with atrioventricular block. **Sjögren's s.,** keratoconjunctivitis sicca with pharyngitis sicca, enlargement of parotid glands, perostomia, and chronic polyarthritis. **Stein-Leventhal s.,** secondary amenorrhea and absence of ovulation associated with bilateral polycystic ovaries, but normal excretion of follicle-stimulating hormone and 17-ketosteroids. **Stevens-Johnson s.,** a severe form of erythema multiforme in which the lesions may involve the oral and anogenital mucosa, associated with such constitutional symptoms as malaise, headache, fever, arthralgia, and conjunctivitis. **Stewart-Morel s.,** frontal internal hyperostosis. **Stewart-Treves s.,** lymphangiosarcoma occurring as a late complication of severe lymphedema of the arm after excision of the lymph nodes, usually in radical mastectomy. **stiffman s.,** a condition of unknown etiology marked by progressive fluctuating rigidity of axial and limb muscles in the absence of signs of cerebral and spinal cord disease but with continuous electromyographic activity. **stroke s.,** stroke; a condition with sudden onset due to acute vascular lesions of the brain (hemorrhage, embolism, thrombosis, rupturing aneurysm), which may be marked by hemiplegia or hemiparesis, vertigo, numbness, aphasia, and dysarthria, and often followed by permanent neurologic damage. **Sturge-Kalischer-Weber s.,** nevoid amentia. **Sturge-Weber s.,** a congenital syndrome of nevus flammeus of the face, angiomas of the leptomeninges and choroid, and late glaucoma, frequently associated with intracranial calcification, mental retardation, contralateral hemiplegia, and epilepsy. **subclavian steal s.,** cerebral or brain stem ischemia resulting from diversion of blood flow from the basilar artery to the subclavian artery, in the presence of occlusive disease of the proximal portion of the subclavian artery. **sudden infant death s.,** sudden and unexpected death of an infant who had previously been apparently well, and which is unexplained by careful postmortem examination. **tarsal tunnel s.,** a complex of symptoms resulting from compression of the posterior tibial nerve or of the plantar nerves in the tarsal tunnel, with pain, numbness, and tingling paresthesia of the sole of the foot. **Taussig-Bing s.,** transposition of the great vessels of the heart and a ventricular septal defect straddled by a large pulmonary artery. **temporomandibular joint s.,** tinnitus, vertigo, discomfort in the ears, and other symptoms due to faulty articulation of the temporomandibular joint. **testicular feminization s.,** an extreme form of male pseudohermaphroditism, with external genitalia and secondary sex characters typical of the female, but with presence of testes and absence of uterus and uterine tubes. **thoracic outlet s.,** compression of the brachial plexus nerve trunks, with pain in arms, paresthesia of fingers, vasomotor symptoms, and weakness and wasting of small muscles of the hand; it may be caused by drooping shoulder girdle, a cervical rib or fibrous band, an abnormal first rib, continual hyperabduction of the arm (as during sleep), or compression of the edge of scalenus anterior muscle. **Treacher Collins s.,** see *mandibulofacial dysostosis.* **trisomy D s.,** holoprosencephaly due to an aberration of the autosomes of the D group, in which central nervous system defects are associated with mental retardation, along with cleft lip and palate, polydactyly, and dermal pattern anomalies, and abnormalities of the heart, viscera, and genitalia. **trisomy E s.,** neonatal hepatitis, mental retardation, scaphocephaly or other skull abnormality, micrognathia, blepharoptosis, low-set ears, corneal opacities, deafness, webbed neck, short digits, ventricular septal defects. Meckel's diverticulum, and other deformities; due to the presence of an extra E group chromosome. **trisomy 21 s.,** Down's s. **Turcot's s.,** familial polyposis of the colon associated with malignant tumors of the central nervous system. **Turner's s.,** short stature, undifferentiated (streak) gonads, and variable abnormalities that may include webbing of neck, low posterior hair line, increased carrying angle of elbow, cubitus valgus, and cardiac defects; associated with a defect or absence of the second sex chromosome. The phenotype is female. **Turner's s., male,** Noonan's s. **van der Hoeve's s.,** see *osteogenesis imperfecta.* **Vernet's s.,** paralysis of the glossopharyngeal, vagus, and spinal accessory nerves due to a lesion in the region of the jugular foramen. **Villaret's s.,** unilateral paralysis of the glossopharyngeal, vagus, spinal accessory, and hypoglossal nerves and sometimes the facial nerve, due to a lesion in the retroparotid space. **Waardenburg's s.,** a congenital hereditary syndrome of cochlear deafness, wide bridge of the nose, lateral displacement of medial canthi, confluent eyebrows, eyes of different color, white lashes and forelock, and leukoderma. **Waterhouse-Friderichsen s.,** the malignant or fulminating form of epidemic cerebrospinal meningitis, with sudden onset, short course, fever, collapse, coma, cyanosis, petechiae on the skin and mucous membranes, and bilateral adrenal hemorrhage. **s. of Weber,** paralysis of the oculomotor nerve on the same side as the lesion, causing ptosis, strabismus, and loss of light reflex and accommodation; also spastic hemiplegia on the side opposite the lesion with increased reflexes and loss of superficial reflexes. **Weber-Christian s.,** nodular nonsuppurative panniculitis. **Werner's s.,** premature senility of an adult, with early graying and some hair loss, cataracts, hyperkeratinization, and scleroderma-like changes in the skin of the limbs, followed by chronic ulceration. **Wernick's s.,** presbyophrenia. **Wilson-Mikity s.,** a rare form of pulmonary insufficiency in low-birth-weight infants, marked by hyperpnea and cyanosis of insidious onset during the first month of life and often resulting in death. Radiographically, there are multiple cystlike foci of hyperaeration throughout the lung with coarse thickening of the interstitial supporting structures. **Wiskott-Aldrich s.,** a hereditary syndrome of chronic eczema, chronic suppurative otitis media, anemia, and thrombocytopenic purpura. **Wolff-Parkinson-White s.,** the association of paroxysmal tachycardia (or atrial fibrillation) and preexcitation, in which the electrocardiogram displays a short P-R interval and a wide QRS complex which characteristically shows an early QRS vector (delta wave). **Zollinger-Ellison s.,** intractable, sometimes fulminating, atypical peptic ulcers associated with extreme gastric hyperacidity and nonbeta-cell, noninsulin-secreting islet cell tumors of the pancreas.

syndromic (sin-dro′mik) occurring as a syndrome.

Syndrox (sin′droks) trademark for preparations of methamphetamine.

synechia (sĭ-nek′e-ah), pl. *synech′iae* [Gr.] adhesion, as of the iris to the cornea or lens. **annular s.,** adhesion of the whole rim of the iris to the lens. **anterior s.,** adhesion of the iris to the cornea. **posterior s.,** adhesion of the iris to the capsule of the lens or to the surface of the vitreous body. **total anterior s.,** adhesion of the entire surface of the iris to the cornea. **s. vul′vae,** a congenital condition in which the labia minora are sealed in the midline, with only a small opening below the clitoris through which urination and menstruation may occur.

synechotomy (sin″ĕ-kot′o-me) incision of a synechia.

synencephalocele (-en-sef′ah-lo-sēl″) encephalocele with adhesions to adjoining parts.

syneresis (sĭ-ner′ĕ-sis) a drawing together of the

particles of the dispersed phase of a gel, with separation of some of the disperse medium and shrinkage of the gel.

synergism (sin′er-jizm) the joint action of agents so that their combined effect is greater than the algebraic sum of their individual effects. **synergist′ic,** adj.

synergist (-er-jist) a muscle or agent which acts with another.

synergy (-er-je) correlated action or cooperation on the part of two or more structures or drugs. In neurology, the faculty by which movements are properly grouped for the performance of acts requiring special adjustments. **synerget′ic, syner′gic,** adj.

synesthesia (sin″es-the′ze-ah) a secondary sensation accompanying an actual perception; the experiencing of a sensation in one place, due to stimulation applied to another place; also, the condition in which a stimulus of one sense is perceived as sensation of a different sense, as when a sound produces a sensation of color.

synesthesialgia (-es-the″ze-al′je-ah) a condition in which a stimulus produces pain on the affected side but no sensation on the normal side.

syngamy (sing′gah-me) 1. sexual reproduction. 2. the union of two gametes to form a zygote in fertilization.

syngeneic (sin″jen-e′ik) in transplantation biology, denoting individuals or tissues having identical genotypes, i.e., identical twins or animals of the same inbred strain, or their tissues.

syngenesis (sin-jen′ĕ-sis) 1. the origin of an individual from a germ derived from both parents and not from either one alone. 2. the state of having descended from a common ancestor.

synizesis (sin″ĭ-ze′sis) 1. occlusion. 2. a mitotic stage in which the nuclear chromatin is massed.

synkaryon (sin-kar′e-on) fertilization nucleus.

Synkayvite (sin′ka-vīt) trademark for preparations of menadiol sodium diphosphate.

synkinesis (sin″ki-ne′sis) an associated movement; an involuntary movement accompanying a volitional movement. **synkinet′ic,** adj.

synnecrosis (-nĕ-kro′sis) symbiosis in which the relationship between populations (or individuals) is mutually detrimental.

synophthalmus (-of-thal′mus) cyclops.

Synophylate (-o-fi′lāt) trademark for preparations of the theophylline sodium glycinate.

synorchidism (sin-or′kĭ-dizm) synorchism.

synorchism (sin′or-kizm) congenital fusion of the testes into one mass.

synoscheos (sin-os′ke-os) adhesion between the penis and scrotum.

synosteotomy (sin″os-te-ot′o-me) dissection of the joint.

synostosis (-os-to′sis), pl. *synosto′ses* [Gr.] 1. a union between adjacent bones or parts of a single bone formed by osseous material. 2. the osseous union of bones that are normally distinct. **synostot′ic,** adj.

synotia (sĭ-no′she-ah) persistence of the ears in their horizontal position beneath the mandible.

synotus (sĭ-no′tus) a fetus exhibiting synotia.

synovectomy (sin″o-vek′to-me) excision of a synovial membrane.

synovia (sĭ-no′ve-ah) the transparent, viscid fluid secreted by the synovial membrane and found in joint cavities, bursae, and tendon sheaths. **syno′vial,** adj.

synovialis (sĭ-no″ve-a′lis) [L.] synovial.

synovialoma (sĭ-no″ve-ah-lo′mah) synovioma.

synovioma (sĭ-no″ve-o′mah) a tumor of synovial membrane origin.

synovitis (sin″o-vi′tis) inflammation of a synovial membrane, usually painful, particularly on motion, and characterized by fluctuating swelling, due to effusion in a synovial sac. **dry s.,** that with little effusion. **purulent s.,** that with effusion of pus in a synovial sac. **serous s.,** that with copious nonpurulent effusion. **s. sic′ca,** dry s. **simple s.,** that with clear or but slightly turbid effusion. **tendinous s.,** inflammation of a tendon sheath.

synovium (sĭ-no′ve-um) a synovial membrane.

synthase (sin′thās) any enzyme, especially a lyase, which catalyzes a synthesis that does not involve the breakdown of a pyrophosphate bond, as opposed to *synthetase.*

synthesis (sin′thĕ-sis) 1. creation of a compound by union of elements composing it, done artifically or as a result of natural processes. 2. the process of bringing back into consciousness activities or experiences that have become split off or disassociated. **synthet′ic,** adj.

synthesize (-thĕ-sīz″) to produce by synthesis.

synthetase (-thĕ-tās) ligase.

Synthroid (-throid) trademark for a preparation of levothyroxine.

Syntocinon (sin-to′sĭ-non) trademark for a solution of synthetic oxytocin.

syntonic (-ton′ik) pertaining to a stable, integrated personality.

Syntropan (sin′tro-pan) trademark for a preparation of amprotropine.

syntrophoblast (sin-trof′o-blast) syncytiotrophoblast.

syntropic (-trop′ik) 1. turning or pointing in the same direction. 2. denoting correlation of several factors, as the relation of one disease to the development or incidence of another. 3. pertaining to a well-balanced personality.

syntropy (sin′tro-pe) the state of being syntropic.

syphilid (sif′ĭ-lid) any of the skin lesions of secondary syphilis.

syphilis (sif′ĭ-lis) a veneral disease caused by *Treponema pallidum,* leading to many structural and cutaneous lesions, transmitted by direct sexual contact or *in utero.* See *primary s., secondary s.,* and *tertiary s.* **syphilit′ic,** adj. **congenital s.,** syphilis acquired *in utero,* manifested by any of several characteristic malformations of teeth or bones and by active mucocutaneous syphilis at birth or shortly thereafter, and by ocular or neurologic changes. **early s.,** the stage comprising primary, secondary, and early latent syphilis. **early latent s.,** the stage following the primary state (or *primary s.*), during which no signs or symptoms are present.

late s., the stage comprising late latent and tertiary syphilis. **late latent s.,** the stage following secondary syphilis, during which there is serologic or historical evidence of syphilis but no other signs or symptoms are detectable; it may last for many decades. **latent s.,** syphilis manifested solely by serologic or historical evidence; see *early latent s.* and *late latent s.* **nonvenereal s.,** a chronic treponemal infection mainly seen in children, occurring in many areas of the world, caused by an organism indistinguishable from *Treponema pallidum,* and transmitted by direct nonsexual contact and indirectly by common use of table and drinking utensils. **primary s.,** syphilis in its first stage, the primary lesion being a chancre, which is infectious and painless; the nearby lymph nodes become hard and swollen. **secondary s.,** syphilis in the second of three stages, with fever, multiform skin eruptions (syphilids), iritis, alopecia, mucous patches, and severe pain in the head, joints, and periosteum. **tertiary s.,** late generalized syphilis, with involvement of many organs and tissues, including skin, bones, joints, and cardiovascular and central nervous systems; see also *tabes dorsalis.*

syphiloma (sif″ĭ-lo′mah) a tumor of syphilitic origin; a gumma.

syphilophyma (sif″ĭ-lo-fi′mah) any syphilitic growth or excrescence.

syring(o)- word element [Gr.], *tube; fistula.*

syringe (sir′inj) an instrument for injecting liquids into or withdrawing them from any vessel or cavity. **chip s.,** a small, fine-nozzled syringe, used to direct an air current into a tooth cavity being excavated, to remove small fragments, or to dry the cavity. **dental s.,** a small syringe used in operative dentistry, containing an anesthetic solution. **hypodermic s.,** one for introduction of liquids through a hollow needle into subcutaneous tissues. **Luer's s., Luer-Lok s.,** a glass syringe for intravenous and hypodermic use.

syringectomy (sir″in-jek′to-me) fistulectomy.

syringitis (sir″in-ji′tis) inflammation of the auditory tube.

syringoadenoma (sĭ-ring″go-ad″ĕ-no′mah) syringocystadenoma.

syringobulbia (-bul′be-ah) the presence of cavities in the medulla oblongata.

syringocarcinoma (-kar″sĭ-no′mah) cancer of a sweat gland.

syringocele (sĭ-ring′go-sēl) a cavity-containing herniation of the spinal cord through the bony defect in spina bifida.

syringocoele (sĭ-ring′go-sēl) the central canal of the spinal cord.

syringocystadenoma (sĭ-ring″go-sist″ad-ĕ-no′-mah) adenoma of the sweat glands.

syringocystoma (-sis-to′mah) cystic tumor of a sweat gland.

syringoma (sir″ing-go′mah) syringocystadenoma.

syringomeningocele (sĭ-ring″go-mĕ-ning′go-sēl) meningocele resembling syringomyelocele.

syringomyelia (-mi-e′le-ah) presence of fluid-filled cavities in the spinal cord substance.

syringomyelitis (-mi″ĕ-li′tis) inflammation of the spinal cord with formation of cavities.

syringomyelocele (-mi′ĕ-lo-sēl″) hernial protrusion of the spinal cord through the bony defect in spina bifida, the mass containing a cavity connected with the central canal of the spinal cord.

syringotomy (sir″ing-got′o-me) fistulotomy.

syrinx (sir′inks) [Gr.] 1. a tube or pipe; a fistula. 2. the lower part of the trachea of birds in which vocal sounds are produced.

syrosingopine (si″ro-sing′go-pēn) an antihypertensive agent, $C_{35}H_{42}N_2O_{11}$.

syrup (sir′up) a concentrated solution of a sugar, such as sucrose, in water or other aqueous liquid, sometimes with a medicinal agent added; usually used as a flavored vehicle for drugs. **simple s.,** one compounded with purified water and sucrose.

systaltic (sis-tal′tik) alternately contracting and dilating; pulsating.

system (sis′tem) 1. a set or series of interconnected or interdependent parts or entities (objects, organs, or organisms) that act together in a common purpose or produce results impossible by action of one alone. 2. a school or method of practice based on a specific set of principles. **alimentary s.,** digestive s. **cardiovascular s.,** the heart and blood vessels, by which blood is pumped and circulated through the body. See Plate VIII. **centimeter-gram-second s.,** see *C.G.S.* **centrencephalic s.,** the neurons in the central core of the brain stem from the thalamus down to the medulla oblongata, connecting the two hemispheres of the brain. **chromaffin s.,** the chromaffin cells of the body (which characteristically stain strongly with chromium salts) considered collectively; they occur along the sympathetic nerves, in the adrenal, carotid, and coccygeal glands, and in various other organs. **circulatory s.,** channels through which nutrient fluids of the body flow; often restricted to the vessels conveying blood. **conduction s., conductive s. (of heart),** the system comprising the sinoatrial and atrioventricular nodes, atrioventricular bundle, and Purkinje fibers. **digestive s.,** the organs concerned with ingestion, digestion, and absorption of food or nutritional elements; see Plate IV. **ecological s.,** ecosystem. **endocrine s.,** the system of glands and other structures that elaborate internal secretions (hormones) which are released directly into the circulatory system, influencing metabolism and other body processes; included are the pituitary, thyroid, parathyroid, and adrenal glands, pineal body, gonads, pancreas, and paraganglia. **extrapyramidal s.,** a functional, rather than anatomical, unit comprising the nuclei and fibers (excluding those of the pyramidal tract) involved in motor activities; they control and coordinate especially the postural, static, supporting, and locomotor mechanisms. It includes the corpus striatum, subthalamic nucleus, substantia nigra, and red nucleus, along with their interconnections with the reticular formation, cerebellum, and cerebrum; some authorities include the cerebellum and vestibular nuclei. **genitourinary s.,** urogenital

s. **haversian s.,** a haversian canal and its concentrically arranged lamellae, constituting the basic unit of structure in compact bone (osteon). **hematopoietic s.,** the tissues concerned in the production of blood, including bone marrow and lymphatic tissue. **heterogeneous s.,** a system or structure made up of parts which cannot be mechanically separated, as a solution. **homogeneous s.,** a system or structure made up of parts which cannot be mechanically separated, as a solution. **hypophyseoportal s.,** the venules connecting the capillaries (gomitoli) in the median eminence of the hypothalamus wih the sinusoidal capillaries of the anterior pituitary. **limbic s.,** a group of brain structures common to all mammals, comprising the phylogenetically old cortex (archipallium and paleopallium) and its primarily related nuclei; it is associated with olfaction, autonomic functions, and certain aspects of emotion and behavior. **lymphatic s.,** the lymphatic vessels and lymphoid tissue, considered collectively. **masticatory s.,** all bony and soft structures of the face and mouth involved in mastication, and the vessels and nerves supplying them. **metric s.,** a decimal system of weights and measures based on the meter; see *Table of Weights and Measures.* **muscular s.,** the muscles of the body considered collectively; generally restricted to the voluntary, skeletal muscles. **nervous s.,** the organ system which, along with the endocrine system, correlates the adjustments and reactions of the organism to its internal and external environment, comprising the central and peripheral nervous systems. See Plates X and XI. **nervous s., autonomic,** the portion of the nervous system concerned with regulation of activity of cardiac muscle, smooth muscle, and glands. **nervous s., central,** the brain and spinal cord. **nervous s., parasympathetic,** the craniosacral portion of the autonomic nervous system, its preganglionic fibers traveling with cranial nerves III, VII, IX, X, and XI, and with the second to fourth sacral ventral roots; it innervates the heart, smooth muscle and glands of head and neck, and thoracic, abdominal, and pelvic viscera. **nervous s., peripheral,** all elements of the nervous system (nerves and ganglia) outside the brain and spinal cord. **nervous s., sympathetic,** the thoracolumbar part of the autonomic nervous system, the preganglionic fibers of which arise from cell bodies in the thoracic and first three lumbar segments of the spinal cord; postganglionic fibers are distributed to the heart, smooth muscle, and glands of the entire body. **portal s.,** an arrangement by which blood collected from one set of capillaries passes through a large vessel or vessels and another set of capillaries before returning to the systemic circulation, as in the pituitary gland and liver. **respiratory s.,** the tubular and cavernous organs that allow atmospheric air to reach the membranes across which gases are exchanged with the blood. See Plates VI and VII. **reticular activating s.,** the system of cells of the reticular formation of the medulla oblongata that receive collaterals from the ascending sensory pathways and project to higher centers; they control the overall degree of central nervous system activity, including wakefulness, attentiveness, and sleep; abbreviated RAS. **reticuloendothelial s.,** a functional system that serves as an important bodily defense mechanism, composed of highly phagocytic cells having both endothelial and reticular attributes and the ability to take up colloidal dye particles. **stomatognathic s.,** structures of the mouth and jaws, considered collectively, as they subserve the functions of mastication, deglutition, respiration, and speech. **urogenital s.,** the organs concerned with production and excretion of urine, together with the organs of reproduction. **vascular s.,** the vessels of the body, especially the blood vessels. **vasomotor s.,** the part of the nervous system that controls the caliber of the blood vessels.

systema (sis-te′mah) system.

systemic (sis-tem′ik) pertaining to or affecting the body as a whole.

systole (sis′to-le) the contraction, or period of contraction, of the heart, especially of the ventricles. **systol′ic,** adj. **aborted s.,** a systole, usually premature, not associated with pulsation of a peripheral artery. **atrial s.,** the contraction of the atria by which blood is propelled from them into the ventricles. **extra s.,** a premature contraction of an atrium or ventricle, or of both, while fundamental rhythm is maintained. **ventricular s.,** the contraction of the cardiac ventricles by which blood is forced into the aorta and pulmonary artery.

systremma (sis-trem′ah) a cramp in the muscles of the calf of the leg.

Sytobex (si′to-beks) trademark for a parenteral preparation of crystalline vitamin B_{12}.

syzygy (siz′ĭ-je) 1. the conjunction and fusion of organs without the loss of identity. 2. the temporary adherence of male and female gregarines prior to encystment and the production of gametes.

T

T. temperature; intraocular tension, normal intraocular tension being indicated by Tn, while T + 1, T + 2, etc., indicate increased tension, and T – 1, T – 2, etc., indicate decreased tension.

T$_m$ tubular maximum (of the kidneys); used in reporting kidney function studies, with inferior letters representing the substance used in the test, as T$_{m_{PAH}}$ (tubular maximum for para-aminohippuric acid).

T.A. toxin-antitoxin.

Ta chemical symbol, *tantalum.*

tabacosis (tab″ah-ko′sis) poisoning by tobacco, chiefly by inhaling tobacco dust; also, a form of pneumoconiosis attributed to tobacco dust (*t. pulmo′num*).

tabanid (tab′ah-nid) any gadfly of the family Tabanidae, including the horseflies and deerflies.

Tabanus (tah-ba′nus) a genus of bloodsucking biting flies (horse or gadflies) which transmit trypanosomes and anthrax to various animals.

tabardillo (tah″bar-dēl′yo) murine typhus.

tabes (ta′bēz) 1. any wasting of the body; progressive atrophy of the body or a part of it. 2. tabes dorsalis. **tabet′ic,** adj. **t. dorsa′lis,** the tertiary (or late) form of syphilis marked by degeneration of the dorsal columns of the spinal cord and sensory nerve trunks, with muscular incoordination, paroxysms of intense pain, visceral crises, disturbances of sensation, and various trophic disturbances, especially of bones and joints. **t. mesenter′ica,** tuberculosis of mesenteric glands in children.

tabescent (tah-bes′ent) growing emaciated; wasting away.

tabetiform (tah-bet′ĭ-form) resembling tabes.

tablature (tab′lah-chur) separation of the chief cranial bones into inner and outer tables, separated by a diploë.

table (ta′b'l) a flat layer or surface. **inner t.,** the inner compact layer of the bones covering the brain. **outer t.,** the outer compact layer of the bones covering the brain. **vitreous t.,** inner t.

tablespoon (-spōōn) a household unit of capacity containing about 4 fl.dr., or 15 ml.

tablet (tab′let) a solid dosage form containing a medicinal substance with or without a suitable diluent. **buccal t.,** one which dissolves when held between the cheek and gum, permitting direct absorption of the active ingredient through the oral mucosa. **enteric-coated t.,** one coated with material that delays release of the medication until after it leaves the stomach. **sublingual t.,** one that dissolves when held beneath the tongue, permitting direct absorption of the active ingredient by the oral mucosa.

taboo (tah-boo′) any of the negative traditions and behaviors generally regarded as harmful to social welfare.

taboparesis (ta″bo-pah-re′sis) dementia paralytica occurring concomitantly with tabes dorsalis.

tabular (tab′u-lar) resembling a table.

Tacaryl (tak′ah-ril) trademark for preparations of methdilazine.

TACE (tās) trademark for preparations of chlorotrianisene.

tache (tahsh) [Fr.] a spot or blemish. **tachet′ic,** adj. **t. blanche** ("white spot"), a white spot on the liver in certain infectious diseases. **t's bleuâtres** ("bluish spots"), maculae caeruleae. **t. cérébrale** ("cerebral spot"), a congested streak produced by drawing the nail across the skin; a concomitant of various nervous or cerebral diseases. **t. motrice** ("motor spot"), a motor nerve ending in which the nerve fibril passes to a muscle cell, where it ends in a slight enlargement. **t. noire** ("black spot"), an ulcer covered with a black crust, a characteristic local reaction at the presumed site of the infective bite in certain tickborne rickettsioses.

tachogram (tak′o-gram) the graphic record produced by tachography.

tachography (tah-kog′rah-fe) the recording of the movement and speed of the blood current.

tachy- word element [Gr.], *rapid; swift.*

tachycardia (tak″e-kar′de-ah) abnormally rapid heart rate. **tachycar′diac,** adj. **atrial t.,** a rapid cardiac rate, usually 160–190 per minute, originating from an atrial locus. **ectopic t.,** rapid heart action in response to impulses arising outside the sinoatrial node. **paroxysmal t.,** rapid heart action that starts and stops abruptly. **ventricular t.,** an abnormally rapid ventricular rhythm with aberrant ventricular excitation, usually above 150 per minute, generated within the ventricle, and most often associated with atrioventricular dissociation.

tachylalia (-la′le-ah) rapidity of speech.

tachymeter (tah-kim′ĕ-ter) an instrument for measuring rapidity of motion.

tachyphagia (tak″e-fa′je-ah) rapid eating.

tachyphasia, tachyphrasia (-fa′ze-ah; -fra′ze-ah) extreme volubility of speech.

tachyphrenia (-fre′ne-ah) mental hyperactivity.

tachyphylaxis (-fi-lak′sis) 1. rapid immunization against the effect of toxic doses of an extract by previous injection of small doses of it. 2. the decreasing responses following consecutive injections made at short intervals. **tachyphylac′tic,** adj.

tachypnea (tak″ip-ne′ah) very rapid respiration.

tachyrhythmia (tak″e-rith′me-ah) tachycardia.

tachysterol (tak-is′tĕ-rol) an isomer of ergosterol produced by irradiation.

Tacosal (tak′o-sal) trademark for a preparation of diphenylhydantoin.

tactile (tak′til) pertaining to touch.

tactometer (tak-tom′ĕ-ter) an instrument for measuring tactile sensibility.

tactus (tak′tus) [L.] touch. **tac′tual,** adj. **t.**

erudi′tus, delicacy of touch acquired by practice.

Taenia (te′ne-ah) a genus of tapeworms. **T. echinococ′cus,** *Echinococcus granulosus.* **T. sagina′ta,** a species 12–25 feet long, found in the adult form in the human intestine and in the larval state in muscles and other tissues of cattle and other ruminants; human infection usually results from eating inadequately cooked beef. **T. so′lium,** a species 6–12 feet long, found in the adult intestine; the larval form most often is found in muscle and other tissues of the pig; human infection results from eating inadequately cooked pork.

taenia (te′ne-ah) 1. tenia (1). 2. a tapeworm of the genus *Taenia.*

taeniacide (-sīd″) 1. lethal to tapeworms. 2. an agent lethal to tapeworms.

taeniafuge (-fūj″) teniafuge.

taeniasis (te-ni′ah-sis) infection with tapeworms of the genus *Taenia.*

Tagathen (tag′ah-then) trademark for a preparation of chlorothen.

Taka-Diastase (tah′kah-di′as-tās) trademark for an amylolytic enzyme produced by action of spores of the fungus *Aspergillus oryzae* on wheat bran; used as a digestant.

talbutal (tal′bu-tal) a hypnotic and sedative, $C_{11}H_{16}N_2O_3$.

talc (talk) a native hydrous magnesium silicate, sometimes with a small amount of aluminum silicate; used as a dusting powder.

talcosis (tal-ko′sis) a condition due to inhalation or implantation in the body of talc.

talcum (tal′kum) talc.

talipes (tal′ĭ-pēz) clubfoot; a congenital deformity of the foot, which is twisted out of shape or position; the foot may be in dorsiflexion (*t. calca′neus*) or plantar flexion (*t. equi′nus*), abducted, everted (*t. val′gus*), abducted, inverted (*t. va′rus*), or various combinations of these (*t. calcaneoval′gus, t. calcaneova′rus, t. equinoval′gus,* or *t. equinova′rus*).

talipomanus (tal″ĭ-pom′ah-nus) clubhand.

talocalcaneal (ta″lo-kal-ka′ne-al) pertaining to the talus and calcaneus.

talocrural (-kroo′ral) pertaining to the talus and the leg bones.

talofibular (-fib′u-lar) pertaining to the talus and fibula.

talonavicular (-nah-vik′u-lar) pertaining to the talus and navicular bone.

talonid (tal′o-nid) the posterior part of a lower molar tooth.

talus (ta′lus), pl. *ta′li* [L.] see *Table of Bones.*

tambour (tam′boor) a drum-shaped appliance used in transmitting movements in a recording instrument.

tampon (tam′pon) [Fr.] a pad or plug made of cotton, sponge, or oakum, variously used in surgery to plug the nose, vagina, etc., for the control of hemorrhage or the absorption of secretions.

tamponade (tam″po-nād′) 1. surgical use of a tampon. 2. pathologic compression of a part.

cardiac t., compression of the heart due to collection of blood in the pericardium.

Tandearil (tan-de′ah-ril) trademark for a preparation of oxyphenbutazone.

tank (tank) an artificial receptacle for liquids. **Hubbard t.,** a tank in which exercises may be performed under water.

tannase (tan′ās) an enzyme that catalyzes the hydrolysis of ester linkages in gallic acid compounds.

tannate (tan′āt) any of the salts of tannic acid, all of which are astringent.

tannin (tan′in) tannic acid.

tantalum (tan′tah-lum) chemical element (*see table*), at. no. 73, symbol Ta; a noncorrosive and malleable metal that has been used for plates or disks to replace cranial defects, for wire sutures, and for making prosthetic appliances.

tantrum (tan′trum) a violent display of temper.

tap (tap) 1. a quick, light blow. 2. to drain off fluid by paracentesis. **spinal t.,** lumbar puncture.

Tapazole (tap′ah-zol) trademark for a preparation of methimazole.

tape (tāp) a long, narrow strip of fabric or other flexible material. **adhesive t.,** a strip of fabric or other material evenly coated on one side with a pressure-sensitive adhesive material.

tapeinocephaly (tah-pi″no-sef′ah-le) flatness of the skull, with a vertical index below 72. **tapeinocephal′ic,** adj.

tapetum (tah-pe′tum), pl. *tape′ta* [L.] 1. a covering structure or layer of cells. 2. a stratum in the human brain composed of fibers from the body and splenium of the corpus callosum sweeping around the lateral ventricle. **t. lu′cidum,** the iridescent epithelium of the choroid of animals which gives their eyes the property of shining in the dark.

tapeworm (tāp′werm) a parasitic intestinal cestode worm having a flattened, bandlike form. **armed t.,** *Taenia solium.* **beef t.,** *Taenia saginata.* **broad t.,** *Dibothriocephalus latum.* **dog t.,** *Dipylidium caninum.* **fish t.,** *Diphyllobothrium latum.* **hydatid t.,** *Echinococcus granulosus.* **pork t.,** *Taenia solium.* **unarmed t.,** *Taenia saginata.*

tapotement (tah-pōt-maw′) [Fr.] a tapping manipulation in massage.

tar (tahr) a dark-brown or black, viscid liquid obtained from various species of pine or from bituminous coal. **coal t.,** a by-product obtained in destructive distillation of bituminous coal; used as a topical antieczematic. **juniper t.,** volatile oil obtained from wood of *Juniperus oxycedrus;* used as a topical antieczematic. **pine t.,** a product of destructive distillation of the wood of various pine trees; used as a local antieczematic and rubefacient.

tarantula (tah-ran′chu-lah) a venomous spider whose bite causes local inflammation and pain, usually not to a severe extent, including *Eurypelma hentzii* (American t.), *Sericopelma communis* (black t.) of Panama, and *Lycosa tarentula* (European wolf spider).

tardive (tahr′div) [Fr.] tardy; late.

tare (tār) 1. the weight of the vessel in which a substance is weighed. 2. to weigh a vessel in order to allow for it when the vessel and a substance are weighed together.

target (tahr′get) an object or area toward which something is directed, as the metal or plate of an x-ray tube on which the electrons impinge and from which the x-rays are sent out; see also under *organ.*

tarichatoxin (tar″ik-ah-tok′sin) a neurotoxin from the newt (*Taricha*), identical with tetrodotoxin.

tars(o)- word element [Gr.], *edge of eyelid; tarsus of the foot; instep.*

tarsadenitis (tahr″sad-ĕ-ni′tis) inflammation of the tarsus of the eyelid and the meibomian glands.

tarsal (tahr′sal) pertaining to a tarsus.

tarsalgia (tahr-sal′je-ah) pain in a tarsus.

tarsalia (tahr-sa′le-ah) the bones of the tarsus.

tarsalis (tahr-sa′lis) [L.] tarsal.

tarsectomy (tahr-sek′to-me) 1. excision of one or more bones of the tarsus. 2. excision of the cartilage of the eyelid.

tarsitis (tahr-si′tis) inflammation of the tarsus of the eyelid; blepharitis.

tarsoclasis (tahr-sok′lah-sis) surgical fracturing of the tarsus of the foot.

tarsomalacia (tahr″so-mah-la′she-ah) softening of the tarsus of an eyelid.

tarsometatarsal (-met″ah-tar′sal) pertaining to the tarsus and metatarsus.

tarsophyma (-fi′mah) any tumor of the tarsus.

tarsoplasty (tahr′so-plas″te) plastic surgery of the tarsus of the eyelid.

tarsoptosis (tahr″sop-to′sis) falling of the tarsus; flatfoot.

tarsorrhaphy (tahr-sor′ah-fe) suture of a portion of or the entire upper and lower eyelids together; done to shorten or entirely close the palpebral fissure.

tarsotomy (tahr-sot′o-me) surgical incision of a tarsus, or an eyelid.

tarsus (tahr′sus) 1. the seven bones—talus, calcaneus, navicular, medial, intermediate and lateral cuneiform, and cuboid—composing the articulation between the foot and leg; the ankle or instep. 2. the cartilaginous plate forming the framework of either (upper or lower) eyelid.

tartar (tahr′tahr) 1. the lees, or sediment, of a wine cask; crude potassium bitartrate. 2. dental calculus. **t. emetic,** antimony potassium tartrate.

tartrate (tahr′trāt) a salt of tartaric acid.

taste (tāst) the peculiar sensation caused by the contact of soluble substances with the tongue; the sense effected by the tongue, the gustatory and other nerves, and the gustation center. Four qualities are distinguished: sweet, sour, salty, and bitter.

taster (tās′ter) an individual capable of tasting a particular test substance (e.g., phenylthiocarbamide) used in genetic studies.

tattooing (tah-too′ing) the introduction, by punctures, of permanent colors in the skin. **t. of cornea,** permanent coloring of the cornea, chiefly to conceal leukomatous spots.

taurine (taw′rēn) a crystallized acid, ethylamine sulfonic acid, from the bile; found also in small quantities in lung and muscle tissues.

taurocholate (taw″ro-ko′lāt) a salt of taurocholic acid.

tautomer (taw′to-mer) a chemical compound exhibiting, or capable of exhibiting, tautomerism.

tautomeral (taw-tom′er-al) pertaining to the same part; said especially of neurons and neuroblasts sending processes to aid in formation of the white matter in the same side of the spinal cord.

tautomerase (-ās) an enzyme that catalyzes tautomeric reactions.

tautomeric (taw″to-mer′ik) exhibiting, or capable of exhibiting, tautomerism.

tautomerism (taw-tom′er-izm) stereoisomerism in which the compounds are mutually interconvertible, under normal conditions, forming a mixture that is in dynamic equilibration.

taxis (tak′sis) 1. an orientation movement of a motile organism in response to a stimulus; it may be either toward (positive) or away from (negative) the source of the stimulus; used also as a word ending, affixed to a stem denoting the nature of the stimulus. 2. exertion of force in manual replacement of a displaced organ or part.

taxon (tak′son), pl. *tax′a* [Gr.] a particular group (category) into which related organisms are classified; the main categories (in ascending order) are species, family, order, class, phylum, and kingdom.

taxonomy (tak-son′o-me) the orderly classification of organisms into appropriate categories (taxa), with application of suitable and correct names. **taxonom′ic,** adj.

Tb chemical symbol, *terbium.*

tb tuberculosis; tubercle bacillus.

Tc chemical symbol, *technetium.*

Te chemical symbol, *tellurium.*

TEA tetraethylammonium.

tea (te) 1. the dried leaves of *Thea chinensis,* containing caffeine and tannic acid, or a decoction thereof. 2. any decoction or infusion.

TEAC tetraethylammonium chloride.

tears (tērz) the watery, slightly alkaline and saline secretion of the lacrimal glands, which moistens the conjunctiva. **crocodile t.,** see under *syndrome.*

tease (tēz) to pull apart gently with fine needles to permit microscopic examination.

teaspoon (te′spoon) a household unit of capacity containing about 1 fl.dr., or 4 ml.

teat (tēt) the nipple of the mammary gland.

technetium (tek-ne′she-um) chemical element (*see table*), at. no. 43, symbol Tc.

technic (tek′nik) technique.

technician (tek-nish′an) a person skilled in the performance of technical procedures.

technique (tek-nēk′) the method of procedure and details of a mechanical process or surgical operation.

tectorial (tek-to′re-al) of the nature of a roof or covering.

tectorium (tek-to′re-um) Corti's membrane.

tectospinal (tek″to-spi′nal) extending from the tectum of the midbrain to the spinal cord.

tectum (tek′tum) a rooflike structure. **t. of mesencephalon, t. of midbrain,** the dorsal portion of the midbrain.

teeth (tēth) see *tooth.*

teething (tēth′ing) the entire process resulting in eruption of the teeth.

tegmen (teg′men), pl. *teg′mina* [L.] a covering structure or roof. **t. tym′pani,** 1. the thin layer of bone separating the tympanic antrum from the cranial cavity. 2. the roof of the tympanic cavity, related to part of the petrous portion of the temporal bone.

tegmentum (teg-men′tum), pl. *tegmen′ta*[L.] 1. a covering. 2. the part of the cerebral peduncle dorsal to the substantia nigra. **tegmen′tal,** adj.

Tegretol (teg′rĕ-tol) trademark for preparations of carbamazepine.

teichopsia (ti-kop′se-ah) scintillating scotoma.

T-1824 Evans blue.

tela (te′lah), pl. *te′lae* [L.] any weblike tissue. **t. conjuncti′va,** connective tissue. **t. elas′tica,** elastic tissue. **t. subcuta′nea,** subcutaneous tissue.

telalgia (tel-al′je-ah) referred pain.

telangiectasia (tel-an″je-ek-ta′ze-ah) a vascular lesion formed by dilation of a group of small blood vessels. **telangiectat′ic,** adj. **hereditary hemorrhagic t.,** a hereditary condition marked by multiple small angiomas of the skin and mucous membranes, often with nosebleed or gastrointestinal bleeding and sometimes with arteriovenous fistula of the lung or liver.

telangiectasis (-ek′tah-sis), pl. *telangiec′tases.* Telangiectasia. **spider t.,** vascular spider.

telangiosis (-o′sis) any disease of the capillaries.

tele- word element [Gr.], *far away; operating at a distance; an end.*

telecardiography (tel″ĕ-kar″de-og′rah-fe) the recording of an electrocardiogram by transmission of impulses to a site at a distance from the patient.

telecardiophone (-kar′de-o-fōn″) an apparatus for making heart sounds audible at a distance from the patient.

telecinesia (-si-ne′ze-ah) telekinesis.

telefluoroscopy (-floo″or-os′ko-pe) television transmission of fluoroscopic images for study at a distant location.

telekinesis (-ki-ne′sis) 1. movement of an object produced without contact. 2. the ability to produce such movement. **telekinet′ic,** adj.

telemetry (tĕ-lem′ĕ-tre) the making of measurements at a distance from the subject, the measurable evidence of phenomena under investigation being transmitted by radio signals.

telencephalon (tel″en-sef′ah-lon) endbrain: 1. the paired brain vesicles, which are the anterolateral outpouchings of the forebrain, together with the median, unpaired portion, the terminal lamina of the hypothalamus; from it the cerebral hemispheres are derived. 2. the anterior of the two vesicles formed by specialization of the forebrain in embryonic development. **telencephal′ic,** adj.

teleneurite (tel″ĕ-nu′rīt) an end expansion of an axon.

teleneuron (-nu′ron) a nerve ending.

teleological (te″le-o-loj′ĭ-kal) serving an ultimate purpose in development.

teleology (-ol′o-je) the doctrine of final causes or of adaptation to a definite purpose.

teleomitosis (tel″e-o-mi-to′sis) completed mitosis.

teleorganic (-or-gan′ik) necessary to life.

Telepaque (tel′ĕ-pāk) trademark for a preparation of iopanoic acid.

telepathy (tĕ-lep′ah-the) the communication of thought through extrasensory perception.

teleradiography (tel″ĕ-ra″de-og′rah-fe) teleroentgenography.

telergy (tel′er-je) 1. automatism. 2. a hypothetical action of one brain on another at a distance.

teleroentgenography (tel″ĕ-rent″gen-og′rah-fe) roentgenography with the x-ray tube 6½ to 7 feet away from the plate in order more nearly to secure parallelism of the rays.

telesthesia (tel″es-the′ze-ah) telepathy; perception at a distance.

teletherapy (tel″ĕ-ther′ah-pe) treatment in which the source of the therapeutic agent, e.g., radiation, is at a distance from the body.

telluric (tĕ-lu′rik) 1. pertaining to tellurium. 2. pertaining to or originating from the earth.

tellurium (tĕ-lu′re-um) chemical element (*see table*), at. no. 52, symbol Te.

telo- word element [Gr.], *end.*

telodendron (tel″o-den′dron) any of the fine terminal branches of an axon.

telogen (tel′o-jen) the quiescent or resting phase of the hair cycle, following catagen, the hair having become a club hair and not growing further.

telognosis (tel″og-no′sis) diagnosis based on interpretation of roentgenograms transmitted by telephonic or radio communication.

telolecithal (tel″o-les′ĭ-thal) having a yolk concentrated at one of the poles.

telolemma (-lem′ah) the covering of a motor end-plate.

telomere (tel′o-mēr) an extremity of a chromosome, which has specific properties, one of which is a polarity that prevents reunion with any fragment after a chromosome has been broken.

telophase (-fāz) the last of the four stages of mitosis and of the two divisions of meiosis.

TEM triethylenemelamine.

Temaril (tem′ah-ril) trademark for preparations of trimeprazine.

temperature (tem′per-ah-chur) an expression of heat or coldness in terms of a specific scale. See Table accompanying *thermometer.* **absolute t.,** that reckoned from absolute zero (–273.15° C. or –459.67° F.). **critical t.,** that below which a gas may be converted to a liquid by pressure. **normal t.,** that usually registered by a healthy person (98.6° F. or 37° C.).

template (tem′plat) a pattern or mold. In dentistry, a curved or flat plate used as an aid in setting teeth for a denture. In theoretical immunology, an antigen that determines the configuration of combining (antigen-binding) sites of antibody molecules. In genetics, a strand of DNA which specifies the synthesis of a complementary strand of RNA (mRNA), which in turn serves as a template for the synthesis of nucleic acids or proteins.

temple (tem′p′l) the lateral region on either side of the head, above the zygomatic arch.

tempolabile (tem″po-la′bil) subject to change with time.

tempora (tem′po-rah) [L.] the temples.

temporal (-ral) 1. pertaining to the temple. 2. pertaining to time; limited as to time; temporary.

temporomandibular (tem″po-ro-man-dib′u-lar) pertaining to the temporal bone and mandible.

temporomaxillary (-mak′sĭ-lar″e) pertaining to the temporal bone and maxilla.

temporo-occipital (-ok-sip′ĭ-tal) pertaining to the temporal and occipital bones.

temporosphenoid (-sfe′noid) pertaining to the temporal and sphenoid bones.

tempostabile (tem″po-sta′bīl) not subject to change with time.

Tempra (tem′prah) trademark for preparations of acetaminophen.

tenacious (tĕ-na′shus) viscid; adhesive.

tenaculum (tĕ-nak′u-lum) a hooklike surgical instrument for grasping and holding parts.

tenalgia (ten-al′je-ah) pain in a tendon.

tenderness (ten′der-nes) a state of unusual sensitivity to touch or pressure. **rebound t.,** a state in which pain is felt on the release of pressure over a part.

tendinitis (ten″dĭ-ni′tis) inflammation of tendons of tendon-muscle attachments.

tendinoplasty (ten′dĭ-no-plas′te) tenoplasty.

tendinosuture (ten″dĭ-no-su′chur) tenorrhaphy.

tendinous (ten′dĭ-nus) pertaining to, resembling, or of the nature of a tendon.

tendo (ten′do), pl. *ten′dines*[L.] tendon. **t. Achil′-lis, t. calca′neus,** Achilles tendon.

tendolysis (ten-dol′ĭ-sis) the freeing of a tendon from adhesions.

tendon (ten′don) a fibrous cord of connective tissue continuous with the fibers of a muscle and attaching the muscle to bone or cartilage. **Achilles t., calcaneal t.,** the powerful tendon at the back of the heel, attaching the triceps surae muscle to the calcaneus.

tendonitis (ten″do-ni′tis) tendinitis.

tendovaginal (-vaj′ĭ-nal) pertaining to a tendon and its sheath.

tenectomy (tĕ-nek′to-me) excision of a lesion of a tendon or of a tendon sheath.

tenesmus (tĕ-nez′mus) ineffectual and painful straining at stool or in urinating. **tenes′mic,** adj.

tenia (te′ne-ah), pl. *te′niae* [L.] 1. a flat band or strip of soft tissue. 2. a tapeworm of the genus *Taenia.* **te′niae co′li,** the three thickened bands (*t. li′bera, t. mesocol′ica,* and *t. omenta′-lis*) formed by longitudinal fibers in the muscu-

lar tunic of the large intestine, extending from the root of the vermiform appendix to the rectum.

teniacide (te′ne-ah-sīd″) 1. lethal to tapeworms. 2. an agent lethal to tapeworms.

teniafuge (-fūj″) an agent that expels tapeworms.

teniasis (te-ni′ah-sis) taeniasis.

teno- word element [Gr.], *tendon.*

tenodesis (ten-od′ĕ-sis) suture of the end of a tendon to a bone.

tenodynia (ten″o-din′e-ah) tenalgia.

tenomyoplasty (-mi′o-plas″te) plastic repair of a tendon and muscle.

tenomyotomy (-mi-ot′o-me) excision of a portion of a tendon and muscle.

tenonectomy (-nek′to-me) excision of part of a tendon to shorten it.

tenonitis (-ni′tis) 1. tendinitis. 2. inflammation of Tenon's capsule.

tenonometer (-nom′ĕ-ter) an apparatus for measuring intraocular pressure.

tenontitis (ten″on-ti′tis) tendinitis.

tenonto- word element [Gr.], *tendon.*

tenontodynia (ten″on-to-din′e-ah) tenalgia.

tenontography (ten″on-tog′rah-fe) a written description or delineation of the tendons.

tenontology (ten″on-tol′o-je) sum of what is known about the tendons.

tenontothecitis (ten-on″to-the-si′tis) tenosynovitis.

tenophyte (ten′o-fīt) a growth or concretion in a tendon.

tenoplasty (-plas″te) plastic repair of a tendon. **tenoplas′tic,** adj.

tenoreceptor (ten″o-re-sep′tor) a proprioreceptor in a tendon.

tenorrhaphy (ten-or′ah-fe) suture of a tendon.

tenositis (ten″o-si′tis) tendinitis.

tenostosis (ten″os-to′sis) conversion of a tendon into bone.

tenosuture (ten″o-su′chur) tenorrhaphy.

tenosynovectomy (-sin″o-vek′to-me) excision or resection of a tendon sheath.

tenosynovitis (-sin″o-vi′tis) inflammation of a tendon sheath. **villonodular t.,** a condition marked by exaggerated proliferation of synovial membrane cells, producing a solid tumor-like mass, commonly occurring in periarticular soft tissues and less frequently in joints.

tenotomy (ten-ot′o-me) transection of a tendon. **graduated t.,** partial transection of a tendon.

tenovaginitis (ten″o-vaj″ĭ-ni′tis) tenosynovitis.

Tensilon (ten′sĭ-lon) trademark for a solution of edrophonium.

tension (ten′shun) 1. the act of stretching or the condition of being stretched or strained. 2. the partial pressure of a component of a gas mixture. **arterial t.,** blood pressure within an artery. **intraocular t.,** see under *pressure.* **premenstrual t.,** a complex of symptoms, including emotional instability and irritability, sometimes occurring in the 10 days before menstruation. **surface t.,** tension or resistance which acts to preserve the integrity of a surface.

tissue t., a state of equilibrium between tissues and cells which prevents overaction of any part.

tensor (ten'sor) any muscle that stretches or makes tense.

tent (tent) 1. a fabric covering designed to enclose an open space, especially such a covering over a patient's bed for administering oxygen or vaporized medication by inhalation. 2. a conical, expansible plug of soft material for dilating an orifice or for keeping a wound open, so as to prevent its healing except at the bottom. **sponge t.,** a conical plug made of compressed sponge used to dilate the os uteri.

tentacle (ten'tah-k'l) a slender whiplike appendage in animals that may function in prehension and feeding or as a sense organ.

tentorium (ten-to're-um), pl. *tento'ria* [L.] an anatomical part resembling a tent or covering. **tento'rial,** adj. **t. cerebel'li,** the process of the dura mater supporting the occipital lobes and covering the cerebellum.

tephromyelitis (tef"ro-mi"ĕ-li'tis) inflammation of the gray substance of the spinal cord.

tepor (te'por) [L.] gentle heat.

ter- word element [L.], *three; three-fold.*

tera- a word element ([Gr.] *monster*) used in naming units of measurement to designate a quantity 10^{12} (a trillion, or million million) times the unit specified by the root to which it is joined, as teracurie; symbol T.

teras (ter'as), pl. *ter'ata* [L., Gr.] a monster. **terat'ic,** adj.

teratism (ter'ah-tizm) an anomaly of formation or development; the condition of a monster.

terato- word element [Gr.], *monster; monstrosity.*

teratoblastoma (ter"ah-to-blas-to'mah) a neoplasm containing embryonic elements, differing from a teratoma in that its tissue does not represent all germinal layers.

teratogen (ter'ah-to-jen) an agent or influence that causes physical defects in the developing embryo. **teratogen'ic,** adj.

teratogenesis (ter"ah-to-jen'ĕ-sis) the production of deformity in the developing embryo, or of a monster. **teratogenet'ic,** adj.

teratogenous (ter"ah-toj'ĕ-nus) the production of deformities in offspring *in utero.*

teratogeny (ter"ah-toj'ĕ-ne) teratogenesis.

teratoid (ter'ah-toid) resembling a monster.

teratology (ter"ah-tol'o-je) that division of embryology and pathology dealing with abnormal development and congenital deformations. **teratolog'ic,** adj.

teratoma (ter"ah-to'mah) a true neoplasm made up of different types of tissue, none of which is native to the area in which it occurs; usually found in the ovary or testis.

teratomatous (ter"ah-tom'ah-tus) pertaining to or of the nature of teratoma.

teratosis (ter"ah-to'sis) the condition of a monster.

terbium (ter'be-um) chemical element (*see table*), at. no. 65, symbol Tb.

terebene (ter'ĕ-bēn) an antiseptic and expectorant terpene, $C_{10}H_{16}$, from turpentine oil.

terebration (ter"ĕ-bra'shun) an act of boring or trephining; also, a boring pain.

teres (te'rēz) [L.] long and round.

ter in die (ter in de'a) [L.] three times a day.

term (term) a definite period, especially the period of gestation, or pregnancy.

terminal (ter'mĭ-nal) 1. forming or pertaining to an end; placed at the end. 2. a termination, end, or extremity; see *ending.*

terminatio (ter"mĭ-na'she-o), pl. *terminatio'nes* [L.] an ending; the site of discontinuation of a structure, as the free nerve endings (*termina'tiones nervo'rum li'berae*), in which the peripheral fiber divides into fine branches that terminate freely in connective tissue or epithelium.

terminology (ter"mĭ-nol'o-je) 1. the vocabulary of an art of science. 2. the science dealing with the investigation, arrangement, and construction of terms.

terminus (ter'mĭ-nus), pl. *ter'mini* [L.] an ending.

ternary (ter'nah-re) 1. third in order. 2. made up of three distinct chemical elements.

terpene (ter'pēn) any hydrocarbon of the formula $C_{10}H_{16}$.

terpin (ter'pin) a product obtained by the action of nitric acid on oil of turpentine and alcohol; used as an expectorant in the form of the hydrate salt.

Terramycin (ter'ah-mi"sin) trademark for preparations of oxytetracycline.

tertian (ter'shan) recurring every three days (every second day); see under *malaria.*

tertiary (ter'she-a"re) third in order.

tertigravida (ter"she-grav'ĭ-dah) a woman pregnant for the third time; gravida III.

tertipara (ter-tip'ah-rah) a woman who has had three pregnancies which resulted in viable offspring; para III.

Tessalon (tes'sah-lon) trademark for a preparation of benzonatate.

tessellated (tes'ĕ-lāt"ed) divided into squares, like a checker board.

test (test) 1. an examination or trial. 2. a significant chemical reaction. 3. a reagent. **acetic acid t.,** one for albumin in urine; acetic acid is added to boiled urine and a white precipitate forms. **alkali denaturation t.,** a spectrophotometric method for determining the concentration of fetal (F) hemoglobin. **Allen-Doisey t.,** one for detection of estrogenic activity. **Almén t's,** tests for detection of albumin, blood, blood pigment, or dextrose in solutions, such as urine. **aptitude t.,** one designed to measure the capacity for developing general or specific skills. **Aschheim-Zondek t.,** one for pregnancy, based on the effects on the ovaries of immature female mice produced by injection of the patient's urine. **association t.,** one based on associative reaction, usually by mentioning words to a patient and noting what other words the patient will give as the ones called up in his mind. **Babcock's t.,** one for determination of the fat content of milk. **barium t.,** roentgenographic examination using a barium sulfate mixture as opaque contrast medium to locate digestive tract disorders. **Benedict's t.,** a qualitative or quantitative test for the determination of dextrose content of solutions. **Binet's t., Binet-Simon t.,** a method of ascertaining a child's or youth's mental age by asking a series of questions adapted to, and standardized on, the capacity of normal children at various ages. **Calmette t.,** ophthalmic reaction. **caloric t.,** Bárány's symptom (2). **Casoni's t.,** intradermal injection of hydatid fluid followed by production of wheal-flare reaction denotes hydatid infection. **cephalin-cholesterol flocculation t.,** Hanger's t. **Chautard's t.,** one for acetone in the urine. **chromatin t.,** determination of genetic sex of an individual by examination of body cells for the presence of sex chromatin. **cis-trans t.,** a test in microbial genetics to determine whether two mutations that have the phenotypic effect, in a haploid cell or a cell with single phage infection, are located in the same gene or in different genes; the test depends on the independent behavior of two alleles of a gene in a diploid cell or in a cell infected with two phages carrying different alleles. **coin t.,** a silver coin held flat on the anterior chest wall is struck with the edge of another silver coin; a clear, bell-like sound heard by stethoscope on the posterior chest wall indicates air in the pleural space. **complement fixation t.,** see *fixation of complement.* **conjunctival t.,** 1. see *ophthalmic reaction.* 2. the local reaction occurring after instillation of a pollen or pollen extract into the conjunctiva of a person sensitive to that pollen. **Coombs' t.,** one using various antisera, usually employed to detect the presence of proteins (usually antibodies) on the surface of red cells, as in the test of erythroblastosis fetalis. **Dick t.,** an intracutaneous test for determination of susceptibility to scarlet fever. **double-blind t.,** a study of the effects of a specific agent in which neither the administrator nor the recipient, at the time of administration, knows whether the active or an inert substance is being used. **finger-nose t.,** one for coordinated movements of the extremities; with the arm extended to one side the patient is asked to try to touch the end of his nose with the tip of his index finger. **Fishberg concentration t.,** determination of the ability of the kidneys to maintain excretion of solids under conditions of reduced water intake and a high protein diet, in which urine samples are collected and tested for specific gravity. **Frei t.,** intracutaneous injection of antigen derived from infected chick embryos, used in the diagnosis of lymphogranuloma venereum. **Friedman t.,** one for pregnancy, based on the effects on the ovaries of a mature, nonpregnant female rabbit, produced by injection of the patient's urine. **galactose tolerance t.,** a test of carbohydrate tolerance of the liver by measuring the amount of galactose eliminated in the urine after oral or intravenous administration of galactose. **Galli Mainini t.,** one for pregnancy, based upon the presence of spermatozoa in the urine of a male frog or toad after injection of the patient's urine. **glucose tolerance t.,** a test of the body's ability to utilize carbohydrates by measuring the blood sugar level at stated intervals after ingestion or intravenous injection of a large quantity of glu-

cose. **guaiac t.,** one for determination of blood in a stain. **Ham t.,** one for paroxysmal nocturnal hemoglobinuria, performed by incubating red cells in an acid environment; a positive test may be obtained in other forms of anemia. **Hanger's t.,** a test for liver cell disease based on the flocculation of a cephalin-cholesterol emulsion by the patient's serum. **Heller t's,** tests for detection of albumin, blood, or dextrose in the urine. **Hinton's t's,** serologic tests performed for the diagnosis of syphilis. **histamine t.,** 1. subcutaneous injection of 0.1% solution of histamine to stimulate gastric secretion. 2. after rapid intravenous injection of histamine phosphate, normal persons experience a brief fall in blood pressure, but in those with pheochromocytoma, after the fall, there is a marked rise in blood pressure. **Holmgren t.,** one for detection of imperfect perception of color, based on matching various strands of yarn. **Huhner t.,** determination of the number and condition of spermatozoa in mucus aspirated from the cervical canal within two hours after intercourse. **inkblot t.,** Rorschach t. **Kahn t.,** a precipitation test for syphilis. **Kline t.,** a microscope slide precipitation test for syphilis. **Kolmer's t.,** a modification of the Wassermann test for syphilis. 2. a specific complement-fixation test for various bacterial diseases. **Kveim t.,** an intracutaneous test for the diagnosis of sarcoidosis. **latex agglutination t., latex-fixation t.,** a serologic test for rheumatoid arthritis. **Mantoux t.,** an intracutaneous tuberculin test. **Master "2-step" exercise t.,** a test of coronary circulation, electrocardiograms being recorded while and after the subject repeatedly ascends and descends two steps, each 9 inches high. **Moloney t.,** one for detection of delayed hypersensitivity to diphtheria toxoid. **multiple-puncture t.,** an intracutaneous test in which the material used (e.g., tuberculin) is introduced into the skin by pressure of several needles or pointed tines or prongs. **neutralization t.,** one for the bacterial neutralization power of a substance by testing its action on the pathogenic properties of the organism concerned. **Nickerson-Kveim t.,** Kveim t. **Pándy t.,** one for globulin in cerebrospinal fluid. **Pap t., Papanicolaou t.,** an exfoliative cytological staining procedure for detection and diagnosis of various conditions, particularly malignant and premalignant conditions of the female genital tract; also used in evaluating endocrine function and in diagnosis of malignancies of other organs. **patch t.,** a test for hypersensitivity, performed by observing the reaction to application to the skin of filter paper or gauze saturated with the substance in question. **Patrick's t.,** thigh and knee of the supine patient are flexed, the external malleolus rests on the patella on the opposite leg, and the knee is depressed; production of pain indicates arthritis of the hip. Also known as *fabere sign,* from the initial letters of movements necessary to elicit it, i.e., *f*lexion, *a*bduction, *e*xternal *r*otation, and *e*xtension. **Paul-Bunnell t.,** a method of testing for the presence of heterophil antibodies in the blood for diagnosis of infectious mononucleosis, based on the agglutination of sheep erythrocytes by the inactivated serum of patients with the disease. **phlorhizin t.,** a test of kidney function based on injection of phlorhizin and sodium carbonate. **plasmacrit t.,** a rapid screening test for syphilis, using plasma from microhematocrit tubes. **precipitation t., precipitin t.,** any test in which the positive reaction consists in the formation and deposit of a precipitate in the fluid being tested. **prothrombin consumption t.,** a test to measure the formation of intrinsic thromboplastin by determining the residual serum prothrombin after blood coagulation is complete. **Queckenstedt's t.,** see under *sign.* **Quick's t.,** 1. a test for liver function based on excretion of hippuric acid after administration of sodium benzoate. 2. (*one-stage prothrombin time*) by adding an extrinsic thromboplastin to oxalated blood the integrity of the prothrombin complex, composed of Factors II, V, VII, X, may be defined; used to control administration of coumarin-type anticoagulants. **Quick tourniquet t.,** estimation of capillary fragility by counting the number of petechiae appearing in a limited area on the flexor surface of the forearm after obstruction to the circulation by a blood pressure cuff applied to the upper arm. **Rinne t.,** a test of hearing made with tuning forks of 256, 512, and 1024 cycle frequency, comparing the duration of perception by bone and by air conduction. **Roberts' t's,** tests for detecting albumin or dextrose in the urine. **Rorschach t.,** one for disclosing disorders of emotion by the patient's response to 10 cards bearing symmetrical ink blots in various colors and shading. **Rosenbach t.,** detection of cold hemolysins by hemoglobinuric response to immersion of the hands or feet in ice water. **Rubin t.,** one for patency of the uterine tubes, made by transuterine inflation with carbon dioxide gas. **Rubner's t.,** 1. one for carbon monoxide in the blood. 2. one for lactose, dextrose, maltose, and levulose in the urine. **Schick t.,** an intracutaneous test for determination of susceptibility to diphtheria. **Schiller t.,** one for early carcinoma, performed by painting the uterine cervix with a solution of iodine and potassium iodide, diseased areas being revealed by a failure to take the stain. **Schilling t.,** one for diagnosis of primary pernicious anemia. **Schirmer's t.,** a test of tear production in keratoconjunctivitis sicca, performed by measuring the area of moisture on a piece of filter paper inserted over the conjunctival sac of the lower lid, with the end of the paper hanging down on the outside. **Schwabach t.,** a test of hearing made with tuning forks of 256, 512, 1024, and 2048 cycle frequency, the duration of perception of the patient by bone conduction being compared with that of the examiner. **scratch t.,** cutireaction. **sickling t.,** one for demonstration of abnormal hemoglobin and the sickling phenomenon in erythrocytes. **single-blind t.,** a study of the effects of a specific agent in which the administrator, but not the recipient, knows whether the active or an inert substance is being used. **Strauss t.,** one for the presence of lactic acid in stomach contents. **Thorn t.,** a test for adrenal cortical response after injection of ACTH or of epinephrine. **three-glass t.,** on

arising in the morning, the patient urinates successively in three containers (I, II, III): in acute anterior urethritis, only the urine in I will be turbid from pus or will contain blood; in posterior urethritis the urine in all three will be turbid or contain blood; shreds in III point to chronic prostatitis. **tine t.,** four 2 mm.-long tines or prongs attached to a handle and coated with dip-dried Old tuberculin are pressed into the skin of the volar surface of the forearm; 48–72 hours later the skin is checked for palpable induration around the wounds. **tourniquet t.,** one involving application of a tourniquet to an extremity, as in determination of capillary fragility or status of the collateral circulation. **treponemal hemagglutination (TPHA) t., Treponema pallidum complement fixation (TPCF) t., Treponema pallidum cryolysis complement fixation (TPCP) t., Treponema pallidum immobilization (TPI) t.,** serologic tests related directly to the causative organism, used in the diagnosis of syphilis. **tuberculin t.,** a test for the existence of tuberculosis, consisting in the injection subcutaneously of 5 mg. of tuberculin. **tuberculin t., Sterneedle,** an intracutaneous test for tuberculosis, 1 or 2 drops of tuberculin P.P.D. being forced to penetrate the outer layer of the skin by pressure of the six needle points of the Sterneedle. **Uffelmann t.,** one for detection of hydrochloridic acid and lactic acid in the gastric contents. **van den Bergh t.,** one for determination of the level of bilirubin in the blood serum. **Wassermann t.,** see under *reaction.* **Watson-Schwartz t.,** one used in the diagnosis of acute porphyria. **Weber t.,** a hearing test made by placing a vibrating tuning fork at some point on the midline of the head and noting whether it is perceived as heard in the midline or referred to either ear. **Widal t.,** one for typhoid fever, based on agglutination of *Salmonella typhosa* by dilutions of the patient's serum.

testalgia (tes-tal′je-ah) testicular pain.

test type (test tīp) printed letters of varying size, used in the testing of visual acuity.

testectomy (tes-tek′to-me) orchiectomy.

testicle (tes′tĭ-k′l) testis.

testicular (tes-tik′u-lar) pertaining to the testis.

testis (tes′tis), pl. *tes′tes* [L.] the male gonad; either of the paired egg-shaped glands normally situated in the scrotum, in which the spermatozoa develop. Specialized interstitial cells secrete testosterone. **Cooper's irritable t.,** a testis affected with neuralgia. **inverted t.,** one so positioned in the scrotum that the epididymis is attached anteriorly. **retained t., undescended t.,** one that has failed to descend into the scrotum, but remains within the abdomen or the inguinal canal.

testitis (tes-ti′tis) orchitis.

testoid (tes′toid) a term applied to testicular hormones and other natural or synthetic compounds having a similar effect.

testolactone (tes″to-lak′tōn) an antineoplastic steroid, $C_{19}H_{24}O_3$, prepared from testosterone or progesterone by microbial synthesis; used in postmenopausal breast cancer.

testosterone (tes-tos′tĕ-rōn) a hormone secreted by the interstitial cells of the testes, which functions in the induction and maintenance of male secondary sex characters; a pharmaceutical compound is produced synthetically from cholesterol and certain other sterols or isolated from bull testes. Testosterone and its cypionate, enanthate, and propionate esters are used in replacement therapy of testicular deficiency, palliative therapy in inoperable carcinoma of the female breast, and certain gynecologic conditions. ethinyl t., ethisterone. methyl t., methyltestosterone.

Testryl (tes′tril) trademark for a suspension of pure crystalline testosterone.

tetanic (tĕ-tan′ik) pertaining to tetanus.

tetaniform (tĕ-tan′ĭ-form) resembling tetanus.

tetanigenous (tet″an-nij′ĕ-nus) producing tetanic spasms.

tetanism (tet′ah-nizm) persistent muscular hypertonicity, as in the newborn.

tetanization (tet″ah-ni-za′shun) the induction of tetanic convulsions or symptoms.

tetanize (tet′ah-nīz) to induce tetanic convulsions or symptoms.

tetanode (tet′ah-nōd) the unexcited stage of tetany.

tetanoid (tet′ah-noid) resembling tetanus.

tetanolysin (tet″ah-nol′ĭ-sin) the hemolytic fraction of the exotoxin formed by the tetanus bacillus (Clostridium tetani).

tetanospasmin (tet″ah-no-spaz′min) the neurotoxic component of the tetanus toxin, of primary importance in the pathogenesis of tetanus.

tetanus (tet′ah-nus) 1. an acute, often fatal disease marked by tonic muscular spasm and hyperreflexia, resulting in trismus (lockjaw), generalized muscle spasm, opisthotonus, glottal spasm, and seizures; it is caused by the neurotoxin (tetanospasmin) of Clostridium tetani, whose spores enter the body through a wound. 2. continuous tonic contraction of a muscle; steady contraction of a muscle without distinct twitching. idiopathic t., that in which a portal of entry cannot be located. infantile t., t. neonato′rum, tetanus of very young infants, usually due to umbilical infection. puerperal t., that occurring postpartum. traumatic t., that which follows wound infection with Clostridium tetani.

tetany (tet′ah-ne) 1. a syndrome manifested by sharp flexion of the wrist and ankle joints (carpopedal spasm), muscle twitchings, cramps, and convulsions, sometimes with attacks of stridor; due to abnormal calcium metabolism and occurring in parathyroid hypofunction, vitamin D deficiency, alkalosis, and as a result of ingestion of alkaline salts. 2. tetanus (2). duration t., a continuous tetanic contraction in response to a strong continuous current, occurring especially in degenerated muscles. gastric t., a severe form due to disease of the stomach, attended by difficult respiration and painful tonic spasms of the extremities. hyperventilation t., tetany produced by forced inspiration and expiration continued for a considerable time. latent t., tet-

any elicited by the application of electrical and mechanical stimulation. parathyroid t., parathyroprival t., tetany due to removal or hypofunctioning of the parathyroids.

tetarcone (tet′ar-kōn) tetartocone.

tetartanopia (tet″ar-tah-no′pe-ah) 1. quadrantanopia. 2. perception of red and green only, with blue and yellow perceived as an achromatic (gray) band.

tetartanopsia (-nop′se-ah) tetartanopia.

tetartocone (tet-ar′to-kōn) the posterior internal cusp of a lower bicuspid tooth.

tetra- word element [Gr.], four.

tetrabasic (tet″rah-ba′sik) having four replaceable hydrogen atoms.

tetrabrachius (-bra′ke-us) a double monster having four arms.

tetracaine (tet′rah-kān) a local and spinal anesthetic, $C_{15}H_{24}N_2O_2$, used in the form of the hydrochloride salt.

tetrachloride (tet″rah-klo′rīd) a compound of a radical with four atoms of chlorine.

tetrachloroethylene (-klōr″o-eth′ĭ-lēn) an anthelmintic, C_2Cl_4.

tetracrotic (-krot′ik) having four sphygmographic elevations to one beat of the pulse.

tetracycline (-si′klēn) an antibiotic, $C_{22}H_{24}N_2O_8$, isolated from elaboration products of certain species of Streptomyces; the base and the hydrochloride salt are used as an antiamebic, antibacterial, and antirickettsial.

Tetracyn (tet′rah-sin) trademark for preparations of tetracycline.

tetrad (tet′rad) a group of four similar or related entities, as (1) any element or radical having a valence, or combining power, of four; (2) a group of four chromosomal elements formed in meiosis; (3) a square of cells produced by division into two planes of certain cocci (Sarcina). Fallot's t., tetralogy of Fallot.

tetradactyly (tet″rah-dak′tĭ-le) the presence of four digits on the hand or foot.

tetraethylammonium (-eth″il-ah-mo′ne-um) the radical $(C_2H_5)_4N$, used in the form of the bromide or chloride salt as a ganglionic blocking agent.

tetraethylthiuram disulfide (-thi′u-ram) disulfiram.

tetragonum (-go′num) [L.] a four-sided figure. t. lumba′le, the quadrangle bounded by the four lumbar muscles.

tetrahydrocannabinol (-hi″dro-kah-nab′ĭ-nol) the active principle of cannabis, occurring in two isomeric forms, both considered psychomimetically active.

tetrahydrozoline (-hi-dro′zo-lēn) an adrenergic, $C_{13}H_{16}N_2$, used topically in the form of the hydrochloride salt to reduce nasal congestion.

tetraiodophthalein (-i″o-do-thal′e-in) iodothalein.

tetraiodothyronine (-i″o-do-thi′ro-nēn) thyroxine.

tetralogy (tĕ-tral′o-je) a group or series of four. t. of Fallot, a complex of congenital heart defects consisting of pulmonic stenosis, interventricular septal defect, hypertrophy of right ventricle, and dextroposition of the aorta.

tetramastigote (tet″rah-mas′tĭ-gōt) 1. having four flagella. 2. an organism having four flagella.

tetrameric (-mer′ik) having four parts.

tetramethylenediamine (-meth″ĭ-lēn-di-am′-ēn) putrescine.

tetranitrol (-ni′trol) erythrityl tetranitrate.

tetranopsia (-nop′se-ah) quadrantanopia.

tetraparesis (-pah-re′sis) muscular weakness affecting all four extemities.

tetrapeptide (-pep′tīd) a peptide which, on hydrolysis, yields four amino acids.

tetraplegia (-ple′je-ah) quadriplegia.

tetraploid (tet′rah-ploid) 1. characterized by tetraploidy. 2. an individual or cell having four sets of chromosomes.

tetraploidy (-ploi″de) the state of having four sets of chromosomes (4n).

tetrapus (-pus) a monster with four feet.

tetrasaccharide (tet″rah-sak′ah-rīd) a carbohydrate composed of four monosaccharide groups.

tetrascelus (tĕ-tras′ĕ-lus) a monster with four legs.

tetrasomy (tet′rah-so″me) the presence of two extra chromosomes of one type in an otherwise diploid cell. **tetraso′mic,** adj.

tetraster (tĕ-tras′ter) a figure in mitosis produced by quadruple division of the nucleus.

tetratomic (tet″rah-tom′ik) 1. containing four atoms in the molecule. 2. containing four replaceable hydrogen atoms. 3. containing four hydroxyl groups.

tetravalent (-va′lent) having a valence of four.

tetrodotoxin (tet″ro-do-tok′sin) a highly lethal neurotoxin, $C_{11}H_{17}N_3O_3$, present in numerous species of puffer fish (suborder Tetraodontoidea) and in newts of the genus *Taricha* (tarichatoxin); ingestion results, within minutes, in malaise, dizziness, and tingling about the mouth, which may be followed by ataxia, convulsions, respiratory paralysis, and death.

tetrodotoxism (-tok′sizm) the most severe form of ichthyosarcotoxism; see *tetrodotoxin.*

tetroquinone (tet″ro-kwĭ-nōn) a systemic keratolytic, $C_6H_4O_6$.

tetroxide (tĕ-trok′sīd) a compound of an element or a radical with four oxygen atoms.

textiform (teks′tĭ-form) formed like a network.

textoblastic (teks″to-blas′tik) forming adult tissue; regenerative; said of cells.

texture (teks′chur) the structure or constitution of tissues. **tex′tural,** adj.

Th chemical symbol, *thorium.*

thalamencephalon (thal″ah-men-sef′ah-lon) the part of the diencephalon comprising the thalamus, metathalamus, and epithalamus.

thalamocoele (thal′ah-mo-sēl″) the third ventricle.

thalamocortical (thal″ah-mo-kor′tĭ-kal) pertaining to the thalamus and cerebral cortex.

thalamolenticular (-len-tik′u-lar) pertaining to the thalamus and lenticular nucleus.

thalamotomy (thal″ah-mot′o-me) surgical destruction of selected areas of the thalamus.

thalamus (thal′ah-mus), pl. *thal′ami* [L.] the portion of the thalamencephalon forming part of the lateral wall of the third ventricle, and lying between the hypothalamus and epithalamus; it is a relay center for sensory impulses to the cerebral cortex.

thalassemia (thal″ah-se′me-ah) a heterogeneous group of hereditary hemolytic anemias marked by a decreased rate of synthesis of one or more hemoglobin polypeptide chains, classified according to the chain involved (α, β, δ); the two major categories are α- and β-thalassemia. α-t., **alpha-t.,** that caused by diminished synthesis of alpha chains of hemoglobin. The *homozygous* form is incompatible with life, the stillborn infant displaying severe hydrops fetalis. The *heterozygous* form may be asymptomatic or marked by mild anemia. β-t., **beta-t.,** that caused by diminished synthesis of beta chains of hemoglobin. The *homozygous* form (Cooley's, Mediterranean, or erythroblastic anemia; t. major), in which hemoglobin A is completely absent, appears in the newborn period and is marked by hemolytic, hypochromic, microcytic anemia, hepatosplenomegaly, skeletal deformation, mongoloid facies, and cardiac enlargement. The *heterozygous* form (t. minor) is usually asymptomatic, but there is mild anemia. **t. major,** see *beta-t.* **t. minor,** see *beta-t.* **sickle cell–t.,** a hereditary anemia involving simultaneous heterozygosity for hemoglobin S and thalassemia.

thalassoposia (thah-las″o-po′ze-ah) the drinking of sea water.

thalassotherapy (-ther′ah-pe) treatment of disease by sea bathing, sea voyages, or sea air.

thalidomide (thah-lid′o-mīd) a sedative and hypnotic, $C_{13}H_{10}N_2O$, commonly used in Europe in the early 1960's, and discovered to cause serious congenital anomalies in the fetus, notably amelia and phocomelia, when taken during early pregnancy.

thallium (thal′e-um) chemical element (*see table*), at. no. 81, symbol Tl. It may be absorbed from the gut and from the intact skin, causing a variety of neurologic and psychic symptoms and liver and kidney damage.

thallus (thal′us) 1. a simple plant body not differentiated into root, stem, and leaf, characteristic of mycelial fungi and some algae. 2. the actively growing vegetative organism as distinguished from reproductive or resting portions, as in fungi.

thanato- word element [Gr.], *death.*

thanatobiologic (than″ah-to-bi″o-loj′ik) pertaining to life and death.

thanatognomonic (than″ah-tog″no-mon′ik) indicating the approach of death.

thanatoid (than′ah-toid) resembling death.

thanatophidia (than″ah-to-fid′ĕ-ah) the venomous snakes, collectively.

thebaine (the-ba′in) a crystalline, poisonous, and anodyne alkaloid from opium, having properties similar to those of strychnine.

theca (the′kah), pl. *the′cae* [L.] a case or sheath.

the′cal, adj. **t. cor′dis,** pericardium. **t. follic′-uli,** an envelope of condensed connective tissue surrounding a vesicular ovarian follicle, comprising an internal vascular layer (*t. interna*) and an external fibrous layer (*t. externa*).

thecitis (the-si′tis) tenosynovitis.

thecodont (the′ko-dont) having the teeth inserted in sockets or alveoli.

thecoma (the-ko′mah) theca cell tumor.

thecostegnosis (the″ko-steg-no′sis) contraction of a tendon sheath.

Theileria (thi-le′re-ah) a genus of minute intra-erythrocytic protozoan parasites.

theileriasis (thi″lĕ-ri′ah-sis) infection with *Theileria*.

theine (the′in) the alkaloid of tea, isomeric with caffeine.

thelalgia (the-lal′je-ah) pain in the nipples.

thelarche (the-lar′ke) beginning of development of the breast at puberty.

Thelazia (the-la′ze-ah) a genus of nematode worms parasitic in the eyes of mammals.

thelaziasis (the″la-zi′ah-sis) infection of the eye with *Thelazia*.

theleplasty (the′lĕ-plas″te) a plastic operation on the nipple.

thelerethism (thel-er′ĕ-thizm) erection of the nipple.

thelitis (the-li′tis) inflammation of a nipple.

thelium (the′le-um) 1. a papilla. 2. a nipple.

thelorrhagia (the″lo-ra′je-ah) hemorrhage from the nipple.

thelygenic (thel″ĭ-jen′ik) producing only female offspring.

thenar (the′nar) 1. the fleshy part of the hand at the base of the thumb. 2. pertaining to the palm.

thenyldiamine (then″il-di′ah-mēn) an antihistaminic, $C_{14}H_{19}N_3S$, used as the hydrochloride salt.

Thenylene (then′ĭ-lēn) trademark for a preparation of methapyrilene.

thenylpyramine (then″il-pir′ah-mēn) methapyrilene.

theobromine (the″o-bro′min) an alkaloid prepared from dried ripe seed of the tropical American tree *Theobroma cacoa* or made synthetically from xanthine; it has properties similar to those of caffeine, and is used as a smooth muscle relaxant, as a diuretic, and as a myocardial stimulant and vasodilator. Available as t. calcium salicylate, t. sodium salicylate, t. sodium formate, and t. salicylate.

Theoglycinate (-gli′sĭ-nāt) trademark for a preparation of theophylline sodium glycinate.

theophylline (-fil′in) an alkaloid, $C_7H_8N_4 \cdot H_2O$, occurring in tea or produced synthetically, used as a smooth muscle relaxant, myocardial stimulant, and diuretic; available as t. ethanolamine, t. methylglucamine, t. sodium acetate, and t. sodium glycinate. **t. cholinate,** oxtriphylline. **t. ethylenediamine,** aminophylline.

theory (the′o-re) 1. the doctrine or the principles underlying an art as distinguished from the practice of that particular art. 2. a formulated hypothesis or, loosely speaking, any hypothesis or opinion not based upon actual knowledge. **cell t.,** all organic matter consists of cells, and cell activity is the essential process of life. **clonal-selection t. of immunity,** immunologic specificity is preformed during embryonic life and is mediated through cell clones. **Cohnheim's t.,** 1. the emigration of leukocytes is the essential feature of inflammation. 2. tumors develop from embryonic rests which do not participate in formation of normal surrounding tissue. **Ehrlich's side-chain t.** (of immunity and cytolysis), the protoplasm of body cells contains highly complex organic molecules consisting of a tolerably stable central group to which are attached less stable lateral (side) chains of atoms or atomic groups (*receptors*) which carry on the ordinary chemical transformations in the protoplasm, the stable center of the molecule remaining unaffected. The lateral chains contain a group of atoms (*haptophore group*) capable of uniting with similar groups in toxins, bacteria, and other foreign cells. See also *amboceptor* and *complement.* **germ t.,** 1. all organisms are developed from a cell. 2. infectious diseases are of microbial origin. **Hering's t.,** color perception depends on a visual substance in the retina which is variously modified by anabolism for black, green, and blue, and by catabolism for white, red, and yellow. **Lamarck's t.,** acquired characteristics may be transmitted. **Metchnikoff's t.,** bacteria and other harmful elements in the body are attacked and destroyed by phagocytes, and inflammation is produced by this contest between the phagocytes and harmful elements. **Planck's t.,** quantum t. **preformation t.,** the outmoded theory that the individuals of successive generations are contained, completely formed, within the reproductive cell of one of the parents. **quantum t.,** radiation and absorption of energy occur in quantities (quanta) which vary in size with the frequency of the radiation. **recapitulation t.,** ontogeny recapitulates phylogeny, i.e., an organism in the course of its development goes through the same successive stages (in abbreviated form) as did the species in its evolutionary development. **Young-Helmholtz t.,** color vision depends on three sets of retinal receptors, corresponding to the colors red, green, and violet.

Thephorin (thef′o-rin) trademark for preparations of phenindamine.

theque (tĕk) [Fr.] a round or oval collection, or nest, of melanin-containing nevus cells occurring at the dermoepidermal junction of the skin or in the dermis proper.

therapeutic (ther″ah-pu′tik) pertaining to therapeutics, or treatment of disease; curative.

therapeutics (-pu′tiks) 1. the science and art of healing. 2. a scientific account of the treatment of disease.

therapeutist (-pu′tist) therapist.

therapist (ther′ah-pist) a person skilled in the treatment of disease or other disorder. **physical t.,** a person skilled in the techniques of physical therapy and qualified to administer treatment prescribed by a physician.

therapy (ther′ah-pe) the treatment of disease;

therapeutics. See also *treatment*. **anticoagulant t.,** the use of drugs to render the blood sufficiently incoagulable to discourage thrombosis. **aversion t.,** therapy directed at associating an undesirable behavior pattern with unpleasant stimulation. **collapse t.,** collapse and immobilization of the lung in treatment of pulmonary disease. **electroconvulsive t., electroshock t.,** the induction of convulsions by the passage of an electric current through the brain, as in the treatment of affective disorders. **fever t.,** treatment of disease by induction of high body temperature by physical means or by induction of fever-producing vaccines. **group t.,** psychotherapy carried out with a group of patients under the guidance of a single therapist. **immunosuppressive t.,** treatment with agents, such as x-rays, corticosteroids, and cytoxic chemicals, which suppress the immune response to antigen(s); used in organ transplantation, autoimmune disease, allergy, multiple myeloma, etc. **inhalation t.,** treatment of pathophysiologic alterations of gas exchange in the cardiopulmonary system by the use of respirators, aerosols, oxygen, gas mixtures, etc. **insulin shock t.,** induction of hypoglycemic coma by the administration of insulin in the treatment of affective disorders. **milieu t.,** daily participation in group psychiatric therapy at a hospital, providing for observation and utilization of the patients' interpersonal relationships in a social setting, as well as occupational, physical, and individual psychotherapy. **nonspecific t.,** treatment of disease by agents which produce a general effect on cellular activity. **occupational t.,** the use of any occupation for remedial purposes. **physical t.,** use of physical agents and methods in rehabilitation and restoration of normal bodily function after illness or injury; it includes massage and manipulation, therapeutic exercises, hydrotherapy, and various forms of energy (electrotherapy, actinotherapy, and ultrasound). **replacement t.,** treatment to replace deficient formation or loss of body products by administration of the natural body products or synthetic substitutes. **serum t.,** serotherapy. **shock t.,** treatment of affective disorders by induction of coma or convulsions by various means, including insulin injection, electroshock, etc. **specific t.,** measures which are effective against the organism causing the disease. **substitution t.,** the administration of a hormone to compensate for glandular deficiency. **vaccine t.,** injection of killed cultures of an organism to produce immunity to or modify the course of a disease.

theriogenology (the″re-o-jen-ol′o-je) the branch of veterinary medicine that deals with reproduction in all its aspects. **theriogenolog′ic,** adj.

therm (therm) a unit of heat. The word has been used as equivalent to (a) large calorie; (b) small calorie; (c) 1000 large calories; (d) 100,000 British thermal units.

therm(o)- word element [Gr.], *heat.*

thermaerotherapy (therm-a″er-o-ther′ah-pe) treatment by the application of hot air.

thermal (ther′mal) pertaining to heat.

thermalgesia (ther″mal-je′ze-ah) painful sensation produced by heat.

thermalgia (ther-mal′je-ah) causalgia.

thermanalgesia (therm″an-al-je′ze-ah) absence of sensibility to heat.

thermanesthesia (-es-the′ze-ah) inability to recognize heat and cold.

thermatology (ther″mah-tol′o-je) the study of heat as a therapeutic agent.

thermelometer (ther″mel-om′ĕ-ter) an electric thermometer for measuring small temperature changes.

thermesthesia (therm″es-the′ze-ah) perception of heat or cold.

thermesthesiometer (-es-the″ze-om′ĕ-ter) an instrument for measuring sensibility to heat.

thermhyperesthesia (-hi-pes-the′ze-ah) increased sensibility to high temperatures.

thermhypesthesia (-hi-pes-the′ze-ah) decreased sensibility to high temperatures.

thermic (ther′mik) pertaining to heat.

thermistor (ther-mis′tor) a thermometer whose impedance varies with ambient temperature and so is able to measure extremely small temperature changes.

thermocautery (ther″mo-kaw′ter-e) cauterization by a heated wire or point.

thermochemistry (-kem′is-tre) the aspect of physical chemistry dealing with temperature changes that accompany chemical reactions.

thermocoagulation (-ko-ag″u-la′shun) tissue coagulation with high-frequency currents.

thermocouple (ther′mo-kup″'l) a pair of dissimilar electrical conductors so joined that they may be used for measuring temperature differences.

thermodiffusion (ther″mo-dĭ-fu′zhun) diffusion influenced by a temperature gradient.

thermoduric (-du′rik) able to endure high temperatures.

thermodynamics (-di-nam′iks) the branch of science dealing with heat and energy, their interconversion, and problems related thereto.

thermoexcitory (-ek-si′tor-e) stimulating production of bodily heat.

thermogenesis (-jen′ĕ-sis) the production of heat, especially within the animal body. **thermogenet′ic, thermogen′ic,** adj.

thermogenics (-jen′iks) the science of heat production.

thermogram (ther′mo-gram) 1. a graphic record of temperature variations. 2. the visual record obtained by thermography.

thermograph (-graf) 1. an instrument for recording temperature variations. 2. thermogram (2). 3. the apparatus used in thermography.

thermography (ther-mog′rah-fe) a technique wherein an infrared camera photographically portrays the body's surface temperature, based on self-emanating infrared radiations; sometimes used as a means of diagnosing underlying pathologic conditions, such as breast tumors.

thermohyperalgesia (ther″mo-hi″per-al-je′ze-ah) extreme thermalgesia.

thermohyperesthesia (-es-the′ze-ah) extreme sensitiveness to heat.

thermoinhibitory (ther″mo-in-hib′ĭ-tor″e) retarding generation of bodily heat.

thermolabile (-la′bil) easily affected by heat.

thermology (ther-mol′o-je) the science of heat.

thermolysis (ther-mol′ĭ-sis) 1. chemical dissociation by means of heat. 2. dissipation of bodily heat by radiation, evaporation, etc. **thermolyt′ic,** adj.

thermomassage (ther″mo-mah-sahzh′) massage with heat.

thermometer (ther-mom′ĕ-ter) an instrument for determining temperatures, in principle making use of a substance with a physical property that varies with temperature and is susceptible of measurement on some defined scale. **Celsius t.,** one on which the melting point of ice is 0 and the boiling point of water is 100 degrees; *see table.* **centigrade t.,** one (e.g., the Celsius thermometer), having the interval between two established reference points divided into 100 units. **clinical t.,** one used to determine the temperature of the human body. **Fahrenheit t.,** one on which the freezing point of water is 32 and the boiling point is 212 degrees; *see table.* **Kelvin t.,** one employing the Kelvin scale. **Rankine t.,** one employing the Rankine scale. **Réaumur's t.,** one on which the freezing point of water is 0 and the boiling point is 80 degrees. **recording t.,** a temperature-sensitive instrument by which the temperature to which it is exposed is continuously recorded. **resistance t.,** one which uses the electric resistance of metals for determining temperature. **self-registering t.,** recording t.

thermometry (ther-mom′ĕ-tre) measurement of temperature.

thermophile (ther′mo-fīl) an organism that grows best at elevated temperatures. **thermophil′ic,** adj.

thermophore (-fōr) 1. a device or apparatus for retaining heat. 2. an instrument for estimating heat sensibility.

thermopile (-pīl) a number of thermocouples in series, used to increase sensitivity to change in temperature or for direct conversion of heat into electric energy.

thermoplacentography (ther″mo-plas″en-tog′-rah-fe) use of thermography for determination of the site of placental attachment.

thermoplegia (-ple′je-ah) heatstroke or sunstroke.

thermopolypnea (-pol″ip-ne′ah) quickened breathing due to great heat.

thermoreceptor (-re-sep′tor) a nerve ending sensitive to stimulation by heat.

thermoregulation (-reg″u-la′shun) heat regulation.

thermostabile (-sta′bil) not affected by heat.

thermostat (ther′mo-stat) a device interposed in a heating system by which temperature is automatically maintained between certain levels.

thermosteresis (ther″mo-stĕ-re′sis) deprivation of heat.

thermosystaltic (-sis-tal′tik) contracting under the stimulus of heat.

thermotaxis (-tak′sis) 1. normal adjustment of bodily temperature. 2. movement of an organism in response to the stimulation of a temperature gradient. **thermotac′tic, thermotax′ic,** adj.

thermotherapy (-ther′ah-pe) therapeutic use of heat.

thermotics (ther-mot′iks) the science of heat.

thermotonometer (ther″mo-to-nom′ĕ-ter) an instrument for measuring the amount of muscular contraction produced by heat.

thermotropism (ther-mot′ro-pizm) the orientation of a living cell in response to a heat stimulus. **thermotrop′ic,** adj.

thesaurismosis (the-saw″riz-mo′sis) storage disease.

thesaurosis (the″saw-ro′sis) storage disease.

thi(o)- a word element [Gr.], *sulfur.*

thiabendazole (thi″ah-ben′dah-zol) a broad-spectrum anthelmintic, $C_{10}H_7N_3S$.

thiamazole (thi-am′ah-zōl) methimazole.

thiaminase (-am′ĭ-nās) an enzyme that catalyzes the splitting of thiamine into a pyrimidine and a thiazole derivative.

thiamin, thiamine (thi′ah-min) vitamin B_1; a component of the B complex group of vitamins, found in various foodstuffs and present in the free state in blood plasma and cerebrospinal fluid. Deficiency results in neurological symptoms, cardiovascular dysfunction, edema, and reduced intestinal motility. **t. hydrochloride,** a vitamin supplement used in prophylaxis and treatment of thiamine deficiency. **t. mononitrate,** $C_{12}H_{17}N_5O_4S$, used like thiamine hydrochloride. **phosphorylated t., t. pyrophosphate,** the active form of thiamine, serving as a cofactor in certain reactions in carbohydrate metabolism.

thiamylal (thi-am′ĭ-lal) an ultrashort-acting barbiturate; the sodium salt is used intravenously as a general anesthetic.

thiazole (thi′ah-zōl) C_3H_3NS, occurring in two isomers.

thiethylperazine (thi-eth″il-per′ah-zēn) a phenothiazine derivative, $C_{22}H_{29}N_3S_2$, useful as an antiemetic and antinauseant.

thiemia (-e′me-ah) sulfur in the blood.

thigh (thi) the portion of the leg above the knee; the femur.

thigmesthesia (thig″mes-the′ze-ah) tactile sensibility.

thigmotaxis (thig″mo-tak′sis) movement of an organism in response to contact. **thigmotac′tic, thigmotax′ic,** adj.

thigmotropism (thig-mot′ro-pizm) the orientation of an organism in response to the stimulus of contact. **thigmotrop′ic,** adj.

thihexinol (thi-hek′sĭ-nol) an anticholinergic, $C_{18}H_{26}BrNOS_2$, used to inhibit intestinal hypermotility.

thimerosal (-mer′o-sal) a local anti-infective, $C_9H_9HgNaO_2S$.

thinking (thingk′ing) the formulation of images or concepts in one's mind. **dereistic t.,** dereism.

thiobarbital (thi″o-bahr′bĭ-tahl) a salt of thiobarbituric acid, used as a thyroid depressant.

TABLE OF TEMPERATURE EQUIVALENTS
CELSIUS (CENTIGRADE) : FAHRENHEIT SCALE

CELSIUS : FAHRENHEIT $°F = (°C \times \frac{9}{5}) + 32$				FAHRENHEIT : CELSIUS $°C = (°F - 32) \times \frac{5}{9}$					
C°	F°	C°	F°	F°	C°	F°	C°	F°	C°
−50	−58.0	49	120.2	−50	−46.7	99	37.2	157	69.4
−40	−40.0	50	122.0	−40	−40.0	100	37.7	158	70.0
−35	−31.0	51	123.8	−35	−37.2	101	38.3	159	70.5
−30	−22.0	52	125.6	−30	−34.4	102	38.8	160	71.1
−25	−13.0	53	127.4	−25	−31.7	103	39.4	161	71.6
−20	−4.0	54	129.2	−20	−28.9	104	40.0	162	72.2
−15	−5.0	55	131.0	−15	−26.6	105	40.5	163	72.7
−10	14.0	56	132.8	−10	−23.3	106	41.1	164	73.3
−5	23.0	57	134.6	−5	−20.6	107	41.6	165	73.8
0	32.0	58	136.4	0	−17.7	108	42.2	166	74.4
+1	33.8	59	138.2	+1	−17.2	109	42.7	167	75.0
2	35.6	60	140.0	5	−15.0	110	43.3	168	75.5
3	37.4	61	141.8	10	−12.2	111 `	43.8	169	76.1
4	39.2	62	143.6	15	−9.4	112	44.4	170	76.6
5	41.0	63	145.4	20	−6.6	113	45.0	171	77.2
6	42.8	64	147.2	25	−3.8	114	45.5	172	77.7
7	44.6	65	149.0	30	−1.1	115	46.1	173	78.3
8	46.4	66	150.8	31	−0.5	116	46.6	174	78.8
9	48.2	67	152.6	32	0	117	47.2	175	79.4
10	50.0	68	154.4	33	+0.5	118	47.7	176	80.0
11	51.8	69	156.2	34	1.1	119	48.3	177	80.5
12	53.6	70	158.0	35	1.6	120	48.8	178	81.1
13	55.4	71	159.8	36	2.2	121	49.4	179	81.6
14	57.2	72	161.6	37	2.7	122	50.0	180	82.2
15	59.0	73	163.4	38	3.3	123	50.5	181	82.7
16	60.8	74	165.2	39	3.8	124	51.1	182	83.3
17	62.6	75	167.0	40	4.4	125	51.6	183	83.8
18	64.4	76	168.8	41	5.0	126	52.2	184	84.4
19	66.2	77	170.6	42	5.5	127	52.7	185	85.0
20	68.0	78	172.4	43	6.1	128	53.3	186	85.5
21	69.8	79	174.2	44	6.6	129	53.8	187	86.1
22	71.6	80	176.0	45	7.2	130	54.4	188	86.6
23	73.4	81	177.8	46	7.7	131	55.0	189	87.2
24	75.2	82	179.6	47	8.3	132	55.5	190	87.7
25	77.0	83	181.4	48	8.8	133	56.1	191	88.3
26	78.8	84	183.2	49	9.4	134	56.6	192	88.8
27	80.6	85	185.0	50	10.0	135	57.2	193	89.4
28	82.4	86	186.8	55	12.7	136	57.7	194	90.0
29	84.2	87	188.6	60	15.5	137	58.3	195	90.5
30	86.0	88	190.4	65	18.3	138	58.8	196	91.1
31	87.8	89	192.2	70	21.1	139	59.4	197	91.6
32	89.6	90	194.0	75	23.8	140	60.0	198	92.2
33	91.4	91	195.8	80	26.6	141	60.5	199	92.7
34	93.2	92	197.6	85	29.4	142	61.1	200	93.3
35	95.0	93	199.4	86	30.0	143	61.6	201	93.8
36	96.8	94	201.2	87	30.5	144	62.2	202	94.4
37	98.6	95	203.0	88	31.0	145	62.7	203	95.0
38	100.4	96	204.8	89	31.6	146	63.3	204	95.5
39	102.2	97	206.6	90	32.2	147	63.8	205	96.1
40	104.0	98	208.4	91	32.7	148	64.4	206	96.6
41	105.8	99	210.2	92	33.3	149	65.0	207	97.2
42	107.6	100	212.0	93	33.8	150	65.5	208	97.7
43	109.4	101	213.8	94	34.4	151	66.1	209	98.3
44	111.2	102	215.6	95	35.0	152	66.6	210	98.8
45	113.0	103	217.4	96	35.5	153	67.2	211	99.4
46	114.8	104	219.2	97	36.1	154	67.7	212	100.0
47	116.6	105	221.0	98	36.6	155	68.3	213	100.5
48	118.4	106	222.8	98.6	37.0	156	68.8	214	101.1

thiobarbiturate (-bahr-bich-ŭ-rāt) a salt or derivative of thiobarbituric acid.

thiocyanate (-si'ah-nāt) a salt analogous in composition to a cyanate, but containing sulfur instead of oxygen.

thiodiphenylamine (-di-fen″il-am′ēn) phenothiazine.

thioglucosidase (-glu-ko′sĭ-dās) an enzyme found in mustard seed that catalyzes the hydrolysis of thioglycosides to a thiol and a sugar.

thioguanine (-gwah′nēn) an antineoplastic (2-aminopurine-6-thiol) used in leukemia.

Thiomerin (-mer′in) trademark for a preparation of mercaptomerin.

thiomersalate (-mer′sah-lāt) thimerosal.

thionin (thi′o-nin) a dark-green powder, purple in solution, used as a metachromatic stain in microscopy.

thiopental (thi″o-pen′tal) an ultrashort-acting barbiturate, $C_{11}H_{17}N_2O_2S$; the sodium salt is used intravenously or rectally to induce general anesthesia.

thiopentone (-pen′tōn) thiopental.

thiopropazate (-pro′pah-zāt) a phenothiazine derivative, $C_{23}H_{28}ClN_3O_2$, used as a major tranquilizer in the form of the hydrochloride salt.

thioridazine (-rid′ah-zēn) a tranquilizer, $C_{21}H_{26}N_2S_2$, used as the hydrochloride salt.

thiosulfate (-sul′fāt) any salt of thiosulfuric acid.

thiotepa (-te′pah) a neoplastic suppressant, $C_6H_{12}N_3PS$.

thiothixene (-thiks′ēn) a tranquilizer, $C_{23}H_{29}N_3O_2S_2$.

thiouracil (-u′rah-sil) a thiourea derivative, $C_4H_4N_2OS$, which adversely affects thyroid hormone synthesis.

thiourea (-u′re-ah) urea with its oxygen replaced by sulfur, $CS(NH_2)_2$; it inhibits thyroid function.

thirst (therst) a sensation, often referred to the mouth and throat, associated with a craving for drink; ordinarily interpreted as a desire for water.

thixotropism (thik-sot′ro-pizm) thixotropy.

thixotropy (thik-sot′ro-pe) the property of certain gels of becoming fluid when shaken and then becoming semisolid again. **thixotrop′ic,** adj.

thlipsencephalus (thlip″sen-sef′ah-lus) a monster with a defective skull.

thonzylamine (thon-zil′ah-min) an antihistaminic, $C_{16}H_{22}N_4O$, used as the hydrochloride salt.

thorac(o)- word element [Gr.], *chest.*

thoracalgia (thor″rah-kal′je-ah) pain in the chest wall.

thoracectomy (thor″rah-sek′to-me) thoracotomy with resection of part of a rib.

thoracentesis (thor″rah-sen-te′sis) thoracocentesis.

thoracic (tho-ras′ik) pertaining to the chest.

thoracoacromial (tho″rah-ko-ah-kro′me-al) pertaining to the chest and acromion.

thoracoceloschisis (-se-los′kĭ-sis) congenital fissure of the thorax and abdomen.

thoracocentesis (-sen-te′sis) paracentesis of the chest wall.

thoracocyllosis (-sĭ-lo′sis) deformity of the thorax.

thoracocyrtosis (-sir-to′sis) abnormal curvature of the chest wall.

thoracodelphus (-del′fus) a double monster with one head, two arms, and four legs, the bodies being joined above the navel.

thoracodidymus (-did′ĭ-mus) thoracopagus.

thoracodynia (-din′e-ah) pain in the thorax.

thoracogastroschisis (-gas-tros′kĭ-sis) congenital fissure of the thorax and abdomen.

thoracolumbar (-lum′bar) pertaining to thoracic and lumbar vertebrae.

thoracolysis (tho″rah-kol′ĭ-sis) the freeing of adhesion of the chest wall.

thoracomelus (tho″rah-kom′ĕ-lus) a monster with a supernumerary limb attached to the thorax.

thoracometer (tho″rah-kom′ĕ-ter) stethometer.

thoracomyodynia (tho″rah-ko-mi″o-din′e-ah) pain in the muscles of the chest.

thoracopagus (tho″rah-kop′ah-gus) conjoined twins united at the thorax.

thoracopathy (tho″rah-kop′ah-the) any disease of the thoracic organs or tissues.

thoracoplasty (tho′rah-ko-plas″te) surgical removal of ribs, allowing the chest wall to collapse a diseased lung.

thoracoschisis (tho″rah-kos′kĭ-sis) congenital fissure of the chest wall.

thoracoscope (tho-ra′ko-skōp) an endoscope for examining the pleural cavity through an intercostal space.

thoracoscopy (tho″rah-kos′ko-pe) examination of the pleural space with a thoracoscope.

thoracostenosis (tho″rah-ko-stě-no′sis) abnormal contraction of the thorax.

thoracostomy (tho″rah-kos′to-me) incision of the chest wall, with maintenance of the opening for drainage.

thoracotomy (tho″rah-kot′o-me) incision of the chest wall.

thorax (tho′raks) the chest; the part of the body between the neck and the respiratory diaphragm, encased by the ribs. **Peyrot's t.,** an obliquely oval thorax associated with massive pleural effusions.

Thorazine (thor′ah-zēn) trademark for preparations of chlorpromazine.

thorium (tho′re-um) chemical element (*see table*), at. no. 90, symbol Th.

thoron (tho′ron) a radioactive isotope of radon.

thoroughpin (thur′o-pin) distention of the synovial sheaths at the upper portion and back of the hock joint of a horse.

thozalinone (tho-zal′ĭ-nōn) an antidepressant, $C_{11}H_{12}N_2O_2$.

threadworm (thred′werm) any oxyurid, especially *Enterobius vermicularis.*

threonine (thre′o-nin) a naturally occurring

amino acid, one of those essential for human metabolism.

threpsology (threp-sol′o-je) the scientific study of nutrition.

threshold (thresh′old) the level which must be reached for an effect to be produced, as the degree of intensity of a stimulus which just produces a sensation, or the concentration that must be present in the blood before certain substances are excreted by the kidney (*renal t.*).

thrill (thril) a vibration felt by the examiner on palpation. **diastolic t.,** one felt over the precordium during diastole in advanced aortic insufficiency. **hydatid t.,** one sometimes felt on percussing over a hydatid cyst. **presystolic t.,** one felt just before the systole over the apex of the heart. **systolic t.,** one felt over the precordium during systole in aortic stenosis, pulmonary stenosis, and ventricular septal defect.

thrix (thriks) hair.

-thrix word element [Gr.], *hair.*

throat (thrōt) 1. pharynx. 2. fauces. 3. anterior aspect of the neck. **sore t.,** see under S.

throb (throb) a pulsating movement or sensation.

thromb(o)- word element [Gr.], *clot; thrombus.*

thrombase (throm′bās) thrombin.

thrombasthenia (throm″bas-the′ne-ah) a platelet abnormality characterized by defective clot retraction and impaired ADP-induced platelet aggregation; clinically manifested by epistaxis, inappropriate bruising, and excessive posttraumatic bleeding. **Glanzmann's t.,** thrombasthenia.

thrombectomy (throm-bek′to-me) surgical removal of a clot from a blood vessel.

thrombi (throm′bi) plural of *thrombus.*

thrombin (throm′bin) an enzyme resulting from activation of prothrombin, which catalyzes the conversion of fibrinogen to fibrin; a preparation from prothrombin of bovine origin is used as a topical hemostatic.

thromboangiitis (throm″bo-an″je-i′tis) inflammation of a blood vessel, with thrombosis. **t. oblit′erans,** Buerger's disease; that affecting and obliterating the blood vessels of the limbs, primarily the legs, leading to ischemia and gangrene.

thromboarteritis (-ar″ter-i′tis) thrombosis associated with arteritis.

thromboclasis (throm-bok′lah-sis) the dissolution of a thrombus. **thromboclas′tic,** adj.

thrombocyst, thrombocystis (throm′bo-sist; throm″bo-sis′tis) a sac formed around a thrombus.

thrombocyte (throm′bo-sīt) a blood platelet. **thrombocyt′ic,** adj.

thrombocythemia (throm″bo-si-the′me-ah) a fixed increase in the number of circulating blood platelets. **essential t.,** a clinical syndrome with repeated spontaneous hemorrhages, either external or into the tissues, and greatly increased number of circulating platelets.

thrombocytocrit (-si′to-krit) the volume of packed blood platelets in a given quantity of

blood; also, the instrument used to measure platelet volume.

thrombocytolysis (-si-tol′ĭ-sis) destruction of blood platelets (thrombocytes).

thrombocytopathy (-si-top′ah-the) any qualitative disorder of blood platelets.

thrombocytopenia (-si″to-pe′ne-ah) decrease in number of platelets in circulating blood.

thrombocytopoiesis (-si″to-poi-e′sis) the production of blood platelets (thrombocytes). **thrombocytopoiet′ic,** adj.

thrombocytosis (-si-to′sis) increase in number of platelets in circulating blood.

thromboembolism (-em′bo-lizm) obstruction of a blood vessel with thrombotic material carried by the blood from the site of origin to plug another vessel.

thromboendarterectomy (-end″ar-ter-ek′to-me) excision of an obstructing thrombus together with a portion of the inner lining of the obstructed artery.

thromboendarteritis (-end″ar-ter-i′tis) inflammation of the innermost coat of an artery, with thrombus formation.

thromboendocarditis (-en″do-kar-di′tis) 1. formation of a thrombus on a heart valve which has previously been eroded. 2. an infectious disease of rabbits.

thrombogenesis (-jen′ĕ-sis) clot formation. **thrombogen′ic,** adj.

thromboid (throm′boid) resembling a thrombus.

thrombokinase (throm″bo-ki′nās) activated coagulation Factor X.

thrombolymphangitis (-lim″fan-ji′tis) inflammation of a lymph vessel due to a thrombus.

thrombolysis (throm-bol′ĭ-sis) dissolution of a thrombus. **thrombolyt′ic,** adj.

thrombon (throm′bon) the circulating blood platelets and their precursors.

thrombopathy (throm-bop′ah-the) thrombocytopathy.

thrombopenia (throm″bo-pe′ne-ah) thrombocytopenia.

thrombophilia (-fil′e-ah) a tendency to the occurrence of thrombosis.

thrombophlebitis (-fle-bi′tis) inflammation of a vein associated with thrombus formation. **t. mi′grans,** a recurrent condition involving different vessels simultaneously or at intervals. **postpartum iliofemoral t.,** thrombophlebitis of the iliofemoral vein following childbirth.

thromboplastic (-plas′tik) causing or accelerating clot formation in the blood.

thromboplastid (-plas′tid) a blood platelet.

thromboplastin (-plas′tin) a substance in blood and tissues which, in the presence of ionized calcium, aids in the conversion of prothrombin to thrombin. **tissue t.,** coagulation Factor III.

thrombopoiesis (-poi-e′sis) 1. thrombogenesis. 2. thrombocytopoiesis. **thrombopoiet′ic,** adj.

thrombosed (throm′bōsd) affected with thrombosis.

thrombosis (throm-bo′sis) the formation or presence of a thrombus. **thrombot′ic,** adj. **cerebral t.,** thrombosis of a cerebral vessel, which may result in cerebral infarction. **coro-**

nary t., thrombosis of a coronary artery, often leading to myocardial infarction.

thrombosthenin (throm″bo-sthe′nin) a contractile protein of platelets, active in clot formation.

thrombostasis (throm-bos′tah-sis) stasis of blood in a part with formation of thrombus.

thrombus (throm′bus), pl. *throm′bi.* A solid mass formed in the living heart or vessels from constituents of the blood. **mural t.,** one attached to the wall of the endocardium in a diseased area. **occluding t.,** one that occupies the entire lumen of a vessel and obstructs blood flow. **parietal t.,** one attached to a vessel or heart wall.

thrush (thrush) candidiasis of the oral mucous membranes, usually affecting infants, with formation of whitish spots (aphthae), which are followed by shallow ulcers; it is caused by *Candida albicans.*

thrypsis (thrip′sis) a comminuted fracture.

thulium (thoo′le-um) chemical element (*see table*), at. no. 69, symbol Tm.

thumb (thum) the radial or first digit of the hand. **tennis t.,** tendinitis of the tendon of the long flexor muscle of the thumb, with calcification.

thym(o)- word element [Gr.], *thymus; mind, soul, or emotions.*

thymectomize (thi-mek′to-mīz) to excise the thymus.

thymectomy (thi-mek′to-me) excision of the thymus.

thymelcosis (thi″mel-ko′sis) ulceration of the thymus.

thymergasia (thi″mer-ga′ze-ah) an affective or reaction-type psychosis, such as manic-depressive psychosis. **thymergas′ic, thymergas′tic,** adj.

-thymia word element [Gr.], *condition of mind.* **-thy′mic,** adj.

thymic (thi′mik) pertaining to the thymus.

thymicolymphatic (thi″mĭ-ko-lim-fat′ik) pertaining to the thymus and lymphatic nodes.

thymidine (thi′mĭ-dēn) a nucleoside of DNA.

thymine (thi′min) a pyrimidine base, $C_5H_6N_2O$, in DNA.

thymitis (thi-mi′tis) inflammation of the thymus.

thymocyte (thi′mo-sīt) a lymphocyte arising in the thymus.

thymogenic (thi″mo-jen′ik) of affective or hysterical origin.

thymokinetic (-ki-net′ik) tending to stimulate the thymus.

thymol (thi′mol) a phenol, $C_{10}H_{14}O$, obtained from thyme oil and other volatile oils or produced synthetically; used as a topical antifungal and antibacterial, and as an antimicrobial agent in trichloroethylene.

thymoma (thi-mo′mah) a tumor derived from the epithelial or lymphoid elements of the thymus.

thymopathy (thi-mop′ah-the) any disease of the thymus. **thymopath′ic,** adj.

thymoprivic, thymoprivous (thi″mo-priv′ik; thi-mop′rĭ-vus) pertaining to or resulting from removal or atrophy of the thymus.

thymosin (thi′mo-sin) a humoral factor secreted by the thymus, which promotes the growth of peripheral lymphoid tissue.

thymus (thi′mus) a ductless glandlike body in the anterior mediastinal cavity, usually having two longitudinal lobes joined across the median plane; it reaches its maximum development during childhood and then undergoes involution. It is the site of lymphopoiesis and plays a role in immunologic competence.

thyro- word element [Gr.], *thyroid.*

thyroadenitis (thi″ro-ad″ĕ-ni′tis) inflammation of the thyroid.

thyroaplasia (-ah-pla′ze-ah) defective development of the thyroid with deficient activity of its secretion.

thyroarytenoid (-ar″ĭ-te′noid) pertaining to the thyroid and arytenoid cartilages.

thyrocalcitonin (-kal′sĭ-to″nin) calcitonin.

thyrocardiac (-kar′de-ak) pertaining to the thyroid and heart.

thyrocele (thi′ro-sēl) tumor of the thyroid gland; goiter.

thyrochondrotomy (thi″ro-kon-drot′o-me) surgical incision of the thyroid cartilage.

thyrocricotomy (-kri-kot′o-me) incision of the cricothyroid membrane.

thyroepiglottic (-ep″ĭ-glot′ik) pertaining to the thyroid and epiglottis.

thyrogenic, thyrogenous (thi″ro-jen′ik; thi-roj′ĕ-nus) originating in the thyroid.

thyroglobulin (thi″ro-glob′u-lin) an iodized glycoprotein characteristically present in the colloid of the thyroid follicles.

thyroglossal (-glos′al) pertaining to the thyroid and tongue.

thyrohyal (-hi′al) pertaining to the thyroid cartilage and the hyoid bone.

thyrohyoid (-hi′oid) pertaining to the thyroid gland or cartilage and the hyoid bone.

thyroid (thi′roid) 1. resembling a shield. 2. the thyroid gland; see under *gland.* 3. a pharmaceutical preparation of cleaned, dried, powdered thyroid gland, obtained from those domesticated animals used for food by man.

thyroidectomize (thi″roi-dek′to-mīz) to excise the thyroid.

thyroidectomy (thi″roi-dek′to-me) excision of the thyroid.

thyroidism (thi′roid-izm) hyperthyroidism; also, a morbid condition due to excessive doses of thyroid.

thyroiditis (thi″roi-di′tis) inflammation of the thyroid. **Hashimoto's t.,** struma lymphomatosa.

thyroidotomy (thi″roi-dot′o-me) incision of the thyroid.

thyroiodine (thi″ro-i′o-dīn) iodine as it exists in the hormones of the thyroid gland.

thyrolysin (thi-rol′ĭ-sin) a substance destructive to thyroid tissue. **thyrolyt′ic,** adj.

thyromegaly (thi″ro-meg′ah-le) goiter.

thyromimetic (-mi-met′ik) producing effects

similar to those of thyroid hormones or the thyroid gland.

thyroparathyroidectomy (-par″ah-thi″roi-dek′to-me) excision of thyroid and parathyroids.

thyroprival, thyroprivic (-pri′val; -priv′ik) pertaining to, marked by, or due to deprivation or loss of thyroid function.

thyroptosis (thi″rop-to′sis) downward displacement of a goitrous thyroid.

thyrosis (thi-ro′sis) any disease based on disordered thyroid action.

thyrotherapy (thi″ro-ther′ah-pe) treatment with preparations of thyroid.

thyrotomy (thi-rot′o-me) 1. surgical division of the thyroid cartilage. 2. the operation of cutting the thyroid gland.

thyrotoxic (thi″ro-tok′sik) marked by toxic activity of the thyroid.

thyrotoxicosis (-tok″si-ko′sis) a morbid condition due to overactivity of the thyroid gland; see *Graves' disease.*

thyrotoxin (-tok′sin) a toxic substance produced in the thyroid gland.

thyrotrophic (-trof′ik) thyrotropic.

thyrotrophin (-trof′in) thyrotropin.

thyrotropic (-trop′ik) 1. pertaining to or marked by thyrotropism. 2. having an influence on the thyroid gland.

thyrotropin (-trop′in) a hormone of the anterior pituitary gland having an affinity for and specifically stimulating the thyroid gland.

thyrotropism (thi-rot′ro-pizm) affinity for the thyroid gland.

thyroxine (thi-rok′sin) an iodine-containing hormone, 3,5,3′,5′-tetraiodothyronine, secreted by the thyroid gland; its chief function is to increase the rate of cell metabolism. A synthetic preparation is used in treating hypothyroidism.

Ti chemical symbol, *titanium.*

tibia (tib′e-ah) see *Table of Bones.* **tib′ial,** adj. **t. val′ga,** bowing of the leg in which the angulation is away from the midline. **t. va′ra,** osteochondrosis deformans tibiae.

tibialis (tib″e-a′lis) [L.] tibial.

tibiofemoral (tib″e-o-fem′o-ral) pertaining to the tibia and femur.

tibiofibular (-fib′u-lar) pertaining to the tibia and fibula.

tibiotarsal (-tar′sal) pertaining to the tibia and tarsus.

tic (tik) any spasmodic movement or twitching, as of the face. **t. douloureux** (doo-loo-roo′), trigeminal neuralgia. **facial t.,** spasm of the facial muscles.

tick (tik) a bloodsucking acarid parasite of the superfamily Ixodoidea, divided into *soft-bodied ticks* (family Argasidae) having no scutum in any developmental stage; and *hard-bodied ticks* (family Ixodidae), having a scutum in all developmental stages. Some ticks are vectors and reservoirs of disease-causing agents.

t.i.d. [L.] *ter in di′e* (three times a day).

tide (tīd) a physiological variation or increase of a certain constituent in body fluids. **acid t.,**
temporary increase in the acidity of the urine which sometimes follows fasting. **alkaline t.,** temporary increase in the alkalinity of the urine during gastric digestion. **fat t.,** the increase of fat in the lymph and blood after a meal.

Tigan (ti′gan) trademark for a preparation of trimethobenzamide.

tigrolysis (ti-grol′i-sis) chromatolysis (2).

timbre (tim′ber, tam′br) [Fr.] musical quality of a tone or sound.

time (tīm) a measure of duration. **bleeding t.,** the duration of bleeding after controlled, standardized puncture of the earlobe or forearm; a relatively inconsistent measure of capillary and platelet function. **circulation t.,** the time required for blood to flow between two given points. **clotting t., coagulation t.,** the time required for blood to clot in a glass tube. **inertia t.,** the time required to overcome the inertia of a muscle after reception of a stimulus from a nerve. **prothrombin t.,** the time required for clot formation after tissue extract (brain) and calcium have been added to blood plasma. **reaction t.,** the time elapsing between the application of a stimulus and the resulting reaction.

Timovan (tim′o-van) trademark for a preparation of prothipendyl.

tin (tin) chemical element (*see table*), at. no. 50, symbol Sn.

tinct. tincture.

tinctorial (tingk-to′re-al) pertaining to dyeing or staining.

tincture (tingk′chur) an alcoholic or hydroalcoholic solution prepared from an animal or vegetable drug or a chemical substance. **belladonna t.,** a preparation of belladonna leaf in a menstruum of alcohol and water; an anticholinergic. **benzoin t., compound,** a mixture of benzoin, aloes, storax, and tolu balsam in alcohol; used as a topical protectant. **cardamom t., compound,** a preparation of powdered cardamom seed, cinnamon, caraway, and cochineal in glycerin and diluted alcohol; used as a flavoring agent. **digitalis t.,** finely powdered digitalis in a menstruum of alcohol and water; a cardiotonic. **green soap t.,** a mixture of green soap, lavendar oil, and alcohol; a skin detergent. **iodine t.,** a mixture of iodine and sodium iodide in a menstruum of alcohol and water; an anti-infective for the skin. **lemon t.,** a flavoring agent prepared by maceration of outer yellow rind of fresh ripe fruit of *Citrus limon* in alcohol. **nitromersol t.,** nitromersol, sodium hydroxide, and alcohol in hydroalcoholic solution; a local anti-infective. **opium t.,** an alcoholic solution of opium, each 100 ml. of which yields 0.95–1.05 gm. of anhydrous morphine; an antiperistaltic. **sweet orange peel t.,** a flavoring agent prepared by maceration of the outer rind of natural colored fresh ripe fruit of *Citrus sinensis* in alcohol. **thimerosal t.,** thimerosal, monoethanolamine, acetone, ethylenediamine solution, with alcohol and water; a local anti-infective. **tolu balsam t.,** tolu balsam in alcohol; a flavoring agent. **vanilla t.,** vanilla and sucrose in equal parts of diluted alcohol and water; a flavoring agent.

Tindal (tin′dal) trademark for a preparation of acetophenazine.

tinea (tin′e-ah) ringworm; a name applied to many different superficial fungal infections of the skin, the specific type (depending on appearance, etiology, or site) usually designated by a modifying term. **t. bar′bae,** infection of the bearded parts of the face and neck caused by *Trichophyton.* **t. cap′itis,** fungal infection of the scalp, due to species of *Trichophyton microsporum.* **t. circina′ta,** tinea corporis marked by the presence of annular lesions. **t. cor′poris,** fungal infection of glabrous skin, usually due to species of *Trichophyton* or *Microsporum.* **t. cru′ris,** fungal infection starting in the crural or perineal folds, extending onto the upper inside of the thighs, due to *Epidermophyton floccosum* or species of *Trichophyton.* **t. imbrica′ta,** a form of tinea corporis seen in the tropics, due to *Trichophyton concentricum;* the early lesion is annular with a circle of scales at the periphery. **t. ke′rion,** a highly inflammatory, suppurative form of tinea barbae or of tinea capitis, due to *Trichophyton mentagrophytes* or *T. verrucosum.* **t. pe′dis,** athlete's foot; a chronic superficial fungal infection of the skin of the foot, especially between the toes and on the soles, due to species of *Trichophyton* or to *Epidermophyton floccosum.* **t. profun′da,** trichophytic granuloma. **t. syco′sis,** an inflammatory, deep type of tinea barbae, due to *Trichophyton violaceum* or *T. rubrum.* **t. un′guium,** onychomycosis. **t. versico′lor,** a chronic, noninflammatory, usually asymptomatic disorder due to *Pityrosporon orbiculare,* marked only by multiple macular patches.

tingible (tin′jĭ-b'l) stainable.

tinnitus (tĭ-ni′tus) a noise in the ears, which may at times be heard by others than the patient. **t. au′rium,** a subjective sensation of noise in the ears.

tintometer (tin-tom′ĕ-ter) an instrument for determining the relative proportion of coloring matter in a liquid.

tintometry (tin-tom′ĕ-tre) the use of the tintometer.

tirefond (tēr-faw′) [Fr.] an instrument like a corkscrew for raising depressed portions of bone.

tissue (tish′u) a group or layer of similarly specialized cells which together perform certain special functions. **adenoid t.,** lymphoid t. **adipose t.,** connective tissue made of fat cells in meshwork of areolar tissue. **areolar t.,** connective tissue made up largely of interlacing fibers. **bony t.,** bone. **brown adipose t., brown fat t.,** a peculiar type of fat found in certain body regions in various mammals and in the human fetus. **cancellous t.,** the spongy tissue of bone. **cartilaginous t.,** the substance of cartilage. **chromaffin t.,** a tissue composed largely of chromaffin cells, well supplied with nerves and vessels; it occurs in the adrenal medulla and also forms the paraganglia of the body. **cicatricial t.,** the dense fibrous tissue forming a cicatrix, derived directly from granulation tissue.

connective t., the stromatous or nonparenchymatous tissues of the body; that which binds together and is the ground substance of the various parts and organs of the body. **elastic t.,** connective tissue made up of yellow elastic fibers, frequently massed into sheets. **endothelial t.,** endothelium. **epithelial t.,** epithelium. **erectile t.,** spongy tissue that expands and becomes hard when filled with blood. **extracellular t.,** the total of tissues and body fluids outside the cells. **fatty t.,** adipose t. **fibrous t.,** the common connective tissue of the body, composed of yellow or white parallel fibers. **gelatinous t.,** mucous t. **glandular t.,** an aggregation of epithelial cells that elaborate secretions. **granulation t.,** the newly formed vascular tissue normally produced in healing of wounds of soft tissue, ultimately forming the cicatrix. **indifferent t.,** undifferentiated embryonic tissue. **interstitial t.,** connective tissue between the cellular elements of a structure. **lymphadenoid t.,** tissue resembling that of lymph nodes, found in the spleen, bone marrow, tonsils, and other organs. **lymphoid t.,** a lattice work of reticular tissue, the interspaces of which contain lymphocytes. **mesenchymal t.,** mesenchyma. **mucous t.,** a jelly-like connective tissue, as occurs in the umbilical cord. **muscular t.,** the substance of muscle. **myeloid t.,** red bone marrow. **nerve t., nervous t.,** the substance of which the nerve centers are composed. **osseous t.,** the specialized tissue forming the bones. **reticular t., reticulated t.,** connective tissue consisting of reticular cells and fibers. **scar t.,** cicatricial t. **sclerous t's,** the cartilaginous, fibrous, and osseous tissue. **skeletal t.,** the bony, ligamentous, fibrous, and cartilaginous tissue forming the skeleton and its attachments. **splenic t.,** red pulp. **subcutaneous t.,** the layer of loose connective tissue directly under the skin.

titanium (ti-ta′ne-um) chemical element (*see table*), at. no. 22, symbol Ti; used for fixation of fractures. **t. dioxide,** TiO_2, used as a topical protectant in ointment or lotion.

titer (ti′ter) the quantity of a substance required to react with or to correspond to a given amount of another substance.

titrate (ti′trāt) to analyze by titration.

titration (ti-tra′shun) determination of a given component in solution by addition of a liquid reagent of known strength until a given reaction is produced.

titrimetry (ti-trim′ĕ-tre) analysis by titration. **titrimet′ric,** adj.

titubation (tit″u-ba′shun) the act of staggering or reeling; a staggering gait with shaking of the trunk and head, commonly seen in cerebellar disease.

Tl chemical symbol, *thallium.*

TLC tender loving care; thin layer chromatography; total lung capacity.

Tm chemical symbol, *thulium.*

Tn see *T.*

TNT trinitrotoluene.

tobacco (to-bak′o) the dried prepared leaves of the plant *Nicotiana tabacum,* the source of various alkaloids, the principal one being nicotine.

tobramycin (to″brah-mi′sin) an aminoglycoside antibiotic produced by *Streptomyces tenebrarius.*

Toclase (to′klās) trademark for preparations of carbetapentane.

toco- word element [Gr.], *childbirth; labor.* See also words beginning *toko-.*

tocology (to-kol′o-je) obstetrics.

tocometer (to-kom′ĕ-ter) tokodynamometer.

tocopherol (to-kof′er-ol) an alcohol having the properties of vitamin E; it is isolated from wheat germ oil or produced synthetically. **alpha t.,** vitamin E.

toe (to) a digit of the foot. **hammer t.,** deformity of a toe, most often the second, in which the proximal phalanx is extended and the second and distal phalanges are flexed, giving a clawlike appearance. **Morton's t.,** metatarsalgia. **pigeon t.,** permanent toeing-in position of the feet. **webbed t's,** toes abnormally joined by strands of tissue at their base.

Tofranil (to-fra′nil) trademark for preparations of imipramine.

togavirus (to″gah-vi′rus) a subgroup of arboviruses, including mosquito-borne and tickborne viruses that cause hemorrhagic fever; they are RNA viruses with envelopes (or "togas").

toilet (toi′let) the cleansing and dressing of a wound.

toko- word element [Gr.], *childbirth; labor.* See also words beginning *toco-.*

tokodynagraph (to″ko-di′nah-graf) a tracing obtained by the tokodynamometer.

tokodynamometer (-di″nah-mom′ĕ-ter) an instrument for measuring and recording the expulsive force of uterine contractions.

tolazamide (tol-az′ah-mīd) a hypoglycemic, C_{14}-$H_{21}N_3O_3S$.

tolazoline (tol-az′o-lēn) a smooth muscle relaxant and peripheral vasodilator, $C_{10}H_{12}N_2$, used as the hydrochloride salt.

tolbutamide (tol-bu′tah-mīd) an oral hypoglycemic agent, $C_{12}H_{18}N_2O_3S$.

tolerance (tol′er-ans) the ability to endure without effect or injury. **tol′erant,** adj. **drug t.,** decrease in susceptibility to the effects of a drug due to its continued administration. **immunologic t.,** specific nonreactivity of lymphoid tissues to a particular antigen capable under other conditions of inducing immunity.

tolerogen (tol′er-o-jen) an antigen that induces a state of specific immunological unresponsiveness to subsequent challenging doses of the antigen.

tolnaftate (tol-naf′tāt) a topical antifungal, C_{19}-$H_{17}NOS$.

toluene (tol′u-ēn) the hydrocarbon C_7H_8.

toluidine (tol-u′ĭ-din) a compound made by reducing nitrotoluene.

tomatin (to-ma′tin) an antifungal antibiotic isolated from tomato plants affected with wilt.

-tome word element [Gr.], *an instrument for cutting; a segment.*

tomo- word element [Gr.], *a section; a cutting.*

tomogram (to′mo-gram) a radiograph produced by the tomograph.

tomograph (-graf) an apparatus for moving the x-ray tube through an arc during exposure, thus showing in detail a predetermined plane of tissue while blurring details of other planes.

tomography (to-mog′rah-fe) body section radiography by means of the tomograph. **tomograph′ic,** adj.

-tomy word element [Gr.], *incision; cutting.*

tone (tōn) 1. normal degree of vigor and tension; in muscle, the resistance to passive elongation or stretch. 2. a healthy state of a part; tonus. 3. a particular quality of sound or of voice.

tongue (tung) the movable muscular organ on the floor of the mouth; it is the chief organ of taste, and aids in mastication, swallowing, and speech. **bifid t.,** one with an anterior lengthwise cleft. **black t.,** the presence of a brown furlike patch on the dorsum of the tongue, composed of hypertrophied filiform papillae with microorganisms and some pigment. **blue t.,** a viral disease of cattle and sheep in South Africa, with hyperemia and edema of the lips, tongue, and oral mucosa. **cleft t.,** bifid t. **coated t.,** one covered with a whitish or yellowish layer consisting of desquamated epithelium, debris, bacteria, fungi, etc. **fissured t., furrowed t.,** a tongue with numerous furrows or grooves on the dorsal surface, often radiating from a groove on the midline. **geographic t.,** a tongue with denuded patches surrounded by thickened epithelium. **hairy t.,** one with the papillae elongated and hairlike. **raspberry t.,** a red, uncoated tongue, with elevated papillae, as seen a few days after the onset of the rash in scarlet fever. **scrotal t.,** fissured t. **strawberry t.,** a coated tongue with enlarged red fungiform papillae, seen 24 hours after onset of the rash in scarlet fever. **trombone t.,** involuntary movement of the tongue, consisting of vigorous alternating protrusion and retraction.

tongue-tie (tung′ti) abnormal shortness of the frenum of the tongue, interfering with its motion; ankyloglossia.

tonic (ton′ik) 1. producing and restoring normal tone. 2. characterized by continuous tension.

tonicity (to-nis′ĭ-te) the state of tissue tone or tension; in body fluid physiology, the effective osmotic pressure equivalent.

tono- word element [Gr.], *tone; tension.*

tonoclonic (ton″o-klon′ik) both tonic and clonic; said of muscular spasms.

tonofibril (ton′o-fi″bril) an organoid in the form of a fine fibril seen especially in epithelial cells.

tonogram (-gram) the record produced by tonography.

tonograph (-graf) a recording tonometer.

tonography (to-nog′rah-fe) recording of changes in intraocular pressure due to sustained pressure on the eyeball.

tonometer (to-nom′ĕ-ter) an instrument for measuring tension or pressure, especially intraocular pressure.

tonometry (to-nom′ĕ-tre) measurement of tension or pressure, e.g., intraocular pressure. **digital t.,** estimation of the degree of intraocular pressure by pressure exerted on the eyeball by the examiner's finger.

tonoplast (ton′o-plast) the limiting membrane of an intracellular vacuole.

tonoscope (-skōp) 1. an apparatus for rendering sound visible by registering the vibrations on a screen. 2. a device for examining the head or brain by means of sound. 3. tonometer.

tonsil (ton′sil) a small, rounded mass of tissue, especially of lymphoid tissue; generally used alone to designate the palatine tonsil. **ton′sillar,** adj. **t. of cerebellum,** a rounded mass of tissue on the inferior surface of the cerebellum. **faucial t.,** palatine t. **lingual t.,** an aggregation of lymph follicles at the root of the tongue. **Luschka's t.,** pharyngeal t. **palatine t.,** a small mass of lymphoid tissue between the pillars of the fauces on either side of the pharynx. **pharyngeal t.,** the diffuse lymphoid tissue and follicles in the roof and posterior wall of the nasopharynx.

tonsilla (ton-sil′ah), pl. *tonsil′lae* [L.] tonsil.

tonsillectomy (ton″sĭ-lek′to-me) excision of a tonsil.

tonsillitis (ton″sĭ-li′tis) inflammation of the tonsils, especially the palatine tonsils. **follicular t.,** tonsillitis especially affecting the crypts. **parenchymatous t., acute,** that affecting the whole substance of the tonsil. **pustular t.,** a variety characterized by formation of pustules.

tonsillolith (ton-sil′o-lith) a calculus in a tonsil.

tonsillotomy (ton″sĭ-lot′o-me) incision of a tonsil.

tonus (to′nus) tone or tonicity; the slight, continuous contraction of a muscle, which in skeletal muscles aids in the maintenance of posture and in the return of blood to the heart.

tooth (tooth), pl. *teeth.* One of the small, bonelike structures of the jaws for the biting and mastication of food. **accessional teeth,** those having no deciduous predecessors; the permanent molars. **artificial t.,** one made of porcelain or other synthetic compound in imitation of a natural tooth. **auditory teeth,** toothlike projections in the cochlea. **bicuspid t.,** one of the premolar teeth. **canine t., cuspid t.,** the third tooth on either side from the midline in each jaw. **deciduous teeth,** the 20 teeth of the first dentition in man which are supplanted by the 32 teeth of the second dentition. **eye t.,** a canine tooth of the upper jaw. **Hutchinson teeth,** notched, narrow-edged permanent incisors; regarded as a sign of congenital syphilis, but not always of such origin. **impacted t.,** one so placed in the jaw that it is unable to erupt or to attain its normal position in occlusion. **incisor teeth,** the four front teeth, two on each side of the midline, in each jaw. **milk teeth,** deciduous teeth. **molar teeth,** the three (in the permanent dentition, two in the deciduous) posterior teeth on either side in each jaw; see Plate XV. **peg t.,** a tooth whose sides converge or taper together incisally. **permanent teeth,** the 32 teeth of the second dentition. **premolar teeth,** the two permanent teeth on either side in each jaw, between the canine and the molar teeth. **primary teeth,** deciduous teeth. **stomach t.,** a canine

tooth of the lower jaw. **temporary teeth,** deciduous teeth. **wisdom teeth,** the last molar tooth on either side in each jaw.

top(o)- word element [Gr.], *particular place or area.*

topagnosia (top″ag-no′ze-ah) 1. loss of touch localization. 2. loss of ability to recognize familiar surroundings.

topalgia (to-pal′je-ah) fixed or localized pain.

topectomy (to-pek′to-me) ablation of a small and specific area of the frontal cortex in the treatment of mental illness.

topesthesia (top″es-the′ze-ah) ability to recognize the location of a tactile stimulus.

tophaceous (to-fa′shus) gritty or sandy.

tophus (to′fus), pl. *to′phi* [L.] 1. a deposit of urates in the tissues about the joints in gout. 2. dental calculus.

topical (top′ĭ-kal) pertaining to a particular area, as a topical anti-infective applied to a certain area of the skin and affecting only the area to which it is applied.

Topitracin (top″ĭ-tra′sin) trademark for a preparation of bacitracin.

topoanesthesia (top″o-an″es-the′ze-ah) inability to recognize the location of tactile stimuli.

topographic (-graf′ik) describing or pertaining to special regions.

topography (to-pog′rah-fe) the description of an anatomic region or a special part.

toponarcosis (top″o-nar-ko′sis) local anesthesia.

torcular Herophili (tor′ku-lar he-rof′ĭ-li) confluence of sinuses.

torpor (tor′por) [L.] sluggishness. **tor′pid,** adj. **t. ret′inae,** sluggish response of the retina to the stimulus of light.

torque (tork) a rotary force; in dentistry, the rotation of a tooth on its long axis, especially the movement of the apical portions of the teeth by use of orthodontic appliances.

torsion (tor′shun) 1. act of twisting; state of being twisted; in dentistry, the condition of a tooth when it is turned on its long axis. 2. in ophthalmology, any rotation of the vertical corneal meridians. **tor′sive,** adj.

torsiversion (tor″sĭ-ver′zhun) turning of a tooth on its long axis out of normal position.

torso (tor′so) the body, exclusive of the head and limbs.

torticollis (tor″tĭ-kol′is) wryneck; a contracted state of the cervical muscles, with torsion of the neck.

tortipelvis (-pel′vis) dystonia musculorum deformans.

tortuous (tor′choo-us) twisted; full of twists and turns.

torulus (tor′u-lus), pl. *tor′uli* [L.] a small elevation; a papilla. **t. tac′tilis,** a tactile elevation in the skin of the palms and soles.

torus (to′rus), pl. *to′ri* [L.] a swelling or bulging projection.

totipotential (to″tĭ-po-ten′shal) characterized by the ability to develop in any direction; said of cells that can give rise to cells of all orders.

touch (tuch) 1. the sense by which contact of an

object with the skin is recognized. 2. palpation with the finger.

tourniquet (tōōr′nĭ-ket) a band to be drawn tightly around a limb for the temporary arrest of circulation in the distal area.

tox(o)- word element [Gr.; L.], *toxin; poison.*

Toxascaris (tok-sas′kah-ris) a genus of nematode parasites, including *T. leoni′na,* found in lions, tigers, and other large Felidae, as well as dogs and cats.

toxemia (tok-se′me-ah) 1. a general intoxication sometimes due to absorption of bacterial products (toxins) formed at a local source of infection. 2. t. of pregnancy. **toxe′mic,** adj. **alimentary t.,** toxemia due to absorption from the alimentary canal of chemical poisons generated therein; a form of autointoxication. **t. of pregnancy,** a group of pathologic conditions, essentially metabolic disturbances, occurring in pregnant women, manifested by preeclampsia and fully developed eclampsia.

toxic (tok′sik) poisonous; pertaining to poisoning.

toxic(o)- word element [Gr.], *poison; poisonous.*

toxicant (tok′sĭ-kant) 1. poisonous. 2. a poison.

toxicity (tok-sis′ĭ-te) the quality of being poisonous, especially the degree of virulence of a toxic microbe or of a poison.

toxicodendron (tok″sĭ-ko-den′dron) *Rhus toxicodendron.*

toxicogenic (-jen′ik) producing or elaborating toxins.

toxicoid (tok′sĭ-koid) resembling a poison.

toxicologist (tok″sĭ-kol′o-jist) a specialist in toxicology.

toxicology (tok″sĭ-kol′o-je) the science or study of poisons. **toxicolog′ic,** adj.

toxicomania (tok″sĭ-ko-ma′ne-ah) intense desire for poisons or intoxicants.

toxicopathy (tok″sĭ-kop′ah-the) toxicosis. **toxicopath′ic,** adj.

toxicopexis (tok″sĭ-ko-pek′sis) the fixation or neutralization of a poison in the body. **toxicopec′tic, toxicopex′ic,** adj.

toxicophidia (-fid′e-ah) thanatophidia.

toxicophobia (-fo′be-ah) morbid dread of poisons.

toxicosis (tok″sĭ-ko′sis) any diseased condition due to poisoning.

toxiferous (tok-sif′er-us) conveying or producing a poison.

toxigenic (tok″sĭ-jen′ik) toxicogenic.

toxigenicity (-jĕ-nis′ĭ-te) the property of producing toxins.

toxin (tok′sin) a poison, especially a protein or conjugated protein produced by some higher plants, certain animals, and pathogenic bacteria, that is highly poisonous for other living organisms. **animal t.,** zootoxin. **bacterial t's,** toxins produced by bacteria, including exotoxins, endotoxins, and toxic enzymes. **botulinus t.,** one of five type-specific, immunologically differentiable exotoxins (types A to E) produced by *Clostridium botulinum.* **dermonecrotic t.,** an exotoxin produced by certain bacteria that causes extensive local necrosis on intradermal inoculation. **Dick t.,** erythrogenic t. **diphtheria t.,** a protein exotoxin produced by *Corynebacterium diphtheriae* that is primarily responsible for the pathogenesis of diphtheritic infection; it is an enzyme that activates transferase II of the mammalian protein synthesizing system. **erythrogenic t.,** an exotoxin produced by many strains of *Streptococcus pyogenes,* which produces an erythematous reaction on intradermal inoculation in man, and is responsible for the scarlatiniform rash of scarlet fever. **extracellular t.,** exotoxin. **fatigue t.,** kenotoxin. **intracellular t.,** endotoxin. **plant t.,** phytotoxin.

toxin-antitoxin (tok″sin-an′tĭ-tok″sin) a nearly neutral mixture of diphtheria toxin with its antitoxin; used for diphtheria immunization.

toxipathy (tok-sip′ah-the) toxicosis.

toxisterol (tok-sis′ter-ol) a poisonous isomer of ergosterol, produced by ultraviolet irradiation of the latter.

Toxocara (tok″so-ka′rah) a genus of nematode parasites found in the dog (*T. ca′nis*) and cat (*T. ca′ti*); both species are sometimes found in man.

toxocariasis (-ka-ri′ah-sis) infection by worms of the genus *Toxocara.*

toxoid (tok′soid) a toxin treated by heat or chemical agent to destroy its deleterious properties without destroying its ability to stimulate antibody production. **diphtheria t.,** a sterile preparation of formaldehyde-treated products of the growth of *Corynebacterium diphtheriae,* used as an active immunizing agent. **tetanus t.,** a sterile preparation of formaldehyde-treated products of the growth of *Clostridrium tetani,* used as an active immunizing agent.

toxophilic (tok″so-fil′ik) easily susceptible to poison; having affinity for toxins.

toxophore (tok′so-fōr) the group of atoms in a toxin molecule which produces the toxic effect.

toxophorous (tok-sof′o-rus) bearing poison; producing the toxic effect.

Toxoplasma (tok″so-plaz′mah) a genus of sporozoa that are intracellular parasites of many organs and tissues of birds and mammals, including man. *T. gon′dii* is the etiologic agent of toxoplasmosis.

toxoplasmin (-plaz′min) an antigen prepared from mouse peritoneal fluids rich with *Toxoplasma gondii;* injected intracutaneously as a test for toxoplasmosis.

toxoplasmosis (-plaz-mo′sis) a disease due to *Toxoplasma gondii.* The *congenital* form is marked by central nervous system lesions, which may lead to blindness, brain defects, and death. The acquired form is of two types: *lymphadenopathic t.,* closely resembling mononucleosis, and *disseminated t.,* with lesions involving the lungs, liver, heart, skin, muscle, brain, and meninges. Chorioretinitis invariably occurs in the congenital form, and often in the chronic form.

trabecula (trah-bek′u-lah), pl. *trabec′ulae* [L.] a little beam; in anatomy, a general term for a supporting or anchoring strand of connective tissue, e.g., a strand extending from a capsule into the substance of the enclosed organ. **trabec′ular,** adj.

trabeculate (trah-bek′u-lāt) marked with cross bars or trabeculae.

tracer (trās′er) a means by which something may be followed, as (*a*) a mechanical device by which the outline or movements of an object can be graphically recorded, or (*b*) a material by which the progress of a compound through the body may be observed. **radioactive t.,** a radioactive isotope replacing a stable chemical element in a compound introduced into the body, enabling its metabolism, distribution, and elimination to be followed.

trachea (tra′ke-ah) windpipe; the cartilaginous and membranous tube descending from the larynx and branching into the left and right main bronchi. **tra′cheal,** adj.

trachealgia (tra″ke-al′je-ah) pain in the trachea.

tracheitis (-i′tis) inflammation of the trachea.

trachel(o)- word element [Gr.], *neck; necklike structure,* especially the uterine cervix.

trachelagra (tra″kĕ-lag′rah) gout in the neck.

trachelectomy (-lek′to-me) cervicectomy.

trachelematoma (-lem″ah-to′mah) a hematoma on the sternocleidomastoid muscle.

trachelism, trachelismus (tra′kĕ-lizm; tra″-kĕ-liz′mus) spasm of the neck muscles; spasmodic retraction of the head in epilepsy.

trachelitis (tra″kĕ-li′tis) cervicitis.

trachelocystitis (tra″kĕ-lo-sis-ti′tis) inflammation of the neck of the bladder.

trachelodynia (-din′e-ah) pain in the neck.

trachelomyitis (-mi-i′tis) inflammation of the muscles of the neck.

trachelopexy (tra′kĕ-lo-pek″se) fixation of the uterine cervix.

tracheloplasty (-plas″te) plastic repair of the uterine cervix.

trachelorrhaphy (tra″kĕ-lor′ah-fe) suture of the uterine cervix.

trachelotomy (-lot′o-me) incision of the uterine cervix.

tracheo- word element [Gr.], *trachea.*

tracheoaerocele (tra″ke-o-a′er-o-sēl″) a tracheal hernia containing air.

tracheobronchial (-brong′ke-al) pertaining to the trachea and bronchi.

tracheobronchitis (-brong-ki′tis) inflammation of the trachea and bronchi.

tracheobronchoscopy (-brong-kos′ko-pe) inspection of the interior of the trachea and bronchi.

tracheocele (tra′ke-o-sēl″) hernial protrusion of tracheal mucous membrane.

tracheoesophageal (tra″ke-o-ĕ-sof′ah-je-al) pertaining to the trachea and esophagus.

tracheolaryngeal (-lah-rin′je-al) pertaining to the trachea and larynx.

tracheolaryngotomy (-lar″ing-got′o-me) incision of the larynx and trachea.

tracheomalacia (-mah-la′she-ah) softening of the tracheal cartilages.

tracheopathy (tra″ke-op′ah-the) disease of the trachea.

tracheopharyngeal (tra″ke-o-fah-rin′je-al) pertaining to the trachea and pharynx.

tracheophony (tra″ke-of′o-ne) sound heard in auscultation over the trachea.

tracheoplasty (tra′ke-o-plas″te) plastic repair of the trachea.

tracheopyosis (tra″ke-o-pi-o′sis) purulent tracheitis.

tracheorrhagia (-ra′je-ah) hemorrhage from the trachea.

tracheoschisis (tra″ke-os′kĭ-sis) fissure of the trachea.

tracheoscopy (-os′ko-pe) inspection of interior of the trachea. **tracheoscop′ic,** adj.

tracheostenosis (tra″ke-o-stĕ-no′sis) constriction of the trachea.

tracheostomize (tra″ke-os′to-mīz) to perform tracheostomy upon.

tracheostomy (-os′to-me) creation of an opening into the trachea through the neck, with the tracheal mucosa being brought into continuity with the skin; also, the opening so created. The term is also used to refer to a tracheotomy done for insertion of a tube.

tracheotome (tra′ke-o-tōm″) an instrument for incising the trachea.

tracheotomy (tra″ke-ot′o-me) incision of the trachea through the skin and muscles of the neck. **inferior t.,** performed below, and **superior t.,** above, the isthmus of the thyroid.

trachitis (trah-ki′tis) tracheitis.

trachoma (trah-ko′mah) a contagious disease of the conjunctiva and cornea, producing photophobia, pain, and lacrimation, caused by a strain of *Chlamydia trachomatis.* Clinically, it progresses from a mild infection with tiny follicles on the eyelid conjunctiva to invasion of the cornea, with scarring and contraction which may result in blindness.

trachomatous (-tus) pertaining to or of the nature of trachoma.

trachychromatic (tra″ke-kro-mat′ik) strongly or deeply staining.

trachyphonia (-fo′ne-ah) roughness of the voice.

tracing (trās′ing) a graphic record produced by copying another, or scribed by an instrument capable of making a visual record of movements.

tract (trakt) a longitudinal assemblage of tissues or organs, especially a bundle of nerve fibers having a common origin, function, and termination, or a number of anatomic structures arranged in series and serving a common function. **alimentary t.,** see under *canal.* **biliary t.,** the organs, ducts, etc., participating in secretion (the liver), storage (the gallbladder), and delivery (hepatic and bile ducts) of bile into the duodenum. **digestive c.,** alimentary canal. **dorsolateral t.,** a group of nerve fibers in the lateral funiculus of the spinal cord dorsal to the posterior column. **extrapyramidal t.,** see under *system.* **Flechsig's t.,** spinocerebellar t., posterior. **gastrointestinal t.,** the stomach and intestine in continuity. **Gowers' t.,** spinocerebellar t., anterior. **iliotibial t.,** a thickened longitudinal band of fascia lata extending from the tensor muscle downward to the lateral condyle of the tibia. **intestinal t.,** the small and large intestines in continuity. **optic t.,** the nerve tract proceeding backward from the optic chiasm, around the cerebral peduncle, and dividing into a lateral and medial root, which end in the superior colliculus and lateral geniculate body, respectively. **pyramidal t's,** collections of nerve fibers arising in the brain and passing down through the spinal cord to motor cells in the anterior horns. **respiratory t.,** the organs which allow entrance of air into the lungs and exchange of gases with the blood, from air passages in the nose to the pulmonary alveoli. See Plate VI. **spinocerebellar t., anterior,** a group of nerve fibers in the lateral funiculus of the spinal cord, arising mostly in the gray matter of the opposite side, and ascending to the cerebellum through the superior cerebellar peduncle. **spinocerebellar t., posterior,** a group of nerve fibers in the lateral funiculus of the spinal cord, arising mostly from the nucleus thoracicus, and ascending to the cerebellum through the inferior cerebellar peduncle. **urinary t.,** the organs concerned with the elaboration and excretion of urine: kidneys, ureters, bladder, and urethra. **uveal t.,** the vascular tunic of the eye, comprising the choroid, ciliary body, and iris.

traction (trak′shun) the act of drawing or pulling. **axis t.,** traction along an axis, as of the pelvis in obstetrics. **elastic t.,** traction by an elastic force or by means of an elastic appliance. **skeletal t.,** traction applied directly upon long bones by means of pins, wires, etc., **skin t.,** traction on a body part maintained by an apparatus affixed by dressings to the body surface.

tractotomy (trak-tot′o-me) transection of a nerve tract in the central nervous system.

tractus (trak′tus), pl. *trac′tus* [L.] tract.

tragacanth (trag′ah-kanth) dried gummy exudation from *Astragalus gummifer* or other species of *Astragalus;* used as a suspending agent for drugs.

tragomaschalia (trag″o-mas-kal′e-ah) odorous perspiration from the axilla.

tragus (tra′gus), pl. *tra′gi* [L.] the cartilaginous projection anterior to the external opening of the ear; used also in the plural to designate hairs growing on the pinna of the external ear, especially on the tragus. **tra′gal,** adj.

trait (trāt) 1. any genetically determined condition; also, the condition prevailing in the heterozygous state of a recessive disorder, as the sickle cell trait. 2. a distinctive behavior pattern. **sickle cell t.,** the condition, usually asymptomatic, due to heterozygosity for hemoglobin S.

Tral (tral) trademark for preparations of hexocyclium methylsulfate.

tramazoline (trah-maz′o-lēn) an adrenergic, $C_{13}H_{17}N_3$.

trance (trans) a state of diminished activity and consciousness, resembling sleep.

Trancopal (tran′ko-pal) trademark for a preparation of chlormezanone.

tranquilizer (tran″kwĭ-li′zer) an agent that calms or quiets an anxious or agitated patient without affecting clarity of consciousness. **major t.,** a drug used to reduce psychotic symptoms. **minor t.,** one that is useful in the treatment of milder symptoms of anxiety, tension, or neuroses.

trans- word element [L.], *through; across; beyond;* in names of chemical compounds it indicates certain atoms or radicals on opposite sides of the molecule.

transabdominal (trans″ab-dom′ĭ-nal) across the abdominal wall or through the abdominal cavity.

transacetylation (trans-as″ĕ-til-a′shun) a chemical reaction involving the transfer of the acetyl radical.

transacylase (-as′ĭ-lās) an enzyme that catalyzes transacylation.

transacylation (-as″ĭ-la′shun) a chemical reaction involving the transfer of the acyl radical between acetic and higher carboxylic acids.

transamidase (-am′ĭ-dās) an enzyme which catalyzes the transfer of an amide group from one molecule to another.

transamidinase (-am′ĭ-din-ās) an enzyme that catalyzes the transfer of amidine, as from arginine to ornithine.

transaminase (-am′ĭ-nās) an enzyme that catalyzes transamination. **glutamic-oxalacetic t., (GOT),** an enzyme normally present in serum (SGOT) and various tissues, especially the heart and liver; it is released into serum as a result of tissue injury and is present in increased concentration in myocardial infarction or acute damage to liver cells. **glutamic-pyruvic t.,** an enzyme normally present in serum and body tissues, especially the liver; it is released into serum as a result of tissue injury and is present in higher concentration in the serum of patients with acute damage to liver cells.

transamination (-am″ĭ-na′shun) the reversible exchange of amino groups between different amino acids.

transanimation (-an″ĭ-ma′shun) mouth-to-mouth resuscitation.

transaortic (trans″a-or′tik) performed through the aorta.

transatrial (trans-a′tre-al) performed through the atrium.

transaudient (-aw′de-ent) penetrable by sound waves.

transaxial (-ak′se-al) directed at right angles to the long axis of the body or a part.

transcalent (-ka′lent) penetrable by heat rays.

transcortical (-kor′tĭ-kal) connecting two parts of the cerebral cortex.

transcortin (-kor′tin) an α-globulin that binds and transports biologically active, unconjugated cortisol in plasma.

transcription (-krip′shun) the process by which genetic information contained in DNA produces a complementary series of bases in an RNA chain.

transduction (-duk′shun) the transfer of a genetic fragment from one microorganism to another by bacteriophage.

transection (tran-sek′shun) a cross section; division by cutting transversely.

transferase (trans′fer-ās) any enzyme that catalyzes the transfer, from one molecule to another, of a chemical group that does not exist in free state during the transfer.

transference (trans-fer′ens) 1. the passage of a symptom or affection from one part to another. 2. in psychiatry, the shifting of an affect from one person to another or from one idea to another; especially the transfer by the patient to the analyst of emotional tones, of either affection or hostility, based on unconscious identification.

transferrin (-fer′rin) a serum globulin that binds and transports iron.

transfix (-fiks′) to pierce through or impale.

transfixion (-fik′shun) a cutting through from within outward, as in amputation.

transforation (trans″fo-ra′shun) perforation of the fetal skull.

transformation (-for-ma′shun) change of form or structure; conversion from one form to another. In oncology, the change that a normal cell undergoes as it becomes malignant.

transfusion (trans-fu′zhun) the introduction of whole blood or blood components directly into the blood stream. **direct t.,** immediate t. **exchange t.,** repetitive withdrawal of small amounts of blood and replacement with donor blood, until a large proportion of the original volume has been replaced. **immediate t.,** transfer of blood directly from a vessel of the donor to a vessel of the recipient. **indirect t., mediate t.,** introduction of blood which has been stored in a suitable container after withdrawal from the donor. **placental t.,** return to an infant after birth, through the intact umbilical cord, of the blood contained in the placenta. **replacement t., substitution t.,** exchange t.

transiliac (-il′e-ak) across the two ilia.

transillumination (trans″ĭ-lu″mĭ-na′shun) the passage of strong light through a body structure, to permit inspection by an observer on the opposite side.

translation (trans-la′shun) the formation of a polypeptide chain in the sequence directed by messenger RNA.

translocation (trans″lo-ka′shun) the attachment of a fragment of one chromosome to a nonhomologous chromosome. **reciprocal t.,** the mutual exchange of fragments between two broken chromosomes, one part of one uniting with part of the other.

translucent (trans-lu′sent) slightly penetrable by light rays.

transmethylase (-meth′ĭ-lās) an enzyme that catalyzes transmethylation.

transmethylation (trans″meth-ĭ-la′shun) the transfer of a methyl group (CH—) from the molecules of one compound to those of another.

transmigration (-mi-gra′shun) 1. diapedesis. 2. change of place from one side of the body to the other.

transmission (trans-mish′un) the transfer, as of a disease, from one person to another.

transmutation (trans″mu-ta′shun) 1. evolutionary change of one species into another. 2. the change of one chemical element into another.

transorbital (trans-or′bĭ-tal) performed through the bony socket of the eye.

transpeptidase (-pep′tĭ-dās) an enzyme which catalyzes the transfer of an amino or peptide group from one molecule to another.

transphosphorylase (-fos′for-ĭ-lās) an enzyme that catalyzes transphosphorylation.

transphosphorylation (-fos″for-ĭ-la′shun) the exchange of phosphate groups between organic phosphates, without their going through the stage of inorganic phosphates.

transpiration (trans″pĭ-ra′shun) discharge of air, vapor, or sweat through the skin.

transplacental (-plah-sen′tal) through the placenta.

transplant 1. (trans′plant) tissue used in grafting or transplanting. 2. (trans-plant′) to transfer tissue from one part to another.

transplantation (trans″plan-ta′shun) the grafting of tissues taken from one part of the body to another part, or to another individual.

transport (trans′port) movement of materials in biological systems, particularly into and out of cells and across epithelial layers. **active t.,** movement of materials in biological systems resulting directly from expenditure of metabolic energy.

transposition (trans″po-zish′un) 1. displacement of a viscus to the opposite side. 2. the operation of carrying a tissue flap from one situation to another without severing its connection entirely until it is united at its new location. 3. The exchange of position of two atoms within a molecule. **t. of great vessels,** a congenital cardiovascular malformation in which the position of the chief blood vessels of the heart is reversed. Life then depends on a crossflow of blood between the right and left sides of the heart, as through a ventricular septal defect.

transsegmental (-seg-men′tal) extending across segments.

transseptal (trans-sep′tal) extending or performed through or across a septum.

transsexual (-seks′u-al) 1. a person affected by transsexualism. 2. a person whose external anatomy has been changed to resemble that of the opposite sex.

transsexualism (-seks′u-al-izm″) a disturbance of gender identity in which the person has an overwhelming desire to be of the opposite sex, often seeking hormonal and surgical treatment to achieve this goal.

transthalamic (trans″thah-lam′ik) across the thalamus.

transthoracic (-tho-ras′ik) through the thoracic cavity or across the chest wall.

transtympanic (-tim-pan′ik) across the tympanic membrane or cavity.

transudate (tran′su-dāt) a fluid substance that has passed through a membrane or has been extruded from a tissue; in contrast to an exudate, it is of high fluidity and has a low content of protein, cells, or solid materials derived from cells.

transudation (tran″su-da′shun) 1. passage of a transudate. 2. transudate.

transurethral (trans″u-re′thral) performed through the urethra.

transvaginal (trans-vaj′ĭ-nal) through the vagina.

transversalis (trans″ver-sa′lis) [L.] transverse.

transverse (trans-vers′) extending from side to side; at right angles to the long axis.

transversectomy (trans″ver-sek′to-me) excision of a transverse process of a vertebra.

transversus (trans-ver′sus) [L.] transverse.

transvesical (-ves′ĭ-kal) through the bladder.

transvestism (-ves′tizm) the condition of being a transvestite.

transvestite (-ves′tīt) a person who derives sexual pleasure from dressing in the attire of the opposite sex.

tranylcypromine (tran″il-si′pro-mēn) a monoamine oxidase inhibitor, $(C_9H_{11}N)_2$; the sulfate salt is used as an antidepressant.

trapezium (trah-pe′ze-um) an irregular, four-sided figure; see *Table of Bones.*

Trasentine (tras′en-tin) trademark for preparations of adiphenine.

trauma (traw′mah) a wound or injury, whether physical or psychic. **birth t.,** an injury to the infant during the process of being born. In some psychiatric theories, the psychic shock produced in an infant by the experience of being born. **psychic t.,** an emotional shock that makes a lasting impression.

traumat(o)- word element [Gr.], *trauma.*

traumatic (traw-mat′ik) pertaining to, resulting from, or causing trauma.

traumatism (traw′mah-tizm) 1. the physical or psychic state resulting from an injury or wound. 2. a wound.

traumatology (traw″mah-tol′o-je) the branch of surgery dealing with wounds and disability from injuries.

traumatopnea (-top-ne′ah) passage of air through a wound in the chest wall.

travail (trah-vāl′) childbirth; see *labor.*

tray (tra) a flat-surfaced utensil for the conveyance of various objects or material. **impression t.,** a contoured container to hold the material for making an impression of the teeth and associated structures.

treatment (trēt′ment) management and care of a patient or the combating of disease or disorder. **active t.,** that directed immediately to the cure of the disease or injury. **Banting t.,** treatment of obesity by a low carbohydrate diet rich in nitrogenous matter. **causal t.,** treatment directed against the cause of a disease. **conservative t.,** that designed to avoid radical medical therapeutic measure or operative procedures. **dietetic t.,** treatment of disease by regulation of the diet. **empiric t.,** treatment by means which experience has proved to be beneficial. **expectant t.,** treatment directed toward relief of untoward symptoms, leaving cure of the disease to

natural forces. **Karell t.,** treatment of heart and kidney disease by keeping the patient in bed and giving only 800 ml. of milk daily for 4 or 5 days, the diet then being gradually increased until, on the thirteenth day the regular diet is resumed. **Kenny's t.,** treatment of poliomyelitis by wrapping the patient in woolen cloths wrung out of hot water and re-educating muscles by passive exercise after pain has subsided. **light t.,** phototherapy. **palliative t.,** treatment designed to relieve pain and distress with no attempt to cure. **preventive t., prophylactic t.,** that in which the aim is to prevent the occurrence of the disease; prophylaxis. **rational t.,** that based upon knowledge of disease and the action of the remedies given. **shock t.,** see under *therapy.* **specific t.,** treatment particularly adapted to the disease being treated. **supporting t.,** that which is mainly directed to sustaining the strength of the patient. **symptomatic t.,** expectant t.

tree (tre) 1. a perennial of the plant kingdom having a main stem or trunk and numerous brances. 2. an anatomic structure with branches resembling a tree. **bronchial t.,** the bronchi and their branching structures. **tracheobronchial t.,** the trachea, bronchi, and their branching structures.

trehalose (tre-ha′lōs) a disaccharide from the cocoons of the beetle *Trehala manna* and yeast.

Trematoda (trem″ah-to′dah) a class of Platyhelminthes, including the flukes; they are parasitic in man and animals, infection usually resulting from ingestion of inadequately cooked fish, crustaceans, or vegetation containing their larvae.

trematode (trem′ah-tōd) an individual of the class Trematoda.

trembles (trem′belz) poisoning in cattle and sheep feeding on the white snakeroot (*Eupatorium rugosum*), in which the animal has muscular tremors and becomes weak and may suddenly stumble and fall; see also *milk sickness* (1).

tremor (trem′or, tre′mor) an involuntary trembling or quivering. **coarse t.,** that involving large groups of muscle fibers contracting slowly. **fibrillary t.,** rapidly alternating contraction of small bundles of muscle fibers. **fine t.,** one in which the vibrations are rapid. **flapping t.,** asterixis. **Hunt's t.,** the tremor attending every voluntary movement, characteristic of cerebellar lesions. **intention t.,** that occurring when the patient attempts voluntary movement. **senile t.,** that due to the infirmities of old age. **volitional t.,** trembling of entire body during voluntary effort; seen in multiple sclerosis.

tremulous (trem′u-lus) shaking, trembling, or quivering.

trepan (trĕ-pan′) to trephine.

trepanation (trep″ah-na′shun) trephination.

trephination (tref″ĭ-na′shun) the operation of trephining.

trephine (trĕ-fīn′, trĕ-fēn′) 1. a crown saw for removing a circular disk of bone, chiefly from the skull. 2. an instrument for removing a circular area of cornea. 3. to remove with a trephine.

trepidation (trep″ĭ-da′shun) 1. a trembling or oscillatory movement. 2. nervous anxiety and fear. **trep′idant**, adj.

Treponema (trep″o-ne′mah) a genus of spirochetes (family Treponemataceae), some of them being pathogenic and parasitic for man and other animals, and including the etiologic agents of pinta (*T. carate′um*), syphilis (*T. pal′lidum*), and yaws (*T. perten′ue*).

treponema (-ne′mah) an organism of the genus *Treponema*. **trepone′mal**, adj.

Treponemataceae (-ne″mah-ta′se-e) a family of bacteria (order Spirochaetales), commonly occurring as parasites in vertebrates, some of them causing disease.

treponematosis (-ne″mah-to′sis) infection with organisms of the genus *Treponema*.

treponemicidal (-ne″mĭ-si′dal) destroying treponemas.

trepopnea (tre″pop-ne′ah) more comfortable respiration with the patient turned in a definite recumbent position.

treppe (trep′ĕ) [Ger.] the gradual increase in muscular contraction following rapidly repeated stimulation.

tresis (tre′sis) perforation.

tri- word element [Gr., L.], *three*.

triacetate (tri-as′ĕ-tāt) an acetate which contains 3 molecules of the acetic acid radical.

triacetin (-as′ĕ-tin) an antifungal agent, $C_9H_{14}O_6$.

triacetyloleandomycin (-as″ĕ-til-o″le-an″do-mi′sin) troleandomycin.

triad (tri′ad) 1. any trivalent element. 2. a group of three associated entities or objects. **Beck's t.,** rising venous pressure, falling arterial pressure, and small quiet heart; characteristic of cardiac compression. **Hutchinson's t.,** diffuse interstitial keratitis, labyrinthine disease, and Hutchinson's teeth, seen in congenital syphilis. **Saint's t.,** hiatus hernia, colonic diverticula, and cholelithiasis.

triage (tre-ahzh′) [Fr.] the sorting out and classification of casualties of war or other disaster, to determine priority of need and proper place of treatment.

triamcinolone (tri″am-sin′o-lōn) an anti-inflammatory glucocorticoid, $C_{21}H_{27}FO_6$.

triamterene (tri-am′ter-ēn) a diuretic, $C_{12}H_{11}N_7$, which increases sodium and chloride excretion, but not potassium excretion.

triangle (tri′ang-g'l) a three-cornered object, figure, or area, as such an area on the surface of the body capable of fairly precise definition. **carotid t., inferior,** the part of the carotid trigone medial to the omohyoid muscle. **carotid t., superior,** the part of the carotid trigone lateral to the omohyoid muscle. **cephalic t.,** one on the anteroposterior plane of skull, between lines from the occiput to the forehead and to the chin, and from the chin to the forehead. **Codman's t.,** a triangular area visible roentgenographically where the periosteum, elevated by a bone tumor, rejoins the cortex of normal bone. **digastric t.,** submandibular t. **t. of elbow,** in front,

the supinator longus on the outside and pronator teres inside, the base toward the humerus. **t. of election,** superior carotid t. **facial t.,** its angles—basion, and alveolar and nasal points. **Farabeuf's t.,** one in the upper part of the neck bound by the internal jugular vein, the facial nerve, and the hypoglossal nerve. **femoral t.,** the area formed superiorly by the inguinal ligament, laterally by the sartorius muscle, and medially by the adductor longus muscle. **frontal t.,** one bounded by the maximum frontal diameter and the lines to the glabella. **Hesselbach's t.,** inguinal t. (1). **iliofemoral t.,** one formed by Nélaton's line, another line through the superior iliac spine, and a third from this to the greater trochanter. **infraclavicular t.,** one formed by the clavicle above, upper border of the pectoralis major on the inside, and the anterior border of the deltoid on the outside. **inguinal t.,** 1. the area on the inferoanterior abdominal wall bounded by the rectus abdominis muscle, the inguinal ligament, and inferior epigastric vessel. 2. femoral t. **Langenbeck's t.,** one whose apex is the anterior superior iliac spine, its base the anatomic neck of the femur, and its external side the external base of the greater trochanter. **Lesser's t.,** one formed by the hypoglossal nerve above, and the two bellies of the digastricus on the two sides. **lumbocostoabdominal t.,** one between the obliquus externus, the serratus posticus inferior, the erector spinae, and the obliquus internus. **Macewen's t.,** mastoid fossa. **t. of necessity,** inferior carotid t. **occipital t.,** one having the sternomastoid in front, the trapezius behind, and the omohyoid below. **occipital t., inferior,** one having the bimastoid line as its base and the inion its apex. **Pawlik's t.,** an area on the anterior vaginal wall corresponding to the trigone of the bladder. **Petit's t.,** the space bounded by the crest of the ilium, the latissimus dorsi, and the external oblique muscle of the abdomen. **Scarpa's t.,** femoral t. **subclavian t.,** the triangular area bounded by the clavicle, sternocleidomastoid, and omohyoid. **submaxillary t.,** lower jaw bone above, posterior belly of the digastric, and the stylohyoid below, and the median line of the neck in front. **suboccipital t.,** one between the rectus capitis posterior major and superior and inferior oblique muscles. **suprameatal t.,** mastoid fossa.

triangular (tri-ang′gu-lar) having three angles or corners.

triangularis (-ang″gu-la′ris) [L.] triangular.

Triatoma (tri″ah-to′mah) a genus of bugs (order Hemiptera), the cone-nosed bugs, important in medicine as vectors of *Trypanosoma cruzi*.

triatomic (-ah-tom′ik) containing three atoms in the molecule.

tribe (trīb) a taxonomic category subordinate to a family (or subfamily) and superior to a genus (or subtribe).

triboluminescence (tri″bo-lu″mĭ-nes′ens) luminescence produced by mechanical energy, as by the grinding, rubbing, or breaking of certain crystals.

tribrachius (tri-bra′ke-us) a monster with three arms.

tribromoethanol (-bro″mo-eth′ah-nol) C_2H_3-Br_3O, used in amylene hydrate solution as a basal anesthetic.

Triburon (trib′u-ron) trademark for preparations of triclobisonium.

TRIC *trachoma-inclusion* conjunctivitis (group); see *Chlamydia trachomatis.*

tricephalus (tri-sef′ah-lus) a monster with three heads.

triceps (tri′seps) three-headed, as a triceps muscle. **t. su′rae,** see *Table of Muscles.*

trich(o)- word element [Gr.], *hair.*

trichiasis (trĭ-ki′ah-sis) 1. a condition of ingrowing hairs about an orifice, or ingrowing eyelashes. 2. appearance of hairlike filaments in the urine.

trichina (trĭ-ki′nah), pl. *trichi′nae* [Gr.] an individual organism of the genus *Trichinella.*

Trichinella (trik″ĭ-nel′ah) a genus of nematode parasites, including *T. spira′lis,* the etiologic agent of trichinosis, found in the muscles of the rat, pig, and man.

trichinosis (-no′sis) a disease due to eating inadequately cooked meat infected with *Trichinella spiralis,* attended by diarrhea, nausea, colic, and fever, and later by stiffness, pain, muscle swelling, fever, sweating, eosinophilia, circumorbital edema, and splinter hemorrhages.

trichinous (trik′ĭ-nus) affected with or containing trichinae.

trichloride (tri-klo′rīd) any combination of three atoms of chloride with one of another element.

trichlormethiazide (-klor″mĕ-thi′ah-zīd) a diuretic and antihypertensive, $C_8H_8ClN_3O_4S_2$.

trichloroethylene (-klo″ro-eth′ĭ-lēn) a clear, mobile liquid used as an inhalation analgesic for short operative procedures.

trichoanesthesia (trik″o-an″es-the′ze-ah) loss of hair sensibility.

trichobezoar (-be′zōr) hairball; a bezoar composed of hair.

trichocardia (-kar′de-ah) cor villosum.

trichoclasia (-kla′se-ah) trichorrhexis nodosa.

Trichodectes (-dek′tēz) a genus of parasitic insects of the order Mallophaga, the biting lice.

trichoepithelioma (-ep″ĭ-the″le-o′mah) a benign skin tumor originating in the follicles of the lanugo; it may occur as an inherited condition marked by multiple tumors (*t. papillo′sum mul′tiplex*).

trichoesthesia (-es-the′ze-ah) sensibility of the hair to touch.

trichoglossia (-glos′e-ah) hairy tongue.

trichoid (trik′oid) resembling hair.

trichologia (trik″o-lo′je-ah) the pulling out of the hair by delirious patients; trichotillomania.

trichomadesis (-mah-de′sis) abnormally rapid or premature loss of the scalp hair.

trichome (tri′kōm) a filamentous or hairlike structure.

trichomonacide (trik″o-mo′nah-sīd) an agent destructive to trichomonads.

trichomonad (trĭ-kom′o-nad) a parasite of the genus *Trichomonas.*

trichomonal (trĭ-kom′o-nal) pertaining to *Trichomonas.*

Trichomonas (trĭ-kom′o-nas) a genus of flagellate protozoa parasitic in animals and birds and in man; it includes *T. homi′nis,* a common intestinal parasite of man, *T. te′nax,* a nonpathogenic species found in the human mouth, and *T. vagina′lis,* found in the vagina, which produces a refractory vaginal discharge and pruritus; it has been found in the male bladder and urethra.

trichomoniasis (trik″o-mo-ni′ah-sis) infection by organisms of the genus *Trichomonas.*

trichomycosis (-mi-ko′sis) any disease of the hair caused by fungi. **t. axilla′ris,** infection of the axillary and sometimes of the pubic hair, due to *Corynebacterium tenuis* and not a fungus, with development of clumps of bacteria on the hairs, appearing as red, yellow, or black nodules. **t. favo′sa,** favus.

trichonodosis (-no-do′sis) a condition characterized by apparent or actual knotting of the hair.

trichopathy (trĭ-kop′ah-the) disease of the hair.

trichophytid (trĭ-kof′ĭ-tid) a secondary skin eruption that is the expression of an allergic reaction to a trichophyton infection and that occurs in an area remote from the site of infection.

trichophytin (trĭ-kof′ĭ-tin) a filtrate from cultures of *Trichophyton;* used in testing for trichophytosis.

trichophytobezoar (trik″o-fi″to-be′zōr) a bezoar composed of animal hair and vegetable fiber.

Trichophyton (trĭ-kof′ĭ-ton) a genus of fungi, species of which attack skin, hair, and nails; common species include *T. mentagrophy′tes, T. ru′brum, T. ton′surans, T. schoenlei′ni, T. concen′tricum, T. ferrugin′eum,* and *T. viola′ceum.*

trichophytosis (trik″o-fi-to′sis) infection with fungi of the genus *Trichophyton.* **trichophyt′ic,** adj.

trichoptilosis (-tĭ-lo′sis) splitting of hairs at the end.

trichorrhexis (-rek′sis) the condition in which the hairs are split and feather-like. **t. nodo′sa,** a condition marked by fracture and splitting of the cortex of a hair into strands, giving the appearance of white nodes at which the hair is easily broken.

trichoschisis (trĭ-kos′kĭ-sis) trichoptilosis.

trichoscopy (trĭ-kos′ko-pe) examination of the hair.

trichosiderin (trik″o-sid′er-in) an iron-containing brown pigment found in normal human red hair.

trichosis (trĭ-ko′sis) any disease or abnormal growth of the hair.

Trichosporon (trĭ-kos′po-ron) a genus of fungi that are normal flora of the respiratory and digestive tracts of man and animals, and may infect the hair.

trichosporosis (trik″o-spo-ro′sis) infection with *Trichosporon;* see *piedra.*

trichostasis spinulosa (trĭ-kos′tah-sis spin″u-lo′sah) obstruction of the hair follicles with a spinulous dark plug, consisting of many lanugo hairs in a horny mass, affecting the skin of the alae nasi and other facial areas, or of the arms, chest, abdomen, or interscapular area.

trichostrongyliasis (trik″o-stron″jĭ-li′ah-sis) infection with *Trichostrongylus.*

trichostrongylosis (-stron″jĭ-lo′sis) trichostrongyliasis.

Trichostrongylus (-stron′jĭ-lus) a genus of nematodes parasitic in animals and man.

trichotillomania (-til″o-ma′ne-ah) compulsion to pull out one's hair.

trichotomous (trĭ-kot′o-mus) divided into three parts.

trichroism (tri′kro-izm) the exhibition of three different colors in three different aspects. **trichro′ic,** adj.

trichromatopsia (tri″kro-mah-top′se-ah) normal color vision for all three primary colors.

trichromic (tri-kro′mik) 1. pertaining to or exhibiting three colors. 2. able to distinguish only three of the seven colors of the spectrum.

trichuriasis (trik″u-ri′ah-sis) infection with *Trichuris.*

Trichuris (trik-u′ris) a genus of intestinal nematode parasites, including *T. trichiu′ra* (whipworm), the species principally infecting man.

tricipital (tri-sip′ĭ-tal) 1. three-headed. 2. relating to the triceps muscle.

triclobisonium (tri″klo-bi-so′ne-um) an anti-infective, $C_{36}H_{74}N_2$, used topically as the chloride salt in superficial infections of the skin and vagina, and in vulvitis, vaginitis, and related infections due to *Trichomonas vaginalis, Candida albicans,* and *Hemophilus vaginalis.*

triclofos (tri′klo-fōs) a hypnotic and sedative, $C_2H_3Cl_3NaO_4P.$

Tricofuron (tri″ko-fu′ron) trademark for preparations of furazolidone.

Tricoloid (tri′ko-loid) trademark for preparations of tricyclamol.

tricornute (tri-kor′nūt) having three horns, cornua, or processes.

tricrotism (tri′krot-izm) quality of having three sphygmographic waves or elevations to one beat of the pulse. **tricrot′ic,** adj.

tricuspid (tri-kus′pid) having three points or cusps, as a valve of the heart.

tricyclamol (-si′klah-mol) a procyclidine derivative, $C_{20}H_{32}NO$, used to inhibit gastrointestinal hypermotility and to reduce gastric juice secretion.

tridactylism (-dak′tĭ-lizm) presence of only three digits on the hand or foot.

tridentate (-den′tāt) having three prongs.

tridermic (-der′mik) derived from the ectoderm, endoderm, and mesoderm.

tridihexethyl (tri″di-heks-eth′il) an anticholinergic, $C_{21}H_{36}NO$, used as the chloride salt in the treatment of gastrointestinal disturbances.

Tridione (tri-di′ōn) trademark for preparations of trimethadione.

triethanolamine (-eth″ah-nol′ah-mēn) a compound used as an alkalizing agent.

triethylamine (-eth″il-am′in) a ptomaine from putrefying fish.

triethylenemelamine (tri-eth″ĭ-lēn-mel′ah-mēn) an antineoplastic, $C_9H_{12}N_6.$

triethylenethiophosphoramide (-thi″o-fos-for′ah-mīd) thiotepa.

trifid (tri′fid) split into three parts.

trifluoperazine (tri″floo-o-per′ah-zēn) a phenothiazine derivative, $C_{21}H_{24}F_3N_3S$; its hydrochloride salt is used as a major tranquilizer.

triflupromazine (-pro′mah-zēn) a phenothiazine derivative, $C_{18}H_{19}F_3N_2S$; its hydrochloride salt is used as a major tranquilizer.

trifluromethylthiazide (tri-floor″o-meth″il-thi′ah-zīd) flumethiazide.

trifurcation (tri″fer-ka′shun) division, or the site of separation, into three branches.

trigeminy (tri-jem′ĭ-ne) the condition of occurring in threes, especially the occurrence of three pulse beats in rapid succession.

triglyceride (-glis′er-īd) a compound consisting of three molecules of fatty acid esterified to glycerol; a neutral fat that is the usual storage form of lipids in animals.

trigonal (tri′go-nal) 1. triangular. 2. pertaining to a trigone.

trigone (tri′gōn) a triangular area. **t. of bladder,** vesical t. **carotid t.,** the triangular area bounded by the posterior belly of the digastric muscle, the sternocleidomastoid muscle, and the anterior midline of the neck. **olfactory t.,** the triangular area of gray matter between the roots of the olfactory tract. **vesical t.,** the smooth triangular portion of the mucosa at the base of the bladder, bounded behind by the interureteric fold, ending in front in the uvula of the bladder.

trigonectomy (tri″gon-ek′to-me) excision of the vesical trigone.

trigonid (tri-gon′id) the first three cusps of a lower molar tooth.

trigonitis (tri″go-ni′tis) inflammation or localized hyperemia of the vesical trigone.

trigonocephalus (trig″o-no-sef′ah-lus) an individual exhibiting trigonocephaly.

trigonocephaly (-sef′ah-le) triangular shape of the head due to sharp forward angulation at the midline of the frontal bone. **trigonocephal′ic,** adj.

trigonum (tri-go′num), pl. *trigo′na* [L.] trigone.

trihexyphenidyl (tri-hek″se-fen′ĭ-dil) an anticholinergic, $C_{20}H_{31}NO$, used as the hydrochloride salt in parkinsonism.

trihybrid (-hi′brid) a hybrid offspring of parents differing in three mendelian characters.

triiodothyronine (tri″i-o″do-thi′ro-nēn) one of the thyroid hormones, an organic iodine-containing compound liberated from thyroglobulin by hydrolysis. It has several times the biological activity of thyroxine.

trilabe (tri′lāb) a three-pronged lithotrite.

Trilafon (-lah-fon) trademark for preparations of perphenazine.

trilaminar (tri-lam′ĭ-nar) three-layered.

Trilene (tri′lēn) trademark for a preparation of trichloroethylene.

trilobate (tri-lo′bāt) having three lobes.

trilocular (-lok′u-lar) having three loculi or cells.

trilogy (tril′o-je) a group or series of three. **t. of Fallot,** a term sometimes applied to concurrent pulmonic stenosis, atrial septal defect, and right ventricular hypertrophy.

trimanual (tri-man′u-al) accomplished by use of three hands.

trimeprazine (-mep′rah-zēn) a drug, (C₁₈H₂₂N₂-S)₂, with mild central nervous depressant, moderate antiemetic and anticonvulsant, and powerful antihistaminic action; used as an antipruritic in the form of the tartrate salt.

trimester (-mes′ter) a period of three months.

trimethadione (tri″meth-ah-di′ōn) an anticonvulsant, C₆H₈NO₃.

trimethaphan camsylate (tri-meth′ah-fan) a short-acting ganglionic blocking agent, C₃₂H₄₀-N₂O₅S₂, used as an antihypertensive.

trimethidinium (-meth″ĭ-din′e-um) a ganglionic blocking agent; **t. methosulfate,** is used as an antihypertensive.

trimethobenzamide (-meth″o-ben′zah-mīd) an antiemetic, C₂₁H₂₈N₂O₅, used as the hydrochloride salt.

trimethylene (-meth′ĭ-lēn) cyclopropane.

Trimeton (tri′me-ton) trademark for preparations of pheniramine.

trimorphous (tri-mor′fus) existing in three different forms.

trinitroglycerol (tri-ni″tro-glis′er-ol) nitroglycerin.

trinitrophenol (-fe′nol) a substance, C₆H₂-(NO₂)₃OH, used as dye, tissue fixative, antiseptic, astringent, and stimulant of epithelialization; it can be detonated on percussion or by heating above 300° C.

trinitrotoluene (-tol′u-ēn) TNT: a high explosive, C₆H₂(NO₂)₃CH₃, derived from toluene; it sometimes causes poisoning in those who work with it, marked by dermatitis, gastritis, abdominal pain, vomiting, constipation, and flatulence.

triocephalus (tri″o-sef′ah-lus) a monster with no organs of sight, hearing, or smell.

triolism (tri′o-lizm) sexual interests or practices involving three persons of both sexes.

triorchidism (tri-or′kĭ-dizm) the presence of three testes.

triose (tri′ōs) a monosaccharide containing three carbon atoms in a molecule.

trioxsalen (tri-ok′sah-len) a psoralen, C₁₄H₁₂O₃, used in conjunction with ultraviolet exposure in treatment of vitiligo and psoriasis.

tripara (trip′ah-rah) tertipara.

tripelennamine (tri″pĕ-len′ah-min) an antihistaminic, C₁₆H₂₁N₃, used orally, parenterally, and topically in the symptomatic treatment of various allergic disorders.

tripeptide (tri-pep′tīd) a peptide formed from three amino acids.

triphalangism (-fal′an-jizm) three phalanges in a digit normally having only two.

triphasic (-fa′zik) having three phases.

triphenylmethane (-fen″il-meth′ān) a substance from coal tar, the basis of various dyes

and stains, including aurin, rosaniline, basic fuchsin, and gentian violet.

triplegia (-ple′je-ah) paralysis of three extremities.

triplet (trip′let) 1. one of three offspring produced at one birth. 2. a combination of three objects or entities acting together, as three lenses or three nucleotides.

triplex (tri′pleks) triple or threefold.

triploid (trip′loid) having triple the haploid number of chromosomes (3n).

triplokoria (trip″lo-ko′re-ah) the presence of three pupils in an eye.

triplopia (trĭ-plo′pe-ah) defective vision, objects being seen as threefold.

triprolidine (tri-pro′lĭ-dēn) an antihistaminic, C₁₉H₂₂N₂, used as the hydrochloride salt.

-tripsy word element [Gr.], *crushing;* used to designate a surgical procedure in which a structure is intentionally crushed.

tripus (tri′pus) a conjoined twin monster having three feet.

trisaccharide (tri-sak′ah-rīd) a carbohydrate composed of three saccharide groups.

trismus (triz′mus) motor disturbance of the trigeminal nerve, especially spasm of the masticatory muscles, with difficulty in opening the mouth (lockjaw); a characteristic early symptom of tetanus.

trisomy (tri′so-me) the presence of an additional (third) chromosome of one type in an otherwise diploid cell (2n + 1). See also under *syndrome.* **triso′mic,** adj.

trisplanchnic (tri-splangk′nik) pertaining to the three great visceral cavities.

tristearin (-ste′ah-rin) a white crystalline fat, C₃H₅(C₁₈H₃₅O₂)₃, found in harder fats, such as tallow.

tristichia (-stik′e-ah) the presence of three rows of eyelashes.

tristimania (tris″tĭ-ma′ne-ah) melancholia.

trisulcate (tri-sul′kāt) having three furrows.

trisulfate (-sul′fāt) a binary compound containing three sulfate (SO₄) groups in the molecule.

trisulfide (-sul′fīd) a sulfur compound containing three atoms of sulfur to one of the base.

tritanope (trit′ah-nōp) a person exhibiting tritanopia.

tritanopia (tri″tah-no′pe-ah) blue-yellow blindness, marked by imperfect perception of blue and yellow, with perception of only red and green. **tritanop′ic,** adj.

tritiate (trit′e-āt) to treat with tritium.

tritium (trit′e-um, trish′e-um) see *hydrogen.*

tritocone (tri′to-kōn) the distobuccal cusp of a mammalian upper premolar tooth.

tritoconid (tri″to-ko′nid) the distobuccal cusp of a mammalian lower premolar tooth.

triturable (trich′er-ah-b'l) susceptible of being triturated.

triturate (trich′ĕ-rāt) 1. to reduce to powder by rubbing. 2. a substance powdered fine by rubbing.

trituration (trich″ĕ-ra′shun) 1. reduction to powder by friction or grinding. 2. a finely powdered substance. 3. the creation of a homogeneous whole by mixing, as the combining of particles of an alloy with mercury to form dental amalgam.

triturator (-ra′tor) an apparatus in which substances can be continuously rubbed.

trivalent (tri-va′lent) having a valence of three.

tRNA transfer RNA; see *ribonucleic acid.*

trocar (tro′kar) a cannula with a sharp-pointed obturator for piercing the wall of a cavity.

trochanter (tro-kan′ter) a broad, flat process on the femur, at the upper end of its lateral surface (*greater t.*), or a short conical process on the posterior border of the base of its neck (*lesser t.*). **trochanter′ic, trochanter′ian,** adj.

troche (tro′ke) a medicinal preparation for solution in the mouth, consisting of an active ingredient incorporated in a mass made of sugar and mucilage or fruit base.

trochlea (trok′le-ah), pl. *troch′leae* [L.] a pulley-shaped part or structure; used in anatomic nomenclature to designate various bony or fibrous structures through or over which tendons pass or with which other structures articulate. **troch′lear,** adj.

trochocephaly (tro″ko-sef′ah-le) a rounded appearance of the head due to synostosis of the frontal and parietal bones.

trochoid (tro′koid) pivot-like, or pulley-shaped.

trochoides (tro-koi′dēz) a pivot joint.

Troglotrema (trog″lo-tre′mah) a genus of flukes, including *T. salmin′cola* (salmon fluke), a parasite of various fish, especially salmon and trout, which is a vector of *Neorickettsia helminthoeca.*

troleandomycin (tro″le-an″do-mi′sin) the triacetyl ester of oleandomycin, $C_{41}H_{67}NO_{14}$, used as an antibacterial.

trolnitrate (trol-ni′trāt) a vasodilator, $C_6H_{12}N_4O_9$, used as an antianginal agent in the form of the phosphate salt.

Trombicula (trom-bik′u-lah) a genus of acarine mites (family Trombiculidae), including *T. akamu′shi, T. delien′sis, T. fletch′eri, T. pal′lida,* and *T. scutella′ris,* whose larvae (chiggers) are vectors of *Rickettsia tsutsugamushi,* the cause of scrub typhus.

trombiculiasis (trom-bik″u-li′ah-sis) infestation with mites of the genus *Trombicula.*

Trombiculidae (trom-bik′u-li″de) a family of mites cosmopolitan in distribution, whose parasitic larvae (chiggers) infest vertebrates.

tromethamine (tro-meth′ah-mēn) an alkalizing agent, $C_4H_{11}NO_3$, used intravenously in metabolic acidosis.

Tromexan (tro-mek′san) trademark for a preparation of ethyl biscoumacetate.

Tronothane (tron′o-thān) trademark for preparations of pramoxine.

troph(o)- word element [Gr.], *food; nourishment.*

trophectoderm (trof-ek′to-derm) the earliest trophoblast.

trophedema (trof″ĕ-de′mah) a chronic disease with permanent edema of the feet or legs.

trophesy (trof′ĕ-se) defective nutrition due to disorder of the trophic nerves.

trophic (trof′ik) pertaining to nutrition.

-trophic, -trophin word element [Gr.], *nourishing; stimulating.*

trophoblast (trof″o-blast) the peripheral cells of the blastocyst, which attack the fertilized ovum to the uterine wall, become the placenta, and the membranes that nourish and protect the developing organisms. **trophoblas′tic,** adj.

trophoblastoma (trof″o-blas-to′mah) choriocarcinoma.

trophodermatoneurosis (-der″mah-to-nu-ro′sis) acrodynia.

trophology (tro-fol′o-je) the science of nutrition of the body.

trophoneurosis (trof″o-nu-ro′sis) any trophic disorder of a part due to deficiency of its nerve supply. **trophoneurot′ic,** adj.

trophonosis (-no′sis) any disease due to nutritional causes.

trophonucleus (-nu′kle-us) macronucleus.

trophopathy (tro-fop′ah-the) any derangement of nutrition.

trophoplast (trof″o-plast) a granular protoplasmic body.

trophotaxis (trof″o-tak′sis) taxis in relation to nutritive materials.

trophotherapy (-ther′ah-pe) treatment of disease by dietary measures.

trophozoite (-zo′īt) the active, motile feeding stage of a sporozoan parasite.

tropia (tro′pe-ah) strabismus.

-tropic word element [Gr.], *turning toward; changing; tending to turn or change.*

tropicamide (tro-pik′ah-mīd) an anticholinergic, $C_{17}H_{20}N_2O_2$, applied topically to the conjunctiva to produce mydriasis and cycloplegia.

tropine (tro′pēn) a crystalline alkaloid from atropine and various plants.

tropism (tro′pizm) a growth response in a non-motile organism elicited by an external stimulus, either toward (*positive t.*) or away from (*negative t.*) the stimulus; used as a word element combined with a stem indicating the nature of the stimulus (e.g., phototropism) or material or entity for which an organism (or substance) shows a special affinity (e.g., neurotropism).

tropocollagen (tro″po-kol′ah-jen) the molecular unit of all forms of collagen; it is a helical structure of three polypeptides.

tropomysin (-mi′o-sin) a muscle protein of the I band that inhibits contraction by blocking the interaction of actin and myosin, except when influenced by troponin.

troponin (tro′po-nin) a complex of muscle proteins which, when combined with Ca^{++}, influence tropomyosin to initiate contraction.

troxidone (trok′sĭ-dōn) trimethadione.

T.R.U. turbidity reducing unit.

truncate (trung′kāt) 1. to amputate; to deprive of limbs. 2. having the end cut squarely off.

truncus (trung′kus), pl. *trun′ci* [L.] trunk.

trunk (trungk) the main part, as the part of the body to which the head and limbs are attached, or a larger structure (e.g., vessel or nerve) from which smaller divisions or branches arise, or which is created by their union. **trun′cal,** adj.

brachiocephalic t., a vessel arising from the arch of the aorta and giving rise to the right common carotid and right subclavian arteries. **celiac t.,** the arterial trunk arising from the abdominal aorta and giving origin to the left gastric, common hepatic, and splenic arteries. **lumbosacral t.,** a trunk formed by union of the lower part of the ventral branch of the fourth lumbar nerve with the ventral branch of the fifth lumbar nerve. **pulmonary t.,** a vessel arising from the conus arteriosus of the right ventricle and bifurcating into the right and left pulmonary arteries. **sympathetic t.,** two long ganglionated nerve strands, one on each side of the vertebral column, extending from the base of the skull to the coccyx.

truss (trus) an elastic, canvas, or metallic device for retaining a reduced hernia within the abdominal cavity.

trypaflavine (trip″ah-fla′vin) acriflavine hydrochloride.

trypanocidal (tri-pan″o-si′dal) destructive to trypanosomes.

trypanolysis (tri″pan-ol′ĭ-sis) the destruction of trypanosomes. **trypanolyt′ic,** adj.

Trypanosoma (tri″pan-o-so′mah) a multispecies genus of protozoa parasitic in the blood and lymph of invertebrates and vertebrates, including man; most species live part of their life cycle in the intestines of insects and other invertebrates, the typical adult stage being found only in the vertebrate host. Trypanosomal infections of man include Gambian and Rhodesian forms of African trypanosomiasis (caused by *T. gambien′se* and *T. rhodesien′se,* respectively) and Chagas' disease (caused by *T. cru′zi*). Other species cause serious diseases of domestic animals, including *T. bru′cei, T. congolen′se, T. evan′si,* etc.

trypanosome (tri-pan′o-sōm) an individual of the genus *Trypanosoma.* **trypanoso′mal, trypanoso′mic,** adj.

trypanosomiasis (tri-pan″o-so-mi′ah-sis) infection with trypanosomes. **African t.,** a disease common among natives of tropical Africa, due to infection with *Trypanosoma gambiense* (Gambian t.) or *T. rhodesiense* (Rhodesian t.); it is transmitted by the bite of various species of *Glossina,* and in the advanced stage involves the central nervous system, producing sleeping sickness. In this stage, the patients become depressed, tremulous, lethargic, and somnolent, until they want to sleep all the time, become emaciated, and eventually die. **American t., Brazilian t., South American t.,** Chagas' disease.

trypanosomicide (-so′mĭ-sīd) 1. lethal to trypanosomes. 2. an agent lethal to trypanosomes.

trypanosomid (-so′mid) a skin eruption occurring in trypanosomiasis.

tryparsamide (trip-ar′sah-mīd) an antitrypanosomal agent, $C_8H_{10}AsN_2NaO_4$, used in African trypanosomiasis.

trypsin (trip′sin) an enzyme that catalyzes the hydrolysis of practically all types of proteins, produced in the intestine by activation of trypsinogen. **tryp′tic,** adj. **crystallized t.,** a proteolytic enzyme crystallized from an extract of the pancreas of the ox; used in the débridement of necrotic wounds and ulcers.

trypsinogen (trip-sin′o-jen) the inactive precursor of trypsin, secreted by the pancreas and activated to trypsin by contact with enterokinase.

tryptic (trip′tik) relating to or resulting from digestion by trypsin.

tryptophan (trip′to-fān) a naturally occurring amino acid, existing in proteins and essential for human metabolism.

tryptophanase (trip′to-fan″ās) an enzyme that catalyzes the cleavage of tryptophan into indole, pyruvic acid, and ammonia.

tryptophanuria (trip″to-fān-u′re-ah) excessive urinary excretion of trytophan.

T.S. test solution.

tsetse (tset′se) an African fly of the genus *Glossina,* which transmits trypanosomiasis.

T.S.H. thyroid-stimulating hormone.

T.U. tuberculin unit.

Tuamine (too′ah-min) trademark for preparations of tuaminoheptane.

tuaminoheptane (tu-am″ĭ-no-hep′tān) an adrenergic, $C_7H_{17}N$, used as a nasal decongestant in the form of the base (for inhalation) and sulfate salt (topical solution).

tuba (tu′bah), pl. *tu′bae* [L.] tube.

Tubadil (too′bah-dil) trademark for a preparation of tubocurarine.

Tubarine (too′bah-rin) trademark for a preparation of tubocurarine.

tube (tūb) a hollow cylindrical organ or instrument. **tu′bal,** adj. **auditory t.,** eustachian tube; the narrow channel connecting the middle ear and the nasopharynx. **Chaoul t.,** a tube used in x-ray therapy. **Coolidge t.,** an x-ray tube with a cathode consisting of a tungsten spiral enclosed in a molybdenum tube. **drainage t.,** a tube used in surgery to facilitate escape of fluids. **Durham's t.,** a jointed tracheotomy tube. **endobronchial t.,** a double-lumen tube inserted into the bronchus of one lung, permitting complete deflation of the other lung; used in anesthesia and thoracic surgery. **endotracheal t.,** an airway catheter inserted in the trachea in endotracheal intubation. **eustachian t.,** auditory t. **fallopian t.,** uterine t. **feeding t.,** one for introducing high-caloric fluids into the stomach. **fermentation t.,** a U-shaped tube with one end closed, for determining gas production by bacteria. **Geissler's t.,** an x-ray tube containing a highly rarefied gas. **intubation t.,** a breathing tube introduced into the air passage after tracheotomy. **Levin t.,** a gastroduodenal catheter of sufficiently small caliber to permit transnasal passage. **Miller-Abbott t.,** a double-channel intestinal tube with an inflatable balloon at its distal end, for use in treatment of obstruction of the small intestine, and occasionally as a diagnostic aid. **nasogastric t.,** a soft tube to be inserted through a nostril and into the stomach, for instilling liquids or other substances, or for withdrawing gastric contents. **neural t.,** the epithelial tube produced by folding of the neural plate in the early embryo. **otopharyngeal t.,** auditory t. **Ryle's t.,** a thin rubber tube for giving a test meal. **Schacho-wa's spiral t's,** renal tubules. **Sengstaken-Blakemore t.,** an instrument used for tamponade of bleeding esophageal varices. **stomach t.,** one which is passed through the esophagus to the stomach, for introduction of nutrients or for gastric lavage. **test t.,** a tube of thin glass, closed at one end; used in chemical tests and other laboratory procedures. **tracheotomy t.,** a curved tube that is inserted into the trachea through the opening made in the neck at tracheotomy. **uterine t.,** a slender tube extending laterally from the uterus toward the ovary on the same side, conveying ova to the cavity of the uterus and permitting passage of spermatozoa in the opposite direction. **vacuum t.,** a glass tube from which gaseous contents have been evacuated. **Wangensteen t.,** a small nasogastric tube connected with a special suction apparatus to maintain gastric and duodenal decompression.

tubectomy (tu-bek′to-me) excision of a portion of the uterine tube.

tuber (tu′ber), pl. *tubers* or *tu′bera*[L.] a swelling or protuberance. **t. cine′reum,** a layer of gray matter forming part of the floor of the third ventricle, to which the infundibulum of the hypothalamus is attached.

tubercle (tu′ber-k'l) 1. any small, rounded mass produced by infection with *Mycobacterium tuberculosis.* 2. a nodule or small eminence, especially one on a bone, for attachment of a tendon. **tuber′cular,** adj. **anatomic t.,** tuberculosis verrucosa. **auricular t., darwinian t.,** a small projection sometimes found on the edge of the helix; conjectured by some to be a relic of simioid ancestry. **dissection t.,** a warty growth often occurring on the hand in persons performing dissection. **Farre's t's,** masses beneath the capsule of the liver in certain cases of hepatic cancer. **fibrous t.,** one of bacillary origin which contains connective-tissue elements. **genial t's,** mental t. **Ghon's t.,** the primary lesion of tuberculosis of the lungs in children, consisting of a localized parenchymal area of disease and enlargement of regional hilar or mediastinal lymph nodes. **gracile t.,** an enlargement of the fasciculus gracilis in the medulla oblongata, produced by the underlying nucleus gracilis. **intervenous t.,** a ridge across the inner surface of the right atrium between the openings of the venae cavae. **Lisfranc's t.,** an eminence on the first rib, for attachment of the scalenus anticus. **Lower's t.,** intervenous t. **mental t.,** a prominence on the inner border of either side of the mental protuberance of the mandible. **miliary t.,** one of the many minute tubercles formed in many organs in acute miliary tuberculosis. **pubic t.,** a prominent tubercle at the lateral end of the pubic crest. **scalene t.,** Lisfranc's t. **supraglenoid t.,** one on the scapula for attachment of the long head of the biceps.

tuberculate, tuberculated (tu-ber′ku-lāt″; tu-ber′ku-lāt″ed) covered or affected with tubercles.

tuberculid (tu-ber′ku-lid) a papular skin eruption usually attributed to allergy to tuberculosis. **papulonecrotic t.,** an eruption of crops of deep-seated papules or nodules, with central necrosis or ulceration.

tuberculigenous (tu-ber″ku-lij′ĕ-nus) causing tuberculosis.

tuberculin (tu-ber′ku-lin) a sterile liquid containing the growth products of, or specific substances extracted from, the tubercle bacillus; used in various forms in the diagnosis of tuberculosis; see also under *test.* **New t.,** a suspension of the fragments of tubercle bacilli, freed from all soluble materials and with glycerin added. **Old t.,** a sterile solution of concentrated, soluble products of the growth of the tubercle bacillus, adjusted to standard potency by addition of glycerin and isotonic sodium chloride solution, final glycerin content being about 50 per cent. **purified protein derivative (P.P.D.) of t.,** a sterile, soluble, partially purified product of the growth of the tubercle bacillus in a special liquid medium free from protein.

tuberculitis (tu-ber″ku-li′tis) inflammation of or near a tubercle.

tuberculocele (tu-ber′ku-lo-sēl″) tuberculous disease of a testis.

tuberculofibroid (tu-ber″ku-lo-fi′broid) characterized by a tubercle that has undergone fibroid degeneration.

tuberculoid (tu-ber′ku-loid) resembling a tubercle or tuberculosis.

tuberculoma (tu-ber″ku-lo′mah) a tumor-like mass resulting from enlargement of a caseous tubercle.

tuberculosilicosis (tu-ber″ku-lo-sil″ĭ-ko′sis) silicosis complicated by pulmonary tuberculosis.

tuberculosis (tu-ber″ku-lo′sis) any of the infectious diseases of man and other animals due to species of *Mycobacterium* and marked by formation of tubercles and caseous necrosis in tissues of any organ; in man, the lung is the major seat of infection and the usual portal through which infection reaches other organs. **avian t.,** a form affecting various birds, due to *Mycobacterium avium,* which may be communicated to man and other animals. **bovine t.,** an infection of cattle due to *Mycobacterium bovis,* transmissible to man and other animals. **disseminated t.,** acute miliary t. **hematogenous t.,** that carried through the blood stream to other organs from the primary site of infection. **t. of lungs,** pulmonary tuberculosis; infection of the lungs due to *Mycobacterium tuberculosis;* characteristically, the course of the untreated disease is: tuberculous pneumonia, formation of tuberculous granulation tissue, caseous necrosis, calcification, and cavity formation. Symptoms may include weight loss, fatigue, night sweats, purulent sputum, hemoptysis, and chest pain. **t. lupo′sa,** lupus vulgaris. **miliary t., acute,** an acute form in which minute tubercles are formed in a number of organs, due to dissemination of the bacilli through the body by the blood stream. **open t.,** 1. that in which there are lesions from which tubercle bacilli are being discharged out of the body. 2. tuberculosis of the lungs with cavitation. **pulmonary t.,** t. of lungs. **t. of spine,** Pott's disease. **t. verruco′sa, warty t.,** a condition usually resulting from external inoculation of the tubercle bacilli into the skin, with wartlike papules coalescing to form distinctly verrucous patches with an inflammatory, erythematous border.

tuberculostatic (tu-ber″ku-lo-stat′ik) 1. inhibiting the growth of *Mycobacterium tuberculosis*. 2. a tuberculostatic agent.

tuberculotic (tu-ber″ku-lot′ik) pertaining to or affected with tuberculosis.

tuberculous (tu-ber′ku-lus) pertaining to or affected with tuberculosis; caused by *Mycobacterium tuberculosis*.

tuberculum (tu-ber′ku-lum), pl. *tuber′cula*[L.] a tubercle, nodule, or small eminence; in anatomy, used principally to designate a small eminence on a bone. **t. acus′ticum,** area vestibularis. **t. arthrit′icum,** a gouty concretion in a joint. **t. doloro′sum,** a painful nodule or tubercle.

tuberosis (tu″ber-o′sis) a condition characterized by the presence of nodules.

tuberositas (tu″ber-os′ĭ-tas), pl. *tuberosita′tes* [L.] tuberosity; in anatomy, an elevation on a bone to which a muscle is attached.

tuberosity (tu″bĕ-ros′ĭ-te) an elevation or protuberance.

tuberous (tu′ber-us) covered with tubers; knobby. See also under *sclerosis*.

tubo- word element [L.], *tube*.

tubocurarine (tu″bo-ku-rah′rēn) an alkaloid from the bark and stems of *Chondrodendron tomentosum;* it is the active principle of curare, used as a skeletal muscle relaxant.

tuboligamentous (-lig″ah-men′tus) pertaining to the uterine tube and broad ligament.

tubo-ovarian (-o-va′re-an) pertaining to the uterine tube and ovary.

tuboperitoneal (-per″ĭ-to-ne′al) pertaining to the uterine tube and the peritoneum.

tubouterine (-u′ter-in) pertaining to the uterine tube and uterus.

tubule (tu′būl) a small tube. **tu′bular,** adj. **collecting t's,** the terminal channels of the nephrons which open on the summits of the renal pyramids in the renal papillae. **dentinal t's,** dental canaliculi. **Henle's t's,** the straight ascending and descending portions of a renal tubule forming Henle's loop. **mesonephric t's,** the tubules comprising the mesonephros, or temporary kidney, of amniotes. **metanephric t's,** the tubules comprising the permanent kidney of amniotes. **renal t's,** the minute reabsorptive canals made up of basement membrane and lined with epithelium, composing the substance of the kidney and secreting, collecting, and conducting the urine; see also *nephron*. **seminiferous t's,** the tubules of the testis. **uriniferous t's,** renal t's.

tubulin (tu′bu-lin) the constituent protein of microtubules; thought to be involved in phagocyte motility.

tubulorrhexis (tu″bu-lo-rek′sis) rupture of the renal tubules.

tubulus (tu′bu-lus), pl. *tu′buli* [L.] tubule; a minute canal.

tuft (tuft) a small clump or cluster; a coil. **malpighian t.,** renal glomerulus.

tugging (tug′ing) a pulling sensation, as a pulling sensation in the trachea (*tracheal t.*), due to aneurysm of the arch of the aorta.

tularemia (tu″lah-re′me-ah) a plaguelike disease of rodents, caused by *Francisella* (*Pasteurella*) *tularensis,* which is transmissible to man.

tumefacient (tu″mĕ-fa′shent) producing tumefaction.

tumefaction (-fak′shun) a swelling; the state of being swollen, or the act of swelling; puffiness; edema.

tumescence (tu-mes′ens) 1. the condition of being swollen. 2. a swelling.

tumid (tu′mid) swollen; edematous.

tumor (tu′mor) 1. swelling, one of the cardinal signs of inflammation; morbid enlargement. 2. neoplasm; a new growth of tissue in which cell multiplication is uncontrolled and progressive. **Abrikossoff's t.,** myoblastoma. **benign t.,** one lacking the properties of invasion and metastasis and showing a lesser degree of anaplasia than do malignant tumors; it is usually surrounded by a fibrous capsule. **Brenner t.,** a benign fibroepithelioma of the ovary. **carotid body t.,** a firm, round mass at the bifurcation of the common carotid artery. **connective tissue t.,** any tumor arising from a connective tissue structure, e.g., a fibroma or sarcoma. **desmoid t.,** a hard fibrous tumor. **erectile t.,** cavernous hemangioma. **Ewing's t.,** a malignant tumor of bone, arising in medullary tissue and more often in cylindrical bones. **false t.,** structural enlargement due to extravasation, exudation, echinococcus, or retained sebaceous matter. **fibroid t.,** a fibroma. **fibroplastic t.,** a fibroma or a fibrosarcoma. **giant cell t.,** 1. a bone tumor, ranging from benign to frankly malignant, composed of cellular spindle cell stroma containing multinucleated giant cells resembling osteoclasts. 2. a benign, small, yellow, tumor-like nodule of tendon sheath origin, most often of the wrist and fingers or ankle and toes, laden with lipophages and containing multinucleated giant cells. **glomus t.,** glomangioma. **granular cell t.,** a benign, circumscribed, tumor-like lesion of soft tissue, particularly of the tongue, skin, and muscle, composed of large cells with prominent granular cytoplasm; considered by some to arise from myoblasts (myoblastoma) and by others from neurogenic elements (granular cell schwannoma); still others regard it as a manifestation of lipid storage cell disease. **granulosa t., granulosa cell t.,** an ovarian tumor originating in the cells of the membrana granulosa. **granulosa-theca cell t.,** an ovarian tumor composed of granulosa (follicular) cells and theca cells; either form may predominate. **heterologous t.,** one made up of tissue differing from that in which it grows. **homoiotypic t., homologous t.,** one resembling the surrounding parts in its structure. **Hürthle cell t.,** a new growth of the thyroid gland composed wholly or predominantly of large cells (Hürthle cells) having abundant granular, eosinophilic cytoplasm. Such tumors are usually benign (Hürthle cell adenoma) but on occasion may be locally invasive or may rarely metastasize (Hürthle cell carcinoma, or malignant Hürthle cell tumor). **islet cell t.**, a tumor of the islands of Langerhans, which may result in hyperinsulinism. **Krompecher's t.**, rodent ulcer. **Krukenberg's t.**, carcinoma of the ovary, usually metastatic from gastrointestinal cancer, marked by areas of mucoid degeneration and by the presence of signet-ring–like cells. **Leydig cell t.**, a tumor of the Leydig cells of the testis. **lipoid cell t. of ovary**, a usually benign ovarian tumor composed of eosinophilic cells or cells with lipoid vacuoles; it causes masculinization. **malignant t.**, one having the properties of invasion and metastasis and showing a high degree of anaplasia. **mast cell t.**, a benign, local aggregation of mast cells forming a nodulous tumor. **melanotic neuroectodermal t.**, a benign, rapidly growing, dark tumor of the jaw and occasionally of other sites; almost always seen in infants. **mixed t.**, one composed of more than one type of neoplastic tissue. **mucous t.**, myxoma. **muscular t.**, myoma. **organoid t.**, teratoma. **papillary t.**, papilloma. **pearl t.**, cholesteatoma. **phantom t.**, abdominal or other swelling not due to structural change. **sand t.**, psammoma. **simple t.**, one containing a single type of cells. **teratoid t.**, teratoma. **theca cell t.**, a fibroid-like ovarian tumor containing yellow areas of lipoid material derived from theca cells. **true t.**, a neoplasm. **turban t's**, multiple benign epitheliomas of the scalp grouped together so as to cover the entire scalp. **Warthin's t.**, papillary adenocystoma lymphomatosum. **Wilms' t.**, a rapidly developing malignant mixed tumor of the kidneys, made up of embryonal elements, usually affecting children before the fifth year.

tumoricidal (tu″mor-ĭ-si′dal) destructive to cancer cells.

tumorigenesis (-jen′ĕ-sis) the production of tumors. **tumorigen′ic**, adj.

tumultus (tu-mul′tus) excessive organic action or motility.

Tunga (tun′gah) a genus of fleas, including _T. pen′etrans,_ the chigoe (q.v.).

tungsten (tung′sten) chemical element (_see table_), at. no. 74, symbol W.

tunic (tu′nik) a covering or coat. **Bichat's t.**, tunica intima.

tunica (tu′nĭ-kah), pl. _tu′nicae_ [L.] a tunic; in anatomy, a general term for a membrane or other structure covering or lining a body part or organ. **t. adventi′tia**, the outer coat of various tubular structures. **t. albugin′ea**, a dense, white, fibrous sheath enclosing a part or organ. **t. conjuncti′va**, the conjunctiva. **t. ex′terna**, an outer coat, especially the fibroelastic coat of a blood vessel. **t. in′tima**, the innermost coat of blood vessels. **t. me′dia**, the middle coat of blood vessels. **t. muco′sa**, mucous membrane. **t. muscula′ris**, the muscular coat or layer surrounding the tela submucosa in most portions of the digestive, respiratory, urinary, and genital tracts. **t. pro′pria**, a proper coat or layer of a part, as distinguished from an investing membrane. **t. sero′sa**, the membrane lining the external walls of body cavities and reflected over the surfaces of protruding organs; it secretes a watery exudate. **t. vagina′lis**, the serous membrane covering the front and sides of the testis and epididymis. **t. vasculo′sa**, a vascular coat, or a layer well supplied with blood vessels.

tunicin (tu′nĭ-sin) a substance resembling cellulose, from the tissues of certain low forms of animal life.

tunnel (tun′el) a passageway of varying length through a solid body, completely enclosed except for the open ends, permitting entrance and exit. **carpal t.**, the osseofibrous passage for the median nerve and the flexor tendons, formed by the flexor retinaculum and the carpal bones. **Corti's t.**, see under _canal._ **flexor t.**, carpal t. **tarsal t.**, the osseofibrous passage for the posterior tibial vessels, tibial nerve, and flexor tendons, formed by the flexor retinaculum and the tarsal bones.

turbidimeter (ter″bĭ-dim′ĕ-ter) an apparatus for measuring turbidity of a solution.

turbidimetry (-dim′ĕ-tre) the measurement of the turbidity of a liquid.

turbidity (ter-bid′ĭ-te) cloudiness; disturbance of solids (sediment) in a solution, so that it is not clear. **tur′bid**, adj.

turbinal (ter′bĭ-nal) turbinate.

turbinate (-nāt) 1. shaped like a top. 2. turbinate bone (concha nasalis ossea).

turbinectomy (-nek′to-me) excision of a turbinate bone (nasal concha).

turbinotomy (-not′o-me) incision of a turbinate bone.

turgescence (ter-jes′ens) distention or swelling of a part.

turgescent (ter-jes′ent) becoming swollen.

turgid (ter′jid) swollen and congested.

turgor (ter′gor) condition of being turgid; normal, or other fullness.

turista (tu-rēs′tah) Mexican name for traveler's diarrhea.

turnsick, turnsickness (tern′sik; -sik-nes) gid.

turpentine (ter′pen-tīn) the concrete oleoresin from _Pinus palustris_ and other species of _Pinus;_ its volatile oil is used as a counterirritant and rubefacient.

turricephaly (tur″ĭ-sef′ah-le) oxycephaly.

tussis (tus′is) [L.] cough. **tus′sal, tus′sive**, adj. **t. convulsi′va**, pertussis.

tutamen (tu-ta′men), pl. _tutam′ina_ [L.] a protective covering or structure. **tutam′ina oc′uli**, the protecting appendages of the eye, as the lids, lashes, etc.

Tween 80 (twēn) trademark for polysorbate 80.

twig (twig) a final ramification, as of branches of a nerve or blood vessel.

twin (twin) one of two offspring produced in one pregnancy. **allantoidoangiopagous t's**, twins united by the umbilical vessels only. **conjoined t's**, monozygotic twins whose bodies are joined to a varying extent. **dizygotic t's**, twins developed from two separate ova fertilized at the same time. **enzygotic t's**, monozygotic t's. **fraternal t's, heterologous t's**, dizygotic t's. **identical t's**, monozygotic t's. **impacted t's**, twins so situated during delivery that pressure of one against the other produces incomplete simultaneous engagement of both. **monozy-**

gotic t's, two individuals developed from one fertilized ovum. **omphaloangiopagous t's,** allantoidoangiopagous t's. **Siamese t's,** conjoined t's. **similar t's,** monozygotic t's. **unequal t's,** twins of which one is incompletely developed. **uniovular t's,** monozygotic t's.

twinning (twin′ing) 1. the production of symmetrical structures or parts by division. 2. the simultaneous intrauterine production of two or more embryos.

twitch (twich) a brief, contractile response of a skeletal muscle elicited by a single maximal volley of impulses in the neurons supplying it.

tybamate (ti′bah-māt) a minor tranquilizer, $C_{13}H_{26}N_2O_4$.

Tylenol (ti′lĕ-nol) trademark for preparations of acetaminophen.

tylion (til′e-on) a point on anterior edge of the optic groove in the median line.

tyloma (ti-lo′ma) a callus or callosity.

tylosis (ti-lo′sis) formation of callosities. **tylot′ic,** adj.

tympanal (tim′pah-nal) pertaining to the tympanum or to the tympanic membrane.

tympanectomy (tim″pah-nek′to-me) excision of the tympanic membrane.

tympanic (tim-pan′ik) 1. of or pertaining to the tympanum. 2. bell-like; resonant.

tympanism (tim′pah-nizm) tympanites.

tympanites (tim″pah-ni′tēz) abnormal distention due to the presence of gas or air in the intestine or the peritoneal cavity.

tympanitic (tim″pah-nit′ik) 1. pertaining to or affected with tympanites. 2. bell-like; tympanic.

tympanitis (tim″pah-ni′tis) otitis media.

tympanomastoiditis (tim″pah-no-mas″toi-di′-tis) inflammation of the middle ear and the pneumatic cells of the mastoid process.

tympanoplasty (tim′pah-no-plas″te) surgical reconstruction of the tympanic membrane and establishment of ossicular continuity from the tympanic membrane to the oval window.

tympanosclerosis (tim″pah-no-sklĕ-ro′sis) a condition characterized by the presence of masses of hard, dense connective tissue around the auditory ossicles in the tympanic cavity.

tympanotomy (tim″pah-not′o-me) myringotomy.

tympanous (tim′pah-nus) distended with gas.

tympanum (tim′pah-num) the cavity of the middle ear, in the temporal bone, located just medial to the tympanic membrane.

tympany (tim′pah-ne) 1. tympanitis. 2. a tympanic, or bell-like, percussion note. **t. of stomach,** a kind of indigestion in cattle and sheep, marked by abnormal collection of gas in the first stomach.

type (tīp) the general or prevailing character of any particular case of disease, person, substance, etc. **asthenic t.,** a type of physical constitution, with long limbs, small trunk, flat chest, and weak muscles. **athletic t.,** a type of physical constitution, with broad shoulders, deep chest, flat abdomen, thick neck, and good muscular development. **blood t's,** see *blood group.* **phage t.,** an intraspecies type of bacte-

rium demonstrated by phage typing. **pyknic t.,** a type of physical constitution marked by rounded body, large chest, thick shoulders, broad head, and short neck. **sympathetico-tonic t.,** a type of physical constitution characterized by sympathicotonia. **vagotonic t.,** a physical type characteristic of deficient adrenal activity: there are slow pulse, low blood pressure, localized sweating, high sugar tolerance, and oculocardiac reflex.

typhl(o)- word element [Gr.], *cecum; blindness.*

typhlectasis (tif-lek′tah-sis) distention of the cecum.

typhlitis (tif-li′tis) inflammation of the cecum.

typhlodicliditis (tif″lo-dik″lĭ-di′tis) inflammation of the ileocecal valve.

typhlolexia (-lek′se-ah) word blindness.

typhlolithiasis (-lĭ-thi′ah-sis) calculi in the cecum.

typhlosis (tif-lo′sis) blindness.

typhlotomy (tif-lot′o-me) cecotomy.

typhoid (ti′foid) 1. resembling typhus. 2. typhoid fever.

typhoidal (ti-foi′dal) resembling typhoid fever.

typhopneumonia (ti″fo-nu-mo′ne-ah) pneumonia with typhoid fever.

typhus (ti′fus) any of a group of arthropod-borne rickettsial diseases, with high fever, macular or maculopapular eruption appearing from the third to seventh day, malaise, and severe headache. Often used in English-speaking countries to refer to epidemic typhus, and in several European languages to typhoid fever. **ty′phous,** adj. **endemic t.,** murine t. **epidemic t.,** the classic form, due to *Rickettsia prowazekii* and transmitted from man to man by body lice. **Kenya t.,** a rickettsial disease occurring in Kenya, believed to be identical with boutonneuse fever, except that tache noire is absent. **murine t.,** an infectious disease due to *Rickettsia typhi,* transmitted from rat to man by the rat flea and rat louse. **recrudescent t.,** Brill's disease. **t. recur′rens,** relapsing fever. **scrub t.,** a self-limited, febrile disease due to *Rickettsia tsutsugamushi* and transmitted by chiggers; characterized by sudden onset of fever with a primary skin lesion and development of rash about the fifth day. **tropical t.,** scrub typhus.

tyramine (ti′rah-mēn) a decarboxylation product of tyrosine, which may be converted to cresol and phenol, found in decayed animal tissue, ripe cheese, and ergot. Closely related structurally to epinephrine and norepinephrine, it has a similar but weaker action.

tyrocidin, tyrocidine (ti″ro-si′din) a polypeptide antibiotic substance, the major component of tyrothricin.

tyrogenous (ti-roj′ĕ-nus) originating in cheese.

tyroid (ti′roid) of cheesy consistency; caseous.

tyroma (ti-ro′mah) a caseous tumor.

tyromatosis (ti″ro-mah-to′sis) a condition characterized by caseous degeneration.

tyrosine (ti′ro-sēn) a naturally occurring amino acid present in most proteins; it is a product of phenylalanine metabolism and a precursor of melanin, epinephrine, and thyroxine.

tyrosinemia (ti″ro-sĭ-ne′me-ah) a hereditary disorder marked by excess of tyrosine in the blood and by tyrosyluria; it results in liver failure or severe nodular cirrhosis, with renal tubular involvement similar to Fanconi syndrome, and hypoglycemia.

tyrosinosis (-sĭ-no′sis) a condition characterized by faulty metabolism of tyrosine in which an intermediate product, para-hydroxyphenyl pyruvic acid, appears in the urine and gives it an abnormal reducing power.

tyrosinuria (-sĭ-nu′re-ah) presence of tyrosine in the urine.

tyrosis (ti-ro′sis) caseation (2).

tyrosyluria (ti″ro-sil-u′re-ah) increased urinary

secretion of para-hydroxyphenyl compounds derived from tyrosine, as in tyrosinemia.

tyrothricin (-thri′sin) an antibiotic substance produced by growth of a soil bacillus, *Bacillus brevis,* consisting principally of gramicidin and tyrocidin; used as a topical antibacterial.

tyrotoxism (-tok′sizm) poisoning from a toxin present in milk or cheese.

tyvelose (ti″vel-ōs) an unusual sugar that is a polysaccharide somatic antigen of *Salmonella* species.

Tyvid (ti′vid) trademark for a preparation of isoniazid.

tzetze (tset′se) tsetse.

U

U chemical symbol, *uranium.*

U. unit.

ubiquinone (u-bik′kwĭ-nōn) coenzyme Q.

udder (ud′er) the mammary organ of cattle and certain other mammals; within the large baglike envelope are two or more glands, each having a teat.

UDP uridine diphosphate.

ulcer (ul′ser) a local defect, or excavation of the surface of an organ or tissue, produced by sloughing of necrotic inflammatory tissue. **Curling's u.,** an ulcer of the duodenum seen after severe burns of the body. **decubitus u.,** bedsore; an ulceration due to prolonged pressure from lying too still in bed for too long a time. **dental u.,** a lesion on the oral mucosa due to trauma inflicted by the teeth. **duodenal u.,** a peptic ulcer situated in the duodenum. **gastric u.,** one of the gastric mucosa. **Hunner's u.,** one involving all layers of the bladder wall, occurring in chronic interstitial cystitis. **marginal u.,** a gastric ulcer in the jejunal mucosa near the site of a gastrojejunostomy. **peptic u.,** an ulceration of the mucous membrane of the esophagus, stomach, or duodenum, due to action of the acid gastric juice. **perforating u.,** one involving the entire thickness of an organ or of the wall of an organ creating an opening on both surfaces. **phagedenic u.,** a necrotizing lesion in which tissue destruction is prominent. **rodent u.,** ulcerating basal cell carcinoma of the skin. **stercoraceous u., stercoral u.,** one caused by pressure of impacted feces; also, a fistulous ulcer through which fecal matter escapes. **stress u.,** peptic ulcer, usually gastric, resulting from stress; possible predisposing factors include changes in the microcirculation of the gastric mucosa, increased permeability of the gastric mucosa barrier to H^+, and impaired cell proliferation. **trophic u.,** one due to imperfect nutrition of the part. **tropical u.,** a chronic, sloughing ulcer usually on the lower extremities, occurring in tropical regions. **varicose u.,** an ulcer due to varicose veins. **venereal u.,** a

condition marked by formation of ulcers resembling chancre or chancroid about the vulvae of women not exposed to venereal disease.

ulcerate (ul′sĕ-rāt) to undergo ulceration.

ulceration (ul″sĕ-ra′shun) 1. the formation or development of an ulcer. 2. an ulcer.

ulcerative (ul′ser-ah-tiv) pertaining to or characterized by ulceration.

ulcerogangrenous (ul″ser-o-gang′grĕ-nus) characterized by both ulceration and gangrene.

ulcerogenic (-jen′ik) causing ulceration; leading to the production of ulcers.

ulceromembranous (-mem′brah-nus) characterized by ulceration and a membranous exudation.

ulcerous (ul′ser-us) 1. of the nature of an ulcer. 2. affected with ulceration.

ulcus (ul′kus), pl. *ul′cera* [L.] ulcer. **u. cancro′sum,** rodent ulcer. **u. ventric′uli,** gastric ulcer. **u. vul′vae acu′tum,** a rapidly growing nonvenereal ulcer of the vulva.

ulectomy (u-lek′to-me) 1. excision of scar tissue. 2. gingivectomy.

ulerythema (u″ler-ĭ-the′mah) an erythematous skin disease with formation of cicatrices and atrophy. **u. ophryog′enes,** a hereditary form in which keratosis pilaris involves the hair follicles of the eyebrows.

ulitis (u-li′tis) gingivitis.

ulna (ul′nah), pl. *ul′nae* [L.] the inner and larger bone of the forearm; see *Table of Bones.* **ul′nar,** adj.

ulnad (ul′nad) toward the ulna.

ulnaris (ul-na′ris) [L.] ulnar.

ulnocarpal (ul″no-kar′pal) pertaining to the ulna and carpus.

ulnoradial (-ra′de-al) pertaining to the ulna and radius.

ulocace (u-lok′ah-se) ulceration of the gums.

ulocarcinoma (u″lo-kar″sĭ-no′mah) carcinoma of the gums.

uloglossitis (-glos-si′tis) gingivoglossitis.

uloncus (u-long'kus) swelling of the gums.

ulorrhagia (u''lo-ra'je-ah) a sudden or free discharge of blood from the gums.

ulotomy (u-lot'o-me) 1. incision of scar tissue. 2. incision of the gums.

Ultandren (ul-tan'dren) trademark for a preparation of fluoxymesterone.

ultra- word element [L.], *beyond; excess.*

ultrabrachycephalic (ul''trah-brak''e-sĕ-fal'ik) having a cephalic index of more than 90.

ultracentrifugation (-sen-trif''u-ga'shun) subjection of material to an exceedingly high centrifugal force, which will separate and sediment the molecules of a substance.

ultracentrifuge (-sen'trĭ-fūj) the centrifuge used in ultracentrifugation.

ultrafilter (-fil'ter) the filter used in ultrafiltration.

ultrafiltration (-fil-tra'shun) filtration through a filter capable of removing very minute (ultramicroscopic) particles.

ultramicroscope (-mi'kro-skōp) a special darkfield microscope for examination of particles of colloidal size.

ultramicroscopic (-mi''kro-skop'ik) 1. pertaining to the ultramicroscope. 2. too small to be seen with the ordinary light microscope.

ultramicroscopy (-mi-kros'ko-pe) use of the ultramicroscope.

Ultran (ul'tran) trademark for preparations of phenaglycodol.

ultrasonic (ul''trah-son'ik) beyond the audible range; relating to sound waves having a frequency of more than 20,000 cycles per second.

ultrasonics (-son'iks) the science dealing with ultrasonic sound waves.

ultrasonogram (-son'o-gram) the record obtained by ultrasonography.

ultrasonography (-son-og'rah-fe) the visualization of the deep structures of the body by recording the reflection of ultrasonic waves directed into the tissues. **ultrasonograph'ic,** adj.

ultrasound (ul''trah-sownd) mechanical radiant energy of a frequency greater than 20,000 cycles per second.

ultrastructure (-struk''chur) the structure visible only under the ultramicroscope and electron microscope.

ultraviolet (ul''trah-vi'o-let) denoting electromagnetic radiation of wavelength shorter than that of the violet end of the spectrum, having wavelengths of 4–400 nanometers.

ululation (ul''u-la'shun) the loud crying or wailing of hysterical patients.

umbilical (um-bil'ĭ-kal) pertaining to the umbilicus.

umbilicated (um-bil'ĭ-kāt''ed) marked by depressed spots resembling the umbilicus.

umbilication (um-bil''ĭ-ka'shun) a depression resembling the umbilicus.

umbilicus (um-bil'ĭ-kus, um''bĭ-li'kus) the navel; the scar marking the site of attachment of the umbilical cord in the fetus.

umbo (um'bo), pl. *umbo'nes* [L.] 1. a rounded elevation. 2. the slight projection at the center of the outer surface of the tympanic membrane.

uncal (un'kal) of or pertaining to the uncus.

unciform (un'sĭ-form) hooked shaped.

Uncinaria (un''sĭ-na're-ah) a genus of hookworms, including *U. stenoceph'ala,* commonly causing hookworm disease in dogs, and also parasitic in foxes, cats, and other carnivores.

uncinariasis (-nah-ri'ah-sis) infection with *Uncinaria;* see also *hookworm disease.*

uncinate (un'sĭ-nāt) 1. unciform. 2. relating to or affecting the uncinate gyrus.

uncipressure (-presh''ur) pressure with a hook to stop hemorrhage.

unconscious (un-kon'shus) 1. insensible; incapable of responding to sensory stimuli and of having subjective experiences. 2. that part of the mental activity which includes primitive or repressed wishes, concealed from consciousness by the psychic censor. **collective u.,** the portion of the unconscious which is theoretically common to mankind.

uncovertebral (un''ko-ver'tĕ-bral) pertaining to the uncinate processes of a vertebra.

unction (ungk'shun) 1. an ointment. 2. application of an ointment or salve; inunction.

unctuous (ungk'chu-us) greasy or oily.

uncus (ung'kus) the medially curved anterior end of the parahippocampal gyrus.

undifferentiated (un''dif-er-en'she-āt''ed) not differentiated; primitive.

undine (un'dēn) a small glass flask for irrigating the eye; a vibration.

undulation (un''du-la'shun) a wavelike motion in any medium.

ung. [L.] *unguen'tum* (ointment).

ungual (ung'gwal) pertaining to the nails.

unguent (ung'gwent) an ointment.

unguentum (ung-gwen'tum), pl. *unguen'ta* [L.] ointment.

unguiculate (ung-gwik'u-lāt) having claws or nails; clawlike.

unguinal (ung'gwĭ-nal) pertaining to a nail.

unguis (ung'gwis), pl. *un'gues* [L.] nail (2).

ungula (ung'gu-lah) [L.] an animal's hoof.

ungulate (ung'gu-lāt) hoofed mammal; see also *unguligrade.*

unguligrade (ung'gu-lĭ-grād'') walking or running on the tips of one or two digits of each limb; characteristic of certain quadrupeds known as ungulates.

uni- word element [L.], *one.*

uniaxial (u''ne-ak'se-al) 1. having only one axis. 2. developing in an axial direction only.

unicameral (u''nĭ-kam'er-al) having only one cavity or compartment.

unicellular (-sel'u-lar) made up of a single cell, as the bacteria.

unicornous (-kor'nus) having only one cornu.

uniglandular (-glan'du-lar) affecting only one gland.

unigravida (-grav'ĭ-dah) primigravida.

unilateral (-lat'er-al) affecting only one side.

unilocular (-lok'u-lar) monolocular.

uninucleated (-nu'kle-āt''ed) mononuclear (1).

uniocular (u''ne-ok'u-lar) monocular.

union (ūn′yun) the renewal of continuity in a broken bone or between the edges of a wound.

uniovular (u″ne-ov′u-lar) arising from one ovum.

unipara (u-nip′ah-rah) primipara.

uniparous (u-nip′ah-rus) 1. producing only one ovum or offspring at a time. 2. primiparous.

unipolar (u″nĭ-po′lar) having a single pole or process, as a nerve cell.

unipotent (u-nip′o-tent) unipotential.

unipotential (u″nĭ-po-ten′shal) having only one power, as giving rise to cells of one order only.

unit (u′nit) 1. a single thing; one segment of a whole that is made up of identical or similar segments. 2. a specifically defined amount of anything subject to measurement, as of activity, dimension, velocity, volume, or the like. **Allen-Doisy u.,** see *mouse u.* and *rat u.* **Angström u.,** the unit of wavelength, equal to 10^{-10} meter; symbol A, Å, or A.U. **atomic mass u.,** the unit mass equal to $\frac{1}{12}$ the mass of the nuclide of carbon-12. **Bodansky u.,** the quantity of phosphatase in 100 ml. of serum that will liberate 1 mg. of phosphorus as phosphate ion from sodium β-glycerophosphate in 1 hour under standard conditions. **British thermal u.,** a unit of heat, being the amount necessary to raise the temperature of 1 lb. of water from 39° to 40° F.; abbreviated B.T.U. **cat u.,** that amount of digitalis per kilogram of weight of a cat which is just sufficient to kill when slowly and continuously injected into the vein. **C.G.S. u.,** any unit in the centimeter-gram-second system. **Clauberg u.,** a unit of measurement of progestin activity. **Collip u.,** a unit of dosage of parathyroid extract. **coronary care u.,** a specially designed and equipped hospital area containing a small number of private rooms, with all facilities necessary for constant observation and possible emergency treatment of patients with severe heart disease. **electrostatic u's,** that system of units based on the fundamental definition of a unit charge as one which will repel an equal and like charge with a force of 1 dyne when the two charges are 1 cm. apart in a vacuum. **Hanson u.,** a unit of measurement of parathyroid activity. **intensive care u.,** a hospital unit in which are concentrated special equipment and skilled personnel for the care of seriously ill patients requiring immediate and continuous attention; abbreviated ICU. **International u.,** a unit of biological material, as of enzymes, hormones, vitamins, etc., established by the International Conference for the Unification of Formulas. **Kienböck's u.,** a unit of x-ray exposure equal to 0.1 erythema dose; symbol X. **motor u.,** the unit of motor activity formed by a motor nerve cell and its many innervated muscle fibers. **mouse u.,** the least amount of estrus-producing hormone which will cause a characteristic change in the vaginal epithelium in a spayed mouse. **Oxford u.,** a unit of penicillin dosage, being that amount which, dissolved in 50 ml. of meat extract broth, just inhibits completely a test strain of *Staphylococcus aureus.* **rat u.,** the highest dilution of an estrus-producing hormone which, in three injections at four-hour intervals during the first day, will produce cornification and desquamation of the vaginal epithelium in a mature spayed rat. **SI u.,** any of the base units (meter, kilogram, second, ampere, kelvin, candela, and mole), supplementary units (radian and steradian), and derived units (newton, pascal, and joule) adopted by the General Conference of Weights and Measures and called the "Système International d'Unités." **Somogyi u.,** that amount of amylase which will destroy 1.5 mg. of starch in 8 minutes at 37° C. **Svedberg u.,** a unit of time (10^{-13} seconds) and velocity used in measuring the sedimentation constant of a colloid solution. **Thayer-Doisy u.,** a unit of vitamin K activity, equivalent to that of 1 microgram of pure vitamin K_1. **toxic u., toxin u.,** the smallest dose of a toxin which will kill a guinea pig weighing about 250 gm. in three to four days. **U.S.P. u.,** one used in the United States Pharmacopeia in expressing potency of drugs and other preparations.

unitary (u′nĭ-ter″e) composed of or pertaining to a single object or individual.

United States Pharmacopeia see *U.S.P.*

Unitensen (u″nĭ-ten′sen) trademark for preparations of cryptenamine.

univalent (-va′lent) having a valence of one.

unmyelinated (un-mi′ĕ-lin-a′ted) not having a myelin sheath.

unphysiologic (un″fiz-e-o-loj′ik) not in harmony with the laws of physiology.

unsaturated (un-sach′ŭ-rāt″ed) 1. not having all affinities of its elements satisfied. 2. not holding all of a solute which can be held in solution by the solvent. 3. denoting compounds in which two or more atoms are united by double or triple bonds.

unsex (-seks′) to deprive of the gonads.

unstriated (-stri′āt-ed) having no striations, as smooth muscle.

urachus (u′rah-kus) a fetal canal connecting the bladder with the allantois, persisting throughout life as a cord (median umbilical ligament). **u′rachal,** adj.

uracil (u′rah-sil) pyrimidine component found in nucleic acid.

uracrasia (u″rah-kra′ze-ah) disordered state of urine.

uragogue (u′rah-gog) diuretic.

uran(o)- word element [Gr.], *palate.*

uraniscus (u″rah-nis′kus) the palate.

uranium (u-ra′ne-um) chemical element (*see table*), at. no. 92, symbol U.

uranoplasty (u-ran′o-plas″te) palatoplasty. **uranoplas′tic,** adj.

uranorrhaphy (u″rah-nor′ah-fe) staphylorrhaphy.

uranoschisis (u″rah-nos′kĭ-sis) cleft palate.

uranostaphyloschisis (u″rah-no-staf″ĭ-los′kĭ-sis) fissure of the soft and hard palates.

uranyl (u′rah-nil) the UO^{++} ion, as in uranyl sulfate.

urarthritis (u″rar-thri′tis) gouty arthritis.

urate (u′rāt) a salt of uric acid.

uratemia (u″rah-te′me-ah) urates in the blood.

uratic (u-rat′ik) pertaining to urates or to gout.

uratoma (u″rah-to′mah) a concretion made up of urates; tophus.

uratosis (-to′sis) the deposit of urates in the tissues.

uraturia (-tu′re-ah) urates in the urine.

urceiform (er-se′ĭ-form) pitcher-shaped.

ur-defense (er″de-fens′) a belief essential to the psychological integrity of the individual.

urea (u-re′ah) 1. the diamide of carbonic acid found in urine, blood, and lymph, the chief nitrogenous constituent of urine, and the chief nitrogenous end-product of protein metabolism; it is formed in the liver from amino acids and from ammonia compounds. 2. a pharmaceutical preparation of urea occasionally used to lower intracranial pressure. **ure′al,** adj. **u. nitrogen,** the nitrogen component of urea; measurement of the urea nitrogen content of the blood (*blood urea nitrogen*, BUN) is used as a test of kidney function.

ureametry (u-re″am′ĕ-tre) measurement of urea in urine.

ureapoiesis (u-re″ah-poi-e′sis) formation of urea. **ureapoiet′ic,** adj.

urease (u′re-ās) an enzyme which catalyzes the decomposition of urea to ammonia and carbon dioxide.

urecchysis (u-rek′ĭ-sis) an effusion of urine into cellular tissue.

Urecholine (u″rĕ-ko′lin) trademark for preparations of bethanechol.

uredema (u″rĕ-de′mah) swelling from extravasated urine.

ureide (u′re-īd) a compound of urea and an acid or aldehyde formed by the elimination of water.

urelcosis (u″rel-ko′sis) ulceration in the urinary tract.

uremia (u-re′me-ah) the retention of excessive by-products of protein metabolism (urea, etc.) in the blood, and the toxic condition produced thereby, marked by nausea, vomiting, vertigo, convulsions, and coma. **ure′mic,** adj.

uremigenic (u-re″mĭ-jen′ik) 1. caused by uremia. 2. causing uremia.

ureometry (u″re-om′ĕ-tre) ureametry.

ureotelic (-o-tel′ik) having urea as the chief excretory product of nitrogen metabolism.

uresiesthesis (u-re″se-es-the′sis) the normal impulse to pass the urine.

uresis (u-re′sis) the passage of urine; urination.

-uresis word element [Gr.], *urinary excretion of.* **-uret′ic,** adj.

ureter (u-re′ter) the tubular organ through which urine passes from kidney to bladder. **ure′teral, ureter′ic,** adj.

ureter(o)- word element [Gr.], *ureter.*

ureteralgia (u-re″ter-al′je-ah) pain in the ureter.

ureterectasis (-ek′tah-sis) distention of the ureter.

ureterectomy (-ek′to-me) excision of a ureter.

ureteritis (-i′tis) inflammation of a ureter.

ureterocele (u-re′ter-o-sēl″) intravesical ballooning of the lower end of the ureter.

ureterocelectomy (u-re″ter-o-se-lek′to-me) excision of a ureterocele.

ureterocolostomy (-ko-los′to-me) anastomosis of a ureter to the colon.

ureterocystoscope (-sis′to-skōp) a cystoscope with a catheter for insertion into the ureter.

ureterocystostomy (-sis-tos′to-me) ureteroneocystostomy.

ureterodialysis (-di-al′ĭ-sis) rupture of a ureter.

ureteroenterostomy (-en″ter-os′to-me) anastomosis of one or both ureters to the wall of the intestine.

ureterography (u-re″ter-og′rah-fe) roentgenography of the ureter, after injection of a contrast medium.

ureteroheminephrectomy (u-re″ter-o-hem″ĭ-nĕ-frek′to-me) excision of the diseased portion of a reduplicated kidney and its ureter.

ureteroileostomy (-il″e-os′to-me) anastomosis of the ureters to an isolated loop of the ileum drained through a stoma on the abdominal wall.

ureterolith (u-re′ter-o-lith″) a calculus in the ureter.

ureterolithiasis (u-re″ter-o-lĭ-thi′ah-sis) formation of a calculus in the ureter.

ureterolithotomy (-lĭ-thot′o-me) incision of ureter for removal of calculus.

ureterolysis (u-re″ter-ol′ĭ-sis) 1. rupture of the ureter. 2. paralysis of the ureter. 3. the operation of freeing the ureter from adhesions.

ureteroneocystostomy (u-re″ter-o-ne″o-sis-tos′to-me) surgical transplantation of a ureter to a different site in the bladder.

ureteroneopyelostomy (-pi′ĕ-los′to-me) ureteropyeloneostomy.

ureteronephrectomy (u-re″ter-o-nĕ-frek′to-me) excision of a kidney and ureter.

ureteropathy (u-re″ter-op′ah-the) any disease of the ureter.

ureteropelvioplasty (u-re″ter-o-pel′ve-o-plas″-te) surgical reconstruction of the junction of the ureter and renal pelvis.

ureteroplasty (u-re′ter-o-plas″te) plastic repair of a ureter.

ureteropyelitis (u-re″ter-o-pi″ĕ-li′tis) inflammation of a ureter and renal pelvis.

ureteropyelography (-pi-ĕ-log′rah-fe) roentgenography of the ureter and renal pelvis.

ureteropyeloneostomy (-pi″ĕ-lo-ne-os′to-me) surgical creation of a new communication between a ureter and the renal pelvis.

ureteropyelonephritis (-pi″ĕ-lo-nĕ-fri′tis) inflammation of ureter, renal pelvis, and kidney.

ureteropyeloplasty (-pi′ĕ-lo-plas″te) plastic repair of a ureter and renal pelvis.

ureteropyelostomy (-pi″ĕ-los′to-me) ureteropyeloneostomy.

ureteropyosis (-pi-o′sis) suppurative inflammation of a ureter.

ureterorrhagia (-ra′je-ah) discharge of blood from a ureter.

ureterorrhaphy (u-re″ter-or′ah-fe) suture of the ureter.

ureterosigmoidostomy (u-re″ter-o-sig″moid-os′to-me) anastomosis of a ureter to the sigmoid colon.

ureterostomy (u-re″ter-os′to-me) creation of a new outlet for a ureter.

ureterotomy (-ot′o-me) incision of a ureter.

ureteroureterostomy (u-re″ter-o-u-re″ter-os′-to-me) end-to-end anastomosis of the two portions of a transected ureter.

ureterovaginal (-vaj′ĭ-nal) pertaining to or communicating with a ureter and the vagina.

ureterovesical (-ves′ĭ-kal) pertaining to a ureter and the bladder.

urethan (u′rĕ-than) an antineoplastic, $C_3H_7NO_2$, formed by esterification of carbamic acid.

urethr(o)- word element [Gr.], *urethra.*

urethra (u-re′thrah) the passage through which urine is discharged from the bladder to the exterior or the body. **ure′thral,** adj.

urethralgia (u″re-thral′je-ah) pain in the urethra.

urethratresia (u-re″thrah-tre′ze-ah) imperforation of the urethra.

urethrectomy (u″re-threk′to-me) excision of the urethra.

urethremphraxis (u″re-threm-frak′sis) obstruction of the urethra.

urethrism (u-re′thrizm) irritability or chronic spasm of the urethra.

urethritis (u″re-thri′tis) inflammation of the urethra. **u. cys′tica,** inflammation of the urethra with formation of multiple submucosal cysts. **nonspecific u.,** simple u. **u. petrif′icans,** urethritis with formation of calcareous matter in the urethral wall. **simple u.,** that not due to a specific infection. **specific u.,** that due to gonorrheal infection of the urethra. **u. vene′rea,** gonorrhea.

urethrobulbar (u-re″thro-bul′bar) pertaining to the urethra and the bulb of the penis.

urethrocele (u-re′thro-sēl) prolapse of the female urethra.

urethrocystitis (u-re″thro-sis-ti′tis) inflammation of the urethra and bladder.

urethrodynia (-din′e-ah) urethralgia.

urethrography (u″re-throg′rah-fe) radiography of the urethra.

urethrometry (u″re-throm′ĕ-tre) 1. determination of the resistance of various segments of the urethra to retrograde flow of fluid. 2. measurement of the urethra.

urethropenile (u-re″thro-pe′nīl) pertaining to the urethra and penis.

urethroperineal (-per″ĭ-ne′al) pertaining to the urethra and perineum.

urethroperineoscrotal (-per″ĭ-ne″o-skro′tal) pertaining to the urethra, perineum, and scrotum.

urethrophraxis (-frak′sis) obstruction of the urethra.

urethrophyma (-fi′mah) a tumor or growth in the urethra.

urethroplasty (u-re′thro-plas″te) plastic repair of the urethra.

urethroprostatic (u-re″thro-pros-tat′ik) pertaining to the urethra and prostate.

urethrorectal (-rek′tal) pertaining to the urethra and rectum.

urethrorrhagia (-ra′je-ah) flow of blood from the urethra.

urethrorrhaphy (u″re-thror′ah-fe) suture of a urethral fistula.

urethrorrhea (u-re″thro-re′ah) abnormal discharge from the urethra.

urethroscope (u-re′thro-skōp) an instrument for viewing the interior of the urethra.

urethroscopy (u″re-thros′ko-pe) visual inspection of the urethra. **urethroscop′ic,** adj.

urethrospasm (u-re′thro-spazm) spasm of the urethral muscular tissue.

urethrostaxis (u-re″thro-stak′sis) oozing of blood from the urethra.

urethrostenosis (-stĕ-no′sis) constriction of the urethra.

urethrostomy (u″re-thros′to-me) creation of a permanent opening of the urethra in the perineum.

urethrotome (u-re′thro-tōm) an instrument for cutting a urethral stricture.

urethrotomy (u″re-throt′o-me) incision of the urethra.

urethrotrigonitis (u-re″thro-tri″go-ni′tis) inflammation of the urethra and the trigone of the bladder.

urethrovaginal (-vaj′ĭ-nal) pertaining to the urethra and vagina.

urethrovesical (-ves′ĭ-kal) pertaining to the urethra and bladder.

urhidrosis (ur″hĭ-dro′sis) the presence in the sweat of urinous materials, chiefly uric acid and urea.

-uria word element [Gr.], *condition of the urine.* **-u′ric,** adj.

uricacidemia (u″rik-as″ĭ-de′me-ah) the accumulation of uric acid in the blood.

uricaciduria (-as″ĭ-du′re-ah) excess of uric acid in the urine.

uricase (u′rĭ-kās) an enzyme that catalyzes the conversion of uric acid into allantoin.

uricemia (u″rĭ-se′me-ah) uricacidemia.

uricolysis (u″rĭ-kol′ĭ-sis) the cleavage of uric acid or urates. **uricolyt′ic,** adj.

uricometer (u″rĭ-kom′ĕ-ter) an instrument for measuring uric acid in urine.

uricosuria (u″rĭ-ko-su′re-ah) excretion of uric acid in the urine.

uricosuric (-su′rik) 1. pertaining to, characterized by, or promoting uricosuria. 2. an agent that promotes uricosuria.

uricotelic (-tel′ik) having uric acid as the chief excretory product of nitrogen metabolism.

uridine (u′rĭ-dēn) a ribonucleoside containing uracil. **u. diphosphate (UDP),** a nucleotide that participates in glycogen metabolism and in some processes of nucleic acid synthesis.

uriesthesis (u″re-es-the′sis) uresiesthesis.

urin(o)- word element [Gr., L.], *urine.*

urina (u-ri′nah) [L.] urine.

urinal (u′rĭ-nal) a receptacle for urine.

urinalysis (u″rĭ-nal′ĭ-sis) analysis of the urine.

urinate (u′rĭ-nāt) to void urine.

urination (u″rĭ-na′shun) the discharge of urine from the bladder.

urine (u′rin) the fluid excreted by the kidneys, stored in the bladder, and discharged through the urethra. **u′rinary,** adj. **residual u.,** urine remaining in the bladder after urination.

urinemia (u″rĭ-ne′me-ah) uremia.

uriniferous (u″rĭ-nif′er-us) transporting or conveying urine.

uriniparous (u″rĭ-nip′ah-rus) excreting urine.

urinogenital (u″rĭ-no-jen′ĭ-tal) urogenital.

urinogenous (u″rĭ-noj′ĕ-nus) of urinary origin.

urinology (u″rĭ-nol′o-je) urology.

urinoma (u″rĭ-no′mah) a cyst containing urine.

urinometer (u″rĭ-nom′ĕ-ter) an instrument for determining the specific gravity of urine.

urinometry (u″rĭ-nom′ĕ-tre) determination of the specific gravity of urine.

urinoscopy (u″rĭ-nos′ko-pe) uroscopy.

urinous (u′rĭ-nus) pertaining to or of the nature of urine.

uriposia (u″rĭ-po′ze-ah) the drinking of urine.

Uritone (u′rĭ-tōn) trademark for preparations of methenamine.

uro- word element [Gr.], *urine* (urinary tract, urination).

uroacidimeter (u″ro-as″ĭ-dim′ĕ-ter) an instrument for measuring the acidity of urine.

uroanthelone (-an′thĕ-lōn) urogastrone.

urobilin (-bi′lin) a brownish pigment formed by oxidation of urobilinogen.

urobilinemia (-bi″lĭ-ne′me-ah) urobilin in the blood.

urobilinogen (-bi-lin′o-jen) a colorless compound formed in the intestines by reduction of bilirubin.

urocele (u′ro-sēl) distention of the scrotum with extravasated urine.

urochezia (u″ro-ke′ze-ah) the discharge of urine in the feces.

urochrome (u′ro-krōm) a breakdown product of hemoglobin related to the bile pigments, found in the urine and responsible for its yellow color.

uroclepsia (u″ro-klep′se-ah) the involuntary escape of urine.

urocrisia (-kriz′e-ah) diagnosis by examining the urine.

urocyanogen (-si-an′o-jen) a blue pigment of urine, especially of cholera patients.

urocyanosis (-si″ah-no′sis) indicanuria.

urocyst (u′ro-sist) the urinary bladder. **urocys′tic,** adj.

urocystitis (u″ro-sis-ti′tis) inflammation of the urinary bladder.

urodynia (-din′e-ah) pain on urination.

uroedema (-ĕ-de′mah) edema due to infiltration of urine.

uroenterone (-en′ter-ōn) urogastrone.

uroerythrin (-er′ĭ-thrin) a reddish pigment of the urine.

uroflavin (-fla′vin) a fluorescent compound closely related to riboflavin, excreted in the urine.

urofuscohematin (-fus″ko-hem′ah-tin) a red-brown pigment of urine in certain diseases.

urogastrone (-gas′trōn) anthelone U; a polypeptide from normal and pregnancy urine of man and other mammals, which inhibits gastric secretion.

urogenital (-jen′ĭ-tal) pertaining to the urinary apparatus and genitalia.

urogenous (u-roj′ĕ-nus) 1. producing urine. 2. produced from or in the urine.

uroglaucin (u″ro-glaw′sin) indigo blue occurring in the urine.

urogram (u′ro-gram) a film obtained by urography.

urography (u-rog′rah-fe) radiography of any part of the urinary tract. **ascending u., cystoscopic u.,** retrograde u. **descending u., excretion u., excretory u., intravenous u.,** urography after intravenous injection of an opaque medium which is rapidly excreted in the urine. **retrograde u.,** urography after injection of a contrast medium into the bladder through the urethra.

urogravimeter (u″ro-grah-vim′ĕ-ter) urinometer.

urohematin (-hem′ah-tin) the pigmentary substance of the urine.

urohematoporphyrin (-hem″ah-to-por′fĭ-rin) hematoporphyrin found in the urine.

urokinase (-ki′nās) an enzyme in the urine of man and other mammals which converts plasminogen to plasmin and activates the fibrinolytic system.

urolith (u′ro-lith) a calculus in the urine or the urinary tract. **urolith′ic** adj.

urolithiasis (u″ro-lĭ-thi′ah-sis) the formation of urinary calculi, or the condition associated with urinary calculi.

urologist (u-rol′o-jist) a specialist in urology.

urology (u-rol′o-je) the branch of medicine dealing with the urinary system in the female and genitourinary tract in the male. **urolog′ic,** adj.

urolutein (u″ro-lu′te-in) a yellow pigment of the urine.

uromelanin (-mel′ah-nin) a black pigment from urine.

uromelus (u-rom′ĕ-lus) a fetus with fused limbs and one foot.

urometer (u-rom′ĕ-ter) urinometer.

uroncus (u-rong′kus) a swelling caused by retention or extravasation of urine.

uronephrosis (u″ro-nĕ-fro′sis) distention of the renal pelvis and tubules with urine.

uropathy (u-rop′ah-the) any disease of the urinary tract.

uropepsin (u″ro-pep′sin) a pepsin-like enzyme occurring in urine.

urophanic (-fan′ik) appearing in the urine.

urophein (-fe′in) an odoriferous gray pigment of urine.

uroplania (-pla′ne-ah) urine in, or its discharge from, organs not of the urogenital tract.

uropoiesis (-poi-e′sis) the formation of urine. **uropoiet′ic,** adj.

uroporphyria (-por-fir′e-ah) porphyria with excessive excretion of uroporphyrin.

uroporphyrin (-por′fĭ-rin) one of a group of porphyrins produced during biosynthesis of natural porphyrins and excreted in urine.

uroporphyrinogen (-por″fĭ-rin′o-jen) a precursor of uroporphyrin and coproporphyrinogen.

uropsammus (-sam′us) urinary gravel.

urorrhagia (-ra′je-ah) excessive secretion of urine.

urorrhea (-re′ah) involuntary flow of urine.

urorrhodin (-ro′din) a rose-colored pigment found in the urine in typhoid fever, tuberculosis, and other diseases.

urorrhodinogen (-ro-din′o-jen) a urinary chromogen that is decomposed to urorrhodin.

urorubin (-roo′bin) a red pigment from urine.

urorubrohematin (-roo″bro-hem′ah-tin) a red pigment rarely found in the urine in certain constitutional diseases, as in leprosy.

uroscheocele (u-ros′ke-o-sēl″) urocele.

uroschesis (u-ros′kĕ-sis) retention or suppression of the urine.

uroscopy (u-ros′ko-pe) diagnostic examination of the urine. **uroscop′ic,** adj.

urosemiology (u″ro-se″me-ol′o-je) uroscopy.

urosepsin (-sep′sin) a septic poisoning from urine in the tissues.

urosepsis (-sep′sis) septic poisoning from retained and absorbed urinary substances. **urosep′tic,** adj.

urostealith (ste″ah-lith) a urinary calculus having fatty constituents.

urotoxia (-tok′se-ah) 1. the toxicity of the urine. 2. the toxic substances of the urine. 3. the unit of the toxicity of the urine or a quantity sufficient to kill 1 kg. of living substance. **urotox′ic,** adj.

urotoxin (-tok′sin) the toxic constituents of urine.

Urotropin (u-rot′ro-pin) trademark for a preparation of methenamine.

uroureter (u″ro-u-re′ter) distension of the ureter with urine.

uroxanthin (-zan′thin) a yellow pigment of normal urine convertible into indigo blue.

ursone (ur′sōn) a crystallizable compound, C_{30}-$H_{48}O_3$, found in the waxlike coatings of various fruits and leaves.

Urtica (er-ti′kah) a genus of plants, the true nettles, which are covered with stinging hairs and secrete a poisonous fluid. *U. dio′ica,* of temperate regions, has stimulant, diuretic, and hemostatic properties.

urticant (er′tĭ-kant) producing urticaria.

urticaria (er″tĭ-ka′re-ah) hives; a vascular reaction of the skin marked by transient appearance of slightly elevated patches (wheals) which are redder or paler than the surrounding skin and often attended by severe itching; the exciting cause may be certain foods or drugs, infection, or emotional stress. **urtica′rial,** adj. **u. bullo′sa, bullous u.,** a rare form marked by the presence of bullae. **giant u., u. gigan′tea,** angioneurotic edema. **u. hemorrhag′ica,** purpura with urticaria. **u. medicamento′sa,** that due to use of a drug. **papular u., u. papulo′sa,** an allergic reaction to the bite of various insects, with appearance of lesions that evolve into inflammatory, increasingly hard, red or brownish, persistent papules. **u. pigmento′sa,** mastocytosis manifested as persistent pink to brown macules or soft plaques of various size; pruritus and urtication occur on stroking the lesions. **u. pigmento′sa, juvenile,** urticaria pigmentosa present at birth or in the first few weeks of life, usually disappearing before puberty, taking the form of a single nodule or tumor or of a disseminated eruption of yellowish brown to yellowish red macules, plaques, or bullae. **solar u.,** a rare form produced by exposure to sunlight.

urtication (er″tĭ-ka′shun) 1. the development or formation of urticaria. 2. a burning sensation as of stinging with nettles.

urushiol (u-roo′she-ol) the toxic irritant principle of poison ivy and various related plants.

USAN United States Adopted Names, non-proprietary designations for compounds used as drugs, established by negotiation between their manufacturers and a council sponsored jointly by the American Medical Association, American Pharmaceutical Association, United States Pharmacopeial Convention, Inc., and The National Formulary.

U.S.P. United States Pharmacopeia, a legally recognized compendium of standards for drugs, published by the United States Pharmacopeial Convention, Inc., and revised periodically; it also includes assays and tests for determination of strength, quality, and purity.

U.S.P.H.S. United States Public Health Service.

ustilaginism (us′tĭ-laj′ĭ-nism) a condition resembling ergotism due to ingestion of maize containing *Ustilago maydis.*

Ustilago (us′tĭ-la′go) the smuts, a genus of fungi parasitic on plants. *U. may′dis* causes corn smut and ustilaginism.

uter(o)- word element [L.], *uterus.*

uteralgia (u″ter-al′je-ah) pain in the uterus.

uterine (u′ter-in, u′ter-īn) pertaining to the uterus.

uteroabdominal (u″ter-o-ab-dom′ĭ-nal) pertaining to the uterus and abdomen.

uterocervical (-ser′vĭ-kal) pertaining to the uterus and cervix uteri.

uterofixation (-fik-sa′shun) hysteropexy.

uterogestation (-jes-ta′shun) uterine gestation; normal pregnancy.

uterography (u″ter-og′rah-fe) hysterography.

uterolith (u′ter-o-lith″) hysterolith.

uterometer (u″ter-om′ĕ-ter) hysterometer.

utero-ovarian (u″ter-o-o-va′re-an) pertaining to the uterus and ovary.

uteropexy (u′ter-o-pek″se) hysteropexy.

uteroplacental (u″ter-o-plah-sen′tal) pertaining to the placenta and uterus.

uteroplasty (u′ter-o-plas″te) plastic repair of the uterus.

uterorectal (u″ter-o-rek′tal) pertaining to or communicating with the uterus and rectum.

uterosacral (-sa′kral) pertaining to the uterus and sacrum.

uterosalpingography (-sal″ping-gog′rah-fe) hysterosalpingography.

uteroscope (u'ter-o-skōp'') hysteroscope.

uterotomy (u''ter-ot'o-me) hysterotomy.

uterotonic (u''ter-o-ton'ik) 1. increasing the tone of uterine muscle. 2. a uterotonic agent.

uterotubal (-tu'bal) pertaining to the uterus and oviducts.

uterovaginal (-vaj'ĭ-nal) pertaining to the uterus and vagina.

uterovesical (-ves'ĭ-kal) pertaining to the uterus and bladder.

uterus (u'ter-us) the hollow muscular organ in female mammals in which the fertilized ovum normally becomes embedded and in which the developing embryo and fetus is nourished. Its cavity opens into the vagina below and into a uterine tube on either side. **u. bicor'nis,** one with two cornua. **u. cordifor'mis,** a heart-shaped uterus. **u. du'plex,** a double uterus, normal in marsupials but rarely seen in humans. **gravid u.,** one containing a developing fetus. **u. masculi'nus,** prostatic utricle. **u. unicor'nis,** one with a single cornu.

utricle (u'tri-k'l) 1. any small sac. 2. the larger of the two divisions of the membranous labyrinth of the internal ear. **prostatic u., urethral u.,** a small blind pouch in the substance of the prostate.

utricular (u-trik'u-lar) 1. pertaining to the utricle. 2. bladder-like.

utriculitis (u-trik''u-li'tis) inflammation of the prostatic utricle or the utricle of the ear.

utriculosaccular (u-trik''u-lo-sak'u-lar) pertaining to utricle and saccule of the labyrinth.

utriculus (u-trik'u-lus) utricle. **u. masculi'nus, u. prostat'icus,** prostatic utricle.

uve(o)- word element, *uvea.*

uvea (u've-ah) the iris, ciliary body, and choroid together. **u'veal,** adj.

uveitis (u''ve-i'tis) inflammation of the uvea. **uveit'ic,** adj. **heterochromic u.,** see under *iridocyclitis.* **sympathetic u.,** see under *ophthalmia.*

uveoparotitis (u''ve-o-par''o-ti'tis) uveoparotid fever.

uveoscleritis (-skle-ri'tis) scleritis due to extension of uveitis.

uviform (u'vĭ-form) shaped like a grape.

uviofast (u've-o-fast'') uvioresistant.

uviometer (u''ve-om'ĕ-ter) an instrument for measuring ultraviolet emanation.

uvioresistant (u''ve-o-re-zis'tant) resistant to or unaffected by ultraviolet rays.

uviosensitive (-sen'sĭ-tiv) sensitive to ultraviolet rays.

uvula (u'vu-lah), pl. *u'vulae* [L.] a pendant, fleshy mass, specifically the palatine uvula. **u'vular,** adj. **u. of bladder,** u. vesicae. **u. cerebel'li, u. of cerebellum,** u. vermis. **u. palati'na, palatine u.,** the small, fleshy mass hanging from the soft palate above the root of the tongue. **u. ver'mis,** the part of the vermis of the cerebellum between the pyramid and nodule. **u. vesi'cae,** a rounded elevation at the neck of the bladder, formed by convergence of muscle fibers terminating in the urethra.

uvulectomy (u''vu-lek'to-me) excision of the uvula.

uvulitis (u''vu-li'tis) inflammation of the uvula.

uvuloptosis (u''vu-lop-to'sis) a relaxed, pendulous state of the uvula.

uvulotomy (u''vu-lot'o-me) the cutting off of the uvula or a part of it.

V

V chemical symbol, *vanadium.*

V. *Vibrio;* vision; visual acuity.

v. *vein,* or [L.] *vena;* volt.

vaccigenous (vak-sij'ĕ-nus) producing vaccine.

vaccina (vak'si-nah) vaccinia.

vaccinable (vak-sin'ah-b'l) susceptible of being successfully vaccinated.

vaccinal (vak'sĭ-nal) 1. pertaining to vaccinia, to vaccine, or to vaccination. 2. having protective qualities when used by way of inoculation.

vaccinate (vak'sĭ-nāt) to inoculate with vaccine to produce immunity.

vaccination (vak''sĭ-na'shun) the introduction of vaccine into the body to produce immunity.

vaccine (vak'sēn) a suspension of attenuated or killed microorganisms (viruses, bacteria, or rickettsiae), administered for prevention, amelioration, or treatment of infectious diseases. **autogenous v.,** a bacterial vaccine prepared from cultures of material derived from a lesion of the patient to be treated. **bacterial v.,** a preparation of attenuated or killed bacteria, used to increase immunity to the organisms injected, or sometimes for pyrogenetic effects in treatment of certain noninfectious diseases. **BCG v.,** a preparation used as an active immunizing agent against tuberculosis, consisting of a dried, living, avirulent culture of the Calmette-Guerin bacillus. **cholera v.,** a preparation of killed cholera vibrios, used in immunization against cholera. **diphtheria and tetanus toxoids and pertussis v.,** a preparation of killed *Bordetella pertussis* in a mixture of diphtheria and tetanus toxoids; used as an active immunizing agent. **inactivated v.,** a vaccine containing nonreplicating microorganisms which are noninfectious but which retain their protective antigens. **influenza virus v.,** a preparation of inactivated influenza virus prepared from the extraembryonic fluid of influenza virus–infected chick embryo, used to produce immunity. **measles virus v.,** a preparation from the causative virus, used to produce active immunity to the disease; the attenuated type is grown on chick embryo or canine kidney tissue culture, and the inactivated type on chick embryo or monkey kidney tissue culture. **mixed v.,** polyvalent v. **mumps v.,** a sterile suspension of mumps virus, inactivated and used to produce active immunity against mumps (epidemic parotitis). **pertussis v.,** a preparation of killed pertussis bacilli, used to immunize against whooping cough. **plague v.,** a preparation of killed plague bacilli, used as an active immunizing agent. **poliomyelitis v.,** one used to immunize against poliomyelitis, prepared from killed polioviruses (*Salk v.*) and injected subcutaneously, or from live poliovirus(es) (*Sabin oral v.*) and given orally. **poliovirus v., live oral,** see *poliomyelitis v.* **polyvalent v.,** a vaccine prepared from more than one strain or species of microorganisms. **rabies v.,** a preparation of rabies virus that has been treated with a virucidal agent, used to prevent developmnt of rabies in an exposed person. **Rocky Mountain spotted fever v.,** a preparation of killed *Rickettsia rickettsii,* grown in monkey kidney tissue, used as an active immunizing agent. **Sabin oral v.,** see *poliomyelitis v.* **Salk v.,** see *poliomyelitis v.* **smallpox v.,** a preparation of vaccinia virus, grown by various methods, used to produce immunity to smallpox. **tuberculosis v.,** BCG v. **typhoid and paratyphoid v.,** a preparation of killed typhoid bacilli, used to immunize against typhoid fever. **typhus v.,** a preparation of killed rickettsial organisms of a strain(s) of *Rickettsia prowazeki,* derived from an aqueous suspension of infected yolk sac membrane of chick embryos; used to immunize against epidemic typhus. **yellow fever v.,** a preparation of attenuated yellow fever virus, used to immunize against yellow fever.

vaccinia (vak-sin′e-ah) a viral disease of cows (see *cowpox*). In humans, a localized pustular eruption produced by inoculation of vaccinia virus is used to induce antibody formation against smallpox. Vaccinia is also transmissible by contact with a vaccinated person or an infected cow. **vaccin′ial,** adj. **v. gangreno′sa,** generalized vaccinia marked by failure to develop antibodies against the virus (due to agammaglobulinemia), with spreading necrosis at the site and metastasis of lesions throughout the body. **generalized v.,** a benign systemic infection sometimes occurring after smallpox vaccination, marked by a widespread papular rash, which later vesiculates but leaves no scars. **progressive v.,** v. gangrenosa.

vacciniform (vak-sin′ĭ-form) resembling vaccinia.

vacciniola (vak″sĭ-ne-o′lah) generalized vaccinia.

vaccinotherapy (vak″sĭ-no-ther′ah-pe) therapeutic use of vaccines.

vacuolar (vak′u-o″lar) containing, or of the nature of, vacuoles.

vacuolated (vak′u-o-lāt″ed) containing vacuoles.

vacuolation (vak″u-o-la′shun) the process of forming vacuoles; the condition of being vacuolated.

vacuole (vak′u-ōl) a space or cavity in the protoplasm of a cell. **contractile v.,** a small fluid-filled cavity in the protoplasm of certain unicellular organisms; it gradually increases in size and then collapses, its function is thought to be respiratory and excretory.

vacuolization (vak″u-o-li-za′shun) vacuolation.

vacuome (vak′u-ōm) the system of vacuoles in a cell which stain with neutral red.

vacuum (vak′u-um) [L.] a space devoid of air or of other gas.

vagal (va′gal) pertaining to the vagus nerve.

vagina (vah-ji′nah) 1, a sheath or sheathlike structure. 2. the canal in the female, from the vulva to the cervix uteri, that receives the penis in copulation.

vaginal (vaj′ĭ-nal) pertaining to the vagina, to the tunica vaginalis, or to any sheath.

vaginalectomy (vaj″ĭ-nal-ek′to-me) vaginectomy.

vaginalitis (vaj″ĭ-nal-i′tis) inflammation of the tunica vaginalis testis.

vaginate (vaj′ĭ-nāt) enclosed in a sheath.

vaginectomy (vaj″ĭ-nek′to-me) 1. resection of the tunica vaginalis testis. 2. excision of the vagina.

vaginismus (vaj″ĭ-niz′mus) painful spasm of the vagina.

vaginitis (vaj″ĭ-ni′tis) 1. inflammation of the vagina. 2. inflammation of a sheath. **adhesive v.,** that in which ulceration and exfoliation of the mucosa results in adhesions of the membranes. **atrophic v.,** that in postmenopausal women, with thinning and, often, ulceration of the vaginal epithelium; it may progress to adhesive vaginitis. **desquamative inflammatory v.,** a form resembling atrophic vaginitis but affecting women with normal estrogen levels. **emphysematous v.,** a variety marked by the formation of gas in the meshes of the connective tissue. **senile v.,** atrophic v.

vaginoabdominal (vaj″ĭ-no-ab-dom′ĭ-nal) pertaining to the vagina and abdomen.

vaginocele (vaj″ĭ-no-sēl″) vaginal hernia.

vaginodynia (vaj″ĭ-no-din′e-ah) colpodynia.

vaginofixation (-fik-sa′shun) colpopexy.

vaginolabial (-la′be-al) pertaining to the vagina and labia.

vaginomycosis (-mi-ko′sis) any fungal disease of the vagina.

vaginopathy (vaj″ĭ-nop′ah-the) any disease of the vagina.

vaginoperineal (vaj″ĭ-no-per″ĭ-ne′al) pertaining to the vagina and perineum.

vaginoperineorrhaphy (-per″ĭ-ne-or′ah-fe) colpoperineorrhaphy.

vaginoperineotomy (-per″ĭ-ne-ot′o-me) incision of the vagina and perineum.

vaginoperitoneal (-per″ĭ-to-ne′al) pertaining to the vagina and peritoneum.

vaginopexy (vah-ji′no-pek″se) colpopexy.

vaginoplasty (-plas″te) colpoplasty.

vaginoscopy (vaj″ĭ-nos′ko-pe) colposcopy.

vaginotomy (vaj″ĭ-not′o-me) colpotomy.

vaginovesical (vaj″ĭ-no-ves′ĭ-kal) pertaining to the vagina and bladder.

vagitus (vah-ji′tus) [L.] the cry of an infant.

v. uteri′nus, the cry of an infant in the uterus.

vagolysis (va-gol′ĭ-sis) surgical lysis of the vagus nerve.

vagolytic (va″go-lit′ik) having an effect resembling that produced by interruption of impulses transmitted by the vagus nerve.

vagomimetic (-mi-met′ik) having an effect resembling that produced by stimulation of the vagus nerve.

vagotomy (va-got′o-me) surgical transection of the fibers of the vagus nerve. **medical v.,** that accomplished by administration of suitable drugs.

vagotonia (va″go-to′ne-ah) irritability of the vagus nerve, characterized by vasomotor instability, sweating, disordered peristalsis, and muscle spasms. **vagoton′ic,** adj.

vagotonin (va-got′o-nin) a preparation of hormone from the pancreas which increases vagal tone, slows the heart, and increases the store of glycogen in the liver.

vagotropic (va″go-trop′ik) having an effect on the vagus nerve.

vagovagal (-va′gal) arising as a result of afferent and efferent impulses mediated through the vagus nerve.

vagus (va′gus), pl. *va′gi* [L.] the vagus nerve; see *Table of Nerves.*

vagusstoff (va′gus-stof) a substance liberated by the vagus nerve endings that inhibits cardiac activity; probably identical to acetylcholine.

valence (va′lens) the numerical measure of the capacity to combine; in chemistry, an expression of the number of atoms of hydrogen (or its equivalent) that one atom of a chemical element can hold in combination, if negative, or displace in a reaction, if positive; in immunology, an expression of the number of antigenic determinants with which one molecule of a given antibody can combine.

valethamate (val-eth′ah-māt) an anticholinergic, $C_{19}H_{32}NO_2$; *v. bromide* is used as an antispasmodic in hypermotility and spasm of the gastrointestinal, genitourinary, and biliary tracts.

valgus (val′gus) [L.] bent out, twisted; denoting a deformity in which the angulation is away from the midline of the body, as in talipes valgus.

valine (va′lēn) a naturally occurring amino acid, essential for human metabolism.

valinemia (val″ĭ-ne′me-ah) elevated levels of valine in the blood and urine.

Valium (val′e-um) trademark for a preparation of diazepam.

vallate (val′āt) having a wall or rim; rim-shaped.

vallecula (vah-lek′u-lah), pl. *vallec′ulae* [L.] a depression or furrow. **v. cerebel′li,** the longitudinal fissure on the inferior cerebellum, in which the medulla oblongata rests. **v. syl′vii,** a depression made by the fissure of Sylvius at base of the brain. **v. un′guis,** the sulcus of the matrix of the nail.

Vallestril (val-les′tril) trademark for a preparation of methallenestril.

Valmid (val′mid) trademark for a preparation of ethinamate.

value (val′u) a measure of worth or efficiency; a quantitative measurement of the activity, concentration, etc., of specific substances. **normal v′s,** the range in concentration of specific substances found in normal healthy tissues, secretions, etc.

valva (val′vah), pl. *val′vae* [L.] a valve.

valve (valv) a membranous fold in a canal or passage that prevents backward flow of material passing through it. **aortic v.,** that guarding the entrance to the aorta from the left ventricle. **atrioventricular v′s,** the valves between the right atrium and right ventricle (tricuspid v.) and the left atrium and left ventricle (mitral v.). **Bauhin's v.,** ileocecal v. **Béraud's v.,** a fold at the beginning of the nasolacrimal duct. **bicuspid v.,** mitral v. **cardiac v′s,** those controlling the flow of blood through and from the heart. **coronary v.,** that at the entrance of the coronary sinus into the right atrium. **Hasner's v.,** lacrimal fold. **Heister's v.,** spiral fold. **Houston's v.,** the middle one of three transverse folds of the rectum. **ileocecal v., ileocolic v.,** that guarding the opening between the ileum and cecum. **Kerckring's v′s,** circular folds. **mitral v.,** that between the left atrium and left ventricle, usually having two cusps (anterior and posterior). **pulmonary v.,** that at the entrance of the pulmonary trunk from the right ventricle. **pyloric v.,** a prominent fold of mucous membrane at the pyloric orifice of the stomach. **semilunar v.,** one having semilunar cusps, i.e., the aortic and pulmonary valves; sometimes used to designate the semilunar cusps composing these valves. **thebesian v.,** coronary v. **tricuspid v.,** that guarding the opening between the right atrium and right ventricle. **v. of Varolius,** ileocecal v. **v. of Vieussens,** superior medullary velum.

valvotomy (val-vot′o-me) incision of a valve.

valvula (val′vu-lah), pl. *vul′vulae* [L.] a small valve.

valvular (val′vu-lar) pertaining to, affecting, or of the nature of a valve.

valvulitis (val-vu-li′tis) inflammation of a valve, especially of a heart valve.

valvuloplasty (val′vu-lo-plas″te) plastic repair of a valve, especially a heart valve.

valvulotome (-tōm) an instrument for cutting a valve.

valvulotomy (val″vu-lot′o-me) valvotomy.

vanadate (van′ah-dāt) any salt of vanadic acid.

vanadium (vah-na′de-um) chemical element (*see table*), at. no. 23, symbol V. Its salts have been used in treating various diseases. Absorption of its compounds, usually via the lungs, causes chronic intoxication, the symptoms of which include respiratory tract irritation, pneumonitis, conjunctivitis, and anemia.

vanadiumism (-izm″) poisoning by vanadium (q.v.).

Vancocin (van′ko-sin) trademark for a preparation of vancomycin.

vancomycin (van″ko-mi′sin) an antibiotic produced by *Streptomyces orientalis,* highly effective against gram-positive bacteria, especially against staphylococci; used as the hydrochloride salt.

vanilla (vah-nil′ah) cured, full-grown, unripe fruit of species of *Vanilla;* used as a flavoring agent.

vanillin (vah-nil′in) a flavoring agent, C_8H_8O, derived from vanilla and other plants or produced synthetically.

vanillism (vah-nil′izm) dermatitis, coryza, and malaise seen in raw vanilla handlers, due to the mite *Acarus siro.*

Vanogel (van′o-jel) trademark for an aqueous suspension of aluminum hydroxide gel.

vapor (va′por) [L.] steam, gas, or exhalation.

vaporization (va″por-i-za′shun) 1. the conversion of a solid or liquid into a vapor without chemical change; distillation. 2. treatment by vapors; vapotherapy.

vaporize (va′por-īz) to convert into vapor or to be transformed into vapor.

vapotherapy (va″po-ther′ah-pe) therapeutic use of vapor, steam, or spray.

varication (var″ĭ-ka′shun) 1. the formation of a varix. 2. a varicose condition; a varicosity.

variceal (var″ĭ-se′al) of or pertaining to a varix or varices.

varicella (var″ĭ-sel′ah) chickenpox.

varicelliform (var″i-sel′ĭ-form) resembling varicella.

varices (var′ĭ-sēz) [L.] plural of *varix.*

variciform (vah-ris′ĭ-form) resembling a varix; varicose.

varicoblepharon (var″ĭ-ko-blef′ah-ron) a varicose swelling of the eyelid.

varicocele (var′ĭ-ko-sēl) varicosity of the pampiniform plexus of the spermatic cord, forming a scrotal swelling that feels like a "bag of worms."

varicocelectomy (var″ĭ-ko-se-lek′to-me) excision of a varicocele.

varicography (var″ĭ-kog′rah-fe) x-ray visualization of varicose veins.

varicomphalos (var″ĭ-kom′fah-los) a varicose tumor of the umbilicus.

varicophlebitis (var″ĭ-ko-fle-bi′tis) varicose veins with inflammation.

varicose (var′ĭ-kōs) of the nature of or pertaining to a varix; unnaturally and permanently distended (said of a vein); variciform.

varicosity (var″ĭ-kos′ĭ-te) 1. a varicose condition; the quality or fact of being varicose. 2. a varix, or varicose vein.

varicotomy (var″ĭ-kot′o-me) excision of a varix or of a varicose vein.

varicula (vah-rik′u-lah) a varix of the conjunctiva.

Varidase (var′ĭ-dās) trademark for preparations of streptokinase and streptodornase.

variety (vah-ri′ĕ-te) in taxonomy, a subcategory of a species.

variola (vah-ri′o-lah) smallpox. **vari′olar, vari′olous,** adj. **v. hemorrha′gica,** hemorrhagic smallpox. **v. ma′jor,** severe smallpox, such as the hemorrhagic or malignant form, with a high fatality rate. **v. milia′ris,** smallpox with an eruption of small vesicles. **v. mi′nor,** a mild form of smallpox having a low fatality rate.

variolate (va′re-o-lāt) 1. having the nature or appearance of smallpox. 2. to inoculate with smallpox virus.

variolation (var″re-o-la′shun) deliberate inoculation with unmodified smallpox virus to produce immunity to the naturally occurring disease.

varioliform (va″re-o′lĭ-form) resembling smallpox.

varioloid (va′re-o-loid″) a modified and mild form of smallpox occurring in a person who has had a previous attack or has been vaccinated.

variolovaccinia (vah-ri″o-lo-vak-sin′e-ah) cowpox in the heifer due to inoculation with smallpox.

varix (vār′iks), pl. *var′ices* [L.] an enlarged tortuous vein, artery, or lymphatic vessel. **aneurysmal v.,** a markedly dilated tortuous vessel; sometimes used to denote a form of arteriovenous aneurysm in which the blood flows directly into a neighboring vein without the intervention of a connecting sac. **arterial v.,** a racemose aneurysm or varicose artery. **esophageal varices,** varicosities of branches of the azygous vein which anastomose with tributaries of the portal vein in the lower esophagus, due to portal hypertension in cirrhosis of the liver. **lymph v., v. lymphat′icus,** a soft, lobulated swelling of a lymph node, due to obstruction of lymphatic vessels.

varolian (vah-ro′le-an) pertaining to the pons varolii.

varus (va′rus) [L.] bent inward; denoting a deformity in which the angulation of the part is toward the midline of the body, as in talipes varus.

vas (vas), pl. *va′sa* [L.] a vessel. **va′sal,** adj. **v. aber′rans,** 1. a blind tubule sometimes connected with the epididymus; a vestigial mesonephric tubule. 2. any anomalous or unusual vessel. **va′sa afferen′tia,** vessels that convey fluid to a structure or part. **va′sa bre′via,** short gastric arteries. **v. capilla′re,** a capillary. **v. def′erens,** ductus deferens. **va′sa efferen′tia,** vessels that convey fluid away from a structure or part. **v. lymphat′icum,** lymphatic vessels. **va′sa pre′via,** presentation, in front of the fetal head during labor, of the blood vessels of the umbilical cord where they enter the placenta. **va′sa rec′ta,** long U-shaped vessels arising from the efferent glomerular arterioles of juxtamedullary nephrons and supplying the renal medulla. **va′sa vaso′rum,** the small nutrient arteries and veins in the walls of the larger blood vessels. **va′sa vortico′sa,** vorticose veins.

vas(o)- word element [L.], *vessel; duct.*

vascular (vas′ku-lar) pertaining to blood vessels or indicative of a copious blood supply.

vascularity (vas″ku-lar′ĭ-te) the condition of being vascular.

vascularization (vas″ku-lar-i-za′shun) the formation of new blood vessels in tissues.

vascularize (vas′ku-lar-īz) to supply with vessels.

vasculature   700

vasculature (vas'ku-lah-chūr) 1. the vascular system of the body, or any part of it. 2. the supply of vessels to a specific region.

vasculitis (vas"ku-li'tis) inflammation of a vessel; angiitis.

vasculopathy (vas"ku-lop'ah-the) any disorder of blood vessels.

vasectomy (vah-sek'to-me) excision of the vas (ductus) deferens, or a portion of it.

vasifactive (vas"ĭ-fak'tiv) vasoformative.

vasiform (vas'ĭ-form) resembling a vessel.

vasitis (vas-i'tis) inflammation of the vas (ductus) deferens.

vasoactive (vas"o-ak'tiv) exerting an effect on the caliber of blood vessels.

vasoconstriction (-kon-strik'shun) decrease in the caliber of blood vessels. **vasoconstric'tive,** adj.

vasoconstrictor (-kon-strik'tor) 1. causing constriction of the blood vessels. 2. a vasoconstrictive agent.

vasodentin (-den'tin) dentin provided with blood vessels, as in the teeth of some fishes.

vasodepression (-de-presh'un) decrease in vascular resistance with hypotension.

vasodepressor (-de-pres'sor) 1. having the effect of lowering the blood pressure through reduction in peripheral resistance. 2. an agent that causes vasodepression.

Vasodilan (-di'lan) trademark for a preparation of isoxsuprine.

vasodilatation (-dil"ah-ta'shun) a state of increased caliber of the blood vessels. **vasodi'lative,** adj.

vasodilation (-di-la'shun) increase in the caliber of blood vessels.

vasodilator (-di-la'tor) 1. causing dilatation of blood vessels. 2. a nerve or agent which causes dilatation of blood vessels.

vasoepididymostomy (-ep"ĭ-did"ĭ-mos'to-me) anastomosis of the vas (ductus) deferens and the epididymis.

vasoformative (-for'mah-tive) pertaining to or promoting the formation of blood vessels.

vasoganglion (-gang'gle-on) a vascular ganglion or rete.

vasography (vas-og"rah-fe) radiography of the blood vessels.

vasohypertonic (vas"o-hi"per-ton'ik) vasoconstrictor.

vasohypotonic (-hi"po-ton'ik) decreasing the tone of blood vessels.

vasoinhibitor (-in-hib'ĭ-tor) an agent which inhibits vasomotor nerves. **vasoinhib'itory,** adj.

vasoligation (-li-ga'shun) ligation of the vas (ductus) deferens.

vasomotion (-mo'shun) change in caliber of blood vessels.

vasomotor (-mo'tor) 1. affecting the caliber of blood vessels. 2. a vasomotor agent or nerve.

vasoneuropathy (-nu-rop'ah-the) a condition caused by combined vascular and neurologic defect.

vasoneurosis (-nu-ro'sis) angioneurosis.

vaso-orchidostomy (-or"kĭ-dos'to-me) anasto-

mosis of the epididymis to the severed end of the vas (ductus) deferens.

vasoparesis (pah-re'sis) paralysis of vasomotor nerves.

vasopressin (-pres'in) a hormone secreted by cells of the hypothalamic nuclei and stored in the posterior pituitary for release as necessary; it constricts blood vessels, raising the blood pressure, and increases peristalsis, exerts some influence on the uterus, and influences resorption of water by the kidney tubules, resulting in concentration of the urine. Also prepared synthetically or obtained from the posterior pituitary of domestic animals; used as an antidiuretic.

vasopressor (-pres'or) 1. stimulating contraction of the muscular tissue of the capillaries and arteries. 2. a vasopressor agent.

vasopuncture (-pungk'chur) puncture of the vas (ductus) deferens.

vasoreflex (-re'fleks) a reflex of blood vessels.

vasorelaxation (-re"lak-sa'shun) decrease of vascular pressure.

vasorrhaphy (vas-or'ah-fe) suture of the vas (ductus) deferens.

vasosection (vas"o-sek'shun) the severing of a vessel or vessels, especially of the ductus deferentes (vasa deferentia).

vasosensory (-sen'sor-e) supplying sensory filaments to the vessels.

vasospasm (vas'o-spazm) spasm of blood vessels, decreasing their caliber. **vasospas'tic,** adj.

vasostimulant (vas"o-stim'u-lant) stimulating vasomotor action.

vasostomy (vah-sos'to-me) surgical formation of an opening into the ductus (vas) deferens.

vasotomy (vah-sot'o-me) incision of the vas (ductus) deferens.

vasotonia (vas"o-to'ne-ah) tone or tension of the vessels.

vasotonic (-ton'ik) pertaining to, characterized by, or increasing vasotonia.

vasotrophic (-trof'ik) affecting nutrition through alteration of blood vessel caliber.

vasotropic (-trop'ik) tending to act on blood vessels.

vasovagal (-va'gal) vascular and vagal; see also under *attack.*

vasovasotomy (-vah-sot'o-me) anastomosis of the ends of the severed vas (ductus) deferens.

vasovesiculectomy (-vě-sik"u-lek'to-me) excision of the vas (ductus) deferens and seminal vesicle.

Vasoxyl (vas-ok'sil) trademark for preparations of methoxamine.

vastus (vas'tus) [L.] great; said of muscles.

V.C. acuity of color vision.

V-Cillin (ve-sil'in) trademark for a preparation of phenoxymethyl penicillin.

V.D. venereal disease.

V.D.G. venereal disease–gonorrhea.

V.D.H. valvular disease of the heart.

V.D.R.L. Venereal Disease Research Laboratory.

V.D.S. venereal disease–syphilis.

vection (vek′shun) the carrying of disease germs from an infected person to a well person.

vectis (vek′tis) a curved lever for making traction on the fetal head in labor.

vector (vek′tor) 1. a carrier, especially the animal (usually an arthropod) which transfers an infective agent from one host to another. 2. a quantity possessing magnitude, direction, and sense (positivity or negativity), and commonly represented by a straight line resembling an arrow: the length of the line denotes magnitude, the arrowhead denotes direction, and the position of the line with respect to an axis of reference denotes sense. **vecto′rial**, adj. **biological v.**, an anthropod vector in whose body the infecting organism develops or multiplies before becoming infective to the recipient individual. **mechanical v.**, an arthropod vector which transmits an infective organism from one host to another but which is not essential to the life cycle of the parasite.

vectorcardiogram (vek″tor-kar′de-o-gram″) the record, usually a photograph, of the loop formed on the oscilloscope in vectorcardiography.

vectorcardiography (-kar″de-og′rah-fe) the registration, usually by formation of a loop display on an oscilloscope, of the direction and magnitude (vector) of the moment-to-moment electromotive forces of the heart during one complete cycle. **vectorcardiograph′ic**, adj.

vegan (vej′an) a vegetarian who excludes from his diet all protein of animal origin.

veganism (vej′ah-nizm) strict adherence to a vegetable diet, with exclusion of all protein of animal origin.

vegetable (vej′ĕ-tah-b′l) 1. pertaining to or derived from plants. 2. any plant or species of plant, especially one cultivated as a source of food.

vegetal (vej′ĕ-tal) 1. pertaining to plants or to a plant. 2. vegetative.

vegetarian (vej″ĕ-ta′re-an) one who eats only foods of vegetable origin.

vegetarianism (vej″ĕ-ta′re-ah-nizm″) the restriction of one's food to substances of vegetable origin.

vegetation (vej″ĕ-ta′shun) any plantlike fungoid neoplasm or growth; a luxuriant fungus-like growth of pathologic tissue.

vegetative (vej″ĕ-ta″tiv) 1. concerned with growth and nutrition. 2. functioning involuntarily or unconsciously. 3. resting; denoting the portion of a cell cycle during which the cell is not replicating.

vegetoanimal (vej″ĕ-to-an′ĭ-mal) common to plants and animals.

vehicle (ve′ĭ-k′l) 1. an excipient. 2. any medium through which an impulse is propagated.

veil (vāl) 1. a covering structure. 2. a caul or piece of amniotic sac occasionally covering the face of a newborn child. 3. slight huskiness of the voice.

Veillonella (va″yon-el′ah) a genus of gram-negative bacteria (family Neisseriaceae), found as nonpathogenic parasites in the mouth, intestines, and urogenital and respiratory tracts of man and other animals.

vein (vān) a vessel in which blood flows toward the heart, in the systemic circulation carrying blood that has given up most of its oxygen. For names of veins of the body, *see the table*, and see Plates VIII and IX. **afferent v's**, veins that carry blood to an organ. **allantoic v's**, paired vessels that accompany the allantois, growing out from the primitive hindgut and entering the body stalk of the early embryo. **cardinal v's**, embryonic vessels that include the precardinal and postcardinal veins and the ducts of Cuvier (*common cardinal v's*). **emissary v.**, one passing through a foramen of the skull and draining blood from a cerebral sinus into a vessel outside the skull. **postcardinal v's**, paired vessels in the early embryo caudal to the heart. **precardinal v's**, paired venous trunks in the embryo cranial to the heart. **pulp v's**, vessels draining the venous sinuses of the spleen. **subcardinal v's**, paired vessels in the embryo, replacing the postcardinal veins and persisting to some degree as definitive vessels. **sublobular v's**, tributaries of the hepatic veins that receive the central veins of hepatic lobules. **supracardinal v's**, paired vessels in the embryo, developing later than the subcardinal veins and persisting chiefly as the lower segment of the inferior vena cava. **trabecular v's**, vessels coursing in splenic trabeculae, formed by tributary pulp veins. **varicose v.**, a dilated, tortuous vein, usually in the subcutaneous tissues of the leg; incompetency of the venous valve is associated. **vesalian v.**, an emissary vein connecting the cavernous sinus with the pterygoid venous plexus. **vitelline v's**, veins that return the blood from the yolk sac to the primitive heart of the early embryo.

Velacycline (vel″ah-si′klen) trademark for preparations of rolitetracycline.

velamen (ve-la′men), pl. *velam′ina* [L.] a membrane, meninx, or velum.

velamentous (vel″ah-men′tus) membranous and pendent; like a veil.

Velban (vel′ban) trademark for a preparation of vinblastine.

vellus (vel′us) the fine hair that succeeds the lanugo over most of the body.

velopharyngeal (vel″o-fah-rin′je-al) pertaining to the soft palate and pharynx.

velum (ve′lum), pl. *ve′la* [L.] a covering structure or veil. **ve′lar**, adj. **v. interpos′itum**, membranous roof of the third ventricle. **medullary v.**, one of the two portions (*superior medullary v.* and *inferior medullary v.*) of the white substance that form the roof of the fourth ventricle. **v. palati′num**, soft palate.

ven-, vene-, veni-, veno- word element [L.], *vein*.

vena (ve′nah), pl. *ve′nae* [L.] vein. **v. ca′va**, see *Table of Veins*.

venectasia (ve″nek-ta′ze-ah) phlebectasia.

venectomy (ve-nek′to-me) phlebectomy.

venenation (ven″ĕ-na′shun) poisoning; a poisoned condition.

venenous (ven′ĕ-nus) venomous.

venereal (vĕ-ne′re-al) due to or propagated by sexual intercourse.

venereologist (vĕ-ne″re-ol′o-jist) a specialist in venereology.

venereology (vĕ-ne″re-ol′o-je) the study and treatment of venereal diseases.

venery (ven′er-e) coitus.

venesection (ven″ĕ-sek′shun) phlebotomy.

venipuncture (ven″ĭ-pungk′chur) surgical puncture of a vein.

venisuture (-su′chur) phleborrhaphy.

venoclysis (ve-nok′lĭ-sis) phleboclysis.

venogram (ve′no-gram) phlebogram.

venography (ve-nog′rah-fe) phlebography.

venom (ven′om) poison, especially a toxic substance normally secreted by a serpent, insect, or other animal. **Russell's viper v.,** the venom of the Russell viper (*Vipera russelli*), which acts *in vitro* as an intrinsic thromboplastin and is useful in defining deficiencies of blood coagulation Factor X.

venomization (ven″om-i-za′shun) treatment of a substance with snake venom.

venomotor (ve″no-mo′tor) controlling dilation of constriction of the veins.

venomous (ven′o-mus) secreting poison; poisonous.

veno-occlusive (ve″no-ŏ-kloo′siv) characterized by obstruction of the veins.

venoperitoneostomy (-per″ĭ-to″ne-os′to-me) anastomosis of the saphenous vein with the peritoneum for drainage of ascites.

venosclerosis (-sklĕ-ro′sis) phlebosclerosis.

venosity (ve-nos′ĭ-te) 1. excess of venous blood in a part. 2. a plentiful supply of blood vessels or of venous blood.

venostasis (ve″no-sta′sis) retardation of the venous outflow in a part; see *phlebostasis.*

venotomy (ve-not′o-me) phlebotomy.

venous (ve′nus) pertaining to the veins.

venovenostomy (ve″no-ve-nos′to-me) phlebophlebostomy.

vent (vent) an opening or outlet, such as an opening that discharges pus, or the anus.

venter (ven′ter), pl. *ven′tres* [L.] 1. any belly-shaped part; a fleshy contractible part of a muscle. 2. the abdomen or stomach. 3. a hollowed part or cavity.

ventilation (ven″tĭ-la′shun) 1. the process or act of supplying a house or room continuously with fresh air. 2. the process of exchange of air between the lungs and the ambient air. 3. in psychiatry, the open discussion of grievances.

ventr(i)-, ventr(o)- word element [L.], *belly; front (anterior) aspect of the body; ventral aspect.*

ventrad (ven′trad) toward a belly, venter, or ventral aspect.

ventral (ven′tral) 1. pertaining to the abdomen or to any venter. 2. directed toward or situated on the belly surface; opposite of dorsal.

ventralis (ven-tra′lis) [L.] ventral.

ventricle (ven′trĭ-k'l) a small cavity or chamber, as in the brain or heart. **ventric′ular,** adj. **v. of Arantius,** 1. the rhomboid fossa, especially its lower end. 2. fifth v. **fifth v.,** the median cleft between the two laminae of the septum pellucidum. **fourth v.,** a median cavity in

the hindbrain, containing cerebrospinal fluid. **v. of larynx,** the space between the true and false vocal cords. **lateral v.,** the cavity in each cerebral hemisphere, derived from the cavity of the embryonic tube, containing cerebrospinal fluid. **left v.,** the lower chamber of the left side of the heart, which pumps oxygenated blood out through the aorta to all the tissues of the body. **Morgagni's v.,** v. of larynx. **pineal v.,** an extension of the third ventricle into the stalk of the pineal body. **right v.,** the lower chamber of the right side of the heart, which pumps venous blood through the pulmonary trunk and arteries to the capillaries of the lung. **third v.,** a narrow cleft below the corpus callosum, within the diencephalon between the two thalami. **Verga's v.,** an occasional space between the corpus callosum and fornix.

ventricornu (ven″trĭ-kor′nu) the anterior horn of gray matter in the spinal cord. **ventricor′nual,** adj.

ventriculitis (ven-trik″u-li′tis) inflammation of a ventricle, especially a cerebral ventricle.

ventriculo- word element [L.], *ventricle* (of heart or brain).

ventriculoatriostomy (ven-trik″u-lo-a″tre-os′to-me) introduction of a catheter with a one-way valve to drain cerebrospinal fluid from a cerebral ventricle to the right atrium via the jugular vein, for relief of hydrocephalus.

ventriculocisternostomy (-sis″ter-nos′to-me) surgical creation of a communication between the third ventricle and the interpeduncular cistern, for drainage of cerebrospinal fluid.

ventriculocordectomy (-kor-dek′to-me) punch resection of the vocal cords.

ventriculogram (ven-trik′u-lo-gram″) a radiograph of the cerebral ventricles.

ventriculography (ven-trik″u-log′rah-fe) 1. radiography of the cerebral ventricles after introduction of air or other contrast medium. 2. radiography of a ventricle of the heart after injection of a contrast medium.

ventriculometry (ven-trik″u-lom′ĕ-tre) measurement of intracranial pressure.

ventriculonector (ven-trik″u-lo-nek′tor) bundle of His.

ventriculopuncture (-pungk′chur) surgical puncture of a lateral ventricle of the brain.

ventriculoscopy (ven-trik″u-los′ko-pe) endoscopic or cystoscopic examination of cerebral ventricles.

ventriculostomy (ven-trik″u-los′to-me) surgical creation of a free communication between the third ventricle and the interpeduncular cistern for relief of hydrocephalus.

ventriculosubarachnoid (ven-trik″u-lo-sub″-ah-rak′noid) pertaining to the cerebral ventricles and subarachnoid space.

ventriculotomy (ven-trik″u-lot′o-me) incision of a ventricle of the heart.

ventriculus (ven-trik′u-lus), pl. *ventric′uli* [L.] 1. a ventricle. 2. the stomach.

ventricumbent (ven″trĭ-kum′bent) prone; lying on the belly.

ventriduct (ven′trĭ-dukt) to bring or carry ventrad.

COMMON NAME*	NA TERM†	REGION*	RECEIVES BLOOD FROM*	DRAINS INTO*
accompanying v. of hypoglossal nerve	v. comitans nervi hypoglossi	accompanies hypoglossal nerve	formed by union of profunda linguae v. and sublingual v.	facial, lingual, or internal jugular
adrenal v's. See suprarenal v., left and right.				
anastomotic v., inferior	v. anastomotica inferior	interconnects superficial middle cerebral v. and transverse sinus		
anastomotic v., superior	v. anastomotica superior	interconnects superficial middle cerebral v. and superior sagittal sinus		
angular v.	v. angularis	between eye and root of nose	formed by union of supratrochlear v. and supraorbital v.	continues inferiorly as facial v.
antebrachial v., median	v. mediana antebrachii	forearm between cephalic v. and basilic v.	a palmar venous plexus	cephalic v. and/or basilic v., or median cubital v.
appendicular v.	v. appendicularis	accompanies appendicular artery		joins anterior and posterior cecal v's to form ileocolic v.
v. of aqueduct of vestibule	v. aqueductus vestibuli	passes through aqueduct of vestibule	internal ear	superior petrosal sinus
arcuate v's of kidney	vv. arcuatae renis	a series of complete arches across the bases of the renal pyramids, formed by union of interlobular v's and straight venules of kidney		interlobar v's
auditory v's, internal. See labyrinthine v's.				
auricular v's, anterior	vv. auriculares anteriores	anterior part of auricle		superficial temporal v.
auricular v., posterior	v. auricularis posterior	passes down behind auricle	a plexus on side of head	joins retromandibular v. to form external jugular v.
axillary v.	v. axillaris	the upper limb	formed at lower border of teres major muscle by junction of basilic v. and brachial v.	at lateral border of first rib is continuous with subclavian v.
azygos v.	v. azygos	intercepting trunk for right intercostal v's as well as connecting branch between superior and inferior venae cavae; it ascends in front of and on right side of vertebrae	ascending lumbar v.	superior vena cava

*v. = vein; v's = (pl.) veins. †v. = [L.] vena; vv. = [L.(pl.)] venae.

COMMON NAME*	NA TERM†	REGION*	RECEIVES BLOOD FROM*	DRAINS INTO*
azygous v., left. *See* hemiazygos v.				
azygos v., lesser superior. *See* hemiazygos v., accessory.				
basal v.	v. basalis	passes from anterior perforated substance backward and around cerebral peduncle	anterior perforated substance	internal cerebral v.
basilic v.	v. basilica	forearm, superficially	ulnar side of dorsal rete of hand	joins brachial v's to form axillary v.
basilic v., median	v. mediana basilica	sometimes present as medial branch of a bifurcation of median antebrachial v.		basilic v.
basivertebral v's	vv. basivertebrales	venous sinuses in cancellous tissue of bodies of vertebrae, which communicate with venous plexus on anterior surface of vertebrae and with external and internal vertebral plexuses		
brachial v's	vv. brachiales	accompany brachial artery		join basilic v. to form axillary v.
brachiocephalic v's	vv. brachiocephalicae (dextra et sinistra)	thorax	head, neck, and upper limbs; formed at root of neck by union of ipsilateral internal jugular and subclavian v's	unite to form superior vena cava
bronchial v's	vv. bronchiales		larger subdivisions of bronchi	azygos v. on left; hemiazygos or superior intercostal v. on right
v. of bulb of penis	v. bulbi penis		bulb of penis	internal pudendal v.
v. of bulb of vestibule	v. bulbi vestibuli		bulb of vestibule of vagina	internal pudendal v.
cardiac v's, anterior	vv. cordis anteriores		anterior wall of right ventricle	right atrium of heart, or lesser cardiac v.
cardiac v., great	v. cordis magna		anterior surface of ventricles	coronary sinus
cardiac v., middle	v. cordis media		diaphragmatic surface of ventricles	coronary sinus
cardiac v., small	v. cordis parva		right atrium and ventricle	coronary sinus

cardiac v's, smallest	vv. cordis minimae	numerous small veins arising in myocardium, draining independently into cavities of heart and most readily seen in the atria		
carotid v., external. *See* retromandibular v.				
cavernous v's of penis	vv. cavernosae penis		corpora cavernosa	deep v's and dorsal v. of penis
central v's of liver	vv. centrales hepatis	in middle of hepatic lobules	liver substance	hepatic v.
central v. of retina	v. centralis retinae	eyeball	retinal v's	superior ophthalmic v.
central v. of suprarenal gland	v. centralis glandulae suprarenalis	the large single vein into which the various veins within the substance of the gland empty, and which continues at the hilus as the suprarenal v.		
cephalic v.	v. cephalica	winds anteriorly to pass along anterior border of brachioradial muscle; above elbow, ascends along lateral border of biceps muscle and pectoral border of deltoid muscle	radial side of dorsal rete of hand	axillary v.
cephalic v., accessory	v. cephalica accessoria	forearm	dorsal rete of hand	joins cephalic v. just above elbow
cephalic v., median	v. mediana cephalica	sometimes present as lateral branch formed by bifurcation of median antebrachial v.		cephalic v.
cerebellar v's, inferior	vv. cerebelli inferiores		inferior surface of cerebellum	transverse, sigmoid, and inferior petrosal sinuses, or occipital sinus
cerebellar v's, superior	vv. cerebelli superiores		upper surface of cerebellum	straight sinus and great cerebral v., or transverse and superior petrosal sinuses
cerebral v., anterior	v. cerebri anterior	accompanies anterior cerebral artery		basal v.
cerebral v., great	v. cerebri magna	curves around splenium of corpus callosum	formed by union of the 2 internal cerebral veins	continues as or drains into straight sinus
cerebral v's, inferior	vv. cerebri inferiores	veins that ramify on base and inferolateral surface of brain, those on inferior surface of frontal lobe draining into inferior sagittal sinus and cavernous sinus; those on temporal lobe into superior petrosal sinus and transverse sinus; and those on occipital lobe into straight sinus		
cerebral v's, internal (2)	vv. cerebri internae	pass backward from interventricular foramen through tela choroidea	formed by union of thalamostriate v. and choroid v.; collect blood from basal ganglia	unite at splenium of corpus callosum to form great cerebral v.
cerebral v., middle, deep	v. cerebri media profunda	accompanies middle cerebral artery in floor of lateral sulcus		basal v.

COMMON NAME*	NA TERM+	REGION*	RECEIVES BLOOD FROM*	DRAINS INTO*
cerebral v., middle, superficial	v. cerebri media superficialis	follows lateral cerebral fissure	lateral surface of cerebrum	cavernous sinus
cerebral v's, superior	vv. cerebri superiores	about 12 veins draining superolateral and medial surfaces of cerebrum toward longitudinal fissure	superolateral and medial surfaces of	superior sagittal sinus
cervical v., deep	v. cervicalis profunda	accompanies deep cervical artery down neck	a plexus in suboccipital triangle	vertebral v. or brachiocephalic v.
cervical v's, transverse	vv. transversae colli	accompany transverse cervical artery		subclavian v.
choroid v.	v. choroidea	runs whole length of choroid plexus	choroid plexus, hippocampus, fornix, corpus callosum	joins thalamostriate v. to form internal cerebral v.
ciliary v's	vv. ciliares	anterior vessels follow anterior ciliary arteries; posterior follow posterior ciliary arteries	arise in eyeball by branches from ciliary muscle; anterior ciliary v's also receive branches from sinus venosus, sclerae, episcleral v's and conjunctiva of eyeball	superior ophthalmic v.; posterior ciliary v's empty also into inferior ophthalmic v.
circumflex femoral v's, lateral	vv. circumflexae femoris laterales	accompany lateral circumflex femoral artery		femoral v. or profunda femoris v.
circumflex femoral v's, medial	vv. circumflexae femoris mediales	accompany medial circumflex femoral artery		femoral v. or profunda femoris v.
circumflex iliac v., deep	v. circumflexa ilium profunda	a common trunk formed by veins accompanying deep circumflex iliac artery	accompanying deep cir-	external iliac v.
circumflex iliac v., superficial	v. circumflexa ilium superficialis	accompanies superficial circumflex iliac artery		great saphenous v.
v. of cochlear canal	v. canaliculi		cochlea	superior bulb of internal jugular v.
colic v., left	v. colica sinistra	accompanies left colic artery		inferior mesenteric v.
colic v., middle	v. colica media	accompanies middle colic artery		superior mesenteric v.
colic v., right	v. colica dextra	accompanies right colic artery		superior mesenteric v.
conjunctival v's	vv. conjunctivales		conjunctiva	superior ophthalmic v.
coronary v's. *See* entries under cardiac v's.				
cubital v., median	v. mediana cubiti	the large connecting branch passing obliquely upward across cubital fossa	cephalic v., below elbow	basilic v.

Term	Latin	Regional	Drains into / connects
cutaneous v.	v. cutanea	one of the small veins that begin in papillae of skin, form subpapillary plexuses, and open into the subcutaneous veins	
cystic v.	v. cystica	gallbladder	right branch of portal v.
deep v's of clitoris	vv. profundae clitoridis	clitoris	vesical venous plexus
deep v's of penis	vv. profundae penis	penis	dorsal v. of penis
digital v's of foot, dorsal	vv. digitales dorsales pedis	dorsal surfaces of toes	unite at clefts to form dorsal metatarsal v's
digital v's, palmar	vv. digitales palmares	accompany proper and common palmar digital arteries	superficial palmar venous arch
digital v's, plantar	vv. digitales plantares	plantar surfaces of toes	unite at clefts to form plantar metatarsal v's
diploic v., frontal	v. diploica frontalis	frontal bone	supraorbital v. externally, or superior sagittal sinus internally
diploic v., occipital	v. diploica occipitalis	occipital bone	occipital v. or transverse sinus
diploic v., temporal, anterior	v. diploica temporalis anterior	lateral portion of frontal bone, anterior part of parietal bone	sphenoparietal sinus internally, or a deep temporal v. externally
diploic v., temporal, posterior	v. diploica temporalis posterior	parietal bone	transverse sinus
dorsal v. of clitoris, deep	v. dorsalis clitoridis profunda	accompanies dorsal artery of clitoris	vesical plexus
dorsal v's of clitoris, superficial	vv. dorsales clitoridis superficiales	clitoris, subcutaneously	external pudendal v.
dorsal v. of penis, deep	v. dorsalis penis profunda	the single median vein lying subfascially in penis between the dorsal arteries; it begins in small veins around corona of glans, is joined by deep veins of penis as it passes proximally, and passes between arcuate pubic and transverse perineal ligaments, where it divides into a left and a right vein to join prostatic plexus	
dorsal v's of penis, superficial	vv. dorsales penis superficiales	penis, subcutaneously	external pudendal v.
dorsal v's of tongue. See lingual v's, dorsal.	vv. dorsales linguae		
emissary v., condylar	v. emissaria condylaris	a small vein running through condylar canal of skull, connecting sigmoid sinus with vertebral v. or internal jugular v.	
emissary v., mastoid	v. emissaria mastoidea	a small vein passing through mastoid foramen of skull, connecting sigmoid sinus with occipital v. or posterior auricular v.	
emissary v., occipital	v. emissaria occipitalis	an occasional small vein running through a minute foramen in occipital protuberance of skull, connecting confluence of sinuses with occipital v.	

TABLE OF VEINS (*Continued*)

COMMON NAME*	NA TERM†	REGION*	RECEIVES BLOOD FROM*	DRAINS INTO*
emissary v., parietal	v. emissaria parietalis	a small vein passing through parietal foramen of skull, connecting superior sagittal sinus with superficial temporal v's		
epigastric v., inferior	v. epigastrica inferior	accompanies inferior epigastric artery		external iliac v.
epigastric v., superficial	v. epigastrica superficialis	accompanies superficial epigastric artery		great saphenous v. or femoral v.
epigastric v's, superior	vv. epigastricae superiores	accompany superior epigastric artery		internal thoracic v.
episcleral v's	vv. episclerales	around cornea		vorticose v's and ciliary v's
esophageal v's	vv. esophageae		esophagus	hemiazygos v. and azygos v., or left brachiocephalic v.
ethmoidal v's	vv. ethmoidales	accompany anterior and posterior ethmoidal arteries and emerge from ethmoidal foramina		superior ophthalmic v.
facial v.	v. facialis	the vein beginning at medial angle of eye as angular v., descending behind facial artery, and usually ending in internal jugular v.; sometimes joins retromandibular v. to form a common trunk		
facial v., deep	v. faciei profunda		pterygoid plexus	facial v.
facial v., posterior. *See* retromandibular v.				
facial v., transverse	v. transversa faciei	passes backward with transverse facial artery just below zygomatic arch		retromandibular v.
femoral v.	v. femoralis	follows course of femoral artery in proximal two thirds of thigh	continuation of popliteal v.	at inguinal ligament becomes external iliac v.
femoral v., deep	v. profunda femoris	accompanies deep femoral artery		femoral v.
fibular v's. *See* peroneal v's.	vv. fibulares (NA alternative for vv. peroneae)			
gastric v., left	v. gastrica sinistra	accompanies left gastric artery		portal v.
gastric v., right	v. gastrica dextra	accompanies right gastric artery		portal v.
gastric v's, short	vv. gastricae breves		left portion of greater curvature of stomach	splenic v.
gastroepiploic v., left	v., gastroepiploica sinistra	accompanies left gastroepiploic artery		splenic v.

708

gastroepiploic v., right *v. gastroepiploica dextra*	accompanies right gastroepiploic artery	superior mesenteric v.
genicular v's *vv. genus*	accompany genicular arteries	popliteal v.
gluteal v's, inferior *vv. gluteae inferiores*	accompany inferior gluteal artery; unite into a single vessel after passing through greater sciatic foramen	internal iliac v.
gluteal v's, superior *vv. gluteae superiores*	accompany superior gluteal artery and pass through greater sciatic foramen	internal iliac v.
hemiazygos v. *v. hemiazygos*	an intercepting trunk for lower left posterior intercostal v's; ascends on left side of vertebrae to eighth thoracic vertebra, where it may receive accessory branch, and crosses vertebral column	azygos v.
hemiazygos v., accessory *v. hemiazygos accessoria*	the descending intercepting trunk for upper, often fourth through eighth, left posterior intercostal v's; it lies on left side and at eighth thoracic vertebra joins hemiazygos v. or crosses to right side to join azygos v. directly; above, it may communicate with left superior intercostal v.	
hemorrhoidal v's. *See* entries under rectal v's.		
hepatic v's *vv. hepaticae*	2 or 3 large veins in an upper group and 6 to 20 small veins in a lower group, forming successively larger vessels	inferior vena cava on posterior aspect of liver
hypogastric v. *See* iliac v., internal.		
ileal v's. *See* jejunal and ileal v's.		
ileocolic v. *v. ileocolica*	accompanies ileocolic artery	superior mesenteric v.
iliac v., common *v. iliaca communis*	ascends to right side of fifth lumbar vertebra	arises at sacroiliac joint by union of external and internal iliac v's
		unites with fellow of opposite side to form inferior vena cava
iliac v., external *v. iliaca externa*	extends from inguinal ligament to sacroiliac joint	continuation of femoral v.
		joins internal iliac v. to form common iliac v.
iliac v., internal *v. iliaca interna*	extends from greater sciatic notch to brim of pelvis	formed by union of parietal branches
		joins external iliac v. to form common iliac v.
iliolumbar v. *v. iliolumbalis*	accompanies iliolumbar artery	internal iliac v. and/or common iliac v.
innominate v's. *See* brachiocephalic v's.		

Table of Veins (Continued)

COMMON NAME*	NA TERM†	REGION*	RECEIVES BLOOD FROM*	DRAINS INTO*
intercapital v's	vv. intercapitales	veins at clefts of fingers that pass between heads of metacarpal bones and establish communication between dorsal and palmar venous systems of hand		
intercostal v's, anterior (12 pairs)	vv. intercostales anteriores	accompany anterior thoracic arteries		internal thoracic v's
intercostal v., highest	v. intercostalis suprema	first posterior intercostal vein of either side, which passes over apex of lung		brachiocephalic, vertebral, or superior intercostal v.
intercostal v's, posterior, IV and XI	vv. intercostales posteriores (IV et XI)	accompany posterior intercostal arteries IV and XI		azygos v. on right; hemiazygos or accessory hemiazygos v. on left
intercostal v., superior, left	v. intercostalis superior sinistra	crosses arch of aorta	formed by union of second, third, and sometimes fourth posterior intercostal v's	left brachiocephalic v.
intercostal v., superior, right	v. intercostalis superior dextra		formed by union of second, third, and sometimes fourth posterior intercostal v's	azygos v.
interlobar v's of kidney	vv. interlobares renis	pass down between renal pyramids	venous arcades of kidney	unite to form renal v.
interlobular v's of kidney	vv. interlobulares renis		capillary network of renal cortex	venous arcades of kidney
interlobular v's of liver	vv. interlobulares hepatis	arise between hepatic lobules	liver	portal v.
interosseous v's of foot, dorsal. See metatarsal v's, dorsal.				
intervertebral v.	v. intervertebralis	vertebral column	vertebral venous plexuses	in neck, vertebral v.; in thorax, intercostal v's; in abdomen, lumbar v's; in pelvis, lateral sacral v's
jejunal v's. See jejunal and ileal v's.				

English name	Latin name	Description	Region	Drains into
jejunal and ileal v's	vv. jejunales et ilei		jejunum and ileum	superior mesenteric v.
jugular v., anterior	v. jugularis anterior	arises under chin and passes down neck		external jugular v., or subclavian v., or jugular venous arch
jugular v., external	v. jugularis externa	begins in parotid gland behind angle of jaw and passes down neck	formed by union of retromandibular v. and posterior auricular v.	subclavian v., internal jugular v., or brachiocephalic v.
jugular v., internal	v. jugularis interna	from jugular fossa, descends in neck with internal carotid artery and then with common carotid artery	begins as superior bulb, draining much of head and neck	joins subclavian v. to form brachiocephalic v.
labial v's, anterior	vv. labiales anteriores		anterior aspect of labia in female	external pudendal v.
labial v's, inferior	vv. labiales inferiores		region of lower lip	facial v.
labial v's, posterior	vv. labiales posteriores		labia in female	vesical venous plexus
labial v., superior	v. labialis superior		region of upper lip	facial v.
labyrinthine v's	vv. labyrinthi	pass through internal acoustic meatus	cochlea	inferior petrosal sinus or transverse sinus
lacrimal v.	v. lacrimalis		lacrimal gland	superior ophthalmic v.
laryngeal v., inferior	v. laryngea inferior		larynx	inferior thyroid v.
laryngeal v., superior	v. laryngea superior		larynx	superior thyroid v.
lingual v.	v. lingualis	a deep vein, following distribution of lingual artery		internal jugular v.
lingual v., deep	v. profunda linguae		deep aspect of tongue	joins sublingual v. to form accompanying v. of hypoglossal nerve
lingual v's, dorsal	vv. dorsales linguae	veins that unite with a small vein accompanying lingual artery and join main lingual trunk		
lumbar v's, I and II	vv. lumbales (I et II)	accompany first and second lumbar arteries		ascending lumbar v.
lumbar v's, III and IV	vv. lumbales (III et IV)	accompany third and fourth lumbar arteries		usually, inferior vena cava
lumbar v., ascending	v. lumbalis ascendens	an ascending intercepting vein for lumbar v's of either side; it begins in lateral sacral region and ascends to first lumbar vertebra, where by union with subcostal v. it becomes on right side the azygos v. and on left the hemiazygos v.		
maxillary v's	vv. maxillares	usually form a single short trunk with pterygoid plexus		joins superficial temporal v. in parotid gland to form retromandibular v.
mediastinal v's	vv. mediastinales		anterior mediastinum	brachiocephalic v., azygos v., or superior vena cava

TABLE OF VEINS (Continued)

COMMON NAME*	NA TERM†	REGION*	RECEIVES BLOOD FROM*	DRAINS INTO*
meningeal v's	vv. meningeae	accompany meningeal arteries	dura mater (also communicate with lateral lacunae)	regional sinuses and veins
meningeal v's, middle	vv. meningeae mediae	accompany middle meningeal artery		pterygoid venous plexus
mesenteric v., inferior	v. mesenterica inferior	follows distribution of inferior mesenteric artery		splenic v.
mesenteric v., superior	v. mesenterica superior	follows distribution of superior mesenteric artery		joins splenic v. to form portal v.
metacarpal v's, dorsal	vv. metacarpeae dorsales	veins arising from union of dorsal veins of adjacent fingers and passing proximally to join in forming dorsal venous network of hand		deep palmar venous arch
metacarpal v's, palmar	vv. metacarpeae palmares	accompany palmar metacarpal arteries		deep palmar venous arch
metatarsal v's, dorsal	vv. metatarseae dorsales		arise from dorsal digital v's of toes at clefts of toes	dorsal venous arch
metatarsal v's, plantar	vv. metatarseae plantares	deep veins of foot	arise from plantar digital v's at clefts of toes	plantar venous arch
musculophrenic v's	vv. musculophrenicae	accompany musculophrenic artery	parts of diaphragm and wall of thorax and abdomen	internal thoracic v's
nasal v's, external	vv. nasales externae	small ascending branches from nose		angular v., facial v.
nasofrontal v.	v. nasofrontalis		supraorbital v.	superior ophthalmic v.
oblique v. of left atrium	v. obliqua atrii sinistri	left atrium of heart		coronary sinus
obturator v's	vv. obturatoriae	enter pelvis though obturator canal	hip joint and regional muscles	internal iliac v. and/or inferior epigastric v.
occipital v.	v. occipitalis	scalp; follows distribution of occipital artery		opens under trapezius muscle into suboccipital venous plexus, or accompanies occipital artery to end in internal jugular v.
ophthalmic v., inferior	v. ophthalmica inferior	a vein formed by confluence of muscular and ciliary branches, and running backward either to join superior ophthalmic v. or to open directly into cavernous sinus; it sends a communicating branch through inferior orbital fissure to join pterygoid venous plexus		

ophthalmic v., superior	v. ophthalmica superior	a vein beginning at medial angle of eye, where it communicates with frontal, supraorbital, and angular v's; it follows distribution of ophthalmic artery, and may be joined by inferior ophthalmic v. at superior orbital fissure before opening into cavernous sinus	
ovarian v., left	v. ovarica sinistra	pampiniform plexus of broad ligament on left	left renal v.
ovarian v., right	v. ovarica dextra	pampiniform plexus of broad ligament on right	inferior vena cava
palatine v., external	v. palatina externa	tonsils and soft palate	facial v.
palpebral v's	vv. palpebrales	small branches from eyelids	
palpebral v's, inferior	vv. palpebrales inferiores	lower eyelid	superior ophthalmic v. facial v.
palpebral v's, superior	vv. palpebrales superiores	upper eyelid	angular v.
pancreatic v's	vv. pancreaticae	pancreas	splenic v., superior mesenteric v.
pancreaticoduodenal v's	vv. pancreaticoduodenales	4 veins that drain blood from pancreas and duodenum, closely following pancreaticoduodenal arteries, a superior and an inferior vein originating from an anterior and a posterior venous arcade; anterior superior v. joins right gastroepiploic v., and posterior superior v. joins portal v.; anterior and posterior inferior v's join, sometimes as one trunk, uppermost jejunal v. or superior mesenteric v.	
paraumbilical v's	vv. paraumbilicales	veins that communicate with portal v. above and descend to anterior abdominal wall to anastomose with superior and inferior epigastric and superior vesical v's in region of umbilicus; they form a significant part of collateral circulation of portal v. in event of hepatic obstruction	
parotid v's	vv. parotideae	parotid gland	superficial temporal v.
perforating v's	vv. perforantes	accompany perforating arteries of thigh	profunda femoris v.
pericardiac v's	vv. pericardiaceae	pericardium	brachiocephalic, inferior thyroid, and azygos v's, superior vena cava
pericardiacophrenic v's	vv. pericardiacophrenicae	pericardium and diaphragm	left brachiocephalic v.
peroneal v's	vv. peroneae	accompany peroneal artery	posterior tibial v.
pharyngeal v's	vv. pharyngeae	pharyngeal plexus	internal jugular v.
phrenic v's, inferior	vv. phrenicae inferiores	accompany inferior phrenic arteries	on right, enters inferior vena cava; on left, enters left suprarenal or renal v., or inferior vena cava

COMMON NAME*	NA TERM†	REGION*	RECEIVES BLOOD FROM*	DRAINS INTO*
phrenic v's, superior. *See* pericardiacophrenic v's.				
popliteal v.	v., poplitea	follows popliteal artery	formed by union of anterior and posterior tibial v's	at adductor hiatus becomes femoral v.
portal v.	v. portae	a short, thick trunk formed by union of superior mesenteric and splenic v's behind neck of pancreas; it ascends to right end of porta hepatis, where it divides into successively smaller branches, following branches of hepatic artery, until it forms a capillary-like system of sinusoids that permeates entire substance of liver		
posterior v. of left ventricle	v. posterior ventriculi sinistri cordis		posterior surface of left ventricle	coronary sinus
prepyloric v.	v. prepylorica	accompanies prepyloric artery, passing upward over anterior surface of junction between pylorus and duodenum		right gastric v.
profunda femoris v. *See* femoral v., deep.				
profunda linguae v. *See* lingual v., deep.				
v. of pterygoid canal	v. canalis pterygoidei	passes through pterygoid canal		pterygoid plexus
pudendal v's, external	vv. pudendae externae	follow distribution of external pudendal artery		great saphenous v.
pudendal v., internal	v. pudenda interna	follows course of internal pudendal artery		internal iliac v.
pulmonary v., inferior, left	v. pulmonalis inferior sinistra		lower lobe of left lung	left atrium of heart
pulmonary v., inferior, right	v. pulmonalis inferior dextra		lower lobe of right lung	left atrium of heart
pulmonary v., superior, left	v. pulmonalis superior sinistra		upper lobe of left lung	left atrium of heart
pulmonary v., superior, right	v. pulmonalis superior dextra		upper and middle lobes of right lung	left atrium of heart
pyloric v. *See* gastric v., right.				
radial v's	vv. radiales	accompany radial artery		brachial v's
ranine v. *See* sublingual v.				
rectal v's, inferior	vv. rectales inferiores		rectal plexus	internal pudendal v.

Term	Latin			
rectal v's, middle	vv. rectales mediae		rectal plexus	internal iliac and superior rectal v's
rectal v., superior	v. rectalis superior	establishes connection between portal and systemic systems	upper part of rectal plexus	inferior mesenteric v.
renal v's	vv. renales	short, thick trunks, one from either kidney, the one on the left being longer than that on the right	kidneys	inferior vena cava
retromandibular v.	v. retromandibularis	the vein formed in upper part of parotid gland behind neck of mandible by union of maxillary and superficial temporal v's; it passes downward through the gland, communicates with facial v. and, emerging from the gland, joins with posterior auricular v. to form external jugular v.		
sacral v's, lateral	vv. sacrales laterales	follow lateral sacral arteries		help form lateral sacral plexus; empty into internal iliac v. or superior gluteal v's
sacral v., median	v. sacralis mediana	follows median sacral artery		common iliac v.
saphenous v., accessory	v. saphena accessoria		when present, medial and posterior superficial parts of thigh	great saphenous v.
saphenous v., great	v. saphena magna	extends from dorsum of foot to just below inguinal ligament		femoral v.
saphenous v., small	v. saphena parva	from behind ankle passes up back of leg to knee		popliteal v.
scrotal v's, anterior	vv. scrotales anteriores		anterior aspect of scrotum	external pudendal v.
scrotal v's, posterior	vv. scrotales posteriores		scrotum	vesical venous plexus
v. of septum pellucidum	v. septi pellucidi		septum pellucidum	thalamostriate v.
sigmoid v's	vv. sigmoideae		sigmoid colon	inferior mesenteric v.
spinal v's	vv. spinales	anastomosing networks of small veins that drain blood from spinal cord and its pia mater into internal vertebral venous plexuses		
spiral v. of modiolus	v. spiralis modioli		modiolus	labyrinthine v's
splenic v.	v. lienalis	passes from left to right of neck of pancreas	formed by union of several branches at hilus of spleen	joins superior mesenteric v. to form portal v.
stellate v's of kidney	venulae stellatae renis		superficial parts of renal cortex	interlobular v's of kidney
sternocleidomastoid v.	v. sternocleidomastoidea	follows course of sternocleidomastoid artery		internal jugular v.
striate v.	v. striata		anterior perforated substance of brain	basal v.

TABLE OF VEINS (*Continued*)

COMMON NAME*	NA TERM†	REGION*	RECEIVES BLOOD FROM*	DRAINS INTO*
stylomastoid v. subclavian v.	v. stylomastoidea v. subclavia	follows stylomastoid artery follows subclavian artery	continues axillary v. as main venous channel of upper limb	retromandibular v. joins internal jugular v. to form brachiocephalic v.
subcostal v.	v. subcostalis	accompanies subcostal artery		joins ascending lumbar v. to form azygos v. on right, hemiazygos v. on left
subcutaneous v's of abdomen	vv. subcutaneae abdominis	superficial layers of abdominal wall		
sublingual v. submental v. supraorbital v.	v. sublingualis v. submentalis v. supraorbitalis	follows sublingual artery follows submental artery passes down forehead lateral to supratrochlear v.		lingual v. facial v. joins supratrochlear v. at root of nose to form angular v.
suprarenal v., left suprarenal v., right suprascapular v.	v. suprarenalis sinistra v. suprarenalis dextra v. suprascapularis	accompanies suprascapular artery (sometimes as 2 veins that unite)	left suprarenal gland right suprarenal gland	left renal v. inferior vena cava usually into external jugular v., occasionally into subclavian v.
supratrochlear v's (2)	vv. supratrochleares		venous plexuses high up on forehead	join supraorbital v. at root of nose to form angular v.
temporal v's, deep	vv. temporales profundae		deep portions of temporal muscle	pterygoid plexus
temporal v., middle	v. temporalis media	descends deep to fascia to zygoma	arises in substance of temporal muscle	joins superficial temporal v.
temporal v's, superficial	vv. temporales superficiales	veins that drain lateral part of scalp in frontal and parietal regions, the branches forming a single superficial temporal v. in front of ear, just above zygoma; this descending vein receives middle temporal and transverse facial v's and, entering parotid gland, unites with maxillary v. deep to neck of mandible to form retromandibular v.		
testicular v., left testicular v., right thalamostriate v.	v. testicularis sinistra v. testicularis dextra v. thalamostriata		left pampiniform plexus right pampiniform plexus corpus striatum and thalamus	left renal v. inferior vena cava joins choroid v. to form internal cerebral v's

Term	Latin (NA)	Description	Drains into
thoracic v's, internal	vv. thoracicae internae	2 veins formed by junction of the veins accompanying internal thoracic artery of either side; each continues along the artery to open into brachiocephalic v.	
thoracic v., lateral	v. thoracica lateralis	accompanies lateral thoracic artery	axillary v.
thoracoacromial v.	v. thoracoacromialis	follows thoracoacromial artery	subclavian v.
thoracoepigastric v's	vv. thoracoepigastricae	long, longitudinal, superficial veins in anterolateral subcutaneous tissue of trunk	superiorly into lateral thoracic v.; inferiorly into femoral v.
thymic v's	vv. thymicae	thymus	left brachiocephalic v.
thyroid v., inferior	v. thyroidea inferior	either of 2 veins, left and right, that drain thyroid plexus into left and right brachiocephalic v's; occasionally they may unite into a common trunk to empty, usually, into left brachiocephalic v.	
thyroid v's, middle	vv. thyroideae mediae	thyroid gland	internal jugular v.
thyroid v., superior	v. thyroidea superior	arises from side of upper part of thyroid gland	internal jugular v., occasionally in common with facial v.
tibial v's, anterior	vv. tibiales anteriores	accompany anterior tibial artery	join posterior tibial v's to form popliteal v.
tibial v's, posterior	vv. tibiales posteriores	accompany posterior tibial artery	join anterior tibial v's to form popliteal v.
tracheal v's	vv. tracheales	trachea	brachiocephalic v.
tympanic v's	vv. tympanicae	small veins from middle ear that pass through petrotympanic fissure and open into the plexus around temporomandibular joint	retromandibular v.
ulnar v's	vv. ulnares	accompany ulnar artery	join radial v's at elbow to form brachial v's
umbilical v.	v. umbilicalis (formerly)	in the early embryo, either of the paired veins that carry blood from chorion to sinus venosus and heart; they later fuse and become left umbilical v. of fetus	
umbilical v. of fetus, left	v. umbilicalis sinistra	the vein formed by fusion of atrophied right umbilical v. with the left umbilical v., which carries all the blood from placenta to ductus venosus	
uterine v's	vv. uterinae	uterine plexus	internal iliac v's
vena cava, inferior	vena cava inferior	the venous trunk for the lower limbs and for pelvic and abdominal viscera; it begins at level of fifth lumbar vertebra by union of common iliac v's and ascends on right of aorta	right atrium of heart
vena cava, superior	vena cava superior	the venous trunk draining blood from head, neck, upper limbs, and thorax; it begins by union of 2 brachiocephalic v's and passes directly downward	right atrium of heart

717

TABLE OF VEINS (*Concluded*)

COMMON NAME*	NA TERM†	REGION*	RECEIVES BLOOD FROM*	DRAINS INTO*
vertebral v.	v. vertebralis	passes with vertebral artery through transverse foramina of upper 6 cervical vertebrae	suboccipital venous plexus	brachiocephalic v.
vertebral v., accessory	v. vertebralis accessoria	descends with vertebral v. and emerges through transverse foramen of seventh cervical vertebra	a plexus formed around vertebral artery by vertebral v.	brachiocephalic v.
vertebral v., anterior	v. vertebralis anterior		venous plexus around transverse processes of upper cervical vertebrae	vertebral v.
vesical v's	vv. vesicales		vesical plexus	internal iliac v.
vestibular v's	vv. vestibulares		vestibule of labyrinth	labyrinthine v's
vorticose v's (4)	vv. vorticosae	eyeball	choroid	superior ophthalmic v.

ventrimeson (ven″trĭ-mes′on) the median line on the ventral surface. **ventrime′sal,** adj.

ventrofixation (ven″tro-fik-sa′shun) fixation of a viscus, e.g., the uterus, to the abdominal wall.

ventrohysteropexy (-his′ter-o-pek″se) ventrofixation of the uterus.

ventrolateral (-lat′er-al) both ventral and lateral.

ventroscopy (ven-tros′ko-pe) illumination of the abdominal cavity for purposes of examination.

ventrose (ven′trōs) having a belly-like expansion.

ventrosuspension (ven″tro-sus-pen′shun) ventrofixation.

ventrotomy (ven-trot′o-me) celiotomy.

venula (ven′u-lah), pl. *ven′ulae* [L.] venule.

venule (ven′ūl) any of the small vessels that collect blood from the capillary plexuses and join to form veins. **ven′ular,** adj. **stellate v's of kidney,** see *Table of Veins*.

Veralba (ver-al′bah) trademark for a mixture of protoveratrines A and B.

Veratrum (ver-a′trum) a genus of poisonous liliaceous plants, including *V. al′bum* (European white hellebore) and *V. vir′ide* (American green hellbore), both of which are a source of antihypertensive alkaloids.

verbigeration (ver-bij″er-a′shun) abnormal repetition of meaningless words and phrases.

verge (verj) a circumference or ring. **anal v.,** the opening of the anus on the surface of the body.

vergence (ver′jens) disjunctive movement of the eyes in opposite directions.

Veriloid (ver′ĭ-loid) trademark for a preparation of alkavervir.

vermicide (ver′mĭ-sīd) an agent lethal to intestinal animal parasites.

vermicular (ver-mik′u-lar) wormlike in shape or appearance.

vermiculation (ver-mik″u-la′shun) peristaltic motion; peristalsis.

vermiculous (ver-mik′u-lus) 1. wormlike. 2. infested with worms.

vermiform (ver′mĭ-form) worm-shaped.

vermifugal (ver-mif′u-gal) expelling worms or intestinal animal parasites.

vermifuge (ver′mĭ-fūj) an agent that expels worms or intestinal animal parasites; an anthelmintic.

vermilionectomy (ver-mil″yon-ek′to-me) excision of the vermilion border of the lip.

vermin (ver′min) an external animal parasite; such parasites collectively.

vermination (ver″mĭ-na′shun) infestation with worms or with vermin.

verminous (ver′mĭ-nus) pertaining to, due to, or abounding in worms or in vermin.

vermis (ver′mis) [L.] 1. a worm, or wormlike structure. 2. v. cerebelli. **v. cerebel′li,** the median part of the cerebellum, between the two hemispheres.

vernix (ver′niks) [L.] varnish. **v. caseo′sa,** an unctuous substance composed of sebum and desquamated epithelial cells.

verruca (vĕ-ru′kah), pl. *verru′cae* [L.] 1. a wart. 2. one of the wartlike elevations on the endocardium in various types of endocarditis. **ver′rucose, verru′cous,** adj. **v. acumina′ta,** condyloma acuminatum. **v. necrogen′ica,** tuberculosis verrucosa. **v. perua′na, v. peruvia′na,** verruga peruana. **v. pla′na,** a small, smooth, usually skin-colored or light brown, slightly raised wart sometimes occurring in great numbers; seen most often in children. **v. planta′ris,** a viral epidermal tumor on the sole of the foot.

verruciform (vĕ-roo′sĭ-form) wartlike.

verruga (vĕ-roo′gah) [Sp.] wart. **v. perua′na,** a hemangioma-like tumor or nodule occurring in Carrión's disease.

version (ver′zhun) the act of turning; especially the manual turning of the fetus in delivery. **bipolar v.,** turning effected by acting upon both poles of the fetus, either by external or combined version. **cephalic v.,** turning of the fetus so that the head presents. **combined v.,** external and internal versions together. **external v.,** turning effected by outside manipulation. **internal v.,** turning effected by the hand or fingers inserted through the dilated cervix. **pelvic v.,** version by manipulation of the breech. **podalic v.,** conversion of a more unfavorable presentation into a footling presentation. **spontaneous v.,** one which occurs without aid from any extraneous force.

vertebr(o)- word element [L.], *vertebra; spine.*

vertebra (ver′tĕ-brah), pl. *ver′tebrae* [L.] any of the 33 bones of the vertebral (spinal) column, comprising 7 *cervical,* 12 *thoracic,* 5 *lumbar,* 5 *sacral,* and 4 *coccygeal* vertebrae. See *Table of Bones.* **ver′tebral,** adj. **basilar v.,** the lowest lumbar vertebra. **cervical vertebrae,** the seven vertebrae closest to the skull, constituting the skeleton of the neck. **coccygeal vertebrae,** the three to five segments of the vertebral column most distant from the skull, which fuse to form the coccyx. **cranial v.,** the segments of the skull and facial bones regarded by some as modified vertebrae. **v. denta′ta,** the second cervical vertebra, or axis. **dorsal vertebrae,** thoracic vertebrae. **false vertebrae,** those vertebrae which normally fuse with adjoining segments: the sacral and coccygeal vertebrae. **lumbar vertebrae,** the five segments of the vertebral column between the twelfth thoracic vertebra and the sacrum. **v. mag′num,** the sacrum. **odontoid v.,** the second cervical vertebra, or axis. **v. pla′na,** a condition of spondylitis in which the body of the vertebra is reduced to a sclerotic disk. **sacral vertebrae,** the segments (usually five) below the lumbar vertebrae, which normally fuse to form the sacrum. **sternal v.,** sternebra. **thoracic vertebrae,** the 12 segments of the vertebral column between the cervical and the lumbar vertebrae, giving attachment to the ribs and forming part of the posterior wall of the thorax. **true vertebrae,** those segments of the vertebral column that normally remain unfused throughout life: the cervical, thoracic, and lumbar vertebrae.

vertebrarium (ver″tĕ-bra′re-um) [L.] the vertebral column.

Vertebrata (ver″tĕ-bra′tah) a subphylum of the

Chordata, comprising all animals having a vertebral column, including mammals, birds, reptiles, amphibians, and fishes.

vertebrate (ver′tĕ-brāt) 1. having a spinal column (vertebrae). 2. an animal with a vertebral column; any member of the Vertebrata.

vertebrectomy (ver″tĕ-brek′to-me) excision of a vertebra.

vertebrobasilar (ver″te-bro-bas′ĭ-lar) pertaining to or affecting the vertebral and basilar arteries.

vertebrochondral (-kon′dral) pertaining to a vertebra and a costal cartilage.

vertebrocostal (-kos′tal) pertaining to a vertebra and a rib.

vertebrosternal (-ster′nal) pertaining to a vertebra and the sternum.

vertex (ver′teks) the summit or top, especially the top of the head (*v. cra′nii*).

vertical (ver-tĭ-kal) 1. perpendicular to the plane of the horizon. 2. relating to the vertex.

verticalis (ver″tĭ-ka′lis) [L.] vertical.

verticillate (ver-tis′ĭ-lāt) arranged in whorls.

vertigo (ver′tĭ-go) a sensation of rotation or movement of one's self (*subjective v.*) or of one's surroundings (*objective v.*) in any plane. **vertig′inous,** adj. **auditory v., aural v.,** Meniere's disease. **central v.,** that due to disorder of the central nervous system. **cerebral v.,** due to some brain disease. **epileptic v.,** that which attends or follows an epileptic attack. **gastric v.,** that associated with disease or disorders of the stomach. **labyrinthine v.,** a form associated with disease of the labyrinth of the ear. **objective v.,** see *vertigo*. **ocular v.,** a form due to eye disease. **organic v.,** that due to vestibular brain disease or to tabes dorsalis. **peripheral v.,** vestibular v. **positional v., postural v.,** that associated with a specific position of the head in space or with changes in position of the head in space. **subjective v.,** see *vertigo*. **toxemic v.,** that due to poisoning, alcoholism, uremia, or lithemia. **vestibular v.,** vertigo due to disturbances of the vestibular centers or pathways in the central nervous system.

vertigraphy (ver-tig′rah-fe) see *body-section roentgenography*.

verumontanitis (ver″u-mon″tah-ni′tis) inflammation of the colliculus seminalis.

verumontanum (ver″u-mon-ta′num) colliculus seminalis.

vesalianum (vĕ-sa″le-a′num) a sesamoid bone in the tendon of origin of the gastrocnemius muscle, or in the angle between the cuboid and fifth metatarsal.

vesic(o)- word element [L.], *blister; bladder.*

vesica (vĕ-si′kah), pl. *vesi′cae* [L.] bladder. **v. fel′leae,** gallbladder. **v. urina′ria,** urinary bladder.

vesical (ves′ĭ-k′l) pertaining to the urinary bladder.

vesicant (ves′ĭ-kant) 1. producing blisters. 2. an agent that produces blisters.

vesication (ves″ĭ-ka′shun) 1. the process of blistering. 2. a blistered spot or surface.

vesicle (ves′ĭ-k′l) 1. a small bladder or sac containing liquid. 2. a small circumscribed elevation of the epidermis containing a serous fluid; a small blister. **allantoic v.,** internal hollow portion of allantois. **auditory v.,** a detached ovoid sac formed by closure of the auditory pit in the early embryo, from which percipient parts of the ear develop. **blastodermic v.,** blastocyst. **brain v's,** the five divisions of the closed neural tube in the developing embryo, including the telencephalon, diencephalon, mesencephalon, metencephalon, and myelencephalon. **brain v's, primary,** the three earlier subdivisions of the embryonic neural tube, including the forebrain, midbrain, and hindbrain. **brain v's, secondary,** the four brain vesicles formed by specialization of the forebrain and of the hindbrain in later embryonic development. **cerebral v's,** brain v's. **chorionic v.,** the developing ovum at the time of its invasion of the endometrium of the uterus. **compound v.,** multilocular v. **encephalic v's,** brain v's. **germinal v.,** the fluid-filled nucleus of an oocyte toward the end of prophase of its meiotic division. **lens v.,** a vesicle formed from the lens pit of the embryo, developing into the crystalline lens. **multilocular v.,** one with multiple chambers or compartments. **optic v.,** an evagination on either side of the forebrain of the early embryo, from which the percipient parts of the eye develop. **otic v.,** auditory v. **seminal v's,** paired sacculated pouches attached to the posterior urinary bladder; the duct of each joins the ipsilateral ductus deferens to form the ejaculatory duct. **umbilical v.,** the pear-shaped expansion of the yolk sac growing out into the cavity of the chorion, joined to the midgut by the yolk stalk.

vesicocele (ves′ĭ-ko-sēl″) hernia of bladder.

vesicocervical (ves″ĭ-ko-ser′vĭ-kal) pertaining to the bladder and cervix uteri.

vesicoclysis (ves″ĭ-kok′lĭ-sis) introduction of fluid into the bladder.

vesicoenteric (ves″ĭ-ko-en-ter′ik) vesicointestinal.

vesicointestinal (-in-tes′tĭ-nal) pertaining to or communicating with the urinary bladder and intestine.

vesicoprostatic (-pros-tat′ik) pertaining to the bladder and prostate.

vesicopubic (-pu′bik) pertaining to the bladder and pubes.

vesicosigmoidostomy (-sig″moi-dos′to-me) creation of a permanent communication between the urinary bladder and the sigmoid flexure.

vesicospinal (-spi′nal) pertaining to the bladder and spine.

vesicotomy (ves″ĭ-kot′o-me) cystotomy.

vesicoureteral (ves″ĭ-ko-u-re′ter-al) pertaining to the bladder and ureter.

vesicouterine (-u′ter-īn) pertaining to the bladder and uterus.

vesicovaginal (-vaj′ĭ-nal) pertaining to the bladder and vagina.

vesicula (vĕ-sik′u-lah), pl. *vesic′ulae* [L.] vesicle.

vesicular (vĕ-sik′u-lar) 1. composed of or relating to small, saclike bodies. 2. pertaining to or made up of vesicles on the skin.

vesiculated (vĕ-sik′u-lāt″ed) marked by vesicles.

vesiculation (vĕ-sik″u-la′shun) formation of vesicles.

vesiculectomy (vĕ-sik″u-lek′to-me) excision of a vesicle, especially the seminal vesicle.

vesiculiform (vĕ-sik′u-lĭ-form″) shaped like a vesicle.

vesiculitis (vĕ-sik″u-li′tis) inflammation of a vesicle, especially a seminal vesicle (*seminal v.*).

vesiculocavernous (vĕ-sik″u-lo-kav′er-nus) both vesicular and cavernous.

vesiculogram (vĕ-sik′u-lo-gram″) a roentgenogram of the seminal vesicles.

vesiculography (vĕ-sik″u-log′rah-fe) radiography of the seminal vesicles.

vesiculopapular (vĕ-sik″u-lo-pap′u-lar) marked by or having characteristics of vesicles and papules.

vesiculopustular (-pus′tu-lar) marked by or having characteristics of vesicles and pustules.

vesiculotomy (vĕ-sik″u-lot′o-me) incision into a vesicle, especially the seminal vesicles.

vesiculotympanic (vĕ-sik″u-lo-tim-pan′ik) having both a vesicular and tympanic quality; said of percussion sounds.

Vesprin (ves′prin) trademark for preparations of triflupromazine.

vessel (ves′sel) any channel for carrying a fluid, such as blood or lymph. **absorbent v's,** lymphatic v's. **blood v.,** one of the vessels conveying the blood, comprising arteries, capillaries, and veins. **chyliferous v's,** lacteal v's. **collateral v's,** 1. a vessel that parallels another vessel, nerve, or other structure. 2. a vessel important in establishing and maintaining a collateral circulation. **great v's,** the large vessels entering the heart, including the aorta, the pulmonary arteries and veins, and the venae cavae. **lacteal v's,** those that take up chyle from the intestinal wall during digestion. **lymph v's, lymphatic v's,** the capillaries, collecting vessels, and trunks that collect lymph from the tissues and carry it to the blood stream. **nutrient v's,** vessels supplying nutritive elements to special tissues, as arteries entering the substance of bone or the walls of large blood vessels.

vestibule (ves′tĭ-būl) a space or cavity at the entrance to a canal. **vestib′ular,** adj. **v. of aorta,** a small space at root of the aorta. **v. of ear,** an oval cavity in the middle of the bony labyrinth. **v. of mouth,** the portion of the oral cavity bounded on the one side by teeth and gingivae, or residual alveolar ridges, and on the other by the lips (*labial v.*) and cheeks (*buccal v.*). **v. of nose,** the anterior part of the nasal cavity. **v. of pharynx,** 1. fauces. 2. oropharynx. **v. of vagina,** the space between the labia minora into which the urethra and vagina open.

vestibuloplasty (ves-tib′u-lo-plas″te) surgical modification of gingival–mucous membrane relationships in the vestibule of the mouth.

vestibulotomy (ves-tib″u-lot′o-me) incision into the vestibule of the ear.

vestibulourethral (ves-tib″u-lo-u-re′thral) pertaining to the vestibule of the vagina and the urethra.

vestibulum (ves-tib′u-lum), pl. *vestib′ula* [L.] vestibule.

vestige (ves′tij) the remnant of a structure that functioned in a previous stage of species or individual development. **vestig′ial,** adj.

vestigium (ves-tij′e-um), pl. *vestig′ia* [L.] vestige.

veterinarian (vet″er-ĭ-na′re-an) a person trained and authorized to practice veterinary medicine and surgery; a doctor of veterinary medicine.

veterinary (vet′er-ĭ-ner″e) 1. pertaining to domestic animals and their diseases. 2. veterinarian.

V.F. vocal fremitus.

V.f. visual field.

via (vi′ah), pl. *vi′ae* [L.] way; channel.

viability (vi″ah-bil′ĭ-te) the state or quality of being viable.

viable (vi′ah-b'l) able to maintain an independent existence; able to live after birth.

Viadril (vi′ah-dril) trademark for a preparation of hydroxydione.

vial (vi′al) a small bottle.

vibesate (vi′bĕ-sāt) a modified polyvinyl plastic applied topically as a spray to form an occlusive dressing for surgical wounds and other surface lesions.

vibex (vi′beks), pl. *vib′ices* [L.] a narrow linear mark or streak; a linear subcutaneous effusion of blood.

vibratile (vi′brah-tīl) swaying or moving to and fro; vibratory.

vibration (vi-bra′shun) 1. a rapid movement to and fro; oscillation. 2. the shaking of the body as a therapeutic measure. 3. a form of massage.

vibrator (vi′bra-tor) an apparatus used in vibratory treatment.

vibratory (vi′brah-tor″e) vibrating or causing vibration.

Vibrio (vib′re-o) a genus of gram-negative bacteria (family Spirillaceae), including *V. chol′erae* (*V. com′ma*), or cholera vibrio, the cause of Asiatic cholera.

vibrio (vib′re-o) an organism of the genus *Vibrio* or other spiral motile organism. **cholera v.,** *Vibrio cholerae.* **El Tor v.,** a biotype of *Vibrio cholerae.*

vibriocidal (vib″re-o-si′dal) destructive to *Vibrio,* especially *V. cholerae.*

vibrion (ve″bre-on′) a vibrio, or spiral motile organism. **v. septique,** *Clostridium septicum.*

vibriosis (vib″re-o′sis) infection with *Vibrio,* especially *V. fetus,* a causative agent of infectious abortion of cattle, sheep, and goats.

vibrissa (vi-bris′ah), pl. *vibris′sae* [L.] one of the hairs growing in the vestibule of the nose in man or about the muzzle of an animal.

vibrocardiogram (vi″bro-kar′de-o-gram″) the record produced by vibrocardiography.

vibrocardiography (-kar″de-og′rah-fe) graphic recording of chest wall vibrations produced by action of the heart.

vibrotherapeutics (-ther″ah-pu′tiks) the therapeutic use of vibrating appliances.

Vicia (vish′e-ah) a genus of herbs, including *V.*

fa′ba (*V. fa′va*), the fava or broad bean, whose beans or pollen contain a component capable of causing favism in susceptible persons.

videognosis (vid″e-og-no′sis) diagnosis based on the interpretation of roentgenograms transmitted by television techniques to a radiologic center.

vigilambulism (vij″il-am′bu-lizm) a state resembling somnambulism, but not occurring in sleep; double or multiple personality.

villi (vil′i) plural of *villus*.

villikinin (vil″ĭ-ki′nin) a hypothetical hormone said to stimulate intestinal villus movement.

villitis (vĭ-li′tis) inflammation of the villous tissue of the coronet and plantar substance of the horse's foot.

villoma (vĭ-lo′mah) a papilloma, chiefly of the rectum.

villose (vil′ōs) shaggy with soft hairs; covered with villi.

villositis (vil″o-si′tis) a bacterial disease with alterations in the villi of the placenta.

villosity (vĭ-los′ĭ-te) 1. condition of being covered with villi. 2. a villus.

villus (vil′us), pl. *vil′li* [L.] a small vascular process or protrusion, as from the free surface of a membrane. **arachnoid v.,** microscopic projections of the arachnoid into some of the venous sinuses; see *arachnoid granulations.* **chorionic villi,** threadlike projections growing in tufts on the external surface of the chorion. **intestinal villi,** multitudinous threadlike projections covering the surface of the mucous membrane lining the small intestine, serving as the sites of absorption of fluids and nutrients. See Plates V and XV. **synovial villi,** slender projections from the surface of the synovial membrane into the cavity of a joint.

villusectomy (vil″ŭ-sek′to-me) synovectomy.

Vinactane (vin-ak′tān) trademark for a preparation of viomycin.

vinbarbital (vin-bar′bĭ-tal) a short- to intermediate-acting barbiturate, $C_{11}H_{16}N_2O_3$, used orally as a sedative; the sodium salt is used for parenteral administration.

vinblastine (vin-blas′tēn) an antineoplastic alkaloid, $C_{46}H_{58}N_4O_9$, extracted from *vinca rosea;* used as the sulfate salt, especially for supplemental or alternative therapy in the treatment of Hodgkin's disease.

Vinca (vin′kah) a genus of apocynaceous woody herbs, including *V. ro′sea* (Madagascar periwinkle), which contains many alkaloids, such as vinblastine and vincristine.

vincristine (vin-kris′tēn) an antineoplastic alkaloid, $C_{46}H_{56}N_4O_{10}$, extracted from *Vinca rosea;* used as the sulfate salt.

vinculum (ving′ku-lum), pl. *vin′cula* [L.] a band or bandlike structure. **vin′cula ten′dinum,** filaments which connect the phalanges with the flexor tendons.

vinegar (vin′ĕ-gar) 1. a weak and impure dilution of acetic acid. 2. a medicinal preparation of dilute acetic acid.

Vinethene (vin′ĕ-thēn) trademark for vinyl ether.

vinleurosine (vin-loor′o-sēn) an antineoplastic alkaloid from *Vinca rosea.*

vinyl (vi′nil) the univalent group, CH_2CH, from vinyl alcohol.

Viocin (vi′o-sin) trademark for a preparation of viomycin.

Vioform (vi′o-form) trademark for preparations of iodochlorhydroxyquin.

violet (vi′o-let) 1. the reddish-blue color produced by the shortest rays of the visible spectrum. 2. a dye which produces a reddish-blue color. **crystal v.,** gentian v. **gentian v., methyl v.,** a dye derived from triphenylmethane, used as a topical anti-infective, stain, and internal anthelmintic.

viomycin (vi″o-mi′sin) an antibiotic, $C_{23}H_{36}N_{12}O_8$, produced by *Streptomyces puniceus, S. floridae,* and *Actinomyces vinaceus,* or by other means; the sulfate salt is used as a tuberculostatic.

viosterol (vi-os′ter-ol) ergocalciferol.

viper (vi′per) any venomous snake of the *Vipera,* including the sand viper (*V. ammodytes*), the adder or European viper (*V. berus*), and Russell's viper (*V. russelli*).

viral (vi′ral) pertaining to or caused by a virus.

Virales (vi-ra′lēz) the taxonomic order comprising the viruses.

viremia (vi-re′me-ah) the presence of viruses in the blood.

virgin (vir′jin) a female who has not had coitus.

viridin (vir′ĭ-din) an oily principle, $C_{12}H_{19}N$, distilled from bone oil and coal tar.

virile (vir′il) 1. peculiar to men or the male sex. 2. possessing masculine traits, especially copulative power.

virilescence (vir″ĭ-les′ens) the development of male secondary sex characters in the female.

virilism (vir′ĭ-lizm) the presence of male characteristics in women.

virility (vĭ-ril′ĭ-te) possession of normal primary sex characters in a male.

virilization (vir″ĭ-li-za′shun) induction or development of male secondary sex characters, especially appearance of such changes in the female.

virion (vi′re-on) the complete viral particle, found extracellullarly and capable of surviving in crystalline form and infecting a living cell; it comprises the nucleoid (genetic material) and the capsid.

virologist (vi-rol′o-jist) a microbiologist specializing in virology.

virology (vi-rol′o-je) the study of viruses and virus diseases.

virucidal (vi″rŭ-si′dal) capable of neutralizing or destroying a virus.

virucide (vi′rŭ-sīd) an agent which neutralizes or destroys a virus.

virulence (vir′u-lens) the degree of pathogenicity of a microorganism as indicated by case fatality rates and/or its ability to invade the tissues of the host; the competence of any infectious agent to produce pathologic effects. **vir′ulent,** adj.

viruliferous (vir″u-lif′er-us) conveying or producing a virus or other noxious agent.

viruria (vi-roo′re-ah) the presence of viruses in the urine.

virus (vi′rus) a minute infectious agent which, with certain exceptions, is not resolved by the light microscope, lacks independent metabolism and is able to replicate only within a living host cell; the individual particle (virion) consists of nucleic acid (nucleoid)—DNA or RNA (but not both)—and a protein shell (capsid), which contains and protects the nucleic acid and which may be multilayered. **animal v's,** viruses that produce diseases of man and animals. **arbor** (arthropod-borne) **v.,** arbovirus. **attenuated v.,** one whose pathogenicity has been reduced by serial passage or other means. **bacterial v.,** bacteriophage; one that is capable of producing transmissible lysis of bacteria. **CELO** (chicken-embryo lethal orphan) **v.,** an orphan virus which is lethal for chicken embryos and induces tumors in newborn and weanling hamsters. **Coxsackie v.,** coxsackievirus. **defective v.,** one that cannot be completely replicated or cannot form a protein coat; in some cases replication can proceed if missing gene functions are supplied by other viruses; see helper v. **ECHO** (enteric cytopathogenic human orphan) **v.,** echovirus. **encephalomyocarditis v.,** an enterovirus that causes mild aseptic meningitis and encephalomyocarditis. **enteric v.,** enterovirus. **enteric orphan v's,** orphan viruses isolated from the intestinal tract of man and various other animals; they include such viruses isolated from cattle (ecboviruses), dogs (ecdoviruses), man (echoviruses), monkeys (ecmoviruses), and swine (ecsoviruses). **Epstein-Barr v.,** a herpesvirus believed to be the etiologic agent of infectious mononucleosis or closely related to it. **filterable v., filtrable v.,** a pathogenic agent capable of passing through fine filters of diatomite or unglazed porcelain; ultravirus. **v. fixé, fixed v.,** rabies virus whose virulence and incubation period have been stabilized by serial passage and remained fixed during further transmission; used for inoculating animals from which rabies vaccine is prepared. **Friend v.,** a murine leukemia virus causing malignant reticulopathy in mice. **Graffi v.,** a murine leukemia virus which causes chloroleukemia in mice. **Gross v.,** a virus resembling the Rous sarcoma virus, which causes many kinds of leukemia in newborn mice and rats. **helper v.,** one that aids in the development of a defective virus by supplying or restoring the activity of the viral gene or enabling it to form a protein coat. **herpes v.,** herpesvirus. **latent v., masked v.,** one which ordinarily occurs in a noninfective state and is demonstrable by indirect methods which activate it. **lytic v.,** one that is replicated in the host cell and causes death and lysis of the cell. **Moloney v.,** a murine leukemia virus which causes lymphoid leukemia in mice. **murine leukemia v.,** any of a group of leukoviruses causing leukemia and solid tumors in rats, mice, hamsters, and other animals; the group includes the Gross, Rauscher, Friend, Moloney, and Graffi viruses. **orphan v's,** viruses isolated in tissue culture but not found specifically associated with any illness. **parainfluenza v.,** one of a group of viruses isolated from patients with upper respiratory tract disease of varying severity. **plant v's,** viruses that replicate in and may cause diseases of higher plants. **polyoma v.,** any of a subgroup of papovaviruses capable of causing experimental neoplastic disease in laboratory animals. **pox v.,** poxvirus. **Rauscher leukemia v.,** a murine leukemia virus that causes lymphoid leukemia in mice. **respiratory syncytial v.,** a virus isolated from children with bronchopneumonia and bronchitis, which causes syncytium formation in tissue culture. **Rous-associated v. (RAV),** a helper virus in whose presence a defective Rous sarcoma virus is able to form a protein coat. **Rous sarcoma v.,** see Rous sarcoma. **street v.,** Pasteur's name for rabies virus derived from a dog with a naturally acquired case of the disease. **tickborne v.,** one transmitted by ticks.

vis (vis), pl. vi′res [L.] force, energy. **v. a ter′go,** the factor of pressure transmitted through the capillaries to the veins by the blood pumped into the arteries by the heart. **v. formati′va,** energy manifesting itself in formation of new tissue. **v. medica′trix natu′rae,** the power of recovery inherent in an organism.

viscer(o)- word element [L.], viscera.

viscera (vis′er-ah) plural of viscus.

viscerad (vis′er-ad) toward the viscera.

visceral (vis′er-al) pertaining to a viscus.

visceralgia (vis″er-al′je-ah) pain in any viscera.

visceroinhibitory (vis″er-o-in-hib′ĭ-tor″e) inhibiting the essential movements of any viscus.

visceromegaly (-meg′ah-le) splanchnomegaly.

visceromotor (-mo′tor) concerned in the essential movements of the viscera.

visceroparietal (-pah-ri′ĕ-tal) pertaining to the viscera and the abdominal wall.

visceroperitoneal (-per″ĭ-to-ne′al) pertaining to the viscera and peritoneum.

visceropleural (-ploo′ral) pertaining to the viscera and the pleura.

visceroptosis (vis″er-op-to′sis) splanchnoptosis.

viscerosensory (vis″er-o-sen′sor-e) pertaining to sensation in the viscera.

visceroskeletal (-skel′ĕ-tal) pertaining to the visceral skeleton.

viscerosomatic (-so-mat′ik) pertaining to the viscera and the body.

viscerotonia (-to′ne-ah) a group of traits characterized by general relaxation, and love of comfort, sociability, and conviviality; considered typical of an endomorph.

viscerotropic (-trop′ik) primarily acting on the viscera; having a predilection for the abdominal or thoracic viscera.

viscid (vis′id) glutinous or sticky.

viscidity (vĭ-sid′ĭ-te) the quality of being viscid.

viscosimeter (vis″ko-sim′ĕ-ter) an apparatus used in measuring viscosity of a substance.

viscosity (vis-kos′ĭ-te) resistance to flow; a physical property of a substance that is dependent on the friction of its component molecules as they slide by one another.

viscous (vis′kus) sticky or gummy; having a high degree of viscosity.

viscus (vis′kus), pl. *vis′cera*[L.] any large interior organ in any of the four great body cavities, especially those in the abdomen.

vision (vizh′un) faculty of seeing; sight. **vis′ual,** adj. **achromatic v.,** vision characterized by lack of color vision. **binocular v.,** the use of both eyes together, without diplopia. **central v.,** that produced by stimulation of receptors in the macula lutea. **chromatic v.,** 1. color v. 2. chromatopsia. **color v.,** perception of the different colors making up the spectrum of visible light. **day v.,** visual perception in the daylight or under conditions of bright illumination. **dichromatic v.,** that in which color perception is restricted to a pair of primaries, either blue and yellow or (rarely) red and green. **direct v.,** central v. **double v.,** diplopia. **half v.,** hemianopia. **indirect v.,** peripheral v. **monocular v.,** vision with one eye. **multiple v.,** polyopia. **night v.,** visual perception in the darkness of night or under conditions of reduced illumination. **oscillating v.,** oscillopsia. **peripheral v.,** that produced by stimulation of receptors in the retina outside the macula lutea. **solid v., stereoscopic v.,** perception of the relief of objects or of their depth; vision in which objects are perceived as having three dimensions. **tunnel v.,** a condition of concentric reduction in the visual field, as though the subject were looking through a long tunnel or tube.

visualization (vizh″u-al-i-za′shun) the act of viewing or of achieving a complete visual impression of an object.

visuoauditory (vizh″u-o-aw′dĭ-tor″e) pertaining to sight and hearing.

visuognosis (vizh″u-og-no′sis) recognition and interpretation of visual impressions.

visuopsychic (vizh″u-o-si′kik) visual and psychic; applied to the area of the cerebral cortex concerned in judgment of visual sensations.

visuosensory (-sen′so-re) pertaining to perception of visual impressions.

vital (vi′tal) pertaining or necessary to life.

vitalism (vi′tah-lizm) the theory that biological functions are produced by a distinct principle called vital force. **vitalis′tic,** adj.

vitalist (vi′tah-list) a believer in vitalism.

Vitallium (vi-tal′e-um) trademark for a cobalt-chromium alloy used for cast dentures and surgical appliances.

vitamer (vi′tah-mer) a substance or compound which has vitamin activity.

vitamin (vi′tah-min) any of a group of unrelated organic substances occurring in many foods in small amounts and necessary for normal metabolic functioning of the body; they may be water- or fat-soluble. **antihemorrhagic v.,** see *v. K.* **antineuritic v.,** thiamine. **antipellagra v.,** niacin. **antiscorbutic v.,** ascorbic acid. **permeability v.,** a substance necessary to ensure integrity of the capillary walls.

v. A, a fat-soluble vitamin occurring in nature in two forms: *retinol* and *dehydroretinol*. It is found in fish liver oils, liver, butter, egg yolk, cheese, and many vegetables, in most of which it exists as its precursor, carotene; deficiency in the diet causes (*a*) inadequate production and regeneration of rhodopsin with resultant nightblindness, and (*b*) epithelial tissue disturbances resulting in keratomalacia, xerophthalmia, and lessened resistance to infection through epithelial surfaces.

v. A₁, retinol.

v. A₂, dehydroretinol.

v. B, any member of the *vitamin B complex,* a group of water-soluble substances including thiamine, riboflavin, niacin, niacinamide, the vitamin B₆ group, biotin, pantothenic acid, folic acid, possibly para-aminobenzoic acid, inositol, cyanocobalamine (vitamin B₁₂), and possibly choline.

v. B₁, thiamine.

v. B₂, riboflavin.

v. B₆, a group of substances (including pyridoxine, pyridoxal, and pyridoxamine) widely distributed in animal and plant tissues, concerned in amino acid metabolism, in degradation of tryptophan, and in breakdown of glycogen to glucose-1-phosphate.

v. B₁₂, cyanocobalamine.

v. Bᴄ, folic acid.

v. C, ascorbic acid.

v. D, any of several related antirachitic compounds, including cholecalciferol and ergocalciferol; they are present in fish liver oils and in butter and egg yolk and produced in the body on exposure to sunlight, and may be produced artificially by irradiation of ergosterol and a few related sterols. Deficiency tends to cause rickets in children and osteomalacia and osteoporosis in adults. Known collectively as *calciferol.*

v. D₂, ergocalciferol.

v. D₃, cholecalciferol.

v. E, a vitamin necessary in the diet of many species for normal reproduction, normal muscular development, normal resistance of erythrocytes to hemolysis, and various other biochemical functions; chemically, it is α-tocopherol (q.v.), found in wheat germ oil, cereals, egg yolk, and beef liver, or produced synthetically.

v. G, riboflavin.

v. H, biotin.

v. K, a group of vitamins found in alfalfa, spinach, cabbage, putrefied fish meal, hog-liver fat, egg yolk, and hempseed, which promote clotting of blood by increasing the synthesis of prothrombin by the liver.

v. K₁, one of the oil-soluble vitamins, $C_{31}H_{46}O_2$, found in green plants and prepared synthetically; used as a prothrombinogenic agent and in veterinary medicine as an antidote for warfarin poisoning.

v. K₂, a naturally occurring vitamin, $C_{41}H_{56}O_2$, first isolated from putrefied fish meal; used in veterinary medicine.

v. K₃, menadione.

v. L, a factor necessary for lactation in rats; L_1 is found in beef-liver extract, L_2 in yeast.

v. M., folic acid.

vitellin (vi-tel′in) the phosphoprotein found in egg yolk.

vitelline (vi-tel′in) resembling or pertaining to the yolk of an egg or ovum.

vitellolutein (vi″tel-o-lu′te-in) yellow pigment obtainable from egg yolk.

vitellorubin (-roo′bin) reddish pigment obtainable from egg yolk.

vitellus (vi-tel′us) the yolk of egg.

vitiligines (vit″ĭ-lij′ĭ-nēz) depigmented areas of the skin.

vitiligo (vit″ĭ-li′go) a condition in which destruction of melanocytes in small or large circumscribed areas results in patches of depigmentation often having a hyperpigmented border, and often enlarging slowly. **vitilig′inous,** adj.

vitrectomy (vĭ-trek′to-me) extraction via the pars plana of the contents of the vitreous chamber and their replacement by a physiological solution.

vitreodentin (vit″re-o-den′tin) an usually hard and glasslike form of dentin.

vitreous (vit′re-us) 1. glasslike or hyaline. 2. vitreous body. **persistent hyperplastic v.,** a congenital anomaly, usually unilateral, due to persistence of embryonic remnants of the fibromuscular tunic of the eye and part of the hyaloid vascular system. Clinically, there is a white pupil, elongated ciliary processes, and often microphthalmia; the lens, although clear initially, may become completely opaque.

vitriol (vit′re-ol) any crystalline sulfate. **blue v.,** copper sulfate. **green v.,** ferrous sulfate. **white v.,** zinc sulfate.

vitrum (vit′rum) [L.] glass.

vivi- word element [L.], *alive; life.*

vividialysis (viv″ĭ-di-al′ĭ-sis) dialysis through a living membrane.

vividiffusion (-dĭ-fu′zhun) circulation of the blood through a closed apparatus in which it is passed through a membrane for removal of substances ordinarily removed by the kidneys.

vivification (-fi-ka′shun) conversion of lifeless into living protein matter by assimilation.

viviparous (vi-vip′ah-rus) giving birth to living young which develop within the maternal body.

vivisection (viv″ĭ-sek′shun) surgical procedures performed upon a living animal for purpose of physiologic or pathologic investigation.

vivisectionist (-ist) one who practices or defends vivisection.

VLDL very low-density lipoproteins.

vocal (vo′kal) pertaining to the voice.

voice (vois) sound produced by the speech organs and uttered by the mouth.

void (void) to cast out as waste matter, especially the urine.

vola (vo′lah) a concave or hollow surface. **v. ma′nus,** the palm. **v. pe′dis,** the sole.

volar (vo′lar) pertaining to sole or palm; indicating the flexor surface of the forearm, wrist, or hand.

volaris (vo-la′ris) palmar.

volatile (vol′ah-til) evaporating rapidly.

volatilization (vol″ah-til-ĭ-za′shun) conversion into a vapor or gas without chemical change.

volition (vo-lish′un) the act or power of willing. **voli′tional,** adj.

volley (vol′e) a rhythmical succession of muscular twitches artificially induced; the aggregate of nerve impulses set up by a single stimulus.

volsella (vol-sel′ah) vulsella.

volt (vōlt) the unit of electromotive force; 1 ampere of current against 1 ohm of resistance. **electron v.,** the energy acquired by an electron when accelerated by a potential of 1 volt, being equivalent to 3.82×10^{-20} small calories, or 1.6×10^{-12} ergs; usually expressed in million electron volts or Mev.

voltage (vōl′tij) electromotive force measured in volts.

voltaism (vōl′tah-izm) galvanism. **volta′ic,** adj.

voltmeter (vōlt′me-ter) an instrument for measuring electromotive force in volts.

volume (vol′ūm) the space occupied by a substance or a three-dimensional region; the capacity of such a region or of a container. **expiratory reserve v.,** the maximal amount of gas that can be expired from the resting end-expiratory level. **inspiratory reserve v.,** the maximal amount of gas that can be inspired from the end-inspiratory position. **mean corpuscular v.,** see *MCV.* **minute v.,** the volume of air expelled from the lungs per minute. **packed-cell v.,** the volume of packed red cells in milliliters per 100 ml. of centrifuged blood. **residual v.,** the amount of gas remaining in the lung at the end of a maximal expiration. **stroke v.,** the volume of blood ejected from a ventricle at each beat of the heart. **tidal v.,** the volume of gas inspired and expired during one respiratory cycle.

volumetric (vol″u-met′rik) pertaining to or accompanied by measurement in volumes.

volumometer (vol″u-mom′ĕ-ter) an instrument for measuring volume or changes in volume.

voluntary (vol′un-tār″e) accomplished in accordance with the will.

volute (vo-lūt′) rolled up.

volvulosis (vol″vu-lo′sis) onchocerciasis due to *Onchocerca volvulus.*

volvulus (vol′vu-lus) [L.] torsion of a loop of intestine, causing obstruction.

vomer (vo′mer) [L.] see *Table of Bones.* **vo′mer-ine,** adj.

vomeronasal (vo″mer-o-na′zal) pertaining to the vomer and the nasal bone.

vomica (vom′ĭ-kah), pl. *vom′icae* [L.] 1. the profuse and sudden expectoration of pus and putrescent matter. 2. an abnormal cavity in an organ, especially in the lung, caused by suppuration and the breaking down of tissue.

vomit (vom′it) 1. matter expelled from the stomach by the mouth. 2. to eject stomach contents through the mouth. **black v.,** vomit consisting of blood which has been acted upon by the gastric juice, seen in yellow fever and other conditions in which blood collects in the stomach. **coffee-ground v.,** vomit consisting of dark altered blood mixed with stomach contents.

vomiting (-ing) forcible ejection of contents of stomach through the mouth. **cyclic v.,** recurring attacks of vomiting. **dry v.,** attempts at vomiting, with the ejection of nothing but gas. **pernicious v.,** vomiting in pregnancy so severe as to threaten life. **v. of pregnancy,** that occurring in pregnancy, especially early morning vomiting (morning sickness). **projectile v.,** vomiting with the material ejected with great force. **stercoraceous v.,** vomiting of fecal matter.

vomitory (vom′i-to″re) an emetic.

vomiturition (vom″ĭ-tu-rish′un) repeated ineffectual attempts to vomit; retching.

vomitus (vom′ĭ-tus) [L.] 1. vomiting. 2. matter vomited.

vortex (vor′teks), pl. *vor′tices* [L.] a whorled or spiral arrangement or pattern, as of muscle fibers, or of the ridges or hairs of the skin.

vox (voks) [L.] voice. **v. choler′ica,** the peculiar suppressed voice of true cholera.

voyeurism (voi′yer-izm) a sexual aberration in which gratification is derived from looking at sexual objects or acts.

V.R. vocal resonance.

V.S. volumetric solution.

v.s. vibration seconds (the unit of measurement of sound waves).

vuerometer (vu″er-om′ĕ-ter) an instrument for measuring distance between the eyes.

vulgaris (vul-ga′ris) [L.] ordinary; common.

vulnerary (vul′ner-er″e) 1. pertaining to wounds or the healing of wounds. 2. an agent that promotes wound healing.

vulnus (vul′nus), pl. *vul′nera* [L.] a wound.

vulsella, vulsellum (vul-sel′ah; vul-sel′um) a forceps with clawlike hooks at the end of each blade.

vulva (vul′vah) [L.] the external genital organs of the female, including the mons pubis, labia majora and minora, clitoris, and vestibule of the vagina. **vul′val, vul′var,** adj. **fused v.,** synechia vulvae.

vulvectomy (vul-vek′to-me) excision of the vulva.

vulvismus (vul-viz′mus) vaginismus.

vulvitis (vul-vi′tis) inflammation of the vulva.

vulvocrural (vul″vo-kroo′ral) pertaining to the vulva and thigh.

vulvouterine (-u′ter-in) pertaining to the vulva and uterus.

vulvovaginal (-vaj′ĭ-nal) pertaining to the vulva and vagina.

vulvovaginitis (-vaj″ĭ-ni′tis) inflammation of the vulva and vagina.

vv. venae (L. pl.); veins.

v/v volume (of solute) per volume (of solvent).

W

W chemical symbol, *tungsten* (*wolfram*).

W. wehnelt (a unit of hardness of x-rays).

w. watt.

waist (wāst) the portion of the body between the thorax and the hips.

wall (wawl) a structure bounding or limiting a space or a definitive mass of material. **cell w.,** a structure outside of and protecting the cell membrane, present in all plant cells and in many bacteria and other types of cells. **nail w.,** a fold of skin overlapping the sides and proximal end of a fingernail or toenail. **parietal w.,** somatopleure. **splanchnic w.,** splanchnopleure.

walleye (wawl′i) 1. leukoma of the cornea. 2. exotropia.

ward (ward) a large room in a hospital, with beds for the accommodation of many patients. **isolation w.,** one for isolation of persons having or suspected of having infectious disease. **psychopathic w.,** one in a general hospital for temporary reception of psychiatric patients.

warfarin (war′fer-in) an anticoagulant, $C_{19}H_{16}$-O_4, usually used as the sodium salt.

wart (wort) verruca; an epidermal tumor of viral origin; also loosely applied to any of various benign, wartlike, epidermal proliferations of nonviral origin. **anatomic w.,** the wart in tuberculosis verrucosa. **fig w.,** condyloma acuminatum. **moist w.,** condyloma latum. **mosaic w.,** an irregularly shaped lesion on the sole, with a granular surface, formed by an aggregation of

contiguous plantar warts. **necrogenic w.,** tuberculosis verrucosa. **Peruvian w.,** verruga peruana. **pitch w's,** precancerous, keratotic, epidermal tumors occurring in those working with pitch and coal tar derivatives. **plantar w.,** verruca plantaris. **pointed w.,** condyloma acuminatum. **postmortem w., prosector's w.,** tuberculosis verrucosa. **soot w.,** chimney-sweeps' cancer. **tuberculous w.,** tuberculosis verrucosa. **venereal w.,** condyloma acuminatum.

wash (wosh) a solution used for cleansing or bathing a part, as an eye or the mouth.

Wassermann-fast (wos′er-man-fast″) showing a positive Wassermann reaction despite antisyphilitic treatment.

waste (wāst) 1. a gradual loss, decay, or diminution of bulk. 2. useless and effete material, unfit for further use within the organism. 3. to pine away or dwindle.

water (wot′er) 1. clear, colorless, odorless, tasteless liquid, H_2O. 2. an aqueous solution of a medicinal substance. 3. purified w. **aromatic w.,** a solution, usually saturated, of a volatile oil or other aromatic or volatile substance in purified water, prepared by distillation or solution. **chlorine w.,** a saturated solution of chlorine in water. **cinnamon w.,** a clear, saturated solution of cinnamon oil in purified water; used as a flavored vehicle. **w. of crystallization,** that which is an ingredient of many salts, forming a structural part of a crystal. **distilled w.,** water purified by distillation. **egg w.,** 1. water that has bathed eggs of various invertebrates and acquired one or another substance detectable by a physiological reaction; e.g., oyster egg water may stimulate spawning of male oysters. 2. water containing fertilizin exuded from ripe eggs of sea urchins and other aquatic animals by which spermatozoa are agglutinated. **ground w.,** water lying deep to the surface of the earth, maintained at its level by a layer of impervious material. **heavy w.,** a compound analogous to water but containing the mass 2 isotope of hydrogen (deuterium), differing from ordinary water in having a higher freezing point (3.8° C.) and boiling point (101.4° C.), and in being incapable of supporting life. **w. for injection,** water that has been purified by distillation and contains no added substance. **w. for injection, bacteriostatic,** sterile water for injection, containing one or more suitable antimicrobial agents. **w. for injection, sterile,** water for injection that has been sterilized. **lime w.,** calcium hydroxide solution. **orange flower w.,** a saturated solution of odoriferous principles of fresh flowers of *Citrus aurantium,* separated from excess volatile oil; used as a flavor, vehicle, and perfume in pharmaceutical preparations. **peppermint w.,** a clear, saturated solution of peppermint oil in purified water; used as a vehicle in pharmaceutical preparations. **purified w.,** water obtained by either distillation or ion-exchange treatment; used when mineral-free water is required. **rose w., stronger,** a saturated solution of odoriferous principles of fresh flowers of *Rosa centifolia,* separated from excess volatile oil; used as a perfume in pharmaceutical preparations.

water-borne (wot'er-born) spread or transmitted by drinking water.

water brash (-brash) pyrosis.

waters (wot'erz) popular name for *amniotic fluid.*

watt (wot) a unit of electric power, being the work done at the rate of 1 joule per second. It is equivalent to 1 ampere under pressure of 1 volt.

wattage (wot'ij) the output or consumption of an electric device expressed in watts.

wattmeter (wot'me-ter) an instrument for measuring wattage.

wave (wāv) a uniformly advancing disturbance in which the parts moved undergo a double oscillation; any wavelike pattern. **alpha w's,** see under *rhythm.* **beta w's,** see under *rhythm.* **brain w's,** the fluctuations of electric potential in the brain, as recorded by electroencephalography. **delta w's,** 1. an early QRS vector in the electrocardiogram in Wolff-Parkinson-White syndrome. 2. see under *rhythm* (1). **electromagnetic w's,** the entire series of ethereal waves which are similar in character, and which move with the velocity of light, but which vary enormously in wavelength. The unbroken series is known from the hertzian waves used in radio transmission which may be miles in length (one mile equals 1.6×10^5 cm.) through heat and light, the ultraviolet, roentgen rays, and the gamma rays of radium to the cosmic rays, the wavelength of which may be as short

as 0.0004 of an Angström unit (4×10^{-12} cm.). **hertzian w's,** electromagnetic waves resembling light waves, but having greater wavelength; used in wireless telegraphy. **light w's,** the electromagnetic waves that produce sensations on the retina; see *light.* **P w.,** a deflection in the electrocardiogram produced by excitation of the atria. **pulse w.,** the elevation of the pulse felt by the finger or shown graphically in a recording of pulse pressure. **Q w.,** in the QRS complex, the initial downward (negative) deflection, related to the initial phase of depolarization. **R w.,** the initial upward deflection of the QRS complex, following the Q wave in the normal electrocardiogram. **radio w's,** electromagnetic radiation of wavelengths between 10^{-1} and 10^6 cm. and frequency of about 10^{11} to 10^4 cps. **S w.,** a downward deflection of the QRS complex following the R wave in the normal electrocardiogram. **T w.,** the second major deflection of the normal electrocardiogram, reflecting the potential variations occurring with repolarization of the ventricles. **theta w's,** see under *rhythm.* **U w.,** a potential undulation of unknown origin immediately following the T wave, seen in the normal electrocardiogram and accentuated in hypokalemia. **ultrashort w's,** electromagnetic waves of wavelength of less than 10 meters. **ultrasonic w's,** waves similar to sound waves but of such high frequency that the human ear does not perceive them as sound.

wavelength (wāv'length) the distance between the top of one wave and the identical phase of the succeeding one.

wax (waks) a plastic substance deposited by insects or obtained from plants. **wax'y,** adj. **ear w.,** cerumen. **grave w.,** adipocere. **white w.,** bleached, purified wax from the honeycomb of the bee, *Apis mellifera;* used as an ingredient of several ointments. **yellow w.,** beeswax; purified wax from the honeycomb of the bee, *Apis mellifera;* used as a stiffening agent, and as an ingredient of yellow ointment.

waxing (wak'sing) the shaping of a wax pattern or the wax base of a trial denture into the contours desired.

W.B.C. white blood cell; white blood (cell) count.

wean (wēn) to discontinue breast feeding and substitute other feeding habits.

weanling (wēn'ling) an animal newly changed from breast feeding to other forms of nourishment.

webbed (webd) connected by a membrane.

weight (wāt) heaviness; the degree to which a body is drawn toward the earth by gravity. See *Table of Weights and Measures.* **apothecaries' w.,** a system of weights used in compounding prescriptions based on the grain (equivalent 64.8 mg.). Its units are the scruple (20 grains), dram (3 scruples), ounce (8 drams), and pound (12 ounces). **atomic w.,** the weight of an atom of a substance as compared with the weight of an atom of carbon-12, which is taken as 12.00000. Abbreviated at. wt. **avoirdupois w.,** the system of weight commonly used for ordinary commodities in English-speaking countries; its units are the dram (27.344 grains),

Tables of Weights and Measures

Measures of Mass

Avoirdupois Weight

GRAINS	DRAMS	OUNCES	POUNDS	METRIC EQUIVALENTS, GRAMS
1	0.0366	0.0023	0.00014	0.0647989
27.34	1	0.0625	0.0039	1.772
437.5	16	1	0.0625	28.350
7000	256	16	1	453.5924277

Apothecaries' Weight

GRAINS	SCRUPLES (℈)	DRAMS (ʒ)	OUNCES (℥)	POUNDS(lb.)	METRIC EQUIVALENTS, GRAMS
1	0.05	0.0167	0.0021	0.00017	0.0647989
20	1	0.333	0.042	0.0035	1.296
60	3	1	0.125	0.0104	3.888
480	24	8	1	0.0833	31.103
5760	288	96	12	1	373.24177

Troy Weight

GRAINS	PENNYWEIGHTS	OUNCES	POUNDS	METRIC EQUIVALENTS, GRAMS
1	0.042	0.002	0.00017	0.0647989
24	1	0.05	0.0042	1.555
480	20	1	0.083	31.103
5760	240	12	1	373.24177

Measures of Mass

Metric Weight

MICROGRAM	MILLIGRAM	CENTIGRAM	DECIGRAM	GRAM	DECAGRAM	HECTOGRAM	KILOGRAM	EQUIVALENTS	
								AVOIRDUPOIS	APOTHECARIES'
1	...	...	...	...	...	...	...		0.000015 grains
10^3	1	...	...	...	...	...	...		0.015432 grains
10^4	10	1	...	...	...	...	...		0.154323 grains
10^5	10^2	10	1	...	...	...	...		1.543235 grains
10^6	10^3	10^2	10	1	...	...	...		15.432356 grains
10^7	10^4	10^3	10^2	10	1	...	...	5.6438 dr.	7.7162 scr.
10^8	10^5	10^4	10^3	10^2	10	1	...	3.527 oz.	3.215 oz.
10^9	10^6	10^5	10^4	10^3	10^2	10	1	2.2046 lb.	2.6792 lb.
10^{12}	10^9	10^8	10^7	10^6	10^5	10^4	10^3	2204.6223 lb.	2679.2285 lb.

MINIMS	FLUID DRAMS	FLUID OUNCES	GILLS	PINTS	QUARTS	GALLONS	EQUIVALENTS		
							CUBIC INCHES	MILLI-LITERS	CUBIC CENTIMETERS
1	0.0166	0.002	0.0005	0.00013	...	...	0.00376	0.06161	0.06161
60	1	0.125	0.0312	0.0078	0.0039	...	0.22558	3.6966	3.6967
480	8	1	0.25	0.0625	0.0312	0.0078	1.80468	29.5729	29.5737
1920	32	4	1	0.25	0.125	0.0312	7.21875	118.2915	118.2948
7680	128	16	4	1	0.5	0.125	28.875	473.167	473.179
15360	256	32	8	2	1	0.25	57.75	946.333	946.358
61440	1024	128	32	8	4	1	231	3785.332	3785.434

MEASURES OF CAPACITY

METRIC MEASURE

MICROLITER	MILLILITER	CENTILITER	DECILITER	LITER	DEKALITER	HECTOLITER	KILOLITER	MYRIALITER	EQUIVALENTS (APOTHECARIES' FLUID)
1	...	...	...	...	...	...	...	...	0.01623108 min.
10^3	1	...	...	...	...	...	...	...	16.23 min.
10^4	10	1	...	...	...	...	...	...	2.7 fl. dr.
10^5	10^2	10	1	...	...	...	...	...	3.38 fl. oz.
10^6	10^3	10^2	10	1	...	...	...	...	2.11 pts.
10^7	10^4	10^3	10^2	10	1	...	...	...	2.64 gal.
10^8	10^5	10^4	10^3	10^2	10	1	...	...	26.418 gal.
10^9	10^6	10^5	10^4	10^3	10^2	10	1	...	264.18 gal.
10^{10}	10^7	10^6	10^5	10^4	10^3	10^2	10	1	2641.8 gal.

1 liter = 2.113363738 pints (Apothecaries').

Measures of Length

Metric Measure

MICRON	MILLI-METER	CENTI-METER	DECI-METER	METER	DEKA-METER	HECTO-METER	KILO-METER	MYRIA-METER	MEGA-METER	EQUIVALENTS
1	0.001	10^{-4}	...	...	...	...	...	...	...	0.000039 inch
10^3	1	10^{-1}	...	...	...	...	...	...	...	0.03937 inch
10^4	10	1	...	...	...	...	...	...	...	0.3937 inch
10^5	10^2	10	1	...	...	...	...	...	...	3.937 inch
10^6	10^3	10^2	10	1	...	...	...	...	...	39.37 inch
10^7	10^4	10^3	10^2	10	1	...	...	...	...	10.9361 yards
10^8	10^5	10^4	10^3	10^2	10	1	...	...	...	109.3612 yards
10^9	10^6	10^5	10^4	10^3	10^2	10	1	...	...	1093.6121 yards
10^{10}	10^7	10^6	10^5	10^4	10^3	10^2	10	1	...	6.2137 miles
10^{11}	10^8	10^7	10^6	10^5	10^4	10^3	10^2	10	1	62.1370 miles

CONVERSION TABLES

AVOIRDUPOIS—METRIC WEIGHT

Ounces	Grams
1/16	1.772
1/8	3.544
1/4	7.088
1/2	14.175
1	28.350
2	56.699
3	85.049
4	113.398
5	141.748
6	170.097
7	198.447
8	226.796
9	255.146
10	283.495
11	311.845
12	340.194
13	368.544
14	396.893
15	425.243
16 (1 lb.)	453.59

Pounds	
1 (16 oz.)	453.59
2	907.18
3	1360.78 (1.36 kg.)
4	1814.37 (1.81 ")
5	2267.96 (2.27 ")
6	2721.55 (2.72 ")
7	3175.15 (3.18 ")
8	3628.74 (3.63 ")
9	4082.33 (4.08 ")
10	4535.92 (4.54 ")

METRIC—AVOIRDUPOIS WEIGHT

GRAMS	OUNCES
0.001 (1 mg.)	0.000035274
1	0.035274
1000 (1 kg.)	35.274 (2.2046 lb.)

APOTHECARIES'—METRIC LIQUID MEASURE

Minims	Milliliters
1	0.06
2	0.12
3	0.19
4	0.25
5	0.31
10	0.62
15	0.92
20	1.23
25	1.54
30	1.85
35	2.16
40	2.46
45	2.77
50	3.08
55	3.39
60 (1 fl.dr.)	3.70

Fluid drams	
1	3.70
2	7.39
3	11.09
4	14.79
5	18.48
6	22.18
7	25.88
8 (1 fl.oz.)	29.57

Fluid ounces	
1	29.57
2	59.15
3	88.72
4	118.29
5	147.87
6	177.44
7	207.01
8	236.58
9	266.16
10	295.73
11	325.30
12	354.88
13	384.45
14	414.02
15	443.59
16 (1 pt.)	473.17
32 (1 qt.)	946.33
128 (1 gal.)	3785.32

METRIC—APOTHECARIES' LIQUID MEASURE

MILLILITERS	MINIMS	MILLILITERS	FLUID DRAMS	MILLILITERS	FLUID OUNCES
1	16.231	5	1.35	30	1.01
2	32.5	10	2.71	40	1.35
3	48.7	15	4.06	50	1.69
4	64.9	20	5.4	500	16.91
5	81.1	25	6.76	1000 (1 L.)	33.815
		30	7.1		

CONVERSION TABLES

APOTHECARIES'—METRIC WEIGHT		METRIC—APOTHECARIES' WEIGHT	
Grains	Grams	Milligrams	Grains
1/150	0.0004	1	0.015432
1/120	0.0005	2	0.030864
1/100	0.0006	3	0.046296
1/80	0.0008	4	0.061728
1/64	0.001	5	0.077160
1/50	0.0013	6	0.092592
1/48	0.0014	7	0.108024
1/30	0.0022	8	0.123456
1/25	0.0026	9	0.138888
1/16	0.004	10	0.154320
1/12	0.005	15	0.231480
1/10	0.006	20	0.308640
1/9	0.007	25	0.385800
1/8	0.008	30	0.462960
1/7	0.009	35	0.540120
1/6	0.01	40	0.617280
1/5	0.013	45	0.694440
1/4	0.016	50	0.771600
1/3	0.02	100	1.543240
1/2	0.032		
1	0.065	Grams	
1 1/2	0.097 (0.1)	0.1	1.5432
2	0.12	0.2	3.0864
3	0.20	0.3	4.6296
4	0.24	0.4	6.1728
5	0.30	0.5	7.7160
6	0.40	0.6	9.2592
7	0.45	0.7	10.8024
8	0.50	0.8	12.3456
9	0.60	0.9	13.8888
10	0.65	1.0	15.4320
15	1.00	1.5	23.1480
20 (1ʒ)	1.30	2.0	30.8640
30	2.00	2.5	38.5800
Scruples		3.0	46.2960
1	1.296 (1.3)	3.5	54.0120
2	2.592 (2.6)	4.0	61.728
3 (1ʒ)	3.888 (3.9)	4.5	69.444
Drams		5.0	77.162
1	3.888	10.0	154.324
2	7.776		
3	11.664		Equivalents
4	15.552	10	2.572 drams
5	19.440	15	3.858 "
6	23.328	20	5.144 "
7	27.216	25	6.430 "
8 (1ℨ)	31.103	30	7.716 "
Ounces		40	1.286 oz.
1	31.103	45	1.447 "
2	62.207	50	1.607 "
3	93.310	100	3.215 "
4	124.414	200	6.430 "
5	155.517	300	9.644 "
6	186.621	400	12.859 "
7	217.724	500	1.34 lb.
8	248.828	600	1.61 "
9	279.931	700	1.88 "
10	311.035	800	2.14 "
11	342.138	900	2.41 "
12 (1 lb.)	373.242	1000	2.68 "

METRIC DOSES WITH APPROXIMATE APOTHECARY EQUIVALENTS*

These *approximate* dose equivalents represent the quantities usually prescribed, under identical conditions, by physicians trained, respectively, in the metric or in the apothecary system of weights and measures. In labeling dosage forms in both the metric and the apothecary systems, if one is the approximate equivalent of the other, the approximate figure shall be enclosed in parentheses.

When prepared dosage forms such as tablets, capsules, pills, etc., are prescribed in the metric system, the pharmacist may dispense the corresponding *approximate* equivalent in the apothecary system, and vice versa, as indicated in the following table.

Caution—For the conversion of specific quantities in a prescription which requires compounding, or in converting a pharmaceutical formula from one system of weights or measures to the other, *exact* equivalents must be used.

LIQUID MEASURE		LIQUID MEASURE	
METRIC	APPROX. APOTHECARY EQUIVALENTS	METRIC	APPROX. APOTHECARY EQUIVALENTS
1000 ml.	1 quart	3 ml.	45 minims
750 ml.	1 1/2 pints	2 ml.	30 minims
500 ml.	1 pint	1 ml.	15 minims
250 ml.	8 fluid ounces	0.75 ml.	12 minims
200 ml.	7 fluid ounces	0.6 ml.	10 minims
100 ml.	3 1/2 fluid ounces	0.5 ml.	8 minims
50 ml.	1 3/4 fluid ounces	0.3 ml.	5 minims
30 ml.	1 fluid ounce	0.25 ml.	4 minims
15 ml.	4 fluid drams	0.2 ml.	3 minims
10 ml.	2 1/2 fluid drams	0.1 ml.	1 1/2 minims
8 ml.	2 fluid drams	0.06 ml.	1 minim
5 ml.	1 1/4 fluid drams	0.05 ml.	3/4 minim
4 ml.	1 fluid dram	0.03 ml.	1/2 minim

WEIGHT		WEIGHT	
METRIC	APPROX. APOTHECARY EQUIVALENTS	METRIC	APPROX. APOTHECARY EQUIVALENTS
30 Gm.	1 ounce	30 mg.	1/2 grain
15 Gm.	4 drams	25 mg.	3/8 grain
10 Gm.	2 1/2 drams	20 mg.	1/3 grain
7.5 Gm.	2 drams	15 mg.	1/4 grain
6 Gm.	90 grains	12 mg.	1/5 grain
5 Gm.	75 grains	10 mg.	1/6 grain
4 Gm.	60 grains (1 dram)	8 mg.	1/8 grain
3 Gm.	45 grains	6 mg.	1/10 grain
2 Gm.	30 grains (1/2 dram)	5 mg.	1/12 grain
1.5 Gm.	22 grains	4 mg.	1/15 grain
1 Gm.	15 grains	3 mg.	1/20 grain
0.75 Gm.	12 grains	2 mg.	1/30 grain
0.6 Gm.	10 grains	1.5 mg.	1/40 grain
0.5 Gm.	7 1/2 grains	1.2 mg.	1/50 grain
0.4 Gm.	6 grains	1 mg.	1/60 grain
0.3 Gm.	5 grains	0.8 mg.	1/80 grain
0.25 Gm.	4 grains	0.6 mg.	1/100 grain
0.2 Gm.	3 grains	0.5 mg.	1/120 grain
0.15 Gm.	2 1/2 grains	0.4 mg.	1/150 grain
0.12 Gm.	2 grains	0.3 mg.	1/200 grain
0.1 Gm.	1 1/2 grains	0.25 mg.	1/250 grain
75 mg.	1 1/4 grains	0.2 mg.	1/300 grain
60 mg.	1 grain	0.15 mg.	1/400 grain
50 mg.	3/4 grain	0.12 mg.	1/500 grain
40 mg.	2/3 grain	0.1 mg.	1/600 grain

Note—A milliliter (ml.) is the equivalent of a cubic centimeter (cc.).

*Adopted by the latest Pharmacopeia, National Formulary, and New and Nonofficial Remedies, and approved by the Federal Food and Drug Administration.

ounce (16 drams), and pound (16 ounces). **equivalent w.**, the weight in grams of a substance that is equivalent in a chemical reaction to 1.008 gm. of hydrogen. **molecular w.**, the weight of a molecule of a substance as compared with that of an atom of carbon-12; it is equal to the sum of the atomic weights of its constituent atoms. Abbreviated mol. wt.

wen (wen) a sebaceous or epidermal inclusion cyst.

wet-nurse (wet′ners) a woman who suckles infants other than her own.

wheal (hwēl) a localized area of edema on the body surface, often attended with severe itching and usually evanescent; it is the typical lesion of urticaria.

wheeze (hwēz) a whistling respiratory sound.

whiplash (hwip′lash) see under *injury.*

whipworm (-werm) *Trichuris trichiura.*

whistle (hwis′l) 1. a shrill musical breath sound. 2. an instrument for making a shrill whistling sound. **Galton's w.**, a whistle used in hearing tests.

whitlow (hwit′lo) felon. **melanotic w.**, a malignant tumor of the nail bed characterized by formation of melanotic tissue.

W.H.O. World Health Organization, an international agency associated with the United Nations and based in Geneva.

whoop (hōōp) the sonorous and convulsive inspiration of whooping cough.

whooping cough (hōōp′ing kof) an infectious disease caused by *Bordetella pertussis,* marked by catarrh of the respiratory tract and peculiar paroxysms of cough, ending in a prolonged crowing or whooping respiration.

whorl (hwerl) a spiral arrangement.

window (win′do) a circumscribed opening in a plane surface. **aortic w.**, a transparent region below the aortic arch, formed by the bifurcation of the trachea, visible in the left anterior oblique radiograph of the heart and great vessels. **oval w.**, fenestra vestibuli. **round w.**, fenestra cochleae.

windpipe (wind′pīp) the trachea.

wing (wing) a winglike structure or part; see *ala.*

winking (wingk′ing) quick opening and closing of the eyelids. **jaw w.**, involuntary closing of the eyelids occasionally associated with jaw movements.

wire (wīr) a slender, elongated, flexible structure of metal. **Kirschner w.**, a steel wire for skeletal transfixion of fractured bones and for obtaining skeletal traction in fractures.

withdrawal (with-draw′al) 1. pathological retreat from external reality. 2. abstention from drugs to which one is habituated or addicted. Also, denoting the symptoms occasioned by such withdrawal.

witzelsucht (vit′sel-zōōkt) [Ger.] a mental condition marked by the making of poor jokes and puns and the telling of pointless stories at which the speaker is intensely amused; a characteristic frontal lobe lesions.

Wohlfahrtia (vōl-fahr′te-ah) a genus of flies. The larvae of *W. magnif′ica* produce wound myiasis; those of *W. o′paca* and *W. vig′il* cause cutaneous myiasis.

wolfram (wool′fram) tungsten (symbol W).

womb (wōōm) uterus.

worm (werm) 1. any of the soft-bodied, naked, elongated invertebrates of the phyla Annelida, Acanthocephala, Aschelminthes, and Platyhelminthes. 2. The spiral tube of a distilling apparatus. **eye w.**, *Loa loa.* **flat w.**, any of the Platyhelminthes. **guinea w.**, *Dracunculus medinensis.* **Medina w.**, *Dracunculus medinensis.* **spiny-headed w.**, **thorny-headed w.**, any of the Acanthocephala.

wound (wōōnd) a bodily injury caused by physical means, with disruption of the normal continuity of structures. **contused w.**, one in which the skin is unbroken. **incised w.**, one caused by a cutting instrument. **lacerated w.**, one in which the tissues are torn. **open w.**, one having a free outward opening. **penetrating w.**, **puncture w.**, one caused by a sharp, usually slender object, which passes through the skin into the underlying tissues.

W.R. Wassermann reaction.

wrist (rist) the region of the joint between the forearm and hand; the carpus. Also, the corresponding forelimb joint in quadrupeds. **drop w.**, wristdrop.

wristdrop (rist′drop) a condition resulting from paralysis of the extensor muscles of the hand and fingers.

wryneck (ri′nek) torticollis.

wt. weight.

Wuchereria (voo″ker-e′re-ah) a genus of filarial nematodes indigenous to the warmer regions of the world, including *W. bancrof′ti,* which causes elephantiasis, lymphangitis, and chyluria by interfering with the lymphatic circulation.

wuchereriasis (voo″ker-ĕ-ri′ah-sis) infestation with worms of the genus *Wuchereria.*

w./v. weight (of solute) per volume (of solvent).

Wyamine (wi′ah-min) trademark for preparations of mephentermine.

Wydase (wi′dās) trademark for preparations of hyaluronidase for injection.

X

X symbol, *Kienböck's unit* (of x-ray exposure).

xanth(o)- word element [Gr.], *yellow*.

xanthate (zan′thāt) any salt of xanthic acid.

xanthelasma (zan″thel-az′mah) xanthoma affecting the eyelids, marked by soft yellowish spots or plaques; see *planar xanthoma*.

xanthematin (zan-them′ah-tin) a yellow substance derivable from hematin.

xanthemia (zan-the′me-ah) yellow coloring matter in the blood; carotenemia.

xanthic (zan′thik) 1. yellow. 2. pertaining to xanthine.

xanthine (zan′thēn) a compound, $C_5H_4N_4O_2$, found in most bodily tissues and fluids; it is a precursor of uric acid. **dimethyl x.,** theobromine. **trimethyl x.,** caffeine.

xanthinuria (zan″thin-u′re-ah) excess of xanthine in the urine, due to a hereditary disorder of purine metabolism.

xanthochromatic (zan″tho-kro-mat′ik) yellow-colored.

xanthochromia (-kro′me-ah) yellowish discoloration, as of the skin or spinal fluid.

xanthochromic (-kro′mik) yellow-colored; applied almost exclusively to cerebrospinal fluid.

xanthocyanopsia (-si″ah-nop′se-ah) inability to perceive red or green tints, vision being limited to yellow and blue.

xanthogranuloma (-gran″u-lo′mah) a tumor having histologic characteristics of both granuloma and xanthoma. **juvenile x.,** a dermatosis in which groups of yellow, yellow-brown, reddish yellow, or brown papules occur on the extensor surfaces of the extremities, sometimes involving the eye, meninges, and testes, typically beginning in infancy or early childhood, usually with spontaneous remission in one to three years.

xanthoma (zan-tho′mah) a yellow papule, nodule, or plaque in the skin due to lipid deposits; microscopically the lesions show light cells with foamy protoplasm (foam cells). **diabetic x., x. diabetico′rum,** xanthomatosis associated with diabetes. **x. dissemina′tum,** chronic, benign normolipoproteinemic xanthomatosis, with small, yellowish red to brown papules and nodules chiefly affecting the flexural and intertriginous surfaces and the mucous membranes of the oropharynx, larynx, and bronchi. **eruptive x., x. erupti′va,** a form marked by sudden eruption of crops of small, yellow or yellowish brown papules encircled by an erythematous halo. **generalized x.,** see *planar x.* **x. mul′tiplex,** x. disseminatum. **x. palpebra′rum,** xanthelasma. **planar x., plane x., x. pla′num,** xanthomatosis marked by yellowish to orange, flat macules or slightly elevated plaques, localized to the eyelids (*xanthelasma*) or distributed over large areas of the skin (*generalized planar x.*). **x. tubero′sum, tuberous x.,** a hereditary lipid storage disease, with groups of flat, or elevated and rounded, yellowish or orangish nodules on the skin over joints, especially the el-

bows and knees; it may be associated with certain types of hyperlipoproteinemia, biliary cirrhosis, and myxedema.

xanthomatosis (zan″tho-mah-to′sis) an accumulation of excess lipids in the body. **x. bul′bi,** fatty degeneration of the cornea due to disorder of lipid metabolism, marked by xanthomas.

xanthomatous (zan-tho′mah-tus) pertaining to xanthoma.

xanthophose (zan′tho-fōz) a yellow phose.

xanthophyll (-fil) a yellow pigment of plants.

xanthoprotein (zan″tho-pro′te-in) an orange pigment produced by heating proteins with nitric acid.

xanthopsia (zan-thop′se-ah) chromatopsia in which objects are seen as yellow.

xanthopsin (zan-thop′sin) all-*trans* retinal; see *retinal* (2).

xanthopterin (zan-thop′ter-in) a yellow pigment from wasps, hornets, and butterflies, having hematopoietic activity in anemic animals.

xanthosine (zan′tho-sēn) a nucleoside composed of xanthine and ribose.

xanthosis (zan-tho′sis) yellowish discoloration; degeneration with yellowish pigmentation.

Xe chemical symbol, *xenon*.

xeno- word element [Gr.], *strange; foreign*.

xenodiagnosis (zen″o-di″ag-no′sis) 1. diagnosis by means of finding, in the feces of clean laboratory-bred bugs fed on the patient, the infective forms of the organism causing the disease; used in the early stages of Chagas' disease. 2. diagnosis of trichinosis by means of feeding laboratory-bred rats or mice on meat suspected of being infected with *Trichinella*, and then examining the animals for the parasite.

xenogeneic (-jen-e′ik) in transplantation biology, denoting individuals or tissues from individuals of different species and hence of disparate cell type.

xenogenesis (-jen′ě-sis) 1. heterogenesis (1). 2. production of offspring unlike either parent.

xenogenous (ze-noj′ě-nus) caused by a foreign body, or originating outside the organism.

xenograft (zen′o-graft) a graft of tissue transplanted between animals of different species.

xenomenia (zen″o-me′ne-ah) vicarious menstruation.

xenon (ze′non) chemical element (*see table*), at. no. 54, symbol Xe.

xenoparasite (zen″o-par′ah-sīt) an organism not usually parasitic on a particular species, but which becomes so because of a weakened condition of the host.

xenophobia (-fo′be-ah) morbid dread of strangers.

xenophonia (-fo′ne-ah) alteration in the quality of the voice.

xenophthalmia (zen″of-thal′me-ah) inflammation caused by a foreign body in the eye.

Xenopsylla (zen″op-sil′lah) a genus of fleas, many species of which transmit pathogens; *X.*

737

cheo'pis, the rat flea, transmits plague and murine typhus.

xero- word element [Gr.], *dry; dryness.*

xerocheilia (ze″ro-ki′le-ah) dryness of the lips.

xeroderma (-der′mah) a mild form of ichthyosis; excessive dryness of the skin. **x. pigmento′sum,** a rare and often fatal hereditary pigmentary and atrophic disease in which the skin and eyes are extremely sensitive to light, beginning in childhood and progressing to early development of freckles, telangiectases, keratoses, papillomas, and malignancy.

xerography (ze-rog′rah-fe) xeroradiography.

xeroma (ze-ro′mah) abnormal dryness of the conjunctiva; xerophthalmia.

xeromenia (ze″ro-me′ne-ah) the appearance of constitutional symptoms at the menstrual period without any flow of blood.

xerophagia (-fa′je-ah) the eating of dry food.

xerophthalmia (ze″rof-thal′me-ah) abnormal dryness and thickening of the conjunctiva and cornea due to vitamin A deficiency or to local disease.

xeroradiography (ze″ro-ra″de-og′rah-fe) the making of radiographs by a dry, totally photoelectric process, using metal plates coated with a semiconductor, such as selenium.

xerosis (ze-ro′sis) abnormal dryness, as of the eye (*xerophthalmia*), skin, or mouth. **xerot′ic,** adj.

xerostomia (ze″ro-sto′me-ah) dryness of the mouth due to lack of normal secretion.

xiph(o)- word element [Gr.], *xiphoid process.*

xiphisternum (zif″ĭ-ster′num) xiphoid process. **xiphister′nal,** adj.

xiphocostal (zif″o-kos′tal) pertaining to the xiphoid process and ribs.

xiphoid (zif′oid, zi′foid) 1. sword-shaped; ensiform. 2. xiphoid process.

xiphoiditis (zif″oi-di′tis) inflammation of the xiphoid process.

xiphopagus (zi-fop′ah-gus) symmetrical conjoined twins united in the region of the xiphoid process.

X-linked (eks′linkt) transmitted by genes on the X chromosome; sex-linked.

x-ray (eks′ra) roentgen ray; see under *ray.*

xylene (zi′lēn) dimethylbenzene, C_8H_{10}; used as a solvent in microscopy.

xylenol (zi′lĕ-nol) any of a series of colorless crystalline substances resembling phenol.

Xylocaine (zi′lo-kān) trademark for preparations of lidocaine.

xylol (zi′lol) xylene.

xylometazoline (zi″lo-met″ah-zo′lēn) an adrenergic, $C_{16}H_{24}N_2$, used as a topical nasal decongestant in the form of the hydrochloride salt.

xylose (zi′lōs) a pentose occurring in mucopolysaccharides of connective tissue and sometimes in the urine; also obtained from vegetable gum, beechwood, and jute.

xylulose (zi′lu-lōs) a pentose sugar occurring as L-xylulose, one of the few L sugars found in nature and sometimes excreted in the urine (see *pentosuria*), and D-xylulose.

xylyl (zi′lil) the hydrocarbon radical $CH_3C_6H_4$-CH_2.

xysma (zis′mah) material resembling bits of membrane in stools of diarrhea.

xyster (zis′ter) a file-like instrument used in surgery.

Y

Y chemical symbol, *yttrium.*

yaw (yaw) a lesion of yaws. **mother y.,** the initial cutaneous lesions of yaws.

yawn (yawn) a deep, involuntary inspiration with the mouth open, often accompanied by the act of stretching.

yaws (yaws) a usually nonvenereal, systemic infectious disease caused by the spirochete *Treponema pertenue,* most commonly affecting children in the tropics, initially manifested by a granulomatous lesion (mother yaw), which ulcerates and heals leaving a scar, followed weeks to months later by successive crops of granulomatous papules distributed over the body. Bone involvment may occur also.

Yb chemical symbol, *ytterbium.*

yeast (yēst) a general term including single-celled, usually rounded fungi that produce by budding, some of which transform to a mycelial stage under certain environmental conditions, while others remain single-celled. They are fermenters of carbohydrates, and a few are pathogenic for man. **brewer's y.,** *Saccharomyces cerevisiae,* used in brewing beer, making alcoholic liquors, and baking bread. **dried y.,** dried cells of any suitable strain of *Saccharomyces cerevisiae,* usually a by-product of the brewing industry; used as a natural source of protein and B-complex vitamins.

yellow (yel′o) 1. the primary color of wavelength of 571.5–578.5 mμ. 2. a dye or stain which produces a yellow color. **visual y.,** all-*trans* retinal; see *retinal* (2).

yellows (yel′ōz) 1. a form of canine leptospirosis resembling leptospiral jaundice in man, due to *Leptospira icterohaemorrhagica.* 2. photosensitization and jaundice after ingestion of clover or alfalfa followed by exposure to sunlight, seen in cattle and sheep in Scotland during June and July.

Yersinia (yer-sin′e-ah) a genus of gram-negative bacteria. *Y. pseudotuberculosis* causes pseudotuberculosis in rodents and mesenteric lymphadenitis in man.

yogurt (yo′gert) a form of curdled milk produced

by fermentation with organisms of the genus *Lactobacillus*.

yoke (yōk) a connecting structure; a depression or ridge connecting two structures.

yolk (yōk) the stored nutrient of the ovum.

ytterbium (ĭ-ter′be-um) chemical element (*see table*), at no. 70, symbol Yb.

yttrium (ĭ′tre-um) chemical element (*see table*), at. no. 39, symbol Y.

Z

Z symbol, *atomic number*.

Zactane (zak′tān) trademark for a preparation of ethoheptazine.

Zarontin (zah-ron′tin) trademark for a preparation of ethosuximide.

zeatin (ze′ah-tin) a cytokinin or growth-stimulating factor of plants.

zeaxanthin (ze″ah-zan′thin) a carotenoid from yellow corn, egg yolk, and the seaweed *Fucus vesiculosis*.

zein (ze′in) a yellowish prolamin from corn.

zeoscope (ze′o-skōp) an apparatus for determining the alcoholic strength of a liquid by means of its boiling point.

Zephiran (zef′ĭ-ran) trademark for a preparation of benzalkonium chloride.

zero (ze′ro) the point on a thermometer scale at which the graduation begins; zero of the Celsius (centigrade) scale is the ice point, and that of the Fahrenheit scale is 32 degrees below the ice point. **absolute z.,** the lowest possible temperature, designated as 0 on the Kelvin or Rankine scale, the equivalent of $-273.15°$ C. or $-459.67°$ F.

zinc (zingk) chemical element (*see table*), at. no. 30, symbol Zn; its salts are often poisonous when absorbed by the system, producing a chronic poisoning. **z. acetate,** $Zn(C_2H_3O_2)2\cdot 2H_2O$, an astringent and styptic. **z. bacitracin,** the zinc salt of bacitracin, used as a topical antibacterial. **z. carbonate,** $2ZnCO_3\cdot 3Zn(OH)_2$; used as a dusting powder or in the form of a cerate, and as an ingredient of medicinal zinc peroxide. **z. chloride,** a salt used topically as an astringent, desensitizer for dentin, caustic antiseptic, and deodorant. **z. hydroxide,** $Zn(OH)_2$, an ingredient of medicinal zinc peroxide. **z. oxide,** ZnO, a topical astringent and protectant. **z. peroxide,** ZnO_2, used in pharmaceuticals. **z. peroxide, medicinal,** a mixture of zinc peroxide, zinc carbonate, and zinc hydroxide, used topically in 40% solution as a local anti-infective and oxidant, and as an astringent and deodorant. **z. stearate,** a compound of zinc with stearic and palmitic acids, used as a water-repellent protective powder in dermatoses. **z. sulfate,** $ZnSO_4$, an ophthalmic astringent. **z. undecylenate,** $C_{22}H_{38}O_4Zn$, used topically in a 20% ointment as an antifungal. **white z.,** z. oxide.

zirconium (zir-ko′ne-um) chemical element (*see table*), at. no. 40, symbol Zr.

Zn chemical symbol, *zinc*.

zo(o)- word element [Gr.], *animal*.

zoacanthosis (zo″ak-an-tho′sis) a dermatitis caused by penetration into the skin of bristles, hairs, etc., of lower animals.

zoanthropy (zo-an′thro-pe) delusion that one has become a beast. **zoanthrop′ic,** adj.

zoetic (zo-et′ik) pertaining to life.

zoetrope (zo′ĕ-trōp) an apparatus affording pictures of objects apparently moving as in life.

zona (zo′nah), pl. *zo′nae* [L.] 1. zone. 2. herpes zoster. **z. arcua′ta,** canal of Corti. **z. cartilagin′ea,** limbus laminae spiralis. **z. cilia′ris,** ciliary zone. **z. denticula′ta,** the inner zone of the lamina basilaris ductus cochlearis with the limbus of the osseous spiral lamina. **z. fascicula′ta,** the thick middle layer of the adrenal gland. **z. glomerulo′sa,** the outermost layer of the adrenal cortex. **z. hemorrhoida′lis,** that part of the anal canal extending from the anal valves to the anus and containing the rectal venous plexus. **z. incer′ta,** a narrow band of gray matter between the subthalamic nucleus and thalamic fasciculus. **z. ophthal′mica,** herpetic infection of the cornea. **z. orbicula′ris,** a ring around the neck of the femur formed by circular fibers of the articular capsule of the hip joint. **z. pectina′ta,** the outer part of the lamina basilaris ductus cochlearis running from the rods of Corti to the spiral ligament. **z. pellu′cida,** the transparent, noncellular secreted layer surrounding an ovum. **z. perfora′ta,** the inner portion of the lamina basilaris ductus cochlearis. **z. radia′ta,** a zona pellucida exhibiting conspicuous radial striations. **z. reticula′ris,** the innermost layer of the adrenal cortex. **z. stria′ta,** a zona pellucida exhibiting conspicuous striations. **z. tec′ta,** canal of Corti. **z. vasculo′sa,** a region in the supramastoid fossa containing many foramina for the passage of blood vessels.

zone (zōn) an encircling region or area; by extension, any area with specific characteristics or boundary. **ciliary z.,** the outer of the two regions into which the anterior surface of the iris is divided by the angular line. **comfort z.,** an environmental temperature between 13° and 21° C. (55°–70° F.) with a humidity of 30 to 55 per cent. **epileptogenic z.,** an area which when stimulated may bring on an epileptic attack. **erogenous z's, erotogenic z's,** areas of the body whose stimulation produces erotic desire. **Lissauer's marginal z.,** a bridge of white substance between the apex of the posterior horn and the periphery of the spinal cord. **transitional z.,** the circle in the equator of the lens of the eye in which epithelial fibers are developed into lens fibers.

zonesthesia (zo″nes-the′ze-ah) a sensation of constriction, as by a girdle.

zonifugal (zo-nif′u-gal) passing outward from a zone or region.

zoning (zōn′ing) the occurrence of a stronger fixation of complement in a lesser amount of suspected serum.

zonipetal (zo-nip′ĕ-tal) passing toward a zone or region.

zonula (zōn′u-lah), pl. *zon′ulae* [L.] zonule.

zonule (zōn′ūl) a small zone. **zon′ular,** adj. **ciliary z., z. of Zinn,** a series of fibers connecting the ciliary body and lens of the eye.

zonulitis (zōn″u-li′tis) inflammation of the ciliary zonule.

zonulolysis (zon″u-lol′ĭ-sis) dissolution of the ciliary zonule by use of enzymes, to permit surgical removal of the lens.

zonulotomy (zon″u-lot′o-me) incision of the ciliary zonule.

zoo- word element [Gr.], *animal.*

zoobiology (zo″o-bi-ol′o-je) the biology of animals.

zoochemistry (-kem′is-tre) chemistry of animal tissues.

zoodermic (-der′mik) performed with the skin of an animal, as in skin grafting.

zoodynamics (-di-nam′iks) animal physiology.

zoogenous (zo-oj′ĕ-nus) 1. acquired from animals. 2. viviparous.

zoogeny (zo-oj′ĕ-ne) the development and evolution of animals.

zoogeography (zo″o-je-og′rah-fe) the scientific study of the distribution of animals.

zooglea (-gle′ah) a colony of bacteria embedded in a gelatinous matrix.

zoogony (zo-og′o-ne) the production of living young from within the body. **zoog′onous,** adj.

zoografting (zo′o-graft″ing) the grafting of animal tissue.

zooid (zo′oid) 1. animal-like. 2. an animal-like object or form. 3. an individual in a united colony of animals.

zoolagnia (zo″o-lag′ne-ah) sexual attraction toward animals.

zoology (zo-ol′o-je) the biology of animals.

Zoomastigophora (zo″o-mas″tĭ-gof′o-rah) a class of protozoa (subphylum Mastigophora), including all the flagellates that parasitize higher animals.

zoonosis (-no′sis), pl. *zoono′ses.* Disease of animals transmissible to man. **zoonot′ic,** adj.

zooparasite (-par′ah-sīt) any parasitic animal organism or species. **zooparasit′ic,** adj.

zoopathology (-pah-thol′o-je) the science of the diseases of animals.

zoophagous (zo-of′ah-gus) carnivorous.

zoophilia (zo″o-fil′e-ah) abnormal fondness for animals.

zoophobia (-fo′be-ah) abnormal fear of animals.

zoophyte (zo′o-fīt) any plantlike animal.

zooplankton (zo″o-plangk′ton) minute animal organisms floating free in practically all natural waters.

zooplasty (zo′o-plas″te) zoografting.

zoopsia (zo-op′se-ah) hallucination with vision of animals.

zoospore (zo′o-spōr) a motile reproductive spore.

zoosterol (zo-os′ter-ol) a sterol of animal origin.

zootechnics (zo″o-tek′niks) the art of breeding, keeping, and handling animals in domestication or captivity.

zootherapeutics (-ther″ah-pu′tiks) veterinary medicine.

zootomy (zo-ot′o-me) the dissection or anatomy of animals.

zootoxin (zo″o-tok′sin) a toxic substance of animal origin, e.g., venom of snakes, spiders, and scorpions.

zoster (zos″ter) herpes zoster.

zosteriform (zos-ter′ĭ-form) resembling herpes zoster.

zosteroid (zos′ter-oid) zosteriform.

Z-plasty (ze′plas-te) repair of a skin defect by the transposition of two triangular flaps, for relaxation of scar contractures.

Zr chemical symbol, *zirconium.*

zwitterion (tsvit′er-i″on) an ion that has both positive and negative regions of charge.

zyg(o)- word element [Gr.], *yoked; joined; a junction.*

zygal (zi′gal) shaped like a yoke.

zygapophysis (zi″gah-pof′ĭ-sis) the articular process of a vertebra.

zygion (zij′e-on) the most lateral point on the zygomatic arch.

zygodactyly (zi″go-dak′tĭ-le) union of digits by soft tissues (skin), without bony fusion of the phalanges.

zygoma (zi-go′mah) 1. the zygomatic process of the temporal bone. 2. zygomatic arch. 3. a term sometimes applied to the zygomatic bone. **zygomat′ic,** adj.

zygomaticofacial (zi″go-mat″ĭ-ko-fa′shal) pertaining to the zygoma and face.

zygomaticotemporal (-tem′por-al) pertaining to the zygoma and temporal bone.

zygomaxillare (zi″go-mak′sĭ-lār″e) a craniometric point at the lower end of the zygomatico-maxillary suture.

zygon (zi′gon) the stem connecting the two branches of a zygal fissure.

zygosity (zi-gos′ĭ-te) the condition relating to conjugation, or to the zygote, as (*a*) the state of a cell or individual in regard to the alleles determining a specific character, whether identical (homozygosity) or different (heterozygosity); or (*b*) in the case of twins, whether developing from one zygote (monozygosity) or two (dizygosity).

zygote (zi′gōt) the cell resulting from union of a male and a female gamete; the fertilized ovum. More precisely, the cell after synapsis at the completion of fertilization until first cleavage. **zygot′ic,** adj.

zygotene (zi′go-tēn) the synaptic stage of meiosis.

Zyloprim (zi′lo-prim) trademark for preparations of allopurinol.

zym(o)- word element [Gr.], *enzyme; fermentation.*

zymase (zi′mās) enzyme.

zymic (zi′mik) pertaining to enzymes or fermentation.

zymogen (zi′mo-jen) proenzyme; an inactive precursor that is converted to an active enzyme by action of an acid, another enzyme, or by other means. **zymogen′ic,** adj.

zymogram (-gram) a graphic representation of enzymatically active components of a material separated by electrophoresis.

zymohexase (zi″mo-hek′sās) an enzyme that catalyzes the splitting of fructose 1,6-diphosphate into dihydroxy acetone phosphate and phosphoglyceric aldehyde.

zymoid (zi′moid) resembling an enzyme.

zymolysis (zi-mol′ĭ-sis) fermentation or digestion by means of an enzyme. **zymolyt′ic,** adj.

zymophore (zi′mo-fōr) the group of atoms in a molecule of an enzyme responsible for its specific effect; the active site of an enzyme. **zymoph′orous,** adj.

zymoprotein (zi″mo-pro′te-in) any of a class of proteins having catalytic powers.

zymosan (zi′mo-san) a mixture of polysaccharides, proteins, and ash, derived from the cell walls or the entire cell of yeast. It is anticomplementary, and is used in assaying properdin.

zymoscope (-skōp) an apparatus for determining the fermenting power of yeast.

zymose (zi′mōs) β-fructofurosidase.

zymosis (zi-mo′sis) 1. fermentation. 2. the development of any zymotic disease. 3. any infectious or contagious disease. **zymot′ic,** adj.

zymosterol (zi-mos′ter-ol) a sterol occurring in fungi and molds.